NURSING CARE
OF THE
CRITICALLY ILL CHILD

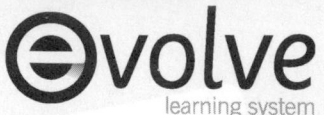 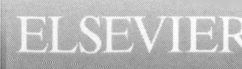
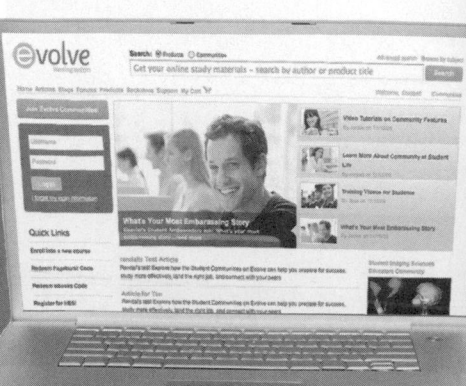
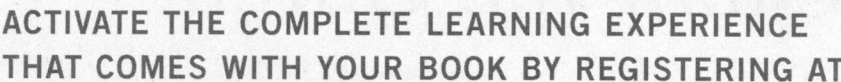

Third Edition 3

NURSING CARE
OF THE
CRITICALLY ILL CHILD

Mary Fran Hazinski, RN, MSN, FAAN, FAHA, FERC
Professor
Vanderbilt University School of Nursing
Assistant, Departments of Surgery and Pediatrics
Vanderbilt University School of Medicine
Clinical Nurse Specialist, Pediatric Critical Care
Monroe Carell, Jr. Children's Hospital at Vanderbilt
Nashville, Tennessee

LIS LIBRARY	
Date	Fund
29/6/15	Q-Chat
WITHDRAWN	
Order No	
2614698	
University of Chester	

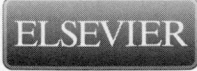

With approximately 270 illustrations

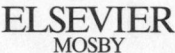

3251 Riverport Lane
St. Louis, Missouri 63043

NURSING CARE OF THE CRITICALLY ILL CHILD, THIRD EDITION ISBN: 978-0-323-02040-4

Notices

Knowledge and best practice in this field are constantly changing. As new research and experience broaden our understanding, changes in research methods, professional practices, or medical treatment may become necessary.

Practitioners and researchers must always rely on their own experience and knowledge in evaluating and using any information, methods, compounds, or experiments described herein. In using such information or methods they should be mindful of their own safety and the safety of others, including parties for whom they have a professional responsibility.

With respect to any drug or pharmaceutical products identified, readers are advised to check the most current information provided (i) on procedures featured or (ii) by the manufacturer of each product to be administered, to verify the recommended dose or formula, the method and duration of administration, and contraindications. It is the responsibility of practitioners, relying on their own experience and knowledge of their patients, to make diagnoses, to determine dosages and the best treatment for each individual patient, and to take all appropriate safety precautions.

To the fullest extent of the law, neither the Publisher nor the authors, contributors, or editors, assume any liability for any injury and/or damage to persons or property as a matter of products liability, negligence or otherwise, or from any use or operation of any methods, products, instructions, or ideas contained in the material herein.

Library of Congress Cataloging-in-Publication Data
Nursing care of the critically ill child / [edited by] Mary Fran Hazinski. – 3rd ed.
 p. ; cm.
 Includes bibliographical references and index.
 ISBN 978-0-323-02040-4 (hardcover : alk. paper)
 I. Hazinski, Mary Fran.
 [DNLM: 1. Pediatric Nursing–methods. 2. Critical Care–methods. 3. Critical Illness–nursing. WY 159]

618.92′00231–dc23
                 2012002172

Senior Content Strategist: Tamara Myers
Senior Content Development Specialist: Linda Thomas
Publishing Services Manager: Jeff Patterson
Project Manager: Tracey Schriefer
Design Direction: Maggie Reid

Printed in the United States of America

Last digit is the print number: 9 8 7 6 5 4 3 2 1

*In memory of Tom,
with appreciation to Ames,
to Millie and Bob Gorman, my wonderful parents,
and to Michael and Stephanie, with love and admiration*

Contributors

Kate Amond, RN, MS, CPNP
Pediatric Nurse Practitioner
Department of Pediatric Cardiothoracic Surgery
American Family Children's Hospital
Madison, Wisconsin
*Chapter 21, Bioinstrumentation: Principles
    and Techniques*

Nick G. Anas, MD
Director, Pediatric Intensive Care
Children's Hospital of Orange County
Orange County, California
Clinical Professor of Pediatrics
David Geffen School of Medicine
University of California Los Angeles
Los Angeles, California
Chapter 9, Pulmonary Disorders

Alisha Armstrong, RN, MSN, PNP-BC
Pediatric Nurse Practitioner
Pediatric Trauma/Surgery
Monroe Carell, Jr. Children's Hospital at Vanderbilt
Nashville, Tennessee
Chapter 19, Pediatric Trauma

William Banner, Jr., MD, PhD
Adjunct Clinical Professor
College of Pharmacy
University of Oklahoma
Oklahoma City, Oklahoma
*Chapter 4, Pharmacokinetics and
    Pharmacodynamics*

Marc D. Berg, MD, FAAP
Associate Professor of Pediatrics
Medical Director, University Physician's Healthcare
Pediatric Critical Care Medicine
College of Medicine
University of Arizona
Tucson, Arizona
*Chapter 6, Shock, Cardiac Arrest,
    and Resuscitation*

Frances Blayney, BSN, RN-C, MS, CCRN
Education Manager
Pediatric Intensive Care Unit
Children's Hospital Los Angeles
Los Angeles, California
Chapter 13, Renal Disorders

Carolyn M. Blume-Odom, BSN, RN, CSPI
Certified Specialist in Poison Information
Missouri Poison Center
SSM Cardinal Glennon Children's Medical Center
St. Louis, Missouri
Chapter 18, Toxicology and Poisonings

Ronald A. Bronicki, MD
Associate Medical Director
Cardiovascular Intensive Care Unit
Texas Children's Hospital
Associate Professor of Pediatrics
Baylor College of Medicine
Houston, Texas
Chapter 9, Pulmonary Disorders

Michelle Lynn Burke, MSN, ARNP, CPN, CPON
Clinical Specialist
Department of Hematology Oncology
Miami Children's Hospital
Miami, Florida
*Chapter 15, Hematologic and Oncologic Emergencies
    Requiring Critical Care*

Dai H. Chung, MD
Professor and Chairman
Janie Robinson & John Moore Lee Endowed Chair
Department of Pediatric Surgery
Vanderbilt University Medical Center
Nashville, Tennessee
Chapter 20, Care of the Child with Burns

Susan E. Coffin, MD, MPH
Hospital Epidemiologist
Medical Director, Infection Prevention and Control
Associate Professor of Pediatrics, Division of Infectious
    Diseases
The Children's Hospital of Philadelphia
University of Pennsylvania School of Medicine
Philadelphia, Pennsylvania
Chapter 16, Immunology and Infectious Disorders

Allan R. de Caen, MD, FRCP(C)
Medical Director, PICU
Clinical Professor
Division of Pediatric Critical Care Medicine
Department of Pediatrics
Stollery Children's Hospital/University of Alberta
Edmonton, Alberta, Canada
Chapter 6, Shock, Cardiac Arrest, and Resuscitation

Valarie Furgeison Eichler, RN, MSN, CPNP-PC/AC
Acute Care Pediatric Nurse Practitioner
Critical Care Services
Children's Medical Center
Dallas, Texas
Chapter 11, Neurologic Disorders

Susan M. Fernandes, MHP, PA-C
Assistant Director of Clinical Research
Boston Adult Congenital Heart Service
Department of Cardiology
Children's Hospital Boston
Boston, Massachusetts
Chapter 8, Cardiovascular Disorders

Gwen Paxson Fosse, RN, BSN, MSA
Clinical Outreach Nurse Specialist
Pediatric Administration
Helen DeVos Children's Hospital
Grand Rapids, Michigan
Chapter 8, Cardiovascular Disorders

Mary Jo Gilmer, PhD, MBA, RN-BC, FAAN
Professor of Nursing, Vanderbilt University School of Nursing
Professor of Pediatrics, Monroe Carell Jr Children's Hospital
    at Vanderbilt
Co-Director, Pediatric Palliative Care Research Team
Vanderbilt University School of Nursing
Nashville, Tennessee
*Chapter 3, Care of the Child with Life-Limiting Conditions
    and the Child's Family in the Pediatric Critical Care Unit*

Punkaj Gupta, MBBS
Assistant Professor
Department of Pediatric Cardiology
University of Arkansas for Medical Sciences
Little Rock, Arkansas
Chapter 8, Cardiovascular Disorders

Debra Hanisch, RN, MSN, CPNP, FHRS, FAHA
Nurse Practitioner
Division of Pediatric Cardiology
Lucile Packard Children's Hospital at Stanford
Palo Alto, California
Chapter 8, Cardiovascular Disorders

Stephen R. Hays, MD, FAAP
Associate Professor
Anesthesiology and Pediatrics
Vanderbilt University School of Medicine
Director, Pediatric Pain Services
Monroe Carell Jr. Children's Hospital at Vanderbilt
Nashville, Tennessee
Chapter 5, Analgesia, Sedation, and Neuromuscular Blockade

Mary Fran Hazinski, RN, MSN, FAAN, FAHA, FERC
Professor
Vanderbilt University School of Nursing
Assistant, Departments of Surgery and Pediatrics
Vanderbilt University School of Medicine
Clinical Nurse Specialist
Monroe Carell, Jr. Children's Hospital at Vanderbilt
Nashville, Tennessee
Chapter 1, Children are Different
Chapter 6, Shock, Cardiac Arrest, and Resuscitation
Chapter 8, Cardiovascular Disorders
Chapter 10, Chest X-Ray Interpretation

Cindy L. Kerr, MSN, CPNP-AC/PC
Nurse Practitioner
Department of Interventional Radiology
Children's Hospital Boston
Boston, Massachusetts
Chapter 14, Gastrointestinal and Nutritional Disorders

Laura A. Klee, RNC, MSN
ECMO Coordinator
Critical Care Services
Children's Hospital Los Angeles
Los Angeles, California
*Chapter 7, Mechanical Support of Cardiopulmonary
    Function: Extracorporeal Membrane Oxygenation,
    Ventricular Assist Devices, and the Intraaortic
    Balloon Pump*

Andrea Kline-Tilford, MS, RN, CPNP-AC/PC, FCCM
Pediatric Nurse Practitioner and Instructor
Department of Women, Children and Family Nursing
College of Nursing
Rush University
Chicago, Illinois
Chapter 9, Pulmonary Disorders

Lisa M. Kohr, BSN, MSN, MPH, PhD(c)
Pediatric Nurse Practitioner
Cardiac Intensive Care Unit
The Children's Hospital of Philadelphia
Philadelphia, Pennsylvania
Chapter 8, Cardiovascular Disorders

Bradley A. Kuch, BS, RRT-NPS, FAARC
Director of Transport
Clinical Research Associate
Department of Critical Care Medicine
Children's Hospital of Pittsburgh of the University of
    Pittsburgh Medical Center
Pittsburgh, Pennsylvania
Chapter 21, Bioinstrumentation: Principles and Techniques

Kelly Lankin, MSN, RN, CCRN
Staff Nurse
Pediatric Intensive Care Unit
Ann & Robert H. Lurie Children's Hospital of Chicago
Chicago, Illinois
Chapter 17, Overview of Solid Organ Transplantation

Daniel L. Levin, MD
Professor of Pediatrics and Anesthesia
Department of Pediatrics
Children's Hospital at Dartmouth
Dartmouth Medical School
Lebanon, New Hampshire
Chapter 9, Pulmonary Disorders

Twila R. Luckett, BSN, RN-BC
Nurse Clinician
Pediatric Pain Service
Monroe Carell Jr. Children's Hospital at Vanderbilt
Nashville, Tennessee
Chapter 5, Analgesia, Sedation, and Neuromuscular Blockade

Maureen A. Madden, RN, MSN, CPNP-AC, CCRN, FCCM
Assistant Professor
Pediatric Critical Care Nurse Practitioner
Department of Pediatrics, Division of Critical Care
UMDNJ-Robert Wood Johnson Medical School
Bristol Myers Squibb Children's Hospital
Robert Wood Johnson University Hospital
New Brunswick, New Jersey
Chapter 10, Chest X-Ray Interpretation

Erin L. Marriott, RN, MS, CPNP
Pediatric Cardiology Nurse Practitioner
Department of Pediatric Cardiology
American Family Children's Hospital
Madison, Wisconsin
Chapter 8, Cardiovascular Disorders

Sarah A. Martin, RN, MS, CPNP-PC/AC, CCRN
Advanced Practice Nurse
Division of Pediatric Surgery
Ann & Robert H. Lurie Children's Hospital of Chicago
Chicago, Illinois
Chapter 14, Gastrointestinal and Nutritional Disorders

Lisa M. Milonovich, RN, MSN, PCCNP
Pediatric Critical Care Nurse Practitioner, Team Leader
Critical Care Services
Children's Medical Center Dallas
Dallas, Texas
Chapter 11, Neurologic Disorders

Jodi E. Mullen, MS, RN-BC, CCRN, CCNS
Clinical Nurse Specialist
Pediatric Intensive Care Unit
The Children's Medical Center of Dayton
Dayton, Ohio
Chapter 21, Bioinstrumentation: Principles and Techniques

Jo Ann Nieves, MSN, CPN, ARNP, PNP-BC, FAHA
Pediatric Nurse Practitioner
Department of Cardiology
Miami Children's Hospital
Miami, Florida
Chapter 8, Cardiovascular Disorders

Linda Nylander-Housholder, ARNP, MSN, CCRN
Advanced Care Educator
Department of Staff and Community Education
Miami Children's Hospital
Miami, Florida
Chapter 21, Bioinstrumentation: Principles and Techniques

Neal R. Patel, MD, MPH
Associate Professor
Pediatrics, Anesthesiology and Biomedical Informatics
Chief Medical Informatics Officer
Division of Pediatric Critical Care
Vanderbilt University Medical Center
Nashville, Tennessee
Chapter 23, Clinical Informatics

Ronald M. Perkin, MD, MA
Professor and Chairman
Department of Pediatrics
Brody School of Medicine
East Carolina University
Greenville, North Carolina
Chapter 6, Shock, Cardiac Arrest, and Resuscitation
Chapter 24, Ethical Issues in Pediatric Critical Care

John B. Pietsch, MD
Associate Professor
Department of Pediatric Surgery
Co-Director, Junior League Fetal Center at Vanderbilt
Director, ECMO Program
Vanderbilt University School of Medicine
Nashville, Tennessee
Chapter 17, Overview of Solid Organ Transplantation
Chapter 19, Pediatric Trauma
Chapter 20, Care of the Child with Burns

Nancy A. Pike, PhD, RN, CPNP-AC, FAHA
Assistant Professor
School of Nursing
University of California Los Angeles
Nurse Practitioner - Cardiothoracic Surgery
Children's Hospital Los Angeles
Los Angeles, California
*Chapter 7, Mechanical Support of Cardiopulmonary
    Function: Extracorporeal Membrane Oxygenation,
    Ventricular Assist Devices, and the Intraaortic
    Balloon Pump*
Chapter 21, Bioinstrumentation: Principles and Techniques

Caroline A. Rich, RN, MSN, CPNP, AC/PC
Pediatric Hospitalist
Helen DeVos Children's Hospital
Wayne State University
Grand Rapids Community College
Grand Rapids, Michigan
Chapter 8, Cardiovascular Disorders

Kathryn E. Roberts, RN, MSN, CCRN, CCNS
Critical Care Clinical Nurse Specialist
Pediatric Intensive Care Unit
The Children's Hospital of Philadelphia
Philadelphia, Pennsylvania
Chapter 12, Fluid, Electrolyte, and Endocrine Problems
Chapter 16, Immunology and Infectious Disorders

Nancy A. Rudd, RN, MS
Pediatric Nurse Practitioner
Herma Heart Center
Children's Hospital of Wisconsin
Department of Pediatrics
Medical College of Wisconsin
Milwaukee, Wisconsin
Chapter 8, Cardiovascular Disorders

Mary Rummell, MN, RN, CPNP, CNS
Clinical Nurse Specialist
Pediatric Cardiology
Professional Practice Leader
Pediatric Intermediate Care Unit
Doernbecher Children's Hospital
Portland, Oregon
Chapter 8, Cardiovascular Disorders

Deborah Salani, MSN, ARNP, CPON, BC-NE
Director
Pediatric Intensive Care Unit
Miami Children's Hospital
Miami, Florida
*Chapter 15, Hematologic and Oncologic Emergencies
    Requiring Critical Care*

Ricardo A. Samson, MD
Chief, Cardiology Section
Professor of Pediatrics
College of Medicine
University of Arizona
Tucson, Arizona
Chapter 8, Cardiovascular Disorders

Anthony J. Scalzo, MD, FAAP, FACMT, FAACT
Professor of Toxicology and Emergency Medicine
Director, Division of Toxicology
Department of Pediatrics
Saint Louis University School of Medicine
Medical Director, Missouri Poison Center
SSM Cardinal Glennon Children's Medical Center
St. Louis, Missouri
Chapter 18, Toxicology and Poisonings

Stephen M. Schexnayder, MD, FAAP, FACP, FCCM
Oakley Chair in Critical Care Medicine
Professor and Vice Chair for Education
Department of Pediatrics
University of Arkansas for Medical Sciences
Chief, Critical Care Medicine
Arkansas Children's Hospital
Little Rock, Arkansas
Chapter 6, Shock, Cardiac Arrest, and Resuscitation
Chapter 8, Cardiovascular Disorders

Patricia Ann E. Schlosser, RN, MS, CPNP, CCRN
Clinical Nurse Specialist, Pediatric Nurse Practitioner
Pediatric Critical Care Nursing
American Family Children's Hospital
University of Wisconsin
Madison Wisconsin
Chapter 8, Cardiovascular Disorders
Chapter 21, Bioinstrumentation: Principles and Techniques

Margaret C. Slota, DNP, RN, FAAN
Associate Professor
Director, DNP and Nursing Leadership Graduate Programs
School of Nursing
Carlow University
Pittsburgh, Pennsylvania
Chapter 2, Psychosocial Aspects of Pediatric Critical Care
Chapter 21, Bioinstrumentation

Lauren Sorce, RN, MSN, CPNP-AC/PC, FCCM
Pediatric Nurse Practitioner
Department of Pediatric Critical Care
Ann & Robert H. Lurie Children's Hospital of Chicago
Chicago Illinois
Chapter 9, Pulmonary Disorders

Sandra Staveski, RN, MS, CPNP-AC/PC, CNS, CCRN
Cardiovascular ICU Nurse Practitioner
Assistant Clinical Professor
Cardiology/Family Health Care Nursing
Lucile Packard Children's Hospital at Stanford
University of California at San Francisco
Palo Alto/San Francisco, California
Chapter 8, Cardiovascular Disorders

Gail L Stendahl, DNP, RN, CPNP-PC/AC, CCTC
Heart Transplant Nurse Practitioner
Herma Heart Center
Children's Hospital of Wisconsin
Milwaukee, Wisconsin
Chapter 8, Cardiovascular Disorders

Tara Trimarchi, MSN, RN, CRNP
Manager, Quality Improvement
Office of Patient Safety and Quality
The Children's Hospital of Philadelphia
Philadelphia, Pennsylvania
*Chapter 22, Fundamentals of Patient Safety and Quality
    Improvement*

Dawn Tucker, MSN, RN, CPNP PC/AC
Cardiovascular Acute Care Nurse Practitioner
Heart Center
Children's Mercy Hospitals and Clinics
Kansas City, Missouri
Chapter 9, Pulmonary Disorders

Purnima Unni, MPH, CHES
Pediatric Trauma Injury Prevention Program Coordinator
Pediatric Trauma Program
Monroe Carell Jr. Children's Hospital at Vanderbilt
Nashville, Tennessee
Chapter 19, Pediatric Trauma

Ruby L. Whalen, RN, BN, CCRC
Nurse Clinician
Department of Cardiology
Miami Children's Hospital
Miami, Florida
Chapter 8, Cardiovascular Disorders

Winnie Yung, MN, RN, CCRN
Clinical Specialist/Nurse Educator
Cardiovascular Intensive Care Unit
Lucile Packard Children's Hospital at Stanford
Palo Alto, California
Chapter 8, Cardiovascular Disorders

Beth Zemetra, RN, BSN
Education Manager
Cardiothoracic Intensive Care Unit
Children's Hospital Los Angeles
Los Angeles, California
*Chapter 7, Mechanical Support of Cardiopulmonary
    Function: Extracorporeal Membrane Oxygenation,
    Ventricular Assist Devices, and the Intraaortic
    Balloon Pump*

Reviewers

SPECIAL REVIEWER

Margaret C. Slota, DNP, RN, FAAN
Associate Professor
Director, DNP and Nursing Leadership Graduate Programs
School of Nursing
Carlow University
Pittsburgh, Pennsylvania

Nick G. Anas, MD
Director, Pediatric Intensive Care
Children's Hospital of Orange County
Orange County, California
Clinical Professor of Pediatrics
David Geffen School of Medicine
University of California Los Angeles
Los Angeles, California

Nancy Blake, RN, CCRN, NEA-BC, PhDc
Director, Critical Care Services
Patient Care Services
Children's Hospital Los Angeles
Los Angeles, California

Jeanne Braby, RN, MSN, CCRN
Unit Based Advanced Practice Nurse
Cardiac Intensive Care Unit
Children's Hospital of Wisconsin
Milwaukee, Wisconsin

Margaret-Ann Carno, PhD, MBA, CPNP, D, ABSM, FAAN
Assistant Professor of Clinical Nursing and Pediatrics
School of Nursing
University of Rochester
Rochester, New York

Tracy B. Chamblee, PhD, RN
Clinical Nurse Specialist
Critical Care Services
Children's Medical Center Dallas
Dallas, Texas

Leon Chameides, MD
Emeritus Director of Pediatric Cardiology
Connecticut Children's Medical Center
Clinical Professor of Pediatrics
University of Connecticut School of Medicine
Hartford, Connecticut

Arthur Cooper, MD, MS
Professor of Surgery
Director of Trauma and Pediatric Surgical Services
Columbia University Medical Center at Harlem Hospital
New York, New York

Amy F. Dittmer, MSN, PNPc
Pediatric Critical Care Nurse Practitioner
Pediatric Intensive Care Unit
St. Joseph's Children's Hospital
Tampa, Florida

Jessica Strohm Farber, DNP, CRNP, PNP-BC
Pediatric Critical Care Nurse Practitioner
Division of Pediatric Critical Care
University of Maryland Medical System
Baltimore, Maryland

Joyce Foresman-Capuzzi, MSN, RN, CCNS, CEN, CPN, CTRN, CCRN, CPEN, SANE-A, EMT-P
Clinical Nurse Educator
Emergency Department
Lankenau Medical Center
Wynnewood, Pennsylvania

Kathleen M. Leack, MS, RN
Clinical Nurse Specialist
Pediatric General Surgery
Children's Hospital of Wisconsin
Milwaukee, Wisconsin

Daniel L. Levin, MD
Professor of Pediatrics and Anesthesia
Department of Pediatrics
Children's Hospital at Dartmouth
Dartmouth Medical School
Lebanon, New Hampshire

Kelly Keefe Marcoux, MSN, CPNP-AC
Director, APN Services
Nursing
Bristol-Myers Squibb Children's Hospital
Robert Wood Johnson University Hospital
New Brunswick, New Jersey

Judith M. Marshall, MS
Advanced Practice Nurse
Ambulatory Services
Ann & Robert H. Lurie Children's Hospital of Chicago
Chicago, Illinois

Jodi E. Mullen, MS, RN-BC, CCRN, CCNS
Clinical Nurse Specialist
Pediatric Intensive Care Unit
The Children's Medical Center of Dayton
Dayton, Ohio

Jennifer L. Najjar, MD
Assistant Professor of Pediatrics
Ian M. Burr Division of Endocrinology and Diabetes
Department of Pediatrics
Vanderbilt University School of Medicine
Nashville, Tennessee

Tracy Ann Pasek, RN, MSN, CCNS, CCRN, CIMI
Clinical Nurse Specialist
Pain/Pediatric Intensive Care Unit
Children's Hospital of Pittsburgh of UPMC
Pittsburgh, Pennsylvania

John B. Pietsch, MD
Associate Professor
Department of Pediatric Surgery
Co-Director, Junior League Fetal Center at Vanderbilt
Director, ECMO Program
Vanderbilt University School of Medicine
Nashville, Tennessee

Devon Plumer, BSN, MSM, CPNP-AC/PC
Pediatric Specialty Services
SEAHEC
New Hanover Regional Medical Center
Wilmington, North Carolina

William E. Russell, MD
Professor of Pediatrics
Professor of Cell and Developmental Biology
Ian M. Burr Division of Pediatric Endocrinology and Diabetes
Department of Pediatrics
Vanderbilt University School of Medicine
Nashville, Tennessee

Stephen M. Schexnayder, MD, FAAP, FACP, FCCM
Oakley Chair in Critical Care Medicine
Professor and Vice Chair for Education
Department of Pediatrics
University of Arkansas for Medical Sciences
Chief, Critical Care Medicine
Arkansas Children's Hospital
Little Rock, Arkansas

Melanie Jacobson Schuster, RN, MSN, PCCNP, CNS
Pediatric Critical Care Nurse Practitioner
Pediatric Intensive Care Unit
Cook Children's Medical Center
Fort Worth, Texas

Eva Sheets, RN, BSN, MBA, CCRN, RNC
Adjunct Nursing Instructor
Hillsborough Community College
Tampa, Florida

Kerry Shields, RN, MSN, MBE
Anesthesia and Critical Care
Pediatric Critical Care Nurse Practitioner Program
The Children's Hospital of Philadelphia
The University of Pennsylvania
Philadelphia, Pennsylvania

Sharon M. Stein, MD
Associate Professor of Radiology and Radiological Sciences
Associate Professor of Pediatrics
Monroe Carell, Jr. Children's Hospital at Vanderbilt
Vanderbilt University School of Medicine
Nashville, Tennessee

Patricia A. Trangenstein, PhD, RN-BC
Professor of Nursing Informatics
Frist Nursing Informatics Center
School of Nursing
Vanderbilt University
Nashville, Tennessee

Tara Trimarchi, MSN, RN, CRNP
Manager, Quality Improvement
Office of Patient Safety and Quality
The Children's Hospital of Philadelphia
Philadelphia, Pennsylvania

Holly Webster, BSN, MS, PNP
Pediatric Critical Care Nurse Practitioner
Pediatric Intensive Care Unit
Primary Children's Medical Center
Salt Lake City, Utah

Sandra L. Wesolowski, RN
Pediatric Nurse II, CCRN
Pediatric CICU
Children's Hospital of Wisconsin
Milwaukee, Wisconsin

James Whitlock
Division Head, Haematology/Oncology
Women's Auxiliary Millennium Chair in Haematology/
    Oncology
Director, Garron Family Cancer Centre
Senior Associate Scientist
Child Health Evaluative Sciences Program, Research Institute
The Hospital for Sick Children
Professor of Paediatrics, University of Toronto
Toronto, Ontario, Canada

Michele Wilson, MS, RN, PCCNP, CNS, CCRN
Clinical Nurse Specialist
Pediatric Intensive Care Unit
Loma Linda University Children's Hospital
Loma Linda, California

Martha Yee, MSN
Pediatric Critical Care Nurse Practitioner
Pediatric Intensive Care Unit
NP's On Demand, Inc.
El Paso, Texas

Tresa E. Zielinski, MSN
Manager, Advanced Practice Nursing
Cardiac Services
Ann & Robert H. Lurie Children's Hospital of Chicago
Chicago Illinois

Preface

"Although tables, equations, and technology can increase the efficiency of care or the precision of its delivery, they cannot take the place of the astute observations, skilled interventions, and personal warmth provided by a competent, compassionate pediatric critical care nurse."

Mary Fran Hazinski
Preface to *Nursing Care of the Critically Ill Child*, edition 2

This third edition of *Nursing Care of the Critically Ill Child* is intended to be a reference for nurse students, teachers, and clinicians of every level who are involved in the care of critically ill or injured children and their families. It provides information in both printed form and online resources (via the *Evolve* website).

As in past editions, the chapters include detailed information about anatomy and physiology, pathophysiology, clinical signs and symptoms, and management of the most common problems and diseases encountered in pediatric critical care. The 58 contributors to this edition have been selected for their expertise, experience, and ability to present even the most complex information clearly and concisely, with practical applications to patient care.

All chapters from previous editions have been substantially rewritten and expanded. Many new chapters have been added, including Care of the Child with Life-Limiting Conditions and the Child's Family in the Pediatric Critical Care Unit; Pharmacokinetics and Pharmacodynamics; Shock, Cardiac Arrest, and Resuscitation; Mechanical Support of Cardiopulmonary Function; Fluid, Electrolyte, and Endocrine Problems; Immunology and Infectious Disorders; Overview of Solid Organ Transplantation; Toxicology and Poisonings; Fundamentals of Patient Safety and Quality Improvement; Clinical Informatics; and Ethical Issues in Pediatric Critical Care.

This is the first edition to be published with the *Evolve* website resource (see inside front pages). The essential information helpful to the bedside nurse is included in the printed book pages. The *Evolve* website is a companion to this textbook available at no cost at http://evolve.elsevier.com/Hazinski/nursingcare/. It contains additional in-depth information for many of the chapters and provides many links to additional on-line resources. The reader is alerted to the availability of this information with cross-references throughout the book.

An abbreviated Table of Contents can be found inside the front cover. As in previous editions, the most frequently used tables (normal vital sign ranges, daily fluid and caloric requirements, estimation of circulating blood volume, the Glasgow Coma Scale, and Pediatric Emergency Department Supplies based on the Broselow length-based tape) and the nomogram for estimation of body surface area can be found on pages included inside the front and back covers.

This book would not have been possible without the support of my family and my colleagues at Vanderbilt University School of Nursing and the Monroe Carell, Jr. Children's Hospital at Vanderbilt and the support of many mentors and colleagues, including the contributors and the reviewers listed on the preceding pages. Linda Thomas, Tracey Schriefer, and Tamara Myers at Elsevier were especially helpful in getting this book to press. F.G. Stoddard and Brenda Schoolfield provided a great deal of assistance during manuscript preparation. Peggy Slota assisted with review and proofing of the final chapter versions.

I am constantly impressed by the knowledge and dedication of pediatric nurses and physicians and the many members of the pediatric critical care team. As healthcare becomes more complex and providers are challenged to improve quality and reduce costs of care, the role of the pediatric critical care nurse becomes more crucial. I began this preface with a quote from the last edition because it still rings true today. On a daily basis, we work with heroic patients, families, and colleagues, intervening when lives truly hang in the balance—I can't imagine anything more challenging, rewarding, or inspiring.

Mary Fran Hazinski, RN, MSN, FAAN, FAHA, FERC

Contents

APPENDICES

Children Are Different

Mary Fran Hazinski

PEARLS

- Children are not "little adults." They are physically, physiologically, and emotionally immature. Critical care equipment, assessment techniques, and therapies must be appropriate for the child's anatomy and physiology.
- The skilled critical care nurse is able to determine at a glance whether the child "looks good" or "looks bad." This rapid evaluation includes visual and tactile assessment of the child's color, perfusion, level of activity, and position. This assessment is similar to that described as the pediatric initial impression[8a]: level of consciousness, breathing, and color.
- Normal vital signs are not always appropriate vital signs in the seriously ill or injured patient. Tachycardia and tachypnea are usually appropriate when the child is in distress. Hypotension may be only a late sign of shock in children.

INTRODUCTION

Children are physically, physiologically, and emotionally immature and differ from adults in several important ways. This chapter summarizes the general assessment of critically ill children, highlighting clinically significant anatomic and physiologic differences between children and adults.

Although many of the clinical signs and symptoms of disease and organ system failure are the same in patients of all ages, some diseases or complications of disease are more likely to occur in the child than in the adult. In addition, the manifestations of distress or organ failure can differ in children. The child is smaller, with immature respiratory and cardiovascular systems that have fewer reserves than those of the adult. As a result, the child in cardiopulmonary distress can decompensate more quickly than the adult with similar illness.

The child's metabolic rate is more rapid than that of the adult, so the child requires higher cardiac output, greater gas exchange, and higher fluid and caloric intake per kilogram of body weight than the adult. However, because children are smaller than adults, their absolute cardiac output, minute ventilation, fluid requirement, and urine volume are lower. Normal serum electrolyte, calcium and glucose concentrations, and arterial blood gases are identical for children (beyond the neonatal period) and adults, but some imbalances are more likely to occur in the critically ill child than in the critically ill adult.

Any nurse caring for the seriously ill or injured child must modify assessment skills and intervention techniques so they are suitable for the child. The nurse must be aware of the signs of organ system dysfunction and failure in the child and must be able to respond quickly when deterioration occurs.

PSYCHOSOCIAL DEVELOPMENT

Children are emotionally and cognitively immature, and this will affect their comprehension of and response to critical illness. The child's communication skills are not well developed until later school age, so the nurse must be able to anticipate the child's needs and concerns and must be sensitive to the child's nonverbal communication.

The family constitutes an essential part of the child's support system, so it is important to assess family dynamics and establish effective communication with family members. It is important for the nurse to provide support for all family members because the family's anxiety can be communicated quickly to the child.

The child and parents or primary caretaker must be treated as a unit, and the parents should be allowed to remain with the child as much as possible. Visitation hours should be liberal, if not unlimited. Communication with the parents must be clear, frequent, and consistent. Joint nurse-physician rounds (involving all caregivers) that include the patient and family will help establish open and consistent communication within the healthcare team and with the family. Specific information about the child's emotional and intellectual development and the response of the child and family to the child's illness is included in Chapters 2 and 3.

GENERAL ASSESSMENT

Initial Impression: "Looks Good" vs. "Looks Bad"

Every skilled critical care nurse and physician develops a systematic method for determining the severity of the patient's condition, making both qualitative and quantitative assessments. Often, the initial, general impression of how the patient looks is more important than any single vital sign or clinical measurement.[8a]

The skilled critical care clinician can determine at a glance whether the patient "looks good" or "looks bad." This determination requires a rapid visual evaluation of the child's color, skin perfusion, level of consciousness (activity and responsiveness), breathing, and position of comfort (Box 1-1). Each portion of this assessment is reviewed in detail in this section.

Assessment of General Appearance: "Looks Good" Versus "Looks Bad"

Color (trunk, extremities)
Skin perfusion
Level of consciousness (activity, responsiveness)
Breathing
Position of comfort

The child's color is normally consistent over the trunk and extremities. The child's mucous membranes, nail beds, palms, and soles are normally pink. When cardiorespiratory distress is present, the skin is often mottled and extremities and mucous membranes can be pale. Although the mucous membranes of the adult with hypoxemia often become dusky, such central cyanosis (best observed in the mucous membranes) is not consistently detected in the hypoxemic child. The observation of cyanosis requires the presence of at least 3 to 5 g of desaturated hemoglobin per deciliter of blood, so the anemic child might never appear cyanotic despite the presence of profound hypoxemia. In addition, some healthcare providers have difficulty perceiving subtle color changes.

The child's extremities are normally warm, with brisk capillary refill (2 s or less). When poor perfusion or stress is present, extremities are cool and capillary refill is often sluggish. Cold stress can also cause peripheral vasoconstriction and cooling of skin, particularly in extremities, so the environmental temperature should be considered when evaluating perfusion. If poor capillary refill is attributed to a cool environment, warm the patient and frequently recheck perfusion to determine whether the compromise in peripheral perfusion was caused by cold stress or if is actually caused by inadequate cardiac output.

A change in the child's level of activity and responsiveness is often noted when systemic perfusion or neurologic function is compromised. Beyond a few weeks of age, the healthy infant will demonstrate good eye contact, orient preferentially to faces, and visually track brightly colored objects. The healthy infant should move all extremities spontaneously. In contrast, the infant in mild distress may hold all extremities flexed and demonstrate a facial grimace. The critically ill infant often will not sustain eye-to-eye contact and can be more irritable than usual, with a high-pitched or a very weak cry. As the infant deteriorates further, extremities will be flaccid, and the infant may be unresponsive.

The healthy toddler should protest vigorously when separated from the parents and should demonstrate stranger anxiety toward unfamiliar hospital personnel. The seriously ill toddler initially can be extremely irritable and comforted only by parents. With further deterioration, the toddler will be lethargic and unresponsive. The toddler normally will protest when the parents leave the bedside; lack of such protest is abnormal.

The healthy preschooler is typically distrustful or afraid of hospital personnel, but should be curious about equipment and tasks performed by the nurse or physician. At this age the child is usually able to localize and describe pain and symptoms. The school-aged child should be able to cooperate with procedures and answer questions about health, symptoms, and activities of daily living. The healthy school-aged child and adolescent are extremely self-conscious during physical examination. Initially, critical illness can make the child more irritable and uncooperative. As further deterioration occurs, the child will become lethargic and then unresponsive.

The healthy child of any age should respond to a painful stimulus (such as a venipuncture), and most children will attempt to withdraw from the stimulus. Therefore, a decreased response to painful stimuli is abnormal and usually indicates serious cardiorespiratory or neurologic deterioration.

The healthcare provider should evaluate the child's breathing rate and effort, forming an opinion of the degree of distress that the child is demonstrating. The provider is reassured if the child is breathing at a regular rate that is appropriate for the child's age and clinical condition. By contrast, the provider should be concerned about the child who is breathing rapidly, irregularly, or at a rate that is too slow for the child's clinical condition, or if the child demonstrates significant effort (e.g., retractions, nasal flaring).

Most children prefer to sit upright in the hospital bed, particularly if strangers are present. The upright position is typically the position of comfort if respiratory distress is present, and the child will probably resist placement in the supine position. If the child reclines quietly in bed, then fear, pain, and serious illness are probably present. Young infants can't assume a position of comfort, but may demonstrate less respiratory distress when the head of the bed is elevated.

Evaluation of Vital Signs

In the critical care unit, clinicians constantly evaluate the child's general appearance (including breathing) and vital signs. Whenever possible the nurse should obtain "resting" information or measurements, including evaluation of heart rate and respiratory rate and effort, before disturbing the child. This resting information can be compared with information obtained when the child is awake and active. The child with upper airway obstruction can breathe comfortably when asleep, but demonstrate increased respiratory rate and effort while awake and active. Alternatively, if the child exhibits tachypnea with severe retractions even during sleep, more significant respiratory distress is present.

Normal vital signs are not always appropriate vital signs when the child is critically ill. The critically ill or stressed child should exhibit tachycardia and tachypnea; a "normal" heart rate and respiratory rate in such a child can indicate deterioration, and cardiorespiratory arrest might be imminent.

The child normally has a faster heart rate and respiratory rate and a lower arterial blood pressure than does an adult. As a result, smaller quantitative changes in the vital signs may be qualitatively more significant in the child than in the adult, particularly if they constitute a trend.

If the adult's systolic blood pressure falls approximately 15 mm Hg, from 140/80 to 125/80 mm Hg, the mean arterial blood pressure has fallen 5%. However, if the infant's systolic blood pressure falls 15 mm Hg, from 72/42 to 57/42 mm Hg, the infant's mean arterial pressure has fallen about 10% and this change may be associated with a compromise in perfusion.

Normal vital signs ranges are provided in Tables 1-1 to 1-3. Evaluation of vital signs requires consideration of normal values for the child's age,[14a] trends in the individual patient's vital signs, and appropriate vital signs for the child's condition. Remember that in children, shock can be present despite the observation of a normal blood pressure. Hypotension is often a late sign of shock in the pediatric patient.

The child's heart rate and respiratory rate normally increase during stress and when the child is frightened or in pain, and they normally decrease when the child is sleeping. If vital signs are obtained when the child is crying, this should be indicated with the vital signs. Attempts should be made to comfort the frightened child, so that resting vital signs can be documented and evaluated.

Assessment Format

Consistent use of a familiar format will facilitate the nurse's recall of important assessment information. The American Heart Association uses an ABC format to indicate assessment and support of airway, breathing, and circulation, and these priorities are still appropriate for assessment of the critically ill child.[8a] In addition, all pediatric life support courses teach an initial assessment by determining the general impression of the child's consciousness, breathing, and color; this text uses the "looks good versus looks bad" assessment. The skilled critical care clinician repeatedly performs these fundamental assessments.

An additional alphabetical format may be useful for pediatric critical care nurses. This format uses the first seven letters of the alphabet to help the nurse recall the steps in a seven-point check (Box 1-2). The seven essential assessment points include the child's airway (and aeration), brain (neurologic function),

Table 1-1 Normal Heart Rates in Children*

Age	Awake Heart Rate (beats/min)	Sleeping Heart Rate (beats/min)
Neonate	100-205	90-160
Infant	100-180	90-160
Toddler	98-140	80-120
Preschooler	80-120	65-100
School-aged child	75-118	58-90
Adolescent	60-100	50-90

*Always consider the patient's normal range and clinical condition. Heart rate will normally increase with fever or stress.

Table 1-2 Normal Respiratory Rates in Children*[14a]

Age	Rate (breaths/min)
Infant	30-53
Toddler	22-37
Preschool	20-28
School age	18-25
Adolescent	12-20

*Consider the patient's normal range. The child's respiratory rate is expected to increase in the presence of fever or stress.

Box 1-2 Seven-, Eight-, or Nine-Point Check

A. Airway and aeration
B. Brain
C. Circulation
D. Drips, drugs
E. Electrolytes
F. Fluids
G. Genitourinary/gastrointestinal and growth and development
H. Heat (thermoregulation)
I. Immunologic immaturity

Table 1-3 Normal Blood Pressures in Children

Age	Systolic Pressure (mm Hg)*	Diastolic Pressure (mm Hg)*	Mean Arterial Pressure (mm Hg)[†]	Systolic Hypotension (mm Hg)[‡]
Birth (12 h, <1000 g)	39-59	16-36	28-42[§]	<40-50
Birth (12 h, 3 kg)	60-76	31-45	48-57	<50
Neonate (96 h)	67-84	35-53	45-60	<60
Infant (1-12 mo)	72-104	37-56	50-62	<70
Toddler (1-2 yr)	86-106	42-63	49-62	<70 + (2 × Age in years)
Preschool (3-5 yr)	89-112	46-72	58-69	<70 + (2 × Age in years)
School age (6-7 yr)	97-115	57-76	66-72	<70 + (2 × Age in years)
Preadolescent (10-12 yr)	102-120	61-80	71-79	<90
Adolescent (12-15 yr)	110-131	64-83	73-84	<90

Data from Gemelli M, et al. Longitudinal study of blood pressure during the 1st year of life. *Eur J Pediatr* 149:318-320, 1990; Versmold H, et al. Aortic blood pressure during the first 12 hours of life in infants with birth weight 610-4220 gms. *Pediatrics* 67:107, 1981; Haque IU, Zaritsky AL. Analysis of the evidence for the lower limit of systolic and mean arterial pressure in children. *Pediatr Crit Care* 8:138-144; and National Heart, Lung and Blood Institute: *Fourth report on the diagnosis, evaluation, and treatment of high blood pressure in children and adolescents*, National Heart, Lung and Blood Institute, Bethesda, MD, May, 2004 (available on line: http://www.nhlbi.nih.gov/guidelines/hypertension/child.tbl.htm).
*Systolic and diastolic blood pressure ranges assume 50th percentile for height for children 1 year and older, and are consistent with the Pediatric Advanced Life Support Course. (Chameides, L et al: Pediatric advanced life support provider manual. Dallas, 2011, American Heart Association).
[†]Mean arterial pressures (Diastolic pressure + [Difference between systolic and diastolic pressures ÷ 3]) for 1 year and older, assuming 50th percentile for height.
[‡]Threshold for hypotension in children 1-10 years old from Pediatric Advanced Life Support Course. (Chameides, L et al: Pediatric advanced life support provider manual. Dallas, 2011, American Heart Association).
[§]Approximately equal to postconception age in weeks (may add 5 mm Hg).

circulation, drips or drugs administered, electrolyte balance, fluids (including fluid balance and fluid administration rate), genitourinary and gastrointestinal function, and growth and development.[17a] When caring for the critically ill neonate, this format can be modified to create a nine-point check, with the addition of the letter *H* for heat, or thermoregulation, and the letter *I* for immunologic immaturity.

GENERAL CHARACTERISTICS

Thermoregulation

Infants and young children have large surface area-to-volume ratios, so they lose more heat to the environment through evaporation, conduction, and convection than do adults. In addition, the small child can lose heat if large quantities of intravenous or dialysis fluids are administered without warming.

Cold-stressed neonates and infants younger than 6 months cannot shiver to generate heat. When the environmental temperature falls, these infants maintain body temperature through nonshivering thermogenesis. This process begins with the secretion of norepinephrine and results in the breakdown of brown fat and creation of heat. Nonshivering thermogenesis is an energy-requiring process, so the infant's oxygen consumption will increase whenever it develops. Regeneration of brown fat requires adequate nutrition; if the infant's caloric intake is inadequate, brown fat will not be made to replace that used, and the infant will be less able to maintain body temperature in a cool environment.

Although the healthy infant is able to increase oxygen delivery in response to increased oxygen consumption during nonshivering thermogenesis, the critically ill infant may not be able to increase oxygen delivery effectively. As a result, cold stress can produce hypoxemia, lactic acidosis, and hypoglycemia. Cooling of the neonate also can stimulate pulmonary vasoconstriction, resulting in increased right ventricular afterload. For these reasons, cold stress can worsen existing cardiovascular dysfunction, causing increased heart failure or right-to-left intracardiac shunting.

The nurse can reduce cold stress by maintaining a neutral thermal environment for the neonate. A neutral thermal environment is the environmental temperature at which the infant maintains a rectal temperature of 37° C with the lowest oxygen consumption. This neutral temperature should be maintained during all aspects of the infant's care, especially during transport and diagnostic tests. Over-bed radiant warmers can help maintain the infant's temperature without interfering with observation and care. The beds are equipped with servo-control devices to adjust heat output in response to changes in the infant's skin temperature. Adjustable alarms indicate when excessive warming is required to maintain the infant's temperature or when the infant's temperature varies from the selected range. (For further information regarding warming devices, see Chapter 21)

Unless there are contraindications (e.g., severe thrombocytopenia), nurses typically monitor both skin (e.g., axillary or via infant skin probe) and central (e.g., oral, esophageal, bladder) temperatures of critically ill infants and young children, because changes in these temperatures may be observed when systemic perfusion is compromised. Bladder temperature monitored via urinary catheter is an additional method of monitoring core body temperature.

Peripheral vasoconstriction and cooling of the skin is often an early sign of cardiovascular dysfunction and low cardiac output. The very young infant also can demonstrate a fall in core body temperature. The older infant or child with low cardiac output can demonstrate a low skin temperature with a normal or increased core body temperature, because heat generated by metabolism cannot be lost through the diminished skin blood flow.

Fluid Requirements and Fluid Therapy

The child's daily fluid requirement is larger per kilogram body weight than that of the adult, because the child has a higher metabolic rate and greater insensible and evaporative water losses per kilogram body weight. Estimation of these fluid requirements is frequently based on the child's body weight. However, evaporative water losses are affected directly by the child's body surface area (BSA), determined by height and weight using a nomogram (see inside back cover), so calculations of fluid requirements are most accurate when based on the BSA.

If a BSA nomogram is not readily available, the BSA can be estimated using body weight and the following formula:

$$\frac{(4 \times \text{Weight [kg]}) + 7}{90 + \text{Weight (kg)}} = \text{BSA (m}^2)$$

The weight can be estimated from body length using a length-based tape (see section, Cardiac Arrest and Resuscitation) such as the Broselow resuscitation tape (Fig. 1-1; see also Evolve Fig. 1-1 in the Chapter 1 Supplement on the Evolve Website.)

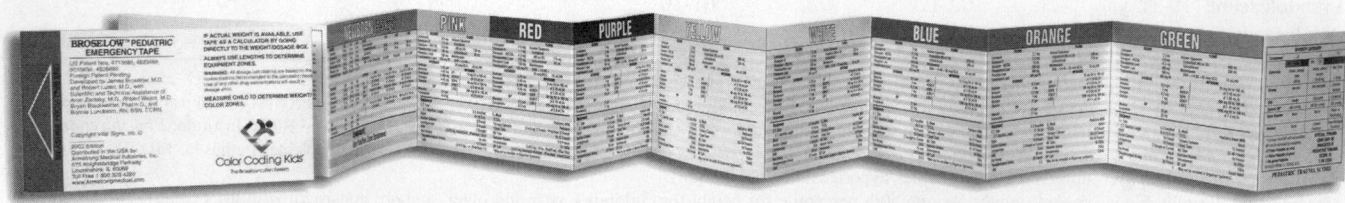

A

FIG. 1-1 Broselow Pediatric Emergency Tape. **A,** The two-sided tape allows for rapid identification of doses of emergency drugs, appropriate equipment sizes, and estimated body weight based on child's body length.

PINK / RED

B

PINK

RESUSCITATION		RAPID SEQUENCE INTUBATION	
		PREMEDICATIONS	
Epinephrine (1:10,000)	0.065 mg (0.65 mL)	Atropine	0.13 mg
Epinephrine ET (1:1,000)	0.65 mg (0.65 mL)	Pan/Vecuronium (Defasiculating Agent)	N/A; N/A < 20 kg
Atropine (0.1 mg/mL)	0.13 mg (1.3 mL)	Lidocaine	10 mg
Atropine ET (0.4 mg/mL)	0.2 mg (0.5 mL)	Fentanyl	20 mcg
Sodium Bicarbonate	6.5 mEq	**INDUCTION AGENTS**	
Lidocaine	6.5 mg	Etomidate	2 mg
Lidocaine ET	13-20 mgs	Ketamine	13 mg
Defibrillation		Midazolam	2 mg
1st/2nd Dose (may repeat)	13J/26J	Propofol	20 mg
Cardioversion		**PARALYTIC AGENTS**	
1st/2nd Dose	7J/13J	Succinylcholine (give atropine prior)	13 mg
Adenosine		Pancuronium	1.3 mg
1st Dose	0.65 mg	Vecuronium	1.3 mg
2nd Dose If Needed	1.3 mg	Rocuronium	7 mg
Amiodarone	32 mg	**MAINTENANCE**	
Calcium Chloride	130 mg	Pancuronium/Vecuronium	0.7 mg
Magnesium Sulfate	325 mg	Lorazepam	0.3 mg

6 KG   **7 KG**

RED

RESUSCITATION		RAPID SEQUENCE INTUBATION	
		PREMEDICATIONS	
Epinephrine (1:10,000)	0.085 mg (0.85 mL)	Atropine	0.17 mg
Epinephrine ET (1:1,000)	0.85 mg (0.85 mL)	Pan/Vecuronium (Defasiculating Agent)	N/A; N/A < 20 kg
Atropine (0.1 mg/mL)	0.17 mg (1.7 mL)	Lidocaine	13 mg
Atropine ET (0.4 mg/mL)	0.26 mg (0.65 mL)	Fentanyl	25 mcg
Sodium Bicarbonate	8.5 mEq	**INDUCTION AGENTS**	
Lidocaine	8.5 mg	Etomidate	2.5 mg
Lidocaine ET	17-26 mgs	Ketamine	17 mg
Defibrillation		Midazolam	2.5 mg
1st/2nd Dose (may repeat)	17J/34J	Propofol	25 mg
Cardioversion		**PARALYTIC AGENTS**	
1st/2nd Dose	9J/17J	Succinylcholine (give atropine prior)	17 mg
Adenosine		Pancuronium	1.7 mg
1st Dose	0.85 mg	Vecuronium	1.7 mg
2nd Dose If Needed	1.7 mg	Rocuronium	9 mg
Amiodarone	42 mg	**MAINTENANCE**	
Calcium Chloride	170 mg	Pancuronium/Vecuronium	0.9 mg
Magnesium Sulfate	425 mg	Lorazepam	0.4 mg

8 KG   **9 KG**

C

PINK

SEIZURE		FLUIDS	
Lorazepam	0.7 mg	**Volume Expansion**	
Diazepam IV	1.3 mg	Crystalloid (NS or LR)	130 mL
Diazepam — RECTAL	3.3 mg	Colloid/blood	65 mL
Phenobarbital Load	130 mg	**Maintenance**	
Phenytoin Load	100 mg	D5W + 1/2 NS +	
Fosphenytoin Load	100 mg-PE	20 meq KCl/L	27 mL/HR
OVERDOSE			
Dextrose	3.25 g		
Naloxone	0.65 mg	**Infusion:** Pursuant to JCAHO's National Patient Safety Goal 3b - "Rule of 6" for Infusions should be converted to Standardized Concentrations.	
Flumazenil	0.065 mg		
Glucagon	0.5 mg		
Charcoal	6.5 g		
ICP			
Mannitol	6.5 g		
Furosemide	6.5 mg		

Equipment	
E.T. Tube	3.5 Uncuffed
E.T. Insertion Length(Pink/Red)	10.5-11 cm
Stylet	6 French
Suction Catheter	8 French
Laryngoscope	1 Straight
BVM	Infant/Child
Oral Airway	50 mm
*Nasopharyngeal Airway	14 French
*LMA	(3-4-5 kg) 1, (Pink/Red) 1.5

RED

SEIZURE		FLUIDS	
Lorazepam	0.9 mg	**Volume Expansion**	
Diazepam IV	1.7 mg	Crystalloid (NS or LR)	170 mL
Diazepam — RECTAL	4.2 mg	Colloid/blood	85 mL
Phenobarbital Load	170 mg	**Maintenance**	
Phenytoin Load	130 mg	D5W + 1/2 NS +	
Fosphenytoin Load	130 mg-PE	20 meq KCl/L	35 mL/HR
OVERDOSE			
Dextrose	4.25 g		
Naloxone	0.85 mg	**Infusion:** Pursuant to JCAHO's National Patient Safety Goal 3b - "Rule of 6" for Infusions should be converted to Standardized Concentrations.	
Flumazenil	0.085 mg		
Glucagon	0.5 mg		
Charcoal	8.5 g		
ICP			
Mannitol	8.5 g		
Furosemide	8.5 mg		

O₂ Mask	Pediatric NRB
*ETCO₂	Pediatric
*Urinary Catheter	(3-4-5 kg) 5 French, (Pink/Red) 8 French
*Chest Tube	10-12 French
NG Tube	5-8 French
Vascular Access	22-24Ga
Intraosseous	18Ga/15Ga
BP Cuff	(3-4-5 kg) Neonatal #5/Infant, (Pink/Red) Infant/Child
*May not be included in Organizer System(s).	

FIG. 1-1, cont'd B, One side of the tape displays appropriate doses and administration volumes of resuscitation and rapid sequence intubation drugs and estimated weight (determined from child's length). C, The second (color-coded) side of the tape indicates appropriate sizes of emergency equipment and additional fluid and drug information based on child's length. (See also Evolve Fig. 1-1 in the Chapter 1 Supplement on the Evolve Website.) (Used with permission of James Broselow and Vital Signs. Copyright Vital Signs, Inc. All Rights Reserved.)

Table 1-4 Formulas for Estimating Daily Maintenance Fluid and Electrolyte Requirements for Children

	Daily Requirements	Hourly Requirements
Fluid Requirements Estimated from Weight*		
Newborn (up to 72 hr after birth)	60-100 mL/kg (newborns are born with excess body water)	–
Up to 10 kg	100 mL/kg (can increase up to 150 mL/kg to provide caloric requirements if renal and cardiac function are adequate)	4 mL/kg
11-20 kg	1000 mL for the first 10 kg + 50 mL/kg for each kg over 10 kg	40 mL for first 10 kg + 2 mL/kg for each kg over 10 kg
21-30 kg	1500 mL for the first 20 kg + 25 mL/kg for each kg over 20 kg	60 mL for first 20 kg + 1 mL/kg for each kg over 20 kg
Fluid Requirements Estimated from Body Surface Area (BSA)		
Maintenance	1500 mL/m^2 BSA	–
Insensible losses	300-400 mL/m^2 BSA	–
Electrolytes		
Sodium (Na)	2-4 mEq/kg	–
Potassium (K)	1-2 mEq/kg	–
Chloride (Cl)	2-3 mEq/kg	–
Calcium (Ca)	0.5-3 mEq/kg	–
Phosphorous (Phos)	0.5-2 mmol/kg	–
Magnesium (Mg)	0.4-0.9 mEq/kg	–

*The "maintenance" fluids calculated by these formulas must only be used as a starting point to determine the fluid requirements of an individual patient. If intravascular volume is adequate, children with cardiac, pulmonary, or renal failure or increased intracranial pressure should generally receive less than these calculated "maintenance" fluids. The formula utilizing body weight generally results in a generous "maintenance" fluid total.

The estimate of maintenance fluid requirements (Table 1-4) provides a baseline for tailoring the fluid administration rate for each patient. Actual fluid administration is tailored to the child's clinical condition. Normal insensible water losses average 300 to 400 mL/m^2 BSA per day. Fever increases insensible water losses by approximately 0.42 mL/kg per hour per degree Celsius elevation in temperature above 37° C.[40] Radiant warmers, phototherapy, and the presence of diaphoresis or large burns also will increase a child's insensible water loss. Fluid retention can diminish fluid requirements postoperatively and fluid retention typically develops in the presence of congestive heart failure, respiratory failure, or renal failure.

Although the child's fluid requirements per kilogram body weight are higher than those of an adult, the absolute amount of fluid required by the child is small. Excessive fluid administration is avoided through careful regulation and tabulation of all fluids administered to the child. Unrecognized sources of fluid intake can include fluids used to flush monitoring lines or to dilute medications.

When the child is critically ill, hourly (or more frequent) evaluation of the child's fluid balance is needed to enable rapid modification of fluid therapy in response to changes in the child's condition. All intravenous and irrigation fluids should be administered through volume-controlled infusion pumps.

Many infusion pumps are programmable, and with entry of the child's weight and drug concentration, the pumps will calculate drug dose administered by continuous infusion. Each nurse is responsible for all drugs administered during that nurse's shift, so the accuracy of all infusion devices must be verified at the beginning of each shift and when changes are made in infusion rates, to avoid perpetuation of programming or other errors.

If hydration and fluid intake are adequate, the infant's urine volume should average 2 mL/kg per hour. The normal urine volume will be 1 to 2 mL/kg per hour in the child and 0.5 to 1 mL/kg per hour in the adolescent. A small reduction in urine volume can indicate significant compromise in renal perfusion or function.

It is important to monitor and document all sources of fluid loss in the critically ill child. Unrecognized fluid loss can result from phlebotomy, nasogastric or pleural drainage, vomiting, diarrhea, or intestinal drainage. If fluid output exceeds intake, notify the appropriate provider; adjustment in fluid administration may be indicated.

Measurement of the child's weight on a regular basis will aid in evaluation of the child's fluid balance. You should ideally weigh the child using the same method (e.g., in-bed scale or the same external scale) at the same time each day, and at the same time in relation to diuretic administration, to avoid even small errors in measurement. Small daily weight changes can be significant, particularly if a trend is observed. A weight gain or loss of 50 g/day in the infant, 200 g/day in the child, or 500 g/day in the adolescent should be discussed with a physician or appropriate provider.

If the patient bed incorporates a scale, the bed scale should be zeroed before patient admission with a recorded list of the linens that are on the bed at the time of zeroing. If the linens and weights are not recorded, similar linens can be weighed, but this will obviously introduce error from one measurement to the next. If the bed does not incorporate a scale, sling scales are used. If possible, weigh bulky dressings and equipment before they are placed on the child. If this is impossible, record the weight of similar dressings and equipment to estimate their contribution to the child's weight.

Children have proportionally more body water than do adults. Total body water constitutes approximately 75% to 80% of the full-term infant's weight and 60% to 70% of the body weight of the adult. During the first weeks of life, most body water is located in the extracellular compartment, and much of this water is exchanged daily. For this reason and because the infant kidney is less able to concentrate urine (see section, Renal Function), dehydration can develop rapidly if the infant's fluid intake is compromised or fluid losses are excessive.

Signs of dehydration are approximately the same in patients of any age and include dry mucous membranes, decreased urine volume with increased urine concentration, and poor skin turgor. The dehydrated infant usually will have a sunken fontanelle. Mild dehydration produces weight loss; moderate and severe dehydration generally produce signs of circulatory compromise. Peripheral circulatory compromise will be observed in the infant or child with moderate isotonic dehydration, but it may develop following mild dehydration in patients with hyponatremia. Moderate dehydration is typically associated with a 7% to 10% weight loss in children and a 5% to 7% weight loss in the adolescent or adult.

Oral intake often is compromised during serious illness, so the critically ill child depends on uninterrupted delivery of intravenous fluids. Because small intravenous catheters can easily kink and become obstructed, they must be handled carefully, anchored securely, and flushed regularly. When intravenous access is difficult to establish during resuscitation, intraosseous access provides a readily accessible and reliable route to administer fluids and medications.

Intravenous fluids are provided to flush monitoring lines, dilute medications, replace volume loss, or provide nutrition. In the past, hypotonic crystalloids (e.g., 5% dextrose with 0.2% sodium chloride) were routinely used for pediatric maintenance and replacement fluids, with the assumption that critically ill patients are likely to retain sodium and water. However, children are much more likely to develop hyponatremia if hypotonic rather than isotonic solutions are used, and isotonic fluids do not increase risk of hypernatremia.[2,9] At this time there is insufficient evidence to identify a single optimal intravenous fluid for pediatric maintenance therapy, so practitioners will need to individualize intravenous fluid selection for each patient.

Providers should monitor serum electrolytes and clinical status during parenteral fluid therapy to enable rapid detection and treatment of any imbalances that develop. The nurse should verify that the volume and content of each infusion is appropriate. If the patient's status changes, it is often necessary to change the volume and content of the patient's intravenous infusions.

The nurse should regularly inspect intravenous infusion sites and routinely touch every fluid administration system from beginning to end. With this careful inspection, the nurse will detect any loose connection or leak and can verify correct position of clamps and stopcocks; this inspection can prevent inadvertent interruption of or errors in fluid infusion.

Electrolyte, Glucose, and Calcium Balance

Normal serum electrolyte, glucose, and calcium concentrations are the same for both adults and children, as are renal and cellular mechanisms for maintaining serum electrolyte balance. However, some forms of electrolyte, glucose, and calcium imbalance are more likely to occur or cause complications in children than in adults. In addition, abnormalities of sodium, potassium, glucose, calcium, and magnesium occur frequently in critical care, so the nurse should monitor laboratory values and assess for clinical manifestations of these imbalances. It is important to anticipate the effect of therapy on the child's electrolytes (e.g., correction of acidosis will be associated with a fall in serum potassium concentration) and attempt to prevent electrolyte imbalances.

Sodium is the major intravascular ion, and acute changes in serum sodium concentration will affect serum osmolality and free water movement. Hyponatremia in the critically ill child can result from antidiuretic hormone excess (i.e., the syndrome of inappropriate antidiuretic hormone secretion) and liberal water administration in excess of sodium, including administration of hypotonic fluids.[4] Hyponatremia can also result from excess sodium losses, such as those occurring with adrenocortical insufficiency (see Chapter 12).

An acute fall in serum sodium will typically produce an acute fall in serum osmolality; this will produce an osmotic gradient from the extracellular compartment (including the vascular space) to the intracellular compartment, so free water shifts into the cells. A significant intracellular fluid shift can produce cerebral edema, seizures, and coma. The volume of water shift and the severity of clinical manifestations with hyponatremia are directly related to the acuity and the magnitude of the fall in serum sodium and osmolality. As in the adult, hyponatremia associated with neurologic symptoms is a neurologic emergency. In children it is treated with hypertonic saline (3% sodium chloride, 2-4 mL/kg).

Hypernatremia can result from excessive sodium administration or free water loss, such as that occurring with diabetes insipidus or vomiting. Hypernatremia in infants and young children is most frequently observed as a complication of dehydration. Cerebral hemorrhage and cerebral dysfunction have been reported after abrupt correction of hyponatremia in adults (i.e., rapid rise in serum sodium concentration),[18] and similar complications are thought to occur in children. Rapid correction of hypernatremia can produce an acute fall in serum osmolality, with resultant intracellular free water shift and cerebral edema. In general, when correcting hyponatremia or hypernatremia the child's serum sodium concentration should be changed at a maximum rate of 10 to 12 mEq/24 h (or an average of 0.5 mEq/h).

Changes in the serum potassium concentration occur with changes in acid-base status, use of cardiopulmonary bypass, and administration of diuretics. Hypokalemia can produce cardiac arrhythmias and perpetuate digitalis toxicity. However, cardiac arrhythmias related solely to potassium imbalance rarely occur in children until the serum potassium is extremely low (<3 mEq/L) or high (>7 mEq/L).

The serum potassium should be expected to fall as the child's pH rises, and it will rise as the pH falls because hydrogen ion moves intracellularly in exchange for potassium. A low serum potassium concentration in a patient with acidosis is problematic, because it will drop even lower as the acidosis is corrected (see Chapter 12).

During periods of stress in adults, epinephrine and cortisol are secreted, resulting in glycogen breakdown and increased serum glucose levels; thus, the critically ill adult often demonstrates hyperglycemia. However, infants have continuously high glucose needs and low glycogen stores, so they often develop hypoglycemia during periods of stress. Hypoglycemia can depress the infant's cardiovascular or neurologic function. Hypoglycemia or hyperglycemia can be an early sign of sepsis in the infant, and glycosuria can be an early sign of infection in the child.

All critical care clinicians will closely monitor the critically ill infant's serum glucose concentration and treat hypoglycemia. If point-of-care testing is available, perform heel-stick glucose testing routinely, and treat and repeat as necessary during stabilization of the critically ill infant. A constant glucose infusion is preferable to frequent bolus administration of glucose; the infusion will prevent the wide fluctuations in glucose levels that can result from intermittent bolus glucose administration and reactive hyperinsulinemia. In many critical care units, 10% glucose solutions are used for intravenous maintenance fluid therapy for neonates.

Several case series in adult[38] and pediatric patients suggested that uncontrolled hyperglycemia, whether it is endogenous or exogenous in origin, can be harmful to critically ill patients and can increase complication rates and decrease survival. Although this is a significant concern, other studies have found contradictory evidence, and additional studies are underway to clarify these issues. Use of insulin infusion to prevent hyperglycemia was associated with reduced critical care unit mortality in adult studies[38] and one multicenter pediatric study,[39] but was also associated with increased hypoglycemic episodes.

The relative risk of hyperglycemia and potential harm from hypoglycemia must be considered and are currently being evaluated. If insulin is administered by continuous infusion to control hyperglycemia, it is typically used during the first 12 to 18 hours of pediatric critical care, with careful monitoring of serum glucose concentration using point-of-care testing, if possible. A glucose infusion can be added and titrated to prevent significant hypoglycemia during the insulin infusion.

The serum ionized calcium concentration (normal value is approximately 4.8 to 5.2 mg/dL or 1.2 to 1.38 mmol/L) is the "working" calcium, involved in nerve and muscle function.[12] Therefore, the healthcare team monitors ionized and total calcium concentration during critical illness and provides supplementary calcium for documented hypocalcemia.

A fall in total or ionized calcium is observed frequently in critically ill infants and children. Ionized hypocalcemia has been reported after cardiac arrest in children with septic shock or renal failure.[41] The phosphate in citrate phosphate dextran-preserved blood will precipitate with ionized calcium, so some transfusions may produce ionized hypocalcemia.

The serum ionized calcium concentration is affected by the serum albumin concentration and by the serum pH. The ionized calcium concentration falls when the serum albumin or serum pH rise (both increase binding of calcium to albumin), and the ionized calcium concentration will rise when serum albumin or pH fall.

Abnormalities in magnesium balance are observed frequently in critically ill patients. Magnesium affects parathyroid function and contributes to control of the intracellular potassium concentration. As a result, hypomagnesemia can contribute to refractory hypocalcemia or hypokalemia. In addition, it can be associated with increased neuromuscular excitability, gastrointestinal dysfunction, and arrhythmias.[18]

Hypomagnesemia (<1.3 to 2.0 mEq/dL) in the critically ill child is most commonly caused by inadequate magnesium intake, particularly if the child is nutritionally compromised or receiving intravenous fluids without magnesium supplement. Hypomagnesemia is also observed in the child with increased magnesium losses, such as those that occur with chronic congestive heart failure or renal failure or following administration of osmotic diuretics.

Renal Function

Kidney weight doubles in the first 10 months of life, more as the result of proximal tubular growth than from an increase in glomerular size. The glomerular filtration rate (GFR) also increases significantly after birth; the GFR of the full-term neonate (per square meter of BSA) is approximately one third that of an adult. Renal blood flow and the GFR double during the first 2 weeks of life, and the GFR continues to increase during the first year. The GFR approaches adult values by approximately 3 years of age (Table 1-5).[3,36] Until that time, the relatively low GFR and reduced tubular secretion can prolong the half-life of administered drugs (see Chapters 4 and 13).

Immediately after birth, the neonate normally has a high urine volume with low osmolality. This is thought to result from the immaturity of renal sodium and fluid regulatory mechanisms. The normal newborn typically demonstrates diuresis of excess body water during the first 72 hours of life. After that time, urine volume normally falls and urine concentration gradually rises.

The newborn kidney is able to conserve sodium and glucose as well as the adult kidney. The newborn kidney is less able to excrete free water and to concentrate urine than the adult kidney, however. As a result, the infant kidney may be less able to excrete a large water load and may be unable to concentrate urine in response to dehydration.

Regulation of acid-base balance by the newborn kidney is relatively efficient, although the infant kidney has less ability to secrete hydrogen ions or fixed acid than the adult kidney (this is exacerbated by limited dietary protein intake). As a result, renal compensation for metabolic acidosis may be

Table 1-5	Changes in Glomerular Filtration Rate with Age	
Age	**Glomerular Filtration Rate (mL/min per 1.73 m²)**
Premature infant	6
Full-term newborn	8-60
1 month	26-90
1 year	63-150
3 years	89-179
6 years	79-170
Adult male	110-152

Consistent with values from Barakat AY, Ichikawa I: Laboratory data. In Ichikawa I, editor: *Pediatric textbook of fluids and electrolytes*, Baltimore, 1990, Williams and Wilkins; and Tan JM: Nephrology. In Custer JW, Rau RE, editors: *The Johns Hopkins Hospital Harriet Lane Handbook*, ed 18, Philadelphia, 2009, Mosby-Elsevier.

limited in the neonate. Dehydration, hypotension, and hypoxemia all produce a marked fall in the infant's GFR, so renal function can become compromised quickly during critical illness (for further information, see Chapter 13).

Pediatric Pharmacokinetics

Drug absorption, distribution, and elimination will be affected by age and clinical condition. Drug absorption is influenced by maturation of the gastrointestinal tract, liver, and kidney. Because the gastric pH is higher (less acidic) during the first 2 years of life, bioavailability of weak acids administered orally (e.g., phenytoin and phenobarbital) may be reduced in this age group, so higher doses (per kilogram body weight) may be required to achieve target serum concentrations of such drugs.[1]

Drug distribution is affected by cardiac output, organ blood flow, composition and relative size of body compartments, pH of body fluids, and extent of drug binding to plasma proteins and tissues. The higher proportion of water in the body during the first years of life increases the volume of distribution for hydrophilic drugs during these years.[1] Even if a drug has a consistent volume of distribution (mg/kg body weight) for patients of all ages, the neonate has limited ability to eliminate some drugs, so those drugs will have longer half-lives and lower clearances when administered to neonates than to older children and adults. Even when loading doses for drugs are similar (per kilogram body weight) for neonates and adults, neonates will likely require lower maintenance doses of the drugs than will be required by adults.

Drug clearance is affected by metabolic, hepatic, and renal blood flow and function.[1] Developmental changes associated with hepatic metabolism and renal secretion or filtration can slow down or speed up drug elimination. Several metabolic processes mature during the first months of life (see Fig. 4-7), and many drug elimination pathways continue to mature during the first years of life. Failure to recognize these developmental changes in children can lead to drug dosing errors and complications. By the end of the first year of life, liver metabolism and drug clearance are similar to those reported in older children and adults.

The nurse should be familiar with the pharmacokinetics and pharmacodynamics of all drugs administered to the patient (see also Chapter 4) and should evaluate drug dose in light of the patient's organ perfusion and function and in light of clinical factors, such as drugs or conditions that may alter protein binding.

Nutrition and Gastrointestinal Function

The child has a higher metabolic rate than does the adult, and the child requires more calories per kilogram body weight (Table 1-6). Most of a child's maintenance calories are needed for basal metabolism and growth, so the child typically requires a caloric intake that approaches the typical maintenance caloric intake even if the child is inactive.

Critical illness, trauma, or burns will increase the child's caloric requirements significantly, and fever will increase caloric requirements 12% per hour per degree Celsius elevation in temperature above 37° C.[40] Unless intolerably large quantities of fluids are administered, maintenance calories cannot be

Table 1-6	Estimated Normal Maintenance Caloric Requirements for Infants and Children	
Age	**Kcal/kg per 24 hours**
0-6 months	90-110
6-12 months	80-100
12-36 months	75-90
4-10 years	65-75
>10 years, male	40-55
>10 years, female	38-50

Nutrient	Percent of total daily calories
Carbohydrates	40-70 ⎫
Fat	20-50 ⎬ Combined 85-88
Protein	7-15

provided through 5% or 10% dextrose intravenous fluids. Therefore, provision of parenteral nutrition or tube feedings must be planned early in the child's hospitalization.

Liver enzymatic synthesis and degradation are immature in the newborn, and they typically mature during the first months and years of life. The neonatal liver is less able to metabolize toxic substances, which can result in prolongation of beneficial or toxic effects of drugs during the first months of life.

Gastric motility is reduced, but gastric emptying is more rapid in neonates. Although nasogastric or orogastric feeding can be a useful method of providing nutrition during the first weeks of life, some gastroesophageal reflux should be anticipated.

CARDIOVASCULAR FUNCTION

Cardiac Output

Normal cardiac output is higher per kilogram body weight in the child than in the adult. The cardiac output at birth is 400 mL/kg per minute; it falls to approximately 200 mL/kg per minute within the first weeks of life and to 100 mL/kg per minute during adolescence.[32]

To allow direct comparison of cardiac outputs for patients of different ages and sizes, the cardiac index is usually calculated. The cardiac index is equal to the cardiac output per square meter of BSA (cardiac output ÷ BSA in m^2); normal values are 3.5 to 4.5 L/min per m^2 BSA in the child and 2.5 to 3.5 L/min per m^2 BSA in the adult. A cardiac index of less than 2.1 to 2.5 L/min per m^2 BSA is considered low cardiac output in a patient of any age.[32]

When the child is critically ill, cardiac output should be evaluated as either *adequate* or *inadequate* to meet metabolic demands; shock can be present despite a normal or high cardiac output. For example, in a patient with high oxygen requirements (e.g., septic shock) and a normal rather than increased cardiac output, metabolic acidosis can develop, indicating inadequate tissue oxygen delivery.

Heart Rate and Rhythm

Cardiac output is the product of heart rate and stroke volume (volume of the blood ejected by the ventricles in each minute). In the child, heart rate is more rapid and stroke volume is smaller than in the adult, so pediatric cardiac output is directly proportional to heart rate.

Tachycardia is the most efficient method of increasing cardiac output in any patient, and it is the chief method of increasing cardiac output in the child. Tachycardia is normally observed when the child is frightened, febrile, or stressed. However, an increase in heart rate to extremely high levels may reduce cardiac output. If the ventricular rate exceeds 180 to 220 beats/min, ventricular diastolic filling time and coronary artery perfusion time are severely compromised, so stroke volume and cardiac output usually fall.[30]

Transient bradycardia may be normal in the infant or child, particularly during periods of sleep or times of vagal stimulation (such as that produced by suctioning, defecation, or feeding). Profound or persistent bradycardia, however, usually results in a fall in cardiac output and systemic perfusion. The most common cause of bradycardia in the child is hypoxia, so the initial treatment of bradycardia requires assessment and support of airway and ventilation. Symptomatic bradycardia (i.e., bradycardia associated with signs of poor perfusion) despite adequate oxygenation and ventilation is an ominous sign of deterioration and requires immediate resuscitation.[8a,20,30]

Many neonatal and pediatric arrhythmias are clinically benign, because they do not compromise systemic perfusion, and they are unlikely to convert to malignant arrhythmias. The significance of any arrhythmia is determined by its effects on the child's systemic perfusion—the heart rhythm is either stable or unstable.[8a,20,30]

Unstable arrhythmias include those in which the ventricular rate is too slow to maintain effective perfusion, too fast to maintain systemic perfusion, or the rhythm results in ineffective perfusion (with loss of pulses). The most common clinically significant unstable arrhythmias observed in children are bradycardia and supraventricular tachycardia; children with cardiovascular disease and some with channelopathies or left ventricular outflow tract obstruction may demonstrate ventricular arrhythmias (see section, Cardiac Arrest and Resuscitation).

Factors Influencing Stroke Volume

Cardiac output can be affected by changes in the stroke volume. The stroke volume in the neonate is extremely small, averaging 1.5 mL/kg, or 5 mL, in the full-term newborn. This stroke volume increases with age and averages approximately 75 to 90 mL in the adolescent or adult.[32]

As in the adult, the child's stroke volume is affected by cardiac preload, contractility, and afterload. Ventricular preload is increased by increasing myocardial fiber length before ventricular contraction; this is accomplished in the critical care unit with intravenous volume administration.

There is not a linear relationship between volume administered and preload (ventricular end-diastolic pressure [VEDP]) produced. The effect of volume administration on VEDP is influenced by ventricular compliance (i.e., the distensibility of the ventricle); compliance varies from patient to patient and can vary in the same patient. Neonatal myocardium is less compliant and has a smaller response to volume loading than the myocardium of older children and adults.[27] When treating

shock with bolus fluid administration, the critical care provider will titrate volume administration to patient response.

Early studies of isolated and nonhuman myocardium led to the conclusion that the neonate and young infant are incapable of increasing stroke volume in response to volume administration. We now know, however, that infants and children can increase stroke volume and cardiac output in response to increases in preload, provided that ventricular function remains adequate and ventricular afterload is normal or low. The heart rate, however, is the major factor that determines cardiac output in infants and children.

Cardiac contractility refers to efficiency of myocardial fiber shortening. Contractility can be impaired in postoperative patients or patients with ischemia, electrolyte or acid-base imbalance, coronary artery insufficiency, or infection. Neonatal myocardium is less compliant and contains less contractile mass than does adult myocardium, and the neonatal ventricle is thought to require higher VEDP to maximize stroke volume. Infant myocardium, however, actually has a higher ejection fraction than that of the older child or adult.[32]

Ventricular afterload is ventricular wall stress, commonly considered as impedance to ventricular ejection. Infants and children tolerate mild increases in ventricular afterload (such as may result from mild pulmonary or aortic stenosis), provided the afterload does not develop acutely. As in the adult, significant increases in ventricular afterload can produce heart failure and decreased cardiac output (see Chapters 6 and 8 for more information).

Response to Catecholamines

The developmental response to exogenous catecholamine administration is still under investigation. Published studies of catecholamine administration in children have used heterogeneous groups of patients (many ages, sizes, and clinical conditions), so it is difficult to generalize observations. The response of the myocardium and vascular tone to exogenous catecholamine administration will probably be affected more by the child's clinical condition (e.g., whether downgrading or upgrading of receptors or in hepatic and renal dysfunction) than by the child's age (see Chapters 6 and 8). Therefore, the correct dose of any vasoactive drug must be determined at the patient's bedside with careful titration according to patient response. This drug titration requires ongoing assessment to maximize therapeutic effects and minimize side or toxic effects.

Signs of Shock

Signs of low cardiac output or poor systemic perfusion are generally the same in any patient, regardless of age. Most patients develop tachycardia, pallor, cool skin, and decreased urine output. Peripheral pulses are usually diminished in intensity, and metabolic acidosis develops. In patients with sepsis, the skin may be warm with brisk capillary refill and pulses may be bounding.

As noted previously, the infant with poor systemic perfusion can demonstrate temperature instability, and the child can develop a high core temperature in the face of profound reduction in skin blood flow. Subtle signs of poor systemic perfusion in the infant or young child include a change in level of

---

Box 1-3 Signs of Poor Systemic Perfusion

Tachycardia
Mottled color, pallor
Cool skin, prolonged capillary refill
Oliguria (urine volume <1-2 mL/kg per hour)
Diminished intensity of peripheral pulses
Metabolic acidosis
Change in responsiveness
LATE: hypotension, bradycardia

Table 1-7 Estimated Circulating Blood Volume in Children

Age	Blood Volume (mL/kg)
Neonate	80-85
Infant	75-80
Child	70-75
Adolescent, adult	65-70

---

consciousness or responsiveness and hypoglycemia (Box 1-3). Unlike in adults, however, hypotension is usually only a late sign of poor systemic perfusion in the child.

The American Heart Association (AHA) Pediatric Advanced Life Support Guidelines[20] define hypotension as a systolic blood pressure less than 60 mm Hg in term neonates (up to 28 days of age), and a systolic blood pressure less than 70 mm Hg in infants (1 to 12 months of age). In children 1 to 10 years old, systolic hypotension is present if the systolic pressure is less than 70 mm Hg plus twice the age in years.[8a,20] This estimate corresponds to slightly higher than the fifth percentile systolic blood pressure for children of median height.[17] For the same age group, the critically low mean arterial pressure (the fifth percentile mean arterial pressure for children of median height) can be estimated by the following formula[17]:

$$\text{Mean arterial pressure} = (1.5 \times \text{Age in years}) + 40 \text{ mm Hg}$$

For children 10 years of age and older, a systolic blood pressure less than 90 mm Hg is considered hypotensive.[8a,20,30]

Signs of congestive heart failure, similar in the adult and the child, include the signs of adrenergic stimulation and evidence of high systemic and pulmonary venous pressures. Pulmonary venous congestion will produce tachypnea and increased respiratory effort, and in infants it can result in difficulty feeding.

Treatment of congestive heart failure in any patient requires eliminating excess intravascular fluid and improving myocardial function. Diuretic therapy and limitation of fluid intake will eliminate excess intravascular fluid. Administration (and titration) of inotropic agents, inodilators or vasodilators can improve cardiovascular function. Digoxin derivatives are used less often in children than in adults, and potential benefits of use must be weighed against risk of toxicity. Because risk of toxicity is high in premature infants, digoxin is less likely to be used in this population. Digoxin can be used in infants with large ventricular septal defects and preoperative congestive heart failure and in older children who have structurally normal hearts and cardiomyopathy (see section, Congestive Heart Failure in Chapter 8).

Circulating Blood Volume

The child's circulating blood volume is larger per kilogram body weight than that of the adult (Table 1-7). However, the child's absolute blood volume is small, so quantitatively small blood loss can significantly reduce blood volume and systemic perfusion. A 25-mL blood loss in a 70-kg adult would represent loss of only 0.5% to 0.6% of blood volume. The same 25-mL blood loss in the 3-kg neonate constitutes a 10% hemorrhage.

Calculate the child's total circulating blood volume on admission, and consider all blood lost or drawn for laboratory analysis as a percentage of this blood volume. Unit protocols should establish a consistent technique for withdrawing blood samples from indwelling lines to minimize blood loss and net fluid administration (particularly for neonates). When frequent blood sampling is required, include a running total of blood lost or drawn in the patient record. Notify a provider if acute blood loss totals 5% to 10% of the child's circulating blood volume; blood administration may be necessary.

As in the adult, systemic oxygen delivery is a product of arterial oxygen content and cardiac output. A threshold hemoglobin concentration for red blood cell (RBC) transfusion of approximately 7 g/dL (typically associated with a hematocrit of 20% to 21% or less) was found to be sufficient in stable critically ill children with adequate cardiovascular function.[22] However, there are insufficient data to recommend a threshold hemoglobin concentration for premature infants or children with conditions such as severe hypoxemia, hemodynamic instability, or heart disease. The healthcare team must individualize transfusion approach, weighing the potential risks of transfusion and the need to optimize the hemoglobin concentration to support the child's systemic oxygen delivery and cardiac output (see Chapter 15).

Cardiac Arrest and Resuscitation

Although there are differences in the epidemiology of out-of-hospital versus in-hospital pediatric cardiac arrest, most episodes of cardiac arrest in infants and children are associated with a terminal rhythm of bradycardia or pulseless electrical activity which, if untreated, progresses to asystole. Sudden arrhythmic arrest is much less common in infants and children than in adults.[30]

Recent analysis of in-hospital pediatric resuscitation data from the American Heart Association National Registry of Cardiopulmonary Resuscitation (NRCPR) in the United States,[26] and data downloaded from automated external defibrillators in the prehospital setting[33] support many of the widely held concepts regarding the epidemiology of pediatric arrest, reinforce the need to prevent arrest, and raise questions for additional studies.

In-hospital cardiac arrest often develops as a progression of respiratory failure and shock. Typically half or more of pediatric victims of in-hospital arrest have preexisting respiratory failure, and one third or more have shock, although these figures vary somewhat among reporting hospitals.[25,26] When pediatric in-hospital respiratory failure or arrest with bradycardia is treated before the development of (pulseless) cardiac arrest, survival is generally high.[14,25]

Bradycardia, asystole, or pulseless electrical activity were recorded as initial rhythms in half or more of recent reports of in-hospital pediatric cardiac arrest, with survival to hospital discharge ranging from 22% to 40%.[25,26] In the NRCPR analysis of first rhythm in cardiac arrest, children who received chest compressions for severe bradycardia with pulses had a significantly higher rate of survival to hospital discharge than those who had a pulseless arrest (60% versus 27%).[14,26] In addition, children with bradycardia who received chest compressions had a higher survival rate than adults who arrested with a terminal bradycardic rhythm.[26]

An analysis of the initial rhythm of in-hospital cardiac arrest in the NRCPR confirmed age-related differences in initial in-hospital arrest rhythms and outcomes. Pediatric patients were more likely than adults to exhibit asystole and only about half as likely to exhibit ventricular fibrillation (VF). Pulseless electrical activity was also less common in children than in adults.[26]

Although VF and pulseless ventricular tachycardia (VT) are uncommon presenting rhythms for pediatric patients with in-hospital pulseless arrest, a "shockable" rhythm was present sometime during the course of one fourth of attempted in-hospital resuscitations in children.[26] This report confirms the importance of training pediatric resuscitation team members in coordination of high-quality chest compressions with shock delivery.

Pediatric advanced life support includes accurate and rapid preparation of appropriate drugs. Use of emergency drug and supply tables and tapes (see Fig. 1-1 earlier in chapter) will improve accuracy and eliminate the need for rapid calculations at a stressful time.[23]

Although retrospective pediatric arrest series have provided important information about the epidemiology of pediatric cardiac arrest, many uncontrolled factors (e.g., definitions of arrest, patient comorbidities, quality of cardiopulmonary resuscitation [CPR], and system factors) can influence outcome. The quality of prearrest, arrest, and postarrest care influences survival. Rapid response teams can reduce the incidence of cardiac arrests outside the pediatric critical care unit, particularly respiratory arrests, although success rates of rapid response teams vary based on activation criteria, team members, and hospital type.

Outcome of in-hospital pediatric resuscitation is undoubtedly influenced by the quality of CPR provided, including duration of "hands off" intervals, and specific periarrest interventions such as extracorporeal membrane oxygenation support, cardiorespiratory support and attempted defibrillation (including technique and dose). Each healthcare system that provides resuscitation is responsible for monitoring outcome and identifying areas for improvement (see Chapter 6).

There are limited data to characterize pediatric out-of-hospital cardiac arrest, although existing data (most recently obtained with automated external defibrillators) support the long-held belief that brady-asystolic rhythms are far more common than "shockable rhythms."[33] VF and VT are not common pediatric arrest rhythms in the out-of-hospital setting, especially in children 7 years of age and younger. Shockable rhythms are more likely to be present with sudden, witnessed collapse, particularly among adolescents.[33]

Although the frequency of sudden cardiac arrest in athletes is not known, extrapolation from a statewide survey in Minnesota suggests the annual incidence is approximately 1 per 200,000 athletes, with more than half of deaths attributed to hypertrophic cardiomyopathy (the leading cause), commotio cordis, or coronary artery anomalies.[24] More recently, channelopathies causing long-QT syndrome have been identified as causes of sudden cardiac arrest.[20] Sudden cardiac arrest in athletes is likely associated with VF or VT, and many episodes are witnessed. Immediate bystander CPR and early defibrillation with an automated external defibrillator can improve the chance of survival. Infants with congenital heart disease often develop ventricular arrhythmias. More data are needed regarding any modifications in resuscitation approach that these children might require.[29]

For adults with a return of spontaneous circulation after cardiac arrest, therapeutic hypothermia and protocols for hemodynamic support and respiratory care improved outcomes of patients admitted after cardiopulmonary arrest and return of spontaneous circulation.[35] Although similar studies have not been reported in children, it is likely that improving post-resuscitation care can increase the rates of survival following cardiopulmonary arrest.

RESPIRATORY FUNCTION

The five major components of the respiratory system and their functions are listed in Table 1-8. Every component of the respiratory system is immature in the child, and this immaturity may contribute to the development of respiratory failure when respiratory dysfunction is present.

Central Nervous System Control of Breathing

Although central and peripheral respiratory chemoreceptors for response to hypoxemia and hypercarbia are present at birth, infants possess fewer peripheral chemoreceptors than do adults. Healthy infants and children typically develop tachypnea and hyperpnea in response to hypoxemia. Premature infants, however, often demonstrate a biphasic response to hypoxemia, with initial hyperpnea followed by a slowing of the respiratory rate and apnea. Careful monitoring of the

Table 1-8   Major Components of Respiratory System

Component	Function
Central nervous system	Control ventilation
Airways	Conduct gas to and from respiratory surface
Chest wall	Enclose lungs
Respiratory muscles	Contribute to expansion of chest wall and lung, stabilize chest wall, and maintain airway patency
Lung tissue	Surface for gas diffusion

infant's rate and effort is needed to detect early evidence of deterioration.

If central nervous system depression results from trauma, disease, narcotic administration, or cerebral edema, the nurse must be prepared to support the child's airway and respiratory function. It is always better to initiate support of ventilation while the patient's respiratory effort is adequate than to delay support until respiratory failure or arrest occur and the patient exhibits apnea or is gasping.

Airways

At birth, the full "adult" complement of conducting airways is present and the airway branching pattern is complete. These airways grow in size and length during childhood. Alveoli and respiratory bronchioles multiply after birth. The number of alveoli increases by more than 10-fold by adulthood, and the alveolar surface area increases by a factor of 20.[6,37]

Supporting airway cartilage and small airway muscles are incompletely developed until school age, so laryngospasm and bronchospasm can produce airway obstruction in the young child. Although it was previously thought that the lack of small airway muscle development contributed to the lack of infant response to bronchodilator therapy, this concept has generally been dispelled.

All airways of infants and children are smaller than airways of adults. Because resistance to air flow (R) is inversely related to 1/radius $(r)^4$ during quiet breathing (laminar air flow), reduction in airway radius will increase resistance to air flow exponentially, and will increase work of breathing.

$$R \propto \frac{1}{r^4}$$

Small amounts of accumulated mucus, edema or airway constriction can have a minimal effect on the adult airway, but will often produce critical reduction in airway radius and critical increase in resistance to air flow and work of breathing in infants and young children (Fig. 1-2). Pediatric artificial airways are also small; they provide greater resistance to airflow than a normal natural airway and can quickly become obstructed by mucus.

The position and shape of the pediatric larynx is different from that of the adult. The pediatric larynx is more anterior and cephalad, and the articulation of the epiglottis with the larynx is more acute in children than in adults. These differences make the upper airway of infants more funnel-shaped than columnar. Pediatric intubation is often difficult for these reasons, and application of slight pressure on the cricoid cartilage may be necessary to displace the larynx posteriorly to facilitate intubation (although excessive pressure may make intubation more difficult).[8a,20,30]

Until a child is approximately 8 years old, the smallest diameter of the pediatric larynx is at the level of the cricoid cartilage, and maximum endotracheal tube size is limited by the size of this area. By comparison, the cricoid area of the adult larynx is relatively wide, so maximal adult endotracheal tube size usually is limited by the diameter of the adult larynx at the level of the vocal cords (Fig. 1-3). In the past, fear of tracheal injury prevented the use of cuffed endotracheal tubes

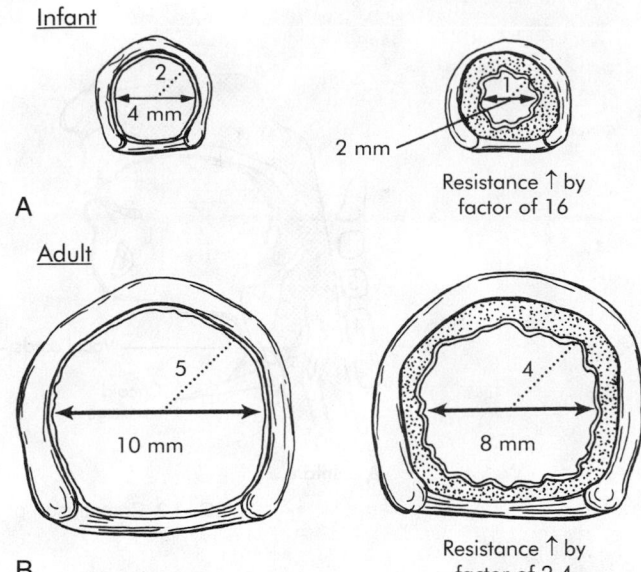

FIG. 1-2 Effects of 1 mm of circumferential edema in neonates and young adults. **A,** The diameter of the larynx of the neonate is approximately 4 mm in diameter. If 1 mm of circumferential edema develops, it will halve the airway radius and increase resistance to airflow by a factor of 16 during quiet breathing (and more if airflow is turbulent). **B,** The larynx of the young adult is approximately 10 mm in diameter and 5 mm in radius. If the young adult develops 1 mm of circumferential edema, it will reduce the radius by about 20% (from 5 to 4 mm), and increase resistance to air flow by a factor of 2.4 during quiet breathing (more if airflow is turbulent).

in children. However, cuffed tubes are now used for children in the prehospital and hospital settings, and may be preferable to uncuffed tubes, particularly when there is a high risk of aspiration or when it is difficult to maintain sufficient airway pressures during assisted ventilation in a child with poor lung compliance or when a large glottic leak is present.[20] The tube cuff pressure must be monitored and maintained per manufacturer's recommendation (usually less than 20 to 25 cm H_2O).[30]

There are several formulas to estimate pediatric endotracheal tube size, depth of insertion, and suction catheter size (Box 1-4). However, body length provides the most reliable parameter for selection of accurate endotracheal tube size.[23]

After an endotracheal tube is inserted, the provider should verify correct position (using clinical assessment and a device such as an exhaled carbon dioxide detector or end-tidal carbon dioxide capnography) and appropriate size. If an uncuffed endotracheal tube is of appropriate size, positive pressure ventilation should produce an air leak when 25 cm H_2O is provided during hand ventilation. If no leak is detected, it might be necessary to replace the tube (when patient condition allows) with a tube that is 0.5 mm (internal diameter) smaller. Cuffed tubes should still allow a slight glottic air leak.

The pediatric trachea is much shorter than the adult trachea. The slightest downward or upward displacement of a pediatric endotracheal tube can move the tube into a mainstem bronchus or out of the trachea. Artificial airways must be securely taped in place, and nurses and therapists should monitor the tube insertion depth at the lip or nares, verifying position with auscultation and exhaled CO_2 tension hourly and with any change in patient condition. Continuous monitoring

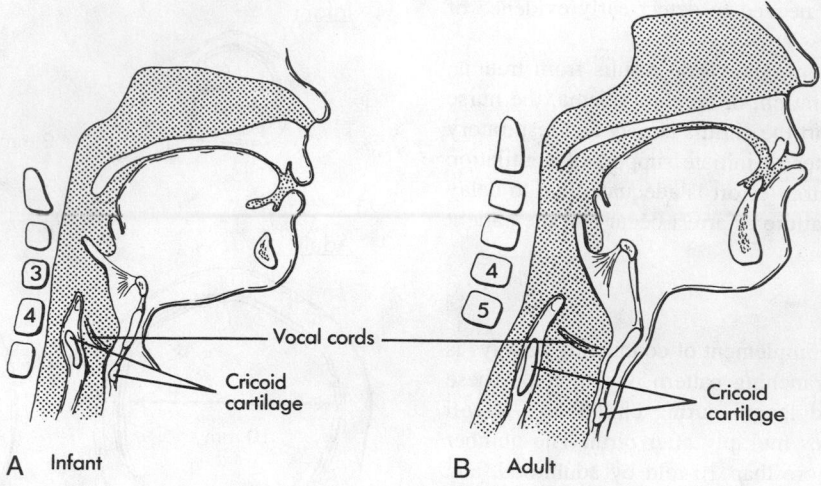

FIG. 1-3 Comparison of infant A, and adult B, larynx.

Box 1-4	**Formulas for Estimating Endotracheal (ET) Tube Size, Depth of Insertion, and Suction Catheter Size[8a,20,30]**

Cuffed ET tubes
- Children 1-2 years of age = 3.5 mm
- Children 2-10 years = $\dfrac{(\text{Age in years})}{4} + 3.5$

Uncuffed tubes
- Children 1-2 years of age = 4.0 mm
- Children 2-10 years = $\dfrac{(\text{Age in years})}{4} + 4$

DEPTH OF INSERTION (cm) = Endotracheal ID* × 3
FRENCH SUCTION CATHETER SIZE = Endotracheal ID* × 2; then increase to next French size

*Use the number only (not the units) for this calculation.
ID, Internal diameter.

---

of waveform capnography will enable immediate detection of inadvertent extubation (see Chapter 9) and may assist in evaluating the quality of resuscitation (see Chapter 6).

The tip of an orotracheal tube will move with changes in the child's head position. Flexion of the neck will displace an orotracheal tube further into the trachea, and extension of the neck will move the tip of the orotracheal tube further out of the trachea (see Fig. 10-19).

The cartilage supporting the infant's larynx is compliant and can be easily compressed anteriorly or posteriorly when the neck is flexed or extended, respectively. When respiratory distress develops during spontaneous breathing, slight neck extension (with or without a jaw lift) can improve airway patency. It is important to avoid neck flexion or hyperextension when distress is present.

During childhood, growth of the peripheral airways lags behind growth of the larger airways, so peripheral airway resistance constitutes a greater portion of total airway resistance than in adults. Because the smaller bronchioles provide high resistance to air flow, the alveolar units served by these bronchioles require long filling and emptying times. If inadequate

exhalation time is provided during mechanical ventilation, air trapping and alveolar distension can develop, producing complications such as increased positive end-expiratory pressure and pneumothorax. During pediatric mechanical ventilation, an optimal inspiratory:expiratory time ratio of 1:3 is usually provided. Mechanical ventilators must be capable of delivering small tidal volumes in short inspiratory times at low peak airway pressures.

Chest Wall

The cartilaginous chest wall of the infant and child is twice as compliant as the chest wall of the adult. As a result, during episodes of respiratory distress the chest wall can retract, compromising the child's ability to maintain functional residual capacity or increase tidal volume. Chest retractions will also increase the work of breathing.

The shape of the infant's chest and the orientation of the ribs also reduce the efficiency of ventilation during episodes of respiratory distress. The ribs are horizontal in orientation, and they articulate linearly with the vertebrae and sternum, so the intercostal muscles do not have the leverage to lift the ribs effectively. After the child reaches school age, the 45-degree orientation of the ribs enables the intercostal muscles to lift the ribs with a lever effect to elevate the chest wall.

During effective positive pressure ventilation, the child's chest should expand easily outward. Positive pressure ventilation is ineffective if the child's chest does not rise bilaterally. When evaluating effectiveness of positive pressure ventilation, if the nurse stands at the head or the foot of the bed and compares chest expansion bilaterally it will be easy to see if chest expansion is inadequate. If one side of the chest is not expanding, endotracheal tube migration, pneumothorax, or atelectasis may be present.

The chest wall is extremely thin in children, so respiratory sounds are easily transmitted throughout all lung fields. As a result, respiratory sounds from other areas of the lung can be heard over an area of atelectasis or pneumothorax. When assessing respiratory sounds and aeration, the nurse should auscultate all lung fields, and compare respiratory sounds heard over one side of the chest with those heard over the contralateral chest. Unilateral pathologic findings (e.g., atelectasis, pneumothorax, pleural effusion) can produce a change in pitch rather than a change in intensity of respiratory sounds.

Respiratory Muscles

Respiratory muscles consist of the diaphragm, the chest wall muscles, and the muscles of the upper and lower airways. These muscles contribute to expansion of the lung and to maintenance of airway patency. Loss of tone, power, and coordination in respiratory muscles will contribute to respiratory failure.

The diaphragm is the chief muscle of respiration. Diaphragm contraction results in an increase in intrathoracic volume and a fall in intrathoracic pressure, so that air enters the lungs. In neonates, the diaphragm is located higher in the thorax and has a smaller radius of curvature than in adults, and so it contracts less efficiently.

The diaphragm inserts obliquely in adults but horizontally in infants. Contraction of the infant diaphragm will tend to draw the lower ribs inward especially if the infant is supine. During episodes of respiratory distress, diaphragm movement will likely be optimized if the infant is placed prone or on the side, with the head of the bed elevated.

Anything that impedes diaphragm contraction or movement, such as abdominal distension, decreased abdominal wall compliance or diaphragm paralysis or paresis can contribute to respiratory failure in children. Paradoxic abdominal motion during inspiration (retraction of the chest wall and expansion of the abdomen) can indicate severe respiratory distress and usually results in rapid fatigue and decompensation.

In adults, the intercostal muscles function as accessory muscles of respiration and can lift the ribs if diaphragm function is impaired. In children, however, the intercostal muscles are not fully developed, so they function largely to stabilize rather than to lift the chest wall.

Lung Tissue

Lung compliance is low in neonates but increases during childhood. Low lung compliance and high chest wall compliance make respiratory function inefficient during episodes of respiratory distress. During childhood, respiratory efficiency improves as chest wall compliance decreases (i.e., the chest wall becomes more stiff) and lung compliance increases.

Closing volume (the minimum lung volume required to maintain peripheral airway patency) constitutes a higher percentage of total lung volume in children than in adults. Some infant airways remain closed during normal breathing; this can render the infant more susceptible to atelectasis.

Elastic tissue in the septae of the alveoli that surround smaller airways contributes to the maintenance of airway patency. There is a smaller amount of elastic and collagen tissue in the pediatric lung than in the adult lung; this can contribute to the increased incidence of pulmonary edema, pneumomediastinum, and pneumothorax in infants and young children. The relative paucity of elastic fibers, in combination with the low elastic recoil of the thorax and lung in the infant

Box 1-5	Signs of Respiratory Distress

Tachypnea, tachycardia
Retractions
Nasal flaring
Grunting
Stridor or wheezing
Mottled color
Change in responsiveness
Hypoxemia, hypercarbia, decreased oxyhemoglobin saturation
LATE: poor air entry, weak cry, apnea or gasping, deterioration in systemic perfusion, bradycardia

and toddler, can contribute to premature airway closure and atelectasis.

Collateral pathways of ventilation, including the intraalveolar Kohn's pores and bronchoalveolar canals of Lambert, are incompletely developed during infancy. As a result, small airway obstruction can produce significant respiratory distress, because collateral pathways cannot ensure ventilation of alveoli distal to the obstruction.

Neonates may be more susceptible to pulmonary edema than older children or adults. Pulmonary edema may be observed frequently during episodes of respiratory distress, even when pulmonary capillary pressure is low. As a result, limitation of fluid intake and possible diuresis is often advisable when caring for euvolemic infants with respiratory failure.

Signs of Respiratory Distress

Signs of respiratory distress in children include: tachypnea, tachycardia, retractions, nasal flaring, grunting, mottled color, and change in responsiveness (Box 1-5). The infant may also demonstrate a weak cry. Hypercarbia, hypoxemia, or a fall in oxyhemoglobin saturation may also be documented. Apnea or gasping, decreased air movement, and alteration in perfusion can be late signs of respiratory distress, indicating impending arrest.

NEUROLOGIC FUNCTION

Brain and Skull Growth

All major structures of the brain and all cranial nerves are present and developed at birth. The infant's neurologic system functions largely at a subcortical level. Brainstem functions and spinal cord reflexes are present, but cortical functions (e.g., memory and fine motor coordination) are incompletely developed. The autonomic nervous system is intact but immature; the infant has limited ability to control body temperature in response to changes in environmental temperature.

At birth, the brain is 25% of its mature adult weight. By 2½ years of age, the brain has achieved 75% of its mature adult weight.[13] The growth in brain size is largely due to the development of fiber tracts and myelinization of neurons. This tremendous central nervous system growth during the first years of life adds uncertainty to the prediction of long-term consequences of early neurologic insults or injury. The child may recover with fewer sequelae than anticipated, because other areas of the brain begin to compensate for the injured areas;

this is called *plasticity*. Subtle signs of unsuspected neurologic sequelae can manifest as learning disabilities when the child enters school.

Mortality is approximately the same following similar head injury in adults and children. However, children who survive head injury often demonstrate more complete recovery than do adult victims with similar injury. The Glasgow Coma Scale is less accurate in predicting the outcome of severe head injury in children than it is in adults, so modified pediatric coma scales have been published (see Chapter 11). A poor prognosis is indicated following head injury in children by the absence of spontaneous respiration, cardiovascular instability despite adequate volume resuscitation, flaccid paralysis, and fixed and dilated pupils. The presence of diabetes insipidus or disseminated intravascular coagulation can also indicate a poor prognosis.

The infant's skull is not rigid during infancy, and the bones of the cranium normally fuse at approximately 16 to 18 months old. As a result, to a point, gradual increases in intracranial volume can be accommodated by skull expansion. Cranial enlargement can indicate the presence of a slow-growing tumor, hydrocephalus, or other mass lesions. Skull expansion does not, however, prevent the development of increased intracranial pressure.

The infant's head circumference is documented on admission to the hospital. If the infant has central nervous system disease or injury (e.g., meningitis, head trauma), the head circumference is recorded frequently (intervals to be determined by protocol or by the healthcare team), and an increase should be reported to a physician or other on-call provider.

Because the fontanelles are not covered by the skull, palpation of the fontanelles can provide information about intracranial pressure or volume. The anterior fontanelle should feel flat and firm but not tense. It will typically bulge with any condition that increases superior vena cava pressure (including congestive heart failure) or intracranial volume or pressure (such as meningitis). If the anterior fontanelle is sunken, significant dehydration may be present.

Normal cerebral blood flow and cerebral perfusion pressure in the infant have not been definitively established. Adult cerebral blood flow averages approximately 50 mL/100 g brain tissue per minute, and the infant's cerebral blood flow is thought to approximate 60% of that amount.[19] The normal volume of cerebrospinal fluid production in children is unknown.

Criteria for brain death pronouncement in children require the use of accepted pediatric brain death criteria that are fundamentally the same as those used for adult. Clinical brain death criteria include absence of reversible cause and complete cessation of brain function (e.g., absence of cranial nerve function and absence of brainstem function, including absence of spontaneous respirations). For further information, see Chapter 11.

Neurologic Evaluation

Because infants demonstrate primarily reflexive behavior, a large part of the infant neurologic examination consists of evaluation of reflexes. It is important to note that some reflexes (e.g., a positive Babinski's reflex) that are pathologic in the older child or adult may be normally present in the infant. Examination of cranial nerve function—especially the presence of pupil response to light, blinking, coughing, and gag reflex—is possible during routine nursing care of the critically ill or injured child.

Evaluation of the infant's level of consciousness is based largely on evaluation of the infant's alertness, response to the environment and parents, level of activity, and cry. Extreme sensitivity to stimuli usually indicates irritability, and extreme irritability or lethargy is abnormal. Infants with neurologic disease or injury often demonstrate a high-pitched cry.

Once the child is sufficiently mature to comprehend and answer questions, it will be possible to assess level of consciousness, orientation to time and place, and ability to follow commands. If the names of the child's family members and favorite pets and friends are recorded in the care plan, every member of the healthcare team will be able to question the child about familiar people and quickly determine the accuracy of the child's responses. The child's responsiveness must also be evaluated in light of the child's fatigue and clinical condition. A 5-year old might be sleepy after spending most of the night in the emergency department, but should still respond to a painful procedure.

Decreased response to painful stimuli is abnormal and can indicate deterioration in neurologic function. When assessing the child's response, provide a central pain stimulus over the trunk. Withdrawal of extremities from a peripheral pain stimulus can be mediated by a spinal reflex; such reflex withdrawal does not enable verification of higher brain activity.

The neurologic examination includes evaluation of the child's muscle tone. The term newborn and infant usually demonstrate dominance of flexor muscles, so extremities will be flexed even during sleep. Hypotonia or paralysis is abnormal in a patient of any age. When evaluating muscle strength, discrepancies can be appreciated most easily when antigravity muscles are used (e.g., instruct the child to simultaneously extend both arms with eyes closed; unilateral weakness is present if one arm falls). Small tremors may be normal during infancy, but tonic-clonic movements are abnormal.

Assessing the child's ability to follow commands is a critical part of the assessment of responsiveness and motor function. Ask the child to raise two fingers, stick out his or her tongue or wiggle toes; these movements cannot be accomplished reflexively. Reflex curling of the fingers in response to palmar pressure may be misinterpreted as a voluntary hand squeeze, so this is not a reliable method to evaluate response to commands.

When using the Glasgow Coma Scale to score motor function, withdrawal of extremities is evaluated by pinching the medial aspect of each extremity in turn. Appropriate withdrawal occurs if the child adducts extremities (i.e., moves them away from the stimulus, away from midline).

Signs of increased intracranial pressure (Box 1-6) are the same in patients of all ages and include change in level of consciousness; decrease in spontaneous movement, movement in response to commands, and movement in response to painful stimulus; and pupil dilation with decreased constriction to light. In children, bradycardia, systolic hypertension, and altered breathing pattern are usually late signs of increased intracranial pressure and often indicate impending cerebral herniation.

Box 1-6	**Signs of Increased Intracranial Pressure in Children**

Decreased responsiveness (irritability, lethargy)
Inability to follow commands
Decreased spontaneous movement and movement in response to commands
Decreased response to painful stimulus
Pupil dilation with decreased response to light
LATE: change in heart rate (tachycardia or bradycardia), hypertension, altered breathing pattern

IMMUNE FUNCTION AND INFECTION

Extremely young and old patients are particularly susceptible to infection. Neonates and infants are immunologically immature, are deficient in immunoglobulin stores, and lack previous antigen exposure to infectious agents.

Passive immunity is normally conveyed from the mother to the fetus during the last trimester of gestation, through transfer of antibodies, such as immunoglobulin (Ig) G. As a result, premature infants can be deficient in maternally transmitted immunoglobulin. IgG levels normally fall after birth, so young infants are relatively deficient in IgG. During late infancy and early childhood, intrinsic production of IgG begins to rise, with adult levels achieved at approximately 4 years of age. Synthesis of IgM begins during fetal life, but adult levels of IgM are not reached until 2 years of age.

Neonates have a decreased ability to synthesize new antibodies, and both polymorphonuclear leukocyte function and small polymorphonuclear leukocyte storage pools are deficient during the first weeks of life. In general, infants do not have robust antibody response to pathogens, particularly gram-negative organisms (e.g., pneumococcus, meningococcus, *Escherichia coli*). Infants have decreased ability to mount the IgG_2 subclass of antibodies necessary to eliminate *Haemophilus influenzae,* so they are particularly susceptible to infection from this organism during the first 2 years of life. Fortunately, the development and widespread use of the *H. influenza* vaccine dramatically reduced the incidence of meningitis and epiglottitis caused by this organism.

During early childhood, endogenous antibody formation is inadequate, and the child has not yet developed immunity to common viruses. Immature T cell function further increases the risk of respiratory and viral infections.

Healthcare-Acquired (Nosocomial) Infections

Nosocomial infections can develop in as many as 12% of pediatric critical care patients.[16] The sources of nosocomial infections in children differ from those reported in adults. Whereas the most common nosocomial infections observed in adult patients are urinary tract and wound infections, the most common nosocomial infections in pediatric patients are bloodstream infections (including catheter-related bloodstream infections [CRBSIs]) and ventilator-associated pneumonias (VAPs).[8,31] The risk of pediatric nosocomial infection and sepsis increases with increased length of stay, each invasive device day, illness severity at admission, and depressed immune status.[7]

As in adults, nosocomial infections are reduced by strict hand washing before and after every patient contact, strict attention to aseptic technique, and specific bundled care to target common causes of infection such as CRBSIs and VAP (see section, Care of Vascular Monitoring Lines, and Chapters 16 and 22).[8,15,28,31]

Care of Vascular Monitoring Lines

CRBSIs are among the most common nosocomial infections in pediatric critical care. Risk factors include parenteral nutrition and antimicrobial therapy.[34] Risk factors for patients in the pediatric cardiac critical care unit include unscheduled medical admission, noncardiac comorbidities, prolonged device use, and medical therapies such as extracorporeal membrane oxygenation.[11]

Although there is limited evidence to support specific strategies to prevent CRBSI in children, bundled therapies have been effective. Most multifaceted approaches are based on adult studies and include: (1) use of maximal sterile barrier precautions (e.g., cap, mask, sterile gown, sterile gloves, large sterile drape) during catheter placement; (2) use of 2% to 3% chlorhexidine gluconate/70% isopropyl alcohol or other appropriate antiseptic agents to prepare the skin before catheter placement and during routine care of the catheter insertion site; (3) prompt removal of catheters as soon as they are no longer required; and (4) strict adherence to appropriate hand hygiene practices, with annual handwashing campaigns.[21,28,34] For additional information, see Chapters 16.

In studies performed in adult intensive care units, antiseptic impregnated catheters were associated with reduced rates of CRBSI (see Chapter 22). Studies performed in children have described delayed time to infection, but not reduced infection rate associated with the use of antibiotic-impregnated catheters.

Catheters should be taped or secured to prevent inadvertent dislodging. Use of volume-controlled infusion pumps to provide continuous irrigation of each vascular catheter allows precise regulation of the volume of fluids administered hourly. Arterial catheters should be irrigated gently, especially in neonates and young infants, because forceful irrigation in small patients can result in retrograde delivery of air or particulate matter into the arch of the aorta and cerebral arteries.

Ventilator-Associated Pneumonia

Although the incidence of VAP is lower in children than adults, VAP remains the second most common cause of nosocomial infections children. The pathogenesis is poorly understood, but in children it is likely related to aspiration and immunodeficiency.[15] VAP is a significant cause of increased critical care length of stay, increased mechanical ventilation days, and mortality in pediatric and adult critical care.

As with prevention of CRBSIs, the use of a multidisciplinary approach with bundled care protocols has been associated with a decreased prevalence of VAP. Strategies documented to reduce the risk of VAP in children include hand hygiene, elevation of the head of the bed, scheduled mouth care, and changing the ventilator circuit only when soiled.[5] Use of heated ventilator circuits can reduce the pooling of water within the circuit.[5] Additional factors associated with reduction of VAP in adults include: avoidance of nasotracheal intubation and the use of in-line suctioning to prevent the aspiration of pooled tracheal sections.[10]

SUMMARY

The child differs from the adult in several important ways. With knowledge of these differences the pediatric critical care nurse can best adapt assessment techniques and priorities of care to detect patient changes and tailor therapy.

References

1. Anderson GD, Lynn AM: Optimizing pediatric dosing: a developmental pharmacologic approach. *Pharmacotherapy* 29(6):680–690, 2009.
2. Armon K, et al: Hyponatremia and hypokalemia during intravenous fluid administration. *Arch Dis Child* 93(4):285–287, 2008, [Epub 2007, Jan 9].
3. Barakat AY, Ichikawa I: Laboratory data. In Ichikawa I, editors: *Pediatric textbook of fluids and electrolytes*, Baltimore, 1990, Williams and Wilkins.
4. Beck CE: Hypotonic versus isotonic maintenance intravenous fluid therapy in hospitalized children: a systematic review. *Clin Pediatr* 46(9):764–770, 2007.
5. Bigham MT, et al: Ventilator-associated pneumonia in the pediatric intensive care unit: characterizing the problem and implementing a sustainable solution. *J Pediatr* 154(4):582–587, 2009.
6. Boyden EA: Development and growth of the airways. In Hodson WA, editors: *Development of the lung*, New York, 1977, Marcel Dekker.
7. Carcillo J, et al: Rationale and design of the pediatric critical illness stress-induced immune suppression (CRISIS) Prevention Trial. *J Parenter Enteral Nutr* 33:368–374, 2009.
8. Centers for Disease Control and Prevention (CDC): National nosocomial infections surveillance (NNIS) system report: data summary from January 1992 through June 2003; Atlanta, Georgia: US Department of Health and Human Services, CDC: August, 2003.
8a. Chameides LC, Samson RA, Schexnayder SM, Hazinski MF, editors: *Pediatric advanced life support provider manual*, Dallas, 2011, American Heart Association.
9. Choong K, et al: Hypotonic versus isotonic saline in hospitalized children: a systematic review. *Arch Dis Child* 91:828–835, 2006.
10. Coffin SE, et al: Strategies to Prevent Ventilator-Associated Pneumonia in Acute Care Hospitals. *Infect Control Hosp Epidemiol* 29: S31–S40, 2008.
11. Costello JM, et al: Risk factors for central line-associated bloodstream infection in a pediatric cardiac intensive care unit. *Pediatr Crit Care Med* 10(4):453–459, 2009.
12. Custer JW: Blood chemistries and body fluids. In Custer JW, Rau RE, editors: *The Harriet Lane handbook*, ed 18, Philadelphia, 2009, Mosby Elsevier.
13. Dobbing J, Sands J: Quantitative growth and development of human brain. *Arch Dis Child* 48:757, 1973.
14. Donoghue A, et al: Cardiopulmonary resuscitation for bradycardia with poor perfusion versus pulseless cardiac arrest. *Pediatrics* 124(6): 1541–1548, 2009.
14a. Felming S, et al: Normal ranges of heart rate and respiratory rate in children from birth to 18 years of age: a systematic review of observational studies. *Lancet* 377:1011–1018, 2011.
15. Foglia E, Meier MD, Elward A: Ventilator-associated pneumonia in neonatal and pediatric intensive care unit patients. *Clin Microbiol Rev* 20(3):409–425, 2007.
16. Grohskopf LA, et al: A national point-prevalence survey of pediatric intensive care unit-acquired infections in the United States. *J Pediatr* 140:432–438, 2002.
17. Haque IU, Zaritsky AL: Analysis of the evidence for the lower limit of systolic and mean arterial pressure in children. *Pediatr Crit Care* 8:138–144, 2007.
17a. Hazinski MF: Nursing care of the critically ill child: the 7-point check. *Pediatric Nursing*. 11:453, 1985.
18. Huether SE: The cellular environment; fluids and electrolytes, acids and bases. In Mc Cance KL, Huether SE, editors: *Pathophysiology: the biologic basis for disease in adults and children*, Philadelphia, 2009, Elsevier.
19. Kirsch JR, Traystman RF, Rogers MC: Cerebral blood flow measurement techniques in infants and children. *Pediatrics* 75:887, 1985.
20. Kleinman ME, Chameides L, Schexnayder SM, Samson RA, et al: Part 14: pediatric advanced life support: 2010 American Heart Association Guidelines for Cardiopulmonary Resuscitation and Emergency Cardiovascular Care. *Circulation* 122:S876–S908, 2010.
21. Kline AM: Pediatric catheter-related bloodstream infections; latest strategies to decrease risk. *AACN Clin Issues* 16:185–198, 2005.
22. Lacroix J, et al: Transfusion strategies for patients in pediatric intensive care units. *New Engl J Med* 356:1609–1619, 2007.
23. Luten R, Zaritsky A: The sophistication of simplicity…optimizing emergency dosing. *Acad Emerg Med* 15(5):461–465, 2008.
24. Maron BJ: Sudden death in young athletes. *N Engl J Med* 349 (11):1064–1075, 2003.
25. Meaney PA, et al: Higher survival rates among younger patients after pediatric intensive care unit cardiac arrests. *Pediatrics* 118(6): 2424–2433, 2006.
26. Nadkarni VM, et al: First documented rhythm and clinical outcome from in-hospital cardiac arrest among children and adults. *JAMA* 295(1):50–57, 2006.
27. Notterman DA: Pediatric pharmacotherapy. In Chernow B, editors: *The Pharmacologic approach to the critically III patient*, ed 3, Philadelphia, 1994, Williams and Wilkins.
28. O'Grady NP, et al: Guidelines for the Prevention of Intravascular Catheter-Related Infections. *Clin Infect Dis* 35:1281–1307, 2009.
29. Peddy SB, et al: Cardiopulmonary resuscitation: special considerations for infants and children with cardiac disease. *Cardiol Young* 17(Suppl. 2):116–126, 2007.
30. Ralston M, et al: *PALS provider manual*. Dallas, 2006, American Heart Association.
31. Rowin ME, Patel VV, Christenson JC: Pediatric intensive care unit nosocomial infections. *Crit Care Clin* 19:473–487, 2003.
32. Rudolph AM: The changes in the circulation after birth. *Circulation* 41:343, 1970.
33. Smith BT, Rea TD, Eisenberg MS: Ventricular fibrillation in pediatric cardiac arrest. *Acad Emerg Med* 13(5):525–529, 2006.
34. Smith MJ: Catheter-related bloodstream infections in children. *Am J Infect Control* 36(S173):e1–e3, 2008.
35. Sunde K, et al: Implementation of a standardised treatment protocol for post resuscitation care after out-of-hospital cardiac arrest. *Resuscitation* 73(1):29–39, 2007.
36. Tan JM: Nephrology. In Custer JW, Rau RE, editors: *The Johns Hopkins Hospital. The Harriet Lane Handbook*, ed 18, Philadelphia, 2009, Mosby Elsevier.
37. Tooley WH: Lung growth in infancy and childhood. In Rudolph AM, editors: *Pediatrics*, ed 18, Norwalk, 1987, Appleton-Century-Crofts.
38. Van den Berghe G, et al: Outcome benefit of intensive insulin therapy in the critically ill; insulin dose versus glycemic control. *Crit Care Med* 31:359–366, 2003.
39. Vlasselaers D, et al: Intensive insulin therapy for patients in paediatric intensive care: a prospective, randomised controlled study. *Lancet* 373:547–556, 2009.
40. Winters RW: Maintenance fluid therapy. In Winters RW, editors: *The body fluids in pediatrics*, Boston, 1973, Little, Brown, & Co.
41. Zaritsky A, Nadkarni V, Getson P, Kuehl K: CPR in children. *Ann Emerg Med* 10(16):1107–1111, 1987.

Psychosocial Aspects of Pediatric Critical Care

2

Margaret C. Slota

- The environment and dynamics of a pediatric critical care unit (PCCU) create many challenges for the child, family, and staff members.
- Focused skills and attention are required to prevent psychosocial considerations from being lost in the demanding requirements of technology, treatment interventions, and physical care.
- A pediatric critical care unit stay can result in short- or long-term psychosocial sequelae, including emotional and behavioral disorders, which may be decreased by efforts to reduce stress and promote coping.
- The knowledgeable and caring nurse is in a key position to encourage and support the child's and family's coping strategies and to teach more effective strategies to make the critical care experience a growth-producing experience for the child and family.
- Pediatric critical care nursing is a rewarding career option, offering the opportunity to influence the lives of critically ill or injured children and their families.

INTRODUCTION

"Real isn't how you are made," said the Skin Horse. "It's a thing that happens to you. When a child loves you for a long, long time, not just to play with, but REALLY loves you, then you become Real... It doesn't happen all at once... You become. It takes a long time. That's why it doesn't often happen to people who break easily, or have sharp edges, or who have to be carefully kept."

From The *Velveteen Rabbit* by Margery Williams

The birth of a child brings many dreams, but the thought of a critical care hospitalization probably never enters parents' minds. Hospitalization for even a minor illness is stressful for both child and family, but when the child is critically ill, the experience can be overwhelming. Empathetic and caring nurses can mitigate some of the most stressful aspects so that the patient and extended family can cope effectively. The experience of caring for a critically ill or injured child is challenging, but produces exponential growth in a nurse over time. To survive and thrive in the PCCU, the nurse has to be flexible and must not "break" easily. The very real

connection between the family, the child, and an experienced nurse can be a life-changing experience for all.

Increasingly, children are enduring and surviving critical care hospitalization as the result of improved diagnostic, therapeutic, and supportive modalities and care.[63,100] The child and the parents have unique emotional needs in addition to their medical needs. A critical care unit stay can produce short- or long-term deleterious effects, including emotional and behavioral disorders.[65] Children and their parents may be at risk for anxiety, depression, or post-traumatic stress disorder after a PCCU stay.[38,41,57–59,97]

An essential part of managing the child in a critical care unit is assessing the developmental milestones that the child has achieved, recognizing responses and reactions to the illness and hospitalization, and intervening when necessary to support and promote coping. Although the experience is undoubtedly challenging, hospitalization in a critical care unit can be managed to promote physical and psychological healing and reduce post-hospitalization sequelae. Using evidence-based assessment criteria before discharge to identify children at the highest risk for sequelae can help to ensure appropriate follow-up after discharge.[90] Lack of attention to special abilities, needs, and fears can result in a negative experience for the child and family and contribute to deleterious psychological effects. However, with strong support the experience can be psychologically and emotionally beneficial for a child and family.[103] Thoughtful interventions aimed at enhancing a child's and family's coping skills can help the child and family grow from this demanding event and acquire skills that can be used again in future stressful situations.[57] It is important for nurses to recognize the significance of the potential sequelae and the role that nurses play in preventing undesired outcomes.

In addition to pain and other physical stressors that the child may be experiencing, psychological stress can lead to physiologic complications.[84] The release of catecholamines and their metabolites is one of the most reliable indicators of stress, evidenced by an immediate cardiovascular response of increased blood pressure and heart rate. Cardiac glycogen tends to be depleted during stress, and release of vasopressin can result in a decrease in urine output. Stress can stimulate the coagulation cascade and increase fibrinolysis. Because the basal metabolic rate may increase, body temperature regulation is challenged by the increase in heat production and concomitant increase in heat loss. Adrenocorticotropic hormone is released, causing increased secretion of glucocorticoids, which in turn can lead to hyperglycemia, suppressed immune and inflammatory reactions, thymus shrinkage, and atrophy of lymph nodes. Stress ulcers, increased catabolism, and loss of body weight can occur.[79] Critical illness or injury poses more than enough physiologic problems for the child without the added physiologic effects that accompany acute stress—effects that could be decreased by efforts to reduce the child's stress and increase the ability to cope. Although the hospital environment itself can induce further psychological stress, even traumatized children and siblings in a hospital setting can benefit from the coordination of care and treatment and thoughtful planning for discharge.[50]

The pediatric critical care nurse is in a key position to encourage and support the child's coping strategies and to teach the child and family more effective strategies. Nurses spend more time with the child and family than any other healthcare provider and thus have many opportunities for assessment and intervention. Nurses can also influence the approaches of other members of the healthcare team to the child and family. PCCU nurses who focus on only the physiologic and technologic aspects of critical care will meet only part of their responsibilities.

This chapter explores the psychosocial, emotional, and developmental aspects to be considered when caring for critically ill children in each age group and interventions to enable the child, parents, extended family, and pediatric critical care nurse to understand and effectively cope with the events that occur. It also reviews the child's major fears, requirement for play, concepts of death, and methods to support the parents, siblings, and extended family. The chapter reviews both challenging and rewarding aspects of the role of the nurse in a PCCU.

THE CRITICALLY ILL INFANT

Much has been discovered regarding the amazing and exciting capabilities of neonates. At one time, infants were regarded as passive recipients of care, deficient in abilities to see, hear, or interact. However, healthy infants are able to establish eye contact, respond to and discriminate among various sounds, and initiate social interactions. Investigators have documented a wide range of individual differences regarding neurobehavioral maturity and control and styles of behavior and communication.[3,4,14,15]

Developmental Tasks of the Infant

Erikson identified eight crises that must be resolved at major stages of human development.[27] He theorized that the developing infant, child, or young adult leaves each crisis with both positive and negative aspects. The developmental crisis of infancy is to acquire a sense of basic trust while overcoming a sense of mistrust. To acquire a sense of trust, the infant must develop a sense of physical safety and confidence that physical needs will be met. The quality of the parent-infant interaction and the parents' ability to interpret the infant's cues are important to the development of trust. When an infant is frustrated repeatedly in attempts to make needs known and have them met, distrust and pessimism can develop. Once a sense

of trust is achieved, unfamiliar or unknown situations can be tolerated with minimal fear.

Both Erikson[27] and Freud[31] have identified infancy as the oral phase of development. Sucking is of primary importance to the infant, because it is the infant's major source of gratification and tension release.

When an infant is hospitalized in a critical care unit, the potential for frustration is high. Illness disrupts many of the infant's physiologic processes and normal routines and rhythms, such as eating, sleeping, and exercise. The infant is in an unfamiliar environment, with care provided by strangers who are not as sensitive as the parents were to the infant's cues. The presence of an endotracheal tube or restraints can prevent the infant from sucking, eliminating a major source of gratification and comfort.

The infant's affective experience is determined largely by the emotional reactions of significant caregivers. This social referencing can be seen, for example, in a situation in which an infant looks to the mother after a surprise event to determine by her reaction whether to laugh or cry. This example further indicates the important role that parents play in their infant's life.[42] Because the parents typically know the infant very well, they can to teach the nurse about the infant's unique cues, needs, and responses; their presence during the infant's hospitalization is essential to help meet the baby's needs.

Although infants are unable to express their feelings and needs with language, they can indicate their need for more attention or stimulation in other ways.[76,93,99] Perhaps more important, they communicate when they are becoming overstimulated and need rest. It is crucial that nurses constantly assess the infant's tolerance during planning and provision of nursing care. In older children, it may be useful to group procedures and then to allow longer periods of uninterrupted rest, but this approach may not be optimal for infants. Too much stimulation at one time can diminish the infant's coping resources, resulting in adverse physiologic reactions such as vomiting, respiratory distress, apnea, or bradycardia. Gaze aversion is a behavioral cue of fatigue or overstimulation that nurses and parents sometimes miss.

Three-month-old Jamie underwent surgery for ligation of a patent ductus arteriosus. On the second postoperative day, the nurse was holding Jamie after feeding. The nurse repeatedly tried to establish eye contact with Jamie, but he continued to look away from her. Each time Jamie looked away, the nurse spoke encouragingly to him and turned his body or bent her head so that they were again in a position to have eye contact. After several gaze aversion attempts on Jamie's part, he vomited.

Because the nurse was not sensitive to early indications that Jamie was becoming overstimulated and could not tolerate eye contact at that point in time, the stimulation continued and led to a more extreme response.

States of Consciousness in the Infant

The infant's state of consciousness exerts a powerful influence on the infant's response at any given time. Two sleep states (deep and light) and four awake states have been identified in full-term infants (drowsy, quiet alert, active alert, and crying).[10,14,89]

During deep sleep the infant is motionless except for occasional startles or twitches. There are no eye or facial movements except for occasional sucking movements at regular intervals. The infant's threshold to stimuli is high; only intense and disturbing stimuli will arouse infants in this state. Although it is possible to arouse the infant with gentle shaking or stimulation, usually the infant will return to sleep. Generally, the nurse will be frustrated in attempts to feed an infant in this state or to arouse the infant to an alert state. It is more effective to wait until the baby cycles to a more responsive state. It is important for the nurse to be aware that this deep sleep state exists normally. Although inability to arouse an infant can result from neurologic abnormalities, it requires strong stimuli to arouse infants from this normal deep sleep state.

Light sleep accounts for the highest proportion of an infant's sleep. During this state, the infant may demonstrate some body movement, rapid eye movements (fluttering of eyes beneath closed eyelids), and irregular breathing. Infants are more responsive to stimuli and more easily aroused during this period.

During the drowsy state, the infant has a variable activity level, irregular breathing, and delayed response to sensory stimuli. The infant's eyes appear heavy-lidded and have a dull, glazed appearance. Infants in this state can often be aroused to the more interactive quiet alert state by providing visual or auditory or oral stimulation. Such intervention can be helpful in facilitating parent-infant interaction in the critical care unit.

It is during the quiet-alert state that the infant can be the most interactive and provide the most positive feedback to parents or other caretakers. Infants in this state have wide, bright eyes, regular breathing, and minimal body activity. They are interested in their environment and focus attention on their caretakers, moving objects, or other stimuli. It can be gratifying and comforting for parents to be able to smile at and talk to the baby in this state.

Infants in a critical care unit may spend a large portion of their awake time in an active-alert state. This state is characterized by significant body activity with periods of fussiness. Breathing is irregular. The infant's eyes are open but are not as bright as in the quiet alert state, and there is frequent facial movement. The infant can become sensitive to and upset by disturbing stimuli such as hunger, background noise in the critical care unit, and excessive handling. As the infant becomes more active and upset, intervention is often necessary to bring the infant to a lower (i.e., quiet-alert) state and avoid escalation to a crying state. Many critical care units have attempted to reduce excessive background noise and other auditory and visual stimulation.

Crying is one of the infant's major methods of communication.[10] Crying is associated with increased body activity, grimaces, wide-open or tightly closed eyes, and irregular breathing. Although the infant's color can change to bright red, very sick patients or those with cyanotic heart disease may demonstrate peripheral or more generalized cyanosis. Infants may be able to bring themselves to a quieter state by instituting self-consoling behaviors such as sucking on their fingers, fist, or endotracheal tube or by paying attention to voices or faces nearby. However, ill infants often need consolation from their caregivers and are often unable to provide self-consoling maneuvers, or such maneuvers may be ineffective. The nurse should attempt soothing maneuvers such as changing the infant's diaper, feeding the infant, moving close to the infant, making eye contact, or talking to the infant in a calm, soft voice. The infant may also be comforted if held closely, swaddled, or rocked with a pacifier. Infants frequently are highly upset when uncovered or wrapped loosely, but become calm and drowsy when they are swaddled. A combination of verbal and tactile stimuli, such as patting, stroking, holding, or rocking is generally more effective in alleviating distress in hospitalized infants than verbal stimuli alone. Rocking seems to bring comfort and build trust and may relax the parent or nurse as well as the patient.

Touch is extremely important to infants, who need to be caressed, stroked, cuddled, held, hugged, and loved to feel secure and develop normally, and detrimental long-term effects from lack of tactile stimulation during infancy have been documented.[92,99] Therapeutic touch is a potentially useful therapeutic modality to relax the patient and enhance recovery.[43,46] However, premature and severely stressed infants can exhibit negative responses to excessive handling and stimulation.[99] The nurse must identify a therapeutic balance between too much and too little handling for each infant and modify the nursing approach based on the infant's cues (e.g., gaze aversion, respiratory effort).

Cognitive Development in the Infant

Cognitive or intellectual development in normal children has been observed and described in detail by the Swiss psychologist Jean Piaget, who identified five major phases in a child's development of logical thought.[69,71,72] The nurse is more likely to communicate effectively with children by understanding these phases and the basis of the child's perceptions, fears, and misunderstandings.

Piaget named the period of infancy and early toddlerhood, from birth to approximately 2 years, the *sensorimotor phase*. There are six stages in this phase of intellectual development. From birth to 1 month, the infant generally uses reflexes such as sucking, grasping, and crying. The infant is completely self-centered and cannot differentiate self from others. Infants in this stage show little or no tolerance for frustration or delayed gratification.

In the second stage, approximately 1 to 4 months, the use of reflexes is gradually replaced by voluntary activity. Infants begin to recognize familiar faces and objects such as a bottle, and they show awareness of strange surroundings. They begin to differentiate themselves from others and discover parts of their own bodies. Young infants delight in playing with their fingers, hands, and feet. These infants seem to believe that an object or person exists only while within their sight. If an object falls to the floor or is hidden, the infant immediately loses interest and will not search for it. If a person leaves the room or moves out of sight, the infant acts as if that person no longer exists. Infants in this stage show no anxiety around strangers and may become bored when left alone for more than a few minutes.

In sensorimotor stage three, approximately 4 to 8 months, causality, time, deliberate intention, and appreciation of separateness from the environment are beginning to develop. During this stage the infant begins to develop the concept of object permanence—that is, objects and people still exist even when they cannot be seen. The infant will search for partially hidden objects and will look for objects that have disappeared from view, realizing that parents are present even when they are not in sight. Once the infant develops object permanence, attachment to parents or primary caretakers is obvious and strong. The baby demonstrates stranger anxiety and will likely protest when the parents depart. In this stage, infants begin to be able to postpone gratification and await anticipated routines with eager expectation. The baby develops an association between objects and events. For example, an infant may cry in response to nursing interventions related to insertion of an intravenous catheter, but may not yet be able to take constructive action, such as withdrawal, to try to prevent the painful event.

During the fourth sensorimotor stage, approximately 9 to 12 months, the infant's concept of object permanence develops further. The baby learns that hidden objects still exist, and that he or she can take action, such as retrieving an object from under a blanket, to make the object reappear. This is the beginning of intellectual reasoning. The infant begins to understand the meaning of some words and simple commands and begins to associate gestures with events. For example, waving means someone is leaving. The presence of the infant's mother is extremely important to the infant's sense of security, and the threat of her departure is met with protest. The infant is developing a sense of independence in feeding and locomotion and begins to venture away from the mother for short periods to explore the surroundings. The infant now responds when addressed by name and inhibits behavior when told "no." By the end of this stage, the infant is jabbering expressively, verbalizing words that refer to the parents, and saying a few other simple words.

During this period the infant may adopt a favorite blanket, pillow, or stuffed animal as a transitional object[101] that provides comfort and a sense of security during the parents' absence. Absence of the transitional object, particularly during times of stress, will increase the infant's anxiety. Thumb sucking, genital play, and transitional objects are all potential mechanisms of self-consolation when parents are absent. The last two stages in the sensorimotor phase are discussed in the section, Emotional and Psychosocial Development of Toddlers, in The Critically Ill Toddler part of this chapter, below.

The Infant in the Critical Care Environment

Young infants admitted to a critical care unit may be most affected by the strange environment and disruption of normal routines. The infant's usual sleep-wake cycles are interrupted by procedures, lights, alarms, or other noxious stimuli. Providers often attempt to arouse the infant regardless of the infant's sleep state. Ironically, the critical care unit may also produce sensory deprivation with a lack of meaningful stimulation. Some characteristics of a stress-enhancing intensive-care environment—one that adds to the demands placed on the ill infant or child—and those of a more growth-enhancing unit are shown in Box 2-1.

The nurse must maintain a soothing and reassuring environment. Providers should attempt to interrupt constant, rhythmic sounds (e.g., the whooshing of a ventilator or beeping of a cardiac monitor) by introducing more meaningful, varying sounds such as talking, humming, or singing to the infant or by playing soft, soothing music. Providers should be aware that noises such as loud laughing or talking at the nurses' desk, loud music, music with a rapid beat or uninterrupted music can be highly disturbing. Infants and children who receive pharmacologic paralytic agents are hypersensitive to bright lights, loud music, and voices. Because they are not able to move, they may become extremely anxious.

The often stark, sterile environment of the critical care unit can be made more comforting by the use of natural lighting, colorful walls and curtains, and bright mobiles. Pictures, blankets, or toys from home can help make the environment more attractive. The infant's parents can personalize the environment by mounting pictures of themselves or other family members on the crib in the infant's line of sight to give the infant something to look at.

From approximately 6 months of age through the preschool period, separation anxiety is the infant's major source of fear. Separation from parents is extremely stressful.[12,87] Because separation is so traumatic, it is helpful for a parent to stay with the hospitalized infant as much as possible. Most hospitals have facilities for parents to stay with young children. If it is not possible for a parent to remain with the child throughout the hospitalization, it is beneficial to maintain flexible visiting opportunities at all hours for parents.

Robertson[77] has identified three distinct phases in the crisis of separation: protest, despair, and denial. Although shorter length of stay and more liberal visiting hours have reduced the separation of children from parents during hospitalization, some aspects of this crisis of separation may still be observed. During the protest phase the child cries loudly and screams for the parents while visually searching for them. The infant will tightly cling to the parent if the parent shows signs of leaving. Attention from others is rejected and may even intensify the protest of a child who is experiencing stranger anxiety. The child may seem inconsolable, sometimes quieting only when exhausted. This anxiety, which can last from hours to days depending on the child's energy and degree of illness, adds to the child's stress in the critical care unit. It can be frustrating to care for the infant who is protesting, but the nursing staff should still attempt to provide comfort, with consoling gestures, conversation, and objects (such as a pacifier or transitional object). If the nurse takes the time to interact with the infant while the parent is present, that nurse may seem safe to the infant, and the infant may be more receptive to that nurse's interactions. It can also be helpful to attempt to distract the infant with a colorful toy or musical mobile.

The second phase of the separation crisis is the phase of despair. In this phase the child continues the mourning process, but becomes more passive and withdrawn. The child seems disinterested in play, food, or the environment and looks lonely, apathetic, or even depressed. Some of the child's activities during this phase may be thumb sucking, head banging, rocking, sitting quietly and sadly, or clutching objects. The child continues to watch for the parents' return. When they do come,

---

Box 2-1 **Environmental Characteristics of PCCUs**

Characteristics of a Stress-Enhancing Critical Care Unit

Children are denied periods of undisturbed sleep.

Human contact usually involves painful stimuli, sometimes inflicted without warning.

Holding, cuddling, and social behaviors are discouraged.

Lighting is constant and uncomfortably bright.

Background noise is loud and continuous.

Use of physical restraints is common.

Examination and treatment times are based on staff convenience or hospital routines or schedules.

There is little consistency among the child's caretakers.

Conversations, often involving a large number of people, are held at or near the child's bed.

Families are deprived of continuous access to their child, togetherness, and privacy.

Parents must seek out information about their child and are not welcomed and sought out by caregivers.

Treatment is depersonalized.

Characteristics of a Growth-Enhancing Critical Care Unit

Consideration, concern, and gentleness are the basic tenets from which all care flows.

Caregivers introduce themselves with name and role and address the child and family members by name.

Care and examinations are organized with consideration of patient needs and priorities.

Caregivers are always alert to identify signs of pain and/or discomfort in the child; methods of relief are promptly initiated.

Caregivers use every opportunity to comfort and reassure patients as a way to counterbalance harsh therapies.

Positive contacts occur with the child between treatments and procedures.

Whenever possible, the child is taught and/or assisted in using positive coping strategies and techniques.

The child is acknowledged as an individual during necessary bedside conversations and is included in an age-appropriate manner.

Colorful pictures, mobiles, toys, and stuffed animals are used; parents are encouraged to bring the child's transitional object, special pillow, or other favorite comforting objects from home.

Parents are rarely asked to leave their child's bedside; caregivers greet them warmly and make them feel welcome.

If the parents are not present when a child is dying, a caregiver holds and/or speaks lovingly to the child. A dying child is never left alone.

The centers of attention and concern for all caregivers are the unique needs of the children and their families.

Psychological and emotional needs are given the same priority as physical concerns.

Adapted from Weibley TT: Inside the incubator. *MCN Am J Matern Child Nurs* 14:96–100, 1989.

---

the child may ignore them or act angry, but will usually cling ferociously to them if they show signs of leaving again.

The last phase of the separation crisis is denial, or detachment. The child seems to have adjusted at last, appearing friendly and interested in the environment and other people. More receptive to strangers, the child accepts caretaking from many people. This phase may be interpreted by inexperienced staff as a positive sign that the child is adjusting and is no longer anxious. This behavior may not be a sign of contentment, however, but of resignation. The child detaches from the parent to escape the pain of separation and denies longing for the parent's presence.[77] The child may react with indifference when the parent returns or may seem to prefer the nurse or another staff member.

If the parents do not understand the basis of the child's distress, they can become extremely upset. They may restrict their time with the child in an attempt to minimize the child's distress; however, this will only reinforce the child's fears. It is important for the nurse to explain the child's behavior to the parents and encourage them to spend as much time as they can with their child. The nurse should assure the parents that they are helping their child to cope effectively with the frightening environment in the critical care unit. By minimizing the parents' distress, the nurse will be helping to maintain the child's best support system.

Preparation of the Infant for Procedures and Surgery

Older infants react intensely to potentially painful situations (Box 2-2). They are uncooperative and may refuse to lie still, attempting to push the threatening person away or to escape. Distraction is not as effective as it is with younger infants. The best technique to decrease fear and resistance is to familiarize the older infant with some of the equipment beforehand (e.g., let the older infant play with a stethoscope), to perform the procedure as quickly as possible, and to maintain parent-child contact. Advance warning of a painful procedure is essential. Painful procedures should never be initiated while the child is asleep, unless the child is anesthetized.

The Infant and Play

Play is critical for development, providing an important opportunity for infants to learn about themselves and the world.[47] Six features differentiate play from other behaviors[53]:

1. Play is intrinsically motivated, needing no external stimulus.
2. Play behaviors are purposeless with no concern for efficiency.
3. Play is focused on discovery of what the child can do with an object as distinguished from exploration, which allows the child to determine what an object is.

Box 2-2 Preparation of Infants, Children and Adolescents for Procedures and Surgery

Infants

Major fears: Separation and strangers
Preparation:

Provide consistent caretakers.
Decrease parents' anxiety, because it is transmitted to infant.
Minimize separation from parents.

Toddlers

Major fears: Separation and loss of control
Characteristics of toddlers' thinking:

Egocentric, primitive, magical, unable to recognize views of others
Little concept of body integrity

Preparation:

Prepare the child a few hours or even minutes before some procedures, because preparation too far in advance produces even more intense anxiety.
Keep explanations simple, and choose wording carefully, avoiding words with double meanings (homophones or homonyms) and other connotations.
Let the toddler play with equipment, such as putting a mask on a teddy bear.
Minimize separation from parents; keep security objects at hand.
Recognize that any intrusive procedure, such as rectal temperature or ear examination, is likely to provoke an intense reaction related to fear of injury.
Use restraints judiciously, because being held down can provoke more fear or protest than the actual procedure.

Preschoolers

Major fears: Bodily injury and mutilation; loss of control; the unknown; the dark; being left alone
Characteristics of preschoolers' thinking:

Preoperational: egocentric, magical, animistic, transductive
Tendency to repeat and use words they do not really understand, providing their own explanations and definitions
Highly literal interpretation of words
Inability to abstract
Primitive ideas about their bodies, such as fearing that all their blood will leak out if a bandage is removed
Difficulty in differentiating a "good" hurt (beneficial treatment) from a "bad" hurt (illness or injury)

Preparation:

Prepare the preschooler days in advance for major events (hours for minor ones), because advance preparation is important.
Keep explanations simple and concrete, and choose wording carefully; try not to use words such as cut or take out, or homophones such as dye; explain intended meanings of any major terms.
Emphasize that the child will wake up after surgery, because anesthesia described as "being put to sleep" may be frightening if the child has had experience with euthanizing family pets.
Use pictures, models, actual equipment, or hospital play and behavioral rehearsal because verbal explanations are usually insufficient.

Emphasize that the procedure or surgery is to help the child be more healthy. Do not tell children that they will feel "better" after surgery, because they will typically feel worse in the immediate postoperative period.
Repeat many times that the child has not done anything wrong and is not being punished.
Use explanations that include what the child will see, hear, feel, smell, and taste.
To assess comprehension, ask the child to explain the information to another person or doll.
Re-explain things every time they happen; do not assume the child remembers; anxiety can interfere with memory.
Listen to what the child says when playing; look at what the child draws.
Be honest. Explain deviations from routines, unfulfilled promises, and changes in plans.
Because children have a limited concept of time, tie explanations to known events, such as a nap or lunch.
Give the child choices whenever possible.
Reassure the child that the room will not be dark and that there will always be someone nearby.
Do not tie evaluations of the child to behavior during the procedures; for example, he is not "a good boy" for holding still, but rather, "You helped us finish faster because you were holding still!".
Teach the child some simple coping skills such as distraction techniques in advance of the procedure, and then guide the child in their use during the procedures.
Postprocedure play sessions are important to help the child understand and integrate the experience, especially for children for whom advance preparation is not possible.

School-aged children

Major fears: Loss of control, bodily injury and mutilation, failure to live up to expectations of important others, death
Characteristics of thinking in school age:

Concrete operational period
Beginning of logical thought, but continuing tendency to be literal
Vague, false, or nonexistent ideas about illness and body construction and functioning
A tendency, particularly in older children, to nod with understanding when in reality they do not understand
Ability to listen attentively to all that is said without always comprehending
Reluctance to ask questions or admit not knowing something they think they are expected to know
Better ability to understand relationship between illness and treatment
Increased awareness of the significance of various illnesses, potential hazards of treatments, lifelong consequences of injury, and the meaning of death

Preparation:

Prepare days to weeks in advance for major events, because it is extremely important to the child's ability to cope effectively, to cooperate, and to comply with treatment; in addition, preparation gives the child a greater sense of control.
Ask children to explain what they understand.

Box 2-2 **Preparation of Infants, Children and Adolescents for Procedures and Surgery—cont'd**

Use body diagrams, pictures, and models; these children enjoy learning scientific terminology and handling actual equipment because their thinking is concrete, although some older school-aged children object to being seen handling a doll.

Because child is beginning to assert more independence, let child choose whether parents will be present during the procedure (if you can honor the choice the child makes).

Because the peer group is important, stress that contact with friends can be maintained.

Because children do not want to be seen as different, emphasize the "normal" things the child will be able to do.

Give as many choices as possible to increase the child's sense of control.

Reassure children that they have done nothing wrong and that necessary procedures and surgery are not punishments.

Coping techniques and the use of standardized narrated slides, interactive computer programs, or videos can be helpful.

Anticipate and answer questions regarding the long-term consequences, such as what the scar will look like and how long activities may be curtailed.

Conduct sessions after the procedure to help the child work through and master the experience.

Adolescents

Major fears: Loss of control, altered body image, separation from peer group

Characteristics of adolescents' thinking:

Beginning of formal operational thought and ability to think abstractly

Existence of some magical thinking, such as feeling guilty for illness, and egocentrism

Tendency toward hyperresponsiveness to pain, reaction not always in proportion to the event; minor injuries and illnesses usually magnified

Little understanding of the structure and functions of the body.

Preparation:

Allow adolescents to be an integral part of decision-making about their care, because they can project into the future and see long-term consequences and are able to understand.

Because advance preparation is vital to ability to cope, cooperate, and comply, prepare the adolescent in advance—preferably weeks before major events.

Give information sensitively, because adolescents react not only to what they are told but to the manner in which they are told.

Explore tactfully what adolescents know and what they do not know, because they are extremely concerned that others will think they are not knowledgeable or will discover their feelings of inadequacy, dependency, and confusion.

Stress how much adolescents can do for themselves and how important their compliance and cooperation are to their treatment and recovery; be honest about the consequences.

Allow the adolescent as many choices and as much control as possible.

Respect adolescents' need to exert independence from parents, and remember that they may alternate between dependence and a wish to be independent.

Because their peer group is important, stress that this contact can be maintained.

Because adolescents do not want to be seen as different, emphasize the normal things they will be able to do.

Modeling films or computer programs may be helpful.

These children may benefit from being taught coping techniques such as relaxation, deep breathing, self-comforting talk and/or the use of imagery.

Note: It is important to remember that the child's psychosocial developmental stage may not always match the child's chronologic age. Development may be delayed, particularly in chronically ill children. For example, an adolescent who is delayed in development may need to be approached more like a school-age child. In addition, preparation of children and their parents should include preparation of siblings. Siblings may have fantasies about what is happening, and they may fear that they caused what happened (the illness or injury) or that the same thing will happen to them. It is vital to discuss these issues with parents who might not realize what the siblings are experiencing.

---

4. Play is make-believe or without pretense and is not guided by externally imposed rules.
5. During play, the infant or child is actively engaged.
6. Play is also pleasurable and internally real to the child.

Three types of infant play have been described. The earliest type of play, appearing at a young age, is social-affective play. The infant interacts with people, imitating adult actions, such as coughing or sticking out his tongue. The second type is sense-pleasure play, during which the infant derives pleasure from objects in the environment such as lights and colors, tastes and odors, textures and consistencies. Body motion—such as rocking, swinging, or bouncing— and pleasant sounds also provide pleasurable experiences. Sensorimotor activity is the third category of infant play. Infants initially play with body parts,

bringing hands and feet into their mouths; oral testing is an important means of exploration. Motor activity is highly enjoyable for infants, and they take great pleasure in kicking their feet and waving their arms. Between 7 and 10 months of age, infants are able to enjoy throwing things out of the crib onto the floor. This game seems to be an endless source of fun. At approximately 9 months old, infants show a newly developed sense of object permanence. Games such as peek-a-boo and toys that go away and come back, such as a jack-in-the-box, provide enjoyable ways for the infant to work through fears associated with separation anxiety.[53]

Infants can become highly frustrated if their feet and arms are restrained, particularly if they are accustomed to being active. Restraints should be used in the critical care unit only when medically necessary. When restraints are necessary for safety, they should still allow the infant as much movement as possible.

Pediatric critical care nurses should be creative when facilitating the play of these very ill patients. Toys that are appropriate for the baby's age should be available, and the nurse should encourage the parents to bring toys from home. The older infant may benefit from observing as the nurse plays with puppets or dolls or punches a balloon. This form of passive play can provide the infant with a pleasant distraction from discomfort and fear.

The Infant and Death

The infant's reactions to fatal illness and dying will be based on the degree of discomfort involved and on the parents' reactions. Emotional expression in an infant is at a primitive level that is directly linked to impulse and sensation.[44]

Emotional empathy exists between parents and children; this enables special communication that makes the feelings of each transparent to the other. Parents serve as the frame of reference for the child, and parental attitudes and feelings are clearly transmitted, even when the child does not fully understand the words being used. If the parents are helped to cope with their anxiety, they will be more calm and supportive and can decrease the infant's anxiety. Because separation from parents is the most stressful event that can happen, even highly anxious parents should not be kept away from their child; instead they should be supported to promote effective coping.

THE CRITICALLY ILL TODDLER

In an ideal world, hospitalization of older infants and toddlers (ages 1 to 3) would be avoided, because this is the age group at greatest risk for emotional sequelae related to the experience of hospitalization.[77] The pediatric critical care nurse can be instrumental in making this experience less traumatic and more productive for the toddler and the parents.

Emotional and Psychosocial Development of Toddlers

The major developmental task for toddlers is beginning the development of autonomy and self-control,[27] so toddlers typically become more independent as the months pass. They can be a bountiful source of enjoyment and satisfaction as they take delight in exploring and discovering new things. They are often liberal with expressions of affection such as engaging smiles, hugs, and kisses. However, the reputation of this period as the "terrible twos" is well deserved, and caregivers must have a great deal of patience and understanding.

This is the "no" stage, and toddlers often adamantly state this newly learned word even when the toddler may want to say "yes"—a concept not learned until later. Parents and caregivers see resistive behavior as the toddler struggles to assert independence and gain control of the environment. Frequent temper tantrums can result from the toddler's low frustration tolerance and need to test the limits of acceptable behavior. Dawdling behavior is common, particularly at mealtimes.

The toddler is extremely attached to and dependent on the parents. Parents represent safety and security. The toddler is typically more aware of separation from the mother and seeks more attention and greater closeness to her. The child forms relationships with the parents, rather than simply requiring their presence. Although a toddler can tolerate some physical distance from a parent and ventures away to explore and play, the toddler needs to find the parent or call to the parent at short intervals. Separation from the parents for prolonged or unexpected periods is difficult, especially when other stresses are present. Older toddlers are more able to accept symbols, such as a parent's keys, as an indication that the parent will return. The toddler also may be more able to accept care and consolation from another caregiver if given an opportunity to become familiar with that caregiver over a period of time, particularly if the toddler sees that the caregiver has the parents' approval.

Freud refers to the toddler years as the anal stage, because elimination and retention are important skills developed during this period.[31] Toilet training begins during these years. Because bowel and bladder control are newly acquired skills, they may be lost when the toddler is stressed. Toddlers who have been toilet trained find it distressing to be placed in diapers. They also may find it confusing and anxiety-provoking to be told that it is acceptable to wet in their diaper or go to the bathroom in their bed after being told the opposite so frequently during toilet training. Toddlers require sensitivity and reassurance from parents and staff to help them feel less anxious. If possible, the child should be allowed to use a bedside potty chair.

Cognitive Development of the Toddler

The toddler makes massive strides in intellectual development, beginning to think and reason, although in a way that is different from adult cognition. During Piaget's fifth sensorimotor stage of intellectual development, from approximately 13 to 18 months, the toddler further differentiates the self from other objects and will search for an object where it was last seen.[69] Early traces of memory also begin to develop during this period.

The child in this stage is beginning to be aware of causal relationships and can understand that flipping one switch will cause a machine to make noise, and flipping another switch may turn on a light. However, the child is not able to transfer that knowledge to new situations; for example, may not be aware that turning a switch of another machine may cause it to make noise. The toddler must continuously examine the same object every time it appears in a new place or under changed conditions. For this reason the toddler is likely to want to examine each stethoscope brought to the bedside by a different person.

During the final stage of the sensorimotor period, from approximately 19 to 24 months, egocentric and magical thinking begin. Toddlers view themselves as the center of the universe and can appreciate no point of view but their own. As toddlers become aware of their thoughts, they believe that others must also be aware of them and that events happen because of their activity, thoughts, and wishes. For example, they may think that their parents went away or hospitalization occurred because they misbehaved.

The toddler is extremely ritualistic and takes comfort from consistency of environment and daily activities. The global organization of thought that is characteristic of this period causes the child to recognize experiences or events as parts of a whole. As a result, if even small changes in the environment or schedule are made, the child may require time for readjustment.

The toddler is beginning to develop a sense of time and understands some temporal terms and relationships, such as "in a minute" or "after lunch," although specific time intervals, such as "3 hours" are meaningless. The toddler's attention span, which is limited, is characterized by a sense of immediacy and concern for the present. Language abilities increase and the toddler can understand simple directions or requests.

From approximately 2 to 4 years of age, children demonstrate the preoperational or preconceptual phase of cognitive development. Vocabulary and language development markedly increase during this period. Magical thinking and egocentricity are still prevalent during this phase, giving the child feelings of omnipotence and supreme authority. This ideation also causes the child to feel guilty, assuming that bad thoughts are responsible for events. The child's inability to reason the cause and effect of illness or injuries makes these events especially stressful.

The toddler will begin to demonstrate animism, a process in which lifelike qualities are attributed to inanimate objects. For example, the child may blame a glass of milk for falling or believe that an x-ray machine or elevator is a monster.

Toddlers do not use deductive reasoning (from the general to the particular) or inductive reasoning (from the particular to the general); instead they reason transductively (from the particular to the particular). Children frequently will believe that there is a causal relationship between any two events that occur at the same time or are contiguous to each other in time and space. For example, the color of a balloon can explain why it is floating, or the need for sleep makes it dark outside.

The Toddler in the Critical Care Environment

Toddlers can become terrified in a critical care unit. They are in a new place where they see, hear, smell, and feel frightening things. There are many strangers around who sometimes do scary and painful things, and the toddler is unable to freely move about. Gone is the security of familiar surroundings and routines. The toddler may be separated from parents, and may be uncomfortable or in pain. As a result of egocentric thinking, toddlers may think their bad behavior caused their illness or hospitalization. Because most of the direct contacts in the PCCU are intrusive instead of comforting, interactions with staff can create fear.

Parental presence and support are more crucial than ever to the toddler during this period. When a parent is not present, a toddler may believe that punishment through abandonment is occurring. The toddler is terrified of complete desertion, and fears that the parent is angry; therefore, cries of "I want my mommy; I be good!" may be heard. The toddler can exhibit the same three stages of protest, despair, and denial that the infant does, but is able to be more verbal and assertive in protest.[77] Toddlers may call for their parents and may verbally reject consolation and care from others. Physical aggression,

hostility, fighting, kicking, hitting, pinching, and biting may be displayed during this period. If nurses are not familiar with a child's particular rituals for comfort, provision of different comfort measures can add to the child's confusion and distress.

The best way to minimize the toddler's anxiety is to minimize separation from the parents. During the toddler years, perhaps more than any other, every effort should be made to arrange for one parent or another familiar adult to stay with the child as much as possible. It is important for the nurse to convey to the parents that they are welcome in the unit to provide necessary support for their child. The PCCU is no place for restrictive visiting hours that might benefit the staff but add to the anxiety of the child or parents.

Rooming-in or frequent regular visiting by the parent decreases the possibility that the child will enter the despair phase of separation crisis. Children who progress to the despair state may become listless, anorexic, uncommunicative, and withdrawn. Regression to an earlier stage of development usually is demonstrated as loss of sphincter control, reduced verbal communication, or passivity. When the parent returns, the toddler often cries or expresses anger, distrust, or rejection. If the parent attempts to depart again, however, the child may cling tightly, crying and begging the parent to remain. If toddlers progress to denial, they can appear to be more accepting and interactive, but might actually be more disturbed.

It is helpful when a small number of nurses consistently care for the hospitalized toddler, to minimize the variety of schedules and personalities to which the child must adapt. In addition, the child who has the opportunity to build trust in a few nurses may be able to take comfort from them when a parent is not present.

Physical restraint or restriction, altered routines and rituals, and enforced dependency represent a loss of bodily control to the toddler who is striving for more autonomy. This loss can make the toddler frightened and resistant. By allowing toddlers as much movement and independence as possible, the nurse can increase their cooperation and decrease their fears and frustrations. The toddler often can be allowed to sit upright or remain on a parent's lap during frightening procedures. Less physical restraint may be required if the child is given the opportunity to handle the equipment being used. For example, toddlers often enjoy listening to their chest (or to that of a toy or another person) with the stethoscope. When physical restraint is necessary, lost activity should be replaced with another form of activity whenever possible.

Loss of familiar rituals and routines decreases the toddler's the sense of control, predictability, and security.

Terry's mother always put him to bed at night at home by laying him on the bed, stroking him while she quietly sang a lullaby, then kissing both cheeks, pulling his favorite blanket up against his cheek, and then turning out the light—in that order. This routine was part of going to sleep for 2-year-old Terry.

If the toddler's mother or nurse can continue some home routines in the hospital, it will help the toddler's sense of familiarity and security. Routines and rituals that are most important to the toddler must be recorded as part of the child's history and incorporated into the plan of care, when possible.

All children need limits to feel secure and may be more frightened without them. This is particularly true of toddlers who have not yet mastered a great deal of control over their own impulses. They need to feel that there is someone close who will protect them from injuring themselves, others, or their environment. Setting limits can help children channel strong feelings into safe, socially acceptable, pleasurable activities. To prevent children from hurting themselves, others, or property, they should be restrained temporarily or removed from the situation with an explanation of why they cannot continue the behavior. Adults should acknowledge the child's feelings and then direct the youngster into acceptable behavior for dealing with these strong emotions.

Carrie, age 2½ years, began angrily thrashing about and kicking after her nurse checked her blood pressure. Her actions threatened the safety of the intravascular lines and other tubes. Carrie's nurse gently but firmly restrained Carrie's legs and told her: "No, Carrie, I know that you are very angry, but I can't let you kick and move all over like this. You'll hurt yourself. I know what you can do, though. I have something fun for you to play with. Stop kicking and I'll show you." After about a minute, Carrie stopped trying to kick and looked expectantly at the nurse. The nurse then produced a hammering board and showed Carrie how she could pound on it—a much more constructive way for Carrie to discharge her anger and one that she seemed to enjoy.

The immature thought processes of toddlers can contribute to their anxiety. Egocentricity, magical thinking, transductive logic, and animism can magnify fears of known events and make unknown or unfamiliar situations terrifying. Sinister characteristics may be attributed to machines and hospital personnel. Toddlers, thinking that their misbehavior caused their illness, might not understand their parents' inability or unwillingness to rescue them. Toddlers need frequent reassurance that they are not bad, are not being punished, are loved, will get better (if true), and will be able to walk and talk and go home again. The toddler might not understand the concept of returning home, but will be comforted by gentle reassurance.

Preparation of the Toddler for Procedures and Surgery

Any real or perceived painful experience will be met with extreme emotional distress and physical resistance. Because toddlers have a poorly defined concept of body integrity, any intrusive procedures—even painless ones such as measuring body temperature or examining of the ears—can provoke an intense reaction. Toddlers can understand only very simple explanations. Prolonged or detailed explanations or explanations given too far in advance may create more anxiety (see Box 2-2, earlier in chapter). When it is necessary to perform painful procedures, lengthy discussions or provisions of choices are best avoided. It is best to provide a brief explanation, assure the child that you will be there, perform the procedure as quickly as possible, and then comfort the child. Offer choices when you are able to do so.

The Toddler and Play

Most of the toddler's time is normally spent in some type of play activity. Play is a major component in learning about the world, communicating feelings, overcoming boredom, developing motor skills and independence, and working through anxieties.[23] The toddler's need for play continues during periods of illness. Through play the toddler can find a constructive, acceptable outlet for fears, frustrations, anxieties, and anger. Familiar toys can be comforting and provide a sense of security. Play can serve as a diversion from pain and fear and can become a replacement for mobility. It also can provide some feeling of autonomy and independence by providing control over something.[11]

Play might have to be passive when the child is critically ill; creativity is needed to find activities that are meaningful and provide positive sensory stimulation. Bright, colorful mobiles, posters, stuffed animals, and toys can provide visual stimulation. Musical mobiles, CDs, talking story books, radios, tape recordings made by the child's parents or other family members, and visits from the music therapist can help substitute pleasant and meaningful sounds for hospital noises. Favorite television shows or movies can help bring a sense of familiarity into the critical care unit. A book of fabrics and other materials with various textures can be stimulating for the child. Any of these activities will be especially comforting when initiated by the child's parents.

When the toddler is recovering, more active play can be introduced. Hammering or pounding boards, punching balloons, water play, and active toys such as a "busy box" are all meaningful outlets for toddlers who are immobilized or confined to bed rest. Peek-a-boo is still enjoyed at this age and reinforces the toddler's learning that things and people go away but come back. The child may also enjoy "talking" puppets or dolls or listening to tapes of books read by parents or siblings.

The Toddler and Death

The toddler's egocentrism, lack of a concept of infinite time, and inability to distinguish between fact and fantasy prevent comprehension of the absence of life and the permanence of death. The toddler is developing cognitive concepts of consistency and permanence, and presence and absence, and does so through games such as hide and seek and peek-a-boo. Although toddlers can repeat what sounds like a definition of death, such as "people who die go to heaven," they are unable to comprehend what this means. Death may mean separation from the love objects and people the toddler needs and depends on.[9] The most frightening aspects of hospitalization for the toddler usually include pain, anxiety, and separation from parents, but they do not include anxiety about death. Rather than fear of death, the dying toddler will respond to comforting support offered by the parents and will also respond with fear or sadness to the anxiety, sadness, depression, or anger expressed by parents.

THE CRITICALLY ILL PRESCHOOL CHILD

Emotional and Psychosocial Development of the Preschooler

The preschooler, at 3 to 5 years old, has come a long way in the development of motor, verbal, and social skills. This is a time of enthusiastic and energetic learning and exploration.

The chief developmental task of the preschooler is creating a sense of initiative.[27] Tolerance of frustration is still limited, but is better developed. Guilt feelings result when the child is not able to live up to the child's own or other's expectations of appropriate behavior. The preschooler's conscience is fairly primitive, is likely to be overzealous and uncompromising, and can be unnecessarily cruel.[27,30] Thoughts about "being bad" or wishing for "bad things" to happen to other people can also lead to feelings of guilt and anxiety. Painful treatments, isolation, separation from parents, loss of autonomy, and immobilization are likely to be interpreted as deserved punishments for real or imagined wrongdoing.

During the preschool years, the child begins the process of sex-role identification. Freud has termed this period the *phallic stage*.[31] Initially, in the oedipal phase, the child is drawn to the parent of the opposite sex. Late in the preschool period, the child begins to strongly identify with and seeks to imitate the parent of the same sex. It is during this time that children discover that boys and men have penises and girls and women do not. For some children, seeing another child naked in the critical care unit (however briefly) may be the child's first experience with this discovery. During this period, boys have a fear of castration as punishment for real or imagined misdeeds. Urinary catheterization or other procedures near the genital area may cause a great deal of anxiety, provoking frantic resistance. It is important to provide careful explanation of exactly what will and will not happen during such procedures in order to decrease the child's fear and increase cooperation. In addition, protecting modesty by keeping the genital area covered and asking permission to look, listen, and touch conveys respect for the child.[73]

The development of the superego or conscience is also a major task for the preschooler. The child begins to learn right from wrong and good from bad. Although preschoolers cannot comprehend all of the reasons why something is acceptable or not acceptable, they learn appropriate behavior through reward and punishment and from examples set by parents or other adults. Preschoolers are more aware of danger and will usually obey simple limits or rules that have been explained to them.

The preschooler is generally able to tolerate brief separations from the parents if given explanations of where the parents will be and when they will return. The preschooler is also less frightened and more trusting of strangers and thus is often able to relate well to unfamiliar people. Serious illness is likely to cause regression in the preschooler, however, and the need for parents may once again become very strong. The preschooler can manifest some or all of the stages of separation anxiety experienced by the infant and toddler, but the older child's protest behaviors are usually more passive and subtle than those of the infant or toddler. The preschool child may ask parents repeatedly when they will return, cry for them, refuse to eat, demonstrate sleeplessness, throw things, break toys, or refuse to cooperate in activities or care. The critical care staff must be alert to these signs and reassure the child regarding the parents' return, providing other comforts and interventions as necessary.

Cognitive Development of the Preschooler

The preschooler continues in the preoperational phase of intellectual development until approximately 4 years old. An egocentric view of the world continues, and magical thinking remains. As the imagination develops, the preschooler has a difficult time differentiating reality from fantasy, thus increasing the potential for misunderstanding. Transductive reasoning remains.

The preschooler's magical, egocentric, and transductive thinking, combined with a developing conscience, strengthens the child's view that illness and hospitalization are punishments for misbehavior. This view presents a special problem if the child received an injury while engaged in a forbidden activity, such as playing with matches or crossing the street alone. If the child was injured with others, particularly family members, the patient may feel inordinate guilt and anxiety regarding the event. This is particularly true if the child had preinjury fantasies or wished for injury to or death of parents or siblings. The child might be terrified when it appears that such fantasies have come true. If these fears are extreme, the child could require psychiatric evaluation and counseling.

Global organization of thought still ties the early preschooler to rigid routines. The familiar patterns of the rituals of daily activities provide the child with a sense of security. Preschoolers want to know both the cause and the purpose of everything; to them, nothing happens by chance. Questions such as, "Why am I here?" and "Why are you doing that?" or "Why is she crying?" may be incessant. Because preschoolers believe there must be a reason for everything that happens, they are troubled by the purposes of or explanations for many events. They are beginning to generalize in thinking. For example, after being stuck with a needle by a person in a white coat, the child might believe that everyone in a white coat is going to stick him with a needle. Although the preschool child can perceive an event correctly, the interpretation of the event might be inaccurate.

During ages 4 to 6 years, the child is in the stage of intellectual development called the *intuitive phase*. *Why* questions persist. The child has a larger vocabulary, but tends to define objects in terms of their functions, such as "a bed is to sleep in." When the preschooler asks "why?" simple answers beginning with *to* and followed by the function may be best understood. The child's attention span and concept of time are increasing. Toward the end of this period the preschooler's rigidity and ritualism begin to decrease, allowing more flexibility and fewer negative reactions to changes in environment and routines.

The Preschooler in the Critical Care Environment

Five-year-old Timmy had been in the PCCU for 3 days and was intubated and in need of peritoneal dialysis. Timmy was restrained and literally surrounded by equipment, but without toys or other comforts. Although he was receiving analgesia, he was fairly alert. Two nurses talked over Timmy's bed about the equipment needed to start his dialysis as he moved about restlessly on the bed and occasionally set off his ventilator alarm. His nurse put a blood pressure cuff on Timmy's arm and started to pump it up, increasing the child's activity. The nurse's reassurance did not calm Timmy. A resident took Timmy's other arm and began locating a vein from which to draw blood while explaining Timmy's case to a medical student. Timmy's protest activity markedly increased as the resident placed the tourniquet, saying to Timmy, "There's going to be a stick now." Those were the only words spoken to Timmy during the procedure. While Timmy continued fighting the ventilator, his restraints, and his situation, the two nurses conferred about the dialysis procedure. A few minutes later the resident returned, watched Timmy for a short time, and told the nurse, "His last gas wasn't terrific, and he's really agitated. Let's paralyze him." The nurse agreed that would be a good idea and administered the drug. Timmy was not told that he would soon be unable to move. Very shortly, Timmy lay quietly in his bed with only his increased heart rate to indicate his anxiety.

In this disturbing scenario, none of the staff members showed empathy for Timmy or tried to decrease his anxiety before deciding to administer neuromuscular blockers—a solution that makes care easier for the staff but terrifying to the child. Use of neuromuscular blockers without adequate sedation and analgesia and communication is inappropriate and intensifies fear. It is sometimes too easy for busy professionals to forget that the struggling patient in the bed in front of them is a frightened child.

For the preschooler who has difficulty separating fantasy from reality, the critical care unit can provide plenty of material for an active imagination. The environment and personnel in the critical care unit can appear threatening or hostile to a child who is already frightened, in pain, and sleep deprived. The preschooler believes in supernatural beings such as ghosts, monsters, and cartoon characters and may develop an explanation for a strange sight or noise involving one of these fantasies. Fears can be reinforced by the alarms and other frightening noises, smells, behaviors, bright or flashing lights, or overheard snatches of conversation.

The preschooler also has fears of the unknown, the dark, and being left alone. The nurse can eliminate some of the child's fears by reminding the child that a light will be on and a nurse will always be nearby. Creativity and understanding are necessary on the part of staff and parents if the preschooler is to feel safe and secure in the critical care unit.

Because preschoolers have primitive ideas about their bodies,[34] major fears of bodily injury and mutilation can cause many misconceptions and a great deal of anxiety about hospitalization. Any intrusive procedure, whether painful or not, is highly threatening to the preschool child. The child not only fears the pain of an injection, but also may worry that the puncture site will not close and that all the body "insides" will leak out. Bandages are sources of comfort, because many preschoolers feel that they will "hold everything in." The nurse should anticipate the child's concern if dressings or stitches are removed, especially in the child who believes that a large dressing or many stitches are holding a large part of him together. Assuring the child that the dressing will be replaced or showing the child that the skin has healed may decrease fear and resistance. Bandaging and unbandaging a doll or stuffed animal may help the child work through such fears.

It is highly stressful for critically ill preschoolers to lose control of their bodies or emotions. Although the critically ill child cannot be offered control for most aspects of care, realistic choices should be offered whenever possible to provide the child with a sense of some control.

Because the preschooler has a great need for movement and large muscle exercise, immobility at this age presents a special problem. The preschooler can use various coping strategies to deal with the stress of critical illness. Regression is most common because young children usually abandon their most recently acquired skills first. The reappearance of self-comforting behaviors such as thumb sucking, a loss of previously acquired body control, or increased need for physical comfort may be upsetting to the child's family. Parents will require reassurance that such behavior is the child's temporary way of coping with a stressful situation and that the child will regain lost skills after recovery. It is important to accept the regressive behavior and support the child rather than pressing the child to "act his age" or admonishing the child for behavior such as thumb sucking.

Preschool children can display additional coping strategies, including projection (attributing their own feelings, wishes, or behavior to other people or objects), repression, denial, withdrawal, aggression, fantasy, and motor activity. Children also may identify with the aggressor during play and assume the role of the nurse or physician or other perceived aggressor. In this way they attempt to reduce fear and anxiety by assuming some of the characteristics of these all-powerful adults to vicariously feel more control over their situation.

Preparation of the Preschooler for Procedures and Surgery

Explanations in advance are vital to decrease the preschooler's anxiety about a procedure and to increase the child's cooperation (see Box 2-2, earlier in chapter). When explaining surgical procedures to preschoolers, it may be best to tell them that something will be "fixed" rather than "removed" or "taken out," because the threat of losing a part of the body might be frightening. If anesthesia is described as "being put to sleep," it might invoke images of the way the neighborhood dog died. To decrease the child's fear, it is important to assure the child that he or she will wake up after the procedure.

Honesty is needed when explaining procedures to children. It is unfair to tell the child that a painful treatment will not hurt, because this approach deprives the child of an opportunity to prepare in advance. It is better to avoid use of analogies when describing the sensations the child will experience during a procedure, such as "this will feel like a bee sting," because the analogy may mean something different to the child. Instead, the nurse can tell the child something like "now this is going to hurt, but we're going to do this very fast, start counting with me, 1—2—3... almost done... 4—5—6... OK, done! It's all done." Honesty about the pain of the procedure strengthens the effectiveness of the nurse's reassurance that the procedure is over. Dishonest explanations, changes in plans, unfulfilled promises, and deviations from the procedure as explained also can threaten the child's trust in the staff. When changes are unavoidable, they must be acknowledged and explained to the child. Explanations also should emphasize that staff members care about the child and that the purpose of the procedure is not to punish the child but to help the child get well.

After the procedure has occurred, assess the child's perception of what happened, explain any misconceptions, and give the child an opportunity to work through feelings about what occurred.[8] Children who are admitted to the unit on an emergency basis also can benefit from such retrospective review.

The Preschooler and Play

During therapeutic play, stressful situations, fears, and disturbing facts of life can be dramatized repeatedly until the experience is assimilated and the fear or strong feeling is mastered. This type of play is a way for children to communicate what they cannot yet verbally express, and it is an acceptable outlet for negative feelings. Play also serves an important normalizing function; regardless of what is happening in terms of the illness or injury and treatments, the child is still able to play and to have fun. The preschool child may assume the roles of others and involve other people, often adults, assigning roles.

The preschooler's play reflects more fine motor coordination and verbalization, and a longer attention span than a toddler's play. The preschooler has a need for large muscle movement during play. Therapeutic play periods are an important part of any stable critically ill child's plan of care. Some guidelines for helping critically ill children play are listed in Table 2-1.

The nurse can serve an important role in creating an environment that makes play possible. Several factors influence the child's ability to play: the availability of physical space, permission from adults, safety during play, and the child's condition and physical limitations.[23] Children can learn about their environment through hands-on experiences and imaginative play that help them describe and integrate new sights, sounds, and experiences.

Robby, a 4½-year-old boy, was admitted to the critical care unit after a motor vehicle crash. His lower extremities were paralyzed. He was free to move only his head and arms. Robby's nurse recognized his anger and need for activity. She suspended a beach ball on a string from the curtain bar above Robby's bed. She told Robby that he could punch the ball if he wanted to whenever he felt like it. While the nurse stood at his bedside, he hesitantly touched the ball, then withdrew and diverted his eyes from the nurse. While the nurse was occupied across the room, Robby began to hit the ball slowly. After a few minutes he was punching the ball with more vigorous strokes. Thereafter, Robby spent a great deal of time punching his ball and its location was switched occasionally so that he could punch it with his other arm and hand.

The Preschooler and Death

For many years, incorrect assumptions were used to justify failure to discuss death with children. One such assumption was that children could not comprehend death and if they did, it would be harmful to discuss it with them. However, young children are aware of death, and their understanding of death follows a developmental progression based on their cognitive development.[45]

The preschooler is aware that death exists, but views death as an altered form of life[9] and as a temporary, reversible condition. Magical thinking and egocentrism dominate preschool children's views of death and lead preschoolers to believe that their naughtiness, anger, or bad thoughts are responsible for what is happening to them.[70] Preschoolers have difficulty understanding causality (i.e., the intent or reasons behind events) and tend to attribute magical or supernatural causes to

---

Table 2-1 Guidelines for Helping the Critically Ill Child Play

Guidelines	Intervention Suggestions
Use knowledge of child development to guide clinical judgment.	Target play activities to child's developmental level, not just chronologic age. Utilize expertise of child life or play therapists or advanced practice nurses. Make appropriate referrals for children who seem particularly troubled.
In general, reflect only what the child expresses; but determine when it is appropriate to go beyond child's expression.	Be nondirective. Do not try to interpret children's play for them. Use a puppet, doll, or the opening line "some children" to talk about feelings or fears the child might be experiencing.
Supply materials that stimulate play.	Use age-appropriate materials. Give choices of hospital equipment and other toys so children can play out or withdraw from direct hospital play. Provide art materials because they allow nonverbal expression of emotions and thoughts.
Allow enough time for the child to play without interruption.	Allot specific time periods for undisturbed play. Ensure that other staff members respect the child's play time, barring emergencies.
Permit the child to proceed at his or her own pace.	Do not push the child to deal with difficult or frightening issues before the child is ready; the child might not feel safe enough to handle some topics until after hospital discharge.
Play for the child who physically or emotionally cannot play.	Engage in active play and involve the child to whatever extent possible. Use puppets or dolls as before. Involve parents or visiting siblings in this way.
Allow direct play for the child who initiates it.	Support children who directly play out themes such as death or abusive or traumatic experiences. Answer questions as they arise.

Adapted from Petrillo M, Sanger S: *Emotional care of hospitalized children: an environmental approach*, ed 2, Philadelphia, 1980, JB Lippincott.

what they see and cannot understand. For example, preschoolers may believe that people die because they misbehaved.

It is important to recognize that it is not bad—or good—that a preschooler thinks of death in these ways; it simply is fact. Interventions delivered at an inappropriate developmental level, such as attempting to teach the preschooler about the permanence of death, will be ineffective and may provoke anxiety. Caregivers instead must use reassurance and explanations to clarify frightening misconceptions. Children need a great deal of reassurance that they are not being punished and that they are not responsible for their illness or condition.

Much of a preschool child's experience with death consists of the sight of dead birds, dogs, cats, or other animals that are often mutilated in death. In addition, the child has fears regarding bodily injury during this period. As a result, the preschooler may view death as mutilation or prolonged torture.[25] Pain, restraints, and intrusive procedures that the critically ill child experiences can lend credence to these fantasies. It is important to explore the child's view of death, to dispel misconceptions, and to decrease the patient's anxiety. Simple reassurances are often not helpful. It is often difficult or even impossible for an adult to think at a preoperational level and thus anticipate and fully understand the child's misconceptions without first exploring the child's beliefs.

The child's view of death is also affected by past experiences, such as the death of a family member. The child may identify with the illness or death of characters portrayed on television programs or the evening news and may come to view death as being killed or murdered. The family and child's cultural and religious beliefs also will play important roles in how the young child thinks about death and must be taken into account when planning explanations and interventions. Such beliefs might be shared by the family only after the nurse has demonstrated support and compassion.

Preschool children think of death more often than most adults are aware. Death should be discussed with the preschooler in a simple, honest way, with consideration given to the child's cognitive development and previous experiences. Children often understand *how* things are said better than *what* is said; therefore, the mood and amount of anxiety conveyed may be more important than the actual words used. When children ask whether they are going to die, it is important to discover what the term *die* means to the child and the child's perception of her prognosis. The nurse might ask, "What do you think?" or "What do you think is going to happen?" Lengthy explanations are rarely necessary or helpful at this age. If the child asks a direct question, a direct response is appropriate, such as reassurance and description of the care and support that will be provided.

THE CRITICALLY ILL SCHOOL-AGED CHILD

Emotional and Psychosocial Development of the School-Aged Child

During the school-age period of 6 to 12 years old, the child develops a sense of industry.[27] This is the age of accomplishment, increasing competence, and mastery of new skills. The child takes pride in the ability to assume new responsibilities, set goals, and complete tasks; with increasing independence comes increasing self-esteem. If the child experiences repeated failure or frustration in attempts at achievement during this period, a sense of inadequacy or inferiority may develop instead.

As peer relationships and peer-group approval become important, the child becomes less dependent on the family. In the course of the school year, the child often becomes a member of a clique, club, or gang and frequently has a best friend. Most peer-group interactions take place with members of the same sex, and the opposite sex may be viewed with distaste. This attitude often begins to change as the child enters preadolescence at approximately 11 to 13 years of age.

Rejection by a peer group can be devastating to the child during this stage of development. Chronic illness, injury, or conditions causing visible disability can set the child apart as different from peers and can make the child the object of ridicule. Separation from the peer group is often a significant and challenging consequence of illness and hospitalization during school years. Visits, letters, telephone calls, or e-mail messages from peers that help the child to maintain contact will help the child to cope. Because school is a significant part of the child's life, the parents might encourage the child's teacher and classmates to send cards and letters to the hospital. Occasionally, children are able to read or complete some uncomplicated schoolwork while in the critical care unit. Some children will be comforted by the fact that they can still do their homework, whereas others might prefer the freedom from schoolwork to reduce pressures during hospitalization.

The school-aged child is also an integral part of a family. Because separation from siblings can be particularly difficult at this time, every attempt should be made to continue contact with the child's siblings through visits, phone calls, emails, or exchange of photographs. School-aged children are able to tolerate separation from their parents and usually do not react to such separations with the intensity of the younger child. Older school-aged children might even enjoy periods away from their parents. During periods of critical illness and hospitalization, however, the child's need for parental support and involvement may be increased.

The school-age period marks the beginning of a major change in the parent-child relationship. Children begin to realize that the parent is not the omnipotent, omniscient being consistent with their images from early childhood. They discover that the parent is sometimes wrong and will not always be able to protect them from injury or pain. As a result, they can begin to question their parents' judgment. Relationships with other authority figures during this period influence future parent-child relationships.

The child is trying to find a balance between increased need for independence and control and continued desire for parental support and guidance. This conflict will intensify as the child approaches adolescence. For these reasons, it is important to ask for the child's opinion and understand the child's viewpoint, especially when caring for children with chronic or terminal illnesses.[80]

Parents might have difficulty relinquishing some of their control of the child during this period. They need to be patient and sensitive to support the child appropriately during illness and hospitalization, yet avoid forcing the child into a dependent role. The parents' response may be complicated if the child alternates unpredictably between dependent and independent behavior. The parents may require assistance in understanding their child's behavior in order to decrease potential feelings of hurt, anger, or frustration. Older, school-aged children often will criticize the parents in an attempt to declare independence.

Cognitive Development in the School-Aged Child

At approximately 7 years of age, the child enters the period of concrete operations, marking the beginning of logical thought.[69] Although still functioning very much in the present, the child is able to use deductive reasoning and to see the relationship of parts to the whole. As a result, the child becomes more flexible and may no longer require absolute consistency in daily routine. However, the school-age period still involves magical rituals that help children cope with stressful situations and give them security. Rituals such as "crossing fingers and toes" and incantations such as "step on a crack and break your mother's back" help school-aged children feel some sense of control over the world and their situations.

The child's concepts of time, space, and causality are more sophisticated and realistic during these years. True cooperation becomes possible because children are now able to differentiate their viewpoint from those of peers and authority figures and are able to value and respect viewpoints and opinions of others. As they learn to tell time, read, write, and do arithmetic, a new world is opened. They are able to understand events happening in the past, present, and future and are receptive to the acquisition of knowledge and learning new things.

The child's moral judgment becomes more developed during this period. Preschool and early school-aged children follow rules because they believe rules are unalterable and imposed from above. They learn to judge the rightness or wrongness of an act by its consequences, rewards, or punishment rather than by its motives. Although young school-aged children know the rules and what they may or may not do, they do not understand the reasons behind them. They see behavior as either totally right or totally wrong and think that everyone else believes the same. Children of 6 or 7 years of age can interpret accidents and illness as punishment.

Older school-aged children no longer view rules as rigid and unchangeable, but recognize that rules are established and maintained through social agreement. They also realize that rules may be flexible and based on circumstances. They no longer judge an act solely on its consequences, but on the motivation and intentions behind the act and the context in which it appears. Although older school-aged children can view rule violation in relation to the total situation and the perceived morality of the rule itself, it is not until adolescence or later that they will be able to view morality on an abstract basis, using reasoning and principled thinking.

The school-age period has been described by Freud as the period of latency.[31] During this period, there is less concern over physical issues. The child who is hospitalized for a serious illness or injury, however, finds attention centered on the body and its functions. School-aged children generally take an active interest in their condition, but may be self-conscious when the attention of the healthcare team is focused on their bodies.

The School-Aged Child in the Critical Care Environment

School-aged children are keenly aware of the critical care environment and sensitive to noise, activities, behaviors of staff, and sleep deprivation. They are susceptible to fear, confusion, anger, and disorientation. Fears during the school-age period are more realistic, although elements of magic and fantasy can still contribute to anxiety. Because school-aged children are struggling to become independent, loss of control is a major concern. The critical care unit is an unfamiliar place, and the child is subjected to many procedures and examinations by many unfamiliar people. Physical examinations in open areas without privacy can lead to feelings of resentment and anxiety, because the child has acquired feelings of modesty and shame concerning nakedness.[73] The hospitalized child is forced to depend on strangers for assistance with basic personal needs such as taking a bath, voiding, and having a bowel movement. It is important to respect the child's privacy and modesty and to give the child choices in scheduling care activities if possible.

Fears regarding possible mutilation and bodily injury or harm are prevalent during this period. School-aged children are typically concerned about the benefits, hazards, and techniques of procedures such as anesthesia and surgery. They may fear that the physician will start the operation before they are asleep or that they will awaken during the surgery. In addition, they usually fear the helplessness of anesthetized sleep, afraid that they may not wake up again and that they may die.[64] Older school-aged children are usually concerned about the consequences of the procedure or operation, including the postoperative appearance of the wound.

If the child is unable to communicate verbally, the child needs an alternative means of conveying requests, questions and feelings. For younger (prereading) children, pictures such as faces with different expressions (such as happy, sad, and crying) or common conversational objects can be used. For older children, a variety of electronic devices (particularly hand-held computers or telephones with text messaging) can be helpful.

Tools, such as the Children's Critical Illness Impact Scale, a self-report measure, can be useful in measuring psychological outcomes for 6 to 12 year olds after hospitalization in a PCCU.[75] Domains such as worries, fears, friends and family, sense of self, and behaviors were analyzed in initial studies of this scale.

Preparation of the School-Aged Child for Procedures and Surgery

To help school-age children cope and cooperate during procedures and to comply with the prescribed treatment regimen (see Box 2-2 in preceding pages), nurses should provide advance preparation for each procedure plus explanations during the procedure. Such explanations increase the chances that the child will gain confidence from the procedure rather than be overwhelmed by it.

At this age, the child's ideas about illness and body function are often nonexistent, vague, or false. The nurse cannot assume that the child actually understands the location or function of organs and body parts. Older school-aged children and adolescents will often nod and appear to understand explanations or words when in reality they have either no idea or a distorted idea of body functions and may not understand the explanations given. Note that explanations provided to the child by the parents may be inaccurate. Children are often reluctant to ask questions or admit that they do not know something they believe they are expected to know. To verify the child's comprehension, the nurse should ask the child to explain his or her illness or to draw a picture of his or her body and note any illness, injury, or problem present.

Children may be able to repeat information about their condition after listening attentively to all that is said around them; however, their interpretations of what they overhear may not always be accurate. Children are quick to pick up contradictions and often will request factual information. Cognitive mastery provides a way to maintain a sense of control over what is happening to them. With their newly acquired ability for logical thought and deductive reasoning, they are better able to understand the relationships between their illness or injury and its symptoms, and the need for and effects of treatments. The school-aged child also is more aware of the prognosis of illness, indispensability of certain body parts, potential hazards of treatments, life-long consequences of permanent injury, and the meaning of death.

A doll or human figure outlines can be used to discuss the functions of the body and explain procedures and operations. Some older children object to handling a doll, even if it is described as a teaching doll or dummy, and in those cases, body outlines can be used. School-age children enjoy learning scientific terminology and manipulating equipment that will be used in their treatment. Various coping techniques such as relaxation, imagery, deep breathing, and self-comforting talk have been found to be helpful for some children.[17,66]

The school-aged child might not always wish the parents to be present during procedures, and healthcare providers should respect the child's preference for parental support or privacy. If their presence is not desired by the child, the parents might require help to understand this assertion of their child's growing independence. The child's preference and needs may change, however, and will have to be ascertained on an ongoing basis.

The school-aged child may fear disgracing himself or disappointing parents or other significant adults by losing control. School-aged children, especially boys, are often given the message that they are expected to be brave and not cry. It is important to realize that school-aged children frequently exhibit the greatest amount of bravado when they are feeling the most helpless and most in need of support and reassurance. Parents and staff members should let the child know that it is all right to be frightened, angry, or upset and that crying can help decrease some anxiety.[73]

David, a 10-year-old boy, was hospitalized in a critical care unit with the possible diagnosis of meningitis. It was obvious how frightened he was during a lumbar puncture procedure and how much difficulty he was having maintaining control of his emotions. The nurse told him that she realized how frightening this all was for him, that he hurt and was uncomfortable, and that it was okay for him to cry if he felt like it. David loudly responded, "No, I can't. My dad told me not to!" David's father had deprived his son (most likely unwittingly and unintentionally) of a constructive outlet for his pain, fear, and anger. Instead he had given David another major stress factor—that is, his father's expectation that David should be stoic.

Parents sometimes need help understanding that crying and protest behavior are healthy and often helpful outlets for the child facing extremely stressful situations. Parents might need reassurance that such outlets do not indicate weakness or failure on the part of the child or parents.

The School-Aged Child and Play

Unstructured play gives the child an opportunity to gain diverse skills and a greater sense of competence. It also enhances the child's feelings of control and predictability.[11] When a school-aged child begins to recover from a critical illness, boredom can result. Play can serve as a means of entertainment and distraction, as a temporary escape from stress, and as a vehicle for resolving emotions. School-aged children have a longer attention span and increased cognitive abilities. They particularly enjoy playing with hospital equipment, and their own accurate use of this equipment reflects their keen observations of protocol, procedure, and technique. Role reversal with members of the healthcare team provides the child with the opportunity to exert some control and can give the team members valuable insight into the child's interpretations of and feelings about his illness and care. School-aged children also enjoy books, storytelling, and word games, and they may enjoy reading about their disease or procedure. It is often difficult to arrange peer interaction in a critical care unit, but it might be possible for a visiting sibling or young friend to play with the patient. Competitive games are particularly enjoyable during the school-age years and it is important to the child that rules, often made up by the child, be obeyed. School-aged children also enjoy ordering and collecting things. Older school-aged children begin to engage in daydreaming.

The School-Aged Child and Death

Early school-aged children often have a real understanding of the seriousness of their illness, although their understanding of death is still influenced by their cognitive development. The child relies less on magical explanations to explain happenings and is less egocentric. However, during these years death is often personified as a ghost, skeleton, boogeyman, or the devil, and the child may believe that death will come to take him away from his parents and friends. Nightmares and fear of the dark are common, and it is helpful for the nurse to leave a dim light on at night. If the child is convinced that there will be nurses nearby throughout the night to provide protection, the child often will be able to relax and fall asleep more confidently. The finality of death is not appreciated in young school-aged children. At approximately age 7, however, children are beginning to suspect that they themselves will die one day.

After the ages of 8 or 9 years, children begin to develop a more permanent view of death because they have a more complete concept of time. Children realize that their parents are not omnipotent, that they are powerless to avert death, and that ultimately everyone will die. Children at this age often use symbolic methods such as drawings or stories to express needs and fears. In the next few years, the child's concept of death is elaborated by cultural and religious experiences. The adult concept of death as final, irreversible, and inevitable is reached during the late school-age years.

Terminally ill school-aged children are often aware of their fatal prognosis without being told, because they understand nonverbal cues and often overhear more than staff and parents realize. Although attempts to shield the child from knowing a fatal prognosis may be made with good intention, such an approach is rarely beneficial for the child. Open communication allows the child an opportunity to discuss fears and apprehensions and minimizes risks of incomplete information or erroneous assumptions. The child then can be helped to work through fears, find more effective coping strategies, and ultimately accept the inevitable.

Deaths of other patients in the critical care unit may be a source of stress for the child. Older children may identify with the deceased child, particularly if their diagnoses are similar. Children need honest explanations if they ask what happened to the other child, because nervous or evasive answers will only heighten anxiety. If accurate, children should be reassured that the deceased child did not have the same medical problems. Staff members should answer the child's questions as simply and honestly as possible. If staff members or parents feel uncomfortable answering the child's questions, an advanced practice nurse, palliative care specialist, social worker, chaplain, or physician with particular skill in discussing death with children should be asked to help the child work through some of the anxiety. Parents often feel frustrated and helpless when faced with the child's questions about death and may need assistance in addressing their own needs.

THE CRITICALLY ILL ADOLESCENT

Adolescence is a time of profound physiologic, physical, and psychological change. Because the adolescent years are characterized by emotional turmoil, critically ill adolescents are often the most challenging patients. Supporting them and meeting their needs require patience, creativity, and understanding on the part of the critical care unit staff. Although a highly stressful time for adolescents, four benefits of hospitalization that have been identified by hospitalized adolescents are: improved physical well-being or appearance, positive perceptions of self as a result of attention received from others, an expansion of their social network, and a respite from responsibilities.[94,95]

Emotional and Psychosocial Development of the Adolescent

The major sources of anxiety during adolescence include separation from parents, adaptation to a rapidly changing body, the development of a sexual identity, and acquisition of a

sense of identity and autonomous function.[27] The behavior of adolescents is frequently inconsistent and unpredictable, and it is often as bewildering to the adolescent as it is to others. Behaviors such as mood swings, depression, periodic regression, and mild antisocial behavior that are normal during adolescence would likely be viewed with more concern if exhibited by children of other ages.

Adolescence can be divided into three stages—early, middle, and late adolescence—although the boundaries of these stages are imprecise. Early adolescence extends from approximately 12 to 15 years in girls and approximately 13 to 16 years in boys. During this period, body image issues are of primary concern. Younger teenagers are extremely preoccupied with body changes and sensations. Because they are aware of every possible individual flaw or imperfection, they worry that others are also aware. The peer group grows in importance and becomes the standard against which adolescents measure acceptability. The most intense relationships outside the home are with best friends of the same sex. Separation from parents normally increases and the teenager spends more time away from home, but is still willing to adhere to parental wishes, communicate with parents, and be accountable to them. The parent-child relationship still remains relatively intact. Young adolescents who become ill are primarily concerned with how the illness or injury will affect appearance, function, mobility, and peer relationships.

Mid-adolescence is often the most difficult and trying time. Conflicts over issues of autonomy, accountability, and self-determination can create tension between teenagers and parents. Teenagers often reject and rebel against parental support and control while continuing to depend on the parents. Mid-adolescents are still highly egocentric, narcissistic, and preoccupied with appearance, attraction to the opposite sex, and ability to meet gender role expectations. Peer reactions and relationships determine the teenager's body image and behavior and become the venue for experimentation with new roles and behaviors. Because illness or injury results in forced dependency and perceived loss of control, hospitalization is highly stressful for a mid-adolescent. Hospitalized mid-adolescents will be extremely anxious about changes in physical appearance that could make them different from or unacceptable to their peer group.

The late adolescent, aged approximately 17 to 22 years, is normally fairly secure in self-esteem, inner controls, independence, and relationships. Late adolescents function at a highly independent level; they listen to parental advice but then make their own decisions. During this period the primary concern is role definition in terms of education, career, marriage, or lifestyle. Serious illness or injury during this period is most threatening in its potential for affecting the realization of career and lifestyle goals or forcing changes in vocational plans.

Cognitive Development in the Adolescent

During adolescence, Piaget's fourth and last stage of cognitive development is attained—formal operations.[69] Most adolescents develop the ability to think abstractly and are able to project to the future and see the potential, long-term consequences of actions and illnesses. Although they are able to understand others' opinions, feelings, and points of view, adolescents are still fairly self-absorbed. The adolescent discovers the ability to interpret observations, understand broad concepts, and develop new insights and opinions. Increased cognitive abilities allow adolescents to have a greater understanding of their condition, treatment, and prognosis. It is appropriate and important to include teenagers in the planning of and decisions about medical therapy.

The adolescent perception of illness and its significance can be distorted. Illness or injury is often viewed in terms of how it will alter appearance or level of activity. An adolescent may react more negatively to an insignificant but visible or restrictive illness or injury than to an invisible but potentially life-threatening one.

Magical thinking still exists to some degree during the adolescent years. Teenagers often believe that they are to blame for an illness or injury and sometimes believe that they are being punished for rebellion against parents, forbidden fantasies, or for sexual activities. As a result, they also may be dealing with feelings of guilt and shame while coping with the physical aspects of their illness. Adolescents may, in fact, be responsible for injuries they receive, because they often take enormous risks and engage in dangerous behaviors to convince themselves and others of their bravery and invincibility. When such behavior results in serious injury to the adolescent or to others, the resulting guilt, grief, and mourning may cause depression or other serious reactions.

The Adolescent in the Critical Care Environment

When first admitted to a critical care unit after a serious injury or sudden illness, the adolescent may be in a state of emotional and physical shock and concerned about bodily functions and pain. Occasionally the teenager feels protected in the critical care unit and has little or no anxiety about being there. However, as this initial shock phase subsides, the critical illness may become terrifying or humiliating. The major threats to seriously ill adolescents are loss of control and of identity, altered body image, and separation from peer group.

Illness and hospitalization constitute a major situational crisis for the adolescent. Helplessness is much more threatening to adolescents than to younger children, although adolescents have more sophisticated coping mechanisms. They are extremely concerned that others will discover their inadequacy, dependency, and confusion; therefore, they hide it from everyone, including themselves. Because they have heightened body awareness and developing sexuality, privacy is of paramount importance to teenagers. Every attempt should be made to keep the adolescent covered, particularly over the genital areas (and, in females, over the breasts), during examinations and treatments. If the critical care unit does not contain private rooms, many adolescents will prefer to keep the curtains drawn around the bed to maintain privacy. It is embarrassing and traumatic for adolescents to lie exposed while several members of the healthcare team examine and discuss them. Lack of respect for and inattention to these needs can cause the adolescent even greater stress than experienced from physical pain.

Although separation from parents may be welcomed and appreciated during this time, separation from peer group support can be extremely disturbing. Healthcare providers should facilitate peer group contact as much as possible. However, while some adolescents benefit greatly from peer visits, others may not wish to be seen by friends if they believe they look disfigured or will be seen as being different. Such determinations need to be made individually.

Although the adolescent often uses denial to cope with stress, regression also may be used. The adolescent can become demanding of staff and parents and may be afraid to be alone. Such regression enables adolescents to return to the more dependent state of early childhood, allowing them to set aside the burden of dealing with tasks they are physically and emotionally unable to handle.

The teenager may also use other coping strategies, such as varying degrees of withdrawal. In addition, intellectualization may be useful to adolescents who wish to deal with the objective facts about their condition rather than the emotional aspects. High scholastic achievers in particular may use this strategy, requesting information and reading material to supplement their knowledge. Intellectualization can be a helpful coping strategy unless the information provided is distorted by the adolescent's fears and fantasies. The staff should support the patient's attempts at cognitive mastery, while frequently verifying the accuracy of perceptions. Other coping strategies include reaction formation, projection, and displacement of hospitalization-related anxiety into complaints concerning less significant aspects of care. Some adolescent behaviors that are distressing to staff members include manipulation, verbal abuse, physical attacks, sexual suggestiveness, and refusal to cooperate with the plan of care. Staff members should establish consistent limits, particularly for physical attacks and sexual suggestions.

Preparation of the Adolescent for Procedures and Surgery

Adolescents do not wish to be passive recipients of healthcare, but rather, active participants in planning and implementing their care. Preparation for procedures reduces fear of the unknown and helps the teenager maintain some feelings of control (see Box 2-2, earlier in chapter).

Adolescents react not only to what they are told but also to the manner in which the information is given. They are often reluctant to admit that they do not understand explanations, and their fears may be manifested as overconfidence, conceit, or pretentiousness. Many adolescents have little understanding of the structure and workings of the body. Therefore, the nurse must carefully and tactfully evaluate the adolescent's knowledge and individualize each teaching program.

Minor injuries and illnesses are often magnified and can affect a teenager's body image; consequently, a critical illness can be terrifying. Adolescents need assistance and reassurance in trying to gain a more realistic view of their illness. Because they are facing many unique problems during hospitalization, they need help identifying their strengths and effective coping mechanisms. Four types of stressful situations have been identified by adolescents hospitalized for minor surgical procedures[94]:

1. The anticipated surgery and its associated risks
2. Pain
3. Visible and handicapping consequences of surgery
4. Socially disruptive consequences of hospitalization and surgery

Pain was reported as the most frequently anticipated and distressing aspect of hospitalization. Therefore, it is important to teach coping strategies before performing painful procedures and to later review the adolescent's perceptions of and responses to the procedure. Provide analgesics when necessary and assess and document their effectiveness.

The Adolescent and Play

Although the idea of play may seem more appropriately applied to the care of younger children, adolescents also need the opportunity for a temporary escape, an outlet for strong feelings, and meaningful stimulation that will decrease the possibility of sensory deprivation or overload. Familiar activities, such as television or video games, personal music selections, e-mail, text messaging, and other peer communications may be appropriate and meaningful activities for a critically ill adolescent. As the adolescent recovers, reading, schoolwork, and other activities can be helpful diversions. Music therapists are often helpful in engaging adolescents in familiar activities. Some adolescents may use journaling as a way of venting thoughts and feelings in a private way. Others can benefit from the opportunity to share thoughts and feelings with an adult they trust and admire, with other adolescents, or through blogs. Daydreaming is a useful occupation for adolescents. It helps them decrease feelings of loneliness, master fears, safely establish a new identity, solve current problems, test themselves imaginatively in situations they have never experienced, and focus on the future.

The Adolescent and Death

Although adolescents have the intellectual capacity to understand death on the adult level, they usually do not view death in the same way as adults do. They can understand cognitively that death is permanent and that it will happen to everyone one day. However, they do not accept death as a believed reality, but may fantasize that death can be defied.[9] Adolescents may be unable to totally accept the finality of death, because they believe they are invincible. This belief can lead to self-destructive or daring behavior, resulting in injury, drug use and abuse, and suicide. Because remnants of magical thinking persist, the adolescent may view fatal illness as punishment; this can create guilt and remorse. Reassurance and open discussions of feelings, concerns, and fears are important.

Adolescents have a great deal of difficulty coping with the idea of their death. At a time when they are striving to establish their own identity and make plans for their future, it is extremely difficult to face the fact they have no future. Such a realization of death before fulfillment adds further turmoil to the challenges of adolescence.

Adolescents need to be highly involved in decisions about their care and treatment, even if it requires preparation for their own death. The critical care nurse must be alert to nonverbal cues and unasked questions when caring for critically ill adolescents, particularly if the patient is unable to speak as the result of intubation or other interventions. These patients may need to write, draw, or use electronic communication devices to express feelings and questions. Some adolescents might request that treatment be discontinued and that they be allowed to die. Each situation must be handled individually. Adolescents can have the cognitive understanding of death without the emotional maturity that is necessary to make final decisions regarding withholding or withdrawing medical care. They may be highly aware, however, that prolongation of life will increase suffering. Certainly, all adolescents who are conscious and able should be involved in decisions about treatment.

FAMILY MEMBERS AND THE CRITICAL CARE UNIT

A child's admission to a critical care unit is a major family event. Family-centered care includes a parent-professional partnership in the delivery of the child's care. The nurse must assess each family to understand their perceptions of the impact of the critical care admission and to meet each family's individual needs. Some questions that the nurse might include in a family assessment are presented in Box 2-3. The term *parents* is used in this chapter to denote the child's significant caretakers.

A child is a member of a family and has roles to play as a child, sibling, grandchild, niece or nephew, cousin, or friend. A child's critical illness can cause massive disruption in the established roles and functions of the family system. The way in which the family and staff members respond to this potential crisis can drastically affect the outcomes. Family

---

Box 2-3 **Helpful Questions about Family**

Who are the significant family members?

Who is identified as the family leader? Spokesman? Contact member?

Who makes the decisions regarding care for family members?

What is the family's religious and ethnic orientation? Do these play important roles in the family?

What is the developmental level of the patient?

What are the expected times and days when family members will visit?

Where does the family live in relationship to the hospital? How far must they travel?

What is the educational level of family members?

What information do family members need to or want to know?

What emotional support do the family members need?

Which significant family members need to be consulted in decision making?

Has the family experienced something like this before? How did they cope? What resources did they use?

What are the family members' expectations regarding patient outcome? What are their goals for the patient?

From Caine RM: Families in crisis: making the critical difference. *Focus Crit Care* 16:184, 1989.

members often feel frustrated because they are unable to meet the child's needs. If allowed to remain with the child, the parents can continue to provide significant and different emotional support for the child than the staff does. To restrict or prohibit the parents' presence with the child is not consistent with family-centered care.[22,88]

Parents and children need one another. Disruption of the parent-child relationship can be more anxiety-provoking than the critical care unit stimuli or the illness or injury.[20] There is an emotional linkage or empathy between the child and significant adults.[13,40,59] Evidence of emotional contagion presents long before the child comprehends emotional expression. High anxiety in the parents will lead to high anxiety in the child. However, if the parents are able to adopt a calm, nurturing, and supportive attitude, it will help the child to cope effectively.[66] Mothers who participated in a study (based on self-regulation,[48] control,[21] and emotional contagion theories) to increase their knowledge of behaviors and emotions resulting from a critical care unit stay and interventions to support coping were able to have a positive effect on their own and their child's outcomes.[58] They were better able to support their child during distressing procedures and experienced improved functional and emotional coping outcomes compared with the control group. Their children demonstrated improved mental health and psychological outcomes after discharge. Therefore, the child's parents and significant others, such as siblings, must also be a focus of nursing care and concern. Nursing support is important for the sake of the family members and because such support affects the child's stress level and recovery.

Children belong to their families, not to the staff members. No matter how caring and attentive the nursing staff is, they cannot replace the love and support of the child's own family. Parents are not visitors; they have the right to be involved in their child's care. Family members may need to see the ill child to be reassured or to realize that the child's prognosis is grave. Relatives of critically ill patients need to be near the patient and feel that there is hope. A grandparent, favorite aunt or uncle, sibling, or baby-sitter can also provide special comfort and security.

The description of who is considered a family member is no longer as clear as it once was. Single-parent families, stepfamilies, and nontraditional families are common. It is important to determine who constitutes family for each patient, record this in the medical record, and tailor visitation to each child. Visiting policies should be liberal and geared to the requirements of the child and family. The critical care unit should be open 24 hours a day to relatives and friends who are significant to the child. Certainly, space limitations can affect the number of people who can visit at one time, but restrictions should be flexible and serve the best interests of the children in the unit. In some cases, parents are grateful for a break or the opportunity to rest away from the critical care unit, and the support of staff members, family and friends is helpful.

Although staff members often expect and encourage parents to be involved in their child's care, parents often need clarification of staff expectations.[102] Expectations can vary with the child's clinical condition and diagnosis. Nurses often establish positive relationships with families, but the family may not necessarily view it as a collaborative partnership.[28] Nurses can have ambivalent feelings about the patients' families. Although nurses recognize that families are an important source of support, nurses may feel that visits increase the child's or family's anxiety. In fact, separation can increase anxiety. Although knowledge and observation of their child's discomfort is difficult for parents, separation from the child and exclusion from their child's care is less desirable.

At times, nurses may find the care of the critically ill child so demanding that they have limited energy left to support family members. Staff nurses, especially novices, may feel uncomfortable performing procedures while family members watch or having the family present during emergency procedures.[24,98] However, parents who are allowed to remain at the bedside are reassured by the competence of the nurse; if asked to leave, they may feel the nurse lacks self-confidence or confidence in the validity of the procedure. Some procedures, such as endotracheal suctioning, are very difficult for family members to observe. The nurse must be sensitive to their cues and help them make the best decision for them *and* the child. In most instances, parents should be given the option of remaining at the bedside during procedures because their presence is comforting and participation will help them feel more involved in their child's care. The older child may be given the option of asking parents to remain (or not).

Since the nurses' attitudes toward family presence may be influenced by their own experiences and ideas, department protocols and guidelines may help to promote positive approaches for both staff and families.[98] Nurses may develop attitudes about family members based on inadequate information about family relationships. Nurses' subjective feelings about patients and families have been reported to be influential factors in determining their level of involvement with the patient's family.[39] Factors such as a family member's age, sex, demeanor, or appearance may trigger a range of feelings in the nurse. Judgmental feelings about family members serve no useful purpose and are detrimental to the nurse-family relationship. Although nurses often cannot prevent such feelings, they can be aware of the feelings and try to keep them from interfering in the child's care. Strong negative feelings are almost impossible to hide from the family members, because so much of what we communicate is nonverbal. In these cases, it may be better that another nurse care for the child—one who is better able to establish a therapeutic relationship with the family.

Parenting Children of Different Ages in the PCCU

Some of the concerns and reactions of parents of critically ill children will vary depending on the child's age. Parents of the critically ill neonate have awaited the arrival of their child with such high hopes that feelings of inadequacy, failure, and guilt can accompany the parents' discovery that they have failed to keep their child healthy. They may need assistance in developing their parenting roles and in recognizing their importance to their child's care. Parents should be encouraged to participate in their infant's care as much as possible. Activities in which the family can participate, such as stroking, holding, calming, singing, diapering, and feeding, are all important aspects of care. In one study, maternal optimism was found to be reflected in the use of active, cognitive coping strategies during the infant's stay in the critical care unit.[51] Staff members can intervene with patients who are not as optimistic by encouraging active involvement in care.

Parents of toddlers need to be encouraged to continue their central role in their child's life. Their presence is extremely important, because it can help alleviate much of the child's distress. If the toddler has been hospitalized following injury or ingestion, parents may have to cope with guilt. Parents sometimes blame one another for an unintentional injury and require support and assistance in resolving anger. They often will benefit from performing purposeful activities that will help the child. Parents of toddlers are also valuable interpreters of the child's beginning verbal and nonverbal communication, routines, and rituals. Parents should be asked to make a list of the child's likes and dislikes, favorite toys and games, nicknames, special words for body parts and functions, and routines at home. This helps the parents to be involved in and contribute to their child's care and provides important information for individualizing care.

During the preschool period, attitudes about discipline and beginning sexual curiosity can influence parental concerns. The parents also may be anxious about their child's regression during hospitalization. In general, parents of preschool children are helpful in explaining procedures and treatments in language the child can understand, and parental participation in comforting and caretaking activities remains important to the child.

During the school-age period, the parent-child relationship changes as the child develops independence and relationships outside the home. Parents may feel guilt for allowing independent activity that led to an injury. The child's regression may be difficult for the parents to accept, particularly for fathers who want sons to be brave. Parents may need assistance in interpreting their child's demanding or rejecting behavior. Family members can dispel some of the child's loneliness and boredom by engaging in activities within the limits placed by the illness or injury. Parents can help the patient keep abreast of news from home, school, and friends during this period and can assist in providing comfort and explanations for the child. However, older school-aged children may prefer that care be performed by the nurse.

Adolescence is often a trying time for the parent-child relationship. Any disagreements or arguments that preceded the adolescent's hospitalization may cause the parents guilt and remorse when the adolescent becomes critically ill. If the adolescent was injured in an accident, the parents may feel guilty or frustrated because they could not prevent the injury. The adolescent often demonstrates both dependent and independent behavior, which can be confusing to parents. Parents often do not expect regression from their teenagers and need to be prepared for this behavior and reassured that it is normal and temporary. Parents should be encouraged to include the adolescent in decisions about care. Visits from other family members and friends should be encouraged so that the adolescents will maintain contact with their peer groups.

Parental Stressors

The admission of a child to a critical care unit meets the criteria for a "traumatic stressor," an event that reflects "actual or threatened death or serious injury or a threat to the physical integrity of self or others."[6] When the diagnosis, injury or treatment will result in body disfigurement or when the hospitalization is unplanned, dramatic, or far from home, it is even more stressful.[1,65] The effects are more significant for a family without previous exposure to critical illness or medical settings.

The child's critical illness or injury can produce monumental stressors, particularly if sudden or unexpected. The hospital environment may provide other sources of stress, such as lack of privacy in the waiting room, unfamiliar people who might be crying or talking loudly, an unfamiliar location, and disrupted sleeping and eating patterns.

Sources of stress from outside the hospital, such as financial, social, or personal costs, can add to the parents' burden.[1,32] Parents may be worried about the care or problems of other children at home or the cost of lodging, transportation, babysitters, food, hospitalization, and time lost from work. They may incur personal losses, such as loss of autonomy and privacy.[32] Other family members may be ill or injured at the same time as the child. If the child is hospitalized at a great distance from family and friends, the parents will be forced to stay in a strange city, away from support systems. At such times, relatively small associated stresses, such as trying to find a parking place, can become intolerable.[49] Family problems that existed before the hospitalization are often exacerbated during this time, particularly if one member is believed to be responsible for the child's illness or injury.

Of all the stressors the parents face, the critical care unit itself may be the most significant. If the child requires critical care, most people assume that this means that the child is seriously ill or even close to death. However, most nonmedical family members cannot imagine how complex or busy the unit is. Simply entering a critical care unit can be overwhelming for lay people who may already have emotional overload; the unit then adds sensory stimuli from alarms or other noises, unfamiliar sights, and unpleasant smells. Parents often are shocked at the first sight of their child in the critical care unit. Characteristics of the critical care experience that were reported to be important to parents included privacy, proximity to their child, adequate space, reduced sensory stimuli, cleanliness, and safety.[56] When the child dies in the critical care unit, positive connections and memories can be a source of comfort to bereaved parents, whereas negative memories contribute to the devastation felt by the parents.[55]

Responses to Stress

It may be therapeutic to help parents acknowledge that their child's critical care hospitalization is a traumatic stressor.[65] Families who are not in denial are better able to engage themselves and their child in active problem solving and mobilize supportive resources.[65] When events are too overwhelming to process immediately, the mind may alternate between denial and awareness until the information can be processed in sufficiently small segments to manage.[65] Staff members can help by listening to the parents' feelings and communicating acceptance that the parents' feelings are both understandable and manageable.[65]

People under stress are often unable to function at normal levels. Sedgwick[83] identified seven responses to stress that are important to understand when working with families of critically ill children. Behavior that would otherwise be inappropriate can reflect a normal response to stress.

1. *Reduced ability to use incoming information.* The parent may ask the same questions repeatedly of different staff members. It is essential that staff members use consistent content and wording of information. Parents may think they are being given inconsistent information when staff members use different words to describe the same condition. Consistency in communication between the healthcare team and the family is important. Thus, a primary communicator can be helpful, if feasible. If parents are provided with short summaries of important information composed by the primary nurse and physician and documented in the child's care plan, the parents can refer to this information later when they are able to digest it. This documentation will also ensure that consistent terms are used in explanations.

   Under stress, it is only possible to absorb a small amount of threatening information at any one time. When explaining treatments and equipment, the nurse should give brief explanations about their typical use for particular types of patients and problems. Family members sometimes act surprised when hearing information that was previously provided, denying that the doctor and nurses informed them. Before reacting to the parents' denials, it is important to realize that even if family members were told the information, they were likely unable to assimilate it.

   A parent may unconsciously cause or aggravate nursing staff discord by comparing information or nursing care provided by different nurses. If inconsistencies in the quality of care are present, these should be investigated and corrected. However, nurses should avoid discussion or criticism of minor variations in staff members' personalities or styles with parents.

   To facilitate effective communication of medical information, familiar staff members should establish frequent and consistent methods of communication with the family. In some units, parents participate during medical rounds. An observation of parental presence on rounds found that it did not interfere with education and communication, parents were satisfied with participation, medical staff found it beneficial, and privacy was not a concern despite implementation in an open unit.[68]

2. *Decreased ability to think clearly and solve problems.* Families of critically ill or injured children are often confused about the child's condition and medical plan of care. Parents will have limited ability to organize thoughts or questions and to draw conclusions from obvious evidence. The parent may be unable to sort or prioritize information and may respond identically to small and large stresses. The mother can appear to be as distressed about the fact that the infant's head was shaved for insertion of an intravenous catheter as about the infant's sudden need for intubation and emergency medical treatment. This inability to prioritize reflects extreme stress.

3. *Reduced ability to master tasks.* This response is related to an altered perception of the environment, a narrowed perceptual field, and an inability to mobilize resources. Even simple tasks such as completing the admission process may be beyond the parent's ability. The nurse should assess the parent's ability to function and provide assistance as needed.

4. *Decreased sense of personal effectiveness.* This can be reflected by feelings of loss, bewilderment, incompetence, failure, worthlessness, helplessness, or humiliation. Parents may feel guilty because they did not prevent their child's illness or injury.[65] Relationships with others can suffer. A sense of personal ineffectiveness is perhaps the most frustrating consequence. All parents feel a sense of helplessness when their child is critically ill. They need to be told what they can do to help with small tasks, such as reading to the child, before progressing to more difficult ones.

5. *Reduced ability to make effective, constructive decisions.* Often parents are asked to give consent for emergency procedures or surgery before they see their child or clearly understand the extent of the child's illness or injury. The parents' perceptions of events are often distorted, with gaps in memory filled with information that is only partially accurate. It is important to help parents identify the significant facts required to make an informed decision and then provide them with adequate time to assimilate this information.

   Although guidelines for obtaining informed consent are clear legally, the degree of involvement of parents in medical decision making varies with the decision, location, and parental abilities.[65] Parents are more likely to support interventions if they have been involved in the discussions and decision-making and in the formulation of the plan of care.[36] In a study comparing parents of children in PCCUs in different countries, the authors noted that in some cases, the quality of communication was more important than whether ultimate decisional authority rested with the parents, and that some degree of medical paternalism was unavoidable, regardless of existing legal or ethical norms.[19]

   Communication concerning serious events or decisions should be held in a location where parents can listen and ask questions without disruptions. They need a quiet, private space to hear upsetting news and time to assimilate information before they are required to respond or make decisions. In a study of physician communication with parents of critically ill children, the most significant issue identified by parents was the physician's availability to meet their need for information.[55] Parents noted that it was important to receive honest information presented in a straightforward manner in understandable language at a comprehensible pace. Nurses can facilitate conferences between physicians and parents and ensure that the parents understand the information provided.

6. *Heightened or decreased sensitivity to self.* Often the parents' body functions become a preoccupation, and somatic symptoms such as constipation, headache, or backache develop. People under a large amount of stress are easily distracted and annoyed and may be generally irritable.

Benign events such as the sound of a tapping pencil in the waiting room or the smell of certain foods can become disproportionately annoying. On the other hand, some parents become completely involved in their child and completely oblivious to themselves. They may need to be reminded to eat, take a break, or get some rest.

7. *Decreased sensitivity to the environment.* Stress can make parents somewhat oblivious to things happening around them. Because of this, they can miss cues from their child, spouse, or the staff. Because parents are less able to process subtleties in words or messages, straightforward communication is best.

Anyone who is overwhelmed by a stressful life event may enter a crisis state, characterized by an inability to cope with actual or perceived problems.[18,29] A crisis for one person will not necessarily be a crisis for another or, for that matter, may not be a crisis for the same person at another time. Difficulty arises when previously used strategies are not sufficient to solve the current challenge. Aguilera[2] identified balancing factors that modulate vulnerability to crisis: a realistic perception of the events, adequate coping strategies, and adequate situational support and support systems.

To help support family members during the crisis, it is important to determine the member's perception of the stressful event. Family members must have a realistic perception of the situation in order to manage it. Problem solving will probably not be successful until the real issue is identified, so nurses should correct any important misconceptions as tactfully as possible.

Coping describes ongoing efforts to manage a problem or situation. Coping strategies are behaviors that an individual typically demonstrates when stressed. They are highly individual, may be subconscious, and are subject to change depending on the context and demands of the situation. It is important to remember that the behavior you are viewing indicates the individual's strategy for coping with that specific situation at that specific moment. Coping strategies can include behavior that is inappropriate under normal circumstances but appropriate during periods of stress. Although nurses tend to see positive behaviors and affect as coping,[26] more negative responses, such as a toddler crying in protest when his mother leaves the room, can also be adaptive coping responses. In fact, in resilient children (i.e., children who have come through stressful experiences with a healthy adaptation), the actual coping behavior is not the most important factor in determining long-term outcome.[78] Longitudinal studies of children who have experienced stressful situations have identified three major processes or factors that led to more positive outcomes[33]:

1. The child's personality—outgoing and engaging children seem to do better
2. A supportive family
3. An outside support system that encourages and reinforces coping efforts and strengthens them with positive values

Parents may demonstrate various stages in coping with their child's admission to a critical care unit, particularly if the admission is unexpected. These stages are similar to the stages of the grieving process. Initially, most parents experience a period of shock, disbelief, and denial. These reactions are characterized by comments such as "This can't be happening to us" or "It's not that serious, she'll be OK." This initial stage may be brief for some families, but can last longer if the child remains unstable. Denial is often necessary for the parents to be able to function. While unrealistic expectations should not be supported, the staff should not remove all hope. Parents often understand the seriousness of the situation, but may not initially be able to admit it to themselves or others. As this stage progresses, the parents may feel helpless and guilty as they blame themselves or each other for the child's illness or injury.

Anger is another frequent reaction. Although parents may be angry at the child for injuring himself or at God for allowing this to happen, these are not acceptable targets for some parents. Other family members may not be safe targets for anger if the parent feels a need for support from them. Parents can turn against each other, particularly if they had previous disagreements or if they differ in coping styles or priorities. Although some parents are afraid to criticize staff members for fear of reprisals against the child, anger may also be displaced onto the staff, resulting in complaints about the child's care. Parents may need help in recognizing the source of their anger and finding constructive outlets for strong feelings. Some parents feel anger that has no simple target, so it results in negative behaviors such as angry outbursts, blaming, and desire for revenge.[65]

Depression is common and can indicate that the parent is attempting to handle the strong feelings the situation has triggered. A supportive listener is usually helpful to the parent during this stage. Eventually, the parents may reach a stage of resolution and acceptance in which they are able to make plans and decisions and can discuss the child's condition realistically.

Rarely do both parents react in the same way at the same time during a child's critical care; differing reactions can add to their stress. Staff members can help by including the parents in decision-making, engaging them in the care of their child, and referring them to appropriate resources to enable them to work together to support their child. Parents may not be able to return their lives and their child's life to the way it was before, but may find some benefit in the adaptation that the crisis required.[65] For example, they may find comfort and strength from having revised priorities. "Parents who are helped to survive and thrive have much to teach us if we are open to listening."[65]

The presence of adequate situational supports is important. A person experiencing a crisis is more dependent than usual. It is important that the nurse obtain information about the family structure and relationships, religious affiliations and beliefs, and other possible support systems. If family members are too stressed to support the patient or one another, the assistance of the healthcare team and outside resources (e.g., social services, chaplain, community support) will be vital to the family's constructive resolution of the crisis.

Strategies to Support Families

Preparation for the Impact of the Critical Care Environment

Whether the admission is planned or unplanned, it is important to try to assess the parents' potential reaction to the sights and sounds of the PCCU by discussing their expectations before they enter the unit. Advance preparation is useful for parents when the critical care admission is planned, such as for major surgery. Verbal explanation is the most common method of preparation. Some parents who have been prepared verbally emphasize that no matter how much they were told about the critical care unit, they still did not feel prepared for actually seeing it.[49] Audio-visual tours that show the hospital staff members and equipment in a critical care unit can be a useful supplement to verbal explanations. With the use of standardized media, the parents have an opportunity to see and hear actual sights and sounds from the critical care unit. A standardized approach ensures that all important information is included, and staff members are aware of all information the parents receive. It is helpful when a staff member views the program with the parents, because some of the sights and information can be upsetting, and may generate questions. Specific information presented should be documented and reinforced. Demonstrations using miniature or full-sized equipment on a doll or teddy bear are useful for preparing children, but do not give the parents a realistic idea of what to expect.

Tours of the critical care unit are helpful in familiarizing the parents with the physical characteristics of the unit and in giving them a more accurate idea of how their child will appear. The tour can be most effective if the parents are able to see a stable child (with the permission of that child's parents) with equipment similar to that planned for their child. If such stable patients are not present, it may be difficult to provide an effective demonstration. In addition, parents often are reluctant to look at other patients and invade the privacy of other children and families.

The parents' first visit to the child in the critical care unit is often reflective of how the parents will cope with the critical care stay. It is extremely important for the parents to visit their child as soon as possible, even if only briefly, after the child's arrival. The thought of seeing the child can be extremely frightening. When the child is unconscious or unresponsive, this first visit is particularly difficult. Parents should never be brought into a critical care unit without preparation for what they are about to see. Even in emergency situations, some on-the-spot preparation at the door can provide information about the most striking aspects of the unit and the equipment surrounding the child. These explanations will necessarily be brief, and all of the information given may not be heard or absorbed at that time.

During the first visit to the child in the critical care unit, family members should always be accompanied by a staff member who is available to answer questions, explain ongoing therapy, and correct major misconceptions about the child's care or equipment. The nurse at the bedside can react quickly to correct the problem if a monitor or other alarm should sound and to reassure the parents that everything is all right. Parents can be saved some ongoing and unnecessary anxiety if they realize that alarms can sound even when there is no problem.

The child and the area around the bed should be neat and clean before the parents enter, if possible. When time is short, a clean sheet can be placed over the child or the bed. The most important function of the first visit for the parents is to reaffirm that their child is still alive. A brief check of the child with an explanation of the next steps often gives the parents sufficient information and reassurance to enable them to contact family and friends for additional support.

Initially it may be most helpful to the parents if the nurse simply provides silent support at the child's bedside, allowing the parents time to digest the sights and sounds of the critical care unit. Supportive gestures can be far more helpful at that moment than information about the child's equipment. The nurse should allow time after the parents' initial visit to assess their response to the environment and to answer additional questions.

Supporting Parental Coping

During their visits in the critical care unit, parents may use a variety of coping strategies. Silent observation may be the first reaction. The parents may stop a few feet from the child's bed and simply stare at the child and equipment to reduce the initial impact of what they are seeing. Parents may need time to pull their thoughts together before they can move in and support their child. A nurse with good intentions may take parents by the arm and bring them closer, saying, "It's OK for you to move up closer to the bed and hold his hand," but this action can actually increase the parents' stress if they are not ready to approach the child. Because some parents need time to be able to accept the situation, restricting bedside visits to short periods may not allow time during a single visit for the parents to relax enough to approach, touch and interact with their child.

Visual survey is another way of becoming familiar with new situations. Some parents seem to pay attention to everything but their child, because they may be too frightened to actually look at their child, supine on the bed with a great deal of equipment. The parents may need to become familiar with the environment before they are able to focus on their child. The nurse must wait before giving explanations until the parents are able to focus on what the nurse is saying.

The parents may also use withdrawal as a coping strategy. Some parents withdraw emotionally and seem to be unresponsive or detached; others may leave the PCCU after a brief visit of 1 or 2 minutes. These parents may need intervention and explanation, or they may simply need more time to adapt. Parents often must be encouraged to take breaks during the child's stay in the critical care unit.

The parents may restrict their reaction to the child's complex situation and focus on only small details, such as a piece of tape that seems too tight or a small area of blood on the sheet. Such concerns may seem to be inappropriate in light of the child's condition, but they may be the only things the parents feel they can change. Response to the parents' expressed concerns can help parents cope by giving them some feeling of control over their child's care.

Parents may also use intellectualization as a coping strategy. The equipment or numbers are factors that are often easier to deal with than their child's appearance. Although parents may not really understand what a number means, they may realize that it is higher or lower than before and such information may be easier to handle than other possibilities. Answering the parents' questions on an intellectual level can help them to master some anxiety. This method of coping is sometimes carried to an extreme, however. One father used a stopwatch to time his child's ventilator and hurriedly informed the nurse when it delivered 39 rather than the selected 40 breaths per min. Intervention was necessary to assist this father in identifying and discussing his actual fears and concerns.

In a study of staff behaviors and parental coping patterns helpful to parents during their child's PCCU stay, a number of problem-focused coping strategies were identified.[60] The following strategies were used by all of the parents in the study: (1) believing the child is getting the best care possible, (2) receiving as much information about the situation as possible, (3) asking questions of the staff, (4) being near the child as much as possible, (5) praying, and (6) ensuring that the child is getting proper care.

Some families adopt hypervigilance to cope, never leaving the bedside, requesting information about minute details of care, delaying consents to medications and treatments in order to perform exhaustive research, and demanding reviews of medical records and nursing assignments. Because an overly vigilant family's behavior can seem threatening, staff members might respond with defensiveness, withholding details, avoiding contact, or restricting visitation. Those responses typically increase the family's vigilance. It is more effective to include the family in planning care, provide consistent and frequent information sharing, and acknowledge the value of the parent-child relationship.[88]

It is difficult to imagine how terrifying it can be to have a child in a critical care unit. Sympathetic statements such as "I know how you feel" are untrue and inappropriate unless, in fact, the nurse's child has been critically ill. What nurses say to parents is usually not as important to them as the attitude conveyed. The nurse should not attempt to say something profound during each parental interaction; it is more important that the nurse demonstrate a caring demeanor through actions and nonverbal communication.

A study examining parents' perceptions of caregiver behavior found that nurses who engaged in "nurturing and vigilant" behaviors that complemented the parental role reinforced family integrity during the crisis.[37] Collaboration between parents and nurses that addresses the needs and preferences of parents is one of the most satisfying aspects of nursing caring practices.[22,54] Research has shown that parents used the relationship with the nurse to help cope and assure them that their needs and their child's needs were being met.[96] A parent does not expect staff members to have all answers at all times, but the parent has a right to expect staff members to be honest and demonstrate compassion.

Many times, the stress of the child's illness destabilizes the family or the parents' relationships. Families that have experienced multiple crises and life changes in the months preceding hospitalization are most susceptible.[65] If nurses identify such crises during the family assessment, the information can be used to plan interventions that emphasize support groups, strategies for coping, and professional mental health referrals as needed.[65]

Siblings

A child's illness or injury can have a profound effect on other siblings in the family. When a critical illness or injury strikes one child and requires that parents spend a large amount of time at the hospital, the other healthy children in the family often feel excluded or forgotten. Young siblings may fear that their behavior or wishes caused the ill child to get sick. Their response to stress can manifest in different ways, such as negative behavior, mood changes, eating or sleeping disturbances, and loss of interest in favorite activities. School performance, peer relationships, and behavior at school or home can be affected. Alternatively, siblings may concentrate on academic pursuits as a way of escaping stresses at home or as a way of demonstrating competence in an effort to win attention from parents or combat feelings of hopelessness. The sibling's peer relationships can be affected if the sibling must frequently be absent from school, spends time with family members instead of friends or becomes irritable and preoccupied. Siblings can develop somatic complaints as a way of seeking parental attention or as a way of identifying with the ill sibling.

Attempts to shelter siblings from unpleasant information will likely increase—rather than decrease—the siblings' fears and fantasies. They know something is wrong with their brother or sister but, without explanations from trusted adults, they have only their own imaginations. Often the situation imagined by the sibling is much more distressing than a visit to the PCCU would be. Such visits should occur, however, only after an assessment of the sibling and the family coping styles and relationships, and only after the sibling has been prepared for the sights and sounds in the unit. After the visit, a debriefing session with the sibling is important to allow the nurse and the parents to assess the sibling's reaction, answer questions, and clarify misconceptions.[86]

Often the parents are extremely concerned about the effect of one child's critical illness on their other children, but are not sure what to do or say to support the children at home. Nurses should help parents identify ways to reduce sibling anxiety. Parents may also need encouragement to remain at home for several hours per day to spend time with other family members or to split responsibilities between the hospitalized child and siblings, especially during lengthy hospitalizations. If the hospitalized child is unstable, close family members, such as grandparents, can bring siblings to the hospital to visit parents and the child. Child life therapists can help both siblings and parents.

CHALLENGES OF PEDIATRIC CRITICAL CARE NURSING

Challenges involved in critical care nursing in general, and in particular in a PCCU, are well documented in the literature. Beyond the stresses of a critical care environment and critically ill children, the concepts of toxic or hostile work environments and horizontal violence are discussed in the literature, with recommended strategies for recognition, prevention, and management.[74]

Some factors that contribute to stress, such as abusive language and screaming, are obvious, but others are more subtle (e.g., unilateral decision making, abuse of power, lack of respect, inequitable reward structures, intimidation, imbalance between work and personal life). Longstanding interdependencies can make the healthy and toxic behaviors more difficult to untangle in organizations.[74] When those who wield more power, such as nursing executives and physicians, model disruptive behavior, the workplace stressors can be intensified.

Nursing leaders are responsible for providing appropriate role models and monitoring the work environment. The American Association of Critical-Care Nurses has made a commitment to promote a healthy work environment and has published standards to establish such environments.[5] Working collaboratively, leaders and staff can implement standards for a healthy environment that address the key factors in the PCCU environment, such as interpersonal relationships, systems issues, and patient care situations that are known to generate stress.[85] The Evolve Website contains excellent information regarding Burnout and Compassion Fatigue Among Caregivers (see the Chapter 24 Supplement on the Evolve Website).

Interpersonal Relationships

Interpersonal conflict has been identified as one of the greatest sources of stress for critical care nurses, and it can affect patient outcomes.[52,81,82,91] The most frequently cited and intense stressors are nurse-physician conflicts. Nurse-management and nurse-nurse conflicts are additional identified stressors. If the team is not cohesive and supportive, it is likely that the helplessness felt around traumatic events in the unit or inability to cure the patient will erupt into inappropriate staff behavior. Another type of interpersonal conflict, nurse-family conflict, has been addressed above.

Nurse-Physician Relationships

Critical care nurses have an expanded level of knowledge and they perform interventions that have traditionally been performed by physicians. With experience, the critical care nurse's knowledge and skills often exceed those of the beginning resident. The complex and potentially life-threatening situations found in the PCCU require good communication, respect, support, cooperation, and collaboration among all members of the healthcare team. However, this high level of functioning may not always be achieved.

Lack of collaboration, trust, and respect for the expertise and contributions of others can lead to conflict and disharmony, ultimately reducing the quality of care delivered to children and their families. In some cases, nurses do not believe that a collegial relationship exists between nurses and physicians; they may feel that some physicians neither respect nor listen to them. This source of stress can be intensified when the nurse believes that the physician is ineffectively or incorrectly managing the patient's care. Because several consulting services often are involved in the care of the critically ill child, they can provide conflicting orders, leaving the nurse caught in the middle and forced to arbitrate differences between services or to choose which orders to follow.

Healthcare systems can create barriers to effective collaboration, such as hierarchical, paternalistic, and traditional lines of authority and accountability in patient care matters.[91] In addition, nurses are accountable for providing a quality of care consistent with their expertise. The nurse is responsible for questioning physicians' orders that appear to be incorrect. The nurse is held to legal standards of expertise, capable of observing and assessing medical procedures and making judgments about appropriateness of care. This paradox of the nurse's substantial responsibility but limited authority, status, and power highlights one of the primary sources of potential role conflict and impedance to communication between nurses and physicians.

Frustration with the nurse-physician relationship is not unique to the nurse. Physicians may believe that experienced nurses are too critical of new physicians and are resistant to change. An intimidating nurse can make a highly competent resident feel insecure and appear hesitant and indecisive. When nurses bypass house staff members and seek the advice of senior physicians, the fellows and residents may be unaware of the patient's status. At times, nurses are territorial about the critical care unit, discouraging the involvement of rotating physicians.

Mutual respect and cooperation among all members of the healthcare team are necessary to provide high quality care. Effective collaboration requires mutual support and open communication, with free sharing of knowledge and information between nurses and physicians.[91] Guidelines or policies can exist, but management, medical directors, and nurse educators must consistently model and enforce appropriate professional behavior. Both nursing and medical directors must be strong and supportive leaders who are able to solve actual and potential conflicts. Staff meetings attended by nursing and medical staff and other professionals should be scheduled regularly and as needed to facilitate communication and mutual support. Differing ideas about treatment plans can be discussed so that all members of the team are able to contribute to decisions.

Nurse-Management Relationships

Nurse managers may find it difficult to meet staff nurse expectations. If managers are heavily involved in direct patient care, they might be criticized for a lack of organization and vision. If the manager spends most time at an administrative level to negotiate better working conditions for staff, the manager might be criticized for being absent from the unit too often. In addition, managers are often required to defend unpopular administrative decisions to the nursing staff.

Some of the anger and criticism directed at management by staff nurses is scapegoating. The intense feelings of anger and frustration the critical care nurse experiences can sometimes be directed more safely toward nursing managers than toward patients, families, co-workers, or physicians. Staff-development instructors, preceptors, and charge nurses are also perceived as safer targets, because they usually do not have line authority or responsibility for nursing staff performance evaluations.

Although it is exciting to work with intelligent, independent, and assertive critical care nurses, it is challenging to manage such nurses. Critical care nurses are expected to take a lot of responsibility for the quality of patient care, so they wish to participate in the decisions being made about that care. Because critical care units usually require high standards of care, greater autonomy, and specialized skills, a participative management style is usually more effective than a hierarchical structure. If a manager seeks to impose a more hierarchical structure, staff stress and resentment can result.

Chaos theory reflects on the similarity between the disorder, confusion, and change felt in the work setting and the forces occurring in nature.[35,74] Nature reorders itself after turmoil and, in a similar fashion, that reordering occurs in the workplace as well. Managers can use the strength and ideas of the workforce to develop transformational changes in clinical practice. A collaborative nursing management approach can foster nursing growth in an era of continuous change.[35]

Conflict can be prevented or reduced if front line managers maintain close communication with staff members and share ideas, problems, and solutions with them. It is vital to identify the root causes of dissatisfaction. Often, apparently minor complaints provide clues to more serious problems. For example, staff complaints about the unit orientation may actually represent frustration with high staff turnover and nursing shortages. The frequent presence of managers in the patient care areas conveys the managers' desire to identify problems.

Lack of positive feedback is a source of stress for nurses, particularly when they are working under demanding conditions. Too often, mistakes are widely discussed, while positive behaviors go unnoticed. Feedback is necessary and important, but leaders are not the only source of feedback. Both positive and negative feedback can be shared directly among members of the healthcare team. A good method for receiving feedback is to begin by giving supportive feedback to others.

The types of behaviors for which a nurse is rewarded indicate the value system of the person or system providing the feedback; behavior that is reinforced will be repeated. Often nurses are rewarded for attention to and knowledge of pure tasks, such as knowing a particular laboratory result when a physician asks, recognizing an arrhythmia, or functioning appropriately in an emergency. Hospitals are less likely to recognize nurses for innovative interventions and "thinking out of the box" that truly affect the child's and family's special needs. Nurse managers must be aware of the behaviors that are rewarded in their units and make sure that those are the behaviors they want repeated. Recognition is important to everyone, but it is essential to new staff members who are insecure in their new roles and want to be accepted and respected by their co-workers and leadership.

Nurse-Nurse Relationships

Peer conflicts frequently are additional sources of stress for nurses. Competitive feelings and envy are often present among staff. Nurses can compete for mastery of technical skills or the most challenging patient assignments. Sometimes the nurse who asks too many questions or admits fears can be viewed as incompetent by peers. Some nurses view offers of help as threats to their competence. A critical care unit, however, is a place where mutual assistance, support, and interdependence are crucial to the delivery of high-quality care. Staff and leadership nurses in critical care units must be identify occasions when competition is winning over cooperation, and they should take steps to discuss and remedy such situations. Disruptive behavior and horizontal violence should not be tolerated under any circumstances.

Systems Issues

The current shortage of qualified nurses means that many critical care units remain understaffed. The critical care nurse must bear the increased work load, double shifts, and the stress of working with reassigned staff and registry/traveler nurses who may not be familiar with all the skills and activities required in critical care. Staffing shortages may necessitate frequent schedule changes and postponement of vacations; these factors further increase stress.

Even moderate nursing turnover demands ongoing orientation, which is challenging for the experienced staff, who may already be overburdened. An organized preceptor orientation program helps ensure that preceptors for new staff are enthusiastic, educated, and committed to the process. Many departments have also found that pairing new staff with mentors after the orientation process helps to continue the supportive environment for newer staff.

If well-developed continuing education programs in the critical care unit are not available, nurses may feel insecure about their own knowledge and dissatisfied with the lack of opportunity. Creative ongoing educational programs include many resources, such as advanced practice nurses, physicians, educators, administrators, and staff nurses. Involved physicians have the opportunity to explain their philosophy and preferences for patient care and better appreciate the nurses' knowledge of and interest in specific patient care problems. The participating nurses can raise questions or suggest alternative care techniques in an environment conducive to an exchange of ideas. When patient census is low, the staff nurse may be relieved of patient care responsibilities to research a clinical problem and deliver a brief summary of the findings to other staff. This allows each staff member to develop specific areas of expertise and helps staff nurses to gain respect for and respect from colleagues.

From a human factors engineering standpoint, the PCCU is a demanding environment, making staff susceptible to physical and workload stresses in addition to the emotional stressors. Evidence indicates that the combination of fatigue, workload, and the sensory-overloaded environment can be a factor in less than optimal staff performance, potentially contributing to errors.[62] Equipment malfunctions, cramped facilities, a noisy environment, and lack of supplies can add to stressful working conditions and compassion fatigue (for system factors contributing to caregiver burnout and compassion fatigue, see Burnout and Compassion Fatigue Among Caregivers and Evolve Table 24-4 in the Chapter 24 Supplement on the Evolve Website).

Patient Care Issues

If the patient's clinical course is unpredictable, disturbing, or out of control, or the nurse feels helpless, vulnerable, exhausted, closely bonded to the child, or identifies similar characteristics in the patient and his or her own child, then PCCU nurses may experience primary or secondary traumatization.[65] Primary traumatization occurs when the medical event itself is highly traumatic for the staff member. Secondary traumatization can occur in the caregiver who empathizes closely with the pain of the child and family and allows the intense feelings to accumulate, often resulting in burnout.[65]

The pediatric critical care nurse is faced with many challenges and stressful situations with which he or she must cope. Caring for any unresponsive child for several days can lead to feelings of vulnerability, exhaustion, frustration, sorrow, and anxiety. Caring for neurologically impaired children can raise questions about the quality of patient life that is being salvaged. Pediatric nurses described caring for a child in a persistent vegetative state as emotionally stressful and ethically challenging.[61] The decision to withdraw life support, regardless of the circumstances, is always difficult for the healthcare team.

Nurses may feel frustrated and powerless when their views are not considered or they may feel a share in the heavy responsibility if they participate in the decision. Enormous amounts of emotional energy are required to support family members through this experience. It can also be particularly stressful to care for children who have been abused or are victims of violent crimes, because the nurse may have strong feelings of revulsion or anger. Staff members must try to avoid the temptation to assign guilt, take sides, and express anger they feel toward abusive parents.

The pediatric critical care nurse has frequent encounters with death. These nurses not only have to deal with their feelings about the child's death, but may receive the brunt of parental anger and anxiety. Each patient requires an investment of time, energy, and technical skills. The nurse often becomes attached to and involved with patients, and this emotional bond makes it difficult for the nurse when the child dies, although it is this same emotional bond that allows the nurse to provide compassionate support to the family. It is also important that the nurse be able to maintain a therapeutic relationship with the family. If the nurse becomes overly involved, she or he will be unable to effectively support the family. Benner and Wrubel[7] note that the remedy for over-involvement is not avoiding involvement, but identifying the right level and kind of involvement.

Trusted colleagues, managers, and other social support can assist traumatized staff by acting as an outlet for emotions. Staff members also need to develop a lifestyle outside of work that involves personal life-affirming activities and nurturing relationships.[65] Unit leaders and managers should assess staff members' responses to dramatic events and look for chronic "numbing," which occurs when staff members exhibit decreased emotion or growing irritability.[65] Some longtime PCCU nurses grow weary of the pain of too many suffering or dying children, too many traumatized families, and too much of everything. These nurses need a break.

Strategies for Coping

Supportive relationships with colleagues are by far the most significant factors in reducing stress in the critical care unit. When nurses have close, positive relationships in a unit, that unit usually has high morale. Shared intense, emotional, and stressful experiences can foster camaraderie, closeness, and an understanding for the feelings of other members of the healthcare team. If a co-worker is extremely frustrated, it might be necessary to relieve that nurse from patient care responsibilities for a short period.

Emotional empathy and reassurance from those with whom one works closely is highly meaningful. Sometimes people need to hear that someone realizes how they feel and recognizes the intensity of their efforts. Physical contact is important, too. Supportive physical contact, such as hugs, can be beneficial in the professional setting. Praise from co-workers can also be especially satisfying. It is important to take a moment to tell a co-worker when he or she does something especially well.

After the death of a child, the child's nurse will need time to grieve and regroup and will typically not be ready to received another assignment the moment the grieving family leaves the critical care unit. It is important to allow for such time, even when the patient census is high and another child is waiting in the emergency department for a critical care bed. If the nurse has empathized with the family's sorrow, it will be difficult to abandon or suppress those feelings and immediately form a new relationship with another child and family. Nurses need to be sensitive to the feelings and needs of those with whom they work and be sure that they are giving their colleagues time, understanding, and support.

Coping strategies such as the use of laughter, bravado, detachment, and other self-protecting maneuvers have been recognized as being temporarily helpful for the intense feelings of pain and threat that critical care staff members experience.[7] Although acknowledgment of feelings and colleague support are the most beneficial long-term coping strategies,[7] the use of humor can sometimes provide short-term relief and a feeling that the situation is not too overwhelming. Tears of laughter are much less threatening than tears of grief and frustration. Because staff members' use of humor can be perceived by families as insensitive, its use is best reserved for locations where family members are not present.

Group meetings or debriefings can provide a constructive outlet for feelings and can be a means of sharing and discovering mutual concerns. A staff psychologist or employee assistance personnel can be invited to coordinate the meetings. After dramatic or distressing events, critical incident stress debriefing has been shown to be helpful.[29] Such meetings can foster open communication and can be used for problem solving and conflict resolution or can even facilitate the use of humor in an appropriate setting.

The use of regular physical activity and relaxation techniques can reduce stress on a long-term basis. Each nurse should recognize when his or her own breathing is rapid and shallow and should learn to concentrate on slow diaphragmatic breathing. Doing so will help to decrease the level of physiologic arousal and lead to a decrease of anxiety and restlessness. In addition, staff members should have a location where they can find a few moments of quiet and peace to relax and defuse. It is important that the nurse has a balance between work life and personal life. See the Chapter 24 Supplement on the Evolve Website, for more information about Burnout and Compassion Fatigue Among Caregivers.

REWARDS OF PEDIATRIC CRITICAL CARE NURSING

We often focus on the stressors of critical care nursing and forget the reasons that nurses thrive in this environment. The major rewards of critical care nursing are often the same as the major stressors: the nature of direct patient care, interpersonal relationships, and personal growth and development. It is exciting to watch a critically ill child progress and recover, especially because knowledgeable nursing care contributes to such recovery. It is gratifying to visit children after they have been transferred from the critical care unit, seeing the child who was close to death now resuming normal activities.

Pediatric critical care nurses experience a lot of gratification from assisting children and their families through an extremely difficult and sometimes devastating experience and sharing personal, intense feelings. Supporting a family through a child's death can be an opportunity to help someone through one of the most difficult challenges they will experience. The nurse may find more prolonged, intense, and positive relationships with these families than with any other. Such opportunities are highly rewarding.

The critical care nurse is able to deliver total patient care and to have close involvement with one or two patients and families. Such intense involvement is not always possible with larger assignments in less acute nursing care units. The nurse is often able to take more initiative and to make more independent decisions in the critical care unit. The close working relationships and teamwork that occur among nurses, physicians, and other co-workers in the critical care unit can be highly satisfying.

Critical care nurses are usually recognized for their specialized knowledge and competence. The PCCU is an environment that is rich with learning opportunities, and it provides excellent opportunities for professional growth and development. The challenges, fast pace, excitement, stimulation, and opportunities for learning are all positive aspects of the critical care setting. Although fewer words were used to describe the rewards compared with the challenges, one can aptly summarize the rewards of PCCU nursing: it is rare to have the opportunity to make a difference in the life of a special child and family, yet pediatric critical care nurses do that every single day.

CONCLUSIONS

The environment and dynamics of a PCCU may create many challenges for the child, family, and staff. This chapter has summarized some of the psychosocial and emotional considerations that are important aspects of pediatric critical care. Focused skills and attention are required to prevent these considerations from being lost in the requirements of technology, treatment interventions, and physical care. A knowledgeable, empathetic, and caring nurse can help to turn the critical care experience from a stress-filled to a growth-producing one for the child, family, and nurse.

References

1. Agazio JB, Ephraim P, Flaherty NJ, Gurney CA: Effects of nonlocal geographically separated hospitalizations upon families. *Mil Med* 168(10):778–783, 2003.
2. Aguilera DC: *Crisis intervention: theory and methodology*, ed 7, St Louis, 1994, CV Mosby.
3. Als H: Assessing infant individuality. In Brown CC, editor: *Infants at risk*, Skillman, NJ, 1981, Johnson & Johnson.
4. Als H, et al: Individualized behavioral and environmental care for the very low birth weight infant at high risk for bronchopulmonary dysplasia: neonatal intensive care unit and developmental outcome. *Pediatrics* 78:1123, 1986.
5. American Association of Critical-Care Nurses. *AACN Standards for establishing and sustaining health work environments*, Aliso Viejo, Calif, 2005, AACN.
6. American Psychiatric Association: *Diagnostic and statistical manual of mental disorders*, ed. 4, Text revision, Washington, DC, 2000, American Psychiatric Association.
7. Benner P, Wrubel J: *The primacy of caring: stress and coping in health and illness*, Menlo Park, Calif, 1989, Addison-Wesley.
8. Betz CL: After the operation—postprocedural sessions to allay anxiety. *Am J Matern Child Nurs* 7:260, 1982.
9. Betz CL, Poster EC: Children's concepts of death: implications for pediatric practice. *Nurs Clin North Am* 19:341, 1984.
10. Blackburn S: Sleep and awake states of the newborn. In Barnard KE, et al., editors: *Early parent-infant relationships*, White Plains, NY, 1978, The National Foundation for March of Dimes.
11. Bolig R, Fernie DE, Klein EL: Unstructured play in hospital settings: an internal locus of control rationale. *Child Health Care* 15:101, 1986.
12. Bowlby J: *Attachment and loss,* vol 2, Separation, New York, 1973, Basic Books.
13. Brazelton TB: *Infants and mothers: differences in development,* New York, 1969, Dell Publishing.
14. Brazelton TB: *Neonatal behavior assessment scale*, ed 2, Philadelphia, 1984, JB Lippincott.
15. Brazelton TB: Behavioral competence of the newborn infant. *Semin Perinatol* 3:35, 1979.
16. Caine RM: Families in crisis: making the critical difference. *Focus Crit Care* 16:184, 1989.
17. Caire JB, Erickson S: Reducing distress in pediatric patients undergoing cardiac catheterization. *Child Health Care* 14:146, 1986.
18. Callahan J: Crisis theory and crisis in emergencies. In Kleepsies PM, editor: *Emergencies in mental health practice: evaluation and management*, New York, 2000, Guilford Press.
19. Carnevale FA, Canoui P, Cremer R, et al: Parental involvement in treatment decisions regarding their critically ill child: A comparative study of France and Quebec. *Pediatr Crit Care Med* 8(4):337–342, 2007.
20. Carter M, et al: Parental environmental stress in pediatric intensive care units. *Dimens Crit Care Nurs* 4:180, 1985.
21. Carver CS, Scheier MF: Control theory: a useful conceptual framework for personality-social, clinical and health psychology. *Psychol Bull* 92:111–135, 1982.
22. Curley MA, Meyer EC: Caring practices: the impact of the critical care experience on the family. In Curley MA, Moloney-Harmon PA, editors: *Critical care nursing of infants and children*, ed 2, Philadelphia, 2001, WB Saunders.
23. D'Antonio IJ: Therapeutic use of play in hospitals. *Nurs Clin North Am* 19:351, 1984.
24. Dingeman RS, Mitchell EA, Meyer EC, Curley MA: Parent presence during complex invasive procedures and cardiopulmonary resuscitation: A systematic review of the literature. *Pediatrics* 120 (4):842–854, 2007.
25. Duton HD: The child's concept of death. In Schoenberg B, et al., editors: *Loss and grief*, New York, 1970, Columbia University Press.
26. Ellerton ML, Ritchie JA, Caty S: Nurses' perceptions of coping behaviors in hospitalized preschool children. *J Pediatr Nurs* 4:197, 1989.
27. Erikson EH: *Children and society*, ed 2, New York, 1963, WW Norton & Co, Inc.
28. Espezel HJ, Canamc J: Parent-nurse interactions: care of hospitalized children. *J Adv Nurs* 44(1):34–41, 2003.
29. Flannery RB, Everly GS: Crisis intervention: a review. *Int J Emerg Ment Health* 2(2):119–125, 2000.
30. Fraiberg SH: *The magic years*, New York, 1968, Charles Scribner and Sons.
31. Freud A: The role of bodily illness in the mental life of children. *Psychoanalytic study of the child*, vol 7, New York, 1952, International Universities Press.
32. Gallery P: Paying to participate: financial, social and personal costs to parents of involvement in their children's care in hospital. *J Adv Nurs* 25:746–752, 1997.
33. Garmezy N: Stress, competence, and development: continuities in the study of schizophrenic adults, children vulnerable to

psychotherapy, and the search for stress-resistant children. *Am J Orthopsychiatry* 57:159, 1987.

34. Gellert E, Gircus JS, Cohen J: Children's awareness of their bodily appearance: a developmental study of factors associated with the body percept. *Genet Soc Gen Psychol Monogr* 84:109, 1971.
35. Grossman SC, Valiga TM: *The new leadership challenge: creating the future of nursing,* ed 3, Philadelphia, 2009, F. A. Davis.
36. Hallström I, Runeson I, Elander G: An observational study of the level at which parents participate in decisions during their child's hospitalization. *Nurs Ethics* 9(2):202–208, 2002.
37. Harbaugh BL, Tomlinson PS, Kirschbaum M: Parents' perceptions of nurses' caregiving behaviors in the pediatric intensive care unit. *Issues Compr Pediatr Nurs* 27:163–178, 2004.
38. Heiney SP, Neuberg RW, Myers D, Bergman LH: The aftermath of bone marrow transplant for parents of pediatric patients: a post-traumatic stress disorder. *Oncol Nurs Forum* 21:843–847, 1994.
39. Hickey M, Lewandowski LA: Critical care nurses' role with families: a descriptive study. *Heart Lung* 17:670, 1988.
40. Jimerson SS: Patterns of anxiety. In Haber J, Hoskins PP, Leach AM, Sideleau BF, editors: *Comprehensive psychiatric nursing,* ed 3, New York, 1987, McGraw-Hill.
41. Jones SM, Fiser DH, Livingston RL: Behavioral changes in pediatric intensive care. *Am J Dis Chil* 146:375–379, 1992.
42. Klinnert MD, et al: Emotions as behavior regulators: social referencing in infancy. In Plutchick R, Kellerman A, editors: *Emotion: theory, research, and experience,* vol 2, New York, 1983, Academic Press.
43. Kolcaba K, DiMarco A: Comfort theory and its application to pediatric nursing. *Pediatr Nurs* 31(3):187–194, 2005.
44. Koocher G: Childhood, death, and cognitive development. *Dev Psychol* 9:369, 1973.
45. Kübler-Ross E: *On children and death,* New York, 1983, MacMillan.
46. Leduc E: The healing touch. *Am J Matern Child Nurs* 14:41, 1989.
47. Lee JL, Fowler MD: Merely child's play? Developmental work and playthings. *J Pediatr Nurs* 1:260, 1986.
48. Leventhal H, Johnson JE: Laboratory and field experimentation: development of a theory of self-regulation. In Woolridge PJ, Schmitt MH, Skipper JK, Leonard RC, editors: *Behavioral science and nursing theory,* St. Louis, 1983, Mosby.
49. Lewandowski LA: Stresses and coping styles of parents of children undergoing open-heart surgery. *Crit Care Nurs Q* 3:77, 1980.
50. McGarvey TP, Haen C: Intervention strategies for treating traumatized siblings on a pediatric inpatient unit. *Am J Orthopsychiatry* 75(3):395–408, 2005.
51. McIntosh BJ, Stern M, Feguson KS: Optimism, coping, and psychological distress: maternal reactions to NICU hospitalization. *Child Health Care* 33(1):59–76, 2004.
52. Manojlovich M, DeCicco B: Health work environments, nurse-physician communication, and patients' outcomes. *Am J Crit Care* 16(6):536–543, 2007.
53. Marino BL: Assessments of infant play: applications to research and practice. *Issues Compr Pediatr Nurs* 11:227, 1988.
54. Marino BL, Marine EK, Hayes JS: Parents' report of children's hospital care: what it means for your practice. *Pediatr Nurs* 26(2):97–98, 2000.
55. Meert KL, et al: Parents' perspectives on physician-parent communication near the time of a child's death in the pediatric intensive care unit. *Pediatric Critical Care Medicine* 9(1):2–7, 2008.
56. Meert KL, et al: Exploring parents' environmental needs at the time of a child's death in the pediatric intensive care unit. *Pediatr Crit Care Med* 9(6):623–628, 2008.
57. Melnyk BM, Small L, Carno MA: The effectiveness of parent-focused interventions in improving coping/mental health outcomes of critically ill children and their parents: an evidence base to guide clinical practice. *Pediatr Nurs* 30:143–148, 2004.
58. Melnyk BM, et al: Creating opportunities for parent empowerment: program effects on the mental health/coping outcomes of critically ill young children and their mothers. *Pediatrics* 113(6):e597–e607, 2004.
59. Melnyk BM, Feinstein NF: Mediating functions of maternal anxiety and participation in care on young children's posthospital adjustment. *Res Nurs Health* 24:18–26, 2001.

60. Miles M, Carter M: Coping strategies used by parents during their child's hospitalization in an intensive care unit. *Child Health Care* 14:14, 1985.
61. Montagnino BA, Ethier AM: The experiences of pediatric nurses caring for children in a persistent vegetative state. *Pediatr Crit Care Med* 8(5):440–446, 2007.
62. Montgomery VL: Effect of fatigue, workload, and environment on patient safety in the pediatric intensive care unit. *Pediatr Crit Care Med* 8(2 Suppl.):S11–S16, 2007.
63. Odetola FO, et al: A national survey of pediatric critical care resources in the United States. *Pediatrics* 115(4):e382–e386, 2005.
64. OrsutoSr J Sr, Corbo BH: Approaches of health care-givers to young children in a pediatric intensive care unit. *Matern Child Nurs J* 16:157, 1987.
65. Peebles-Kleiger MJ: Pediatric and neonatal intensive care hospitalization as traumatic stressor: implications for intervention. *Bull Menninger Clin* 64(2). 2000.
66. Peterson L, Shigetomi C: The use of coping techniques to minimize anxiety in hospitalized children. *Behav Ther* 12:1, 1981.
67. Petrillo M, Sanger S: *Emotional care of hospitalized children: an environmental approach,* ed 2, Philadelphia, 1980, JB Lippincott Company.
68. Phipp LM, et al: Assessment of parental presence during bedside pediatric intensive care unit rounds: effect on duration, teaching, and privacy. *Pediatr Crit Care Med* May 8(3):220–224, 2007.
69. Piaget J: *The origins of intelligence in children,* New York, 1952, International Universities Press, Inc.
70. Piaget J: *The moral judgment of the child,* New York, 1965, The Free Press.
71. Piaget J: *The language and thought of the child,* ed 3, New York, 1967, Humanities Press International, Inc.
72. Piaget J, Inelder B: *The psychology of the child,* New York, 1964, Basic Books, Inc, Publishers.
73. Popovich DM: Clinical practice: preserving dignity in the young hospitalized child. *Nurs Forum* 38(2):12–17, 2003.
74. Porter-O'Grady T, Malloch K: *Quantum leadership: a resource for health care innovation,* ed 2, Sudbury, MA, 2007, Jones and Bartlett Publishers.
75. Rennick JE, et al: Developing the children's critical illness impact scale: capturing stories from children, parents, and staff. *J Pediatr Crit Care Med* 9(3):252–260, 2008.
76. Riese ML: Temperament in full-term and preterm infants: stability over ages 6 to 24 months. *J Dev Behav Pediatr* 9:6, 1988.
77. Robertson J: *Young children in hospitals,* New York, 1969, Basic Books, Inc, Publishers.
78. Rutter M: Psychosocial resilience and protective mechanisms. *Am J Orthopsychiatry* 57:317, 1987.
79. Sapolsky RM, Romero LM, Munck AU: How do glucocorticoids influence stress responses? Integrating permissive, suppressive, stimulatory, and preparative actions. *Endocr Rev* 21:5589, 2000.
80. Sartain SA, Clarke CL, Heyman R: Hearing the voices of children with chronic illness. *J Adv Nurs* 32(4):913–921, 2000.
81. Schmalenberg C, Kramer M: Types of intensive care units with the healthiest, most productive work environments. *Am J Crit Care* 16(5):458–468, 2007.
82. Schmalenberg C, Kramer M: Clinical units with the healthiest work environments. *Crit Care Nurse* 28(3):65–77, 2008.
83. Sedgwick R: Psychological responses to stress. *J Psychiatr Nurs* 13:20, 1975.
84. Selye H: *Stress in health and disease,* Boston, 1976, Butterworth Publishers.
85. Shirey MR, Fisher ML: Leadership agenda for change toward health work environments in acute and critical care. *Crit Care Nurse* 28(5):66–78, 2008.
86. Shonkwiler MA: Sibling visits in the pediatric intensive care unit. *Crit Care Q* 8:67, 1985.
87. Skerrett K, Hardin SB, Puskar KR: Infant anxiety. *Matern Child Nurs J* 12:51, 1983.
88. Slota MC, et al: Perspectives on family-centered, flexible visitation in the intensive care unit setting. *Crit Care Med* 31(5 Suppl.):S1–S5, 2003.
89. Slota MC: Implications of sleep deprivation in the pediatric critical care unit. *Focus Crit Care* 15(3):35–44, 1988.

90. Small L: Early predictors of poor coping outcomes in children following intensive care hospitalization and stressful medical encounters. *Pediatr Nurs* 28(4):393–401, 2002.
91. Stein-Parbury J, Liaschenko J: Understanding collaboration between nurses and physicians as knowledge at work. *Am J Crit Care* 16 (5):470–477, 2007.
92. Stepp-Gilbert E: Sensory integration: a reason for infant enrichment. *Issues Compr Pediatr Nurs* 11:319, 1988.
93. Stern DN: *The interpersonal world of the infant,* New York, 1985, Basic Books.
94. Stevens M: Adolescents' perception of stressful events during hospitalization. *J Pediatr Nurs* 1:303, 1986.
95. Stevens MS: Benefits of hospitalization: the adolescents' perspective. *Issues Compr Pediatr Nurs* 11:197, 1988.
96. Stratton KM: Parents experiences of their child's care during hospitalization. *J Cult Divers* 11(1). 2004.
97. Wallen K, et al: Symptoms of acute posttraumatic stress disorder after intensive care. *Am J Crit Care* 17(6):534–543, 2008.
98. Weber MD: Family presence protocols: a nurse's perspective. *Crit Connect* 7(6):1–7, 2008.
99. Weibley TT: Inside the incubator. *Am J Matern Child Nurs* 14:96–100, 1989.
100. Wilson DF, et al: Collaborative Pediatric Critical Care Research Network (CPCCRN). *Pediatr Criti Care Med* 7(4):301–307, 2006.
101. Winnicott DW: Transitional objects and transitional phenomena: a study of the first "not me" possession. *Int J Psychoanal* 34:89, 1953.
102. Ygge BM, Lindholm C, Arnetz J: Hospital staff perceptions of parental involvement in paediatric hospital care. *J Adv Nurs* 53 (5):534–542, 2006.
103. Zastowny T, Krischenbaum DS, Meng AL: Coping skills training for children: effects on distress before, during, and after hospitalization for surgery. *Health Psychol* 5:231, 1986.

Care of the Child with Life-Limiting Conditions and the Child's Family in the Pediatric Critical Care Unit

3

Mary Jo Gilmer

Ⓔvolve Be sure to check out the supplementary content available at http://evolve.elsevier.com/Hazinski.

To cure sometimes
To relieve often
To comfort always

Sir William Osler

Thoughts of a pediatric critical care unit (PCCU) conjure sounds of cardiac monitor alarms, ventilators with rhythmic inspiratory/expiratory cycles, gurgling suction machines, and nurses engaged in animated conversations with residents and hospitalists. A look around reveals postoperative dressings, exposed torsos, and intravenous solutions, blood and parenteral alimentation finding their way through carefully secured catheters into tiny veins.

The PCCU is also a place for palliative care. How can the seemingly disparate approaches of high technology and high compassion work in concert for the benefit of children and families? The answer to this dilemma requires understanding the objectives of palliative care.[32]

PEARLS

- Palliative care is a holistic approach to the care of the child and family when the child has a life-threatening or life-limiting condition.
- Palliative care is not the withdrawal of support, rather it is the active, total care of the child and family, with an emphasis on management of physical and emotional pain and suffering rather than on a cure for the child's disease or condition.
- Healthcare providers need to be just as aggressive in providing palliative care as they are in providing curative therapies. Providers should begin plans to provide palliative care as soon as the life-threatening or life-limiting condition is diagnosed.
- There is never "nothing more we can do." We can always support families as they navigate the difficult challenges of life-threatening or life-limiting conditions.

DEFINITION

The most frightening news parents can receive is that their child has a life-threatening condition. Even more frightening and painful is the death of that child. These experiences often take place in a PCCU, where comprehensive palliative care is essential. Pediatric palliative care embraces a holistic approach to the care of a child with a life-threatening or life-limiting condition and the child's family; it involves active, total care of the child's body, mind, and spirit. Palliative care begins at the time of diagnosis and involves evaluating and alleviating a child's physical, psychological, and social distress.[57] To help support the best quality of life for these children, nurses need to have a clear understanding of the patients and families served, and must comprehensively address the needs of children with life-threatening conditions and their families. Nurses must provide care that responds to the anguish and suffering of patients and families, supports caregivers and healthcare providers, and cultivates educational programs.[33]

In the past, palliative care was not initiated until cure was no longer thought to be possible. However, many of the goals of cure-oriented and palliative care are the same, including interdisciplinary collaboration, clear and timely communication with families, and careful management of physical and emotional pain and suffering. Experts now believe that palliative care should begin whenever a potentially life-limiting condition is diagnosed.[57] Unfortunately, children and families are often deprived of the benefits of palliative care because healthcare providers are reluctant to even discuss aggressive provision of comfort measures until all attempts to cure have been exhausted.

Death in the PCCU can be perceived as a failure, leaving the staff, parents, and other family members stunned and helpless because they were unable to prevent the child's death. Palliative care is an affirmation of life itself, dealing with dying as a natural process in the life course. Palliative care can be provided with aggressive curative treatments or it can take precedence over a curative approach as a child's death becomes imminent. Many healthcare professionals choose to work in critical care because they take satisfaction from aggressively treating complex life-threatening conditions. Nurses might not understand that palliative care can also be aggressive care, providing comfort and compassion while managing physical and emotional pain. When the healthcare provider is unable to cure the physical condition, the provider can always offer support to the child and family though their difficult physical and emotional journeys.

Pediatric palliative care focuses on the maintenance of quality of life for children and families, including a physical dimension that involves management of pain and distressing symptoms.[26] Nurses who provide care to these children face many challenges. Physical care is important, but nurses must also address the emotional and psychological needs. A holistic family-centered model of care encourages family involvement in a mutually beneficial and supportive partnership.[22] This chapter explores the needs of children with life-limiting conditions and their families in the PCCU setting, and it presents nursing interventions designed to meet the needs of the whole family.

INDICATIONS

Each year, approximately 54,000 children die in the United States, many after a lengthy illness.[38] Most of these children die in hospitals, most often in neonatal and pediatric critical care units.[11] The death of a child is an intensely painful experience, both emotionally and physically. In the United States, it is estimated that 1 million children are living with a serious, chronic illness that impacts their quality of life. In the PCCU, most diagnoses are potentially life-threatening or life-limiting and include trauma, cardiovascular conditions, respiratory compromise, congenital defects, and neurodegenerative disorders. Palliative care services can be beneficial at many times in the illness trajectory including diagnosis, treatment, survivorship, or end-of-life.

Historically, palliative care has been provided at the end-of-life in homes or hospice residences, but a need to integrate palliative care principles from the time of diagnosis throughout critical care interventions is becoming increasingly common. A growing number of patients with complex medical problems are alive as the result of PCCU technology, but now are dependent on that technology to continue living. These children often have residual cardiorespiratory or neurologic problems and require technologic support that is unavailable in or impractical for the home care setting. For some of these children, survival outside the hospital might not be the best option.[10] Therefore, many of these children ultimately die in the PCCU. The PCCU staff might find it difficult to switch from life-saving interventions to care that focuses predominantly on addressing the comfort and psychological needs common to dying children and their families. Some children's hospitals are developing pediatric palliative care teams or centers to ensure seamless continuity of care from critical care units to the home, and to assist the team in providing the best possible care for children with life-limiting conditions and their families.

APPROACHES TO A FAMILY-CENTERED MODEL OF CARE

Nothing can realistically prepare parents or children to face a child's life-threatening illness or injury, but experienced nurses can provide invaluable guidance and support. Palliative care services are appropriately applied to both curable and incurable conditions, and children's lives may be enhanced when many of the services are applied early in the course of disease treatment. Most, if not all, children with life-threatening conditions fear death or reoccurrence and pain and suffering. Caring for these children presents unique challenges for parents

and for healthcare providers. Key ethical concepts include distinctions between withholding and withdrawing treatment and possible consequences such as double effect. The doctrine of double effect is used to describe giving medications with the intention of making a child comfortable, knowing one possible consequence is hastening the child's death.[51] Inherent in illness is the potential for pain and suffering that may be eased through appropriate family-centered palliative care. Strategies that enable children and their families to express their feelings, to identify realistic hopes and expectations, and to focus on using their strengths to their best advantage can facilitate optimal coping and adaptation. Family-centered care that incorporates the child's social structure and relationships is regarded as a comprehensive ideal for end-of-life care.[51]

The Child's Needs
Admission and Diagnosis

The most common condition requiring PCCU admission is respiratory distress requiring intubation. A conscious child with a life-threatening illness or injury will probably be extremely frightened by the PCCU environment, equipment, and interventions such as intubation, establishment of IV access, and insertion of additional catheters. The child may be especially bewildered when regaining consciousness.

Nurses in the PCCU should help assess the child's and family's feelings about a decision to intubate the child. However, if a child deteriorates suddenly and unexpectedly, resuscitation and intubation may be performed emergently before there is an opportunity to assess the family's wishes. In some cases, the family is not ready to make a decision regarding attempted resuscitation, or allowing natural death. In any case, nurses in the PCCU must be prepared to respond to the child and family's anxiety, fear, and anticipatory grief. It is important to talk with the child and family and offer explanations for therapy and procedures, even if it appears the child cannot hear.

Nurses can help families by providing careful explanations of events necessitating PCCU admission, the equipment present, and the care provided by the nursing staff. If the child is responsive, the child can be taught to communicate with the nursing staff. The child might be told, for example, that, because he has been very sick, he developed a problem in breathing, and that a soft tube (or airway or breathing tube) was put into his lungs (or into the windpipe) to help him breathe. The nurse might add that the staff is doing everything they can to help the child feel better, and the child's parents and nurses will be close to his bed to care for him. Such communication is important even if the child appears to be unconscious. Call bells, alphabet and phrase boards, pointing, writing, and drawing can all help facilitate communication with the conscious intubated child.[39,55]

If intubation is not necessary, verbal communication is possible. The child's questions can be more spontaneous, and the child's answers can be more detailed and less influenced by the answer options provided by the parents or staff (i.e., not limited to *yes* or *no*). Conversations related to the PCCU environment may be stifled while the child remains in the PCCU. The child should be given many opportunities to express concerns, fears, questions, and preferences regarding care and

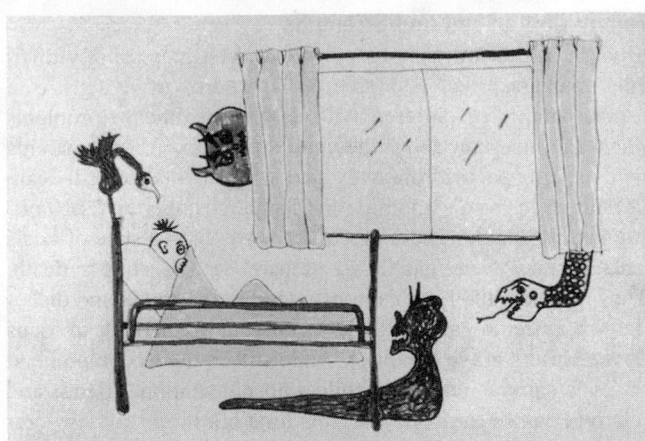

FIG. 3-1 The child's view of the PCCU. Art can provide valuable insight into the child's fears and concerns in the PCCU. This picture was created by a young school-age child. (Drawing courtesy of Julie Wall.)

termination of care (see Chapter 24; also see Special Considerations: Care of the Dying Adolescent in the Chapter 24 Supplement on the Evolve Website). Art and play therapy can provide a means of communication about the child's fears, and discussion of the child's art provides an opportunity to explore the child's feelings (Fig. 3-1). Child life specialists can be particularly helpful in advocating for children's wishes and assisting patients with self-expression (see also Table 2-1).

Physical Needs

Often the single most important aspect of physical care for the child with a life-limiting condition is the reduction or elimination of pain; however, studies have shown that many children are not adequately medicated to relieve their pain.[16,32,56] While physicians and nurse practitioners will prescribe analgesics, nurses have a major role in recognizing and relieving pain. To identify and quantify pain and to evaluate the effectiveness of analgesics, the nurse should assess both physiologic and behavioral manifestations of pain (see Chapter 5 for further information).[26,40,44] Although it can be extremely difficult to determine whether a preverbal, intubated, or obtunded child is in pain, the nurse can identify signs of distress through close observation of the child's heart rate, respiratory rate, breathing effort, pupil size, muscle tone, and facial expression. The presence of a facial grimace or guarding, tension or flexion of muscles, pupil dilation, tachycardia, tachypnea, and diaphoresis all can indicate the presence of pain. If the nurse is unsure whether symptoms of pain are present, the nurse should ask the parents to assist in the determination of the child's level of comfort.

Pain control uses both pharmacologic and psychologic measures (see Chapter 5 for further information about assessment and relief of pain). Although administration of analgesics can result in double effect, pain relief should be the most important physical consideration when death is inevitable.[23] When healthcare team members are able to acknowledge that the child may be dying, the dying child is more likely to receive adequate analgesics

Specific treatment for dyspnea and respiratory distress in the PCCU are highly variable and need to be individualized, based on the underlying source of the dyspnea and the child's level of consciousness and needs (see Principles of Withdrawing Life-Sustaining Treatments in the Chapter 24 Supplement on the Evolve Website). Supplementary oxygen, corticosteroids, diuretics, and bronchodilators may be useful approaches to care. Another relatively common symptom seen in dying children in the PCCU is delirium, which can be calm or agitated. Delirium decreases a child's ability to receive, process, and recall information and can be mitigated with the reduction of noise and lights and by the presence of family members or familiar staff.[51]

Comfort measures are often as important as life-saving measures to a child with a life-limiting condition and to the child's family. These measures can include but are not limited to soothing baths and backrubs, opportunities to be held and to play with favorite toys and pets, and diversional activities such as computers, movies, and favorite music. Such activities can reduce anxiety and pain and relieve the impersonal atmosphere of the PCCU environment.[23]

Establishing and maintaining a daily schedule, including times for rest and sleep, is extremely important. Meticulous skin care, comfortable positioning and frequent repositioning, hygiene, and the preservation of optimal bowel and bladder function are all components of good nursing care. This care assures the child and family that the staff members remain committed to the child's care.

Emotional Needs

Establishment of effective communication is often challenging for family members, even when all are in good health. It can be especially challenging to establish effective communication for the child with a life-threatening condition, the child's family members, and the child's healthcare providers, because the child's condition, treatment, and prognosis introduce additional stresses and fears (see Fig. 3-1). There are several critical points during the continuum of care when communication is especially important: at diagnosis, during exacerbations, and at the end of life. Frequently these critical points occur in a PCCU. Initiation of palliative care services might be delayed because it is difficult for families and healthcare providers to accept the fact that further curative treatment will be futile.

Open and honest communication among healthcare professionals and families is difficult but essential, especially when confronted with uncertainties. Families are frequently overwhelmed, and nurses may need to take an active role in identifying the family's wishes and desires and ensuring that the patient, family members and healthcare providers communicate effectively.

Parents will likely find it especially difficult to talk with the child about the severity of the child's condition and poor or fatal prognosis. In a recent survey of parents after the death of a child with cancer, none of the parents who discussed death with their children regretted the discussions, while many of those who did not have such conversations wished they had.[31] Parents were most likely to regret their failure to discuss death if they sensed that their child was aware that death was imminent.[31] The nurse is often the best person to help the parents begin such discussions at appropriate times, and the nurse can help the parents to answer the child's questions, reduce the child's fears, and address the child's concerns.

Jason, aged 8 years, was critically ill and awaiting a heart transplant. Several days before Christmas, he was hospitalized in the PCCU with severe heart failure and low cardiac output. As the days passed, Jason became more agitated, and it was clear that something was bothering him. Jason's mother was initially reluctant to ask Jason what was wrong, because she was afraid he would want to talk about dying. She was concerned that her grief and sadness would overwhelm her during the conversation and she would be unable to give Jason the support he needed. After discussions with the nurse, Jason's parents agreed that they needed to talk honestly with Jason so he would know that he and his parents were working together. When Jason's parents asked Jason what was wrong, Jason stated that he knew he might die before Christmas, and he was concerned that Santa would not know what to do with his new toys. Jason's mother asked Jason what he would want Santa to do, and Jason asked if he could leave Santa a list, so Santa could give Jason's toys to cousins and friends based on Jason's wishes. The nurse gave Jason's mother a piece of paper and a pen, and Jason's mother wrote the list as Jason dictated it. Once the list was complete, Jason was peaceful, with no further signs of agitation. He died that night, with his mother and father at his side.

Spiritual Needs

Spiritual needs such as love, faith, hope, and beauty motivate human experiences, emotions, and relationships, and suffering can occur when these needs are not met.[5] Palliative care attempts to address spiritual needs, bringing the child and family together around personal and private attempts to cope with questions about life and meaning that frequently result from feelings of powerlessness and helplessness.

It is important for healthcare providers to listen to families without using religious platitudes. Nurses and other members of the healthcare team can provide psychosocial and spiritual guidance consistent with family values, ideals, and choices.[41] Nurses can provide a safe place where spiritual needs, uncertainty, and hope can be expressed. If hope for cure is no longer realistic, nurses can assist families in realizing other wishes, such as hoping the child does not experience pain or that the child is not alone when death comes.[22] As a need for palliative care becomes apparent, parents may have intense spiritual needs. Nurses can support families through caring presence, words, and actions to foster trust.[35]

The Family's Needs

One of the most important needs of children who are dying or have life-limiting conditions is the need to have ongoing, close contact with their families. Parents should be encouraged to remain with the child as much as possible, given their other responsibilities as parents and providers and their emotional ability to be present. Visiting regulations should be altered (if needed) to ensure that dying children have a private place to see their siblings and say good-bye. The child also may need to see grandparents and other close family members or friends. Because these visits could be the last contact between a critically ill child and family members, they are extremely important and should be facilitated.

Family Challenges and Strengths

Modern healthcare technology has made it increasingly difficult to characterize and predict the course of dying. As a result, parents of children with serious healthcare problems often are uncertain about the child's prognosis. Some parents will experience the relatively sudden and unexpected death of their child from acute illness, trauma, postoperative complications, or suicide. These parents are usually in a state of crisis because they were unable to prepare for the child's death. They are most likely to demonstrate extreme shock and disbelief and extreme guilt. Often they will find it difficult to focus on the child's grave condition while still trying to comprehend the events precipitating the child's hospitalization. Friends and relatives can be supportive at this time but they may also create constant interruptions and distractions. The family requires frequent opportunities to speak with the hospital staff to help them assimilate the explanations provided, determine the best timing for visitors and to be with the child.

Parents of chronically ill children, on the other hand, have experienced the child's long, intense, and often complicated illness. They have likely experienced many crises during the course of the child's illness and may have prepared repeatedly for the child's death. Such a continuous roller-coaster of emotional stress can compromise the family's ability to cope effectively with the child's ultimate deterioration and death. When a child has a chronic illness and has recovered from many near-death experiences, families and healthcare professionals may be reluctant to abandon curative efforts and allow natural death. Such reluctance can result in missed opportunities for resolution and spiritual healing.[27] Other family members and friends can provide valuable support, although occasionally such support people may refuse to believe that the child is really dying.

Communication and Planning

Nurses can assess the effects of the child's illness and admission to the PCCU through a relatively short, directed nursing interview with the parents that focuses on them, their child, their history, experiences with the child's illness, and their concerns and abilities for present and future care for both themselves and their child. Many times, the simple question of "What do you understand about how [child's name] is doing?" will reveal a wealth of information that can be useful to improve communication and address anxieties. The nurse must also assess the cultural and religious differences that will influence the family's ability to cope with death and loss. The nurse should be direct in discussing and planning to meet the family's need to be involved in the child's care. Once the nurse has gathered information about the family's strengths, stresses and wishes, the healthcare team can plan to optimize support for the family. This information should be recorded and shared with other health team members so the family is not asked to answer the same questions repeatedly. Nursing reports, team meetings, family conferences, and rounds should be scheduled on a regular basis to communicate this information. Consistent caregivers, consistent updates, and frequent care conferences that include family members, and involved disciplines and specialties are key elements in supporting a family's adjustment and coping.

Emotional Needs

Parents may respond to a life-limiting condition or predicted death of the child with anticipatory grief. Anticipatory grief is a coping mechanism that is sometimes used when the death of a loved one is perceived as inevitable; the grieving process may begin before the death occurs, in anticipation of that loss. Parents may begin to grieve over their child's condition at the time of diagnosis or at any time the child experiences a serious setback or relapse. Anticipatory grief has been shown to facilitate the grieving process because it provides time to prepare for loss, the opportunity to complete unfinished business and resolve conflicts, and time to say good-bye.[8]

Parental anticipation of a child's death is evident when the parents talk about the seriousness of the child's illness and demonstrate awareness that recovery or stabilization is not likely. The parents often will begin to talk with the staff about the possibility of death, sharing memories of the child's life and talking about what life will be like without the child. If the child's death does not occur for several days, the parents may plan the child's funeral. These discussions indicate that the parents may be accepting the reality of the child's death and preparing emotionally for that death.

Grief responses of parents also can result in expressions of anger and guilt about the child's impending death and the parents' increasing sorrow. The nurse can assist parents with their anticipatory grief by listening to their expressed feelings of loss and encouraging parents to talk about what their child means to them. It may be helpful to encourage the family's participation in the child's care, with inclusion of siblings and extended family members as desired. Nurses can help family members stay connected with their child until death occurs.

In the case of the sudden death of the child, parents will not have time to prepare. For these parents, the healthcare team must rapidly yet compassionately help the parents to understand the gravity of the child's condition to enable the parents to have even a brief time to anticipate the child's death.

Parents use a variety of strategies in response to the stress of a child's illness. Coping involves conscious efforts to regulate emotion, behavior, and the environment through one's response to a stressful event. Coping has been described in work with adolescents as either voluntary engagement coping or voluntary disengagement coping.[14] Voluntary engagement coping includes primary control coping with direct attempts to influence stressors (e.g., problem solving, emotional expression, emotional regulation) and secondary control coping with attempts to adapt to the stressor (e.g., acceptance, cognitive restructuring, positive thinking, distraction). Parents and siblings can use either type of coping in dealing with a stressful situation, but when a situation is out of their control, evidence shows that secondary control coping seems to work best.[15]

Some parents might withdraw or simply avoid visiting the child. This is an example of voluntary disengagement coping, which is described as efforts to distance oneself emotionally, cognitively, and physically from the stressor. There is little evidence that disengagement coping is helpful in the grieving process.

Michael, a 6-month-old infant with congenital heart disease, Down's syndrome, and choanal atresia was mortally ill, but his parents rarely visited, and refused to discuss a "do-not-attempt resuscitation" status. The staff became increasingly frustrated because Michael continued to suffer with no hope of recovery. An interview with the parents revealed their lack of insight regarding his medical condition, their unrealistic expectations for his recovery, and their belief that his life was in God's hands. They stated that if Michael was going to die, he would, but meanwhile treatment must continue. To help the parents understand the gravity of Michael's condition, the staff began to consistently make observations about his deterioration during daily telephone calls to the parents. In addition, a home-health nurse began to visit the parents to help them share their feelings of hope and loss. Eventually, Michael's parents were able to return to the hospital and discuss the removal of mechanical ventilation. They held Michael in their arms as he died.

SPECIAL SITUATIONS AFFECTING TIMING OF DEATH

Withholding or Withdrawing Treatment

Nurses often play an important role in helping parents make decisions about withholding treatments or attempted resuscitation or withdrawing therapy. The nursing staff members continuously observe the extent of the child's suffering and its effects on the child and family, so nurses are often the best people to speak on behalf of the child and family. However, nurses must be able to objectively represent the concerns of the family during discussions with the healthcare team and must encourage parents to express preferences regarding treatment. The nurse must avoid adoption of a crusading approach during these discussions. If the nurse assumes a spokesperson role, that nurse is obligated to speak only for the child and family; the nurse's personal opinions must be clearly distinguished from the expressed preferences of the child and family. Families benefit from and value a healthcare team that provides clear information and that hears and respects the family's decisions.[40]

Usually a decision to withhold or withdraw life support, such as ventilators, extracorporeal membrane oxygenation (ECMO) and other life-extending therapies, is made before the child dies in an intensive care setting. It may be difficult for the healthcare team to broach the subject of treatment limitations or withdrawal or establishment of do-not-attempt resuscitation orders. It is even more difficult for parents to participate in such decisions. Some states have legislation to address "allow natural death" decisions, which may be much easier for parents to affirm.

Emotional, religious, philosophical, legal, and ethical considerations are involved in these complex decisions. If such decisions are avoided, the terminally ill or dying child might be subjected to futile resuscitation attempts or might be forced to endure painful treatment, intubation, or surgical procedures. Often these treatments carry the risk of the most feared aspects of death: pain, loneliness, separation from parents, and loss of control. Nurses can help the child and family plan elements of a child's last hours or days by facilitating decisions about who should be present, the location, and the timing for withdrawal of life support (see Plan for Withdrawal in the section on Principles of Withdrawing Life-Sustaining Treatments in the Chapter 24 Supplement on the Evolve Website).

If staff members and parents are unable to reach a decision about treatment termination or limitation, outside consultants may be needed to help the family and healthcare team consider the treatment options available. Historically, the federal government,[43] medical[13] and nursing[3] disciplines, bioethics groups, and the courts[4,12] have all played a part in addressing controversial issues. In the 1980s, federal legislation recommended formation of infant care review committees; in many hospitals these groups evolved into multidisciplinary ethics committees. Consultation with these committees can provide extremely helpful insight into the options available for the child. However, most decisions regarding treatment termination must still be made in consultation with the parents and the child's primary physician, in accordance with state laws (see Chapter 24 for further information).

Futility legislation authorizes a healthcare team to withdraw suggested treatment if further life support is deemed medically inappropriate by the ethics committee and the hospital gives the family 10 days' notice and attempts to transfer a child to an alternative provider.[50] Because this legislation was passed in Texas, it is not recognized everywhere. In addition, laws can vary by state. A court order may be requested by a child-protective agency before life support is terminated for a severely ill child who is under protective custody (see Chapter 24; also see Foregoing Life-Sustaining Treatment in Children with Inflicted Trauma in the Chapter 24 Supplement on the Evolve Website). Such requests are based on individual agency policy rather than state or federal law. A court order is not required to remove ventilatory support when a child has been pronounced brain dead. These patients have died, and treatment should be discontinued (unless organ donation is pursued).

Occasionally parents continue to deny the child's death after brain death declaration and may require a few hours to accept the diagnosis; under these conditions, the ventilator may continue to provide ventilation for a few hours (or overnight) to allow the family time to come to terms with the child's death. The child is considered legally dead, however, when brain death is pronounced.

Limitation (or prevention) of attempted resuscitation requires a written document signed by a physician. Because verbal orders regarding resuscitation can be subject to confusion or misinterpretation, they should not be accepted. In the absence of a written order to the contrary, resuscitation must be initiated in the event of an in-hospital patient respiratory or cardiac arrest. However, an unsuccessful resuscitation attempt can be discontinued at any time by the physician in charge of the resuscitative efforts. If the family agrees with withdrawal of support—and only after they have made the decision to withdraw support—they should be offered the option of organ donation after cardiac death (DCD).[30]

Organ Donation

Although discussion of organ donation can be difficult, parents might initiate the discussion. Federal law requires that hospitals have protocols for identification of potential organ donors. In the United States and Puerto Rico, organ procurement organizations coordinate organ acquisition in designated service areas (these areas can cover all or part of a state), evaluate potential donors, discuss donation with family members,

arrange for the surgical removal of donated organs, and preserve organs and arrange for their distribution according to national organ sharing policies.[52]

The Joint Commission also requires hospital protocols for determination of brain death and identification of potential organ donors.[28] If solid organ transplantation is desired, the patient must be declared dead before these organs can be used; brain death or cardiopulmonary death criteria can be used. The coroner should be consulted if the circumstances of the child's death necessitate a postmortem coroner's examination. Most coroners will still allow organ donation.

When a child dies suddenly, shock, disbelief, and denial can prevent parents from focusing on decisions regarding organ donation. The staff member who is closest to the parents is usually the best provider to introduce the possibility of organ donation as soon as the healthcare team realizes that the child will die and determines that organ donation is feasible, but a healthcare team conference is generally indicated to determine the best family approach. Because parents need time to absorb the reality of the child's impending death and to address the issue of organ donation, the idea should be introduced early, and the parents must be given sufficient time to make a decision.

Parents will benefit from hearing about the positive aspects of organ donation, and they will require information about the logistics of the surgery involved. Solid organ donation will require several hours of preparation and surgery, and incisions will be made in the child's body. However, most organ donation can be accomplished without delaying typical funeral arrangements. A coordinator from the local organ procurement agency should be contacted whenever a potential organ donor is identified; these coordinators can be extremely valuable resources for the hospital staff and family. They also will communicate with the family (if the family agrees) after organ donation has occurred, to keep the family informed in general terms of the results of organ transplantation.

Regardless of the parents' decision about organ donation, the child's body should always be treated with respect and sensitivity. Any movement or treatments should be performed gently. Parents often have expressed satisfaction in seeing that their child looked clean and well cared for, even after pronouncement of death.

Organ Donation after Brain Death

The concept of brain death is poorly understood by the general public, and most parents have misconceptions about the process and the outcomes of organ donation. Following death, many parents have stated that donation of their child's organs helped them to find meaning in their own child's sudden and untimely death. Surveys have shown that parents from lower socioeconomic and educational backgrounds may be less likely to consent to organ donation as a result of religious beliefs and personal attitudes.[1]

Organ donation should not interfere with the parents' need to see and hold their child for a final time. Despite the fact that the child will be intubated and mechanically ventilated, it is beneficial to offer the parents the opportunity to hold the child, because this will be the last time they will be able to feel the child's warmth in their arms. It is a vital step in grief resolution.

Alex, a 2-year-old child, was killed suddenly when he darted across the street into the path of an oncoming car. His parents, trying to find meaning in their sudden tragedy, agreed to donation of Alex's kidneys and liver to enable another child to live. Alex's mother asked to hold her son before he went to the operating room. The PCCU nurse in this small community hospital was upset by the death and insecure in caring for the child. She refused to move the child from the bed, for fear of displacing the endotracheal tube. The parents said good-bye to Alex standing at the side of his bed. Weeks later, the mother remained inconsolable about that last memory, and felt that she was robbed of the opportunity to embrace her son one last time.

Once the child is pronounced brain dead, it is imperative that the entire healthcare team understand that the child has, in fact, died, so that the parents are not confused by the team's use of inconsistent terminology. The staff should not refer to a ventilator as *life support*, because it cannot support the child's life. The ventilator is continuing to oxygenate the blood, so that the heart will continue beating and organs will continue to receive oxygen until donation occurs. However, the ventilator cannot support life, because the child died when the brain ceased to function.

Organ Donation After Cardiac Death (DCD)

Organ DCD, previously called *nonheartbeating organ donation*, allows families to donate organs after cardiac arrest. Although this method of organ donation was first described in the 1960s, the process has become more refined and more common in recent years. It is important to note that the patient considered for DCD is not dead and does not become a donor until cardiac arrest occurs.

Uncontrolled DCD is a less common form of DCD that can occur if family members consent to immediate organ donation after the patient dies following a sudden cardiopulmonary arrest and an unsuccessful resuscitation attempt.[46] After death pronouncement, the donor is moved to the operating suite or ECMO is rapidly instituted to allow organ recovery under more controlled conditions.

Controlled DCD is the most common form of DCD currently used. In this form of DCD, withdrawal of support is planned in advance. Controlled DCD occurs when a patient has catastrophic, unrecoverable brain injury or insult that does not meet criteria for pronouncement of brain death, but does result in a family and medical decision to withdraw support. The patient then becomes eligible for organ donation and, if the family consents, support is withdrawn in a sequence that will allow rapid organ recovery within minutes of cardiac arrest and pronouncement of death. During withdrawal of support, at the discretion of the child's primary physician and according to end-of-life hospital protocols, opioids and sedatives are typically administered to minimize patient discomfort.[46] In some cases, heparin is also administered to minimize formation of thrombi in the donated organs.[29,46] When support is withdrawn and cardiac arrest occurs, the child's primary medical team makes the pronouncement of death. A waiting period of 2 to 5 minutes is required either between cardiac arrest and pronouncement of death or immediately after

pronouncement of death. Organ recovery cannot begin until after both the pronouncement of death and the waiting period have been completed.[46]

ECMO support can be used as part of the DCD protocol to allow controlled, unhurried organ recovery and improve the perfusion of donor organs before procurement.[34] Premortem ECMO cannulation can occur in the PCCU to facilitate institution of ECMO immediately after the pronouncement of death and the waiting period of 2 to 5 minutes have elapsed.

DCD requires careful planning and coordination.[29] All members of the healthcare team should be aware of the protocol and the precise sequence of actions, and the team should rehearse the complete sequence before it is actually implemented. When discussing the parents' final visit with their child, the nurse should discuss the timing and sequence of all important steps, the equipment likely to be present, whether surgical drapes will be placed before death, and when the child is likely to move from the PCCU. If it is necessary to rapidly move the child to the operating suite after cardiac arrest, the parents should be aware that such movement will occur. The parents should be assured that the child's primary healthcare team will care for the child until the child dies and the primary physician makes the pronouncement of death.[46] The physicians should explain the comfort measures that they will provide for the child during withdrawal of care and before death. Parents should also be aware that they have the option of stopping the donation process if it becomes too uncomfortable or upsetting for them.[30]

Although members of the organ procurement agency will explain the process to the family before it begins, no member of the organ procurement team has responsibility for or involvement in the care of the child (i.e., before pronouncement of death); they will assume responsibility for the donor after pronouncement of death. Minor exceptions to this policy can include pretrieval blood sampling or administration of medications to enhance organ viability.[46]

Parents should be prepared for the possibility that attempts for DCD can fail because the interval between withdrawal of support and cardiac arrest is unpredictable. If the interval is too long, the organs may become ischemic and unsuitable for donation. In general, if cardiac arrest does not develop within 60 to 90 minutes[29,34] after withdrawal of support, the patient is no longer considered a candidate for DCD. In such instances, care will continue to be provided by the child's primary care team.[29] Tissue donation may still be possible after the child dies.

INTERDISCIPLINARY COLLABORATIVE CARE

Interdisciplinary collaboration is essential to provide the highest quality of care for children and their families. Social workers can provide support and access resources for the family. Child life specialists are particularly adept at helping children express themselves, even when children are nonverbal. Occupational therapists, physical therapists, recreational therapists, pharmacists, chaplains, ethicists, and volunteers all can add to the richness of care and compassion available to critically ill children and their families. If there is a need to transition to outside resources such as hospice, it is important to discuss the transition as early as feasible to allow parents time to adjust to changes in the goals of care. Hospice services can be introduced as resources in the community, available to address physical and emotional pain if and when a child is able to go home.

Professionals in each discipline need to be aware of verbal and nonverbal communication styles. Healthcare providers should be aware of their own spiritual and cultural beliefs and should be careful to avoid imposing them on the child or family. Providers should also identify potential barriers to communication, learn and practice effective communication skills, and remain attentive to intrateam communication styles, skills, and needs. Providers must also develop conflict resolution skills. They should avoid professional insensitivity (e.g., interrupting, patronizing) and avoid physical or emotional distancing. They should cultivate empathy, compassion, humility, and altruism.

Nurses must address their grief needs to avoid the effects of cumulative grief. They should create opportunities to debrief after an intense experience, sharing feelings and brainstorming about what went well and what should be improved. In some hospitals, palliative care teams or crisis intervention teams may be called to support the staff.

SUPPORT OF THE FAMILY AT OR NEAR THE TIME OF DEATH

Talking about Death

Despite great strides in the treatment of life-threatening conditions, many of the characteristics of childhood conditions create significant challenges to parents and healthcare professionals who are communicating with a sick child about the child's illness.[54] Features that make communication challenging include the complex nature of the disease, the aversive nature of some treatments, the probability of adverse side effects, and the possibility that treatment will be unsuccessful or that the child could die from the condition. From the time of initial diagnosis and throughout the course of treatment, parents often need to talk with their children about their feelings. Parents bear the primary responsibility of filtering information and making decisions for their children. They must assimilate enormous amounts of information during an intensely emotional time, and then facilitate their child's understanding of this information. When treatment is not successful and a child is in the terminal phase, these difficulties can be magnified.

The National Cancer Institute recommends that parents and healthcare professionals communicate openly with children about cancer, even when children are being treated palliatively.[37] Because the death of a child is an intensely painful experience, few studies have examined communication strategies in families dealing with end-of-life circumstances. Thus, parents receive relatively little evidence-based guidance about the optimal ways to communicate with their child about cancer or the possibility of death.

There is general agreement that terminally ill adolescents are anxious about and aware of their severity of illness and prognosis. Studies of ill school-aged children have demonstrated that terminally ill children 6 to 12 years of age demonstrate more hospital-related anxiety, a greater awareness about hospitalization, more preoccupation with intrusive procedures,

and more concerns about death and mutilation than do similar chronically ill children who are not terminally ill.[42] Thus, even if the child has not been informed of the fatal prognosis, the child may be aware of and anxious about impending death.

The nurse should consider the child's psychosocial developmental level and the ability of the child to understand when discussing concepts such as terminal illness and death. Examples of questions frequently asked by children and some suggested responses are included in Table 3-1.

The child may express anger at parents or hospital staff; this anger may reflect the child's inability to discuss impending death or the child's perception that such discussion is not acceptable. Anger and frustration are also understandable responses to painful and invasive therapy. It is important that the nurse explain the child's reaction to the family, so the family's feelings of guilt are not compounded. The family (when they are able) and the healthcare team must communicate receptiveness to the child's questions about death. The family also should have the opportunity to remain with the child to communicate their love and support, so the child does not feel abandoned. In addition, the nursing staff must avoid reacting defensively to the child's fears and frustrations. It is important to reassure the child that he or she will not be alone.

Hope can seem to be elusive when a child is confronted with impending death. There are, however, many flavors and colors of hope. When asked what they hope for, most parents will respond, "We hope for a miracle." The nurse might respond, "I certainly do too, but if that's not possible, what else do you hope for?" At that juncture, parents may respond that they hope their child is not in pain or that they are with their child when the child dies. Those are hopes that nurses can realistically help meet.

Table 3-1	Potential Responses to a Dying Child's Questions About Death
Question or comment	**Response**
Am I dying?	"You are very sick and I am worried about you. It is possible that you might die, but we are doing everything we can to help you. Are you afraid of dying?" Following the child's answer, the nurse can explore the child's specific fears.
I'm afraid to die	"Can you tell me what scares you the most?" The nurse can explore the child's perceptions of death and reinforce the positive concepts and reduce the negative concepts. At all times, it is important to tell the child that he or she will not die alone; someone will always be with the child.
I don't want to die	"I can understand that—I don't want to die either. What is the worst thing about dying to you?" or, "What does dying mean to you?" The nurse then can explore the child's concerns.

Angela, a 6 year old with severe cardiomyopathy, had been intubated in the PCCU for a month. As her condition worsened, she became less communicative and appeared uninterested in her surroundings. The nurse mentioned this to Angela's mother, and together they agreed that Angela might be concerned about dying. The nurse and the mother asked Angela if she ever thought about dying. When Angela nodded, the mother, with the nurse's support, asked Angela about things that might make her sad. "Are you afraid to die? Are you wondering what it will be like? Are you worried about what will happen to me?" Angela pointed to her mother and indicated that her main concern revolved around how her mother would handle her death. The mother told Angela that she would be very sad and would miss her. She then emphasized that she would have many happy memories and would be all right. The nurse promised to continue to help Angela's mother after Angela's death. Angela died peacefully the next day.

While parents are key participants in the discussion of death with a dying child, they often will require assistance from healthcare professionals. Children may express their awareness of the seriousness of their illness, their concerns about dying, or their premonitions of their own death.[54] This can pave the way for open discussion with the parents.[7]

Maria had been terminally ill with cancer for several months when she shared a special dream with her father. In the dream, angels came and asked her to play with them. After describing the dream, Maria asked her father if it was all right to join the angels. The father was upset about the dream, and told Maria not to talk about such things. Two days later, Maria suffered a respiratory arrest and was intubated and transferred to the PCCU. It was then that the father discussed Maria's dream with a nurse. The nurse helped the father explore the potential meaning of the dream and his own feelings of dread about Maria's impending death. The father then was able to talk to Maria again about the dream, and told her that it was OK to play with the angels whenever she was ready. Maria died the next day.

Not all families can sustain or endure open communication about death, because family members are dealing with their own anxiety, grief, fear, and coping strategies. Nurses should assess the family's level of grief and philosophical and emotional response to the impending death. The nurse can gather information about the family's views of death by asking about religious backgrounds, values, beliefs and previous experiences with death and loss. The nurse also must determine the specific information provided to the dying child and to other family members. This will enable the nurse to assess the family's beliefs about and ability to cope with the child's death and to support the child.

When family members have difficulty expressing their fears and concerns about death, a physician, primary nurse, clinical nurse specialist or nurse practitioner who has an ongoing relationship with the child and family may be able to help the child and family discuss the child's potential death. The nurse can keep the family and the healthcare team informed about information provided to or by the child, so that the child's fears can be addressed in a consistent fashion. The nurse should observe the child's responses closely, help the child communicate concerns, and be prepared to answer the child's questions honestly while maintaining an element of hope. Nurses may wish to tell children and their families that the healthcare team is hoping for the best, but preparing for anything that could happen. Children who are dying may express anxiety about pain, loneliness, separation from parents, and loss of control, so these issues should be addressed. It is important to help the child understand the reaction of family members; too often, the child interprets the family's anxiety and depression as rejection or loss of love.

Support During Attempted Resuscitation

When a child suffers an unexpected cardiopulmonary arrest and resuscitation is attempted, healthcare providers must be clear and compassionate when communicating with the family. Most family members prefer to be present during the attempted resuscitation of a family member. Family members who were present during an attempted resuscitation reported that it was helpful to the (surviving) child and to the family members.[21] In addition, standardized psychological tests suggest that family members who are present during an unsuccessful resuscitation attempt demonstrate more constructive grieving behavior than those who are not given the option to be present.[47] In a recent prospective, alternate day study, family presence did not affect the efficiency of 283 pediatric trauma resuscitations; there was no difference in time to milestones such as computed tomography scan or time to complete the resuscitation when family members were present, compared with time required in 422 resuscitations without family presence.[21] Since 2000, the *American Heart Associations Guidelines for Cardiopulmonary Resuscitation and Emergency Cardiovascular Care* have recommended that family members be offered the option of remaining with their loved one during attempted resuscitation whenever possible.[2,6] If family members remain at the bedside, the resuscitation team must be sensitive to their presence, and one staff member (e.g., nurse, chaplain, social worker) should remain with the family to answer their questions, explain what is happening, and assess and address the needs of the family members.[25]

If parents are not able or choose not to be present during the attempted resuscitation, they should not have to wait for long periods with little or no information. Such waits will increase their anxiety and frustration. At least one staff member should act as a liaison to communicate with and support the parents while the resuscitation is in progress. This liaison should keep the resuscitation team aware of the parents' questions and the information provided to the parents, including specific terms used.

Parents should be asked whether there is anyone they would like to contact, such as clergy, members of their church, special friends or family. The family should have access to a telephone so they can make local or long-distance calls to contact family and friends. Note that cell phones might not function well inside hospitals, so staff members should be sure to offer a working telephone, as needed.

Throughout the resuscitation attempt, the parents should be informed about the child's condition and the treatment measures provided. Although it is important to provide some hope until the child's condition is determined to be hopeless, the possibility of the child's death should be discussed. This discussion will allow the parents to begin to prepare themselves. One of the major challenges in communicating with parents of critically ill children is the need to balance hope with reality. Statements about the child's condition must be direct and sensitive and should involve the use of carefully chosen terms, rather than use of medical jargon or clichés. Phrases such as "He is seriously ill and may die" are more appropriate than "His condition is deteriorating," "He just fell apart," or "We couldn't get him back." Word choices are extremely important when talking with families and even carefully selected words can be misinterpreted, especially when a family is stressed (Table 3-2). The American Heart Association *Pediatric Advanced Life Support Course* has an excellent supplementary module to help teach healthcare providers to discuss a child's death with parents.[24]

If the child suffers a cardiac arrest, the parents should be told that the heart is not beating and that it may be difficult to help the heart start beating again. Such information is clear and concise. Parents should not be expected to understand the difference between cardiac arrest and respiratory arrest or the meaning of medical terms such as ventricular fibrillation or asystole.

Communication should be provided at regular intervals, and the family should always know when they will speak to the physician or nurse again. Usually, quarter-hour intervals are appropriate for periodic reports. Of course, any changes in the patient's condition also should be communicated immediately to the parents. During these reports, the parents should be given progressively more pessimistic information as the child's prognosis becomes more grave. For example, the parents may initially be told that the child "stopped breathing," but that the nurse was "providing breaths using a mask and bag and oxygen." On a second visit, the parents may be told that "despite the help of the nurses and doctors, the heart slowed and stopped beating," and that this is "usually a sign

that the heart is suffering from lack of oxygen." Each time the parents should be assured that the doctors and nurses are helping to give oxygen and circulate the blood with CPR (this term is likely familiar to most parents, and more familiar than *resuscitation*).

If interventions such as extracorporeal circulation are considered or will be provided, the staff should describe the therapy in simple terms, focusing on what the family will see and emphasizing that the child is unconscious and is not afraid or in pain. This is not the time for comprehensive discussion of the technology or risks and benefits, but family members will require a brief overview of the rationale for and goals of the therapy. As soon as the child is more stable, the child's physician should discuss any procedures or treatments, including risks and benefits, in more detail.

If a child does not respond to continued resuscitative efforts, parents can be told that "the longer the heart is unresponsive, the more worried the doctors are that the heart will not start beating on its own." At this time the parents often voice concerns about the futility of the resuscitation, or the worry that the child has suffered damage to all organs. By the time resuscitative efforts are discontinued, the parents may be better prepared to hear that the child has died.

Expected Death

If, after consultation among family and healthcare providers, a decision is made to allow a child's natural death without attempted resuscitation or other intervention, the healthcare team should continue to keep the family informed of changes and provide aggressive management of symptoms, including pain. The healthcare team should describe how the child's breathing and appearance may change just prior to death. The amount of sedation and analgesia the child receives also should be discussed with the parents. All parents will want the child's death to be pain-free; some parents will wish that the child remain as alert as possible, while other parents will

Table 3-2 Language Matters

Health Provider Statement	What the Family May Hear
He's stable. (Child is supported by vasopressors, ventilator, dialysis.)	He is getting better.
She gained weight. (Child's heart failure is worsening.)	She is growing well like a healthy child.
Do you want us to do CPR?	She may survive if we do CPR
Do you want us to intubate him?	He has a chance if we place a breathing tube and provide mechanical ventilatory support.

Ambiguous Terms	Clear Description
Do you want us to do everything?	Although we've tried many treatments for several days, unfortunately, Jason is too sick and they are not helping him to get better.
It's time we talk about pulling back.	We want to provide the care that Allison needs now. Her comfort is now our highest priority.
I think we should stop aggressive therapy	We will change our goals of care to respect her wishes.
There is nothing more we can do	Let's stop treatments that are not helping him.

Helpful Language	
I wish things were different.	
I hope he gets better, too, but I think it is very unlikely.	
How do you and your family usually deal with difficult conversations?	
We hope for the best, but we need to prepare for whatever may happen.	

request that the child be sedated. The child's wishes should also be determined, if possible.

The child and family should be moved to a private area of the unit. However, this privacy should not isolate the child from the nursing staff. If a private room is available, any limits to visitation time and number of visitors can be relaxed, allowing several family members to visit at the same time. Nurses should encourage parents to continue to eat and to rest in order to maintain physical strength, but should not force parents to leave the bedside if the parents are reluctant to do so. The healthcare team can order food trays for the parents, if they desire to stay with their child. If the parents leave the bedside, they should be reassured that they will be summoned back if there is any change in the child's condition. Healthcare providers should record the family's cell phone and pager numbers (the devices may be supplied by the hospital), and the family should know how to call the child's nurse and physician directly.

The family might ask that a clergy member be summoned, or the nurse can suggest that a hospital chaplain be called. In addition, the nurse should provide adequate analgesia to the child and ensure that the parents are aware that the child is comfortable. A nurse should remain with the child and family (or be present in the immediate vicinity to meet the family's needs), and cardiac monitoring alarms should be silenced if at all possible. When any child dies, a physician should be present to confirm that the child has died, to offer support to the family, and to answer any questions that the parents may have.

Informing Parents of a Child's Death

If parents are not present when the child dies, it is ideal that news of the child's death be conveyed by a physician and nurse whom the parents know and trust. Ideally, the parents should be told in a private room, where they can react without worrying about the presence of strangers. Buckman's six-stage protocol for communicating difficult news describes communication, decision making, and building relations.[9] This approach includes three steps to prepare for the discussion of important information (i.e., prepare for the discussion, establish what the patient and family know, and determine how information is to be handled), one step to deliver the information, and three steps to respond to the family's reaction and planning (i.e., respond to emotions, establish goals and priorities, and establish a plan).[53]

If the parents must be told of the child's death over the telephone, they should be prepared to hear bad news before they are told that the child died. If possible, the physician or nurse should ensure that the parents are not alone at home, and that supportive friends or family are with the parents. If the child dies peacefully and in no apparent pain, it is important to share this information with the parents, which usually provides some comfort to the family.

Support of the Parents at the Time of Child's Death

Sensitive and compassionate nursing care is needed to help the parents cope at the time of the child's death.[35] Parents benefit from an opportunity to express their pain and sorrow in a private place and with the supportive presence of healthcare professionals. The responses of the parents will be determined by the family's unique method of coping with the child's death. Nursing staff should avoid labeling or attempting to suppress grief behavior, because this is unproductive and can hinder parental progress in the grief process.

Most healthcare professionals feel insecure about what to say to parents who are deeply distressed and grieving. Listening is often the most important form of support that the staff can provide. This can be difficult, especially when the parents express their painful feelings of loss. Each nurse must be in touch with his or her own feelings about the death of the child, because these feelings can interfere with therapeutic communication.

Staff members should avoid platitudes and should not tell parents "I know how you feel." Even if a staff member has experienced the death of a child, it is impossible to know how each parent feels, so such remarks seem to minimize the parents' pain and rejects its uniqueness. Religious pronouncements, such as "It was God's will," are usually inappropriate, because it is presumptuous to interpret the meaning of life or death for the family. One mother's response to just this remark was quick: "That's ridiculous—I can't believe that God started this morning by deciding He wanted to take my baby!" Another phrase that many parents find unsettling is "At least..."—for example, "At least you had 3 years with her," "At least she didn't suffer," or "At least you have three other healthy children." Such remarks are generally not comforting.

Members of the healthcare team may cry with the parents when the child dies. Such emotions can be appropriate and will help the parents realize that their child's death has touched many people. However, such emotional displays by a healthcare provider are inappropriate if the provider is unable to continue to function as a support to the parents, or if the parents end up comforting the provider. If the parents begin comforting the nurse, the nurse has abdicated the supportive role that the parents need. If a nurse feels overwhelmed by grief, that nurse should be excused to grieve privately, and another nurse should be available to support the parents.

Family members might express anger, rage, and other violent emotions when a child dies. It is difficult but important for the nurse and additional support staff to remain with the family members who are expressing strong emotions or who have lost control. Too often when the parents express strong emotion, they are suppressed verbally or quickly offered medication. Sedation should not be used without careful consideration of the purpose of the medication. Too often sedatives are prescribed to meet the needs of the hospital staff or uncomfortable family members and friends, rather than to meet the needs of the parents. As a bereaved parent, Schiff wrote an honest portrayal of what the death of her son felt like. "On that bright sunny March morning we were told that Robby had died. I screamed. A nurse, tears suddenly coming to her eyes, offered me a tranquilizer and I thought, how inane. Robby was dead and I was being given a pill to make it go away. Impossible."[48]

A number of bereaved parents, especially mothers, have described a lethargy or "fog" that enveloped them for days following sedation after the child's death. Sedation may only postpone the painful reactions to a time when the parent is alone and unsupported.[26] In addition, it can separate the parent from decisions about the child's funeral or burial, and the parent might later regret lack of participation in these plans or decisions.

At the time of the child's death, most parents experience a period of acute distress. They may feel numb and have a sense of disbelief and denial. If the child dies suddenly, however, the response of the parents can be intensified and last for a longer period of time than if the parents were able to prepare for the child's death. The nursing staff members who work with families during this time will play a crucial role in helping the family to cope with the immediate effects of the child's death. Parents often remember in minute detail how they were told of the child's death, who was present, and how the parents were treated by the nursing staff. Both positive and negative responses are recalled for months and years afterward.

Some parents will demonstrate a temporary lack of affect, including a sense of apparent calmness; parents may demonstrate evidence of relief, or even a period of euphoria. These parents might understand the child's death at a cognitive level, but deny their deep and painful feelings. Such behavior can lead the healthcare team to the mistaken conclusion that the parents did not really care about the child, or that they are coping well.

Emotions such as anger, rage, frustration, and guilt can overwhelm the parents. Behavioral responses are varied and might include intense crying, wailing, hysteria, physical acting-out, or stoicism. These behavioral and emotional responses of parents are determined by the personality and cultural background of each parent, the relationship between the child and the parents, and the circumstances of the death.

In time, parents may share their feelings of helplessness and begin to explore the unanswerable question "Why?" It is important to avoid suppressing these questions or negating or dismissing them. The nurse should listen to the parents concerns and indicate that feelings of guilt are normal. In addition, the nurse should reinforce the positive aspects of the parents' role.[36] The nurse can make observations about the child, such as "Everyone has mentioned that Jimmy was always smiling and happy—he certainly must have known he was loved." When a parent is responsible in any way for the death of the child (e.g., death due to inflicted trauma), the staff members must be careful to avoid expressions of anger.

Parents need support and guidance related to the many decisions required after the child's death (e.g., autopsy consent, informing friends and relatives, funeral and burial decisions). For many young couples, the death of their child is their first experience with the death of a loved one. Parents may need help informing siblings (see Support for Siblings).

The Final Visit

Parents and other family members should have an opportunity to see the child after death. This final visit with the child may enable the parents to say good-bye, to realize that the child has died, and to begin the grief process. Many parents who are unable or unwilling to see their child for a final visit have expressed regret at missing this visit; they may later find it difficult to believe that the child is actually dead.

A child died of head injuries when the go-cart he was riding was hit by a truck. Although his mother was present at the scene of the crash, the child's body was covered, and the mother saw only the child's shoes and the go-cart. For many weeks, the mother thought over and over that perhaps another child was killed, and her child was really unhurt. As a result she searched for him on the school bus and looked for him in crowds. The child's father viewed the child's body in the funeral home and reported fewer problems in believing that his son had died.

Parents should be asked separately about their desire to see the child after death, so that each parent can make an individual decision. It is not necessary for the parents to agree in their decision; the visit may be important for one parent, but repugnant to the other. Spouses should be helped to accept each other's decision.

The healthcare team often wonders whether parents should be encouraged to view the body of a child who has died following massive injuries. There is no universal answer to this question, and the parents' wishes should be considered in making the decision. If the parents do not see the child, however, their fantasies about the child's mutilation can exceed reality. In addition, denial of the death and difficulty in accepting it can be prolonged when the parents do not see the child's body and have that final contact.

Before the final visit, the room and the child's body should be cleaned and prepared, to reduce the emotional impact of any injuries or treatments on the child's appearance. This final bath also provides the nursing staff with an opportunity to say good-bye to the child and to begin to accept the child's death. The nurse should be sensitive to the cultural mores of the family. Occasionally, a family member wishes to participate in this final preparation of the child's body. All blood, betadine, or adhesive is removed, and lotion is often applied to the child's skin. Clean sheets and covers should be placed on the bed, and the child should be dressed in clean pajamas or a gown. The child's hair should be washed or brushed neatly. Incisions and wounds can be covered with clean, dry dressings.

If a postmortem examination will be performed, it may be necessary for invasive catheters and tubes to remain in place; if the tubes must remain, fresh tape should be used to cover any blood-stained or discolored tape. If a postmortem examination will not be performed and organ donation is not possible, equipment is typically removed. It can be comforting for the parents to see the child at peace, without intravenous lines or other invasive equipment. If the child died suddenly, the parents might need reassurance that everything possible was done to save the child. In this case, some equipment may remain in the room with the child.

If the child sustained severe, visible injuries, the child's appearance should be described to the parents before their visit. Unless the child's head and face are seriously injured, most injuries will be effectively covered by dressings and sheets. The nurse must determine whether the parents need privacy or support while seeing their child after death. If possible, the parents should be asked whether they would like to hold their child, because few parents are able to express this request.

The length of the final visit varies widely; some parents may wish to stay for an hour or more. Parents cope with loss in different ways, and some parents use this time to sort out many of their feelings and struggles.

One emergency department nurse reported helping a mother hold her infant daughter who had died of sudden infant death syndrome. The mother rocked the baby and sang to her for over 20 min. When the mother put her infant down, she was ready to phone her husband and help him with his grief.

Some parents may want to leave the hospital as soon as possible after the final paperwork is completed. If, however, the child has been hospitalized for a long time, the parents might be reluctant to leave the hospital because they feel that the hospital staff will best understand their grief. In addition, the hospital staff members share common recent memories of the child. Departure from the hospital for these parents may represent the final separation from their child.

Parents have reported that it is extremely traumatic to receive their child's possessions, because this action symbolizes the full reality of the child's death. Too often a plastic garbage sack is the most readily available container for the belongings, but use of such a sack is insensitive and possibly offensive to the parents. Special containers should be available for this purpose. If the child is an infant, the nurse should ask if the mother was nursing the infant. If so, the mother will require information about delactation (members of the local LaLeche League can be helpful).

Some children's hospitals now give parents a handmade book that can include items such as a lock of hair, notes from nurses, hand and foot prints, and drawings of the child. This can be assembled before a child dies (when death is anticipated), so healthcare providers have opportunities to reflect and comment on their memories of the child, or it may be initiated at the time of death.

Support for Siblings

Parents sometimes unintentionally neglect the important needs of siblings during support of the dying child. When providing information to parents about support of the siblings, the nurse must consider the siblings' age and maturity level and the circumstances of the child's death.[53] If possible, parents should prepare siblings throughout the child's critical illness or in the days preceding the death of the child.

Siblings of preschool age or older may be given the opportunity to come to the hospital when a child is critically ill, and to say good-bye and to be with the parents during the final visit after the child's death. Toddlers also can be brought to visit with the dying child, particularly if the dying child wishes to see the toddler. Decisions regarding the presence of the sibling must be individualized, and consideration must be given to sleep and meal times for very young siblings (e.g., infants and toddlers). Even young siblings can provide comfort to the patient and the parents during this time.

Most siblings have indicated that it was helpful to have an open discussion with their parents about a child's death. Frequently, siblings can feel responsible for the death of their brother or sister or can feel guilty for surviving. Parents should be aware of these potential responses of the siblings and should signal their willingness to discuss the child's death frequently with the siblings. Siblings report that if the parents become emotional or avoid discussion of the child's death, the siblings are made to feel that the subject should not be discussed. As a result, the sibling is forced to deal with grief and fear alone.

As a rule, if the sibling is old enough to know and love the child who has died, the sibling probably should be allowed to attend and even contribute in some way to the funeral. Siblings may want to select a flower arrangement or choose music for the service, or release a balloon following the service. When siblings are prevented from attending the funeral, they often have difficulty coping with the child's death. They also may resent being separated from the rest of the family during this important time.

Books can be helpful in facilitating discussions with siblings about death.[17,18] Siblings can benefit from involvement in group therapy with other children who have experienced the death of a family member. The local chapter of Compassionate Friends or a hospital nurse or physician specialist, chaplain, or social worker may be aware of such groups.

GRIEF AFTER DEATH

The grief response observed in the hospital is only the beginning of a long phase of sorrow and pain. As the shock and numbness dissipate, parents and other family members experience a number of distressing emotions that continue for months and even years.[26,45] In fact, family members are changed forever by the experience of a child's death. Hospice and palliative care programs may speak of and try to contribute to a "good death," but parents facing the death of their child have no perception of a "good" death and are not ever truly prepared for the child's death.[20]

Parents report a sense of emptiness, yearning, loneliness, and the intense desire to hold, caress, touch, and talk with the child who has died. There may be preoccupation with thoughts about the child, a sense of the child's presence in a room, fleeting visions of the child in a crowd, or experiences of hearing the child cry or talk. Parents suddenly may find themselves setting the table for the child, or preparing for some other parenting task that involves the child. It might be painful for the parents even to walk past the child's room. It can be helpful to discuss these potential experiences with the parents, because if the parents are not prepared for them, the experiences can be particularly stressful.

One mother reported that, following the child's death, she would have several good days and would begin to think that she was coping well with the child's death. Then, without warning, she would find a toy of her child's or a small sock under the cushion of the sofa. These chance encounters would be so painful that the mother was unable to function for hours afterward.

Parents should know that it can be therapeutic to reminisce about the child and recall happy memories. Too often in an attempt to prevent grief, these memories are suppressed, so that the parents deprive themselves of a potential source of comfort. Research has shown that continuing bonds may be a coping strategy that can increase the quality of life for bereaved families and decrease negative consequences such as marital disruptions, mental illnesses, and behavior problems.[19,49]

Parents often are devastated after the child dies because they were unable to protect their child from death. This feeling is based on the protective parental role in society and often produces feelings of intense helplessness and guilt. Guilt is one of the most painful and persistent emotions experienced by bereaved parents. Following a child's death, parents evaluate their parenting experiences. This process often involves identification of discrepancies between their ideal standards of parenting and their perceived performance. This evaluation also can reinforce feelings of guilt.[36]

Helplessness can cause anger about the child's death. Healthcare professionals who failed to save the child's life can become the target for this anger. If the child died following an injury, the drunken driver or the municipality that failed to deal with an unsafe intersection also may be targets for anger. Anger also may be directed toward family members and friends who fail to understand and those who do not support the parents adequately. Anger toward God and confusion over religious beliefs can be another difficult component of grief.

Fear about the potential death of other family members can be especially powerful when the child dies suddenly after an unintentional injury. The remaining children in the family may be overprotected for a time, and family routines may be altered and activities curtailed.

Grieving parents often find themselves increasingly disorganized in activities of daily living and in work activities. They have difficulty concentrating, and thought processes become confused. Typically the parent is unable to make decisions and depression is common, so job performance often deteriorates. This disorganization is typically apparent months after the child's death. At this time the parents may think they are failing to deal effectively with the child's death, and counseling can be helpful.

Bereaved parents are helped gradually by the passage of time and the concern of others who listen to their expressions of pain. In time, sometimes years, the pain becomes less intense, although it can be reawakened by unexpected memories. Anniversaries of the child's birth and death and other milestones (e.g., date of the child's injury or the graduation of the child's class) are painful for many years.

Grief following the death of a child is intense, with long-lasting effects on parents and other family members. Someone from the healthcare team should be available to the parents and responsible for contacting the parents after the child's death. This contact person can make telephone calls, send letters and reference material about parental grief and sibling support, and provide information about bereavement support groups. Some families may wish to return to the hospital for visits or counseling sessions and perhaps to discuss postmortem findings with the child's physician; others will find it extremely difficult to return to the place where their child died. Some hospitals have an annual "Time for Remembering" service, inviting families of children who have died to return to meet with healthcare providers and other families to support one another and reflect on positive memories.

Nursing staff will often grieve after the death of the child. For further information, please refer to Chapter 24, and Burnout and Compassion Fatigue Among Caregivers in the Chapter 24 Supplement on the Evolve Website.

ADVANCED PRACTICE CONCEPTS

- Apply palliative care concepts from the time of diagnosis.
- For many years after the child's death, parents will remember the healthcare providers who were with them when their child died and what the healthcare providers said.
- Be sensitive to spiritual and cultural perspectives.
- Care for yourself as well as those around you.
- Listen.

CONCLUSIONS

Professionals who work in critical care settings have a vital contribution to make in supporting children with life-limiting conditions and their families. The care of critically ill and dying children is challenging and emotionally draining, and the family requires a great deal of support. Societal attitudes about childhood death reinforce the feeling of failure when a child's life cannot be saved. This can have a tremendous impact on the professional staff. Such experiences raise many philosophical, spiritual, and professional questions about suffering, death, and the meaning of life. Debriefings with staff after the death of a child can be beneficial in several ways. Such debriefings can provide nurses with administrative and peer support, allow time for remembering a child and family, and help nurses learn useful strategies for improving end-of-life care. Staff members who are able to handle their own feelings are better able to help parents adequately during this tragic experience.

References

1. Alden DL, Cheung AHS: Organ donation and culture: a comparison of Asian American and European American beliefs, attitudes, and behaviors. *J Appl Soc Psychol* 30(2):293–314, 2000.
2. American Heart Association: American Heart Association Guidelines for CPR and ECC, Part 12. Pediatric Advanced Life Support—family presence during resuscitation. *Circulation* 112(Suppl. IV):181, 2005.
3. American Nurses Association: American Nurses Association position statement on foregoing artificial nutrition and hydration. *Ky Nurse* 41(2):16, 1993.
4. Annas GJ: Asking the courts to set the standard of emergency care—the case of Baby K. *N Engl J Med* 330(21):1542–1545, 1994.
5. Bartel M: What is spiritual? What is spiritual suffering? *J Pastoral Care Counsel* 58(3):187–201, 2004.
6. Berg MD, Schexnayder SM, Chameides L, Terry M, et al: Part 13: pediatric basic life support. *Circulation* 122:S862–S875, 2010.
7. Bluebond-Langner M: *The private worlds of dying children*, Princeton, NJ, 1978, Princeton University Press.
8. Bonanno GA, Kaltman S: The varieties of grief experience. *Clin Psychol Rev* 21(5):705–734, 2001.
9. Buckman R, Kason Y: *How to break bad news: a guide for health care professionals*, Baltimore, 1992, Johns Hopkins University Press.
10. Carnevale FA, et al: Daily living with distress and enrichment: the moral experience of families with ventilator-assisted children at home. *Pediatrics* 117(1):e48–e60, 2006.
11. Carter BS, et al: Circumstances surrounding the deaths of hospitalized children: opportunities for pediatric palliative care. *Pediatrics* September 1, 114(3):e361–e366, 2004.

12. Clayton EW: What is really at stake in Baby K: a response to Ellen Flannery [Commentary]. *J Law Med Ethics* 23(1):13–14, 1995.

13. Committee on Bioethics: Guidelines on forgoing life-sustaining medical treatment. *Pediatrics* 93(3):532–536, 1994.

14. Compas BE, Champion JE, Reeslund K: Coping with stress: Implications for preventive interventions with adolescents. *Prev Res* 12:17–20, 2005.

15. Compas BE, et al: Coping with stress during childhood and adolescence: problems, progress, and potential in theory and research. *Psychol Bull* 127(1):87–127, 2001.

16. Contro N, et al: Family perspectives on the quality of pediatric palliative care. *Arch Pediatr Adolesc Med* 156(1):14–19, 2002.

17. Corr CA: Selected literature for adolescents: Annotated descriptions. In Corr CA, Nabe CM, Corr DM, editors: *Death and dying, life and living*, ed 5, Belmont, CA, 2006, Thomson Wadsworth, pp. 602–609.

18. Corr CA: Selected literature for children: annotated descriptions. In Corr CA, Nabe CM, Corr DM, editors: *Death and dying, life and living*, ed 5, Belmont, CA, 2006, Thomson Wadsworth, pp. 588–601.

19. Davies DE: Parental suicide after the expected death of a child at home. *Br Med J* 332(7542):647–648, 2006.

20. Davies G, et al: Bereavement. In Carter BS, Levetown M, editors: *Palliative care for infants, children, and adolescents: a practical handbook*, Baltimore, MD, 2004, Johns Hopkins University Press, pp. 196–219.

21. Dudley NC, et al: The effect of family presence on the efficiency of pediatric trauma resuscitations. *Ann Emerg Med* 53:777–784, 2009.

22. Gilmer MJ: Pediatric palliative care. *Crit Care Nurs Clin North Am* 14(2):207–214, 2002.

23. Gregoire MC, Frager G: Ensuring pain relief for children at the end of life. *Pain Res Manag* 11(3):163–171, 2006.

24. Hazinski MF, Zaritsky AL, Nadkarni VM, Hickey RW, et al: *Coping with the death of a child*, Dallas, 2003, American Heart Association.

25. Henderson DP, Knapp JF: Report of the national conference on family presence during pediatric resuscitation and procedures. *J Emerg Nurs* 32:23–29, 2006.

26. Himelstein BP, et al: Pediatric palliative care. *N Engl J Med* 350 (17):1752–1762, 2004.

27. Hutton N: Pediatric palliative care: the time has come. *Arch Pediatr Adolesc Med* 156(1):9–10, 2002.

28. Joint Commission on Accreditation of Healthcare Organizations: *Health care at the crossroads: Strategies for narrowing the organ donation gap*, 2008, Available from: http://www.jointcommission.org/nr/rdonlyres/e4e7dd3f-3fdf-4acc-b69e-aef3a1743ab0/0/organ_donation_white_paper.pdf. Accessed 05-19-10.

29. Kelso CMcV, et al: Palliative care consultation in the process of organ donation after cardiac death. *J Palliat Med* 10:118–126, 2007.

30. Kolovos NS, Webster P, Bratton SL: Donation after cardiac death in pediatric critical care. *Pediatric Critical Care Medicine* 8:47–49, 2007.

31. Kreicbergs U, et al: Talking about death with children who have severe malignant disease. *N Engl J Med* 351(12):1175–1186, 2004.

32. Levetown M, Liben S, Audet M: Palliative care in the pediatric intensive care unit. In Carter BS, Levetown M, editors: *Palliative care for infants, children, and adolescents: a practical handbook.*, Baltimore, MD, 2004, Johns Hopkins University Press, pp. 273–291.

33. Liben S, Papadatou D, Wolfe J: Paediatric palliative care: challenges and emerging ideas. *Lancet* 371(9615):852–864, 2008.

34. Magliocca JF, et al: Extracorporeal support or organ donation after cardiac death effectively expands the donor pool. *J Trauma* 58:1095–1102, 2005.

35. Meert KL, Thurston CS, Briller SH: The spiritual needs of parents at the time of their child's death in the pediatric intensive care unit and during bereavement: a qualitative study. *Pediatr Crit Care Med* 6 (4):420–427, 2005.

36. Miles MS, Demi AS: Guilt in bereaved parents. In Rando TA, editors: *Parental loss of a child*, Champaigne, IL, 1986, Research Press Company, pp. 97–118.

37. National Cancer Institute: *Young people with cancer: A handbook for parents*, Washington, DC, 2002, National Institutes of Health.

38. National Vital Statistics Reports: *Mortality data*, 2008, National Center for Health Statistics.

39. Noyes J: Enabling young 'ventilator-dependent' people to express their views and experiences of their care in hospital. *J Adv Nurs* 31 (5):1206–1215, 2000.

40. Oakes LL: Assessment and management of pain in the critically ill pediatric patient. *Crit Care Nurs Clin North Am* 13(2):281–295, 2001.

41. Orloff SF, et al: Psychosocial and spiritual needs of the child and family. In Carter BS, Levetown M, editors: *Palliative care for infants, children, and adolescents: a practical handbook*, Baltimore, MD, 2004, Johns Hopkins University Press, pp. 141–162.

42. Poltorak DY, Glazer JP: The development of children's understanding of death: cognitive and psychodynamic considerations. *Child Adolesc Psychiatr Clin N Am* 15(3):567–573, 2006.

43. President's Commission for the Study of Ethical Problems in Medicine and Biomedical and Behavioral Research: *Deciding to forego life-sustaining treatment*, Washington, DC, 1983, U.S. Government Printing Office.

44. Ramelet AS, Abu-Saad HH, Bulsara MK, Rees N, McDonald S: Capturing postoperative pain responses in critically ill infants aged 0 to 9 months. *Pediatric Critical Care Medicine* 7(1):19–26, 2006.

45. Rando TA: An investigation of grief and adaptation in parents whose children have died from cancer. *J Pediatr Psychol* 8(1):3–20, 1983.

46. Reich DJ, et al: ASTS recommended practice guidelines for controlled donation after cardiac death organ procurement and transplantation. *Am J Transplant* 9:1–8, 2009.

47. Robinson SM, et al: Psychological effect of witnessed resuscitation on bereaved relatives. *Lancet* 352:614–617, 1998.

48. Schiff HS: *The bereaved parent*, New York, 1977, Penguin Books.

49. Silverman P, et al: The effects of negative legacies on the adjustment of parentally bereaved children and adolescents. OMEGA. *J Death Dying* 46(4):335–352, 2002.

50. Truog R: Tackling medical futility in Texas. *N Engl J Med* 357:1–3, 2007.

51. Truog R, et al: Recommendations for end-of-life care in the intensive care unit: A consensus statement by the American College of Critical Care Medicine. *Crit Care Med* 36(3):953–963, 2008.

52. U.S. Government Organization on Organ and Tissue Donation and Transplantation: *Procurement Organ Procurement Organizations*, 2008, Available from: http://www.organdonor.gov/. Accessed 06-02-08.

53. von Gunten CF, Ferris FD, Emanuel LL: Ensuring competency in end-of-life care: communication and relational skills. *JAMA* 284 (23):3051–3057, 2000.

54. Way P: Michael in the clouds: Talking to very young children about death. *Bereave Care* 27(1):7–9, 2008.

55. Wojnicki-Johansson G: Communication between nurse and patient during ventilator treatment: patient reports and RN evaluations. *Intensive Crit Care Nurs* 17(1):29–39, 2001.

56. Wolfe J, Grier HE, Klar N, et al: Symptoms and suffering at the end of life in children with cancer. *N Engl J Med* 342(5):326–333, 2000.

57. World Health Organization: *WHO definition of palliative care for children*, Geneva, 2008, World Health Organization.

Pharmacokinetics and Pharmacodynamics

William Banner, Jr.

PEARLS

- *Pharmacokinetics* describes how the body alters drug concentration, including how the drug is dispersed in and removed from the body; it is the effect that the body has on the drug. Pharmacokinetics involves drug absorption, distribution, and elimination.
- *Pharmacodynamics* describes the relationship between drug concentration and drug effect; it is the effect the drug has on the body.
- The steady state is a state of equilibrium between how much of the drug is administered and how much is being removed from the body. In drugs with first-order kinetics (i.e., the systems that eliminate the drug are not saturated), steady state can be predicted from the drug half-life ($t_{1/2}$).
- The drug half-life is the time it takes for half of the drug to be eliminated from the body. In each half-life, the drug concentration in the blood will fall by half. You can use the half-life to predict the time to steady state and to know when to anticipate drug effects or changes in effects.
- In general, when administering a drug by continuous infusion, a blood concentration of 90% of steady-state value is achieved in approximately four to five half-lives of the drug. Drugs with long half-lives will require a longer time to achieve steady state unless a loading dose is provided.

INTRODUCTION

Many drugs used in critical care, particularly vasoactive and sedative agents, must be titrated based on patient response, and both pharmacokinetics and pharmacodynamics influence that response. *Pharmacokinetics* describes how the body alters drug concentration, including how the drug is dispersed in and removed from the body; it is the effect that the body has on the drug. *Pharmacodynamics* describes the relationship between drug concentration and drug effect; it is the effect the drug has on the body.

The purpose of this chapter is to highlight principles governing both pharmacokinetic and pharmacodynamic processes and how they affect clinical decisions. This chapter is not intended to be a drug reference; it is a reference regarding principles of drug therapy.

PRINCIPLES OF PHARMACOKINETICS

The effects of drug administration vary with both the drug and the patient. There have been many attempts to model these processes using mathematical equations to guide clinical therapy. In addition, understanding of developmental changes in drug metabolism and excretion and emerging information about pharmacogenetics enable more accurate prediction of pediatric drug dosing and effects.[2-5]

Paths of Drugs in the Body

The path of a drug in the body from administration and distribution to elimination is complex. We can break this path into individual components for better understanding (Fig. 4-1).

Drug Absorption

Drugs are administered and absorbed by several routes. *Bioavailability* refers to the fraction of administered drug that reaches the circulation (blood); it is affected by the route of administration. The bioavailability of drugs administered orally can be altered in pediatric patients by developmental changes in the gastric pH. The gastric pH is relatively neutral in the neonate and it becomes more acidic as the child grows. In addition, some drugs (e.g., meperidine) when taken orally, are rapidly metabolized by the liver before they reach the general circulation; this is termed *first pass* metabolism and it reduces drug bioavailability.

Drugs administered intravenously can also be affected by the site of administration. Drugs administered through an umbilical vein catheter can flow directly into the portal circulation, where they can damage the liver. Administration of a drug into an umbilical artery catheter can cause drug precipitation in the kidneys or lower extremity vascular damage.

Drug Distribution

Drug distribution is affected by factors such as protein binding, lipid solubility, and ionization state, and by conditions such as blood pH, temperature, and other substances in the blood (e.g., blood urea nitrogen [BUN], other drugs). The *volume of distribution* is the ratio of the concentration of drug in the blood to the total amount of drug in the body. For example, gentamicin has a small volume of distribution; it is principally found in the blood. In contrast, digoxin undergoes widespread distribution to tissues, so the concentration in the blood represents only a fraction of the total body stores (i.e., it has a large volume of distribution). Gentamicin and digoxin are both removed by similar processes in the kidney, but the rates of elimination of the two drugs differ because the amount that is present in the blood affects how quickly the kidneys can remove the drug.

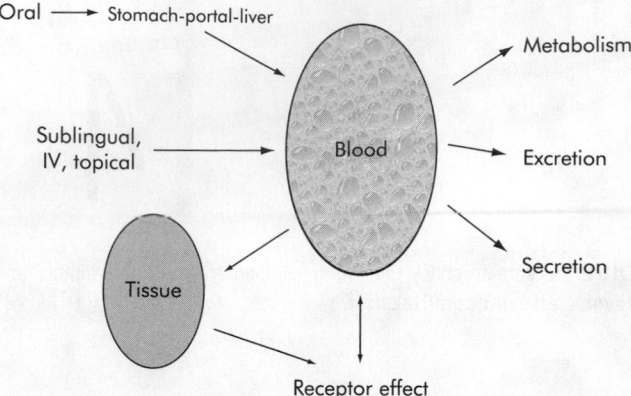

FIG. 4-1 Possible paths of drugs in the body from entry to distribution and elimination. A drug will follow some of these pathways. Drug effects are caused by blood concentration, tissue concentrations, or both. (Courtesy William Banner, Jr.)

The drug's site of action can also help predict how drug distribution will affect its efficacy and safety. Shortly after the intravenous administration of digoxin, blood concentrations can be extremely high, but the patient will not exhibit toxicity because digoxin acts on the cardiac muscle. As the blood drug concentration decreases and concentrations in the tissue (including the heart muscle) increase, the likelihood of a toxic effect increases. It is only after the drug is distributed into tissue that blood concentrations can be used to predict the likelihood of a beneficial or toxic effect.

Drug Elimination
Drugs are eliminated from the body in several ways. Some drugs such as ethyl alcohol can be exhaled through the lungs. The most common routes of elimination, however, are through the kidney and the liver. In the kidney, drugs can be filtered in the glomerulus or secreted by tubular cells. The most common method of renal excretion is through filtration. In general, the liver metabolizes drugs to change their solubility so they can be excreted through the biliary tract or the kidney.

A small number of drugs are broken down by enzymes present in plasma. These drugs, including succinylcholine, produce very short-term effects. A few drugs, such as cisatracurium, spontaneously degrade in the blood.

MATHEMATICAL MODELING OF DRUG PATHS

Mathematical models of drug kinetics (including elimination), called *kinetic modeling*, have identified several general patterns of drug behavior. The Michaelis-Menten equation describes drug kinetics, including drug elimination. According to the Michaelis-Menten equation, when the enzyme that metabolizes a drug is not saturated (i.e., there is plenty of enzyme still available to metabolize even more drug than is present), drug elimination will vary based on how quickly the drug is presented to the enzyme. If the enzyme is fully saturated (i.e., all available enzyme is being used to metabolize the drug), then drug elimination will occur at a fixed rate.

Michaelis-Menten Kinetics
A common drug governed by Michaelis-Menten kinetics is phenytoin. With even a single dose of phenytoin, the enzymes that metabolize the drug (the cytochrome P450 enzymes) are typically saturated, so the phenytoin blood concentration will initially fall slowly after administration. However, once the blood concentration falls sufficiently, the enzymes responsible for metabolism are no longer saturated and the blood concentration will then fall quickly (Fig. 4-2, curve A). Giving too much of a drug initially or giving additional doses too soon can increase the drug concentration and risk of toxicity and prolong effects and elimination time. Implications of phenytoin kinetics with repeated dosing are discussed in the next section.

First Order Kinetics
One extreme of the Michaelis-Menten equation occurs when the kidney or the liver is functioning well below its capacity to remove the drug and there is little risk of overloading the system. This extreme is referred to as *first-order kinetics*.

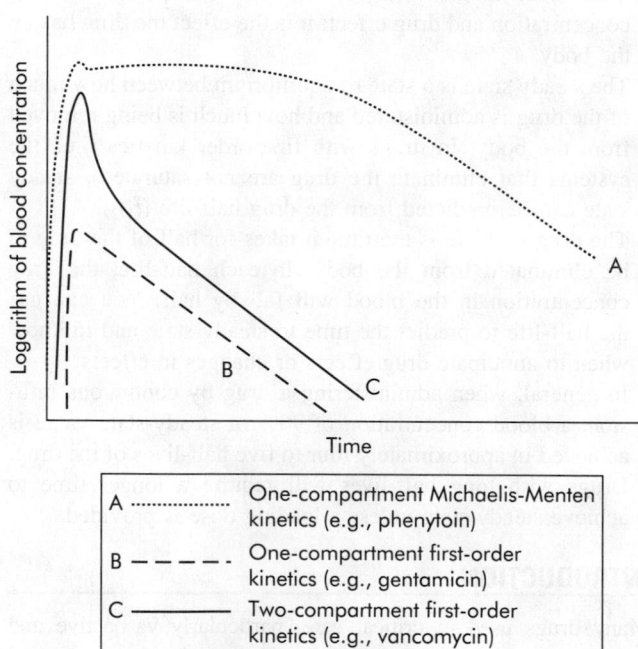

A	⋯⋯⋯⋯	One-compartment Michaelis-Menten kinetics (e.g., phenytoin)
B	– – – –	One-compartment first-order kinetics (e.g., gentamicin)
C	————	Two-compartment first-order kinetics (e.g., vancomycin)

FIG. 4-2 Three general models of drug elimination. After a single dose of a drug is given, the graph of the logarithm (log) of blood concentration produced over time varies based on drug distribution and elimination (kinetics). *Curve A:* If the drug is primarily distributed in the blood (e.g., phenytoin) and is eliminated by enzyme systems, it demonstrates one-compartment Michaelis-Menten kinetics as shown. The log of the blood concentration over time initially declines slowly until some enzyme systems are no longer saturated. From that time, the concentration will fall more rapidly. *Curve B:* If the drug is largely distributed in the blood (one compartment) and the elimination systems have plenty of capacity (first-order kinetics), the graph of the log of blood concentration over time will be an inverted V. The concentration rises in a straight line and then declines in a straight line. The log of the drug concentration will fall by half during each half-life of the drug. *Curve C:* Drugs distributed in the tissues (e.g., vancomycin) typically demonstrate two-compartment kinetics. Immediately after administration the concentration rises. As the drug is distributed into the tissues the drug concentration falls rapidly (the first part of the downward curve). As the drug is eliminated, the drug level falls more gradually. (Courtesy William Banner, Jr.)

Box 4-1 Metaphor for Understanding First Order and Zero-Order Kinetics

Another way to conceptualize first-order kinetics for drug elimination is to compare drug metabolism to customers going through checkout lanes at a store. A group of cashiers has a certain capacity to process customers, much as the liver processes or metabolizes a drug. If the number of cashiers is sufficiently high, when a customer appears that customer will be processed immediately. As long as the number of cashiers exceeds the number of customers presenting at the checkout lanes, the number of customers processed through the checkout lanes will be determined by the number of customers who are present at the checkout lanes. Renal filtration or excretion and liver metabolism typically have sufficient capacity, so they have capacity ("cashiers") available at all times to eliminate many drugs. This is called first-order kinetics.

If the capacity to process or metabolize the drug is saturated, then the rate of drug metabolism will become constant and if drug administration exceeds the rate of metabolism, the drug will begin to accumulate. Using the cashier metaphor, if the number of customers exceeds the available cashiers, the rate that customers are processed will become constant (for example, 10 customers/h), regardless of how many customers are waiting. The customers will accumulate if the number of customers exceeds the number of cashiers and the customers appear at the checkout line at a rate that is faster than they can be processed. If the capacity to metabolize the drug is saturated (zero-order kinetics) drug concentrations will increase in a manner similar to customer accumulation at the cashiers.

With first-order kinetics, drugs behave similarly to radioactive decay, and elimination is described in terms of the drug's half-life ($t_{1/2}$). The drug half-life is the time it takes for half of the drug to be eliminated from the body. When a half-life is listed in a drug database, the drug has first-order kinetics (see section, Half-life). See Box 4-1 for a metaphor to further explain first- and zero-order kinetics. Many of the principles described in the following sections (e.g., time to study state, volume of distribution, filtration rates) apply chiefly to drugs with first-order kinetics.

Volume of Distribution

Volume of distribution can be used to predict the drug concentration achieved with a drug loading dose. As noted previously, a drug like gentamicin has a low volume of distribution (it remains in the blood), so effective blood concentrations are quickly established without the need for a loading dose. By comparison, when administering a drug like digoxin, with a high volume of distribution, a relatively large initial loading dose must be given to achieve reasonable blood concentration after tissue distribution.

The volume of distribution is generally expressed as a liquid volume per body weight, such as liters per kilogram (L/kg) or milliliters per kilogram (mL/kg). The volume of distribution is used to calculate loading doses for drugs such as phenytoin, for which a loading dose of 20 mg/kg is administered to occupy the volume of distribution

(0.7 L/kg) and achieve a therapeutic blood (serum) concentration.

Although it is tempting to relate anatomic places to the mathematical concept of compartments for drug distribution, the characterization is not entirely accurate. In general, we consider the group of tissues into which the drug distributes at a similar rate as occupying the same compartment, because the tissues all receive the drug at the same time.

Generally speaking, when injecting an intravenous drug, the first compartment it occupies is the blood. If the drug is primarily distributed in the blood (e.g., gentamicin), that is where the drug remains until it is eliminated; these kinetics are described as *one-compartment kinetics*. The graph of the logarithm of blood concentration over time shows a rise when the drug is administered and a straight line as the drug is eliminated (see Fig. 4-2, curve B).

If a drug is distributed in the blood and the tissues (e.g., vancomycin), intravenous administration temporarily increases the concentration of the drug in the blood. Initially, blood levels decline rapidly as the drug moves into tissue, and then a more gradual decline occurs as the drug is eliminated. This drug activity is called *two-compartment kinetics* (see Fig. 4-2, curve C).

Implications of Multicompartment Distribution

Drugs can disappear rapidly from the blood if they are distributed in the tissue. The best example of this is sodium thiopental (Pentothal). In clinical practice, a single dose of intravenous thiopental has a short effect. However, the drug has a long final half-life. The explanation for this apparent contradiction is that most thiopental elimination occurs after the drug concentration is below the level needed to keep the patient asleep (i.e., anesthetized). If several doses of thiopental are administered in a short period of time in an attempt to produce anesthesia, the tissues will become saturated and no distribution will occur. If the drug concentration increases to sufficiently high levels, the clinical effect (i.e., anesthesia) may last a long time (see Fig. 4-3).

Fentanyl also has a relatively short clinical half-life when administered as a single injection. However, if continuous infusions are used over a period of days, the drug will soon have an elimination half-life of 24 hours, meaning that it will take an extended period of time for the drug levels to decrease sufficiently so the patient wakes up. This long ultimate half-life is sometimes referred to as the *beta half-life*.

Drug Clearance

The clearance of a drug is a measure of how quickly the drug is eliminated. Whereas half-life describes the rate of decline in drug concentration, and volume of distribution indicates where the drug is located in the body, the overall drug clearance is mathematically related to both half-life and volume of distribution. In clinical practice, half-life and clearance are used almost interchangeably, because it is unusual for the volume of distribution of a drug to change for any given drug, but many changes in development and disease states affect the drug half-life and therefore drug elimination. When comparing different drugs, it is appropriate to speak of clearance as a true measure of how a drug is eliminated from the body.

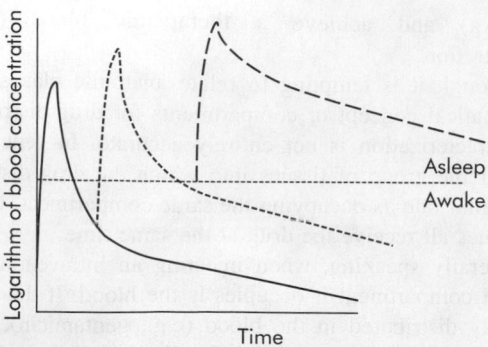

FIG. 4-3 Thiopental accumulation in body compartments: single versus multiple doses. Drugs that appear to have a short duration of action may simply be rapidly distributed into tissue, allowing patients to recover from the drug effects. When pentothal is given in a single dose (*solid curve*), the drug concentration rises rapidly and then falls rapidly as the drug is distributed into the tissues; as a result, the patient will wake in a short time. If an additional dose is given within a short time (*dotted curve*), the drug effects last for a longer time. If several doses are administered over a short time, the tissues can become saturated and the drug does not have a rapid distribution phase (*dashed curve*). The drug accumulates in the blood (i.e., concentration is high), elimination takes more time, and the patient will take much longer to wake. The kinetics of fentanyl are similar. (Courtesy William Banner, Jr.)

Frequently Used Terms

Drug concentration is affected by drug administration rate and dose, drug absorption and drug elimination. To evaluate a drug concentration, providers must be familiar with common terms such as *half-life*, *steady state*, and *loading dose*, and they must be familiar with drug metabolism and excretion patterns.

Half-Life

As noted previously, the drug half-life is the time required for half of the drug to be eliminated from the body. In each half-life, the drug concentration in the blood will fall by half. For example, if gentamicin has a 2-hour half-life, this means that the blood concentration will halve in 2 hours; and halve again in 2 more hours, and halve again 2 hours later. Six hours after administration, the blood concentration of a drug with a 2-hour half-life will be 12.5% of the initial drug concentration. The half-life of a drug can be found in many drug data bases.

Steady State

When multiple doses of any medication are given, there is a period of accumulation before the drug reaches what is referred to as *steady state*. The steady state is a state of equilibrium between the amount of drug administered and the amount of drug being removed from the body. In drugs with first-order kinetics (i.e., the systems that eliminate the drug are not saturated), steady state can be predicted from the drug half-life. When a drug is administered as a continuous infusion, 50% of steady state is achieved during the first half-life of the drug. By the end of the second half-life of the drug, 75% of steady state will be achieved. If there is a need to achieve steady state more rapidly, administer a bolus prior to initiation of the drug infusion (see section, Bolus Plus Infusion Kinetics). Note that the average blood concentration

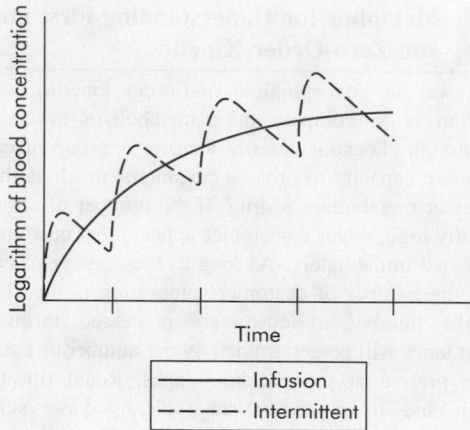

FIG. 4-4 Time to steady-state concentration. Steady-state concentration is achieved after four to five half-lives of the drug (each *vertical hatch mark* on the time line represents one half-life of the drug) whether the drug is administered by continuous infusion (*solid line*) or intermittently (*dashed line*). The time to equilibrium and the blood concentration associated with steady state varies as the result of the drug actions, distribution, interactions, and factors affecting drug elimination. (Courtesy William Banner, Jr.)

at which steady state ultimately is achieved is the same regardless of whether the drug is given by continuous infusion or intermittent dosing (see Fig. 4-4).

Clinical Examples. Several clinical examples demonstrate the range of time to steady state in drugs given by continuous infusion. Dopamine has a half-life of 1 to 2 minutes. During continuous infusion, dopamine reaches a steady-state value in the first 4 to 10 minutes of administration (four to five times the half-life of 1 to 2 minutes). By comparison, phenobarbital has a half-life of approximately 30 to 60 hours. Therefore, if phenobarbital is given by continuous infusion without a loading dose, it may take days or weeks to reach a steady-state concentration.

In patients with normal renal function, drugs such as aminoglycosides (e.g., gentamicin) have a half-life of approximately 2 hours; such drugs reach a steady state at around 8 to 10 hours, or by about the time of the second dose. However, in a patient with renal failure, the half-life of gentamicin can increase beyond 10 hours; it may take several days to achieve steady state.

Loading Doses

A loading dose is a dose administered to help achieve steady state of a drug. As stated above, loading doses are based on the volume of distribution of the drug. A loading dose is more likely to be recommended for drugs that have long half-lives, such as phenobarbital, because it would take too long (four to five half-lives of such a drug) to achieve steady state. The drug effects and side effects also influence whether and how a loading dose should be administered. For example, when digoxin is administered intravenously, patients will not tolerate administration of the entire digitalizing loading dose at one time, because such a loading dose would produce extremely high serum concentrations that could cause adverse effects.

The loading dose and maintenance dose are mathematically distinct and do not predict one another. As noted previously, the maintenance dose is the dose needed to maintain the blood level required to produce clinical effect.

Many drugs have a similar volume of distribution (L/kg or mL/kg body weight) for neonates and for adults. However, because neonates have limited ability to eliminate drugs, drugs given to the neonate will have longer half-life and lower clearance than when the same drugs are administered to adults. Although loading doses for some drugs can be similar (per kilogram body weight) for neonates and adults, neonates will likely require lower maintenance doses.

Bolus Plus Infusion Kinetics

Critical care nurses often administer analgesics, sedatives, and vasoactive agents by continuous infusion, and these drugs are titrated to clinical effect. As a result, nurses should be familiar with the effects of continuous infusions and loading doses on drug concentration, as shown in Fig. 4-5.

As noted previously, if a drug is administered by either loading dose or continuous infusion, drug concentration will increase over time and achieve 90% of steady state over approximately four to five half-lives of the drug.

To avoid a delay in the onset of effective therapy by continuous infusion, a bolus dose can be given. The bolus dose is followed by the continuous infusion. Note that the same steady-state concentration will ultimately be achieved whether or not a bolus is given; the bolus shortens the time required to achieve this steady state.

A continuous infusion may be erroneously referred to as a *maintenance dose*. However, the continuous infusion will not maintain the therapeutic level if the infusion is not correctly calculated in light of elimination and other factors affecting blood concentration.

If the patient is unable to eliminate a drug normally (i.e., the patient has a decrease in clearance), a continuous infusion can contribute to drug accumulation (i.e., an elevated steady-state concentration) and toxicity. This can occur, for example, when a neonate is given the same bolus plus infusion dose as an older child. See section, Additional Factors Affecting Drug Elimination for further information.

Michaelis-Menten or Non-linear Kinetics and Dosing

A few common drugs do not obey the basic rules of steady-state equilibrium and can produce toxicity in unexpected ways. The most common of these is phenytoin and its precursor fosphenytoin. At low concentrations, phenytoin has a predictable relationship of dose to steady-state concentration (Fig. 4-6). However, as the dose increases, enzymes that normally inactivate the drug eventually become saturated. At that point, the steady-state concentration begins to rise out of proportion to the increase in dose, and even small increases in dose are then likely to substantially increase drug concentration and produce toxicity.

TOTAL VERSUS FREE CONCENTRATION

The drug concentration typically measured in the clinical laboratory is the total concentration of drug present in blood (actually in the serum). For most drugs it is adequate to monitor the blood/serum concentration when monitoring effects and when toxicity is a concern. Some drugs, however, bind avidly to protein binding sites in the serum. For these drugs, the drug level that most closely correlates with drug

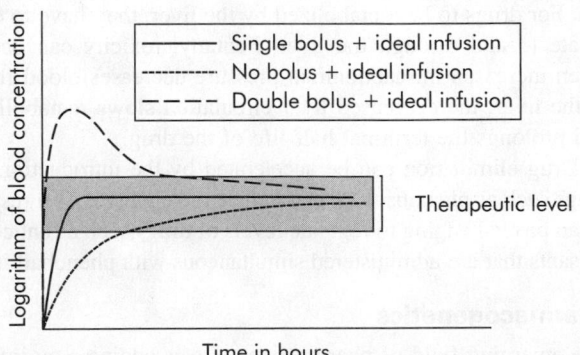

FIG. 4-5 Bolus plus infusion kinetics. The concentration of drug reaches steady state (in this case, synonymous with therapeutic level shaded in grey) in several different ways over different time courses. When a continuous infusion is provided without a loading dose (*dotted line*), the drug will achieve steady state over approximately four to five half-lives of the drug. The *solid line* depicts the relationship of the logarithm (log) of blood concentration over time when a bolus dose plus continuous infusion is provided. The bolus dose helps to rapidly achieve steady state (in this example, synonymous with therapeutic drug concentration), and the continuous infusion has been calculated to keep the blood concentration within the therapeutic ranges. If two boluses are given (such as in the operating room to produce deep sedation) before the continuous infusion is provided (see *dashed line*), the initial concentration will be higher than after a single dose, and it will remain elevated for a longer period of time. The final steady-state concentration is the same whether one or more boluses are administered, provided the clearance is equal. (Courtesy William Banner, Jr.)

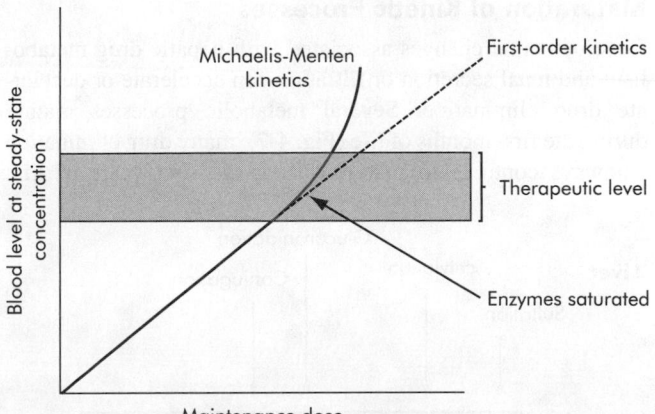

FIG. 4-6 Phenytoin Michaelis-Menten kinetics. This graph depicts the relationship between maintenance dose and steady state dose with phenytoin, a drug with Michaelis-Menten kinetics. For drugs with first-order kinetics (i.e., enzymes or systems that metabolize or inactivate the drug are not saturated), an increase in maintenance dose will produce a linear increase in steady-state concentration (see initial portion of *solid line* and continuation in *dashed line*). This is not the case for phenytoin and other drugs that demonstrate Michaelis-Menten kinetics. Once the enzymes that metabolize the drug are fully saturated (*arrow*), any increase in maintenance dose will produce a significant rise in steady-state concentration (*solid line* above grey therapeutic level). Other drugs such as salicylate and theophylline demonstrate similar kinetics. (Courtesy William Banner, Jr.)

benefits and side effects is the "free" concentration of drug—that is, the concentration of drug that is not bound to protein.

Anticonvulsants, particularly phenytoin, have a high degree of protein binding; typically approximately 10% of the drug is free in the serum. It is only this unbound fraction that passes through the blood brain barrier and produces effects in the brain. For these drugs, at a blood concentration of x, the actual active amount of drug available is only 10% of x.

If protein binding sites are diminished (e.g., in hypoalbuminemia) or protein binding sites are occupied by another substance (e.g., BUN), the percent of free or unbound drug available at a given total concentration can be higher than normal. Thus, a patient with a normal amount of protein binding can exhibit therapeutic effects at a given concentration, but that same patient can develop toxic effects at the same total concentration if they develop conditions producing a higher amount of free drug (see Evolve Fig. 4-1 in the Chapter 4 Supplement on the Evolve Website).

When evaluating the concentration of drugs such as phenytoin, providers can request that the laboratory measure only the free, or unbound, concentration if conditions such as a low albumin or high BUN are present. This free portion is interpreted with a different therapeutic scale, usually available from the clinical laboratory.

ADDITIONAL FACTORS AFFECTING DRUG ELIMINATION

The rate of drug excretion can accelerate or decelerate and still be considered a first-order (nonsaturated) model. Many developmental factors, diseases, and additional drugs can affect enzyme and organ function and influence the rate of drug metabolism

Maturation of Kinetic Processes

Developmental changes associated with hepatic drug metabolism and renal secretion or filtration can accelerate or decelerate drug elimination. Several metabolic processes mature during the first months of life (Fig. 4-7); many drug elimination pathways continue to mature during the first years of life.

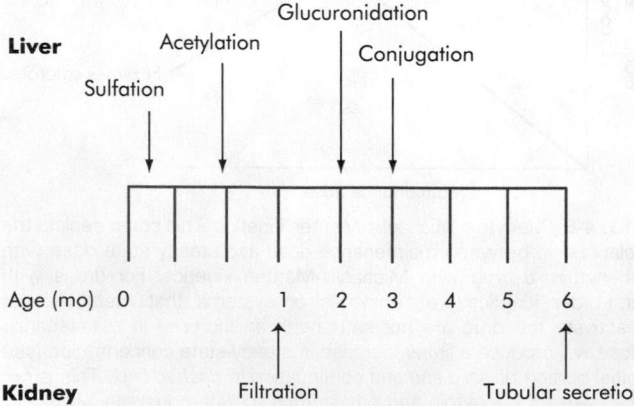

FIG. 4-7 Maturation of drug elimination in infants. Drug elimination in newborns changes rapidly as a result of maturation in liver and kidney function. Providers must consider the immaturity of the newborn's drug elimination systems when drugs are prescribed. (Courtesy William Banner, Jr.)

Table 4-1	Changes in Glomerular Filtration Rate with Age

Age	Glomerular Filtration Rate (mL/min per 1.73 m^2)
Premature infant	6
Full-term newborn	8-60
1 month	26-90
1 year	63-150
3 years	89-179
6 years	79-170
Adult male	110-152

Consistent with values from Barakat AY, Ichikawa I: Laboratory data. In Ichikawa I, editor: *Pediatric textbook of fluids and electrolytes*, Baltimore, 1990, Williams and Wilkins; and Tan JM: Nephrology. In Custer JW, Rau RE, editors: *The Johns Hopkins Hospital Harriet Lane Handbook*, ed 18, Philadelphia, 2009, Mosby-Elsevier.

Failure to recognize these developmental changes in children can lead to drug complications.

By the end of the first year of life, liver metabolism and drug clearance is similar to that reported in older children and adults. The child's glomerular filtration rate does not reach adult levels (in mL/min per m^2 body surface area) until approximately 3 years of age (Table 4-1)[1,6].

Clinical Factors Affecting Drug Metabolism

Many factors affect drug metabolism. Metabolism of one drug can slow when other drugs interact or interfere with the enzyme systems that normally inactivate that drug. Drug metabolism is also likely to be slowed if the liver is injured or if it is involved in other processes, such as handling bilirubin. For drugs to be metabolized by the liver, they have to circulate to and through the liver. Fentanyl toxicity can occur when increased intraabdominal pressure decreases blood flow to the liver; the decreased liver circulation slows metabolism and prolongs the terminal half-life of the drug.

Drug elimination can be accelerated by the introduction of drugs such as phenobarbital that induce metabolism. As a result, it can be challenging to regulate levels of drugs such as anticonvulsants that are administered simultaneous with phenobarbital.

Pharmacogenetics

The emerging field of pharmacogenetics is adding new information that is critical to our understanding of drugs. Cells of the liver use the cytochrome P450 system to metabolize drugs. This cytochrome P450 system collaborates with many other systems, such as glucuronidation and acetylation, to metabolize drugs, and it initially breaks down a drug to allow the other enzymes to attack it.

Because the cytochrome P450 system works in the first stage of drug metabolism, its activity can become a critical rate-limiting step in drug metabolism. The capacity and characteristics of the cytochrome P450 system are determined by genetics; many genetically determined subtypes of the system can cause variability in drug kinetics and elimination. Dosing of warfarin can be predicted by monitoring one genetic variant of the cytochrome P450 system, and further individualization of drug therapy might be possible in the future.

Drug Excretion

The kidney can remove drugs from the body through either filtration or secretion. The most common method of renal elimination is filtration through the glomerulus, with passive elimination in the urine. Drugs removed by filtration demonstrate first-order kinetics—the more filtration that occurs, the more drug is removed.

Active transport mechanisms in the renal tubules can secrete some drugs (e.g., penicillin) directly into the urine. Cells lining the tubules actively transport the drug from the blood into the urine. This tubular active transport system is inhibited by a drug called *probenecid*, which can be used to prolong the effects of penicillin and ampicillin.

Altered renal function will change elimination kinetics for drugs that are filtered or secreted by the kidney. The dose of aminoglycosides such as gentamicin has to be based on the clearance or filtration of these drugs, as estimated by serum creatinine or calculated creatinine clearance.

The premature infant has markedly reduced renal function, glomerular filtration rate, and drug clearance, even when compared with a full-term infant. These renal dynamics improve significantly during the first 3 years of life (see Table 4-1). Dosing requirements for a number of drugs change during infancy, even from week to week during the first months of life. In general, for seriously ill or injured infants, the combination of immature renal function and disease state will likely slow drug elimination.

PRACTICAL CLINICAL CONSIDERATIONS

Dosing Changes

Providers must be aware of drug kinetics and elimination when adjusting drug dose. For a drug with first-order kinetics, an increase in dose will increase steady-state concentration proportionately. Providers can use that proportional increase to calculate a change in drug dose to reach a given drug concentration: to increase the drug concentration by 20%, increase the dose by 20%.

If the drug has Michaelis-Menten kinetics, any increase in dose will result in a more substantial increase in the drug concentration. For example, a 20% increase in dose may produce a 50% increase in concentration.

Drugs often demonstrate a variety of kinetics and compartments of distribution. Table 4-2 includes a short list of common pediatric critical care drugs with different kinetics and distribution.

Table 4-2 Common Drugs and Kinetic Models

Drug	Kinetics	Distribution
Gentamicin	First order	One compartment
Vancomycin	First order	Two compartment
Phenytoin	Michaelis-Menten	One compartment
Phenobarbital	First order	One compartment
Fentanyl	First order	Two compartment
Midazolam	First order	Two compartment
Digoxin	First order	Multicompartment
Pentobarbital	First order	Two compartment

Bayes' Theorem

Bayes' theorem is used to analyze complex clinical situations to give more credibility or weight to the most important variables that will influence the situation. When interpreting any laboratory value, providers make judgments based on the absolute value in addition to other patient variables. One example is analysis of the serum potassium concentration. The clinician should react differently to an elevated potassium concentration obtained from a heelstick sample in a child with a normal electrocardiogram (ECG) than to an elevated potassium concentration obtained by venipuncture in the child with acute renal failure, an elevated serum creatinine, and peaked T waves on the ECG. In the child with the heelstick sample, providers should give less weight to potassium concentration and more weight to the clinical findings and the conditions under which the sample was obtained. The provider should be concerned, however, about the elevated potassium concentration in the child with renal failure, because other indicators suggest that it is clinically significant. Drug level monitoring should use such analysis. Computer programs using mathematical regression analysis models are available to aid in the interpretation of drug levels.

Drug Monitoring and Dosing

Although it is important to understand principles of pharmacokinetics to interpret drug concentrations, few clinicians understand the actual mathematical theories and calculations underpinning the kinetics. Fortunately, most drug databases provide relatively simple dosing recommendations and equations that factor in the kinetics. Recommended drug doses often differ based on postconceptual age, weight, and parameters of renal function.

There are two basic reasons to determine drug levels or concentration: to judge safety or efficacy, and to predict future dosing. Drug levels are most often used to monitor for safety and efficacy and are rarely used to attempt to calculate future dosing.

When a sample is obtained to evaluate drug concentration, it is critical to know the timing of the sampling in regard to drug administration. For drugs that require a timed infusion, failure to accurately time both the drug administration and the blood sampling can yield a falsely high or low drug concentration that can cause erroneous decisions about future dosing. The following general approaches to drug dosing and monitoring form a basis for drug use.

Start from the Expected

Determine the dose based on variables listed in standard databases, which should factor in the postconceptual age of a child, weight range, and actual body weight.

Wait Until Steady State

Identify the time to steady state for a drug. In general, 90% of the steady-state concentration will be achieved in four to five half-lives for a drug. The drug concentration after the third dose will only approximate steady state if the drug (e.g., aminoglycosides or vancomycin) has a relatively short half-life. Drugs with long half-lives will require a longer time to achieve steady state unless a loading dose is provided.

It may be appropriate to evaluate a drug concentration before steady state, to provide additional safety in situations where drug elimination is likely to be compromised by immaturity of the drug elimination system, disease, or organ failure. The best example is a small newborn or infant with renal insufficiency. In this patient, the drug kinetics might be markedly altered, so evaluation of the drug concentration after a small number of doses could provide useful information.

It may also be reasonable to check a drug concentration after a loading dose if a desired drug effect (pharmacodynamic) has not been achieved. For example, if a loading dose of phenytoin does not stop seizure activity, the phenytoin drug level can be checked to predict the benefit of administering an additional loading dose, and to determine the size of such a dose. For phenytoin, a loading dose of 20 mg/kg usually creates a blood concentration of 15 to 20 mcg/mL. A drug level of 12 mcg/mL the day after a loading dose might prompt administration of an additional 10 mg/kg loading dose to raise the concentration to 20 mcg/mL. Note that the drug levels from samples drawn before achieving the predicted steady state are not useful to predict maintenance dosing.

Make Conservative Changes in Dose

When drug concentrations are obtained in the clinical setting, the nurse must interpret the concentrations in light of the patient's condition. It is particularly dangerous to overinterpret a low drug concentration and make a large increase in dose. Many variables in the patient's condition and in the blood sampling process in a critical care unit can introduce error and create a falsely low value. A substantial increase in the dose of a drug such as phenytoin can markedly increase the drug concentration (see Fig. 4-6, earlier).

Monitor for Changes in Clinical Condition

In general, once steady-state concentrations have been achieved and appropriate drug levels are documented, providers might expect that levels will remain fairly constant unless organ dysfunction develops. Providers must also consider the effect of organ development on drug excretion as the infant grows. Unless drug doses are increased as the infant's glomerular filtration rate increases, the concentration of a drug will likely fall if the drug is administered continuously over the first months of life. Such a concentration decline should not be attributed to noncompliance or failure of drug effect.

Determine Whether Another Loading Dose is Indicated

Drugs with long half-lives may require hours or days to reach steady state. If a monitored drug level is low, an additional partial loading dose may be needed to increase the concentration.

DRUG INFORMATION IN DATABASES

Several well-researched databases are available to guide pediatric drug therapy. These databases contain core information that will be useful to guide therapy.

Indications, Contraindications, and Mechanisms of Action

Nurses should be aware of a drug's mechanism of action and contraindications, particularly if such contraindications are designated by a black box (indicating a warning from the U.S. Food and Drug Administration). The nurse should discuss concerns regarding potential contraindications with the provider who has ordered the drug.

Pharmacokinetic Parameters

The drug's volume of distribution, protein binding, clearance, and drug half-life may be listed. A drug with a volume of distribution less than 1 L/kg is chiefly distributed in the blood, with only a small amount of tissue distribution. Larger volumes of distribution (>1 L/kg) reflect greater tissue distribution. The greater the tissue distribution, the more likely that administration of a loading dose will be needed, if it can be tolerated. If a loading dose is recommended, it should be listed with the dosing information.

Protein binding (listed as a percent of total) and its clinical importance may be noted in this section. Highly bound drugs can be displaced from proteins by other drugs or in some clinical conditions (e.g., a high BUN). Providers should consider the degree of protein binding when evaluating drug levels; measurement of the free (unbound) drug concentration may be needed.

The drug clearance reflects changes that occur with disease and maturation of organ function. Such data should also be included with dosing information. If a drug's clearance is altered by disease states or organ function, it may be necessary to alter initial doses to avoid toxicity.

As noted previously, the drug half-life is an extremely useful piece of information. The nurse can use the half-life to predict time to steady state and to know when to anticipate drug effects or changes in effects. Estimates of time of achievement of steady state (typically four to five half-lives of the drug, unless a bolus is administered), will help determine when to obtain blood levels and when to expect a response to therapy.

The drug half-life can be used to help the nurse anticipate clinical changes when drugs are initiated or discontinued. Intravenous milrinone has a half-life of approximately 3 hours in infants, whereas dopamine has a half-life of approximately 2 minutes. If milrinone is discontinued, the drug concentration will decrease by half every 3 hours in the infant (and more rapidly in children and adults), so the benefits of the milrinone will likely decrease over the same time period. By comparison, if a dopamine infusion is discontinued, the drug concentration will halve in approximately 2 minutes, so clinical changes can be observed in that time.

Some databases will list a half-life for short-term administration and a half-life for long-term administration; these may also be termed the distributional effect (or $t_{1/2}$-alpha) and terminal elimination (or $t_{1/2}$-beta), respectively. The terminal elimination half-life will ultimately determine the time to steady state and may be responsible for prolonged effects observed in children after long-term use of sedatives.

Dosing Information

Dosing information is a critical component of any database. Loading dose, if needed, is typically the first parameter listed. The database may list a rapid loading dose, such as with some anticonvulsants, or a divided loading dose to be given over 24 h, such as with digoxin. In general, the loading dose is based on weight and does not factor in disease state or other patient parameters. To determine the loading dose for a patient, providers must identify any constraints (e.g., irritation to veins or maximum rate of infusion) to drug administration.

The initial dosing recommendations are generally divided by age group. For some drugs, dosing can be based on both development (e.g., postconceptual age) and weight (e.g., premature infant weight <1000 g). Note that to increase accuracy, drug orders should include the dose in milligrams per kilogram and the final dose (amount) to be given.

Disease-dependent variables will affect the maintenance but not the loading dose. The database may provide specific recommendations regarding alteration of dose in renal failure or in hepatic dysfunction, but databases often provide only general guidelines. Some drug dosing (e.g., fentanyl) can be affected by technology such as continuous renal replacement therapy or extracorporeal membrane oxygenation (ECMO), so ECMO loading doses and need for increased infusion rates during ECMO therapy may be noted.

Drug Interactions

Most databases list known interactions with food or disease states or other drugs. For example, enteral feedings that are high in calcium concentration (e.g., infant formulas) can interact with and change the bioavailability of some oral medications. Databases can list precautions regarding intravenous administration rate or problems with admixture with other drugs.

Sampling for Monitoring Drug Concentrations

Most drug databases suggest timing for blood sampling to monitor drug concentration. It is important to consider the primary purpose in determining the drug concentration. When monitoring for safety, a blood sample is typically obtained at the end of a dosing interval (i.e., immediately before a dose), and is called a *trough level*. When monitoring for efficacy, the sample is typically obtained to identify the concentration immediately after a dose (e.g., 30 minutes after a dose is infused), and is called the *peak level*.

If providers want to perform rigorous pharmacokinetic predictions, both peak and trough levels are evaluated to calculate a half-life and predict future dosing of drugs. Peak and trough levels are evaluated less commonly than in previous years to predict drug dosing, because more accurate information is now available to guide drug dosing.

PHARMACODYNAMICS

Pharmacodynamics is the description of the effects of the drug on the body. Mathematically there is a sigmoidal (S-shaped) relationship between the receptor activation causing a drug response (i.e., clinical effects) and the logarithm of its blood concentration. This relationship is relatively flat at low concentrations, until enough of the drug is present to produce effects. The relationship is also flat at high concentrations, once receptors are saturated and maximal effects are obtained. At moderate doses (i.e., the center part of this *S*), there is a nearly direct relationship between drug concentration and drug effects. In other words, increasing the dose increases the effects (see Pharmacodynamics in the Chapter 4 Supplement on the Evolve Website for more information and Chapter 6 for additional information about titration of vasoactive infusions).

Critical care providers monitor pharmacodynamics in both concrete and subtle ways. Many of the drugs used in critical care have fairly solid endpoints that are used to titrate a dose (e.g., a target systolic blood pressure when titrating vasopressors such as norepinephrine). However, other drugs can be used to produce more qualitative clinical effects. For example, during milrinone therapy, nurses cannot readily monitor the child's cardiac output at the bedside, but they monitor quality of systemic perfusion by evaluating a variety of subjective factors including signs of end-organ function (e.g., urine output).

One of the most complex drugs that requires pharmacodynamic assessment is dopamine. Dopamine interacts with three different receptors: the dopamine receptor, the beta-1 receptor, and the alpha receptor. It has a different range of affinities for binding to these three receptors. For each receptor there is a typical S-shaped relationship between the logarithm of dopamine concentration and receptor binding that produces drug effects (Fig. 4-8). As dopamine blood concentration increases, one receptor nears saturation; at the same time, dopamine begins to bind with another receptor, producing additional clinical effects. The net effect on a variable such as systemic vascular resistance is not a typical *S* because stimulation of different receptors will produce different effects. The key to

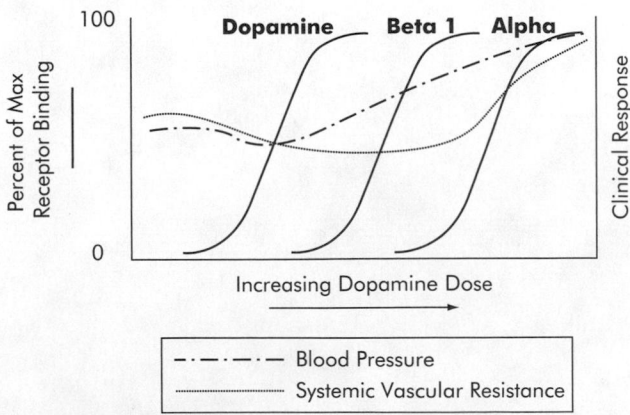

FIG. 4-8 Pharmacodynamics of dopamine. Dopamine has a complex pharmacodynamic model because it acts on three separate receptor systems and will produce effects that change with increasing dose. The net effect on clinical response is indicated by a curve depicting likely changes in systemic vascular resistance (*dotted line*) and blood pressure (*dot and dash line*). Of course, individual patient responses vary and the drug must be titrated according to the patient's response. (Courtesy William Banner, Jr.)

dopamine titration is understanding that dopamine's pharmacodynamic effect is modulated by three receptor systems (see Chapter 6).

SUMMARY

The more that critical care nurses understand the potential effects of drug distribution and the child's age and other factors (e.g., clinical condition) that influence drug elimination, the more they will be able to avoid the problems of drug side effects and toxicities. Through knowledge of basic principles of pharmacokinetics and pharmacodynamics in clinical practice, the nurse can better titrate drugs to maximize therapeutic effects and minimize adverse or toxic drug effects.[2-5]

References

1. Barakat AY, Ichikawa I: Laboratory data. In Ichikawa I, editor: *Pediatric textbook of fluids and electrolytes*, Baltimore, 1990, Williams and Wilkins.
2. Bauer L: *Applied clinical pharmacokinetics*, ed 2, New York, 2008, McGraw-Hill.
3. Birkett DJ: *Pharmacokinetics made easy*, North Ryde NSW Australia, 2002, McGraw-Hill Australia.
4. Burton ME, et al., editors: *Applied pharmacokinetics and pharmacodynamics, principles of therapeutic drug monitoring*, Baltimore, 2006, Lippincott Williams & Wilkins.
5. Potts AL, et al: Dexmedetomidine pharmacokinetics in pediatric intensive care—a pooled analysis. *Paediatr Anaesth* 19(11):1119–1129, 2009.
6. Tan JM: Nephrology. In Custer JW, Rau RE, editors: *The Johns Hopkins Hospital Harriet Lane Handbook*, ed 18, Philadelphia, 2009, Mosby-Elsevier.

Analgesia, Sedation, and Neuromuscular Blockade

5

Twila R. Luckett • Stephen R. Hays

evolve Be sure to check out the supplementary content available at http://evolve.elsevier.com/Hazinski.

PEARLS

- Analgesia entails assessment and treatment of pain; sedation entails assessment and treatment of agitation; neuromuscular blockade entails pharmacologic inhibition of voluntary muscle movement.
- Analgesia often improves agitation, but does not necessarily provide sedation; sedation often improves pain, but does not necessarily provide analgesia; neuromuscular blockade provides neither analgesia nor sedation, and should never be induced without first ensuring adequate levels of both analgesia and sedation.
- Most critically ill children experience some degree of pain and agitation: optimal nursing care of critically ill children asks how best to provide appropriate analgesia and sedation, not whether analgesia or sedation should be provided.
- Pain and agitation are usually dynamic processes. Nurses should perform appropriate assessments to monitor pain, agitation, and effectiveness of interventions; reassess patients regularly using consistent tools and modify interventions as needed.
- Change in pharmacologic analgesia and sedation to different agents, or to different routes of administration, requires equipotent conversion to ensure ongoing efficacy and to prevent inadequate or excessive dosing.
- All opioid analgesics and many systemic sedatives can induce physiologic tolerance, and should be weaned gradually after prolonged administration to prevent withdrawal. Appropriate use of these agents does not cause addiction, and they should not be avoided because of such concern.

INTRODUCTION

Pain and agitation are common in critically ill patients. As our understanding of these processes in critically ill children has evolved, we now recognize the vital importance of appropriate analgesia and sedation in such patients.[48] In 1986, the World Health Organization first published its Analgesic Ladder for the management of cancer pain (Fig. 5-1). This paradigm and others like it are now widely accepted as guidelines for analgesia and sedation in all patients. Despite such advances, considerable progress remains to be made. Caregiver education should enhance awareness of the crucial need for appropriate analgesia and sedation in critically ill children. Practice patterns must continue to change to include appropriate analgesia and sedation as essential components of pediatric critical care.

Ongoing research must continue to explore the nature of these complex processes and their optimal management.

In the past, many caregivers mistakenly assumed the immature pediatric nervous system rendered children incapable of experiencing pain or agitation, or caregivers mistakenly believed that children could not safely tolerate analgesics or sedatives. Particularly in pediatric patients, caregivers often interpreted lack of request for analgesia or sedation as indicating lack of pain or agitation, so pediatric patients often received inadequate analgesia. We now know that children of all ages can feel pain and experience pain without expressing the need for analgesia and they can safely receive a wide variety of analgesic interventions. We also know that agitation is common in pediatric patients, and children often receive inadequate sedation.

Assessment of pain and agitation is especially challenging when patients are unable to articulate their experiences and feelings, and analgesia and sedation may be particularly inadequate in these patients. Critically ill children are at risk for significant pain and agitation, and pediatric critical care providers must be vigilant in providing appropriate analgesia and sedation.

Appropriate analgesia and sedation have been shown to attenuate the stress response associated with critical illness, hastening recovery while lessening incidence and severity of complications. Nurses should assess each patient individually, and interventions including pharmacologic agents should be tailored to the patient and the setting. Nurses should regularly assess patient status, including response to interventions, and modify interventions as appropriate.

All pharmacologic agents used to provide analgesia, sedation, and neuromuscular blockade have potential side effects and complications, particularly a risk of respiratory depression and cardiovascular compromise. Risk may be higher in pediatric patients, especially when they are developmentally immature or medically fragile.[54] Ongoing patient monitoring is essential.

ANATOMY, PHYSIOLOGY, AND EMBRYOLOGY OF PAIN

Pain is a complex phenomenon, representing the interaction of many anatomic pathways, physiologic processes, and psychosocial factors. Pain has thus proven remarkably difficult to define, particularly in children. A widely accepted definition of pain is that suggested by the International Association for

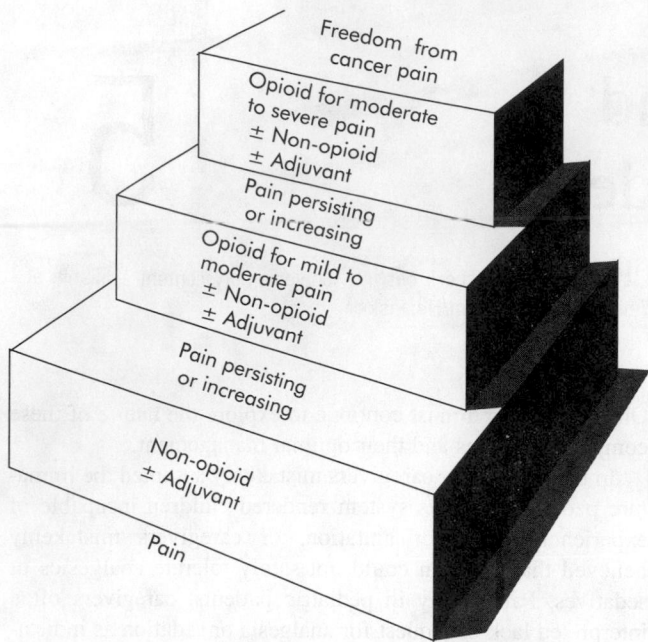

FIG. 5-1 The World Health Organization Analgesic Ladder. First described in 1986 for management of cancer pain, the World Health Organization Analgesic Ladder has since become a widely accepted paradigm for analgesia and sedation in patients of all ages and in all clinical settings. Interventions are provided concordant to severity of pain and agitation, with openness to adjuvant measures including nonpharmacologic interventions throughout. (With permission from: *Cancer pain relief and palliative care in children.* Companion volume to: *Cancer pain relief, with a guide to opioid availability.* Geneva 1998, World Health Organization. Available from: http://whqlibdoc.who.int/publications/9241545127.pdf. Accessed October 23, 2010.)

the Study of Pain: an unpleasant sensory and emotional experience associated with actual or potential tissue damage, or described in terms of such damage. This definition underscores the degree to which pain is a highly personal and subjective experience.

Clinical care of patients in pain is complicated by lack of objective indicators: no vital sign, radiologic study, or laboratory value can reliably quantify or even indicate pain.

FIG. 5-2 Simplified diagram of the neuroanatomy of nociception. 1, Transduction of painful stimuli occurs with activation of peripheral nociceptors. 2, Transmission along first-order primarily A-delta (δ) and c-fibers carries nociceptive input to the dorsal horn of the spinal cord, and from there via second- and third-order neurons, chiefly to the contralateral thalamus and cerebral cortex. 3, Perception occurs when pain becomes a conscious subjective experience. 4, Modulation can affect nociception at any point in this process, for example via descending inhibitory pathways. (From Lewis SM. *Medical-surgical nursing: assessment and management of clinical problems,* ed. 8, St. Louis, 2011, Mosby.)

Except perhaps in the setting of malingering or drug-seeking, rare in pediatric practice, the best clinical approach is usually to accept the patient's description or indication of pain as truthful and accurate, and to provide analgesia as appropriate.

Nociception

Nociception is the normal process through which pain is experienced (Fig. 5-2). Nerve pathways underlying pain sensation in humans are fully developed at term (see Anatomy, Physiology and Embryology of Pain in the Chapter 5 Supplement on the Evolve Website). Most pain in critically ill children is nociceptive in nature and tends to respond to conventional antinociceptive analgesics.

Nociception appears to involve four steps: transduction, transmission, perception, and modulation. *Transduction* refers to the initiation of pain sensation through activation of sensory nerve endings, or nociceptors. Stimulation above the nociceptor activation threshold causes depolarization of the nerve cell membrane, with subsequent propagation of a nerve impulse, or action potential, along the sensory nerve fiber. Nerve cell depolarization, propagation of the action potential, and subsequent repolarization all result from transmembrane flow of ions through channels in the nerve cell membrane.

Transmission refers to the propagation of a nerve impulse, or action potential, along sensory nerve fibers of the peripheral nervous system to the dorsal horn of the spinal cord, and from there to other locations in the central nervous system. Peripheral transmission relies primarily on two types of sensory nerve fibers, A-delta (δ) and c-fibers. A-delta fibers are larger, high-threshold, myelinated fast fibers that transmit fairly localized, acute, sharp pain. The c-fibers are smaller generalized-stimulus unmyelinated slow fibers that transmit less well-localized dull or aching pain. The c-fibers can remain stimulated, even after cessation of painful stimuli, and can play an important role in chronic pain.

Nociceptive sensory nerve fibers terminate in the dorsal horn of the spinal cord, where they synapse with dorsal horn nerve cells. The pain impulse is then carried toward the brain primarily via the spinothalamic tracts. These tracts receive input from sensory nerve fibers in laminae of the dorsal horn

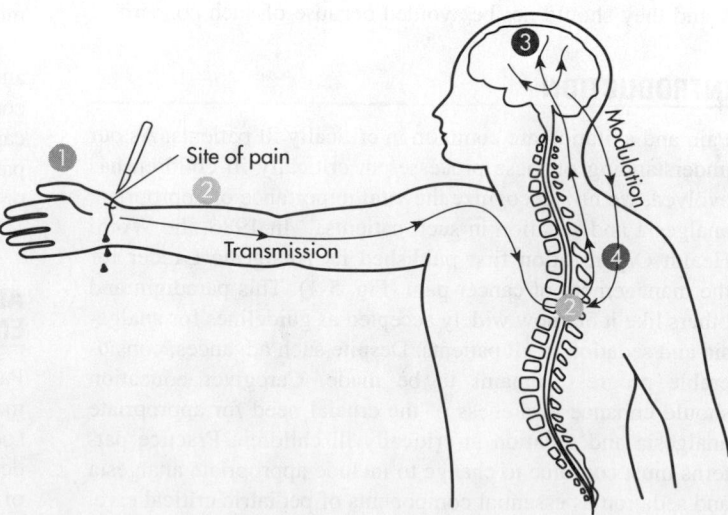

of the spinal cord, cross to contralateral spinal cord laminae, and ascend to the thalamus and other higher centers. Further transmission then occurs from the thalamus to the cerebral cortex with extensive cross-connections throughout the central nervous system.

Perception refers to the complex and poorly understood process by which pain becomes a conscious experience. Perception includes the physical sensation of noxious stimuli and the entire conscious experience of such stimuli with attendant emotional and behavioral components.[22] Perception is a unique process in each patient and is affected by age, developmental maturity, and underlying medical condition. Perception is also a highly dynamic process, varying among patients and in the same patient at different times.

Modulation refers to modification of pain by other nervous system input. Modulation can ameliorate or exacerbate pain and may explain some of the tremendous variability in subjective pain experience, especially in children. Modulation is a highly complex process and can take place at any point in transduction, transmission, and perception. A particularly important modulatory pathway is the descending pain system, with nerve axons projecting from the brainstem and other supraspinal centers to various laminae of the spinal cord. These descending fibers inhibit transmission of painful sensory stimuli, enhancing analgesia. Anxiety can also modulate pain, causing increased sensitivity to pain and resultant pain-related disability, particularly in chronic pain.[40]

Hypersensitization and Preemptive Analgesia

Acute pain warns of actual or potential tissue injury. Persistent or severe pain, however, can contribute to adverse processes. Inadequately treated surgical pain may impair breathing and compromise pulmonary toilet, promoting inadequate ventilation, atelectasis, and pneumonia. Pain also induces a neuroendocrine stress response, increasing sympathetic activity and releasing stress hormones and inflammatory mediators. The resultant hypermetabolic, catabolic state may be complicated by impaired immune function that can increase morbidity and mortality.

Tissue injury and inflammation potentiate nociceptor activity, leading to hypersensitivity to painful stimuli. Dorsal horn neurons respond to sustained afferent stimulation with neurophysiologic and morphologic changes consistent with increased excitability. Hypersensitization can alter normal sensory perception, accentuate pain caused by stimuli, and even produce pain in response to normally innocuous stimuli, suggesting that hypersensitization at the cellular level correlates with clinical hypersensitivity to pain.

Administration of preemptive analgesia before tissue injury can inhibit nociception, blunting neuroendocrine stress response and preventing development of peripheral and central hypersensitization. General anesthesia alone is not sufficient for such purposes; nonsteroidal antiinflammatory drugs (NSAIDs), opioids, and a variety of regional anesthetic techniques have been used with variable results. Although animal models suggest that preemptive analgesia decreases overall pain severity and duration, clinical human studies have yielded conflicting and frequently negative results, particularly in children. As a result, preemptive analgesia as a strategy for blunting hypersensitization and reducing pain remains a subject of ongoing investigation. Timing of analgesia appears less important than its administration.

Classification of Pain

Pain is often classified temporally as acute or chronic, anatomically as somatic or visceral, and pathophysiologically as nociceptive or neuropathic (Table 5-1). Such classifications are not mutually exclusive; clinical presentations may suggest considerable overlap, and clear distinctions are not always possible.

Temporal Classification of Pain

Pain can be classified temporally as acute or chronic. Acute pain persists for an expected duration, often hours to days. Many medical illnesses and surgical procedures are associated with acute pain of fairly predictable duration with subsequent resolution. Acute pain can be somatic or visceral (see section, Anatomic Classification of Pain). Acute pain in children is most commonly nociceptive, although acute neuropathic pain may be encountered.

Chronic pain refers to any pain of prolonged duration, often weeks to months or greater. Chronic pain can persist after apparent resolution of any underlying painful process; it can be somatic or visceral. Chronic pain may be nociceptive or neuropathic, although it is often considered more likely to include a neuropathic component. Particularly with ongoing duration, chronic pain often evolves from a symptom to a syndrome in and of itself.

Anatomic Classification of Pain

Pain can be classified anatomically as somatic or visceral. Somatic pain arises in the periphery, for example in cutaneous or musculoskeletal structures, and is transmitted to the dorsal horn of the spinal cord primarily by peripheral A-delta (δ) or

Table 5-1 **Classifications of Pain**

Temporal Classification*

Acute Pain	Chronic Pain
Expected duration, often hours to days	Prolonged duration, often weeks to months
Somatic or visceral	Somatic or visceral
More commonly nociceptive	Nociceptive or neuropathic

Anatomic Classification

Somatic Pain	Visceral Pain
Originates in somatic innervation of periphery	Originates in autonomic innervation of viscera
Acute or chronic	Acute or chronic
Nociceptive or neuropathic	Nociceptive or neuropathic

Pathophysiologic Classification

Nociceptive Pain	Neuropathic Pain
Result of normal nervous system function	Associated with nervous system dysfunction
Acute or chronic	More commonly chronic
Somatic or visceral	More commonly somatic
Typically responds to conventional analgesics	Responds poorly to conventional analgesics

*Classifications are not mutually exclusive: clinical presentations frequently suggest considerable overlap, and clear distinctions are not always possible.

c-fibers. Given the precise topography of somatic nerve fibers, somatic pain is typically fairly well localized. Superficial somatic pain originates in more external structures such as skin (cutaneous pain), and is more often described as sharp or stabbing. Deep somatic pain originates in more internal structures such as bone and is more often described as throbbing or aching. Somatic pain can be acute or chronic and nociceptive or neuropathic.

Visceral pain arises in visceral organs, particularly capsules or mesentery, and is transmitted to the dorsal horn of the spinal cord by autonomic c-fibers. Topography of visceral sympathetic innervation is less precise than for somatic structures, and visceral parasympathetic innervation projects to the central nervous system through parasympathetic ganglia. Visceral pain thus tends to be more diffuse than somatic pain; precise localization may be difficult, particularly in children. Visceral pain is more often described as dull, throbbing, squeezing or gnawing. Visceral pain may be acute or chronic and nociceptive or neuropathic.

Pathophysiologic Classification of Pain

Pain can be classified pathophysiologically as nociceptive or neuropathic. Nociceptive pain typically begins as an acute process, but can become chronic. It can be somatic or visceral. Most pain in critically ill children is nociceptive.

Temporally, neuropathic pain is more commonly considered a chronic process, but acute neuropathic pain may occur. Neuropathic pain is typically somatic, although visceral neuropathic pain is possible. Neuropathic pain may be localized to a recognizable peripheral nerve or dermatomal distribution, or it may involve multiple areas.

Neuropathic Pain

Neuropathic pain is thought to arise from nervous system dysfunction, although underlying pathophysiologic mechanisms are incompletely understood. Hypersensitivity of sensory nerve fibers causing repetitive depolarization has been proposed, as has wind-up hyperexcitability of dorsal horn neurons secondary to prolonged noxious stimuli. Subjective reporting of neuropathic pain is frequently disproportionate to observed physical findings and to objective assessment of patient comfort. Neuropathic pain can be described as a more intermittent shock-like, shooting, radiating, or stabbing pain, or a more constant burning, prickling, tingling, or aching pain. These descriptors often overlap.

Neuropathic pain often responds poorly to conventional antinociceptive analgesics, but may respond favorably to other medications, particularly some anticonvulsants and some antidepressants. Aggressive physical rehabilitation services and ongoing mental healthcare are often helpful, particularly for chronic neuropathic pain.

Phantom or deafferentation pain is a variant of neuropathic pain associated with central nervous system dysfunction following disruption of peripheral sensory input. Phantom pain can occur long after denervation of affected areas and may persist chronically or even permanently. Phantom pain may be seen following traumatic or surgical amputation and has even been described after dental extraction.[46] The pathophysiology of phantom pain is complex and incompletely understood.

Complex regional pain syndrome (CRPS) is a variant of neuropathic pain associated with autonomic dysfunction. Signs can include changes in skin color or appearance, alterations in hair distribution or texture, and eventually musculocutaneous atrophy. CRPS pain may be associated with prior nerve injury (CRPS type 2, formerly referred to as *causalgia*) or may be idiopathic (CRPS type 1, formerly referred to as *reflex sympathetic dystrophy*). The pathophysiology of CRPS is complex and poorly understood, and a significant psychosocial component is often present.

PATIENT ASSESSMENT

Recognition and treatment of pain and agitation can be particularly challenging in the absence of reliable objective quantitative assessments on which to base clinical decisions. Patient descriptions can guide analgesic and sedative interventions. However, even verbal children may find it difficult to express this information, particularly in the setting of critical illness. Children may be nonverbal or otherwise incommunicative secondary to age, developmental immaturity, medical illness, surgical procedures, or interventions such as intubation. Caregivers must recognize patient behaviors or behavioral patterns that provide clues to the presence, location, severity, and even cause of pain and agitation, and must monitor changes to guide therapy. No single objective assessment strategy will be sufficient or appropriate for every patient in every setting.[31]

Pain, particularly when acute, may produce evidence of increased sympathetic tone, the so-called fight-or-flight response. This response includes pupil dilation, tachycardia, hypertension, alteration in respiratory pattern, hyperglycemia, and change in emotional state. These indicators, however, are not sensitive in discriminating pain from other sources of distress, and do not reliably quantify or even indicate pain. Limited evidence supports the use of vital signs as indicators of pain, but only in the context of acute onset or acute increase in pain. Significant pain may be present without physiologic evidence of distress.

A common cause of inadequate analgesia and sedation is failure of the caregiver to accept and act on the patient report of pain and agitation. Although the patient report must always be taken in context, it is the most reliable assessment of patient experience and should be considered the standard for patient assessment. Caregivers must respect any patient report of pain and agitation, performing timely assessment and providing appropriate treatment.

In the absence of a patient report, caregivers must perform regular and appropriate objective assessments. Caregiver reliance on subjective impression, gut feeling, or personal belief introduces significant potential for variation and bias among caregivers, often leading to inconsistent or inadequate analgesia and sedation.

Patient or family fears and beliefs can hinder adequate analgesia and sedation. Patients or families may not wish to bother busy nursing staff. Children may deny distress, fearing painful injections or unpalatable oral preparations. Patients or families may hope to facilitate early discharge by minimizing reports of pain or agitation, or by limiting requests for analgesia and sedation. Distress may be regarded as a sign of weakness or failure. Fear of side effects, in particular addiction, leads many patients and families to avoid even appropriate analgesia and sedation. Nurses should address these concerns directly and provide education as necessary.

Caregiver fears and beliefs may also hinder adequate analgesia and sedation. Caregivers may fear providing unnecessary analgesia or sedation, particularly controlled substances. They may misinterpret regulations and legal requirements associated with these medications, or may fear promoting patient addiction. In terminal or palliative care settings, caregivers may fear hastening or even causing death. These issues must be addressed within the healthcare team (see Chapter 3).

Nurses should seek accurate and thorough information from the patient, family, and other caregivers to clarify onset, nature, severity, and time course of pain and agitation, as well as response to interventions. This history is particularly important when patients receive significant pharmacologic analgesia or sedation that can produce tolerance. What has helped? What has been ineffective or made things worse? Do interventions provide complete or only partial relief? How long does relief persist? Incomplete relief can suggest a need for additional interventions or increased medication dose, whereas complete but transient relief may suggest a need for more frequent or longer-acting interventions. The psychosocial component of pain and agitation can be significant, and nurses should assess available social and emotional support systems.

Regulatory guidelines and legal mandates require that patient care regimens be reviewed and reconciled at admission, at transfer of location or level of care, and at discharge. This helps ensure accuracy and efficacy of interventions, and it is particularly important when critically ill children transition to care settings where previous interventions may be unavailable. Continuation of medications at equipotent doses without inadvertent omission or unnecessary addition helps maintain analgesia and sedation while minimizing the risk of inadequate or excessive dosing.

Pediatric Pain Behavior

Patient behaviors or behavioral patterns can provide powerful clues to the presence, location, severity, and even cause of pain and agitation. Changes in patient behaviors or behavioral patterns may help guide analgesic and sedative interventions. Pain and agitation can be difficult to recognize even in healthy children who are young or developmentally immature; recognition in critically ill children may be complicated by the child's illness or interventions.

Agitation itself can indicate pain. Children in pain are often restless and cannot be easily distracted. They may cry or fuss, have a short attention span, or fail to respond to previously effective interventions. Facial expression can indicate pain; infants in particular may fail to make or hold eye contact. Children often hold or guard painful body parts rigidly. Pain can produce sleep disturbance, anxiety, nausea, anorexia, and lethargy. Pain—particularly when chronic—may precipitate profound changes in affect and emotional state. Formal psychiatric diagnoses such as anxiety disorder, acute or posttraumatic stress disorder, and major depression are frequently associated with chronic pain. Critical illness itself can produce many of these same behaviors.

Pediatric pain behaviors may be affected by psychosocial stressors and other factors, varying considerably among children or in the same child over time. Children in pain may be frightened or may exhibit developmental regression. Some children may seek attention through dramatic or disruptive behavior; others may be conditioned by gender or parental admonishment to be stoic. Children may fear upsetting or disappointing family and caregivers by admitting distress, or may feel they are being punished. Parents and other caregivers can be valuable interpreters of pediatric behavior.

Sedation or sleep can be mistaken for comfort. Patients of all ages may sleep despite severe pain, particularly if the pain is chronic. Pain itself can induce a state of decreased interaction that inaccurately suggests adequate analgesia. Critical illness and its treatment often exact a tremendous physiologic and emotional toll on patients. The resultant fatigue can produce decreased responsiveness to stimuli including pain. The nurse must consider overall patient status, combining data from assessment tools and other behavioral evaluation as appropriate.

Assessment Tools

Assessment tools typically are scales that can help to quantify pain and agitation in many clinical settings. However, the numeric scores generated must not be taken in isolation; they represent one component of comprehensive patient evaluation, just as vital signs represent one component of physical assessment. Any score must be considered in overall clinical context.

Assessment tools generally rely on subjective patient report, or on objective caregiver evaluation of patients who are unable to provide subjective report. Many assessment tools of both types have been developed for and validated in children. Scores generated using one tool will not necessarily correlate directly with those obtained using another. Caregivers should select an assessment tool appropriate for the patient and use it consistently over time.

Subjective Patient Report

Assessment tools relying on a subjective patient report ask the patient to indicate status on a continuum. Pain scales commonly range from 0 (no pain) to 10 (maximum possible pain); sedation scales vary more widely. Verbal children who are able to count may simply be asked to indicate their pain score on a 0-10 scale. Interactive but nonverbal children, or children unable to count, may be asked to indicate their pain score on a continuum scale using colors, pictures of children, or drawings of faces that represent degrees of distress. Three such pain assessment tools commonly used in pediatric practice are the Oucher! (see Evolve Fig. 5-1 in the Chapter 5 Supplement on the Evolve Website), the McGrath Faces Pain Scale, and the Hicks Faces Pain Scale-Revised (Fig. 5-3). See Patient Assessment in the Chapter 5 Supplement on the Evolve Website.

Tools are also available to help children quantify their pain experience through activities such as counting poker chips (the Hester Poker Chip Scale) or coloring an outline drawing of a child (the Eland Color Tool). Use of such activity tools requires patient interaction and caregiver time that may be impractical in the critical care setting.

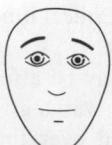 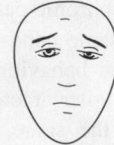 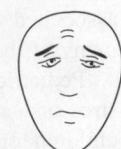 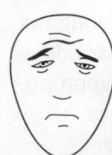 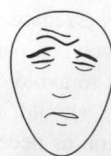 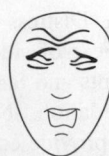

FIG. 5-3 A recently revised version of a faces scale for use in pediatric patients. Children are asked to point to the face best representing their pain, or for young children, how much they hurt. The six faces can be given scores (from left to right) of 0-2-4-6-8-10 or 0-1-2-3-4-5. Faces represented as more anatomically accurate oval cartoons have improved consistency in scores across diverse ethnic groups when compared to previous versions. The no-pain face is affect-neutral, reducing discrepancies between pain and agitation. (With permission from Hicks CL, et al: The Faces Pain Scale-Revised: toward a common metric in pediatric pain measurement. *Pain* 93:173–83, 2001. With permission from the International Association for the Study of Pain (IASP).)

Objective Caregiver Evaluation

When patients are unable to provide subjective reports, objective caregiver evaluation may be necessary. Although intrinsically less reliable than subjective patient report, objective caregiver evaluation may be the only means available to assess pain and agitation in many critically ill children. Objective caregiver evaluation may also be used judiciously to complement confusing or inconsistent patient reports.

Many assessment tools for objective caregiver evaluation of pain and agitation have been developed for and validated in the pediatric setting. Examples include the FLACC scale (characterizing the patient's *F*ace, *L*egs, *A*ctivity, *C*ry, *C*onsolability using specific options) for assessment of pain in nonverbal children (Table 5-2), the COMFORT scale (assessing overall comfort by evaluating specific physical characteristics) for assessment of agitation in critically ill children, and the State Behavioral Scale for assessment of agitation in infants and children during mechanical ventilation.[19] Examples of these tools may be found in Evolve Fig. 5-2 in the Chapter 5 Supplement on the Evolve Website. Additional tools have been reported for use in specific patient populations or particular clinical settings.[50]

Management Planning

With appropriate intervention, most critically ill children should experience little pain and minimal distress. Following comprehensive patient assessment, an appropriate management plan is developed to address patient pain and agitation.[48] The goals of any management plan should be to maximize analgesia and sedation, minimize side effects and complications, and if possible aid in diagnosis and treatment of underlying critical illness. Ideally, all caregivers should be involved in development of this plan and should be aware of planned interventions. During and after interventions, caregivers must perform regular and periodic patient reassessment to evaluate patient response and guide further interventions. Management must be individualized for each patient, combining nonpharmacologic and pharmacologic interventions as appropriate.

NONPHARMACOLOGIC INTERVENTIONS

Nonpharmacologic interventions are important adjuncts in pediatric analgesia and sedation. Because pain and agitation include significant cognitive and affective components, the child often

Table 5-2   FLACC Scale: Used for Assessment of Pain in Nonverbal Children

	SCORING		
Categories	**0**	**1**	**2**
Face	No particular expression or smile	Occasional grimace or frown; withdrawn, disinterested	Frequent to constant frown, clenched jaw, wavering chin
Legs	Normal position or relaxed	Uneasy, restless, tense	Kicking or legs drawn up
Activity	Lying quietly, normal position, moves easily	Squirming, shifting back and forth, tense	Arched, rigid, or jerking
Cry	No cry (awake or asleep)	Moans or whimpers, occasional complaint	Crying steadily, screams or sobs; frequent complaints
Consolability	Content, relaxed	Reassured by occasional touching, hugging, or being talked to; distractible	Difficult to console or comfort

Each of the five categories is scored from 0 to 2, resulting in a score between 0 and 10.
Original validation: Merkel S, et al: The FLACC: a behavioral scale for scoring postoperative pain in young children. *Pediatr Nurs* 23:293–297, 1997.
Validation in children with cognitive impairment: Voepel–Lewis T, et al: Reliability and validity of the FLACC observational tool as a measure of pain in children with cognitive impairment. *Anesth Analg* 95:1224–1229, 2002.
Revised FLACC validation: Malviya S, et al: The revised FLACC observational pain tool: improved reliability and validity for pain assessment in children with cognitive impairment. *Pediatr Anesthesia* 6:258–265, 2006.
Copyright © 2002, The Regents of the University of Michigan.

responds to cognitive interventions that invoke the child's imagination, suggestibility, and sense of play. Behavioral interventions help the child focus on relaxation and deep breathing rather than on the pain or painful stimulus. Biophysical modalities may affect nociceptive transmission and have a significant psychological component. Noninvasive and generally inexpensive, nonpharmacologic interventions can provide patients and families a sense of personal involvement in their care.

Family involvement in nonpharmacologic interventions often increases their effectiveness. Although the child may appear more distressed when family members are present, this may indicate that the child is more willing to express pain, fear and agitation in their presence. Children should receive positive reinforcement for engagement in nonpharmacologic interventions, but should never be punished or ridiculed for being frightened or uncooperative. Child Life specialists and other trained professionals, if available, provide valuable support.

Analgesia and sedation are generally optimized when appropriate treatment modalities are combined. For mild to moderate pain and agitation, nonpharmacologic interventions alone may suffice. For moderate to severe pain, nonpharmacologic interventions should complement, but not necessarily replace, pharmacologic therapy. Comprehensive care of critically ill children uses suitable nonpharmacologic techniques in combination with appropriate medications to optimize analgesia and sedation, minimize side effects, and facilitate recovery.

Cognitive and Behavioral Modalities

Cognitive and behavioral modalities are likely to enhance analgesia and sedation by influencing perception and modulation of pain at the supraspinal level. They also address cognitive and affective causes of anxiety. Cognitive modalities include distraction, relaxation and guided imagery, music therapy and hypnosis. Behavioral modalities include deep breathing and relaxation techniques. Cognitive and behavioral interventions are used most successfully in combination with other nonpharmacologic techniques and in conjunction with appropriate medications.

Preparation for Procedures

Preparation for and explanation of procedures will increase patient and family understanding, can help reduce fear of the unknown, and can enhance analgesia and sedation. Use may be limited by time and clinical conditions.

Honest and straightforward information should be provided in a manner and at a level appropriate for the child's age and psychosocial development. Anticipatory activities such as tours, coloring books, dolls, puppets, and play therapy may be used as time and clinical context allow. Suggestions for coping strategies should be provided, allowing children to practice such strategies and families to rehearse supportive roles. Children should be encouraged to express fears and concerns, and parents and other family members should be involved as appropriate.

Distraction

Simple distraction may significantly enhance analgesia and sedation. Distraction engages children in other activities, refocusing attention on something more pleasant. Distraction does not reduce intensity of noxious stimuli, but can modulate pain and lessen agitation, enhancing analgesia and sedation during the distracting activity. Pain and agitation will likely increase again when distraction ceases.

Distraction can take many forms, such as listening to music, talking about pets or school, blowing bubbles, squeezing hands, and singing or counting. The activity should be appropriate to patient age, developmental level, and interests. Children can be distracted by parents and other family members, in person or on recordings, or by favorite toys, books, and activities. Interactive computer and video games can provide distraction for children able to use them.

Relaxation and Guided Imagery

Relaxation and guided imagery can augment analgesia and sedation, and need not be complex to be effective. Bright lights, loud noises, and other potentially noxious stimuli should be minimized, although this can be challenging in the critical care setting. Soothing music and talking in a soft, calm voice can promote relaxation. Muscle tension intensifies distress and can be alleviated in older children by deep breathing and progressive relaxation exercises. Controlled breathing can be used alone or in combination with other techniques. Such techniques can enhance the child's feelings of control and involvement in care.

As a relaxation strategy, imagery encourages children capable of abstract thinking to focus on something unrelated to their pain and agitation. Imagery is a form of guided self-distraction, and is considered to be a variant of self-hypnosis. Children may also imagine medication traveling through the body to help them, super heroes attacking the source of distress, or other therapeutic scenarios. Imagery can be more effective if it enlists several senses. Guided imagery of playing at the beach might include imagining the touch of sand, the sound of waves, the warmth of sunshine, the smell of the ocean, and the taste of favorite foods as combined sensations.

Music Therapy

Music therapy can provide both distraction and relaxation in children. It has been used effectively in the operating room, postanesthesia care unit, neonatal critical care unit,[4,32] and oncology ward. Music choice should be based on patient age, culture, and preference, guided as necessary by parents, other family members, and friends. Listening to music through headphones offers the added benefit of masking chaotic auditory stimuli.

Hypnosis

Hypnosis capitalizes on a child's prolific imagination and high degree of suggestibility to induce a hypnotic state in which pain and agitation are lessened. Hypnosis has been successful with pediatric oncology patients, in pediatric emergency departments, and for treatment of children with burns or sickle cell disease. When combined with guided imagery, hypnosis has been shown to decrease pain scores, reduce patient anxiety, and shorten duration of hospitalization in pediatric surgical patients. Hypnosis requires specific training and expertise. Sufficient time and an appropriate setting can be elusive in the critical care setting.

Biophysical Modalities

Biophysical modalities are thought to affect nociceptive transmission at or below the level of the spinal cord, although precise mechanisms of action are incompletely understood. These modalities may also have a significant psychological component. Many modalities may be more effective when combined. Use of biophysical modalities is limited by time and logistical constraints, and some require specific training or equipment.

Cutaneous and Oral Stimulation

Many children respond positively to touch, particularly from parents or other loved ones. Positioning family members as close to the bedside as feasible will facilitate ongoing physical contact. Some parents may need to be encouraged to hold or touch their critically ill child. Pleasant cutaneous stimulation, such as stroking, patting, or massaging produces muscle relaxation and may reduce pain and agitation. Massage therapy has been shown to reduce pain associated with dressing changes in pediatric burn patients. Infants can be soothed with pleasant cutaneous stimulation such as gentle rubbing of the head, and they respond particularly well to pacifiers and other oral stimulation. Sugar water provides analgesia for infants undergoing painful procedures such as heel stick blood collection, and is synergistic with pacifier use. When family members perform these techniques, they provide emotional benefits and promote family-centered care.

Cold and Heat Therapy

Cold and heat therapy are cutaneous stimulation techniques. Cooling enhances analgesia by reducing inflammation and slowing nociceptive transmission. Examples include rubbing ice above and below an injury and applying ice or ethyl chloride spray before injection or venipuncture. Monitor the treated area and the child's response, and avoid excessive cooling that can cause skin irritation, cellular injury, and frostbite.

Heat promotes circulation, relaxes muscles, and reduces stiffness. Heat application before venipuncture promotes vasodilation and can reduce pain. Hydrotherapy, often used by physical therapists, combines the benefits of heat with those of water immersion, but can be difficult to provide in the critical care setting. Monitor the treated area, and avoid excessive heating that can cause skin irritation, cellular injury, and burns.

Transcutaneous Electrical Nerve Stimulation (TENS)

TENS delivers weak electrical current to the skin through superficial electrodes. TENS may modulate nociceptive transmission at the spinal cord level, and may also induce release of endorphins and other endogenous neurotransmitters, similar to acupuncture. TENS has been used effectively for children undergoing venipuncture or dressing changes, and it has been used as an adjunctive modality in pediatric chronic pain management. TENS may be particularly useful for treatment of musculoskeletal and myofascial pain. Physical therapists typically oversee TENS therapy and provide instruction for patients and families. TENS is usually well tolerated by patients old enough to understand its use, although some children may find the tingling sensation unpleasant.

Acupuncture

Acupuncture is gaining acceptance and is practiced by both physicians and licensed acupuncturists in the United States. The precise mechanisms of action are incompletely understood. Acupuncture may precipitate release of endorphins, encephalins, serotonin, and other endogenous neurotransmitters, inhibiting nociceptive pathways and enhancing analgesia. Pediatric acupuncture has been used primarily as adjunctive therapy to treat chronic pain. The practice of acupuncture requires specific training.

SYSTEMIC ANALGESICS

Numerous systemic analgesics are available for use in children (Table 5-3). Systemic analgesics can have a wide range of physiologic effects, particularly in critically ill children. Knowledge of the agents being administered is essential for optimal efficacy and patient safety. Nurses must be aware of expected clinical effect, usual time of onset, likely duration, and potential side effects of each agent administered. Medications ordered on an as-needed basis are effective only when given appropriately with ongoing and recurring patient assessment. Frequent requirement for a drug ordered only on an as needed basis should prompt consideration of scheduled administration and additional interventions. Intramuscular injection is painful and absorption variable; it should be avoided except perhaps in the setting of difficult intravenous access. Although

Table 5-3 Systemic Analgesics

Drug	Dose	Comments
Acetaminophen		
Acetaminophen and NSAIDs are generally synergistic and may be given together without need to alternate or stagger doses.		
Acetaminophen	Load: 20 mg/kg PO (maximum 1000 mg), then	Good antipyretic; hepatic toxicity with overdose
	Main: 15 mg/kg PO (maximum 1000 mg) q4-6 h	Loading dose especially useful for procedural or perioperative analgesia
	Load: 40 mg/kg PR (maximum 1300 mg), then	FDA now advises maximum single adult dose of 650 mg
	Main: 20 mg/kg PR (maximum 1300 mg) q4-6 h	for over-the-counter use
	Maximum 4 g/24 h PO/PR	
Nonsteroidal Antiinflammatory Drugs (NSAIDs)		
Acetaminophen and NSAIDs are generally synergistic, and may be given together without the need to alternate or stagger doses.		
Choline magnesium trisalicylate	10 mg/kg PO/PR (maximum 1500 mg) q6-8 h	Only NSAID without platelet dysfunction
	Maximum 4 g/24 h PO/PR	No association with Reye syndrome

Table 5-3 **Systemic Analgesics—cont'd**

Drug	Dose	Comments
Ibuprofen	10 mg/kg PO/PR (maximum 800 mg) q6-8 h IV: 10 mg/kg (for pain) Maximum 3200 mg/24 h PO/PR	Good antipyretic (IV dose: 5 mg/kg may be used for antipyretic) IV formula recently approved analgesic in adults
Ketorolac	0.5 mg/kg IM/IV (maximum 30 mg) q6 h Total therapy must be <5 days	Potentially significant platelet dysfunction

Lower Potency Oral Opioids

Recommended doses are for initial administration in opioid-naïve patients: titration to clinical effect is required; recommended initial opioid doses should typically be reduced 35% to 50% in neonates and young infants.

Drug	Dose	Comments
Codeine	1 mg/kg PO q4 h (adult dose, 30-60 mg)	Tablet and liquid preparations typically in combination with acetaminophen High incidence of gastrointestinal side effects
Hydrocodone	0.2 mg/kg PO q4 h (adult dose, 10-15 mg)	Tablet and liquid preparations typically in combination with acetaminophen or NSAID Moderate incidence of gastrointestinal side effects Sustained-release product available as antitussive, under study as analgesic
Oxycodone	0.1 mg/kg PO q4 h (adult dose, 5-10 mg)	Tablet preparations with or without acetaminophen or NSAID Liquid preparations contain only oxycodone Low incidence of gastrointestinal side effects Sustained-release product available for chronic therapy

Higher Potency Opioids

Recommended doses are for initial administration in opioid-naïve patients: titration to clinical effect is required; recommended initial opioid doses should typically be reduced 25% to 50% in neonates and young infants; PCA demand dose typically q 8-10 min for patient-controlled analgesia, q 15-60 min for nurse or parent-controlled analgesia.

Drug	Dose	Comments
Fentanyl	5-15 mcg/kg PO (adult dose 400 mcg) 0.5-2 mcg/kg IV (adult dose 100 mcg) q 1 h Infusion 0.5-2 mcg/kg per hour (adult dose 100 mcg/h) Patch 25 mcg = 1 mg/h IV morphine PCA demand dose 0.5-1 mcg/kg IV (adult dose 50-100 mcg) PCA basal 0.5-1 mcg/kg per hour IV (adult dose 50-100 mcg/h)	Dosing interval for oral preparation not well defined Rapid IV infusion may cause chest wall rigidity in infants Tachyphylaxis common Transdermal patch not for acute management
Hydromorphone	20-40 mcg/kg PO (adult dose 2-4 mg) q 3 h 10-20 mcg/kg IM/IV/SC (adult dose 1-2 mg) q 3 h Infusion 4 mcg/kg per h (adult dose 0.2-0.3 mg/h) PCA demand dose 4 mcg/kg IV (adult dose 0.2-0.3 mg) PCA basal 4 mcg/kg per hour IV (adult dose 0.2-0.3 mg/h)	Sustained-release oral product under study as analgesic Less histamine release than morphine
Meperidine	0.25-0.5 mg/kg IM/IV/SC (adult dose 12.5-25 mg) Infusion/PCA not recommended	Doses for treatment of shivering Neurotoxic metabolite may induce seizures No hepatobiliary advantage over any other opioid No longer recommended as primary analgesic
Methadone	0.1 mg/kg PO (adult dose 5-10 mg) q6-12 h 0.05 mg/kg IV (adult dose 2.5-5 mg) q6-12 h Infusion/PCA not generally used	Useful for chronic therapy Treatment of addiction must be in federally licensed facility
Morphine	0.3 mg/kg PO (adult dose 15-30 mg) q3 h 0.05-0.1 mg/kg IM/IV/SC (adult dose: 5-10 mg) q3 h Infusion 0.02 mg/kg per h (adult dose 1-1.5 mg/h) PCA demand dose, 0.02 mg/kg IV (adult dose 1-1.5 mg) PCA basal 0.02 mg/kg per hour IV (adult dose 1-1.5 mg/h)	Sustained-release oral product available for chronic therapy Potentially significant histamine release

FDA, U.S. Food and Drug Administration; *h*, hour; *IM*, intramuscular; *IV*, intravenous; *Load*, loading dose; *Main*, maintenance dose; *mcg*, microgram; *PCA*, patient-controlled analgesia; *PO*, by mouth; *PR*, by rectum; *q*, every; *SC*, subcutaneous.

many systemic analgesics can produce sedation, they should not be used primarily for this purpose.

Nonopioid Analgesics

Often overlooked, nonopioid analgesics are important pharmacologic options. Nonopioid analgesics alone may be adequate for mild to moderate pain and generally reduce opioid requirement in moderate to severe pain. Nonopioid analgesics generally demonstrate a ceiling effect: exceeding recommended doses does not significantly improve analgesia, but will increase risk of side effects and toxicity. As with nonpharmacologic interventions, nonopioid analgesics are most effective in the context of a comprehensive management plan. Commonly used nonopioid analgesics include acetaminophen and NSAIDs; ketamine is discussed with other systemic sedatives.

Acetaminophen

Acetaminophen is widely used as an analgesic and an antipyretic. It can provide complete analgesia for mild to moderate pain and may reduce opioid requirement in moderate to severe pain, particularly when given on a scheduled basis. Acetaminophen is not an NSAID. Although it is a cyclooxygenase inhibitor, it has virtually no antiinflammatory activity, and therefore has few gastrointestinal, renal, or hematologic side effects. The primary toxicity of acetaminophen is hepatic, seen with both acute and chronic overdose, although renal toxicity has been described.[42]

Acetaminophen is at least as effective an analgesic as codeine,[12] and it is synergistic with NSAIDs.[52] Acetaminophen and NSAIDs can be given simultaneously without need to alternate or stagger doses. As with most nonopioid analgesics, acetaminophen demonstrates a ceiling effect: exceeding recommended doses does not significantly improve analgesia and increases risk of side effects and toxicity. Recently, an FDA advisory committee recommended the maximum single adult dose for over-the-counter products be reduced to 650 mg because of risk of hepatic injury.[24]

Rectal acetaminophen is useful for a patient who is unwilling or unable to tolerate an oral dose. Because rectal absorption is slower and bioavailability is more variable than with oral administration, higher rectal doses are needed for adequate analgesia. Rectal acetaminophen with a loading dose of at least 40 mg/kg has been shown to reduce pain scores and reduce opioid requirement following surgery in children.

Nonsteroidal Antiinflammatory Drugs

Like acetaminophen, NSAIDs can provide complete analgesia for mild to moderate pain and can reduce opioid requirement in moderate to severe pain, particularly when given on a scheduled basis. NSAIDs are often particularly effective for musculoskeletal pain. Because NSAIDs have significant antiinflammatory activity, they can produce gastrointestinal, renal, and hematologic side effects. Risk of side effects is greater with higher dose or prolonged administration, and with certain agents. NSAIDs reduce splanchnic and renal perfusion, potentially predisposing to gastrointestinal ulcers and renal insufficiency. Most NSAIDs impair platelet function and may increase risk of bleeding. Acetaminophen and NSAIDs are generally synergistic and can be given simultaneously without need to stagger doses. As with most nonopioid analgesics, NSAIDs demonstrate a ceiling effect: exceeding recommended doses does not significantly improve analgesia and does increase the risk of side effects and toxicity.

Aspirin is no longer considered a routine primary analgesic in children. Aspirin induces potent inhibition of platelet function through irreversible acetylation of platelet cyclooxygenase. Anticoagulation persists for several days in patients with normal hepatic and hematopoietic function, until synthesis of new functional platelet cyclooxygenase. Pediatric aspirin use has declined dramatically in recent decades because of a described association with Reye syndrome in children with primary varicella and influenza. Although varicella vaccination has probably lessened such risk, aspirin use in infants and children is largely reserved for long-term anticoagulation, and in some cases for management of rheumatic disease.

The most widely used oral NSAID in children in the United States is ibuprofen, available in a variety of liquid, tablet, and capsule preparations. Intravenous ibuprofen, like intravenous indomethacin, is approved only for medical closure of patent ductus arteriosus in infants. Ibuprofen is a moderate potency analgesic and excellent antipyretic with an impressive pediatric safety record; it is underused for procedural and perioperative pain management in children. Ibuprofen is at least as effective an analgesic as acetaminophen, and it is superior to codeine.[12] Ibuprofen and acetaminophen are synergistic.[52] The liquid preparation can be given rectally at similar doses to patients unwilling or unable to tolerate oral doses.

Ketorolac is the only intravenous NSAID approved in the United States for use as an analgesic. Ketorolac is the most potent and most effective NSAID analgesic, with efficacy approaching that of many opioids. It provides superior postoperative analgesia compared with acetaminophen and other NSAIDs. However, it also has the highest incidence of side effects. Ketorolac is most commonly administered intravenously; oral ketorolac has not been approved for use in children. Total duration of ketorolac therapy must not exceed 5 days to avoid potentially serious gastrointestinal ulceration and renal insufficiency.

Significant platelet dysfunction can develop after a single dose of ketorolac, and its use in patients with risk for bleeding is controversial. Although initial experience suggested greater blood loss during tonsillectomy in children receiving perioperative ketorolac, prospective randomized trials showed only nonsignificant trends toward increased bleeding without clinical complications.[51a] It may be prudent to avoid ketorolac in patients at risk for bleeding until more definitive information is available.

Choline magnesium trisalicylate is unique among NSAIDs in not causing significant platelet dysfunction, and it can be useful in patients at risk for bleeding. Although it is an aspirin derivative, choline magnesium trisalicylate has no known association with Reye syndrome. Despite this apparent safety, it may be prudent to limit use of choline magnesium trisalicylate to children who have had documented varicella or received appropriate immunization. Choline magnesium trisalicylate is available in liquid and tablet preparations. The liquid preparation can be given rectally at similar dose to patients unwilling or unable to tolerate oral doses.

Opioid Analgesics

Opioids remain the mainstay of pharmacologic analgesia in patients of all ages. Acting on opioid receptors in the central nervous system and elsewhere, opioids cause dose-dependent analgesia and respiratory depression. Other side effects include somnolence, pupil constriction, decreased gastrointestinal motility, nausea, and urinary retention. Many opioids induce histamine release, causing urticaria, pruritus, nausea, bronchospasm, and occasionally hypotension. Pruritus is more common and typically more intense with neuraxial administration, likely caused by central nervous system opioid effect rather than histamine release. Opioid side effects can be managed with a variety of agents (Table 5-4).

The opioid antagonist naloxone rapidly reverses opioid effects. Naloxone may precipitate withdrawal in opioid-dependent patients, and pulmonary edema has been reported with higher doses. Low-dose naloxone infusion has been described for prevention and treatment of side effects secondary to ongoing opioid administration.[41] For treatment of opioid overdose, support of effective ventilation before naloxone administration may prevent excessive adrenergic response.

Several agents with mixed opioid agonist-antagonist activity are available; their ceiling effect theoretically limits side effects and improves safety, but also limits analgesia. Opioid agonists and antagonists, particularly nalbuphine, are often used for management of opioid-induced side effects, but are of limited utility as primary analgesics.

Opioid analgesics do not generally have maximum effective doses. Recommended doses are for initial administration in opioid-naive patients and must be titrated to clinical effect. Increasing dose requirement, also known as *tolerance* or *tachyphylaxis*, is often observed with ongoing administration. Opioid therapy longer than 7 to 10 days can result in physical dependence, requiring weaning to avoid withdrawal. Tolerance and dependence are separate phenomena. Addiction, a formal psychopathologic diagnosis of volitional drug-seeking behavior, rarely develops in children receiving appropriate opioid analgesia and is not a valid reason to withhold therapy.

Opioid analgesics are commonly administered in conjunction with systemic sedatives; this increases the risk of side effects, especially respiratory depression. Nurses should carefully titrate doses, provide appropriate monitoring, and keep resources to manage complications (including appropriate reversal agents) readily available.

Opioid use in neonates and young infants has generated much controversy. Historical studies in rats and humans suggested increased permeability of the neonatal blood-brain barrier to opioids, particularly morphine, producing greater respiratory depression (see additional references in the Chapter 5 Supplement on the Evolve Website). It is now clear that pharmacologic properties and clinical effects of opioids in human neonates are highly variable. In general, opioid clearance is decreased and elimination is prolonged in neonates, particularly premature infants, with values approaching adult levels by several months of life. Opioid-naive neonates and young infants receiving opioids should be monitored closely and initial doses generally reduced by 25% to 50%. There is no reason to withhold opioid therapy from any child on the basis of age, provided that doses are individualized and regimens titrated to clinical effect.

Meperidine (Demerol) is no longer recommended as a primary analgesic, although low-dose meperidine is useful for treatment of shivering. Meperidine otherwise offers no advantages over other opioids and causes similar hepatobiliary spasm at equipotent doses. Use of the lytic cocktail of meperidine, promethazine (Phenergan), and chlorpromazine (Thorazine), historically given by intramuscular injection to provide analgesia and sedation for minor procedures, is no longer recommended.

Table 5-4 **Agents for Management of Opioid Side Effects**

Side Effect	Agent	Dose	Comments
Apnea, coma	Naloxone	10-100 mcg/kg IV/IM q 1-2 min PRN Usual initial maximum 400 mcg	Resedation may occur Withdrawal in opioid-dependent patients Higher doses may cause pulmonary edema
Respiratory depression, mild sedation	Naloxone	1-2 mcg/kg IV/IM q 1-2 min PRN Usual initial maximum 400 mcg	Resedation may occur
Constipation	Docusate	5 mg/kg PO (maximum 100 mg) bid	Stool softener
Nausea	Metoclopramide	0.1 mg/kg IV (maximum 10 mg) q6 h PRN	Extrapyramidal side effects
	Ondansetron	0.1 mg/kg IV (maximum 4 mg) q6 h PRN (note: higher doses may be administered for chemotherapy-induced nausea and vomiting)	Relatively nonsedative
	Promethazine	0.25-0.5 mg/kg PO/PR/IV (maximum 25 mg) q6 h PRN	Avoid in children <2 years of age (FDA caution) Extravasation can cause severe tissue injury
Pruritus	Diphenhydramine	0.5-1 mg/kg PO/IV (maximum 50 mg) q6 h PRN	May induce somnolence
	Hydroxyzine	0.5-1 mg/kg PO/IM (maximum 50 mg) q6 h PRN	May induce somnolence
	Nalbuphine	0.05 mcg/kg IV (maximum 5 mg) q4 h PRN	With neuraxial opioid
	Naloxone	0.25-1 mcg/kg per hour IV infusion	With neuraxial opioid

bid, Twice per day; *IM*, intramuscular; *IV*, intravenous; *mcg*, microgram; *PO*, by mouth; *PR*, by rectum, *PRN*, as needed; *q*, every.

Oral Opioids

When analgesic requirements allow and gastrointestinal function permits, oral opioids offer freedom from parenteral therapy. Onset of action is generally slower than with IV administration, rendering oral opioid therapy generally unsuitable for acute management of severe pain. Several lower potency oral opioids are used commonly for management of mild to moderate pain in children. Higher potency opioids may also be given orally, particularly in patients with oncologic or other life-limiting disease.

Codeine is available in liquid and pill forms that commonly include acetaminophen. Codeine requires hepatic conversion to morphine for its analgesic effect and frequently causes considerable gastrointestinal upset. Most patients reporting allergy to codeine actually have gastrointestinal intolerance.

Immediate-release hydrocodone is available in liquid and pill forms, commonly in combination with acetaminophen or an NSAID. Sustained-release hydrocodone is available in liquid form as an antitussive cough suppressant, and a pill form is being evaluated as an analgesic. Hydrocodone tends to cause less gastrointestinal upset than codeine.

Immediate-release oxycodone is available in liquid form alone, and in pills with or without acetaminophen or an NSAID. Sustained-release oxycodone is available in pill form for chronic therapy. Oxycodone is generally well tolerated and causes little gastrointestinal upset, but has been associated with high rates of inappropriate use and diversion.

Immediate-release morphine is available in liquid and pill forms. Sustained-release morphine is available in pill forms for chronic therapy. Morphine induces histamine release and may cause nausea, urticaria, pruritus, bronchospasm, and even hypotension at higher doses, although these are more common with IV administration.

Immediate-release hydromorphone is available in liquid or pill form. Sustained-release hydromorphone in pill form is being evaluated as an analgesic. Hydromorphone causes less histamine release than morphine, and it is generally associated with fewer and less severe histamine-mediated side effects.

Methadone has prolonged onset and duration of action, making it poorly suited for management of acute or dynamic pain, but well suited for chronic therapy in patients with stable analgesic requirements. Use of methadone as an analgesic, or for weaning in the setting of tolerance or dependence, is appropriate and legal. Use of methadone for treatment of psychopathologic addiction is restricted to federally licensed facilities. Although methadone may cause Q-T prolongation and ventricular arrhythmias, particularly at higher doses, recent suggestions to consider screening electrocardiogram before and at intervals during methadone therapy[35,36] remain controversial.[27]

Fentanyl is available for oral administration as a lozenge attached to a stick, the so-called fentanyl lollipop. Oral fentanyl has been used for pre-anesthetic sedation in children, although it is no longer marketed for this indication. Oral fentanyl has more recently been used to provide analgesia and sedation for painful procedures, and for patients with breakthrough acute and chronic pain.[5] Nausea and emesis are fairly common. Intranasal fentanyl is increasingly used for management of acute pain in the emergency department[9] and for treatment of breakthrough pain in opioid-dependent oncology patients.[37] Onset of action is rapid with either route: analgesia and respiratory depression may develop quickly.

Intravenous Opioids

Intravenous opioids remain the mainstay of pharmacologic analgesia for moderate to severe pain in patients of all ages. Because subcutaneous and intramuscular administration can cause additional pain and distress, particularly in children, these routes are typically avoided unless there is difficulty in obtaining IV access. Side effects are more common and potentially more serious with intravenous opioids. Nurses must provide appropriate monitoring and promptly manage complications. Equipotent opioid doses entail similar risk of side effects; no single opioid is intrinsically superior or safer than another.

Morphine is the traditional intravenous opioid analgesic. Morphine induces histamine release and may cause nausea, urticaria, pruritus, bronchospasm, and even hypotension at higher doses, particularly with rapid administration. Hydromorphone tends to induce less histamine release than morphine. Methadone is generally more appropriate for chronic therapy in patients with stable analgesic requirements than for management of acute or dynamic pain, although intravenous methadone has been used successfully in pediatric surgical patients.

Fentanyl tends to cause little histamine release and has few hemodynamic effects, and it is widely used in the critical care setting. Fentanyl may induce mild bradycardia, and may cause potentially significant chest wall and abdominal rigidity, particularly with high dose or rapid administration and in infants. Opioid reversal or neuromuscular blockade may be required if chest wall rigidity prevents adequate ventilation. Fentanyl is highly lipophilic; high dose, repeated, or sustained administration results in significant tissue accumulation which may markedly prolong clinical effect.

Fentanyl is available as a transdermal patch providing continuous absorption that mimics intravenous infusion. Use in smaller patients is limited by dose, because the patches cannot be cut. Onset is slow (approximately 18 hours), and absorption may be variable. Like methadone, transdermal fentanyl is not indicated for acute analgesia, but is well suited for chronic therapy in patients with stable analgesic requirements.

Opioid infusion is an effective means of providing analgesia to patients requiring more than occasional doses of intravenous opioid. Respiratory depression is uncommon in healthy patients at suggested doses; opioid infusion should not prevent spontaneous ventilation or delay weaning from mechanical ventilatory support.

Nurses should frequently and regularly assess patients receiving opioid infusion. Nurses should evaluate adequacy of analgesia, level of sedation, and presence of respiratory depression or other side effects and titrate the infusion appropriately. Continuous pulse oximetry is recommended for patients receiving opioid infusion, at least when initiating the infusion and with any significant increase in regimen. Consider continuous cardiorespiratory monitoring for opioid-naive neonates and young infants.

Patient-Controlled Analgesia (PCA)

If an opioid is administered only after a patient reports pain, this can create a vicious cycle of suffering, a delay in drug administration, and resultant persistent pain or excessive sedation. Optimal opioid administration provides pain relief, but avoids respiratory depression or excessive sedation, preserving a balance between desired efficacy and undesired side effects (Fig. 5-4). Intermittent dosing is time-consuming for providers and frequently upsets this analgesic balance. Continuous infusion eventually establishes a drug level steady state, but is independent of patient request. A safe, effective, and readily titratable modality for ongoing opioid administration in children is PCA. PCA modalities maximize analgesia, minimize side effects, and reduce overall opioid consumption in patients of all ages.

Drug delivery in PCA is controlled by a microprocessor providing dose administration in response to patient or proxy request, usually with the press of a button. Appropriate lockout intervals and maximum doses are programmed to prevent overdose. Analgesia is generally excellent. With adequate instruction, most developmentally appropriate school-aged children can safely and effectively manage their own PCA. Nurse- or parent-controlled PCA, so-called PCA by proxy, can be used for children who are unable or unwilling to control their own pump, although the risk of respiratory depression increases if dosing intervals are not adjusted, particularly in combination with basal infusions. Prevalence of complications during PCA by proxy is similar to that during conventional PCA, although serious complications may be more common.[60]

Morphine is the most common opioid for PCA, but hydromorphone and fentanyl are also used. Meperidine PCA is not recommended. Methadone PCA has been described in pediatric cancer patients with significant opioid requirement and tolerance to other agents. PCA regimens typically allow demand dose administration every 8 to 10 minutes for patient-controlled administration, or every 15 to 60 minutes for PCA by proxy. Longer dosing intervals may be safer in younger or medically fragile patients. Simultaneous basal infusion can be provided to ensure ongoing analgesia, but does not reliably improve analgesia in most patients. PCA basal infusions in adults increase the risk of respiratory complications, but this has not been observed in children. Basal infusion, if used, should be concordant with demand dose.

Nurses should assess patients receiving opioid via PCA frequently and regularly. The nurse should evaluate adequacy of analgesia, level of sedation, and presence of respiratory depression and other side effects and titrate the regimen appropriately. Consider pulse oximetry for all patients and continuous cardiorespiratory monitoring for opioid-naive neonates and young infants. Instruct patients, families, and caregivers regarding appropriate PCA use.

LOCAL ANESTHETICS

Local anesthetics impair nerve conduction through the blockade of nerve cell sodium channels. Local anesthetics are potentially neurotoxic, altering level of consciousness or inducing seizures if therapeutic levels are exceeded. Local anesthetics are also potentially cardiotoxic and may induce arrhythmias including ventricular tachycardia, ventricular fibrillation, and cardiac arrest. Prolonged resuscitation after local anesthetic overdose may be required, particularly with long-acting agents. Recent reports suggest that administration of intravenous lipid emulsion increases the likelihood of successful resuscitation after local anesthetic toxicity, perhaps by serving as a binding reservoir.[25]

Lidocaine and bupivacaine are the most commonly used local anesthetics in pediatric practice. Lidocaine provides dense analgesia, but has a relatively short duration of action and often induces motor block. In topical preparations, lidocaine is commonly combined with prilocaine, which can cause methemoglobinemia, particularly in large doses or small patients. Bupivacaine is widely used because of its long duration of action and relative selectivity for sensory over motor block. Bupivacaine is highly cardiotoxic, with similar thresholds for cardiac and neurologic toxicity: arrhythmias can occur before obtundation or seizures are noted.

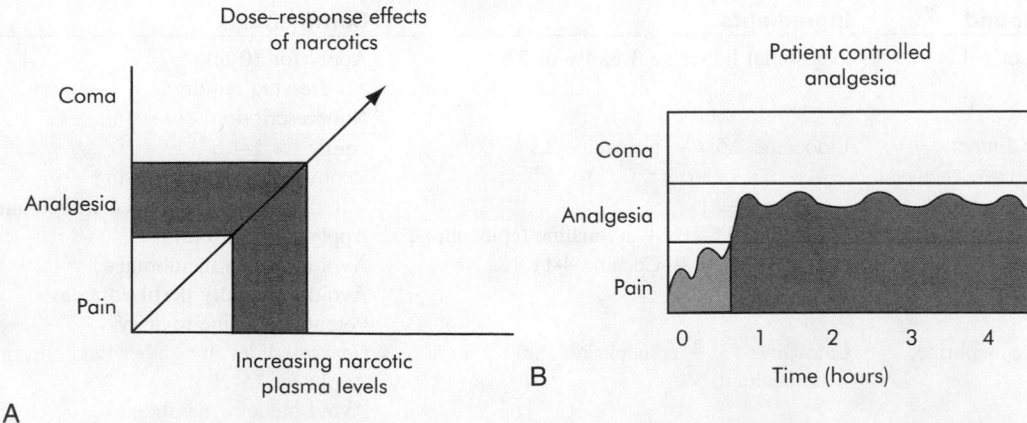

FIG. 5-4 Opioid analgesic window. **A,** Idealized illustration of continuum of opioid effect from pain to analgesia to coma. **B,** Optimal therapy, as in patient-controlled analgesia, maintains plasma opioid levels within the middle (Analgesia) third of the graph representing the analgesic window between inadequate analgesia (Pain) and excessive sedation (Coma). (With permission from Berde CB: Pediatric postoperative pain management. *Pediatr Clin North Am* 36:921–940, 1989. Copyright Elsevier 1989.)

Two newer agents, levobupivacaine and ropivacaine, are potentially less toxic alternatives to bupivacaine. Levobupivacaine, the L-isomer of bupivacaine, induces conduction block similar to bupivacaine, with a somewhat higher threshold for cardiotoxicity. Ropivacaine has somewhat greater selectivity for sensory over motor block than does bupivacaine, also with a somewhat higher threshold for cardiotoxicity. The use of these newer agents is limited primarily by cost.

Local anesthetics provide analgesia by blocking conduction in sensory nerve fibers; they are given through direct infiltration, topical application, or regional anesthetic techniques. Local anesthetics can reduce or even eliminate the need for systemic analgesics, and may be particularly useful in patients with increased sensitivity to opioids, including neonates and children with underlying neurologic or respiratory disease. In pediatric practice, this theoretical advantage is somewhat offset by the frequent requirement for sedation or general anesthesia to tolerate local anesthetic administration. Some children will require supplementary systemic analgesia despite apparently successful local anesthesia. This may result from apprehension and variability in developmental and emotional maturity.

Infiltration

Direct infiltration of local anesthetic is technically straightforward and provides rapid onset of analgesia. Use in children is limited largely by their fear of needles and pain associated with injection. Nonpharmacologic interventions and systemic sedatives may be used as appropriate. Initial cutaneous analgesia may be obtained by topical application if time and clinical context permit. The acidic pH of many local anesthetic solutions enhances solubility and prolongs shelf life, but is largely responsible for injection pain. Simple pH buffering with small volumes of sodium bicarbonate added to local anesthetic solutions immediately before use helps reduce such pain and may increase efficacy.

Topical Application

Many local anesthetics are formulated to provide cutaneous analgesia without the need for potentially painful injections (Table 5-5). Such preparations enhance usefulness of topical anesthetics for minor procedures, and in many instances they reduce or eliminate the need for supplementary systemic analgesia and sedation. The use of topical formulas is limited primarily by cost and time of onset. Specific agents are discussed in Local Anesthetics, Topical Application in the Chapter 5 Supplement on the Evolve Website.

Regional Anesthetic Techniques

The use of regional anesthetic techniques is expanding in the operating room and beyond. These techniques enhance surgical anesthesia and can provide excellent procedural and perioperative pain management for children, potentially reducing the requirement for systemic analgesia and sedation. Regional anesthesia may have a lower risk of adverse effects (e.g., nausea, sedation, respiratory depression) than systemic opioids; in some settings they have been shown to improve outcomes. Analgesia may persist for hours to days or more depending on the medications and technique. Regional anesthetic techniques commonly used in children include a variety of peripheral nerve, plexus, and neuraxial blocks.

Peripheral Nerve Blocks

Virtually any peripheral nerve can be blocked with appropriate equipment and sufficient provider interest. Typically, a small volume of local anesthetic is injected adjacent to the appropriate nerve or nerves to provide anesthesia in the desired distribution. For additional information about these blocks, please see Regional Anesthetic Techniques in the Chapter 5 Supplement on the Evolve Website.

Plexus Blocks

Pediatric providers are gaining experience with plexus blocks, including brachial plexus,[21] lumbosacral, and paravertebral blocks. Intravenous regional anesthesia of the extremities, or

Table 5-5   Topical Local Anesthetics

Product/Compound	Ingredients	Comments
Lidocaine cream or gel	Liposomal lidocaine 3%, 4% or 5%	Apply for 30 min No dressing required Nonprescription
EMLA (generic): Eutectic mixture of local anesthetics	Lidocaine 2.5% + prilocaine 2.5%	Apply for 1-4 h Requires occlusive dressing Prilocaine may cause methemoglobinemia
TAC: tetracaine, adrenaline, cocaine	Tetracaine 0.5-1% + adrenaline (epinephrine 1:2000-4000) + Cocaine 4-11.8%	Apply for 15-20 min Avoid mucous membranes Avoid terminally perfused areas Potential cocaine toxicity
LET: lidocaine, epinephrine, tetracaine	Lidocaine 4% + epinephrine 1:2000 + tetracaine 0.5%	Contains lidocaine rather than cocaine Apply for 15-20 min Avoid mucous membranes Avoid terminally perfused areas
Synera	70 mg lidocaine/70 mg tetracaine in a topical patch	FDA-approved for children 3 years of age and older Apply for 20-30 min Erythema common; monitor for allergic reaction

Bier block, has been described in children, but widespread use has been limited by the theoretical risk of local anesthetic toxicity. Although rare in clinical practice, systemic local anesthetic toxicity may warrant observation in the critical care setting given risk for neurologic and cardiac compromise. Plexus blocks are discussed in greater detail in Regional Anesthetic Techniques in the Chapter 5 Supplement on the Evolve Website.

Neuraxial Blocks

Neuraxial blocks include spinal and epidural techniques. Anesthetic is administered by single injection, repeated injections, or continuous infusion through an indwelling catheter. Spinal (i.e., subarachnoid) block entails injection of anesthetic directly into cerebrospinal fluid, and is performed in pediatric practice primarily in infants at high risk of apnea following general anesthesia. Epidural (i.e., peridural) block entails injection of anesthetic into the potential epidural space between the ligamentum flavum and dura mater surrounding the spinal cord, and is considerably more common in pediatric practice.

Epidural block in children is most commonly performed as a caudal block, a variant of epidural block in which the epidural space is accessed through the sacral hiatus over the posterior aspect of the lower sacrum. Caudal block is most commonly performed as a single injection, providing reliable analgesia below the umbilicus in patients weighing 30 kg or less. The technique is straightforward, success rate is high, and complication rate is low. Specific agents for caudal block are discussed in greater detail in the Chapter 5 Supplement on the Evolve Website.

Excellent analgesia may be provided by repeated injection or continuous infusion of anesthetic through indwelling epidural catheters. Epidural catheters can be inserted caudally and threaded to the desired vertebral level, particularly in infants and young children. Epidural catheters can also be placed directly at the desired vertebral level. As with other invasive access, skin preparation with chlorhexidine rather than iodine confers a lower risk of subsequent epidural catheter colonization. Many combinations of local anesthetic, opioid, and adjuvant agents are commonly used for epidural administration in the United States (Table 5-6). Placement of epidural catheters and selection of agents for epidural injection or infusion are discussed in greater detail in the Chapter 5 Supplement on the Evolve Website.

Nurses should assess patients receiving epidural infusion frequently and regularly, monitoring adequacy of analgesia, degree of motor and sensory block, level of sedation, and presence of respiratory depression and other side effects. Patients receiving epidural opioid should be placed on continuous pulse oximetry, at least on initiation of epidural infusion and with any significant increase in regimen. Continuous cardiorespiratory monitoring may be considered for opioid-naive neonates and young infants. Patients receiving a more hydrophilic opioid, such as hydromorphone or morphine, may need more intensive monitoring. Instruction of patients, families, and caregivers regarding epidural infusion is essential.

SYSTEMIC SEDATIVES

Sedation comprises a continuum ranging from mild anxiolysis to general anesthesia. Definitions of stages of sedation along this continuum are imprecise, particularly in children. Light sedation, or anxiolysis, is less helpful in children, given their often vigorous response to interventions. Moderate (formerly *conscious*) sedation is commonly preferred for increased depth of sedation with preservation of airway reflexes and spontaneous ventilation. Even moderate sedation, however, may be inadequate for many pediatric patients, and its usefulness in children has been questioned. Deep sedation produces greater depression of consciousness and diminished response to stimuli, and it may be required for invasive procedures. Deep sedation can also obtund airway reflexes, compromise ventilation, and impair cardiovascular function, so it requires continuous and close monitoring of cardiorespiratory status.

Because of the variability of individual responses, particularly in children, administration of systemic sedatives with intent to provide light or moderate sedation can rapidly and unexpectedly induce deep sedation or general anesthesia. All sedation depresses level of consciousness and increases risk of airway obstruction, respiratory depression, aspiration, and cardiovascular depression; any of these complications can produce significant morbidity and potential mortality. Because children are particularly prone to such complications, nurses caring for children receiving systemic sedatives must be extremely vigilant.[1-3,16,17]

Sedative-Hypnotic Agents

Systemic sedatives produce a wide range of physiologic effects. Knowledge of the agents being administered is essential for optimal efficacy and greatest patient safety. Nurses

Table 5-6 Agents for Epidural Infusion

Local Anesthetic*	Opioid/Adjuvant	Infusion Rates
Bupivacaine 0.0625-0.1% (maximum dose 0.4 mg/kg per h)	Fentanyl 0.5-1 mcg/kg per h (adult dose 50-100 mcg/h)	Thoracic typically 0.2-0.3 mL/kg per h (maximum 5-10 mL/h)
-OR-	-OR-	
Levobupivacaine 0.0625-0.1% (maximum dose 0.4 mg/kg per h)	Hydromorphone 2-4 mcg/kg per h (adult dose 150-300 mcg/h)	Lumbar typically 0.3-0.4 mL/kg per h (maximum 10-15 mL/h)
-OR-	-OR-	
Lidocaine 0.1-0.5% (maximum dose 3 mg/kg per h)	Morphine 3-6 mcg/kg per h (adult dose 250-500 mcg/h)	Caudal typically 0.4-0.5 mL/kg per h (maximum 15-20 mL/h)
-OR-	-AND/OR-	
Ropivacaine 0.1-0.2% (maximum dose 0.5 mg/kg per h)	Clonidine 0.1-0.5 mcg/kg per h (adult dose 25-50 mcg/h)	

*Recommended local anesthetic and initial opioid doses should typically be reduced 25-50% in neonates and young infants.

Table 5-7   Sedative-Hypnotic Agents

Drug	Indication	Dose
Chloral hydrate	Procedural sedation	25-100 mg/kg PO/PR (maximum 2 g)
Pentobarbital	Procedural sedation	1-2 mg/kg IV (adult dose 50-100 mg) initial dose; 0.25-0.5 mg/kg IV (adult dose 25-50 mg) q5-10 min
	Ongoing sedation	1-2 mg/kg IV (adult dose 50-100 mg) q1-2 h
	Infusion	1-2 mg/kg per h IV (adult dose 50-100 mg/h)
Midazolam	Premedication	0.25-0.5 mg/kg PO/PR (maximum 20 mg) 0.2-0.4 mg/kg SL/nasally (maximum 10 mg)
	Procedural sedation	0.05-0.1 mg/kg IV (adult dose 5 mg) initial dose; 0.025-0.05 mg/kg IV (adult dose 2 mg) q5-10 min
	Ongoing sedation	0.05-0.1 mg/kg IV (adult dose 2-5 mg) q1-2 h
	Infusion	0.05-0.1 mg/kg per h IV (adult dose 2-5 mg/h)
Ketamine	Procedural sedation	4-10 mg/kg PO (adult dose 300-500 mg) 3-4 mg/kg IM (150-300 mg) 0.5-1 mg/kg IV (adult dose 50-100 mg)
	Ongoing sedation	0.5-1 mg/kg IV (adult dose 50-100 mg) q1-2 h
Propofol	Procedural sedation	0.5-2 mg/kg IV (adult dose 50-100 mg) initial dose; 0.5 mg/kg IV (adult dose 25-50 mg) q5-10 min
	Infusion	50-150 mcg/kg per min IV
Dexmedetomidine	Premedication	1-2 mcg/kg nasally
	Procedural sedation	1-2 mcg/kg IV over 10 min
	Infusion	0.2-1 mcg/kg per h IV

Recommended doses are for initial administration: titration to clinical effect is required. Appropriate analgesia should be provided in settings entailing significant pain. *IM*, Intramuscular; *IV*, intravenous; *PO*, by mouth; *PR*, by rectum; *q*, every; *SL*, sublingual.

must be aware of expected clinical effect, usual time of onset, likely duration, and potential side effects of each agent. Medications ordered on an "as needed" basis are effective only when given appropriately in response to ongoing and recurring patient assessment. If a drug ordered on an "as needed" (PRN) basis is required frequently, the healthcare team should consider a change to scheduled administration and other interventions to improve patient comfort. Intramuscular injection is painful and should be avoided if possible, except perhaps in the setting of difficult intravenous access. Most systemic sedatives lack analgesic efficacy and should not be used primarily for analgesia. Many sedative-hypnotic agents are used in children; selection is determined by anticipated depth and duration of sedation desired, risk of potential side effects, and available routes of administration (Table 5-7).

Many systemic sedatives do not have maximum effective doses. Recommended doses are for initial administration in agent-naive patients. Titration to clinical effect is required, and higher doses may be necessary. Increasing dose requirement, also known as *tolerance* or *tachyphylaxis*, is often observed with ongoing administration. Systemic sedative therapy longer than 7 to 10 days can result in physical dependence, requiring weaning before discontinuation to avoid withdrawal. Tolerance and dependence are separate phenomena. Addiction, a formal psychopathologic diagnosis of volitional drug-seeking behavior, rarely develops in children receiving appropriately dosed systemic sedatives, and it is not a valid reason to withhold therapy.

Chloral Hydrate

Chloral hydrate is a sedative-hypnotic agent without specific analgesic efficacy. Rapidly metabolized in the liver to trichloroethanol, chloral hydrate induces a state of intoxication likely through a combination of gamma-aminobutyric acid (GABA) agonism and N-methyl-d-aspartate (NMDA) antagonism. Available in liquid and suppository forms, chloral hydrate has been widely used for sedation in infants and children, primarily because of its low risk of serious complications.

Chloral hydrate has hepatotoxic metabolites and a structural similarity to several known carcinogens, which has prompted concern. Continued administration has been associated with increased risk of malignancy in rodents. No similar observation has been made in humans despite decades of widespread use. Disadvantages of chloral hydrate include pungent preparations, slow onset of action, prolonged recovery, lack of a reversal agent, and significant rates of inadequate sedation and paradoxical agitation. Risk of respiratory and hemodynamic depression with higher doses warrants continuous cardiorespiratory monitoring.

Chloral hydrate remains a popular systemic sedative for non-painful pediatric procedures such as computed tomography scanning and magnetic resonance imaging. It is not indicated for repeated or continued administration. Because chloral hydrate lacks specific analgesic efficacy, appropriate analgesia should be provided in settings entailing significant pain.

Barbiturates

Barbiturates are sedative-hypnotic agents without specific analgesic efficacy. Barbiturate mechanism of action likely derives from stimulation of GABA-ergic inhibitory pathways in the central nervous system. All barbiturates produce dose-dependent respiratory and cardiovascular depression in addition to sedation. Because barbiturates lack analgesic properties, appropriate analgesia should be provided in settings entailing significant pain.

The intermediate-acting barbiturate pentobarbital is a useful agent for pediatric sedation, particularly for pain-free radiologic studies, or for rescue sedation when other agents prove inadequate. Pentobarbital lends itself well to titrated intravenous administration and can be given orally, rectally, or intramuscularly at similar doses. Larger doses may be required in patients with significant barbiturate tolerance. Continuous infusion may be useful if repeated dosing becomes necessary or if ongoing sedation is anticipated. Side effects of pentobarbital infusion, including respiratory and cardiovascular depression are common, requiring meticulous hemodynamic monitoring in critical care settings. Children may demonstrate agitation during recovery from pentobarbital.

Benzodiazepines

Benzodiazepines, among the most widely used systemic sedatives in critical care, are sedative-hypnotic agents without specific analgesic efficacy. Unlike other systemic sedatives, benzodiazepines also have specific anxiolytic and amnestic effects. Acting on the benzodiazepine receptor of the GABA receptor complex, benzodiazepines induce sedation, reduce anxiety, and prevent recall. The principal significant adverse effect of benzodiazepines is respiratory depression; risk increases with higher or repetitive doses, or with concomitant administration of other agents. Because benzodiazepines lack analgesic efficacy, appropriate analgesia should be provided in settings entailing significant pain.

Flumazenil, a specific benzodiazepine receptor antagonist, can provide rapid reversal of benzodiazepine effects. Flumazenil is a proconvulsant and should be used cautiously in patients at risk of seizure.

Given its rapid onset and short duration of action, midazolam is widely used in pediatric practice. Oral, rectal, and nasal administration are commonly used for perioperative and procedural sedation. Currently available preparations often have a bitter taste and sting the nasal mucosa, and children may find oral or nasal administration unpleasant. Intravenous midazolam produces rapid onset of sedation, anxiolysis, and amnesia, and is well suited to incremental titration or continuous infusion. Larger doses may be required in patients with significant benzodiazepine tolerance.

Many other benzodiazepines are available, although relatively few are commonly used in children. Lorazepam has a longer time of onset than midazolam, and it is less likely to induce acute respiratory depression. Lorazepam also has a longer duration of action than midazolam and may be useful when longer-term sedation is desired. Lorazepam is also widely used as an acute anticonvulsant. Diazepam has even slower time of onset and longer duration of action, and it can be useful for maintenance therapy in patients with significant benzodiazepine tolerance or when ongoing prolonged sedation is desired.[34] Commercial preparations of lorazepam and diazepam contain propylene glycol as a solvent and benzyl alcohol as a preservative. Higher or repetitive doses or continuous infusion should be administered with caution to neonates and other patients susceptible to benzyl alcohol toxicity. Although significant propylene glycol accumulation has been documented in critically ill children receiving lorazepam infusion, other laboratory abnormalities were not noted. Peripheral intravenous administration of diazepam can cause significant discomfort and chemical phlebitis; intramuscular administration is not recommended.

Ketamine

Ketamine is a sedative-hypnotic agent similar to the now illicit drug phencyclidine. Unlike other systemic sedatives, ketamine is a potent dissociative analgesic, producing in lower doses a state in which pain is felt but not perceived as unpleasant. Ketamine is an NMDA receptor antagonist with weak agonist activity at opioid receptors and many other sites. Ketamine produces dose-dependent analgesia and sedation, inducing general anesthesia at higher doses; amnesia is variable. As with other phencyclidine derivatives, hallucinations and delirium may occur, but may be less frequent and less severe in younger patients. Ketamine induces bronchodilation, but also potentially significant salivation. Ketamine promotes release of endogenous catecholamines; tachycardia and hypertension may be significant. Although ketamine increases pulmonary arterial pressure, a concomitant increase in inotropy (strength of myocardial contraction) generally preserves cardiovascular function. Ketamine increases intracranial pressure and is a proconvulsant, so it should be used cautiously in patients with intracranial pathology or seizures.

Ketamine is most commonly administered intravenously to induce general anesthesia in medically fragile infants and children, and intramuscularly in patients who are unable to cooperate or who have no reliable intravenous access. Ketamine is used as an analgesic for children with burns[44] or receiving palliative care[13] and when other analgesics prove inadequate. PCA with ketamine has been described.[62] Ketamine is widely used for procedural sedation in children and has become particularly popular in pediatric emergency departments given its favorable safety profile. Continuous infusion may be useful if repeated dosing becomes necessary or if a need for ongoing sedation is anticipated. Emergence may be prolonged after oral administration, particularly with a higher dose, and emergence delirium is common. Although an anticholinergic agent such as atropine or glycopyrrolate can be given to prevent excessive salivation, the effectiveness of this practice has been questioned, as has concomitant administration of benzodiazepines to decrease the likelihood of hallucinations and delirium.[28]

Propofol

Propofol is a sedative-hypnotic agent without specific analgesic effect; it is commonly used for induction and maintenance of sedation and anesthesia. Chemically unrelated to other systemic sedatives, its mechanisms of action are unknown, although propofol likely has significant GABA agonism. Propofol is available only for intravenous administration. It is supplied in a lipid emulsion with an alkaline pH and may cause significant pain on injection. Propofol has considerable antiemetic efficacy,[23] and like ketamine it promotes bronchodilation. Propofol has an extremely rapid onset of action, and with relatively prompt hepatic conjugation and renal excretion it allows for rapid recovery after intermittent dosing or brief infusion. Propofol is also highly lipophilic, leading to significant tissue accumulation and potentially prolonged emergence after repeated administration or prolonged infusion. Because propofol lacks analgesic efficacy, appropriate analgesia should be provided for significant pain.

Prolonged propofol infusion is associated with a rare but often fatal syndrome of metabolic acidosis and cardiovascular failure. Current recommendations suggest propofol infusion in children not exceed 48 hours, although death from apparent propofol infusion syndrome has been reported with shorter duration or with reexposure to the drug. The etiology of this life-threatening reaction to propofol infusion in some patients is unknown, although impairment of mitochondrial oxidative phosphorylation and altered lipid metabolism have been suggested.[26]

Propofol induces dose-dependent sedation, loss of airway reflexes, hypoventilation, apnea, and cardiovascular depression. Higher doses of propofol induce general anesthesia. Although there has been considerable concern over the safety of propofol administration by nonanesthesiologists,[39] current evidence suggests that such use is safe under controlled circumstances.[18] Propofol has been safely and successfully used for pediatric procedural sedation in numerous settings, including the pediatric critical care unit, burn unit, radiology suite, emergency department, ambulatory procedure center, and dental clinic. Although such success is impressive, patient safety was protected by the restriction of propofol use to appropriately trained personnel working in the context of a dedicated sedation team, following carefully designed protocols and adhering to appropriate standards for patient monitoring and management. Propofol infusion may be used in the critical care setting during weaning from mechanical ventilation or for rescue sedation when other agents prove inadequate.[59]

Dexmedetomidine

Dexmedetomidine is a newer sedative-hypnotic agent that is becoming popular in pediatric practice,[18] although the drug is formally approved only for use in adults. As an alpha (α)-2 adrenergic agonist similar to clonidine, dexmedetomidine induces potentially profound sedation with little associated respiratory depression. Dexmedetomidine can cause significant bradycardia and hypotension, particularly at high dose or with rapid administration. Heart rate and blood pressure during anesthesia with dexmedetomidine infusion tend to be lower and recovery more prolonged than during anesthesia with propofol infusion.[30]

Dexmedetomidine is marketed for intravenous use, although the commercially available form can be given nasally, and subcutaneous administration in children has been described.[57] Nasal dexmedetomidine lacks unpleasant taste or odor, it provides preoperative sedation comparable to[56] or greater than[64] oral midazolam, and it may enhance postoperative analgesia.[53]

Dexmedetomidine is often used for pediatric procedural and perioperative sedation[45] and for weaning mechanical ventilation.[11,20] Dexmedetomidine is also used to treat postoperative shivering in children[8] and to facilitate weaning from opioids[58] and benzodiazepines. Although officially approved for use up to 24 hours, prolonged dexmedetomidine infusion for days or even weeks for sedation of critically ill infants and children,[51] including pediatric cardiothoracic surgical patients,[7] has been described. Dexmedetomidine provides little direct analgesia and is useful as a sole agent only when significant analgesia is not required.[6] Appropriate analgesia should be provided when significant pain is present.[45]

Procedural Sedation

Diagnostic and therapeutic procedures requiring sedation in children have increased dramatically in recent years. Although anesthesiologists provide care for many such interventions, procedural sedation for children is also administered by other healthcare providers, including those in the pediatric critical care setting.[18,38]

The American Academy of Pediatrics has established guidelines for the monitoring and management of children undergoing procedural sedation,[1-3] and different guidelines have been published by other organizations.[16] This has created considerable debate, occasional confusion, and some inconsistency, but all guidelines share the common goal of fostering safe and efficient practice.

Supervision of pediatric procedural sedation by knowledgeable and competent personnel is mandatory. Many practice guidelines recommend that the provider performing the procedure (often referred to as the "operator") not also supervise sedation. Guidelines by the American Academy of Pediatrics and American Society of Anesthesiologists stipulate that an appropriate provider be assigned specifically to supervise sedation of pediatric patients, with only intermittent additional duties during administration of light or moderate sedation and no additional duties while conducting deep sedation. Adherence to these guidelines has been shown to reduce complications.

Because of the small but real risk of serious adverse events associated with pediatric procedural sedation, equipment and medications for emergency resuscitation should be readily and rapidly available. Equipment and medications should be appropriate for the ages and sizes of children receiving care, and providers should be skilled in their use. Providers supervising pediatric procedural sedation should, at a minimum, be trained in basic pediatric life support, and training in pediatric advanced life support is recommended. Serious complications associated with pediatric procedural sedation may be avoided by adequate evaluation and preparation of patients prior to sedation, and by close monitoring and early detection of changes in patient status during and after administration of systemic sedatives. Evaluation and monitoring of pediatric patients undergoing procedural sedation is discussed in Procedural Sedation in the Chapter 5 Supplement on the Evolve Website.

To minimize the risk of aspiration of gastric contents, oral intake should be suspended before any elective procedure for which sedation is planned, as for any elective procedure entailing anesthesia (Table 5-8). If sedation must be provided despite recent oral intake, urgency of the intervention should be documented and systemic sedatives administered cautiously to minimize depression of airway reflexes and risk of aspiration. Agents such as metoclopramide, ranitidine, and sodium bicitrate may be considered to augment gastric motility, decrease gastric volume, and increase gastric pH. When appropriate fasting intervals cannot be observed and deep sedation is anticipated, airway protection with induction of anesthesia and rapid sequence intubation may be advisable.

NEUROMUSCULAR BLOCKADE

Neuromuscular blockade, or muscle relaxation, entails pharmacologic inhibition of voluntary muscle movement. Description as *paralysis* should be avoided because of negative

Table 5-8	Recommended Fasting Intervals Before Elective Sedation or Anesthesia

Type of Intake*	Recommended Fasting Interval (h)
Clear liquids, including water, juice without pulp, carbonated beverages, clear tea, black coffee	2
Human breast milk	4
Nonhuman milk, infant formula, light meal without significant protein or fat content	6
Heavy meal with significant protein or fat content, including particularly fried foods or meat	8

Adapted from American Society of Anesthesiologists Task Force on Preoperative Fasting: Practice guidelines for preoperative fasting and the use of pharmacologic agents to reduce the risk of pulmonary aspiration: application to healthy patients undergoing elective procedures: a report by the American Society of Anesthesiologists Task Force on Preoperative Fasting. *Anesthesiology* 90:896–905, 1999.

*These recommendations apply regardless of patient age.

connotations for patients and families. Neuromuscular blockade has no effect on level of consciousness and provides neither analgesia nor sedation. Neuromuscular blockade should be used only when clinically essential,[14,29] and never in isolation. Neuromuscular blockade should never be used simply to keep patients from moving. Appropriate airway and ventilatory support are mandatory. Neuromuscular blockade may be used to facilitate endotracheal intubation, provide surgical relaxation, and allow mechanical ventilation. Prolonged neuromuscular blockade may be necessary in some settings, as after surgical airway reconstruction.[29]

Normal neuromuscular function relies on the release of acetylcholine from motor nerve terminals at the neuromuscular junction (Fig. 5-5). Acetylcholine crosses the synaptic cleft between motor nerve and skeletal muscle fiber, transiently binding to and briefly opening nicotinic acetylcholine receptors on the myocyte motor end plate. The resultant transmembrane flow of ions, primarily sodium, potassium, and calcium depolarizes the surrounding muscle cell membrane, eventually causing myocyte contraction if an appropriate action potential is achieved. Acetylcholine is subsequently metabolized by acetylcholinesterase within the junctional folds.

Throughout infancy and early childhood, the neuromuscular junction matures physically and biochemically, the contractile properties of skeletal muscle change, and the amount of muscle in proportion to body weight increases. Age-related changes in volume of distribution, drug redistribution and clearance, and rate of metabolism also profoundly influence pharmacologic profiles of neuromuscular blocking agents. Pediatric patients exhibit wide variability in sensitivity to neuromuscular blockade, so the degree and duration of blockade in children may be unpredictable.

Neuromuscular Blocking Agents

Neuromuscular blockade is achieved through blockade of nicotinic acetylcholine receptors at the neuromuscular junction. Neuromuscular blocking agents are classified according to

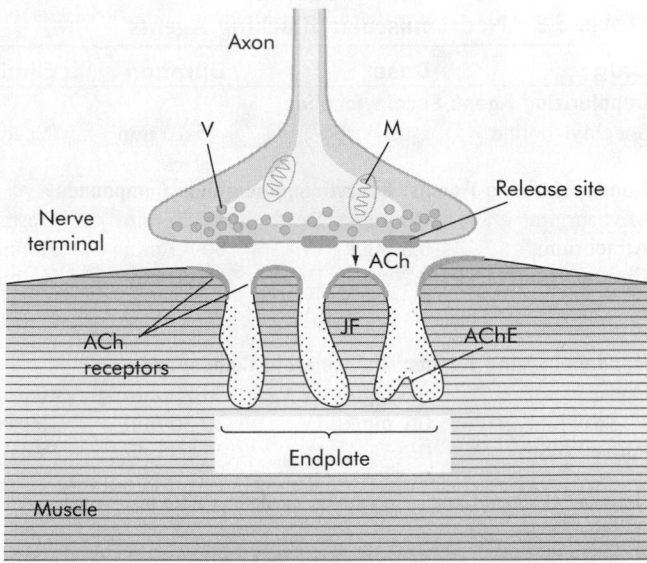

FIG. 5-5 The neuromuscular junction. Diagram of the neuromuscular junction between motor nerve and skeletal muscle fiber. Neuromuscular blocking agents act on acetylcholine receptors at the motor end plate. Ach, acetylcholine; AChE, acetylcholinesterase; JF, junction fold; M, mitochondrion; V, vesicle. (With permission from Drachman DB: Myasthenia gravis. *N Engl J Med* 298:136–142, 1978. Copyright © 1978 Massachusetts Medical Society. All rights reserved.)

their mechanism of action as depolarizing or nondepolarizing agents (Table 5-9). Depolarizing agents activate nicotinic acetylcholine receptors, inducing myocyte depolarization. As long as they persist at the neuromuscular junction, they prevent any further myocyte depolarization, thereby maintaining muscle relaxation. Nondepolarizing agents compete directly with acetylcholine for binding sites on nicotinic acetylcholine receptors, preventing binding of acetylcholine without activating the receptor. Neuromuscular blockade persists as long as sufficient nondepolarizing agent remains to prevent acetylcholine receptor activation. Nondepolarizing agents are eliminated by a wide range of mechanisms. Younger patients, particularly infants, are generally relatively resistant to depolarizing agents but relatively sensitive to nondepolarizing agents.

Depolarizing Agent: Succinylcholine

The only depolarizing neuromuscular blocking agent available in the United States is succinylcholine. Succinylcholine mimics the action of acetylcholine at the neuromuscular junction and at cholinergic sites diffusely, inducing rapid muscle relaxation but also increasing vagal tone and potentially inducing transient bradycardia, particularly in infants and young children. Antimuscarinic agents such as atropine or glycopyrrolate are typically given before administration of succinylcholine to prevent bradycardia in susceptible patients.

Succinylcholine is the most rapid-acting of all currently available muscle relaxants, used when rapid onset of neuromuscular blockade is desired. Administration of succinylcholine may induce transient muscle fasciculations secondary to myocyte depolarization, less so in infants and young children, and in older patients may predispose to significant subsequent myalgias. Succinylcholine causes modest increases

Table 5-9 Neuromuscular Blocking Agents

Drug	Dose*	Duration	Elimination	Comments
Depolarizing Agent: Succinylcholine				
Succinylcholine	1 mg/kg IV	<5-10 min	Pseudocholinesterase	Not for routine use; multiple contraindications
Nondepolarizing Agents: Benzylisoquinolonium Compounds				
Mivacurium	0.2 mg/kg IV	10-20 min	Plasma cholinesterase	Potentially significant histamine release
Atracurium	0.5 mg/kg IV	30-45 min	Hofmann degradation	Histamine release; metabolized to laudanosine
Cisatracurium	0.2 mg/kg IV	45-60 min	Hofmann degradation	Histamine release; metabolized to laudanosine
Doxacurium	0.05 mg/kg IV	45-60 min	Renal excretion	Little histamine release
Nondepolarizing Agents: Aminosteroid Compounds				
Rocuronium	0.6 mg/kg IV	20-30 min	Hepatobiliary excretion	Rapid onset but longer duration at higher doses
Vecuronium	0.1 mg/kg IV	20-30 min	Hepatobiliary excretion	Few hemodynamic effects
Pancuronium	0.1 mg/kg IV	45-60 min	Renal excretion	Vagolytic, may cause significant tachycardia

*Repeated dosing or continuous infusion should be guided by neuromuscular monitoring.
IV, Intravenous.

in intraocular and intracranial pressure, and it is often avoided in the setting of open globe injury or critical intracranial pathology. Increases in intraocular and intracranial pressure can be attenuated by pretreatment with a low-dose nondepolarizing agent. Succinylcholine is rapidly metabolized by plasma pseudocholinesterase; patients with pseudocholinesterase deficiency may demonstrate prolonged neuromuscular blockade up to several hours after even a single dose of succinylcholine.

Succinylcholine-induced myocyte depolarization causes efflux of intracellular potassium, increasing serum potassium in healthy patients by approximately 0.5 mEq/L. Such an increase may be poorly tolerated in patients with preexisting hyperkalemia. In some settings, the release of intracellular potassium following succinylcholine administration is excessive and can rapidly induce life-threatening hyperkalemia, even in patients with a previously normal serum potassium concentration. Risk is increased in several central nervous system and neuromuscular diseases, in addition to injuries associated with significant tissue destruction. Settings associated with increased risk of succinylcholine-induced hyperkalemia are discussed in Depolarizing Agents: Succinylcholine in the Chapter 5 Supplement on the Evolve Website.

Nondepolarizing Agents

Common nondepolarizing neuromuscular blocking agents are classified as either benzylisoquinolinium or aminosteroid compounds. Benzylisoquinolinium compounds, of which curare can be considered the historical prototype, generally include *-urium* in their generic nomenclature. Benzylisoquinolinium compounds tend to promote histamine release, potentially inducing urticaria, bronchospasm, and even hypotension, particularly with high dose or rapid administration. Aminosteroid compounds are structurally similar to glucocorticoids, and generally include *-onium* in their generic nomenclature. Some aminosteroid compounds have vagolytic effects potentially inducing tachycardia.

Mivacurium is a short-acting benzylisoquinolinium compound rapidly metabolized by plasma cholinesterase. Metabolism may be impaired in the setting of severe hepatic disease, but is

independent of renal function. As with succinylcholine, patients with atypical pseudocholinesterase variants demonstrate impaired metabolism of mivacurium and will generally experience prolonged neuromuscular blockade following its administration. Histamine release may be significant, particularly with large dose or rapid administration.

Atracurium and its isomer cisatracurium are intermediate-acting benzylisoquinolinium compounds notable for elimination through Hofmann degradation; under physiologic conditions they degrade spontaneously, independent of hepatic or renal function. Atracurium and cisatracurium are frequently chosen for use in patients with significant hepatic or renal disease. Laudanosine, a hepatically excreted breakdown product of both compounds, is neurotoxic and can cause seizures, although clinical laudanosine toxicity has not been reported. Histamine release may be significant, particularly with large dose or rapid administration.

Doxacurium is a long-acting benzylisoquinolinium compound causing relatively little histamine release; it is a useful alternative to aminosteroid compounds for ongoing neuromuscular blockade.

Rocuronium is a short-acting aminosteroid compound with particularly rapid onset, and it is generally regarded as the most reasonable alternative to succinylcholine when the latter should be avoided. Elimination of rocuronium is primarily through hepatobiliary excretion of the parent compound; duration of action may be prolonged in patients with significant hepatic disease.

Vecuronium is an intermediate-acting aminosteroid compound similar in potency to pancuronium but with a shorter duration of action. Vecuronium has virtually no vagolytic effects and causes little change in hemodynamic parameters. Elimination of vecuronium is largely through hepatobiliary excretion of the parent compound, although renal excretion also occurs. Duration of action may be markedly prolonged in patients with significant hepatic disease, and modestly prolonged in patients with significant renal disease.

Pancuronium is a long-acting aminosteroid compound with significant vagolytic effects. Pancuronium is a popular choice in pediatric practice because it can induce tachycardia, helping to preserve cardiac output. Elimination of pancuronium is largely through renal excretion of the parent compound. Duration of action may be prolonged in patients with significant renal disease.

Neuromuscular blockade can be maintained with repeated dosing or continuous infusion of any agent.[10] Repeated dosing typically requires 25% to 50% of the usual initial dose, whereas continuous infusion typically requires 25% to 50% of the usual initial dose per hour, depending on drug pharmacology and underlying patient disease. Whenever neuromuscular blockade is maintained through repeated dosing or continuous infusion, nurses should monitor the degree of neuromuscular blockade (see section, Neuromuscular Monitoring) to prevent unnecessary and excessive dosing.[15,49] Neuromuscular monitoring is discussed in greater detail in the Chapter 5 Supplement on the Evolve Website.

Reversal of Neuromuscular Blockade

Neuromuscular blockade induced by succinylcholine cannot be pharmacologically reversed. The return of neuromuscular function relies on metabolism of succinylcholine by pseudocholinesterase, and it may be prolonged in patients with atypical pseudocholinesterase variants. In contrast, neuromuscular blockade induced by nondepolarizing agents may be pharmacologically reversible.

Pharmacologic reversal of nondepolarizing neuromuscular blockade has traditionally been accomplished through administration of cholinesterase inhibitors, which are discussed in greater detail in the Chapter 5 Supplement on the Evolve Website. These agents inhibit metabolism of acetylcholine, increasing its concentration in the synaptic cleft and out-competing any remaining nondepolarizing agent. Currently available cholinesterase inhibitors are nonspecific, potentiating acetylcholine at the neuromuscular junction and at cholinergic sites throughout the body. An antimuscarinic agent such as atropine or glycopyrrolate is typically given before the cholinesterase inhibitor to prevent cholinergic side effects, particularly bradycardia.

Sugammadex is a recently developed gamma (γ)-cyclodextrin capable of binding an aminosteroid nondepolarizing agent. The sugammadex molecule encapsulates or traps the aminosteroid compound within a central pore, and the resultant complex is renally excreted.[55] Initial experience with sugammadex has been encouraging,[43] although pediatric experience is limited[47] and the drug is not yet approved for use in the United States. Preliminary data suggest that this agent may increase the safety of longer acting, nondepolarizing neuromuscular blockers.

Critical Illness Polyneuropathy and Myopathy

Prolonged muscle weakness after pharmacologic neuromuscular blockade in critically ill patients is common, affecting many adults requiring mechanical ventilation.[63] Although a similar syndrome of prolonged muscle weakness following critical illness in children is increasingly recognized, particularly after pharmacologic neuromuscular blockade,[33] the condition is thought to be much less common in the pediatric setting, reportedly affecting approximately 1% of critically ill children. The condition has recently been termed *critical illness polyneuropathy and myopathy*, and it is increasingly recognized in pediatric patients.[63]

Critical illness, particularly sepsis, is associated with prolonged subsequent muscle weakness, as well as with immobility and muscle atrophy. Many drugs, particularly aminoglycoside antibiotics and high-dose steroids, are known to cause a predisposition to prolonged muscle weakness. Many other agents, including diuretics such as furosemide and sedatives such as benzodiazepines, may also contribute. Pharmacologic neuromuscular blockade is highly associated with subsequent prolonged muscle weakness, particularly after prolonged blockade, and the risk appears greater with aminosteroid compounds.[10] Concomitant administration of multiple agents predisposing to prolonged muscle weakness likely heightens risk. The etiology of critical illness polyneuropathy and myopathy is likely multifactorial.

Critical illness polyneuropathy and myopathy can vary in clinical presentation from mild diffuse muscle weakness to profound flaccid quadriplegia with respiratory failure. The condition appears to be associated with neuromuscular pathology, including muscle atrophy with denervation and axonal neuropathy, even in the absence of significant inflammation. Clinical weakness may persist for months or years, with neurodiagnostic abnormalities lasting even longer.[61] Pediatric patients generally seem to have a somewhat more favorable prognosis than do adults, although recovery is less likely in very young patients, particularly neonates and premature infants in whom neuromuscular development is still incomplete.

Critical illness polyneuropathy and myopathy is best treated through prevention, although the condition can develop despite all such efforts. All drugs, in particular agents predisposing the patient to prolonged muscle weakness, should be administered at appropriate doses and intervals, with monitoring of drug levels as necessary. Providers should avoid concomitant administration of multiple agents predisposing the patient to prolonged muscle weakness, in particular combinations of steroids, aminoglycoside antibiotics, and neuromuscular blocking agents. Risk appears to be greater with aminosteroid compounds, which are perhaps best avoided for prolonged administration or for concomitant administration with steroid or aminoglycoside.

Neuromuscular Monitoring

During repeated dosing or continuous infusion of any neuromuscular blocking agent, providers should consider neuromuscular monitoring to prevent unnecessary and excessive dosing.[49] Neuromuscular monitoring can be challenging in many patients,[15] particularly small infants, and findings can be influenced by factors such as peripheral edema, level of hydration, electrolyte and acid-base balance, and hemodynamic status. Ideally, providers should evaluate response to "train-of-four" stimulation (i.e., response to provision of 4 pulses in sequence from a nerve stimulator)[49] at least once every 24 hours. If monitoring proves unreliable and patient safety permits, providers may consider daily discontinuation of neuromuscular blockade to assess for respiratory effort and spontaneous movement. Neuromuscular monitoring is reviewed in more detail in the Chapter 5 Supplement on the Evolve Website. Ongoing physical rehabilitation services should be provided to all patients with ongoing critical illness, particularly those receiving pharmacologic neuromuscular blockade.

SUMMARY

Children often experience pain and anxiety during critical illness. Pediatric critical care nurses must anticipate and assess patient pain and anxiety, administer appropriate analgesia and sedation, and when necessary provide neuromuscular blockade. Although institutional practices and provider preferences vary, all share the common goal of optimal patient care.

Pain and anxiety in children are complex developmental and physiologic processes. Assessment requires interpretation of pediatric behaviors, quantified as necessary with assessment tools. Optimal treatment requires a multidisciplinary management plan.

Nonpharmacologic interventions can enhance both analgesia and sedation and are particularly amenable to patient, family, and nurse involvement. Optimal analgesia and sedation use these techniques with pharmacologic agents to maximize patient comfort, minimize side effects, and facilitate recovery.

Systemic analgesics are titrated according to the level of pain: opioid analgesics remain the mainstay of pharmacologic therapy for moderate to severe pain in all patients. Systemic analgesics do not necessarily provide sedation. Local anesthetics provide analgesia through nerve cell conduction blockade and may reduce the requirement for systemic agents.

Sedation is often provided to critically ill children using a variety of sedative-hypnotic agents, most of which lack analgesic effect. Pediatric procedural sedation requires supervision by competent personnel using appropriate procedures, monitoring, and management.

Neuromuscular blockade, although providing neither analgesia nor sedation, is at times necessary in critical care. Neuromuscular blockade should never be administered without first ensuring adequate analgesia and sedation, and then only when necessary. Care should be taken to minimize risk of subsequent prolonged neuromuscular weakness. For additional information about pharmacokinetics and pharmacodynamics in pediatric critical care, see Chapter 4.

References

1. American Academy of Pediatrics, American Academy on Pediatric Dentistry: Guideline for monitoring and management of pediatric patients during and after sedation for diagnostic and therapeutic procedures. *Pediatr Dent* 30(7 Suppl.):143–159, 2008–2009.
2. American Academy of Pediatrics, American Academy of Pediatric Dentistry, Coté CJ, Wilson S, Work Group on Sedation: Guidelines for monitoring and management of pediatric patients during and after sedation for diagnostic and therapeutic procedures: an update. *Pediatrics* 118(6):2587–2602, 2006.
3. American Academy of Pediatrics, American Academy of Pediatric Dentistry, Coté CJ, Wilson S, Work Group on Sedation: Guidelines for monitoring and management of pediatric patients during and after sedation for diagnostic and therapeutic procedures: an update. *Paediatr Anaesth* 18(1):9–10, 2008.
4. Arnon S, et al: Live music is beneficial to preterm infants in the neonatal intensive care unit environment. *Birth* 33(2):131–136, 2006.
5. Aronoff GM, et al: Evidence-based oral transmucosal fentanyl citrate (OTFC) dosing guidelines. *Pain Med* 6(4):305–314, 2005.
6. Barton KP, et al: Dexmedetomidine as the primary sedative during invasive procedures in infants and toddlers with congenital heart disease. *Pediatr Crit Care Med* 9(6):612–615, 2008.
7. Bejian S, et al: Prolonged use of dexmedetomidine in the paediatric cardiothoracic intensive care unit. *Cardiol Young* 19(1):98–104, 2009.
8. Blaine Easley R, Brady KM, Tobias JD: Dexmedetomidine for the treatment of postanesthesia shivering in children. *Paediatr Anaesth* 17(4):341–346, 2007.
9. Borland ML, Clark LJ, Esson A: Comparative review of the clinical use of intranasal fentanyl versus morphine in a paediatric emergency department. *Emerg Med Australas* 20(6):515–520, 2008.
10. Burmester M, Mok Q: Randomised controlled trial comparing cisatracurium and vecuronium infusions in a paediatric intensive care unit. *Intensive Care Med* 31(5):686–692, 2005.
11. Carroll CL, et al: Use of dexmedetomidine for sedation of children hospitalized in the intensive care unit. *J Hosp Med* 3(2):142–147, 2008.
12. Clark E, et al: A randomized, controlled trial of acetaminophen, ibuprofen, and codeine for acute pain relief in children with musculoskeletal trauma. *Pediatrics* 119(3):460–467, 2007.
13. Conway M, et al: Use of continuous intravenous ketamine for end-stage cancer pain in children. *J Pediatr Oncol Nurs* 26(2):100–106, 2009.
14. Cools F, Offringa M: Neuromuscular paralysis for newborn infants receiving mechanical ventilation. *Cochrane Database Syst Rev* 18 (2):CD002773, 2005.
15. Corso L: Train-of-four results and observed muscle movement in children during continuous neuromuscular blockade. *Crit Care Nurse* 28 (3):30–38, 2008.
16. Coté CJ: Round and round we go: sedation—what is it, who does it, and have we made things safer for children? *Paediatr Anaesth* 18 (1):3–8, 2008.
17. Coté CJ: Strategies for preventing sedation accidents. *Pediatr Ann* 34 (8):625–633, 2005.
18. Cravero JP, et al: Pediatric Sedation Research Consortium: The incidence and nature of adverse events during pediatric sedation/anesthesia with propofol for procedures outside the operating room: a report from the Pediatric Sedation Research Consortium. *Anesth Analg* 108 (3):795–804, 2009.
19. Curley MA, et al: State Behavioral Scale: a sedation assessment instrument for infants and young children supported on mechanical ventilation. *Pediatr Crit Care Med* 7(2):107–114, 2006.
20. Czaja AS, Zimmerman JJ: The use of dexmedetomidine in critically ill children. *Pediatr Crit Care Med* 10(3):381–386, 2009.
21. De José María B, et al: Ultrasound-guided supraclavicular vs infraclavicular brachial plexus blocks in children. *Paediatr Anaesth* 18 (9):838–844, 2008.
22. Derbyshire SW, Osborn J: Modeling pain circuits: how imaging may modify perception. *Neuroimaging Clin N Am* 17(4):485–493, 2007.
23. Erdem AF, et al: Subhypnotic propofol infusion plus dexamethasone is more effective than dexamethasone alone for the prevention of vomiting in children after tonsillectomy. *Paediatr Anaesth* 18 (9):878–883, 2008.
24. FDA Joint Advisory Committee Meeting; Drug Safety and Risk Management Committee, Anesthetic and Life Support Drugs Advisory Committee and Nonprescription Drugs Advisory Committee: *Acetaminophen overdose and liver injury—background and options for reducing injury,* June 29-30, 2009.
25. Felice K, Schumann H: Intravenous lipid emulsion for local anesthetic toxicity: a review of the literature. *J Med Toxicol* 4(3):184–191, 2008.
26. Fudickar A, Bein B: Propofol infusion syndrome: update of clinical manifestation and pathophysiology. *Minerva Anestesiol* 75 (5):339–344, 2009.
27. Gourevitch MN: First do no harm… Reduction? *Ann Intern Med* 150(6):417–418, 17. 2009.
28. Green SM, et al: Emergency Department Ketamine Meta-Analysis Study Group: Predictors of emesis and recovery agitation with emergency department ketamine sedation: an individual-patient data meta-analysis of 8,282 children. *Ann Emerg Med* 54(2):171–180, 2009. e1-4. Epub 2009 Jun 6.
29. Hammer GB: Sedation and analgesia in the pediatric Intensive Care Unit following laryngotracheal reconstruction. *Otolaryngol Clin North Am* 41(5):1023–1044, 2008. x-xi.
30. Heard C, et al: A comparison of dexmedetomidine-midazolam with propofol for maintenance of anesthesia in children undergoing magnetic resonance imaging. *Anesth Analg* 107(6):1832–1839, 2008.
31. Herr K, et al: American Society for Pain Management Nursing. Pain assessment in the nonverbal patient: position statement with clinical practice recommendations. *Pain Manag Nurs* 7(2):44–52, 2006.
32. Hunter BC, Sahler OJ: Music for very young ears. *Birth* 33 (2):137–138, 2006.
33. Iodice F, et al: Acute quadriplegic myopathy in a 16-month-old child. *Paediatr Anaesth* 15(7):611–615, 2005.

34. Kost-Byerly S, et al: Perioperative anesthetic and analgesic management of newborn bladder exstrophy repair. *J Pediatr Urol* 4(4):280–285, 2008.

35. Krantz MJ, et al: QTc interval screening in methadone treatment: the CSAT consensus guideline. *Ann Intern Med* Dec 1 [Epub ahead of print], 2008.

36. Krantz MJ, et al: QTc interval screening in methadone treatment. *Ann Intern Med* 150(6):387–395, 2009.

37. Kress HG, et al: Efficacy and tolerability of intranasal fentanyl spray 50 to 200 microg for breakthrough pain in patients with cancer: a phase III, multinational, randomized, double-blind, placebo-controlled, cross-over trial with a 10-month, open-label extension treatment period. *Clin Ther* 31(6):1177–1191, 2009.

38. Leroy PL, Gorzeman MP, Sury MR: Procedural sedation and analgesia in children by non-anesthesiologists in an Emergency Department. *Minerva Pediatr* 61(2):193–215, 2009.

39. Litman RS: Sedation by non-anesthesiologists. *Curr Opin Anaesthesiol* 18(3):263–264, 2005.

40. Martin AL, et al: Anxiety sensitivity, fear of pain and pain-related disability in children and adolescents with chronic pain. *Pain Res Manag* 12(4):267–272, 2007.

41. Maxwell LG, et al: The effects of a small-dose naloxone infusion on opioid-induced side effects and analgesia in children and adolescents treated with intravenous patient-controlled analgesia: a double-blind, prospective, randomized, controlled study. *Anesth Analg* 100(4):953–958, 2005.

42. Mazer M, Perrone J: Acetaminophen-induced nephrotoxicity: pathophysiology, clinical manifestations, and management. *J Med Toxicol* 4(1):2–6, 2008.

43. Mirakhur RK: Sugammadex in clinical practice. *Anaesthesia* 64 (Suppl. 1):45–54, 2009.

44. Owens VF, et al: Ketamine: a safe and effective agent for painful procedures in the pediatric burn patient. *J Burn Care Res* 27(2):211–216, 2006.

45. Phan H, Nahata MC: Clinical uses of dexmedetomidine in pediatric patients. *Paediatr Drugs* 10(1):49–69, 2008.

46. Pinto A, Balasubramaniam R, Arava-Parastatidis M: Neuropathic orofacial pain in children and adolescents. *Pediatr Dent* 30(6):510–515, 2008.

47. Plaud B, et al: Reversal of rocuronium-induced neuromuscular blockade with sugammadex in pediatric and adult surgical patients. *Anesthesiology* 110(2):284–294, 2009.

48. Playfor S, et al: Consensus guidelines on sedation and analgesia in critically ill children. *Intensive Care Med* 32(8):1125–1136, 2006.

49. Playfor S, et al: Consensus guidelines for sustained neuromuscular blockade in critically ill children. *Paediatr Anaesth* 17(9):881–887, 2007.

50. Razmus I, Wilson D: Current trends in the development of sedation/analgesia scales for the pediatric critical care patient. *Pediatr Nurs* 32 (5):435–441, 2006.

51. Reiter PD, Pietras M, Dobyns EL: Prolonged dexmedetomidine infusions in critically ill infants and children. *Indian Pediatr* Apr 1 [Epub ahead of print], 2009.

51a. Romsing J, Ostergaard D, Walther-Larsen S, Valentin N: Analgesic efficacy and safety of preoperative versus postoperative ketorolac in paediatric tonsillectomy. *Acta Anaesthesiol Scand* 42:770–775, 1998.

52. Sarrell EM, Wielunsky E, Cohen HA: Antipyretic treatment in young children with fever: acetaminophen, ibuprofen, or both alternating in a randomized, double-blind study. *Arch Pediatr Adolesc Med* 160 (2):197–202, 2006.

53. Schmidt AP, et al: Effects of preanesthetic administration of midazolam, clonidine, or dexmedetomidine on postoperative pain and anxiety in children. *Paediatr Anaesth* 17(7):667–674, 2007.

54. Sorce LR: Adverse responses: sedation, analgesia and neuromuscular blocking agents in critically ill children. *Crit Care Nurs Clin North Am* 17(4):441–450, 2005.

55. Sparr HJ, Booij LH, Fuchs-Buder T: Sugammadex. New pharmacological concept for antagonizing rocuronium and vecuronium. *Anaesthesist* 58(1):66–80, 2009.

56. Talon MD, et al: Intranasal dexmedetomidine premedication is comparable with midazolam in burn children undergoing reconstructive surgery. *J Burn Care Res* Jun 5 [Epub ahead of print], 2009.

57. Tobias JD: Subcutaneous dexmedetomidine infusions to treat or prevent drug withdrawal in infants and children. *J Opioid Manag* 4(4):187–191, 2008.

58. Tobias JD: Dexmedetomidine to treat opioid withdrawal in infants following prolonged sedation in the pediatric ICU. *J Opioid Manag* 2(4):201–205, 2006.

59. Tobias J: Sedation and analgesia in the pediatric intensive care unit. *Pediatr Ann* 34(8):636–645, 2005.

60. Voepel-Lewis T, et al: The prevalence of and risk factors for adverse events in children receiving patient-controlled analgesia by proxy or patient-controlled analgesia after surgery. *Anesth Analg* 107 (1):70–75, 2008.

61. Vondracek P, Bednarik J: Clinical and electrophysiological findings and long-term outcomes in paediatric patients with critical illness polyneuromyopathy. *Eur J Paediatr Neurol* 10(4):176–181, 2006.

62. White M, et al: Pain management in fulminating ulcerative colitis. *Paediatr Anaesth* 16(11):1148–1152, 2006.

63. Williams S, et al: Critical illness polyneuropathy and myopathy in pediatric intensive care: a review. *Pediatr Crit Care Med* 8 (1):18–22, 2007.

64. Yuen VM, et al: A comparison of intranasal dexmedetomidine and oral midazolam for premedication in pediatric anesthesia: a double-blinded randomized controlled trial. *Anesth Analg* 106(6):1715–1721, 2008.

Shock, Cardiac Arrest, and Resuscitation

6

Ronald M. Perkin • Allan R. de Caen •
Marc D. Berg • Stephen M. Schexnayder •
Mary Fran Hazinski

Ꮛvolve Be sure to check out the supplementary content available at http://evolve.elsevier.com/Hazinski.

This chapter includes information about the epidemiology, pathophysiology, clinical presentation, and management of shock and cardiac arrest. The chapter is divided into these two major sections.

SHOCK

SHOCK PEARLS

- Shock is a common cause of morbidity and mortality in pediatric patients with acute illness and injury.
- Early recognition of shock is essential for survival. Signs of shock in children may be more subtle than those in the adult and hypotension may not develop until late in the clinical course, when cardiovascular collapse is imminent.
- Treatment focuses on restoration of adequate oxygen delivery. Fluid therapy, inotropes, vasodilators, vasopressors, hydrocortisone, thyroid replacement, and extracardiac support devices may be required to accomplish this goal.
- Further shock treatment depends on the cause of the cardiovascular dysfunction and complications caused by the period of inadequate oxygen delivery.

INTRODUCTION

Shock is commonly defined as a clinical state characterized by an inadequate delivery of oxygen and metabolic substrates to meet the metabolic demands of the cells and tissues of the body.[53,245,246] Inadequate delivery of oxygen results in cellular hypoxia, anaerobic metabolism, lactic acidosis, activation of the host inflammatory response, and eventual vital organ dysfunction.

CARDIOVASCULAR PHYSIOLOGY AND SHOCK PATHOPHYSIOLOGY

Cellular Basis of Shock

Adenosine triphosphate (ATP) is the energy currency of the cell. Shock is a state of acute energy failure in which there is insufficient ATP production to support systemic cellular function.[53] During stress and periods of increased energy demand, glucose is produced from glycogenolysis and gluconeogenesis. Fat metabolism is the secondary source of energy in this state. Long-chain fatty acids are oxidized, and carnitine is used to shuttle acetyl coenzyme A (CoA) into mitochondria. Protein catabolism can also contribute acetyl CoA to the Krebs cycle for energy production. However, this method of energy production is inefficient; aerobic metabolism provides 20-fold the energy produced by anaerobic metabolism. Glucose is oxidized to pyruvate via glycolysis (also called the *Embden-Meyerhof pathway*), generating only two molecules of ATP in the process.

When oxygen supply is adequate, pyruvate enters the mitochondria and is converted to acetyl CoA by the pyruvate dehydrogenase enzyme complex; it is then completely oxidized to CO_2 and H_2O via the Krebs cycle (also known as the *tricarboxylic acid* or *citric acid cycle*) and oxidative phosphorylation, generating a net total of 36 to 38 moles of ATP for every mole of glucose. Conversely, when oxygen supply is inadequate, pyruvate is reduced by nicotinamide adenine dinucleotide and lactate dehydrogenase to lactate, a relatively inefficient process that generates considerably less ATP.

Cells do not have the means to store oxygen and are therefore dependent on a continuous supply that closely matches the changing metabolic needs during normal metabolism and cellular function. If the oxygen supply is not sufficient for metabolic requirements, hypoxia will ensue, eventually resulting in cellular injury or death. As defined previously, shock is a state characterized by an inadequate delivery of oxygen and substrates to meet the metabolic demands of the cells and tissues of the body. Alterations in cellular function and structure result directly from the consequent derangements in cellular metabolism and energy production. Eventually, these derangements lead to cellular necrosis, with subsequent release of proteolytic enzymes and other toxic products that produce a systemic inflammatory response.

In practical terms, using this operational definition, a state of shock may result from inadequate substrate delivery (glycopenia) or mitochondrial dysfunction (cellular dysoxia).[53] Oxygen delivery to the cells and tissues depends primarily on three factors: hemoglobin (Hb) concentration, cardiac output (CO), and the relative proportion of oxygenated hemoglobin (i.e., percent saturation [SaO_2]). Oxygen is transported in the blood combined with hemoglobin, although a relatively small amount is freely dissolved in the plasma fraction of the blood. When fully saturated at normal body temperature, each gram of hemoglobin can carry about 1.34 to 1.36 mL of oxygen. The normal arterial oxygen content is calculated as follows:

$$CaO_2 \text{ (mLO}_2/\text{dL blood)} = (\text{Hb g/dL} \times 1.34 \text{ mL/g} \times SaO_2) + (0.003 \text{ mL} \times PaO_2)$$

Oxygen delivery (DO_2) is a product of arterial oxygen content and CO:

$$DO_2 = CO \times CaO_2$$

Generally, more oxygen is delivered to the cells of the body than the cells actually require for normal metabolism. However, a low CO (stagnant hypoxia), low hemoglobin concentration (anemic hypoxia), or low hemoglobin saturation (hypoxic hypoxia) will result in inadequate delivery of oxygen unless the other factors can increase commensurately.

Adequate glucose delivery depends on the presence of adequate blood glucose concentration, normal blood flow (or CO), and an adequate concentration of insulin for cells with insulin-responsive glucose transporters (e.g., cardiomyocytes). Glycopenic shock can be caused by hypoglycemia and by extreme insulin resistance.[53] Finally, even when oxygen delivery and glucose delivery are adequate, shock may occur as a result of mitochondrial dysfunction. For example, cyanide poisons the oxidative phosphorylation chain, preventing production of ATP. Cellular dysoxia (also known as *cytopathic hypoxia*) may theoretically occur from one or a combination of several mechanisms, including diminished delivery of a key substrate (e.g., pyruvate) to the Krebs cycle of the electron transport chain or uncoupling of oxidative phosphorylation.

Determinants of Oxygen Delivery

Normal CO

As defined previously, oxygen delivery is the product of CO and arterial oxygen content (CaO_2). CO is the product of heart rate (HR) and stroke volume (SV; Fig. 6-1). SV, in turn, is dependent on preload, afterload, and contractility. Furthermore,

blood pressure (BP) is determined by the product of CO and systemic vascular resistance (SVR).

Myocardial performance can be affected by changes in oxygenation, perfusion, serum ionized calcium concentration, acid-base, and electrolyte balance, sympathetic or vagal stimulation, and drugs.[244] These factors can affect CO by altering either HR or SV.

Sympathetic nervous system β-adrenergic stimulation increases myocardial calcium release and influx, enhancing myocardial contraction. In addition, because calcium reuptake is more rapid, the ventricular systolic time is shorter. Shortening of ventricular systolic time results in prolongation of the diastolic filling time at the same HR, so SV improves. Many of these effects are mediated by cyclic adenosine monophosphate (cAMP), an intracellular messenger that promotes phosphorylation of sarcolemmal proteins and increases the opening of calcium channels in myocardial cell membranes. Phosphodiesterase then converts the cAMP to an inactive compound, ending the cAMP and sympathetic effects. Phosphodiesterase inhibitors (such as milrinone) prevent the inactivation of cAMP; therefore they prolong any adrenergic effects that are mediated by cAMP.

Contractility is enhanced by any conditions or factors that increase intracellular calcium. Alpha-adrenergic stimulation and cardiac glycosides all increase intracellular ionized calcium. The intracellular sodium concentration can influence the free calcium levels in the myocyte, because sodium and calcium ions share storage sites and compete for space in the sodium-potassium pump. When the intracellular sodium concentration is increased (e.g., during digitalis therapy), sodium occupies space in the exchange pump. As a result, calcium ions accumulate in the myocardial cell, and myocardial contractility increases.

FIG. 6-1 A, Relationships of factors determining cardiac output and systemic perfusion. **B,** Relationships of factors determining systemic oxygen delivery.

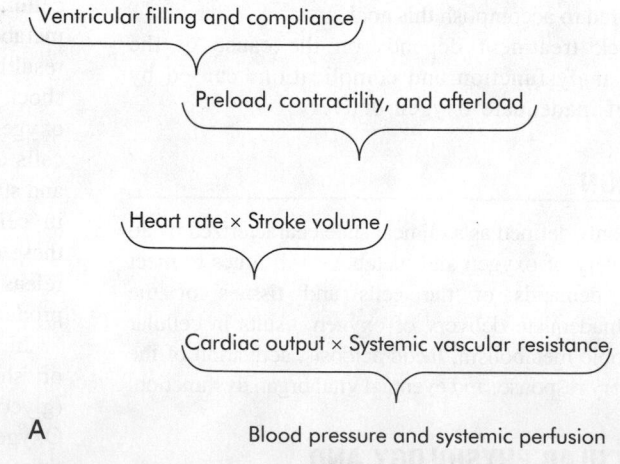

A

Ventricular filling and compliance

Preload, contractility, and afterload

Heart rate × Stroke volume

Cardiac output × Systemic vascular resistance

Blood pressure and systemic perfusion

B

(Hgb concentration × 1.34 mL O_2/Saturated gm Hgb) × [Oxyhemoglobin saturation]) + Dissolved O_2

Arterial oxygen content × Cardiac output

Systemic oxygen delivery

Factors Influencing SV

Three terms first defined in the physiology laboratory are used clinically to describe several important factors influencing myocardial function. These terms—*preload, contractility,* and *afterload*—can be defined precisely in the physiology laboratory using isolated normal myocardial preparations. Their application to the clinical setting, however, where it may be impossible to separate the effects of each factor, has been less precise. The common usage and clinical application of these terms are provided here.

Ventricular Preload. Preload is the amount of myocardial fiber stretch that is present before contraction. The significance of ventricular preload was first appreciated by Howell (in 1894), Frank (in 1894), and Starling (in 1914)[242] in a series of experiments performed on isolated normal myocardial muscle preparations. Howell, Frank, and Starling observed that normal myocardium generates greater tension during contraction if it is stretched before contraction. This increase in the force of contraction occurs as a result of optimization of overlap between actin and myosin filaments in the sarcomere. These observations became known as the Frank-Starling law of the heart, which states that an increase in ventricular work, systolic tension, and SV results from an increase in presystolic stretch (preload). The graphic representation of the relationship between ventricular end-diastolic myocardial fiber length (usually approximated by ventricular end-diastolic pressure [VEDP]) and SV is the Frank-Starling curve, which is a ventricular (myocardial) function curve (Fig. 6-2).

The Frank-Starling law of the heart applies to dysfunctional and normal myocardium, although the appearance (i.e., the position and slope) of each function curve will differ. Optimal stretch of any myocardial fiber should improve myocardial performance, but it will be necessary to tailor the approach to the patient with shock to attempt to identify the optimal preload that yields the best CO and systemic perfusion.

Myocardial fiber length is not readily measured in the clinical setting; therefore VEDP is monitored as an indirect measure of the stretch placed on the myocardial fibers before contraction. VEDP is increased by intravenous volume administration. The relationship between ventricular end-diastolic volume (and fiber length) and VEDP is not a linear one, however. The rise in VEDP that occurs as end-diastolic volume is increased is determined by ventricular compliance (see "Ventricular Compliance") and by venous return; both of these factors may be altered by disease or therapy.

To a point, as VEDP is increased, the force of contraction and myocardial fiber shortening should increase, and SV should rise.[98] If, however, the ventricle is filled beyond a critical point, overlap of actin and myosin filaments is no longer optimal; ventricular dilation can result, and stroke volume decreases.[47] Extremely high VEDPs (higher than approximately 25 cm H_2O pressure when capillary permeability is normal, and lower pressures when capillary permeability is increased) result in pulmonary and systemic edema, and high pressures will compromise coronary and subendocardial blood flow.

If SV or CO can be estimated reliably (e.g., using Doppler, Fick, or thermodilution calculations) a ventricular function curve can be constructed for any patient. CO or SV (CO

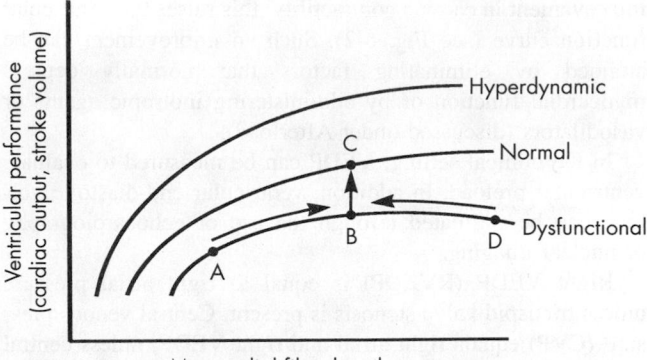

FIG. 6-2 Frank-Starling curve. In the laboratory description of the Frank-Starling law (using isolated normal myocardial fibers), an increase in the end-diastolic myocardial fiber length increased the tension generated by the myocardial fiber. In the clinical setting, measurement of end-diastolic fiber length is impossible, so the ventricular end-diastolic pressure (VEDP) is increased to produce improvement in SV or cardiac output. To a point, an increase in VEDP will produce an improvement in cardiac output. (A → B), This increase in VEDP is accomplished through judicious titration of intravenous fluid. The clinician must also recognize that a family of myocardial function curves exist. The patient's myocardial function can be characterized as normal, dysfunctional, or hyperdynamic. If the myocardium is dysfunctional, it generally requires a higher VEDP than the normal myocardium to maximize cardiac output. In addition, excessive volume administration can produce a decrease in cardiac output and myocardial performance if the ventricle is dysfunctional (B → D). In this case, administration of a diuretic or vasodilator may improve cardiac output (D → B). Correction of acid-base imbalances, reduction in afterload, or administration of inotropic medications may improve myocardial function so that cardiac output increases without need for further increase in VEDP (B → C). If the patient's myocardial function is hyperdynamic, cardiac output will be high even at low VEDP. (Courtesy William Banner, Jr.)

divided by HR) are plotted on the vertical axis of the graph, and VEDP is plotted on the horizontal axis. As fluid administration is titrated and the SV is determined at various VEDPs, the optimal VEDP is identified as the peak point on the curve.

A family of ventricular function curves can be constructed to illustrate the response of normal, depressed, or enhanced myocardial response to increased VEDP (see Fig. 6-2). If the patient demonstrates poor myocardial function, the ventricular function curve will be relatively flat, and a high VEDP will be required to produce even a modest improvement in myocardial function. If myocardial function is normal, a small increase in VEDP can produce a significant rise in SV or CO. If ventricular function is hyperdynamic, even nominal increases in VEDP will produce significant increases in SV or CO.

A goal of the treatment of any patient with cardiovascular dysfunction is to maximize SV and CO while minimizing adverse effects of fluid administration, such as pulmonary edema. An increase in SV and CO can be achieved by moving the patient to the highest point of an individual ventricular function curve (see Fig. 6-2) through judicious fluid administration. Improvement in SV and CO also can be achieved by altering the ventricular compliance, using vasodilator therapy. Further increase in SV and CO also can be achieved through improvement in cardiac contractility; this raises the ventricular function curve (see Fig. 6-2). Such an improvement can be attained by eliminating factors that normally depress myocardial function or by administering inotropic agents or vasodilators (discussed under Afterload).

In the clinical setting, VEDP can be measured to evaluate ventricular preload. In addition, ventricular end-diastolic volume can be estimated through the use of echocardiography or nuclear imaging.

Right VEDP (RVEDP) is equal to right atrial pressure unless tricuspid valve stenosis is present. Central venous pressure (CVP) equals right atrial and right VEDP, unless central venous obstruction is present.

RVEDP and CVP often can be estimated with careful clinical assessment of the level of hydration, liver size, palpation of the infant's fontanelle, determination of presence (or absence) of systemic edema, and evaluation of the cardiac size on chest radiograph.[275] Dry mucous membranes, a sunken fontanelle, and the absence of hepatomegaly are findings consistent with a normal or low central venous pressure. Hepatomegaly and periorbital edema usually are present once the CVP is elevated significantly. Systemic edema also may be noted despite a normal or low CVP if capillary leak or hypoalbuminemia is present. A high RVEDP and heart failure is often associated with cardiac enlargement on chest radiograph.

Left VEDP (LVEDP) is equal to left atrial pressure unless mitral valve disease is present. Reliable estimation of LVEDP is not possible through clinical assessment alone.[275] Although the presence of pulmonary edema frequently is assumed to indicate the presence of a high LVEDP (exceeding 20 to 25 mm Hg), pulmonary edema may be observed at any (even a low) LVEDP if capillary leak is present.

A left atrial catheter or pulmonary artery catheter must be inserted to measure LVEDP, because this pressure cannot be estimated from clinical examination. In the absence of pulmonary venous constriction or obstruction, a pulmonary artery wedge pressure will approximate left atrial pressure. In the absence of mitral valve disease or extreme tachycardia, left atrial pressure should reflect LVEDP. However, the pulmonary artery catheter must be placed appropriately and the transducer must be zeroed, leveled, and calibrated correctly.

VEDP directly affects the resting length of the ventricular myocardial cells before contraction. Although VEDP is increased through the administration of intravenous fluids, VEDP is not related linearly to fluid volume administered. VEDP also will be affected by ventricular compliance. Ventricular compliance is in turn affected by ventricular function, ventricular relaxation, wall thickness, ventricular size, pericardial pressures, and HR.

Ventricular Compliance. *Ventricular compliance* refers to the distensibility of the ventricle. It is defined as the change in ventricular volume (in milliliters) for a given change in pressure (in millimeters of mercury), or $\Delta V/\Delta P$, and can be depicted graphically by a ventricular compliance curve (Fig. 6-3). The opposite of compliance is stiffness ($\Delta P/\Delta V$).

If the ventricle is extremely compliant, a large volume of fluid may be administered without producing a significant

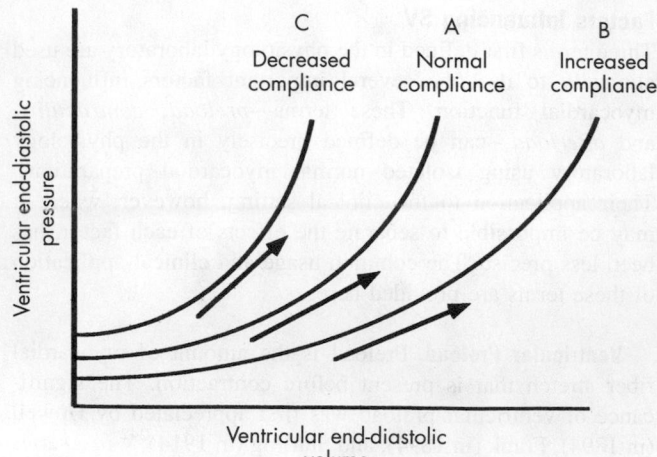

FIG. 6-3 Ventricular compliance is illustrated by a ventricular end-diastolic pressure (VEDP)-volume curve. The slope of a tangent to the curve (*arrows*) indicates the change in pressure/change in volume ($\Delta P/\Delta V$), representing the stiffness of the ventricle at a given filling pressure. Ventricular compliance changes with age (compliance is lower, or the compliance curve is shifted to the left in the fetus or young infant), cardiovascular disease, and drug therapy. In the normal ventricle (*curve A*), a low ventricular end-diastolic volume is associated with a low VEDP. As the ventricle is filled, smaller changes in volume produce exponentially greater rises in end-diastolic pressure. When the ventricle is dysfunctional or hypertrophied (*curve C*), ventricular compliance is reduced, and even a small increase in ventricular end-diastolic volume will produce a rise in VEDP. Vasodilator therapy can increase ventricular compliance (*curve B*), so that greater ventricular volume can be tolerated without a rise in VEDP. In this manner, the stroke volume can be increased without increasing the VEDP. (Courtesy William Banner, Jr.)

increase in VEDP (see Fig. 6-3, *curve B*). If the ventricle is dysfunctional (as occurs with restrictive cardiomyopathy) or hypertrophied, ventricular compliance usually is reduced (see Fig. 6-3, *curve C*). In this case, even a small volume of administered intravenous fluids will produce a significant rise in VEDP.[268] The more dysfunctional and noncompliant the ventricle, the higher the resting VEDP and the VEDP needed to optimize SV and ventricular performance (see Fig. 6-2).

Ventricular compliance is not constant over all ranges of VEDP. Any ventricle is maximally compliant at low filling pressures. As the ventricle is filled, compliance is reduced because ventricular stretch may be maximal.[55,169] Rapid volume infusion tends to raise VEDP more rapidly than gradual volume infusion. Compliant ventricles usually demonstrate a substantial improvement in SV when an intravenous fluid bolus is administered.

Vasodilator therapy will improve ventricular compliance. When these drugs are administered the compliance curve is altered, so a greater end-diastolic volume may be present without a substantial increase in VEDP (see Fig. 6-3). SV may then be increased without a rise in VEDP.

Compliance also is affected by ventricular size, pericardial space, and HR.[55] Infants have small and relatively noncompliant ventricles, so the infant's VEDP may rise sharply with minimal fluid volume administration. If the same volume (on a per-kilogram basis) is administered to an older child, a smaller change in VEDP will result because the ventricles are larger and more compliant in older children.

Constrictive pericarditis and tamponade will decrease ventricular compliance, because ventricular expansion cannot occur in response to volume administration. Diastolic filling will be impaired and SV often is reduced. As a result, if pericarditis or tamponade is present, VEDP usually will be elevated and will rise significantly with even modest fluid volume infusion. SV and CO may not improve despite the rise in VEDP.

Extreme tachycardia (such as supraventricular tachycardia, SVT) can produce a rise in VEDP. A rapid HR is associated with reduced ventricular diastolic time and incomplete relaxation. As a result the VEDP rises.

Because VEDP is affected by a variety of factors, it is important to attempt to determine the VEDP associated with optimal systemic perfusion for each patient on each day. Obviously this optimal pressure can change frequently during the patient's clinical course. Throughout therapy, evidence of systemic perfusion always should be assessed as VEDP is manipulated.

Ventricular Contractility. The term *contractility* refers to the strength and efficiency of contraction; it is the force generated by the myocardium, independent of preload and afterload. Contractility is estimated by velocity of fiber shortening; this can be determined using echocardiography. If myocardial function is good, the ventricular fibers shorten rapidly. As a result, at the same HR, systole requires less time, leaving more time for diastole (filling time). SV will increase if circulating blood volume is adequate and ventricular afterload is unchanged.

Although contractility can be measured in the laboratory, it is not easily isolated and measured in the clinical setting. The most common method of evaluating contractility at the bedside is echocardiographic evaluation of fiber-shortening times and measurement of the shortening fraction of left ventricular diameter. Shortening fraction is calculated by determining the difference between the end-diastolic and end-systolic dimensions. Normal shortening fraction is approximately 28% to 44%.[206]

If a thermodilution CO pulmonary artery catheter is in place, or if reliable Doppler CO estimations can be obtained, the nurse can create a ventricular function curve (see Fig. 6-2). If CO improves with no change in VEDP or HR, ventricular contractility or compliance has probably improved.

Although evaluation of contractility considers the effectiveness of ventricular systolic function, ventricular filling, SV, and CO may also be impaired by a compromise in ventricular diastolic function. Diastolic function can be evaluated by echocardiography, but this evaluation will also be influenced by HR, ventricular preload, and ventricular systolic function.

Afterload. Afterload is any impediment to ventricular ejection; it is the sum of all forces opposing ventricular emptying and is described as ventricular wall stress. If ventricular wall stress is increased, there will be a significant impediment to ventricular ejection, and the ventricle will be required to generate higher pressure to eject the same amount of blood. If the higher pressure cannot be generated, the amount of blood ejected by the ventricle will fall. With any increase in afterload, oxygen consumption and the work of the ventricle increase. Even a normal afterload may be excessive when myocardial function is poor.

The major determinants of ventricular afterload or wall stress are: ventricular lumen radius, ventricular wall thickness (note that hypertrophy decreases afterload), and the ventricular intracavitary ejection pressure (Fig. 6-4). In the absence of left ventricular outflow tract obstruction (e.g., aortic stenosis), left ventricular ejection pressure will equal aortic and systemic arterial pressure. In the absence of right ventricular outflow tract obstruction (e.g., pulmonary stenosis), right ventricular ejection pressure will equal pulmonary arterial pressure. Systemic and pulmonary artery pressures in turn are determined by blood flow and resistance. Therefore in the absence of ventricular outflow tract obstruction or significant alterations in ventricular size or wall thickness, ventricular afterload is related primarily to the impedance provided by the pulmonary and systemic arterial circulations.

The ventricle of the infant or child can usually adapt to increases in ventricular afterload, provided that the increases are neither severe nor acute. For example, if the left ventricular muscle thickness increases and the diameter of the left ventricular chamber is reduced, wall stress (afterload) may be normalized. If, however, afterload increases severely or acutely—such as occurs with acute, reactive pulmonary vasoconstriction in response to severe alveolar hypoxia—CO may fall.

Afterload cannot be measured in the clinical setting. Resistances in the pulmonary and systemic circulations can be calculated using a thermodilution pulmonary artery catheter. SVR can also be calculated using estimations of CO obtained by Doppler calculations, and PVR can be estimated using echocardiography. It is important to note that, at best, SVR and PVR are calculated or estimated numbers, not measurements.

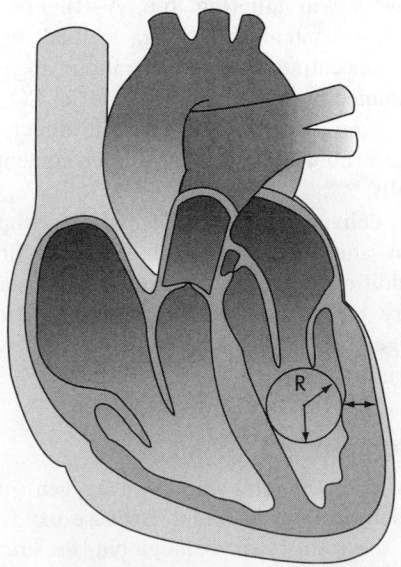

FIG. 6-4 Factors influencing ventricular wall stress. According to Laplace's law, Wall stress = (Ventricular pressure × Ventricular radius) ÷ (2 × Ventricular wall thickness). R, Radius.

Oxygen Delivery

The ultimate function of the heart and lungs is to deliver oxygenated blood to the tissues. Systemic DO_2 is the volume of oxygen (in milliliters) delivered to the tissues per minute. $DO_2(I)$ is the volume of oxygen delivered to the tissues per minute, indexed to body surface area (BSA), so that the units are milliliters per minute per square meter. DO_2 is the product of arterial oxygen content (the amount of oxygen in arterial blood in milliliters per deciliter) the CO (in liters per minute), and a factor of 10. $DO_2(I)$ is the product of arterial oxygen content (in milliliters per deciliter), the cardiac index (in liters per minute per square meter), and a factor of 10 (see Fig. 6-1).

Under resting conditions with normal distribution of CO, oxygen delivery is more than adequate to meet the total oxygen requirements the tissues need to maintain aerobic metabolism, which is referred to as *oxygen consumption* (VO_2). Excess oxygen delivery or oxygen reserve serves as a buffer, so a modest reduction in oxygen delivery will be more than adequately compensated by increased extraction of the delivered oxygen, without any significant reduction in oxygen consumption. During stress or vigorous exercise, oxygen consumption markedly increases, as does oxygen delivery. Therefore, under most conditions, the metabolic demands of the cells and tissues of the body dictate the level of oxygen delivery. However, little oxygen is stored in the cells and tissues of the body; therefore as oxygen delivery falls with critical illness, oxygen extraction must necessarily increase to meet metabolic demands, and oxygen consumption remains relatively constant (i.e., it is delivery independent; Fig. 6-5). However, there is a critical level of oxygen delivery at which the body's compensatory mechanisms are no longer able to meet metabolic needs (i.e., the point at which oxygen extraction is maximal). Once oxygen delivery falls below this level, oxygen consumption must also fall and is said to become delivery dependent (see Fig. 6-5, Normal critical delivery threshold).

If either arterial oxygen content or CO falls without a commensurate and compensatory increase in the other component, oxygen delivery will fall (Fig. 6-6, A–H). For example, if arterial oxygen content falls (e.g., caused by a fall in hemoglobin concentration or its saturation), oxygen delivery can be maintained by a commensurate rise in CO. If CO falls, however, oxygen delivery will fall in direct correlation, because there is no way for arterial oxygen content to increase when CO falls.

If oxygen delivery falls significantly, the sympathetic nervous system attempts to redistribute blood flow to vital organs. In addition, tissue oxygen extraction increases. If these compensatory mechanisms fail to maintain adequate blood flow or oxygen delivery, anaerobic metabolism will result in lactic acidosis.

Oxygen Content

Oxygen content is the total amount of oxygen (in milliliters) carried in each deciliter of blood. Because oxygen is carried primarily in the form of oxyhemoglobin, the arterial oxygen content essentially is determined by the hemoglobin concentration and its saturation, although a small amount of oxygen is carried dissolved in the blood.

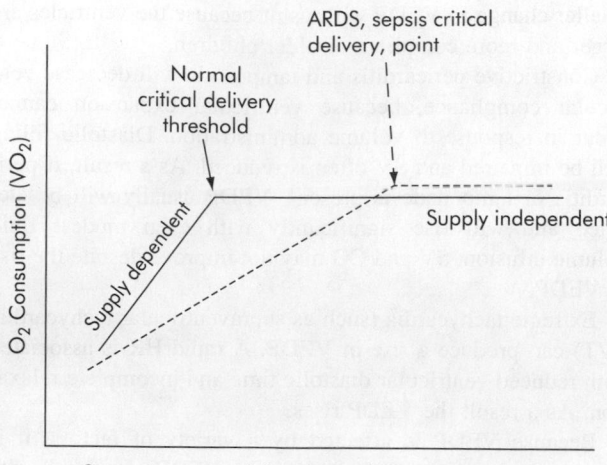

FIG. 6-5 Theoretical relationship between oxygen delivery and oxygen consumption. In normal tissues (horizontal portion of *solid line*, labeled *supply-independent*), oxygen delivery far exceeds oxygen consumption, so a significant fall in systemic oxygen delivery can be tolerated without any change in oxygen consumption (tissue oxygen extraction merely increases). However, eventually a profound fall in oxygen delivery will reach a critical delivery threshold. Further compromise in oxygen delivery will then result in a proportional fall in oxygen consumption (slope of *solid line*, labeled *supply-dependent*); the oxygen consumption is supply-dependent. In patients with adult respiratory distress syndrome and patients with sepsis (*broken line*), oxygen consumption is thought to be far more supply dependent than in the normal population (*dotted arrow* indicates critical delivery threshold for patients with acute respiratory distress syndrome [ARDS] and sepsis—note that oxygen consumption becomes supply dependent at a much higher level of oxygen delivery than in normal patients). In these patients, even a small reduction in oxygen delivery can force a fall in oxygen consumption. For this reason, medical therapy may target increasing oxygen delivery to ranges above normal during the treatment of ARDS or sepsis. (Modified with permission from Schumaker PT, Samuel RW: Oxygen delivery and uptake by peripheral tissues. *Crit Care Clin* 5:255, 1989.)

Arterial oxygen content will be decreased by anemia or a fall in the oxyhemoglobin saturation. For this reason, anemia should be avoided in patients with compromised cardiorespiratory function, and transfusion therapy should be considered if anemia develops.

There is no "magic" hemoglobin concentration that is perfect for all patients. A low hemoglobin value decreases the oxygen-carrying capacity of the blood. An extremely high hemoglobin value is also undesirable, because it increases blood viscosity and resistance to blood flow in small vessels. In the presence of sluggish systemic, pulmonary, or cerebral perfusion, the hemoglobin may be maintained at 10 to 11 g/dL, despite the fall in oxygen content that results.

The optimal hemoglobin threshold for erythrocyte (red blood cell) transfusion in critically ill children is unknown.[160] Whereas transfusion is indicated in conditions of hemodynamic instability and anemia (hemoglobin <10 g/dL), once stability is achieved the threshold hemoglobin level for transfusion may need to be lowered. A recent multicenter trial demonstrated that in stable, critically ill children a hemoglobin threshold of 7 g/dL for red blood cell transfusion decreased transfusion requirements without increasing adverse outcome.[160]

The oxyhemoglobin saturation will fall in the presence of an intrapulmonary shunt or a right-to-left intracardiac shunt (cyanotic congenital heart disease [CHD]). If an intrapulmonary shunt is causing the hypoxemia, the oxyhemoglobin saturation and the arterial oxygen content can usually be increased through the administration of supplementary inspired oxygen. It may be necessary to provide mechanical ventilation with positive end-expiratory pressure to maximize oxyhemoglobin saturation.

The child with cyanotic CHD is always hypoxemic (i.e., has low arterial oxyhemoglobin saturation). As a compensatory mechanism, these children develop polycythemia; this maintains their arterial oxygen content at near normal levels despite oxyhemoglobin desaturation. These children cannot tolerate a fall in hemoglobin concentration, such as can occur after a minor surgical procedure, because it will result in a significant fall in oxygen content. If possible, in these children the hemoglobin concentration should be maintained at approximately 15 to 16 g/dL. The child with cyanotic CHD and polycythemia cannot be allowed to become dehydrated and hemoconcentrated. Once the hemoglobin concentration exceeds 20 to 25 g/dL and the hematocrit exceeds 60% to 70%, the blood becomes too viscous, and the risk of thromboembolic complications is high. Pheresis (removal of whole blood and

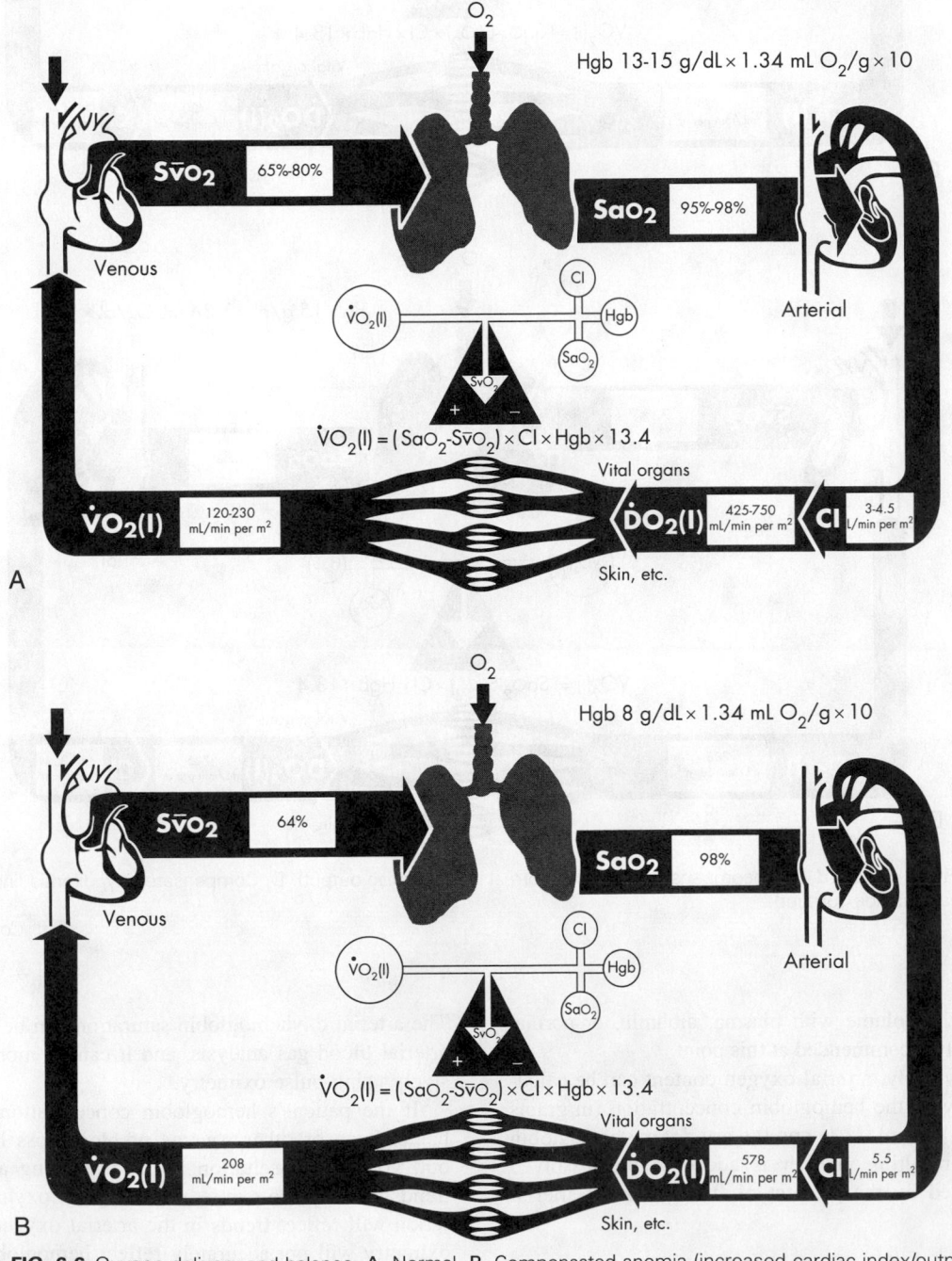

FIG. 6-6 Oxygen delivery and balance. **A,** Normal. **B,** Compensated anemia (increased cardiac index/output).

Continued

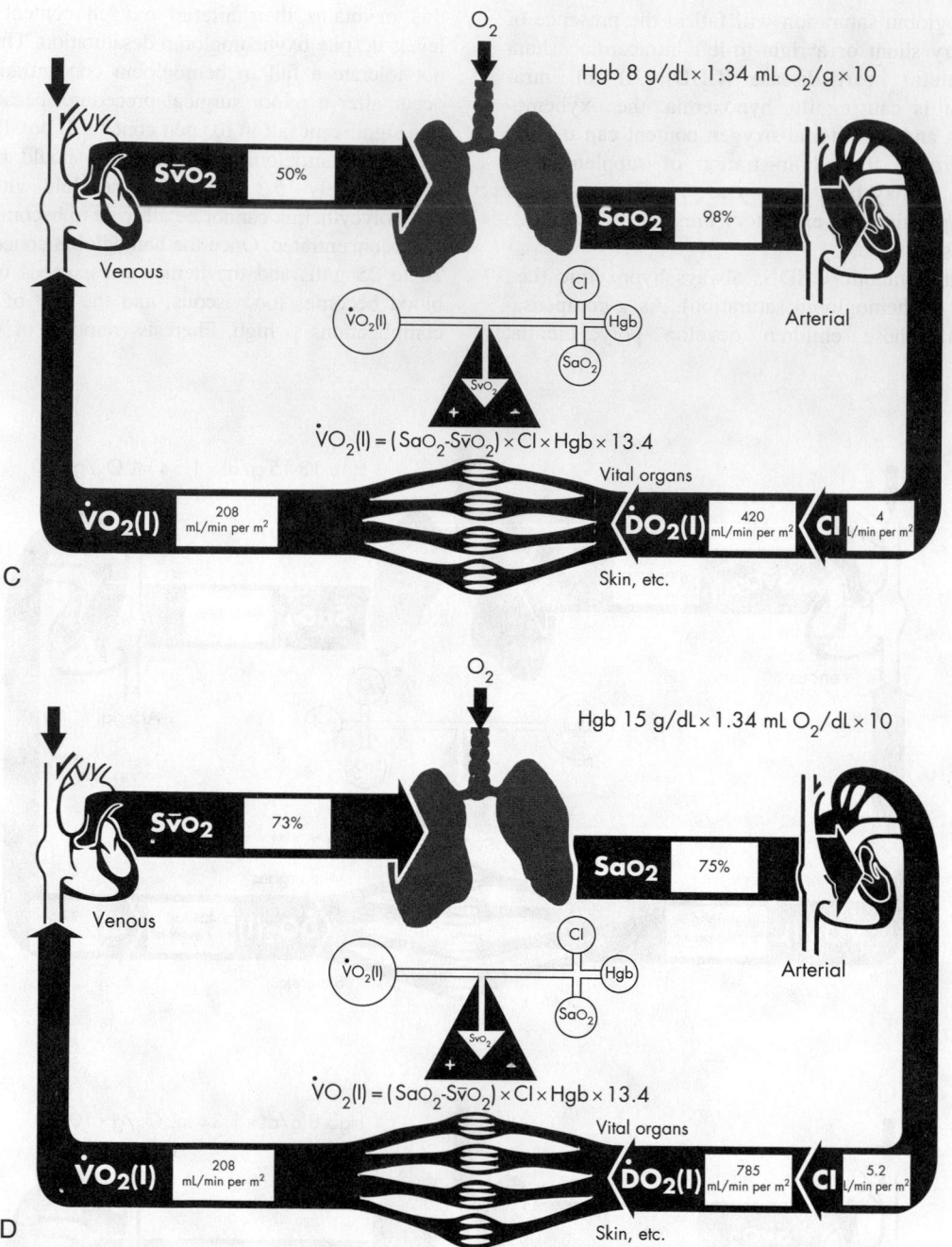

O_2

Hgb 8 g/dL × 1.34 mL O_2/g × 10

$S\bar{v}O_2$ 50%

Venous

SaO_2 98%

Arterial

CI

Hgb

$\dot{V}O_2(I)$

SaO_2

$S\bar{v}O_2$

$\dot{V}O_2(I) = (SaO_2 - S\bar{v}O_2) \times CI \times Hgb \times 13.4$

Vital organs

$\dot{V}O_2(I)$ 208 mL/min per m²

$\dot{D}O_2(I)$ 420 mL/min per m²

CI 4 L/min per m²

Skin, etc.

C

O_2

Hgb 15 g/dL × 1.34 mL O_2/dL × 10

$S\bar{v}O_2$ 73%

Venous

SaO_2 75%

Arterial

CI

Hgb

$\dot{V}O_2(I)$

SaO_2

$S\bar{v}O_2$

$\dot{V}O_2(I) = (SaO_2 - S\bar{v}O_2) \times CI \times Hgb \times 13.4$

Vital organs

$\dot{V}O_2(I)$ 208 mL/min per m²

$\dot{D}O_2(I)$ 785 mL/min per m²

CI 5.2 L/min per m²

Skin, etc.

D

FIG. 6-6, cont'd **C,** Uncompensated anemia (normal index/cardiac output). **D,** Compensated hypoxemia (increased cardiac index/output).

Continued

replacement of the volume with plasma, albumin, or normal saline) is generally recommended at this point.

As noted previously, arterial oxygen content can be calculated by multiplying the hemoglobin concentration (in grams per deciliter) by 1.34 mL O_2/g and the arterial oxyhemoglobin saturation. The resulting number is added to the dissolved oxygen, calculated by the product of 0.003 and the arterial oxygen tension:

$$CaO_2 = (\text{Hgb concentration [g/dL]} \times 1.34\ \text{mL/g} \times SaO_2) + (0.003 \times PaO_2)$$

The arterial oxyhemoglobin saturation can be evaluated using arterial blood gas analysis, and it can be monitored noninvasively using pulse oximetry.

If the patient's hemoglobin concentration is stable (e.g., hemorrhage or other sources of blood loss have been ruled out, volume resuscitation is not producing a hemodilution), trends in the pulse oximeter readings of oxyhemoglobin saturation will reflect trends in the arterial oxygen content. Pulse oximetry will not accurately reflect hemoglobin saturation in the presence of methemoglobinemia or carbon monoxide poisoning, and it is important to note that in the presence of

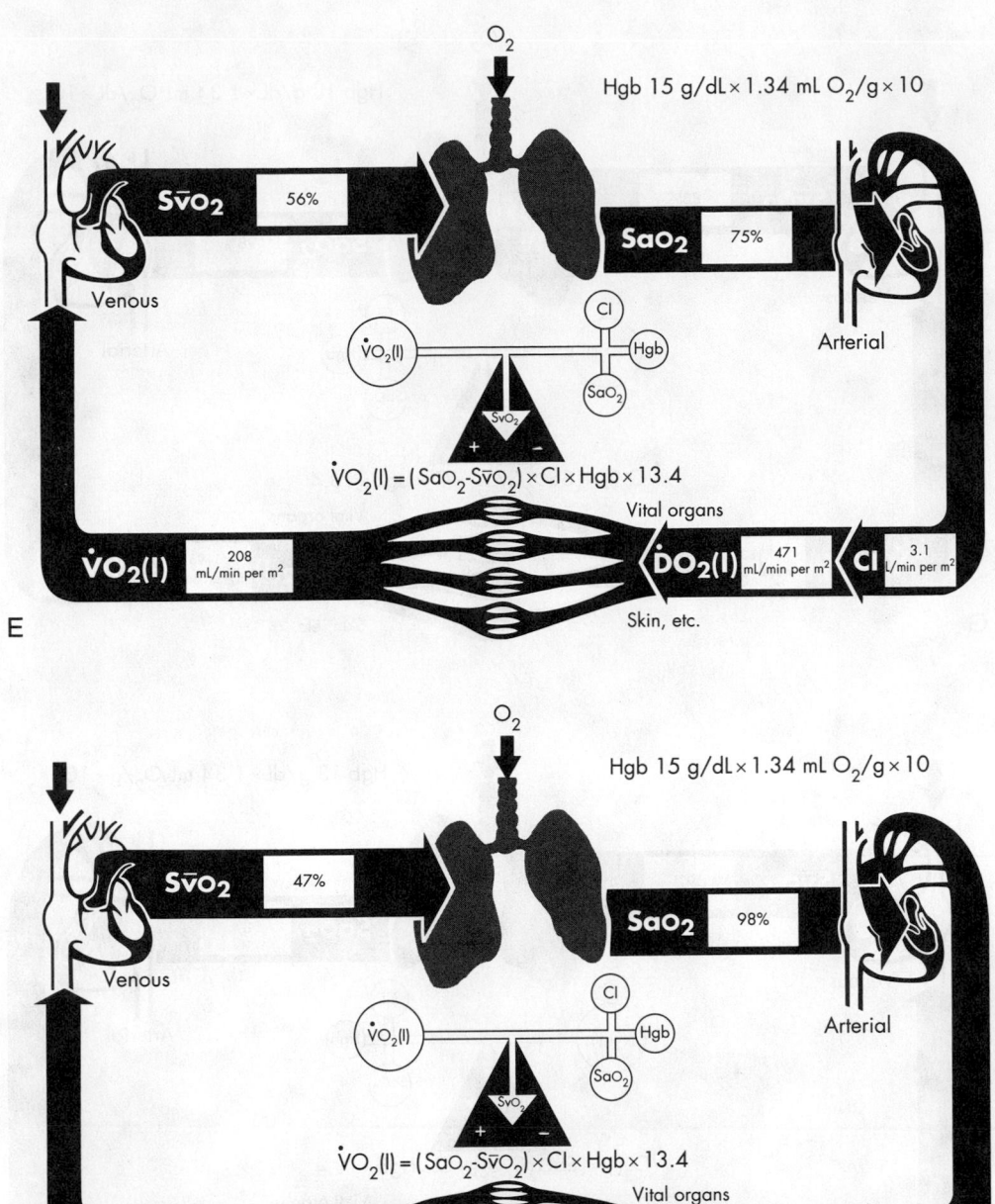

FIG. 6-6, cont'd E, Uncompensated hypoxemia (normal cardiac index/output). F, Shock with low cardiac index/output.
Continued

severe anemia, oxygen delivery will be inadequate despite a normal oxyhemoglobin saturation.

Cardiac Output

CO is the volume of blood ejected by the heart in 1 minute. CO is the product of HR and SV. CO may be recorded in liters per minute or milliliters per minute, although in children it is often normalized to BSA and recorded as the cardiac index (in milliliters per minute per square meter BSA). Normal cardiac index averages 3 to 4.5 mL/min per m² BSA (Table 6-1).

The child's CO or index should be evaluated in light of the child's clinical condition, to determine whether the CO or index is adequate or inadequate to maintain oxygen and substrate delivery and aerobic metabolism. A normal or even elevated CO or index can be inadequate if it is maldistributed (e.g., sepsis) or if metabolic demands are high (e.g., malignant hyperthermia).

CO can be affected by factors that alter HR or SV. If either factor decreases without a commensurate and compensatory increase in the other factor, CO will fall. Children are highly dependent on an adequate HR to maintain an adequate CO or index. If the HR falls, SV may not increase sufficiently; thus bradycardia often produces a fall in CO. Tachycardia is an efficient method of increasing CO during episodes of stress and increased oxygen requirements, such as fever, pain, or cardiorespiratory failure. In fact, tachycardia should be present under these conditions. However, an extremely rapid HR (ventricular

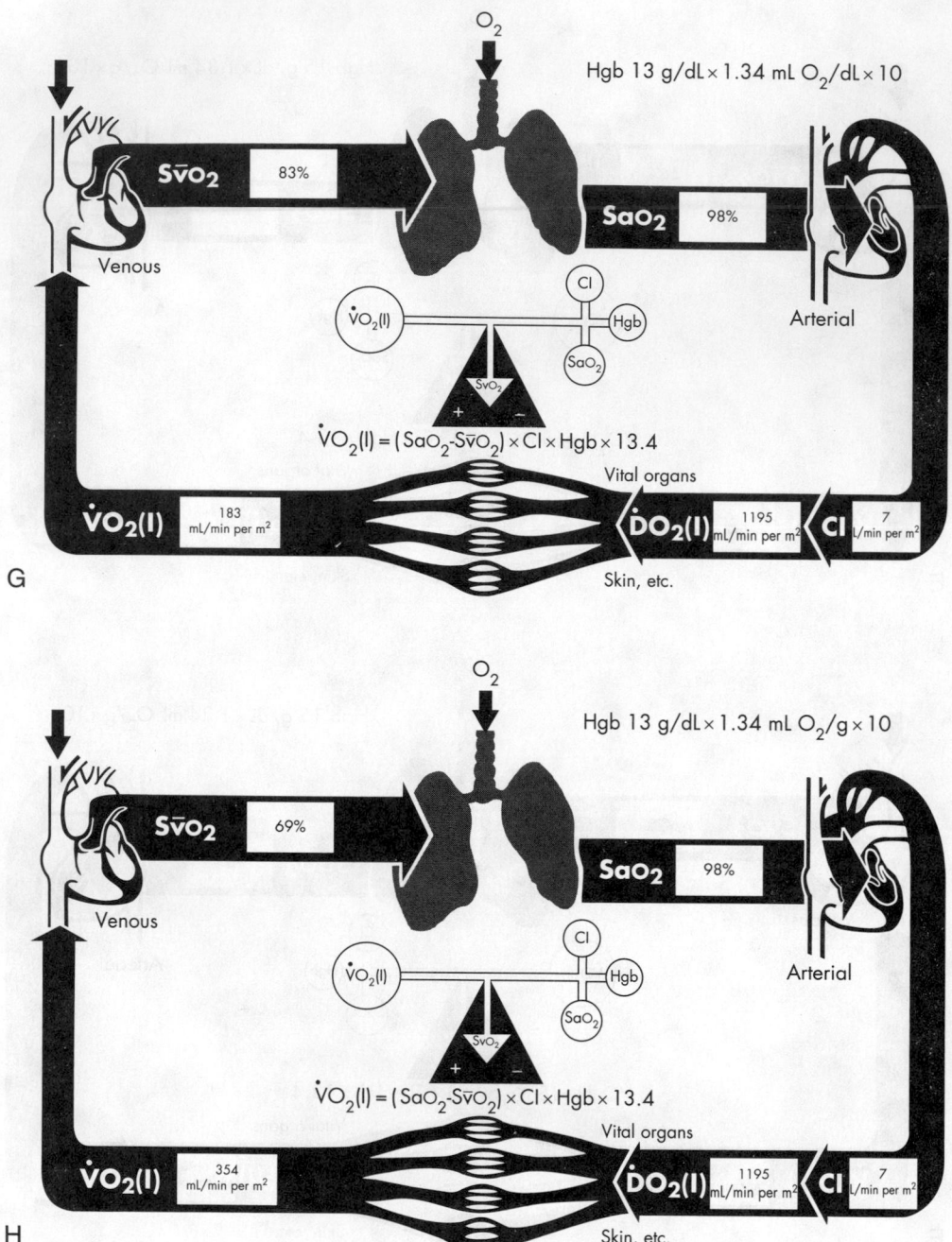

FIG. 6-6, cont'd **G,** Sepsis with low oxygen extraction (high oxygen delivery). **H,** Sepsis with improved oxygen extraction (treated sepsis with high oxygen delivery).

rate exceeding 180 to 220 per min) can produce a fall in CO if ventricular filling time or coronary artery perfusion time is severely compromised. SV averages 1.5 mL/kg. SV will be influenced by HR and by ventricular preload, contractility, and afterload. These factors have been described previously.

Clinical Assessment of CO

CO is evaluated clinically through assessment of systemic and organ perfusion and function. When CO is inadequate to maintain sufficient oxygen delivery and aerobic metabolism, signs of poor systemic perfusion, metabolic acidosis, and organ system failure develop. These signs include tachycardia, mottled or pale color, decreased urine output, alteration in the quality of peripheral pulses, and metabolic (lactic) acidosis. The child's responsiveness and level of consciousness may be compromised.

If hypovolemic or cardiogenic shock are present, adrenergic compensatory mechanisms will attempt to redistribute blood flow, diverting it away from the skin, gut, and kidneys to maintain vital blood flow to the heart and brain. This diversion results in peripheral vasoconstriction with cooling of the extremities, delayed capillary refill, and diminished peripheral pulses.

Table 6-1 Normal Cardiac Output, Oxygen Delivery, and Oxygen Consumption in Children

Age	Weight (kg)	BSA (m²)	Cardiac output* (mL/min)	OXYGEN DELIVERY†		OXYGEN CONSUMPTION	
				DO₂ (mL/min)	DO₂(I) (mL/min per m²)	VO₂ (mL/min)	VO₂(I) (mL/min per m²)
Newborn	3.2	0.2	700-800	133-200	665-1000	36-54	180-270
6 mo	8	0.42	1000-1600	200-280	476-667	70-100	167-238
1 yr	10	0.5	1300-1500	260-300	520-600	85-110	170-220
2 yr	13	0.59	1500-2000	300-400	508-678	91-123	154-208
4 yr	17	0.71	2300-2375	460-475	648-669	110-150	155-211
5 yr	19	0.77	2500-3000	500-600	649-779	115-170	149-221
8 yr	28	0.96	3400-3600	680-720	708-750	150-208	156-200
10 yr	35	1.1	3800-4000	760-800	690-727	190-250	122-227
15 yr	50	1.4	5000-6000	1200	857	300-400	120-200

From Hazinski MF: Cardiovascular disorders. In Hazinski MF, editor: *Manual of pediatric critical care*, St Louis, 1999, Mosby-Year Book, p. 112.
*Cardiac index for children: 3.0-4.5 L/min per m².
†Assuming a hemoglobin concentration of 15 G per dL and normal oxygenation.
BSA, Body surface area; *DO₂*, oxygen delivery; *VO₂*, oxygen consumption.

Compensatory vasoconstriction can initially maintain BP (BP = CO × SVR). In fact, infants and children have high SVR and vasoactive capacity such that hypotension is a late sign of shock.[53,245] This survival mechanism is designed to counterbalance the limited cardiac reserve in children.

Perfusion of the myocardium and endocardium occurs primarily during diastole. Coronary artery perfusion pressure is the difference between aortic end-diastolic pressure and mean right atrial pressure, and it varies inversely with HR (a reflection of diastolic filling time). Under conditions of hypovolemia, an adult can easily double HR from 70 to 140 per min to maintain an adequate CO (cardiac reserve); however, if the newborn or infant doubles HR from 140 to 280 or 120 to 240 per min, respectively, these HRs will often not allow adequate cardiac perfusion. Indeed, SVT with HRs of 240 per min or higher frequently leads to inadequate cardiac filling and subsequent poor tissue perfusion.

During states of shock, newborns, infants, and children compensate by peripheral vasoconstriction to maintain adequate perfusion to the heart, brain, and kidney. Hypotension is an extremely late and poor prognostic sign; therefore shock must be recognized and treated long before hypotension occurs. The hallmark of the care of critically ill children at risk for shock is early recognition and resuscitation before hypotension develops. Time-sensitive and aggressive fluid resuscitation, inotropic support, systemic and pulmonary vasodilator therapy, and extracardiac mechanical support are more commonly used in children than in adults.

When distributive shock is present, compensatory diversion of blood flow cannot occur; therefore the skin may remain warm, and peripheral pulses may actually be bounding. However, shock is still present because some tissue beds have excessive blood flow, whereas others have inadequate blood flow.

Calculation and Estimation of CO

CO can be calculated using a thermodilution catheter placed in the pulmonary artery. Injection of an iced quantity of fluid into the right atrium will produce a temperature change in the pulmonary artery that is inversely related to the CO. Such thermodilution CO calculations can be performed using a pulmonary artery catheter with thermistor or a separate thermistor placed into the pulmonary artery at the time of cardiac surgery. Additional information about thermodilution CO calculation can be found in Chapter 21.

The CO can be continuously evaluated if the pulmonary artery catheter contains an oximeter for continuous evaluation of pulmonary artery (mixed venous) oxyhemoglobin saturation. Pulmonary artery catheterization is not commonly performed in pediatric critical care, although it may be indicated in certain situations that complicate shock resuscitation.[276]

Pulse contour intermittent and continuous CO (PiCCO®) monitoring is possible using a femoral or axillary arterial catheter and a central venous catheter. Algorithms use pulse contour analysis combined with intermittent thermodilution calculations. The arterial waveform contours are analyzed to assess SV and thereby cardiac index (CI). In a pediatric validation study, the PiCCO system provided continuous calculation of CI without the need to perform thermodilution injections with every calculation.[90]

Esophageal Doppler studies of blood flow velocity in the descending aorta have been used in adults for many years, and pediatric probes are now available. In the past, the higher HRs in children compromised reliability of this technique of CO evaluation. Fairly reliable CO calculations have recently been reported in children,[270] although this method of CO evaluation is very operator dependent.[3]

CO and blood volume can be calculated from a form of ultrasound dilution. This technology uses a computer and arterial and venous sensors attached to a specialized extracorporeal tubing loop that is placed between an indwelling central venous and arterial catheter. A small bolus (0.5 to 1.0 mL/kg) of isotonic saline is injected into the central venous catheter to create a dilution curve. The saline dilutes the total blood protein concentration and alters blood velocity detected by the arterial sensor in the extracorporeal loop. The change in blood velocity over time can be graphed, and results in a dilution curve that is similar to that created during thermodilution CO calculations. In addition to calculating the CO and index, the ultrasound dilution computer calculates SV index, active circulating volume, SVR, and ejection fraction. This technology has been validated in neonates and children.[157]

Noninvasive measurement of CO in children is novel and evolving.[128] Doppler ultrasonography is a simple, noninvasive method of assessing blood flow and is an accepted noninvasive method of deriving CO.[118] Data obtained with Doppler ultrasonography correlate well with accepted standard hemodynamic methods in animal studies, adults, and neonates; formal validation is underway in children.[37,65,128]

Because adequate organ perfusion is the goal of supportive and therapeutic critical care, monitors that directly assess organ oxygenation offer the best possibility of improved recognition and treatment of circulatory abnormalities to reduce multiorgan dysfunction and related morbidity and mortality.[260] Some of these monitors are presented in the next several sections

Relationship of Mixed Venous Oxygen Saturation to CO

A true mixed venous oxygen saturation is evaluated from blood in the pulmonary artery, because it includes a true mixed sample of systemic venous blood from the superior vena cava, inferior vena cava, and coronary circulations. The mixed venous oxygen saturation can be continuously monitored through the use of a pulmonary artery catheter that contains a pulmonary artery oximeter. If hemoglobin concentration and saturation and oxygen consumption or extraction are stable (these assumptions often cannot be made about the critically ill patient), the mixed venous oxygen saturation will vary directly with the CO (see Fig. 6-6).

When oxygen delivery falls, tissues compensate by increasing the amount of oxygen extraction from circulating blood.[196] Mixed venous oxygen saturation is thus used as a measure of the balance between oxygen delivery and oxygen demand, and it will fall as the result of either decreased oxygen delivery (i.e., decreased arterial oxygen content; decreased CO, index, or both) or increased oxygen extraction (from increased demand, decreased delivery, or both). The normal mixed venous oxygen saturation is greater than 70%.[196] Mixed venous oxygen saturation levels between 50% and 75% reflect compensatory increased extraction in cases of increased oxygen demand or decreased oxygen delivery, whereas levels between 30% and 50% reflect the beginning of lactic acidosis indicating exhaustion of compensatory extraction. A further decline to levels between 25% and 30% is indicative of severe lactic acidosis, and levels less than 25% probably reflect cellular death.[196]

The mixed venous oxygen saturation has been shown to be an effective indicator of the balance between oxygen supply and demand, and it is a useful guide for management in adults. However, its use is limited in pediatrics by the need for a pulmonary artery or central venous catheter for intermittent or continuous measurement; this is often not feasible, especially early in resuscitation.[183]

Use of Central Venous Oxygen Saturation Monitoring

The desire for easier venous oxygen saturation measurement has led to an assessment of central venous oxygen saturation ($ScvO_2$). Unlike the pulmonary artery catheter samples that are composed of blood from all parts of the systemic venous circulation, including blood from the coronary sinus, $ScvO_2$ is obtained from the superior vena cava, so it assesses only the oxygen delivery-oxygen consumption balance in the upper body.[196] Many studies have examined how the two are related. Oxygen saturation of superior vena cava blood is approximately 70%, which is slightly lower than the saturation of blood in the inferior vena cava (75%). Coronary sinus blood, with an oxygen saturation of approximately 30% to 40%, is then added to the combined superior vena cava and inferior vena cava blood, so that a true mixed venous sample in the pulmonary artery (after mixing is complete) averages approximately 70% to 75% and corresponds to a mixed venous oxygen tension of 38 to 40 mm Hg. Thus the $ScvO_2$ is normally approximately 2% to 3% higher than mixed venous oxygen saturation in healthy individuals.[183] In shock states, however, the difference can range from 5% to 18%.[37,183] Some studies have shown that although the two are not interchangeable, there is a good correlation in the trending of one to the other, and the $ScvO_2$ correlates well with changes in systemic perfusion.[81,132,183]

Limitations of continuous $ScvO_2$ monitoring are significant. Because sympathetic tone raises vascular resistance in splanchnic-mesenteric beds as CO falls, in shock states the effects of desaturated blood from those regions on $ScvO_2$ may be blunted. As an extreme example, the renal blood flow may fall to 20% of its normal value because of intense renal vasoconstriction, with renal vein saturation falling from 85% to 25% while the $ScvO_2$ remains above 60%.[132]

Near-Infrared Spectroscopy (NIRS)

NIRS is relatively new technology that is used to access regional tissue oxygenation as an indicator of tissue perfusion. Near-infrared light (700 to 1000 nm bandwidth) is transmitted through muscle, bone, tissue, and skin, and reflected light is then read by a sensor.[183] The technology is similar to that used for pulse oximetry and continuous monitoring of $ScvO_2$. This technology uses the difference in light absorption between deoxygenated hemoglobin versus oxygenated hemoglobin to calculate a percent saturation level. Because most blood is not in arteries but in capillaries and veins, the greatest quantitative contribution to the calculated light absorption of hemoglobin is from venous and capillary blood. Pulse oximeters attempt to subtract the nonpulsatile component of the light signal (i.e., contributed from veins and capillaries) to examine the absorption spectrum of arterial blood, whereas NIRS technology focuses on the total light signal. An NIRS device approved by the U.S. Food and Drug Administration (INVOS; Somanetics, Troy, MI) uses a dual-detector system to subtract a shallow light path from a deep light path, theoretically allowing the derivation of the average oxyhemoglobin saturation in a volume of tissue approximately 2.5 to 3.0 cm deep under the skin and the sensor. The device displays an approximation of venous-weighted hemoglobin saturation in tissue deep below the sensor. The parameter is displayed as a relative number from 0% to 100% using an algorithm calibrated from in vivo and in vitro cerebral models, and is termed *regional oxygen saturation* (rSO$_2$).[132]

Because venous-weighted capillary blood represents the limiting oxygen tension for diffusion, NIRS provides a window to evaluate the oxygen economy in the monitored tissue bed or regional tissue oxyhemoglobin saturation.[91,132] The use of NIRS technology to monitor oxygenation in the brain, muscle, liver, and kidney has been extensively described.[91,132,133,228] Changes in tissue oxygen tension monitored by NIRS are sensitive indicators of perfusion-metabolism coupling, and regional NIRS monitoring can guide resuscitation from shock.[66,132]

The indication approved by the U.S. Food and Drug Administration for the INVOS device is for trend monitoring of regional saturation in the cerebral circulation, which has been widely modeled as a compartment with 75% venous blood, thus allowing validation of the device in an accepted clinical model. In animal models, brain rSO$_2$ less than 40% is associated with intracellular anaerobic metabolism and depletion of high-energy phosphates.[158] Clinical data in children and adults support the hypothesis that cerebral rSO$_2$ less than 40% to 50%, or a change in baseline of more than 20%, is associated with hypoxic-ischemic neural injury.[132,133,228]

Blood Pressure

Arterial BP may be the most widely used and most widely misinterpreted parameter related to CO. Arterial BP is generated by the kinetic energy imparted by the heart and the interaction of blood flow, viscosity, systemic vascular tone, and downstream (venous) pressure. The major determinants of mean arterial BP are the SVR and CO. Peripheral and central arterial pressure differences result from differential impedances in the vascular system and are increased with nonuniform vasoconstriction. Noninvasive BP measurement by auscultation using a cuff and sphygmomanometer (mercury manometer) and noninvasive oscillometric BP measurements correlate well with indwelling intraarterial measurements under conditions of normal vascular resistance and blood flow, but "cuff" and invasive pressures frequently diverge under conditions of low and high SVR.[132] Automated determination by cuff oscillometry shows good reproducibility and allows for determination of the mean pressure.

Although BP is rapidly and routinely measured, its relationship to CO or systemic perfusion is confounded by simultaneous changes in SVR. SVR tends to change in the opposite direction from CO; the sympathetic nervous system is activated by a falling BP, and sympathetic outflow is reduced and the parasympathetic system is activated with a rising BP. These responses are designed to minimize the variability in BP, making this parameter a late indicator of failing circulation. Similarly, resuscitation to a BP end point is often incomplete if the goal is to restore adequate CO and perfusion.[276]

Blood flow through a regional vascular bed is directly proportional to the organ perfusion pressure (ΔP), which is calculated as the difference between the arterial inflow pressure (P_a) and the venous outflow pressure (P_v): $\Delta P = P_a - P_v$.[53] With reasonable approximation and ignoring local extravascular effects, the inflow arterial pressure can be estimated to be

the mean arterial pressure (MAP), and the outflow venous pressure can be estimated to be CVP:

$$\Delta P = MAP - CVP$$

For any given ΔP, the blood flow is determined by the resistance to blood flow according to the following equation, analogous to Ohm's law, where Q is arterial blood flow and R is vascular resistance:

$$Q = (MAP - CVP)/R$$

Under ideal laminar flow conditions, vascular resistance is independent of flow and pressure; therefore an increase in vascular resistance will decrease blood flow, and a decrease in vascular resistance will increase blood flow for any given ΔP. Control mechanisms in the body generally maintain arterial and venous BPs within a narrow range; therefore changes in organ and tissue blood flow are primarily regulated by changes in vascular resistance. Resistance to blood flow within a vascular network is determined by the size of the vessels, the organization of the vascular network, physical characteristics of the blood, and extravascular forces acting on the vasculature.[53]

The relationship between flow (i.e., CO), perfusion pressure (i.e., MAP − CVP), and SVR is vital to the understanding of the pathophysiologic principles of shock. The perfusion pressure may be more important than BP alone. According to the equation, a patient can theoretically have a normal MAP but no forward flow (i.e., CO)—for example, if CVP is equal to MAP. Importantly, when fluid resuscitation is used to improve BP, the increase in MAP must be greater than the increase in CVP. If the increase in MAP is less than the increase in CVP, then the perfusion pressure is actually reduced, and CO is reduced. Inotropic agents, and not additional fluid resuscitation, are indicated to improve CO in this scenario.

Understanding the perfusion pressure helps guide the management of blood flow reflected as CO. CO can be decreased when perfusion pressure (MAP − CVP) is decreased, but it can also be decreased when the perfusion pressure is normal and vascular resistance is increased. Therefore children with normal BP can have inadequate CO, because systemic vascular tone is too high. CO can be improved in this scenario with the use of inotropes, vasodilators, and volume loading. The cardiovascular pathophysiology of shock can therefore be attributed to reduced CO, reduced perfusion pressure, or both. Reduced CO is caused by either reduced HR or reduced SV caused by hypovolemia (inadequate preload), decreased contractility (insufficient inotropy), or excess vascular resistance (increased afterload). Reduced perfusion pressure can be caused by reduced MAP or increased CVP.

SHOCK STATES

Shock is a progressive condition of circulatory failure that results in inadequate CO and oxygen and substrate delivery to the tissues. Shock may be present in the patient with a low, normal, or high CO or index.[245]

Shock frequently is classified according to its cause. The four major types of shock are hypovolemic, cardiogenic, septic (or distributive), and obstructive. Hypovolemic shock results from inadequate intravascular volume relative to the vascular space. Cardiogenic shock results from myocardial dysfunction. Septic shock is the most common form of distributive shock; it is induced by infectious agents or their by-products with resultant myocardial dysfunction and aspects of cardiogenic shock. Obstructive shock results from severe obstruction to ventricular filling or outflow, such as results from cardiac tamponade, tension pneumothorax, ductal-dependent congenital heart disease (when ductus begins to close), or pulmonary embolus.

Although the patient may demonstrate one type of shock, many patients have combined causes of shock. For example, the patient in early septic shock may demonstrate elements of hypovolemic and cardiogenic shock. A relative hypovolemia is present, and myocardial depression develops rapidly and is associated with maldistribution of blood flow. Therefore it is important to access and support all aspects of cardiovascular function when caring for the patient in shock.

Hypovolemic Shock

Etiology

Hypovolemia is the most common cause of shock in infants and children.[245] *Hypovolemic shock* is best defined as a sudden decrease in the intravascular (blood) volume, relative to vascular capacity (i.e., inadequate intravascular volume relative to the vascular space), to such an extent that effective tissue perfusion cannot be maintained. Causes include hemorrhage from gastrointestinal disease or trauma, fluid and electrolyte loss, endocrine disease, and plasma loss.

Intravascular volume loss can also result from a shift of fluid into a third space. Third space fluid comprises a pool of water, electrolytes, and protein that is not available for incorporation into the intravascular space. Examples include fluids found in pleural effusions, ascites, and intraluminal fluid in the gastrointestinal tract. Surgical bowel manipulation or trauma can produce a shift of fluid into this potential fluid space. When the fluid shift is substantial, it can contribute to the development of hypovolemic shock.

Pathophysiology

Hypovolemia causes a decrease in preload that reduces SV and CO. Activation of peripheral and central baroreceptors produces an outpouring of catecholamines; the resulting tachycardia and peripheral vasoconstriction are usually initially adequate to support the BP, with little or no evidence of hypotension. Another aspect of the body's compensatory mechanism for dealing with hypovolemia is through the activation of the renin-angiotensin-aldosterone system. Angiotensin (a potent vasoconstrictor) promotes the release of aldosterone, which increases the kidney's sodium resorption; this, combined with an increase in antidiuretic hormone secretion, results in increased water resorption in the kidney.

Clinical Signs and Symptoms

Reliable indicators of early, compensated hypovolemic shock in children are persistent tachycardia, cutaneous vasoconstriction, and diminution of the pulse pressure (difference between

systolic and diastolic BPs). Clinical evidence of decreased tissue perfusion includes skin mottling, prolonged capillary refill, and cool extremities. Systemic arterial BP is frequently normal, which is the result of increased SVR, making BP monitoring of limited value in managing the patient with compensated hypovolemic shock.[132,245] Neurologic status is initially normal or only minimally impaired.

Although capillary refill has long been advocated as an important means of quickly and reliably assessing the level of hydration and circulatory status of acutely ill or injured children, there are several important limitations to the use of capillary refill in the assessment of circulatory status in children.[23,112,297] It is necessary to account for the ambient temperature, in addition to the site of measurement, when interpreting the results.

On rare occasions, BP may be paradoxically elevated in children with hypovolemia.[33] Recognition of this phenomenon is extremely important because some healthcare providers may be reluctant to provide appropriate fluid resuscitation for these patients because of fear of exacerbating the hypertension. Treatment of the hypertension, especially with β-blockers or calcium channel antagonists, may precipitate hypotension. Dehydrated, volume-depleted children with paradoxic hypertension should be given a trial of volume expansion; such therapy will cause little harm and could ameliorate the hypertension.

With continued loss of intravascular volume or with delayed or inadequate intravascular volume replacement, the intravascular fluid losses surpass the body's compensatory abilities, causing circulatory failure and organ dysfunction. Pronounced systemic vasoconstriction and hypovolemia produce ischemia and hypoxia in the visceral and cutaneous circulations. Cellular metabolism and function are altered in these areas, resulting in damage to the blood vessels, kidneys, liver, pancreas, and bowel. SV and CO are decreased. The patient ultimately becomes hypotensive, acidotic, lethargic, or comatose, and oliguric or anuric. It is important to emphasize that arterial BP falls only after compensatory mechanisms are exhausted; this may be long after the precipitating event and only after a severe reduction in CO.[243] Terminal phases of hypovolemic shock are characterized by myocardial dysfunction and widespread cell death.

Ischemia can develop in nonvital organs as a result of reduced circulating blood volume and preferential vasoconstriction. In skeletal muscle during shock, the normal intermittent perfusion pattern in capillary networks has been observed to transform to a marked maldistribution of flow, with cessation of blood flow in most capillaries.[198,199] In addition to a low and irregular flow state in capillaries, recent findings have demonstrated a progressive narrowing of the capillary lumen during shock. The nearly 25% decrease in lumen diameter after 1 hour of shock principally results from swelling of endothelial cells; this significantly increases the capillary resistance to flow and contributes to further flow retardation.[198,199] In addition, in a variety of organs impaired microcirculatory blood flow has been observed with reperfusion after a period of ischemia (no reflow or slow reflow). The causes of no reflow include red blood cell aggregation, leukocyte trapping, and edema of tissue and capillary endothelial cells.[199]

In any form of shock, including hypovolemic shock, the end result of hypoperfusion and tissue ischemia is cellular oxygen and nutrient deficiency that can affect the integrity of cell function and structure. Anaerobic metabolism results from the decrease in oxygen delivery, leading to glycogen depletion and lactate production. An increase in cytosolic calcium is also evident, which leads to an increase in membrane phospholipid hydrolysis and lysosomal membrane damage.[295] This process eventually progresses to irreversible cellular injury and a host of inflammatory responses, which stimulate further tissue inflammation and injury. Ischemia or reperfusion can also induce expression of inflammatory genes in endothelial cells. In some hypovolemic animal models, fluid resuscitation leads to a decrease in the inflammatory cascade that was triggered by organ ischemia secondary to hypoperfusion.[295] Because this inflammatory response is not likely to protect or repair organs from hypovolemic insult, downregulation of this inflammation seen with fluid resuscitation is likely to be beneficial.

Serum tonicity is important in both the presentation and the management of dehydration. In approximately 80% of cases of dehydration, patients have normal serum osmolality; 15% are hyperosmolar, and 5% are hypoosmolar.[243] The serum sodium concentration can be used as a rough estimate of serum osmolality and dehydration, which is classified as hyponatremic, isonatremic, or hypernatremic (Box 6-1).

Hyponatremic dehydration occurs secondary to a disproportionate loss of solute to fluid (i.e., proportionately more sodium lost than water). There is depletion of extracellular (including intravascular and interstitial) fluid volume relative to intracellular fluid volume, producing characteristic physical findings of dry mucous membranes, reduced skin turgor, cool extremities, compromised perfusion, and in severe cases, hemodynamic collapse.

Hypernatremic dehydration is the result of fluid loss out of proportion to solute loss (i.e., proportionately more water lost than sodium). There is relative preservation of the extracellular volume, but at the expense of water drawn into the extracellular (including vascular space) compartment from the intracellular compartment. Physical findings include a doughy consistency of the skin and subcutaneous tissues and the apparent maintenance of good hemodynamic function and BP, even in the face of large volume losses.

The approach for infants or children with diarrheal dehydration can be organized using the five-point assessment[141,243] (Table 6-2). Initial management is guided by a simple history and physical examination, followed by assignment of the patient to one of three groups based on severity of illness.

Table 6-3 lists the signs and symptoms that can be used to group patients by severity of dehydration. Of the 10 findings listed, none is sufficiently accurate to be used in isolation.[113] The presence of fewer than three signs corresponds with a fluid deficit of less than 5%, whereas children with a deficit of 5% to 9% generally have three or more clinical findings. At least six or seven findings should be present to diagnose a deficit of 10% or more.

A recent study has suggested that it may be possible to rely on a relatively restricted subset of clinical indicators: general appearance, capillary refill, mucous membranes, and tears. Of these four findings, the presence of any two indicates a deficit of 5% or more, and three or more findings indicates a deficit of at least 10%.[113]

Children usually have healthy compensatory mechanisms that initially maintain peripheral perfusion and BP despite volume loss. HR increases to maintain CO despite deceased SV (see table of Normal Blood Pressures in Children on pages

Box 6-1	**Classification of Hypovolemic Shock Based on Serum Sodium**

Hyponatremic: serum sodium <130 mEq/dL
Isonatremic: serum sodium 130-150 mEq/dL
Hypernatremic: serum sodium >150 mEq/dL

Table 6-2 **Rapid Assessment of Dehydration**

Point of Assessment	Method
Volume deficit	History and physical
Osmolar disturbance	Serum sodium
Acid-base disturbance	Serum pH, PCO_2, bicarbonate
Potassium disturbance	Serum potassium
Renal function	Serum blood urea nitrogen, creatinine Urine analysis, specific gravity, sodium

Adapted from Kallen RJ: The management of diarrheal dehydration in infants using parenteral fluids. *Pediatr Clin North Am* 37:265, 1990.

Table 6-3 **Severity of Dehydration Based on History and Physical Examination**

Assessment Characteristic	Mild	Moderate	Severe
General appearance	Alert, restless, thirsty	Lethargic, postural dizziness	Limp, coma, cold and cyanotic extremities
Radial pulse	Full	Thready, weak, rapid	Feeble, inpalpable
Respiration	Normal	Deep	Deep, rapid
Skin elasticity	Pinch retracts immediately	Pinch retracts slowly	Pinch retracts very slowly (>2 s)
Eyes	Normal	Sunken	Very sunken
Tears	Present	Diminished	Absent
Mucous membrane	Moist	Dry	Very dry
Urine output	Normal	↓	↓ or absent
Capillary refill time	<2 s	>2 s	Prolonged
Heart rate	Varies with age	Varies with age	Varies with age

Table 6-4	Classification of Hemorrhage by Blood Volume Lost	
Degree of Hemorrhage	Blood Volume Lost (%)	Signs
Class I	<15	Minimal tachycardia; normal respiration, BP, capillary refill
Class II	15-30	Tachycardia; tachypnea; diminished pulse pressure; systolic BP unchanged; prolonged capillary refill; minimal decrease in urine output; anxiety
Class III	30-40	Tachycardia; tachypnea; decreased BP; decreased urine output; mental status changes
Class IV	>40	Hypotension; anuria; loss of consciousness

Adapted from Morgan WM 3rd, O'Neill JA Jr: Hemorrhagic and obstructive shock in pediatric patients. *New Horiz* 6:150–154, 1998.
BP, Blood pressure.

inside front cover). For this reason, tachycardia is an early sign of acute blood loss with impending shock. Total blood volume in children is generally estimated as 7% to 8% of body weight or 70 to 80 mL/kg. With blood loss of 10% to 15% (class I hemorrhage as defined by Advanced Trauma Life Support), the injured child easily compensates with a 10% to 20% increase in HR (Table 6-4). BP and peripheral capillary refill are usually unchanged. Even with a 20% to 25% loss of blood volume (class II hemorrhage), there is often little change in the systolic BP as increasing tachycardia and peripheral vasoconstriction mediated through the sympathetic nervous system and other mechanisms serve to maintain perfusion pressure. It is for this reason that one must avoid the tendency to equate hypotension with shock in the pediatric trauma patient. Hypotension is a late finding with ongoing hemorrhage and often signals that the child is near the point of complete decompensation.[243] Furthermore, studies in adults and children with trauma showed that systolic BP is a predictor of mortality and that prehospital hypotension is associated with an increased risk of mortality.[120,185,274] There is a need for studies to validate the appropriate BP target and to better define hypotension in critically ill children.[120]

Management

Initial treatment of the child in hypovolemic shock is the same, regardless of the cause. Therapy begins with establishing adequate oxygenation and ventilation. Oxygen should always be the first drug administered. Once a patent airway is ensured or established (intubation may be required) and ventilation is adequate, measures to restore an effective circulating blood volume should begin. The most important therapeutic maneuvers are establishing adequate intravenous or intraosseous access and rapid volume replacement.

Vascular access is achieved using the largest, most easily accessible vein. Peripheral venotomy can be performed in the veins of the hand, foot, arm, leg, or scalp, but these vessels tend to be small and difficult to cannulate in the hypovolemic child, so attempts to achieve vascular access should be limited before attempting intraosseous access.[243] If peripheral access is difficult and vascular access is critical, early intraosseous access is encouraged.[57a,259]

If time allows and clinical experts are available, vascular access can be obtained by central venous cannulation or saphenous cutdown; however, the latter route is less frequently used because intraosseous access is so readily available. The femoral vein is often the most easily accessible in an emergency situation.[243]

The amount of volume required to resuscitate a child in hypovolemic shock is variable. However, the most common error made in resuscitation of a child in hypovolemic shock is inadequate or delayed volume administration.[119,271] The variance in disease processes that lead to hypovolemic shock may require different treatment and will be discussed separately.

Fluid Therapy: Diarrhea and Dehydration. Diarrhea can severely disrupt the balance of fluids and electrolytes, and it is a leading cause of infant mortality worldwide.[290] Dehydration and shock as a consequence of diarrhea are more likely to occur in infants or small children than in adults.

Isotonic crystalloid (20 mL/kg), delivered as a rapid infusion, is effective in the resuscitation of all children with shock secondary to dehydration, regardless of the serum osmolality or osmolarity. The use of hypotonic solutions is ineffective (it is distributed in both the intracellular and extracellular—including intravascular—spaces) and can be harmful in hypernatremic dehydration, because it can reduce serum sodium concentration too quickly.

Administering large volumes of isotonic saline (0.9% sodium chloride) frequently can cause the development of hyperchloremic acidosis; this occurs because isotonic saline contains 154 mEq/L of chloride, and its administration results in a dilutional decrease of serum bicarbonate and an increase in serum chloride concentration. Both of these changes will produce metabolic acidosis. Resuscitation with lactated Ringer's solution provides a more balanced electrolyte replacement and is less likely to produce metabolic acidosis. The infusion of lactated Ringer's solution in general does not influence the circulating serum lactate concentration.[74]

The use of colloid is not indicated in the initial resuscitation of the patient with shock secondary to dehydration. Albumin and other colloids have been used effectively for volume replacement in patients who have large volumes of nonfunctional extracellular or third space fluid loss or low albumin states.[123]

The first fluid infusion (20 mL/kg) should be administered rapidly and the HR, pulse pressure, BP, peripheral perfusion, quality of mentation, and volume of urine output should be monitored closely for signs of improvement. Improvement in these measurements suggests that maintenance fluid administration can then be initiated and vital signs can be monitored. The appropriate maintenance fluid to be used is determined by the child's serum electrolyte balance.

The end point of fluid resuscitation should be normalization of HR and respiratory rate, an increase in arterial BP, an increase in pulse pressure and peripheral perfusion, establishing adequate urine output, and a decrease in the metabolic acidosis. However, if shock persists after the first fluid infusion is completed, a second infusion of 20 mL/kg should be started. If the patient does not improve after two or three infusions of isotonic crystalloid solution (40 to 60 mL/kg), more aggressive monitoring and therapy are clearly required and the child must be evaluated for complicating factors. Causes of unresponsive shock in a patient with adequate oxygenation include unrecognized pneumothorax or pericardial effusion, intestinal ischemia (e.g., volvulus, intussusception, necrotizing enterocolitis), sepsis, myocardial dysfunction, adrenocortical insufficiency, pulmonary hypertension, and potential occult bleeding caused by inflicted trauma.[243]

While the initial 60 mL/kg of fluid is infusing, some children require inotropic or vasopressor support to maintain adequate end-organ perfusion. This subset of patients, said to have fluid-refractory shock, may require a combination of fluid resuscitation and catecholamine support. It is important to confirm the diagnosis in these cases, because the clinical signs of different types of shock frequently overlap. In addition, it is important to reassess the patient frequently and thoroughly during the resuscitation to guide additional therapy. For example, if the child with hypovolemic shock secondary to diarrhea does not improve despite significant volume administration, the child may have unrecognized ongoing gastrointestinal losses, requiring further volume administration to keep pace with ongoing output. An analogous situation is the child with diabetic ketoacidosis who continues to lose large amounts of fluid in the urine that, if inadequately replaced, will lead to a further decrease in intravascular volume.

Children with dehydration secondary to burns or septic shock frequently require large amounts of fluid administration, because they have ongoing capillary leak; they often require concurrent inotropic support, vasopressor support, or both.[50] To guide therapy, it is important to determine whether these children have failure of the vasculature, cardiac function, or a combination, leading to requirements for support in addition to volume administration. The cardiac failure seen with thermal injuries, trauma, or sepsis must be evaluated further to distinguish cardiac dysfunction from decreased CO resulting from external compression or obstruction (e.g., pericarditis, tamponade).[92]

Children who have fluid-refractory shock may also have adrenal insufficiency. With the increased use of long-term steroid therapy in children (e.g., transplantation, malignancy, asthma), a relative adrenal insufficiency may be contributing to the patient's fluid-refractory shock state, and exogenous steroid therapy may have a role in treatment of these patients (see the discussion under the section, Septic Shock).

Fluid Therapy in Traumatic or Hemorrhagic Shock. Shock in the injured child is almost always secondary to hypovolemia, so acute blood loss must always be considered first. With hemorrhagic shock, the source of blood loss may be external and readily apparent, such as the laceration of a major vessel in an extremity or a large scalp laceration. The scalp is often a source of significant blood loss in infants and children,

because of its inherent vascularity and because the head is relatively large (with a relatively large percentage of the child's BSA) in young children. More commonly, however, the source of blood loss is internal and therefore less apparent. Extremity (i.e., femur fracture) and intraabdominal injuries are common after blunt trauma in children, especially with motor vehicle crashes,[243] and can result in significant occult blood loss.

Intraabdominal solid organ injury is a common cause of occult blood loss, and such injuries are probably the most common cause of traumatic shock in children.[99,152] Single or complex fractures of the liver and spleen often result in significant hemorrhage. Associated injury to the inferior vena cava is rare, but if present it usually leads to life-threatening hemorrhage. Mesenteric injury is often seen as part of the "lap belt syndrome," but does not usually result in sufficient blood loss to cause shock. Blunt injury of the kidney can also cause significant blood loss into a retroperitoneal hematoma. Fracture of the bony pelvis is relatively common in older children and may lead to massive hemorrhage, at times requiring urgent stabilization.

Occult blood loss may occur in the chest as well, with laceration of the lung or an intercostal vessel. Great vessel injury secondary to blunt trauma in children is, fortunately, rare.

With any signs of hypovolemic shock (e.g., tachycardia), a fluid bolus of 20 mL/kg of isotonic crystalloid solution should be given. Transfusion of packed red blood cells or whole blood is indicated for the patient with hemorrhagic shock who shows signs of persistent intravascular volume depletion despite the rapid administration of 60 mL/kg (three boluses) of crystalloid. Packed red blood cells should be given in boluses of 10 mL/kg. Type-specific blood is used if available, but typing should not delay resuscitation. Un–cross-matched O-negative universal donor blood should be immediately available. Aggressive fluid resuscitation is paramount, even when there is associated closed-head injury, because ongoing hypoperfusion leads to secondary hypoxic end-organ injury, especially in the brain.[5,14,54,60,302]

Although hypovolemia is the most frequent cause of shock, occasionally other causes of hemodynamic compromise may be present. Obstructive shock owing to tension pneumothorax or pericardial tamponade, myocardial confusion, and spinal shock can complicate the management of pediatric trauma.[243] Blunt cardiac injury can cause myocardial contusion, myocardial concussion, aneurysm, septal defects, chamber rupture, valvular rupture, and damage to the pericardium.[40,78,249] Each of these entities has separate presentations, although the lesions are often concurrent. The majority of blunt injuries to the heart are myocardial contusions; devastating events such as ventricular rupture are rare.[78,249]

There are important clinical considerations in the management of children with blunt cardiac injury:
- If a child with a suspected blunt cardiac injury is hemodynamically stable and has a normal sinus rhythm, then the development of serious arrhythmia or cardiac failure is not likely. In other words, high risk for a patient is usually evident immediately.[78]
- Trauma patients with a suspected cardiac injury should receive prompt evaluation of cardiac function with

echocardiography.[40,78] Any patient with unexplained hypotension or diminished peripheral perfusion should be studied using echocardiography.

- Elevated cardiac isoenzyme values and electrocardiography are nonspecific for clinically significant myocardial injury.[78]

Crystalloid Versus Colloid. Volume resuscitation can include the use of crystalloid, colloid, or blood products, or all three. Crystalloids are electrolyte-containing solutions distributed through the body according to their chemical composition and tonicity. Isotonic crystalloid solutions (lactated Ringer's solution, 0.9% sodium chloride) are distributed throughout the extracellular compartment (i.e., the vascular and interstitial spaces). Hypotonic solutions have a proportion of water not associated with sodium and are therefore distributed throughout the entire body water. Hypertonic solutions (sodium concentrations in excess of 180 mEq/L) increase serum osmolality and therefore induce movement of water from the intracellular space to the extracellular space.

Colloids used in the treatment of patients in shock include plasma, prepared plasma fractions, and synthetic plasma substitutes. Colloids consist of large molecules that are generally restricted to the intravascular compartment, exerting an oncotic effect on the distribution of water. In doing so, isooncotic solutions (5% albumin, fresh frozen plasma) result in a greater expansion of the intravascular volume than that achieved with isotonic crystalloid solutions when the same volume is infused. Hyperoncotic solutions, such as 25% albumin, move fluid into the vascular compartment from the interstitial space.

Plasma expanders, such as the dextrans and hydroxyethyl starch, are also available for intravascular volume replacement. The dextrans, dextran-40 and dextran-70, are available as either 0.9% sodium chloride solutions or 5% dextrose solutions. Hetastarch is amylopectin in which hydroxyethyl starch groups are substituted. It is available as a 6% solution in 0.9% sodium chloride. Use may be limited by hypersensitivity reactions; experience with use of dextrans and hetastarch in pediatrics is limited.

There continues to be an ongoing debate as to the most suitable type of fluid to use for resuscitation. Both choices, crystalloid solutions and colloid solutions, have their own advantages and disadvantages.

The advantages of using crystalloids for resuscitation are their ready availability and their cost effectiveness. The cost of 5% albumin is manyfold that of the common crystalloid solutions. The main disadvantage is that crystalloids reduce colloid oncotic pressure and can predispose to pulmonary and peripheral edema.[61]

Colloid solutions are useful because they contain relatively large molecules that are impermeable to the capillary membrane, leading to increased volume remaining in the intravascular space. Disadvantages of colloid infusions are chiefly related to cost and the potential exposure to blood products.

There is now a reasonable evidence base to support the use of isotonic crystalloids (e.g., normal saline) as the best initial choice of fluid for intravenous resuscitation of shock. Two randomized controlled studies of fluid resuscitation in pediatric septic shock failed to demonstrate any difference in outcome, regardless of whether crystalloid or colloid (i.e., albumin) fluid therapy was used in initial resuscitation.[303,319] A well-powered study investigating fluid resuscitation of adults in shock has also failed to show benefit of the use of colloids over crystalloids. Subgroups of patients in the adult study (e.g., patients with traumatic brain injuries) had a better outcome with the use of crystalloids instead of colloids.[96] A physiology-based argument has existed for many years that whereas crystalloids may be clinically effective for fluid resuscitation, their reduced osmolar drag relative to colloid therapy leads to increased capillary leak and movement of water extravascularly. As a result, the "3:1 rule" suggests that a significantly greater volume of crystalloid than colloid would be necessary to replace the depleted intravascular compartment. A consistent finding from all three of the previously cited studies is that there is no difference between the volume of crystalloid and colloid necessary to resuscitate the patient in shock. This is not to say that there is no role for colloids in fluid resuscitation. Children with advanced septic shock might still benefit from colloid therapy, and those with advanced hemorrhagic shock will ultimately require the use of blood products to replace both blood cells and coagulation factors.

Distributive Shock: Definitions

Distributive shock, as the name implies, results from abnormalities in vasomotor tone that lead to the maldistribution of a normally effective blood volume and flow. Peripheral vasodilation and shunting can lead to a state of relative hypovolemia. Distributive shock arises from a variety of disorders and encompasses various states of shock arising from anaphylaxis (anaphylactic shock), central nervous system injury (which includes neurogenic and spinal shock), and sepsis.

Anaphylaxis refers to a systemic, immediate hypersensitivity reaction that is potentially life threatening and characterized by the onset of signs and symptoms within seconds to minutes after exposure to the offending agent (e.g., insect envenomation, medication, food), involvement of multiple organ systems, and involvement of systems distant from the site of exposure. Although the true incidence of anaphylaxis is difficult to define, it is certainly not uncommon, and the most frequent causes of anaphylaxis are foods, hymenoptera stings, and medications.

Anaphylaxis is caused by the release of mediators from mast cells and basophils. Antigen bridging of immunoglobulin (Ig) E antibodies bound to high-affinity IgE receptors on the cell surface leads to the aggregation of the receptors and activation of an enzymatic cascade initiating mediator release. Mast cells and basophils are concentrated near exposed mucosal surfaces, such as the lung and the gastrointestinal tract, and children with anaphylaxis will typically have signs and symptoms affecting these organ systems (e.g., wheezing, respiratory distress, vomiting, hives). Although several mediators are released from the mast cell and basophil, including histamine, platelet activating factor, and the leukotrienes (the so-called slow-reacting substances of anaphylaxis), histamine is the most important mediator of anaphylaxis. Intramuscular administration of epinephrine is the mainstay of the treatment of anaphylaxis. Additional adjunctive therapies include the administration of systemic corticosteroids and parenteral antihistamines.

Neurogenic shock results from autonomic dysfunction occurring secondary to injury to the spinal cord. Loss of peripheral vascular tone and subsequent increased venous capacitance lead to a relative hypovolemia caused by expansion of the vascular space. Children with neurogenic shock often fail to improve with fluid resuscitation, but instead respond to treatment with selective α-adrenergic vasoactive infusions (Table 6-5; see discussion under Cardiogenic Shock, Treatment, later in this chapter).

Septic Shock

Etiology and Definitions

Septic shock is the most complex and controversial type of shock. Septic shock comprises a cascade of metabolic, hemodynamic, and clinical changes resulting from invasive infection and the release of microbial toxins into the bloodstream. Historically, a distinction was made between the clinical findings and the type of invading microorganism (e.g., gram-positive versus gram-negative shock). However, on closer analysis, it became apparent that the systemic response was independent of the type of invading organism (e.g., bacteria, virus, fungus, rickettsia), rather it was a host-dependent response.[51,243] The morbidity and mortality are primarily the result of endogenous proteins and phospholipids synthesized by the patient.[51] Sepsis is the culmination of complex interactions between the infecting microorganism and the host immune, inflammatory, and coagulation responses.[11,46,265]

One of the factors hampering progress in the understanding of sepsis and septic shock has been the variability of definitions used and patient populations studied. As an approach to standardizing the definitions of sepsis and organ failure, the American College of Chest Physicians and the Society of Critical Care Medicine held a consensus conference to define sepsis and organ failure more precisely.[9] This group proposed the term *systemic inflammatory response syndrome* (SIRS), recognizing that the inflammatory response can be precipitated by processes other than infection. The group included in the definition of SIRS abnormalities of temperature, HR, respiratory rate, and white blood cell count. Whereas the definitions used were applied to adults, age-appropriate values must be used to apply the same descriptions to children.

Recently, consensus definitions for the pediatric sepsis continuum were developed and published.[109] The pediatric sepsis continuum includes SIRS, infection, sepsis, severe sepsis, septic shock, and multiple organ dysfunction syndrome.

Initial definitions for these points on the sepsis continuum have been proposed and are listed in Box 6-2. A few comments need to be made concerning the use of these definitions. First, it is important to realize that the definitions are sensitive but not specific screening tools to be used primarily for research purposes, and any direct application to the clinical setting must take into account the dynamic and continuous nature of the sepsis disease process and the static and categorical nature of the definitions.[39]

Second, the definitions of severe sepsis and septic shock in children create challenges. Unlike adults, children may clearly be in a shock state without the presence of systemic hypotension.

Thus, the delineation between severe sepsis and septic shock in children may be artificial, and these two definitions may be describing the same clinical syndrome when applied to children.

Third, the clinical parameters used to define SIRS and organ dysfunction are greatly affected by the normal physiologic changes that occur as children develop,[39,109] and the baseline organ function of children with chronic diseases must be considered. The consensus definitions propose six age groups for age-specific vital signs and laboratory parameters: newborn (0 to 7 days), neonate (1 week to 1 month), infant (1 month to 1 year), toddler and preschooler (2 to 5 years), school-aged child (6 to 12 years), and adolescent and young adult (13 to 18 years). The age groups were determined by a combination of age-specific risks for invasive infections, age-specific antibiotic treatment recommendations, and developmental cardiorespiratory physiologic changes.[39,109] Evidence-based data combined both physiologic and laboratory normative information to support these age groupings. Furthermore, most of the normative data were reported to identify the 5th and 95th percentile ranges. The relationship between values and ranges obtained in normal children and appropriate values and ranges in critically ill children with sepsis is unclear.

Finally, the panel chose not to advocate for the use of a single multiple-organ dysfunction score, but developed criteria for organ dysfunction based on those used in the Pediatric Logistic Organ Dysfunction score or the pediatric multiple organ dysfunction syndrome[39,159,239] (Box 6-3).

These definitions for pediatric sepsis are a significant step forward in facilitating clinical trials in pediatric sepsis, but the definitions go beyond use for research; they can facilitate earlier clinical recognition and treatment of sepsis in children.[239] Further refinements may allow differentiation between morbidity arising from infection and morbidity caused by the host response to infection. The PIRO system stratifies patients on the basis of their predisposing conditions (*P*), the nature and extent of the infection (*I*), the nature and magnitude of the host response (*R*), and the degree of concomitant organ dysfunction (*O*)[164,231] (Table 6-6).

Pathophysiology

The pathophysiology of septic shock is not completely understood. A combination of the direct effects of microbial agents, microbiological toxins, and the patient's inflammatory response to infection results in the cardiovascular instability and multisystem organ failure seen in septic shock.

Organ dysfunction is the final tissue sequelae in response to severe sepsis and is the ultimate determinant of survival. Mortality is much higher in patients with sepsis who develop progressive multiple organ failure than in those who develop a single or no organ dysfunction in response to sepsis.[164,231] What remains unclear is why some patients develop one type of organ dysfunction and others develop another organ dysfunction, despite seemingly similar septic stimuli. Some patients develop profound coagulation abnormalities in the early phases of sepsis, whereas others develop severe acute respiratory dysfunction syndrome, and others experience acute renal failure. The sequence and pattern of organ dysfunction

Table 6-5 **Pediatric Vasoactive Drugs for the Treatment of Shock**[*†]

Dose	Effects	Cautions
Sympathomimetics		
Dobutamine, 2-20 mcg/kg per min	Selective β-adrenergic effects; increases cardiac contractility and also increases heart rate (this latter effect is variable); $β_2$ effects produce peripheral vasodilatation; no dopaminergic or α-adrenergic effects	Extreme tachyarrhythmias have been reported, particularly in infants; hypotension may develop; may produce pulmonary venoconstriction
Dopamine, 1-5 mcg/kg per min	Dopaminergic effects predominate, including increase in glomerular filtration rate and urine volume	Can produce extreme tachyarrhythmias; can result in increase in pulmonary artery pressure; inhibits thyroid-stimulating hormone and aldosterone secretion
Dopamine, 2-10 mcg/kg per min	Dopaminergic effects persist and $β_1$ effects are seen, especially an increase in heart rate	As above
Dopamine, 8-20 mcg/kg per min	α-Adrenergic effects dominate	As above
Epinephrine, 0.05-0.15 mcg/kg per min	Endogenous catecholamine, which produces α, $β_1$, and $β_2$ adrenergic effects; at low doses, $β_1$ effects dominate	Will increase myocardial work and oxygen consumption at any dose; splanchnic constriction will occur at even low doses
Epinephrine, 0.2-0.3 mcg/kg per min	α-Adrenergic (vasoconstrictive) effects dominate	As above
Isoproterenol, 0.05-0.1 mcg/kg per min	β-Adrenergic effects; $β_1$ effects may result in rapid increase in heart rate; $β_2$ effects may produce peripheral vasodilatation and also may effectively treat bronchoconstriction	Monitor for tachyarrhythmias, hypotension; will increase myocardial oxygen consumption
Norepinephrine, 0.05-1.0 mcg/kg per min	Endogenous catecholamine with α- and β-adrenergic effects; produces potent peripheral and renal vasoconstriction; can increase blood pressure	May produce tachyarrhythmias, increased myocardial work, and increased oxygen consumption; may result in hepatic and mesenteric ischemia
Vasopressin		
Vasopressin, 0.2 to 2 milliunits/kg per min (0.0002 to 0.002 unit/kg per min)	Antidiuretic hormone analogue that acts on vasopressin receptors; produces peripheral and splanchnic vasoconstriction; also used to treat GI hemorrhage for this reason	May cause hypertension, bradycardia
Phosphodiesterase inhibitors and inodilators		
Inamrinone, Loading dose: 0.075 to 0.1 mg/kg (75 to 100 mcg/kg) slowly, Infusion: 5-10 mcg/kg per min	Nonadrenergic inotropic agent that produces phosphodiesterase inhibition and increase in intracellular cyclic-adenosine monophosphate cAMP intracellular calcium uptake also is delayed; these effects result in improved cardiac contractility and vasodilatation	Monitor for arrhythmias (especially accelerated junctional rhythm, junctional tachycardia, and ventricular ectopy); may produce hypotension (especially if patient is hypovolemic), liver and gastrointestinal dysfunction, thrombocytopenia, and abdominal pain; experience in children is limited and recent
Milrinone, Loading Dose: 0.05 mg/kg (50 mcg/kg) over 10-60 min, Infusion: 0.25-0.75 mcg/kg per min	As above	Reduce dose when renal dysfunction present
Vasodilators		
Nitroglycerin, 0.25-0.5 mcg/kg per min; increase as tolerated to maximum 10 mcg/kg per min (adolescents, 5 mcg/min; *note,* not per kg per min)	Arterial and venodilator	Is adsorbed by polyvinylchloride tubing; use special infusion set
Nitroprusside, 0.3-0.5 mcg/kg per min; titrate up to 8 mcg/kg per min	Arterial and venodilator	Light-sensitive; use specialized infusion set or cover tubing when infusion slow; may produce thiocyanate and cyanide toxicity, particularly for higher doses or prolonged infusion

*Infusion rate = mL/hr = [Weight (kg) × Dose (mcg/kg per min) × 60 min/h] ÷ Concentration (mcg/mL).
†For additional information, see Cardiogenic Shock, Treatment in this chapter.
GI, Gastrointestinal; *IV,* intravenous.

Box 6-2 **International Consensus Definitions of Systemic Inflammatory Response Syndrome, Sepsis, Severe Sepsis, and Septic Shock in Children**

Systemic Inflammatory Response Syndrome
The presence of at least two of the following four large bulleted criteria, one of which must be abnormal temperature or leukocyte count:
- ALTERATION IN TEMPERATURE: Core body temperature of >38.5°C or <36°C.
- ALTERATION IN HEART RATE (characterized by any of the three open bullets, below):
  ○ Tachycardia in the absence of external stimulus, chronic drugs, or painful stimuli, defined as follows:
    – Newborn to 1 year: HR >180/minute
    – 2-5 years: >140/minute
    – 6-12 years: >130/minute
    – 13 to <18 years: >110/minute
  ○ Otherwise unexplained persistent elevation in heart rate over a 0.5- to 4-hr time period
  ○ For children under 1 yr: bradycardia, in the absence of external vagal stimulus, β-blocker drugs, or congenital heart disease, defined by one of the three dashes below:
    – Newborn to 1 month: <100/minute
    – 1 month to 1 year: <90/minute
    – otherwise unexplained persistent depression over a 30-minute time period.
- ALTERATION IN RESPIRATORY RATE (characterized by either of the open bullets, below):
  ○ Mean respiratory rate >95th percentile normal for age, defined as follows:
    – Newborn-1 week: >50/minute
    – 1 week-1 month: >40/minute
    – 1 month to 1 year: >34/minute
    – 2-5 years: >22/minute
    – 6-12 years: >18/minute
    – 13 to <18 years: >14/minute
  ○ Mechanical ventilation for an acute process not related to underlying neuromuscular disease or the receipt of general anesthesia.
- ALTERATION IN WHITE BLOOD CELL COUNT: Leukocyte count elevated or depressed for age (not secondary to chemotherapy-induced leukopenia) or >10% immature neutrophils.

Infection (one of the following)
- A suspected or proven (by positive culture, tissue stain, or polymerase chain reaction test) infection caused by any pathogen
- A clinical syndrome associated with a high probability of infection.
Note: Evidence of infection includes positive findings on clinical examination, imaging, or laboratory tests (e.g., white blood cells in a normally sterile body fluid, perforated viscus, chest radiograph consistent with pneumonia, petechial or purpuric rash, purpura fulminans)

Sepsis
- SIRS in the presence of or as a result of suspected or proven infection

Severe Sepsis
Sepsis plus one of the following:
- Cardiovascular organ dysfunction
- Acute respiratory distress syndrome
- Two or more other organ dysfunctions; organ dysfunctions are defined in Box 6-3

Septic Shock
- Sepsis and cardiovascular organ dysfunction as defined in Box 6-3

Modified from Goldstein B, et al: International pediatric sepsis consensus conference: definitions for sepsis and organ dysfunction in pediatrics. *Pediatr Crit Care Med* 6:2–8, 2005.

---

after severe sepsis can also vary between patients and provide some insights into the likelihood of survival and response to therapy.

The host inflammatory response to systemic infection is perhaps the key element to understanding severe sepsis and septic shock. The complexities of the host response and the variations between patients in response to microbial challenge present the major hurdle to a comprehensive understanding of the pathophysiology of septic shock. Although there is better understanding of many of the essential cellular and humoral elements that contribute to septic shock than in years past, integration of these disparate processes into a clearly defined and recognizable system has proved to be extremely difficult.

It is now recognized that multiple clinical and laboratory variables have the capacity to alter the host response to infection. Many of these are rather simple and straightforward. The patient's age, nutritional status, sex, genetic background, and underlying disease processes may affect the host innate immune and acquired immune response to invasive infection. The complexity arises from the redundancy of inflammatory networks and the fact that there are many nonlinear, competing negative feedback loops and amplification pathways that occur simultaneously in the septic host. There is also evidence of compartmentalization at the immune response where cellular elements in the systemic circulation can express a different series of immune responses when compared with cells residing in the liver, spleen, lung, or other host tissues.

Some patients have a marked systemic response, often referred to as *hyperinflammation*, induced by certain microbial pathogens.[231] The clearest examples of this occur in previously healthy children who develop meningococcal sepsis or in patients with streptococcal toxic shock syndrome after a relatively mild soft-tissue injury.[232,241] The other extreme exists in febrile, neutropenic patients with cancer or in bone marrow transplant patients who have a markedly impaired systemic host response to microbial infection and often die of overwhelming infection with an inadequate host response.[11,135,231] There are numerous gradations in the spectrum between these two extremes, yet it is often difficult to clinically distinguish between patients with hyperinflammation and those with inadequate inflammatory responses.

A key element in the pathogenesis of sepsis is activation of the cytokine network. Cytokines are host produced, pleomorphic immunoregulatory peptides.[305,316] The most widely investigated cytokines are tumor necrosis factor, interleukin-1, and interleukin-8, which are generally proinflammatory, and

Box 6-3 **Criteria for Organ Dysfunction in Children with Severe Sepsis or Septic Shock**

Cardiovascular dysfunction
Despite administration of isotonic intravenous fluid boluses of more than 40 mL/kg in 1 hour, is described by the characteristics in one or more of the three bullets below:
- Decrease in BP (hypotension) to <5th percentile for age, estimated for children 1-10 years of age as follows:
  – Mean arterial pressure: <40 mm Hg + (1.5 × age in years)
  – Systolic BP < 70 mm Hg + (2 × age in years)
- Need for vasoactive drug to maintain BP in normal range (dopamine >5 μcg/kg per min or dobutamine, epinephrine, or norepinephrine at any dose)
- Two of the following:
  – Unexplained metabolic acidosis: base deficit more severe than −5.0 mEq/L
  – Increased arterial lactate >2 times upper limit of normal
  – Oliguria: urine output <0.5 mL/kg per hr
  – Prolonged capillary refill: >5 seconds
  – Core to peripheral temperature gap >3°C

Respiratory* (one of the following four bulleted conditions)
- $PaCO_2/FiO_2 < 300$ in absence of cyanotic heart disease or preexisting lung disease
- $PaCO_2 > 65$ torr or 20 mm Hg over baseline $PaCO_2$

- Proven need[†] or >50% inspired oxygen to maintain saturation >92%
- Need for nonelective invasive or noninvasive mechanical ventilation[‡]

Neurologic (either of the following)
- Glasgow Coma Score ≤11
- Acute change in mental status with a decrease in Glasgow Coma Score ≥3 points from abnormal baseline

Hematologic (one of the following three bulleted conditions)
- Platelet count <80,000/mm^3
- A decline of 50% in platelet count from highest value recorded over the past 3 days (for chronic hematology/oncology)
- International normalized ratio >2

Renal
- Serum creatinine ≥twofold upper limit of normal for age or twofold increase in baseline creatinine

Hepatic (either of the following)
- Total bilirubin ≥4 mg/dL (not applicable for newborn)
- ALT twofold upper limit of normal for age

Modified from Goldstein B, et al: International pediatric sepsis consensus conference: definitions for sepsis and organ dysfunction in pediatrics. *Pediatr Crit Care Med* 6:2–8, 2005.
*Acute respiratory distress syndrome must include a PaO_2/FiO_2 ratio ≤200 mm Hg, bilateral infiltrates, acute onset, and no evidence of left heart failure. Acute lung injury is defined identically except the PaO_2/FiO_2 ratio must be ≤300 mm Hg.
[†]Proven need assumes oxygen requirement was tested by decreasing flow with subsequent increase in flow if required.
[‡]In postoperative patients, this requirement can be met if the patient has developed an acute inflammatory or infectious process in the lungs that prevents them from being extubated.
ALT, Alanine transaminase; *BP*, blood pressure.

Table 6-6 **Basic Elements of PIRO Stratification of Patients with Sepsis**

P	Predisposing factors	Innate: Genetic polymorphisms and deficiencies of immune response genes affecting innate immune response, coagulation system complement receptors, Toll-like receptors, and intracellular signaling. Acquired: Burns, trauma, acquired immune deficiencies
I	Infection	Site, quantity, intrinsic virulence, and local versus systemic infection caused by specific microbial pathogens
R	Response	Differential responses based on hyperresponsiveness versus hyporesponsiveness-immunosuppression; response modifiers such as age, sex, nutritional status, diabetes, other preexisting diseases, and physiologic status of host
O	Organ dysfunction	Number, severity, and pattern of organ dysfunction in response to systemic infection; primary versus secondary organ injury; and organ injury owing to sepsis versus preexisting organ dysfunction

Modified from Opal SM: Concept of PIRO as a new conceptual framework to understand sepsis. *Pediatr Crit Care Med* 6(3):S55–S60, 2005.

interleukin-6 and interleukin-10, which tend to be antiinflammatory. A trigger, such as a microbial toxin, stimulates the production of tumor necrosis factor and interleukin-1, which in turn promote endothelial cell-leukocyte adhesion, release of proteases and arachidonic acid metabolites, and activation of clotting.[51,316] Interleukin-1 and tumor necrosis factor are synergistic, share many biologic functions, and interact to promote positive feedback cascades that result in fever, vasodilation, cardiovascular failure, and lactic acidosis (see Septic Mediators in the Chapter 6 Supplement on the Evolve Website).[51]

The cytokines stimulate the production of many important effector molecules, including proinflammatory cytokines, antiinflammatory cytokines, and nitric oxide. Increased proinflammatory cytokines, antiinflammatory cytokines, and nitric oxide correlate with outcome and the development of multiple organ failure in pediatric sepsis and septic shock.[51,289,320]

It is now clear that inflammation is just one of the many contributors to septic physiology. Other factors include enhanced coagulation and impaired fibrinolysis (Table 6-7).[8,135,194] Because of the multiple factors involved, the clinical pattern and presentation of septic shock can vary a great deal and depend on the dynamic interplay of the invading organism, elapsing time, and host response.

Clinical Signs and Symptoms
Abnormal hemodynamic responses are the hallmarks of septic shock. The clinical cascade may unfold over several days or a few hours. In many patients, the early stages consist of a

Table 6-7 **Mediators of and Immunotherapy for Sepsis**

Agent	Site of Action
Antiendotoxin antibodies E5 (murine) HA-1A (human)	Neutralize endotoxin
Bactericidal permeability-increasing protein	Neutralize endotoxin
TNF antibodies	Block TNF
IL-1 receptor antagonists	Inhibit action of IL-1 on cellular receptors
IL-1 antibodies	Block IL-1 receptor interaction
IL-6 and IL-8 antibodies	Block IL-6, IL-8 receptor interaction
Bradykinin-receptor antagonists	Prevent vasoactive effects of bradykinin
Platelet activating factor antagonist	Block platelet activation and platelet aggregation
Cyclooxygenase inhibitors (ibuprofen)	Block pyrogen, thromboxane, and prostaglandin production
NO synthase inhibitors	Block production of NO, restore vascular tone
Inhibitors of leukocyte-adhesion molecules	Prevent endothelium-leukocyte interaction
Corticosteroids	Promote and antiinflammatory response
Antiinflammatory cytokines (IL-6, IL-10)	Inhibit inflammatory response; reduce production of proinflammatory cytokines

IL, Interleukin; *NO,* nitric oxide; *TNF,* tumor-necrosis factor.

hyperdynamic state with an elevated CO, decreased SVR, and a widened pulse pressure, with episodic hypotension and warm extremities with brisk capillary refill.[35,37,51,52] In this hyperdynamic stage, the patient may also demonstrate high fever, mental confusion, and hyperventilation. Although these patients are typically tachycardic and tachypneic, the vital signs and clinical examination may not reflect the severity of disease. Mental status changes, a sensitive indicator of hypoperfusion, may present in a clinical spectrum that begins with fussiness, irritability, or hallucinations and, if untreated, evolves to lack of response to parents or noxious stimuli, and eventual coma.[243]

If sepsis is unchecked and uncorrected, cardiovascular function steadily deteriorates, which is characterized by a decline in CO, hypotension, and worsening metabolic acidosis. Paradoxically, hypotension may develop in the presence of normal or elevated CO. One fundamental abnormality in patients with septic shock is an altered relationship of SVR and CO.[292] The patient's status deteriorates when cardiac compensation for falling SVR is lost. Some patients die of refractory hypotension associated with extremely low SVR.[191,292]

A progression from high to low CO can occur over any time period.[35] As CO falls, tissue perfusion worsens, leading to anaerobic metabolism and accumulation of lactic acid.[195] Progressive lactic acidemia can be a sign of impending death.[21,22,292] Infants or children with heart disease and any

other patients with limited cardiac reserve can progress rapidly to this hypodynamic picture.

Survival following septic shock has been related to the host's ability to establish and maintain a hyperdynamic cardiovascular state.[44,253,254] In this hyperdynamic shock, CO is increased and the SVR is low. Clinical studies of adults with septic shock have documented both right and left ventricular dilation with decreased contractility and reduced ejection fraction.[44,238] In these patients, CO is maintained only through ventricular dilation (an increase in end-diastolic volume maintains SV at near-normal levels despite the fall in ejection fraction) and tachycardia (see Fig. 6-6). These septic shock studies in adults have not been replicated in children. Infants and children may not be fully capable of using or maintaining the same compensatory physiologic mechanisms. For example, infants and children have higher resting HRs, which can limit the efficiency of a chronotropic protective response. Because the pediatric ventricle is less compliant than the adult ventricle, the pediatric ventricle may be less able to dilate.

In the early stages of septic shock, hypovolemia or myocardial dysfunction (resulting from preexisting or intercurrent ventricular disease) can blunt or eliminate the hyperdynamic response to sepsis.[191,292] Several factors can contribute to the relative hypovolemia that commonly develops during septic shock. Increased capillary permeability, dilation of arteries and veins with subsequent peripheral pooling of intravascular blood volume, inappropriate polyuria, and poor oral intake all combine to reduce the effective blood volume (i.e., inadequate intravascular volume relative to the vascular space).[243] Fluid loss secondary to fever, diarrhea, vomiting, or sequestered third space fluid also contributes to the relative hypovolemia.

In some patients without complicating preexisting heart disease, a relative depression in left ventricular contractility exists even in early stages.[44,153,238,264,291] Myocardial contractility is most likely depressed because of the inhibitory effects of one or more circulating substances (so-called myocardial depressant factor or factors). In patients who survive, this myocardial depression is transient.

Contrary to adult experience, low CO—not low SVR—is associated with mortality in pediatric septic shock.[51,254] Ceneviva et al.[56] reported outcome data associated with aggressive volume resuscitation and goal-directed therapies in children with septic shock. In this study, 50 children with fluid refractory septic shock were hemodynamically characterized using measurements and calculations obtained through use of pulmonary artery catheters. The majority of children (58%) in septic shock showed a low CO and high SVR state (group I); 20% showed the classic adult high CO and low SVR state (group II); and 22% had decreased CO and SVR (group III).

Patients in group I responded to inotropic therapy with or without a vasodilator. Patients in group II responded to vasopressor therapy, but some needed the addition of an inotrope for evolving myocardial dysfunction. Patients in group III responded to combined vasopressor and inotropic therapy. The overall 28-day survival rate was 80% (group I, 72%; group II, 90%; group III, 91%). This study demonstrates that therapies directed at cardiac dysfunction and systemic vasoconstriction (i.e., vasodilators) are likely to be needed more in pediatric than in adult septic shock.[56]

Cardiovascular abnormalities described in sepsis include alterations of both systolic and diastolic ventricular function.[212,291] Although diastolic performance in sepsis has been less characterized, echocardiographic studies have demonstrated a pattern of abnormal left ventricular relaxation, which is more severe in nonsurvivors.

Septic shock is also characterized by abnormal utilization of oxygen.[122,124,254] Although sepsis causes a hypermetabolic stress associated with increased oxygen demand, deterioration characteristically occurs when oxygen consumption falls during a period of increased cardiovascular function and oxygen delivery. This fall in oxygen consumption is the result of decreased oxygen extraction and reflects a severe impairment of oxidative metabolism at a time of major metabolic and physiologic stress. The pathophysiology of inadequate oxygen consumption in septic shock remains unclear. The most widely accepted theories to account for this oxygen debt are the redistribution of blood flow, with a consequent decrease in nutrient capillary flow, and the development of a cellular metabolic blockade at the mitochondrial level such that delivered oxygen cannot be used. Progressive deterioration in oxygen consumption and oxygen extraction portends a poor prognosis for patients in septic shock.[124]

Management

Primary therapeutic goals for the initial treatment of septic shock are identification and control of the infection and rapid reversal of cardiovascular dysfunction.

Antibiotic Treatment. The removal or control of microorganisms by surgical debridement or drainage and antibiotic therapy is a crucial component of the treatment of septic shock. Antibiotic treatment is appropriate in patients with circulatory shock whenever an infectious etiology is suspected. Antimicrobial drugs are necessary but not sufficient for the treatment of sepsis, and paradoxically, they may precipitate septic changes by liberating microbial products (e.g., release of endotoxin following lysis of gram-negative bacteria).[316]

Airway and Ventilation. The primary goal in the initial management of septic shock is to restore hemodynamic stability. Fundamental aspects of management include increasing the oxygen delivery by maximizing CO and arterial oxygen content while minimizing oxygen requirements.

Detection of septic shock is facilitated by the nearly universal presence of tachypnea.[316] Sepsis places extreme demands on the cardiopulmonary system, requiring a high-minute ventilation precisely when the compliance of the respiratory system is diminished, airway resistance is increased, and muscle efficiency is impaired. Timely intubation and mechanical ventilation reduce respiratory muscle oxygen demand and the risk of aspiration and cerebral anoxia from catastrophic respiratory arrest.

Volume Resuscitation. Restoration of preload by volume resuscitation is the first therapeutic measure for a decreased CO.[38,50–52,72,119] Early and effective expansion of the circulating blood volume may enhance oxygen delivery and

prevent progression of the septic shock state. The American College of Critical Care Medicine-Pediatric Advanced Life Support guidelines recommend rapid, stepwise interventions with the following therapeutic end points in the first hour: reduction in extreme tachycardia, capillary refill of less than 2 s, normal pulses with no differential between peripheral and central pulses, warm extremities, urine output greater than 1 mL/kg per hour, and normal mental status.[38,72] Further hemodynamic optimization using metabolic endpoints to treat global tissue hypoxia include an $ScvO_2$ obtained from the superior vena cava greater than or equal to 70%, a cardiac index greater than 3.3, and less than 6.0 L/min per m^2 BSA with normal perfusion pressure for age.[38,52,72]

Studies in children have shown that early aggressive volume repletion, even without addressing myocardial dysfunction, significantly improves outcome.[72,119,227] More importantly, when resuscitation was inadequate and shock persisted, the odds of mortality doubled with each hour of persistent shock.[137] Goal-directed hemodynamic optimization represents an organized approach to volume repletion, attainment of a target BP (vascular tone) and a more definitive resolution of a pathologic oxygen supply dependency or global tissue hypoxia through the normalization of $ScvO_2$ as a surrogate end point.[72]

A study in adult patients with severe sepsis and septic shock confirmed that global tissue hypoxia, defined by an $ScvO_2$ less than 70%, can still be present even if physical examination, vital signs, central venous pressure, and urinary output are considered adequate.[262] In addressing this global tissue hypoxia using an early goal-directed approach, further reductions in the inflammatory response, morbidity, and mortality were achieved compared with conventional therapy.[262] Whereas the early goal-directed therapy patients received more fluids, red blood cell transfusions, and inotropes over the first 6 hours for a higher rate of attaining an $ScvO_2$ greater than or equal to 70%, there was essentially no difference in these therapies after the first 72 hours. Because of this early hemodynamic optimization, significant reductions in vasopressor, mechanical ventilation, and pulmonary artery catheter use were also realized.[262] Similarly, a pediatric study using a goal-directed approach demonstrated more fluid, more red blood cell transfusion, and more inotropic support in the first 6 hours of treatment in the group using $ScvO_2 \geq 70\%$ as an end point.[72] After 72 hours the amount of crystalloid administered and the percentage of red blood cells in transfusion were not different between the two groups. These observations were similar to those found in adults. These studies support the concept that early resuscitation rather than later resuscitation is beneficial.[52,56,227] In addition, there was a statistically significant reduction in the number of children with $ScvO_2$ less than 70% at 72 hours in the intervention group (i.e., early and aggressive fluid resuscitation produced better oxygen delivery to utilization ratio). This finding supports the concept that goal-directed therapy can reduce global oxygen debt over the long term and the short term in patients with septic shock. In addition to the favorable reduction in mortality, a decrease in pulmonary (increased number of ventilator-free days), neurologic, and renal dysfunction was also seen.

Isotonic crystalloid solutions can be used initially to restore intravascular volume in the presence of septic shock if they increase the blood volume and CO. Debate over the relative advantages and disadvantages of crystalloid and colloid fluids for the treatment of sepsis and septic shock continues.[52] A metaanalysis has shown no difference in mortality between patients resuscitated with normal saline or albumin, and a multidisciplinary consensus statement concluded that crystalloid is the preferred solution in patients with sepsis.[89] Three randomized controlled trials compared the use of colloid to crystalloid resuscitation in children with dengue shock.[82,220,319] No difference in mortality between the colloid or crystalloid resuscitation groups was shown.

Theoretically, transfusion of packed red blood cells to maintain a normal hemoglobin concentration is the most effective means of increasing arterial oxygen content and systemic oxygen availability. Initial guidelines in patients with severe sepsis target a hemoglobin concentration greater than or equal to 10 g/dL.[52]

The optimal hemoglobin for a critically ill child with severe sepsis is not known.[71] A recent multicenter trial reported similar outcomes in stable, critically ill children managed with a transfusion threshold of 7.0 g/dL and those with a threshold of 9.5 g/dL; however, the study excluded children with congenital heart disease or hemodynamic instability.[160] Whether a lower transfusion trigger is safe or appropriate in the initial resuscitation has not been determined.[71]

Excessive tachycardia, severe mixed venous desaturation, cardiac systolic dysfunction, and failure to resolve lactic acidosis or failure to improve gastric intramucosal pH may indicate the need to increase hemoglobin concentration to levels of 10 g/dL.[72,180,243,292]

Although fluid administration and antimicrobial therapy remain the cornerstones of the therapeutic approach to sepsis and septic shock, patients often require therapy with inotropic agents, vasoactive drugs, or both.[38,51] Children can have predominant cardiac failure, predominant vascular failure, or a combination of cardiac and vascular failure.[35,37,52,56,72] Therapeutic approaches differ with each condition.

Myocardial depression complicates septic shock and can prevent the development of optimal CO despite adequate intravascular volume. The catecholamine and noncatecholamine inotropes may both be effective in reversing myocardial depression and improving contractility (see Table 6-5; Figs. 6-7 and 6-8).[38]

Inotropic Support. Children in a normotensive, hypodynamic state after volume resuscitation require an inotrope to increase CO and to reverse shock. Dobutamine or moderate-dose dopamine can be used as the first line of inotropic support. Patients with dobutamine-resistant septic shock often respond to the addition of epinephrine with or without vasodilators. When patients remain in a normotensive low CO state, despite adequate volume resuscitation and epinephrine and vasodilator therapy, then the use of milrinone should be considered.[25,174]

Catecholamines exert their β-adrenergic receptor effects by elevating intracellular calcium transit through increasing production of intracellular cAMP. However, benefits from the application of catecholamines in septic shock may not be sufficient. Myocardial hyporesponsiveness to catecholamine administration during septic shock has been documented by several investigators.[52,247,291] This hyporesponsivity of the myocardium to catecholamines may be due to cytokine-induced

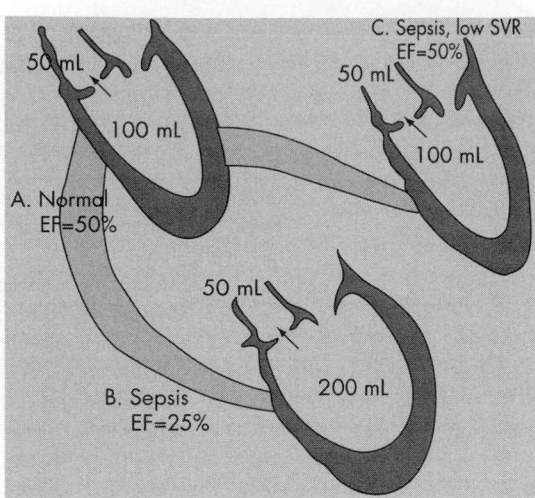

FIG. 6-7 Potential mechanism for maintenance of near-normal stroke volume in septic shock, despite fall in ejection fraction (EF). When ejection fraction falls during septic shock, stroke volume can be maintained at normal or near-normal levels if ventricular dilation results in an increase in ventricular end-diastolic volume. For ease of calculations, simple numbers are used in this illustration. **A,** In the healthy patient with an ejection fraction of 50% and an end-diastolic volume of 100 mL, stroke volume is 50 mL. **B,** If ejection fraction falls to 25% and ventricular dilation results in an increase in ventricular end-diastolic volume of 200 mL, the stroke volume can remain at 50 mL. If the patient then has an increased heart rate, cardiac output and index may be higher than normal. **C,** If the SVR is extremely low, EF and stroke volume may be maintained during septic shock, but hypotension is likely to be present.

uncoupling of the β-adrenergic receptor system or due to deranged intracellular calcium metabolism.[25]

The bipyridines (milrinone, inamrinone) have no interaction with the adrenergic receptors, but exert their effects through the inhibition of phosphodiesterases, which degrade cAMP. Milrinone has been shown to improve cardiovascular function in pediatric patients with hypodynamic septic shock who are adequately volume resuscitated and are being treated with catecholamines.[25,174]

Vasopressors. Vasopressor therapy is commonly required in children with fluid refractory shock and hypotension. Choices for vasopressor effect include dopamine in a dose range of 10-20 mcg/kg per minute, norepinephrine, and epinephrine. Alpha-adrenergic agonists are vasoconstricting drugs that can boost SVR. All the drugs mentioned have marked β-adrenergic properties as well, increasing the HR and myocardial contractility.

Dopamine is an α-adrenergic agonist at higher concentrations. It mediates vasoconstriction indirectly by causing the release of norepinephrine from sympathetic vesicles.[272]

Norephinephrine often reverses dopamine-refractory septic shock.[202] Norephinephrine can also improve urine output and renal function by increasing perfusion pressure in hypotensive patients.

Both high-dose dopamine and norepinephrine have been recommended as the first-line vasopressor agents in the treatment of refractory shock. There is controversy about whether one agent is superior to the other.[70] Dopamine and norepinephrine have different effects on the kidney, the splanchnic region, and the pituitary axis, but the clinical implications of these differences are uncertain. Consensus guidelines and

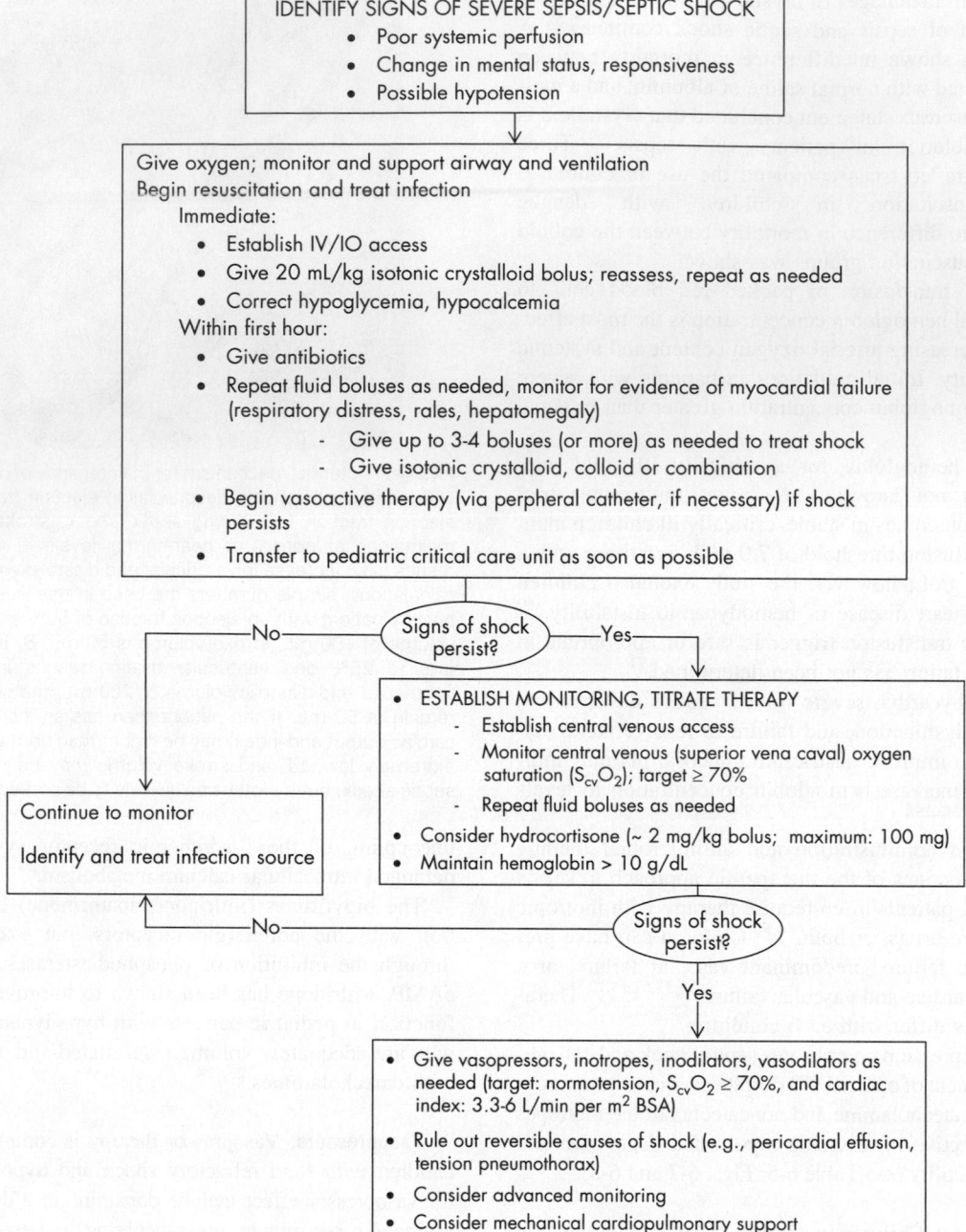

IDENTIFY SIGNS OF SEVERE SEPSIS/SEPTIC SHOCK
- Poor systemic perfusion
- Change in mental status, responsiveness
- Possible hypotension

Give oxygen; monitor and support airway and ventilation
Begin resuscitation and treat infection
  Immediate:
  - Establish IV/IO access
  - Give 20 mL/kg isotonic crystalloid bolus; reassess, repeat as needed
  - Correct hypoglycemia, hypocalcemia
  Within first hour:
  - Give antibiotics
  - Repeat fluid boluses as needed, monitor for evidence of myocardial failure (respiratory distress, rales, hepatomegaly)
    - Give up to 3-4 boluses (or more) as needed to treat shock
    - Give isotonic crystalloid, colloid or combination
  - Begin vasoactive therapy (via perpheral catheter, if necessary) if shock persists
  - Transfer to pediatric critical care unit as soon as possible

Signs of shock persist? —No— Continue to monitor / Identify and treat infection source

Signs of shock persist? —Yes—

ESTABLISH MONITORING, TITRATE THERAPY
  - Establish central venous access
  - Monitor central venous (superior vena caval) oxygen saturation ($S_{cv}O_2$); target $\geq$ 70%
  - Repeat fluid boluses as needed
- Consider hydrocortisone (~ 2 mg/kg bolus; maximum: 100 mg)
- Maintain hemoglobin > 10 g/dL

Signs of shock persist? —No—

Signs of shock persist? —Yes—

- Give vasopressors, inotropes, inodilators, vasodilators as needed (target: normotension, $S_{cv}O_2 \geq$ 70%, and cardiac index: 3.3-6 L/min per m² BSA)
- Rule out reversible causes of shock (e.g., pericardial effusion, tension pneumothorax)
- Consider advanced monitoring
- Consider mechanical cardiopulmonary support

FIG. 6-8 Suggestions for hemodynamic support in pediatric septic shock. Based on recommendations of Brierley J, Carcillo JA, Choong K, Cornell T, et al: Clinical practice parameters for hemodynamic support of pediatric and neonatal septic shock: 2007 update from the American College of Critical Care Medicine. *Crit Care Med* 37:666–688, 2009. *BP,* Blood pressure; *CI,* cardiac index; *SVRI,* systemic vascular resistance index.

expert recommendations suggest that either agent may be used as a first-choice vasopressor in patients with shock.[71]

Recently, a multicenter, randomized trial assigned adult patients with shock to receive either dopamine or norepinephrine as first-line vasopressor therapy to restore and maintain BP.[70] The type of shock present most frequently was septic shock (62.2%), followed by cardiogenic shock (16.7%) and hypovolemic shock (15.7%). The primary outcome was mortality at 28 days after randomization; secondary end points included adverse events and number of days without the need for organ support. Although the mortality did not differ significantly between the group of patients treated with dopamine and the group treated with norepinephrine, this study raises

serious concerns about the safety of dopamine therapy, because dopamine, as compared with norepinephrine, was associated with more arrhythmias and with an increased rate of death in the subgroup of patients with cardiogenic shock.[70]

Although epinephrine is used for resuscitation and to treat anaphylaxis, its β_2-adrenergic effects can cause hyperglycemia, acidosis, and other adverse effects; therefore it may not be ideal for treating shock.[170] However, a recent study reported no difference in clinical in-patient outcomes or safety in a prospective comparison of norepinephrine with or without dobutamine to epinephrine for septic shock.[12]

In children with a warm vasodilated state after volume resuscitation, norepinephrine can be used to increase diastolic

BP while maintaining good perfusion.[51,202] However, these cases of vasodilatory shock are characterized by hypotension caused by peripheral vasodilation and by a poor response to therapy with vasopressor drugs.[162] Vasodilatory shock is caused by the inappropriate activation of vasodilator mechanisms and the failure of vasoconstrictor mechanisms. Unregulated nitric oxide synthesis through activation of soluble guanylate cyclase and generation of cyclic guanosine monophosphate (cGMP) causes dephosphorylation of myosin and hence vasorelaxation. In addition, nitric oxide synthesis and metabolic acidosis activate the potassium channels in the plasma membrane of vascular smooth muscle. The resulting hyperpolarization of the membrane prevents the calcium that mediates norepinephrine- and angiotensin II–induced vasoconstriction from entering the cell. As a result, hypotension and vasodilation persist, despite high plasma concentrations of these hormones. In marked contrast, the plasma concentrations of vasopressin are low, despite the presence of hypotension. This finding is unexpected, because plasma vasopressin concentrations are markedly elevated early in septic shock and hemorrhagic shock. However, the initial massive release of hormone may result in subsequent depletion, such that plasma concentrations of vasopressin are eventually too low to maintain arterial pressure. Although the pressor response to exogenous vasopressin in vasodilatory shock may be due to several different mechanisms, the ability of this hormone to block potassium channels in vascular smooth muscle and interfere with nitric oxide signaling are probably important contributors.

Elucidation of key components of the pathogenesis of vasodilatory shock—potassium channel activation, an increase in nitric oxide synthesis, and vasopressin deficiency—has suggested new possibilities for therapy. Unfortunately, a recent phase-three trial of a nonselective inhibitor of nitric oxide synthase in patients with septic shock was halted because of side effects.[63]

In recent years, vasopressin has been increasingly used to treat the hypotension associated with shock.[24,162,170] Vasopressin can be particularly effective in reversing mediator-induced vasodilatory shock in patients with sepsis or anaphylaxis.[170,173,323]

The use of vasopressin for hypotension in the setting of vasodilatory shock (warm shock) seems appropriate, and the limited use of vasopressin in this setting appears to be safe. However, for both adults and children, the appropriate patient population and dose regimen have not yet been determined.[173]

In a recent report, admission and serial plasma vasopressin levels were appropriately elevated in children with septic shock.[176] These findings are in contrast with those reported in adults, suggesting that the role of vasopressin administration in children with septic shock is limited until prospective studies are performed. Although the addition of vasopressin to norepinephrine therapy in adult patients with septic shock appears to produce mortality rates similar to those of mortality with norepinephrine alone and it is safe, there is no compelling advantage to using vasopressin rather than norephinephrine.[240,266]

Vasopressin could have variable effects depending on the cardiovascular profile of shock in any given patient. For example, vasopressin could produce favorable effects in a high CO and low SVR shock state, but could be deleterious if used alone in a patient with severe left ventricular dysfunction. Other reported adverse effects of vasopressin and norepinephrine include decreased CO,[181,266] mesenteric ischemia,[151,266,306] hyponatremia, skin necrosis, and digital ischemia.[83,125,140]

The use of vasopressors should be titrated to end points of normal perfusion pressure or SVR. Strict end-point measures should be used to avoid unnecessary vasoconstriction to key organs. A frequent adverse affect of α-agonist treatment is localized severe vasoconstriction after extravasation of the infusion; therefore these infusions are best administered into central venous or intraosseous catheters.[272]

When any patient in circulatory shock fails to respond to initial therapy, reversible causes should always be considered. These causes include pneumothorax, pericardial tamponade, and adrenal insufficiency.

Corticosteroid Therapy. Corticosteroid therapy has been used in varied doses for sepsis and related syndromes for more than 50 years, with no clear benefits on mortality.[13] Since 1998, studies in adults have consistently used prolonged low-dose corticosteroid therapy, and analysis of this subgroup suggests a beneficial drug effect on short-term mortality.[13] The Corticosteroid Therapy of Septic Shock (CORTICUS) study group found that hydrocortisone did not improve survival or reversal of shock in patients with septic shock, either overall or in patients who did not have a response to corticotrophin, although hydrocortisone hastened reversal of shock but not survival in those patients in whom shock was ultimately reversed.[283]

Over the past decade the concept of relative adrenal insufficiency has been proposed in the critical care unit (PCCU) setting and generally refers to patients with vasopressor-resistant hypotension.[277] In critically ill adults who had a normal baseline cortisol level (≥20 mcg/dL) and incremental rise of cortisol of less than or equal to 9 mcg/dL after administration of 250 mcg of intravenous adrenocorticotropic hormone (ACTH), treatment with stress doses of hydrocortisone was associated with improved survival.[10]

Pizarro et al.[252] studied the baseline and peak incremental response (increase above baseline) to 250 mcg of ACTH in critically ill children with septic shock to learn whether this test would predict shock resistant to vasopressor in the pediatric setting. All children (18%) with a basal serum cortisol of less than 20 mcg/dL had catecholamine-resistant shock. Eighty percent of those with a low incremental cortisol response to ACTH (≤9 mcg/dL at 30 or 60 min) compared with 20% who had "normal" incremental cortisol response had catecholamine-resistant shock. The study concludes that absolute and relative adrenal insufficiency is common in children with septic shock and may contribute to the development of catecholamine-resistant shock—that is, it is associated with an increased vasopressor requirement.[252] However, doubts still persist regarding the efficacy of replacement therapy with low-dose steroids in children with catecholamine-resistant septic shock, and further study is needed to determine whether treatment of such patients changes morbidity, mortality, or both.[252,327]

The most recent consensus guidelines for treatment of pediatric septic shock suggest that hydrocortisone therapy should be reserved for use in children with catecholamine resistance and suspected or proven adrenal insufficiency.[38] Patients at risk for adrenal insufficiency include children with severe septic shock and purpura, children who have previously received steroid therapies for chronic illness, and children with pituitary or adrenal abnormalities.[71,252,261,327] Children who have clear risk factors for adrenal insufficiency should be treated with stress-dose steroids (hydrocortisone, 50 mg/m^2 BSA per 24 hours).[71]

Children who have received etomidate or ketoconazole may also be at risk for adrenal insufficiency.[327] The use of etomidate as an anesthetic induction agent in critically ill patients is controversial, because this drug inhibits the 11β-hydroxylase enzyme that converts 11β-deoxycortisol into cortisol in the adrenal gland.[190] A single dose of etomidate has been demonstrated to inhibit cortisol production for up to 48 hours, prompting the suggestion of steroid supplementation during this period.[204,307]

Adrenal insufficiency in severe pediatric sepsis is associated with a poor prognosis.[68,71] No strict definitions exist, but absolute adrenal insufficiency in the case of catecholamine-resistant septic shock is assumed at a random total cortisol concentration of less than 18 mcg/dL.[71] Relative adrenal insufficiency has been defined as a peak serum cortisol level increase of 9 mcg/dL or less above baseline, evaluated 30- or 60-minutes after administration of 250 mcg of corticotrophin (a 30- to 60-minutes post-ACTH stimulation test).[71] The treatment of relative adrenal insufficiency in children with septic shock is controversial.[71,327] A retrospective study from a large administrative database recently reported that the use of any corticosteroid in children with severe sepsis was associated with increased mortality.[192] Given the lack of data in children and the potential risk, steroids should not be used in children who do not have risk factors or who do not meet minimal criteria for adrenal insufficiency. A randomized, controlled trial in children is eagerly awaited.

There are potential complications to glucocorticoid administration in critically ill children, including antianabolic effects, attenuated immunity, depressed wound healing, calcium mobilization, impaired insulin action, and hyperglycemia.[327] Although adjunctive corticosteroids for severe sepsis may hasten resolution of unstable hemodynamics, this may occur at the metabolic risk of hyperglycemia.[327] Risk of hyperglycemia and associated increased mortality secondary to the gluconeogenic effects of cortisol deserve close scrutiny in children.[93,284,327]

Immunotherapy. Because septic shock can result from endogenous proteins and phospholipids synthesized by the patient, it has been hypothesized that diminution or elimination of the host response will lessen morbidity and mortality.[243] Although this hypothesis continues to be explored, the results of immunotherapy have, in general, been discouraging.[193,243,258] Some experimental therapies and their targets are listed in Table 6-7.

Administration of polyvalent intravenous immunoglobulin was recently shown to have no effect on outcome in an international, multicenter study of proven or suspected neonatal sepsis.[39a] In a recent randomized controlled study, administration of polyclonal immunoglobulin in pediatric patients with sepsis syndrome ($n = 100$) significantly reduced mortality

and length of stay, also resulting in fewer complications, especially disseminated intravascular coagulation.[87]

Treatment of Coagulation Dysfunction. In patients diagnosed with sepsis, severe sepsis, or septic shock, cytokine-mediated endothelial injury and tissue factor activation initiate a cascade of events that culminate in the development of coagulation dysfunction characterized as procoagulant and antifibrinolytic.[226] This abnormal state predisposes the patient to develop microvascular thrombosis, tissue ischemia, and organ hypoperfusion. Multiple organ dysfunction syndrome may be a product of this perturbation in coagulation regulation. Treatments aimed at correcting this coagulation dysfunction have met with limited success.[226]

Coagulation proteases and their cofactors modify the outcome of severe inflammation by engaging signaling-competent cell surface receptors. The central effector protease of the protein C pathway, activated protein C, interacts with the endothelial cell protein C receptor, protease-activated receptors, and other receptors to affect hemostasis and immune cell function.[311] The immune regulatory capacity of the protein C pathway and its individual components might be at least as important as its well-documented effects on coagulation.[311]

The use of recombinant human activated protein C, although indicated in some adults with sepsis-induced organ dysfunction, is not recommended for use in children with septic shock.[71] A randomized clinical trial of recombinant human activated protein C in pediatric severe sepsis patients was stopped by recommendation of the Data Monitoring Committee for futility, with evidence of increased bleeding complications.[71,213]

The keystone of the treatment of hemostatic abnormalities in patients with sepsis is to treat the underlying infection using appropriate antibiotics and source control.[165,166] However, additional supportive treatment, specifically aimed at the coagulation abnormalities, may be required.

Low levels of platelets and coagulation factors may increase the risk of bleeding. However, plasma or platelet substitution therapy should not be instituted on the basis of laboratory results alone and is indicated only in patients with active bleeding and in those requiring an invasive procedure or otherwise at risk for bleeding complications.[165] The use of agents that are capable of restoring the dysfunctional anticoagulation pathways in patients with disseminated intravascular coagulation has been studied.[165] The use of antithrombin concentrate, activated protein C, and recombinant factor VIIa are not currently recommended for use in pediatric septic shock.[110,200]

Systemic inflammation will invariably lead to activation of the coagulation system, but components of the coagulation system may markedly modulate the inflammatory response. Increasing evidence points to extensive cross-talk between the coagulation and inflammation systems at various points, with tissue factor, thrombin, components of the protein C pathway and fibrinolytic activators, and inhibitors playing pivotal roles. Increased insight into the molecular mechanisms that play a role in the close relationship between inflammation and coagulation could lead to the identification of new targets for therapies that can modify excessive activation or dysregulation of these systems.[166]

Extracorporeal Membrane Oxygenation (ECMO). ECMO is used in septic shock in children but its effect is not clear. Survival from refractory shock or respiratory failure associated with sepsis is 80% in neonates and 50% in children.[71] In one study of 12 ECMO patients with meningococcal sepsis, 8 of 12 patients survived, with six functionally normal at a median of 1 year of follow-up.[108] One multivariate analysis of long-term survivors of ECMO found no significant difference between the performance of children with sepsis and those treated for other causes (i.e., without sepsis).[205]

Cardiogenic Shock

Etiology and Definition

Cardiac shock is the pathophysiologic state in which an abnormality of cardiac function is responsible for failure to maintain adequate tissue oxygenation.[58,245] The final common pathway is depressed CO, which in most instances results from decreased myocardial contractility. Cardiogenic shock or severe congestive heart failure (CHF) during infancy and childhood represents a diagnostic and therapeutic challenge because of its myriad etiologies (Box 6-4). In the following section, the abbreviation CHF is used for severe CHF or cardiogenic shock.

Pathophysiology

In contrast to hypovolemic shock, compensatory responses can have deleterious effects in patients with cardiogenic shock.[45,58,269,273] Compensatory responses are nonspecific and imprecise, and in patients with cardiogenic shock these responses may contribute to the progression of shock by further depressing cardiac function.

The Sympathetic Nervous System. The baroreceptor-mediated increase in sympathetic tone that occurs with ventricular dysfunction has several consequences, including increased myocardial contractility, tachycardia, and arterial vasoconstriction, and it can produce increased cardiac afterload as well as venoconstriction and increased cardiac preload.[269]

Increased local and circulating concentrations of norepinephrine can contribute to myocyte hypertrophy; this can occur directly through stimulation of α1- and β-adrenergic receptors or secondarily by activating the renin-angiotensin-aldosterone system. Norepinephrine is directly toxic to myocardial cells, an effect mediated through calcium overload, the induction of apoptosis, or both.[216,269] Norepinephrine-induced death of myocytes can be prevented by concomitant, nonselective β-adrenergic blockade or combined β- and α-adrenergic blockade. In the past, β-adrenergic blockade was thought to be contraindicated in patients with heart failure. However, if patients can tolerate short-term β-adrenergic blockade, ventricular function subsequently improves.[58,229,273,315] There are few data on the use of β-blockers in children with heart failure.[273]

Renin-Angiotensin-Aldosterone System. The activity of the renin-angiotensin-aldosterone system is increased in most patients with heart failure.[269,273] As with plasma norepinephrine,

---

Box 6-4   Etiologies of Cardiogenic Shock in Infants and Children

Conduction Abnormalities
Supraventricular tachycardia
Ventricular arrhythmias
Bradycardia

Cardiomyopathy
Hypoxic/Ischemic Events
   Cardiac arrest
   Prolonged shock
   Head injury
   Anomalous origin of the coronary arteries
   Excessive catecholamine state
   Cardiopulmonary bypass
   Acute myocardial infarction
Infectious
   Viral
   Bacterial
   Fungal
   Protozoal
   Rickettsial
Metabolic
   Hypothyroid/hyperthyroid
   Hypoglycemia
   Pheochromocytoma
   Glycogen storage disease
   Mucopolysaccharidoses
   Nutritional deficiencies (thiamine, selenium, carnitine)
   Disorders of fatty acid metabolism

   Acidosis
   Hypothermia
   Hypocalcemia, hypophosphatemia
Connective Tissue or Inflammatory Diseases
   Systemic lupus erythematous
   Juvenile rheumatoid arthritis
   Polyarteritis nodosa
   Kawasaki disease
   Acute rheumatic fever
Neuromuscular Disorders
   Duchenne's muscular dystrophy
   Myotonic dystrophy
   Limb-Girdle
   Spinal muscular atrophy
   Friedreich's ataxia
Toxin Hypersensitivity
   Sulfonamides
   Penicillins
   Anthracyclines
   Lead
   Cocaine
   Carbon monoxide
Other
   Familial dilated cardiomyopathy

Congenital Heart Disease

Trauma

the degree of increase in plasma renin activity provides a prognostic index in these patients.[269] Patients with mild heart failure may have little or no increase in either plasma renin activity or the plasma aldosterone concentration. However, normal plasma renin and aldosterone values would be inappropriate in these patients because of their increased intracellular fluid and total blood volumes.[251,310] Among patients with severe heart failure, the concentrations of plasma renin and aldosterone are high.

Through renal vasoconstriction, stimulation of the renin-angiotensin-system, and direct effects on the proximal convoluted tubule, increased renal adrenergic activity contributes to the avid renal sodium and water retention that occurs in patients with heart failure. The kidneys become adversaries of the heart, lungs, and liver.

Aldosterone has an important role in the pathophysiology of heart failure. Aldosterone promotes the retention of sodium, loss of magnesium and potassium, sympathetic activation, parasympathetic inhibition, myocardial and vascular fibrosis, baroreceptor dysfunction, vascular damage, and impaired arterial compliance.[251,310] Many physicians have assumed that inhibition of the renin-angiotensin-aldosterone system by an angiotensin converting enzyme (ACE) inhibitor will adequately suppress the formation of aldosterone. In addition, treatment with an aldosterone-receptor blocker in conjunction with an ACE inhibitor has been considered relatively contraindicated because of the potential for serious hyperkalemia. However, there is increasing evidence to suggest that ACE inhibitors only transiently suppress the production of aldosterone.[251,310] Furthermore, treatment with the aldosterone-receptor blocker spironolactone, in conjunction with an ACE inhibitor, is effective and well tolerated and it does not lead to serious hyperkalemia.[7,251]

Other adverse consequences of long-term activation of the renin-angiotensin-aldosterone system in patients with CHF include a progressive remodeling of the heart and vasculature, which is mediated in part by the induction of various cytokines and growth factors.[310] Most of these actions support or increase arterial BP and maintain glomerular filtration. Vasoconstriction and the release of aldosterone in response to angiotensin occur in seconds or minutes, in keeping with their roles of supporting the circulation after hemorrhage, dehydration, or postural change. Other actions, such as vascular growth and ventricular hypertrophy, require days or weeks.[111]

An ACE inhibitor is now considered first-line therapy for patients with heart failure.[315] These drugs have improved survival in patients with chronic heart failure and all degrees of severity. Moreover, ACE inhibition reverses left ventricular hypertrophy, a common harbinger of heart failure.[43,250] The role of angiotensin-converting enzyme inhibitors in the treatment of heart failure in children is much less clear.[273]

The amino acid sequence of angiotensin II has long been known, and compounds that competitively inhibit its action have been studied almost as long. The recently released angiotensin-receptor antagonist losartan appears to be beneficial in some patients with heart disease.[111]

Nonosmotic Release of Arginine Vasopressin. Water retention in excess of sodium retention can occur in patients with heart failure and lead to hyponatremia. In fact, hyponatremia

is an ominous prognostic indicator in patients with heart failure.[269] Hyponatremia may be partly due to the increased water intake caused by the increased thirst associated with heart failure. However, increased water intake alone rarely causes hyponatremia. In patients with heart failure and hyponatremia, hypoosmolality, which inhibits the release of arginine vasopressin in normal subjects, is associated with persistently high plasma concentrations of arginine vasopressin. This observation suggests a pivotal role for arginine vasopressin in hyponatremia. In preliminary studies of patients with heart failure, a nonpeptide, orally active antagonist of arginine vasopressin proved effective in reversing impaired urinary diluting capacity, increasing solute-free water excretion, and correcting hyponatremia.[269]

Natriuretic Hormone System. The natriuretic hormone system participates in the regulation of fluid balance and vascular resistance in healthy humans and in those afflicted with a variety of disease states.[64] The natriuretic hormone system is composed of several structurally and functionally related peptides, primarily produced by the myocardium, vascular endothelium, and kidneys; they influence volume homeostasis and vascular tone by binding to dedicated receptors throughout the cardiovascular and renal system.[64] These peptides induce natriuresis, diuresis, and vasodilation and specifically act to counter the effects of the renin-angiotensin-aldosterone system.[217]

The cardiac members of these peptides are the atrial or A-type natriuretic peptide (ANP) and the B-type natriuretic peptide (BNP). ANP is secreted primarily from the cardiac atria in response to increased left and right atrial pressures as well as volume loads, and BNP is secreted primarily from the ventricles in response to increased left and right ventricular pressures and volume loads.

The physiologic properties of the natriuretic peptides made them attractive candidates for heart failure therapy. Indeed, BNP (nesiritide) was found to be beneficial, and it was approved for treatment of acute decompensated CHF in the United States in 2001. However, responsiveness to natriuretic peptides decreases as heart failure worsens, even as the plasma concentrations of the peptides rise.[168]

Soon after the discovery of the physiologic role of these peptides, it became clear that the natriuretic peptides serve as biochemical markers for heart disease or shock.[30,75,97,168,186,201,217] In comparative studies, BNP and its terminal prohormone fragment, N-terminal pro-BNP, were found to be superior to ANP as markers in heart failure and myocardial infarction.[217]

Endothelial Hormones. A crucial vascular structure is the endothelium, because it is strategically located between the circulating blood and the vascular smooth muscle and it is a source of a variety of mediators regulating vascular tone and growth as well as platelet function and coagulation.[182] The endothelium is both a target for and a mediator of cardiovascular disease.

Prostacyclin and prostaglandin E are vasodilating hormones produced from arachidonic acid in many cells (see Septic Shock, Mediators of the Septic Cascade, and Evolve Fig. 6-1 in the Chapter 6 Supplement on the Evolve Website).

Angiotensin II, norepinephrine, and renal nerve stimulation increase the synthesis of these vasodilating prostaglandins, which then attenuate the vasoconstrictor effects of these three stimuli.[58] These vasodilatory prostaglandins may thus counterbalance the neurohormone-induced renal vasoconstriction that occurs in heart failure.

Nitric oxide is an even more potent vasodilator than prostacyclin and prostaglandin E. Endothelial cells contain a constitutive nitric oxide synthase, the activity of which may be blunted in heart failure.[182,210] Thus, the constrictor action of the endogenous vasoconstrictors whose concentrations are elevated in heart failure—including angiotensin II, norepinephrine, and arginine vasopressin—may be enhanced by a concomitant decrease in nitric oxide synthesis in endothelial cells.

The endothelins are peptides of 21 amino acids that are produced in a wide variety of cells. Endothelin-1 is the only member produced in endothelial cells, and it is also produced in vascular smooth muscle cells.[167] Hypoxia, shear stress, and hormones associated with the development of CHF stimulate the production of endothelin-1.[167]

Endothelin-1 can stimulate aldosterone secretion and decrease kidney perfusion and function, both of which contribute to the retention of sodium and water and increased intravascular volume. Endothelin-1 also stimulates hypertrophy of the ventricles and increases sympathetic activity and arterial vasoconstriction. Endothelin-1 is one of the most potent vasoconstrictors, and plasma endothelin concentrations are increased in some patients with heart failure.[167,235] High plasma endothelin-1 concentrations are associated with a poor prognosis in patients with heart failure.[235]

Locally produced endothelin-1 has been implicated in closure of the ductus arteriosus at birth.[167] Inhibition of the production and action of endothelin-1 by prostacyclin or prostaglandin E may prevent closure of the ductus.

Cytokines. It is becoming increasingly apparent that proinflammatory cytokines play an important role in modulating the structure and function of the diseased heart.[59] The plasma concentrations of some cytokines, such as tumor necrosis factor alpha (TNF-α), are increased in patients with heart failure.[59] TNF-α, which is produced under a variety of stresses, exerts negative inotropic effects, and can produce left ventricular remodeling, pulmonary edema, cardiomyopathy, and is a major mediator of apoptosis (cell death).[59,318] Various cytokines and TNF-α, in particular, represent new targets for therapeutic intervention in patients with heart failure.

Ventricular Dilation and Hypertrophy. The ventricle responds to abnormal loading conditions by chamber dilation and hypertrophy. Ventricular dilation causes an increase in end-diastolic ventricular volume, which results in an increased SV and an improvement in CO. Another compensatory mechanism is hypertrophy of the myocardium.[100] However, both these mechanisms increase oxygen requirements and make the heart more susceptible to ischemia.

Myocardial hypertrophy is an early milestone during the clinical course of heart failure and is an important risk factor for subsequent cardiac morbidity and mortality.[136] In response to a variety of mechanical, hemodynamic, hormonal, and pathologic stimuli, the heart adapts to increased demands of cardiac work by increasing muscle mass through the initiation of a hypertrophic response. However, initiation of this hypertrophic response can result in heart muscle failure and the loss of myocytes as a result of programmed cell death (apoptosis).[58,318]

Downward Spiral in Cardiogenic Shock. Diminished CO initiates baroreceptor-mediated neurohumoral events, particularly the activation of the sympathetic nervous system, the activation of the renin-angiotensin-aldosterone system, and the nonosmotic release of vasopressin, all of which attempt to maintain arterial perfusion to vital organs. However, over time, these neurohumoral events may have deleterious effects that include pulmonary edema, hyponatremia, increased cardiac afterload and preload, and cardiac remodeling.

As myocardial contractility deteriorates and CO decreases, SVR increases in response to neurohumoral mediators to maintain circulatory stability. However, this increase in afterload adds to the heart's workload and further decreases pump function. Therefore in cardiogenic shock, a vicious cycle is established: ventricular dysfunction is exacerbated by neurohumoral vasoconstriction, which contributes to further ventricular dysfunction.

Because of the self-perpetuating cycle, compensated phases of cardiogenic shock may not be observed; patients are tachycardic, hypotensive, diaphoretic, oliguric, and acidotic. Extremities are cool and mental status is altered. Hepatomegaly, jugular venous distension, rales, and peripheral edema may be observed. CO is depressed, and central venous pressure, pulmonary wedge pressure, and SVR are all elevated.

Diastolic Heart Failure. Another form of CHF and cardiogenic shock (see Fig. 6-3) is caused by diastolic dysfunction.[16,115,312] Impaired myocardial relaxation changes the pressure-to-volume relationship during diastole and increases ventricular pressure at any volume. This lack of myocardial relaxation is hemodynamically unfavorable because increased left VEDP will be transmitted to the lungs and result in pulmonary edema and dyspnea. Such patients exhibit heart failure, but have normal left ventricular systolic function.[100] Heart failure in the presence of a normal cardiac silhouette on the chest radiograph should suggest the possibility of diastolic dysfunction.

Diastolic heart failure is an insidious disease. Insults to the myocardium are followed by a series of compensatory changes that are beneficial in the short run, but have long-term deleterious effects. Structured remodeling and other factors, including myocardial ischemia, left ventricular hypertrophy, increased HR, and abnormal calcium flux can impair diastolic function and cause an increase in left ventricular filling pressure.[16,115,312]

Both ischemia and hypertrophy impair relaxation in early diastole. Ischemia reduces the supply of high-energy phosphates required for rapid removal of calcium from the cytoplasm and hypertrophy slows the rate of actin-myosin dissociation.[312] Hypertrophy also decreases left ventricular compliance in all phases of diastole.[312]

When approaching a patient with cardiogenic shock, it is important to characterize both systolic and diastolic function. Therapy designed to improve systolic function may impair myocardial diastolic function.[312]

Right Ventricular Failure. Right ventricular (RV) failure can be defined as the inability of the right ventricle to provide adequate blood flow through the pulmonary circulation at a normal central venous pressure.[114] RV failure may complicate the management of many pediatric critical care unit (PCCU) patients. Respiratory failure causing hypoxic pulmonary vasoconstriction, pulmonary hypertension, and consequent RV dysfunction is often seen in critically ill patients. Sepsis can cause right-sided heart failure directly by inducing RV dysfunction.[161] Pulmonary embolism (PE) can result in RV failure. RV failure may be an independent risk factor for morbidity and mortality in patients with left ventricular failure.[114] Finally, pulmonary arterial hypertension in children contributes significantly to morbidity and mortality in diverse pediatric cardiac, lung, hematologic, and other diseases.[2] Without therapy, high pulmonary vascular resistance contributes to progressive RV failure, low CO, and death.[2,41] Fundamental management strategies for pulmonary hypertension are listed in Box 6-5 (see also Chapter 8).[225,293]

The bedside nurse is an essential part of the team managing pulmonary hypertension and RV failure. Every member of the healthcare team, and particularly the bedside nurse, must have a thorough understanding of the pathophysiology, clinical signs and symptoms, monitoring modalities, and treatment of pulmonary hypertension.[225]

Molecular Basis for Myocyte Dysfunction. Advances in molecular biology techniques have led to a greater understanding of the precise mechanisms involved in both normal and abnormal myocardial contractions. A large portion of this work has centered on calcium handling by the myocyte.

Contraction is generated by an action potential. Depolarization leads to the opening of ionic channels, causing a small influx of calcium that is amplified by calcium-induced calcium release from the sarcoplasmic reticulum. It is this sarcoplasmic calcium that binds to the contractile apparatus leading to contraction.

The contractile apparatus is composed of actin, myosin, tropomyosin, and troponin. Troponin is a complex of three subunits: troponin I, C, and T.[142,280] The troponin complex acts as the regulatory mechanism in the contraction process. The calcium that is released from the sarcoplasmic reticulum binds to the troponin C subunit, causing a conformational change in the entire troponin complex. This change results in the movement of tropomyosin, allowing crossbridging to occur between actin and myosin, and thus contraction.[280]

In CHF, there appears to be a change in the phosphorylation state of troponin I; less phosphorylation of troponin I was found in failing human hearts versus normal controls. When troponin I is dephosphorylated in the failing heart, it appears to be more sensitive to calcium, producing greater myofilament activation in response to a comparable increase in calcium concentration. This action could be considered an adaptive response as the failing myocardium attempts to

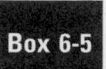

Box 6-5 Fundamental Contributors to and Management Strategies for Pulmonary Hypertension

Avoid factors that cause pulmonary vasoconstriction
Alveolar hypoxia (atelectasis, hypoventilation)
Acidosis/hypercarbia
Agitation/pain
Excessive hematocrit
Hyperinflation
Hypothermia

Promote factors that cause pulmonary vasodilation
Oxygen
Alkalosis/hypocarbia
Sedation/anesthesia
Normal to low hematocrit
Normal functional residual capacity
Nitric oxide

Acute management of pulmonary hypertension
Reduce sympathetic stimulation
    Maintain adequate sedation and analgesia; consider the use of muscle relaxants
    Premedicate before noxious stimuli, such as endotracheal tube suctioning
    Maintain normothermia
Lower pulmonary vascular resistance
    Gas exchange
        ↑Alveolar oxygen tension
        Alkalosis/treat acidosis (metabolic or respiratory)
Mechanical ventilation
    Maintain adequate functional residual capacity
    Avoid hypoinflation or hyperinflation
    Minimize intrathoracic pressure
Vasodilating drugs
    Specific: inhaled nitric oxide
    Aerosolized iloprost (a prostacyclin analogue)
    Nonspecific:
        cGMP system—nitroprusside
        cAMP system: phosphodiesterase type 3 inhibitors (milrinone)
        Phosphodiesterase type 5 inhibitor (sildenafil)
        Isoproterenol
        Prostacyclin I_2, prostaglandin E_1

cAMP, Cyclic adenosine monophosphate; *cGMP*, cyclic guanosine monophosphate.

increase contractility. However, it is unclear whether, similar to the neurohumoral adaptations, this beneficial response eventually becomes deleterious, because the increased calcium sensitivity may lead to impaired myocardial relaxation and produce diastolic dysfunction.

Clinical Signs and Symptoms

Everyone caring for seriously ill or injured infants and children must be aware of the subtle findings associated with cardiogenic failure, such as feeding intolerance, irritability, and respiratory distress. Because each of these findings can easily mimic other, more common diseases, recognition of the child with CHF begins with a careful history and physical examination and is supplemented by chest radiography, electrocardiography, and echocardiography. For further information, see section, Congestive Heart Failure in Chapter 8.

In infancy, poor feeding is one of the important symptoms of CHF. Infants with heart failure can take long a time to feed, with a noticeable increase in respiratory effort; therefore they frequently consume less than their required caloric intake. As a result of inadequate caloric intake and an increased metabolic rate, weight gain is slow. Caregivers may also notice an increase in sweating (diaphoresis), a consequence of increased adrenergic activity. These infants are prone to have recurrent lower respiratory tract infections.

Older children may have a reduced level of exercise tolerance; careful questioning about the degree of physical activity is important. Paroxysmal nocturnal dyspnea may also be a symptom in older children. If there has been a significant degree of fluid retention from CHF, a recent increase in weight may be elicited.

The classic presentation of CHF in infants is a pale and sweaty child with an increased respiratory rate. Other common clinical findings are tachycardia, a gallop rhythm, cardiomegaly, tachypnea, and hepatomegaly.

Cardiomegaly can be difficult to diagnose clinically in infants, because the infant has a small thorax. However, the diagnosis is supported by lateral displacement of the point of maximum impulse and a sternal heave. The definitive method of identifying cardiomegaly is the presence of an enlarged cardiac shadow on chest radiograph or echocardiograph.

With the systemic vasoconstriction caused by the α-adrenergic adaptive response to heart failure, peripheral pulses will be diminished in intensity as compared with central arterial pulses. In addition, the extremities will be cool and mottled with a prolonged capillary refill (>2 seconds). However, in the case of high-output cardiac failure secondary to a large aortic runoff from a patent ductus arteriosus, bounding pulses may be present.

Most of the signs of left-sided heart failure result from pulmonary congestion. Tachypnea is an important early sign reflecting pulmonary venous congestion. As this congestion worsens, breathing becomes more labored, and the child demonstrates intercostal retractions, nasal flaring, grunting, and use of accessory muscles of respiration.

Adventitial lung sounds are usually not diagnostic of heart failure. Wheezing has been associated with pulmonary congestion. This wheezing may be caused by airway edema from an accumulation of lung water or by airway compression from the enlarged left atrium, and it may cause the diagnosis to be confused with viral bronchiolitis in infants. Crackles frequently are not heard during CHF in infants; therefore their absence does not preclude the diagnosis of pulmonary congestion.

Enlargement of the liver reflects systemic venous congestion and usually results from defects producing combined right- and left-sided heart failure. However, hepatomegaly can also be seen with pure right-sided heart failure, such as defects producing pulmonary hypertension or isolated pulmonary stenosis. In older children, distension of the external jugular vein is evidence of systemic venous congestion.

Peripheral edema is rarely seen in children as a consequence of CHF unless the CHF is severe.

Elevated serum level of cardiac troponin, either I or T, is a highly sensitive and specific indicator of myocardial damage. Levels can be elevated within 1-2 hours after acute myocardial injury and remain detectable up to 14 days after myocardial infarction.[4] Cardiac troponin I has a sensitivity and specificity profile in pediatrics similar to that reported in adults.[131] Measurement of serum levels give an indication of ongoing myocardial cell injury and death in the child presenting with cardiogenic shock.[142]

As previously discussed, BNP and its terminal prohormone fragment, N-terminal pro-BNP, may serve as markers for heart disease.[186,217]

Two-dimensional and Doppler echocardiographic studies provide important information about the size, thickness, and performance of the heart, as well as delineation of any cardiac malformations. Doppler investigation of the diastolic mitral inflow pattern is useful in assessing the presence of diastolic dysfunction.

The importance of age at presentation must be stressed. The age at clinical presentation is affected by the anatomic abnormality, the pulmonary vascular resistance, the patency of the ductus arteriosus, and the limited cardiac reserve of the young infant.[58]

CHF in First Weeks of Life. Most cardiac anomalies do not cause heart failure for days to weeks, because they depend on the ductus arteriosus or elevated perinatal pulmonary vascular resistance for palliation. Depressed myocardial function, rather than structural defects, is the more common cause of CHF in the immediate perinatal period. Because the fetal and neonatal myocardium functions at near maximal capacity, the CO is high at rest, and total body and myocardial oxygen consumption are elevated and supply-demand inequity can readily develop. In addition, neonatal myocardium cannot effectively oxidize fatty acids as an energy source and depends on carbohydrates from intake and glycogen stores for energy production.

Heart failure in the first day of life is usually caused by neonatal heart muscle dysfunction resulting from asphyxia, sepsis, hypoglycemia, or myocarditis. Structural abnormalities that can play a role at this early age include tricuspid or pulmonary regurgitation or systemic arteriovenous fistula. Contributing neonatal HR abnormalities that can cause failure include paroxysmal SVT or congenital complete heart block.

A common cause of heart failure in the first week of life is the hypoplastic left heart syndrome. These infants exhibit a sudden onset of a shocklike state when the patent ductus arteriosus closes.[94] Other entities that manifest at this age include critical aortic stenosis, total anomalous pulmonary venous return, and pulmonary stenosis. HR abnormalities and heart muscle dysfunction discussed previously remain possibilities.

The coarctation syndrome can manifest during the first 1 to 6 weeks of life with sudden onset of severe CHF,[94] typically developing when the patent ductus arteriosus constricts. The progressive fall of pulmonary vascular resistance during the first month of life results in the worsening of left-to-right shunts. Examples include large ventricular septal defects and atrioventricular septal defects (atrioventricular canal defects).[79] In addition, anomalous origin of the coronary artery should be considered in an infant exhibiting signs of angina: poor feeding, irritability, and sweating that often occurs during feeding.[187]

CHF Developing Later in Infancy. Most of the conditions noted above may present in this age group, but generally the symptoms will appear before the infant is 6 weeks old. Exceptions include patients with myocarditis or endocardial fibroelastosis and those for whom heart failure is secondary to systemic hypertension or endocrine abnormalities (e.g., hypothyroidism or adrenal insufficiency). Although endocardial fibroelastosis has been decreasing in frequency, a form of familial cardiomyopathy secondary to carnitine deficiency has been described.[49]

One acquired condition that must be kept in mind is Kawasaki disease.[218] Kawasaki disease is an acute vasculitis of unknown etiology that occurs predominantly in infants and young children. Coronary artery aneurysms or ectasia develop in approximately 15% to 25% of untreated children with the disease and can lead to myocardial infarction, CHF, cardiogenic shock, or sudden death.[73,76,143,218] In the United States, Kawasaki disease has surpassed acute rheumatic fever as the leading cause of acquired heart disease in children.[218]

CHF Developing in Childhood and Adolescence. CHF in childhood or adolescence is not common. Older children who have congenital heart disease can develop CHF because of the onset of valvular regurgitation or tachyarrhythmias.

Acquired heart disease causing heart failure is relatively more common at this age. Myocarditis may cause heart muscle dysfunction in this group. In addition, diseases that cause valvular regurgitation, such as rheumatic fever or bacterial endocarditis, can also cause heart failure. Substance abuse, such as cocaine or inhalants, must be added to the differential diagnosis of myocardial infarction and CHF in adolescents.

Management

The appropriate management of CHF and cardiogenic shock in infancy is critically dependent on the specific cause (Box 6-6). Accurate and rapid diagnosis is of prime importance. Additional management is presented in Chapter 8.

It is obvious from the clinical signs and symptoms section, above, that the clinical findings of severe CHF and cardiogenic shock in the child may be very similar to other disease states such as respiratory distress, dehydration, and sepsis.[184,321] The therapy for each, however, can be markedly divergent, yet each needs to be addressed quickly to avoid further morbidity or mortality.

Fluid therapy must be used with caution in the patient with CHF, but it can be life saving in the child with severe dehydration or sepsis. A high index of suspicion of CHF in addition to other entities will allow the provider treating the child to tailor fluid management to the child's need.

Clues obtained from the history and physical examination, such as an absence of increased fluid losses or the presence of hepatomegaly, should raise the suspicion of CHF rather than

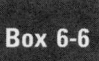

Box 6-6 **General Principles in Management of Severe Congestive Heart Failure or Cardiogenic Shock**

Minimize Myocardial Oxygen Demands
- Intubation, mechanical ventilation
- Maintain normal core temperature; treat fever
- Provide sedation
- Correct anemia

Maximize Myocardial Performance
- Correct arrhythmias
- Optimize preload
  Salt and water restriction
  Augment preload with small fluid boluses
  Diuretics, venodilators for congestion
- Improve contractility
  Provide oxygen
  Support adequate ventilation
  Correct acidosis and other metabolic abnormalities
  Inotropic drugs (see Table 6-5)
- Reduce afterload
  Provide sedation and pain relief
  Correct hypothermia
  Appropriate vasodilator use

Exclude Congenital or Traumatic Heart Disease

Consider Surgical and Other Therapies

dehydration. Administration of small-volume boluses with frequent monitoring of vital signs can lead to a logical treatment plan. Boluses of 5 to 10 mL/kg will allow the provider to gauge the hemodynamic response. If these maneuvers do not decrease the HR, raise the BP, or improve systemic perfusion, then a cardiac source must be considered higher on the list of possibilities.

CVP monitoring can be helpful to evaluate preload, but practitioners must remember that this is a pressure measurement and not a direct measure of ventricular end-diastolic volume (i.e., preload). Many other factors potentially affect a single measured CVP, including intrathoracic pressure (e.g., positive pressure ventilation), tricuspid valve function, and ventricular stiffness or compliance. Measurement and trending of the CVP can be helpful during management.

There is no single optimal CVP for all patients. A given CVP might be optimal filling in the normal heart, but represent under filling in the heart of a child with tetralogy of Fallot and an extremely stiff (i.e., noncompliant) right ventricle. Other clinical signs and symptoms (e.g., signs of right-sided heart failure such as hepatomegaly or left-sided heart failure such as pulmonary edema) can be helpful in putting the CVP in context.

Interpretation of the CVP and preload requires knowledge of the patient's cardiac rhythm. A significant percentage of ventricular filling results from atrial contraction, so the loss of an AV-associated rhythm (e.g., junctional ectopic tachycardia, third-degree heart block) can lead to significant reduction in ventricular filling and SV. Conversion of these arrhythmias with drug therapy or electrical cardioversion, or palliation of an arrhythmia with AV-pacing, can significantly enhance CO. Even an inappropriately fast AV-associated rhythm (e.g., SVT) can be detrimental, because it reduces the time available for ventricular filling. Treatment includes slowing of the HR via drug therapy or patient cooling.

Inappropriate bradycardia can also reduce CO, especially when myocardial contractility is already compromised. Treatment often involves the use of atrial or AV-pacing in the postoperative cardiac patient or the use of catecholamines (e.g., isoproterenol) to increase HR in the nonoperative patient who does not have pacing wires.

Although volume administration and correction of metabolic derangements (e.g., pH, glucose, calcium, magnesium) may enhance cardiac function temporarily, pharmacologic interventions are often necessary to improve cardiac function. This approach to treatment relies on the use of drugs to restore or augment myocardial contractility, improve CO, and restore and maintain blood flow. There is no standard drug or dose for treatment of shock; therapy must be continually tailored to the patient's response. The proper choice of drug or drugs requires knowledge of the child's precise hemodynamic disturbance and drug actions and interactions.

Table 6-5 and Box 6-6 list the general supportive and pharmacologic measures used in the treatment of severe CHF or cardiogenic shock. These measures are designed to increase tissue oxygen supply, decrease tissue oxygen requirements, and correct metabolic abnormalities.

Catecholamines. The catecholamines are the most potent positive inotropic agents available, but it is important to note that effects are not limited to inotropy. Catecholamines also possess chronotropic properties and produce complex effects on vascular beds in many organs. Consequently, the choice of an agent may depend as much on the state of the circulation as it does on the myocardium. The available catecholamines are norepinephrine, epinephrine, isoproterenol, dopamine, and dobutamine.[53,58,273,299,313,324a] These catecholamines have been used extensively in infants and children.

The catecholamines are adrenergic receptor agonists. Adrenergic receptors fall into three primary categories: α-adrenergic, β-adrenergic, and dopaminergic receptors. The receptors responsible for inotropic stimulation are the β_1-adrenoreceptors located in the myocardium. The β_2-receptors are located in vascular and bronchial smooth muscle and mediate vasodilation and bronchodilation, respectively. The α-adrenoreceptors include the α_1-subtype located on peripheral vasculature. Stimulation mediates smooth muscle contraction and, thus, vasopressor effects. Following their initial descriptions, α_2-receptors were identified on the presynaptic terminals of sympathetic nerves; stimulation of these receptors inhibits norepinephrine release. The α_2-receptors have also been identified on postsynaptic smooth muscle where stimulation results in contraction, although the contribution of this mechanism to vasopressor effects of adrenergic agonists is not fully known.[53]

From a pharmacokinetic standpoint, nearly all the inotropes used clinically are cleared by first-order kinetics so that changes in infusion rates linearly correlate to plasma concentrations, making them practical to titrate to clinical effect. In addition, the adrenergic receptor agonists are rapidly metabolized by circulating catechol-*O*-methyltransferase followed by deamination (via monoamine oxidase) or sulfoconjugation (by phenolsulfotransferase); the effective half-lives of these agents are on the order of minutes. Therefore these agents are administered via continuous infusion, most commonly via a central venous catheter.

Dopamine. Dopamine is a naturally occurring endogenous catecholamine. It is a norepinephrine precursor that provides both direct and indirect adrenergic effects. Dopamine administration stimulates dopaminergic, α- and β-adrenergic receptors at increasing doses; effects include stimulation of norepinephrine release from terminal vesicles in sympathetic neurons. Because some dopamine effects are produced by norepinephrine release, a diminished response to this drug may be seen in catecholamine-depleted patients or after chronic dopamine therapy. Dopamine is particularly useful for treatment of the child with mild symptoms of shock, particularly if HR is low (or only mildly elevated) and peripheral vasoconstriction is compromising renal blood flow and urine output.

The use of low-dose or renal-dose dopamine, at doses less than 5 mcg/kg per min (usually 2 to 4 mcg/kg per minute), has been proposed in the past to prevent or treat acute renal failure and to increase urine output in CHF patients who are refractory to loop diuretics. Physiologically, low-dose dopamine increases renal blood flow and increases urine output by stimulating both dopaminergic (DA- and DA-2) and adrenergic (both α and β) receptors. Therefore low-dose dopamine may affect renal blood flow by direct vasodilation (dopamine receptors), by increasing CO (β receptors), or by increasing perfusion pressure via vasoconstriction (α receptors). At low doses, especially less than 2 mcg/kg per minute, dopaminergic receptor effects predominate, resulting in renal vasodilatation and increased renal blood flow. Dopamine also inhibits aldosterone release and inhibits sodium-potassium adenosine triphosphatase at the tubular epithelial cell level, resulting in increased sodium excretion and thereby diuresis.[172,324a]

Several early studies showed significantly increased natriuresis, diuresis, and improved renal function with use of low-dose dopamine.[88,172] However, the overwhelming consensus among studies with more rigorous methodology (e.g., randomized prospective studies with larger sample size) is that there is no convincing scientific evidence of a beneficial effect with low-dose dopamine beyond a possible natriuretic diuresis.[145,172] A large metaanalysis by Kellum and Decker[145] concluded that "the use of low-dose dopamine for the treatment or prevention of acute renal failure cannot be justified on the basis of available evidence and should be eliminated from routine clinical use." Therefore, based on these studies, there is little if any role for "renal dose" dopamine in heart failure therapy in attempts to preserve renal function.[145]

Dobutamine. Dobutamine is the inotropic agent synthetically derived from the catecholamine parent structure that possesses mixed β-receptor agonist activities. Therefore dobutamine possesses both chronotropic and inotropic properties mediated through β_1-adrenergic receptor stimulation and modest vasodilating effects related to its β_2-adrenergic receptor agonist property. The limitation of vasodilating effects relates to its preparation as a racemic mixture where the (+) isomer has potent effects, but conversely the (−) isomer is a selective α_1-adrenergic receptor agonist mediating vasoconstrictor effects.[53]

Dobutamine should maintain its inotropic effects during prolonged administration better than dopamine, because the actions of dobutamine do not depend on the release of norepinephrine. Downregulation of receptors certainly will reduce the effectiveness of a dobutamine dose, however. There may be an age-specific insensitivity to dobutamine; it has been demonstrated that children under the age of 2 years have a reduced response to dobutamine.[247]

Although dobutamine does not have selective vascular actions, SVR and BP often fall during dobutamine administration; therefore this is not the drug of choice for the hypotensive child with cardiogenic or septic shock. Dobutamine may be ideal for the normotensive child with CHF or cardiogenic shock.

Long-term improvement in cardiac function has been reported following short-term dobutamine therapy. Occasionally, children with severe ventricular dysfunction (e.g., a child awaiting a cardiac transplant) are admitted to the PCCU so that short-term dobutamine therapy can be provided. The effectiveness of dobutamine under these conditions seems to be related to improvement in myocardial perfusion and the myocardial oxygen supply-demand relationship.

Epinephrine. Epinephrine is an endogenous hormone released from the adrenal medulla in response to stress. Epinephrine is a potent inotropic and chronotropic agent. It is often the drug of choice for the treatment of bradycardia or hypotension. Epinephrine can exert both β- and α-adrenergic effects: the β effects, including an increase in HR, conduction velocity, and ventricular contractility, generally are observed at lower doses (0.005-0.02 mcg/kg per minute). At doses exceeding 0.3 mcg/kg per minute, α-adrenergic effects predominate, including significant peripheral vasoconstriction.[324a]

Although epinephrine can mediate splanchnic vasoconstriction and theoretically lead to intestinal ischemia, this adverse effect is thought to be less significant in the critical care setting if it is countered by significant augmentation of CO.[53] Patients with heart failure and increased SVR may be harmed by a higher epinephrine dose, unless it is concomitantly administered with a vasodilator. Non–cardiac-related effects of epinephrine include increasing plasma glucose levels, increasing fatty acid levels, and increased renin activity with a concomitant decrease in serum potassium and aldosterone levels.

Norepinephrine. Norepinephrine is an endogenous catecholamine, producing increases in HR and BP through both β- and α-adrenergic effects. Because this drug can produce potent peripheral and renal vasoconstriction at even low doses, its use often has been limited to the treatment of children with profound hypotensive shock refractory to other inotropic agents. Norepinephrine recently has been found to be beneficial in the treatment of adult patients with septic vasodilatory shock refractory to dopamine and dobutamine therapy. Its pressor effects make it a useful agent in treating neurogenic distributive shock states.

In a recent multicenter, randomized trial of adults comparing dopamine to norepinephrine, dopamine was associated with increased mortality in patients with cardiogenic shock.[70] However, it will be necessary to demonstrate that dopamine produces an increased mortality in pediatric patients before the decades of experience with dopamine in critically ill children is abandoned.[53]

Isoproterenol. Isoproterenol is a pure β-adrenergic agonist, increasing HR, atrioventricular conduction velocity, and ventricular contractility. The increase in CO following isoproterenol administration probably is attributable more to an increase in HR than to significant improvement in SV.

Isoproterenol is helpful in the treatment of bradycardia, particularly in the presence of heart block, because it can increase the ventricular rate. However, it produces more profound tachycardia than either dopamine or dobutamine, and it increases myocardial oxygen consumption; these effects limit its usefulness. The vasodilation that results from its use makes it a poor choice for hypotensive shock, especially in patients with associated tachycardia.

The noncatecholamine inotropic drugs used in pediatric CHF and cardiogenic shock include the phosphodiesterase inhibitors and levosimendan and the digitalis glycosides.

Phosphodiesterase Inhibitors. The phosphodiesterase (PDE) inhibitors are a class of drugs called *bipyridines* that mediate both inotropy and vasodilation; these drugs are often referred to as *inodilators*.[53] The effects of PDE inhibitors results from their prevention of hydrolysis of cAMP (type III PDE inhibitors; e.g., milrinone, amrinone, enoximone) and/or cGMP (type V PDE inhibitors; e.g., sildenafil, dipyridamole), and resulting increase in intracellular cAMP. When type III PDE inhibitors are administered alone, the increase of cAMP improves contractility and also causes vasodilation of pulmonary and systemic arteries, resulting in decreased ventricular afterload.

Unique to this class of agents, PDE inhibitors improve ventricular relaxation (so-called lusitropic property). This effect is mediated by decreased breakdown of cAMP, resulting in activation of protein kinase A, which subsequently phosphorylates the sarcoplasmic reticulum protein phospholamban.[53] This phosphorylation modulates the activation of sarcoplasmic reticulum adenosine triphosphatase resulting in more rapid uptake of cytosolic calcium and thus facilitating more rapid and improved myocyte relaxation.[53] As a result of these pharmacologic properties, the main hemodynamic effects of PDE inhibitors are to decrease both systemic and pulmonary vascular resistances, decrease filling pressures, and substantially augment CO, most often with little change in HR.

The interaction of PDE inhibitors with administered inotropes, vasodilators, and even vasopressors can be used to therapeutic advantage in patients with a variety of forms of shock. For example, epinephrine can remain a potent and relatively pure inotrope at higher doses when combined with a type III PDE inhibitor that will prevent breakdown of the cAMP produced by β_1- and β_2-adrenergic stimulation with the result that increased cAMP inhibits the usual effects of epinephrine-mediated α_1-adrenergic stimulation.[53] In a similar manner, norepinephrine may be a more effective inotrope while maintaining vasopressor effectiveness when administered with a type III PDE inhibitor. The hydrolysis of norepinephrine-mediated β_1-receptor cAMP production is inhibited so that increased cAMP improves both contractility and relaxation. In addition, norepinephrine-mediated α_1- and α_2-adrenergic effects remain unopposed, because milrinone possesses no specific β_1-receptor activity and therefore has minimal vasodilatory effect in the face of potent α-adrenergic vasoconstriction.[53] In a related manner, the type V PDE inhibitors (e.g., sildenafil, dipyridamole) may potentiate the pulmonary vasodilator effects of inhaled nitric oxide

Milrinone is a type III phosphodiesterase inhibitor. It has inotropic, vasodilator, and lusitropic (enhancing myocardial diastolic relaxation) properties. It has a longer half-life than continuous infusion catecholamines (hours as opposed to minutes). Consequently, beneficial drug effects have delayed times of onset, whereas adverse effects (e.g., drug accumulation leading to vasodilation and hypotension) can last a long time even after drug administration is halted. The drug will accumulate in the setting of renal insufficiency, leading to a rise in plasma levels and increased vasodilation. The hypotension that occasionally occurs with loading can be mitigated by slowing the infusion rate and with the use of volume expanders.

When milrinone was given prophylactically to children with biventricular congenital heart disease after surgery, it significantly reduced the likelihood of patients progressing to a low CO state.[134] It has been used extensively in the PCCU setting for both univentricular and biventricular heart disease (surgical and nonsurgical patients).

Levosimendan. Levosimendan is a calcium-sensitizing agent, with inotropic, lusitropic, and vasodilatory properties. Levosimendan binds to myocardial troponin C to improve the efficiency of the myocyte contractile apparatus. Unlike catecholamines and the phosphodiesterase inhibitors, its actions are independent of the use of cAMP as an intracellular mediator, and they do not lead to increased intracellular levels of calcium or increased myocardial oxygen demand. Levosimendan has been used in infants and children with CHF and cardiogenic shock, especially after cardiopulmonary bypass.[215] Despite multiple clinical trials, its use in pediatrics is limited.[36,215,301,314]

Digoxin. The digitalis glycosides may augment myocardial contractility. Because of narrow therapeutic to toxic ratio, long half-life, and dependence of clearance on renal (digoxin) or hepatic function, their use in patients with cardiogenic shock should be avoided in the early stages of treatment.

Other Agents. Thyroid hormone secretion is greatly suppressed in children and adults with critical illness and after surgical procedures.[32] After cardiac surgery, low thyroid hormone plasma concentrations and impaired cardiac function resemble the endocrine and cardiovascular alterations associated with hypothyroidism.[32] Postoperative outcomes are affected by poor cardiac performance, such as low CO, left ventricular dysfunction, and increased vascular resistance. Transient suppression of thyroid function after cardiac surgery is well documented, but therapeutic intervention has not yet been uniformly recommended.[32] In adult patients, after coronary artery bypass surgery, infusion of tri-iodothyronine raises plasma tri-iodothyronine concentrations and improves cardiac performance by increasing the cardiac index and lowering SVR.[150]

Transient secondary hypothyroidism has been shown to occur in children with cardiac malformations after cardiopulmonary bypass operations, especially in those who receive dopamine.[32,304] The benefits of tri-iodothyronine supplementation has been demonstrated in these children.[32]

As previously discussed, nesiritide (synthetic human BNP) is a potent vasodilator that has been used to rapidly reduce cardiac filling pressures and improve dyspnea in patients with acute decompensated heart failure.[64] Nesiritide is well tolerated in children with heart failure and is associated with improved diuresis.[188] Further studies will be needed to evaluate the role of nesiritide in the management of CHF and cardiogenic shock (see "Congestive Heart Failure in Common Clinical Problems," in Chapter 8).[19]

Finally, as previously discussed, children and adults may experience vasodilatory shock because of a systemic inflammatory response after cardiopulmonary bypass or septic shock.[197] This vasodilatory shock is usually caused by inappropriate activation of vasodilatory mechanisms and failure of vasoconstrictor mechanisms associated with endogenous deficiency of arginine vasopressin.[62,162,197] Studies have shown a beneficial effect of arginine vasopressin administration in children and adults with extremely low CO after cardiac surgery.[197,263]

More recently terlipressin, a long acting analog of vasopressin, has caused significant improvement in hemodynamic, respiratory, and renal indices in children with extremely low CO after open heart surgery.[197] Further controlled studies are needed to confirm safety and efficacy of the drug in this population.

Vasodilator Drugs. Neurohumoral compensatory mechanisms that initially compensate for a fall in output of the failing heart can ultimately contribute to worsening of the heart failure. The kidney's response to a decrease in CO leads to expansion of extracellular fluid volume and ultimately to circulatory congestion and edema. Systemic vasoconstriction will raise aortic impedance; this may maintain perfusion pressure in the face of declining CO, but it eventually impairs ventricular function. Therefore one of the rationales of vasodilator therapy is to counteract these physiologic responses—for example, vasodilators are used to oppose systemic vasoconstriction, just as angiotensin-converting enzyme inhibitors are used to block the renin-angiotensin system, and diuretics are used to prevent or reverse abnormal fluid retention.[58]

Many vasodilators, representing several different pharmacologic classes, have been shown to improve cardiac performance and lessen clinical symptoms by means of arterial and venous smooth muscle relaxation (see Table 6-5). Arterial relaxation should result in an increase in ejection fraction, an increase in SV, and a decrease in end-systolic left ventricular volume. Some vasodilator drugs may increase left ventricular compliance; this effect should shift blood into the periphery and reduce right and left ventricular end-diastolic volume, with attendant beneficial effects on pulmonary and systemic capillary pressure. This reduction in end-diastolic volume and pressure, in turn, should decrease edema, reduce myocardial wall stress, and improve diastolic myocardial perfusion and myocardial function.

For treatment of cardiogenic shock, intravenous vasodilators with rapid onset of action and short half-life are preferred. Selection of vasodilator agents must be based on the principal hemodynamic effects of the drug and the specific hemodynamic abnormalities of the patient. Factors that increase systemic resistance, such as hypothermia, acidosis, hypoxia, pain, and anxiety, should be treated before considering vasodilator drugs.

The use of vasodilators in shock is generally limited to situations in which cardiac dysfunction is associated with elevated ventricular filling pressures, elevated SVR, and normal or near-normal systemic arterial BP. Occasionally, the combination of vasodilator and inotropic therapy results in hemodynamic improvement not attainable with either drug alone.

As previously outlined, there is a growing awareness that RV dysfunction plays a pivotal role in some of the most frequently encountered and important cardiopulmonary disorders in children, including congenital heart disease, acute respiratory distress syndrome, bronchopulmonary dysplasia, and other chronic pulmonary disorders.[58] The ability of the right ventricle to respond to increased pulmonary vascular resistance in these situations often determines outcome. Measures to decrease pulmonary vascular resistance have, therefore, become more common in the treatment of many seriously ill pediatric patients. Such measures include supplementary oxygen, adequate ventilation, alkalosis, inhaled nitric oxide, prostaglandin E_1, prostacyclin, sildenafil, analgesia, and sedation.[2,225,293] The most commonly used systemic vasodilators in the management of cardiogenic shock are nitroglycerin, nitroprusside, and milrinone (see Pulmonary Hypertension in Chapter 8).

Nitroglycerin. Nitroglycerin is a short-acting venous and arterial vasodilator, acting through its release of nitric oxide, stimulating cGMP production. Venodilator effects predominate at lower doses, whereas arterial dilator effects occur at higher doses. Venodilation can be beneficial in states where the heart is overdistended and preload is excessive, while arterial dilation can benefit the heart where the combination of reduced contractility and elevated SVR impairs overall CO.

Polyvinyl chloride tubing will adsorb nitroglycerin, particularly when the tubing is new or the administration rate is slow. When adsorption occurs, the patient receives an unpredictably reduced drug dose. To minimize adsorption of the drug, nitroglycerin should be administered through an infusion pump with polypropylene or polyethylene tubing. An alternative administration system uses a large (60-mL) disposable polypropylene syringe or a glass syringe with a syringe pump and a short length of microbore tubing. These systems will minimize the adsorption surface for nitroglycerin and ensure more predictable drug delivery. The tubing should not be changed (replaced) frequently (follow institutional protocol).

Nitroprusside. Nitroprusside is a short-acting smooth muscle relaxant that produces both arterial and venous dilation through its release of nitric oxide. A typical initial infusion dose of sodium nitroprusside is approximately 0.3 to 0.5 mcg/kg per minute, titrated to a typical infusion of approximately 0.5 to 8 mcg/kg per minute. Its onset of action is immediate, and its duration of effect is 1 to 3 minutes. This drug is light sensitive, so it is stored in amber vials before use and must be protected from light after mixing. Special opaque tubing may be used with infusion pumps, or the tubing can be covered with opaque (e.g., cloth) tape. If the solution will clear the tubing within a few hours (usually not the case at pediatric infusion rates), the tubing may remain uncovered.

Prolonged infusion (longer than 24 hours) of nitroprusside can result in the formation of thiocyanate and cyanide (byproducts of nitroprusside metabolism) with potentially toxic effects. This toxicity will be more likely in the presence of prolonged high-dose therapy (>2 mcg/kg per minute) and may be more likely in patients with renal or hepatic disease.[209] Thiocyanate levels should be checked every 2 days during prolonged nitroprusside therapy if possible; toxic levels are greater than 10 mg/dL.

Signs of thiocyanate toxicity include confusion, hyperreflexia, weakness, skin rash, tinnitus, and fatigue. Signs of cyanide toxicity include agitation, diminished level of consciousness, tachypnea, incontinence, seizures, and cardiorespiratory arrest. Metabolic (lactic) acidosis is an early sign of cyanide toxicity, because cyanide inhibits aerobic metabolism. Detection of cyanide toxicity can be difficult in infants and children. The signs and symptoms of toxicity may be masked by critical illness or inability to communicate.[209]

Diuretics. Patients with pulmonary edema require immediate measures to support adequate oxygenation and ventilation. Oxygen should be administered by mask or high-flow nasal cannula. The need for intubation and mechanical ventilation should be assessed. Diuretics such as furosemide are frequently used to reduce preload and to improve the congestive symptoms present.[58] Furosemide may be given orally or intravenously, depending on the severity of CHF, with 1 to 2 mg/kg used as a starting dose to be given every 8 hours. With large and repeated doses, fluid depletion or electrolyte abnormalities are possible.

Interventional Cardiology. Over the past decade, transcatheter interventions have become increasingly important in the treatment of patients with congenital heart lesions.[58] These procedures may be broadly grouped as dilations (e.g., septostomy, valvuloplasty, angioplasty, endovascular stenting) or as closures (e.g., vascular embolization, device closure of defects). Balloon valvuloplasty has become the treatment of choice for patients in all age groups with simple valvular pulmonic stenosis and, although not curative, seems at least comparable to surgery for congenital aortic stenosis in newborns to young adults. Balloon angioplasty is successfully applied to a wide range of aortic, pulmonary artery, and venous stenoses. Stents are useful in dilating lesions when the intrinsic elasticity results in vessel recoil after balloon dilation alone. Catheter-delivered coils are used to embolize a wide range of arterial, venous, and prosthetic vascular connections. Although some devices remain investigational, they have been successfully used for closure of abnormal vessels and atrial and ventricular septal defects. For further information, see Chapter 8.

Surgical Intervention. A number of congenital cardiac defects may cause severe CHF and cardiogenic shock. Diagnosis of these defects is critical, because surgery may be required before hemodynamic stability can be achieved.

Cardiac function can be supported temporarily by mechanical means including intraaortic balloon counter-pulsation, use of left-ventricular assist device or ECMO (see Chapter 7).[34,58,257,278] Cardiac transplantation has become an important tool for treating patients with severe myocardial dysfunction who would otherwise succumb to their heart disease.

Etiology-Specific Treatment of Cardiogenic Shock. Management of the pediatric patient in cardiogenic shock requires the general measures described previously and determining the etiology of the cardiac dysfunction. Once the diagnosis is known, management principles specific to the etiology will be required. For the management of the myriad of causes that can result in cardiogenic shock, see Box 6-6.

Obstructive Shock
Etiology, Pathophysiology, Clinical Signs and Management

Obstructive shock is caused by a mechanical obstruction of blood flow to or from the heart. Common causes of obstructive shock include tension pneumothorax, cardiac tamponade, and PE. Also included in this category are the congenital heart lesions characterized by left ventricular outflow tract obstruction, including critical aortic stenosis, coarctation of the aorta, and interrupted aortic arch; these are also discussed in greater detail in Chapter 8.

Tension Pneumothorax. A pneumothorax is defined as an accumulation of air in the pleural space. A tension pneumothorax occurs because of the progressive accumulation of air in the pleural space, causing compression of the ipsilateral lung and resulting in a shift of the mediastinum to the contralateral hemithorax. This produces compression of the great vessels and contralateral lung, compromising both cardiovascular and respiratory function. Whether the air enters the pleural space through a defect in the chest wall, a lacerated or ruptured bronchus, or a ruptured alveolus, a one-way valve effect is created: air enters the pleural space during inhalation, but cannot exit during exhalation. Accumulation of air continues until the intrathoracic pressure of the affected hemithorax equilibrates with atmospheric pressure.[53] At this point, the accumulation of pressure within the thorax leads to depression of the ipsilateral hemidiaphragm and displacement of the mediastinum and associated great vessels toward the contralateral hemithorax. Although the superior vena cava is able to move to some extent, the inferior vena cava is relatively fixed within the diaphragm and will be compressed. Because two thirds of the venous return in children and adults comes from below the diaphragm, compression of the inferior vena cava leads to a drastic and profound reduction in venous return to the heart, leading to cardiovascular collapse and signs and symptoms of obstructive shock.[53] Immediate decompression of the pneumothorax via needle thoracentesis or thoracentesis and thoracostomy tube placement will improve symptoms and is the treatment of choice.

Cardiac Tamponade. The pericardium is relatively noncompliant, so the accumulation of a small amount of fluid (usually <200 mL) is sufficient to produce cardiac tamponade. However, chronic accumulation of fluid can develop with little to no hemodynamic derangements as the pericardium slowly stretches to accommodate the excess volume. There are important therapeutic differences between treatment of an acute versus a chronic pericardial fluid accumulation. If the pericardial effusion or hemopericardium is acute, removal of even a small volume of pericardial fluid will decrease the intrapericardial pressure significantly and relieve symptoms of cardiac tamponade. Conversely, a large volume of pericardial fluid will need to be removed from a symptomatic patient with chronic effusion to attain comparable relief of tamponade symptoms.

Cardiac tamponade is compression of the heart by accumulation of the pericardial fluid beyond a critical threshold. The true filling pressure of the heart is represented by the myocardial transmural pressure (i.e., intracardiac pressure minus intrapericardial pressure).[282] Therefore as intrapericardial pressure rises, the filling pressure of the heart decreases and SV falls. The body attempts to compensate for the increase in intrapericardial pressure (and hence transmural pressure) by increasing systemic CVP and pulmonary venous pressure so that the left and right ventricular filling pressures are higher than the intrapericardial pressure. Left and right atrial pressures increase and equilibrate as the intrapericardial pressure rises. Although this equalization of atrial pressures is often touted as a hallmark of cardiac tamponade, it is more commonly observed with inflammation-induced etiologies and should not be trusted as a pathognomonic sign of cardiac tamponade in the postoperative cardiac patient.[53]

Pericardiocentesis is the life-saving procedure of choice for children with cardiac tamponade. Medical stabilization with fluid administration and inotropic support is temporary at best and somewhat controversial, because fluid resuscitation may precipitate (i.e., in the case of low-pressure tamponade) or worsen tamponade physiology, especially in children who are either normovolemic or hypervolemic.[175] In the latter scenario, fluid administration will increase intracardiac pressures further, hence increasing intrapericardial pressures and worsening tamponade.[53,282]

Pulmonary Embolism. In recent years, there has been an increase in the number of pediatric patients with venous thromboembolism (VTE); some have even called this a new epidemic in pediatric tertiary care.[237,256] Whether there has been a true increase in the occurrence of pediatric VTE, an increase in detection of previously undiagnosed VTE, or both cannot be determined from the studies to date. On the basis of known risk factors for VTE in children, this increase is thought to be related to advancements in the treatment and supportive care of critically ill children who previously would not have survived.[256] The complexity of the medical conditions of pediatric patients in tertiary care hospitals continues to increase, paralleling advances in therapeutic technology and supportive care. The presence of a central venous catheter is the single most common risk factor for VTE in children.[67,138,256] PE after catheter-related thrombosis certainly occurs, but the incidence in children has not been defined.

Acute PE is a major cause of complications and death associated with surgery, injury, and medical illnesses in adult patients.[154] PE is uncommonly diagnosed in children and is often discovered only on autopsy.[18,53,300] In fact, approximately 50% of cases of fatal PE are not diagnosed until autopsy. However, PE occurs more frequently in children than is commonly assumed, and unfortunately PE is frequently difficult to diagnose and fatal.[53,285] The clinical presentation often is confusing, perhaps compounded by the fact that few pediatricians have much experience with this disorder. Results of screening tests, such as oxygen saturation, electrocardiography, and chest radiography, may be normal. As a result, a high index of clinical suspicion is necessary.

A massive PE has a profound effect on gas exchange and hemodynamics. Obstruction to flow through the pulmonary artery results in increased dead space ventilation (i.e., affected lung segments are ventilated but not perfused), which is observed clinically as a substantial decrease in the end-tidal CO_2 ($P_{ET}CO_2$) that no longer reflects the arterial PCO_2. In addition, a widened alveolar-to-arterial O_2 gradient (A-a oxygen tension) is present in most children.[53] The mechanism for hypoxemia is somewhat controversial, although several mechanisms likely play a role. For example, an intracardiac right-to-left shunt through a patent foramen ovale may occur as right atrial pressure increases and eventually exceeds that of left atrial pressure. In addition, $\dot{V}/\dot{Q}$ mismatching is compounded by the accompanying fall in CO that results from massive PE, leading to mixed venous desaturation. There is some evidence that inhibition of cyclooxygenase may improve ventilation-perfusion mismatch in patients with PE.[20]

PE increases the RV afterload, resulting in an increase in the RV end-diastolic volume (RVEDV). The increase in RVEDV adversely affects left ventricular hemodynamics through ventricular interdependence. Specifically, the interventricular septum bows into the left ventricle (LV) and impairs diastolic filling, resulting in decreased LV preload and subsequent hypotension.[41]

Management of PE includes immediate and general support of airway, oxygenation, ventilation, and CO (e.g., volume administration and vasoactive support as needed). If there are no contraindications, fibrinolytic therapy may help dissolve the clot, and anticoagulation therapy may prevent further clot development. Surgical intervention, if immediately available, may be needed. Consultation with a specialist is typically indicated.

CARDIAC ARREST AND RESUSCITATION

CARDIAC ARREST PEARLS

- About 75% of pediatric out-of-hospital cardiac arrests are associated with hypoxia-ischemia resulting from progression of respiratory failure or shock, rather than sudden arrhythmias. In these patients, treatment of respiratory failure or shock may prevent the arrest and ventilation plus compressions are both critical elements of resuscitation.
- About 25% of pediatric out-of-hospital cardiac arrests are sudden arrhythmic events. These events require prompt bystander CPR (especially prompt compressions) and shock delivery.

- A shockable rhythm is present in about one fourth of pediatric in-hospital resuscitations, so providers must be skilled in the integration of CPR with shock delivery.
- High-quality CPR is the foundation of all treatment for cardiac arrest; too often, CPR is performed poorly in both the prehospital and in-hospital settings. Without excellent CPR, all other therapies, including medications or defibrillation, are doomed to fail. Critical elements of high quality CPR include[26,57a,149]:
  - Compressions of sufficient rate (at least 100/min)
  - Compressions of sufficient depth, compressing at least one third the depth of the chest of the infant and child
    - Infants: about 1½ inches (4 cm)
    - Children: about 2 inches (5 cm)
  - Complete chest recoil after each compression
  - Minimal interruptions in chest compressions
  - Appropriate (not excessive) ventilation

CARDIAC ARREST IN CHILDREN

Out-of-hospital and In-hospital Arrest

Etiology

Most children who require resuscitation demonstrate respiratory arrest before cardiac arrest.[57] These children often can be resuscitated successfully if their airway is cleared and oxygenation and ventilation are supported before the development of cardiac arrest.[104,149,171,325]

Primary cardiac arrest is much less common in children than in adults in both the prehospital and the inhospital setting. Out-of-hospital pediatric cardiac arrest usually occurs as a secondary event, following a period of prolonged hypoxia; these arrests are asphyxial arrests, and overall survival in children (particularly for out-of-hospital cardiac arrest) has been poor.[57,85,104,234,325] Survival for infants is approximately 3% and increases to 12.6% for adolescents.[15] For children who experience cardiac arrest in the hospital, survival to hospital discharge is 27%.[214] Survival both for in-hospital and out-of-hospital arrest is higher for a shockable presenting rhythm (ventricular fibrillation and pulseless ventricular tachycardia, so-called arrhythmic or sudden cardiac arrest) than when the presenting rhythm is asystole or pulseless electrical activity.[267]

Respiratory arrest in infants is most commonly the result of airway obstruction, progressive respiratory failure, or sudden infant death syndrome. Cardiopulmonary arrest beyond 1 year of age occurs most commonly as a complication of trauma or submersion injury (i.e., drowning). Sudden cardiac arrhythmias and cardiac arrest may occur in children with congenital heart lesions, myocarditis, cardiomyopathies, or channelopathies.

It is important to note that respiratory arrest should be prevented in the hospital. If the child receives appropriate support of oxygenation and ventilation, a relatively higher proportion of resuscitation required in the PCCU will be necessitated by progressive shock and hemodynamic collapse or arrhythmias.[127,308,309]

Pathophysiology

In adults, out-of-hospital cardiac arrest may be a sudden event related to an arrhythmia or myocardial infarction, whereas in-hospital arrest may occur from arrhythmia or the progression of respiratory failure, shock, or both.[214] As a result, if defibrillation and CPR are instituted promptly and the cardiac rhythm is restored rapidly, the patient may survive neurologically intact.

As noted previously, out-of-hospital cardiopulmonary arrest in the child usually is hypoxic/asphyxial, occurring as a terminal event following progressive deterioration and multisystem ischemia. Resuscitation is often unsuccessful, and survivors may have severe neurologic insult. Survival following most pediatric pulseless cardiac arrest is poor, averaging 9% to 21%, with poor neurologic outcomes for many of the survivors.[178,322] Sudden primary (arrhythmic) cardiac arrest may occur in infants and children, typically caused by conditions such as long QT syndrome, other channelopathies, or underlying congenital heart disease. In these children, perfusion may be normal until the sudden collapse. These children demonstrate higher survival rates, particularly if prompt bystander cardiopulmonary resuscitation (CPR) and defibrillation are provided.[279] Following in-hospital cardiac arrest, pediatric survival is better than adult survival (27% versus 17%, respectively), and many survivors have good neurologic outcomes.[214]

The terminal cardiac rhythm in children is usually bradycardia that progresses to asystole. This bradycardia is associated with extremely poor systemic perfusion and progressive metabolic acidosis. In approximately 7% of in-hospital arrests in children, the initial rhythm is a shockable one (i.e., ventricular fibrillation or pulseless ventricular tachycardia), although a shockable rhythm is present in approximately one fourth of all attempted resuscitations at some time during the attempted resuscitation.[214]

As noted previously, critically ill hospitalized children, particularly those with underlying cardiac pathology or electrolyte disorders, may develop sudden arrhythmias, particularly ventricular tachycardia that may progress to fibrillation. These arrhythmias may be associated with hypoxia (bradycardia is most common) or hypercyanotic spells, or they may be associated with progressive ventricular irritability or heart block. However, they can also be sudden.

The most common cause of symptomatic bradycardia in children is hypoxia. If bradycardia develops, the provider should assess and support airway and ventilation with oxygen. If bradycardia persists despite support of adequate airway, oxygenation, and ventilation, CPR is required. Survival from resuscitation for bradycardia is higher in children than in adults.[77]

Worrisome ventricular arrhythmias include multiform premature ventricular contractions at rest; these premature ventricular contractions are particularly worrisome if they are coupled, especially in the face of structural heart disease or diminished myocardial function. Ventricular fibrillation is extremely rare in neonates.

Any critically ill child should be assessed constantly, because each patient is at risk for the development of progressive shock or respiratory failure that can progress to cardiac or respiratory arrest. Therefore throughout hospitalization the child's airway, breathing, and circulation (ABCs) must be assessed.

Clinical Signs and Symptoms of Prearrest and Arrest

In children, hypoxic/ischemic arrest may be prevented if providers identify and treat respiratory failure and shock. As a result, the clinician will still assess the child's "ABCs," or

airway, breathing, and circulation when the child is not in arrest but is in distress. This assessment is included in the sections immediately below.[149]

Prearrest: Airway. The provider assesses airway patency. This includes determining if the child is capable of maintaining the airway without assistance.[57a] Neurologic dysfunction, sedation, anesthesia, and profound hypoxia can all depress airway protective reflexes. If the child's ability to maintain a patent airway is in doubt, intubation is recommended, before progressive respiratory failure leads to cardiopulmonary arrest. Routine use of cricoid pressure during intubation and during bag-mask ventilation is difficult to teach and may not prevent aspiration.[86,121]

If the child is unconscious the tongue can fall into the pharynx, obstructing the airway. In addition, because the child's upper airway is relatively small, small amounts of mucus accumulation or edema can reduce airway radius critically and severely increase resistance to air flow. Laryngotracheobronchitis (i.e., croup), bacterial tracheitis, or rarely, epiglottitis and other upper airway inflammation may cause upper airway obstruction. In addition, edema or injury to the upper airway following burns, trauma, or surgery can contribute to upper airway obstruction.

Progressive airway obstruction should be anticipated in children with inhalation injuries, with trauma to the head or neck, epiglottitis, or who demonstrate stridor and increased work of breathing immediately after extubation. In these children, the level of consciousness and respiratory effort should be evaluated to determine whether and when intubation is required. Additional signs of airway obstruction include stridor, retractions, nasal flaring, and high-pitched inspiratory sounds. Hypoxemia typically will not be an early sign of airway obstruction, and bradycardia and cyanosis may be only late signs of hypoxia and respiratory failure.

Prearrest: Breathing. Once the child's airway patency is assessed and ensured, the provider determines the effectiveness of the ventilation. Tachypnea will be the first sign of respiratory distress and usually will be accompanied by increased respiratory effort, including retractions, nasal flaring, stridor, wheezing, head bobbing, or grunting. The infant with respiratory failure may have a weak cry. Hypoxemia, despite supplementary oxygen therapy, and hypercarbia are additional signs of respiratory failure.

Children with respiratory failure may demonstrate a change in level of consciousness or responsiveness. A decreased response to painful stimulation usually is associated with severe cardiorespiratory or neurologic deterioration. Poor skeletal muscle tone also may be present, especially in infants. Decreased air movement, apnea or gasping, and bradycardia will be only late signs of severe respiratory distress in children and typically indicate that arrest is imminent. In addition, slowing of the respiratory rate without improvement in other parameters is usually an ominous sign of impending arrest.

Prearrest: Circulation. Terminal rhythms in cardiac arrest include asystole, pulseless electrical activity, ventricular tachycardia, and ventricular fibrillation. Whenever an arrhythmia develops, the nurse should assess the effect of the arrhythmia on the child's systemic perfusion and pulses.

Shock is present when CO is insufficient and oxygen and substrate delivery to tissues is inadequate (see discussion of Shock, earlier in this chapter). The child in shock typically demonstrates tachycardia, with changes in capillary refill, and evidence of reduced organ perfusion (e.g., oliguria, irritability, lethargy, cool extremities). Metabolic acidosis indicates that oxygen and substrate delivery are inadequate to maintain pure aerobic metabolism. Decreased central venous oxygen saturation indicates increased oxygen extraction, demonstrating a reduction in the child's ability to meet metabolic demands. Children with poor systemic perfusion generally demonstrate a mottled color or pallor. Hypotension may be only a late sign of shock in infants and young children. For more complete information regarding the clinical assessment of the patient in shock, see "Shock," earlier in this chapter.

Signs of Arrest. Signs of arrest include unresponsiveness, apnea or gasping (no breathing or only gasping), and absence of a central pulse. The pulse check is not a reliable indicator of the presence or absence of cardiac arrest. Healthcare providers often think a pulse is present when it is not and they often take too long to check a pulse. As a result, the American Heart Association has de-emphasized the pulse check (particularly for basic life support providers) and recommends that providers begin resuscitation if no pulse is definitely felt within 10 seconds in an unresponsive, apneic, or gasping infant, child, or adult.[26]

Management: Prearrest Support

An essential element in the management of critically ill children is the anticipation of deterioration and preparation for necessary support, so arrest is prevented. As part of morning and evening rounds, the critical care team should discuss potential causes and signs of deterioration in every patient and review plans for each potential problem. If and when the child deteriorates, the team will be prepared to respond before the development of cardiac arrest in most cases.

Typically in the PCCU or hospital setting the child's HR and oxyhemoglobin saturation are monitored, so that the monitors provide additional information to determine the type of arrest present. For example, if the child has a respiratory arrest without a cardiac arrest, the provider may see continued regular narrow complexes on a cardiac monitor and evidence of strong and regular pulse signal via oximetry even as the provider is moving to the bedside to verify patent airway and adequate ventilation and palpate a pulse.

Prearrest Support of Airway and Ventilation. Emergency equipment should always be readily available; a hand ventilator bag and mask and an oxygen source with necessary flow meter and tubing should be present at every bedside. When cardiorespiratory distress is present, oxygen should be administered immediately. Next, the child's airway, breathing, and circulation must be assessed and supported rapidly.

If the child has apparent breathing efforts, but stridor or other sounds of airway obstruction are present, a jaw thrust may open the airway and relieve the obstruction. The child may require insertion of an oropharyngeal or nasopharyngeal airway or an advanced airway to maintain a patent upper airway.

If the child has respiratory distress, failure or arrest with pulses (i.e., a respiratory arrest rather than a cardiorespiratory arrest), support of ventilation is required (see Chapter 9).

Prearrest Support of Circulation. If the child has pulses and an adequate HR with poor perfusion, treatment of shock is required. See "Management of Shock" information earlier in this chapter. If bradycardia and poor perfusion develop, hypoxia is likely to be present. Ensure that the airway is patent and support adequate oxygenation and ventilation. If the HR is less than 60 beats/min with signs of poor perfusion despite support of oxygenation and ventilation, then begin CPR.[26,57a]

Management: Resuscitation

Whenever cardiopulmonary arrest occurs, providing high-quality, minimally interrupted CPR is essential to resuscitation. It is important to remember that during cardiac arrest, chest compressions provide all CO (i.e., blood flow) to the patient, and compressions provide a significant percentage of total CO during a bradycardic arrest. Maintenance of an adequate depth ("push hard") and rate ("push fast") during CPR provides the best chance for survival. High-quality CPR is the foundation of all treatment for cardiac arrest; too often, CPR is performed poorly in both the prehospital and in-hospital settings.[1,288,317] Without excellent CPR, all other therapies, including medications or defibrillation, are doomed to fail.

There has been a change in the approach to CPR worldwide during the last decade, with an increased emphasis on chest compressions and decreased emphasis on ventilation.[126] Under some conditions "hands-only" CPR may be appropriate for lay rescuers responding to adult victims of sudden cardiac arrest. However, pediatric cardiac arrest is still most commonly caused by a primary respiratory event or progressive hypoxic-ischemic insult (i.e., progressive respiratory failure or shock). As a result, ventilation is still an essential component of resuscitation in children. In a recent study of out-of-hospital pediatric arrest in Japan, survival was much higher when bystanders used the combination of ventilation with chest compressions rather than compression only.[148]

For the pediatric critical care nurse, cardiac arrest will most likely be encountered in the hospital environment, often the PCCU.[308] In this setting, several trained professional rescuers will usually be available to respond as a team, performing many steps of resuscitation simultaneously. This choreographed approach to resuscitation should be studied and practiced, stressing the importance of the team concept and the coordinated provision of compressions and ventilations with minimal interruptions.[26,57a,149]

Cardiac Compressions. Cardiac compressions should be provided whenever cardiac arrest (asystole or collapse rhythm) develops or when profound symptomatic bradycardia, producing a compromise in systemic perfusion, is unresponsive to oxygenation and ventilation. Children were among the survivors documented in the first published case series of successful closed chest compressions to maintain blood flow during cardiac arrest.[156] The presumed mechanism of blood flow was direct compression of the heart between the sternum and the spine. Later investigations indicated that blood could also be circulated during CPR by the thoracic pump mechanism.[224] In this model, chest compression-induced increases in intrathoracic pressure, and decreases in intrathoracic pressure during the "relaxation phase" of chest compressions, generate a gradient for blood to flow from the pulmonary vasculature, through the heart, and into the systemic circulation.

Regardless of mechanism, CO during CPR seems to be greater in children who have more compliant chest walls than adults.[69,328] This fact of chest wall deformability and improved perfusion during CPR may account for the superior outcomes from in-hospital cardiac arrest seen in infants versus older children.[203]

To best compress the heart directly between the sternum and the spine (i.e., the direct compression model of CPR), the rescuer must compress the sternum directly over the heart. To achieve this, provide compressions just below the intermammary line (i.e., over the lower third of the sternum) in infants or over the lower half of the sternum in older children.[233] Do not compress over the xiphoid process, because thoracic or abdominal injury may result. When two or more rescuers are present and one rescuer provides ventilation, a two-thumb-encircling hands technique should be used to give chest compressions to infants. In children, the heel of one or both hands may be used.[26]

If at all possible, the patient should be placed on a rigid surface such as a backboard during compressions to minimize the effect of the patient bouncing on a soft surface, such as a bed, during CPR. Although the 2010 AHA resuscitation guidelines do not mandate the use of backboards,[26] backboards are often used to provide a firm surface for chest compressions. If the two-thumb-encircling hands technique is used for infants, a backboard is not needed. If the heel of one hand is used for compressions in the child, the rescuer may use the second hand to support the child's back. Bouncing compressions are not effective. However, in the end, the method selected is less important than the provision of hard, fast, minimally interrupted compressions that allow full chest recoil after each compression.[26] If a backboard is used, it should ideally cover the width of the surface on which the child lies. If the child is lying on a mattress or other compressible surface, providers should be aware that accelerometers used to provide feedback regarding depth of compression may overestimate the depth of chest compressions.

Blood Flow during CPR. During untreated cardiac arrest, there is essentially no blood flow. Perfusion of critical organs must be created by chest compressions. This flow, or CO, is the product of stoke volume and rate. The force of compressions, along with heart refilling during the recoil or relaxation phase of compressions, are the major determinants of SV during CPR. SV also depends on preload. Therefore, patients in cardiac arrests associated with circulatory shock (e.g., hypovolemic or septic shock) may need additional intravascular volume to provide adequate SV with chest compressions.

Another important determinant of myocardial blood flow is the chest compression rate. Although the optimal chest compression rate is not known, data from animal and adult studies has shown that coronary perfusion, CO, and survival are superior with chest compression rates of 100 per minute or more compared with rates less than 80 per minute.[95,147,189]

The coronary perfusion pressure (CPP) is the driving force of blood into the coronary arteries and is the difference between the aortic end-diastolic pressure (generated with chest compressions) and the mean right atrial pressure. An adequate CPP is critical to the success of the CPR. If the CPP falls below 15 mm Hg during CPR in adults, the likelihood for a return of spontaneous circulation is greatly decreased.[236] Animal models suggest that outcomes from arrest are improved if the CPP is greater than 22 mm Hg; this is achieved by providing forceful (push hard) and rapid (push fast) compressions and avoiding interruptions. Note that the CPP falls rapidly whenever compressions are stopped. Relatively brief interruptions of chest compressions, such as pauses to provide ventilation, will result in decreases in the CPP, leading to inadequate myocardial perfusion[27] and decreased survival.[146] As noted, an adequate CPP during CPR is critical for successful return of spontaneous circulation.

Survival and good functional outcome following cardiac arrest also require maintenance of adequate cerebral perfusion pressure. Unlike myocardial blood flow, cerebral blood flow is generated during the compression phase of CPR. Because of preferential blood flow to the heart and brain during cardiac arrest, especially with the use of vasoconstrictor medications such as epinephrine, excellent CPR can provide essential blood flow to these critical organs, reducing the risk of brain and heart ischemia.

Vascular Access. Vascular access should be achieved as quickly as possible during resuscitation. However, this may be extremely difficult in the poorly perfused child in shock or cardiac arrest. Central venous access above the level of the diaphragm may be preferable to access below the diaphragm during CPR, because this route may provide the most rapid delivery of drugs to the heart. However, if a central venous catheter is not already in place at the time of cardiac arrest, rapid placement during chest compressions can be difficult. Delay in placement significantly reduces the benefit of the central venous catheter, making a standard peripheral intravenous catheter preferable if vascular access is not in place at the time of the arrest.

If intravenous access cannot be established quickly, intraosseous access should be secured. There is no maximum or minimum age for intraosseous access, and several sites, including the iliac crest, distal radius, and sternum in adolescents, may be used in addition to the traditional tibial approach.[281] Insert an intraosseous needle or a large-bore needle with a stylette into the anterior medial aspect of the tibia.

The intraosseous route provides rapid delivery of fluids and drugs to the heart, as fast as a standard peripheral intravenous catheter.[48,281] The resuscitation team should use a protocol for establishing vascular access during resuscitation so that time is not wasted in a futile attempt to achieve peripheral venous access when the intraosseous route is available.[144]

An additional advantage of intraosseous access is that chest compressions are not interrupted.

There are several new products that allow rapid intraosseous access using a spring-loaded gun or drill-type device. The efficacy of many, but not all, of these instruments has been evaluated in children. As with any medical technology, it is the responsibility of the pediatric care team to be familiar with the particular devices in their clinical setting to ensure their safe and effective use.

With the value of intraosseous vascular access and ease of intraosseous placement now commonly recognized, endotracheal drug administration should be an uncommon event. It is not the preferred route for medication delivery during cardiac arrest. However, some resuscitation medications, including lidocaine, epinephrine, atropine, and naloxone (creating the acronym LEAN) may be administered successfully via the endotracheal tube, but the absorption and efficacy of these drugs when given by this route is uncertain. For example, endotracheal epinephrine has been shown to result in survival that is no better than with intravenous administration,[116] and some studies have shown much worse survival.[223]

Drugs delivered to the trachea should be diluted with normal saline and should be delivered as deeply into the endotracheal tube as possible. The endotracheal tube should then be irrigated with 1 to 2 mL of normal saline, and several positive pressure breaths should be provided. Optimal drug doses for endotracheal administration are not known; it may be necessary to administer larger doses by the endotracheal route than are required for intravenous therapy.

Fluid Therapy. Fluid or blood products should be administered rapidly to the hypovolemic patient in shock. Approximately 20 mL/kg of isotonic crystalloid, colloid, or blood products should be administered as a bolus to attempt to restore adequate intravascular volume. (For further information regarding fluid therapy, please refer to the Management of Shock in the preceding section of this chapter.)

Drug Therapy. The sequence of pediatric advanced life support is depicted in the AHA Pediatric Pulseless Arrest Algorithm (Fig. 6-9). The drugs used during resuscitation are listed in Table 6-8. Emergency drug doses can be calculated prior to the arrest and a list kept at the bedside. Accurate drug doses can also be estimated using a color-coded length-based tape (i.e., the Broselow tape).[130,179] For further information, see Chapter 1 and Fig. 1-1.

Although epinephrine improved initial resuscitation success (i.e., return of spontaneous circulation) after both asphyxial and arrhythmic cardiac arrests in animal models,[208] no single medication has been shown to improve survival to hospital discharge after pediatric cardiac arrest. In fact, the timing of drug delivery and a coordinated systems approach to resuscitation (i.e., early detection, high-quality CPR, aggressive monitoring, and postarrest care) play as large a role or larger than any medication that can be given.[326] These issues may be responsible for results seen in an adult study that showed similar survival for groups with intravascular access and drug administration versus those with no intravascular access (and no intravenous drug administration).[230]

Furthermore, if drug preparation or delivery during resuscitation impairs the quality of the CPR provided, it is harmful, not helpful, to the patient.

The most common medications used for CPR in children (see Table 6-8) are vasopressors (epinephrine) and antiarrhythmics (amiodarone or lidocaine). During CPR, epinephrine has a beneficial α-adrenergic effect by increasing SVR, thereby increasing diastolic BP and CPP. Improved coronary blood flow via high-quality chest compressions and epinephrine increased the likelihood of the return of spontaneous circulation in adults, and similar effects are likely to be present in children. Epinephrine also increases cerebral blood flow during CPR via peripheral vasoconstriction; this can direct a greater proportion of flow to the cerebral circulation. The β-adrenergic epinephrine effects increase myocardial contractility and HR and relax smooth muscle in the skeletal muscle vascular bed and bronchi, although this effect is of less importance.

Epinephrine also changes the character of ventricular fibrillation (i.e., higher amplitude, more coarse) and prolongs fibrillation; these effects increase the likelihood of successful defibrillation.[255,286] For these reasons, epinephrine is the preferred drug in the treatment of bradycardia resulting from hypoxic-ischemic insult or asystolic cardiac arrest. It is also the drug of choice for the patient with ventricular fibrillation or pulseless ventricular tachycardia, and it may enable successful defibrillation if initial defibrillation attempts are unsuccessful by improving myocardial blood flow and ventricular "readiness" for defibrillation. Finally, epinephrine is probably the most effective inotropic and vasoconstrictive agent in the treatment of shock associated with hypotension, bradycardia, or sepsis.[149]

High-dose epinephrine (0.05 to 0.2 mg/kg) can improve myocardial and cerebral blood flow during CPR but may worsen post-resuscitation myocardial dysfunction and survival.[106,107] A prospective, blinded randomized, controlled trial of rescue high-dose epinephrine versus standard-dose epinephrine following failed initial standard dose epinephrine for pediatric in-hospital cardiac arrest demonstrated a worse 24-hour survival in the high-dose epinephrine group.[248] Therefore routine use of high-dose epinephrine for pediatric cardiac arrest is not recommended.[149]

A continuous epinephrine infusion may be provided after return of spontaneous circulation (ROSC) at a dose of 0.1 to 1.0 mcg/kg per minute. This infusion should have chronotropic effects, producing an increase in HR, as well as inotropic effects and should increase systemic arterial pressure, cerebral blood flow, and coronary artery perfusion pressure. Atropine administration is indicated for the child with bradycardia associated with heart block or increased vagal tone.

Buffering Agents. Acidosis results from inadequate oxygen and substrate delivery to tissues and generation of lactic acid. In children with shock or respiratory failure, metabolic acidosis can be complicated by the development of hypercarbia and respiratory acidosis.

During resuscitation the most effective method of treating acidosis is the provision of adequate oxygenation and ventilation and the restoration of effective systemic and pulmonary

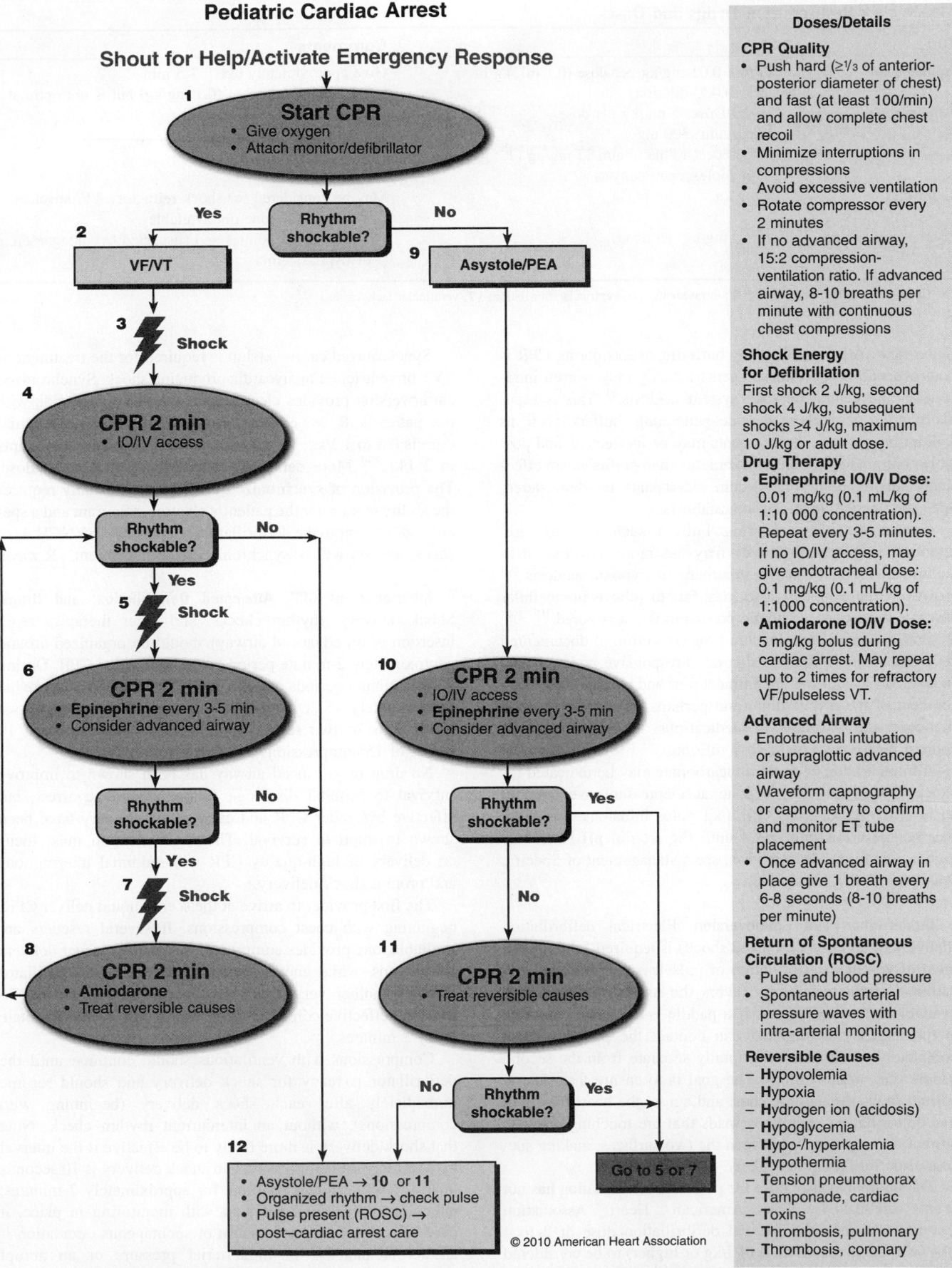

Pediatric Cardiac Arrest

Shout for Help/Activate Emergency Response

1
Start CPR
• Give oxygen
• Attach monitor/defibrillator

Rhythm shockable?

Yes — **2** **VF/VT**

No — **9** **Asystole/PEA**

3 ⚡ **Shock**

4
CPR 2 min
• IO/IV access

Rhythm shockable? — No

Yes

5 ⚡ **Shock**

6
CPR 2 min
• **Epinephrine** every 3-5 min
• Consider advanced airway

Rhythm shockable? — No

Yes

7 ⚡ **Shock**

8
CPR 2 min
• **Amiodarone**
• Treat reversible causes

10
CPR 2 min
• IO/IV access
• **Epinephrine** every 3-5 min
• Consider advanced airway

Rhythm shockable? — Yes

No

11
CPR 2 min
• Treat reversible causes

Rhythm shockable? — Yes

No

Go to 5 or 7

12
• Asystole/PEA → **10** or **11**
• Organized rhythm → check pulse
• Pulse present (ROSC) → post–cardiac arrest care

© 2010 American Heart Association

Doses/Details

CPR Quality
• Push hard (≥1/3 of anterior-posterior diameter of chest) and fast (at least 100/min) and allow complete chest recoil
• Minimize interruptions in compressions
• Avoid excessive ventilation
• Rotate compressor every 2 minutes
• If no advanced airway, 15:2 compression-ventilation ratio. If advanced airway, 8-10 breaths per minute with continuous chest compressions

Shock Energy for Defibrillation
First shock 2 J/kg, second shock 4 J/kg, subsequent shocks ≥4 J/kg, maximum 10 J/kg or adult dose.

Drug Therapy
• **Epinephrine IO/IV Dose:** 0.01 mg/kg (0.1 mL/kg of 1:10 000 concentration). Repeat every 3-5 minutes. If no IO/IV access, may give endotracheal dose: 0.1 mg/kg (0.1 mL/kg of 1:1000 concentration).
• **Amiodarone IO/IV Dose:** 5 mg/kg bolus during cardiac arrest. May repeat up to 2 times for refractory VF/pulseless VT.

Advanced Airway
• Endotracheal intubation or supraglottic advanced airway
• Waveform capnography or capnometry to confirm and monitor ET tube placement
• Once advanced airway in place give 1 breath every 6-8 seconds (8-10 breaths per minute)

Return of Spontaneous Circulation (ROSC)
• Pulse and blood pressure
• Spontaneous arterial pressure waves with intra-arterial monitoring

Reversible Causes
– Hypovolemia
– Hypoxia
– Hydrogen ion (acidosis)
– Hypoglycemia
– Hypo-/hyperkalemia
– Hypothermia
– Tension pneumothorax
– Tamponade, cardiac
– Toxins
– Thrombosis, pulmonary
– Thrombosis, coronary

FIG. 6-9 American Heart Association pediatric advanced life support pediatric pulseless arrest algorithm. (From the American Heart Association; Kleinman M, et al: Pediatric advanced life support. *Circulation* 122 (Suppl. 3):S876–S908, 2010.)

Table 6-8 Resuscitation Drugs and Doses

Drug	Dose	Comments
Epinephrine	IV/IO: 0.01 mg/kg per dose (0.1 mL/kg of 1:10,000 dilution)	Give approximately every 3-5 min ET dose may be given (0.1 mg/kg) but is not optimal
Amiodarone	IV/IO Dose: 5 mg/kg per dose Maximum: 300 mg May repeat to maximum 15 mg/kg (2.2 g in adolescents) per day	Prolongs PR and QT intervals
Lidocaine	1 mg/kg	May be considered for shock-refractory VF/pulseless VT if amiodarone not available
Magnesium sulfate	25-50 mg/kg per dose	For torsades de pointes and suspected hypomagnesemia or hypocalcemia

ET, Endotracheal; *IO,* intraosseous; *IV,* intravenous; *VF,* ventricular fibrillation; *VT,* ventricular tachycardia.

blood flow. Administering any buffering agents during CPR is controversial, because these agents actually may worsen intracellular and central nervous system acidosis.[31] This is especially true of carbon dioxide–generating buffers such as sodium bicarbonate. These agents may be ineffective, and possibly contraindicated, unless ventilation and perfusion are effectively supported. Before sodium bicarbonate is administered, adequate ventilation should be established.

Carbon dioxide–consuming buffers such as carbicarb, although uncommonly used, may be more effective than sodium bicarbonate in the treatment of hypoxic acidosis.[324] However, these buffers also may fail to relieve intracellular acidosis if adequate systemic perfusion is not restored.[101–103]

Buffers may be administered for correction of documented severe acidosis in the unstable or unresponsive arrest victim, in an effort to improve the intracellular and extracellular environment of the myocardium and perhaps the effectiveness of inotropic and vasopressor medications. A typical dose of sodium bicarbonate is 0.5 to 1 mEq/kg.

Administration of sodium bicarbonate may be indicated for shock associated with tricyclic antidepressant overdose. In such an overdose, 1 to 2 mEq/kg bolus infusions of sodium bicarbonate are administered until the arterial pH is 7.45 or higher. For further information, see "Management of Specific Poisonings," in Chapter 18.

Defibrillation and Cardioversion. Electrical defibrillation (delivery of an unsynchronized shock) is required for the treatment of ventricular fibrillation or pulseless ventricular tachycardia. Current technology favors the use of adhesive pads available in pediatric sizes. If a paddle is used, the ideal size is the largest possible that can contact the patient's chest completely while remaining totally separate from the second paddle (i.e., not touching). The goal is to ensure that electric current flows through the chest and across the heart for effective defibrillation. Paddles or pads that are touching result in current flowing simply between the two surfaces, making successful defibrillation less likely.

The optimal energy dose for pediatric defibrillation has not been established. The American Heart Association recommends an initial manual defibrillation dose of 2 to 4 J/kg with an increased dose (4 J/kg or higher) to be considered for the second and subsequent shocks.[149]

Synchronized cardioversion is required for the treatment of SVT or ventricular tachycardia producing shock. Synchronized cardioversion provides electrical stimulation to coincide with the patient's R wave. The consensus recommended initial dose is 0.5 to 1 J/kg, but it is increased in subsequent attempts to 2 J/kg.[149] More data are needed regarding optimal dose. The provision of synchronized cardioversion usually requires the ability to monitor the patient's electrocardiogram and a specific adjustment to the defibrillator (selection of "SYNCH"), so shock delivery will be synchronized with the patient's R wave.

Integration of CPR, Attempted Defibrillation, and Drugs. Shock delivery, rhythm checks, and other therapies (e.g., insertion of an advanced airway) should be organized around approximately 2-minute periods of uninterrupted CPR. During these 2-minute periods of CPR, the single rescuer will provide approximately 5 cycles of 30 compressions and two ventilations or two rescuers will provide approximately 10 cycles of 15 compressions and two ventilations.

No drug or advanced airway has been shown to improve survival to hospital discharge following cardiac arrest, but effective bystander CPR and early shock delivery have been shown to improve survival. Therefore attention must focus on delivery of high-quality CPR with minimal interruptions and prompt shock delivery.

The first provider to arrive at the scene should deliver CPR, beginning with chest compressions. If several rescuers are available, one provides compressions, another rescuer delivers ventilations, while another rescuer prepares the defibrillator and yet another verifies or establishes vascular access. To maintain effective compressions, the compressor should rotate every 2 minutes.

Compressions with ventilations should continue until the defibrillator is ready for shock delivery and should resume immediately after each shock delivery (beginning with compressions), without an intercurrent rhythm check. Note that shock delivery is more likely to be effective if the interval between the last compression and shock delivery is 10 seconds or less.[84] CPR should continue for approximately 2 minutes, although in a critical care unit with monitoring in place, it may be possible to detect return of spontaneous circulation if an abrupt increase in intraarterial pressure or an abrupt increase in exhaled CO_2 (i.e., $P_{ET}CO_2$) is observed.

If ventricular fibrillation is present at the next rhythm check, the second and subsequent shock doses should be 4 J/kg or higher. Epinephrine is generally given and should be administered while compressions are being performed. Providers should also verify effectiveness of oxygenation, ventilation, and compressions.

If ventricular fibrillation persists at the next rhythm check, consideration should be given to administration of amiodarone (5 mg/kg IV) or, if amiodarone is unavailable, lidocaine (1 mg/kg). Ongoing high quality CPR is critical for patients who remain in ventricular fibrillation, because the blood flow generated with chest compressions provides oxygen delivery to the brain and cardiac muscle. High-quality chest compressions and adequate myocardial blood flow can improve the readiness of the fibrillating heart to be defibrillated with a subsequent shock.[42]

If the child's rhythm converts to a perfusing rhythm, postresuscitation care is needed (see section, The Postresuscitation Phase). If the rhythm converts to a nonshockable rhythm, CPR continues with rhythm analysis approximately every 2 minutes and epinephrine administration about every other period of CPR (see description of the 2-minute periods of CPR in the paragraphs above).

If an advanced airway is not in place at the time of cardiac arrest, the resuscitation team leader must weigh the potential benefits of the advanced airway (i.e., an established airway that allows provision of continuous chest compressions without pauses for ventilation) against the risks of intubation, including the need for interruptions of chest compressions.[28] Cuffed endotracheal tubes have been shown to be as safe as uncuffed tubes in children, and may be preferable if the child has noncompliant lungs or a large glottic air leak.[149,219]

Support of the Parents. The parents should be notified when CPR is necessary and, if possible, they should be offered the opportunity to remain in the room during the resuscitation attempt. Although caregivers may hesitate to allow family members to be present during attempted resuscitation, there is evidence that when the family is offered the option to be present during attempted resuscitation, it is helpful to families in their recovery, and it does not negatively affect the care-team's performance.[80,155,298]

If at all possible, one member of the healthcare team should be responsible for communicating with the family to help explain what is happening; the staff member ideally remains with the family if they remain in the room during the resuscitation. During any communication, it is important to refer to the child by name[139] and to relay the information with sensitivity and compassion. It is equally important to listen to the parents' questions and fears. Family presence, or at least regular communication with the family during a cardiac arrest, will often help prepare the parents in stages should resuscitation prove unsuccessful.

Extending or Discontinuing a Resuscitation Attempt

Survival with good outcomes after pediatric cardiac arrest has become increasingly common.[177,211,214,221] Centers with extracorporeal membrane oxygenator-CPR (ECMO-CPR or ECPR) programs can institute mechanical support of blood

flow and oxygenation until the patient can recover. Although ECPR was once considered an extreme measure, reported survival has been relatively high, particularly for patients following cardiovascular surgery. Initial reports of its use are encouraging, with 38% survival to discharge in one study.[294] More encouraging, in 5 of 10 children for whom data were available, there was no change in the neurologic assessment score between admission and after ECPR.[211] It is important to note that using ECPR requires ready availability of a specialized team and equipment. Excellent CPR must be continued without interruption while the ECPR circuit and personnel are assembled, to minimize the chance of hypoxic-ischemic injury before ECMO can support the circulation. Although ECPR is not widely available, it is an area of active interest in the field of resuscitation and pediatric critical care.

Several factors determine the likelihood of survival after cardiac arrest, including the mechanism of the arrest (e.g., traumatic, asphyxial), location (e.g., out-of-hospital versus in-hospital, ward versus PCCU), response (e.g., monitored versus unmonitored, witnessed versus unwitnessed), and underlying pathophysiology (e.g., cardiomyopathy, congenital defect, single ventricle physiology, drug toxicity, or metabolic derangement). These factors should all be considered before deciding to terminate resuscitative efforts.

In the past, continuation of CPR had been considered futile beyond 15 to 20 minutes of CPR or when more than two doses of epinephrine were needed.[325] However, this recommendation is now obsolete, because with improved quality of CPR and better intraresuscitation and postresuscitation care (including ECPR and possible therapeutic hypothermia), intact neurologic survival is often possible despite prolonged CPR. Therefore, a universal or time-based recommendation regarding termination of resuscitation cannot be given.[149]

RESUSCITATION TRAINING AND QUALITY IMPROVEMENT

Every physician and nurse involved in the care of critically ill children must be skilled in providing basic and advanced pediatric life support. Several courses are available through the American Heart Association (the Pediatric Advanced Life Support Course) and the American Academy of Pediatrics (the Advanced Pediatric Life Support Course). All caregivers, including physicians and nurses, should attend such courses and maintain proficiency through recertification and ongoing study and practice. In addition, "mock arrest" situations should be staged frequently by the entire healthcare team. These practice sessions will increase staff familiarity with the principals and essential skills of resuscitation and will improve coordination of efforts during actual resuscitation. A thorough and thoughtful debriefing should occur after any mock arrest session and actual resuscitation to help each team member optimize performance.[149]

Within the hospital setting, systems can be created to provide a rapid response to patient deterioration or an impending arrest before progressing to cardiac arrest. These systems may include medical emergency or rapid response teams. These programs seek to identify patients at particular risk and intervene early to address the underlying condition and reduce the risk of cardiac arrest; they have been proven effective in reducing respiratory arrest, non-PCCU arrest, and mortality.[296] Often the therapy provided is a timely transport to the PCCU, where definitive care can be given and intensive monitoring can be used to reduce the risk of arrest.[214]

Prevention of any arrest is important. Because asphyxial arrest typically follows a prearrest period of progressive hypoxia, hypercarbia, and acidosis, emergency and rapid response teams should focus on detection and treatment of these conditions.[296] Patients with a significant underlying pathologic condition (e.g., cyanotic congenital heart disease), comorbidities (e.g., acute respiratory distress syndrome [ARDS] or renal failure), or abnormal physiology (e.g., shock or anemia) will respond less favorably to resuscitation, so detection and treatment of deterioration in these patients is also important.

For further information about the Pediatric Advanced Life Support courses, contact your local chapter of the American Heart Association. Information about the Advanced Pediatric Life Support Course can be obtained from the American Academy of Pediatrics.

THE POSTRESUSCITATION PHASE

Once circulation is restored, therapeutic hypothermia (i.e., the intentional creation of hypothermia in the patient after cardiac arrest) holds great promise. Although hypothermia after cardiac arrest has been shown to be effective in adults,[29,117] randomized, controlled pediatric studies of this modality are not yet available (studies are underway), and extrapolation of adult studies to children is difficult. Studies of cooling after birth asphyxia in neonatal patients support the potential beneficial effects of cooling on neurologic outcome.[17,105]

Fever following cardiac arrest, brain trauma, stroke, and other ischemic conditions is associated with poor neurologic outcome and hyperthermia following cardiac arrest is common in children.[129] Mild induced systemic hypothermia may benefit children resuscitated from nontraumatic cardiac arrest, and careful prevention of fever is very important.

The postresuscitation (or postcardiac arrest) syndrome is a complex combination of pathophysiologic processes commonly seen after successful resuscitation. This complex includes brain injury, myocardial dysfunction, and systemic ischemia-reperfusion response injury. In addition, the underlying pathology that led to the cardiac arrest may still be present in the postresuscitation phase and will often require correction.

Clinical manifestations of postresuscitation brain injury include coma, seizures, myoclonus, varying degrees of neurocognitive dysfunction (ranging from memory deficits to persistent vegetative state), and brain death. As noted, therapeutic hypothermia may offer the hope of improved neurologic outcome in children as it has adults.[117]

Postresuscitation myocardial dysfunction and hypotensive shock are common[163]; it appears to be pathophysiologically similar to sepsis-related myocardial dysfunction, including increases in inflammatory mediators and endotheliopathy.[6] The condition is typically temporary if the patient survives the period of decreased cardiac function.[163]

Although the optimal management of postcardiac arrest hypotension and myocardial dysfunction has not been defined,

data suggest that aggressive hemodynamic support improves outcomes. Fluid resuscitation and inotropic or vasopressor medications, including epinephrine, dobutamine, dopamine, milrinone, and others, have been used successfully to treat the myocardial dysfunction and hypotension in animals[207,222] and in human clinical studies.[29,287]

How should patients be managed in the postarrest setting? Ideally an organized multidisciplinary postresuscitation protocol begins in the prehospital setting, continues in the emergency department, and is tailored to each patient in the PCCU. Such a protocol includes well-coordinated aggressive critical care, hemodynamic support, induced hypothermia, and percutaneous coronary angioplasty to relieve coronary artery occlusion in adults with sudden cardiac arrest.[287]

Postcardiac arrest myocardial dysfunction and hemodynamic instability are common and should be anticipated. Therefore continuous electrocardiographic and hemodynamic monitoring should be provided for all patients after successful resuscitation from a cardiac arrest. Furthermore, postarrest echocardiography should be considered for quantifying the degree of myocardial dysfunction and tracking any change or response to therapy.

High-quality critical care with hemodynamic goals of supporting adequate BP, CO, and oxygen delivery to the heart and brain are important. The specific goal values for these indices will vary based on patients and clinical situations, but reasonable interventions for vasodilatory shock with low central venous pressure include fluid resuscitation and vasoactive infusions. Standard treatment for LV myocardial dysfunction includes titrating volume administration, inotropic infusions to promote cardiac contractility, and afterload reduction to reduce myocardial work. Much of the evidence that supports these recommendations is taken from the adult critical care literature. The entire field of postresuscitation care, in both adult and pediatric patients, is an area of active current and future study.

References

1. Abella BS, et al: Quality of cardiopulmonary resuscitation during in-hospital cardiac arrest. *J Am Med Assoc* 293(3):305–310, 2005.
2. Abman SH: Pulmonary hypertension in children: a historical overview. *Pediatr Crit Care Med* 11(Suppl.):S4–S9, 2010.
3. Absi MA, Lutterman J, Wetzel GT: Noninvasive cardiac output monitoring in the pediatric cardiac intensive care unit. *Curr Opin Cardiol* 25:77–79, 2010.
4. Adams JEIII, et al: Cardiac troponin I: a marker with high specificity for cardiac injury. *Circulation* 88:101–106, 1993.
5. Adelson PD, et al: Guidelines for the acute management of severe traumatic brain injury in infants, children, and adolescents. *Pediatr Crit Care Med* 4(3 Suppl.):S12–S18, 2003.
6. Adrie C, et al: Successful cardiopulmonary resuscitation after cardiac arrest as a "sepsis-like" syndrome. *Circulation* 106(5): 562–568, 2002.
7. Albert NM, et al: Use of aldosterone antagonists in heart failure. *J Am Med Assoc* 302(15):1658–1665, 2009.
8. Amaral A, Opal SM, Vincent JL: Coagulation in sepsis. *Intensive Care Med* 30(6):1032–1040, 2004.
9. American College of Chest Physicians, and Society of Critical Care Medicine Consensus Conference: Definitions of sepsis and organ failure and guidelines for the use of innovative therapies in sepsis. *Crit Care Med* 20:864–875, 1992.
10. Annane D, et al: Effect of treatment with low doses of hydrocortisone and fludrocortisone on mortality in patients with septic shock. *J Am Med Assoc* 288:862–867, 2002.
11. Annane D, Bellissant E, Cavaillon J: Septic shock. *Lancet* 365:378, 2005.

12. Annane D, et al: Norepinephrine plus dobutamine versus epinephrine alone for management of septic shock: a randomized trial. *Lancet* 360:767–784, 2007.

13. Annane D, et al: Corticosteroids in the treatment of severe sepsis and septic shock in adults: a systematic review. *J Am Med Assoc* 301 (22):2362–2375, 2009.

14. Atabaki SM: Pediatric head injury. *Ped Rev* 28(6):215–223, 2007.

15. Atkins DL, et al: Epidemiology and outcomes from out-of-hospital cardiac arrest in children: the Resuscitation Outcomes Consortium Epistry-Cardiac Arrest. *Circulation* 119(11):1484–1491, 2009.

16. Aurigemma GP, Gaasch WH: Diastolic heart failure. *N Engl J Med* 351(11):1097–1105, 2004.

17. Azzopardi DV, et al: Moderate hypothermia to treat perinatal asphyxial encephalopathy. *N Engl J Med* 361(14):1349–1358, 2009.

18. Babyn PS, Gahunia HK, Massicote P: Pulmonary thromboembolism in children. *Pediatr Radiol* 35:258–274, 2005.

19. Baden HP: Does nesiritide offer something new in the management of pediatric heart failure? *Pediatric Crit Care Med* 6:613, 2005.

20. Baird JS, Greene A, Schleien CL: Massive pulmonary embolus without hypoxemia. *Pediatr Crit Care Med* 6(5):602–603, 2005.

21. Bakker J, et al: Blood lactate levels are superior to oxygen-derived variables in predicting outcome in human septic shock. *Chest* 99:956–962, 1991.

22. Bakker J, et al: Serial blood lactate levels can predict the development of multiple organ failure following septic shock. *Am J Surg* 171:221–226, 1996.

23. Baraff LJ: Capillary refill: is it a useful clinical sign? *Pediatrics* 92:723–724, 1993.

24. Barrett LK, Singer M, Clapp LH: Vasopressin: mechanisms of action on the vasculature in health and in septic shock. *Crit Care Med* 35 (1):33–40, 2007.

25. Barton P, et al: Hemodynamic effects of intravenous milrinone lactate in pediatric patients with septic shock. *Chest* 109:1302–1312, 1996.

26. Berg M, et al: Part 13, pediatric basic life support. In 2010 American Heart Association Guidelines for Cardiopulmonary Resuscitation and Emergency Cardiovascular Care. *Circulation* 122(Suppl. 3): S862–S875, 2010.

27. Berg RA, et al: Adverse hemodynamic effects of interrupting chest compressions for rescue breathing during cardiopulmonary resuscitation for ventricular fibrillation cardiac arrest. *Circulation* 104(20):2465–2470, 2001.

28. Berkowitz ID, et al: Blood flow during cardiopulmonary resuscitation with simultaneous compression and ventilation in infant pigs. *Pediatr Res* 26:558, 1989.

29. Bernard SA, et al: Treatment of comatose survivors of out-of-hospital cardiac arrest with induced hypothermia. *N Engl J Med* 346 (8):557–563, 2002.

30. Bernus A, et al: Brain natriuretic peptide levels in managing pediatric patients with pulmonary atrial hypertension. *Chest* 135:745–751, 2009.

31. Bersin RM, Arieff AI: Use of sodium salts in the treatment of hypoxia-induced acidosis. *Circulation* 77:227, 1988.

32. Bettendorf M, et al: Tri-iodothyronine treatment in children after cardiac surgery: a double-blind, randomized, placebo-controlled study. *Lancet* 356:529–534, 2000.

33. Bissler JJ, Welch TR, Loggie JMH: Paradoxical hypertension in hypovolemic children. *Pediatr Emerg Care* 7:350–352, 1991.

34. Boehmer JP, Popjes E: Cardiac failure: mechanical support strategies. *Crit Care Med* 24(9):S268–S277, 2006.

35. Bratton SL: Patterns of septic shock in children: warm versus cold shock. *AAP Grand Rounds* 21(2):16, 2009.

36. Braun JP, et al: Successful treatment of dilative cardiomyopathy in a 12-year-old-girl using the calcium sensitizer levosimendan after weaning from mechanical biventricular assist support. *J Cardiothorac Vasc Anesth* 18:772–774, 2004.

37. Brierley J, Peters MJ: Distinct hemodynamic patterns of septic shock at presentation to pediatric intensive care. *Pediatrics* 122(4):752–759, 2008.

38. Brierley J, Carcillo JA, Choong K, Cornell T, et al: Clinical practice parameters for hemodynamic support of pediatric and neonatal septic shock: 2007 update from the American College of Critical Care Medicine. *Crit Care Med* 37:666–688, 2009.

39. Brilli RJ, Goldstein B: Pediatric sepsis definitions: past, present and future. *Pediatr Crit Care Med* 6(3):S6–S8, 2005.

39a. Brocklehurst P, and the Neonatal Immunotherapy Study (INIS) Collaborative Group. Treatment of neonatal sepsis with intravenous immune globulin. *N Engl J Med* 365:1201–1211, 2011.

40. Bromberg BI, et al: Recognition and management of nonpenetrating cardiac trauma in children. *J Pediatr* 128:536–541, 1996.

41. Bronicki RA, Anas NG: Cardiopulmonary interaction. *Pediatr Crit Care Med* 10:313–322, 2009.

42. Brown CG, Dzwonczyk R: Signal analysis of the human electrocardiogram during ventricular fibrillation: frequency and amplitude parameters as predictors of successful countershock. *Ann Emerg Med* 27(2):184–188, 1996.

43. Brown NJ, Vaughan DE: Angiotensin-converting enzyme inhibitors. *Circulation* 97:1411–1420, 1998.

44. Bunnell E, Parrillo JE: Cardiac dysfunction during septic shock. *Clin Chest Med* 17:237–248, 1996.

45. Burch M: Heart failure in the young. *Heart* 88:198–202, 2002.

46. Burns JP: Septic shock in the pediatric patient: pathogenesis and novel treatments. *Pediatr Emerg Care* 19(2):112–115, 2003.

47. Burton AL: The law of the heart. In Burton AC, editor: *Physiology and biophysics of the circulation*, Chicago, 1972, Year Book Medical Publishers.

48. Cameron JL, Fontanarosa PB, Passalaqua AM: A comparative study of peripheral to central circulation delivery times between intraosseous and intravenous injection using a radionuclide technique in normovolemic and hypovolemic canines. *J Emerg Med* 7(2):123–127, 1989.

49. Canter CE, Strauss AW: Cardiomyopathies—when to think of congenital causes. *Contemp Pediatr* 12:25–40, 1995.

50. Carcillo JA, David AL, Zaritsky A: Role of early fluid resuscitation in pediatric septic shock. *J Am Med Assoc* 266:1242–1245, 1991.

51. Carcillo JA, Cunnion RE: Septic shock. *Crit Care Clinics* 13:553–574, 1997.

52. Carcillo JA, et al: Clinical practice parameters for hemodynamic support of pediatric and neonatal patients in septic shock. *Crit Care Med* 30:1365–1378, 2002.

53. Carcillo JA, et al: Shock: an overview. In Wheeler DS, et al., editors: *Resuscitation and stabilization of the critically ill child*, London, 2009, Springer-Verlag, pp. 89–113.

54. Carter BG, Butt W, Taylor A: ICP and CPP: excellent predictors of long term outcome in severely brain injured children. *Childs Nerv Syst* 24:245–251, 2008.

55. Casella ES, Rogers ML, Zahka KG: Developmental physiology of the cardiovascular system. In Rogers MC, editor: *Textbook of pediatric intensive care*, Baltimore, 1987, Williams and Wilkins.

56. Ceneviva G, et al: Hemodynamic support in fluid-refractory pediatric septic shock. *Pediatrics* 102:e19, 1998.

57. Chameides L, editor: *Textbook of pediatric advanced life support*, Dallas, 1988, American Heart Association.

57a. Chameides L, Samson R, Schexnayder S, Hazinski MF, editors: *Pediatric advanced life support provider manual*, Dallas, 2011, American Heart Association.

58. Checchia PA, Dietrich A, Perkin RM: Current concepts in the recognition and management of pediatric cardiogenic shock and congestive heart failure. *Ped Emerg Med Reports* 5(5):41–60, 2000.

59. Chen D, et al: Cytokines and acute heart failure. *Crit Care Med* 26 (Suppl.):S9–S16, 2008.

60. Chesnut RM: Avoidance of hypotension: Condition sine qua non of successful severe head-injury management. *J Trauma* 42:S4–S9, 1997.

61. Choi P, et al: Crystalloids vs. colloids in fluid resuscitation: a systematic review. *Crit Care Med* 27:200–210, 1999.

62. Choong K, Kisson N: Vasopressin in pediatric shock and cardiac arrest. *Pediatr Crit Care Med* 9:372–379, 2008.

63. Cobb JP: Use of nitric oxide synthase inhibitors to treat septic shock: the light has changed from yellow to red. *Crit Care Med* 27:855–856, 1999.

64. Costello JM, Goodman DM, Green TP: A review of the natriuretic hormone system's diagnostic and therapeutic potential in critically ill children. *Pediatr Crit Care Med* 7(4):308–318, 2006.

65. Critchley L, Peng Z, Fok B: Testing the reliability of a new ultrasound cardiac output monitor, the USCOM, by using aortic flow probes in anesthetized dogs. *Anesth Analg* 100(3):748–753, 2005.

66. Crookes BA, et al: Noninvasive muscle oxygenation to guide fluid resuscitation after traumatic shock. *Surgery* 135:662–670, 2004.

67. de Jonge RCJ, Polderman KH, Gemke R: Central venous catheter use in the pediatric patient: Mechanical and infectious complications. *Pediatr Crit Care Med* 6:329–339, 2005.

68. De Kleijn ED, et al: Low serum cortisol in combination with high adrenocorticotrophic hormone concentrations is associated with poor

outcome in children with severe meningococcal disease. *Pediatr Infect Dis J* 21:330–336, 2002.

69. Dean JM, et al: Age-related changes in chest geometry during cardiopulmonary resuscitation. *J Appl Physiol* 62(6):2212–2219, 1987.

70. DeBacker D, et al: Comparison of dopamine and norepinephrine in the treatment of shock. *N Engl J Med* 362:779–789, 2010.

71. Dellinger RP, et al: Surviving sepsis campaign: international guidelines for management of severe sepsis and septic shock. *Crit Care Med* 36(1):196–327, 2008.

72. deOliveira CF, et al: ACCM/PALS haemodynamic support guidelines for paediatric septic shock: an outcomes comparison with and without monitoring central venous oxygen saturation. *Intensive Care Med* 34:1065–1075, 2008.

73. Diana MC, et al: Sudden death in an infant revealing atypical Kawasaki disease. *Pediatr Emerg Care* 22(1):35–37, 2006.

74. Didwania A, et al: Effect of intravenous lactated Ringer's solution infusion on the circulating lactate concentration. *Crit Care Med* 25:1851–1854, 1997.

75. Domico M, et al: Elevation of brain natriuretic peptide level in children with septic shock. *Pediatr Crit Care Med* 9:478–483, 2008.

76. Dominquez SR, et al: Kawasaki disease in a pediatric intensive care unit: a case-control study. *Pediatrics* 122:e786–e790, 2008.

77. Donoghue A, et al: Bradycardia in children. *Pediatrics* 124 (6):1541–1548, 2009. Epub 2009 Nov 16.

78. Dowd MD, Krug S: Pediatric blunt cardiac injury: epidemiology, clinical features, and diagnosis. *J Trauma* 40:61–67, 1996.

79. Driscoll DJ: Left-to-right shunt lesions. *Pediatr Clin North Am* 46:355–368, 1999.

80. Dudley NC, et al: The effect of family presence on the efficiency of pediatric trauma resuscitations. *Ann Emerg Med* 53(6):777–784, 2009. e773.

81. Dueck MH, et al: Trends but not individual values of central venous oxy gen saturation agree with mixed venous oxygen saturation during varying hemodynamic conditions. *Anesthesiology* 103(2): 249–257, 2005.

82. Dung NM, et al: Fluid replacement in dengue shock syndrome: a randomized, double-blind comparison of four intravenous-fluid regimens. *Clin Infect Dis* 29:787–794, 1999.

83. Duser MW, et al: Ischemic skin lesions as a complication of continuous vasopressin infusion in catecholamine-resistant vasodilatory shock: incidence and risk factors. *Crit Care Med* 31:1394–1398, 2003.

84. Eftestol T, Sunde K, Steen PA: Effects of interrupting precordial compressions on the calculated probability of defibrillation success during out-of-hospital cardiac arrest. *Circulation* 105(19):2270–2273, 2002.

85. Eisenberg M, Bergner L, Halstrom A: Epidemiology of cardiac arrest and resuscitation in children. *Ann Emerg Med* 12:672, 1983.

86. Ellis DY, et al: Cricoid pressure in emergency department rapid sequence tracheal intubations: a risk-benefit analysis. *Ann Emerg Med* 50(6):653–665, 2007.

87. El-Nawawy A, et al: Intravenous polyclonal immunoglobulin administration to sepsis syndrome patients: a prospective study in a pediatric intensive care unit. *J Trop Pediatr* 51:271–278, 2005.

88. Emory EF, Greenough A: Efficacy of low-dose dopamine infusion. *Acute Paediatr* 82:430–432, 1993.

89. Ernest D, Belzberg AS, Dodek PM: Distribution of normal saline and 5% albumin infusion in septic patients. *Crit Care Med* 27:46–50, 1999.

90. Fakler U, Pauli C, Balling G, Lorenz HP, Eicken A, Hennig M, et al: Cardiac index monitoring by pulse contour analysis and thermodilution after pediatric cardiac surgery. *J Thorac Cardiovasc Surg* 133(1):224–228, 2007.

91. Fadel PJ, et al: Noninvasive assessment of sympathetic vasoconstriction in human and rodent skeletal muscle using near-infrared spectroscopy and Doppler ultrasound. *J Appl Physiol* 96:1323–1330, 2004.

92. Falk JL, O'Brien JF, Kerr R: Fluid resuscitation in traumatic hemorrhagic shock. *Crit Care Clin* 8:323–340, 1992.

93. Faustino EV, Apkon M: Persistent hyperglycemia in critically ill children. *J pediatr* 146:30–34, 2005.

94. Fedderly RT: Left ventricular outflow obstruction. *Pediatr Clin North Am* 46:369–383, 1999.

95. Feneley MP, et al: Influence of compression rate on initial success of resuscitation and 24 hour survival after prolonged manual cardiopulmonary resuscitation in dogs. *Circulation* 77(1):240–250, 1988.

96. Finfer S, et al: A comparison of albumin and saline for fluid resuscitation in the intensive care unit. *N Engl J Med* 350(22):2247–2256, 2004.

97. Fried I, et al: Comparison of N-terminal Pro-B-Type natriuretic peptide levels in critically ill children with sepsis versus acute left ventricular dysfunction. *Pediatrics* 118:e1165, 2006.

98. Friedman WF, George BL: Treatment of congestive heart failure by altering loading conditions of the heart. *J Pediatr* 106:697, 1985.

99. Gaines BA, Ford HR: Abdominal and pelvic trauma in children. *Crit Care Med* 30(11 Suppl.):S416–S423, 2002.

100. Gausch WH: Diagnosis and treatment of heart failure based on left ventricular systolic or diastolic dysfunction. *J Am Med Assoc* 271:1276–1280, 1994.

101. Gazmuri RJ, et al: Cardiac effects of carbon dioxide-consuming and carbon dioxide-generating buffers during cardiopulmonary resuscitation. *J Am Coll Cardiol* 15(2):482–490, 1990.

102. Gazmuri R, et al: Arterial PCO_2 as an indicator of systemic perfusion during CPR. *Crit Care Med* 17:237, 1989.

103. Gazmuri R, et al: Cardiac effects of carbon dioxide-consuming and carbon dioxide-generating buffers during cardiopulmonary resuscitation. *J Am Coll Cardiol* 15:482, 1990.

104. Gillis J, et al: Results of inpatient pediatric resuscitation. *Crit Care Med* 14:469, 1986.

105. Gluckman PD, et al: Selective head cooling with mild systemic hypothermia after neonatal encephalopathy: multicentre randomised trial. *Lancet* 365(9460):663–670, 2005.

106. Goetting MG, Paradis NA: High dose epinephrine in refractory pediatric cardiac arrest. *Crit Care Med* 17:1258, 1989.

107. Goetting MG, Paradis NA: High-dose epinephrine improves outcome from pediatric cardiac arrest. *Ann Emerg Med* 20:22, 1990.

108. Goldman AP, et al: Extracorporeal support for intractable cardiorespiratory failure due to meningococcal disease. *Lancet* 349:466–469, 1997.

109. Goldstein B, et al: International pediatric sepsis consensus conference: definitions for sepsis and organ dysfunction in pediatrics. *Pediatr Crit Care Med* 6:2–8, 2005.

110. Goldstein B, et al: ENHANCE: Results of a global open-label trial of Drotrecogin alfa (activated) in children with severe sepsis. *Pediat Crit Care Med* 7:200–211, 2006.

111. Goodfriend TL, Elliot ME, Catt KJ: Angiotensin receptors and their antagonists. *N Engl J Med* 334:1649–1654, 1996.

112. Gorelick MH, Shaw KN, Baker MD: Effect of ambient temperature on capillary refill in healthy children. *Pediatrics* 92:699–702, 1993.

113. Gorelick MH, Shaw KN, Murphy KO: Validity and reliability of clinical signs in the diagnosis of dehydration in children. *Pediatrics* 99:e6, 1997.

114. Greyson CR: Pathophysiology of right ventricular failure. *Crit Care Med* 36(Suppl.):S57–S65, 2008.

115. Grossman W: Diastolic dysfunction in CHF. *N Engl J Med* 325:1557–1564, 1991.

116. Guay J, Lortie L: An evaluation of pediatric in-hospital advanced life support interventions using the pediatric Utstein guidelines: a review of 203 cardiorespiratory arrests. *Can J Anaesth* 51 (4):373–378, 2004.

117. HACA (HACASG): Mild therapeutic hypothermia to improve the neurologic outcome after cardiac arrest. *N Engl J Med* 346(8):549–556, 2002.

118. Haites NE, et al: Assessment of cardiac output by Doppler ultrasound technique alone. *Br Heart J* 53(2):123–129, 1985.

119. Han YY, et al: Early reversal of pediatric-neonatal septic shock by community physicians is associated with improved outcome. *Pediatrics* 112:793–799, 2003.

120. Haque IU, Zaritsky AL: Analysis of the evidence for the lower limit of systolic and mean arterial pressure in children. *Pediatr Crit Care Med* 8(2):138–144, 2007.

121. Hartsilver EL, Vanner RG: Airway obstruction with cricoid pressure. *Anaesthesia* 55(3):208–211, 2000.

122. Haupt MT: Impaired oxygen extraction in sepsis: is supranormal oxygen delivery helpful? *Crit Care Med* 25:904–905, 1997.

123. Haupt MT, Kaufman BS, Carlson RW: Fluid resuscitation in patients with increased vascular permeability. *Crit Care Clin* 8:341–353, 1992.

124. Hayes MA, et al: Oxygen transport patterns in patients with sepsis syndrome or septic shock: influence of treatment and relationship to outcome. *Crit Care Med* 25:926–936, 1997.

125. Hayes MA, et al: Symmetrical peripheral gangrene: association with noradrenaline administration. *Intensive Care Med* 18:433–436, 1992.

126. Hazinski MF, Nolan JN: Part 1: executive summary. In 2010 International Consensus on CPR Science with Treatment Recommendations. *Circulation* 122(Suppl. 2):S250–S275, 2010.

127. Hazinski MF: Sudden cardiac death in children. *Crit Care Q* 7:59, 1984.

128. Heerman W, et al: Accuracy of non-invasive cardiac monitoring (USCOM). *Crit Care Med* 34(12 Suppl. 2):A61, 2006.

129. Hickey RW, et al: Hypothermia and hyperthermia in children after resuscitation from cardiac arrest. *Pediatrics* 106(pt 1)(1):118–122, 2000.

130. Hinkle AJ: A rapid and reliable method of selecting endotracheal tube size in children. *Anesth Analg* 67:S–592, 1988. (abstract).

131. Hirsch R, et al: Cardiac troponin I in pediatrics: normal values and potential use in the assessment of cardiac injury. *J Pediatr* 130:872–877, 1997.

132. Hoffman GM, Ghanayem NS, Tweddell JS: Noninvasive assessment of cardiac output. *Semin Thorac Cardiovasc Surg Pediatr Card Surg Ann* 8:12–21, 2005.

133. Hoffman GM, et al: Changes in cerebral and somatic oxygenation during stage 1 palliation of hypoplastic left heart syndrome using continuous regional cerebral perfusion. *J Thorac Cardiovasc Surg* 127:223–233, 2004.

134. Hoffman TM, et al: Efficacy and safety of milrinone in preventing low cardiac output syndrome in infants and children after corrective surgery for congenital heart disease. *Circulation* 107:996–1002, 2003.

135. Hotchkiss RS, Karl IE: The pathophysiology and treatment of sepsis. *N Engl J Med* 348:138–150, 2003.

136. Hunter JJ, Chien KR: Signaling pathways for cardiac hypertrophy and failure. *N Engl J Med* 341:1276–1283, 1999.

137. Inwald DP, et al: Emergency management of children with severe sepsis in the United Kingdom: the results of the Paediatric Intensive Care Society sepsis audit. *Arch Dis Child* 94:348–353, 2009.

138. Jacobs BR: Central venous catheter occlusion and thrombosis. *Crit Care Clin* 19:489–514, 2003.

139. Jezierski M: Infant death: guidelines for support of parents in the emergency department. *J Emerg Nurs* 15(6):475–476, 1989.

140. Kahn JM, Kress JP, Hall JB: Skin necrosis after extravasation of low-dose vasopressin administered for septic shock. *Crit Care Med* 30:1899–1901, 2002.

141. Kallen RJ: The management of diarrheal dehydration in infants using parenteral fluids. *Pediatr Clin North Am* 37:265, 1990.

142. Kanaan US, Chiang VW: Cardiac troponins in pediatrics. *Pediatr Emerg Care* 20(5):323–329, 2004.

143. Kanegaye JT, et al: Recognition of a Kawasaki disease shock syndrome. *Pediatrics* 123(5):e783–e789, 2009.

144. Kanter RK, et al: Pediatric emergency intravenous access: evaluation of a protocol. *Am J Dis Child* 140:132, 1986.

145. Kellum JA, Decker J: Use of dopamine in acute renal failure: a meta-analysis. *Crit Care Med* 29:1526–1531, 2001.

146. Kern KB, et al: Importance of continuous chest compressions during cardiopulmonary resuscitation: improved outcome during a simulated single lay-rescuer scenario. *Circulation* 105(5):645–649, 2002.

147. Kern KB, et al: A study of chest compression rates during cardiopulmonary resuscitation in humans. The importance of rate-directed chest compressions. *Arch Intern Med* 152(1):145–149, 1992.

148. Kitamura T, et al: Conventional and chest-compression-only cardiopulmonary resuscitation by bystanders for children who have out-of-hospital cardiac arrests: a prospective, nationwide, population-based cohort study. *Lancet* 375(9723):1347–1354, 2010.

149. Kleinman M, et al: Part 14, pediatric advanced life support in 2010 American heart association guidelines for cardiopulmonary resuscitation and emergency cardiovascular care. *Circulation* 122(Suppl. 3): S876–S908s, 2010.

150. Klemperer JD, et al: Thyroid hormone treatment after coronary-artery bypass surgery. *N Engl J Med* 333:1522–1527, 1995.

151. Klinzing S, et al: High dose vasopressin is not superior to norepinephrine in septic shock. *Crit Care Med* 31:2646–2650, 2003.

152. Knapp JF: Practical issues in the care of pediatric trauma patients. *Curr Probl Pediatr* 28(10):305–328, 1998.

153. Knoester H, et al: Cardiac function in pediatric septic shock survivors. *Arch Pediatr Adolesc Med* 162(12):1164–1168, 2008.

154. Konstantinides S: Acute pulmonary embolism. *N Engl J Med* 359 (26):2804–2813, 2008.

155. Korth SK: Unexpected pediatric death in the emergency department: supporting the family. *J Emerg Nurs* 14:302, 1988.

156. Kouwenhoven WB, Jude JR, Knickerbocker GG: Closed-chest cardiac massage. *J Am Med Assoc* 173:1064–1067, 1960.

157. Krivitski NM, Kislukhin W, Thuramalla NV: Theory and in-vitro validation of a new extracorporeal AV loop approach for hemodynamic assessment in pediatric and neonatal ICU patients. *Pediatr Crit Care Med* 9(4):423–428, 2008.

158. Kurth CD, Levy WJ, McCann J: Near-infrared spectroscopy cerebral oxygen saturation thresholds for hypoxia-ischemia in piglets. *J Cereb Blood Flow Metab* 22:335–341, 2002.

159. Lacroix J, Cotting J: Severity of illness and organ dysfunction scoring in children. *Pediatr Crit Care Med* 6(3):S126–S134, 2005.

160. Lacroix J, et al: Transfusion strategies for patients in pediatric intensive care units. *N Engl J Med* 356:1609–1619, 2007.

161. Lambermont B, et al: Effects of endotoxic shock on right ventricular systolic function and mechanical efficiency. *Cardiovasc Res* 59:412–418, 2003.

162. Landry DW, Oliver JA: The pathogenesis of vasodilatory shock. *N Engl J Med* 345(8):588–595, 2001.

163. Laurent I, et al: Reversible myocardial dysfunction in survivors of -out-of-hospital cardiac arrest. *J Am Coll Cardiol* 40(12):2110–2116, 2002.

164. Leclere F, et al: Cumulative influence of organ dysfunctions and septic state on mortality of critically ill children. *Am J Respir Crit Care Ced* 171:348–353, 2005.

165. Levi M: Disseminated intravascular coagulation. *Crit Care Med* 35:2191–2195, 2007.

166. Levi M, vander Poll T: Inflammation and coagulation. *Crit Care Med* 38(Suppl.):S26–S34, 2010.

167. Levin ER: Endothelins. *N Engl J Med* 333:356–363, 1995.

168. Levin ER, Gardner DG, Samson WK: Natriuretic peptides. *N Engl J Med* 339:321–328, 1998.

169. Levine HF, Gausch WH: Diastolic compliance of the left ventricle. *Med Concepts Cardiovasc Dis* 47:95, 1978.

170. Levy JH: Treating shock—old drugs, new ideas. *N Engl J Med* 362 (9):841–842, 2010.

171. Lewis JK, et al: Outcome of pediatric resuscitation. *Ann Emerg Med* 12:297, 1983.

172. Liang KV, et al: Acute decompensation heart failure and the cardiorenal syndrome. *Crit Care Med* 36(Suppl.):S75–S88, 2008.

173. Liedel JL, et al: Use of vasopressin in refractory hypotension in children with vasodilatory shock: five cases and a review of the literature. *Pediatr Crit Care Med* 3(1):15–18, 2002.

174. Lindsay CA, et al: Pharmacokinetics and pharmodynamics of milrinone lactate in pediatric patients with septic shock. *J Pediatr* 132:329–334, 1998.

175. Little WC, Freeman GL: Pericardial disease. *Circulation* 113:1622–1632, 2006.

176. Lodha R, et al: Serial circulating vasopressin levels in children with septic shock. *Pediatric Crit Care Med* 7:220–224, 2006.

177. Lopez-Herce J, et al: Characteristics and outcome of cardiorespiratory arrest in children. *Resuscitation* 63(3):311–320, 2004.

178. Lopez-Herce JC, et al: Outcome of out-of-hospital cardiorespiratory arrest in children. *Pediatr Emerg Care* 21(12):807–815, 2005.

179. Lubitz DS, et al: A rapid method for estimating weight and resuscitation drug dosages from length in the pediatric age group. *Ann Emerg Med* 17:576, 1988.

180. Lucking SE, et al: Dependence of oxygen consumption on oxygen delivery in children with hyperdynamic septic shock and low oxygen extraction. *Crit Care Med* 18:1316–1318, 1990.

181. Luckner G, et al: Arginine vasopressin in 316 patients with advanced vasodilatory shock. *Crit Care Med* 33:2659–2666, 2005.

182. Luscher TF: The endothelium and cardiovascular disease—a complex relation. *N Engl J Med* 330:1081–1083, 1994.

183. Maar SP: Searching for the Holy Grail: a review of markers of tissue perfusion in pediatric critical care. *Pediatr Emerg Care* 24(12):883–887, 2008.

184. Macicek SM, et al: Acute heart failure syndromes in the pediatric emergency department. *Pediatrics* 124:e898–e904, 2009.

185. MacLeod J, et al: Predictors of mortality in trauma patients. *Am Surg* 70:805–810, 2004.

186. Mahar KO, et al: B-type natriuretic peptide in the emergency diagnosis of critical heart disease in children. *Pediatrics* 121: e1484–e1488, 2008.

187. Mahle WT: A dangerous case of colic: anomalous left coronary artery presenting with paroxysms of irritability. *Pediatr Emerg Care* 14:24–27, 1998.

188. Mahle WT, et al: Nesiritide in infants and children with congestive heart failure. *Pediatr Crit Care Med* 6:543–546, 2005.

189. Maier GW, et al: The physiology of external cardiac massage: high-impulse cardiopulmonary resuscitation. *Circulation* 70(1):86–101, 1984.

190. Marik PE: Critical illness-related corticosteroid insufficiency. *Chest* 135:181–193, 2009.

191. Marik PE, Varon J: The hemodynamic derangements in sepsis: implications for treatment strategies. *Chest* 114:854–860, 1998.

192. Markovitz BP, et al: A retrospective cohort study of prognostic factors associated with outcome in pediatric severe sepsis: what is the role of steroids? *Pediatr Crit Care Med* 6:270–274, 2005.

193. Marshall JC, Charbonney E, Gonzako PD: The immune system in critical illness. *Clin Chest Med* 29:605–616, 2008.

194. Martin JB, Wheeler AP: Approach to the patient with sepsis. *Clin Chest Med* 30:1–16, 2009.

195. Martinot A, et al: Sepsis in neonates and children: definitions, epidemiology, and outcome. *Pediatr Emerg Care* 13:277–281, 1997.

196. Marx G, Reinhart K: Venous oximetry. *Curr Opin Crit Care* 12 (3):263–268, 2006.

197. Matok I, et al: Terlipressin after children with extremely low cardiac output after open heart surgery. *Ann Pharmacother* 43:423–429, 2009.

198. Mazzoni ML, et al: Lumenal narrowing and endothelial cell swelling in skeletal muscle capillaries during hemorrhagic shock. *Circ Shock* 29:27–39, 1989.

199. Mazzoni ML, et al: Capillary narrowing in hemorrhagic shock is rectified by hyperosmotic saline-dextron reinfusion. *Circ Shock* 31:407–418, 1990.

200. McKiernan CA, Liberman SA: Circulatory shock in children: an overview. *Pediatr Rev* 26(12):451–459, 2005.

201. McLean AS, et al: Prognostic values of B-type natriuretic peptide in severe sepsis and septic shock. *Crit Care Med* 35:1019–1026, 2007.

202. Meadows D, et al: Reversal of intractable septic shock with norepinephrine therapy. *Crit Care Med* 16:663–666, 1988.

203. Meaney PA, et al: Higher survival rates among younger patients after pediatric intensive care unit cardiac arrests. *Pediatrics* 118 (6):2424–2433, 2006.

204. Mettauer N, Brierley J: A novel use of etomidate for intentional adrenal suppression to control severe hypercortisolemia of childhood. *Pediatr Crit Care Med* 10:e37–e40, 2009.

205. Meyer DM, Jessen ME: Results of extracorporeal membrane oxygenation in children with sepsis: the Extracorporeal Life Support Organization. *Ann Thorac Surg* 63:756–761, 1997.

206. Meyer RA: Echocardiography. In Admas FH, Emmanouilides GC, Riemenschneider S, editors: *Moss' heart disease in infants, children and adolescents*, Baltimore, 1989, Williams and Wilkins.

207. Meyer RJ, et al: Post-resuscitation right ventricular dysfunction: delineation and treatment with dobutamine. *Resuscitation* 55(2):187–191, 2002.

208. Michael JR, et al: Mechanisms by which epinephrine augments cerebral and myocardial perfusion during cardiopulmonary resuscitation in dogs. *Circulation* 69:822, 1984.

209. Moffett BS, Price JF: Evaluation of sodium nitroprusside toxicity in pediatric cardiac surgical patients. *Ann Pharmacother* 42:1600–1604, 2008.

210. Moncada S, Higgs A: The L-arginine-nitric oxide pathway. *N Engl J Med* 329:2002–2012, 1993.

211. Morris MC, Wernovsky G, Nadkarni VM: Survival outcomes after extracorporeal cardiopulmonary resuscitation instituted during active chest compressions following refractory in-hospital pediatric cardiac arrest. *Pediatr Crit Care Med* 5(5):440–446, 2004.

212. Munt B, et al: Diastolic filling in human severe sepsis: an echocardiographic study. *Crit Care Med* 26:1829–1833, 1998.

213. Nadel S, et al: Drotrecogin alpha (activated) in children with severe sepsis: a multicentre phase III randomized controlled trial. *Lancet* 369:836–843, 2007.

214. Nadkarni VM, et al: First documented rhythm and clinical outcome from in-hospital cardiac arrest among children and adults. *J Am Med Assoc* 295(1):50–57, 2006.

215. Namachivayam P, et al: Early experience with Levosimendan in children with ventricular dysfunction. *Pediatr Crit Care Med* 7:445–448, 2006.

216. Narula J, Kharbandu S, Khan B: Apoptosis and the heart. *Chest* 112:1358–1362, 1997.

217. Nasser N, Bar-Oz B, Nir A: Natriuretic peptides and heart disease in infants and children. *J Pediatr* 248–253, 2005.

218. Newburger JW, et al: Diagnosis, treatment, and long-term management of Kawasaki disease: a statement for health professionals from the committee on rheumatic fever, endocarditis, Kawasaki disease, Council on Cardiovascular Disease in the Young, American Heart Association. *Pediatrics* 114(6):1708–1733, 2004.

219. Newth CJ, et al: The use of cuffed versus uncuffed endotracheal tubes in pediatric intensive care. *J Pediatr* 144(3):333–337, 2004.

220. Ngo NT, et al: Acute management of dengue shock syndrome: a randomized double-blind comparison of 4 intravenous fluid regimens in the first hour. *Clin Infect Dis* 32:204–213, 2001.

221. Nichols DG, et al: Factors influencing outcome of cardiopulmonary arrest in children. *Pediatr Emerg Care* 2:1, 1986.

222. Niemann JT, et al: Milrinone facilitates resuscitation from cardiac arrest and attenuates postresuscitation myocardial dysfunction. *Circulation* 108(24):3031–3035, 2003.

223. Niemann JT, Stratton SJ: Endotracheal versus intravenous epinephrine and atropine in out-of-hospital "primary" and postcountershock asystole. *Crit Care Med* 28(6):1815–1819, 2000.

224. Niemann JT, et al: Pressure-synchronized cine-angiography during experimental cardiopulmonary resuscitation. *Circulation* 64:985, 1981.

225. Nieves J, Kohr L: Nursing considerations in the care of patients with pulmonary hypertension. *Pediatr Crit Care Med* 11(Suppl.): S74–S78, 2010.

226. Nimah M, Brilli RJ: Coagulation dysfunction in sepsis and multiple organ system failure. *Crit Care Clin* 19:441–458, 2003.

227. Ninis N, et al: The role of healthcare delivery in the outcome of meningococcal disease in children: case-control study of fatal and non-fatal cases. *BMJ* 330:1475, 2005.

228. Nollert G, Jonas RA, Reichart B: Optimizing cerebral oxygenation during cardiac surgery: a review of experimental and clinical investigations with near infrared spectrophotometry. *Thorac Cardiovasc Surg* 48:247–253, 2000.

229. O'Connor CM, Gattis WA, Swedberg K: Current and novel pharmacologic approaches in advanced heart failure. *Heart Lung* 28:227–239, 1999.

230. Olasveengen TM, et al: Intravenous drug administration during out-of-hospital cardiac arrest: a randomized trial. *J Am Med Assoc* 302 (20):2222–2229, 2009.

231. Opal SM: Concept of PIRO as a new conceptual framework to understand sepsis. *Pediatr Crit Care Med* 6(3):S55–S60, 2005.

232. Opal SM, Cohen J: Clinical gram-positive sepsis: does it fundamentally differ from gram-negative bacterial sepsis? *Crit Care Med* 1608–1616, 1999.

233. Orlowski JP: Optimum position for external cardiac compression in infants and young children. *Ann Emerg Med* 15:667, 1986.

234. O'Rourke PP: Outcome of children who are apneic and pulseless in the emergency room. *Crit Care Med* 14:466, 1986.

235. Pacher R, et al: Prognostic impact of big endothelin-1 plasma concentrations compared with invasive hemodynamic evaluation in severe heart failure. *J Am Coll Cardiol* 27:633–641, 1996.

236. Paradis NA, et al: Coronary perfusion pressure and the return of spontaneous circulation in human cardiopulmonary resuscitation. *J Am Med Assoc* 263(8):1106–1113, 1990.

237. Parasuraman S, Goldhabar SZ: Venous thromboembolism in children. *Circulation* 113(2):e12–e16, 2006.

238. Parker MM: Pathophysiology of cardiovascular dysfunction in septic shock. *New Horizons* 6:130–138, 1998.

239. Parker MM: Pediatric definitions for sepsis: it's about time. *Pediatr Crit Care Med* 6(1):83, 2005.

240. Parrillo JE: Septic shock—vasopressin, norepinephrine, and urgency. *N Engl J Med* 358(9):954–955, 2008.

241. Pathan N, Faust SN, Levin M: Pathophysiology of meningococcal meningitis and septicaemia. *Arch Dis Child* 88:601–607, 2003.

242. Patterson SW, Starling EH: On the mechanical factors which determine the output of the ventricle. *J Physiol* 48:357, 1914.
243. Perkin RM: Current concepts in the recognition and management of pediatric hypovolemic and septic shock. *Pediatr Emerg Med Rep* 4 (10):95–114, 1999.
244. Perkin RM, Anas NG: Nonsurgical contractility manipulation of the failing circulation. In Swellow DB, Raphaely RL, editors: *Cardiovascular problems in pediatric critical care*, New York, 1986, Churchhill Livingstone, pp. 229–256.
245. Perkin RM: Levin DL. Shock in the pediatric patient. Part I. *J Pediatr* 101:163–169, 1982.
246. Perkin RM, Levin DL: Shock in the pediatric patient. Part II. Therapy. *J Pediatr* 101:319–332, 1982.
247. Perkin RM, et al: Dobutamine: a hemodynamic evaluation in children with shock. *J Pediatr* 100:977–983, 1982.
248. Perondi MB, et al: A comparison of high-dose and standard-dose epinephrine in children with cardiac arrest. *N Engl J Med* 350 (17):1722–1730, 2004.
249. Petre R, Chilcott M: Blunt trauma to the heart and great vessels. *N Engl J Med* 336:626–632, 1997.
250. Pitt B: Blockade of the renin-angiotensin system. *Cardiol Clin* 12:101–113, 1994.
251. Pitt B, et al: The effect of spironolactone on morbidity and mortality in patients with severe heart failure. *N Engl J Med* 334:709–717, 1999.
252. Pizarro CF, et al: Absolute and relative adrenal insufficiency in children with septic shock. *Crit Care Med* 33:855–859, 2005.
253. Pollack MM, Fields AI, Ruttimann UE: Sequential cardiopulmonary variables of infants and children in septic shock. *Crit Care Med* 12:554–559, 1984.
254. Pollack MM, Fields AI, Ruttiman UE: Distributions of cardiopulmonary variables in pediatric survivors and non-survivors of septic shock. *Crit Care Med* 13:454–459, 1985.
255. Pytte M, et al: Haemodynamic effects of adrenaline (epinephrine) depend on chest compression quality during cardiopulmonary resuscitation in pigs. *Resuscitation* 71(3):369–378, 2006.
256. Raffini L, et al: Dramatic increase in venous thromboembolism in Children's Hospitals in the United States from 2001-2007. *Pediatrics* 124:1001–1008, 2009.
257. Rajagopal SK, et al: Extracorporeal membrane oxygenation for the support of infants, children, and young adults with acute myocarditis: a review of the Extracorporeal Life Support Organization registry. *Crit Care Med* 38:382–387, 2010.
258. Ralston DR, St. John RC: Immunotherapy for sepsis. *Clin Chest Med* 17:307–317, 1996.
259. In Ralston M, et al., editors: *PALS provider manual*, Dallas, 2006, American Heart Association, p. 86.
260. Rhodes A, Bennett ED: Early goal-directed therapy: an evidence-based review. *Crit Care Med* 32(Suppl.):S448–S450, 2004.
261. Riordan FA, et al: Admission cortisol and adrenocorticotrophic hormone levels in children with meningococcal disease: evidence of adrenal insufficiency? *Crit Care Med* 27:2257–2261, 1999.
262. Rivers E, et al: Early goal-directed therapy in the treatment of severe sepsis and septic shock. *N Engl J Med* 345:1368–1377, 2001.
263. Rosenweig EB, et al: Intravenous arginine-vasopressin in children with vasodilatory shock after cardiac surgery. *Circulation* 100(19 Suppl.):II182–II486, 1999.
264. Rudiger A, Singer M: Mechanisms of sepsis-induced cardiac dysfunction. *Crit Care Med* 35(6):1599–1608, 2007.
265. Russell JA: Management of sepsis. *N Engl J Med* 355:1699–1713, 2006.
266. Russell JA, et al: Vasopressin versus norepinephrine infusion in patients with septic shock. *N Engl J Med* 358(9):877–887, 2008.
267. Samson RA, et al: Outcomes of in-hospital ventricular fibrillation in children. *N Engl J Med* 354(22):2328–2339, 2006.
268. Schlant RC, Sonnenblick EH, Gorlin R: Normal physiology of the cardiovascular system. In Hurst JW, editor: *The heart, arteries, and veins*, New York, 1990, McGraw-Hill.
269. Schrier RW, Abraham WT: Hormones and hemodynamics in heart failure. *N Engl J Med* 341:577–585, 1999.
270. Schubert S, Schmitz T, Weiss M, Nagdyman N, et al: Continuous non-invasive techniques to determine cardiac output in children after cardiac surgery:evaluatin of transesophageal Doppler and electric velocimetry. *J Clin Monit comput* 22:299–307, 2008.
271. Sebat F, et al: Effect of a rapid response system for patients in shock on time to treatment and mortality during 5 years. *Crit Care Med* 35:2568–2575, 2007.
272. Seri I: Cardiovascular, renal, and endocrine actions of dopamine in neonates and children. *J Pediatr* 126:333–344, 1995.
273. Shaddy RE: Optimizing treatment for chronic congestive heart failure in children. *Pediatr Crit Care Med* 2(4 Suppl.):S69–S72, 2001.
274. Shapiro NI, et al: Isolated prehospital hypotension after traumatic injuries: a predictor of mortality? *J Emerg Med* 25:175–179, 2003.
275. Shippy CR, Appel PL, Shoemaker WC: Reliability of clinical monitoring to assess blood volume in critically ill patients. *Crit Care Med* 12:107, 1984.
276. Shoemaker WC: Relation of oxygen transport patterns to the pathophysiology and therapy of shock states. *Intensive Care Med* 13:231–234, 1987.
277. Shulman DI, et al: Adrenal insufficiency still a cause of morbidity and death in childhood. *Pediatrics* 119(2):e484–e494, 2007.
278. Slaughter MS, et al: Advanced heart failure treated with continuous-flow left ventricular assist device. *N Engl J Med* 361:2241–2251, 2009.
279. Smith BT, Rea TD, Eisenberg MS: Ventricular fibrillation in pediatric cardiac arrest. *Acad Emerg Med* 13:525–529, 2006.
280. Solaro RJ, Rarick HM: Troponin and tropomyosin: proteins that switch on and tune in the activity of cardiac myofilaments. *Circ Res* 83:471–480, 1998.
281. Spivey WHL: Intraosseous infusions. *J Pediatr* 111:639, 1987.
282. Spodick DH: Acute cardiac tamponade. *N Engl J Med* 349(7):684–690, 2003.
283. Sprung CL, et al: Hydrocortisone therapy for patients with septic shock. *N Engl J Med* 358:111–124, 2008.
284. Srinivasan V, et al: Association of timing, duration, and intensity of hyperglycemia with intensive care unit mortality in critically ill children. *Pediatr Crit Care Med* 5:329–336, 2004.
285. Stein PD, Kayali F, Olson RE: Incidence of venous thromboembolism in infants and children: data from the National Hospital Discharge Survey. *J Pediatr* 145:563–565, 2004.
286. Strohmenger HU, et al: Effects of epinephrine and vasopressin on median fibrillation frequency and defibrillation success in a porcine model of cardiopulmonary resuscitation. *Resuscitation* 31(1):65–73, 1996.
287. Sunde K, et al: Implementation of a standardised treatment protocol for post resuscitation care after out-of-hospital cardiac arrest. *Resuscitation* 73(1):29–39, 2007.
288. Sutton RM, et al: Quantitative analysis of CPR quality during in-hospital resuscitation of older children and adolescents. *Pediatrics* 124 (2):494–499, 2009.
289. Symeonides S, Balk RA: Nitric oxide in the pathogenesis of sepsis. *Infect Dis Clin North Am* 13:449–463, 1999.
290. Synder JD: Use and misuse of oral therapy for diarrhea: comparison of U.S. practices with American Academy of Pediatrics recommendations. *Pediatrics* 87:28–33, 1991.
291. Tabbutt S: Heart failure in pediatric septic shock: utilizing inotropic support. *Crit Care Med* 29(10 Suppl.):S231–S236, 2001.
292. Task Force of the American College of Critical Care Medicine and Society of Critical Care Medicine: Practice parameters for hemodynamic support of sepsis in adult patients. *Crit Care Med* 27:639–660, 1999.
293. Taylor MD, Laussen PC: Fundamentals of management of acute postpartum pulmonary hypertension. *Pediatr Crit Care Med* 11 (Suppl.):S27–S29, 2010.
294. Thiagarajan RR, et al: Extracorporeal membrane oxygenation to aid cardiopulmonary resuscitation in infants and children. *Circulation* 116(15):1693–1700, 2007.
295. Thomas NJ, Carcillo JA: Hypovolemic shock in pediatric patients. *New Horiz* 6:120–129, 1998.
296. Tibballs J, Kinney S: Reduction of hospital mortality and of preventable cardiac arrest and death on introduction of a pediatric medical emergency team. *Pediatr Crit Care Med* 10(3):306–312, 2009.
297. Tibby SM, Hatherill M, Murdoch IA: Capillary refill and core-peripheral temperature gap as indicators of hemodynamic status in pediatric intensive care patients. *Arch Dis Child* 80:163–166, 1999.
298. Tinsley C, et al: Experience of families during cardiopulmonary resuscitation in a pediatric intensive care unit. *Pediatrics* 122(4):e799–e804, 2008.
299. Topalian S, Ginsberg F, Parillo JE: Cardiogenic shock. *Crit Care Med* 36(Suppl.):S66–S74, 2008.
300. Truitt AK, et al: Pulmonary embolism: which pediatric trauma patients are at risk? *J Pediatr Surg* 40:124–127, 2005.

301. Turanlahti M, et al: Pharmacokinetics of Levosimendan in pediatric patients evaluated for cardiac surgery. *Pediatr Crit Care Med* 5:457–462, 2004.

302. Udomphorn Y, Armstead WM, Vavilala MS: Cerebral blood flow and autoregulation after pediatric traumatic brain injury. *Pediatr Neurol* 38:225–234, 2008.

303. Upadhyay M: Randomized evaluation of fluid resuscitation with crystalloid (saline) and colloid (polymer from degraded Gelatin) in pediatric septic shock. *Indian Pediatr* 42(3):223–231, 2005.

304. Van den Berghe G, De Zeghar F, Lauwers P: Dopamine suppresses pituitary function in infants and children. *Crit Care Med* 22:1747–1753, 1994.

305. Van der Poll T, van Deventer SJH: Cytokines and anticytokines in the pathogenesis of sepsis. *Infect Dis Clin North Am* 13:413–426, 1999.

306. van Haren FM, Rozendaal FW, vander Hoevan JG: The effect of vasopressin on gastric perfusion in catecholamine-dependent patients in septic shock. *Chest* 124:2256–2260, 2003.

307. Vinclair M, et al: Duration of adrenal inhibition following a single dose of etomidate in critically ill patients. *Intensive Care Med* 34:714–719, 2008.

308. Von Seggern K, Egar M, Fuhrman BP: Cardiopulmonary resuscitation in a pediatric ICU. *Crit Care Med* 14:275, 1986.

309. Walsh CK, Krongrad E: Terminal cardiac electrical activity in pediatric patients. *Am J Cardiol* 51:557, 1983.

310. Weber KT: Aldosterone and spironolactone in heart failure. *N Engl J Med* 341:753–755, 1999.

311. Weiler H: Regulation of inflammation by the protein C system. *Crit Care Med* 38(2 Suppl.):S18–S25, 2010.

312. Weinberger HD: Diagnosis and treatment of diastolic heart failure. *Hosp Pract* 34:115–126, 1999.

313. Wessel DL: Managing low cardiac output syndrome after congenital heart surgery. *Pediatr Crit Care Med* 2(Suppl.):S52–S62, 2001.

314. Wessel DL: Testing new drugs for heart failure in children. *Pediatr Crit Care Med* 7:493–494, 2006.

315. Westaby S, Franklin O, Burch M: New developments in the treatment of cardiac failure. *Arch Dis Child* 81:276–277, 1999.

316. Wheeler AP, Bernard GR: Treating patients with severe sepsis. *N Engl J Med* 340:207–214, 1999.

317. Wik L, et al: Quality of cardiopulmonary resuscitation during out-of-hospital cardiac arrest. *J Am Med Assoc* 293(3):299–304, 2005.

318. Williams RS: Apoptosis and heart failure. *N Engl J Med* 341:759–760, 1999.

319. Wills BA, et al: Comparison of three fluid solutions for resuscitation in Dengue shock syndrome. *N Engl J Med* 353(9):877–889, 2008.

320. Wong HR, et al: Increased serum nitrite and nitrate concentrations in children with sepsis syndrome. *Crit Care Med* 23:835–842, 1995.

321. Woodward GA, et al: Sepsis, septic shock, acute abdomen? The ability of cardiac disease to mimic other medical illnesses. *Pediatr Emerg Care* 12:317–324, 1996.

322. Young KD, Seidel JS: Pediatric cardiopulmonary resuscitation: a collective review. *Ann Emerg Med* 33(2):195–205, 1999.

323. Yunge M, Petros A: Angiotensin for septic shock unresponsive to noradrenaline. *Arch Dis Child* 82:388–389, 2000.

324. Zaritsky A: Controversial issues in pediatric cardio-pulmonary resuscitation. *Crit Care Clin* 4:735, 1989.

324a. Zaritsky A, Chernow B: Use of catecholamines in children. *J Pediatr* 105:341–348, 1984.

325. Zaritsky A, et al: CPR in children. *Ann Emerg Med* 16(10):1107–1111, 1987.

326. Zaritsky A: Subcommittee on Pediatric Resuscitation: *Approach to drug therapy in pediatric advanced life support, pediatric advanced life support, course material*, Dallas, 1990, American Heart Association.

327. Zimmerman JJ: A history of adjunctive glucocorticoid treatment for pediatric sepsis: moving beyond steroid pulp fiction toward evidence-based medicine. *Pediatr Crit Care Med* 8:530–539, 2007.

328. Zuercher M, et al: Leaning during chest compression impairs cardiac output and left ventricular myocardial blood flow in piglet cardiac arrest. *Crit Care Med* 38(4):1141–1146, 2010.

Mechanical Support of Cardiopulmonary Function: Extracorporeal Membrane Oxygenation, Ventricular Assist Devices, and the Intraaortic Balloon Pump

7

Nancy A. Pike • Laura A. Klee •
Beth A. Zemetra

e>volve Be sure to check out the supplementary content available at http://evolve.elsevier.com/Hazinski.

PEARLS

- Signs of critically low cardiac output requiring mechanical circulatory support include: mixed venous oxygen saturation less than 40%, increased ventricular end-diastolic filling pressure, cardiac index less than 2 L/min per m^2 body surface area (BSA), persistent metabolic acidosis, oliguria, poor peripheral perfusion, increased inspired oxygen requirements, and poor ventricular function by echocardiogram.
- Mechanical circulatory support (MCS) is indicated when low cardiac output persists despite maximal medical treatment, including afterload reduction combined with inotropes/catecholamines, diuretics, a phosphodiesterase-III inhibitor, fluid and transfusion management, and mechanical ventilation.
- In the pediatric population, ventricular assist devices (VADs) are used to support the failing heart as a "bridge to recovery" or "bridge to transplant."
- MCS should be anticipated and every attempt should be made to initiate support before the development of end-organ dysfunction or circulatory collapse.
- Persistent low filling of a left ventricular assist device (LVAD) pump with rising right atrial pressure is an indication of right-sided heart failure. An echocardiogram is indicated to evaluate ventricular function and check for a pericardial effusion.
- The oxygen index (OI) is often used to identify possible indication for extracorporeal membrane oxygenation (ECMO) for children with respiratory failure.

  $$OI = [(\text{Mean airway pressure} \times FiO_2 \times 100)/PaO_2].$$

  OI greater than 35 on three or more postductal arterial blood gases 30 to 60 minutes apart is an indication for ECMO support.
- Alveolar-arterial (A-a) gradient of 600 to 624 mm Hg is a clinical indication for ECMO. This is computed as follows (NOTE: 47 mm Hg = partial pressure of water vapor):

  $$\begin{aligned}\text{A-a } O_2 \text{ gradient} &= \text{Alveolar } O_2 \text{ tension} - \text{Arterial } O_2 \text{ tension}\\ &= [FiO_2 \times (\text{Barometric pressure in}\\ &\quad \text{mmHg} - 47) - PaCO_2] - PaO_2\\ &= [FiO_2 \times (760 - 47\text{mmHg}) - PaCO_2] - PaO_2\\ &= \text{normal (at sea level) is } <25 \text{ to } 50 \text{ Torr.}\end{aligned}$$

- Signs to change venovenous (VV) ECMO to venoarterial (VA) ECMO include: persistent hypoxia in the presence of hypotension and poor cardiac output on maximal ventilator and inotropic support, nonperfusing arrhythmias, or cardiac arrest.

INTRODUCTION

The child with life-threatening cardiac or respiratory failure that is refractory to maximal medical support may require MCS. Over the last few years, substantial advances in pediatric MCS have occurred, with expanding indications for use, greater availability of devices suitable for pediatrics, and improved outcomes.[16,20]

ECMO and centrifugal ventricular assist devices remain the mainstay of MCS for children.[23] MCS is not a treatment but rather a therapeutic support to provide adequate tissue oxygen delivery and maintain end-organ perfusion and function while the reversible disease responds to treatment. This support has many potential complications and should be used in appropriate patients with specific criteria for initiation.

Use of MCS in the pediatric population requires knowledge of the pathophysiology and treatment of cardiac and respiratory failure (see Chapters 6 to 9). In addition, the critical care nurse and the ECMO specialist require advanced training in MCS, because they must be familiar with the function of the support device, components of the circuit or console, potential complications, and troubleshooting for the device.

The purpose of this chapter is to provide an overview of MCS options in the pediatric population, with an emphasis on ECMO and VAD physiology, patient selection, indications and contraindications, complications, and postoperative nursing care.

Device Selection

The selection of MCS device is influenced by the indication for the device, the duration of support anticipated, and the devices available. Devices are categorized for short- or long-term support. ECMO, centrifugal VADs, and intraaortic balloon pumps (IABPs) are considered short-term modalities. Pulsatile and rotary-axial devices are typically considered long-term modalities.[11]

Pediatric MCS offers a potential "bridge to transplant" or a "bridge to recovery." The term *destination therapy* is used to describe long-term support for patients who are not heart transplant candidates and those whose heart function is unlikely to recover. Currently, no devices are approved by the U.S. Food and Drug Administration (FDA) for destination therapy in children. Three devices approved by the FDA for destination therapy in adults are the HeartMate VE/XVE LVAS and HeartMate II (Thoratec Corporation, Pleasanton, Calif.), and the AbioCor Implantable replacement heart (Abiomed, Danvers, Mass.).[11,55]

EXTRACORPOREAL MEMBRANE OXYGENATION

ECMO remains the most common form of MCS in the pediatric population. ECMO support evolved directly from cardiopulmonary bypass devices beginning with development of the membrane oxygenator in the 1950s.[13,41] In the 1970s, intraoperative cardiopulmonary bypass was successfully used for infants during surgical correction of congenital heart disease.[3] In 1972, successful ECMO support of a 24-year-old trauma victim with acute respiratory distress syndrome by Hill et al.[37] led to a multicenter National Institutes of Health clinical trial of ECMO versus medical management of adult acute respiratory distress syndrome that failed to show a survival advantage with ECMO support, but did lead to widespread improvement in mechanical ventilation in adults.

In 1976, Bartlett et al.[6] reported the first successful use of ECMO for treatment of severe neonatal respiratory distress. Since that time, ECMO has been used successfully in the treatment of neonates with meconium aspiration, congenital diaphragmatic hernia, pneumonia, sepsis, or persistent pulmonary hypertension.[57] ECMO is now used as rescue therapy for pediatric patients with severe refractory respiratory or heart failure unresponsive to maximal conventional treatment.

In 1989, the ECMO centers formed a national organization, the Extracorporeal Life Support Organization to coordinate clinical research, develop ECMO guidelines, and maintain a national registry of all ECMO centers and cases. ECMO follow-up data have documented the cost effectiveness of ECMO compared with conventional support and improved patient outcomes with the use of ECMO.[49]

ECMO Terminology

Bypass therapy outside of the operating suite has been called extracorporeal carbon dioxide removal, extracorporeal heart assist, extracorporeal lung assist, ECMO, and most recently, extracorporeal life support (ECLS). These terms are often used interchangeably, but the term ECMO will be used in this chapter.

ECMO therapy supports cardiopulmonary function through the use of external cardiopulmonary bypass with an oxygenator. ECMO is designed to deliver well-oxygenated blood to an artery or vein, remove carbon dioxide, and normalize acid-base balance and metabolic processes. This system provides temporary pulmonary and possibly cardiac support for infants or children with severe refractory respiratory failure, heart failure, or cardiorespiratory failure, so the failing organs have time to recover or the child is supported until transplantation.

The two types of ECMO support are VA and VV ECMO. VA ECMO provides both cardiac and respiratory support, whereas VV ECMO provides only pulmonary support. The differences between the VA and VV ECMO are summarized in Table 7-1.

The appropriate ECMO circuit size is determined by the weight of the child; the larger the circuit membrane surface area, the greater the potential gas exchange. However, the larger the surface area of the membrane, the higher the platelet consumption and the larger the circuit priming volume. Because the circuit is not typically primed with blood, a high priming volume relative to the child's circulating blood volume will result in hemodilution.

Venoarterial ECMO

Circuit

The VA ECMO circuit is composed of polyvinyl chloride tubing attached to venous and arterial cannulas (Fig. 7-1). The venous cannula is inserted into the internal jugular vein and advanced through the superior vena cava and right atrium to the tricuspid valve. The arterial cannula is placed into the right common carotid artery with the tip of the cannula advanced to the innominate artery. Postoperative cannulation immediately after cardiac surgery is often accomplished through the median sternotomy incision with direct cannulation of the right atrial appendage and the aorta. In adolescent or adult patients, the femoral artery and vein are often used for VA ECMO cannulation.

Table 7-1 Differences Between VA and VV ECMO

VA ECMO	VV ECMO
Achieves higher PaO_2	Achieves lower PaO_2
Requires lower perfusion rates	Requires higher perfusion rates
Bypasses pulmonary circulation	Maintains pulmonary blood flow
Decreases pulmonary artery pressures	Elevates mixed venous PO_2
Provides cardiac support to assist systemic circulation	Does not provide cardiac support to assist systemic circulation
Requires arterial cannulation	Requires only venous cannulation

ECMO, Extracorporeal membrane oxygenation; *PaO₂*, partial pressure of arterial oxygenation; *PO₂*, partial pressure of oxygen; *VA*, venoarterial; *VV*, venovenous.

Venoarterial ECMO Circuit

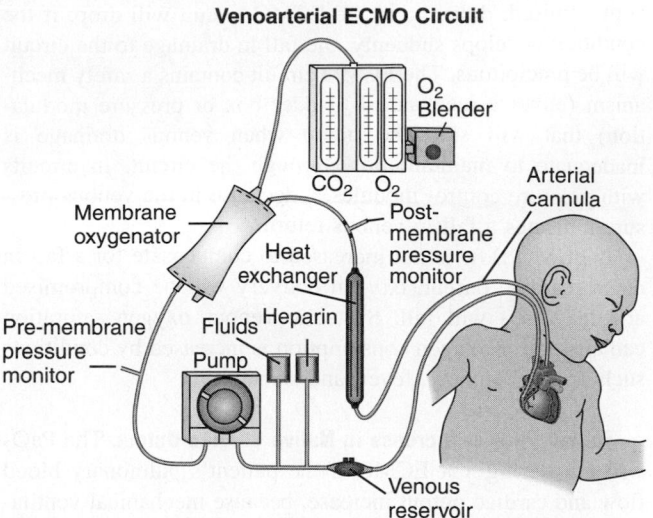

FIG. 7-1 Venoarterial extracorporeal membrane oxygenation circuit. (From Biddle M, Gulanick M, Berra K: Interdisciplinary team in cardiac rehabilitation. In Moser DK, Riegel B, editors: *Cardiac nursing: a companion to Braunwald's heart disease.* Philadelphia, 2008, Saunders.)

The bridge connects the arterial and venous lines and is located near the cannula. The bridge is routinely clamped during ECMO support with brief periods of unclamping to prevent clot formation caused by stagnation of blood in the bridge. If the patient must be separated from ECMO for mechanical complications or for trial periods off ECMO support, the open bridge isolates the patient from the circuit while allowing blood flow to continue through the circuit to prevent stagnation and circuit thrombosis.

Blood from the venous cannula drains passively into a small reservoir called the *bladder.* The ECMO pump draws blood from the bladder, which works like the right atrium. The function of this bladder is to prevent negative pressure from pulling the vessel wall into the cannula, so it reduces risk of damage to the vena cava. The bladder is connected to a servo regulator mechanism that reduces or stops the pump flow if venous return decreases below a minimum threshold.

The tubing from the bladder joins to the ECMO pump, which is either a roller pump or a centrifugal pump. For the past few decades, the roller pump has been used most commonly for ECMO. However, centrifugal pumps are becoming more popular, especially in cardiac ECMO programs and for extracorporeal cardiopulmonary resuscitation. The roller pump functions on the principles of compression and displacement; blood is displaced as rollers travel the length of the raceway (the segment of tubing contained within the pump head). A strong polymer tubing, called *Tygon,* is used in the raceway because it is resistant to creasing and erosion.

Blood leaving the pump enters the membrane oxygenator. The membrane consists of a thin silicon rubber sheath with a plastic screen spacer inside to create a semipermeable membrane separating the gas compartment from the compartment containing the patient's blood. As the patient's blood flows past one side of the membrane, oxygen diffuses from the gas side across the membrane into the blood, and carbon dioxide from the blood diffuses through the membrane into the gas

compartment. The carbon dioxide is then removed, or "swept out" of the system, by the ventilating gas. This ventilating gas is also referred to as the *sweep gas,* and it is regulated by a flow meter from an oxygen blender. The amount of oxygen in the sweep gas and the available surface area for diffusion determines the amount of oxygen delivered to the patient's blood as it flows through the oxygenator. The rate of carbon dioxide removal is also dependent on the amount of sweep gas flow and the surface area. The movement of both oxygen and carbon dioxide are dependent on the pressure gradients for the gases across the membrane.

As the blood moves through the ECMO circuit, heat is lost, so ECMO systems use a heat exchanger to keep the blood warm. The heat exchanger is located either between the oxygenator and the patient or integrated into the oxygenator. When the heat exchanger is placed between the oxygenator and the patient, it also serves as a bubble trap.

The blood returns to the patient from the heat exchanger through an arterial cannula inserted into the right common carotid artery. The tip of the cannula is just proximal to the junction of the brachiocephalic artery and the aorta. With this type of cannulation, ECMO becomes essentially a cardiopulmonary bypass system. The greater the ECMO pump flow, the greater the oxygen delivery.

Venoarterial ECMO Flow and Function

In VA ECMO, blood is drained from the right side of the heart and is returned to the arterial side of the circulation, so that it bypasses the heart. Highly oxygenated blood is returned to the arterial circuit, where it mixes with the blood that the native heart is ejecting into the arterial circulation. Ventilator support is minimal, so blood returning from the lungs is relatively desaturated. As ECMO flow increases, the relative percentage of highly oxygenated blood in the arterial circulation is increased. Therefore, the patient's partial pressure of arterial oxygen (PaO_2) increases with increased ECMO flow. With inadequate ECMO flow, the relative percentage of desaturated blood is increased, so the PaO_2 is low.

Flow from the ECMO circuit delivered into the aorta is continuous and nonpulsatile. As a result, as ECMO flow increases the patient's native (intrinsic) cardiac output decreases and the systemic arterial blood pressure waveform is dampened by the nonpulsatile blood flow into the aorta. At 100% ECMO flow, the arterial pressure waveform is flat with only an occasional pulse that may result when slow ventricular filling triggers occasional ventricular systole. Such complete bypass is not typically provided if the patient has some cardiac function.

Typically VA ECMO is run at 80% bypass, so approximately 80% of the patient's total cardiac output is diverted to the ECMO circuit and then returned to the arterial circulation. At this level of flow, the blood pressure waveform is dampened but preserved, with a pulse pressure of approximately 10 to 15 mmHg. At 80% bypass, the resulting admixture of saturated blood (80% of normal cardiac output) and desaturated blood (from intrinsic cardiac activity) will create sufficient arterial oxygen tension (PaO_2), hemoglobin saturation and oxygen delivery. The PaO_2 can be expected to be normal or even high.

One method to assess adequacy of oxygen delivery is monitoring of the oxygen saturation of blood in the venous side of the circuit; this oxygen saturation is the effective mixed venous oxygen saturation (SvO_2). An SvO_2 of approximately 70% to 75% indicates that the ECMO flow is providing sufficient oxygen delivery. Because the normal range of cardiac output varies widely between and within pediatric age ranges, the typical ECMO flow rate varies widely. Approximations of flow are 100 for infants, 80 for children, and 50 mL/kg per minute for adults.

Hemodynamic Changes During Venoarterial ECMO

During VA ECMO, the patient's PaO_2, SvO_2, and blood pressure will be affected by changes in the ECMO flow and the patient's intrinsic (native) cardiac output and differences between the two.

Extremely High PaO_2 or Fall in Native Cardiac Output. During ECMO support, an extremely elevated PaO_2 typically indicates deterioration rather than improvement in the patient's cardiac output. Any decrease in native cardiac output is likely to increase the relative percentage of arterial flow that consists of highly oxygenated blood from the ECMO circuit. As a result, the PaO_2 rises.

The patient's cardiac output may fall as the result of hypovolemia and decreased preload, hypertension, and increased afterload or myocardial dysfunction. Hypovolemia can result from hemorrhage, frequent blood sampling that is not replaced, diuresis, and capillary leak (e.g., with septic shock). Hypertension and increased afterload can also worsen myocardial dysfunction and reduce native cardiac output, so these conditions can also cause the PaO_2 to rise substantially. If hypertension develops during VA ECMO, aggressive treatment with vasodilators is indicated because hypertension increases the risk of intracranial hemorrhage.

Myocardial dysfunction can cause a fall in native cardiac output. An extreme form of myocardial dysfunction during VA ECMO is known as *cardiac stun*. When cardiac stun develops, the ventricles barely contract. The electrocardiogram (ECG) and heart rate may be normal, but with little contractility observed by echocardiogram. The blood pressure waveform is severely dampened and pulse pressure approaches zero because the mean arterial pressure is generated almost completely from the ECMO flow.

The etiology of cardiac stun is multifactorial, including increased ventricular wall stress, inadequate coronary perfusion, coronary hypoxia from poorly oxygenated left ventricular output during partial ECMO flow, reperfusion injury, and potential hypocalcemia from the use of older or citrated blood products to prime the ECMO circuit. Calcium is precipitated by the phosphate in the citrate-phosphate-dextrose anticoagulant in bank blood. Cardiac stun is usually reversible with time and adequate VA support. ECMO flow must be adjusted to maintain adequate mean arterial pressure while reversible causes such as acid-base and electrolyte imbalances are corrected and myocardial function recovers.

Native cardiac output can also be reduced by cardiac tamponade, hemothorax, or pneumothorax. These problems decrease venous return to the heart and reduce pulmonary blood flow and native cardiac output so the patient's PaO_2 rises because most flow in the aorta is directly from the ECMO pump. If venous return to the right atrium is severely compromised, drainage to the ECMO circuit will drop; if the condition develops suddenly, the fall in drainage to the circuit will be precipitous. The ECMO circuit contains a safety mechanism (either a mechanical bladder box or pressure modulation) that will stop the pump when venous drainage is inadequate to maintain flow through the circuit. In circuits with pressure control modules, a decrease in the venous pressure indicates a fall in venous return.

If ECMO flow is not increased to compensate for a fall in native cardiac output, oxygen delivery will be compromised and the SvO_2 will fall. Systemic venous oxygen saturation can also fall if oxygen consumption is increased by conditions such as pain, anxiety, fever, and seizures.

Falling PaO_2 or Increase in Native Cardiac Output. The PaO_2 will fall during VA ECMO if the patient's pulmonary blood flow and cardiac output increase, because mechanical ventilation support is minimal and the lungs do not oxygenate the blood effectively. Thus, pulmonary venous return and blood ejected by the left ventricle will be relatively hypoxemic or desaturated. Anything that increases pulmonary blood flow and native cardiac output will increase the proportion of aortic flow that is provided by this relatively hypoxemic/desaturated blood, so the PaO_2 falls. Hyperdynamic heart function and hypervolemia secondary to increased volume administration or decreased urine output can increase cardiac output and pulmonary blood flow.

When the PaO_2 falls, ECMO flow is usually increased to maintain systemic oxygen delivery while hypervolemia is treated with diuretic therapy or hemofiltration as appropriate. If the ECMO flow is increased appropriately, the systemic venous oxygen saturation should return to previous levels.

ECMO Support with Single Ventricle Physiology

In patients with single ventricle physiology or shunt-dependent pulmonary blood flow, controversy exists about management of the shunt during MCS. There is debate regarding whether the shunt should be completely closed, partially closed, or left open during MCS. The challenge is to maintain balance between systemic and pulmonary circulation. If the shunt is completely closed during support, there is a risk of pulmonary infarction. If the shunt is open during ECMO, increased ECMO flow may be needed to maintain adequate pulmonary and systemic blood flow and systemic oxygen delivery.[53]

There are limited data regarding the role of ECMO after stage 1 palliation (and its variants) for hypoplastic left heart syndrome. ECMO is a useful tool for treatment of potentially reversible conditions, such as acute shunt thrombosis and transient depressed ventricular function[53]; ECMO may be used electively in the immediate postoperative period. However, the use of ECMO after the Norwood procedure remains controversial because the infant's anatomy is complicated, the therapy is expensive, and survival rate is low.[18,51,53,57]

Venovenous ECMO
Circuit

VV ECMO is an alternative to VA ECMO that may be preferred for treatment of respiratory failure. In VV ECMO, venous blood is drained, sent through the circuit for oxygenation and carbon dioxide removal (ventilation), and returned to the venous side of the circulation.

The VV ECMO circuit has the same major components and flow pattern as the VA ECMO circuit (described previously), but blood is infused back into the venous circulation by a second venous cannula or a double-lumen single venous cannula. In infants, a double-lumen cannula is placed in the right internal jugular vein and blood is withdrawn through this catheter and returned to the right atrium. In older patients, two or more venous cannulas are placed, often in the right internal jugular vein, the femoral vein, or both.

Venovenous ECMO Flow and Function

Because VV ECMO delivers highly oxygenated/saturated blood to the venous side of the heart, the right heart cannula must be carefully positioned and rotated, and native cardiac function must be adequate. The range of PaO_2 typical during VV ECMO is 50 to 70 mmHg, lower than during VA ECMO.

Because both the venous drainage and reinfusion cannula are in the venous system, some blood will be cycled through the ECMO circuit over and over again. This phenomenon is known as *recirculation*. As ECMO flow increases, so does the percentage of blood that will be recirculated. The greater the volume of blood that is recirculated, the lower the amount of blood flow that is sent forward through the tricuspid valve, into the lungs, left heart, and to the body, and the lower the efficiency of gas transfer between the oxygenator and the patient. The degree of recirculation is monitored by comparing the oxygen saturation of the venous drainage (SvO_2) with the arterial saturation (SaO_2). If the SvO_2 is higher than normal and the SaO_2 is low, the volume of recirculation is excessive and either the blood flow rate or cannula placement requires adjustment.

Hemodynamic Changes during Venovenous ECMO

Venous cannula position can impede forward flow, as can right or left atrial volume, and poor contractility. If forward flow is impeded, PaO_2, cardiac output and oxygen delivery fall.

If the PaO_2 is low or falls during VV ECMO, the cannula position should be checked and the physician should be notified to make any adjustments. In addition, therapy to improve cardiac output may include volume administration with packed red blood cells (to maximize oxygen-carrying capacity) and initiation of inotropic support. Occasionally, conversion from VV ECMO to VA ECMO is needed if hypoxia persists, particularly in the presence of hypotension and poor cardiac output despite maximal ventilator and inotropic support. VA ECMO is also considered if the child develops nonperfusing arrhythmias or cardiac arrest.

Although there is no difference in the rate of survival, or rates of intracranial hemorrhage and infarction, seizures and brain death in pediatric respiratory patients for VV versus VA ECMO, VV ECMO is associated with significantly more cannula problems, higher incidence of CPR on ECMO, and use of inotropic support. In addition, there is also a trend toward more renal failure and use of hemofiltration on VV ECMO.[62]

Advantages and Disadvantages of VA and VV ECMO

The major advantage of VA ECMO is that it provides both cardiac and pulmonary support. The disadvantages of VA ECMO are: the need to ligate the right common carotid artery and internal jugular vein after decannulation, that the blood flow it provides to body organs is nonpulsatile, that it may result in lower oxygen delivery to the coronary arteries, and that there is a potential for emboli directly into the arterial circulation.

The advantages of VV ECMO are that the carotid artery is spared, pulsatile flow is maintained, and potential emboli from the circuit are trapped in the pulmonary vascular bed. The major disadvantage of VV ECMO is lack of cardiac support. However, the most common cause of myocardial dysfunction in the neonate is respiratory failure. VV ECMO delivers high concentrations of oxygen to both the lungs and the coronary arteries. The high oxygen levels can produce pulmonary vasodilation, decreasing pulmonary hypertension and reversing hypoxic myocardial dysfunction.

Indications and Contraindications of ECMO Support

The indications and contraindications differ for neonatal, pediatric, and cardiac ECMO. Although specific inclusion and exclusion criteria exist, the use of ECMO remains a center specific decision and has to be considered on a case-by-case basis. The inclusion criteria for neonatal and pediatric ECMO are summarized in Box 7-1.

Box 7-1 | **Inclusion Criteria for Neonatal and Pediatric Respiratory ECMO Support**

Neonatal
- Gestational age >34 weeks
- Weight >2 kg
- Mechanical ventilation <14 days
- Reversible lung injury
- Oxygenation index >35
- No major congenital heart disease
- No lethal malformations or congenital anomalies
- No evidence of irreversible brain injury

Pediatric
- Potentially reversible etiology for pulmonary failure
- Oxygenation index >40 and worsening respiratory failure despite maximal ventilator support
- Hypercarbia and pH <7.1
- PaO_2/FiO_2 ratio <100
- Ventilator support for <14 days
- No other major contraindication to ECMO support such as severe central nervous system abnormality, ongoing hemorrhagic condition or coagulopathy, or multiple organ system failure in >3 organ systems

ECMO, Extracorporeal membrane oxygenation; *FiO₂*, fraction inspired oxygen; *PaO₂*, arterial partial pressure of oxygen.

Neonatal Respiratory Failure

Neonatal ECMO has generally been considered an invasive rescue therapy with an identified set of risks; it is reserved for patients with a high predicted mortality who fail to respond to optimal conventional therapies. In newborns, a predicted mortality rate of 80% or greater was historically the main indication for ECMO. Much work was done in the early years of ECMO therapy to establish criteria for 80% predicted mortality. The most commonly used variable is the OI. An OI greater than 35 on three or more postductal arterial blood gases, 30 to 60 minutes apart, is consistent with an 80% predicted mortality. In addition, a single OI of 60 is a significant predictor of mortality.

Some centers used the A-a oxygen difference (A-a DO_2), also known as the *A-a O_2 gradient*. An A-a difference or gradient of more than 600 for a period between 4 and 12 hours is an accepted indication for ECMO support. However, some centers simply report the use of ECMO in patients with severe hypoxemia (PaO_2 <50 mm Hg), severe acidosis (pH <7.25), and acute deterioration resulting in a PaO_2 of approximately 30 to 40 mm Hg; these are all considered indications for ECMO.

ECMO may be initiated for patients with 50% to 80% predicted mortality if ECMO offers a higher potential for survival than conventional therapy. Examples of such patients include those with meconium aspiration and congenital diaphragmatic hernia with an OI of 25 to 40. The inclusion criteria of a minimum gestational age greater than 34 weeks' gestation and weight greater than 2 kg is somewhat arbitrary, but is based on the increased risk of intraventricular hemorrhage (IVH) and difficult intravenous access in premature neonates.

Contraindications for neonatal ECMO include the presence of irreversible and uncontrolled bleeding or coagulopathy, IVH greater than grade II, birth weight <2 kg, or gestational age <34 weeks, lethal chromosomal abnormality or congenital malformation incompatible with life, and duration of mechanical ventilation >14 days.[43]

With more extensive use of therapies such as high-frequency ventilation, surfactant, and nitric oxide, there has been a marked decline in the need for neonatal ECMO.[38] If patients do not respond to these therapies, ECMO should be offered in a timely manner.

Pediatric Respiratory Failure

There is less consensus regarding indications for ECMO support for pediatric patients than for neonates with respiratory failure. Severe respiratory failure in children has many etiologies. A child is generally considered to be a candidate for ECMO if death is believed to be nearly certain despite maximal conventional therapy, and the lung disease is believed to be reversible and other organ systems are intact.[29] In children, the OI has not been shown to be as predictive of mortality as it is in neonates. Many centers use the criteria of OI >40 and rising, hypercarbia and pH <7.1, a $PaO_2:FiO_2$ ratio less than 100 and falling, ventilator support for less than 14 days, and no contraindications such as significant neurologic or hemorrhagic conditions, or failure of more than three organ systems.[43] With the use of lung protective strategies and adjunctive therapies such as high-frequency ventilation, surfactant, and nitric oxide, it has become harder to establish criteria for initiation of ECMO support. Contraindications for pediatric ECMO are similar to those in the neonatal period; these include diagnoses incompatible with life, intractable hemorrhage or coagulopathy, or severe central nervous system abnormality.

Cardiac Failure

Cardiac ECMO support has steadily increased over the past decade.[24] Although isolated left ventricular failure is relatively rare in children, right ventricular failure, pulmonary hypertension, and hypoxemia are often associated with circulatory collapse in children with congenital heart disease. The most common causes of circulatory failure in infants and children are cardiovascular surgery (postcardiotomy), end-stage cardiomyopathy, and acute myocarditis. The most common indications for ECMO in cardiac patients are severe hypoxia, severe pulmonary artery hypertension, cardiogenic shock, cardiac arrest, and failure to wean from cardiopulmonary bypass after surgical repair.

With ECMO support, postcardiotomy myocardial recovery should occur in approximately 72 hours to 7 days. If there are no signs of myocardial recovery during this time, a cardiac catheterization is needed to assess for residual structural defects. If none exist, the child is listed as a candidate for cardiac transplant. If residual structural defects are identified, surgical reintervention is scheduled.

Contraindications for the use of cardiac ECMO include incurable malignancy, advanced and presumed irreversible multisystem organ failure, extreme prematurity, and severe central nervous system abnormality or hemorrhage.[59] In addition, if a patient will not be a transplant candidate, the patient should be carefully evaluated before ECMO. During the past 10 years, many contraindications have been removed from the list or labeled as relative rather than absolute contraindications.

Weaning from ECMO

There are two basic approaches to weaning patients from VA ECMO. Neither method has been shown to be superior to the other.[32]

In the gradual approach, as lung function improves ECMO is slowly withdrawn and ventilator support is slowly increased. Weaning with this approach may take a period of several days to reach idling flow, or approximately 20 mL/kg per minute. Clinical improvements in pulmonary function and chest radiograph, and loss of edema with a return to pre-ECMO weight faciitate the weaning process.

In the second, more abrupt approach to weaning, ECMO is maintained at full flow of 100 mL/kg per minute with minimal ventilator support until moments before the ECMO circuit is clamped. At that time, the ECMO flow is decreased over a few minutes while ventilator support is simultaneously increased. The circuit is then clamped off and blood gases are obtained to assess pulmonary function. The rationale for this more abrupt termination of ECMO support is that it allows a longer period of low ventilator support to maximize the resting time for lungs to heal.

To discontinue ECMO therapy, the patient must be able to maintain adequate blood pressure, perfusion, acid-base balance, and oxygenation with acceptable ventilator settings without ECMO support. Hypoxia, acidosis, increased serum lactate, decreased cardiac function, and hypotension may be indications to resume ECMO support. During the weaning process, it is not uncommon to increase the ECMO flow or to have more than one unsuccessful attempt to remove ECMO before successful weaning.

Weaning VV ECMO is slightly different than weaning VA ECMO. When weaning VV ECMO, after the ventilator settings are increased, both of the membrane oxygenator gas ports are isolated from ambient air. Eventually, the blood entering and exiting the membrane oxygenator is in equilibrium and reflects typical venous values. This eliminates the need to clamp the venous cannula and allows a longer trial off VV ECMO.[32]

Complications of ECMO

ECMO has historically been reserved for those with the highest predicted mortality, so its use has a favorable benefit-to-risk ratio. There are a number of identified complications of ECMO therapy. Some of these complications are related to the use of ECMO and some are related to the complications of the initial disease process. With any cause of severe cardiorespiratory failure there is the antecedent injury associated with hypoxemia, acidosis, and shock; if ECMO is provided, there are additional potential complications related to altered flow dynamics of ECMO cannulation and bypass. In addition, there are issues of reperfusion injury and heparinization. It can become difficult to separate the complications actually related to ECMO from those related to the initial illness.

The two most common complications of ECMO are bleeding and clot formation in the circuit. Bleeding and hemorrhage are related to the use of heparin for anticoagulation of the circuit; this heparin then anticoagulates the patient too. As blood flows through the circuit, coagulation factors and platelets are activated and clot formation is triggered in the circuit. A consumptive coagulopathy can develop, causing bleeding complications. The tubing and the oxygenator trap platelets, causing thrombocytopenia. A large percentage of the circulating platelets will have reduced function.

During ECMO, patients requiring any surgical intervention (even just chest tube placement) are at increased risk for bleeding at incision sites. Gastrointestinal hemorrhage and IVH are known ECMO complications.

Because the clotting cascade is activated, clots can develop in the ECMO circuit. These clots can obstruct flow if they are sufficiently large. When clots develop in the oxygenator they can cause oxygenator failure.

Once ECMO is initiated, antithrombin III (AT III) replacement is necessary. AT III acts in concert with heparin to provide anticoagulation. Without adequate levels of AT III, the heparin infusing in the patients during ECMO cannot be truly effective as an anticoagulant. Levels of AT III have been shown to be low in most patients requiring ECMO.

The art of managing patients during ECMO involves assessing each patient's activated clotting time (ACT) and other measures of coagulation including AT III levels, platelets, prothrombin time (PT)/activated partial thromboplastin time (aPTT) and international normalized ratio (INR) values, anti Xa heparin activity, and thromboelastrography.

Heparin and blood product administration and factor replacement should be tailored to patient needs.

Other complications of ECMO include neurologic, cardiovascular, and renal complications in addition to infectious and metabolic problems. Neurologic complications include seizures, IVH, cerebral infarction, and the potential for brain death. It is important to note that even before ECMO is initiated, the patient suffers an insult to the central nervous system secondary to hypoxia and poor perfusion. Cannulation for ECMO alters perfusion and can also contribute to reperfusion injury to the brain. It is therefore difficult to identify whether a neurologic complication is related to the use of ECMO, the antecedent injury suffered before ECMO, or a combination of factors.

Cardiovascular complications of ECMO therapy include arrhythmias, hypotension, hypertension, tamponade, and cardiac stun. In addition, newborns are at risk for maintenance or persistence of a patent ductus arteriosus.

Pulmonary complications include pneumothorax or other air leaks as well as pulmonary hemorrhage and hemothoraces. Pneumothoraces are often minimized by the use of rest ventilator settings. However, when increased settings are used to try to wean ECMO support, a spontaneous pneumothorax may develop.

Infectious complications include culture-proven infections and signs of inflammation, such as neutropenia and elevated C-reactive protein that suggest infection. Attachment to an extracorporeal circuit for an extended period provides a portal for potential infection, but these patients are also intubated and have many catheters and tubes that contribute to infection risk. Meticulous attention to aseptic care of the ECMO circuit can diminish the risks of an ECMO-related infection.

Finally, there are a number of metabolic complications of ECMO therapy, including glucose, electrolyte, and acid-base abnormalities. Banked blood may contain high quantities of glucose and citrate, so glucose and calcium imbalances can be problematic. Older blood has a high potassium concentration. In addition, patients may have a high bilirubin level or high plasma-free hemoglobin, indicating significant hemolysis secondary to ECMO.

ECMO Troubleshooting

ECMO Circuit Emergencies

There are many types of ECMO circuit emergencies, so ECMO staff and the bedside nurse must be constantly vigilant to prevent a circuit problem and rapidly respond to and correct any circuit emergency. The following circuit components need to be rapidly assessed in an ECMO emergency:

- Is blood ejecting from the circuit?
- Is air being pumped in the circuit?
- Is the pump delivering forward flow?
- Does the post-oxygenator blood appear red?
- Is the sweep gas being delivered and vented from the oxygenator?
- Are the circuit and equipment functioning properly?

The circuit check can direct the ECMO specialist's immediate response to the emergency. If there is blood ejecting from the circuit and air being pumped, then immediate removal from ECMO is required before the problem can be repaired.

Table 7-2   **Troubleshooting the ECMO Circuit**

Problem	Signs and Symptoms	Response
Clots in circuit	Dark zones or streaks seen; can cause bleeding due to coagulopathy (decreased platelets or fibrinogen unresponsive to transfusion)	Monitor circuit, monitor for coagulopathy, change circuit
Oxygenator failure	Failure to remove CO_2 or add adequate levels of oxygen in spite of increasing sweep gascs and FiO_2; may see blood or serum leaking from gas exhaust port	Remove air and debubble circuit if present; check that all gas lines are intact and not leaking to rule out gas line failure; replace oxygenator if it has failed
Air in venous side of circuit	Bubbles seen	Correct source of problem, remove air
Air in arterial side of circuit	Bubbles seen	Remove patient from ECMO by clamping arterial and venous lines to patient; place patient in Trendelenburg position; replace/repair the component identified as cause; remove all air, recirculate, and then return to ECMO
Power failure	Pump stops with no AC power	Plug into emergency hospital power; use battery or UPS; hand crank
Accidental decannulation	With partial removal on venous side, air entrainment can be seen; with complete decannulation, cannula will be out of the body with bleeding from cannulation site and possible pumping of air or blood	Cease ECMO and stop pump; put direct pressure on site; call surgeon for immediate replacement of cannula and to control bleeding; replace volume losses with available blood products and crystalloid
Water heater failure	Patient exhibits hypothermia; bradycardia with reflex hypertension may be seen with pallor	Obtain new water heater and connect to circuit
Raceway rupture	Blood spurts out of damaged tubing in pump head	Cease ECMO; turn pump off; replace raceway segment with new tubing; clean pump head; place new raceway segment into the pump head and recirculate; return to ECMO
Cracks in tubing or connectors or loose stopcocks	On venous side [negative pressure side] air will entrain into the circuit. On positive pressure side of the circuit, blood will leak out	Tighten connections or replace cracked tubing or connectors; cease ECMO; stop pump; cut out and replace the damaged segments

AC, Alternating current; *ECMO,* extracorporeal membrane oxygenation; *UPS,* universal power source.

The ECMO specialist must identify and fix the pump problem while the patient's nurse and additional critical care unit (PCCU) staff support the patient off ECMO. Immediately clamp the venous line, open the bridge, and clamp the arterial line to remove the patient from the ECMO circuit. Because the patient is dependent on the ventilator, provide ventilation with 100% oxygen or shift the patient back to pre-ECMO ventilator settings. In addition, increased volume and inotropic support may be required, and full cardiopulmonary resuscitation may be needed.

If there is no squirting blood or air being pumped, the patient can be maintained on ECMO while the problem is corrected. ECMO circuit emergencies and problem troubleshooting are summarized in Table 7-2.

VENTRICULAR ASSIST DEVICES

The development and clinical application of circulatory support devices have closely paralleled the development of cardiac transplantation. Denton Cooley and colleagues achieved the first successful bridge to cardiac transplantation with an artificial heart in the late 1960s. Routine bridging to transplantation began in 1984 with the short-term use of the total artificial heart by Jack Copeland, the Pierce-Donachy (Thoratec) VAD by Donald Hill and colleagues, and the Novacor electrical VAD by Oyer and colleagues.

The options for MCS for infants and children with cardiac failure are limited. There are currently no devices approved by the FDA for specific use in infant patients. However, several devices have been used successfully to support infants and children through the following: off-label use of devices approved by the FDA for use in adults, compassionate use of investigational adult VADs, the use of devices that have received an FDA Humanitarian Device Exemption, the use of devices fabricated from FDA-approved components (such as ECMO circuits), and devices that are approved on a case-by-case basis by the FDA for emergency use.[7,8,12,20-22,27,28,31,44,56] Table 7-3 lists ventricular assist devices currently being used in the pediatric population under various exemptions or adult approved devices used in older children.[2,26,30,35,42,45,46,61] Additional information regarding VADs used in children is included in Evolve Table 7-1 in the Chapter 7 Supplement on the Evolve Website.

Components and Function of VAD Support

A VAD is a heart pump that can be used to support the right ventricle (called a *right ventricular assist device* [RVAD]), the left ventricle (called an *LVAD*), or both ventricles (called a *BiVAD*). Most VADs have three major components: a pump (located inside or outside the body), a control system, and an energy source. The control system and energy source are found outside the body. The energy source can be a battery or compressed air (pneumatic).[23]

Table 7-3 **Mechanical Cardiac Support Devices Currently Used in Pediatrics**

Device	Maker	Patient Size	Type
HeartMate LVAD	Thoratec	BSA >0.7 m^2	Pulsatile, implantable
Thoratec VAD	Thoratec	BSA >0.7 m^2	Pulsatile, external
Abiomed BVS 5000	Abiomed	BSA >0.7 m^2	Axial, implantable
DeBakey VAD Child	Micro Med Technology	BSA 0.7-1.5 m^2	Axial, implantable
Excor Pediatrics	Berlin Heart	Weight ≥2.4 kg	Pulsatile, external
Jarvik 2000	Jarvik Heart	BSA* >1.5 m^2	Axial, implantable

*Can be used in patients with BSA <1.5 m^2, but this is not routinely practiced.
BSA, Body surface area.

In the pediatric population, most VAD pumps are extracorporeal (outside the body) and connected to inflow and outflow cannulae (Fig. 7-2). The critical care nurse should understand the components of the VAD and VAD function.

The placement of the VAD cannula differs if the device is a bridge to recovery, compared with a bridge to transplantation. If the VAD support is serving as a bridge to recovery, the inflow cannula is often connected to the patient's atrium.[19] This cannulation is technically easier and spares the ventricle further injury. However, ventricular cannulation enables higher flow rates, so this form of cannulation is used when VAD support is used as a bridge to transplant, because ventricular injury is not a concern.

When an LVAD is used, the inflow cannula (carrying blood from the patient to the pump) is inserted in either the left atrium or the left ventricle. The outflow cannula (carrying blood from the pump to the patient) is inserted in the ascending aorta. When an RVAD is used, the inflow cannula is inserted in either the right atrium or right ventricle, and the outflow cannula is inserted in the pulmonary artery.

Ventricular Assist Device Flow and Function

Most VAD pumps used in children are either displacement pumps (pulsatile or pneumatic devices) or rotary pumps (continuous flow devices). The pulsatile or pneumatic pumps mimic the natural contraction (pumping action) of the heart. Flow rates depend on preload and the size of the external pump. Average flows for an infant-sized pump (12 or 15 mL) are 0.5 to 1.3 L/min and for a child-sized pump (25 or 30 mL) are 1.3 to 3.3 L/min.[4] The external pump size can be changed to accommodate the child's growth and increased stroke volume.

The most common continuous flow devices are axial or centrifugal pumps. Both types have a central rotor containing permanent magnets. Controlled electric currents that run through coils in the pump housing apply forces to the magnets causing the rotors to turn. Axial flow rates vary depending on the size of the device implanted. The child-sized device has been reported to provide an average flow of 0.3 to 2.5 L/min.[4] The pediatric centrifugal Bio-Medicus Bio-pump (Medtronic, Inc. Minneapolis, MN) has both a 50- and 80-mL pump head size to accommodate infants <10 kg and children >10 kg, respectively. The 50-mL pump can provide flow up to 1.5 L/min and the 80-mL pump can provide >2 L/min.[27]

The VAD console and energy source varies depending on the VAD type. Most pneumatic consoles display both left- and right-sided heart support, the pump rate in beats per minute, systolic and diastolic or fill pressures, and vacuum drive pressures. The consoles also have backup units in case of malfunction. These backup units can be automatically or manually converted, depending on the device. In addition, the consoles can be operated by external electrical power as well as internal batteries. Battery life varies by device with an average of 1 to 2 hours. External backup pumping devices should be attached to the console in case of an emergency.

The console of the centrifugal pump displays the speed and blood flow rate, which are manually adjusted by the operator. Inlet and outlet pressure monitors can be used to guide pump speed and prevent tubing collapse. External electrical power and internal batteries operate the console if transport is needed.

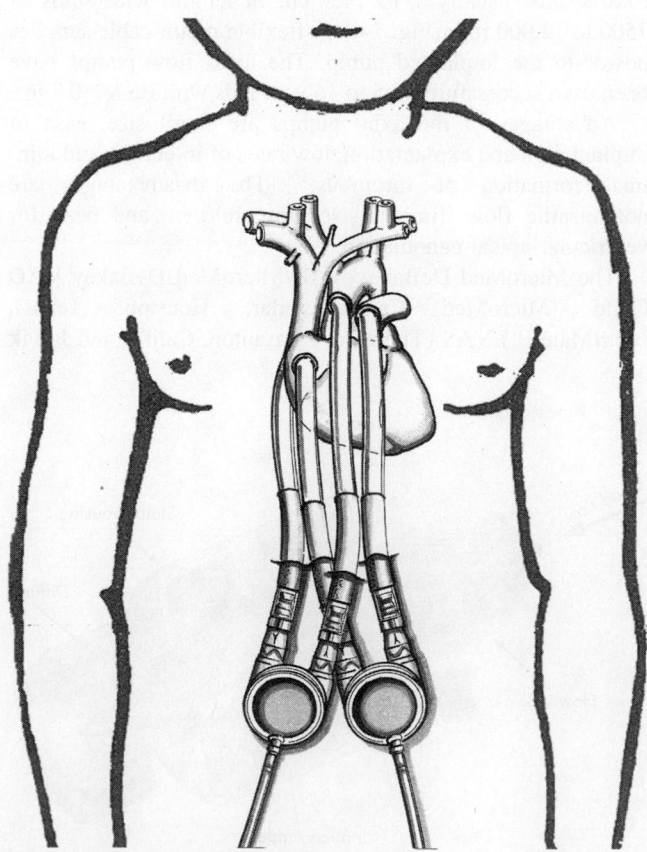

FIG. 7-2 Extracorporeal pneumatic biventricular assist device (Berlin Heart EXCOR). (Redrawn from an illustration of the Berlin EXCOR by Berlin Heart, Berlin, Germany.)

All VADs are preload dependent—the amount of blood returning to the heart is the amount of blood pumped to the body. The VAD is sensitive to impedance to flow, so hypertension and mechanical obstruction must be corrected. Both the LVAD and RVAD allow blood to bypass the failing ventricle. This decompresses that ventricle, decreases myocardial work, and reduces oxygen demand while maintaining adequate systemic perfusion to sustain end-organ function. VAD support has been shown to improve myocardial contractility. It also reverses beta receptor downregulation (documented to occur with heart failure), restoring myocardial response to the inotropic effects of adrenergic stimulation.[48] VAD support can also normalize chamber geometry and reduce myocardial fibrosis, hypertrophy, and disruption in cytoskeletal proteins.[10,34]

Types of Ventricular Assist Device Pumps

Several VAD pumps made for adult patients are available for clinical use. Some are implanted internally and others are external pumps. The VAD pumps can be broadly subdivided into *continuous flow* (nonpulsatile) and *pulsatile pumps*. Both types have a central rotor containing permanent magnets; the magnets cause the rotors to turn.

Continuous Flow Pumps

The continuous flow (nonpulsatile) VADs use either centrifugal or axial flow pumps. Each has advantages and disadvantages.

Centrifugal Pump. The centrifugal pump is external, requires cannulation via a thoracotomy or sternotomy, and can be used for single or biventricular support. The most common centrifugal pump is the Bio-Medicus Bio-Pump (Medtronic, Inc. Minneapolis, Minn). The Bio-Pump uses two magnetically coupled, polycarbonate rotator cones that spin to create centrifugal force along a vertical axis.[11] The rotors are shaped to accelerate the blood circumferentially and thus cause it to move toward the outer rim of the pump. The constrained vortex pump design creates subatmospheric pressure at the tip of the cone, establishing suction in the venous cannula.[40] Blood enters at the apex of the cone and is ejected tangentially at the base of the cone (Fig. 7-3). The cone design retains any small air bubbles.

The pump output is proportional to revolutions per minute and is adjusted according to the venous return. Spins averaging 10,000 to 20,000 rpm will create a blood flow of 5 to 6 L/min in larger pumpheads.[36] This type of pump can support neonates and older children with postoperative cardiac failure but competent lung function.[36,58]

The advantages of the centrifugal pump include: no need for an oxygenator, low priming volume (pediatrics, 50 mL), low requirements for heparin and little hemolysis, adequate decompression of the left ventricle, easy transport, and low cost. However, adequate pulmonary function is required and the chest must remain open, as with ECMO.

The centrifugal VADs include Bio-Medicus Bio-pump, Levitronix CentriMag (Levotronix, Waltham, Mass.), RotaFlow (Jostra, Hirrlingen, Germany), and the Capiox Terumo (Terumo Cardiovascular Systems, Ann Arbor, Mich.). The Levitronix CentriMag is marketed in Europe, but available in the United Stated only as an investigational device.[11] The advantage to this device is that it can be attached to cardiopulmonary bypass cannula already in place. However, cannula adaptors may be needed for smaller patients.

Axial Flow Pump. Axial flow pumps reflect recent industry efforts to develop smaller, lighter, quieter, implantable pediatric VADs. Axial flow pumps are designed to assist the left ventricle as a bridge to transplant or destination therapy. The pump has a magnetically levitated impeller that rotates in a cylindrical chamber so that blood accelerates toward the rotor's axis, usually 7 to 11.5 cm in length, with spins of 7500 to 12,000 rpm (Fig. 7-4). A flexible motor cable supplies power to the implanted pump. The axial flow pumps have been used successfully in 5 to 16 year olds with BSA $\geq$0.7 m^2.

Advantages of the axial pumps are small size, ease of implantation and explantation, low rates of infection, and minimal formation of thrombus.[16] The disadvantages are nonpulsatile flow, limited sizes for children, and need for ventricular apical cannulation.[16]

The MicroMed DeBakey VAD/MicroMed DeBakey VAD Child (MicroMed Cardiovascular, Houston, Texas), HeartMate II LVAS (Thoratec, Pleasanton, Calif.), and Jarvik

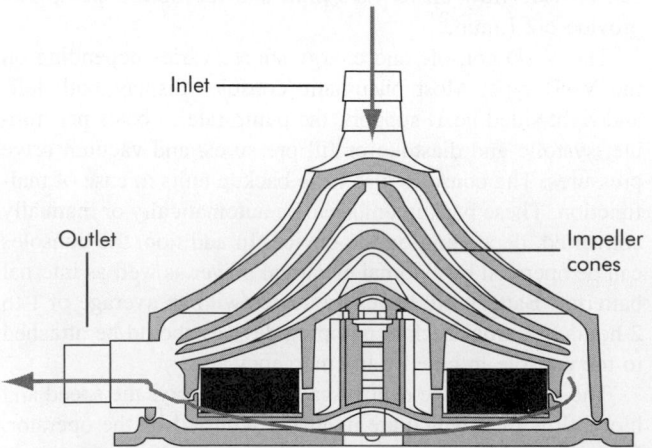

FIG. 7-3 Bio-Medicus centrifugal pump. (From Karl TR, Horton SB, and Brizard C: Postoperative support with the centrifugal pump ventricular assist device (VAD). *Seminars in Thoracic and Cardiovascular Surgery: Pediatric Cardiac Surgery Annual* 9:83–91, 2006.)

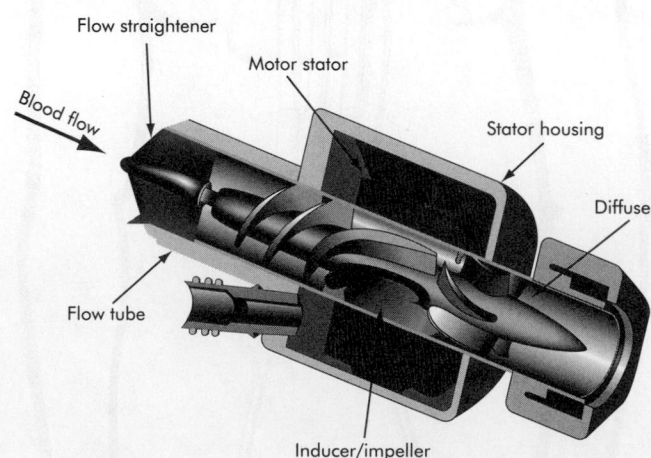

FIG. 7-4 Axial continuous flow pump (Redrawn from an illustration of the Axial Flow Pump, Micromed DeBakey VAD, by Micromed Technology, Houston, Texas.)

2000 (Jarvik Heart, New York,, N.Y.) are currently used axial flow VADs for adults and selected children with a BSA >0.7 m². An infant (3-15 kg) and child (15-25 kg) Jarvik 2000 are being developed through the National Heart, Lung and Blood Institute (NHLBI) Circulatory Assist Program.[4]

Pulsatile Pumps

Pulsatile VADs contain a reservoir. Blood is ejected by the pump either electronically through the movement of pusher plates or with compressed air movement of the bladder. These devices propel blood in synchrony with the patient's ventricular ejection, producing pulsatile arterial blood flow. These devices are paracorporeal systems and consist of a pneumatic compressor-operated diaphragm pump with inflow and outflow valves. A transparent polyurethane pump housing allows inspection for potential thrombus development. The external pump position enables fast and safe pump changes if required.[54]

The Berlin Heart Excor Pediatric VAD (Berlin Heart, Berlin, Germany), Medos HIA-VAD (Medos Medizintechnik, Aachen, Germany) and the Thoratec VAD (Thoratec) provide both single and biventricular support. The Berlin Heart and Medos HIA-VAD are available in the United States under compassionate use appeal to the FDA. The Thoratec device can only be used in patients with BSA >0.8 m².[11]

Adult pulsatile devices used in older children include the HeartMate XVE LVAS (Thoratec), Abiomed BVS 5000 (Abiomed, Danvers, Mass.), and Novacor LVAS (WorldHeart Corp. Oakland, CA). These devices are suitable for patients with BSA >1.2 m² and who require pump flows of more than 2 L/min.

The advantages of pulsatile devices are feasibility for long-term support, potential use without the need for mechanical ventilation, mobility, ability to transition out of the ICU, and need for only low-dose anticoagulation. Disadvantages include thromboembolic complications, infection, and cost.

Indications and Contraindications for Ventricular Assist Device Support

The clinical indications for pediatric VAD support are severe ventricular failure, shocklike state, or the progression of multiorgan failure resulting from acute fulminant myocarditis, cardiomyopathy, postcardiotomy failure, posttransplantation graft failure, and end-stage congenital heart disease.[19] Signs of critically low cardiac output or ventricular failure include: mixed venous oxygen saturation (SvO_2) <40%, increased ventricular end-diastolic filling pressure, cardiac index <2 L/min per m² BSA, persistent metabolic acidosis, oliguria, poor peripheral perfusion, increasing FiO_2 requirement, signs of beginning renal and hepatic failure, and significantly impaired ventricular function by echocardiogram (Box 7-2). VAD support is indicated when all medical treatment options have been exhausted, including afterload reduction combined with catecholamines, diuretics, a phosphodiesterase-III inhibitor, fluid and transfusion management, and mechanical ventilation. In addition, any residual correctable contributing lesion should be ruled out in patients with congenital heart disease.

Before device application, the patient's neurologic status should be evaluated by clinical and cranial ultrasound

---

Box 7-2	Clinical Indications for VAD Support

- Mixed venous saturation <40%
- Cardiac index <2.0 L/min per m²
- Increased filling pressures (CVP, RA)
- Persistent metabolic acidosis
- Increasing FiO_2 requirements
- Poor peripheral perfusion
- Oliguria
- Signs of beginning renal and hepatic failure (elevated LFT results and BUN/creatinine levels)
- Significantly impaired cardiac function by echocardiogram

BUN, Blood urea nitrogen; *CVP*, central venous pressure; *LFT*, liver function test; *RA*, right atrium; *VAD*, ventricular assist device.

---

examination (in neonates and infants) to rule out intracranial bleeding and cerebral damage. However, such evaluation may not be possible when VAD support is initiated in the operating room after cardiotomy. The decision for device application should then be based on the patient's preoperative status and intraoperative course.

Patients are evaluated on an individual basis for VAD support. The overall decision for VAD support should be made earlier rather than later to improve chances for end-organ recovery and survival. Contraindications to VAD support include extreme prematurity, irreversible multisystem organ failure, incurable malignancy, and severe central nervous system damage.[20]

Weaning From VAD Support

Weaning from VAD support is planned for patients with temporary myocardial dysfunction, most commonly associated with acute myocarditis. Before weaning, ventricular recovery and function are assessed.

During use of the centrifugal VAD, the appearance of a pulsatile systemic arterial pressure waveform during full flow is an early sign of improved ventricular function. Transesophageal echocardiogram assessment is helpful to evaluate ventricular contractility and response to volume loading. Once ventricular ejection is verified, the device flow is gradually reduced to a minimum of 150 mL/min. Additional heparin may be required at lower flows, and it may be necessary to flush the cannulae with heparin. Inotropic and pulmonary support should be initiated to maintain adequate perfusion and ventilation during weaning. The device is typically removed in the operating room with sternal closure, if warranted.

Before weaning a pulsatile pneumatic device, improvement in systolic myocardial function is verified by transthoracic echocardiogram or cardiac catheterization. Weaning protocols including the need for additional anticoagulation are device-specific and should be reviewed before initiating the weaning process. The device is removed in the operating suite, with or without the use of temporary cardiopulmonary bypass support. Support can be converted to ECMO support or to a centrifugal VAD pump with later weaning as described previously.[1]

Termination or withdrawal of VAD support may be indicated if myocardial function does not recover. Withdrawal of support requires careful communication with family members (see Chapters 2 and 3).

Complications of Ventricular Assist Device Support

Potential complications of VAD support include: bleeding requiring reoperation, embolism (clot or air), hemolysis, infection, and mechanical failure.[19] Bleeding and embolism are the most common complications following VAD insertion. Mild to moderate bleeding is common and is most often caused by anticoagulation, a coagulopathy, or surgical bleeding. Excessive bleeding requiring massive transfusions often results in pulmonary and multiorgan dysfunction and can be fatal.

Neurologic events such as intracranial hemorrhage and cerebral emboli can result in significant long-term neurologic deficits. Such events are among the major indications for VAD support termination.

Troubleshooting Ventricular Assist Device Support

Troubleshooting VAD support requires knowledge of the type of device (continuous flow or pulsatile), type of support (single or biventricular support), and make of device. Common problems and potential causes are listed in Table 7-4 and are addressed under Nursing Care.

The paracorporeal pneumatic VADs with small pump volumes, designed specifically for infants and children, have been used in Europe since 1992. The Berlin Heart Excor

Table 7-4	Potential Problems and Causes During LVAD Support
Problem	**Potential Cause**
Low LA pressure	• Hypovolemia • RV failure • Excessive mechanical support
High LA pressure	• Inadequate pump support • Volume overload • Obstruction of cannula
Low RA pressure	• Hypovolemia • PFO/ASD
High RA pressure	• Volume overload • RV dysfunction
Inability to maintain adequate pump flow	• Hypovolemia • Cardiac tamponade • Malpositioned cannula • Thrombosis of cannulae or pump • Kinking of cannulae or tubing
Metabolic acidosis	• Inadequate support • Hypovolemia • Organ damage, liver or bowel
Hypoxia	• Pulmonary problem • PFO/ASD
Excessive bleeding	• Heparin overdose, HIT • DIC • Dislodged cannula • Surgical suture line bleeding

(From Reddy M and Hanley FL. Mechanical support of the myocardium. In Chang AC et al., editors. *Pediatric cardiac intensive care*. Baltimore, 1998, Williams and Wilkins, pp. 345–349.)
ASD, Atrial septal defect; *DIC,* disseminated intravascular coagulation; *HIT,* heparin-induced thrombocytopenia; *LA,* left atrium; *LVAD,* left ventricular assist device; *PFO,* patent foramen ovale; *RA,* right atrium; *RV,* right ventricle.

VAD is an extracorporeal device made in a wide range of pump sizes from 10 to 80 mL; it can provide medium- to long-term circulatory support for pediatric patients ranging from 2.5-kg infants to adolescents (see Fig. 7-2).

The Berlin Heart VAD is intended for patients with severe ventricular failure resulting from acute fulminant myocarditis, cardiomyopathy, postcardiotomy failure, posttransplantation graft failure, and end-stage congenital heart disease. In 2007, the FDA approved the use of the Berlin Heart EXCOR Pediatric VAD under a limited conditional investigational device exemption in the United States. The results of the first multisite pediatric clinical trial have been submitted to the FDA. An announcement of approval is pending.

In 2002, the NHLBI recognized the limitations of circulatory support devices in small children. The NHLBI awarded contracts to five research institutes to develop and evaluate circulatory assist devices for children.[4] Information about the devices and program locations is available in Evolve Table 7-1 in the Chapter 7 Supplement on the Evolve Website.

INTRAAORTIC BALLOON PUMP

IABP counterpulsation is frequently used in adults for managing acute left ventricular dysfunction after myocardial infarction or cardiac surgery.[50] The first reported use of an IABP in pediatrics was in 1980.[52] Support for the failing pediatric myocardium has primarily focused on the use of ECMO and VAD. Despite the availability of pediatric-sized catheters, the use of IABP in infants and children is not widespread, with use at a limited number of centers.[14,39,50] The use of IABP in infants and children remains limited for a variety of reasons, including technical difficulty inserting the catheters in the infant or small child, the limited availability of smaller volume catheters, the greater distensibility of the pediatric vasculature, and the difficulty in balloon timing with rapid heart rates in pediatric patients.

Components and Function

The IABP is commonly used for managing acute postoperative or ischemic left ventricular dysfunction in adult patients. However, its use in infants and small children remains limited because of difficulty in catheter insertion and synchronization of the device with the child's rapid heart rate.

The IABP catheter is inserted through a vertical groin incision that provides direct visualization of the common femoral artery. The balloon is inserted until the tip is above the renal artery but distal to (approximately 2 cm below) the origin of the left subclavian artery.

The IABP augments cardiac output by inflating during diastole and by deflating immediately before systole. As the balloon inflates, it displaces a volume equal to the balloon volume, producing augmentation of the diastolic pressure and increased coronary artery perfusion. Counterpulsation requires precise balloon inflation at the onset of diastole and aortic valve closure, to augment diastolic and coronary flow, and rapid balloon deflation at the onset of systole and aortic valve opening so that it produces a fall in left ventricular impedance/afterload as the left ventricle begins to eject (Fig. 7-5).

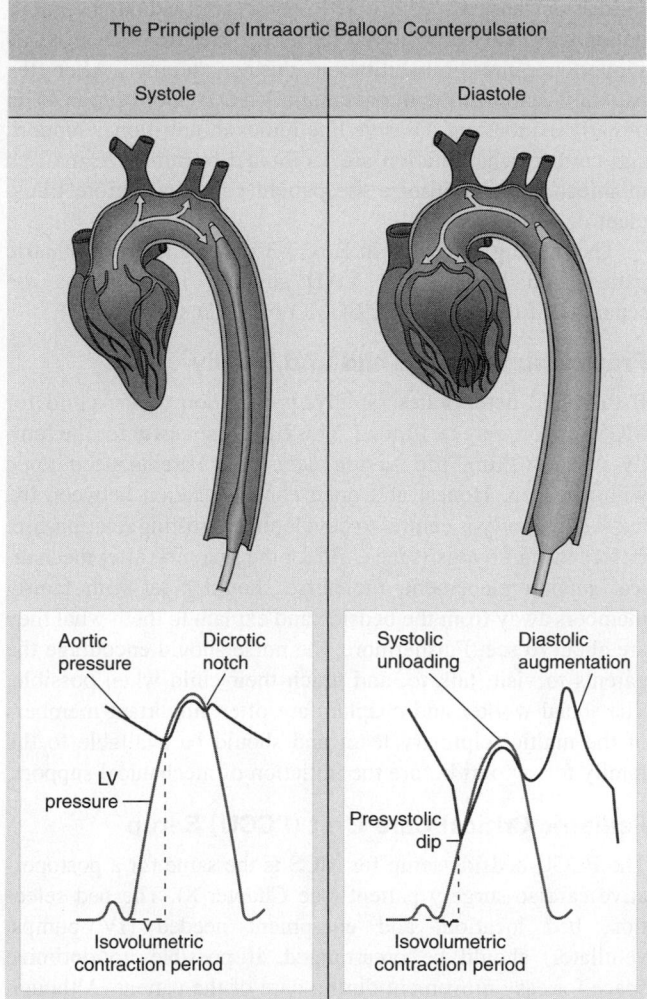

The Principle of Intraaortic Balloon Counterpulsation

Systole | Diastole

Aortic pressure — Dicrotic notch
LV pressure
Isovolumetric contraction period

Systolic unloading — Diastolic augmentation
Presystolic dip
Isovolumetric contraction period

FIG. 7-5 Intraaortic balloon pump. This device includes an elongated balloon that is inserted into the descending aorta. If possible, the tip of the balloon should be distal to the left subclavian artery, to avoid occlusion of the aortic arch vessels. This illustration depicts two counterpulsation cycles. The balloon is rapidly inflated at the beginning of diastole, just after aortic valve closure or at the diacrotic notch, which is timed with the ECG. Balloon inflation augments the aortic diastolic pressure; as a result, arterial diastolic pressure may be higher than arterial systolic pressure (see top right waveform). Rapid deflation of the balloon occurs just before ventricular ejection, producing a systolic unloading effect to augment ventricular ejection. (From Cercek B, Shah PK: Complications of acute myocardial infarction. In Crawford MH, editor: *Cardiology*, ed 3, St Louis, 2009, Mosby.)

Counterpulsation increases cardiac output while decreasing myocardial work and oxygen consumption. Other physiologic benefits of IABP include a reduction in left ventricular end-diastolic pressure, left atrial pressure, and pulmonary artery pressure. To optimize beneficial effects, the balloon size must be optimal and balloon inflation and deflation must be synchronized to the patient's cardiac cycle.

Indications and Contraindications

Indications and contraindications for IABP use have been well established for adults. However, balloon insertion is more invasive in children and requires more consideration and preparation. IABP use is most common in children with left ventricular dysfunction after cardiac surgery or associated with myocarditis, cardiomyopathy, Kawasaki disease, persistent ventricular arrhythmias, or severe sepsis.[33]

Contraindications for IABP therapy in children include the presence of a patent ductus arteriosus, recent coarctation or aortic arch augmentation, significant aortic valve insufficiency, and when left ventricular failure is unlikely to be reversed.

Technique of Balloon Placement

Pediatric intraaortic balloon catheters are generally inserted through a vertical groin incision that provides direct visualization of the common femoral artery. The balloon can also be inserted directly into the aortic arch if the chest is open.

A wide range of pediatric balloon sizes are available. The standard balloon volumes for children are 2.5 to 20 mL (adult capacity, 40 mL), mounted on 4.5- to 7-Fr catheters. The balloon catheter is placed through a 1- to 2-cm section of polytetrafluoroethylene graft material. The balloon is aspirated to remove air, lubricated, and threaded into position in the descending aorta. The balloon is positioned above the renal artery and distal to (approximately 2 cm below) the origin of the left subclavian artery. After insertion, placement is verified by chest radiograph, fluoroscopy, or transesophageal echocardiogram. On the chest radiograph, the tip is roughly at the left second intercostal space. Once placement is confirmed, the polytetrafluoroethylene graft is sutured to the arteriotomy.

Ideally, the balloon occludes 85% to 90% of the aortic lumen during inflation; it should not completely occlude the aorta. Total occlusion could result in aortic wall injury and damage to red blood cells and platelets. After hemostasis is achieved, a heparin infusion is started to maintain an aPTT of 40 to 60 seconds.

Timing of Inflation and Deflation

The IABP uses helium or carbon dioxide to rapidly inflate and deflate the balloon. The balloon inflates at the onset of cardiac diastole and deflates at the onset of systole. The standard method of balloon inflation timing is by triggering the R wave from the ECG while monitoring the arterial waveform pressure. The inflation and deflation points are adjusted to maximize afterload reduction and diastolic augmentation. It is helpful to record an arterial waveform tracing during a 1:2 heart rate-to-counterpulsation ratio, comparing the assisted and unassisted pulse to assess the effectiveness of the timing of counterpulsation.[50] Balloon inflation and deflation can also be timed using M-mode echocardiography.[50] The transducer is positioned parasternal to obtain simultaneous images of both the aortic valve and the balloon. During imaging, the balloon inflation and deflation points are adjusted to coincide with aortic valve closure and opening, respectively.

Weaning

The weaning of the IABP usually begins once systemic perfusion is adequate after pharmacologic support has been substantially reduced or removed. A two-dimensional echocardiogram is often used to aid in the decision to wean. Parameters for weaning generally include improvement in the left ventricular ejection phase indices, such as shortening or ejection fraction. Weaning may occur over a 24- to 48-hour period. The pump is systematically reduced from a 1:1 ratio to 1:2 and then 1:3 over the weaning period.

The IABP catheter is removed at the patient's bedside. Embolectomy catheters may be used once the balloon is removed to evacuate any clot that might remain in the common femoral artery before closure of the artery. Distal pulses should be confirmed before closure of the groin incision and monitored following closure.

Complications

Complications reported during pediatric IABP therapy include limb ischemia, infection, balloon rupture, vessel perforation, thrombocytopenia, aortic dissection, and mesenteric, renal, or cerebral ischemia.[33,50]

The IABP should never remain dormant for longer than 15 minutes, because blood trapped in the folds of the deflated balloon can trigger clot formation. If the IABP is dormant for longer than 15 minutes, manual inflation and deflation is required every 5 minutes until the problem is resolved.

Blood in the driveline or tubing can indicate balloon rupture. Immediately notify a physician if balloon rupture is suspected and prepare for IABP removal. Systemic arterial emboli from the balloon catheter or graft can develop.

Nursing Considerations

The pediatric nurse should be trained and familiar with the IABP console and how to make adjustments to improve timing. Initially, two nurses are usually needed to provide nursing care; one for the care of the patient and one devoted to running the balloon pump. When the patient's condition stabilizes, the critical care nurse will be responsible for both the patient and the IABP.

During IABP therapy, hemodynamic monitoring should be consistent with that required for any patient with LV dysfunction. The nurse may note absent or diminished pulse in the involved extremity following balloon insertion. The nurse should frequently evaluate lower extremity perfusion (including color, temperature, and capillary refill) and notify a provider immediately if evidence of limb ischemia and coolness appears.

NURSING CARE OF THE PEDIATRIC PATIENT REQUIRING MCS

The purpose of this section is to present essential concepts for the nursing care of the postoperative pediatric MCS support patient. General principles of care are similar for all pediatric patients requiring MCS. Most MCS devices should be initiated before the presence of end-organ dysfunction or circulatory collapse. Recently, ECMO or ECLS has been used for rapid resuscitation for children with cardiac arrest. The goal of ECMO or VAD support is the recovery of cardiopulmonary function or provision of MCS as a bridge to transplant.

The multidisciplinary team should prepare the child (if possible) and family regarding the child's clinical condition, expected prognosis, and anticipated support duration (bridge to transplant or bridge to recovery). Although rehabilitation will likely be required for all children after MCS, VAD support requires rehabilitation during therapy. After the patient is stabilized with pneumatic VAD support, progression of early extubation, invasive line removal, nutritional support, and cardiac rehabilitation are facilitated to minimize the risk of infection and optimize the patient condition before transplant or device removal.

The nursing care plan in Box 7-3 is designed for pediatric patients on ECMO and VAD support. Interventions are separated if they differ for ECMO or VAD support.

Preparation of the Child and Family

If the child deteriorates rapidly, preparation of the child for MCS support may be limited. This time is stressful for the family when making life saving decisions. Parents need hope within reason. Honest and open communication between the nurse and family is central to developing a trusting relationship. Before the family visits the child for the first time after mechanical support placement, the nurse should meet with family members away from the bedside and explain to them what they are about to see. Furthermore, the nurse should encourage the parents to visit, talk to, and touch their child when possible. The social worker and chaplain are often important members of the multidisciplinary team and should be available to the family for support before the initiation of mechanical support.

Pediatric Critical Care Unit (PCCU) Setup

The PCCU bedside setup for MCS is the same for a postoperative cardiac surgery patient (see Chapter 8). The bed selection, bed location, and equipment needed (IV pumps, ventilator) should be prearranged, if possible, to optimize space for easy movement during care of the patient. Although equipment for MCS can vary depending on the selected device, all extension cords and drive lines must be well secured to minimize accidental falls or disconnection.

Emergency equipment that should be present at the bedside at all times includes heavy metal tubing clamps, emergency equipment to manually hand crank centrifugal devices, and bulb suction equipment to manually pump the pneumatic device. A backup ECMO machine or VAD console should be plugged, tested, and ready for use if any malfunction requires a circuit or console change. Blood products should be readily available during MCS support.

Admission or Initiation of MCS and Staffing

ECMO support can be initiated in the operating suite, or cannulation can be performed at the bedside. Although there are many variations in staffing, in most ECMO centers two providers are assigned to the patient: a critical care nurse provides all patient care and an ECMO specialist monitors and cares for the ECMO circuit. ECMO specialists are specially trained nurses, respiratory care practitioners, or perfusionists who have attended an ECMO training class. The ELSO published guidelines for the training of these specialists, including detailed knowledge of the pathophysiology of common diseases, ECMO physiology, and immediate treatment for patient events and ECMO emergencies. (For more information, see http://www.elso.med.umich.edu/)

Box 7-3 **Nursing Care of the Pediatric Patient During Mechanical Circulatory Support**

Potential for Hemorrhage and other Complications Related to MCS Malfunction

- ECMO device failure/disruption can result from raceway rupture, inadvertent decannulation, power failure
- VAD device failure/disruption can result from console malfunction or power failure

Expected Outcome

- The patient will not develop bleeding or other complications associated with MCS malfunction.

Nursing Interventions

- Frequently inspect circuits for cracks or stress on the raceway and make planned repairs or replacements.
- Frequently inspect and test alarms and pressure monitors.
- Assess electrical outlets and connections on a routine basis (per hospital protocol).
- Keep emergency resuscitation medications at bedside.
- Keep appropriate emergency equipment (e.g., metal tubing clamps, hand crank, bulb syringes) available
- Have backup ECMO circuit/pump and VAD console available and charged.

Potential Inadquate Cardiac Output Related to

- ECMO/VAD insertion
- Hypovolemia or hemorrhage
- Tamponade or pericardial effusion
- Myocardial dysfunction (cardiac stun)
- Hypoxemia
- Increased systemic or pulmonary vascular resistance
- Arrhythmias

Expected Outcomes

- Patients will demonstrate adequate cardiac output as evidenced by:
  - Appropriate systemic arterial pressure and SVR
  - Adequate NIRS, pH, and lactate level
  - Good peripheral perfusion
  - Appropriate heart rate and rhythm
  - Minimal bleeding (<3 mL/kg per hour)
  - Urine output of 0.5-2 mL/kg per hour
  - Absence of systemic or pulmonary venous congestion
  - No evidence of cardiac tamponade
  - Patient will demonstrate adequate systemic perfusion or pulmonary vascular resistance (PVR) as evidenced by good systemic perfusion, appropriate mean arterial pressure (MAP) per age, and PVR.

Nursing Interventions

- Assess child's systemic perfusion, including temperature, color of mucous membranes, nail beds, skin, quality of peripheral pulses, and capillary refill time.
- Notify provider of signs of poor systemic perfusion.
- Monitor for evidence of bleeding: excessive chest tube output (>3 mL/kg per hour), oozing from cannulation site and sternal patch (if closure delayed).
- Monitor for signs of coagulopathies.
  - Draw blood samples for coagulation studies (ACT, PLT, PT, aPTT) immediately after ECMO/VAD insertion and then as ordered.
  - Adjust heparin infusion per standing orders for VAD and ECMO device.

- If platelet count is low (thrombocytopenia), replace with platelets per order or protocol.
- Keep ACT between 140 and 180 sec for VAD devices and between 200 and 240 sec for ECMO.
- Monitor for signs of cardiac tamponade in patients receiving MCS:
  - Rising central venous pressure (CVP) right atrial (RA) and pulmonary artery end-diastolic pressures, tachycardia, hypotension, decreased SvO_2 or NIRS, decreased MCS device filling, decreased VAD output, and widened mediastinum on chest radiograph.
  - If sternal closure is delayed, sternal patch may bulge.
  - If tamponade is suspected, notify physician immediately and prepare for emergency chest exploration and evacuation of clot, or prepare for the patient to return to the operating suite per institutional policy.
- Measure and record hourly urine output; report output <0.5 mL/kg per hour.
- Monitor heart rate and rhythm; ensure that heart rate is appropriate for the patient's age and condition. Report clinically significant arrhythmias to the provider.
- Monitor patient's arterial blood pressure; report hypotension or hypertension.
- Monitor cardiac index; report decrease and any cardiac index <2.5 L/min per m² BSA.
- Monitor arterial blood gases and serum lactate; report acidosis or abnormalities.
- During ECMO, obtain simultaneous arterial and SvO_2 measurements. If difference is increasing, the child's cardiac output is probably falling; if difference is decreasing, the child's cardiac output probably is rising. Adjust ECMO flow per protocol or order.
- Monitor patient for normal MAP (per age). If SVR or MAP is elevated:
  - Assess for hypervolemia or hypertension related to MCS.
  - Administer continuous vasodilators, such as nitroglycerin or sodium nitroprusside, to keep MAP within normal limits.
  - Ensure adequate intravascular volume before initiation of vasodilators to minimize risk of hypotension.
  - Assess for adequate pain control that may cause hypertension.
- If PVR is elevated on VAD support:
  - Support pulmonary vasodilators (e.g., alkalosis, adequate inspired oxygen) and avoid potential pulmonary vasoconstrictors (alveolar hypoxia, acidosis, hypothermia, agitation)—i.e., provide sedation and analgesia—and administer pulmonary vasodilators such as prostaglandin E1 or inhaled nitric oxide.
  - Assess VAD filling by monitoring console alarms. Patients with elevated PVR will have inadequate VAD filling secondary to decreased venous return.

Potential for Inadequate Intravascular Volume Related to

- Hemorrhage
- Diuresis
- Inadequate volume administration

Continued

Box 7-3   Nursing Care of the Pediatric Patient During Mechanical Circulatory Support—cont'd

Expected Outcome

- Patient demonstrates adequate intravascular volume with adequate ECMO/VAD filling
- Hematocrit within normal limits per age and orders or protocol
- Adequate CVP or RA pressure and pulmonary capillary wedge pressure (PCWP) or left atrial (LA) pressure
- Urine output 0.5-2.0 mL/kg per hour
- Chest tube output <3 mL/kg per hour
- Adequate systemic perfusion, moist mucous membranes, and good skin turgor

Nursing Intervention

- Record and calculate total fluid intake and output, including blood drawn for laboratory analysis.
- Measure CVP/RA and PCWP/LA pressures and support to optimize perfusion per orders.
- Draw blood sample for Hct immediately after ECMO/VAD insertion and then per orders. If Hct is low, administer packed red blood cells (PRBCs) per order.
- Draw blood samples for coagulation studies (ACT, PLT, PT, aPTT) immediately after ECMO/VAD insertion and then per orders. Adjust heparin infusion per standing orders for VAD and ECMO device. If platelet count is low, replace with platelets per orders. Keep ACT between 140 and 180 sec for VAD devices and between 200 and 240 sec for ECMO.
- Milk chest tubes gently and tap firmly to keep free of clots. Notify the provider if chest tube output is >3 mL/kg per hour for 3 h or 5 mL/kg per hour for 1 h.
- For patients with delayed sternal closure, notify the provider if the sternal patch fills or bulges.
- Discuss with a provider the possibility of surgical bleeding in the presence of excessive chest tube output and the absence of coagulopathy.
- Assess patient's hydration and report signs of inadequate hydration. Signs of adequate hydration are
  - Moist mucous membranes
  - Level fontanelle (not sunken or full)
  - Good skin turgor (not tented after pinching)
  - Urine output of 0.5-2 mL/kg per hour
- Avoid any nonessential invasive procedures (e.g., peripheral IV removal) while the patient is receiving heparin therapy, because the procedure may cause uncontrolled bleeding at site.

Potential Impairment in Gas Exchange Related to

- Atelectasis
- Pneumothorax
- Hemothorax
- Plural effusion
- Congestive heart failure
- Low cardiac output
- Pulmonary hypertension
- Inadequate mechanical circulator support
- Inadequate mechanical ventilation

Expected Outcomes

- Patient will demonstrate adequate gas exchange as evidenced by satisfactory clinical appearance and arterial blood gases, appropriate pulse oximetry and exhaled carbon dioxide, and normal lung compliance with full lung expansion and no evidence of atelectasis.

- For the patient requiring VAD/ECMO support, SvO_2 of 70-75% and PaO_2 of 50-70 mmHg will be maintained.

Nursing Interventions

- Monitor for signs of hypoxemia, including tachycardia, increased spontaneous respiratory rate, compromise in systemic perfusion, deterioration in level of consciousness, decreased hemoglobin saturation, rise in exhaled CO_2, deterioration in PaO_2 or pH.
- Long-term VAD use should be weaned to extubation once the patient's condition is stable, with regular pulmonary toilet incorporated into daily routine.
- Draw arterial, venous, and pump (for ECMO) blood gases immediately after ECMO/VAD insertion and then per orders. Venous and arterial pH, PaO_2, and $PaCO_2$ should be within normal limits.
- Adjust sweep gas and ECMO flow per protocol or MD order. Increasing the sweep gas decreases $PaCO_2$ levels, and increasing the ECMO flow rate elevates the PaO_2 levels.
- Auscultate lung sounds and monitor chest expansion.
- Verify appropriate endotracheal tube depth of insertion or adjust if needed.
- Monitor for and notify provider of any change in PIP, PEEP, and exhaled tidal volume.
  - A rise in PIP can indicate reduced lung compliance or pneumothorax.
  - A rise in PEEP can indicate inadvertent PEEP produced by obstruction to exhalation.
  - Loss of PEEP can occur with spontaneous inspiration, a leak around the endotracheal tube, or a leak in the system (see Chapters 9 and 21).
- Suction via endotracheal tube per unit protocol and as needed. Monitor color, consistency and quantity of secretions.
- Change the patient's body position every 1-2 h as tolerated.
- Monitor fluid balance and daily weight.

Potential Alteration in Cerebral Perfusion and Function Related to

- Hypoxia
- Hypotension
- Inadequate systemic perfusion
- Metabolic Acidosis
- Thromboembolism
- Cerebral hemorrhage
- Electrolyte Imbalance
- Prolonged undetected status epilepticus

Expected Outcome

- Patient will demonstrate no signs of increased intracranial pressure and no new neurologic deficit.

Nursing Interventions

- Assess neurologic function before and immediately after initiation of MCS.
- Correct hypotension, hypoxemia, and acidosis as soon as possible.
- Monitor NIRS cerebral tissue oxygenation (normal range >50%). Notify provider of decrease.
- Verify performance and report results of cranial ultrasound examinations daily for first 3 days of ECMO (or per protocol).
- Maintain ACT in desired range for VAD (140-180 sec) or ECMO (200-240 sec)

Box 7-3 **Nursing Care of the Pediatric Patient During Mechanical Circulatory Support—cont'd**

- Monitor ECMO/VAD circuit and tubing for clot or air formation; notify provider if present.
- Check coagulation studies and administer anticoagulation therapy as indicated for MCS.

Potential Alteration in Renal Function and Urine Output Related to
- Hemolysis
- Inadequate systemic perfusion/reperfusion
- Thromboembolus
- Complications of medication

Expected Outcomes
- Patient demonstrates adequate urine output (0.5-2 mL/kg per hour) when fluid intake is adequate
- Patients demonstrates serum creatinine and BUN within normal limits

Nursing Intervention
- Measure urine output every hour and notify provider if hourly total is < 0.5 mL/kg per hour
- If oliguria develops:
  - Administer fluid bolus per order if urine output is inadequate and CVP is low.
  - Initiate fluid restriction and diuretics per order if urine output remains inadequate despite normal to high CVP.
- If urine is red or rust color, provide intravenous fluids to maintain urine flow and prevent RBC accumulation in glomeruli causing acute tubular necrosis or renal failure.
- If hyperkalemia develops during VAD, administer calcium, glucose, and insulin, or sodium polystyrene sulfonate (Kayexalate) enema per orders (see Chapter 12 and Table 12-4).
- Prepare for peritoneal dialysis, hemodialysis, or modified hemofiltration (depending on circulatory support) per orders as indicated (see Chapter 13).
- If renal impairment is suspected, closely monitor serum creatinine, BUN, and K^+ concentrations.
- If renal impairment is present, evaluate doses of drugs that require renal excretion.

Potential Infection Related to
- Cardiovascular surgery
- ECMO/VAD insertion
- Invasive monitoring techniques
- Compromised nutritional status

Expected Outcome
- Patient will demonstrate no signs or symptoms of infection such as fever or hypothermia, leukocytosis or leucopenia, localized infection or inflammation, positive wound or blood culture, or elevated C-reactive protein.

Nursing Interventions
- Ensure that every provider washes hands before and after patient contact.
- Ensure appropriate sterile and aseptic techniques for procedures or dressing changes.
- Maintain occlusive dressings over all invasive monitoring catheters and an open chest.
- Change dressings and intravenous tubing per unit policy.
- Monitor patient for signs and symptoms of infection.

- Administer antibiotics as ordered.
- If infection is present, monitor for evidence of sepsis (tachycardia, blood pressure instability, thrombocytopenia, temperature instability).

Potential Child and Family Knowledge Deficit Related to
- Child's cardiovascular disease
- Initiation and requirement of mechanical circulatory support device
- Prognosis

Expected Outcomes
- Patient and family demonstrate appropriate and accurate knowledge through discussion of the child's disease, purpose of the mechanical support, goals of the mechanical support, and prognosis.

Nursing Interventions
- Ascertain what the patient and family have been told about the disease, therapy, and prognosis.
- Ask parents how they think child can best be prepared for MCS (as appropriate).
- Assess and document the child's and the family's learning needs and barriers to learning.
- Prepare the child and family for clinical course of mechanical circulatory support including:
  - High risk for bleeding and potential need for blood transfusion
  - Potential for decreased cardiac output and possible interventions
  - Sedation and possible neuromuscular blockade
  - Description and explanation of the MCS device
  - Anticipated length of MCS
  - Goals of MCS and anticipated prognosis
- Encourage the child and the family to ask questions and participate in care when appropriate.
- Record specific teaching information (including terminology used) so that the healthcare team can use consistent terms and reinforce identical information.

Potential Child and Family Anxiety Related to
- Child's life-threatening condition
- Long-term prognosis
- Lack of familiarity with MCS device
- Hospitalization and prognosis

Expected Outcomes
- Patient and family demonstrate manageable levels of anxiety as evidenced by:
  - Absence of behavior that interferes with medical care
  - Appropriate family questions
  - Discussion of the disease process
  - Accurate discussion about the need for ECMO/VAD support
  - Family participation in care as appropriate

Nursing Interventions
- Maintain open communication with patient and family.
- Answer all questions honestly at the appropriate level for patient and family understanding.
- Prepare patient (as age appropriate) and family for procedures. Include a child life specialist as appropriate for the child's age and clinical condition.

Continued

- Encourage family participation in patient care as appropriate.
- Encourage the child's expression of feelings and emphasize acceptability of expression.
- Assess the family's resources and refer to appropriate hospital support services (See Chapter 2)

Potential Additional Patient Care Priorities
Potential compromise in nutrition related to
- Inadequate intravenous nutrition

- Impaired gastrointestinal absorption
- Increased metabolic requirements
Impairment in physical mobility related to
- Prolonged supine position connected to ECMO/VAD device
Pain or discomfort related to
- ECMO/VAD cannula site
- Possible open chest
- Surgical incision
- Multiple invasive catheters or procedures

ACT, Activated clotting time; *aPTT*, activated partial thromboplastin time; *BSA*, body surface area; *BUN*, blood urea nitrogen; *CVP*, central venous pressure; *ECMO*, extracorporeal membrane oxygenation; *Hct*, hematocrit; *IV*, intravenous; *LA*, left atrium; *MAP*, mean arterial pressure; *MCS*, mechanical circulatory support; *NIRS*, near-infrared spectroscopy; *PCWP*, pulmonary capillary wedge pressure; *PEEP*, positive end-expiratory pressure; *PIP*, peak inspiratory pressure; *PLT*, platelet count; *PRBC*, packed red blood cells; *PT*, prothrombin time; *PVR*, pulmonary vascular resistance; *RA*, right atrium; *SvO2*, venous oxygen saturation; *VAD*, ventricular assist device.

VADs are placed in the operating suite. Two nurses are initially required to accept the child to the ICU after VAD placement: one nurse cares for the patient and a second nurse monitors the VAD. Once the patient is stabilized, one nurse can care for both the patient and the VAD pneumatic device, provided the nurse is trained in the device type and its operation and components, troubleshooting, and response to emergencies. Some centers that use centrifugal pumps may require a perfusionist to manage the VAD.

Postoperative Care

The postoperative nursing care of patients receiving MCS involves thorough and repeated assessment and support of every organ system, device management and troubleshooting, monitoring of laboratory values, and anticipation and treatment of any complications. Upon initial cannulation or placement of the MCS device, the nurse should perform a primary assessment to provide a baseline to identify any clinical changes.

Neurologic Assessment

The pediatric patient receiving MCS is at risk for cerebral embolism and bleeding, so frequent neurologic assessment is required. Routine cranial ultrasound examinations are performed to assess for the presence of IVH in neonates and infants with an open fontanelle. Clinical neurologic assessment is particularly challenging in patients with centrifugal VAD or ECMO support with open chest cannulation; such cannulation typically requires that patients be sedated with possible neuromuscular blockade. In patients receiving neuromuscular blockade, the only clinical signs of seizures may be abrupt changes in heart rate, blood pressure, skin perfusion, and pupil size. If seizures are suspected, a cranial ultrasound examination or head computed tomography scan will be obtained to look for evidence of bleeding. An electroencephalogram will be required to assess for the presence of seizures and cerebral cortical activity.

When ECMO cannulation uses the internal jugular vein and right common carotid artery, the head is maintained in the midline position to avoid obstruction of the vein or artery. Such compression could compromise cerebral venous drainage or perfusion.

Near-Infrared Spectroscopy (NIRS)

NIRS provides continuous, real-time data regarding tissue oxygenation that can be used in conjunction with clinical and laboratory assessment to evaluate systemic oxygenation and perfusion. The NIRS system uses adhesive sensors placed on the forehead and over the abdomen. Each adhesive sensor contains a light source and two optodes (fiberoptic bundles), often placed at angles from one another to evaluate light absorption and reflection of different tissue depths. As light passes through the skin—and in the case of the brain, through the skull—and into tissue, oxygenated and deoxygenated hemoglobin and oxygenated cell mitochondria affect light absorption and reflection. The NIRS devices calculate the average oxygen saturation of underlying arteries, capillaries, and veins, to reflect a tissue or regional tissue oxygen saturation (rSO_2) that is similar to a mixed venous oxygen saturation. This tissue oxygen saturation is digitally and continuously displayed.

Evaluation of both cerebral and somatic (typically evaluated over the abdomen) oxygenation can help identify changes in regional oxygenation and blood flow. A change in NIRS saturation can indicate declining or inadequate cerebral or somatic oxygenation and allow corrective action to prevent hypoxic injury.

The cerebral rSO_2 value will vary depending on the level of sedation or agitation and the location of the sensor. It will also be affected by factors influencing cerebral blood flow such as increased intracranial pressure (can decrease blood flow), changes in $PaCO_2$ (hypocarbia produces cerebral vasoconstriction and decreased cerebral blood flow, and hypercarbia produces cerebral vasodilation and increased blood flow) and severe hypoxemia (produces cerebral artery dilation and attempts to increase cerebral blood flow). The target cerebral rSO_2 is greater than 50%.[25]

The somatic tissue oxygenation should be higher than cerebral tissue oxygenation, because the kidneys receive 25% of cardiac output at any time. The target difference between somatic and cerebral rSO_2 should be greater than 10%, with somatic readings approximately 10% to 15% points higher than cerebral readings.[25]

NIRS monitoring can be a valuable tool during ECMO support to identify a compromise in tissue oxygenation that may result from reversible problems with cannula placement, and it can assist in the evaluation of systemic oxygen delivery and readiness for decannulation. If a change in cannula position or a circuit malfunction occurs, the flow deficit will produce a fall in rSO_2. Furthermore, if the rSO_2 falls significantly during weaning and clamping of the ECMO circuit, then additional time on ECMO will be needed. If the rSO_2 remains stable in a patient with other signs of adequate systemic perfusion, the patient is likely to be sufficiently stable for decannulation.[25]

Sedation and Analgesia

Sedation and analgesia administration after ECMO or VAD placement will vary depending whether the patient is cannulated through an open or closed chest, and must be titrated to patient response. Continuous sedation and analgesia is maintained with fentanyl (0.5-2 mcg/kg per hour) or morphine sulfate (0.02 mg/kg per hour) and midazolam (0.05-0.1 mg/kg per hour) infusions. Intermittent doses can be provided for agitation, painful procedures, or unexplained hypertension and tachycardia.

Neuromuscular blockade may be needed for the hemodynamically unstable patient receiving MCS. Pancuronium (0.1 mg/kg per dose) or a Cis-atracurium infusion (0.2 mg/kg per hour) can be used. Minimal use of neuromuscular blockade is advantageous to allow spontaneous movement and assess for seizure activity. For further information, see Chapter 5.

Respiratory Assessment

All patients receiving MCS are initially intubated and their lungs are mechanically ventilated. Lung sounds should be auscultated and chest expansion assessed during hand ventilation (with bag). The depth of endotracheal tube insertion should be adjusted if breath sounds are decreased on the left side or if placement is too low or too high on chest radiograph. Patients receiving only left ventricular support via centrifugal devices require full ventilator support. Patients requiring more long-term pneumatic assistance with a VAD should be weaned to extubation once stable.

During VA ECMO, mechanical ventilation settings are generally reduced to an inspired oxygen of 21% to 40%, peak inspiratory pressure of 20 to 25 cm H_2O, positive end-expiratory pressure of 4 to 10 cm H_2O, and respiratory rate of 5 to 10 breaths per minute. The goal of the resting ventilator settings is to maintain functional residual capacity and prevent barotrauma. In patients with minimal lung disease and native cardiac output, gas exchange will then occur within the lungs and through the membrane oxygenator.

Daily chest radiographs and frequent arterial and venous blood gas samples are used to monitor respiratory function. Bilateral opacification of lung fields is generally apparent on chest radiograph within the first 24 hours of ECMO, resulting from a reduction of positive airway pressure and complement activation leading to capillary leak and pulmonary edema. Patients with persistent pulmonary air leaks while receiving ECMO may require very low positive airway pressure to allow the lungs to heal. Pulmonary care should include chest vibration and suctioning of the endotracheal tube as needed to clear secretions. Limitation of suctioning may be needed if bleeding is exacerbated by the procedure.

Potential respiratory complications include pneumothorax or hemothorax, pleural effusions, and pulmonary hemorrhage. Needle aspiration or chest tube insertion are options for emergent decompression of a pneumothorax or hemothorax or drainage of a pleural effusion. If pulmonary hemorrhage develops, management consists of minimizing the target ACT, increasing the platelet count, and minimizing suctioning. If bleeding becomes more severe, epinephrine (0.1 mL/kg of 10,000 dilution) may be instilled into the trachea and positive end expiratory pressure instituted. See Chapter 9 for information regarding mechanical ventilation.

Cardiac Assessment and Support

The patient's cardiac output, hemodynamics, and device flow must be monitored continuously to ensure adequate systemic perfusion. The critical care nurse must understand the device operation and components to interpret hemodynamic changes and ensure effective MCS. Inadequate systemic perfusion can result from inadequate intravascular volume, inappropriate vascular resistance, (native) myocardial dysfunction, arrhythmias, or tamponade.

Inadequate Intravascular Volume. Inadequate intravascular volume can result from hemorrhage, excessive diuresis, or inadequate fluid administration. In the early postoperative period, bleeding following MCS placement can be life-threatening and increase demands on blood resources. Risk factors for bleeding include: low preoperative platelet count, long cardiopulmonary bypass time, hypothermia, preoperative anticoagulation, and hepatic dysfunction. Intraoperative prevention and management require meticulous hemostasis and reversing heparin. Anticoagulation, if indicated for the device, should not be initiated until bleeding from the chest tubes has decreased. Maintaining high filling pressures and treating coagulopathies with blood component therapies (packed red blood cells, fresh frozen plasma, or platelets) is essential. Volume status can be assessed by monitoring central venous pressure, mean arterial or pulse pressure, and indirect indicators such as urine output.

The nurse needs to monitor for excessive fluid loss leading to hypovolemia and inadequate VAD or ECMO filling. If the patient's hematocrit is stable and within normal range for age, colloid or crystalloid solutions can be administered to maintain adequate circulating volume. Maintenance intravenous fluids may need to be added or adjusted until urine output has normalized at 0.5 to 2 mL/kg per hour.

Inappropriate Vascular Resistance. Elevated systemic vascular resistance can result from hypervolemia or from the initiation of MCS. Nonpulsatile device flow leads to the release of renin, which stimulates the renin-angiotensin system, causing arteriolar constriction.[47] Hypertension can cause bleeding in the patient receiving anticoagulation. Vigilant blood pressure control is essential to reduce the incidence of IVH. In addition, the nurse must assess for and treat agitation and pain as potential causes of hypertension.

Neonatal pulmonary hypertension or postoperative elevated pulmonary vascular resistance that is unresponsive to mechanical ventilation, intravenous pulmonary vasodilators, or inhaled nitric oxide may require ECMO support for patient survival, particularly if the increased pulmonary vascular resistance is associated with low cardiac output and acidosis. ECMO can interrupt the cycle of pulmonary hypertension and provides support until the underlying condition resolves or pulmonary vascular resistance falls.

Native Myocardial Dysfunction. Native cardiac output should be optimized on VV ECMO or LVAD support as a bridge to recovery. During VV ECMO, which does not support cardiac function, and occasionally during LVAD support, right ventricular failure develops and requires inotropic support. Inotropic agents such as milrinone, dopamine, and dobutamine are avoided if possible because they increase myocardial oxygen consumption. However, drugs such as epinephrine and norepinephrine may ultimately be required in patients with more severe myocardial dysfunction or overwhelming sepsis.

Native myocardial function will often improve with afterload reduction, particularly when hypertension is present. The most effective antihypertensive drugs are nitroprusside, nitroglycerin, prostaglandin E1, or hydralazine. Before initiation of these vasodilators, volume status is optimized to minimize the risk of hypotension, and abnormal electrolyte concentrations are corrected.

During VA ECMO, the pump provides nonpulsatile flow, so systemic perfusion will improve if the native myocardium ejects some blood.[60] Left ventricular ejection facilitates decompression of the left heart, reducing the need for left atrial venting, and may potentially reduce the risk of intracardiac thrombosis formation from blood stasis. It is challenging to identify the optimal pump flow rate to optimize cardiac output in the presence of right ventricular failure caused by hypoxia and pulmonary hypertension. Before weaning of ECMO support, the native myocardium may require inotropic support.

Arrhythmias. Arrhythmias during MCS can result from hypoxia, from electrolyte imbalance, from irritability caused by atrial cannula position, or as a complication of cardiac surgery. In patients requiring VA ECMO or BiVAD support, atrioventricular synchrony is not crucial because the body is perfused, despite the presence of what are normally nonperfusing arrhythmias. However, synchrony will be critical during weaning from MCS when myocardial function is limited. After cardiotomy, patients with atrial and ventricular epicardial pacing wires may benefit from cardiac pacing if indicated. Antiarrhythmic medication, radiofrequency catheter ablation, or recovery of the underlying myocardial disease may be required before ECMO removal in patients receiving ECMO secondary to lethal arrhythmias.

Tamponade. Pericardial or mediastinal tamponade can develop during MCS. Tamponade inhibits venous return to the MCS device and decreases cardiac output. Signs of cardiac tamponade include a convex or bulging sternotomy patch (if open sternum), increasing right and left atrial pressures with decrease in mean arterial pressure, tachycardia, decreased VAD (cardiac) output, a widened heart size or mediastinum on chest radiograph, cessation of chest tube drainage

(if present), or a pericardial effusion with ventricular compression noted on an echocardiogram. The echocardiogram is the definitive diagnostic test, but treatment should not await the study. Treatments include volume administration, inotropic agents, milking or suctioning (with sterile technique) of chest tubes (if present) to remove clot formation, or immediate reexploration of the chest in the operating suite.

VADs must receive blood from the native heart, so any condition that alters this flow of blood to the device will affect VAD performance and the patient's clinical status. For example, patients receiving LVAD support may have decreased VAD flow despite volume replacement. To improve LVAD flow, the cause of decreased flow (e.g., increased pulmonary vascular resistance, pericardial effusion, decreased native cardiac output) must be identified and treated.

Troubleshooting VAD Pump and Console

As more VADs are placed in children as a bridge to transplant, longer support durations are inevitable. Consequently, VAD dysfunction may become more prevalent. The VAD-trained critical care nurse should examine all external device components such as cannulas, drive lines, battery support, and all mechanical and electrical connections. The nurse should be familiar with the VAD alarms and troubleshooting techniques (see Table 7-4).

The Bio-Medicus centrifugal console has low- and high-flow alarms. Flow can frequently change in response to blood pressure or vascular resistance. Constant visual, auditory, and tactile monitoring is required. Visual and tactile checks of the circuit can detect line "chattering" that would indicate inadequate preload or cannula obstruction. Other visual checks include examination of lines, connector sites, and the centrifugal head for changes in color that could indicate fibrin clot formation. In addition, auditory and tactile checks are needed to detect vibration of the centrifugal head.

The pneumatic console delivers air pressure to compress and empty the blood pump sac delivering pulsatile flow. Each blood pump must fill and eject completely to give the patient an adequate cardiac output. Cardiac output is optimized by adjusting the pressure and vacuum values on the console. Most pneumatic consoles have low-fill alarms, indicating inadequate pump preload before ejection. The nurse should assess the patient's volume status for any changes or signs of right-sided heart failure during single LVAD support.

Use a flashlight daily to assess external pumps for thrombi formation and complete VAD emptying. Illuminate the pump at an angle to verify transmission of a white light through to the opposite side. If a pink light is noted, then the VAD is not completely emptying. The physician should be notified immediately whenever clot formation is noted or suspected in the circuit or pump. The use of heparin-coated pumps and circuits will hopefully reduce the incidence of thromboembolic complications in the future.

Hematologic Assessment

Thrombosis and bleeding are the most common complications of MCS.[60] Patients receiving MCS are susceptible to bleeding from all surgical sites and should be monitored closely (e.g., cannula sites, incisions, chest tubes). All saturated dressings should be measured and included in the total output calculation. All bodily fluids such as stool, urine, gastric drainage, and sputum should be checked for blood. The nurse should monitor the child's abdominal girth and assess for increased abdominal distension and firmness. In addition, the nurse should try to avoid any procedure that may produce bleeding such as heel sticks, venipunctures or injections, insertion of a nasogastric tube, or urinary catheter or rectal probe insertion.

The patient's hematocrit, fibrinogen, and platelet counts are routinely monitored, and appropriate blood products are administered as needed. Blood product replacement protocols may vary among institutions. In general, the target platelet count is >100,000/mm^3, fibrinogen 100 mg/dL, and hematocrit >35%. If possible, blood transfusions should be limited for patients awaiting transplant, because frequent exposure can increase the panel reactive antibody, which can complicate matching for a future transplantation.[11] Blood products should be irradiated, depleted of leukocytes, and negative for cytomegalovirus.[11] If excessive nonsurgical bleeding is encountered, aminocaproic acid, aprotinin, and recombinant factor VII may be administered.

Anticoagulation

Anticoagulation management can be an extremely challenging part of management in patients receiving MCS. The goal of anticoagulation therapy is a balance of preventing pump thrombosis formation and bleeding. Blood exposure to an artificial circuit triggers the coagulation cascade and causes clots to form in the circuit. Anticoagulation is therefore necessary to prevent clot formation and the resultant consumptive coagulopathy that would occur as procoagulants are depleted by the clotting process.

Most anticoagulation regimens begin with intravascular heparin sodium infusion generally titrated in the range of 20 to 60 units/kg per hour to achieve a desired aPTT of 60 to 80 sec or an ACT of 140 to 180 sec (VAD) or 200 to 240 sec (ECMO). These ranges can vary depending on the type of support, the technology used to measure them (e.g., Hemochrons, I Stats), the patient's risk for bleeding, and whether the device circuit is coated with heparin or another bioactive surface. The heparin infusion is usually started once chest tube output has decreased. Patients receiving long-term VAD support can eventually transition to oral anticoagulation, such as warfarin or antiplatelet therapy. Protocols to guide anticoagulation therapy are typically available for specific devices, with recommended INR ranges.

The control of the coagulation system on ECMO is complex. The ACT is followed every hour with titration of the heparin dose. However, AT III levels are low in many patients receiving ECMO, and the combination of AT III and a heparin cofactor is needed for anticoagulant effects. The combination of AT III and a heparin cofactor stops the conversion of fibrinogen to fibrin and ultimately prevents clot formation. A deficiency in AT III can cause heparin to be ineffective, leading to excessive heparin use and the potential for clotting of the circuit. Replacement of AT III or fresh frozen plasma is necessary to restore adequate AT III levels and the anticoagulant effects of heparin.

Patients receiving ECMO also have thrombocytopenia, because platelets are deposited onto artificial surfaces and lost to clot formation in the circuit. In addition, after exposure to the circuit, many remaining platelets are nonfunctional. Thrombocytopenia will ultimately lead to bleeding. Platelet transfusions are given to reverse thrombocytopenia and reduce the risk of hemorrhage.

Consumptive Coagulopathy. Consumptive coagulopathy can develop secondary to clotting in the circuit and inadequate replacement of clotting factors, creating risk of both thromboembolism and risk of bleeding. Replacement with platelet and cryoprecipitate transfusions or use of replacement products, such as factor VII, can precipitate clotting in the circuit. In addition, the use of aminocaproic acid (Amicar) or other fibrinolytic system stabilizers increases the risk of thrombus formation in the device circuit. Fibrinolytics are used before and after surgery in patients receiving ECMO to decrease bleeding from activation of fibrinolysis (clot breakdown), which can increase bleeding. Although stopping lysis of clots is beneficial to control bleeding, the risk is that clot formation is encouraged within the circuit. Monitoring of the circuit and careful titration of heparin can reduce this risk. Patient disorders that cause hypercoagulation or hypocoagulation states can also complicate anticoagulation management.

Heparin-Induced Thrombocytopenia (HIT). A potential problem with the use of heparin is HIT. HIT occurs in approximately 5% of patients who receive heparin.[15] HIT is an immune response with an immune complex (called *heparin-platelet factor IV complex*) formed between administered heparin and platelet factor IV on the surfaces of platelets. The immune system responds to this complex as a foreign substance and forms antibodies, causing platelet aggregation, platelet damage, and ultimately thrombotic complications and thrombocytopenia. Testing for HIT is done by checking the platelet count and serologic or functional assays for heparin-platelet factor 4 (PF 4) antibodies.

The treatment for HIT is removal of all sources of heparin. Because most patients receiving MCS will require anticoagulation, a direct thrombin inhibitor such as argatroban or lepirudin can be used in place of heparin.[5]

Fluid and Electrolyte Replacement and Balance

Patients typically are quite edematous during MCS because they often require fluid resuscitation before device insertion, and often develop capillary leak before and after device insertion. Aggressive diuresis can lead to intravascular volume depletion and cardiac compromise. Diuretic therapy is initiated early to promote the removal of edema fluid. A furosemide infusion (0.2 to 0.3 mg/kg per hour) is commonly used to promote diuresis. Chlorothiazide and bumetanide can be added to promote diuresis, or renal dose dopamine infusion can enhance renal perfusion and glomerular filtration. When the child receives diuretics and requires frequent blood replacement, the child's serum potassium, calcium, and other electrolytes should be closely monitored and replaced as needed.

Renal and Hepatic Function

During the first 24 to 48 hours of MCS therapy, patients often develop acute tubular necrosis with oliguria and rising blood urea nitrogen (BUN) and creatinine. The kidneys and liver may be compromised by low cardiac output, prolonged period of hypoxia or hypotension before initiation of support, prolonged cardiopulmonary bypass (if postoperative), multiple blood transfusions, thromboembolism, antibiotics or other toxic medications, and severe hemolysis.

Monitoring of urine output, BUN and creatinine levels, and liver function studies for worsening or improvement in end-organ perfusion is imperative. Once adequate cardiac output has been restored through the use of MCS, renal and hepatic function should improve. Interventions to minimize renal and hepatic dysfunction include minimizing blood transfusions, providing early nutritional support, monitoring drug levels, and discontinuing of renal or hepatic toxic medications if possible.

If urine output does not improve, the patient may have an open patent ductus arteriosus (PDA) or a combination of inadequate flow, low cardiac output, and low mean arterial pressure compromising renal blood flow. Surgical ligation of the PDA may be warranted if a PDA is documented by echocardiogram.

In the case of rising creatinine levels, hyperkalemia, persistent oliguria, and maximal diuretic support, it may be necessary to perform dialysis via peritoneal dialysis, perform ultrafiltration via the ECMO, or centrifuge VAD circuit. Ultrafiltration is accomplished through the use of a hemofilter connected to the ECMO or centrifuge VAD circuit; water passes through the filter from the plasma, reducing hypervolemia. Ultrafiltration may need to be stopped in the case of low atrial pressure, hypotension, or circuit shutdown from low volume detected by the bladder box.

Nutrition

Infants and children receiving MCS typically have compromised nutritional status secondary to presupport clinical decompensation. Parenteral nutrition and intralipid therapy are usually started within 48 to 72 hours after initiation of MCS with gradual increase to achieve a caloric goal of 80 to 100 kcal/kg per day. Lipid intake should not exceed 1 g/kg per day, or it should be infused through the bladder port to prevent accumulation and embolism within the ECMO circuit. In addition, ranitidine is added in the parenteral nutrition or as a supplementary intravenous medication to inhibit gastric secretions secondary to stress.

Once inotropic support is minimal and bowel sounds have resumed, enteral feedings can be started slowly through a nasogastric tube. Oral feedings can be attempted if the child is extubated. In patients with poor systemic perfusion before MCS, mesenteric artery blood flow is compromised, so feedings should be started slowly with careful monitoring for signs of feeding intolerance such as abdominal distension, high gastric residuals, no stools, or bloody stools. These signs may also be associated with necrotizing enterocolitis in the infant and may not be present until feeding is initiated. The nutritional support service should be involved in the child's care to determine the current nutritional status, recommend age-appropriate diet or formula and caloric goals, and monitor progress through laboratory values such as total protein and albumin.

Infection

Patients receiving MCS support are at high risk for nosocomial infection secondary to surgical incisions or open chest, cannulae sites, invasive monitoring catheters, drainage tubes, mechanical ventilation, and compromised nutrition and immune status. Early indicators of infection may absent or difficult to detect during MCS. Thrombocytopenia results from platelet destruction by the ECMO circuit or VAD pump. In addition, core body temperature can be affected by the ECMO heat exchanger.[47] The white blood cell count with differential should be obtained daily, and routine blood, urine, and endotracheal tube cultures should be obtained to monitor for infection. Patients with unexplained hemodynamic instability, coagulopathy, elevated white blood cell count, or fever should be promptly treated for suspected sepsis pending culture results (see Chapter 6).[60]

Prophylactic broad-spectrum intravenous antibiotics are administered before mechanical support and are continued after insertion. Cannulation through an open sternum poses a greater risk for mediastinitis. Therefore, in patients with an open sternum, antibiotic coverage is broadened to include a second- or third-generation cephalosporin in combination with a course of vancomycin or oxacillin.[9,60]

The nurse should monitor the patient closely for signs and symptoms of infection during MCS. In addition, the nurse should use meticulous aseptic and sterile technique when required for procedures or direct patient care.

Skin Assessment

Children receiving MCS are at high risk for developing skin breakdown related to suboptimal nutritional status and immobility. Furthermore, the patient with a pneumatic VAD will have external pumps on the surface of the abdomen, and cannulas, and drive line connections may be a potential source for the development of skin breakdown. VAD site dressing care (either the pump or percutaneous components) is performed according to manufacturer's recommendations. Strict sterile technique is preferred until the skin has adhered to the Dacron on the cannulae. The nurse should carefully remove encrustations that result from wound secretions to prevent skin necrosis at the cannulae exit sites.

Exit sites should be covered at all times, and the use of age-appropriate binders or pouches is recommended to stabilize pumps or components. Several VADs use proprietary materials with guidelines regarding wound care. Many companies do not recommend oil-based products (ointments), alcohol, or acetone that might degrade the pump case or cannula. (e.g., the Thoratec VAD outer pump casing is sensitive to acetone).

Frequent skin assessment is critical to early detection and prevention of skin breakdown. Early initiation of enteral nutrition and mobility (if requiring long-term use of a pneumatic VAD) can prevent the development of skin breakdown. However, infants or children receiving ECMO might not tolerate position changes. In such patients, low air-flow beds can be used to maintain skin integrity. A gel pillow under the occiput is often used to prevent skin breakdown. Pressure points should be assessed routinely, and passive range-of-motion exercises should be performed to maintain skin integrity and prevent muscle contractures.

Activities of Daily Living and Rehabilitation

For children receiving ECMO or centrifugal VAD support, activities of daily living are limited to passive range-of-motion exercises throughout the duration of support. For the child requiring long-term use of a pneumatic VAD, the goal is extubation and rehabilitation. The primary nurse and multidisciplinary care team facilitate early extubation, discontinuation of invasive catheters, and early ambulation. Patient, parent, and physical therapist involvement are crucial to successful rehabilitation. Allowing the patient to gain independence in activities of daily living and device management (if age appropriate) encourages both functional and psychological well-being. The patient's family should participate in the rehabilitation phase of recovery.

The multidisciplinary team should develop and follow a daily schedule of activity or exercise plan, rest periods, and sleep during the night. If the child is of school age, daily class work is incorporated into the schedule with input from the hospital or local school district teacher.

Psychological Support

One of the most stressful experiences for any parent is a child's critical illness. Psychological support in addition to patient and family education are essential components of postoperative MCS care. If emergent VAD placement occurs, patients may wake from anesthesia unaware of the device, and the family often has no time to prepare.

Parents often face overwhelming feelings of anxiety, fear, and helplessness, yet can remain hopeful for successful therapy.[17] Age-appropriate explanations of components and functions can gradually introduce the device to the patient and family. The nurse also provides crucial emotional support during the recovery period.

When the child's condition is stable, visits from classmates and friends are encouraged, provided that visitors are screened for infection. Visits from other VAD recipients can be a positive experience for the patients requiring support as a bridge to transplant and for their families.

COMMONLY USED DRUGS

The most commonly used drugs during MCS are ones that optimize cardiac and pulmonary function, such as inotropes, antihypertensive or afterload reducing agents, and pulmonary vasodilators. A balance between hemostasis and anticoagulation is required after initiation of MCS. Multiple antifibrinolytics and anticoagulants can be used depending on postinsertion bleeding, development of coagulopathies, and device-specific coagulation to prevent thrombus formation. Other commonly used drugs during MCS include analgesics, sedatives, antibiotics, diuretics, electrolyte replacement, and resuscitation drugs (in case of mechanical failure and emergent removal from ECMO). Table 7-5 includes a list of commonly used drugs with doses and cautions. See Chapter 6 for further description of resuscitation.

MCS FOR SPECIFIC DISEASES

The Chapter 7 Supplement on the Evolve Website provides detailed information about common diseases requiring MCS support. Many of the specifics can be reviewed in more depth in Chapters 6 to 9. It is important to remember that the specific diseases discussed are at end-stage and require MCS for survival.

DIAGNOSTIC TESTS DURING MCS

The following diagnostic tests are the most commonly used to assess cardiac and respiratory function and to evaluate for possible postoperative MCS complications. Refer to Chapters 8 to 10 for more detailed descriptions of the tests.

Echocardiogram

The echocardiogram is often used during ECMO and VAD support to assess for myocardial recovery (by measuring the ejection fraction) and to check cannula placement. The ECMO and VAD flows are reduced to allow the heart to eject blood while receiving minimal inotropic support to best assess readiness for ECMO decannulation or VAD removal.

Cardiac Catheterization

The use of cardiac catheterization is rare during mechanical support because of the risk of bleeding. However, select cases may require cardiac catheterization to obtain muscle biopsy for rejection status in the patient requiring mechanical support after heart transplantation, before heart or lung transplant to assess pulmonary artery pressure, or after a cardiotomy to identify any residual defects that can be corrected surgically to improve ventricular function.

Chest Radiograph

The chest radiograph is frequently used to assess endotracheal tube, invasive catheter, chest tube, and ECMO/VAD cannula placement. Chest radiographs should be evaluated for clinical deterioration or unexplained changes in the patient's condition caused by pleural effusion, hemothorax, pneumothorax, or lobe collapse. General opacification of lung fields within the first 24 hours of ECMO is common and results from complement activation, leading to capillary leak syndrome and withdrawal of distending airway pressure.

Arterial and Venous Blood Gas Assessment

Arterial and venous blood samples are used to assess oxygenation and mixed venous saturation. The preoxygenator blood gas samples are from the right atrium and considered the venous blood gas. The postoxygenator blood gas assesses the oxygenator function, and the child's blood gas represents the arterial blood gas sample. Venous and arterial pH, PaO_2 and $PaCO_2$ should be within normal limits. Increasing the sweep gas decreases $PaCO_2$ levels and increasing the ECMO flow rate elevates the PaO_2 levels.

Cranial Ultrasound

IVH is a possible complication of anticoagulation associated with MCS. The risk of IVH is higher in the neonate and infant because of the continued development of the cerebral vasculature and germinal matrix that are highly sensitive to changes in pH, PaO_2, and intracranial pressure. In patients with an open fontanelle, cranial ultrasound examination is routinely performed before support is initiated, and routine surveillance is per institutional protocol. Development of a large IVH may preclude continuation of ECMO or VAD support.

Table 7-5   **Drugs Commonly Used During MCS**

Drug	Dose	Caution
Anticoagulation*		
Heparin sodium	IV infusion: 20 units/kg per hour Adjust dose by 2-4 units/kg per hour every 4-8 h as required	May cause thrombocytopenia or HIT; hemorrhage is the most common complication; monitor platelet count, PTT, hematocrit, and ACT
Aspirin	For Blalock-Taussig (subclavian to pulmonary artery) shunts: 3-5 mg/kg per day up to 40-81 mg/day For prosthetic heart valves: 6-20 mg/kg per day	At high serum concentrations, may cause GI intolerance, respiratory alkalosis, and pulmonary edema
Aminocaproic acid (Amicar)	IV infusion: 33.3 mg/kg per hour	May cause hypotension, bradycardia, and arrhythmias
Argroban	Initial dose: 2 mcg/kg per minute Measure aPTT after 2 h; adjust dose until aPTT is 1.5-3 times baseline	May be used for anticoagulation in patients diagnosed with HIT; may cause hypotension, ventricular tachycardia, and bradycardia
Recombinant activated factor VII (rFVIIa; NovoSeven)	90 mcg/kg q2 h until hemostasis is achieved or judged ineffective	May cause hypertension or hemorrhage; monitor for signs/symptoms of thrombosis
Warfarin sodium (Coumadin)	Maintenance dose: 0.05-0.34 mg/kg per day Titrate based on INR	For long-term use in stable patient with a VAD; monitor INR or PT and signs/symptoms of hemorrhage
Aprotinin (Trasylol)	40 mL/m² per hour	May cause renal impairment, heart attack, and stroke
Inotropes†		
Dopamine (Inotropin)	2-20 mcg/kg per minute (titrate to desired effect)	May produce extreme tachycardia or result in increased pulmonary artery pressure
Dobutamine (Dobutrex)	2-20 mcg/kg per minute (titrate to desired effect)	May produce extreme tachycardia and pulmonary vasoconstriction; patients with atrial fibrillation or flutter are at risk of developing a rapid ventricular response
Epinephrine (Adrenalin)	0.2-0.3 mcg/kg per minute	May produce tachycardia, hypertension, cardiac arrhythmias, increased myocardial oxygen consumption, decreased renal, and splenic blood flow
Norepinephrine	0.05-1 mcg/kg per minute	May produce arrhythmias, bradycardia, tachycardia, hypertension, or organ ischemia caused by vasoconstriction of renal and mesenteric arteries
Vasopressin (Pitressin)	0.2 to 2 milliunits/kg per minute (0.0002-0.002 units/kg per minute	Can produce venous thrombosis, vasoconstriction, bradycardia, heart block, and distal limb ischemia
Phosphodiesterase-III inhibitor‡		
Milrinone (Primacor)	Loading dose of 0.05 mg/kg (50 mcg/kg) slowly (over 10-60 min). Infusion dose: 0.25-0.75 mcg/kg per minute	Can produce ventricular and supraventricular arrhythmias and bronchospasm
Vasodilators/Antihypertensives§		
Nitropresside (Nipride)	IV: 0.3-8 mcg/kg per minute	Can produce excessive hypotensive response, tachycardia, and elevated serum creatinine
Enalapril (Vasotec)	PO: 0.1-0.5 mg/kg per day in 1-2 doses IV: 5-10 mcg/kg per dose q8-24 h	Can produce hypotension, angioedema, anaphylactic reactions, neutropenia, proteinuria, and hepatic failure
Captopril (Capoten)	PO: 0.1-0.5 mg/kg per dose q8-24 h Maximum: 6 mg/kg per day	Can produce hypotension hepatic failure, anaphylactoid reactions, agranulocytosis, proteinuria
Esmolol (Brevibloc)	IV: 75-150 mcg/kg per minute Titrate dose by 50 mcg/kg per min q10 min Maximum dose: 1000 mcg/kg per minute	May cause bradycardia, hypotension, peripheral ischemia
Propranolol (Inderal)	PO: 0.5 mg/kg per day IV: 0.15-0.25 mg/kg	May cause hypotension and bradycardia.

Table 7-5 Drugs Commonly Used During MCS—cont'd

Drug	Dose	Caution
Pulmonary Vasodilators[‖]		
Inhaled Nitric Oxide (INOmax)	In the ventilated patient: 5-20 ppm	Abrupt discontinuation may lead to worsening hypotension, oxygenation, and increasing pulmonary artery pressure; doses >20 ppm increase the risk of methemoglobinemia and elevated nitrogen dioxide levels
Sildenafil (Viagra)	PO: 0.25-2 mg/kg per dose q4-8 h	May cause hypotension, tachycardia, ventricular arrhythmia, cerebrovascular hemorrhage, pulmonary hemorrhage, sudden hearing loss
Diuretics[¶]		
Furosemide (Lasix)	PO, IV: 1-2 mg/kg per dose q4-12 h IV continuous infusion: 0.1-0.4 mg/kg per hour	May cause hypokalemia and hyponatremia necessitating electrolyte monitoring
Chlorothiazide (Diuril)	PO: 10-40 mg/kg per day divided in 2 doses IV: 2-8 mg/kg per day divided into 1-2 doses	May cause hypokalemia, hyperglycemia, and hyperuricemia
Spironolactone (Aldactone)	PO: 1-3.5 mg/kg per day; may be given as single dose or total dose can be divided into 2 or 4 doses (given twice a day or every 6 h)	Potassium-sparing diuretic; may cause hyponatremia, hyperkalemia, and dehydration
Bumetanide (Bumex)	PO: 0.04-0.8 mg/kg per day; dose is divided and given every 6-8 h	Can have profound diuresis with fluid and electrolyte loss; close supervision and dose evaluation are required.
Electrolyte Replacement[#]		
Potassium chloride	Normal requirement: 2-3 mEq/kg per day Prevention of hypokalemia: 1-2 mEq/kg per day above maintenance IV intermittent infusion for severe depletion: 0.5-1 mEq/kg per dose, typically over 1-3 hours	May cause cardiac arrhythmias, heart block, hypotension, and bradycardia; patients have a cardiac monitor during intermittent infusions
Calcium chloride	IV: 10-20 mg/kg per dose Repeat q4-6 h if needed	May cause vasodilation, hypotension, bradycardia, and cardiac arrhythmias; avoid extravasation
Magnesium sulfate	PO: 100-200 mg/kg per dose q6 h IV: 25-50 mg/kg per dose q4-6 h	May cause hypotension, circulatory collapse, depression of cardiac function, and heart block

*Primary concern related to blood-surface interaction with artificial materials, increasing the risk of clot in the mechanical circulatory support device.
†Indicated for poor systemic perfusion and myocardial function with appropriate oxygenation, ventilation, heart rate, and intravascular volume.
‡Inotropic, chronotropic, and vasodilatory effects.
§Dilate arteries and veins to reduce preload, reduce systemic vascular resistance, and improve ventricular compliance, thus improving cardiac output.
‖To aid in oxygenation and decrease right ventricular afterload.
¶For treatment of oliguria and hypervolemia associated with poor systemic perfusion and CHF as the result of low cardiac output.
#Electrolyte imbalances alter myocardial transmembrane potential, depolarization, and repolarization, thus affecting the excitability of myocardial tissue and conduction of electrical impulses. To ensure optimal myocardial function and cardiac output, electrolytes must be closely monitored and replaced as necessary.
ACT, Activated clotting time; *aPTT,* activated partial thromboplastin time; *GI,* gastrointestinal; *HIT,* heparin-induced thrombocytopenia; *INR,* international normalized ratio; *IV,* intravenous; *PO,* by mouth; *PT,* prothrombin time; *PTT,* partial prothrombin time; *VAD,* ventricular assist device.

References

1. Alexi-Meskishvili V, et al: The use of the Berlin heart in children. In Duncan BW, editors: *Mechanical support for cardiac and respiratory failure in pediatric patients,* New York, 2001, Marcel Dekker.
2. Ashton RC Jr, et al: Left ventricular assist device options in pediatric patients. *ASAIO J* 41:M277–M280, 1995.
3. Baffes TG, et al: Extracorporeal circulation for support of palliative cardiac surgery in infants. *Ann Thorac Surg* 10:354–363, 1970.
4. Baldwin JT, et al: The national heart, lung, and blood institute pediatric circulatory support program. *Circulation* 113:147–155, 2006.
5. Baroletti SA, Goldhaber SZ: Heparin-induced thrombocytopenia. *Circulation* 114:355–356, 2006.
6. Bartlett RH, et al: Extracorporeal membrane oxygenation (ECMO) cardiopulmonary support in infancy. *Trans Am Soc Artif Intern Organs* 22:80–93, 1976.
7. Boneva RS, et al: Mortality associated with congenital heart defects in the United States: trends and racial disparities, 1979-1997. *Circulation* 103:2376–2381, 2001.
8. Boucek MM, et al: Registry for the International Society for Heart and Lung Transplantation: seventh official pediatric report: 2004. *J Heart Lung Transplant* 23:933–947, 2004.
9. Brown KL, et al: Healthcare-associated infection in pediatric patients on extracorporeal life support: the role of multidisciplinary surveillance. *Pediatr Crit Care Med* 7:546–550, 2006.
10. Bruckner BA, et al: Regression of fibrosis and hypertrophy in failing myocardium following mechanical circulatory support. *J Heart Lung Transplant* 20:457, 2001.
11. Carberry KE, et al: Mechanical circulatory support for the pediatric patient. *Crit Care Nurs Q* 30(2):121–142, 2007.
12. Chen YS, et al: Experience and result of extracorporeal membrane oxygenation in treating fulminant myocarditis with shock: what mechanical support should be considered first? *J Heart Lung Transplant* 24:81–87, 2005.
13. Clowes GH, Hopkins AL, Neville WE: An artificial lung dependent upon diffusion of oxygen and carbon dioxide through plastic membranes. *J Thorac Cardiovasc Surg* 32:630–637, 1956.

14. Collison PS, Dager SK: The role of the Intra-aortic balloon pump in supporting children with acute cardiac failure. *Postgrad Med J* 83:308–311, 2007.

15. Comunale ME, Vancott EM: Heparin induced thrombocytopenia. *Int Anesthesiol Clin* 42(3):27–43, 2004.

16. Cooper DS, et al: Cardiac extracorporeal life support: state of the art in 2007. *Cardiol Young* 17(Suppl. 2):104–115, 2007.

17. Curley MA, Meyer EC: Parental experience of highly technical therapy: survivors and nonsurvivors of extracorporeal membrane oxygenation support. *Pediatr Crit Care Med* 4(2):214–219, 2003.

18. De Oliveira NC, et al: Prevention of sudden circulatory collapse after the Norwood operation. *Circulation* 110:II133–II138, 2004.

19. Dickerson HA, Chang AC: Perioperative management of ventricular assist devices in children and adolescents. *Semin Thorac Cardiovasc Surg Pediatr Card Surg Annu* 9:128–139, 2006.

20. Duncan BW, et al: Mechanical circulatory support for the treatment of children with acute fulminant myocarditis. *J Thorac Cardiovasc Surg* 122:440–448, 2001.

21. Duncan BW: Mechanical circulatory support for infants and children with cardiac disease. *Ann Thorac Surg* 73:1670–1677, 2002.

22. Duncan BW: Mechanical circulatory support in infants and children with cardiac disease. In Zwischenberger JB, Bartlett RH, editors: *ECMO Extracorporeal Cardiopulmonary Support in Critical Care*, ed 2, Ann Arbor, MI, 2000, Extracorporeal Life Support Organization.

23. Duncan BW: Pediatric mechanical circulatory support in the United States: past, present, and future. *ASAIO J* 52:525–529, 2006.

24. ECMO Registry of the Extracorporeal Life Support Organization (ELSO). Ann Arbor, Michigan, January 2004.

25. Fenton KN, et al: The significance of baseline cerebral oxygen saturation in children undergoing congenital heart surgery. *Am J Surg* 190 (2):260–263, 2005.

26. Frazier OH, et al: Research and development of an implantable axial-flow left ventricular assist device: the Jarvik 2000 Heart. *Ann Thorac Surg* 71:S125–S132, 2001.

27. Fuchs A, Netz H: Ventricular assist devices in pediatrics. *Images Paediatr Cardiol* 9:24–54, 2002.

28. Goldman AP, et al: The waiting game: bridging to paediatric heart transplantation. *Lancet* 362:1967–1970, 2003.

29. Goodman DM, Green TP: Extracorporeal life support for children with acute respiratory distress syndrome. In Zwischenberger JB, Steinhorn RH, Bartlett RH, editors: *ECMO: extracorporeal cardiopulmonary support in critical care*, Ann Arbor, MI, 2000, Extracorporeal Life Support Organization, pp. 451–460.

30. Griffith BP, et al: HeartMate II left ventricular assist system: from concept to first clinical use. *Ann Thorac Surg* 71:S116–S120, 2001.

31. Grinda JM, et al: Fulminant myocarditis in adults and children: biventricular assist device for recovery. *Eur J Cardiothorac Surg* 26:1169–1173, 2004.

32. Hansell DR: Extracorporeal membrane oxygenation for perinatal and pediatric patients. *Respir Care* 48(4):352–362, 2003.

33. Hawkin JA, Minich LL: Intraaortic balloon counterpulsation for children with cardiac disease. In Duncan BW, editors: *Mechanical support for cardiac and respiratory failure in pediatric patients*, New York, 2001, Marcel Dekker.

34. Heerdt PM, et al: Chronic unloading by left ventricular assist device reverses contractile dysfunction and alters gene expression in end-stage heart failure. *Circulation* 102:2713, 2000.

35. Helman DN, et al: Implantable left ventricular assist devices can successfully bridge adolescent patients to transplant. *J Heart Lung Transplant* 19:121–126, 2000.

36. Hetzer R, Stiller B: Ventricular assist device for children. *Nat Clin Pract Cardiovasc Med* 3(7):377–386, 2006.

37. Hill JD, et al: Prolonged extracorporeal oxygenation for acute post-traumatic respiratory failure (shock-lung syndrome). *N Engl J Med* 286:629–634, 1972.

38. Hintz SR, et al: Decreased use of neonatal extracorporeal membrane oxygenation (ECMO): how new treatment modalities have affected ECMO utilization. *Pediatrics* 106(6):1339–1343, 2000.

39. Kalavrouziotis G, Karunaratne A, Raja S: Intraaortic balloon pumping in children undergoing cardiac surgery: an update on the Liverpool experience. *J Thorac Cardiovasc Surg* 131:1382–1389, 2006.

40. Karl TR, Horton SB: Centrifugal pump ventricular assist device in pediatric cardiac surgery. In Duncan BW, editors: *Mechanical support for cardiac and respiratory failure in pediatric patients*, New York, 2001, Marcel Dekker.

41. Kolobow T, Bowman RL: Construction and evaluation of an alveolar membrane artificial heart-lung. *Trans Am Soc Artif Intern Organs* 9:238–243, 1963.

42. Korfer R, et al: Single-center experience with the Thoratec ventricular assist device. *J Thorac Cardiovasc Surg* 119:596–600, 2000.

43. Lequier L: Extracorporeal life support in pediatric and neonatal critical care: a review. *J Intensive Care Med* 19:243–258, 2004.

44. Lipshultz SE, et al: The incidence of pediatric cardiomyopathy in two regions of the United States. *N Engl J Med* 348:1647–1655, 2003.

45. McBride LR, et al: Clinical experience with 111 Thoratec ventricular assist devices. *Ann Thorac Surg* 67:1233–1239, 1999.

46. Morales DL, et al: Lessons learned from the first application of the DeBakey VAD Child: an intracorporeal ventricular assist device for children. *J Heart Lung Transplant* 24:331–337, 2005.

47. Moynihan PJ, et al: Nursing management of children with cardiac disease on mechanical circulatory support. In Duncan BW, editors: *Mechanical support for cardiac and respiratory failure in pediatric patients*, New York, 2001, Marcel Dekker.

48. Ogletree-Hughes ML, et al: Mechanical unloading restores beta-adrenergic responsiveness and reverses receptor down regulation in the failing human heart. *Circulation* 104:881, 2001.

49. Petrou S, et al: Cost-effectiveness of neonatal extracorporeal membrane oxygenation based on 7-year results from the United Kingdom Collaborative ECMO Trial. *Pediatrics* 117(5):1640–1649, 2006.

50. Pinkney KA, et al: Current results with intraaortic balloon pumping in infants and children. *Ann Thorac Surg* 73:887–891, 2002.

51. Pizarro C, et al: Is there a role for extracorporeal life support after stage I Norwood? *Eur J Cardiothorac Surg* 19:294–301, 2001.

52. Pollock J, Charlton MC, Williams WG: Intraaortic balloon pumping in children. *Ann Thorac Surg* 29:522–528, 1980.

53. Ravishankar C, et al: Extracorporeal membrane oxygenation after staged I reconstruction for hypoplastic left heart syndrome. *Pediatr Crit Care Med* 7:319–323, 2006.

54. Schmid C, et al: Pediatric assist with Medos and Excor systems in small children. *ASAIO J* 52:505–508, 2006.

55. Slaughter MS, et al: Advanced heart failure treated with continuous-flow left ventricular assist device. *N Engl J Med* 361:2241-2251, 2009.

56. Throckmorton AL, et al: Pediatric circulatory support systems. *ASAIO J* 48:216–221, 2002.

57. UK Collaborative ECMO Trial Group: UK collaborative randomised trial of neonatal extracorporeal membrane oxygenation. *Lancet* 348:75–82, 1996.

58. Ungerleider RM, et al: Routine mechanical ventricular assist following the Norwood procedure—improved neurologic outcome and excellent hospital survival. *Ann Thorac Surg* 77:18–22, 2004.

59. Van Meurs KP, et al., editors: *ECMO: extracorporeal cardiopulmonary support in critical care*, ed 3, Ann Arbor, MI, 2005, Extracorporeal Life Support Organization.

60. Wessel DL, Almodovar MC, Laussen PC: Intensive care management of cardiac patients on extracorporeal membrane oxygenation. In Duncan BW, editors: *Mechanical support for cardiac and respiratory failure in pediatric patients*, New York, 2001, Marcel Dekker.

61. Wieselthaler GM, et al: First clinical experience with the DeBakey VAD continuous-axial-flow pump for bridge to transplantation. *Circulation* 101:356–359, 2000.

62. Zahraa JN, et al: Venovenous versus venoarterial extracorporeal life support for pediatric respiratory failure: are there differences in survival and acute complications? *Crit Care Med* 28(2):521–525, 2000.

Cardiovascular Disorders

8

Be sure to check out the supplementary content available at http://evolve.elsevier.com/Hazinski.

INTRODUCTION

Mary Fran Hazinski

Every critically ill or injured child requires thorough assessment of cardiovascular function. Congestive heart failure, arrhythmias, and congenital defects are among the most common cardiovascular problems seen in critically ill children.

This chapter begins with a brief review of essential anatomy and physiology, including a summary of the etiology and genetics of congenital heart disease, cardiac embryologic development, and fetal and perinatal circulation. It includes essential cardiovascular anatomy, physiology, and hemodynamic principles. Care of the child with common clinical problems, including congestive heart failure, altered nutrition and potential gastrointestinal problems, arrhythmias, hypoxemia (caused by intracardiac shunting), pulmonary hypertension, and challenges of adults with congenital heart disease will be presented in the second section of the chapter. The third section addresses the postoperative care of the pediatric cardiovascular surgical patient, including common postoperative complications and postoperative anticoagulation. The fourth section presents specific cardiovascular diseases, including congenital heart defects, coronary artery and vascular anomalies, and infectious and inflammatory diseases and tumors, with information about the etiology, pathophysiology, clinical signs and symptoms, and management of each. The chapter concludes with a discussion of diagnostic tests frequently used in the management of the pediatric cardiovascular patient.

This chapter contains excellent information from expert cardiovascular clinicians. To make it easy to find key references, a list of relevant references appears at the end of the chapter. As with other chapters, additional information is available in the Chapter 8 Supplement on the Evolve Website.

ESSENTIAL ANATOMY AND PHYSIOLOGY

The cardiovascular system delivers oxygenated blood and other nutrients to the tissues of the body, and returns venous blood, carrying carbon dioxide and metabolic byproducts, to the heart and lungs. The blood is propelled by the heart and is carried by the pulmonary arteries to the lungs and by the systemic arteries to the tissues. Systemic veins and pulmonary veins return the blood to the heart.

Effective systemic perfusion requires an appropriate heart rate, adequate intravascular volume relative to the vascular space, effective myocardial function, and appropriate arterial and venous tone. In addition, adequate oxygen and nutrient supply, appropriate cellular use of oxygen, and effective cardiovascular feedback systems are needed. Congenital and acquired cardiovascular anomalies can compromise adequate systemic perfusion and oxygenation.

ETIOLOGIES OF CHD: NONINHERITED AND GENETIC FACTORS

Gwen Paxson Fosse

Congenital heart disease (CHD) encompasses many structural defects or disorders of the heart that are present at birth; they may be diagnosed in utero, at birth, or later in life. Although the general population risk for any birth defect is 4%,[567] the risk of a congenital heart defect is 0.4% to 1%,[264] making the heart the most common organ to be affected by a birth anomaly. Approximately 25% of the children with congenital heart disease, as well as 70% of spontaneous abortions and stillborn fetuses with CHD also have at least one extracardiac anomaly.[506]

In the past quarter century, two population studies, the New England Regional Infant Cardiac Program[290] and the Baltimore-Washington Infant Study,[263,264] increased understanding of the incidence and etiology of CHD. Recent years have brought the human genome project, advances in molecular biology, and expanded capabilities for chromosomal analysis. Small chromosome deletions and duplications can be identified through fluorescence in situ hybridization (FISH) and, more recently, array comparative genomic hybridization (A-CGH), which opens the door to identification of a greater number of genetic diagnoses. All of these factors combined with the epidemiologic results of the population studies mentioned above are contributing to the identification of genes that cause syndromes as well as isolated congenital heart defects, classification of the pathologic processes of embryology that are triggered by genetic abnormalities, and correlation between genotypes and various phenotypes (the characteristic features).[265,657,699] These methods are enabling identification of chromosome anomalies and gene abnormalities that are a result of new or inherited mutations. These and other new developments are leading to better genetic testing, improved diagnostic and prognostic capabilities, future research opportunities, and enhanced care planning and counseling.[932]

Findings about noninherited risk factors for congenital heart disease have also expanded. Knowledge about prescription and nonprescription drugs, environmental influences

181

(chemical, physical, and biologic agents/teratogens), and parental diseases have enhanced our understanding about the etiologies of CHD.

Whether the triggering event is a teratogen, a genetic abnormality, or unknown, the pathogenesis of congenital heart defects follow six mechanisms as proposed by Clark[181,182,506,747]:

I. Ectomesenchymal tissue migration or neural crest abnormalities, resulting in conotruncal (ventricular outflow) and aortic arch anomalies;
II. Abnormalities of intracardiac blood flow, resulting in hypoplasia of structures through which flow was diminished or absent;
III. Cell death abnormalities, resulting in Ebstein malformation and muscular ventricular septal defects;
IV. Extracellular matrix abnormalities, resulting in anomalous formation of the endocardial cushions (atrioventricular septal and canal defects);
V. Abnormal targeted growth, resulting in anomalies of pulmonary venous and left atrium formation; and
VI. Abnormal situs and looping, resulting in malposition of organs, structures, and vascular connections.

An etiologic event triggers abnormal pathogenesis and each of the preceding pathogenetic mechanisms can cause a spectrum of disorders.

Exploration of anomalies in terms of a common pathogenetic mechanism allows researchers to learn more about familial patterns. As more information about the interaction of genes, environment, and proteins involved in developmental pathways is available, our understanding of the biologic basis of normal and abnormal cardiovascular embryologic development (morphogenesis) will be refined.[506] Further information on cardiovascular morphogenesis is provided in the section, Fetal Development of the Heart and Great Vessels.

Although most congenital heart disease was previously believed to be of multifactorial etiology (a combination of a number of genetic factors from both parents, environmental influences, and random events), new information has led to the belief that most human CHDs result from single gene defects[506] and some from exposure to teratogens. Nevertheless, at this point, for most patients with CHD there is not a precise identifiable cause.[506] Congenital heart defects are thought to be related to teratogens in 2% to 4%, genetics in 10% (although this is probably underestimated), and unknown in 85% to 90%.[190,277] As discoveries continue, the percentage with unknown cause should decrease.

This section further describes the teratogens and genetics associated with CHDs as an isolated defect or in association with extracardiac anomalies. These are divided into noninherited and inherited risk factors that lead to CHD.

Noninherited Risk Factors for CHD (Many Potentially Modifiable)

Maternal Disorders or Biologic Teratogens

Maternal disorders or biologic teratogens associated with increased incidence of CHD include phenylketonuria (PKU), diabetes, infections, obesity, systemic lupus erythematosus, and epilepsy.[277] When a mother has untreated PKU during pregnancy, the fetus may have growth and mental retardation

and has a 20% to 25% incidence of CHD. Maternal control of blood phenylalanine concentration and adequate maternal nutrition before and throughout the pregnancy must occur to reduce the risk. All babies conceived when the mother was receiving inadequate nutrition should have an echocardiogram.[558] The most frequently associated defects are tetralogy of Fallot, ventricular septal defect (VSDs), patent ductus arteriosus (PDA), and single ventricle.[414]

Maternal pregestational insulin dependent diabetes increases fetal risk of CHD. The most common defects are malformations with laterality or embryologic heart tube looping defects, transposition of the great arteries, conotruncal defects (e.g., tetralogy of Fallot, interrupted aortic arch, truncus arteriosus), VSDs, atrioventricular septal (AV canal) defects, hypoplastic left heart syndrome, outflow tract defects, PDA, and hypertrophic cardiomyopathy (which may resolve).[414] Less frequently, gestational diabetes also has been associated with CHDs, and these cases may represent women who have undetected type 2 diabetes. Adequate blood sugar control before and during pregnancy does reduce the risk.[414,795]

Maternal infections have long been associated with CHD. Maternal rubella has been associated with PDA, pulmonary valve abnormalities, peripheral pulmonary stenosis, and VSDs. Immunization of women against rubella can eliminate this risk. More recently other maternal febrile illnesses (such as influenza) in the first trimester have been associated with a variety of heart defects, but it is unknown whether the fever, infectious agent, or medication to treat the fever and infection cause the effect.[190,414] Although HIV infection in utero increases the risk of dilated cardiomyopathy and left ventricular hypertrophy, it has not been associated with structural cardiac defects.[414]

Maternal obesity before pregnancy has been associated with CHD, but findings are inconsistent. The many complex variables with obesity and nutrition make this a difficult area for drawing conclusions.[414] Connective tissue disorders such as systemic lupus erythematosus in women are associated with congenital heart block in infant offspring. Maternal connective tissue disorders have not been associated with structural cardiac malformations.[414]

Maternal epilepsy is associated with increased incidence of CHD. The therapy of anticonvulsant drugs and their potential impact on folate metabolism—rather than the seizures themselves—may increase the risk.[414]

Maternal Drug Exposure (Chemical Teratogens)

Of note, use of maternal multivitamins and folic acid in the periconceptual period may reduce the risk of CHDs, but the evidence is not yet conclusive. These supplements may reduce the risk of CHD when used with some other agents that are associated with an increased risk of CHD, for example maternal febrile illness. Further studies are needed.[414]

Exposure to chemical agents can alter cellular development, and the timing of such exposure can influence the effect on risk. Identification of timing related to fetal vulnerability could help ensure counseling about treatment options to avoid critical exposures for a susceptible embryo.[190,277,414] Many therapeutic drugs used preconceptually or during pregnancy have been linked with possible associated risk of congenital heart disease.

(The interested reader can find a list on the Evolve Website. Please see Evolve Box 8-1 in the Chapter 8 Supplement on the Evolve Website.) Because much of the evidence is inconclusive and there are always reports from new studies, research and caution is urged before use of any therapeutic drugs during the periconceptual period and pregnancy.

Nontherapeutic drugs used preconceptually and/or during pregnancy that have been associated with increased risk of CHD include: alcohol, cocaine, marijuana, cigarette smoking, and vitamin A in high doses. Again, the evidence is often inconclusive, so actual risks can be difficult to determine. Many other agents have been studied but the data are insufficient to determine risks for cardiac defects.[414,754]

Environmental Exposures (Chemical, Biologic, and Physical Teratogens) and Influences

Increased risk of a variety of CHDs has been associated with maternal occupational exposure to organic solvents (compositions of solvents can include degreasers, dyes, lacquers, paints, glycol ethers, and mineral oil products); heavy metals; herbicides, pesticides, and rodenticides associated with maternal employment in the agriculture industry; air quality (increased levels of ambient carbon monoxide, ozone, and dioxide); and parental exposure to groundwater contamination with trichloroethylene. There are other environmental exposures, such as hazardous waste sites and occupational exposure to ionized radiation, but no consistent association with CHD has been found.[414,866]

Evaluation of maternal sociodemographic characteristics has shown that maternal age is not associated with nongenetic CHDs as a group. Some specific defects are more likely with advanced maternal age, and young maternal age is associated with tricuspid atresia.[414] Some studies have shown disparity of incidence between white and black infants, with many defects being more prevalent in white infants, whereas pulmonary stenosis is more prevalent in black infants. Other studies have not shown variations in prevalence of birth defects in general among white, black, and Hispanic infants.[414] Reproductive problems (miscarriage, stillbirth, or preterm birth) have been associated with increased incidence of tetralogy of Fallot, nonchromosomal atrioventricular canal defects, ASDs, and Ebstein's anomaly, where the association could represent exposure to teratogens or an inherent susceptibility.[414] Maternal stress associated with job loss, divorce, separation, or death of a close relative or friend, especially in mothers who were not high school graduates, was found to be associated with a greater prevalence of conotruncal heart defects.[414]

Paternal exposures and factors may also play a role in noninherited cardiac defects. Older fathers have been associated with Marfan syndrome. Studies have suggested that increasing paternal age is associated with ASDs, VSDs, PDA, and tetralogy of Fallot, whereas children of men less than 20 years of age were also at higher risk for septal defects.[414] Other paternal exposures have been investigated in a limited number of studies, with the suggestion or trend toward increased risk of CHD associated with paternal exposure to marijuana, cocaine, cigarette smoking, and alcohol.[414]

A unique environmental influence may be present for some monochorionic twins. The smaller twin is more often affected with CHD, which may result from abnormal cord insertion.[373]

Prevention of some CHDs may be accomplished by following these recommendations for mothers who wish to become pregnant: Take a multivitamin with folic acid daily, obtain prenatal and preconceptual care for management of maternal disorders associated with increased risk of CHD, discuss use of any drugs with the healthcare provider, avoid contact with people who have the flu or other febrile illnesses, avoid exposure to organic solvents,[414] and follow any employer guidelines established to avoid exposures that may increase risks.

Genetic Factors Associated with CHD

New findings with molecular genetic studies indicate that the genetic contribution to the etiology of CHD has been underestimated. With the rapid changes in this field it is certain that our understanding will be evolving and the identifiable genetic etiologies of CHD will continue to expand.[700] Review of current literature will always be necessary to have an accurate understanding of these factors.

Humans normally have 46 chromosomes (23 pairs). The first 22 pairs are autosomal (non-sex) chromosomes and the 23rd pair determines gender (XX = female, XY = male). Each chromosome has two arms held together by a centromere—a short arm (p) and a long arm (q). There are more than 35,000 pairs of genes on our chromosomes,[190] and each gene is composed of hundreds or thousands of base pairs. An abnormality in a single base pair can cause a malfunction. Changes in the deoxyribonucleic acid (DNA) sequence (a mutation) in a single gene changes the path of a protein, which is like changing one part of a recipe. (The results can range from asymptomatic to disastrous malformations.) Mutations may occur de novo (a new mutation that is not inherited from a parent) or may result from autosomal-dominant or -negative inheritance. Many gene mutations associated with cardiovascular malformations are now being identified.[190,277,700]

Before advanced cytogenetic tests were available, chromosome abnormalities were found in approximately 8% to 13% of neonates with CHD,[263] but with new testing the prevalence of chromosome aberrations is now estimated to be much higher.[700] These abnormalities can be aneuploidies (abnormal number of chromosomes) such as trisomies (an extra chromosome), or tetrasomies. Other chromosome abnormalities are caused by deletions (a missing piece), duplications (extra genetic material on chromosome), or translocations (genetic material transferred from one chromosome to another).[190,277] Single gene defects have been thought to account for about 3% to 5% of those CHDs with a genetic etiology, but new findings indicate that this range substantially underestimated the problem. Any genetic defect can start an embryonic chain reaction, which can create mild to severe phenotypic expression of the abnormality.[803]

Inheritance of genetic abnormalities associated with CHD can occur in several ways. Deletions, duplications, and single gene defects can all be the result of a mutation (a sporadic change in DNA sequence triggering abnormalities) or Mendelian inheritance from parents with the same gene anomaly. If both parents must contribute the abnormality it is autosomal recessive—both parents carry the genetic difference, but the parents will only have the disorder if they, too, have two genes with the difference. If the anomaly is inherited when only a single parent is a carrier, the inheritance is autosomal dominant, and in this situation that parent also has the condition.

Cardiovascular malformations can occur as a part of a group or pattern of anomalies. A syndrome, a combination of multiple anomalies occurring together resulting from a single cause (the cause is often a genetic error but the cause may be unknown), is thought to cause about 5% of the CHD. More than 400 genetic syndromes list CHD as a possible manifestation.[651,803] Associations, a group of anomalies that occur in a recurrent pattern, may also involve CHDs. There may be no known genetic basis for an association. Inherited metabolic diseases have a variety of genetic etiologies and may include cardiovascular problems.

For more information on characteristics and etiologies of specific defects and conditions see Tables 8-1 and 8-2. There are hundreds of syndromes and conditions with multiple manifestations that involve cardiovascular malformations. Table 8-2 includes an abbreviated table, and a more comprehensive table with genetic associations is provided in Evolve Table 8-1 in the Chapter 8 Supplement on the Evolve Website.

Genetic Testing, Counseling, and Nursing Implications

Genetic testing can reveal important genetic patterns that are critical for identifying other important organ system involvement; gaining prognostic information; learning important

Text continues on p. 190

Table 8-1   Cardiac Defects and Associated Genetics, Teratogens, and Exposures[328,414,700,871,932]

Cardiac Defect	Associated Genetics, Teratogens, and Exposures
Any congenital heart defect	Maternal PKU, pregestational diabetes, febrile illness, influenza, rubella, epilepsy, anticonvulsants, NSAIDS/Ibuprofen, sulfasalazine (antiinflammatory), thalidomide, trimethoprim-sulfonamide, and vitamin A congeners/retinoids. Many illnesses, medical and substance exposures, as well as sociodemographic factors have been studied, but there have been insufficient data to determine risks for CHD with these. Somatic mutations (occur after fertilization and therefore only affect some cells or tissues) are hypothesized to be an important cause of isolated CHDs.
Aortic atresia	See HLHS
Coarctation of the aorta	Turner syndrome. Familial left-sided obstructive heart defects. Deletion of chromosome locus 18p. Duplications in chromosome 4p, 4q, 6q, or 10p. Trisomy 8 or 9. Maternal exposure to organic solvents.
Supravalvular aortic stenosis	Williams-Beuren syndrome. Deletion or translocation (rare) in chromosome locus 7q11. Elastin gene mutations.
Aortic valve or LV outflow tract obstruction	Deletion of chromosome locus 11q or 10q. Trisomy 13 or 18. Duplications of chromosome locus 1q, 2p, 2q, 6q, or 11q. NOTCH 1 gene mutations. Noonan, Turner, or Jacobsen syndromes. Pregestational diabetes. Maternal vitamin A exposure.
Atrial septal abnormalities	Holt Oram, Ellis-van Creveld, Noonan, Rubinstein-Taybi, Kabuki, Williams, Goldenhar, thrombocytopenia-absent radius, Klinefelter, or (rare) Marfan syndrome. Mutations of TBX5 gene on chromosome 12q24.1, NKX2.5 gene on chromosome 5, EVC gene on chromosome 4p16.1, MYH6 gene, or GATA 4 gene. Deletions on chromosome 1, 4, 4p, 5p, 6, 10p, 11,13,17,18, or 22. Trisomy 18 or 21. Pregestational diabetes. Familial ASDs with AV conduction disturbances without extracardiac manifestations (may also have VSD, TOF, and others) has been associated with mutations of NKX2.5 on chromosome 5. Familial ASD without AV conduction disturbances without extracardiac manifestations (may also have VSD and/or PS) has been associated with mutations of GATA 4 gene with variable expression and autosomal dominant inheritance. This condition has also been associated with mutations of NKX2.5 on chromosome 5.
Atrioventricular septal abnormalities/atrioventricular canal/endocardial cushion defects	Trisomy 21, 13 or 18. Deletions of chromosome 3p25, 8p2, or 22q. Duplications of chromosome 10q, 11q, 22q. Holt-Oram, Noonan, Smith-Lemli-Opitz, or Ellis-van Creveld syndrome. Mutation of gene on chromosome 1p21-p31. CRELD1 gene mutations. Chondrodysplasias. Pregestational diabetes. Maternal exposure to organic solvents. Familial AVSD (partial or complete) without extracardiac manifestations has been associated with gene locus on 1p21-p31 mutation with autosomal dominant inheritance.
Bicuspid aortic valve	Turner syndrome. Familial left-sided obstructive heart defects. Deletion of chromosome locus 10p. Duplications in chromosome 6q. Trisomy 13 or 18. BAV without extracardiac manifestations may be associated with other CHDs (especially CoA) and ascending aortic aneurysm is associated with Notch1 gene mutations with autosomal dominant inheritance.
Conotruncal defects (tetralogy of Fallot, truncus arteriosus, interrupted aortic arch and others)	Deletion of chromosome 22q11.2. Mutations of NKX2.5 and 2.6. Pregestational diabetes. Maternal exposure to organic solvents.

Table 8-1 Cardiac Defects and Associated Genetics, Teratogens, and Exposures—cont'd

Cardiac Defect	Associated Genetics, Teratogens, and Exposures
Double-outlet right ventricle	Trisomy 9, 13, or 18. Duplications on chromosome 2p or 12p. Deletion of 22q11 (rare).
Ebstein anomaly	Most cases are sporadic. Chromosome abnormalities are rare. Has been reported with Trisomy 21, abnormalities of 11q with renal malformation, and Pierre Robin sequence. Familial occurrences are rare but are associated with family members with mitral valve abnormalities or with familial atrial conduction problems. Animal studies are suggestive of a genetic connection with genes on chromosome 17q. Maternal marijuana. Maternal exposure to organic solvents.
Heterotaxy syndromes with complex CHD—laterality and looping abnormalities	Chromosome locus 2 (CFC1 gene encoding CRYPTIC protein), 6q (HTX3 gene), LEFTY A gene, or X-linked q26.2 or Xq24-47 (ZIC3 gene). Pregestational diabetes.
Hypoplastic left heart syndrome	Deletion of chromosome locus 11q (Jacobsen syndrome). Turner or Wolf-Hirschhorn (deletion of 4p) syndromes. Trisomy 13 or 18. Familial left-sided obstructive heart defects. Pregestational diabetes. Maternal exposure to organic solvents.
Interrupted aortic arch	Deletion 22q11.
Left-sided obstructive heart disease—familial—CoA, aortic atresia/HLHS, BAV	Increased occurrence of these lesions in first-degree relatives. Inheritance patterns may be multifactorial, autosomal dominant with reduced penetrance, or autosomal recessive.
Left superior vena cava persistence	60% have other anomalies, 87% have other CHD, and 42% syndromes or other conditions (VACTERL, Down's syndrome, CHARGE).
Patent ductus arteriosus	Char syndrome. Mutations of TFAP2B. Pregestational diabetes. Indomethacin tocolysis.
PA branch stenosis	Alagille, congenital rubella, Ehlers-Danlos, Noonan, Costello, Cardiofaciocutaneous, LEOPARD, or Williams-Beuren syndromes. Deletions in chromosome locus 20p12. JAG1 gene mutation. Pregestational diabetes. Maternal vitamin A exposure. Maternal exposure to organic solvents.
Pulmonary Valve Obstruction	Noonan, Alagille, Costello, or LEOPARD syndromes. Mutations of PTPN11, KRAS, SOS1, and HRAS genes. Chromosome deletions of 1p, 8p, 10p, or 22q. Chromosome duplications of 6q, 15q, or 19q. Trisomy 8. Maternal vitamin A exposure. Maternal exposure to organic solvents. Maternal rubella.
Tetralogy of Fallot	Deletion of 22q11, 5p or many other chromosomes. Duplication on chromosome 22 and many other chromosomes. Alagille (JAG1 gene), Noonan (PTNP11), Cat-eye, and nearly 50 other syndromes. Trisomy 18 or 21. Partial trisomy 8q. Translocation 1p36. Maternal exposure to organic solvents. Isolated TOF is associated with NKX2.5 mutations.
Total anomalous pulmonary venous return	Most cases are sporadic. Trisomy 8. Familial cases have been reported with familial scimitar syndrome and a chromosome 4p13-q12 abnormality with autosomal dominant inheritance and variable expression (a large Utah-Idaho family). Maternal exposure to organic solvents.
Transposition of great arteries	Rarely associated with chromosome abnormalities or syndromes. Pregestational diabetes. Maternal exposure to organic solvents.
Tricuspid atresia	Most cases are sporadic. Chromosome abnormalities are rare with tricuspid atresia, but deletions of 22q11 and 4p and duplications of chromosome 22 have been reported. Familial occurrences are rare but have been reported. A gene mutation has been associated in mice, which suggests a genetic basis for this disease.
Truncus arteriosus	Deletion on chromosome 22q11 or 10p. Trisomy 8. An autosomal recessive form has been mapped to chromosome 8p21.
Ventricular septal abnormalities	Holt Oram, Rubinstein-Taybi, Goldenhar, Costello, Williams, Kabuki, Cornelia de Lange, Apert, or Carpenter syndrome. VACTERL association. Familial ASD with or without AV conduction disturbances. TBX5 or GATA 4 mutation. Deletions or duplications of many chromosomes. Trisomy 13, 18, or 21. Pregestational diabetes. Maternal marijuana. Maternal exposure to organic solvents. Septal defects without extracardiac manifestations are associated with mutations in MYH6 and CITED2 genes.

See Table 8-2 for more information on specific genes, syndromes, and conditions.

ADD, Attention deficit disorder; *AS*, aortic stenosis; *ASD*, atrial septal defect; *AV*, atrioventricular; *AVC*, atrioventricular canal; *AVSD*, atrioventricular septal defect; *BAV*, bicuspid aortic valve; *CA*, coronary artery; *CHD*, congenital heart defect; *CNS*, central nervous system; *CoA*, coarctation of aorta; *CV*, cardiovascular; *DCM*, dilated cardiomyopathy; *DORV*, double-outlet right ventricle; *GI*, gastrointestinal; *GU*, genitourinary; *HCM*, hypertrophic cardiomyopathy; *HLHS*, hypoplastic left heart syndrome; *IAA*, interrupted aortic arch; *IVC*, inferior vena cava; *LSVC*, persistent left superior vena cava; *LV*, left ventricular; *LVOTO*, left ventricular outflow tract obstruction; *MV*, mitral valve; *NSAIDs*, nonsteroidal antiinflammatory drugs; *PA*, pulmonary artery; *PAPVR*, partial anomalous pulmonary venous return; *PAtresia*, pulmonary atresia; *PDA*, patent ductus arteriosus; *PKU*, phenylketonuria; *PPS*, peripheral pulmonary stenosis; *PS*, pulmonary stenosis; *RVOTO*, right ventricular outflow tract obstruction; *SVC*, superior vena cava; *SVT*, supraventricular tachycardia; *TAPVR*, total anomalous pulmonary venous return; *TEF*, tracheoesophageal fistula; *TGA*, transposition of great arteries; *TOF*, tetralogy of Fallot; *VSD*, ventricular septal defect.

Table 8-2 Conditions, Cardiac Manifestations, and Genetics

Condition	Cardiac Manifestations	Extracardiac Features	References
Apert syndrome	VSD		
Asplenia syndrome	see Heterotaxy syndrome		
Barth syndrome	Endocardial fibroelastosis, LV noncompaction, DCM, and septal defects.	X-linked disorder of lipid metabolism that affects boys. Skeletal muscle hypoplasia, motor and cognitive disabilities, recurrent infections, hypoglycemia in infancy, methylglutaconic aciduria and acidemia, and other congenital malformations.	462
Brugada syndrome (types 1-4)	Ventricular fibrillation and specific EKG abnormalities—upsloping ST segment, right bundle branch block, and T-wave inversion. In types 3 and 4 there may also be a shortened QT interval. Sudden death that may occur during sleep. Polymorphic ventricular tachycardia and syncope may occur.	Agonal gasps during sleep have been reported. Aborted episodes of sudden death. Sudden infant death syndrome.	120,604,665,666
CHARGE association or syndrome	CHD incidence 50%-70%—conotruncal anomalies (TOF, DORV, aortic arch abnormalities), PDA, AVSD/AVC, VSD, ASD	Findings that make up the acronym are: C-coloboma (congenital hole in one of the structures of the eye) and/or micro-ophthalmia, H-heart, A-atresia (choanal), R-retardation of mental and somatic development, G-genital anomalies, E-ear abnormalities and/or deafness. The most common features: coloboma, choanal atresia, abnormal semicircular canals, arhinencephaly (absence of olfactory lobes of brain), and rhombencephalic (neural tube) dysfunctions. Other commonly associated defects—Facial palsy, cleft palate, dental abnormalities, DiGeorge sequence, omphalocele, and dysphagia. Diagnosis is made when choanal atresia + 2 other cardinal anomalies (heart, ear, or genital) are present.	122,506,604,765
Cri-du-chat syndrome	In 30%-60%: VSD, ASD, PDA	Catlike cry, growth and mental retardation, round face, widely spaced eyes, epicanthal fold, and simian crease	700
DiGeorge sequence (DGS) (see 22q11.2 also)	Conotruncal cardiac anomalies (including right aortic arch)	Abnormalities of thymus (may be absent), immune deficiency, and parathyroid problems (hypocalcemia and hypoparathyroidism)	122,506,541,803
Down syndrome	see Trisomy 21		
Edward syndrome	see Trisomy 18		
Ehlers-Danlos Syndrome	PA branch stenosis	There are types I-VIII, but type I and II are the classic types. The main features are loose-jointedness and fragile, bruisable skin that heals with peculiar "cigarette-paper" scars, premature birth caused by premature rupture of membranes, and internal complications such as rupture of large vessels, hiatus hernia, spontaneous rupture of the bowel, and diverticula of the bowel.	604,700
Elfin facies syndrome	See Williams syndrome		
Ellis-van Creveld syndrome (EVC)	In 50%-60%. ASD or single atrium, AVSD/AVC; other defects are less common	Growth deficiency, short limbs, polydactyly, dental abnormalities, deformity of upper lip, hypoplasia of nails, dwarfism with narrow thorax	328,506,539, 604,700
Fragile X syndrome	MV prolapse, mild dilatation of the ascending aorta	Mental retardation, macroorchidism, distinct facial features (including long face, large ears, and prominent jaw) and connective tissue abnormalities	487
Friedreich's ataxia	In 50%-75%. HCM, subAS, and EKG abnormalities	CNS abnormalities resulting in uncoordinated limb movements, dysarthria, nystagmus, diminished or absent tendon reflexes, Babinski sign, impairment of position and vibratory senses, scoliosis, pes cavus, and hammer toe. Diabetes.	

Syndrome	Cardiovascular features	Other findings	References
Heart block, familial	A variety of types of heart block	Rarely associated with other findings	
Heterotaxy syndromes (hetero = different; taxy = position, arrangement)	Complex cyanotic CHD, systemic and pulmonary venous drainage anomalies, TGA, AVSD/AVC, PS, or atresia, cardiac malposition, AV and/or ventriculoarterial discordance. Asplenia syndrome (associated with more complex CV lesions)—right atrial isomerism, complex conotruncal defects, AVSD/AVC, anomalous location of IVC. Polysplenia syndrome (not as complex CV lesions)—left atrial isomerism, septal defects, interrupted IVC, bilateral SVC, PAPVR, non-sinus pacemaker	Malposition of organs with associated anomalies Situs inversus (mirror image malposition of organs); isomerism—failure of organ system asymmetry; Ivemark syndrome (asplenia/polysplenia sequence) Asplenia: malposition of abdominal viscera (GI malrotation, symmetric liver, right-sided stomach) bilateral right-sidedness—right isomerism, absence of spleen, presence of Howell-Jolly bodies in blood (normally removed by spleen), immunocompromise, and GU, bronchopulmonary, skeletal and CNS abnormalities Polysplenia: multiple nodules of splenic tissue (may be functionally asplenic), malposition of abdominal viscera (symmetric or inverted liver, GI malrotation), cardiac malpositions, bilateral left-sidedness—left isomerism, and GU, bronchopulmonary, skeletal and CNS abnormalities	190,328,363,700
Holt Oram syndrome (Heart hand syndrome)	In 75%. Septal defects (ASD, VSD, AVSD/AVC), conduction disturbances (AV blocks), PAPVR/TAPVR. Complex defects seen in Holt Oram with TBX5 mutations but are rare.	Upper limb anomalies—mild hypoplasia of thumb to variable severity phocomelia—radial aplasia, narrow shoulders, thumb may be absent or may be a triphalangeal, nonopposable, finger-like digit. May have only heart or only hand deformity.	63,122,328,506, 604,700,817
Hunter syndrome	See mucopolysaccharidoses. CV dysfunction related to mucopolysaccharide deposits.	Dysostosis with dwarfism, grotesque facies, hepatosplenomegaly from mucopolysaccharide deposits, deafness, and excretion of large amounts of chondroitin sulfate B and heparitin sulfate in the urine	604
Hurler syndrome	See mucopolysaccharidoses. Cardiovascular dysfunction related to mucopolysaccharide deposits.	Coarse facies, corneal clouding, mental retardation, hernias, dysostosis multiplex, and hepatosplenomegaly. Appear normal at birth and develop the characteristic appearance over the first years of life	463,712
Hypertrophic cardiomyopathy	Progressive disorder of the myocardium that can result in LVOTO leading to potential arrhythmias. Most frequent cause of sudden death in young with strenuous physical exertion.		535,569,604
Hypoplastic left heart syndrome (see Table 8-1, also)	HLHS, often without other anomalies	May be associated with airway problems, GI problems in infancy, or immunologic problems	604
Klinefelter syndrome	In 50%. MV prolapse, venous thromboembolic disease, PDA, and ASD	Typically normal appearing, tall stature, small testes, delayed puberty, emotional and behavioral problems, and variable mental retardation	700
LEOPARD syndrome	In 70%-100%. PS, conduction problems, HCM (asymmetric)	Similar to Noonan syndrome—LEOPARD is an acronym for the manifestations of this syndrome: Lentigines (multiple sun spots on skin), Electrocardiographic conduction abnormalities, Ocular hypertelorism, Pulmonic stenosis, Abnormal genitalia, Retardation of growth, and sensorineural Deafness	328,604,655,700
Long QT syndrome—congenital/familial. Also see Jervell and Lange-Nielsen syndrome.	EKG has prolonged QT interval and polymorphic ventricular arrhythmias causing syncope (may be triggered by acute physical, emotional, or auditory stimulus, and may be misinterpreted as seizures), seizures, and sudden death. A variety of types of long QT syndromes exist and the 2 most common types are listed below.	Rarely associated with other findings. More common in females but males are at higher risk for earlier, life-threatening events.	604

Continued

Table 8-2   Conditions, Cardiac Manifestations, and Genetics—cont'd

Condition	Cardiac Manifestations	Extracardiac Features	References
	Long QT Syndrome 1 (~42% of cases), also known as Romano-Ward syndrome. Ward-Romano syndrome. Question of association with some cases of Sudden Infant Death Syndrome has been raised.		70,604
	Long QT Syndrome 2 (~45% of cases). Mutation in the hERG gene (encodes a protein in the potassium ion channel) has been reported with neonatal long QT syndrome with symptomatic ventricular tachyarrhythmias.		70,604
Marfan syndrome	Aortic root (dilation, aneurysms, dissection) and aortic or mitral valve abnormalities—MV prolapse	Connective tissue disorder (elastin) with variable phenotype. Skeletal manifestations (scoliosis, long thin long bones, joint contractures or laxity, and pectus excavatum), ocular problems (myopia and lens problems), characteristic facial features (long, triangular "droopy" face), oral abnormalities (dental problems and high arched palate), and normal intelligence but neuropsychologic impairment in some (learning disabilities, ADD)	506,604,610, 633,831
Mucopolysaccharidoses (MPS)—see also Hunter and Hurler syndromes	CA changes, cardiomyopathy, cardiac valve dysfunction	Lack of enzymes for breakdown causes accumulation of MPS—organ function affected	604
Neurofibromatosis	In 2%. PS, AS, CoA, HCM	Café au lait spots, optic glioma, scoliosis, pseudarthrosis, neurofibromas	328
Neurofibromatosis-Noonan syndrome	See neurofibromatosis	Features include neurofibromatosis plus short stature, ptosis, midface hypoplasia, webbed neck, learning disabilities, and muscle weakness.	15,549
Noonan syndrome—other names: male Turner syndrome; female pseudo-Turner syndrome	CHD in about 50%-85%. PS, ASD with PS, VSD, AVSD/AVC, mitral regurgitation, LV septal hypertrophy, and other defects are more rare (TOF, CoAo, SubAS, Ebstein's, complex defects, cardiomyopathy)	Short stature, mild mental retardation (25% affected), motor delay, dysmorphic features (short webbed neck, low posterior hairline, hypertelorism, a downward eye slant, and low-set posteriorly rotated ears, epicanthic folds), pectus deformity, coagulation deficiencies, hearing impairment, early feeding difficulties are common (poor suck and refusal to take solids or liquids, tube feedings commonly needed), gastrointestinal dysfunction (vomiting, constipation, abdominal pain and bloating, foregut dysmotility and/or gastroesophageal reflux), and cryptorchidism in males	328,506,604, 655,700
Patau syndrome	see Trisomy 13		
PHACES syndrome	In 90%. CoA, IAA, aortic arch anomalies.	Posterior fossa malformation, hemangiomas, eye anomalies	328
Polysplenia syndrome	see Heterotaxy syndrome		
Pompe disease—acid maltase deficiency (AMD) and glycogen storage disease II	Cardiomegaly caused by muscle degeneration	A glycogen storage disease resulting from a deficiency of the enzyme alpha-glucosidase (GAA) resulting in hypotonia, macroglossia	122,604,830
Potter sequence	Variety of CHDs.	Polycystic kidneys, microbrachycephaly, hypertelorism with telecanthus, large posteriorly angulated and fleshy ears, and various congenital malformations	604
Trisomy 8	In 25%. VSD, PDA, CoA, PS, TAPVR, truncus arteriosus	Skeletal anomalies, widely spaced eyes, broad nasal bridge, small jaw, high arched palate, cryptorchidism, and renal anomalies	700
Trisomy 9	In 65%-80%. PDA, LSVC, VSD, TOF/PAtresia, DORV	Significant growth and mental retardation, microcephaly, deep-set eyes, low-set ears, and 2/3 die in infancy	700

Syndrome	Cardiovascular manifestations	Clinical features	References
Trisomy 13	In 80%-90%. PDA, ASD, VSD, HLHS, laterality defects (atrial isomerism), CoA, abnormal valves, dextrocardia, TOF, complex defects	Cleft lip and palate, holoprosencephaly (midline facial and forebrain hypodevelopment), polydactyly, skin defects, eye abnormalities, apnea, seizures, severe mental deficiency, craniofacial abnormalities, deafness, rib anomalies, genitourinary abnormalities, omphalocele, and death in infancy in 80%	122,190,328, 506,700
Trisomy 18	In 90%-100%. ASD, VSD, AVSD/AVC, PDA, polyvalvular disease, ToF, DORV, BPV, PS, BAV	Polyhydramnios, growth deficiency, feeble at birth, petite facial features, micrognathia, prominent occiput, hypertonia, clenched hands, overlapping digits, short sternum, rocker-bottom feet, tracheoesophageal fistula, diaphragmatic hernia, omphalocele, renal anomalies, biliary atresia, severe retardation, and death in first year of life >90%	122,190,328, 506,700
Trisomy 21	In 40%-50%. AVSD/AVC defects, VSD, ToF, PDA, ASD, DORV (LVOTO lesions are rare)	Microcephaly, flattened occiput, flattened face with characteristic features (epicanthal fold), strabismus, small ears, hypotonia, short neck, small stature, short fingers, simian crease, clinodactyly of fifth finger, brachydactyly, variable mental retardation, premature aging	122,328,380, 463,506,700
Tuberous sclerosis complex (TSC)	CV manifestations reported in childhood—cardiac rhabdomyomas (51%-86% are associated with tuberous sclerosis), aortic aneurysm, and/or rupture of the ascending thoracic aorta	The deletion impacts proteins involved in cell growth causing lesions in multiple organ systems—skin (white macules shaped like a leaf—present at birth in most cases—may be evident only under Wood light), brain (result in epilepsy, learning difficulties, and/or behavioral problems), and renal lesions (hemorrhage or compression and replacement of healthy renal tissue, cysts, polycystic renal disease, and renal carcinoma [Wilms'] can also occur)	604
Turner syndrome—Monosomy X	In 25%-35% CoA, BAV (>50% incidence), AS, IAA, septal defects, MV problems, PAPVR, LSVC, and HLHS. Later—hypertension, aortic dissection/dilation and rupture	Females. May present as a neonate. Webbed neck, lymphedema of hands and feet, unusual chest shape, widely spaced nipples, short stature, triangular face, down-slanting palpebral fissure, low set ears, hormonal effects (streak ovaries, primary amenorrhea, maturation, and growth), normal intelligence	122,190,328, 506,700
VACTERL (VATER) Association	CHD in 10%-70%—ToF, VSD, others	Diagnosed when three or more of the following are present: vertebral anomalies, anal atresia, cardiac defects, tracheo-esophageal fistula, esophageal atresia, renal anomalies, limb defects (humeral hypoplasia, radial aplasia, and proximally placed thumb)	506,604
Williams syndrome—Williams-Beuren syndrome, elfin facies syndrome	CHD in 53%-85%—supravalvar AS, hypoplastic aortic arch, PA stenosis, PPS, CoA, CA stenosis, and/or peripheral vascular disease	Elfin facies (stellate pattern of the iris, short anteverted nose, long philtrum, prominent lips, open mouth, flat nasal bridge, broad forehead), hypercalcemia—infantile, psychosocial and cognitive differences (mild to moderate retardation, "cocktail party" personality, difficulty with numbers—time, money), feeding problems (failure to thrive), skeletal and/or connective tissue anomalies, thyroid disorders, and renal problems (hypertension)	122,190,328, 604,700
Wolff-Parkinson-White syndrome	Short PR interval, prolonged QRS, delta waves: paroxysmal SVT. In some cases there is HCM.	Rarely associated with other findings	604

ADD, Attention deficit disorder; *AS,* aortic stenosis; *ASD,* atrial septal defect; *AV,* atrioventricular; *AVC,* atrioventricular canal; *AVSD,* atrioventricular septal defect; *BAV,* bicuspid aortic valve; *BPV,* bicuspid pulmonary value; *CA,* coronary artery; *CHD,* congenital heart defect; *CNS,* central nervous system; *CoA,* coarctation of aorta; *CV,* cardiovascular; *DCM,* dilated cardiomyopathy; *DORV,* double-outlet right ventricle; *GI,* gastrointestinal; *GU,* genitourinary; *HCM,* hypertrophic cardiomyopathy; *HLHS,* hypoplastic left heart syndrome; *IAA,* interrupted aortic arch; *IVC,* inferior vena cava; *LSVC,* persistent left superior vena cava; *LV,* left ventricle; *LVOTO,* left ventricular outflow tract obstruction; *MV,* mitral valve; *PA,* pulmonary artery; *PAPVR,* partial anomalous pulmonary venous return; *PAtresia,* pulmonary atresia; *PDA,* patent ductus arteriosus; *PPS,* peripheral pulmonary stenosis; *PS,* pulmonary stenosis; *RVOTO,* right ventricular outflow tract obstruction; *SVC,* superior vena cava; *SVT,* supraventricular tachycardia; *TAPVR,* total anomalous pulmonary venous return; *TEF,* tracheoesophageal fistula; *TGA,* transposition of great arteries; *TOF,* tetralogy of Fallot; *VSD,* ventricular septal defect.

reproductive risks for the family; and considering the appropriate testing of other family members.[700] Genetic testing can be performed on blood lymphocytes, cord blood, skin, amniotic fluid, chorionic villi, and bone marrow. Current genetic tests available to be used in assessing CHD include:

- Standard chromosome analysis—reveals standard karyotype and is used to identify many chromosomal disorders, especially those in which there is an abnormal number of chromosomes.[700]
- High resolution banding—better defines chromosomal structure abnormalities such as duplications, deletions, and translocations of genetic material.[700]
- Fluorescence in situ hybridization (FISH)—specific DNA probes can be used to diagnose more subtle structural abnormalities such as microdeletions, tiny duplications, and/or subtle translocations.[700]
- Array comparative genomic hybridization (A-CGH)—even more sensitive than FISH for testing for tiny structural abnormalities of chromosomes.[868]
- Gene discovery—cloning techniques are used to identify genes that produce a protein associated with cardiogenic gene mutations.[700]
- DNA mutation analysis—identifies changes in the coding sequence of a gene to find small deletions, duplications, or substitutions that alter the resulting protein structure. Once a change is found, it must be determined if it constitutes a disease-causing mutation.[700]

As more etiologic genes are identified, progress can be made in determining mechanisms and interactions that cause various phenotypes. That may lead to the development of targeted therapies for patients and fetuses.[871]

Genetic counseling is warranted when there is one major or two minor birth defects and may be employed to attempt to determine exact causes of anomalies in individual situations. Testing must be accurately ordered to direct the proper studies to obtain complete results. Simply ordering a karyotype will not achieve the targeted exploration that can be achieved with FISH or A-CGH studies. Information gathered enables practitioners to counsel the family on problems associated with a condition, allowing them to be proactive in their child's care. Discussions with the family should be informative but not directive so that parents may make their own decisions.[190,651]

At the very least, preconceptual and prenatal counseling of all women of child-bearing age is important to encourage the use of multivitamins and folic acid supplements, avoiding contact with people with flu or other febrile illnesses, and avoiding exposure to organic solvents during pregnancy. Targeted counseling should be done with women who have specific risk factors to discuss any medications that must be considered with pregnancy. Prenatal testing is also available for some conditions, and early diagnoses can affect care management, morbidity, mortality, and family well-being.

Another feature of genetic counseling is providing recurrence risks. With the exception of possibly teratogen exposures, parents can be counseled that their actions did not cause the condition. For chromosomal deletions, duplications, translocations, and gene anomalies, parental testing may be recommended to determine recurrence risks. In cases of gene anomalies,

commercial testing is available for some mutations. Testing capabilities continue to expand so follow-up genetic consultation may be warranted to realize the advantages of new technologies.

Recurrence risks for chromosomal trisomies are low if there are no other birth defects in the family and maternal age is not advanced. For a parent with an autosomal dominant genetic anomaly, there is a 50% risk of recurrence. In parents who have an autosomal negative genetic anomaly (without the evidence of the problem), both parents must have the anomaly to cause the resulting disorder. In these cases the recurrence risk for the couple is 25%. In X-linked recessive anomalies, the risk is 50% for a male to be affected and 50% for a female to be a carrier. In cases of unknown etiology (possibly multifactorial inheritance), if no other child in the family is affected the recurrence risk is presumed to be 3% to 5%, but this changes if a subsequent sibling is affected.[190,651]

Information about genetic conditions is widely available via websites and targeted support groups and associations (e.g., Online Mendelian Inheritance in Man, www.ncbi.nlm.nih.gov/Omim/). Web-based databases and support groups that provide valuable information are provided in the Chapter 8 Supplement on the Evolve Website.

The nursing implications of genetics involvement in congenital heart defects are significant. Nurses who are familiar with the patterns of anomalies can have a heightened index of suspicion when a single malformation is noted and findings can be unmasked. Nursing knowledge can be enhanced by familiarity with the most current scientific statements from the American Heart Association Congenital Heart Defects Committee, Council on Cardiovascular Disease in the Young on both the genetic basis and the noninherited risk factors for congenital heart disease.[414,700]

Nurses are in a unique position to gather information from families and communicate those findings. Facts about previous pregnancies, parents' siblings, childhood deaths, other birth defects, exposures, and much more can be revealing. Nurses are also in a unique position to support families through these challenging situations. Nurses must be prepared to provide families with appropriate resources and encourage referrals.

This quote from *Joey's Journey: Our Life with Lissencephaly*, at http://lfurlotte.tripod.com expresses how parents may feel when they begin a journey with a child affected by anomalies and the support others can provide: "Life will never be the same again. However, with a little different perspective, life does go on and happiness does return."[415]

FETAL DEVELOPMENT OF THE HEART AND GREAT VESSELS

Mary Rummell

Formation of the Heart Tube: Day 22

The cardiovascular system is the first system to function in the embryo. The critical period of cardiovascular growth begins at 15 to 18 days of gestation and is initiated by a period of rapid cell proliferation. During this period, the developing heart is most susceptible to teratogens (factors that can be harmful). Early development of the cardiovascular system is necessary because of the increasing need for nutritional and oxygen requirements by the rapidly growing embryo and for elimination of carbon dioxide and waste products. Moore et al.,[627] Ransom and Srivastava,[723] and Sander et al.,[764] describe heart development as involving five primary steps:

1. Migration of precardiac cells from the primitive streak and assembly of paired cardiac crescents at the myocardial plate
2. Coalescence of the cardiac crescents to form the primitive heart tube, an event that establishes the definitive heart
3. Cardiac looping, a complex process that assures proper alignment of the future cardiac chambers
4. Septation and heart chamber formation
5. Development of the cardiac conduction system and coronary vasculature

The primordial heart and vascular system appear in the middle of the third week. The cardiovascular system is primarily derived from embryonic mesoderm and neural crest cells. The precardiac stem cells (mesoderm) migrate to form the cardiac crescents that fuse to form the single heart tube at 22 days (Fig. 8-1).[627,723,764,902]

At this time (22 days), circulation begins with ebb-and-flow blood flow from the venous to arterial poles. Premyocardial cells and neural crest cells continue to migrate into the region of the heart tube. The regulation of the mesoderm is partially controlled by retinoids, isoforms of vitamin A, that bind to specific nuclear receptors and regulate gene transcription and by extracellular matrix proteins, such as fibronectin, that direct cellular migration. The teratogenic effects caused by interaction of retinoid-like drugs on cell receptors are seen clinically (see Noninherited Risk Factors).[79]

Formation of the Heart Loop: Day 22 to 28

Before and during the looping process, sections of the single heart tube begin to develop specialized cells that will ultimately become the chambers of the mature heart. A cascade of genes is expressed in the anterior (ventricular) and the posterior (atrial) portions of the tube. These genes regulate the cellular processes that transform the heart tube into a four-chambered heart. This transformation occurs through a balance of cell growth, cell differentiation, and cell death (apoptosis). Disruptions in these genetic mechanisms and specific cellular signaling processes result in cardiac malformations seen in congenital heart disease. Problems include defects in cardiac looping, septation, and chamber formation.[764]

The endocardial heart tube begins to expand and elongate and develops areas of dilation: the bulbus cordis (including the truncus arteriosus, conus arteriosus, and conus cordis), ventricle, atrium, and sinus venosus. This expansion and elongation results in coiling of the heart tube *anteriorly and to the right* (this is referred to as "dextral," or "D-looping"), with creation of a bulboventricular loop (see Fig. 8-1, B and C).

Because the venous and arterial poles of the heart tube are fixed during this time of coiling, torsion occurs within the anterior portion of the loop, the truncus arteriosus. This torsion will later contribute to the formation of a spiral septum within the truncus. By the 26th day of gestation, a truncus arteriosus is visible in the center of the anterior portion of the heart, and a common atrium and ventricle are recognizable (see Fig. 8-1, D). By day 28 the looping process is complete.

The embryonic heart begins to contract by day 26 to 28, with cycles that are similar to those in mature hearts.[72] In this "in-series circulation," blood flows from the morphologically right atrium to the morphologically left atrium, left ventricle, right ventricle and then the truncus arteriosus.[902]

As the common atrium and ventricle divide into the chambers of the right and left heart, individual chambers are identified by their structure and appearance, or *morphology*. Structures should be identified by morphology rather than location because the location of the ventricles and great vessels may be abnormal when congenital heart disease is present.

When the ventricles rotate or loop normally to the *right*, a *D-bulboventricular loop* has occurred. The anatomic (i.e., morphologic) right ventricle is anterior (and to the right),

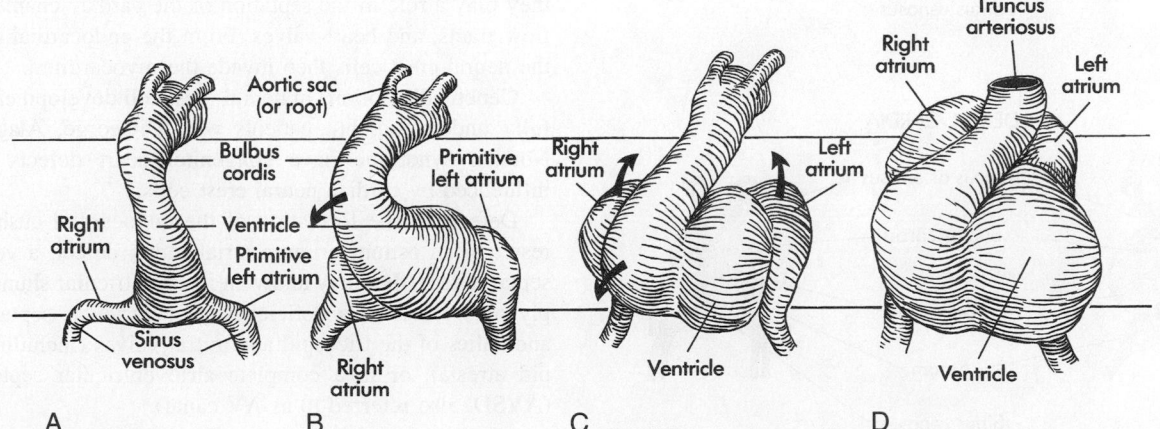

FIG. 8-1 Cardiac embryologic development—coiling of the heart tube. At approximately the 21st to 22nd day of fetal life, the two lateral endothelial heart tubes fuse to form a single endocardial tube. **A,** Between the 22nd and 28th days of life, the heart tube thickens. **B,** and **C,** the tube then coils to the right. **D,** By approximately the 28th day of fetal life, the tube is completely coiled, and major chambers can be identified. At this time, blood is flowing through the heart, and septation of the heart and great vessels can occur. (Illustration by Marilou Kundemueller.)

and the anatomic (i.e., morphologic) left ventricle is posterior (and to the left). Later, normal division of the great vessels will result in location of the aorta posterior and to the *right* of the pulmonary artery. When the great vessels are in normal position and relationship, they are labeled "d-related great vessels" because the aorta is located to the right (dextral) of the pulmonary artery.

Malrotation during the formation of the ventricular loop may cause various cardiac malpositions (such as dextrocardia) and malformations. As noted, the normal direction for the *ventricular loop is to the right,* or D-looping. If the ventricles loop to the *left* instead, *L-looping* has occurred, so the morphologic *left* ventricle is located to the right, and the morphologic *right* ventricle is on the left (Fig. 8-2).

L-looping of the ventricles frequently is associated with transposed great vessels; this combination commonly is referred to as *"corrected transposition of the great arteries."* It is a type of "transposition," because the aorta lies to the left of the pulmonary artery. The great vessels are transposed: the ascending aorta is *anterior* and arises from an anatomic (morphologic or structural) right ventricle, sweeping to the *left,* and the pulmonary artery is *posterior* and arises from the anatomic (or morphologic or structural) left ventricle. The term "corrected" is appropriate because the hemodynamic pathways are not altered; systemic venous return ultimately enters the pulmonary circulation, and pulmonary venous return enters the systemic circulation. The systemic venous return enters the right atrium, flows through a *mitral* valve into

a morphologic left ventricle, and is then ejected into a posterior pulmonary artery. The pulmonary venous return flows into the left atrium, exits through a *tricuspid* valve into a structural right ventricle and is then ejected into an anterior aorta. Although the heart is not normal, the child will be asymptomatic unless a complicating heart lesion is present.

Complete congenital heart block, ventricular septal defect, tricuspid valve anomalies, and cardiac malpositions are common among children with l-transposition. It is important to remember that the mitral valve is located with the morphologic left ventricle in corrected transposition, and that these structures receive *systemic* venous return; the tricuspid valve is associated with the morphologic right ventricle, receiving *pulmonary* venous return. Therefore if tricuspid atresia is present, obstruction to pulmonary venous return occurs (because the tricuspid valve is located abnormally on the left side). Ebstein's malformation, an abnormality of the tricuspid valve, produces signs associated with mitral insufficiency (e.g., pulmonary edema). The use of the phrase *"ventricular inversion with transposed great vessels"* probably would be less confusing than "corrected transposition."

Formation of Cardiovascular Septation: Day 26 to 49

Cardiac septation occurs after the looping process is complete. During the septation process, septae are formed that ultimately close the ostium primum, the central atrioventricular canal, and the interventricular foramen. At the end of this period, the in-series circulation becomes two parallel circulations.[902]

Endocardial Cushion Development: Day 26 to 40

Septation begins on day 26 with the ingrowth of large tissue masses, the endocardial cushions. These cushions form on the dorsal and ventral walls of the atrioventricular (AV) canal separating the primordial atrium from the primordial ventricle.[627] These cushions contain mesenchymal cells, derived from endocardium, and cardiac jelly, derived from endothelium. The endothelial cells line the atrioventricular canal and conotruncal segments. Neural crest cells migrate into the pharyngeal arches and then to the endocardial cushions, where they play a role in the septation of the cardiac chambers, outflow tracts, and heart valves. From the endocardial cushions, the neural crest cells then invade the myocardium.

Genetic disruptions in neural crest cell development are not fully understood, but patients with DiGeorge, Alagille, and Noonan syndrome have congenital heart defects that are influenced by cardiac neural crest cells.[764]

Defects in the formation of the endocardial cushions can result in an ostium primum atrial septal defect, a ventricular septal defect (that may allow an interventricular shunt, or simply may result in a deficiency of ventricular septal tissue), anomalies of the tricuspid and mitral valves (including tricuspid atresia), or in a complete atrioventricular septal defect (AVSD, also referred to as AV canal).

Atrial Septation: Day 30 to 35

Septation of the atria begins around day 30. Two septae develop and are modified to form a flapped orifice, the foramen ovale as illustrated in Fig. 8-3. The first septum to form is the *septum primum,* which grows from the anterior, superior

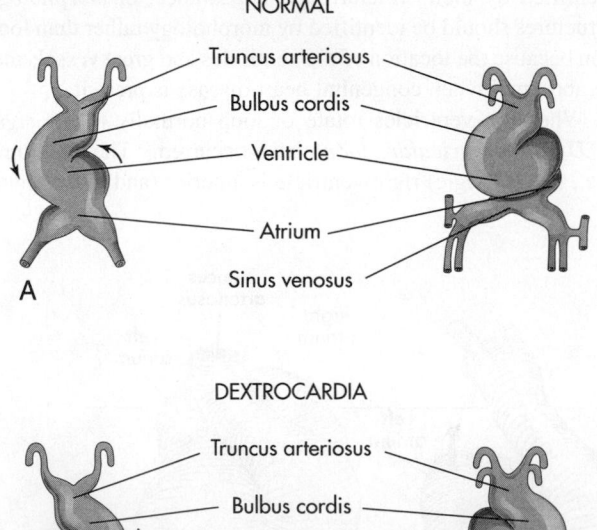

FIG. 8-2 Cardiac loop formation, The primordial heart tube during the fourth week. **A,** Normal looping (bending) to the right. **B,** Abnormal looping (bending) to the left. (From Moore KL, Persaud TVN, Torchia MG: *The cardiovascular system. The developing human: clinically oriented embryology,* ed 8. Philadelphia, 2008, Saunders Elsevier.)

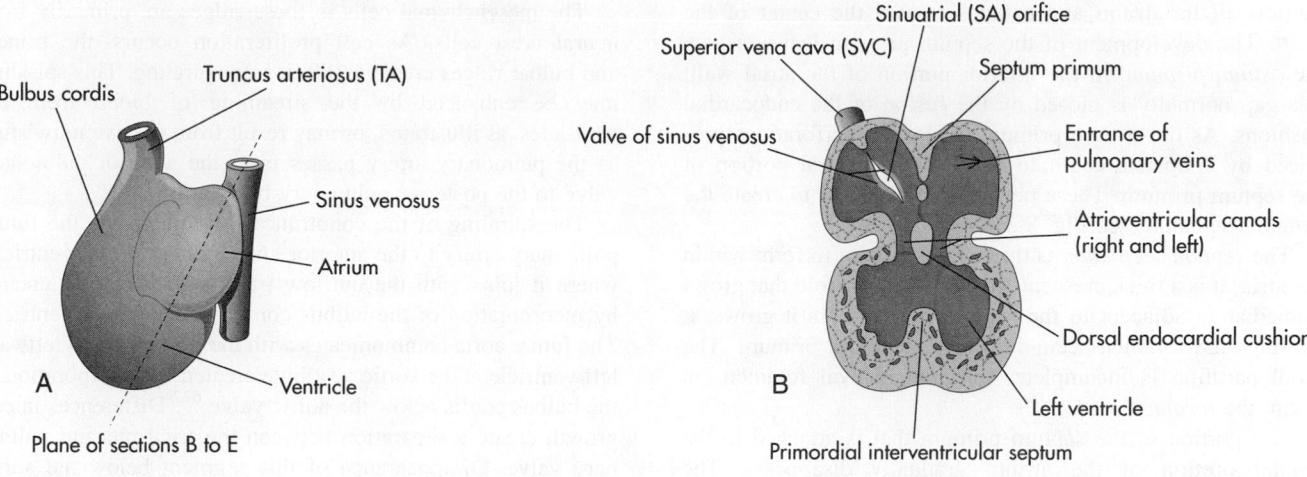

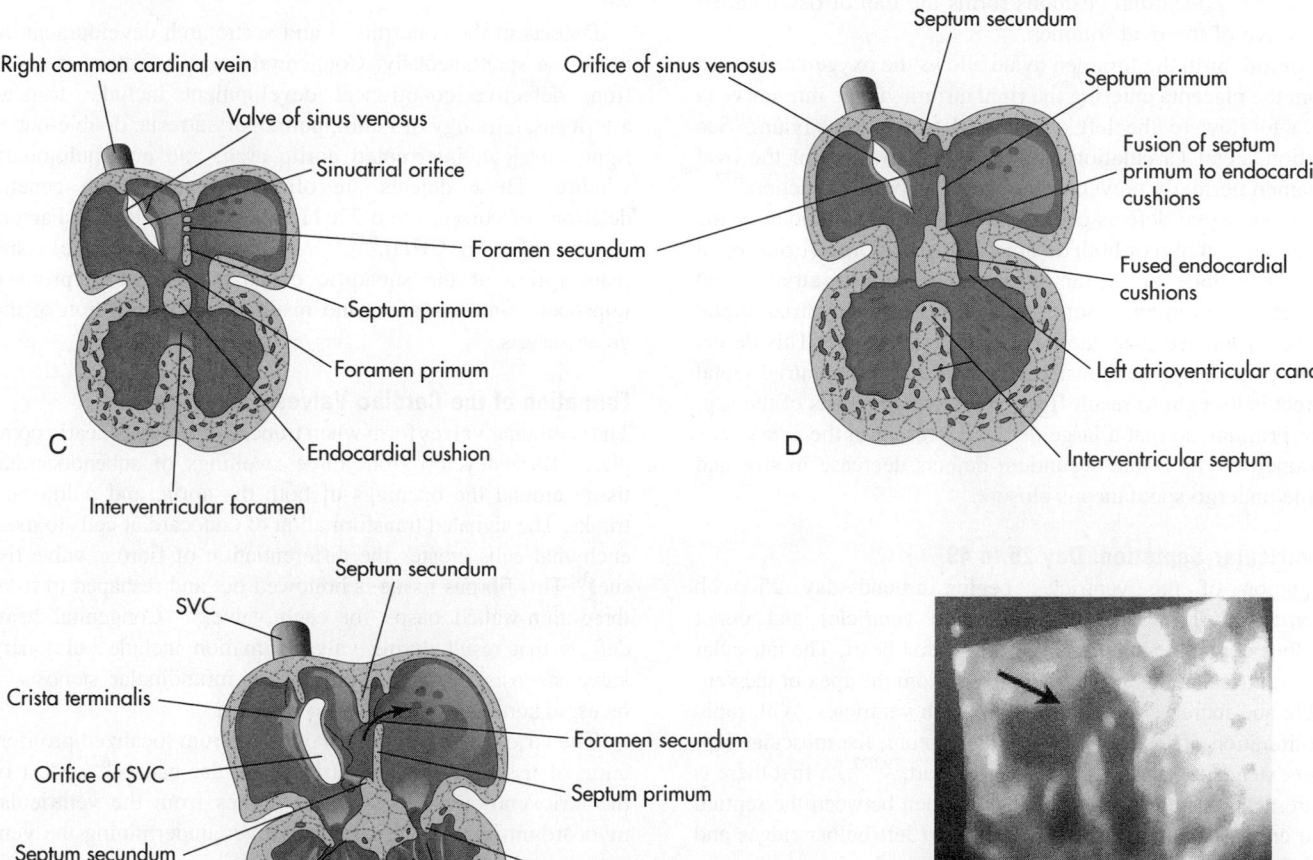

FIG. 8-3 Atrial and ventricular septation. (A-E) Drawings of the developing heart showing partitioning of the atrioventricular canal, primordial atrium and ventricle. **A,** Sketch showing the plane of the sections. **B,** Frontal section of the heart during the fourth week (approximately 28 days) showing the early appearance of the septum primum, interventricular septum, and dorsal endocardial cushion. **C,** Similar section of the heart (approximately 32 days) showing perforations in the dorsal part of the septum primum. **D,** Section of the heart (approximately 35 days) showing the foramen secundum. **E,** At approximately 8 weeks, showing the heart after it is partitioned into four chambers. The *arrow* indicates the flow of well-oxygenated blood from the right to the left atrium. **F,** Sonogram of a second trimester fetus showing the four chambers of the heart. Note the septum secundum (*arrow*) and the descending aorta. (Courtesy of Dr. G. J. Reid, Department of Obstetrics, Gynecology and Reproductive Sciences, University of Manitoba, Women's Hospital, Winnipeg, Manitoba, Canada.) (From Moore KL, Persaud TVN, Torchia MG: *The cardiovascular system. The developing human: clinically oriented embryology,* ed 8. Philadelphia, 2008, Saunders Elsevier.)

portion of the atrium and extends toward the center of the heart. The development of the septum primum leaves a gap, the *ostium primum,* in the inferior portion of the atrial wall; this gap normally is closed by the fusion of the endocardial cushions. As the ostium primum is closing, perforations produced by apoptosis begin to form in the central portion of the septum primum. These perforations coalesce to create the *ostium secundum* (see Fig. 8-3, C and D).[627]

The *septum secundum* is the second septum to form within the atria. It is a thick crescent-shaped muscular fold that grows immediately adjacent to the septum primum. As it grows, it overlaps the foramen secundum in the septum primum. The atrial partition is incomplete, forming an oval foramen (in Latin, the *foramen ovale*).[627]

The portion of the septum primum that is attached to the cranial portion of the atrium gradually disappears. The remaining portion of the primum septum that is attached to the fused endocardial cushions forms the flap of tissue called the valve of the oval foramen.[627]

Before birth the foramen ovale allows the oxygenated blood from the placenta entering the right atrium via the inferior vena cava to flow to the left atrium and to the fetal brain. (See section, Fetal Circulation that follows.) The flap of the oval foramen normally prevents flow in the opposite direction.[627]

Atrial septal defects occur when the primum septum or the secundum septum or both do not completely form. Atrial septal defects include an ostium primum, secundum atrial septal defect, or common atrium. An ostium primum atrial septal defect is located near the atrioventricular valves. This defect will not close spontaneously. An ostium secundum atrial septal defect is thought to result from excessive apoptosis of the septum primum, so that a large defect is present in the area of the foramen ovale. Some secundum defects decrease in size and some undergo spontaneous closure.[723]

Ventricular Septation: Day 25 to 49

Septation of the ventricles begins around day 25 with protrusions from the inlet (primitive ventricle) and outlet (bulbus cordis) segments of the primordial heart. The muscular intraventricular septum initially grows from the apex of the ventricle and increases with dilation of both ventricles. With rapid proliferation of the myoblasts in the septum, the muscular septum extends toward the center of the heart.[79,627] At first there is a crescent-shaped intraventricular foramen between the septum and endocardial cushions. The right and left bulbar ridges and the fused endocardial cushions join with the intraventricular muscular septum to form the membranous septum, obliterating the intraventricular foramen (refer again to Fig. 8-3, B-E).

As the ventricular cavities develop, the walls form a sponge work of muscular bundles. Some of the bundles become the papillary muscles and the tendinous cords (Latin, *chordae tendineae*) of the atrioventricular valves.[627] Ventricular septal defects can occur in any location in the developing ventricular septum. Some muscular defects will close spontaneously.[723]

Septation of the Truncus Arteriosus: Day 26 to 42

Active proliferation of the mesenchymal cells in the walls of the bulbus cordis form the conotruncal or bulbar ridges. Similar ridges form in the truncus arteriosus (Fig. 8-4).

The mesenchymal cells in these ridges are primarily from neural crest cells. As cell proliferation occurs, the truncal and bulbar ridges create a 180-degree spiraling. This spiraling may be enhanced by the streaming of blood from the ventricles, as illustrated, or may result from passive untwisting as the pulmonary artery passes from the anterior pulmonary valve to the posterior pulmonary bifurcation.[902]

The spiraling of the conotruncal septum aligns the future pulmonary artery to the anterior and rightward right ventricle, where it joins with the outflow tract (infundibulum) created by incorporation of the bulbus cordis into the right ventricle. The future aorta communicates with the posterior and leftward left ventricle at the aortic vestibule created by incorporation of the bulbus cordis below the aortic valve.[627] Differences in cell growth create a separation between the tricuspid and pulmonary valve. Disappearance of this segment below the aortic valve provides fibrous continuity between the mitral and aortic valve.[79]

Defects in the conotruncal and aortic arch development do not close spontaneously. Congenital heart defects that result from defective conotruncal development include: truncus arteriosus, tetralogy of Fallot, pulmonary atresia, double-outlet right ventricle, interrupted aortic arch, and aortopulmonary window. These defects are often associated with genetic deletions of chromosome 22q11 (see section, Genetic Factors Associated with CHD).[627,723] Failure of appropriate conal reabsorption of the subaortic conus is thought to produce improper truncal rotation and result in d-transposition of the great vessels.

Formation of the Cardiac Valves: Day 34 to 42

The semilunar valves form when truncal septation is nearly complete. They develop from three swellings of subendocardial tissue around the openings of both the aortic and pulmonary trunks. The signaled transformation of endocardial cells to mesenchymal cells creates the differentiation of fibrous valve tissue.[30] This fibrous tissue is hollowed out and reshaped to form three thin-walled cusps for each valve.[627] Congenital heart defects that result during valve formation include pulmonary valve stenosis or atresia, pulmonary infundibular stenosis, a bicuspid aortic valve, and aortic stenosis.

The atrioventricular valves develop from localized proliferation of tissue around the atrioventricular canals.[627] Most of the atrioventricular valve tissue comes from the ventricular myocardium in a process that involves undermining the ventricular walls. This process is asymmetric and positions the tricuspid valve annulus closer to the apex of the heart than the mitral valve annulus. Physical separation of these two valves creates the atrioventricular septum. Absence of this septum is the common defect in children with atrioventricular septal defects. Ebstein anomaly is thought to result from incomplete undermining of the ventricular wall.[79]

Classification of Complex Cardiac Malpositions and Malformations

Complex cardiac malformations and malpositions can be described according to a labeling system proposed by Van Praagh.[902] This classification included 10 cardiac segments, but three were used most often. The positions of the viscera,

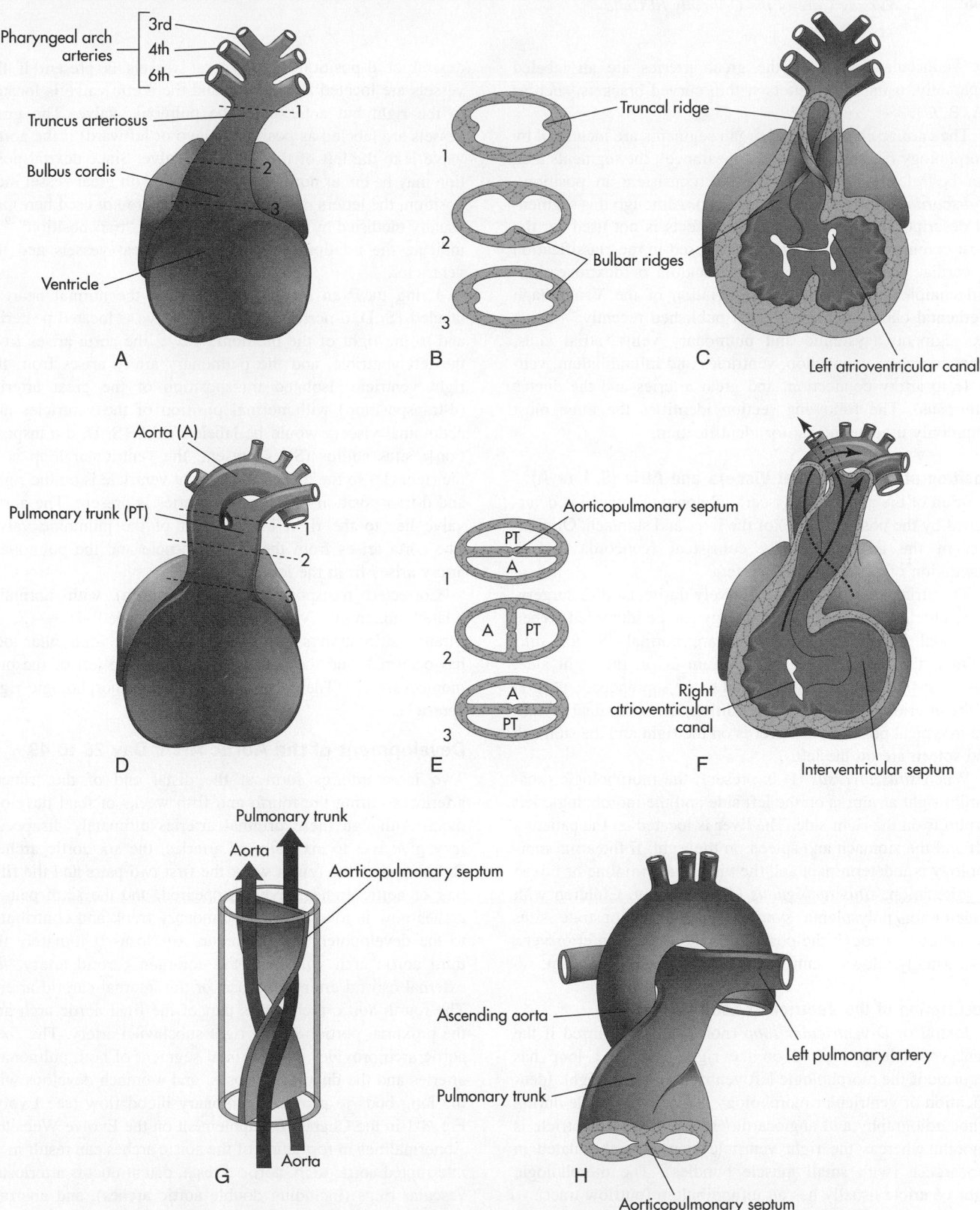

FIG. 8-4 Division of truncus arteriosus into pulmonary artery and aorta. Partitioning of the bulbus cordis and truncus arteriosus. **A,** Ventral aspect of heart at 5 weeks. The *broken lines* and *arrows* indicate the levels of the sections shown in B. **B,** Transverse sections of the truncus arteriosus and bulbus cordis, illustrating the truncal and bulbar ridges. **C,** The ventral wall of the heart and truncus arteriosus has been removed to demonstrate these ridges. **D,** Ventral aspect of heart after partitioning of the truncus arteriosus. The *broken lines* and *arrows* indicate the levels of the sections shown in E. **E,** Sections through the newly formed aorta (A) and pulmonary trunk (PT), showing the aorticopulmonary septum. **F,** 6 Weeks. The ventral wall of the heart and pulmonary trunk has been removed to show the aorticopulmonary septum. **G,** Diagram illustrating the spiral form of the aorticopulmonary septum. **H,** Drawing showing the great arteries (ascending aorta and pulmonary trunk) twisting around each other as they leave the heart. (From Moore KL, Persaud TVN, Torchia MG: *The cardiovascular system. The developing human: clinically oriented embryology,* ed 8. Philadelphia, 2008, Saunders Elsevier.)

the ventricular loop, and the great arteries are all labeled separately, using three letters within curved brackets, such as {A, B, C}.

The cardiac chambers and organ segments are identified by morphology (i.e., structure and appearance); the segments then can be referred to as *concordant* (consistent in position), or *discordant* (inconsistent in position). Although this segmental description of congenital heart defects is not used for the most common forms of defects, it is used in the classification of cardiac malpositions (e.g., dextrocardia or dextroversion) and complex transpositions. A variation of the Van Praagh segmental classification has been published recently[343] using six segments (systemic and pulmonary veins, atrial situs, atrioventricular connection, ventricles and infundibulum, ventricle to artery connection, and great arteries and the ductus arteriosus). The following section identifies the three most commonly used segments for identification.

Position of the Abdominal Viscera and Atria (S, I, or A)

Position of the abdominal viscera (abdominal organs) is determined by the position (side) of the liver and stomach. Orientation of the atria is usually consistent (concordant) with orientation of the abdominal viscera.

The atria can be labeled definitively during cardiac surgery, when characteristic atrial morphology can be identified. When the atrial and visceral positions are normal (S, for *situs solitus*), the morphologic right atrium is on the right side; it is identifiable because it is joined to the suprahepatic portion of the inferior vena cava.[903] In addition, the abdominal viscera are in typical position; the liver is on the right and the stomach and spleen are on the left.

When *situs inversus* (I) is present, the morphologic (anatomic) right atrium is on the left side and the morphologic left atrium is on the right side. The liver is located on the patient's left and the stomach and spleen on the right. If the atrial morphology is indeterminant and the viscera are midline or mixed in orientation, *situs ambiguous* (A) is present. Children with asplenia or polysplenia syndromes may demonstrate situs ambiguous, although the position of the hepatic inferior vena cava usually allows identification of the true right atrium.

Description of the Ventricular Loop (D or L)

A dextral or *D-ventricular loop* (normal) has occurred if the right ventricle is located on the right, and an L-loop has occurred if the morphologic left ventricle is on the right. Identification of ventricular morphology is usually possible during echocardiography and angiocardiography; the left ventricle is smooth, whereas the right ventricle is more trabeculated in appearance (with small muscle bundles). The morphologic right ventricle usually has an infundibulum (outflow tract).

Position of the Great Vessels (*d-* or *l*-Normal, or *d-* or *l*-Transposition). As noted, the position of the great vessels is determined by the relationship of the semilunar valves. Normal (dextral) position of the great vessels is present if the aortic valve is posterior and to the right of the pulmonic valve; this position also is occasionally referred to as the situs position of the great vessels. Abnormal position of the great vessels may be indicated by the letters *d* or *l*. Abnormal

dextral or d-position of the great vessels is present if the vessels are located abnormally and the aortic valve is located to the right but anterior to the pulmonic valve. The great vessels are labeled as position *l* (levo or leftward) if the aortic valve is to the left of the pulmonic valve. Since dextral position may be either normal or associated with great vessel malposition, the letters *d* or *l* (capital letters are *not* used here) are usually modified by the terms "normal" or "transposition"[29] to indicate the relationship between the great vessels and the ventricles.

Using the Van Praagh classification the normal heart is labeled {S, D, d-normal}; the aortic valve is located posterior and to the right of the pulmonic valve, the aorta arises from the left ventricle, and the pulmonary artery arises from the right ventricle. Isolated transposition of the great arteries (d-transposition) with normal position of the ventricles and abdominal viscera would be labeled TGA {S, D, d-transposition}: situs solitus (S) is present, the ventricular loop is to the right (D) so the morphologic right ventricle is on the right, and d-transposition of the great arteries is present. The aortic valve lies to the right but in front of the pulmonic valve. The aorta arises from the right ventricle and the pulmonary artery arises from the left ventricle.

Corrected transposition (l-transposition) with normally related abdominal viscera would be labeled TGA (S, L, l-transposition): situs solitus is present, a left ventricular loop has occurred, and the aortic valve lies to the left of the pulmonic valve.[903] The aorta arises from the morphologic right ventricle.

Development of the Aortic Arch: Day 28 to 49

Two large arteries form at the distal end of the truncus arteriosus during the fourth and fifth weeks of fetal development. Although these original arteries ultimately disappear, they give rise to six pairs of arteries, the six aortic arches. By the end of the fourth week the first two pairs and the fifth pair of aortic arches have disappeared, and the sixth pair of arches now is joined to the pulmonary trunk and contributes to the development of the ductus arteriosus. Ultimately the third aortic arch will form the common carotid artery, the external carotid artery, and part of the internal carotid artery. The fourth aortic arch forms part of the final aortic arch and the proximal portion of the right subclavian artery. The sixth aortic arch provides the proximal segment of both pulmonary arteries and the ductus arteriosus, and a branch develops with the lung buds to provide pulmonary blood flow (see Evolve Fig. 8-1 in the Chapter 8 Supplement on the Evolve Website). Abnormalities in formation of the aortic arches can result in an interrupted aortic arch, aortic atresia, patent ductus arteriosus, vascular rings (including double aortic arches), and aberrant origin of the right subclavian artery.

Development of the Ventricular Myocardium, Conduction System, and Coronary Circulation

After the neural crest cells enter the endocardial cushions, they migrate to the myocardium. The myocardium then develops into a working myocardium and the cardiac conduction system. Originally the atrium acts as the pacemaker of the heart. The sinoatrial node develops during the fifth week. Additional cells from the right atrial wall join with cells from the atrioventricular region to form the atrioventricular node and His bundle located just above the endocardial cushions. Bundle branches are found throughout the ventricular myocardium.[627]

Additional cells develop from a small, transient organ, the proepicardium, on the dorsal thoracic wall. The proepicardial cells contain mesothelial cells that migrate to the heart and form the epicardium that lines the heart. These cells migrate further and differentiate to form the coronary vasculature and cardiac fibroblasts.[764]

In prenatal life myocardial cells undergo significant changes to increase in number (hyperplasia) and size (hypertrophy). The myocardial cells also change shape from round to cylindrical, become more regular in the orientation of the myofibrils (the contractile element), and have increasing proportions of myofibrils. Developmental changes are also seen in the sarcolemma (plasma membrane) and sarcoplasmic reticulum. Both control the ion channels and transmembrane receptors that regulate cardiac function, depolarization, and repolarization. Maturation of these cells and functions continues into the neonatal period.[79]

Fetal Circulation

Fetal circulation differs anatomically and physiologically from postnatal circulation in several important ways. In the fetus, oxygenation of the blood occurs in the placenta, which is a relatively inefficient oxygenator. The fetus is *hypoxemic,* with an aortic arterial oxygen tension of approximately 20 to 30 mm Hg; the saturation of fetal hemoglobin is higher at this oxygen tension than is normal hemoglobin, so oxygen saturation is approximately 60% to 70%. The fact that the oxygen tension is normally much lower in the fetus than postnatally may account for the ability of the neonate to tolerate cyanotic heart disease.[278] Despite this arterial hypoxemia, the fetus does not have *tissue hypoxia* because fetal cardiac output is higher than at any other time in life, averaging approximately 400 to 500 mL/kg per minute. Approximately 20% of the normal fetal oxygen consumption of 8 mL/kg per minute is required to develop new tissue.[278] Fetal cardiac output is constant (at approximately 400 to 500 mL/kg per minute) at a heart rate greater than 120 to 180/min. Changes in preload result in very little change in cardiac output, and changes in afterload are not well tolerated.[278]

Fetal circulation is designed to deliver the best-oxygenated and nutrient rich blood from the placenta to the fetal brain and heart (Fig. 8-5). This blood enters the fetus through the umbilical vein. The blood flow splits in the liver with almost half going through the hepatic veins and portal system of the liver and the rest through the *ductus venosus,* where it joins the inferior vena cava near its junction with the right atrium. In the right atrium the blood from the inferior vena cava (with a PO$_2$ of 32 to 35 mm Hg and an oxygen saturation of 70%— the highest fetal PO$_2$) is divided into two streams. About 40% of this blood passes through the foramen ovale into the left atrium, where it joins the small amount of blood from pulmonary venous return. It then passes through the mitral valve to the left ventricle and then to the ascending aorta where it supplies the coronary, carotid, and subclavian arteries. The preferential streaming of this blood results in an

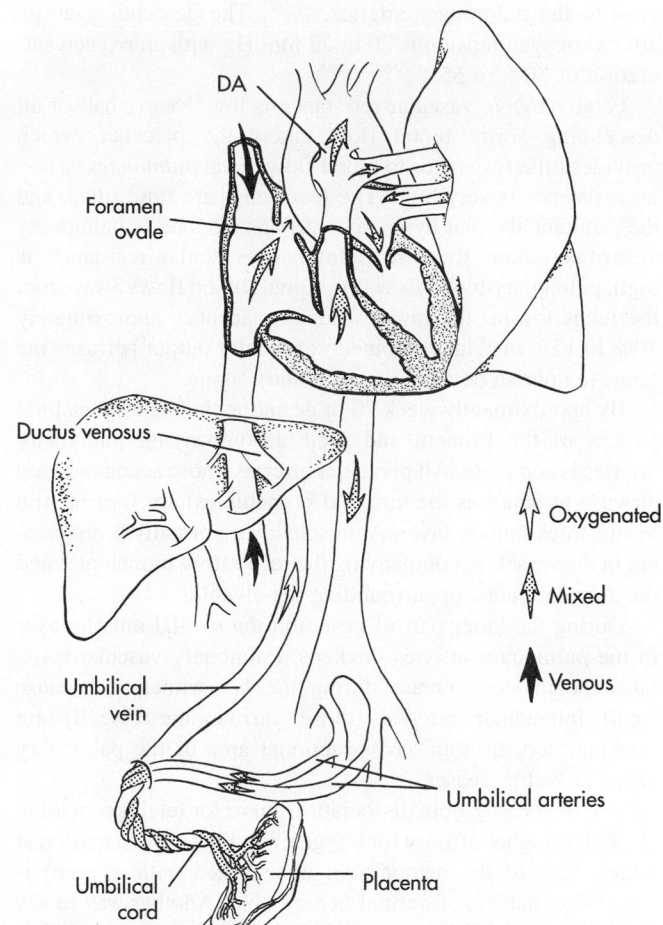

FIG. 8-5 Fetal circulation. Fetal blood is oxygenated in the placenta (which is a less efficient oxygenator than the lungs). The oxygenated blood enters the fetus through the *umbilical vein* and enters the *ductus venosus,* bypassing the hepatic circulation and flowing into the inferior vena cava. When this blood reaches the right atrium, it is diverted by the *crista dividens* toward the atrial septum, and flows through the *foramen ovale* into the left atrium. The blood then passes through the left ventricle and ascending aorta to perfuse the head and upper extremities. This pathway allows the best-oxygenated blood from the placenta to perfuse the fetal brain. Venous blood from the head and upper extremities returns to the fetal heart through the superior vena cava, enters the right atrium and ventricle, and flows into the pulmonary artery. Because pulmonary vascular resistance is high, this blood is diverted through the *ductus arteriosus* into the descending aorta. Ultimately, much of this blood will return to the placenta through the *umbilical arteries.* (Illustration by Marilou Kundemueller.)

ascending aortic arterial oxygen tension (PaO$_2$) of 26 to 28 mm Hg and an oxygen saturation of 65%.[278,686] Ten percent of the blood flow from the left ventricle passes through the aortic arch into the descending aorta, where it joins 90% of the blood leaving the right ventricle. The fetal right ventricle pumps more than two thirds of the combined ventricular output, so the right ventricle is relatively muscular.

Most blood from the right ventricle bypasses the lungs because pulmonary vascular resistance is high; it passes through the *ductus arteriosus* into the descending aorta. (It provides less resistance to flow than pulmonary vascular resistance.) Only 10% to 15% of the right ventricular blood flow goes to the pulmonary arteries.[278,627] The descending aortic arterial oxygen tension is 20 to 22 mm Hg with an oxygen saturation of 50% to 55%.[278,681,686]

Fetal *systemic* vascular resistance is low. Nearly half of all descending aortic blood flow enters the placenta, which provides little resistance to blood flow. Fetal *pulmonary* vascular resistance is very high. The fetal lungs are fluid filled, and the resultant alveolar hypoxia contributes to intense pulmonary vasoconstriction. Because pulmonary vascular resistance is high, pulmonary blood flow is minimal (blood flows away from the lungs toward the low-resistance placenta); approximately 10% to 15% of fetal combined ventricular output perfuses the lungs to nourish developing pulmonary tissue.

By approximately week 20 of gestation the major branching pattern of the bronchi and their accompanying pulmonary arteries is complete. All preacinar arteries (those accompanying airways as small as the terminal bronchioles) are formed, and have a thick muscle layer. A muscle layer normally is *not* present in the vessels accompanying the respiratory bronchioles and the alveolar ducts, or surrounding the alveoli.

During the latter part of gestation the medial muscle layer in the pulmonary arteries thickens. Pulmonary vascular resistance begins to decrease during the last trimester, because small intraacinar arteries (those surrounding alveoli) are forming, and the total cross-sectional area of the pulmonary vascular bed increases.

The oxyhemoglobin dissociation curve for fetal hemoglobin (HbF) has higher affinity for oxygen; it's P_{50} (oxygen tension at which 50% of the hemoglobin is saturated with oxygen) is lower than the P_{50} of normal hemoglobin. Another way to say this is that the HbF oxyhemoglobin dissociation curve is shifted to the left of the normal (postnatal) oxyhemoglobin dissociation curve. This means that at any given PO_2, the fetal hemoglobin will be better saturated than adult hemoglobin would be. Thus, at the same PO_2, oxygen content with fetal hemoglobin will be higher (in mL oxygen/dL blood) than the oxygen content would be with normal hemoglobin. However, because fetal hemoglobin binds more readily to oxygen than normal hemoglobin, fetal hemoglobin does not release oxygen as readily to the tissues. The reason for the difference in oxygen binding is a difference in response to 2,3-diphosphoglycerate (2,3-DPG); in fetal hemoglobin, 2,3-DPG does not alter binding with oxygen, whereas in normal hemoglobin, the 2,3-DPG reduces affinity to oxygen. Fetal hemoglobin normally is replaced by normal hemoglobin within about 3 to 6 months of birth.

NORMAL PERINATAL CIRCULATORY CHANGES

Important circulatory changes occur at birth when oxygenation in the placenta ceases and the lungs expand and begin to oxygenate the blood. At birth, fetal shunts (the foramen ovale, ductus arteriosus, and ductus venosus) and the umbilical vessels are no longer necessary.

Elimination of the placenta causes an immediate fall in the blood pressure in the inferior vena cava and right atrium. Lung expansion with air that includes oxygen causes a dramatic rise in alveolar oxygenation and a fall in the pulmonary vascular resistance. With the decrease in pulmonary vascular resistance, pulmonary artery pressure falls, and blood flow

through the ductus arteriosus is reversed. A rise in arterial oxygen tension and perivascular PO_2 causes vasoconstriction of the ductus arteriosus. This increases pulmonary blood flow, resulting in more pulmonary venous return to the left atrium. This rise in pulmonary venous return increases the left atrial pressure above the inferior vena cava and right atrial pressure and functionally closes the foramen ovale with the flap of the primum septum. Blood pressure increases in the aorta and systemic circulation with removal of the low-resistance placenta from the circulation.[278,385,627,686]

Right ventricular output is reduced to half of the combined ventricular output.[278] The increased workload of the right ventricle during fetal life produced a thickened right ventricular wall that is reflected in the increased RV forces on the neonatal electrocardiogram. The thickness of the right ventricular wall regresses over the first postnatal month because the workload of the right ventricle is reduced. With the reverse in workload and increased systemic vascular resistance, the wall of the left ventricle thickens.[627]

Normal Postnatal Changes in Pulmonary Vascular Resistance

When the lungs fill with air, most of the fluid within the alveoli moves to the pulmonary interstitium, where it is absorbed by the pulmonary capillaries and (to a lesser extent) removed by the lymphatics. As lung fluid is reabsorbed, alveolar hypoxia is eliminated, producing pulmonary vasodilation. Vasoactive substances (including prostaglandins and prostacyclin) mediate pulmonary vasodilation. The medial muscle layer of the pulmonary arteries begins to thin immediately after birth and continues to regress during the first days of life. These changes produce a rapid fall in pulmonary vascular resistance and, consequently, a fall in pulmonary artery pressure.

At sea level, pulmonary vascular resistance falls immediately after birth by approximately 80% and normally reaches near-adult levels during the first weeks of life. Normal pulmonary vascular resistance index (normalized to body surface area) is approximately 7 to 10 Wood units $\times$ m^2 body surface area during the first week of life, but falls to 1 to 3 Wood units $\times$ m^2 body surface area within a few weeks in patients at sea level (Table 8-3). Within 24 hours after birth, mean pulmonary artery pressure has fallen to approximately one half of mean systemic pressure, if the ductus arteriosus has constricted normally. This fall in pulmonary vascular resistance results in a parallel fall in right ventricular systolic and end-diastolic pressure.

The presence of alveolar hypoxia during the first days of life may delay or prevent the normal fall in pulmonary vascular resistance, because the hypoxia stimulates pulmonary vasoconstriction. Alveolar hypoxia is present in premature neonates with severe respiratory distress syndrome; this may delay the perinatal fall in pulmonary vascular resistance. As long as pulmonary vascular resistance remains high, increased pulmonary blood flow through the ductus arteriosus is prevented. Typically the pulmonary vascular resistance falls when the pulmonary disease resolves. This fall in pulmonary vascular resistance often is heralded by symptoms of a large left-to-right shunt through a patent ductus arteriosus. Other factors that may contribute to pulmonary vasodilation and pulmonary vasoconstriction are listed in Box 8-1.

Table 8-3 Calculation of Pulmonary Vascular Resistance

$$Resistance = \frac{Pressure\ drop\ across\ system}{Flow\ through\ system}$$

$$\frac{Pulmonary\ vascular\ resistance}{(in\ Wood\ Units)} = \frac{Mean\ PA\ pressure - LA\ pressure\ (mm\ Hg)}{Cardiac\ output\ (L/min)}$$

Note: This equation yields the *PVR in Wood Units* (units). Normal values are listed below. To convert these units to units of absolute physical resistance (dynes-sec-cm^{-5}), multiply the Wood Units by 80.

To normalize PVR for body surface area, *Pulmonary Vascular Resistance INDEX Units* (PVRI) are calculated. The above equation is utilized, with the substitution of Cardiac Index (L/min per m^2 BSA). In effect, the PVRI is the PVR (in Wood Units) multiplied by the child's body surface area. Normal values are listed below.

Age	Absolute PVR (Wood Units)*	PVR Index*
Newborn infant	25-40 Units	7-10 Index units
Child	0.5-4 Units	1-3 Index units

*To convert these units to dynes-s-cm^{-5}, multiply by 80.

Box 8-1 **Factors Contributing to Pulmonary Vasoconstriction and Vasodilation**

Factors Contributing to Pulmonary Vasoconstriction (the four Hs)
- (Alveolar) hypoxia
- Hydrogen ion (acidosis)
- Hyperinflation (distension of alveoli)
- Hypothermia

Factors Contributing to Pulmonary Vasodilation (Six As)
- Alveolar oxygenation
- Alkalosis
- Analgesia
- Appropriate tidal volume and temperature
- Avoid stimulation
- Administered nitric oxide and other vasodilators

Closure of Fetal Shunts

The rise in the neonate's arterial oxygen tension is thought to be the most potent stimulus to ductal constriction; however, many factors contribute to ultimate ductal closure. The rise in the oxygen tension of the blood bathing the ductus (i.e., the perivascular oxygen tension), the fall in endogenous dilating prostaglandins and adenosine levels, and release of circulating vasoactive substances all promote ductal closure.

Constriction of the ductal medial smooth muscle thickens the ductal wall and shortens the ductus, resulting in an infolding of the intima within the ductal lumen. These changes generally produce functional closure of the ductus within 10 to 24 hours following a full-term birth. The ductus then is converted to the ligamentum arteriosus through fibrous infiltration (Fig. 8-6).

Ductal closure may be delayed or prevented in the very premature infant. Failure of ductal constriction results from a combination of factors, including decreased medial muscle within the ductus, decreased constrictive response to oxygen, and increased levels or heightened effects of circulating

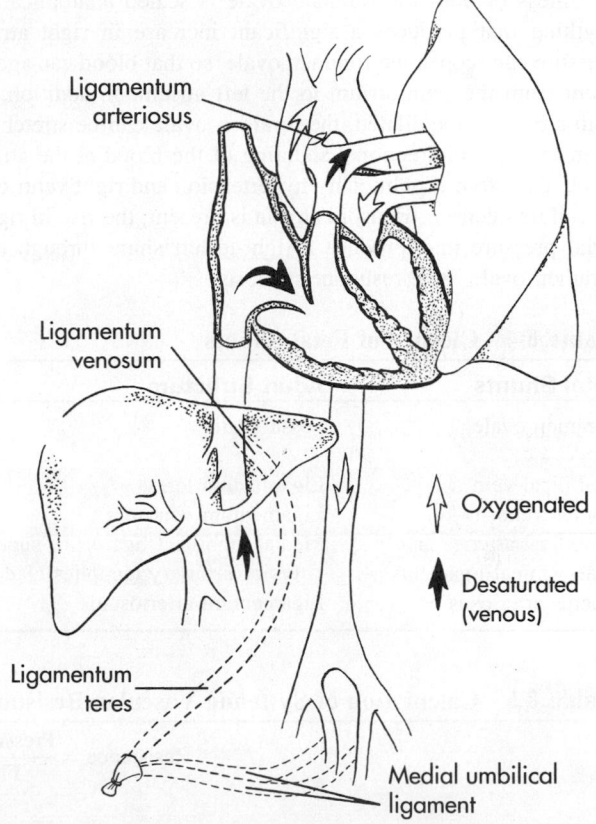

FIG. 8-6 Postnatal circulation. Blood is oxygenated in the lungs, and pulmonary vascular resistance is low. Systemic venous (desaturated) blood returns to the heart through the superior and inferior vena cavae. This blood then flows through the right atrium and right ventricle, into the pulmonary artery, and ultimately into the pulmonary circulation. Oxygenated blood from the lungs returns to the left atrium through the pulmonary veins. This blood passes into the left ventricle and flows into the aorta and systemic arteries to perfuse the body. (Illustration by Marilou Kundemueller.)

vasodilating prostaglandins. Ductal closure also may be delayed in patients living at high altitudes (and therefore exposed to low inspired oxygen tension) and neonates with cyanotic heart disease.

When the umbilical cord is tied and cut, the umbilical arteries and vein constrict. Eventually they undergo fibrous infiltration, becoming the medial umbilical ligament and ligamentum teres, respectively. The ductus venosus ultimately becomes the ligamentum venosum.

The flapped atrial opening, the foramen ovale, closes when left atrial pressure exceeds right atrial pressure. The foramen ovale closes by adherence of two portions of the atrial septum; this form of closure is called *functional* closure of the foramen ovale.

In most individuals the foramen ovale becomes sealed permanently by deposition of fibrin and cell products during the first months of life; this is referred to as *anatomic* closure of the foramen ovale. In approximately 25% of the population, however, the foramen ovale is not sealed anatomically and remains probe-patent beyond adolescence, so that a catheter can be passed from the right to the left atrium during cardiac catheterization or surgery. Table 8-4 provides a summary of the timing of the closure of the fetal shunts.

Unless or until the foramen ovale is sealed anatomically, anything that produces a significant increase in right atrial pressure can reopen the foramen ovale, so that blood can again shunt from the right atrium to the left atrium. In addition, if both atria become dilated, the foramen ovale can be stretched open to allow bidirectional shunting of the blood at the atrial level. Therefore if pulmonary hypertension and right ventricular failure occur or tricuspid atresia is present, the rise in right atrial pressure may produce a right-to-left shunt through the foramen ovale, with resultant cyanosis.

Normal Postnatal Changes in Systemic Vascular Resistance

With separation of the placenta from the circulation the neonate's systemic vascular resistance begins to rise, and continues to increase during childhood. Normal systemic vascular resistance index is approximately 10 to 15 Wood units × m^2 body surface area in the young infant, and is approximately 15 to 30 Wood units × m^2 body surface area in the child and adult (Table 8-5).

GROSS ANATOMY AND FUNCTION

Mary Fran Hazinski

The Right Side of the Heart

Systemic venous blood returns to the right atrium via the superior and inferior vena cavae. The *sinoatrial (SA) node* is located near the junction of the superior vena cava and the right atrium, just under the surface of the epicardium. The right atrium lies just under the sternum and forms the right lateral border of the cardiac silhouette on the anterior-posterior chest radiograph. Much of the inside of the right atrium has a trabeculated appearance, resulting from the presence of pectinate muscles that compose the anterior and lateral walls.

The atrial septum forms the posterior border of the right atrium, extending from right to left. The fossa ovalis (remnant

Table 8-4   Closure of Fetal Shunts

Fetal Shunts	Adult Structure	Closes Functionally	Closes Permanently
Foramen ovale	Fossa ovalis	At birth	3 Months (25% probe patent in adults)
Umbilical vein	Ligamentum teres	With clamping of umbilical cord	
Ductus venosus	Ligamentum venosum	At birth	
Umbilical arteries and abdominal ligaments	Medial umbilical ligaments, superior vesicular artery (supplies bladder)	With clamping of umbilical cord	
Ductus arteriosus	Ligamentum arteriosum	10-15 h	2-3 weeks

Table 8-5   Calculation of Systemic Vascular Resistance

$$\text{Resistance} = \frac{\text{Pressure drop across system}}{\text{Flow through system}}$$

$$\frac{\text{Systemic vascular resistance}}{\text{(in Wood Units)}} = \frac{\text{Mean arterial pressure} - \text{Mean RA pressure (mm Hg)}}{\text{Cardiac output (L/min)}}$$

Note: This equation yields the *SVR in Wood Units* (units). Normal values are listed below. To convert these units to units of absolute physical resistance (dynes-sec-cm^{-5}), multiply the Wood Units by 80.

To normalize SVR for body surface area, *Systemic Vascular Resistance INDEX Units* (SVRI) are calculated. The above equation is utilized, with the substitution of Cardiac Index (L/min per m^2 BSA). In effect, the SVRI is the SVR (in Wood Units) multiplied by the child's body surface area. Normal values are listed below.

Age	Absolute SVR (Wood Units)*	SVR Index*
Infant	35-50 Units	10-15 Index units
Toddler	25-35 Units	20 Index units
Child	15-25 Units	15-30 Index units

*To convert these units to dynes-s-cm^{-5}, multiply by 80.

of the foramen ovale) usually can be visualized high in the septum. The *coronary sinus,* which returns coronary venous blood to the heart, normally lies between the inferior vena cava and the tricuspid valve. The *atrioventricular (AV) node* is located anterior and medial to the coronary sinus and above the tricuspid valve.

Three internodal conduction pathways are thought to provide more rapid conduction between the SA and AV nodes than normal myocardium. Although conduction can occur along any of these three pathways, preferential internodal conduction probably occurs along the anterior internodal pathway, which courses from the sinus node, around the superior vena cava, and along the anterior portion of the atrial septum to the AV node. If these pathways are injured during cardiovascular surgery, AV conduction block can result.

The tricuspid valve is the anterior AV valve. It is positioned so that blood passing through the valve must flow in an anterior, inferior, and leftward direction into the right ventricle. The leaflets of the tricuspid valve are not equal in size, and they are not identifiable immediately as three distinct leaflets. The anterior leaflet extends from the pulmonary infundibulum to the lower anterior portion of the ventricle. The septal (or medial) leaflet attaches to the membranous and muscular portions of the ventricular septum. The posterior leaflet lies along the posterior aspect of the tricuspid ring. Each leaflet is attached to several chordae tendineae, which are in turn attached to one of three papillary muscles in the right ventricle.

The right ventricle is normally the most anterior of the four cardiac chambers, and its inferior border forms much of the left inferior cardiac border on an anteroposterior chest radiograph. The right ventricle receives blood from the right atrium and pumps blood into the low-resistance pulmonary circulation. Because the right ventricle normally generates low pressure, it has a thinner wall and a smaller lumen than the left ventricle. The right ventricle contains muscle bundles, called trabeculations, which give the ventricle a loculated appearance. The *moderator band* is a larger muscle bundle that traverses the right ventricle from the base of the tricuspid valve papillary muscle and joins the septal band of the septum.

The right ventricle is divided functionally into an inflow and an outflow portion by the *crista supraventricularis,* a ridge formed by a combination of septal and parietal bands that extends from the lateral wall of the right ventricle to the anterior leaflet of the tricuspid valve; this defines the pulmonary outflow tract. The pulmonary outflow tract also is called the pulmonary *infundibulum;* blood flows from the right ventricle and is directed posteriorly and superiorly into the pulmonary artery.

The pulmonary valve is a *semilunar valve* that normally is located above, in front of, and to the left of the aortic valve. Its three cusps are labeled the anterior, right, and left cusps.

Beyond the neonatal period, the pulmonary circulation is normally a low-resistance circulatory pathway that carries systemic venous blood to the lungs and then returns oxygenated pulmonary venous blood to the heart. The typical pulmonary branch artery has a thinner wall (with thinner medial muscle layer) and larger lumen than a comparable systemic artery.

The Left Side of the Heart

Oxygenated blood returns from the lungs through four pulmonary veins to the left atrium. The left atrium is the most posterior of the four cardiac chambers and normally does not contribute to the definition of the cardiac border on the anteroposterior chest radiograph. The left atrium has a slightly thicker and smoother wall than the right atrium. The left atrial appendage, a trabeculated extension of the left atrium, abuts the pulmonary artery.

Pulmonary venous blood flows from the left atrium through the mitral valve and into the left ventricle. The mitral valve consists of two leaflets: the septal leaflet extends from the muscular ventricular septum to the anterior wall of the left ventricle, and the posterior leaflet, the larger of the two leaflets, extends across the remaining portion of the valve annulus. The mitral leaflets attach to several chordae tendineae, which in turn attach to two groups of papillary muscles.

The left ventricle is located behind the right ventricle so that pulmonary venous blood passing through the mitral valve must flow inferiorly and laterally. The left ventricle may not form a distinct part of the cardiac border on the anteroposterior chest radiograph. This ventricle is characterized by a thick wall and a large lumen; its walls appear smoother than the trabeculated walls of the right ventricle. The septal leaflet of the mitral valve divides the left ventricle into an inflow and an outflow chamber. This division is only present when the mitral valve is open; the ventricle functions as a single chamber during systole.

The aorta has a thicker wall and a smaller lumen than the pulmonary artery. The aortic valve is a semilunar valve. Because the coronary arteries arise immediately above the aortic valve, the valve cusps are labeled in reference to the coronary arteries. The cusp immediately below the left coronary artery is called the left coronary cusp; the cusp immediately below the right coronary artery is called the right coronary cusp; and the cusp that is not related to any coronary artery is called the noncoronary cusp.

There are normally two coronary arteries: the left coronary artery, which branches into the left anterior descending and left circumflex arteries, and the right coronary artery. Blood flow from the coronary arteries perfuses the heart from epicardium through the myocardium to the endocardium, then coronary venous blood drains into the anterior cardiac veins or the coronary sinus and then into the right atrium.

A systemic artery has a thicker medial muscle layer, a relatively smaller lumen, and more elastic tissue than a pulmonary artery. Systemic arteries normally carry oxygenated blood under relatively high pressure to the tissues.

NORMAL CARDIAC FUNCTION

The Cardiac Cycle

The heart receives systemic venous blood, ejects it into the lungs, and receives pulmonary venous blood and ejects it into the body. In this serial circulation there is sequential relaxation and contraction of the atria, followed by sequential relaxation and contraction of the ventricles. The circulation on the right side of the heart normally is separated from the circulation on the left side of the heart.

Systemic venous return enters the right atrium through the superior and inferior vena cavae. Oxygen saturation of superior vena caval blood is approximately 70%, which is slightly lower than the saturation of blood in the inferior vena cava (75%). Coronary sinus blood, with an oxygen saturation of approximately 30% to 40%, is then added to this venous return, so the mixed venous saturation (best obtained in the pulmonary artery after mixing is complete) usually is approximately 70% to 75%. This corresponds to a mixed venous oxygen tension (PvO_2) of 38 to 40 mm Hg (Fig. 8-7).

During atrial and ventricular diastole the tricuspid valve is open and systemic venous blood flows passively into the right ventricle. Approximately 70% of ventricular filling occurs during this period. Mean right atrial pressure is equal to right ventricular end-diastolic pressure in the absence of tricuspid valve disease. Mean right atrial pressure in spontaneously

breathing infants beyond the neonatal period is approximately 0 to 4 mm Hg; mean right atrial pressure in older children during spontaneous breathing is 2 to 6 mm Hg.[752]

Atrial systole contributes the final 30% of ventricular filling. This volume is not essential for adequate cardiac output in the normal individual. However, loss of atrial systole may compromise stroke volume and cardiac output in a patient with ventricular dysfunction.

The right ventricle fills rapidly at the beginning of ventricular diastole; subsequent ventricular filling is slower until atrial systole occurs (Fig. 8-8, #1). Immediately after atrial contraction, ventricular contraction begins. Initially, ventricular contraction produces only a rise in ventricular pressure (without ejection of blood); this period is called the *isovolumetric phase* of ventricular systole (see Fig. 8-8, #2).

When right ventricular pressure exceeds right atrial pressure, the tricuspid valve closes and ventricular pressure rises rapidly. Once right ventricular pressure exceeds pulmonary artery pressure, the pulmonary valve opens and blood is ejected into the pulmonary artery. This ejection phase of ventricular contraction is called the *isotonic* phase of contraction (see Fig. 8-8, #3). Right ventricular systolic pressure is approximately 15 to 25 mm Hg in normal children and adults; it is typically higher in neonates and young infants. Pulmonary artery diastolic pressure is approximately 4 to 12 mm Hg.[752]

The blood that enters the pulmonary circulation passes through the pulmonary arteries and into the alveolar capillary bed, where it receives oxygen and surrenders carbon dioxide. Oxygenated blood then enters the pulmonary veins and flows into the left atrium. Pulmonary venous blood is normally 97% to 100% saturated with oxygen, unless an intrapulmonary shunt is present. Mean left atrial pressure during spontaneous breathing is normally 3 to 6 mm Hg in infants and 5 to 10 mm Hg in older children.

Because there are no valves between the precapillary pulmonary artery and the left atrium, the pulmonary artery wedge or occlusion pressure (obtained using an end-hole, balloon-tipped, flow-directed pulmonary artery catheter) is roughly equivalent to the left atrial pressure. This assumes that the catheter is placed in a posterior, inferior pulmonary artery branch; the monitoring system is zeroed, leveled, and calibrated correctly; alveolar pressure does not exceed pulmonary end-diastolic pressure (for further information, refer to Chapters 6 and 21); and there is no pulmonary venous constriction or obstruction.

If the mitral valve is normal, left atrial pressure equals left ventricular end-diastolic pressure. Therefore pulmonary artery wedge pressure is approximately equal to left atrial pressure and left ventricular end-diastolic pressure. If pulmonary vascular resistance is normal, pulmonary artery end-diastolic pressure should nearly equal pulmonary artery wedge and left atrial pressures. Conversely, an increased gradient between pulmonary artery end-diastolic pressure and pulmonary artery wedge pressure (or left atrial pressure) indicates that pulmonary vascular resistance is elevated.

As with the right ventricle, left ventricular filling occurs largely during atrial and ventricular diastole (see Fig. 8-8, #5). Left atrial contraction contributes the final 30% of ventricular filling (refer to Fig. 8-8, #1). Immediately after left atrial contraction the left ventricle begins to contract. When

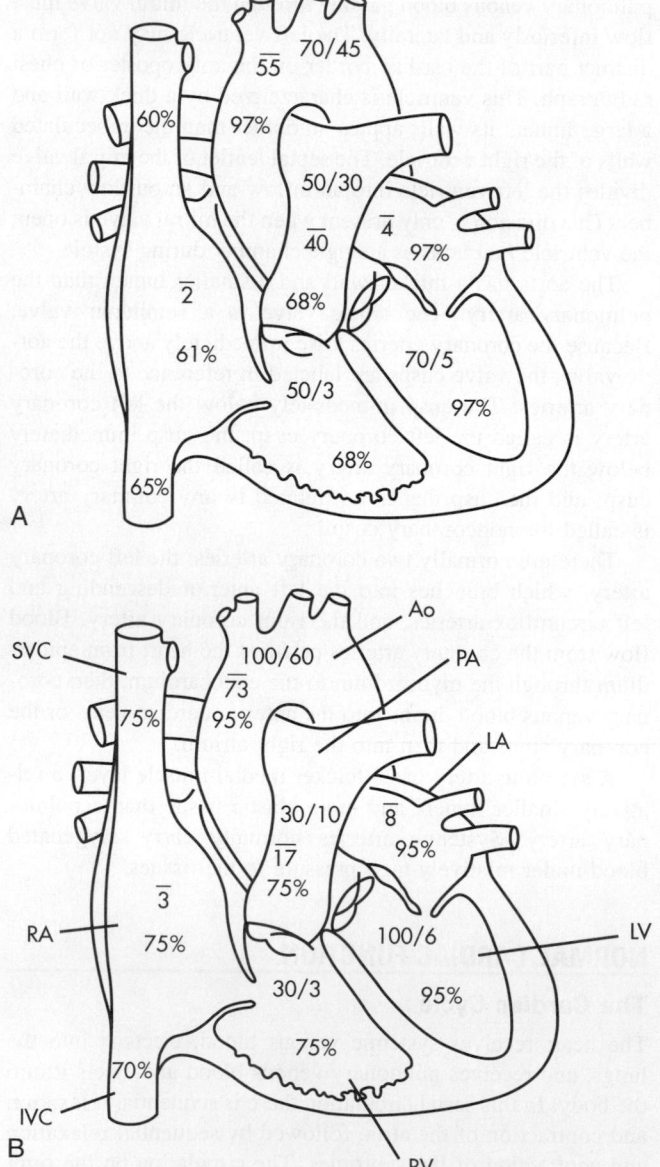

FIG. 8-7 Normal pressures (in mm Hg) and oxygen saturations in the neonatal **A**, and pediatric **B**, heart.

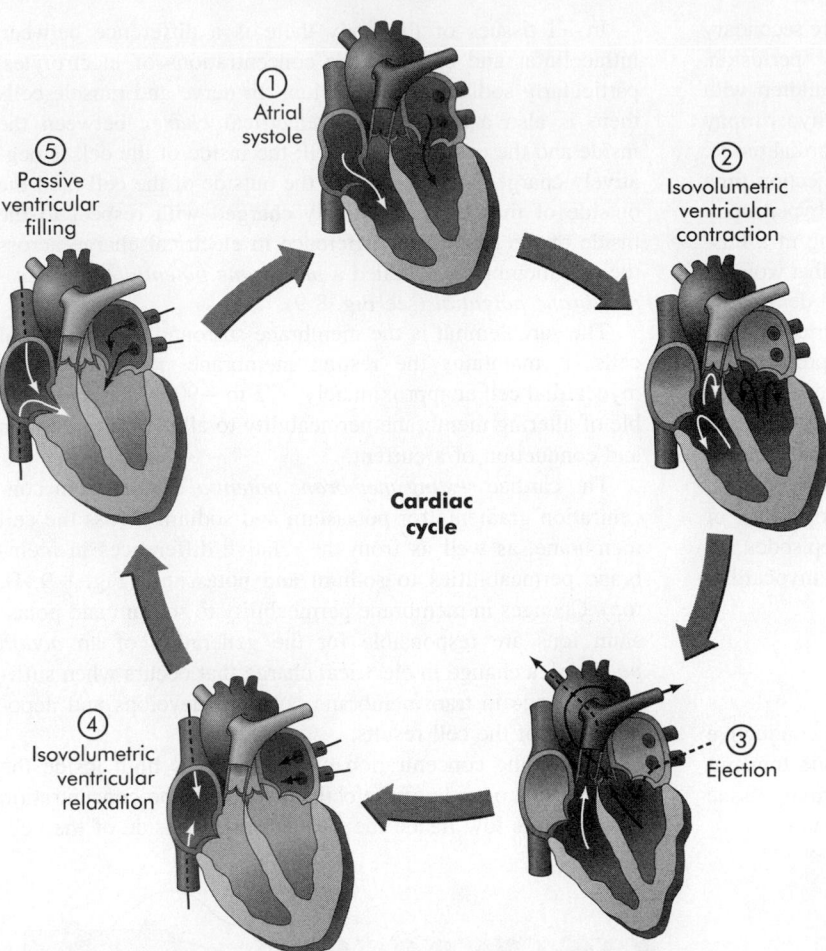

Cardiac cycle

① Atrial systole

② Isovolumetric ventricular contraction

③ Ejection

④ Isovolumetric ventricular relaxation

⑤ Passive ventricular filling

FIG. 8-8 Phases of the cardiac cycle. **1,** Atrial systole. **2,** Isovolumetric ventricular contraction. Ventricular volume remains constant as pressure increases rapidly. **3,** Ejection. **4,** Isovolumetric ventricular relaxation. Both sets of valves are closed, and the ventricles are relaxing. **5,** Passive ventricular filling. The atrioventricular (AV) valves are forced open, and the blood rushes into the relaxing ventricles. (From Patton KT, Thibodeau GA. *Anatomy and physiology,* ed 7. St Louis, 2010, Mosby).

left ventricular pressure exceeds left atrial pressure the mitral valve closes; this initial phase of contraction is called *isovolumetric contraction* (see Fig. 8-8, #2). When left ventricular pressure exceeds aortic pressure the aortic valve opens and blood flows into the aorta and systemic circulation (*isotonic contraction* occurs; see Fig. 8-8, #3). Left ventricular systolic pressure is approximately equal to the child's systemic arterial pressure unless left ventricular outflow tract obstruction is present.

The Coronary Circulation

The distribution of coronary arteries is identical in normal infants and adults, although the structure of the arteries changes continually. The right and left coronary arteries perfuse the heart from epicardium through myocardium to endocardium. The epicardial arteries branch into arterioles that perfuse most of the myocardium and then branch further to perfuse the inner portion of the myocardium. The subendocardium is perfused by a plexus of vessels.

Coronary artery flow occurs predominantly during diastole; left ventricular coronary flow occurs *only* during diastole, whereas right ventricular coronary flow occurs during both systole and diastole. Coronary blood flow constitutes a very small but significant portion of the total cardiac output at rest. Coronary artery flow increases in response to a rise in myocardial oxygen consumption or a significant fall in arterial oxygen content (i.e., severe hypoxemia). Myocardial oxygen supply may be maintained in the presence of compromised flow or reduced oxygen content because oxygen *extraction* increases; however, this increase in extraction will compensate only for a small reduction in coronary artery flow. Typically the myocardium extracts approximately 50% to 60% of the oxygen delivered; if coronary perfusion is compromised, maximal oxygen extraction is approximately 75% of oxygen delivered.

Coronary artery perfusion pressure is the difference between aortic end-diastolic pressure and the mean right atrial pressure. Therefore, if aortic diastolic pressure falls (as a result of hypotension, aortic insufficiency, extreme vasodilation, or a shunt that allows "run off" from the aorta to the pulmonary artery), or mean right atrial pressure rises (such as occurs during right ventricular failure), coronary artery perfusion pressure can fall.

Unlike adults, pediatric patients rarely suffer from anatomic compromise of coronary artery diameter and flow. An example of compromised flow is caused by congenital anomalous origin of the coronary artery from the pulmonary artery. In this case the "stealing" of myocardial blood flow results when blood from the normal coronary artery (arising from the aorta) flows through a fistula, then retrograde through the anomalous coronary artery and into the pulmonary artery. This creates a shunt from the aorta to the pulmonary artery and prevents effective perfusion of the coronary circulation (see Coronary Artery Anomalies).

A variety of congenital heart defects may produce secondary changes that compromise coronary artery perfusion. Subendocardial tissue ischemia may develop in children with severe aortic stenosis. Massive left ventricular hypertrophy increases the time required to perfuse the subendocardial tissue, yet the resistance to aortic ejection increases the ejection time and compromises the diastolic time. In addition, hypertrophy increases myocardial oxygen consumption, resulting in a mismatch between oxygen supply and oxygen demand that worsens during episodes of tachycardia or increased oxygen demand.

Severe aortic insufficiency reduces coronary artery perfusion pressure because aortic end-diastolic pressure is extremely low and mean right atrial pressure is often elevated. Congestive heart failure, like that occurring with critical aortic stenosis or hypertrophic cardiomyopathy, increases mean right atrial pressure and reduces coronary artery perfusion pressure. These conditions can result in the development of subendocardial ischemia, particularly during episodes of tachycardia, when diastolic time is shortened and myocardial oxygen consumption is increased.

Cellular Physiology
Membrane and Action Potentials
The heart contains muscle, connective tissue, and conductive tissue. Both the myocardium and conductive tissue transmit electrochemical impulses, or *current;* conductive tissue transmits current more rapidly than does myocardium.

In all tissues of the body there is a difference between intracellular and extracellular concentrations of electrolytes, particularly sodium and potassium. In nerve and muscle cells there is also a difference in electrical *charge* between the inside and the outside of the cell; the inside of the cell is negatively charged with respect to the outside of the cell (and the outside of the cell is positively charged with respect to the inside of the cell). This difference in electrical charge across the cell membrane is called a *membrane potential* or a *transmembrane potential* (see Fig. 8-9).

The sarcolemma is the membrane surrounding myocardial cells. It maintains the resting membrane potential of the myocardial cell at approximately -75 to -90 mV, but is capable of altering membrane permeability to allow for generation and conduction of a current.

The cardiac *resting membrane potential* results from concentration gradients for potassium and sodium across the cell membrane, as well as from the relative differences in membrane permeabilities to sodium and potassium (Fig. 8-9, B, top). Changes in membrane permeability to sodium and potassium ions are responsible for the generation of an *action potential,* a change in electrical charge that occurs when sufficient change in transmembrane potential develops and depolarization of the cell results.

At rest the concentration of potassium is high inside the cell and low outside of the cell; in contrast, the concentration of sodium is low inside the cell and high outside of the cell.

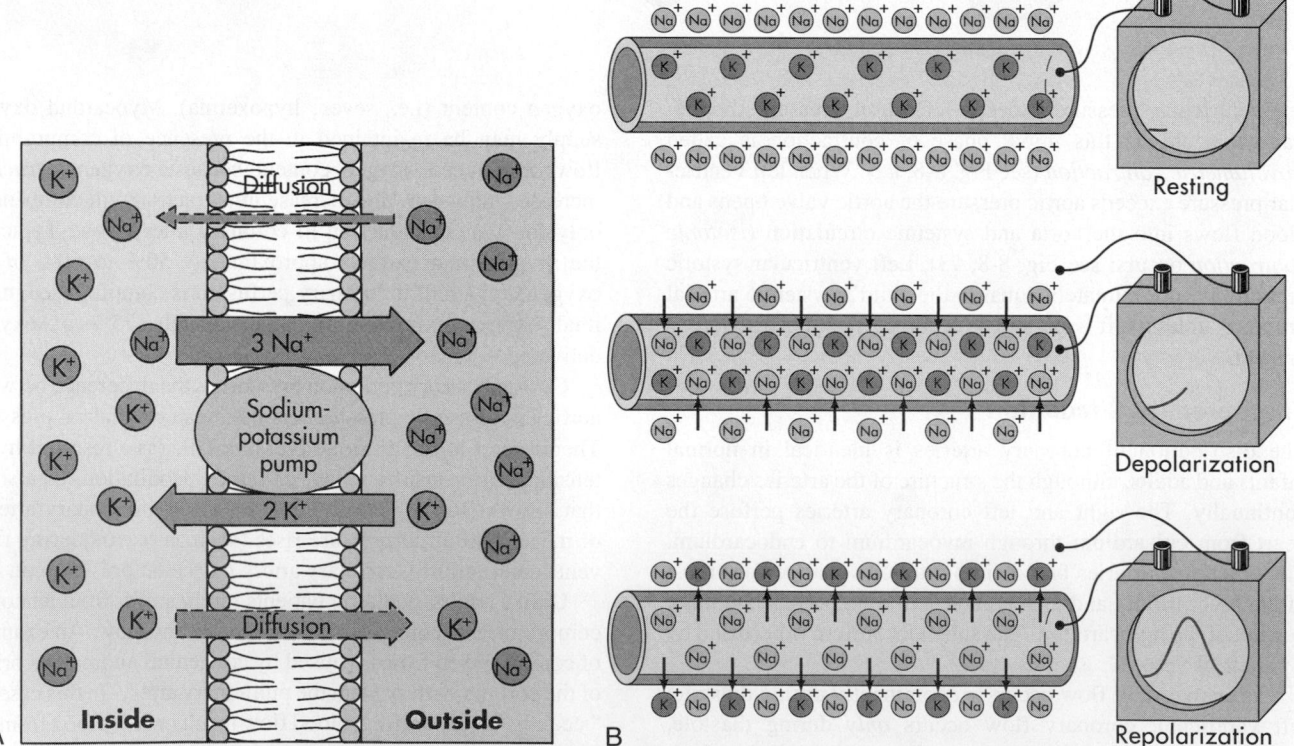

FIG. 8-9 Sodium-potassium pump and propagation of an action potential. **A,** Concentration difference of Na^+ and K^+ intracellularly and extracellularly. The direction of active transport by the sodium-potassium pump is also shown. **B,** Top diagram represents the polarized state of a neuronal membrane when at rest. The lower diagrams represent changes in sodium and potassium membrane permeabilities with depolarization and repolarization. (From Thibodeau GA, Patton KT. *Anatomy and physiology,* ed 6. St Louis, 2007, Mosby.)

Thus, there is a high concentration gradient for potassium to move to the outside of the cell and a concentration gradient for sodium to move to the inside of the cell. An active (energy-requiring) pump moves sodium ions out of the cell and potassium ions into the cell. The hydrolysis of adenosine triphosphate (ATP) provides energy for the pump. For every three sodium ions that are transported out of the cell, two potassium ions are moved into the cell (refer again to Fig. 8-9, *A*); this active pump generates a current (a net positive charge moves out of the cell). Under resting conditions, sodium moved outside the cell remains outside the cell because the sarcolemma is relatively impermeable to sodium.

As noted, the high concentration of potassium inside of the cell (approximately 100 or more mEq/L) and the relatively low potassium concentration outside of the cell (approximately 3.5 to 5.5 mEq/L) creates a large potassium concentration gradient across the cell membrane. Potassium readily diffuses out of the cell in response to this concentration gradient, because the sarcolemma is relatively permeable to potassium. At the same time, large negatively charged proteins remain trapped in the cell, because the membrane is normally impermeable to these large molecules. The exodus of positively charged ions from the cell coupled with the presence of (negatively charged) captured intracellular proteins creates the negative resting membrane potential. The magnitude of the resting membrane potential is linked most closely to the potassium concentration gradient.

Excitation of the myocardium results in altered sarcolemma permeability to sodium, calcium, and potassium and produces a change in intracellular electrical charge (i.e., an *action potential*). For an action potential to develop, the cell must be stimulated sufficiently to increase membrane permeability to sodium. At the same time, membrane permeability to potassium is decreased temporarily. Once the cell is stimulated sufficiently to *threshold potential* (the transmembrane voltage at which an action potential will occur), gating proteins allow sodium ions to enter the cell rapidly through fast channels, producing a *current,* or flow of electrons (depicted in Fig. 8-9, *B,* middle). The inside of the cell rapidly becomes positively charged with respect to the outside of the cell. This sodium influx, then, *depolarizes* the cell.

Depolarization occurs in approximately 300 ms. The fast sodium channels quickly close, but slow channels are then opened that allow calcium to enter the cell. This influx of calcium prolongs the period of time that the inside of the cell is positively charged and prevents immediate repolarization of the cell. The slow calcium channels ultimately close, and membrane permeability to potassium is restored. These two conditions restore the intracellular charge to the negative resting membrane potential.

The development of an action potential is an "all or none" phenomenon—if the cell is stimulated sufficiently (i.e., reaches threshold potential) it will become depolarized. Once membrane permeability to sodium increases at one point in the cell membrane and an action potential is generated, membrane permeability to sodium tends to increase along the length of the cell. This causes a propagation of the action potential throughout the cell. The action potential then spreads from cell to cell in the heart through low-resistance connections, called *intercalated discs*.

As the outside of the cell becomes negative (or depolarized) with respect to the inside of the cell, a *current* is generated. This current can be measured on the surface of a nerve or muscle in the laboratory. At the bedside the net electrical effects of the depolarization and repolarization of myocardial cells is detected and represented graphically by the ECG.

The *cardiac action potential* is a graphic representation over time of changes in the myocardial transmembrane potential of a single myocyte following stimulation. The myocardial action potential is divided into five phases: Phase 0, Phase 1, Phase 2, Phase 3, and Phase 4 (see Fig. 8-10, *A*), which are related to the changes in the transmembrane ion flow discussed in the preceding paragraphs.[77,78,863]

Phase 0. Fast channels are opened, and sodium rushes into the cell. The intracellular charge becomes progressively less negative, then positive with respect to the outside of the cell. Once the transmembrane potential reaches approximately −30 to −40 mV, *slow* calcium channels also open, perpetuating the action potential.

Phase 1. A short phase of rapid partial repolarization occurs as the fast channels are closed abruptly. These gates cannot

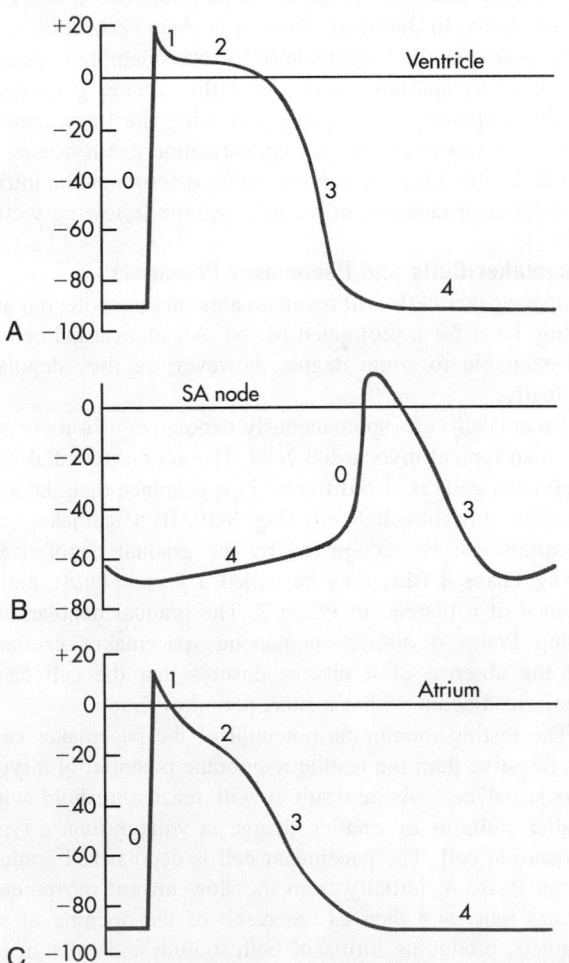

FIG. 8-10 Cardiac action potentials. **A,** Ventricle. **B,** Sinoatrial (SA) node. **C,** Atrium. Sweep velocity in (B) is one half that in (A) or (C) (Modified from Berne RM, Levy MN. *Cardiovascular physiology,* ed 8. St Louis, 2001, Mosby.)

reopen until the cell is repolarized partially during Phase 3, so the cell will be refractory to further excitation until that time. Slow calcium channels remain open at this time.

Phase 2. This plateau is produced when the slow calcium channels remain open, allowing continued diffusion of calcium ions into the cell. This plateau is unique to myocardial cells (it is not a feature of the action potential of skeletal muscle); because it delays repolarization, the plateau lengthens the refractory period of the myocardium, so myocardial tetany cannot occur.

Slow calcium channels not only affect myocardial excitation, they also deliver calcium to the myocardium for contraction and stimulate the sarcoplasmic reticulum to release additional calcium into the intracellular compartment, facilitating contraction. Calcium channels are blocked by specific inhibitor drugs such as verapamil, nifedipine, and diltiazem, and they are activated by sympathomimetic drugs.

Phase 3. Repolarization occurs rapidly when the slow calcium channels close; membrane permeability to potassium is restored. This permeability results in a significant potassium efflux to the outside of the cell.

Phase 4. The resting membrane potential is restored by the sodium-potassium pump and continued potassium efflux from the cell. This phase is the period between two action potentials. In the heart, Phase 4 is characterized by a slow reduction in the magnitude of the transmembrane potential caused by sodium influx; this influx creates *prepotential*. The prepotential ultimately can bring the transmembrane potential to threshold, so depolarization again occurs. The rate of this Phase 4 depolarization determines the intrinsic pacemaker capacity of the cell (see the following section).

Pacemaker Cells and Pacemaker Potentials

Nonpacemaker cells will maintain a membrane potential at the resting level for a prolonged period. All myocardial cells are self-excitable to some degree, however, so they depolarize gradually.

Pacemaker cells spontaneously depolarize at a more rapid rate than typical myocardial cells. The action potential of the pacemaker cells is also different in appearance than the action potential of myocardial cells (Fig. 8-10, B). Pacemaker action potentials can be recognized by the gradual depolarization during Phase 4 (this may be called a *prepotential*), and the absence of a plateau in Phase 2. The gradual depolarization during Phase 4 allows spontaneous pacemaker excitation, and the absence of a plateau ensures that the cell can be depolarized again within a short period of time.

The resting membrane potential of the pacemaker cell is less negative than the resting membrane potential of a typical myocardial cell. As a result it will reach threshold with a smaller stimulus or smaller change in voltage than a typical myocardial cell. The pacemaker cell is depolarized gradually during Phase 4, initially from the slow inward movement of sodium ions, and then as the result of the opening of slow channels, producing influx of both sodium and calcium ions. Under normal circumstances the pacemaker achieves threshold potential in a shorter period of time than the time needed by other myocardial cells. Once the pacemaker depolarizes, it stimulates other myocardial cells to depolarize.

Potential Alterations in Membrane Potentials and Excitability

Anything that increases the magnitude of the pacemaker membrane potential (makes it more negative) may result in slowing of the heart rate, because it will require a longer period of time for the sodium influx to bring the pacemaker membrane potential to threshold. Overdrive pacing (and resultant stimulation of the sodium-potassium pump) and vagal stimulation may result in "hyperpolarization" of pacemaker cells and a fall in intrinsic pacemaker firing rate.

Because the concentration gradients of sodium, potassium, and calcium affect the magnitude of the membrane potential, alterations in the intracellular and extracellular (including serum) concentrations of these electrolytes can influence myocardial excitability and contractility.

Vagal (parasympathetic) stimulation alters myocardial membrane permeability and reduces the excitability of the cell. Sympathetic nervous system stimulation increases intracellular sodium ion movement so that myocardial cells depolarize more rapidly. In addition, adrenergic stimulation increases the movement of calcium out of the cell at the end of Phase 3; these effects produce an increase in heart rate.

Refractory Periods

Myocardium is *absolutely refractory* to further electrical stimulation from the time the action potential begins (Phase 0) until significant repolarization has occurred (near the end of Phase 3). This protects the myocardium from tetany (i.e., continuous stimulation).

The myocardium is then *relatively refractory* to further stimuli from the end of Phase 3 (when the transmembrane potential is approximately -60 mV) until resting membrane potential is nearly reached. During this period a larger stimulus than normal is necessary to depolarize the cell, and conduction of an impulse is not rapid unless fast sodium channels are available.

For a brief period of time before repolarization is complete the myocardium is *more* susceptible than usual to stimulation and depolarization. During this time, called the *supernormal period*, a smaller stimulus than usual will generate an action potential.

Myocardial Contraction

Electrical stimulation of the myocardium should result in mechanical contraction. However, *electrical* depolarization of the myocardium may not result in adequate *mechanical* function if myocardial dysfunction is present.

The myocardium consists of a woven mesh of interconnected myocardial cells or myocytes. Each myocyte is surrounded by a semipermeable membrane, the sarcolemma. The myocyte contains myofibrils, and the myofibrils, in turn, each contain groups of *sarcomeres*. The sarcomere is the contractile element of a myocardial cell that contains thin overlapping protein filaments of *actin* and thicker *myosin* filaments (Fig. 8-11, A). Coupling of these filaments occurs when intracellular ionized calcium is increased.

During depolarization of the myocardium, transcellular calcium influx occurs; calcium enters the cell through calcium channels in the sarcolemma and through invaginations in

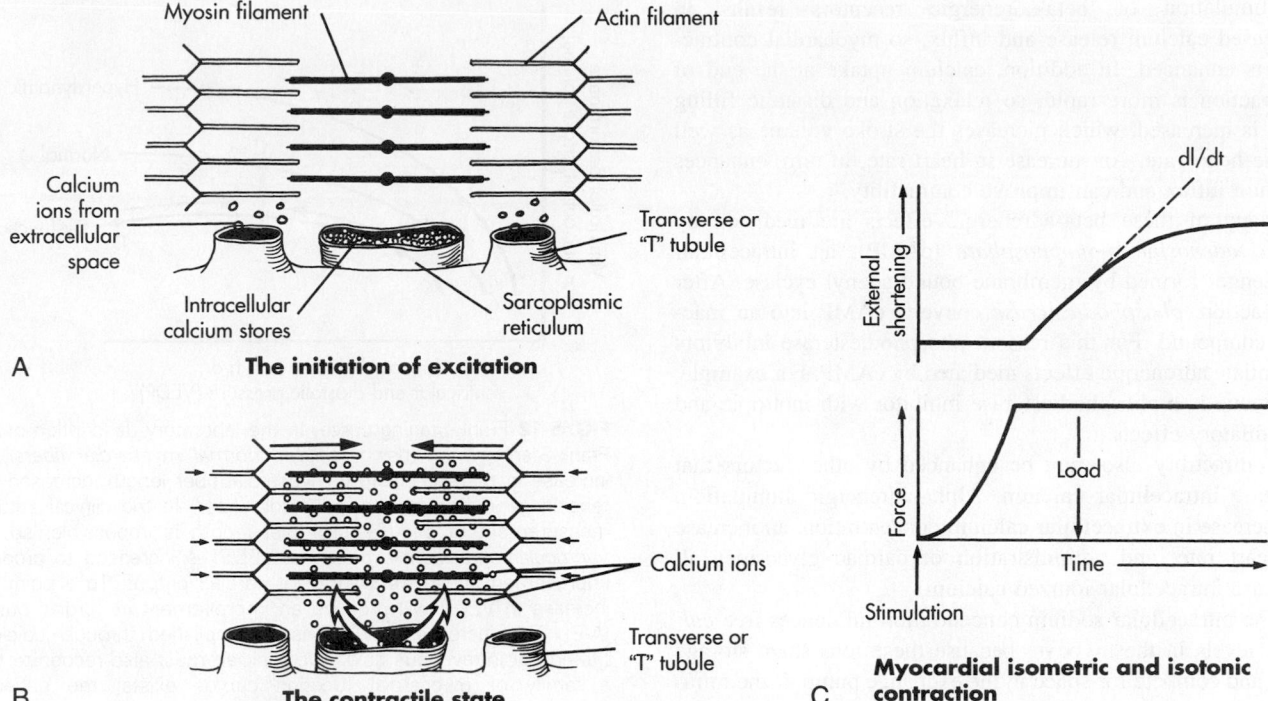

FIG. 8-11 Cardiac excitation and contraction. **A,** Initiation of contraction. Actin and myosin filaments are in the relaxed state, and the sarcoplasmic reticulum contains a store of calcium ions. When depolarization occurs, the wave of excitation is spread rapidly to the inside of the cell via the transverse or "T" tubules. A small amount of free calcium ions then enter the cell from the extracellular space through these T-tubules. The extracellular calcium ion entry alone is not sufficient to produce contraction. **B,** The intracellular entry of calcium then stimulates the release of large quantities of calcium ions from the intracellular stores in the sarcoplasmic reticulum. Calcium then binds to troponin C, enabling cross-linking of actin and myosin filaments and myocardial contraction. **C,** With depolarization and contraction, the myocardium generates tension. Initially, the ventricular fibers generate tension and do not shorten; this is a period of *isometric* contraction, and lasts until the ventricles generate sufficient pressure to open the semilunar valves. Once these valves open, the muscle fibers shorten and blood is ejected. The tangent of the slope of the shortening curve (dl/dt) represents the velocity of initial fiber shortening and can be used as a measure of ventricular contractility. (A and B by Marilou Kundemueller; C From Berne RM, Levy MN. *Cardiovascular physiology,* ed 5. St Louis, 1986, Mosby.)

the sarcolemma, called T-tubules (refer, again, to Fig. 8-11, A and B). This calcium entry into the sarcoplasm stimulates further calcium release from the sarcoplasmic reticulum. The free cytoplasmic calcium reacts with troponin, with the resulting formation of cross-linkages between the actin and myosin filaments. As a result of these linkages, the filaments are pulled together, causing shortening of the myocardial fiber (contraction), so the fibers generate tension. Myocardial relaxation results when calcium uptake by the sarcoplasmic reticulum occurs by means of an energy-requiring pump. Exchange of sodium for calcium ions also occurs during diastole.

Tension generated by the myocardium and velocity of myocardial contraction (or shortening) are inversely related. If the myocardium is restrained, *isometric contraction* will result—the fiber will not shorten, but it will develop tension. If the myocardial fiber is unrestrained, it shortens, or contracts (see Fig. 8-11, B), but it will not develop further tension—this form of contraction is called *isotonic contraction.* During ventricular systole, both isometric and isotonic contractions occur. Isometric contraction occurs before the opening of the semilunar valves, and isotonic contraction occurs after the semilunar valves open. Stroke volume is determined by the amount of

isotonic contraction (or ventricular fiber shortening) that occurs after sufficient tension is developed to overcome resistance to ejection (afterload).[77,78,863]

Myocardial contraction is an energy-requiring process, using ATP and magnesium. Therefore, for contraction to occur, magnesium and effective myocardial aerobic metabolism to generate ATP must be present.

If contraction is to be *effective,* all myocardial cells must contract in synchrony. This requires efficient calcium release and uptake by the sarcoplasmic reticulum. It also requires rapid transmission of action potentials throughout the heart.

FACTORS INFLUENCING NORMAL VENTRICULAR FUNCTION

Myocardial performance can be affected by changes in many conditions, including oxygenation, perfusion, ionized serum calcium concentration, acid-base and electrolyte balance, and drugs. Each of these factors may impair or enhance cardiac output by altering either heart rate (the number of times the ventricles contract per minute) or ventricular stroke volume (the volume of blood ejected by the ventricles with each contraction).

Stimulation of beta-adrenergic receptors results in increased calcium release and influx, so myocardial contraction is enhanced. In addition, calcium uptake at the end of contraction is more rapid, so relaxation and diastolic filling time is increased, which increases the stroke volume as well as the heart rate. An increase in heart rate, in turn, enhances calcium influx and can improve contractility.

Many of these beta-adrenergic effects are mediated by *cyclic adenosine monophosphate* (cAMP), an intracellular messenger formed by membrane-bound adenyl cyclase. After contraction, *phosphodiesterase* converts cAMP into an inactive compound. For this reason, phosphodiesterase inhibitors potentiate adrenergic effects mediated by cAMP. For example, milrinone is a phosphodiesterase inhibitor with inotropic and vasodilatory effects.

Contractility also may be enhanced by other factors that increase intracellular calcium. Alpha-adrenergic stimulation, an increase in extracellular calcium concentration, an increase in heart rate, and administration of cardiac glycosides all increase intracellular ionized calcium.

The intracellular sodium concentration influences free *calcium* levels in the myocyte because these ions share storage sites and compete for space in the exchange pump. If the intracellular sodium concentration is increased (such as occurs during digitalis therapy), sodium occupies space in the exchange pump, so calcium will accumulate in the myocardial cell. The result is that cardiac contractility is enhanced (see further discussion in the Common Clinical Conditions section, under Congestive Heart Failure).

Effects of changes in heart rate and rhythm are discussed in a subsequent section (Arrhythmias). The following review addresses factors that influence ventricular function and stroke volume.

Three terms have been borrowed from the physiology laboratory to describe factors that influence ventricular stroke volume. These terms—preload, contractility, and afterload—have been defined precisely in the laboratory setting using *isolated* myocardial muscle strips. However, they are described only generally in the clinical setting with an intact heart, where it usually is impossible to isolate single variables. Therefore a brief review of the clinical interpretation of these factors is provided. This information is also presented in Chapter 6.

Ventricular Preload

The Frank-Starling Law of the Heart

Preload is the amount of myocardial fiber stretch that is present before contraction. Howell (in 1894), Frank (in 1894), and Starling (in 1914) performed experiments using *isolated normal* myocardial muscle preparations, and observed that normal myocardium generates greater tension during contraction if it is stretched before contraction. The increase in the force of contraction optimizes overlap between actin and myosin filaments in the sarcomere. Their observations became known as the *Frank-Starling law of the heart,* which states that an increase in ventricular end-diastolic myocardial fiber length (manipulated by increasing ventricular end-diastolic *pressure*) will produce an increase in ventricular work, systolic tension, and stroke volume. The graphic representation of the

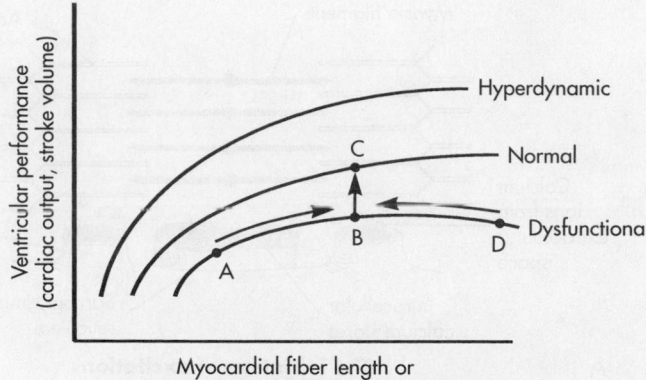

FIG. 8-12 Frank-Starling curve. In the laboratory description of the Frank-Starling Law (using *isolated normal myocardial fibers*), an increase in the end-diastolic myocardial fiber length increased the tension generated by the myocardial fiber. In the clinical setting, measurement of end-diastolic fiber length is impossible, so the *ventricular end-diastolic pressure* (VEDP) is increased to produce improvement in stroke volume or cardiac output. To a point, an increase in VEDP will produce an improvement in cardiac output (A-B). This increase in VEDP is accomplished through judicious titration of intravenous fluid. The clinician must also recognize that a family of myocardial function curves exists; the patient's myocardial function may be characterized as normal, dysfunctional, or hyperdynamic. If the myocardium is dysfunctional, it generally requires a higher VEDP than the normal myocardium to maximize cardiac output. In addition, excessive volume administration can produce a decrease in cardiac output and myocardial performance if the ventricle is dysfunctional (B-D). In this case, administration of a diuretic or vasodilator may improve cardiac output (D-B). Correction of acid-base imbalances, reduction in afterload, or administration of inotropic medications may improve myocardial function so that cardiac output increases without need for further increase in VEDP (B and C). If the patient's myocardial function is hyperdynamic, cardiac output will be high even at low VEDP. (Illustration courtesy of William Banner Jr.)

relationship between ventricular end-diastolic pressure and stroke volume is the Frank-Starling curve, which is a ventricular (myocardial) function curve (Fig. 8-12).[77,78,863]

The Frank-Starling law of the heart is applicable to dysfunctional as well as normal myocardium, although the appearance (specifically, the position and slope) of each function curve will differ. Optimal stretch of any myocardial fiber should improve myocardial performance. Because myocardial fiber length is not readily measured in the clinical setting, *ventricular end-diastolic pressure (VEDP)* is monitored as an indirect indication of the stretch placed on the myocardial fibers before contraction. VEDP is increased through intravenous volume administration. The relationship between ventricular end-diastolic *volume* (and fiber length) and ventricular end-diastolic *pressure* is not a linear one, however, because it is influenced by ventricular *compliance* (see discussion of Compliance, below) and venous return; both of these factors may be altered by disease or therapy.

To a point, as ventricular end-diastolic pressure is increased, the force of contraction and myocardial fiber shortening should increase, and stroke volume should rise. If, however, the ventricle is filled beyond a critical point, overlap of actin and myosin filaments is no longer optimal; ventricular *dilation* can result, and stroke volume can decrease. Extremely high ventricular end-diastolic pressures result in pulmonary and systemic edema, and will compromise coronary and subendocardial blood flow.

If stroke volume or cardiac output can be estimated reliably (e.g., using Doppler, Fick, or thermodilution calculations) a ventricular function curve can be constructed for any patient. Stroke volume (cardiac output divided by heart rate) is plotted on the vertical axis of the graph, and VEDP is plotted on the horizontal axis. As fluid administration is titrated and the stroke volume is determined at various ventricular end-diastolic pressures, the optimal VEDP is identified as the peak point on the curve.

A goal of the treatment of any patient with cardiovascular dysfunction is to maximize stroke volume and cardiac output, while minimizing adverse effects of fluid administration (such as pulmonary edema). An increase in stroke volume and cardiac output can be achieved by moving the patient to the highest point of an individual ventricular function curve (see Fig. 8-12, A to B); this movement may be achieved by judicious fluid administration. Improvement in stroke volume and cardiac output also can be achieved by altering the ventricular compliance, using vasodilator therapy. An increase in stroke volume and cardiac output also can be achieved through improvement in cardiac contractility; this raises the ventricular function curve (see Fig. 8-12, B to C). Such an improvement may be attained by elimination of factors that normally depress myocardial function, or through administration of inotropic agents or vasodilators (see section, Afterload).

Clinical Evaluation of Ventricular Preload

In the clinical setting, ventricular end-diastolic pressure is measured to evaluate ventricular preload. Ventricular end-diastolic volume may also be estimated with echocardiography or nuclear imaging.

Right ventricular end-diastolic pressure (RVEDP) is equal to right atrial pressure unless tricuspid valve stenosis is present. Central venous pressure (CVP) equals right atrial and RVEDP, unless central venous obstruction or positive intrathoracic pressure is present.

RVEDP and CVP often can be estimated with careful clinical assessment of the level of hydration, liver size, palpation of the infant's fontanelle, determination of presence (or absence) of systemic edema, and evaluation of the cardiac size on chest radiograph. Dry mucous membranes, a sunken fontanelle, and absence of hepatomegaly are findings consistent with normal or low central venous pressure; hepatomegaly and periorbital edema usually are present once the CVP is elevated significantly. Systemic edema also may be noted despite a normal or low CVP if capillary leak or hypoalbuminemia is present. A high RVEDP and heart failure is often associated with cardiac enlargement on chest radiograph.

Left ventricular end-diastolic pressure (LVEDP) is equal to left atrial pressure unless mitral valve disease is present. Reliable estimation of LVEDP is not possible through clinical assessment alone. Although the presence of pulmonary edema frequently is assumed to indicate the presence of a high LVEDP (exceeding 20 to 25 mm Hg), pulmonary edema may be observed at *any* (even a low) LVEDP if capillary leak is present.

A left atrial catheter or pulmonary artery catheter must be inserted to measure LVEDP, because this pressure cannot reliably be estimated from clinical examination. In the absence of pulmonary venous constriction or obstruction, a pulmonary artery wedge pressure will approximate left atrial pressure; in the absence of mitral valve disease or extreme tachycardia, left atrial pressure should reflect left ventricular end-diastolic pressure. However, the pulmonary artery catheter must be placed appropriately and the transducer must be zeroed, leveled, and calibrated correctly with appropriate consideration of intrapulmonary pressure. (For information about potential errors in use of pulmonary artery catheters, refer to Chapter 21.)

Factors Affecting Ventricular End-Diastolic Pressure (VEDP)

A change in ventricular end-diastolic pressure affects the resting length of the ventricular myocardial cells before contraction. Although VEDP is increased through the administration of intravenous fluids, *VEDP is not related linearly to fluid volume administered.* VEDP also will be affected by ventricular compliance which is, in turn, affected by ventricular function, ventricular relaxation, wall thickness, ventricular size, pericardial pressures, and heart rate.

Ventricular Compliance

Ventricular *compliance* refers to the *distensibility* of the ventricle. It is defined as the change in ventricular volume (in mL) for a given change in pressure (in mm Hg), or $\Delta V/\Delta P$, and can be depicted graphically by a ventricular compliance curve (see Fig. 6-3). The opposite of compliance is stiffness ($\Delta P/\Delta V$).

If the ventricle is extremely compliant a large volume of fluid may be administered without producing a significant increase in VEDP (see Fig. 6-3, curve B). In contrast, if the ventricle is dysfunctional (as occurs with restrictive cardiomyopathy) or hypertrophied, ventricular compliance usually is reduced (see Fig. 6-3, curve C). In this case, even a small volume of administered intravenous fluids will produce a significant rise in VEDP. The more dysfunctional and noncompliant the ventricle, the higher will be the resting VEDP and the VEDP needed to optimize stroke volume and ventricular performance.

Ventricular compliance is not constant over all ranges of VEDP. Any ventricle is maximally compliant at low filling pressures; as the ventricle is filled, compliance is reduced because ventricular stretch may be maximal. Rapid volume infusion tends to raise VEDP more rapidly than gradual volume infusion. Compliant ventricles usually demonstrate a substantial improvement in stroke volume when intravenous fluid is administered.

Vasodilator therapy will improve ventricular compliance. When these drugs are administered the compliance curve is altered, so a greater end-diastolic volume may be present without a substantial increase in ventricular end-diastolic pressure (see Fig. 6-3). Stroke volume may then be increased without a rise in VEDP.

Compliance also is affected by ventricular size, pericardial space, and heart rate.[141] Infants have very small and relatively noncompliant ventricles, so the infant's VEDP may rise sharply with even small fluid volume administration. If the same volume (on a per kilogram basis) is administered to the older child a smaller change in VEDP will result, because the ventricles are larger and more compliant in the older child.

Constrictive pericarditis and tamponade decrease ventricular compliance because ventricular expansion cannot occur in response to volume administration. Diastolic filling will be impaired and stroke volume often is reduced. Extreme tachycardia (such as supraventricular tachycardia) can produce a rise in VEDP. A rapid heart rate is associated with reduced ventricular diastolic time and incomplete relaxation; as a result the VEDP rises.

Because VEDP is affected by a variety of factors *it is important to attempt to determine the VEDP associated with optimal systemic perfusion for each patient.* Obviously, this optimal pressure may change frequently during the patient's clinical course. Throughout therapy, evidence of systemic perfusion always should be assessed as VEDP is manipulated.

Maturational Changes in Response to Preload Manipulation

Many years ago, studies of newborn animals failed to demonstrate an increase in neonatal stroke volume in response to intravenous volume administration. This led to the conclusion that the human neonate is incapable of increasing stroke volume in response to volume administration. However, in each of these studies, secondary changes in hemodynamics occurred that may have affected stroke volume adversely, thus blunting any positive effect of volume administration.

Research now suggests that neonates are capable of increasing stroke volume in response to volume therapy provided aortic pressure does not rise precipitously, ventricular function is adequate, and systemic vascular resistance is not elevated. In the clinical setting it is always necessary to monitor changes in systemic perfusion as VEDP is manipulated, regardless of the age of the patient. If maximal response to volume infusion is to occur, myocardial contractility must be effective and afterload controlled.

Contractility

Definition

The term *contractility* refers to the strength and efficiency of contraction; it is the *force* generated by the myocardium, independent of preload and afterload. Contractility is estimated by velocity of fiber shortening; if myocardial function is good the ventricular fibers shorten rapidly. As a result, at the same heart rate, systole will require a smaller portion of the cardiac cycle. If systole requires a smaller portion of each cardiac cycle, there will be a longer time for ventricular filling (diastole) and stroke volume will increase (provided that circulating blood volume is adequate and heart rate and ventricular afterload are unchanged).

Clinical Evaluation of Contractility

Although contractility can be measured in the laboratory it is not easily isolated and measured in the clinical setting. The most common method of evaluating contractility at the bedside is echocardiographic evaluation of fiber-shortening times and measurement of the shortening fraction of left ventricular diameter. Shortening fraction is calculated by determining the difference between the end-diastolic and end-systolic dimensions; this difference is then divided by the end-diastolic dimension (see Box 8-2); the normal shortening fraction is approximately 28% to 44%.

If a thermodilution cardiac output pulmonary artery catheter is in place, or if reliable Doppler or other noninvasive cardiac output estimations can be obtained (see Chapters 6 and 21), the nurse may create a ventricular function curve (see Fig. 8-12). If cardiac output improves with no change in VEDP, ventricular contractility or compliance has probably improved.

Other more cumbersome techniques are available to describe *ventricular performance* (i.e., ventricular function in vivo). Ejection fraction [(end-diastolic volume − end-systolic volume)/end-diastolic volume] can be determined with nuclear imaging, angiocardiography, or echocardiography; normal is 65% to 80%. Velocity of circumferential fiber shortening can be calculated using echocardiography, nuclear imaging, or during cardiac catheterization; however, this velocity is influenced by heart rate, preload, contractility, and afterload. The rate of peak pressure development ($\Delta P/\Delta t$—peak pressure development over time) also can be measured in the cardiac catheterization laboratory to monitor changes in contractility.

Another good indicator of contractility is the slope of the left ventricular end-systolic pressure/volume curve. This slope is insensitive to changes in preload but accurately reflects changes in myocardial contractility. To determine this slope, end-systolic pressure is estimated from a carotid pulse tracing or the dicrotic notch of a clear arterial waveform tracing, and the left ventricular end-systolic volume (dimension) is determined by echocardiography. These variables are graphed (pressure on the vertical axis and volume on the horizontal axis); the slope of the curve reflects ventricular contractility. Inotropic drugs shift the curve to the left and increase the slope of the curve. When contractility is depressed, the curve is shifted to the right and has a reduced slope.

When contractility is good, ventricular end-diastolic pressure remains low, ventricular systolic pressure rises sharply, and the rate of preejection period/ejection time is low. In comparison, when ventricular contractility is poor, ventricular end-diastolic pressure is high, ventricular pressure rises slowly during systole, and the ratio of preejection period/ejection time lengthens (i.e., the ejection period shortens), because it takes a longer time for the ventricle to generate sufficient pressure to overcome afterload. These differences often can

---

Box 8-2   **Echocardiographic Calculation of Left Ventricular Shortening Fraction**

$$\text{LV shortening fraction} = \frac{\text{LV end-diastolic dimension} - \text{LV end-systolic dimension}}{\text{LV end-diastolic dimension}} \times 100$$

be appreciated when an electrocardiogram and ventricular pressure curve (or intraarterial pressure curve) are examined simultaneously.

The ventricular pressure curve also may provide information regarding ventricular contractility. This ventricular pressure usually must be examined in the cardiac catheterization laboratory; however, the intraarterial pressure curve may be utilized if the catheter is widely patent and vasoconstriction is not present. The area under the pressure curve correlates with stroke volume. If stroke volume and contractility are good, the slope of the systolic upstroke of the waveform will be steep, and a dicrotic notch clearly visible. If contractility is poor and stroke volume is reduced, the waveform will appear dampened, and the slope of the systolic upstroke of the waveform more horizontal (see Chapter 6).

Contractility can be impaired by electrolyte imbalances, acidosis, and hypoxia. Adrenergic stimulation and resultant tachycardia will improve contractility by increasing intracellular calcium concentration.

Maturational Changes in Cardiac Contractility

Neonatal myocardial fibers have a higher water content and fewer contractile elements (per gram of tissue) than adult myocardial fibers. In addition, immature myocardium is able to generate less tension than adult myocardium. These observations are not necessarily indicative of reduced infant myocardial contractility, however, because infant hearts actually have a higher ejection fraction than adult myocardium.

Afterload

Definition

Afterload is the *impediment* to ventricular ejection. Ventricular afterload is the sum of all forces opposing ventricular emptying and is described as ventricular *wall stress*. If ventricular wall stress is increased, the afterload of the ventricle and the impediment to ventricular ejection are increased. The parallel of ventricular afterload or wall stress in isolated myocardial fibers is myocardial fiber tension.

Because fiber shortening (isotonic contraction) occurs only when the ventricle has generated sufficient tension to equal its afterload, an increase in ventricular afterload reduces the isotonic contraction time and thus the stroke volume of the ventricle. Even a normal afterload may be excessive when myocardial function is poor. With any increase in afterload, oxygen consumption and the work of the ventricle increase (Fig. 8-13).

A simplification of Poiseuille's law states that pressure is a product of flow and resistance:

$$Pressure = Flow \times Resistance$$

From this equation it is clear that an increase in resistance will be associated with a decrease in flow (i.e., cardiac output or stroke volume) unless the driving pressure increases. For example, if aortic stenosis is present, cardiac output will fall unless the left ventricular pressure increases significantly.

The major determinants of afterload or wall stress are: (1) ventricular lumen radius; (2) the thickness of the ventricular wall (hypertrophy decreases afterload); and (3) the ventricular ejection pressure (intracavitary pressure), as indicated in

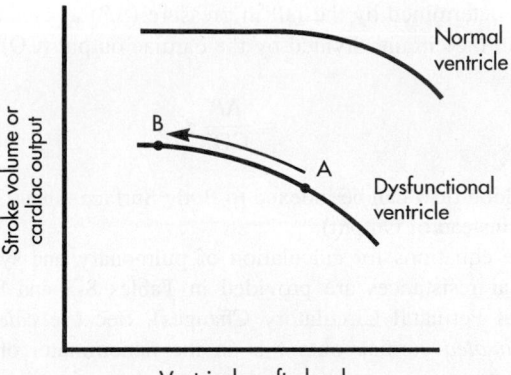

FIG. 8-13 Effects of afterload on ventricular function. The normal ventricle maintains stroke volume despite a moderate rise in afterload (such as an increase in systemic vascular resistance). Severe increases in afterload, however, can ultimately compromise ventricular function and result in a fall in stroke volume and cardiac output (see Normal Ventricle Curve). The dysfunctional ventricle will be much more sensitive to an increase in afterload, and even a relatively small increase in afterload may substantially reduce myocardial performance. Administration of vasodilators may reduce afterload sufficiently so that stroke volume and cardiac output increase (see A and B). (Illustration courtesy of William Banner Jr, MD.)

Box 8-3	**Factors Influencing Ventricular Afterload and Wall Stress**

$$\frac{Ventricular}{wall\ stress} \approx \frac{Intracavitary\ pressure \times Chamber\ lumen\ radius}{2 \times Chamber\ wall\ thickness}$$

Box 8-3. In the normal patient, left ventricular ejection pressure is equal to systemic arterial pressure, and right ventricular ejection pressure is equal to pulmonary artery pressure; systemic and pulmonary artery pressures, in turn, are determined by blood flow and resistance (Poiseuille's law). Therefore, in the absence of ventricular outflow tract obstruction or significant alterations in ventricular size or wall thickness, afterload is determined primarily by the impedance provided by the pulmonary and systemic arterial circulations (respectively, the pulmonary and systemic vascular resistances).

Clinical Evaluation of Afterload

Afterload cannot be measured in the clinical setting. Resistances in the pulmonary and systemic circulation can be *calculated* if a thermodilution pulmonary artery catheter is in place. Systemic vascular resistance also may be estimated if Doppler or other noninvasive estimates or calculations of cardiac output are available. Pulmonary vascular resistance may be estimated with echocardiography. However, it is important to note that systemic and pulmonary vascular resistances represent *calculations* or *estimations* and not direct measurements and each represents one of several factors contributing to right or left ventricular wall stress.

Any calculation of resistance in a circulation is based on *Poiseuille's law*, which states that flow through a system is equal to the change in pressure across the system divided by the resistance in the system (flow = change in pressure/resistance). Resistance in the pulmonary or systemic vascular bed is determined by the fall in pressure (ΔP) as blood flows through the circuit, divided by the cardiac output (CO):

$$R = \frac{\Delta P}{CO^*}$$

*Blood flow can be indexed to Body Surface Area (Cardiac Index instead of Output)

The equations for calculation of pulmonary and systemic vascular resistances are provided in Tables 8-3 and 8-5 (in Normal Perinatal Circulatory Changes). Because *calculated* or *estimated* cardiac output is in the denominator of these equations, *any error in cardiac output determination results in significant error in calculated resistances*. In addition, changes in cardiac output affect calculated resistances. When flow (cardiac output) increases, pressure and calculated resistances in the systemic and pulmonary vascular beds increase, unless dilation of vessels occurs. If cardiac output falls dramatically and blood pressure is unchanged, the calculated SVR and PVR may rise sharply, even in the absence of active vessel constriction. These formulas do not allow determination of cause and effect (i.e., did the cardiac output fall because vascular resistances rose, or did the calculated resistances rise because cardiac output fell?).

Poiseuille's original equation allowed calculation of the effects of blood viscosity and length of major vessels on resistance to blood flow. As blood viscosity or vessel length increases, resistance to blood flow increases. Because most calculations of SVR and PVR are used for the analysis of patient *trends,* blood viscosity, and vessel length are assumed to be constant and have been eliminated from the equation. However, if the patient becomes polycythemic or anemic, pulmonary and systemic vascular resistances are altered, yet are not reflected by the calculation of SVR and PVR from the preceding equations.

Poiseuille's formula also allows consideration of the resistances in all elements of the circulation. The total resistance to flow in a series is the sum of the resistances in the elements of the series. Total pulmonary vascular resistance is the sum of the resistances in all of the pulmonary arteries, pulmonary capillaries, and pulmonary veins.

If the cross-sectional area of a vascular bed *increases* and flow and vessel radius remain the same, resistance to flow decreases proportionately. An increase in the cross-sectional area allows more flow at the same pressure, or reduces the pressure needed to maintain the same flow.

If, on the other hand, the cross-sectional area of the vascular bed *decreases* (as occurs in an infant with hypoplastic lungs), the resistance to blood flow increases in the remaining vessels, even if the diameter of the remaining vessels is unchanged. A reduction in the cross-sectional area of a circulation increases the resistance in the circulation and allows less flow at the same pressure or increases the pressure needed to maintain the same flow.

Because the largest number in the numerator of the Poiseuille's formula is the mean pressure in the vascular bed, changes in that mean pressure often are thought to reflect trends in vascular resistance. For example, if the mean systemic arterial pressure increases, the systemic vascular resistance may be rising. However, such interpretation is subject to error because both mean arterial pressure and mean pulmonary artery pressure are affected by cardiac output, ventricular preload, ventricular contractility, and vascular tone. A better reflection of vascular resistance is the pulmonary or systemic diastolic pressure. Increased vascular tone (i.e., increased pulmonary or systemic vascular resistance) produces a rise in pulmonary or systemic diastolic pressure and a narrowing of the pulse pressure. A fall in pulmonary or systemic vascular resistance produces a fall in pulmonary or systemic diastolic pressure and a widening of the pulse pressure.

Afterload also may be evaluated by determining the velocity of fiber shortening during cardiac catheterization or with echocardiography. This velocity falls in the presence of increased afterload, but also is affected by heart rate, ventricular preload, and ventricular contractility.

Left ventricular end-systolic wall stress can be determined with echocardiography. This determination requires estimation of left ventricular pressure but reflects changes in afterload independent of changes in preload.

The systolic time intervals of a ventricle include the preejection period (PEP), the ventricular ejection time (VET), and the isovolumetric contraction time (ICT); these intervals are determined through echocardiography. The ratio of the preejection period/ventricular ejection time (PEP/VET) correlate linearly with changes in ventricular afterload; the greater the ventricular afterload, the longer the preejection period required for the ventricle to generate sufficient pressure to overcome afterload so that ejection occurs. For example, the ratio of right ventricular preejection period/ventricular ejection time increases in the child who is developing pulmonary vascular disease and pulmonary hypertension.

Maturational Changes in Response to Alterations in Ventricular Afterload

The pediatric ventricle usually can adapt to increases in ventricular afterload provided the increases are not severe or acute. Adaptation may, in fact, be superior to the response of the adult myocardium. For example, if, in the patient with moderate aortic stenosis the left ventricular muscle thickness increases and the diameter of the left ventricular chamber is reduced, wall stress (afterload) may be normalized (refer again to Box 8-3).

If the infant or pediatric myocardium is subjected to extremely high afterload (such as critical aortic stenosis) myocardial dysfunction can quickly develop. *Acute* increases in afterload, such as reactive pulmonary vasoconstriction, are also poorly tolerated during the neonatal period.

Pulmonary vascular resistance is elevated in the neonate and any child with pulmonary vascular disease. Children with elevated PVR or those with a reactive pulmonary vascular bed may demonstrate pulmonary hypertensive "crises." These crises seem to be associated with pulmonary vasoconstriction, an acute rise in right ventricular afterload, and sudden deterioration in cardiac output and systemic perfusion. Factors associated with pediatric hypoxic pulmonary vasoconstriction include alveolar hypoxia, acidosis, alveolar overdistention (by high airway pressures), and hypothermia (refer as needed to Box 8-1).

These factors may be avoided through administration of supplementary oxygen as needed to prevent alveolar hypoxia, maintenance of a mild serum alkalosis, prevention of excessive airway pressures, and sedation. (For further information the reader is referred to the sections Postnatal Changes in Pulmonary and Systemic; Vascular Resistances earlier in the chapter and the section on Common Clinical Conditions, Pulmonary Hypertension, later in the chapter.)

OXYGEN TRANSPORT, CARDIAC OUTPUT, AND OXYGEN CONSUMPTION

Oxygen Transport

The ultimate function of the heart and lungs is to deliver oxygenated blood to the tissues. Systemic oxygen transport or oxygen delivery (SOT or DO_2) is the volume of oxygen (mL/min per m^2 body surface area) delivered to the tissues every minute; it is the product of arterial oxygen content (the amount of oxygen [in mL] per deciliter of arterial blood) and the cardiac index (the volume of blood per meter^2 body surface area delivered to the tissues every minute). Oxygen delivery reflects the quantity of oxygen available to the tissues.

If arterial oxygen content falls, oxygen delivery is maintained only if cardiac output increases commensurately. If cardiac output falls, oxygen delivery falls; SOT often falls in direct correlation to the drop in cardiac output. When SOT falls significantly, there is an attempt to redistribute blood flow to vital organs. In addition, oxygen extraction is increased and anaerobic metabolism results.

Oxygen Content

Oxygen content is the total amount of oxygen (in milliliters) carried in each deciliter of blood. Because oxygen is carried primarily in the form of oxyhemoglobin the arterial oxygen content essentially is determined by the hemoglobin concentration and its saturation.

Factors Affecting Arterial Oxygen Content

Arterial oxygen content will fall in the presence of anemia or if the oxyhemoglobin saturation falls. Anemia should be avoided in the critically ill patient with cardiorespiratory disease because it will compromise arterial oxygen content and may result in a fall in arterial oxygen delivery. Transfusion therapy is one nonventilatory method for improving arterial oxygen content in these patients, and it may improve oxygen delivery. However, the ideal hemoglobin and hematocrit levels for the critically ill patient (and particularly for the critically ill patient with congenital heart disease) have not been determined. Adequate hemoglobin concentration is required to maintain arterial oxygen-carrying capacity and oxygen content; excessive hemoglobin and hematocrit levels, however, increase blood viscosity and resistance to blood flow so that oxygen delivery actually is impaired.

Although the ideal hemoglobin concentration has not been established there are some theoretical differences in the perceived desirable ranges of hemoglobin concentration based on the patient condition. Maintenance of a hemoglobin concentration of 12 to 15 g/dL and a hematocrit of approximately 35% to 40% is probably beneficial for the child with respiratory disease. However, if shock or increased intracranial pressure results in sluggish systemic or cerebral perfusion, a hemoglobin concentration of 10 to 11 g/dL may maintain adequate oxygen content while minimizing blood viscosity.

The child with cyanotic heart disease will require a relatively high hemoglobin concentration to maintain oxygen content in the fact of chronic arterial oxyhemoglobin desaturation. These children generally require hemoglobin of at least 15 g/dL, and anemia will reduce arterial oxygen content. Extreme polycythemia (Hgb concentration >20 g/dL and Hct >55% to 60%) must be avoided, because it will increase blood viscosity and risk of thromboembolic complications.

The oxyhemoglobin saturation will decrease in the presence of an intrapulmonary shunt or a right-to-left intracardiac shunt (cyanotic heart disease); this decrease in saturation will produce a fall in arterial oxygen content and may reduce systemic oxygen transport. If an *intrapulmonary* shunt is causing hypoxemia, arterial oxygen content can be increased through the administration of supplementary oxygen. Mechanical ventilation with the *judicious* use of positive end-expiratory pressure also can increase oxyhemoglobin saturation, arterial oxygen content, and oxygen delivery (see Chapter 9).

If a right-to-left (cyanotic) *intracardiac* shunt produces *mild* or *moderate* arterial oxygen desaturation and hypoxemia (i.e., oxyhemoglobin saturation of 85% to 90% and PaO_2 <50 mm Hg), administration of supplementary inspired oxygen is not likely to be beneficial. Oxygen content in these children increases most effectively when hemoglobin concentration increases and pulmonary blood flow and intracardiac mixing improve (refer to the section, Common Clinical Conditions, Hypoxemia).

Oxygen content *may* improve with oxygen administration in the child with cyanotic heart disease and *severe* hypoxemia (i.e., oxyhemoglobin saturation of 60% to 75%, and PaO_2 <30-45 mm Hg); in these children any small improvement in arterial oxygen tension achieved by oxygen administration may be associated with a relatively significant increase in oxyhemoglobin saturation and arterial oxygen content.

Clinical Evaluation of Arterial Oxygen Content

The most accurate method of determining arterial oxygen content is through measurement of hemoglobin concentration and its saturation, and arterial oxygen tension. The *oxygen content is the product of the hemoglobin concentration, its saturation, and the 1.34 mL (or 1.36 mL according to some sources) of oxygen carried by each gram of saturated hemoglobin per deciliter* (see Box 8-4). In addition, a small amount of oxygen is dissolved in the blood; this amount (mL O_2/dL of blood) is calculated by multiplying 0.003 and the arterial oxygen tension (PaO_2). The dissolved oxygen in the blood usually contributes an inconsequential amount to the oxygen content. However, when severe anemia is present this dissolved oxygen may be very important. Normal *arterial oxygen content is approximately 18 to 20 mL O_2/dL blood*.

Arterial oxygen content is linked most closely to hemoglobin saturation; a pulse oximeter may be used to continuously monitor the oxyhemoglobin saturation. If the hemoglobin concentration is stable the arterial oxygen content is estimated by

---

Box 8-4 **Calculation of Arterial Oxygen Content**

Arterial oxygen content = Oxygen bound to hemoglobin + Dissolved oxygen
= ([Hgb concentration g/dL] × 1.34 mL O_2/g × Hgb saturation) + 0.003 × PaO_2
= (Normal)18 − 20 mL oxygen/dL blood

---

multiplying the oximeter oxyhemoglobin saturation by the known hemoglobin concentration and 1.34 mL O_2/g of hemoglobin. This estimation will be unreliable if the hemoglobin concentration varies widely (e.g., during hemorrhage or transfusion therapy).

Cardiac Output

Cardiac output is the volume of the blood ejected by the heart in 1 min; it is the product of heart rate and stroke volume. Cardiac output often is recorded in L/min or mL/min, although it may be normalized to body weight (mL/kg body weight per min) or to body surface area (mL/m^2 body surface area per min). The normal cardiac output averages approximately 200 mL/kg per minute during infancy, 150 mL/kg per minute during childhood, and 100 mL/kg per minute in the adolescent.[752] Although the cardiac output/kg body weight decreases during childhood, the absolute cardiac output increases as the child grows.

Children of different sizes have different normal ranges of cardiac output, so it is easier to interpret the child's cardiac *index* rather than the cardiac output; the typical cardiac index is the same for children of all ages. *Cardiac index* is equal to the child's cardiac output divided by the child's body surface area in m^2. Normal cardiac index in the child is approximately 3.5-4.5 L/minute per m^2 body surface area.

Although "normal" ranges of cardiac output and index have been established in children these "normal" ranges may not maintain sufficient oxygen delivery to the tissues. *Cardiac output and index always must be evaluated in light of the patient's clinical condition;* the cardiac output or index should be considered as *adequate* to maintain oxygen and substrate delivery to the tissues, or *inadequate,* resulting in tissue and organ ischemia. Therapy is directed at restoring cardiac output that is *adequate* to maintain tissue oxygenation and substrate delivery.

Factors Affecting Cardiac Output

Cardiac output is the product of heart rate and stroke volume. If either component decreases without a commensurate and compensatory increase in the other component, cardiac output falls.

In children the heart rate is rapid and the stroke volume is small. Tachycardia helps to maintain cardiac output during periods of cardiorespiratory distress; any increase in heart rate above normal may improve cardiac output. An extremely rapid heart rate, however, with a ventricular rate exceeding 200 to 220/minute in the infant or 160 to 180/minute in the child results in a compromise in ventricular diastolic filling time and left coronary artery perfusion time, so that stroke volume and cardiac output often fall.

A transient decrease in heart rate may be normal in the infant or child, but significant or sustained bradycardia usually results in a fall in cardiac output or systemic perfusion. Persistent bradycardia may be an ominous clinical finding in the critically ill child and is often associated with hypoxia, or acidosis (refer to Arrhythmias later in this chapter). The bedside nurse should immediately verify that the airway is patent and support oxygenation and ventilation.

Ventricular stroke volume averages approximately 1.5 mL/kg; stroke volume in the 3 kg neonate is approximately 5 mL, and stroke volume in the 50 kg adolescent is approximately 75 mL. Stroke volume is determined by ventricular preload, contractility, and afterload. These factors have been described in the preceding sections. Trends in normal cardiac output and index with age can be found in Chapter 6, Table 6-1.

Clinical Evaluation of Cardiac Output

When cardiac output is inadequate to maintain oxygen and substrate delivery to the tissues, signs of poor systemic perfusion usually are present. Hypotension may not be observed unless acute severe blood loss has occurred or cardiovascular collapse is imminent (see Chapter 6).

The child's cardiac output may be estimated using Doppler studies of flow through the aorta (Box 8-5), or may be calculated using an artoerial/venous oxygen content difference combined with measured or estimated oxygen consumption (the Fick principle), or with thermodilution techniques. Each of these methods involves the application of physiologic principles to biologic systems, so each has potential sources of error that must be eliminated or at least standardized so the techniques can be used to evaluate trends in the patient's condition.

Doppler Echocardiography. Doppler studies use sound waves reflected from red blood cells to evaluate flow *velocity;* Doppler cardiac output determinations measure the velocity of red blood cells as they pass through the ascending aorta. The

---

Box 8-5 **Doppler Cardiac Output Determination**

Doppler Cardiac Output Determination

CO(mL/s) = Mean velocity of RBC (cm/s)
× Area of thoracic aorta (cm^2)

Most Likely Sources of Error
• Determination of area of aorta (estimation of radius or diameter)
• Interobserver and intraobserver variability in determination of velocity

diameter of the thoracic aorta is then calculated based on echocardiographic measurement or normative tables. The cardiac output is the product of the mean red blood cell velocity and the area of the aorta (see Box 8-5). Because the diameter is used to determine the radius (radius = 1/2 measured diameter), and the radius is squared to determine the area of the aorta, any error in the measurement of diameter will be magnified in the ultimate cardiac output determination.

Fick Cardiac Output Calculation. The Fick principle states that the flow of a liquid through a system can be determined if a known quantity of indicator (e.g., oxygen) is added to the fluid, and the quantity of the indicator is measured before and after it passes the site of indicator exchange. Therefore if the patient's oxygen consumption (the amount of oxygen taken up by the body per unit of time) is known and the arterial and venous oxygen content are determined from representative samples, the cardiac output can be calculated.

Calculation of cardiac output using the Fick principle requires calculation, measurement, or estimation of oxygen consumption, careful, simultaneous sampling of arterial and mixed venous blood, and accurate calculation of the arterial and mixed venous oxygen contents (Box 8-6). If the child's cardiorespiratory function is relatively stable and Fick calculations of cardiac output are used for determining trends, the oxygen consumption can be *estimated* and assumed to remain constant. However, oxygen consumption may vary widely during the clinical course of the child with cardiorespiratory failure, so such estimations may introduce significant error in the cardiac output calculation.

The venous sample must be representative of *mixed* systemic venous blood; because the oxygen content varies in the superior and inferior vena cavae and coronary sinus, a central venous or right atrial sample is not ideal for use in this calculation. (Coronary sinus blood has low oxygen content, and inferior vena caval blood has higher oxygen content than superior vena caval blood.) A true mixed venous sample should be obtained from the pulmonary artery. If a central venous or right atrial sample *is* used consistently for the venous sample, the potential error introduced must be considered. *Any* intracardiac or great vessel shunt also introduces significant error into the determination of the true mixed venous oxygen content. (A case study demonstration of the Fick cardiac output calculation is included in Evolve Box 8-3 in the Chapter 8 Supplement on the Evolve Website.)

Mixed Venous Oxygen Saturation. The mixed venous oxygen saturation falls when oxygen delivery decreases in the face of constant oxygen consumption. Oxygen delivery can fall if either cardiac output or arterial oxygen content falls. Mixed venous oxygen saturation also falls if oxygen demand increases at a faster rate than oxygen delivery. *If arterial oxygen content and oxygen demand are stable, the cardiac output is directly related to the mixed venous oxygen saturation.*

Continuous monitoring of mixed venous oxygen saturation is possible using an oximeter placed in the pulmonary artery. These systems analyze the amount of light *reflected* from hemoglobin (as compared with pulse oximeters, which measure the light actually *absorbed* by hemoglobin). The SvO_2 falls in the presence of decreased oxygen transport produced

---

Box 8-6 **Fick Calculation of Cardiac Output**

$$\text{Fick cardiac output (L/min)} = \frac{\text{Oxygen consumption (mL/min)}^*}{\text{Arterial O}_2 \text{ content} - \text{Mixed venous O}_2 \text{ content (mL/L)}^\dagger}$$

To convert the Fick cardiac output to cardiac index

$$\text{Cardiac index L/min per m}^2 = \frac{\text{Fick cardiac output (L/min)}}{\text{Body surface area (m}^2)}$$

Most likely sources of error in Fick cardiac output determination

Determination or estimation of oxygen consumption

If right atrial sample used for mixed venous sample, preferential sampling of SVC, IVC, or coronary sinus blood may yield erroneous results

Mathematical error

Intracardiac or great vessel shunt—a left-to-right shunt can raise the mixed venous oxygen saturation and result in falsely high cardiac output calculation

---

*Determination of oxygen consumption:
- Measurement by calorimeter
- Estimation: 5-8 mL/kg per minute *OR* 150-160 mL/min per m² for child (and 120-130 mL/min per m² for the young neonate).
  Child must be in steady state.

†Calculation of arterial and venous oxygen content:
  Arterial oxygen content = CaO_2 (in mL O_2 per L blood)
  CaO_2 = (Hgb concentration in gm/dl) × 1.34 mL O_2/g × oxyhemoglobin sat′ n × 10
  Mixed venous oxygen content = CvO_2 (in mL O_2 per L blood)
  CvO_2 = (Hgb concentration in gm/dl) × 1.34 mL O_2/gm × oxyhemoglobin sat′ n × 10
To add dissolved oxygen to these figures, multiply 0.003 × PaO_2 and add to arterial oxygen content and multiply 0.003 × PvO_2 and add to mixed venous oxygen content.

by either decreased cardiac output or reduced arterial oxygenation, so the SvO_2 frequently falls despite the presence of a stable cardiac output (see Chapter 21). The superior vena caval (SVC) oxygen saturation ($ScvO_2$) may be sampled as a surrogate for the mixed venous oxygen saturation level. However, it is important to note that the mixed venous oxygen saturation (normally approximately 75%) obtained in the pulmonary artery reflects the mixture of superior vena caval blood (oxygen saturation about 70% to 75%), inferior vena caval blood (oxygen saturation about 80% to 85%) and coronary sinus blood (oxygen saturation typically less than 50%). $ScvO_2$ is, therefore, approximately equal to the mixed venous oxygen saturation, but the location of the catheter tip can alter the venous blood sampled and the saturation obtained.

Thermodilution Cardiac Output Calculation. The thermodilution cardiac output calculation is a form of indicator-dilution calculation. This calculation requires insertion of a pulmonary artery catheter containing a thermistor bead. Cold fluid is injected into the right atrium and acts as a thermal indicator. This cold fluid mixes with right ventricular output and is ejected into the pulmonary artery. A thermistor records the temperature change over time in the pulmonary artery, and a computer calculates the area under the time-temperature curve (Box 8-7).

Box 8-7   **Thermodilution Cardiac Output**

Thermodilution Cardiac Output Calculation

$$CO = \frac{1.08\,(60)C_T V_i\,(T_b - T_i)}{\int_0^\infty \Delta T_b\,(t)dt}$$

Where:

CO = cardiac output

$1.08 = \dfrac{\rho C_p\,(5\%\text{ dextrose in water})}{\rho C_p\,(\text{blood})}$

  = The ratio of the density times the specific heat of D_5W to the density times the specific heat of blood

C_T = Correction factor for the injectate temperature rise as it passes through the catheter and catheter dead space.

60 = s/min

V_i = Injectate volume (in liters)

T_b = Initial blood temperature (°C)

T_i = Initial injectate temperature (°C)

$\displaystyle\int_0^\infty \Delta T_b\,(t)dt$ = Area derived by integration of the time-temperature thermodilution curve (°C-sec).

With thermodilution cardiac output, the *cardiac output is inversely related to the area under the time-temperature curve.* If the temperature change is large and persists for a relatively long period of time the cardiac output must be small (i.e., only a small volume of blood is ejected by the right ventricle to modify the temperature change produced by the cold injectate). If the temperature change is small and is maintained for only a brief period, the cardiac output must be high. (A large right ventricular output will quickly eliminate any effect of the cold injectate on the temperature in the pulmonary artery.)

For thermodilution cardiac output injections to reflect trends in the patient's cardiac output or index, the thermal injections must be standardized. The bedside monitor (or performed calculations) must be coded properly for the volume and temperature of the injectate and the size of the catheter. Usually three injections are performed; the calculation resulting from the first injection is typically discarded, because this injection serves to prime the catheter with cold injectate, and the resultant cardiac output calculation is usually erroneously high. The cardiac output calculated from the second and third injections are averaged, provided they do not differ by more than 10%. A strip chart recorder should be used to provide a hard copy of each injection curve, so that inconsistencies in injection technique can be detected.

Sources of error in the thermodilution cardiac output calculation include inaccurate injectate volume or temperature, inaccurate coding of computer (inappropriate calibration constant or coding for catheter size, or volume or temperature of injectate), excessive dead space in injection system (between the syringe and the right atrial port), or warming of injectate by large-volume central venous infusion.

In general, anything that artificially increases the magnitude of the temperature change in the pulmonary artery (e.g., administration of excessive and inaccurate injectate volume, injection of iced saline when computer is coded for room temperature injectate) results in falsely low cardiac output calculations. Anything that artificially reduces the magnitude of the temperature change in the pulmonary artery (e.g., warming of the injectate in the syringe before administration, injection of erroneously small injectate volume, coding of the computer for iced injections when room temperature injectate is used, or insertion of tubing between the injectate syringe and the right atrial catheter port) results in falsely high cardiac output calculations.

Typically, 3 or 5 mL iced injections are required for thermodilution cardiac output calculations using a flow-directed balloon-tipped pulmonary artery catheter. These injection volumes must be added to the child's total fluid intake. For this reason, injections should be performed only as necessary to calculate the cardiac output, and additional injections to test the temperature of the injectate should be performed into a waste syringe.

Oxygen Consumption

Oxygen consumption (VO_2) is the volume of oxygen consumed by the tissues per unit of time. It is the product of the amount of oxygen extracted from each milliliter of blood and the cardiac output. Oxygen consumption can be calculated, measured, or estimated.

Normally, much more oxygen is delivered to the tissues than is consumed. As a result, mild reductions in oxygen delivery can be tolerated because excess oxygen is available. Oxygen consumption is normally independent of oxygen delivery or supply. Oxygen consumption varies according to need and is increased during fever, exercise, and at times of increased circulating catecholamine levels. If oxygen consumption approaches oxygen delivery, however, or oxygen content falls dramatically, tissue ischemia, anaerobic metabolism, and acidosis can result.

When oxygen delivery is reduced, oxygen consumption may be maintained through an increase in tissue oxygen *extraction*. If oxygen delivery falls precipitously, however, oxygen consumption also falls. At this point, oxygen consumption becomes transport- or delivery-dependent (for further information, see Chapter 6 and Fig. 6-5).

Oxygen consumption may be reduced through administration of analgesics, sedatives, and neuromuscular blockers (during mechanical ventilation), treatment of fever, or use of hypothermia (intentionally produced during some types of cardiovascular surgery). If the patient is cooled and shivering occurs, oxygen consumption will *increase* rather than decrease.

Clinical Evaluation of Oxygen Consumption

To *calculate* oxygen consumption the cardiac output and arterial and mixed venous oxygen saturations must be known. Oxygen consumption is the product of the cardiac output and the difference between arterial and venous oxygen content (Box 8-8). A true mixed-venous oxygen content is determined from a sample of pulmonary artery blood rather than from a central venous or right atrial sample. Normal arteriovenous oxygen content difference is approximately 3 to 5 mL/dL; this is approximately 25% of the total 18 to 20 mL O_2/dL arterial oxygen content.

Because oxygen consumption is maintained at a fairly constant level over a broad range of clinical conditions, *cardiac output is usually inversely proportional to the arteriovenous oxygen difference*. When cardiac output is high, little oxygen is extracted from the tissues and the arteriovenous O_2 difference is small. If cardiac output falls a large amount of oxygen must be extracted from each milliliter of blood, so the arteriovenous O_2 difference widens. Frequently the arteriovenous O_2 difference is evaluated on a regular basis to evaluate trends in cardiac output. However, conditions such as sepsis or malignant hyperthermia can alter this relationship (refer to Shock in Common Clinical Conditions in this chapter and Mixed Venous Oxygen Saturation in Chapter 8).

Oxygen consumption also can be *estimated* from normative data. Oxygen consumption in normal children averages 5 to 8 mL/kg per minute, or 150 to 160 mL/min per m^2 of body surface area. Oxygen consumption in normal infants less than 2 to 3 weeks of age is approximately 120 to 130 mL/min per m^2 body surface area.[752]

AUTONOMIC NERVOUS SYSTEM

The autonomic nervous system controls visceral functions of the body, including blood pressure, cardiovascular function, gastrointestinal motility, and temperature. Autonomic centers are located in the spinal cord and brain stem. The major autonomic center is located in the hypothalamus. These centers closely maintain homeostasis through a balance of closed reflex loops. Afferent signals are received from chemoreceptors and baroreceptors, and efferent signals are transmitted through two major autonomic divisions; the sympathetic and the parasympathetic nervous systems.

Sympathetic Nervous System

Sympathetic nervous system influences are mediated through nerve fibers or the hormonal influences of circulating catecholamines. Sympathetic nerves originate in the spinal cord, between the first thoracic and second lumbar vertebrae. These spinal nerves pass to the chain of *sympathetic ganglion* located adjacent to the spinal column; most spinal sympathetic nerves synapse (contact) with other terminal (or postganglionic) neurons. Ultimately the sympathetic signals are transmitted to effector organs such as the heart or the adrenal medulla.

The terminal sympathetic fibers that travel to effector organs produce localized effects. The adrenal medulla, on the other hand, secretes epinephrine and small amounts of norepinephrine into the bloodstream, producing more global effects.

Sympathetic cardiac nerve fibers are distributed in an epicardial plexus to all chambers of the heart. They accompany the branches of the coronary vessels to innervate the myocardium, and they also are located near the SA node. Sympathetic nerve fibers innervate all arterioles in all systemic organs to enable reflex control of blood flow and pressure.

Adrenergic Neurotransmitters

Norepinephrine is the neurotransmitter that is released from the sympathetic nerves and acts locally at the neuromuscular junction. It is synthesized in the sympathetic nerve fiber and

---

Box 8-8 **Calculation of Oxygen Consumption**

Calculation of Oxygen Consumption

Oxygen consumption = Cardiac output × arteriovenous oxygen content difference × 10
= CO × ([arterial saturation − mixed venous saturation] × [Hgb concentration × 1.34 mL/g]) × 10

Oxygen consumption in infants: 10-14 mL O_2/kg per minute
Oxygen consumption in children: 7-11 mL O_2/kg per minute

is stored in vesicles that are located near the nerve membrane. When an action potential spreads over the terminal sympathetic nerve fiber, norepinephrine is released from the vesicles into the tissue surrounding the effector cells. This norepinephrine normally is active for only a few seconds and then is taken back up by nerve endings, diffuses into other body fluids, or is broken down by enzymes. Norepinephrine release and effects may be modulated by patient condition.

Epinephrine is released chiefly by the adrenal medulla following sympathetic nervous system stimulation; this drug mediates the stress-related metabolic response. The adrenal medulla secretes large quantities of epinephrine and small quantities of norepinephrine into the bloodstream. These circulating neurotransmitters (hormones) produce effects similar to those produced by the terminal nerve fibers (see further discussion later in this section). However, the hemodynamic effects of epinephrine are often more significant and last much longer than the local effects produced by norepinephrine.

The sympathetic nervous system is activated during times of stress, producing a "fight or flight" response; this includes tachycardia, increased cardiac contractility, redistribution of blood flow through arterial vasoconstriction (including peripheral, renal, and splanchnic arterial constriction), diaphoresis, and pupil dilation.

Adrenergic Receptors

Neurotransmitters and exogenous (administered) catecholamines stimulate the effector organs by binding with receptors. *Adrenergic receptors* are glycoproteins associated with cell membranes. They have high specificity and binding affinity for specific catecholamines.[968] Activation of the adrenergic receptor alters intracellular function. Effects of adrenergic receptor activation will be determined by both the type of receptor activated and by the density of receptors on the cell surface. Adrenergic receptors generally are divided into alpha, beta, and dopaminergic (DA) types.

Beta Receptors. Beta receptors are further subdivided into beta-1 and beta-2 subtypes. All beta receptors produce intracellular effects by the stimulation of *adenyl cyclase,* which causes formation of cyclic-AMP. Cyclic-AMP is called a second messenger hormone because it mediates the intracellular effects of hormones.

The beta-1 receptor is the predominant adrenergic receptor in the human heart. Beta-1 receptors are *innervated;* thus, they are activated preferentially by neuronally released norepinephrine. Beta-1 receptor activation results in an increase in heart rate, atrioventricular conduction velocity, and ventricular contractility.

Beta-2 receptors are not innervated; they are activated only by circulating catecholamines (predominantly epinephrine). Beta-2 receptor activation produces peripheral vasodilation and bronchial dilation.

When norepinephrine is secreted from terminal nerve fibers it stimulates only beta-1 (innervated) receptors. Systemically administered norepinephrine, however, stimulates beta-1, beta-2, and alpha-adrenergic receptors. Circulating epinephrine stimulates both beta-1 and beta-2 receptors, and alpha receptors.

Alpha Receptors. Alpha receptors also have been subdivided into alpha-1 and alpha-2 subtypes. Alpha-1 receptor activation affects intracellular function by increasing transcellular calcium flux. Alpha-2 receptor activation stimulates adenyl cyclase and increases intracellular production of cAMP.

Alpha-receptor stimulation results in constriction of vascular and bronchial smooth muscle. This produces peripheral vasoconstriction, including constriction of the skin and mesenteric and renal arteries; venoconstriction also occurs. In mammals, alpha-adrenergic receptor activation increases cardiac contractility, although in humans this effect seems to be produced chiefly by beta-1 receptor activation. Endogenous epinephrine and norepinephrine stimulate both alpha receptor subtypes, but synthetic catecholamines may demonstrate selective stimulation of these receptors.

Dopaminergic Receptors. Dopamine is an endogenous catecholamine that is present in terminal sympathetic nerves as a precursor of norepinephrine. Exogenous dopamine administration produces both direct and indirect actions because it will activate dopaminergic receptors and will stimulate norepinephrine release. At low doses of administered dopamine (approximately 2-5 mcg/kg per minute), DA effects predominate. At moderate infusion rates (approximately 4-10 mcg/kg per minute), both dopaminergic and beta-adrenergic effects may be seen. At high doses (>10 mcg/kg per minute), alpha-adrenergic effects usually dominate. These dose responses can vary, however.

Activation of dopaminergic receptors will result in renal, coronary, mesenteric, and cerebral vasodilation. As a result of renal dilation the glomerular filtration rate and renal sodium excretion increase. When large doses of dopamine are administered these dopaminergic effects may disappear and alpha-adrenergic receptor activation may result in reduction of renal and mesenteric blood flow.

Dopamine also produces noncardiovascular effects. Administration of exogenous dopamine results in decreased aldosterone secretion, inhibition of thyroid stimulating hormone, and reduction in insulin secretion.[968] These effects must be considered when dopamine is administered to critically ill patients.

Modulation of Adrenergic Receptor Activation

The *density* of adrenergic receptors on the cell surface is not static; it is affected by a variety of disease states and conditions. *Downregulation* of a receptor means that there is a *decrease in the number* of that type of receptor on the cell surface. For example, downregulation of beta-adrenergic myocardial receptors occurs with chronic severe congestive heart failure, myocardial ischemia, and hypothyroidism. Alpha-adrenergic receptors are downregulated when sepsis is present.[969] When a beta- or alpha-receptor is down-regulated the cell will be less capable of responding to, respectively, beta- or alpha-adrenergic stimulation from endogenous or exogenous catecholamines.

Upregulation of a receptor means that there is an *increase in the number* of that type of receptor on the cell surface. For example, upregulation of cardiac beta-receptors occurs in patients with mild heart failure and those with hyperthyroidism.

When a receptor is upregulated the cell will be more responsive to stimulation of that receptor by circulating or exogenous catecholamines.

Parasympathetic Nervous System

The parasympathetic nervous system, like the sympathetic nervous system, consists of a series of two to three neurons that begin in the brain or central nervous system and synapse with (contact) other parasympathetic neurons in ganglia located near the spinal cord or effector organs. The cell bodies of the preganglionic parasympathetic nerves are located in the brain stem and in the second, third, and fourth sacral segments of the spinal column. The parasympathetic nerve *fibers* arise from the third, seventh, ninth, and tenth cranial nerves, and from the second, third, and fourth sacral segments of the spinal cord.

Approximately 75% of all parasympathetic nerve fibers are located in the vagus nerves. Although sympathetic nervous system stimulation typically produces effects consistent with a "fight or flight" response, the parasympathetic effects are more consistent with "rest and repair." Parasympathetic (cholinergic) stimulation is associated with a decrease in heart rate, an increase in intestinal motility, and increased enzymatic secretion. Bladder contraction and sphincter relaxation also occur with cholinergic stimulation.

Vagal cardiovascular effects are most pronounced in the presence of active adrenergic (sympathomimetic) stimulation. There may be three possible explanations for this observation. Acetylcholine released from parasympathetic nerves may reduce intracellular levels of cAMP, or accelerate its breakdown, thus reducing beta-adrenergic intracellular effects. In addition, acetylcholine release may inhibit norepinephrine release from sympathetic fibers; this effect would be most pronounced at the sinoatrial (SA) node.

Parasympathetic Neurotransmitter

Acetylcholine is the neurotransmitter identified with the parasympathetic nervous system. It is synthesized in the nerve body and transmitted along the axon to vesicles at the end of the nerve fiber. Stimulation of the parasympathetic nerve results in the liberation of acetylcholine, which binds with a receptor site on the membrane of the effector organ and causes altered intracellular function. Acetylcholine is then broken down into acetate and choline by acetylcholinesterase; the choline is transported back into the neuron and is used in the formation of new acetylcholine.

Acetylcholine is also the neurotransmitter released by the *presynaptic* nerves of the sympathetic nervous system. It is present in skeletal muscle fibers and at neuromuscular junctions.

Cholinergic Receptors

Cholinergic receptors are divided into muscarinic and nicotinic receptors, named after the substances that can activate the specific receptors. Muscarinic receptors are found at all the effector sites of the parasympathetic nervous system, including the heart, viscera, and bladder. Nicotinic receptors are present at the ganglionic junction of preganglionic and terminal (postganglionic) nerves in both the sympathetic and the parasympathetic nervous system. In addition, nicotinic receptors are present in skeletal muscle fibers and at neuromuscular junctions.

Activation of terminal effector cholinergic receptors occurs only following stimulation from a terminal parasympathetic nerve. There are no circulating cholinergic hormones. Parasympathetic stimulation reduces heart rate through a negative chronotropic effect on the sinoatrial node. Cholinergic stimulation has some negative inotropic effect on atrial contractility and a lesser negative inotropic effect on ventricular function.

COMMON CLINICAL CONDITIONS

CONGESTIVE HEART FAILURE

Ricardo Samson

Pearls

- Both congestive heart failure and shock are conditions of cardiac output that is inadequate to meet the metabolic demands of the body.
- Cardiovascular dysfunction is a continuum with no sharp demarcation between severe congestive heart failure and shock.

Etiology

Congestive heart failure refers to a set of clinical signs and symptoms indicative of myocardial dysfunction and cardiac output that is inadequate to meet the metabolic demands of the body. In children it may be caused by increased cardiac workload (imposed by congenital heart defects that alter cardiac preload or afterload, or by severe anemia), impaired cardiac contractility, or alteration in the sequence or rate of cardiac contraction, or a combination of these factors.

Congenital heart disease is the most common cause of congestive heart failure during childhood, particularly during the first year of life. Severe anemia also may produce congestive heart failure at any age. Likewise, congestive heart failure caused by impaired ventricular function (such as cardiomyopathy) may develop at any period during childhood.

Congenital heart defects that most commonly cause congestive heart failure during the newborn period include severe left ventricular outflow tract obstruction (such as hypoplastic left heart, interrupted aortic arch, critical aortic stenosis, or coarctation of the aorta), large arteriovenous fistula, or combined shunt lesions (such as a ventricular septal defect and patent ductus arteriosus). A large patent ductus arteriosus will produce heart failure in the extremely premature neonate. Isolated septal defects (such as a ventricular septal defect) usually do not produce signs of congestive heart failure until pulmonary vascular resistance falls at approximately 2 to 9 weeks of age,[597] and hemoglobin concentration falls.[214a]

Surgical correction of congenital heart defects may cause congestive heart failure as a result of intraoperative cardiac manipulation and resection, with subsequent alteration in pressure, flow, and resistance relationships. Surgical procedures that require a ventriculotomy incision, conduit insertion, or significant ventricular muscle resection (e.g., correction of tetralogy of Fallot or truncus arteriosus) are likely to be associated with postoperative heart failure.

Congestive heart failure may be associated with high or low cardiac output. High cardiac output failure typically is present in the child with congenital heart disease producing a left-to-right shunt, particularly at the level of the ventricles or within the great vessels. This type of shunt produces high pulmonary blood flow, often at systemic pressure. The increased volume of pulmonary venous return results in a tremendous volume load for the left ventricle.

High cardiac output failure also may be caused by severe anemia, such as that resulting from increased red blood cell destruction (e.g., hemolytic anemia) or reduced red blood cell formation (e.g., aplastic anemia, or other bone marrow failure). Mild anemia may be asymptomatic because cardiac output will increase commensurately to maintain oxygen delivery. Severe anemia, however (with a hemoglobin concentration of less than 5 g/dL and a hematocrit of less than 15%), significantly compromises arterial oxygen-carrying capacity and arterial oxygen content, so that only extremely high levels of cardiac output will maintain oxygen delivery. Frequently the child with severe, chronic anemia maintains a compensated state unless or until conditions develop that require further increase in cardiac output (e.g., fever, sepsis).

Low output congestive heart failure typically is seen in children with severe left heart or aortic obstruction (such as critical aortic stenosis or hypoplastic left heart), cardiomyopathy, or tachyarrhythmias.[841] These children demonstrate signs of decreased left ventricular function and poor systemic perfusion. Low cardiac output also may be present in children with severe congestive heart failure and an extremely large left-to-right shunt. The increased work of breathing in children with congestive heart failure (CHF) results in increased blood flow to respiratory muscles, which effectively "steals" systemic blood flow and may contribute to low cardiac output.

Low output congestive heart failure also may be seen in children with elevated pulmonary artery pressures following a Fontan-type correction of tricuspid atresia, hypoplastic left heart, or other single ventricle lesions (see section, Specific Diseases, Single Functioning Ventricle). In these patients, systemic venous return is routed directly into the pulmonary arteries, flowing passively through the lungs to return to the systemic ventricle to be circulated to the body. High pulmonary or systemic venous pressure may be present for days (or longer) following performance of a Fontan-type procedure. In these patients, low cardiac output is exacerbated by mechanical ventilation with high levels of positive end-expiratory pressure (PEEP) or increased pulmonary vascular resistance.[935]

Pathophysiology

Biochemical Alterations. Many primary and secondary genetic and biochemical abnormalities have been described in association with impaired ventricular contractility.[261] In many cases, the final common pathway results in impaired binding or release of calcium or impaired calcium entry into the sarcolemma. These changes lead to abnormalities of excitation-contraction coupling.[438,841] If oxygen demand increases in the presence of limited myocardial oxygen delivery (particularly in children with aortic stenosis, tachyarrhythmias, or

other causes of limited myocardial perfusion, or those with hyperthermia), myocardial perfusion and performance may be inadequate to maintain effective systemic oxygen and substrate delivery. Extreme core hyperthermia may increase oxygen demand significantly. Chronic, severe congestive heart failure also may result in down-regulation (decreased density) of beta-adrenergic receptors.[969] All of these factors may further compromise myocardial function.

Some patients with congestive heart failure develop enhanced calcium influx, prolonged calcium binding, and impaired calcium uptake. When this occurs, the myocardium generates tension effectively but relaxation is impaired. Impaired relaxation, in turn, compromises diastolic filling, and stroke volume falls.[438]

Ventricular Dilation and Hypertrophy. When myocardial dysfunction is present, compensatory ventricular hypertrophy and dilation may enable maintenance of effective systemic perfusion. Ventricular hypertrophy distributes the ventricular load among an increased number of sarcomeres.[438] Ventricular dilation increases ventricular end-diastolic volume and so may improve stroke volume by stretching ventricular fibers, according to the Frank-Starling law of the heart (see section, Essential Anatomy and Physiology).

Afterload is the impedance to ventricular ejection, which can be evaluated by calculating ventricular wall stress. This is accomplished by dividing the product of ventricular pressure and ventricular cavity diameter by twice the ventricular wall thickness (see Box 8-3 and Chapter 6). Uncompensated increases in ventricular cavity diameter (dilation) increase ventricular wall stress and myocardial oxygen consumption, reducing myocardial efficiency.[841]

Ventricular hypertrophy develops early to compensate for increases in ventricular preload and afterload. This increase in ventricular wall thickness may allow ventricular wall stress (afterload) to remain normal in the face of ventricular hypertension and some ventricular dilation. For example, when compensated aortic stenosis is present, ventricular wall stress may be normal if compensatory left ventricular hypertrophy develops. In this case the intraventricular pressure rises, chamber diameter is reduced, and wall thickness increases.

When congestive heart failure develops after a Fontan procedure, systemic venous congestion develops proportional to the impedance to pulmonary venous flow. If pulmonary vascular resistance is high, central venous pressure increases and systemic venous congestion results.

Sympathetic Nervous System Compensation and Redistribution of Blood Volume. When cardiac output becomes insufficient to meet metabolic demands, sympathetic nervous system "fight or flight" compensatory mechanisms are activated. These neural and humeral control mechanisms are designed to improve cardiac output and redistribute blood volume, so that oxygen delivery is maintained to the heart and brain.[543]

Early signs of beta-adrenergic stimulation include an increase in heart rate and ventricular contractility. Alpha-adrenergic effects result in reflex constriction in arterioles of the skin, gut, skeletal muscle, and kidneys so that blood flow is diverted away from nonessential tissues to maintain coronary and cerebral perfusion. Vasoconstriction should improve mean arterial and organ perfusion pressures and enhance systemic venous return.

Compensatory redistribution of blood flow is complicated by the increased work of breathing for the child with congestive heart failure. Under normal conditions, respiratory muscles require a very small portion of cardiac output and oxygen consumption. When congestive heart failure is present, however, the work of breathing increases significantly,[935] and a significant portion of cardiac output may be redistributed to respiratory muscles (see section, Altered Nutrition and Potential Gastrointestinal Complications).

Compensatory mechanisms are compromised in the infant or child with congestive heart failure caused by severe anemia. In these patients, cardiac output is already maximal, and arterial oxygen content is already compromised. As a result, deterioration in these children may be rapid once decompensation occurs.

Renal and Humeral Factors Affecting Blood Volume and Distribution. When renal blood flow is reduced, the renin-angiotensin-aldosterone mechanism is activated, producing renal sodium and water retention. The resulting increase in circulating blood volume should improve systemic venous return and cardiac output, and maximize ventricular function by increasing ventricular end-diastolic volume. Renin release also catalyzes the production of angiotensin I, which is converted to angiotensin II, a potent vasoconstrictor. Angiotensin II crosses the blood-brain barrier and affects the medullary cardiovascular center, stimulating release of further vasoactive substances and affecting blood pressure and volume.[101] Angiotensin II also mediates ventricular hypertrophy, through stimulation of the protein kinase C pathway in cardiac myocytes.[906]

Increased myocardial wall stretch results in release of a family of natriuretic factors—atrial natriuretic peptide (ANP), brain natriuretic peptide (BNP), C-type natriuretic peptide, and dendroaspis natriuretic peptide (DNP). These polypeptides stimulate natriuresis (sodium excretion), diuresis, and vasodilation directly (for additional information, see Evolve Fig. 8-3 in the Chapter 8 Supplement on the Evolve Website); however, in children with congestive heart failure the natriuretic effects seem to be blunted. In addition, these natriuretic peptides interact with renin, aldosterone, and vasopressin to modulate blood volume and distribution.[101]

Renal compensatory mechanisms help to maintain the circulating blood volume despite initial blood loss or chronic hemorrhage. However, they will not succeed in maintaining oxygen delivery in the face of significant or continued red blood cell loss.

Effects on Oxygen Delivery. If cardiac output is compromised significantly or oxygen requirements increase in the presence of limited oxygen delivery, oxygen and nutrient flow to organs may be insufficient to meet the metabolic demands. In addition, increased oxygen consumption (associated with adrenergic stimulation and enhanced work

of breathing) has been documented in children with congenital heart disease and congestive heart failure. Because the young infant has little cardiac output reserve, any increase in oxygen requirements or reduction in oxygen delivery may well result in rapid deterioration.

When chronic congestive heart failure is present, myocardial energy expenditure may exceed myocardial energy production. As a result the heart may develop substrate and energy depletion that contribute to myocardial dysfunction.[438]

Tissue oxygen extraction increases when cardiac output and oxygen delivery fall. This increased extraction occurs as the result of changes in oxygen and capillary diffusion parameters and local metabolic changes. Diffusion parameters for oxygen are altered by the opening of previously closed capillaries and the reduction in velocity of blood traversing the capillary bed. These changes increase the time available for diffusion of oxygen into the tissues. Local tissue acidosis increases levels of red blood cell 2,3-diphosphoglycerate (2,3-DPG), which shifts the oxyhemoglobin dissociation curve to the right. This decreases hemoglobin affinity for oxygen, so oxygen is released more readily to the tissues. The curve shifts back to the normal position when the underlying condition is treated.

Continued severe compromise in oxygen delivery results in anaerobic metabolism and generation of lactic acid. If oxygen delivery remains extremely low, oxygen consumption falls and organ failure may develop.

Clinical Signs and Symptoms

Pediatric congestive heart failure most commonly is observed during infancy and immediately after cardiovascular surgery. Occasionally, children demonstrate chronic congestive heart failure as the result of severe, chronic anemia, inflammatory cardiac disease, or end-stage (inoperable) congenital heart disease.

Clinical signs and symptoms of anemia-induced congestive heart failure include lethargy, weakness, and fatigue. The child is often pale, and a systolic flow murmur is often present. Signs of high cardiac output failure, including tachycardia (with a gallop), pulmonary edema, and hepatosplenomegaly, usually develop once the hematocrit falls below 15% and the hemoglobin concentration is less than 5 g/dL. Signs of shock may develop with acute severe blood loss. If signs of shock are absent, the anemia is probably chronic, and renal sodium and water retention have succeeded in maintaining the circulating blood volume (see Anemia in Chapter 15).

Classic clinical signs and symptoms associated with congestive heart failure result from adrenergic stimulation and redistribution of blood flow and from the effects of right or left ventricular dysfunction. In addition, some infants demonstrate nonspecific signs of respiratory distress and very poor systemic perfusion (Box 8-9). These signs may be used to classify the severity of the congestive heart failure (Table 8-6).

Adrenergic Stimulation. Adrenergic stimulation produces tachycardia and redistribution of blood flow. The increase in heart rate may succeed in maintaining effective cardiac output despite reduced ventricular function. However, tachycardia reduces ventricular diastolic filling time and stroke volume, and decreases left coronary artery myocardial perfusion time. Tachycardia also increases myocardial oxygen consumption.

| Box 8-9 | Signs of Congestive Heart Failure |

Signs and Symptoms of Congestive Heart Failure in Children

Signs of Adrenergic Response
Tachycardia
Tachypnea
Cool skin
Oliguria
Diaphoresis
Signs of Systemic Venous Congestion
Hepatomegaly
Periorbital edema
Ascites (rare)
Pulmonary effusion
Signs of Pulmonary Venous Congestion
Tachypnea
Retractions
Nasal flaring
Pulmonary edema
Nonspecific Signs of Cardiorespiratory Distress
Irritability
Change in responsiveness
Fatigue
Poor feeding, failure to thrive

| Table 8-6 | Ross Classification of Congestive Heart Failure |

Ross Classification System of Pediatric Heart Failure

Class	Symptoms
I	None
II	Mild tachypnea/diaphoresis with feedings in infants Exertional dyspnea in children
III	Marked tachypnea/diaphoresis with feeding in infants Marked exertional dyspnea in children
IV	Symptoms at rest (diaphoresis, tachypnea, tachycardia, retractions)

From Ross RD, Bollinger RO, Pinsky WW: Grading the severity of heart failure in infants. *Pediatr Cardiol* 13:72-75, 1992.

For these reasons a mild increase in heart rate may succeed in maintaining cardiac output, but significant rises in heart rate may contribute to further deterioration.[284] A third heart sound or a summation gallop may be produced by the rapid filling of a noncompliant ventricle. However, extra heart sounds may be difficult to distinguish once the heart rate exceeds 120 to 140/min.

Adrenergic stimulation also produces peripheral vasoconstriction, reduced renal blood flow, and diaphoresis. The child's extremities are often cool (they cool from peripheral to proximal areas), with a pale or mottled color. Decreased renal blood flow results in a urine volume of less than 0.5 to 1.0 mL/kg per hour, despite adequate fluid intake. Urine sodium concentration is usually low, and a microscopic hematuria often is present.[841] Diaphoresis may be observed in infants, particularly over the head and neck.

Systemic Venous Congestion. When right ventricular dysfunction develops, right ventricular end-diastolic pressure increases and right atrial and central venous pressures rise. This produces systemic venous congestion. With hepatic venous hypertension the liver sinusoids fill with blood, so the liver enlarges and becomes palpable below the child's right costal margin; this *hepatomegaly* is one of the earliest signs of systemic venous congestion in children. The infant and child also may demonstrate periorbital edema.

Because jugular venous distension is difficult to perceive in the short, fat neck of the infant, it is not a reliable sign of congestive heart failure until the child is school age or older. Dependent edema, or ascites, is rarely seen in children unless the central venous pressure is extremely high (as may occur after Fontan-type surgical correction of tricuspid atresia), or unless it is associated with other metabolic problems, such as hypoalbuminemia or renal failure.

If ascites does develop it is the result of high central venous and portal venous pressures, and loss of fluid from the surface of the liver or from the surfaces of the gut and mesentery. This high-pressure exudate results in movement of both fluid and protein into the peritoneal cavity. The presence of protein in the ascitic fluid will draw more fluid from the surface of the gut and mesentery, so the ascites often increases.

If ascites is present the child's abdominal girth increases, the abdomen appears full, and the skin is taut and shiny. If two examiners are present a *fluid wave* may be elicited, and areas of shifting dullness may be noted during percussion. (These and other signs and symptoms of ascites are discussed in detail in Chapter 14.)

Pulmonary Venous Congestion. Signs of respiratory distress are often the first and most noticeable signs of congestive heart failure in the infant. Left ventricular failure results in a rise in left ventricular end-diastolic pressure and an increase in pulmonary venous pressure; pulmonary edema develops once pulmonary venous pressure is 20 to 25 mm Hg, but occurs at lower pressure if capillary permeability is increased. Most commonly, children with CHF demonstrate pulmonary *interstitial* (rather than *alveolar*) edema. Pulmonary edema, in turn, reduces lung compliance and increases the work of breathing; these changes result in tachypnea and increased respiratory effort.

Intercostal, subcostal, sternal, supraclavicular, or suprasternal retractions may be noted, and are particularly apparent in the infant. Older children may demonstrate use of accessory muscles of respiration, including use of scapular muscles and the sternocleidomastoid. Because these muscles are inadequately developed in the infant, "head bobbing" may be noted. Nasal flaring is an additional sign of respiratory distress.

The infant or child with severe respiratory distress grunts with expiration. The grunting results from expiration against a closed glottis and is an instinctive attempt to maintain PEEP and prevent atelectasis and collapse of small airways.

Rales (crackles) often are not observed in infants with congestive heart failure, despite the presence of pulmonary interstitial edema. Children with respiratory distress tend to breathe shallowly, so small airway sounds are less likely to be appreciated. In addition, pulmonary *interstitial* edema is cleared rapidly into lymphatics when tachypnea is present.[841] If crackles are noted, the presence of severe congestive heart failure or a concurrent respiratory infection should be suspected. Wheezes may be heard, especially if the child has a large left-to-right shunt. Lobar emphysema or atelectasis occasionally may result from cardiac compression of larger airways.

If the central venous pressure is extremely high, a pleural effusion or chylothorax may develop. These complications produce a decrease in intensity or a change in pitch of breath sounds over the affected chest. Chest expansion (especially that noted during positive pressure ventilation) will be compromised on the involved side, and hypoxemia may be noted.

Nonspecific Signs of Distress. Subtle signs of cardiorespiratory distress in infants and children include a change in disposition or responsiveness; unusual lethargy or irritability is often observed. The infant usually requires prolonged feeding times, sucks poorly, and takes only small amounts of formula. Typically the infant falls asleep during or immediately after the feeding because the work of breathing is significant. The infant usually swallows a large amount of air during feedings, so gastric distension develops. Vomiting is common after feeding.

These infants have high energy requirements and poor caloric intake, therefore failure to thrive is common. Often any weight gain noted results from edema rather than nutrition.

Laboratory Evaluation. The electrocardiogram is not helpful in the diagnosis of congestive heart failure unless associated heart block or an arrhythmia is present. If ventricular dilation is present, cardiomegaly will be apparent on the chest radiograph (see Fig. 10-12). Pulmonary interstitial edema also may be noted. An echocardiogram is helpful in identifying congenital heart disease or pericardial effusion and evaluating cardiac chamber size, ventricular contractility and ejection fraction.

Free water retention (disproportionate to the amount of sodium retention) usually produces a dilutional fall in serum sodium and hemoglobin concentrations. True anemia may result from increased red blood cell destruction or reduced red blood cell production. The bilirubin, lactic dehydrogenase (LDH), and reticulocyte counts are elevated in the patient with accelerated red blood cell destruction. If the anemia is caused by reduced red blood cell production, the reticulocyte count is inappropriately low. Hypoglycemia occasionally is noted in very small infants with congestive heart failure because metabolic needs are high and glycogen stores are minimal.[841]

Serum natriuretic peptides are increasingly being used as biomarkers to aid in the identification and monitoring of congestive heart failure. Although atrial natriuretic peptide (ANP) was the first of these peptides to be described, brain natriuretic peptide (BNP), initially discovered in brain matter, was later found in significantly higher amounts in ventricular myocardium.[713]

BNP is released from the heart as a prohormone (pro-BNP), which is subsequently cleaved into the active 32 amino acid polypeptide, BNP, and a metabolically inactive portion, N-terminal pro-BNP (NT pro-BNP). Consequently, serum assays of serum BNP and NT pro-BNP levels have been shown to be both sensitive and specific for the presence or worsening of heart failure in both adult[205,560,634,790] and pediatric patients.[187,281,345,518]

Management

Care of the child with congestive heart failure targets improvement of cardiac function and elimination of excess intravascular fluid. In addition, oxygen delivery must be supported and oxygen demands controlled or minimized. Reversible causes of congestive heart failure also must be treated.

Improvement in Cardiac Function: Digitalis Derivatives. Digitalis may be extremely effective in the treatment of congestive heart failure. It must, however, be used appropriately with careful monitoring for therapeutic and side and toxic effects.

Therapeutic Effects. Digitalis (administered predominantly as digoxin in children) continues to be used in the treatment of congestive heart failure in children, although evidence of its efficacy in pediatric patients is controversial.[435] The presumed effect of digoxin in older children is inotropic, improving ventricular contractility. Digoxin also affects the excitability of myocardial cells and slows the heart rate. Pediatric digoxin therapy (particularly during infancy) also appears to relieve some symptoms of congestive heart failure through effects on oxygen consumption.

The inotropic effects of digoxin result from inhibition of the sodium-potassium pump, so that sodium accumulates intracellularly. Sodium then competes with calcium for sites on the sodium-calcium exchange mechanism, raising intracellular calcium levels and improving myocardial contractility. Digitalis also interacts with the sarcolemma to sequester calcium, so that intracellular calcium is increased further.[355,841]

Digoxin also slows the heart rate by lowering the resting membrane potential, increasing parasympathetic sensitivity, and reducing sensitivity to norepinephrine. It slows conduction velocity and increases recovery time of the atrioventricular (AV) node. These effects result in a decrease in heart rate but also may contribute to increased ectopic activity.

Digitalis has some direct and indirect peripheral and coronary vasoconstrictive effects, resulting in increased systemic vascular resistance.[355,735] When digitalis is administered to patients with congestive heart failure, it appears to antagonize peripheral effects of catecholamines, thereby reducing oxygen consumption.

The clinical effects of digoxin administration in infants may be variable,[473,789] and positive effects of digoxin may be related to effects on oxygen supply and demand rather than to inotropic effects. Digoxin administration to the premature neonate may not produce significant improvement in contractility, and the incidence of clinical toxicity is significant in these patients.[435] For this reason, digoxin may not be useful in the treatment of congestive heart failure in premature neonates.

Digoxin administration often fails to produce measurable echocardiographic evidence of improvement in cardiac contractility in full-term infants with congestive heart failure caused by a ventricular septal defect. However, demonstrable *clinical* improvement often is noted; this improvement probably is related to a significant fall in oxygen consumption.[435] Studies of digoxin's effects on animals during periods of induced anemia and reduced oxygen transport have documented reduced oxygen consumption and improvement in the match between oxygen supply and oxygen demand.[769]

Dose. When digoxin therapy is initiated, several loading ("digitalizing") doses typically are administered to provide therapeutic serum levels of the drug. Once these levels are achieved, maintenance doses of digoxin are administered to replace the child's estimated daily renal excretion of the drug, so that therapeutic levels are maintained (Table 8-7).

Digoxin doses must be modified based on the child's age and clinical condition. Because digoxin is excreted through the kidneys, neonates who have limited renal tubular function and children with renal failure require reduced dosing. Premature neonates have limited renal tubular function; they

are more sensitive to digoxin and require smaller digoxin doses than full-term neonates or older children.[355] For this reason the risk of digoxin toxicity is highest in premature neonates.

Infants have a larger volume of digoxin distribution than older children because infants have more red blood cell binding sites for digoxin than do older patients. For this reason, higher loading and maintenance doses of digoxin were recommended for neonates and young infants in the past. Although young infants apparently tolerate high doses and high serum digoxin levels better than adults, it is not clear that the higher dosing is beneficial during infancy. Beyond the neonatal period patients normally excrete approximately one third of the daily administered oral dose.[507]

Whenever digoxin is administered to a critically ill child, careful consideration of dose and careful monitoring for evidence of toxicity is required. In any patient the appropriate dose

Table 8-7 Pediatric Digoxin Dose[507]

Age*	Total Digitalizing Dose (mcg/kg) PO[†]	Total digitalizing Dose (mcg/kg) IV or IM[†]	Daily Maintenance Dose (mcg/kg) PO[‡]	Daily Maintenance Dose IV or IM[‡]
Preterm infant*	20-30	15-25	5-7.5	4-6
Full-term infant*	25-35	20-30	6-10	5-8
1 mo to 2 y*	35-60	30-50	10-15	7.5-12
2-5 y*	30-40	25-35	7.5-10	6-9
5-10 y*	20-35	15-30	5-10	4-8
>10 y*	10-15	8-12	2.5-5	2-3
Adults	0.75-1.5 mg	0.5-1 mg	0.125-0.5 mg	0.1-0.4 mg

Treatment of Cardiac Glycoside Intoxication with Digoxin-specific Fab Antibody Fragments (Digibind)

Two formulas may be utilized; the proper dose can be then estimated using the estimated amount of drug ingested or administered, or serum concentration.

A. *Fab dose based on serum concentration of digoxin:*

$$Body\ burden = \frac{Serum\ digoxin\ concentration\ (ng/mL) \times 5.6 \times weight\ (kg)}{1000}$$

Fab dose = 40 Fab fragments per 0.6 *mg* digoxin in body

Note: This formula may be inaccurate following ingestion, because the serum concentration may be only transiently elevated

B. *Fab dose based on estimated dose of digoxin ingested:*
Estimated 80% absorption of orally ingested digoxin

Fab dose = 40 *mg* Fab fragments per 0.6 *mg* digoxin in body

C. *For example:* If serum digoxin level is 5 ng/mL in 10-kg infant:

$$Body\ Burden = \frac{(5ng/mL) \times 5.6 \times 10\ kg}{1000}$$

Body burden = .28 *mg*
Fab dose = 40 *mg*/0.6 *mg* digoxin body burden

$$= 40\ mg \times \left(\frac{.28}{0.6}\right)$$

Fab dose = 18.4 *mg* for the 10 kg child

Therefore, if serum digoxin level is 5-15 ng/mL, Fab dose will be 1.8-5.6 mg/kg.

---

*Based on lean body weight and normal renal function for age. Decrease dose in patients with decreased renal function; digitalizing dose often not recommended in infants and children.
[†]Give one-half of the total digitalizing dose (TDD) in the initial dose, then give one-fourth of the TDD in each of the two subsequent doses at 8- and 12-h intervals. Obtain ECG 6 h after each dose to assess potential toxicity.
[‡]Divided every 12 h in infants and children <10 years of age. Given once daily to children >10 years of age and adults.

of digoxin is the minimum dose necessary to produce therapeutic effects. There is a very small difference between optimal therapeutic levels of digoxin and toxic levels of the drug.

Children with inflammatory cardiac diseases (e.g., myocarditis or cardiomyopathy), chronic hypoxemia, and postoperative cardiovascular patients may demonstrate increased sensitivity to the drug.[355] When providing digoxin therapy for the first time to these patients it is prudent to consider providing lower doses of digoxin, or more gradual loading of the drug. Maintenance doses of digoxin may be administered without previous loading doses; this will result in achievement of therapeutic digoxin levels over 4 to 5 days.[841]

The total *oral* digitalizing dose for children is approximately 25 to 60 mcg/kg (or 0.025-0.060 mg/kg), and the higher doses in these ranges usually are administered to children 2 years of age or less. The digitalizing or loading dose usually is administered in two to four divided oral doses over 24 to 48 hours.

The maintenance digoxin dose is approximately one eighth (12%) of the total loading dose, administered twice a day. The child receives approximately one fourth of the loading dose daily.

Administration. Before administration of the final loading dose, an electrocardiogram or rhythm strip is typically ordered to ensure that arrhythmias have not developed. Because digoxin slows conduction through the AV node, an increased P-R interval often is present following establishment of a therapeutic serum digoxin level. However, second- or third-degree heart block or ectopy should be reported to a physician or the on-call provider before the next dose of digoxin is administered.

In the hospital the child's heart rate usually is checked before administration of any digoxin. If bradycardia is detected the dose usually is held until an electrocardiographic rhythm strip is obtained and toxic heart block or arrhythmias are ruled out. When attempting to determine if digoxin toxicity is present, a particular heart rate is usually less important than assessment of the child's systemic perfusion and evaluation of the electrocardiogram for evidence of heart block (see section, Digoxin Levels).

If the child vomits after administration of an oral dose of digoxin in the hospital, a physician or on-call provider should be consulted before the dose is readministered. It is often difficult to determine how much of the dose was lost, so a repeat dose may result in elevation of serum digoxin levels. In addition, vomiting may be a sign of digoxin toxicity.

It is imperative that the written order for and preparation of the digitalizing doses be double checked before administration because it is very easy to make an error by a factor of 10 or 100 when working with micrograms and milligrams. The order for the digoxin dose should be written (verbal orders should not be used) to avoid miscommunication. The order should be written in both milligrams and micrograms.

Digoxin should be administered with caution to children with decreased renal function, and the dose should be reduced accordingly. Hypokalemia can contribute to the development of clinical signs of digoxin toxicity even in the presence of relatively low serum digoxin levels, so the serum potassium should be monitored and potassium supplementation provided as needed. Hypomagnesemia and hypercalcemia also may aggravate digitalis toxicity, and quinidine may potentiate digoxin toxicity.[355] This is especially pertinent as many patients receiving digoxin are also on concomitant diuretics, which may cause electrolyte disturbances.

Digoxin Levels. A serum digoxin level may be monitored when digoxin therapy is instituted (during the "loading phase"), when the child's response to therapy is suboptimal, when toxicity is suspected, or when the drug dose is changed. Therapeutic serum digoxin levels vary from institution to institution but are in the range of 1.1 to 2.2 ng/mL (nontoxic levels in infants may be as high as 3.5 ng/mL). Serum digoxin levels exceeding 3.5 ng/mL are generally considered toxic.

Blood sampling for serum digoxin levels should be performed at prescribed intervals following digoxin administration (consult with the child's physician or ordering provider and hospital clinical laboratory). These levels must be interpreted with caution. As noted, hypokalemia, hypomagnesemia, and hypercalcemia can aggravate digoxin cardiotoxicity even in the presence of "normal" digoxin levels.[735] Some children exhibit endogenous digitalis-like substances that can influence serum digoxin levels. In addition, premature neonates may demonstrate bradyarrhythmias even in the presence of "therapeutic" levels of digoxin. For these reasons the presence of clinical symptoms compatible with digoxin toxicity usually is interpreted more strongly than the serum digoxin level alone.

Several common critical care drugs are known to affect digoxin levels. Amiodarone, verapamil, diltiazem, spironolactone, carvedilol and indomethacin all increase serum digoxin levels.[735] The digoxin dose should be reduced during concurrent administration of these drugs, and serum digoxin levels should be monitored.

Digoxin Toxicity. The most serious toxic effects of digoxin in children are arrhythmias, which may be observed in the absence of other clinical signs of toxicity. The most common arrhythmia in young children is bradycardia, although heart block and atrial and ventricular premature contractions (ectopy), and ventricular fibrillation have been reported. Virtually any new arrhythmia appearing after initiation of digoxin therapy may be caused by digoxin toxicity.[735]

Less specific and less common signs of digoxin toxicity in children include anorexia, nausea, vomiting, and diarrhea. Drowsiness and lethargy are common signs of toxicity in infants and young children.[356]

If digoxin toxicity is suspected, the physician or on-call provider should be notified; further digoxin usually is held pending the results of serum digoxin-level testing. A blood specimen should be drawn for laboratory analysis. Toxicity may be present at levels as low as 2.5 ng/mL or lower; the serum digoxin level must be evaluated in light of the patient's clinical condition.[355]

If toxicity is discovered in the asymptomatic child, electrocardiographic monitoring should be instituted and the child should be observed closely for the development of arrhythmias. If large amounts of oral digoxin have recently been ingested or administered, induced emesis soon after the ingestion may succeed in recovering 35% to 40% of the ingested drug. Vomiting should only be induced if the child is alert and demonstrates a cough and gag reflex. If massive amounts of digoxin have been ingested, the insertion of temporary transvenous pacing wires is recommended before the development of symptoms.

Treatment of symptomatic digoxin toxicity requires support of cardiovascular function (including treatment of arrhythmias), prevention of further drug absorption, and enhancement of digoxin excretion.[356] Bradycardia usually is treated with atropine or pacemaker therapy. Phenytoin (2-5 mg/kg IV) often is effective in the treatment of digoxin-induced arrhythmias because it increases the sinoatrial node conduction rate and reduces automaticity. Lidocaine does not affect atrial activity but will suppress ventricular automaticity, and so may be effective in the treatment of ventricular tachyarrhythmias.[735,841] Synchronized cardioversion may convert ventricular tachycardia to refractory fibrillation,[365] so it should not be performed.

When renal function is reduced, digoxin excretion is impaired and toxicity may develop more readily. The digoxin level may remain elevated long after the digoxin therapy is stopped in these patients, so support of cardiorespiratory function may be required for several days.

Digoxin excretion is not improved by the administration of furosemide (or other diuretics), exchange transfusion, or dialysis. Hemoperfusion using activated charcoal has had limited effect because the digoxin usually is distributed and bound extensively in tissue.[356,365]

Life-threatening digoxin toxicity associated with malignant arrhythmias, hypotension, and poor systemic perfusion is treated with digoxin-specific Fab antibody fragments.[507] This antibody binds serum digoxin, rendering it inactive.[365] The dose of Fab provided is determined by the total body exposure to digoxin, which can be estimated from the digoxin level or the amount of digoxin ingested (for formulas, see Table 8-7 or package insert). In general, approximately 40 mg of purified digoxin-specific Fab will bind approximately 0.5 mg of digoxin.[507] Note that digoxin elixir is considered to be absorbed totally, while digoxin tablets generally are calculated to be 80% absorbed.

Parent Instruction. If the parents will be administering digoxin at home, the parents must be taught how to administer the drug. In addition, the parents must be taught what to do if a dose is omitted or if the child vomits after the medication is administered. It is usually helpful to provide the parents with a specific approximate administration schedule; for example, the digoxin may be given at 8 AM and 8 PM. If the morning or evening dose is forgotten, but remembered by 12 noon or midnight, respectively, it may be given. However, if the drug is forgotten and not remembered until after 12 noon or midnight, that dose should be omitted and should not be "made up" in subsequent doses. If the parents are unsure whether a specific dose was administered, that dose should be omitted. If the child vomits after receiving the digoxin, the dose probably should not be repeated because it is difficult to predict how much of the drug was absorbed before regurgitation.

Parents should be taught to contact the child's physician or on-call provider if more than one dose of digoxin is omitted or if the child appears ill for any reason, because digoxin toxicity may be present. Parents are typically not taught to count the child's pulse routinely before administration of digoxin doses, because this focuses attention on specific numbers rather than on overall assessment of the child, and it can increase the parents' anxiety. Monitoring of heart rate does not ensure better detection of digoxin toxicity than that resulting from general evaluation of the child's condition.

The parents should be aware that a digoxin overdose may cause serious arrhythmias or death. Digoxin must be kept out of reach of children, and the medication bottle should have a "child-proof" cap.

Improvement in Cardiac Function: Additional Inotropic Agents. Several inotropic agents may effectively improve myocardial contractility during the treatment of congestive heart failure. Dopamine, dobutamine, and epinephrine are adrenergic agonists that may be titrated to provide beta-1 sympathomimetic effects (increased heart rate, atrioventricular conduction velocity, and ventricular contractility). Each of these drugs also may produce peripheral vascular effects that must be considered during drug selection and administration. An additional nonadrenergic inodilator, milrinone, improves myocardial contractility by inhibition of phosphodiesterase, so that intracellular effects of circulating catecholamines are prolonged. (For further information see Shock, Chapter 6.)

Vasodilator Therapy. Vasodilator therapy may improve myocardial function by altering both ventricular preload and afterload. Ventricular preload is reduced as a result of venodilation and displacement of blood volume into venous capacitance vessels. Ventricular afterload is reduced as a result of arterial dilation; in addition, ventricular wall stress decreases when ventricular chamber size is reduced. When vasodilator therapy is provided, the patient's ventricular compliance curve is altered, so that higher ventricular end-diastolic volume (and ultimately, stroke volume) is present at lower ventricular end-diastolic pressure (see Fig. 8-13 earlier in chapter).

Obviously the beneficial effects of vasodilators must be balanced with the potential detrimental effects of reduction in venous return and the potential fall in blood pressure. The hypovolemic patient is particularly likely to become hypotensive during vasodilator therapy. Volume expanders always should be readily available during the initial administration of these drugs.

No vasodilator is a pure arterial or venous dilator. However, these drugs often are classified by their primary sites of action. Vasodilators that dilate both arteries and veins include nitroprusside, phentolamine, prazosin, captopril, and nifedipine. Predominant arterial dilators include hydralazine and minoxidil. The most common venodilator is nitroglycerin. For further information about the dose, administration, and effects of these vasodilators the reader is referred to Shock in Chapter 6.

Angiotensin Converting Enzyme (ACE) Inhibitors. Angiotensin-converting-enzyme (ACE) inhibitors block the conversion of angiotensin I to angiotensin II, resulting in potent vasodilation. ACE inhibitors also block the breakdown of bradykinin,

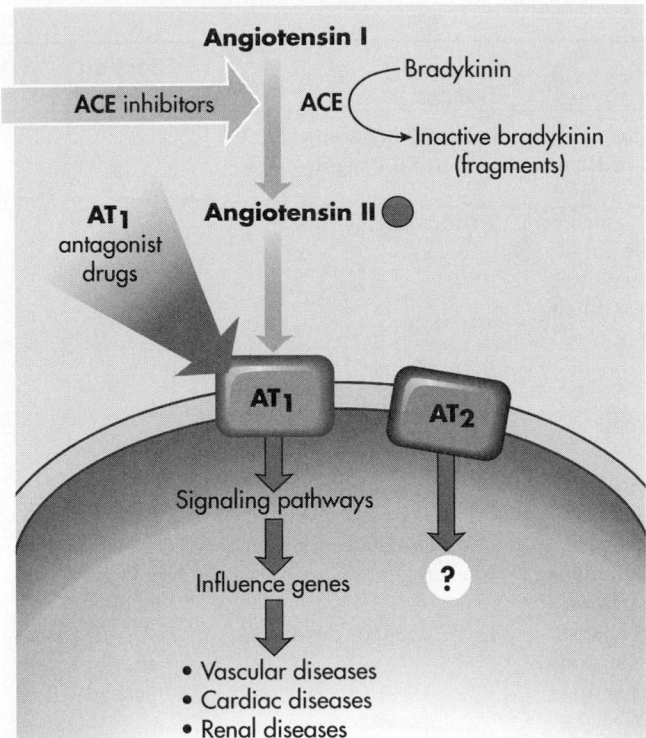

FIG. 8-14 Angiotensins and their receptors, AT1 and AT2. Blocking the angiotensin-converting enzyme (ACE) with ACE inhibitors decreases the amount of angiotensin II. Blocking the receptor AT1 with drugs (AT1 antagonists) blocks the attachment of angiotensin II to the cell, preventing the cellular effects and decreasing the vascular, cardiac, and renal effects. (From McCance KL, Huether SE: *Pathophysiology: The biologic basis for disease in adults and children,* ed 6. St Louis, Mosby, 2009.)

a powerful vasodilator, so it prolongs bradykinin action and augments afterload reduction (Fig. 8-14). In patients with left-to-right shunt lesions, reduction in systemic vascular resistance promotes blood flow into the systemic circulation rather than shunting to the pulmonary vascular bed.[552]

ACE inhibitors also inhibit ventricular remodeling modulated by angiotensin II, thereby preventing the development of ventricular hypertrophy.[697] Ultimately, these drugs have been shown to reduce mortality in adults with CHF and in children with dilated cardiomyopathy.[530,829,850,861] Side effects include hypotension, cough, hyperkalemia, headache, dizziness, fatigue, nausea, and renal impairment.

Careful monitoring of hemodynamic status should be carried out in all patients with CHF when ACE inhibitors are started, because compromised cardiac output increases the risk of significant hypotension. Initial doses of ACE inhibitors are purposely low and then titrated upward to achieve maximal therapeutic effect.

Angiotensin Receptor Blockers. Because of other conversion pathways, ACE inhibitors do not completely prevent the formation of angiotensin II. Therefore, angiotensin receptor blockers (ARBs) are useful for patients who develop side effects from ACE inhibitors. Specifically, the cough associated with ACE inhibitors is caused by elevated bradykinin levels. Because ARBs do not affect bradykinin metabolism, ARBs are a logical choice when this particular side effect is observed (see Table 8-8). Although the benefits of ARBs in adults with heart failure are well described, there is limited information regarding use of ARBs in children with heart failure. Losartan has been used safely in children with Marfan syndrome[113] and is the subject of a current multicenter trial.

Reduction in Intravascular Volume: Diuretic Therapy. Limitation of fluid intake and improvement in systemic perfusion and blood distribution may increase renal perfusion sufficiently in the child with congestive heart failure to prompt a diuresis. However, administration of diuretics is often necessary to aid in the elimination of excess intravascular fluid (Table 8-9).

The most common diuretics used in children are the *loop diuretics.* These drugs block sodium and chloride reabsorption in the ascending limb of the loop of Henle, so that diuresis occurs. However, the increased sodium and chloride excretion may produce hyponatremia and hypochloremia. Potassium excretion in the distal nephron is also typically enhanced by these diuretics, so hypokalemia also may develop.

Hypochloremic or hypokalemic metabolic alkalosis is a significant potential complication of loop-diuretic therapy because either hypokalemia or hypochloremia will enhance renal hydrogen ion excretion and bicarbonate reabsorption. Significant metabolic alkalosis is treated by replacement of potassium and chloride losses. Hypochloremia must be treated effectively because it will prevent sodium excretion and compromise the effectiveness of diuretic therapy. If metabolic

Table 8-8 Angiotensin-Converting Enzyme (ACE) Inhibitors and Angiotensin-Receptor Blockers (ARBs)

A. ANGIOTENSIN-CONVERTING ENZYME INHIBITORS			
Name	Equivalent Daily Dose	Starting Dosage	Maximum Daily Dosage
Captopril	50 mg	0.15-0.3 mg/kg per dose BID-QID	6 mg/kg per day; max. 450 mg
Enalapril	5 mg	0.1 mg/kg divided BID	0.5 mg/kg; max. 40 mg
Lisinopril	10 mg	0.07-0.1 mg/kg once daily; max. starting dose: 5 mg	0.5 mg/kg; max. 40 mg

B. ANGIOTENSIN RECEPTOR BLOCKERS		
Name	Starting Dosage	Maximum Daily Dosage
Losartan	>6 years: 0.7 mg/kg daily; max 50 mg	1.4 mg/kg; max 100 mg
Valsartan	>6 years: 1.3 mg/kg daily; max 40 mg	2.7 mg/kg; max 160 mg

Table 8-9 Diuretic Therapy for Children

Drug (Trade Name)	Peak Effect	Action	Dosage	Effect on Serum [K⁺]
Bumetanide (Bumex)	15-30 min IV 1-2 h PO	Inhibits sodium reabsorption in ascending limb of the loop of Henle; also blocks chloride reabsorption	0.025-0.5 mg/dose every 6 h IV 0.5-1.0 mg/dose PO	↓↓↓
Chlorothiazide (Diuril)	2-4 h	Inhibits tubular reabsorption of sodium primarily in the distal tubule but also in the loop of Henle; also inhibits water reabsorption in cortical diluting segment of ascending limp of loop	20-40 mg/kg per day PO	↓↓
Ethacrynic acid (Edecrin)	5-10 min IV ½-8 h PO	Same as furosemide (below)	1-2 mg/kg per IV dose 2-3 mg/kg per PO dose	↓↓↓
Furosemide (Lasix)	5-20 min IV 1-2 h PO	Inhibits sodium chloride transport in ascending limb of loop of Henle and in proximal and distal tubules	1-2 mg/kg per IV dose 1-4 mg/kg per PO dose	↓↓↓
Hydrochlorothiazide (Hydrodiuril)	2-4 h	Inhibits sodium reabsorption in distal tubule and loop of Henle and inhibits water reabsorption in cortical diluting segment of ascending limb of loop	2-3 mg/kg per day PO given in two divided doses (every 12 h)	↓↓
Hydrochlorothiazide plus Spironolactone (Aldactazide)	2-4 h (prolonged effects)	Hydrochlorothiazide functions as noted above. The spironolactone functions as an aldosterone antagonist and inhibits exchange of sodium for potassium in distal tubule.	1.65-3.3 mg/kg per day PO	— (K⁺ remains approximately unchanged)
Metolazone (Zaroxolyn)	2 h (prolonged effects)	Inhibits sodium reabsorption at the cortical diluting site and in the proximal convoluted tubule. Results in approximately equal excretion of sodium and chloride ions. May increase potassium excretion as a result of increased delivery of sodium to distal tubule (and Na-K exchange)	0.5-2.5 mg per day PO given in divided doses (every 12 h)	↓↓
Nesiritide (Natrecor)	15 min	Recombinant BNP; causes inhibition of rennin-angiotensin system, natriuresis	1 mcg/kg bolus followed by continuous infusion of 0.005-0.02 mcg/kg per minute	No change
Spironolactone (Aldactone)	1-4 days (prolonged effects)	Aldosterone antagonist; inhibits exchange of sodium for potassium in distal tubule	1.3-3.3 mg/kg per day PO	K⁺ is "saved"

alkalosis persists, administration of ammonium chloride (75 mg/kg per day in divided doses) or acetazolamide (Diamox—a carbonic anhydrase inhibitor, administered 5 mg/kg PO or IV once daily) may be indicated.[668]

Electrolyte and acid-base balance must be monitored closely during diuretic therapy. Concurrent administration of a potassium-sparing diuretic may prevent hypokalemia.

Ototoxicity is a potential complication of these diuretics. In addition, the child's renal function should be monitored closely; these drugs usually are not administered if the blood urea nitrogen (BUN) and creatinine levels rise significantly.

Furosemide (Lasix). Furosemide is the most popular loop diuretic. It acts rapidly when administered intravenously (within 5-10 min), and it usually results in significant diuresis. Generally an intravenous dose of 1 mg/kg is effective,

although the dose may be doubled (or more) in children with severe heart failure who require chronic diuretic therapy. Furosemide also may be administered intramuscularly for rapid action, provided the child's systemic perfusion is adequate. Oral furosemide is administered in doses of 1 to 2 mg/kg when less acute diuresis is required (peak action: 1-2 h). This drug should not be administered to children who are allergic to sulfonamides.

Bumetanide (Bumex). This diuretic is extremely potent at doses much smaller (approximately 0.025-0.5 mg/kg IV, PO, or IM every 12 hours) than those required for furosemide. It has a relatively rapid onset of action (approximately 10 minutes), and it has actions similar to furosemide at the loop of Henle. In addition, bumetanide may produce renal and peripheral vasodilation, so that the glomerular filtration rate increases temporarily. This drug also may cause ototoxicity, and diuretic effects can be blunted with concomitant administration of indomethacin. Cross-sensitivity to bumetanide may occur in patients with sulfonamide allergy.

Ethacrynic Acid (Edecrin). This drug is similar in action to furosemide, with a rapid onset of action (1-2 mg/kg IV, slowly). However, it is prescribed less commonly for children because it is associated with a high incidence of gastrointestinal side effects. There is a significant incidence of ototoxicity with pediatric administration of this drug.

Thiazides and Chlorothiazide. Additional diuretics act at the cortical diluting segment, preventing sodium chloride (and water) reabsorption. These drugs include the thiazides, which may be utilized for less acute diuresis. Potassium loss and hypokalemia may result from these diuretics, but not to the degree seen with loop diuretics.

Chlorothiazide (Diuril) is the most popular of the pediatric thiazide diuretics. It is administered orally (20-40 mg/kg over 24 h in divided doses) and has a peak effect within 2 to 4 hours.

Metolazone (Zaroxolyn). This drug also works by blocking sodium chloride and water reabsorption at the cortical diluting segments. It may be particularly effective when administered with furosemide. Relatively small doses (0.5-2.5 mg/kg per day, orally) are usually effective, with a rapid (2-h) onset of action. This drug may produce hepatic dysfunction.

Aldosterone Inhibitors. Aldosterone inhibition also produces diuresis. This prevents sodium reabsorption and inhibits potassium and hydrogen ion loss. These drugs also are known as "potassium-sparing" drugs because potassium loss is minimal; they should not be administered to patients with hyperkalemia. The effects of these drugs are gradual and do not peak for several days; for this reason it is important to anticipate the need for dosage adjustments. If the child is discharged during diuretic therapy, fluid and electrolyte balances should be well regulated before discharge.

Spironolactone (Aldactone) may be administered once daily (1.3-3.3 mg/kg per day orally) and will produce effective diuresis within 1 to 4 days. It is most effective when administered in conjunction with another diuretic that has a different site of renal action. It is often used to counteract the potassium loss brought on by loop diuretics. In addition to its diuretic properties, it is known to have a protective effect for adults with severe congestive heart failure, reducing mortality by up to 30%, and hospitalization rates by up to 35%.[704]

Hydrochlorothiazide and spironolactone (Aldactazide) is a combination of diuretics with differing sites of action that may provide extremely effective diuresis on a chronic basis. The potassium-sparing properties of the spironolactone component may prevent the development of hypokalemia. The dose is similar to spironolactone (1.65-3.3 mg/kg per day). Because this drug has a gradual onset and provides diuresis only several days after beginning therapy, it may be necessary to taper concurrent administration of other (short-acting) drugs.

Nesiritide (Natrecor). Nesiritide is the recombinant form of BNP, the 32 amino acid polypeptide, released from ventricular myocardium. It produces vasodilation and diuresis.

Because of reports of increased renal dysfunction and mortality in adult patients, its use is restricted to intravenous administration for patients in decompensated, severe heart failure with dyspnea at rest. It appears to be well-tolerated in pediatric patients, though hypotension and arrhythmias can occur.[555]

Nursing Implications. When the child receives diuretics it is important for the nurse to monitor the effectiveness of therapy and assess the child carefully for evidence of complications. The precise time of diuretic administration should be noted on the child's medication record and flow sheet, and the timing and quantity of the child's diuretic response also must be noted. It may be helpful to highlight the diuretic response in the nursing record so that it is identified easily. The physician or on-call care provider should be notified immediately if the child fails to respond to a previously effective dose because this may indicate worsening of heart failure (or low cardiac output) or development of renal failure.

Throughout diuretic therapy the child's fluid balance and hydration must be monitored closely. If the child's cardiovascular function is extremely unstable, diuresis may produce acute hypovolemia and a compromise in systemic perfusion. In addition, aggressive diuretic therapy may result in undesirable hemoconcentration.

When the child's congestive heart failure is severe, absorption of and response to oral diuretics may not be satisfactory. It may be necessary to switch to parenteral administration of the drugs until systemic perfusion and gastrointestinal function improve.

Electrolyte balance, particularly serum potassium and chloride ion concentrations, must be monitored during diuretic therapy. Because hypokalemia can potentiate digoxin toxicity, it should be prevented in these children. Potassium replacement of 1 to 4 mEq/kg per day should be sufficient to maintain serum potassium levels of 3.5 to 4.5 mEq/L, despite increased urinary potassium loss. As noted above, potassium-sparing drugs should not be administered in the presence of hyperkalemia, and potassium supplementation should be tapered accordingly when these drugs are added. Acid-base balance also should be monitored, and metabolic alkalosis should be prevented or treated.

If diuretics are administered late in the evening, diuresis may result in sleep disruption (either the child awakens to void, or awakens during diaper or bed-linen change) unless a urinary catheter is in place. Therefore, unless the child's heart failure is severe, some adjustment in scheduling of the evening diuretic dose should be made so that the child experiences diuresis before bedtime.

Parental teaching is required if the child is to receive diuretic therapy at home. Such information should include the technique of administration, potential effects of drug toxicity, flexibility (or lack of it) in administration schedule, and indications for contacting a healthcare provider. If supplementary potassium chloride administration is required the importance of the supplement must be emphasized.

Beta-Adrenergic Blockade. Activation of the sympathetic nervous system and release of catecholamines normally increases cardiac output in acutely ill patients. However, in the setting of chronic congestive heart failure, chronic adrenergic stimulation leads to alterations in myocardial excitation-contraction, gene expression, and eventually, ventricular remodeling and fibrosis.[109,441,748] Beta-blockers prevent these maladaptive changes, while also having antiarrhythmic properties, inducing coronary vasodilation and slowing heart rate.[121,792]

Metoprolol. Metoprolol, a selective beta-1 receptor antagonist, has been shown to be very effective in adults with congestive heart failure.[377,794] Metoprolol improves ejection fraction in children with dilated cardiomyopathy, but sometimes is not well tolerated.[261]

Carvedilol. Carvedilol is a nonselective beta-blocker and alpha-1 blocker. It is gaining acceptance as first line beta-blockade therapy in children with dilated cardiomyopathy. It, too, has been shown to be effective in adults with congestive heart failure,[678] as well as in small case series of pediatric patients. A recent randomized controlled trial showed no difference between carvedilol and placebo, but the study may have been underpowered to show a difference.[793] Subgroup analyses found that single ventricle patients of left ventricular morphology respond better than those of non-LV morphology. A distinguishing feature of carvedilol is its antioxidant activity, which limits both apoptosis (cell death) and cell proliferation (hypertrophy).[32] Similar to ACE inhibitors, carvedilol can cause hypotension and so is started at low doses and cautiously titrated upward. Initial dosing is 0.05 to 0.1 mg/kg per dose given twice daily and is gradually adjusted upward to 0.2 to 0.4 mg/kg per dose twice/day, with a maximum dose of 25 mg.

Fluid Therapy and Nutrition. Accurate measurement and recording of the child's daily weight and intake and output is imperative when congestive heart failure is present. The child should be weighed on the same scale (or in the bed) at the same time of day (preferably by the same nurse) so that weight gain or loss can be evaluated. Significant weight changes (greater than 50 g/24 h in infants, 200 g/24 h in children, or 500 g/24 h in adolescents) should be verified and reported to the on-call provider.

Normal urine output in children should average 1.0 to 2.0 mL/kg body weight per hour if fluid intake is adequate. Sources of fluid loss that are not measured, such as excessive diaphoresis during fever or periods of increased respiratory rate, also should be considered. If a urinary catheter is not in place, all diapers and draw-sheets or pads must be weighed before and after use. One gram of weight increase resulting from urine is counted as 1 mL of urine output.

All sources of fluid intake and output must be totaled to evaluate the child's fluid status and the effectiveness of diuresis. If IV catheters are in place, total IV and oral fluid intake must be considered. Fluids required to flush IV or arterial catheters, to dilute medications, or to obtain cardiac output measurements are often sources of unrecognized fluid intake for the child.

During diuretic therapy the nurse must assess clinical signs of the child's fluid balance. The *hypovolemic* child characteristically demonstrates urine output of less than 0.5 mL/kg body weight per hour and has dry skin and mucous membranes, a flat or sunken fontanelle (in infants less than 18 months of age), and decreased or normal tearing; the child may demonstrate weight loss. The child's central venous or pulmonary artery wedge pressure is usually low when hypovolemia is present, although congestive heart failure or cardiac dysfunction may cause increased systemic and pulmonary venous pressures.

The child with *hypervolemia* usually demonstrates signs and symptoms of systemic and/or pulmonary venous congestion. The central venous and/or pulmonary artery wedge pressure is elevated, and the child usually gains weight. In addition, the child's mucous membranes are moist, and periorbital edema and hepatomegaly usually are noted. If an endotracheal tube is in place, it may be necessary to suction the child's airway more frequently as a result of copious pulmonary secretions.

Infants with congestive heart failure often do not tolerate oral feedings. Small, frequent feedings are usually more successful than infrequent, larger ones. If the infant is breathing faster than 60 times/min or is requiring nearly an hour to ingest 1 to 2 oz of formula, it may be better to provide tube feedings (see section, Altered Nutrition and Potential Gastrointestinal Complications in this chapter and section, Enteral and Parenteral Alimentation in Chapter 14) until the heart failure has improved; continued attempts at oral feedings may cause the infant to use *more* calories breathing and feeding than the child can possibly ingest. The child's daily caloric maintenance requirements should be calculated (Table 8-10), and the nurse should consult with the on-call provider or nutrition therapist if the child's caloric intake is inadequate.

Restriction of fluid intake is often required if heart failure is severe (see Table 8-11 for the formulas necessary for the estimation of daily fluid requirements). If an infant is vigorously demanding more oral fluids than the amount allowed, the nurse should discuss with the healthcare team the possibility of increasing the oral intake and diuretic therapy proportionally.

If congestive heart failure is severe or chronic, consult with the dietician when providing instructions for nutrition after discharge. Low-sodium infant formulas (such as Similac PM 60/40) are available, but their increased cost should be considered when deciding if the infant requires the formula for home

Table 8-10	Calculation of Pediatric Daily Caloric Requirements
Age	**Daily Requirements* (kcal/kg)**
High-risk neonate	120-150
Normal neonate	100-120
1-2 y	90-100
2-6 y	80-90
7-9 y	70-80
10-12 y	50-60

*Ill children (with disease, surgery, fever, or pain) may require additional calories above the maintenance value, and comatose children may require fewer calories (because of lack of movement).

Table 8-11 Formulas for Estimating Daily Maintenance Fluid and Electrolyte Requirements for Children

	Daily Requirements	Hourly Requirements
Fluid Requirements Estimated from Weight*		
Newborn (up to 72 hr after birth)	60-100 mL/kg (newborns are born with excess body water)	–
Up to 10 kg	100 mL/kg (can increase up to 150 mL/kg to provide caloric requirements if renal and cardiac function are adequate)	4 mL/kg
11-20 kg	1000 mL for the first 10 kg + 50 mL/kg for each kg over 10 kg	40 mL for first 10 kg + 2 mL/kg for each kg over 10 kg
21-30 kg	1500 mL for the first 20 kg + 25 mL/kg for each kg over 20 kg	60 mL for first 20 kg + 1 mL/kg for each kg over 20 kg
Fluid Requirements Estimated from Body Surface Area (BSA)		
Maintenance	1500 mL/m^2 BSA	–
Insensible losses	300-400 mL/m^2 BSA	–
Electrolytes		
Sodium (Na)	2-4 mEq/kg	–
Potassium (K)	1-2 mEq/kg	–
Chloride (Cl)	2-3 mEq/kg	–
Calcium (Ca)	0.5-3 mEq/kg	–
Phosphorous (Phos)	0.5-2 mmol/kg	–
Magnesium (Mg)	0.4-0.9 mEq/kg	–

*The "maintenance" fluids calculated by these formulas must only be used as a starting point to determine the fluid requirements of an individual patient. If intravascular volume is adequate, children with cardiac, pulmonary, or renal failure or increased intracranial pressure should generally receive less than these calculated "maintenance" fluids. The formula utilizing body weight generally results in a generous "maintenance" fluid total.

care. The child with chronic congestive heart failure should avoid excessively salty foods, such as bacon, ham, sausage, potato chips, and some soft drinks are to be avoided if the child is requiring diuretic therapy. If a low-sodium diet is absolutely necessary for an older child, the child and the child's primary caretaker must be included in the dietary planning.

Comfort Measures and Thermoregulation. The child with congestive heart failure usually is most comfortable if placed in the semi-Fowler or sitting position so that abdominal contents can drop away from the diaphragm; this allows maximal diaphragm excursion and lung expansion. In addition, placement of a small linen roll under the child's shoulders extends the child's airway and may help the child to breathe with less difficulty.

The child's environment should be kept as quiet as possible to reduce stimulation and encourage rest. The nurse must decide when and how to consolidate nursing care so that the child is allowed periods of uninterrupted sleep yet excessive stimulation is avoided.

Premature infants and neonates with little subcutaneous fat have more difficulty maintaining body temperature when environmental temperature is low. In addition, the neonate's oxygen requirements are increased when the environmental temperature is excessively warm or cold. The "neutral thermal environment" is that environmental temperature at which the neonate maintains a rectal temperature of 37° C with the lowest oxygen consumption. In the critical care unit, a warm environmental temperature is maintained with overbed warmers.

The nurse is responsible for maintaining an appropriate environmental temperature while the infant is in the unit or during diagnostic tests or transport. When an overbed warmer

is used, the infant's insensible fluid loss is increased by approximately 40% to 50%.

Transfusion Therapy to Treat Severe Anemia. If severe congestive heart failure is produced by anemia, improvement in arterial oxygen-carrying capacity through transfusion is usually necessary. This transfusion therapy improves arterial oxygen content, so that oxygen transport can be maintained without the need for an extremely high cardiac output. However, transfusion therapy must be performed with caution when anemia is profound or compensated because hypervolemia may develop and worsen symptoms of congestive heart failure.

Packed red blood cells usually are administered to children with *chronic severe anemia* at a rate of approximately 3 mL/kg per hour. This transfusion rate should be sufficiently gradual so that hypervolemia and worsening of congestive heart failure are avoided. Concurrent administration of a diuretic usually is required. If severe congestive heart failure is already present, a partial exchange transfusion will enable simultaneous removal of red cell-poor blood and replacement with packed red blood cells. Immune-mediated hemolytic anemia may not respond to transfusion therapy; steroid administration or splenectomy may be necessary for these patients (see Anemia, in Chapter 15).

Evaluation of Therapy. The nurse must be aware of the signs and symptoms of increasing heart failure, including continued tachycardia, increased peripheral vasoconstriction, decreased urine output, increased hepatomegaly, and increased respiratory rate and effort. Some of these symptoms may be noted easily by monitoring trends in the vital signs and record of intake and output. However, hepatomegaly and respiratory distress may be described less specifically. It is helpful to

Box 8-10	**Advanced Concepts: Resynchronization Therapy for the Treatment of CHF**

Biventricular pacing and cardiac resynchronization therapy have been shown to be effective in adults with heart failure and prolonged QRS duration of left bundle branch block morphology.[963] The purpose is to restore a more synchronized, "efficient" cardiac contraction in those patients in whom interruption of the ventricular conduction system has caused asynchronous activation and uncoordinated beating of the heart. In pediatric patients, cardiac resynchronization can be successful in decreasing QRS duration, and improving ejection fraction, and ultimately improving NYHA heart failure classification.

mark the edge of the liver at the beginning of the day (with another nurse or provider present to validate) so that changes in liver size can be recognized easily throughout the day. Location and severity of any existing retractions always should be recorded with the vital signs so that an increase in respiratory distress will be apparent to even a new nurse caring for the child.

Care of the child with congestive heart failure requires careful monitoring of clinical condition and careful titration of therapy to maximize therapeutic effects and minimize side effects. Advanced concepts in management of congestive heart failure are included in Box 8-10.

LOW CARDIAC OUTPUT (SHOCK)

This topic is so important to critical care that information was expanded into an entire chapter, Shock, Cardiac Arrest, and Resuscitation (Chapter 6). Postoperative low cardiac output is also addressed in Postoperative Care, later in this chapter.

ALTERED NUTRITION AND POTENTIAL GASTROINTESTINAL COMPLICATIONS

Nancy Rudd

Nutritional challenges are frequently encountered by those caring for critically ill infants and children with cardiac disease. Growth failure is a well-recognized and challenging consequence of congenital heart disease with type and severity of cardiac defect determining the impact on nutritional status and growth. This section reviews the etiology and development of altered nutrition and management strategies. In addition, it summarizes specific gastrointestinal and feeding challenges common to the care of children with cardiovascular problems. The problems addressed include necrotizing enterocolitis, protein-losing enteropathy, chylous effusion, mesenteric arteritis, and vocal cord injury. These conditions and specific nutritional therapy to address each issue are summarized in this section.

Etiology, Pathophysiology and Identification of Growth Failure in Patients with Congenital Heart Disease

Growth failure in children with CHD is multifactoral. A relationship exists between inadequate growth and abnormal hemodynamics in infancy. Physiologic alterations that impact

growth include congestive heart failure, cyanosis, and pulmonary hypertension. The type of cardiac lesion present and the severity of hemodynamic impairment also play a role in the undernutrition of infants with CHD.[9]

The pathology of growth failure in the setting of *congestive heart failure* (CHF) is complex. The diagnosis of CHF often correlates with clinical findings of tachypnea, hepatomegaly, and tachycardia. Growth disturbances are a consequence of increased myocardial and respiratory work, inadequate caloric intake because of anorexia or fatigability during feeding, increased metabolic rate from increased work of breathing, and alterations in gastrointestinal function and absorption. The presence of significant right heart volume overload from left to right intracardiac shunting is a major factor in the development of CHF. Tachypnea results from excessive pulmonary blood flow as seen with cardiac defects resulting in left to right shunting lesions. This increased work of breathing can lead to difficulty for the infant's coordination of sucking, swallowing, and breathing with the result that oral intake is inadequate.

Decreased gastric capacity is caused by pressure on the stomach from an enlarged, congested liver resulting from systemic congestion. Any delay in gastric emptying may predispose the infant to gastroesophageal reflux or may result in premature satiety. Elevated right atrial and systemic venous pressures can cause intestinal protein losses and fat malabsorption from elevated venous pressure in the mesenteric bed. Gastrointestinal perfusion is reduced by catecholamine-mediated redistribution of blood flow away from skin, gut, and kidney to maintain adequate brain and heart perfusion.

Lesions with potential for excessive pulmonary blood flow, increased pulmonary artery pressure, increased blood return to the left heart, and elevation of left ventricular end-diastolic pressure result in high output hemodynamics and can cause hypermetabolism. Lesions with a large left-to-right shunt typically affect weight rather than height in the early stages of infancy. Cardiac lesions that commonly result in CHF in the neonate include hypoplastic left heart syndrome (HLHS), transposition of the great arteries (TGA), patent ductus arteriosus (PDA), total anomalous pulmonary venous return (TAPVR, particularly if associated with obstructed venous return), critical aortic stenosis (AS) or pulmonary stenosis (PS), coarctation of the aorta (CoA) or other obstruction to left heart or aortic flow, and large ventricular septal defect (VSD).

The role of *cyanosis* as a cause of growth failure in children with CHD is unclear. Arterial oxygen desaturation alone does not necessarily result in tissue hypoxia, because tissue aerobic metabolism may not be impaired until arterial PaO_2 falls below 30 mm Hg. In addition, arterial oxygen content and tissue oxygenation may be preserved at near-normal levels if oxygen carrying capacity is increased by elevated hemoglobin.

If hypoxemia and CHF are both present, growth is most severely affected and results in reduced height and weight. Hypoxemia and edema may induce gastroparesis and gut hypomotility. Some have theorized that the duration of hypoxemia in years, not the severity of hypoxemia, plays a significant role in growth retardation.[746] Lesions often resulting in the combination of cyanosis and CHF include double outlet right ventricle (DORV), pulmonary atresia (PA), tricuspid atresia (TA), and hypoplastic left heart syndrome (HLHS).

The presence *of pulmonary hypertension* also plays a critical role in growth disturbances in infants with both cyanotic and acyanotic CHD. Increased resting oxygen consumption has been demonstrated in patients with pulmonary hypertension. In one study, the presence of pulmonary hypertension appeared to be the most significant factor identified in growth impairment in infants with CHD; the combination of cyanosis and pulmonary hypertension had the most severe impact on growth.[907]

Other perioperative factors contributing to growth failure include fever and sepsis. Fever alone can increase the caloric expenditure 12% for each degree Celsius reached above 37°. Sepsis and its resulting influence on energy consumption and increased autonomic tone can increase caloric expenditure 25% to 50%.[566] Gastrointestinal infections such as *Clostridium difficile* and rotavirus can also compromise the child's nutritional status.

Each of these physiologic alterations impacts the ability of a child with hemodynamically significant heart disease to match nutrient intake with metabolic demands. Undernutrition occurs when energy expenditure combined with nutrient losses exceed that of nutrient intake and absorption. There are six classes of nutrients that impact an infant's diet and thus growth: carbohydrates, fats, proteins, vitamins, minerals, and water. All six play an important role in maintaining an optimal nutritional state. However, only three yield energy for the body's use. These three are termed energy nutrients and include carbohydrates, fats, and proteins.

During the first 6 months of life for the *healthy* infant, the suggested level of intake for energy is 91-112 kcal(calories) per kg of body weight to maintain adequate body temperature, growth and activity. Protein needs during infancy are relatively high as a result of rapid skeletal and muscle growth, and average 1.5 g of protein per kilogram of body weight. A neonate weighing less than 3 kg typically requires 120 mL/kg per day of fluids and a 3- to 10-kg infant typically requires 100 mL/kg per day of fluids for maintenance fluid requirements; of course, these requirements must be tailored to the clinical condition.

The infant and child with heart disease may have greater than normal requirements yet have less than normal ability to consume the calories and proper fluid intake. Infants with hemodynamically significant CHD require significantly more nutritional support to sustain growth than their healthy counterparts. Fluid losses in a neonate with congestive heart failure are estimated to be 10% to 15% greater than those of a normal infant because of tachypnea, emesis, diarrhea, and anticongestive management with diuretics. Energy intake required in infants with CHD to sustain normal growth is reported to be between 130 and 150 kcal (calories)/kg per day, and is affected by the type of cardiac lesion and "catch-up" growth needed. Some infants can require as much as 175 to 180 kcal/kg per day.[746] Currently, there are no established growth parameters for infants with hemodynamically significant CHD. Current practice targets a weight gain of 10 to 30 g/day when adequate calories are provided.

Protein balance is another key factor in the management of most infants with CHD because serum protein imbalance may play a role in the development of edema. It is important to ensure adequate protein intake and adequate serum protein in this patient population by monitoring serum albumin, transferrin, or prealbumin levels.

Increased metabolic rate or *energy expenditure* contributes to growth failure particularly when CHF is present. Hypermetabolism is likely related to increased work of respiratory muscles necessary for adequate ventilation in the presence of decreased lung compliance. The basal metabolic rate is elevated in infants with CHD because of cardiac and respiratory work and has been reported to be as much as three to five times higher than the work in infants without heart disease. The presence of dilated or hypertrophied cardiac muscle also increases oxygen consumption. Hypertrophied cardiac muscle uses 20% to 30% of the body's total oxygen consumption instead of the typical 10%.

Nutrient losses also play a role in cardiac undernutrition. Malabsorption significantly limits an infant's tolerance of feedings, compromises the neonate's ability to maximize caloric intake, and decreases nutrient absorption. As noted, nutrient intake is also compromised by altered gastric capacity in the presence of hepatomegaly and by edema of the intestinal wall and mucosal surfaces leading to impaired nutrient absorption. Consequently, the volume of enteral feeding, the caloric concentration, and the delivery time of bolus feedings may need to be adjusted.

Gastroesophageal reflux (GER) describes the movement of gastric contents back into the esophagus. The reflux can be "silent" or it may produce pain or discomfort with signs such as neck arching, coughing, swallowing, or emesis. GER can occur in up to 65% of healthy infants and as many as 40% to 50% of infants age 1-2 months have two episodes of reflux per day.[425] GER also plays a role in CHD. The role of GER in CHD seems most prevalent when the infant has a hemodynamically significant lesion and it likely results from delayed gastric emptying secondary to malabsorption. The presence of a nasogastric tube (NG) to supplement enteral feedings may contribute to GER symptoms because the tube may prevent closure of the gastroesophageal sphincter.

Inadequate *nutrient intake* is felt to be the predominant cause of growth failure in infants with CHD. Oral feeding requires more energy than any other infant activity. For a neonate with symptomatic heart disease, oral feeding can be compared to a "stress test." Tachypnea and resulting fatigue may not allow an infant to consume all of the calories and volume needed to maintain growth. Oral feeding is challenging because the neonate may feel hungry at the start of the feed, feed eagerly initially, then reach early satiety (so the infant stops feeding). The infant may use a lot of energy feeding and may tire quickly, resulting in suboptimal nutrient intake and increased energy expenditure. Other limiting factors include respiratory infections with resulting tachypnea that can impair an infant's coordination of sucking, swallowing and breathing necessary for successful oral feeding. Additional factors leading to inadequate caloric intake may relate to medical management strategies used to treat underlying cardiac pathology. Fluid restriction and anorexia resulting from diuretic use may limit enteral caloric intake.

The physical growth of infants is a direct reflection of their nutritional well-being and is the single most important parameter used in assessing their nutritional status. Assessments of growth are made by periodic determinations of weight, height, and head circumference. Growth charts for each parameter should be utilized to document and evaluate the infant's growth pattern.

Expected weight gain in a term infant during the first 6 months of life should average 20 to 30 g/day with variation based on gender, age in months, and growth percentile.[218] Incremental gain in crown-heel length for full-term infants averages 0.66 cm/week during the first 6 months of life. Healthy infants display rapid increases in head circumference and their head growth correlates well with brain growth. Average gain in head circumference for term infants between birth and 6 months of age is 0.33 cm/week.[480]

Poor nutritional status can negatively impact both preoperative and postoperative outcomes. Inadequate protein and calories can reduce skeletal muscle function and increase the risk of postoperative pneumonia. The immune system is also adversely affected by undernutrition; impaired nutrition can lead to an impaired immune state, predisposing an infant or child to postoperative infection or poor wound healing.

Several studies have focused on the importance of postsurgical nutrition in infants following repair or palliation. Research suggests that weight gain following neonatal surgery is often suboptimal and greater attention should be focused on nutrition in the postoperative period including rapid advancement of enteral feeding to promote optimal growth and nutritional status. One study demonstrated that rapid advancement of calories to higher concentrations significantly improved energy intake and weight gain (20 g/day gain in control group versus 35 g/day loss in the usual care group). In this study enteral feedings were advanced from 20 to 30 calories per ounce over just a 3-day span. Additionally, postoperative hospital stay for the intervention group of infants was significantly decreased.[701]

Management: Strategies to Optimize Nutrition and Growth

With knowledge of the multiple causes of growth deficiency, it is the responsibility of the healthcare team to make nutritional management a high priority in the care of infants and children with congenital heart disease. Many options are available to combat the harm nutritional deficiency can create. Discussion of these treatment options follows.

Gastroesophageal Reflux (GER). To address gastroesophageal reflux and malabsorption issues, several treatment modalities have been used. Smaller, more frequent feedings are recommended along with elevated supine positioning during and after feeding to reduce the reflux of gastric contents into the esophagus. In the past thickening of formula with dry rice cereal was suggested as a means of limiting GER but this practice is somewhat controversial. Although some studies have noted fewer episodes of emesis when thickened formula is introduced, others have shown an increase in gastric emptying time and thus longer interval when reflux episodes were possible. Commercial formulas with added rice have been marketed as a treatment option for infants with symptomatic GER.

Any decision regarding a trial of thickened formula should be left to the individual care provider. Prokinetic agents such as metoclopramide have been used to treat GER during infancy, but there is debate over their effectiveness. Introduction of an antisecretory or acid-neutralizing agent may help prevent erosive esophagitis. Surgical treatment options such as placement of jejunostomy tube, (to bypass the stomach), or the Nissen fundoplication should be reserved for severe GER that does not respond to aggressive medical therapy.

Parenteral Nutrition. Parenteral nutrition is indicated in infants with CHD when the projected time to establish adequate enteral support exceeds the infant's metabolic reserves. Such instances include postoperative patients when oral feedings are not anticipated to commence for more than 1 or 2 days, and infants requiring prolonged intubation, those with marked malnutrition prior to surgery, and infants with any coexisting gastrointestinal abnormalities such as duodenal atresia or gastroschisis.

If enteral nutrition is unlikely to be initiated for greater than 1 or 2 days, a central venous catheter should be placed. This allows maximum dextrose and protein concentrations in the parenteral nutrition as well as administration of intravenous lipid emulsions.[763] To prevent essential fatty acid deficiency, administration of 0.5 g/kg of a 20% lipid solution is needed three times per week.

Enteral Feeding. An important adjunct therapy to parenteral nutrition, when possible, is the use of trophic feeding. Continuous administration of formula or breastmilk at a rate of 0.5 to 2 mL/kg per hour uses the gastrointestinal tract and can lessen the risk of systemic bacterial infection by preventing complications related to intestinal mucosal atrophy and loss of functional intestinal barrier.

Enteral feedings are more physiologic and preferable to parenteral nutrition when gastrointestinal function is adequate. In addition, enteral feedings are more accessible, more cost effective, and safer. The goal of enteral therapies is to sustain growth or enable "catch-up" growth without overburdening cardiovascular function or disturbing fluid and electrolyte balance.

Catch-up growth refers to the velocity of growth following a time period of impaired growth (caused by undernutrition). The nutritional needs to achieve catch-up growth can be as high as 1½ to 2 times the required daily allowances for age.

The total energy expenditure in children with CHD is 22% to 29% greater than that of a healthy, age-matched child, so that caloric intake should be targeted. Optimizing caloric intake to meet increased energy needs may be accomplished enterally by increasing the quantity or volume of feedings or by increasing the caloric density of formula.

Once nutrient requirements have been estimated, an enteral feeding regimen should be determined. Most full-term infants receive breast-milk or a cow's milk-based formula. Soy and hydrolyzed casein formulas are reserved for infants who do not tolerate a milk-based formula. Oral is the preferred route for administration of enteral feeding whenever possible. An on-demand feeding regimen that provides adequate nutrients and results in appropriate weight gain is the optimal outcome. In the infant with CHD who successfully feeds on demand, it is not necessary to restrict or supplement enteral intake and standard formula at 20 cal/oz or 0.67 kcal (calorie)/mL is used.

Bottle feeding is often recommended for infants with CHD because it is speculated to be less strenuous than breastfeeding and the infant's intake can be measured more accurately. Studies in breastfed infants with CHD have included reports of higher oxygen saturations during feedings and more rapid weight gain than in bottle-fed infants.[818] The degree of hemodynamic impairment does not always correlate with an infant's ability to breastfeed. Therefore breastfeeding should not be excluded for infants with hemodynamically significant CHD. However, ad lib breastfeeding requires careful monitoring until evidence of adequate fluid intake and positive growth are demonstrated.[818] Infants being breastfed may be temporarily bottle-fed with expressed breast milk if adequate enteral intake is in question.

The normal diet of an infant consists of either breast milk or commercial formula (with no other supplement needed) for the first months of life. The chemical components found in both breast milk and formula provide two very important benefits; in addition to supplying energy they promote growth and repair of body tissue. Breast milk is low in protein (constituting about 6% of calories) and high in fat (constituting about 52% of calories), compared with formula (about 9% of calories from protein and about 49% from fat). However, the protein types contained in breast milk are more bioavailable than the proteins in formula, so breastmilk actually provides closer to 8% of calories from protein. Once a child is older than 1 year, a 1-kcal/mL formula should be substituted for standard infant formula. Commercially available formulas for this purpose include protein-based PediaSure, and amino-acid based EleCare or Vivonex.

The need to advance feedings to a total volume of 130 to 150 mL/kg per day and goal calories of 120 to 130 kcal/kg per day to achieve target growth is not uncommon in an infant with significant CHD. Noting frequency of emesis, diarrhea, or abdominal distension assists in monitoring for tolerance of enteral feeding. Daily weight, caloric intake, total fluid intake and output, along with laboratory studies are watched closely during the advancement of enteral feedings. If volume intolerance is a limiting factor in meeting caloric requirements, it may be necessary to increase the caloric density of the formula. The caloric density of standard 20 kcal/oz formula or breast milk can be increased to 24, 27, or even 30 kcal/oz by many methods. The simplest method of increasing calories is to add less water to powdered formula than instructions indicate for preparing typical 20 kcal/oz formula. This method results in a higher concentration of calories and nutrients but does reduce free water in the infant's diet. Breast milk contains an estimated 20 kcal/oz and provides nutritional and immunologic advantages over infant formula.

It is important to remember there may be variation in the fat content of breastmilk based on the mother's dietary intake.

Creamatocrit Plus and similar devices are available and used in some clinical settings. This portable centrifuge is designed to measure the caloric and lipid content of breast milk and therefore allows more precise estimation of caloric intake of breastfed infants. If an abundant volume of breast milk is available, hind milk (milk released after several minutes of breast feeding is preferred to foremilk (milk released in the initial minutes of breast feeding), because hind milk has higher fat content and the caloric density may be as high as 30 cal/oz. Foremilk contains higher water content and less fat so will be less calorie dense.

Breast milk can be fortified with a commercial powdered formula to densities of 22, 24, 27, or 30 cal/oz based on nutritional needs. There are multiple recipes for fortification and each is based on the nutrient content of the commercial formula being added. It is important to check with a nutritionist for an appropriate recipe. The use of commercial human milk fortifiers is reserved for preterm infants.[480] Additionally, fortification may be accomplished using commercial glucose polymers, microlipid or MCT oil, or protein supplements. Glucose polymers such as polycose (2 kcal/mL as liquid and 23 kcal/TBSP as a powder) increase carbohydrate concentrations. Medium chain triglycerides such as microlipid (4.5 kcal/mL) or MCT oil (7.7 kcal/mL) increase the fat content. Lastly, Promod, a protein supplement, increases the protein content by 3g/tablespoon.

Concentration of formula is usually the method of choice for increasing caloric content because this method provides a balanced formula that includes all nutrients, rather than simple addition of only fat, carbohydrate, or protein. Some fortification recipes are easier for families to prepare and this can play a role in the method of fortification chosen for a patient. Families must be educated by a nutritionist to ensure the appropriate nutritional composition of formula or breast milk is provided to the infant.

It is important to remember, increasing caloric density may lead to an increased solute load including electrolytes and minerals. Renal solute load refers to excess nitrogen, which is the metabolic end product of protein metabolism, sodium, chloride, and potassium that are excreted in urine by the kidneys. Such a disturbance may cause dehydration as the kidneys react to the excessive solute load and draw too much water from the body into the urine.

The delivery mode of enteral nutrition for the neonate, infant, or child with heart disease must be carefully selected. The preferred route is oral if achievable. However, fatigue, anorexia, or swallowing problems may make exclusive oral feeding unattainable. Initially, enteral feeding may be best managed as a combination of oral (PO) and nasogastric (NG) feedings. This allows the infant to continue to develop oral feeding skills but also receive the necessary energy required for catch-up growth. The advantages of enteral feeding by NG route include delivery of more nutrients with a tube that is minimally invasive and short term. Potential disadvantages are interference with PO feedings resulting from a tube in one nostril and in the esophagus that makes swallowing and breathing potentially more challenging. The NG tube may also make reflux more prevalent and contribute to esophagitis.[566]

Nasojejunal delivery of nutrients is an option when delayed gastric emptying or GER is present. Oral gastric (OG) tubes are sometimes utilized in neonatal feeding strategies. An OG tube may be preferred in infants with respiratory distress, as neonates are primarily nose breathers. Disadvantages of OG tubes include difficulty securing the tube and need for removal and then replacement with oral feeding attempts.

The feeding tube chosen should be the smallest possible to safely deliver feedings. Typically a size 6.5 French in a 2.5- to 3.5-kg neonate is used. Long-dwelling tubes are preferred as they remain soft and flexible up to 30 days.

Initially PO feeding time should be no longer than 20 to 30 min thus limiting the energy expended during prolonged feedings. The remainder of the prescribed volume is given via NG by gravity or with a feeding pump. The goal of bolus feeding is to give the entire oral plus nasogastric feeding in less than 30 to 45 min. This allows adequate gastric emptying before the start of the next feeding. With initial bolus feeding, the duration may be extended to 60 min to monitor for tolerance. As a guideline a trial of removal of the NG tube for an all PO attempt may be considered when the infant has tolerated goal calories and volume for 2 or more days, and is taking greater than 50% of target volumes by mouth.

Enteral feedings can be delivered as intermittent boluses, continuous infusion, or a combination of the two. Bolus feedings are felt to be more physiologic than continuous infusions, although continuous infusions may be the delivery mode of choice in patients unable to tolerate bolus feedings. Practically, for the infant requiring continuous infusion, the duration of feedings should be shortened to 20 or 22 hours per day, allowing brief periods of time for activities with the patient not attached to the feeding pump. Ideally, to help maximize oral motor skills, normalize infant feeding patterns, simplify delivery at home, and still meet nutritional goals, if tolerated, it is most beneficial if the infant receives bolus feedings during the day and a continuous feeding at night.

Long-Term Supplementation. Long-term tube supplementation may be required in patients unable to consume necessary calories or volume despite optimizing caloric density and addressing oral feeding skills. Nonpermanent feeding tube options include NG tubes and NJ (nasojejunostomy) tubes. Some institutions reserve the use of nasogastric tubes for the hospital setting and patients are not discharged home with an NG in place. Concerns include potential dislodgement resulting in aspiration, concern that the tube may interfere with normal function of the upper and lower esophageal sphincters and may contribute to gastroesophageal reflux, impairment of the normal airway protective mechanisms of the pharynx and larynx, resulting in an increased likelihood of aspiration, and need for reinsertion inducing a vasovagal response with cardiac decompensation.

When a permanent source of delivering enteral feeds is required to maintain growth, a percutaneous endoscopic gastrostomy tube (PEG tube) or surgical gastrostomy or gastrojejunostomy tube should be inserted.

Infants experiencing tachypnea and muscle weakness often need specific interventions to achieve oral feeding. Supportive strategies include providing chin support or utilizing a slow-flow nipple allowing the infant to more efficiently sequence and coordinate sucking, swallowing, and breathing. As the infant's oral feeding skills improve, transition to a standard flow nipple can be made.

Although somewhat more challenging to use, the Haberman feeding system can be very effective in promoting successful oral feeding in cardiac infants. The one-way valve system in a Haberman allows for control of fluids (low, medium, and high) when concerns exist regarding an infant's ability to handle fluid flow and regulate breathing pauses without breaking the seal on the nipple.

For attainment of successful growth and nutrition, the goal of any strategy or method used is to set an estimated patient goal, assess growth parameters, and make adjustments as needed until acceptable growth is achieved.

Management: Necrotizing Enterocolitis

The clinical problem of necrotizing enterocolitis (NEC) in patients with cardiovascular problems is presumed to be related to impaired hemodynamics and a low perfusion state. Necrotizing enterocolitis can be seen preoperatively or postoperatively in the neonate with complex CHD and is exhibited by ischemic necrosis of the intestinal mucosa. Nutritional care is supportive and includes discontinuation of enteral feedings with bowel rest, and maintenance of intermittent nasogastric suction for gastrointestinal decompression. Nasogastric suction is recommended until the infant's clinical condition improves, the ileus resolves, and pneumatosis is no longer seen on the abdominal radiograph.[763]

Total parenteral nutrition is used to provide nutritional support during the period of bowel rest. Enteral feedings are cautiously resumed as the infant's clinical condition allows. Breastmilk use is preferable in infants at risk for NEC because of the positive benefits in ease of digestion and absorption as well as added immunologic protection.

Management: Mesenteric Arteritis

Following repair of coarctation of the aorta, infants and children may experience paradoxical hypertension. In severe cases, mesenteric arteritis and even bowel ischemia can develop. Because preoperatively the mesenteric arteries were exposed to a low blood pressure (i.e., typically at a mean pressure rather than pulsatile), the sudden increase in arterial blood pressure is thought to cause acute vessel injury and severe reactive vasoconstriction that can result in inadequate blood flow to the bowel. The clinical occurrence of paradoxical hypertension and mesenteric arteritis are sometimes referred to as postcoarctectomy syndrome.

Older children and adults with severe coarctation of the aorta are felt to be at greatest risk for development of mesenteric arteritis postoperatively. Because of the potential risk of developing mesenteric arteritis, many centers keep patients "NPO" (nothing per os, or nothing by mouth) for the first 48 to 72 h post repair while medically controlling hypertension. Then a clear liquid diet is introduced, with slow advance of diet to solids as tolerated.[44] If clinical concerns of mesenteric arteritis or bowel ischemia arise, enteral feedings must be held, nasogastric decompression initiated, and IV fluids provided until symptoms resolve.

Management: Chylous Effusion

Operative injury to the thoracic duct and lymphatics or postoperative systemic venous hypertension or increased right-sided cardiac pressures can lead to chylous effusions. The development of postoperative chylothorax in infants and children with CHD compromises both nutrition and fluid status.

Traditional treatment of postoperative chylous effusion includes chest tube for drainage and diet modification. Nutrition strategies vary from a low-fat diet to complete enteric rest with total parenteral nutrition.[650] Both options are less than optimal in providing balanced nutrition.

Careful assessment of the child's nutritional state must be ongoing because diet modification therapy is often continued for 4 to 6 weeks as a conservative means of treating chylous effusions. Formulas with a predominant fat source from medium-chain triglycerides (MCTs) are preferred over human milk or standard infant formulas, which are very high in long-chain triglycerides (LCTs). The benefit in managing chylous effusions with MCT formulas is based on the fact that LCTs require absorption via the lymphatic system whereas MCTs bypass the lymphatics and go directly into the portal system.

A variety of MCT formula choices are available for infants and children and include Portagen, a lactose free formula with 85% of its fat as MCT oil, Pregestimil with 55% of fat as MCT oil, Vivonex Pediatric with 68% of fat as MCT oil, and Alimentum with 50% of fat as MCT oil. Because prolonged use of these formulas may result in inadequate intake of essential fatty acids and trace minerals, it is recommended that a nutritionist be consulted in the care of children requiring a low-fat diet. A commercial formula specifically designed for infants with chylothorax, Enfaport, has been developed and reported benefits include 85% of fat as MCT oil, high protein levels, and all the essentially fatty acids to support the nutritional needs of an infant with chylous effusion.

Guidelines for a toddler or child requiring low-fat diet include limiting food choices to those with 3 g or less of fat per serving and restricting calories from fat to 20% to 25% of total daily intake (see, also, Chapter 14).

Management: Protein-Losing Enteropathy

In children with cardiac disease, protein-losing enteropathy is most frequently reported in patients following Fontan-type surgical intervention. Protein-losing enteropathy (PLE) is typified by excessive loss of serum proteins into the gastrointestinal tract resulting in hypoproteinemia detected as abnormally low serum albumin levels. Clinical signs include edema, fatty stools and a change in bowel habits with the development of diarrhea and abdominal discomfort.

Nutritional management focuses on optimizing protein intake and limiting fat to predominantly MCTs. In normal adults, normal protein requirements are 0.6 to 0.8 g/kg desired body weight per day. In protein-losing enteropathy, this value may increase to 1.5 to 3.0 g/kg per day, and protein supplements may be necessary to achieve positive protein balance.[366] Protein intake can be enhanced by consumption of lean meat, low fat milk and cheese, and egg substitutes.

Commercially available protein supplements such as Promod are a reliable source of fat-free dietary protein, but may be expensive and unpalatable. More palatable supplements that provide both protein and nonprotein calories include Ensure, Isocal, Peptamen, and PediaSure.

A reduction in intake of long-chain fatty acids reduces mesenteric lymphatic flow and pressure, thus decreasing the amount of lymph leakage and protein loss. In cases of PLE with severely diminished gastrointestinal motility and absorption, the gastrointestinal tract may not tolerate enteral feedings. Under these circumstances, patients may require parenteral nutrition.

Management: Vocal Cord Injury

Vocal cord, or more appropriately, vocal fold dysfunction, can limit enteral feeding and compromise nutrition. Vocal fold dysfunction is most frequently encountered in children with cardiac disease in the postoperative period and results from surgical intervention. Infrequently, vocal fold injury is caused by endotracheal tube placement. When associated with recent surgery, the vocal fold injury usually results from damage to the left recurrent laryngeal nerve during repair of either coarctation of the aorta or patent ductus arteriosus. Enteral feeding is affected because airway and swallowing problems result from immobility of the affected vocal fold. Vocal fold dysfunction should be suspected if the infant or child has hoarse cry or voice or if coughing and sputtering occur with swallowing of liquids.

Normally the recurrent laryngeal nerve carries signals to the muscles responsible for opening vocal folds during breathing and coughing, and closing vocal folds during swallowing. Damage to the vocal folds can lead to transient or permanent paresis or paralysis. Paresis is the partial interruption of nerve impulses resulting in weak or abnormal motion of laryngeal muscles. Paralysis is the total interruption of nerve impulses resulting in no movement of the muscle.

Direct laryngoscopy is the initial diagnostic method of choice for assessing and documenting vocal cord immobility in the postoperative cardiac patient. Most often the vocal fold immobility is unilateral and involves the left vocal fold, although instances of bilateral injury do occur and can result in significant respiratory difficulty.

The position of the affected vocal fold may vary. A midline position is associated with stridor but adequate swallowing capability. Lateral positioning results in a glottic gap. This puts the child at risk for aspiration because swallowing is not coordinated. Most frequently the affected vocal fold is somewhere between midline and lateral and is in a paramedian position.

Infants with left vocal fold immobility in the paramedian position need to be bottle-fed in a right-side down, side-lying position. Toddlers and children with an affected vocal fold should be taught or instructed to turn their head toward the affected side while swallowing as a way of reducing the risk of aspiration.

In the setting of questionable or documented vocal fold immobility, speech and feeding specialists should be consulted. Their input is essential in addressing the feeding challenges presented by infants with postoperative vocal fold dysfunction. These professionals are skilled in oral-motor assessment and the development of infant-specific feeding strategies designed to promote positive oral feeding outcomes.

ARRHYTHMIAS

Debra Hanisch

Pearls

• When a cardiac arrhythmia is observed or suspected, the nurse's first response must be to quickly assess the effect of the rhythm on the patient's hemodynamic status. A clear recording of the ECG should be obtained as well to document the arrhythmia.

• 90% of arrhythmias in pediatric patients are supraventricular tachycardias.

• 80% of wide QRS tachycardias are supraventricular in origin, but must be regarded as ventricular tachycardias until proved otherwise.

• All antiarrhythmic drugs have the potential to be proarrhythmic and warrant careful monitoring of the patient.

Normal Rhythm and Conduction

The normal conduction system of the heart is depicted in Fig. 8-15. In sinus rhythm, the electrical impulse is initiated by the sinoatrial node, located in the right atrium near the junction of the superior vena cava. From there, the impulse is propagated as a wave of depolarization over the atria, converging at the atrioventricular (AV) node, located

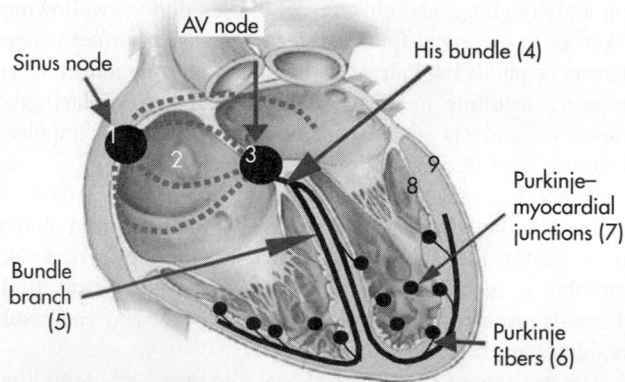

FIG. 8-15 Conduction of the impulse in the heart. The impulse originates in the sinus node (1), continues in the atrial wall (2), and is delayed in the atrioventricular (AV) node (3). Conduction within the ventricles is initially rapid within the rapid conduction system: His bundle (4), right and left bundle branches (5), and Purkinje fibers (6). The impulse is transferred from the rapid conduction system to the working myocardium in the Purkinje-myocardial junctions (7), which are located in the endocardium. Within the slowly conducting working myocardium, the impulse is conducted from endocardium to epicardium. (From Ellenbogen: *Clinical cardiac pacing, defibrillation and resynchronization therapy,* ed 3, Philadelphia, Saunders, 2007.)

at the base of the atrial septum just above the tricuspid valve. Conduction is slowed as it moves through the AV node, allowing time for ventricular filling. From there, the impulse proceeds rapidly down the bundle of His, continues simultaneously down the right and left bundle branches, and finally spreads through the Purkinje fibers to depolarize the ventricles.

Normal components of the ECG are illustrated in Fig. 8-16. The P-wave represents atrial depolarization. The isoelectric segment between the P-wave and QRS complex corresponds to the slowed impulse passing through the AV node. The QRS complex, normally narrow, is produced by rapid ventricular depolarization and is followed by the T-wave, signifying ventricular repolarization. Atrial repolarization occurs but is not visible on the surface ECG.

Analyzing cardiac rhythms involves an assessment of:
• Rhythm
• Heart rate
• P-waves
• QRS complexes
• ST-segments
• P-QRS relationships
• Ectopic and escape beats

Time intervals and heart rate calculations from ECG grid paper are provided in Fig. 8-17, A. Although 12-lead ECG interpretation will not be addressed here, the PR interval, QRS duration, and QT interval are important to note when analyzing rhythm strips. It is also important to identify ST-segment elevation or depression. Table 8-12 displays normal heart rates, and normal PR intervals, and QRS durations in children; these are also depicted in Fig. 8-17, A. QT intervals are corrected (QTc) using Bazett's formula:

$$QT_C = \frac{QT}{\sqrt{RR}}$$

where the measured QT interval (QT) in seconds is divided by the square root of the preceding R-R interval (RR) in seconds. In children and infants older than 6 months, the QTc is normally less than 0.44 s.

Etiology

Arrhythmia substrates can result from congenital heart disease or its surgical correction, hypoxia, electrolyte or acid-base imbalances, metabolic derangements, drug toxicity, genetic disorders, myocardial disease, or injury to cardiac tissue. Arrhythmias can be symptomatic or asymptomatic; they may require urgent treatment or have the potential to deteriorate into symptomatic arrhythmias.

Three common classifications of clinically significant pediatric arrhythmias are bradyarrhythmias, tachyarrhythmias, and arrest (pulseless) rhythms. Hypoxia, sinus node dysfunction and AV block are the most common causes of bradyarrhythmias. Supraventricular tachycardia (SVT) caused by a reentrant conduction pathway is the most common cause of pediatric tachyarrhythmias. Sinus tachycardia is another fast heart rhythm that is not actually an abnormal rhythm but rather an indication that a high heart rate and cardiac output are needed to meet the body's demands. Arrest rhythms

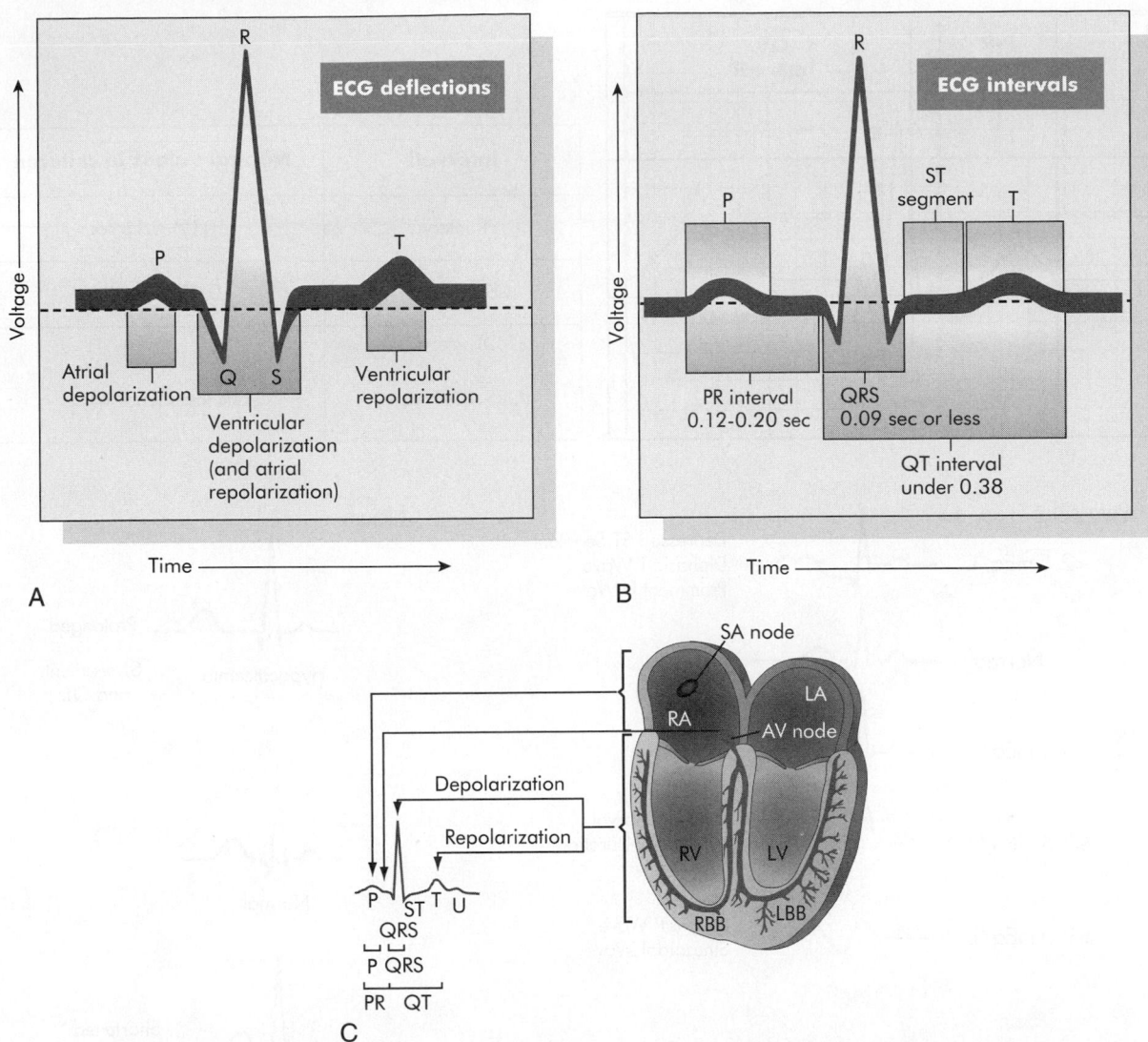

FIG. 8-16 Electrocardiogram (ECG) and cardiac electrical activity. **A,** Normal ECG. Depolarization and repolarization. **B,** ECG intervals among P, QRS, and T waves. **C,** Schematic representation of ECG and its relationship to cardiac electrical activity. AV, Atrioventricular; LA, left atrium; LBB, left bundle branch; LV, left ventricle; RA, right atrium; RBB, right bundle branch. RV, right ventricle. (A and B from Patton KT, Thibodeau GA. *Anatomy & physiology,* ed 7. St Louis, Mosby, 2010. C from Thibodeau GA. *Anatomy & physiology.* St Louis, Mosby, 1987.)

include ventricular fibrillation (VF) and pulseless ventricular tachycardia (VT). These rhythms may indicate ventricular irritability secondary to hypoxia or a severe metabolic derangement, such as acidosis, significant hyperkalemia or hypokalemia, or drug toxicity. Ventricular tachyarrhythmias may also occur as a consequence of a genetic ion channelopathy (i.e., long QT syndrome), myocarditis, cardiomyopathy, myocardial tumor, or scar formation following cardiovascular surgery.

Pathophysiology

Effects of Electrolyte Imbalances, Hypoxia and Acidosis. Electrolyte imbalances, especially potassium, calcium, and magnesium imbalances, alter the myocardial transmembrane potential, which in turn affects depolarization, repolarization, and conduction (Fig. 8-17, B). The cell transmembrane

potential is determined predominantly by the difference in potassium concentration (the concentration gradient) between the inside and the outside of the cell (see section, Essential Anatomy and Physiology).

The child's serum potassium concentration reflects the extracellular potassium concentration. Any significant changes in the serum potassium concentration can increase or decrease myocardial excitability. In severe hypokalemia, ST-segment depression, T-wave flattening, and a prominent U wave (a positive deflection immediately following the T wave) may be observed. In hyperkalemia, tall, narrow, peaked T-waves are observed. When significant hyperkalemia is present, slowing of conduction time can result in a prolonged PR interval and an increased QRS duration. Bradyarrhythmias, tachyarrhythmias, or AV conduction disturbances may be seen. If the child's serum potassium

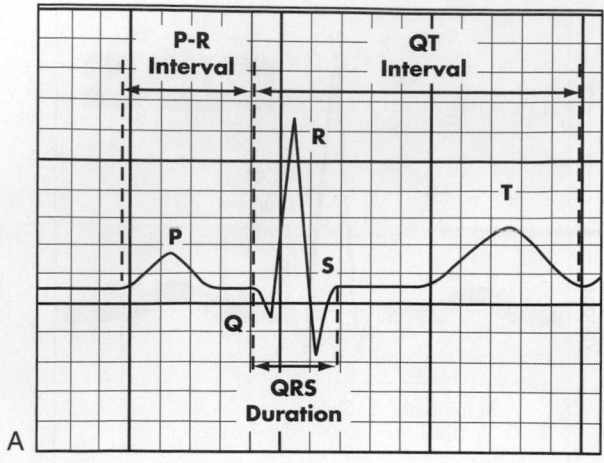

Intervals	Normal values in children
PR interval	0.07–0.18 sec
QRS duration	0.09 sec or less
QT interval (QRS+ST+T-wave)	QTc less than 0.44 sec

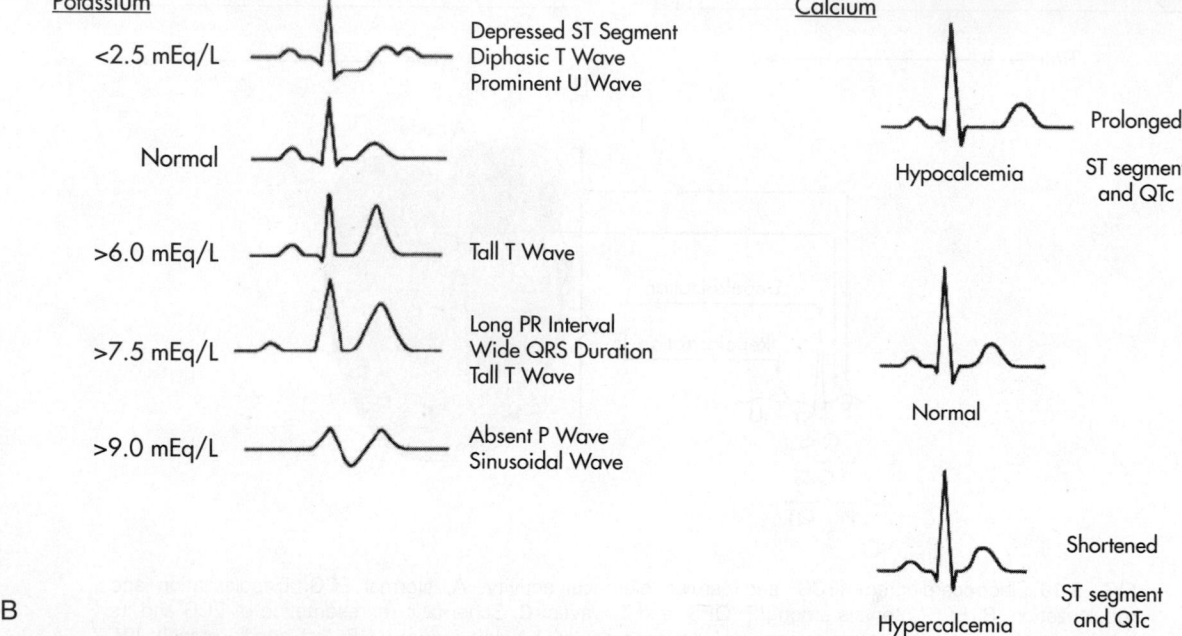

FIG. 8-17 A, ECG intervals. When evaluating an ECG strip, the PR interval and QRS duration should be measured and compared with normal values. In addition, the corrected QT interval, QTc, should be calculated using Bazette's formula: $QT_C = QT/\sqrt{RR}$. B, ECG changes caused by electrolyte imbalance. (Adapted from Park MK, Guntheroth WG. *How to read pediatric ECGs*, ed 4. Philadelphia, Mosby, 2006.)

Table 8-12 Normal Heart Rates, PR Intervals, and QRS Durations in Children

Age	HEART RATE (PER MIN)		PR interval (ms)	QRS Duration (ms)
	Mean	Range		
<1 day	119	94-145	70-120	50-84
1-7 days	133	100-175	70-120	40-79
3-30 days	163	115-180	70-110	40-73
1-3 months	154	124-170	70-130	50-80
3-6 months	140	111-170	70-130	60-80
6-12 months	140	75-190	80-130	50-80
1-3 years	126	60-140	80-150	50-80
3-5 years	98	65-140	90-150	60-84
5-8 years	96	60-140	100-160	50-80
8-12 years	79	60-102	100-170	50-84
12-16 years	75	60-102	110-160	40-80

Modified from Liebman, J. (1982). Tables of normal standards. *Pediatric Electrocardiography*. In Liebman J, Plonsey R, Gillette PC: Baltimore, 1982, Williams & Wilkins, pp. 82-133.

concentration exceeds 7.0 mEq/L, ventricular fibrillation may develop.

Whereas potassium imbalances most notably affect T-waves, calcium imbalances are manifested as changes in the QT interval. Serum hypocalcemia prolongs myocardial repolarization, and can produce ST-segment elevation. Hypercalcemia shortens the ST-segment, decreasing the QT interval. Severe hypercalcemia may cause cardiac conduction abnormalities resulting in bradycardias.[239,832]

No specific ECG changes are identified with magnesium imbalances, but a low magnesium concentration may exacerbate the effects of low calcium. Hypomagnesemia is associated with atrial and ventricular arrhythmias, most commonly torsades de pointes. Magnesium sulfate may be useful as an antiarrhythmic agent because it decreases myocardial cell excitability and conduction. Profound hypermagnesemia (>18 mg/dL) may result in AV block and asystole.[239,601]

A fall in extracellular pH can reduce the rate of spontaneous pacemaker firing and the rate of depolarization. A change in carbon dioxide tension may also affect the ECG; severe hypercapnia has been associated with bigeminy.

Hypoxia/ischemia impairs the function of the sodium-potassium pump, results in a decrease in the magnitude of the transmembrane potential, and slows myocardial conduction time. These changes may contribute to slowing of the heart rate as well as an increased potential for premature ventricular contractions and ventricular tachycardia. Metabolic acidosis and alkalosis are often associated with alterations in potassium or calcium balance. ECG changes reflect these alterations.

Effects of Cardiac Surgery. Arrhythmias may occur during or following cardiovascular surgery either as the result of direct trauma to the conduction tissue, or edema or inflammatory reactions near sutures. Low cardiac output and decreased myocardial perfusion during surgery or in the postoperative period also may produce arrhythmias. Various forms of AV block and escape rhythms often are noted.

Myocardial injury or ischemia can produce ST-segment changes (ST-segment deviation) or an irritable focus that leads to ectopy. Thus, it is important to identify ST-segment changes and treat causes as soon as possible (see section, ST-Segment Deviation).

The arrhythmias that require immediate treatment in the child are those that significantly decrease cardiac output or systemic perfusion, or are likely to deteriorate to rhythms that decrease cardiac output or systemic perfusion. In general these arrhythmias are classified as bradyarrhythmias, tachyarrhythmias, and arrest rhythms. *Any heart rate or rhythm should be evaluated in light of the child's clinical condition and its effect on systemic perfusion.* The rhythm can then be identified as one of the following:

- *Too slow* for clinical condition (bradycardias)
- *Too fast* for clinical condition (tachycardias)
- *Ineffective* (arrest rhythm)

ST-Segment Deviation. ST-segment changes are commonly seen in adult patients but are relatively uncommon in the pediatric population. Precise measurement is needed to reliably identify ST-segment deviations. The isoelectric baseline of the ECG is established by either the P-R segment or by the T-P segment (i.e., the portion of the ECG between the end of the T-wave and the beginning of the next P-wave).[832] ST-segment elevation or depression is defined as the amount (in mm) that the ST segment deviates above or below that baseline respectively. On the 12-lead ECG, ST-segment elevations greater than 1 mm or depressions of 0.5 mm or more are generally considered abnormal.[895] However, ST-segment shifts less than 1 mm in the limb leads or less than 2 mm in the precordial leads may be a normal finding in children, especially in the absence of T-wave changes.[687] This normal finding, referred to as "early repolarization" is a well-described observation, often seen in healthy adolescent males.[833]

Abnormal ST-segment changes are often manifestations of significant pathology. Abnormal ST-segment elevation is indicative of acute myocardial injury, such as infarction, and should prompt immediate attention. Risk factors for myocardial infarction in children include congenital coronary artery anomalies and coronary embolization due to Kawasaki disease or endocarditis. Myocardial ischemia or infarction can also complicate surgery near a coronary artery, such as may occur following an arterial switch procedure for d-transposition of the great arteries.[686] The postoperative team must also be aware of abnormal coronary artery anatomy in patients with congenital heart defects, such as may be present in some patients with tetralogy of Fallot. Close monitoring is needed during postoperative care and *any acute change in the ST segment, whether elevation or depression, should be reported to the on-call provider immediately.*

ST-segment elevation may also result from inflammation as seen with myocarditis or pericarditis. In fact, pericarditis is the most common cause of ST-segment elevation in children.[895] Specific patterns of ST segment elevation have been identified,[89] and certain of these patterns are postulated to be associated with arrhythmias and hypertrophy.[90]

ST-segment depression usually suggests myocardial ischemia. In congenital heart disease, severe aortic valve stenosis or aortic hypoplasia may compromise coronary perfusion. ST-segment depression, along with characteristic T-wave abnormalities, may be present with ventricular hypertrophy or cardiomyopathies.[687] ST-segment depression noted during exercise stress testing indicates coronary blood flow is inadequate to meet increased myocardial oxygen demand during exercise. Other causes of ST-segment depression include hypokalemia and digoxin toxicity. As noted previously, any acute change in the ST segment, whether elevated or depressed, should be reported to the on-call provider immediately.

Bradyarrhythmias. Bradycardia is a heart rate less than 90/min in the infant and less than 60/min in the child. Because tachycardia is the appropriate response to distress and shock, a heart rate that is normal for age in a child with poor systemic perfusion constitutes a relative bradycardia.

Bradycardia can compromise systemic perfusion because it slows the ventricular rate; unless stroke volume increases commensurate with the decrease in heart rate, cardiac output will fall. Bradycardia is often associated with a proportional fall in cardiac output. Because of their low reserve for stroke volume, neonates and young infants are particularly sensitive to changes in heart rate. An additional consequence of a fall in heart rate is that more time is available for ectopic beats to emerge. Bradyarrhythmias occur most commonly as a result of hypoxia, vagal stimulation (e.g., during suctioning), dysfunction of the sinus node, or AV block.

Tachyarrhythmias. Tachycardia is defined as a heart rate greater than 200 to 220/min in the infant and greater than 160 to 180/min in the child over 5 years of age. Although the heart rate can increase transiently during fever or episodes of crying, the term "tachycardia" is reserved for significant and persistent increases in heart rate.

Tachycardia can be a normal response to stress (e.g., pain) or increased oxygen requirements, as in the case of sinus tachycardia. Sinus tachycardia may also be a normal response to a compromise in cardiovascular function, such as CHF. In these cases, the faster heart rate is compensatory and may maintain a normal or even slightly higher cardiac output. However, extremely high heart rates adversely affect ventricular diastolic filling time, causing a decrease in stroke volume and cardiac output. Moreover, coronary artery perfusion occurs almost exclusively during diastole. Tachyarrhythmias result in decreased coronary artery perfusion time in the face of increased myocardial oxygen demand. Cardiogenic shock may ensue if the tachycardia persists.

AV dissociation, if present, may also contribute to a drop in cardiac output. With AV dyssynchrony, "atrial kick," the final 25% to 30% of ventricular filling produced by atrial systole, is lost. This may be associated with a significant fall in stroke volume.

Rhythm Identification and Clinical Signs and Symptoms

Analysis of rhythm strips involves assessment of:
- Rhythm
- Heart rate
- P-waves
- QRS complexes
- ST segments
- P-QRS relationships
- Ectopic and escape beats

The heart rhythm can be described overall as regular, slightly irregular, irregular but with a pattern (regularly irregular as in grouped beating), or irregularly irregular. Whether the rhythm is fast, normal, or slow can be determined by measuring the heart rate and evaluating it in terms of the patient's age, activity, and clinical status.

The heart rate can be calculated by a number of methods. The standard paper speed for ECG recordings is 25 mm per second. At this speed, each small square on the horizontal axis represents 0.04 second; each larger block containing five small squares represents 0.2 second. Sixty (s/min) divided by the R-R interval in seconds will equal the heart rate per minute.

Most ECG paper is marked off in either 1-second (five large blocks) or 3-second (15 large blocks) intervals. An estimated heart rate can be derived by counting the number of R-waves in a 6-second strip (30 large blocks) and multiplying by 10. With fairly regular R-R intervals, the heart rate can be calculated by the 1500 method (based on 1500 small squares = 1 min). This method involves counting the number of small squares (0.04 second intervals) between two consecutive R-waves and dividing 1500 by that number. A simpler method for estimating the heart rate is the 300 method (based on 300 larger squares = 1 min). For this method, the number of larger squares between two consecutive R-waves is counted and divided into 300. Examples of these methods are illustrated in Fig. 8-18.

P-waves, if present, should be regular and they all look the same in terms of size and shape. One P-wave should precede each QRS complex, and a QRS complex should follow each P-wave. In AV dissociation, the P-wave rate should be calculated in addition to the R-wave rate.

R-waves, or QRS complexes, should be regular and narrow, with consistent appearance (size and shape). A wide QRS complex suggests a conduction delay (as in bundle branch block) or origination of the impulse outside the AV node (as seen in AV block or ventricular ectopy). Aberrant AV conduction through an accessory pathway may create a wide QRS as well. The ST segments should be isoelectric (at the same baseline as the T-P segment and the P-R segment).

The ratio of P-waves to QRS complexes should be 1:1 with consistent PR intervals appropriate for the child's age, as described in Table 8-12. Variable PR intervals suggest AV dissociation with the ventricular rate faster than the atrial rate, or second- to third-degree AV block where the ventricular rate is slower than the atrial rate.

Ectopic beats are initiated by a focus outside the sinus node. Premature beats occur early in the rhythm and may originate from an irritable focus from the atria, atrioventricular (AV) junction, or ventricles.

A premature atrial contraction (PAC), caused by an ectopic atrial focus, appears on the ECG as an early-occurring P-wave with a different morphology from the normal sinus P-wave. The PAC typically conducts normally down the AV node to the ventricles, so the QRS complex is unchanged. A compensatory pause results as the sinus node is reset following the interruption. If the PAC occurs very early before ventricular repolarization is complete, it may be blocked from conducting to the ventricles.

A premature junctional contraction (PJC) originates in the AV junction and interrupts the rhythm with its early appearance. From there, the impulse is conducted up to the atria (retrograde) and down to the ventricles (antegrade). On the ECG, an inverted P-wave may be seen just before, within, or after a normal QRS complex. A compensatory pause follows.

A premature ventricular contraction (PVC) is recognizable on the ECG as a wide, bizarre QRS complex occurring early in the rhythm. The PVC is created by an ectopic ventricular focus, from outside the normal conduction system, that initiates ventricular depolarization. As a result, the morphology of the QRS is altered. P-waves tend to march through the PVC, unless a retrograde P-wave is stimulated. In either case, a compensatory pause follows the premature beat before the rhythm resumes.

Escape beats occur late in the rhythm following a pause, or when the underlying rhythm is abnormally slow. When the sinus node fails to act as the dominant pacemaker, a subsidiary pacemaker in the atrium, AV node, or ventricle, enabled by intrinsic automaticity, can initiate impulses. Atrial escape beats have a different P-wave morphology from sinus rhythm but the QRS is unchanged from normal. Junctional and ventricular escape beats look similar to PJCs and PVCs respectively, except they occur late in their timing rather than early.

Rhythms Originating from the Sinus Node. Normal sinus rhythm is initiated by the SA node at a rate within normal limits for the child's age. P-waves and QRS complexes are normal in configuration, occur in a 1:1 ratio (with each P-wave followed by an R-wave), with both P and R waves upright in Leads I and AVF. The PR interval is appropriate for the heart rate and age of the child (see Table 8-12). Though the rhythm is regular, slight beat to beat variation is present. The sinus node's automaticity is influenced by the sympathetic and parasympathetic nervous systems. Circulating catecholamines increase the heart rate while vagal stimulation slows the rate. A balance between these two systems maintains a normal heart rate (Fig. 8-19).

Sinus arrhythmia is an irregular sinus rhythm with respiratory variation (Fig. 8-20, A). The heart rate increases with inspiration and decreases with expiration. This rhythm tends to be more pronounced in children and athletes. Sinus arrhythmia may also be exacerbated by reactive airways disease or increased intracranial pressure. No treatment for this arrhythmia is indicated.

Sinus tachycardia also originates in the sinus node and has all the properties of normal sinus rhythm except the rate is

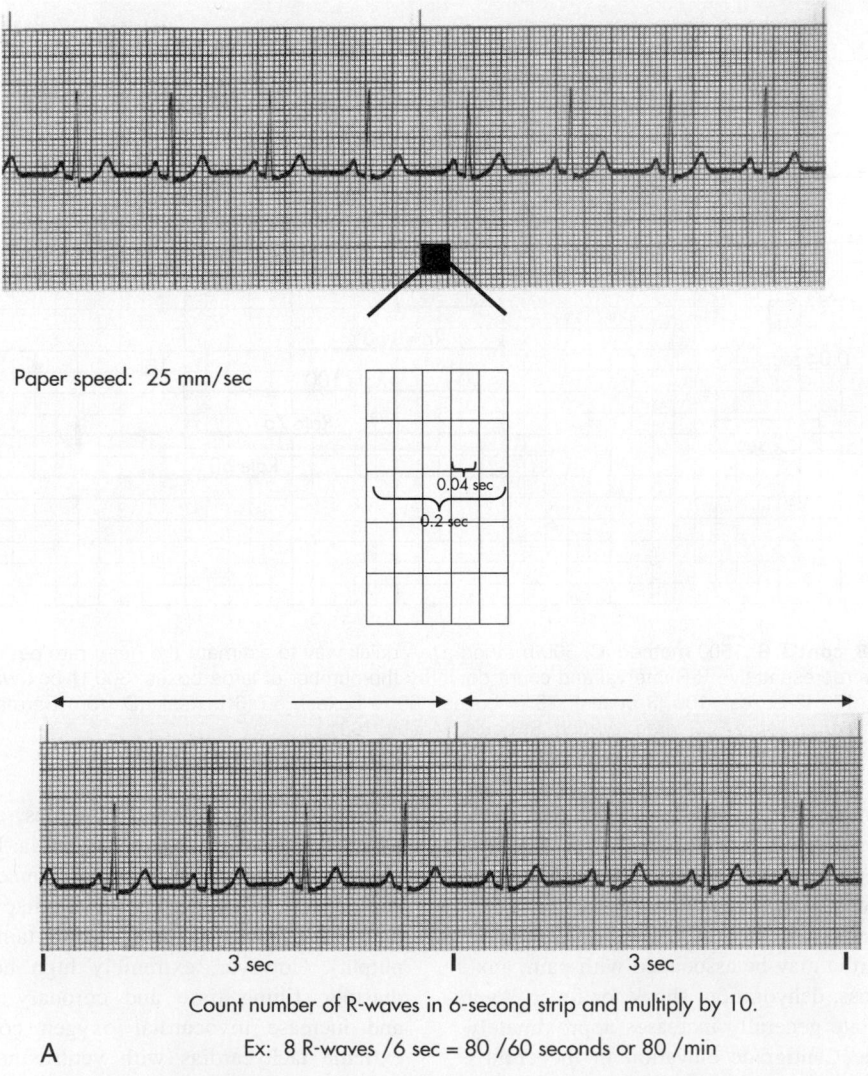

Paper speed: 25 mm/sec

0.04 sec

0.2 sec

3 sec   3 sec

Count number of R-waves in 6-second strip and multiply by 10.

A   Ex: 8 R-waves /6 sec = 80 /60 seconds or 80 /min

FIG. 8-18 How to calculate heart rate. A, Three-slash method.

Continued

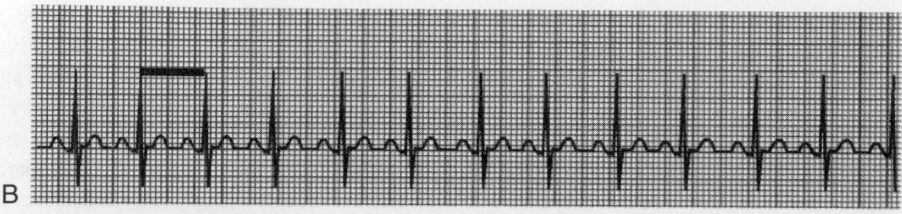

Divide 1500 by the number of small squares in an R-R interval (small square = 0.04 sec).

Ex: 1500 / 12 small squares = 125 /min

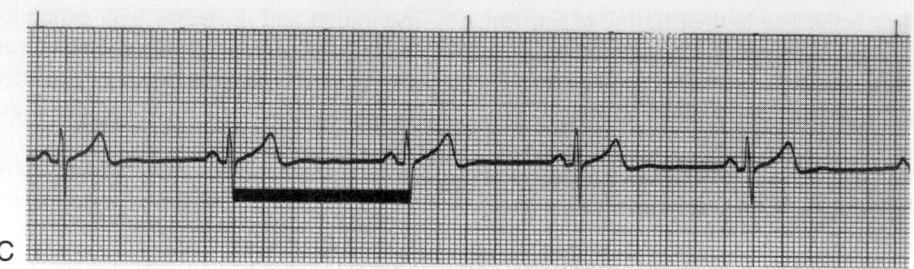

Divide 300 by the number of large squares in an R-R interval (large square = 0.2 sec).

Ex: 300 /6 large squares = 50 /min

Divide 300 by the number of large squares in an R-R interval (large square = 0.2 sec).

Ex: 300 / 6 large squares = 50 /min

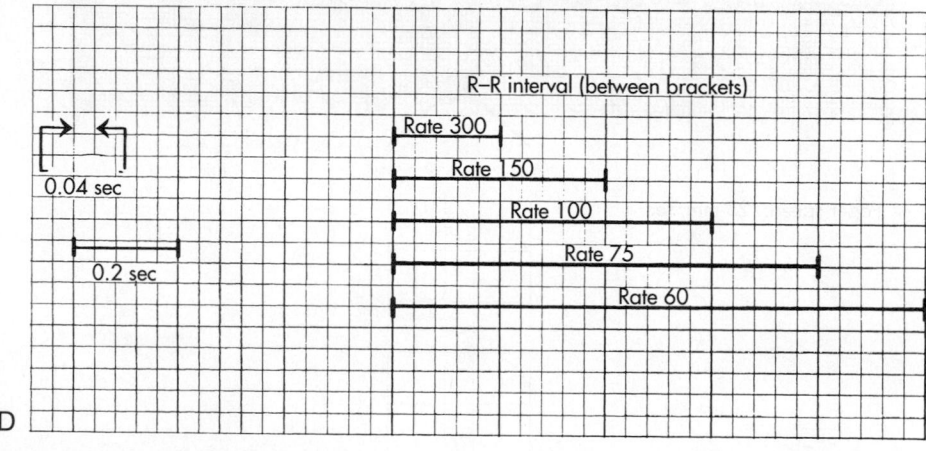

FIG. 8-18, cont'd B, 1500 method. **C,** 300 method. **D,** A quick way to estimate the heart rate per min is to choose a representative R-R interval and count down by the number of large boxes: 300 (1 box within R-R interval), 150 (2 boxes), 100 (3 boxes), 75 (4 boxes), 60 (5 boxes), 50 (6 boxes). (D from Berman W Jr. *Handbook of pediatric ECG interpretation.* St Louis, Mosby, 1991.)

faster than normal for the child's age (see Fig. 8-20, B). Although the heart rate in sinus tachycardia is typically less than 200/min, it can be greater than 220/min in very ill infants, although this is rare. Sinus tachycardia normally occurs during periods of stress or increased oxygen requirement, such as exercise. Sinus tachycardia may be associated with pain, anxiety, anemia, volume loss, dehydration, shock, or fever. As a rule, the child's heart rate generally increases approximately 10/min for each degree Centigrade elevation in the child's temperature above 37° C.

Stimulant drugs, catecholamines, and other chronotropic agents can produce sinus tachycardia. In addition, tachycardia will occur as a compensatory mechanism if ventricular stroke volume decreases or cardiac function is impaired (e.g., with congestive heart failure, tamponade, or low cardiac output). However, extremely high heart rates compromise diastolic filling time and coronary artery perfusion time, and increase myocardial oxygen consumption. Therefore, extreme tachycardias with ventricular rates exceeding 180 to 220/min can result in a significant fall in stroke volume

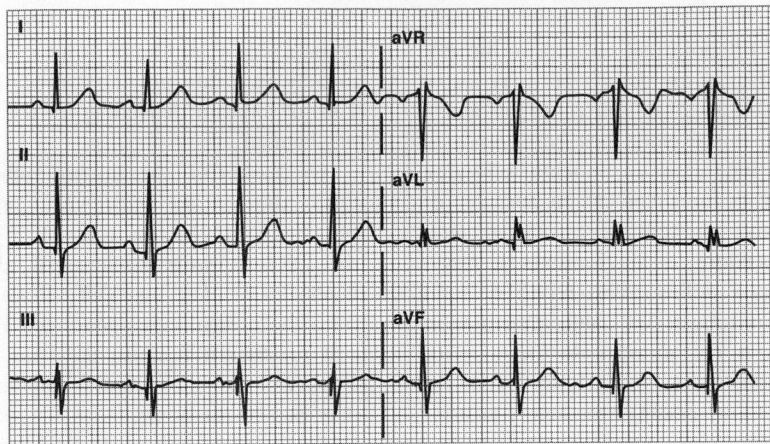

FIG. 8-19 Sinus rhythm at 92 per min in a 6-year-old girl. In normal sinus rhythm, the rate is appropriate for age and the rhythm is fairly regular. P-waves all look the same and are followed in a 1:1 ratio by narrow QRS complexes that all look the same. The PR interval is constant and normal for age. Moreover, P-waves and R-waves are both upright in Leads I and aVF.

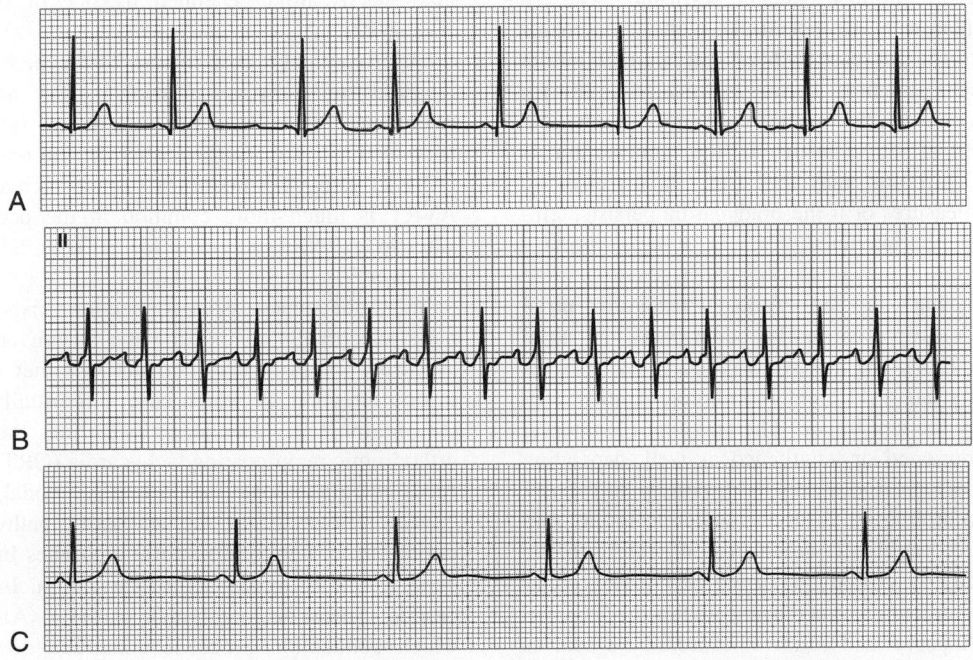

FIG. 8-20 Rhythms originating in the sinus node. **A,** Sinus arrhythmia in a 3-year-old girl. Heart rate varies between 70 and 100/min with respirations. **B,** Sinus tachycardia at 170/min in a 1-year-old boy. **C,** Sinus bradycardia at 50/min in a 13-year-old girl.

and cardiac output. The medical management of sinus tachycardia involves addressing the underlying cause of the tachycardia.

Sinus bradycardia encompasses all of the characteristics of sinus rhythm except the rate is slower than normal for the child's age (see Fig. 8-20, C). In general, heart rates less than 90/min in the infant or less than 60/min in the child are considered slow.

Sinus bradycardia may result from respiratory compromise, hypoxia, or vagal stimulation, as may be observed during suctioning. Hypothermia, hypothyroidism, increased

intracranial pressure, or drugs, such as digoxin or beta-blockers, may produce sinus bradycardia. Trained athletes and adolescents with anorexia nervosa tend to have slower resting heart rates as well.[680] Injury to the sinus node or its arterial supply could result in sinus node dysfunction with resultant bradycardia.

Sinus node dysfunction (SND), sometimes referred to as sick sinus syndrome, may lead to any of a number of bradyarrhythmias, including sinus bradycardia, sinus pauses or arrest, sinoatrial exit block, escape rhythms, and bradycardia-tachycardia syndromes. A junctional escape rhythm may emerge when the atrial rate slows to the point where it is slower than the AV node's depolarization rate, so the AV node takes over. In some cases, slow heart rates may allow certain tachyarrhythmias, such as atrial flutter, to surface.

Surgical injury to the sinoatrial node has been reported with over a 50% incidence long term in patients following the Mustard or Senning procedures for d-transposition of the great arteries.[310,409] Other procedures associated with SND include the Fontan procedure for single ventricle physiology, closure of atrial septal defects, and repair of total anomalous pulmonary venous return. Whenever cannulation for cardiopulmonary bypass is performed near the superior vena cava-right atrial junction, there is a risk for SND. As a surgical complication, SND may occur immediately postoperatively, or may not be manifest for up to 10 years or longer following surgery.[310] Nonsurgical causes of SND include right atrial dilation caused by pressure or volume overload. SND may also be seen in cardiomyopathies or inflammatory conditions, such as myocarditis, pericarditis, and rheumatic fever.[74]

Bradycardia can compromise systemic perfusion because it slows the ventricular rate. Unless stroke volume increases commensurate with the decrease in heart rate, cardiac output will fall. Acute management of hemodynamically significant bradycardia includes adequate ventilation and oxygenation, and administration of epinephrine. If the bradycardia is vagally mediated, atropine may be used. If there is no response to these measures or if the bradycardia persists, temporary pacing should be instituted.

Rhythms Originating in the Atria. Premature atrial contractions (PACs) represent early occurrences of atrial activation. On the ECG, the P-wave will occur early in its timing and typically has a different morphology from the P-waves generated by the sinus node. The resulting PR interval may be slightly shortened or lengthened as well, depending on the site of the ectopic focus and its proximity to the AV node. The QRS morphology is unchanged, except in rare situations where the impulse is conducted aberrantly to the ventricles (Fig. 8-21, A). A PAC occurring before ventricular repolarization is complete (i.e., occurring within the T-wave) will be blocked. A pause will follow the premature beat as the sinus node resets itself. Occasional PACs occur normally in children and may be described as a "skipped beat" because of the pause in the rhythm and the increased stroke volume associated with the subsequent beat. In the critical care environment, PACs may result from stimulant drugs, such as sympathomimetics, digoxin, caffeine, or cocaine. Incisions from atrial surgery or indwelling atrial catheters may cause PACs as well. Hypoxia, hypoglycemia, hypokalemia, and hypercalcemia are other clinical conditions that may be associated with increased PAC activity.[299,501] PACs are generally considered benign but should be monitored for an increase in frequency.

Supraventricular tachycardia (SVT) is the most common abnormal rhythm seen in children, with an estimated incidence in the pediatric population ranging from 0.1% to 0.4%.[491,517,548] The majority of children with SVT (50% to 60%) present within the first year of life.[517] SVT is recognized by an abrupt onset and termination of tachycardia, usually at a rate greater than 220/min, but may range from 130 to 300/min depending on the patient's age and the SVT mechanism.[225]

On the ECG, the rhythm typically appears as a narrow QRS tachycardia with very regular R-R intervals (see Fig. 8-21, B). In less than 10% of recorded SVT rhythms, the QRS is wide because of aberrant conduction to the ventricles.[548] During SVT, P-waves differ in morphology from the normal sinus-generated P-wave, and are often difficult to discern because they are buried within the QRS or T-waves. The tachycardia may last only a few seconds or may persist for hours.

SVT and paroxysmal atrial tachycardia (PAT) are broad terms referring to a sustained tachycardia originating above the bundle of His. Several SVT mechanisms have been identified. The more common ones are described here. Most SVT rhythms are caused by either a reentrant circuit, with or without the use of an accessory pathway, or an automatic tachycardia generated by one or more ectopic foci (Fig. 8-22).

Approximately 90% of SVTs in pediatric patients are reciprocating tachycardias using the AV node as part of the re-entrant circuit.[491] The two major types of re-entrant tachycardias are atrioventricular re-entrant tachycardia (AVRT) and AV nodal re-entrant tachycardia (AVNRT). AVRT is much more common in the pediatric age group, whereas AVNRT accounts for 30% of SVT in adolescents and over 50% of SVT in adults.[491]

In AVRT, an accessory connection exists outside of the AV node, electrically connecting the atrium and ventricle. This accessory pathway may conduct in either direction, or only in one direction, in which case it is usually retrograde from the ventricle to the atrium. During the more common orthodromic reciprocating tachycardia (ORT), conduction proceeds antegrade down the normal AV nodal pathway but then travels retrograde up the accessory pathway back to the atrium. From here, the impulse continues back down the AV node, perpetuating the loop tachycardia. In rare cases, antidromic reciprocating tachycardia (ART) occurs in which conduction proceeds antegrade down the accessory pathway and returns to the atrium retrograde via the AV node. Heart rates for the more common ORT range from 150 to 300/min; neonates average 280/min when in SVT.[224]

A common type of AVRT is Wolff-Parkinson-White syndrome (WPW) in which an accessory connection, called a Kent Bundle, is present. When not in tachycardia, a short PR interval is present, and a characteristic delta wave is visible, appearing as a slurred upstroke to the QRS complex (see Fig. 8-21, C). This delta wave represents preexcitation caused by antegrade conduction traveling down the accessory pathway from atrium to ventricle without the conduction delay normally produced by the AV node. During SVT, the QRS is normal in morphology, without the delta wave. WPW may be found in the absence of congenital heart disease, although in 20% of patients with WPW, structural

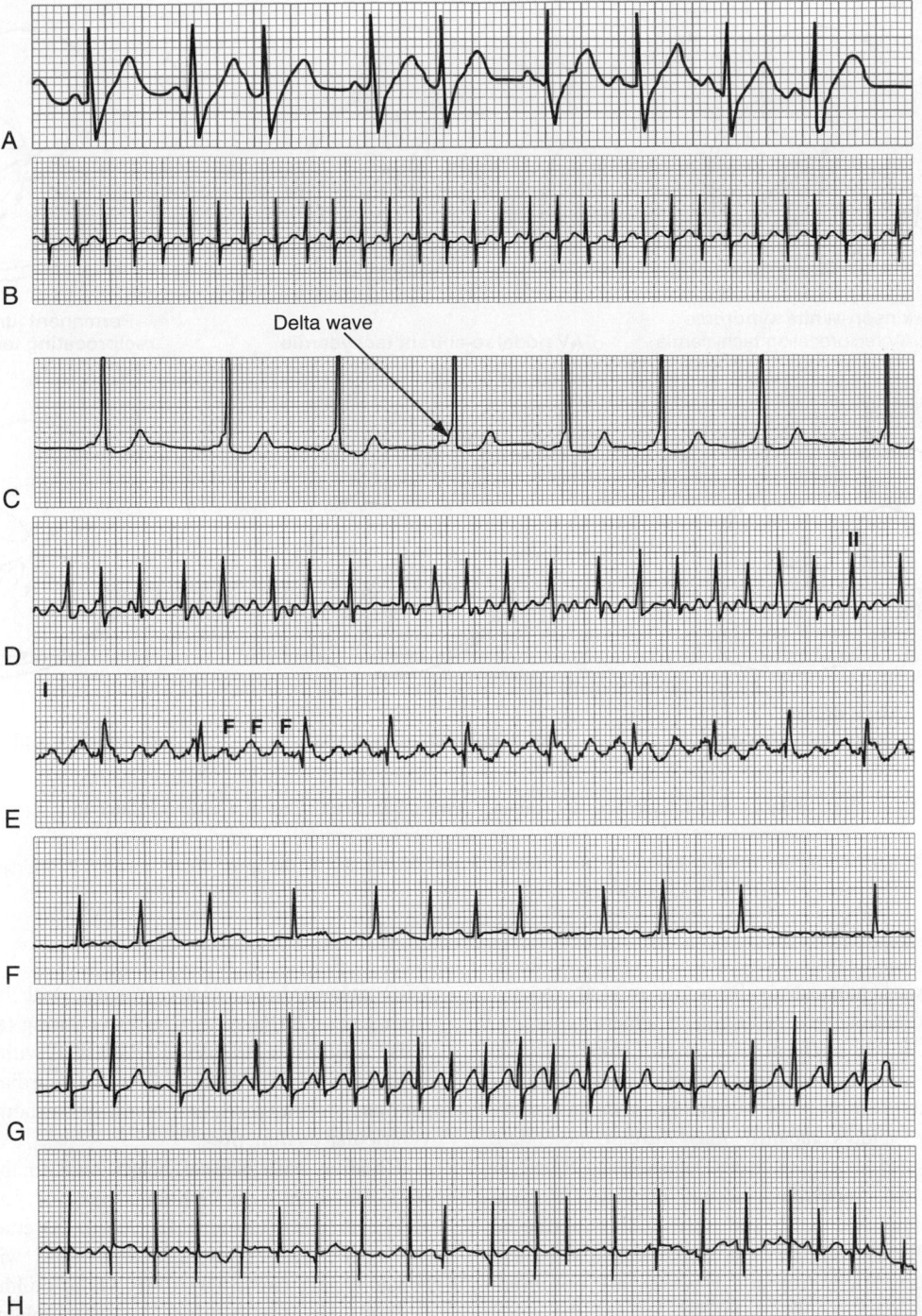

FIG. 8-21 Rhythms originating in the atria. **A,** Two PACs (complexes #3 and #5) in sinus rhythm at 120/min in a 5-year-old boy. The early occurring P-wave falls within the T-wave, appearing as a "bump" in the down slope of the T-wave. Conduction proceeds normally from the atria down through the AV node and across the ventricles, so the morphology of the QRS following a PAC is the same as that seen with a normal beat. **B,** Supraventricular tachycardia at 280/min in a 1-week-old male infant appears as a very rapid, regular, narrow QRS tachycardia with an abrupt onset. **C,** Wolff-Parkinson-White syndrome. The delta wave, a slurred upstroke from the P-wave into the QRS complex, is a manifestation of preexcitation in this 13-year-old girl with WPW. The atrial impulse is conducted across an accessory pathway down to the ventricles without the delay typically produced by the AV node. **D,** Atrial flutter with variable block in a 1-month-old boy. The flutter waves are more easily seen during the longer R-R intervals. The flutter rate in this infant is >400/min. **E,** Intraatrial reentrant tachycardia (IART) in a 17-year-old girl several years following her Fontan procedure for tricuspid atresia. Note the flutter waves, indicated with "F." **F,** Atrial fibrillation in a 16-year-old boy. Note the wavy baseline and irregularly irregular ventricular rhythm characteristic of atrial fibrillation. **G,** Atrial ectopic tachycardia (AET) in a 2-month-old girl. The first complex is a normal sinus beat, followed by a PAC from the ectopic focus. Complex #3 is another normal sinus beat, but then a run of AET begins, "warming up" over the first several complexes. **H,** Multifocal atrial tachycardia in a 1-month-old girl. Note the irregular rhythm and different P-wave morphologies.

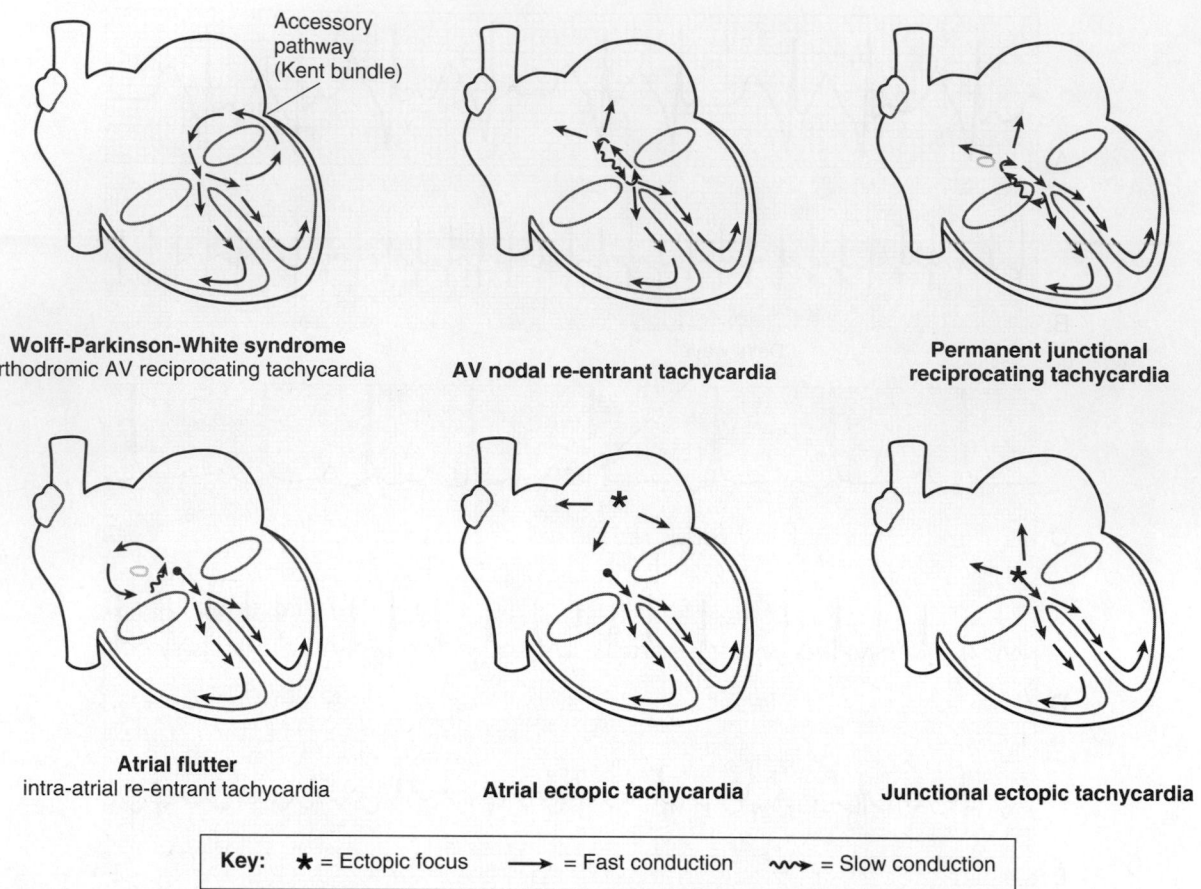

FIG. 8-22 Common mechanisms of supraventricular tachycardia (SVT). (Adapted from Hanisch D. Pediatric arrhythmias. *J Pediatr Nurs* 16(5):351-362, 2001.)

heart disease coexists, particularly Ebstein's anomaly, tricuspid atresia, double-outlet right ventricle, or hypertrophic cardiomyopathy.[225,894] Although not common, some patients with WPW are at risk for sudden death caused by atrial fibrillation with rapid conduction to the ventricles via the accessory pathway. Digoxin and verapamil may further potentiate this risk.

In AVNRT, the reentrant circuit consists of two pathways within the AV node and surrounding perinodal structures, typically a slow, antegrade pathway and a fast, retrograde pathway. The retrograde P-waves are obscured, falling within the QRS or the terminal end of the QRS complex, creating a relatively short RP interval and long PR interval. Heart rates during tachycardia range from 150 to 300/min, with an average of 170/min in the older child.[224] AVNRT accounts for nearly 15% of SVTs in the pediatric population, but rarely appears before the age of 2 years.[491] AVNRT is not associated with congenital heart disease.[224]

The permanent form of junctional reciprocating tachycardia (PJRT) is a less common type of orthodromic reciprocating tachycardia in which the impulse is conducted antegrade through the AV node and retrograde through a slowly conducted accessory pathway. The associated narrow

QRS tachycardia is relatively slow, with heart rates ranging from 130 to 220/min.[224] The ECG during tachycardia characteristically displays a long R-P interval with negative P-waves in leads II, III, and AVF.[243] The tachycardia tends to be incessant and, if untreated, can result in cardiomyopathy with left ventricular dysfunction.[10,243,654]

Children with normal hearts tend to tolerate SVT fairly well, but after 6 to 48 hours, signs of poor cardiac output and heart failure ensue. Infants with extremely fast heart rates will appear pale, restless, and irritable, with tachypnea and hepatomegaly caused by CHF. Older children may verbalize feeling their heart beating fast or complain of chest pain or dizziness. Children with abnormal hearts may quickly develop hemodynamic compromise and require emergent treatment.

To differentiate between sinus tachycardia and supraventricular tachycardia the child's underlying condition should be considered. SVT is generally very rapid and the rhythm is fixed regardless of patient activity. In comparison, sinus tachycardia results in some variability in heart rate if patient activity increases or decreases (e.g., the heart rate may increase to even higher levels when the child is crying, and may fall during sleep). Further distinguishing characteristics are described in Table 8-13.

Table 8-13 **Differentiating Supraventricular Tachycardia from Sinus Tachycardia**

	SVT	ST
History	Nonspecific; lethargy or irritability, poor feeding, tachypnea, diaphoresis, pallor	Suggestive of volume loss (e.g., vomiting, diarrhea, blood loss), shock, or febrile illness
Examination	Signs of congestive heart failure: tachypnea, moist crackles, increased respiratory effort, poor perfusion, hepatomegaly	Consistent with dehydration, blood loss, shock or fever; clear lungs, normal liver; ST may be caused by CHF in congenital heart disease
ECG	Abrupt onset, heart rate >180 to 220/min, regular R-R intervals, P-waves seen in 50%-60% with abnormal axis, narrow QRS in >90% of SVTs	Gradual onset, heart rate usually <180 to 220/min, variable R-R intervals, normal P-wave axis, narrow QRS
Chest x-ray	May have an enlarged heart, signs of pulmonary edema	Small or normal heart, clear lung fields (unless congenital heart disease present)
Echocardiogram	May have ventricular dilation or dysfunction	Usually normal

Adapted from Hanisch DG, Perron L: Complex dysrhythmias in infants and children. *AACN Clin Issues Crit Care Nurs* 3(1),255-269, 1992.

If supraventricular tachycardia is associated with some degree of atrioventricular block the ventricular rate may approximate a normal rate and stroke volume and cardiac output may be adequate (e.g., if atrial flutter with a 2:1 or 3:1 block is present). It is important that the nurse constantly evaluate the child's systemic perfusion, however, so that immediate intervention may be provided if cardiovascular collapse occurs.

The terms atrial flutter and intraatrial reentrant tachycardia (IART) are often used interchangeably. They represent two similar but distinct types of SVT in which the re-entry circuit is confined to the atria. In both entities, zones of slow conduction and anatomic barriers create areas of conduction block that help establish macro-reentrant circuits within the atria. On the ECG, regular saw tooth P-waves, or flutter waves, are seen with either a fixed ratio (e.g., 2:1 or 3:1) or variable AV block. The ventricular rhythm, therefore, may be regular or irregularly irregular.

Atrial flutter (see Fig. 8-21, D) is usually not associated with congenital heart disease, and though relatively common in older adults, is only occasionally observed prenatally and in neonates, and is rarely seen during childhood.[142,433,848] In neonates, atrial rates have been reported to range from 340 to 580/min.[848] The AV node cannot conduct impulses this rapidly, so 2:1 AV block or variable block occurs, resulting in ventricular rates averaging around 200/min. Although significant morbidity is associated with neonatal atrial flutter, most newborns can be treated successfully with a low risk of recurrence.[142,848]

IART is a common sequela following surgery for structural heart disease. ECG findings in IART include flutter waves with a lower amplitude (see Fig. 8-21, E), and therefore less distinct saw tooth pattern than in typical atrial flutter and at slower rates, usually less than 250/min.[464] Procedures, such as the Mustard or Senning operations for transposition of the great arteries, the Fontan procedure for single ventricle physiology, repair of total anomalous pulmonary venous connection, and ASD closures, create the substrate for IART to develop because many atrial incisions are made and subsequent scarring occurs. IART may occur in the early postoperative period or may develop as a late complication years, even decades, following surgery. The coexistence of sinus node dysfunction may result in a bradycardia-tachycardia syndrome. Newer modifications of surgical corrective procedures have been employed in an effort to reduce the risk for long-term arrhythmia complications.[148,194,585,732]

Atrial fibrillation is a common arrhythmia in the adult population, but is quite rare in children. Risk factors include myocarditis, cardiomyopathy, mitral regurgitation, previous atrial surgery, sinus node dysfunction, and WPW.[477,964] The ECG in atrial fibrillation displays a shaky, irregular baseline comprised of fibrillatory waves, along with irregularly irregular R-waves resulting from the variable AV conduction (see Fig. 8-21, F). If the child has been in atrial fibrillation for an undetermined period of time, anticoagulation therapy is instituted prior to attempts at cardioversion to reduce the risk of a thromboembolic event.

Atrial ectopic tachycardia (AET), also known as ectopic atrial tachycardia (EAT) or automatic atrial tachycardia, is another type of SVT. AET is more prevalent in the pediatric population, and accounts for roughly 15% of SVTs in children.[548,919] AET is an automatic tachycardia driven by an irritable focus within the atria but outside of the SA node. Unlike the re-entrant SVT rhythms described above, this automatic tachycardia "warms up" with a gradual acceleration in rate, and conversely, "cools down" (see Fig. 8-21, G). Atrial rates are variable, even within the same patient, and may range from 90 to 330/min.[824,919] The ventricular rhythm may be regular or irregular, depending on the degree of AV block. The incessant nature of AET may lead to a tachycardia-induced cardiomyopathy if uncontrolled.[210,606,964]

Multifocal atrial tachycardia (MAT, MFAT), also known as chaotic atrial tachycardia (CAT) or chaotic atrial rhythm (CAR), is another type of automatic tachycardia originating in the atria. As the name implies, multiple ectopic foci exist producing at least three different P-wave configurations on the ECG (see Fig. 8-21, H). The atrial rhythm is irregular and fast, with variable rates of 200 to 500/min, while the ventricular rhythm is also irregular with rates of 150 to 250/min.[97] MAT is an uncommon rhythm in the pediatric population, affecting mostly infants. As with AET, the incessant tachycardia may lead to cardiomyopathy. Spontaneous resolution has been reported in 50% to 80% of patients by 6 to 18 months of age.[14,97,760,919]

Rhythms Originating at the AV Junction. Junctional rhythms originate in the AV nodal region. From there, the impulse travels up to the atria in a retrograde direction and down to the ventricles in the normal antegrade direction. P-waves are often hidden in the QRS complex. Depending on the speed of conduction, the P-wave may be positioned just before the R-wave, within the R-wave, or immediately after the R-wave, and will be inverted in leads II, III, and AVF. The QRS complexes are usually narrow and normal in configuration. In all cases, the atrial kick and its contribution to cardiac output are compromised as atria and ventricles are depolarized essentially simultaneously (Fig. 8-23). Three types of junctional rhythm occur: junctional escape rhythm, accelerated junctional rhythm, and junctional ectopic tachycardia (JET).

A junctional escape rhythm may be observed when sinus node automaticity is depressed. Sinus slowing results in the "escape" of a junctional rhythm. The rhythm is regular and slower than normal (see Fig. 8-23, A). Hemodynamic compromise may result if the bradycardia is severe, in which case treatment is aimed at correcting the cause of sinus slowing, or increasing the atrial rate with atropine or atrial pacing.

An accelerated junctional rhythm results when automaticity of the AV node is enhanced. The junctional rate exceeds the sinus rate, and the AV node becomes the dominant pacemaker (see Fig. 8-23, B). Rates are typically between 60 and 120/min, but may be as high as 170/min.[195]

Junctional ectopic tachycardia can take two forms: congenital JET and post-operative JET. In each case, enhanced automaticity of the AV node occurs, producing a rapid rhythm that gradually warms up to rates of 170 to 240/min.[433,919] JET is further defined by normal narrow QRS complexes and AV dissociation, in which the ventricular rate is greater than the atrial rate, or less often, 1:1 retrograde VA conduction (see Fig. 8-23, C). During AV dissociation, sinus capture beats may occur when sinus P-waves periodically conduct normally to the ventricles, creating irregularity to the otherwise steady rhythm.[919]

Congenital JET usually presents in the first month of life and is associated with high morbidity and mortality. Tachycardia-induced cardiomyopathy develops in those with incessant tachycardia at heart rates above 200/min.[195,768,919] A mortality rate of 4% to 34% has been reported.[195,909] About half of affected infants appear to have a familial form of JET.[768] In some patients, spontaneous resolution occurs. Medical management consists of antiarrhythmic medications, often amiodarone in combination with another agent, or ablation for those refractory to drug therapy.[195]

Postoperative JET is believed to be related to surgical trauma to the AV nodal area from suturing or stretching. Repairs of VSDs, atrioventricular septal defects (AVSDs), total anomalous pulmonary venous return, and tetralogy of Fallot are associated with a higher incidence of JET.[23,381] The tachycardia usually begins during rewarming in the OR, or shortly after arrival to the critical care unit.[919] The tachycardia tends to only last 24 to 48 hours,[381] but without prompt recognition and treatment, postoperative JET quickly leads to hemodynamic instability by two mechanisms. With the loss of AV synchrony, the atria contract against closed AV valves, resulting in a loss of atrial kick. This, along with the fast

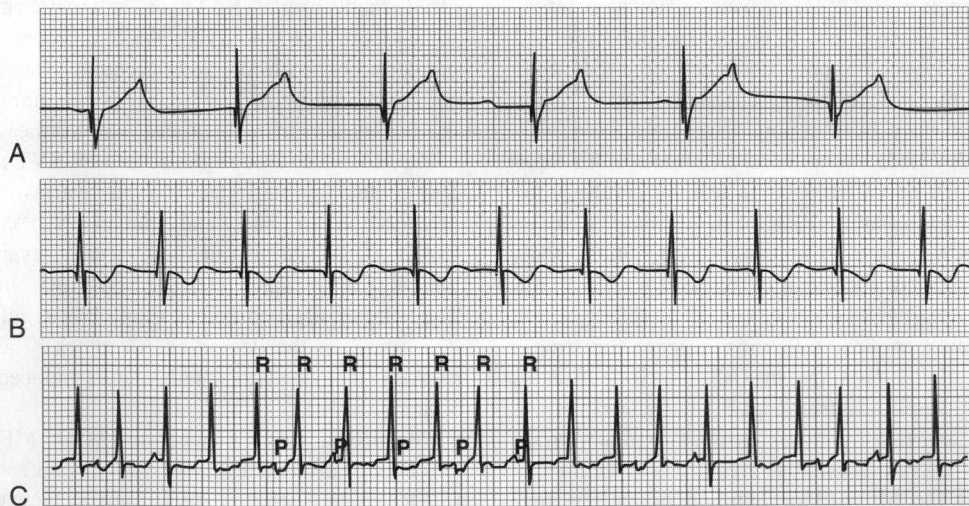

FIG. 8-23 Rhythms originating in the AV node. **A,** Junctional escape rhythm at 54/min in a 15-month-old boy with sinus node dysfunction. The retrograde P-waves are buried within the QRS complex. Because atrial and ventricular activation occur at the same time, ventricular filling is compromised. **B,** Accelerated junctional rhythm at 100/min in a 12-year-old girl. The sinus node is being overdriven by the AV node. The retrograde P-waves are buried in the QRS complex. **C,** Junctional ectopic tachycardia at a rate of 217/min in a 1-month-old boy. AV dissociation is present with a faster ventricular rate than atrial rate. Ventricular filling and cardiac output are compromised by the fast heart rate and AV dyssynchrony. P = P-wave; R = R-wave.

ventricular rate, decreases ventricular diastolic filling so cardiac output falls.

Treatment of postoperative JET consists of maintaining normothermia or slight hypothermia and weaning inotropic infusions because catecholamines further enhance the AV node's automaticity. Atrial pacing is used to establish AV synchrony if the JET rate is slowed to a manageable level. Intravenous antiarrhythmic drugs, particularly amiodarone,[508,773] help to slow the junctional rate. Recently, successful management of JET has been reported with dexmedetomidine, an α-2 adrenoreceptor agonist used primarily for sedation.[177] In life-threatening situations, catheter ablation of the AV node may be necessary.[103,898]

Rhythms Originating in the Ventricles. Abnormal rhythms with a ventricular origin are far less prevalent in children than supraventricular arrhythmias.[433] As discussed previously, premature ventricular contractions (PVCs) are ectopic beats that originate in the ventricle outside of the normal conduction pathway. PVCs are recognized easily because the QRS complex occurs earlier than expected and is wide or bizarre in configuration. The sinus node continues to fire normally, so a P-wave is often buried within the PVC but cannot conduct to the ventricles because they have not completed repolarization. The next P-wave, following the PVC, is conducted to the ventricles normally, so the length of two R-R intervals, including the PVC, is the same as two normal cycles (Fig. 8-24, A).

Rhythms with regularly occurring PVCs are described as bigeminy, trigeminy, or quadrigeminy, referring to a PVC every other beat, every third beat, or every fourth beat respectively (see Fig. 8-24, B). Pairs of PVCs are called couplets. PVCs may be uniform or multiform in configuration.

Isolated PVCs from the same focus may occur normally, especially during times of slower heart rate, such as during

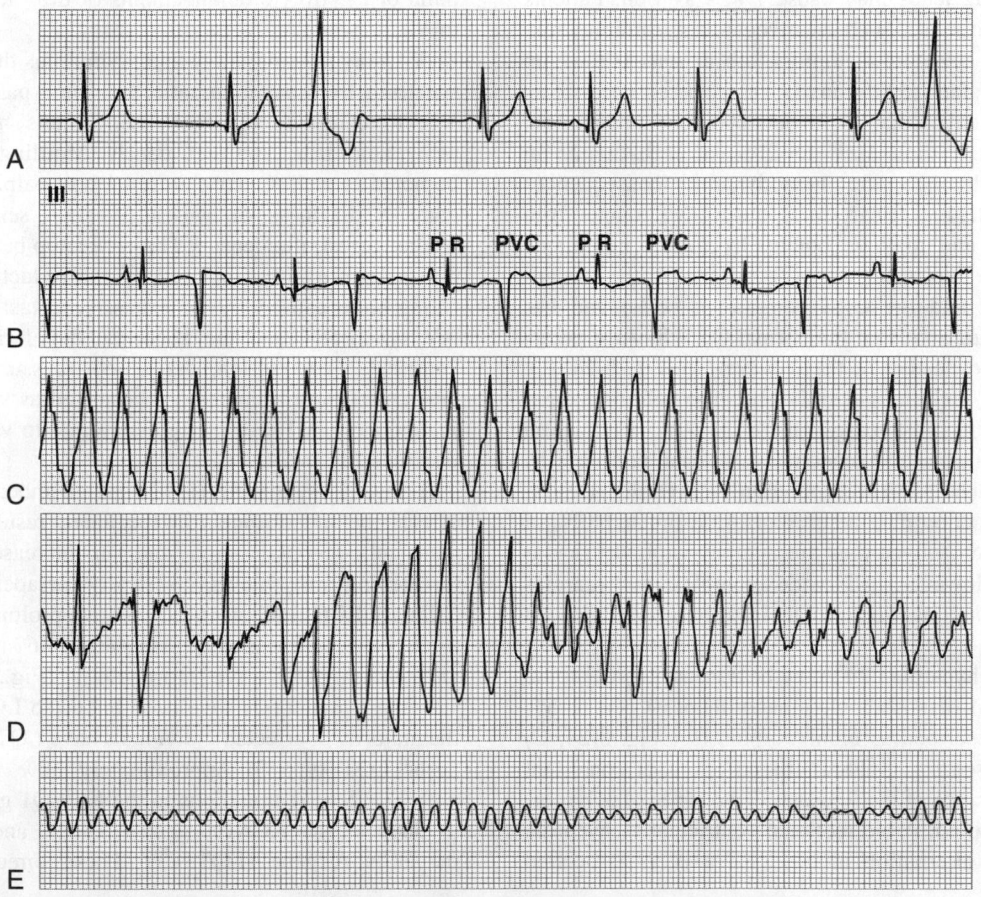

FIG. 8-24 Rhythms originating in the ventricle. **A,** Premature ventricular contractions. Two uniform PVCs demonstrated on this ECG from an 8-year-old boy. Note the early timing of the wide, bizarre complexes, followed by a compensatory pause. **B,** Ventricular bigeminy in a 2-year-old boy. A sinus P-wave (P) followed by a normal QRS (R) alternates with a PVC. There is a slight pause after the PVC, producing a regularly irregular rhythm. (The P-waves here are large because of right atrial enlargement.) **C,** Monomorphic ventricular tachycardia at 227/min in a 4-year-old boy with a cardiac tumor. He decompensated quickly and required immediate DC cardioversion. **D,** Polymorphic ventricular tachycardia, or Torsades de pointes, a type of polymorphic VT, is characterized by undulating ventricular complexes giving the appearance of "twisting (or turning) around a point." **E,** Ventricular flutter/fibrillation. Coarse to fine fibrillatory waves indicative of rapid, chaotic electrical activity characterize this lethal arrhythmia. The ventricles "quiver" rather than contract. Without immediate CPR and defibrillation, death will occur.

sleep, and cause no hemodynamic concern. Because of the early ventricular contraction and AV dyssynchrony, diastolic filling is diminished following a PVC. With this drop in stroke volume, plus the compensatory pause, children will describe the sensation as a "skipped beat." The pulse will feel weaker with the PVC, then stronger with the subsequent beat. *Patients with PVC activity should be monitored closely for an increase in frequency.* Frequent, coupled, or multiform PVCs may reduce cardiac output and should be investigated immediately. They indicate the presence of significant ventricular irritability that may progress to ventricular tachycardia.

In the critical care environment, PVCs may result from electrolyte abnormalities, acid-base imbalances, hypoxia, or hypovolemia. Medications and street drugs, including sympathomimetic drugs, antiarrhythmic agents, digoxin, cocaine, methamphetamine, and psychotropic agents can precipitate PVCs. Postoperative conditions, such as incisions or scars from ventricular surgery or the presence of indwelling catheters or pacing leads may cause PVCs as well. Patients with myocardial disease, such as myocarditis, cardiomyopathy, ischemia, or myocardial tumors, are at risk to develop PVCs and ventricular arrhythmias.

Ventricular tachycardia (VT) is relatively uncommon, accounting for less than 10% to 20% of arrhythmias in children,[237,300] although the hemodynamic consequences can be life-threatening. Heart rates during VT range from 120 to 250/min, and may be potentially higher in infants. By definition, the rate is at least 10% faster than the preceding sinus rhythm and the QRS complex is wider and has a different configuration from the normal QRS. T-wave polarity is usually opposite that of the R-wave (see Fig. 8-24, C). P-waves are difficult to identify because of the rapid heart rate, but in most cases, there is AV dissociation with the ventricular rate exceeding the atrial rate. In the unusual circumstance of slow ventricular tachycardia, 1:1 retrograde VA conduction may be present. An estimated 80% of regular, wide QRS tachycardias are actually supraventricular in origin.[13,75] However, all wide complex tachycardias should be regarded as ventricular in origin until proven otherwise.

Ventricular tachycardia (VT) may be nonsustained (3 to 30 consecutive beats) or sustained (greater than 30 beats). VT may further be described as monomorphic (see Fig. 8-24, C) or polymorphic (see Fig. 8-24, D) based on either consistent or variable appearance of the R-waves. Two types of polymorphic VT are identified. A bidirectional ventricular tachycardia with beat-to-beat alternation in the QRS axis, is associated with a genetic rhythm disorder called catecholaminergic polymorphic ventricular tachycardia (CPVT).[433] The other, more common polymorphic VT is torsades de pointes in which rapid, wide, undulating QRS complexes appear to spiral or turn around an axis. Torsades de pointes is associated with congenital and acquired long QT syndromes. As with atrial tachycardias, the arrhythmic mechanisms for ventricular tachycardias include reentry, enhanced automaticity, and triggered activity. In addition, abnormal repolarization may play a role, as in long QT syndrome.

VT is most commonly seen in patients following congenital heart surgery, such as repair of tetralogy of Fallot, Mustard or Senning repairs of transposition of the great arteries, valve repairs of aortic or pulmonic stenosis, or VSD closures.[13,490] VT may also develop in children with structurally normal hearts and may be associated with ventricular tumors (hamartomas, rhabdomyomas), myocarditis, cardiomyopathy, arrhythmogenic right ventricular dysplasia, or coronary artery anomalies with myocardial ischemia.[13,237,971] Severe metabolic or electrolyte derangements or drug toxicities may lead to VT as well.

VT may present at any age. Symptoms during VT span the spectrum from asymptomatic, for some patients with a slow VT, to cardiovascular collapse. Infants may be lethargic, tachypneic, pale, and feed poorly. Mottling or cyanosis may be noted as well. Older children report palpitations, chest discomfort, dizziness, or nausea. Syncope, seizure activity, and cardiac arrest often ensue. These develop because cardiac output is significantly impaired by the reduction in ventricular filling time caused by an excessively fast rate, the loss of AV synchrony, and the abnormal depolarization that alters ventricular contraction. As blood pressure falls, coronary artery perfusion becomes compromised as well. If not treated immediately, VT will likely deteriorate to ventricular fibrillation (see Fig. 8-24, E).

Long QT syndrome (LQTS) is an inherited disorder that affects the ion channels in the heart, resulting in abnormal ventricular repolarization and an increased risk for life-threatening arrhythmias, classically torsades de pointes. The hallmark ECG findings in LQTS are a prolonged QTc interval, usually measuring greater than 440 to 460 ms (milliseconds), and abnormal T-wave morphology (Fig. 8-25). To date, 12 genetic mutations have been linked to LQTS,[439,847,928] but the majority of affected individuals have LQT type 1, LQT type 2, or LQT type 3. Approximately 30% to 35% of those with LQTS have mutations in the KCNQ1 gene (LQT1), 25% to 30% in the KCNH1 gene (LQT2), and 5% to 10% in the SCN5A gene (LQT3).[847] These three events may be

T-wave

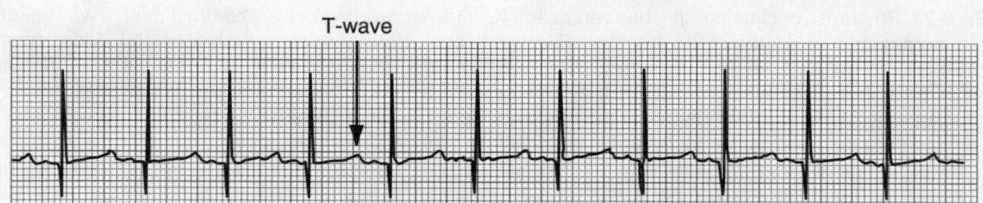

FIG. 8-25 Long QT syndrome. Prolonged QT interval (QTc 521 ms) in a 3-week-old male with congenital deafness. Diagnosed with Jervell and Lange-Nielsen syndrome, the recessive form of long QT syndrome, he received an implanted cardioverter-defibrillator because of his high risk for sudden cardiac death.

recognized by their specific T-wave morphologies and triggers for cardiac events.

Cardiac events associated with LQTS include syncope, torsades de pointes, and sudden death. Exercise, particularly swimming, appears to be a frequent trigger for cardiac events in LQT1. Auditory stimuli or emotional stress are recognized as triggers in LQT2. In LQT3, patients have the highest risk for life-threatening arrhythmias while asleep.[928] A provocative epinephrine challenge may be done in the electrophysiology lab to help identify LQTS in suspect or borderline cases.[913]

Commercially available genetic testing may be performed to confirm the diagnosis and help direct therapy. Treatment consists of beta-blocker therapy for LQT1 and LQT2, sodium channel blocker therapy for LQT3. Implantation of a cardioverter-defibrillator (ICD) is recommended for those at highest risk for sudden cardiac death. In some cases, left sympathetic denervation may be helpful.[56] Once an index case has been identified, genetic testing of first-degree family members is often recommended.

Ventricular flutter, another potentially lethal arrhythmia, is a very rapid ventricular tachycardia; this rhythm does not allow sufficient time for ventricular filling and invariably results in inadequate cardiac output. Ventricular flutter usually deteriorates rapidly to ventricular fibrillation.

Both ventricular flutter and fibrillation are catastrophic rhythms, so that the difference between the two is usually moot.

Ventricular fibrillation is characterized by chaotic myocardial electrical activity. Because organized myocardial depolarization does not occur, organized ventricular contraction is not possible. As a result the ventricles quiver and do not pump blood. Ventricular fibrillation is not a common terminal rhythm in young children. However, it is a collapse rhythm, and cardiac compressions (CPR) and emergency defibrillation must be provided immediately.

AV Blocks. AV block occurs when conduction from the atria through the AV node to the ventricles is delayed, intermittent, or nonexistent, described as first-, second-, or third-degree AV block respectively.

First-degree heart block is defined as prolonged conduction through the AV node. This produces a prolonged PR interval on the ECG, but there is consistent 1:1 AV conduction; every P wave is followed by a QRS complex (Fig. 8-26, A). This form of heart block may be caused by digoxin, calcium channel blockers, beta-blockers, or sotalol therapy.[282] A prolonged PR interval may also be seen in rheumatic heart disease, Lyme disease, myocarditis, or muscular dystrophies.[749] Metabolic abnormalities that can prolong AV conduction include

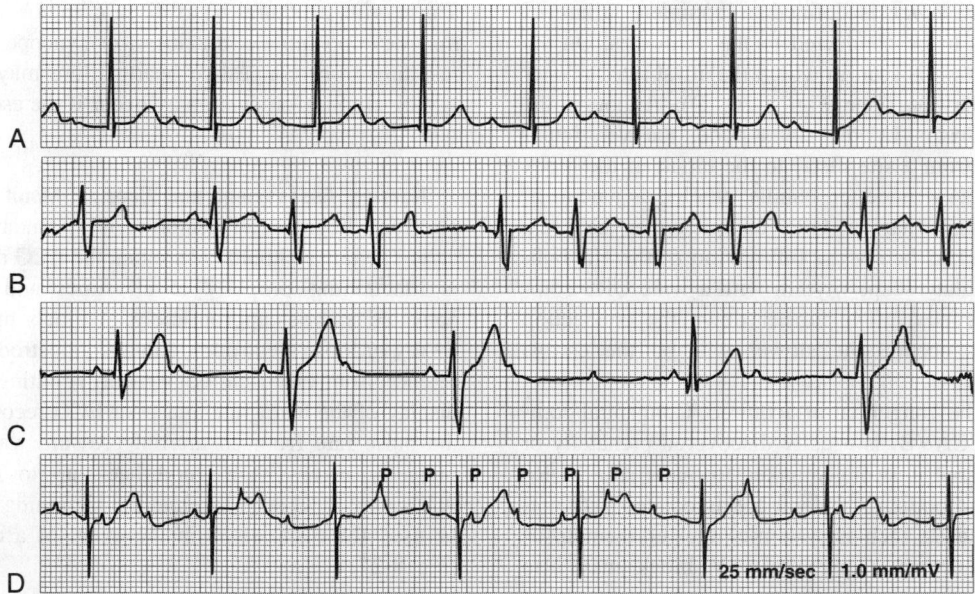

FIG. 8-26 AV blocks. **A,** First degree AV block is defined as a prolonged PR interval with a 1:1 A-V ratio. Conduction is delayed as it travels through the AV node, but never blocked. This rhythm was noted in a 4-year-old girl whose brother has congenital complete AV block. **B,** Second degree Mobitz type I AV block is also known as Wenckebach. There is gradual prolongation of the PR interval (in the second, third and fourth complexes) until a P-wave meets a refractory ventricle and is blocked (so it is not followed by a QRS complex); then the pattern repeats. The appearance of "grouped beating" is the hallmark of Wenckebach. **C,** Second degree Mobitz type II AV block appears as intermittent AV block. The PR intervals, when present, are the same. Often the block occurs as a fixed ratio, i.e., two P-waves for every QRS complex. Sometimes the block is variable, as shown here. **D,** Third degree AV block, or complete heart block, is a dissociated rhythm in which the atria depolarize at one rate and the ventricles, not receiving any impulses through the AV node, are reliant on automaticity to generate impulses to sustain a rhythm. The result is more P-waves than R-waves, each going at a steady but independent rate. This ECG is from a newborn with congenital complete AV block who received a pacemaker on day 2 of life.

hyper- or hypokalemia, hyper- or hypocalcemia, hypomagnesemia, or hypoglycemia.[749,931]

Second-degree heart block is present when there is intermittent failure of conduction of impulses from the atria to the ventricles. Two distinct types of second-degree heart block are identified: Mobitz I and Mobitz II.

Mobitz type I AV block, also known as Wenckebach, is recognized by its characteristic pattern of a gradually lengthening PR interval eventually followed by a nonconducted P-wave, or dropped beat (see Fig. 8-26, B). This pattern gives the appearance of grouped beating. In Mobitz type II AV block, there is intermittent failure of the P-wave to be conducted, but where measureable PR intervals occur, they are consistent and do not lengthen (see Fig. 8-26, C). Generally, Mobitz II AV block produces a fixed ratio of P-waves to QRS complexes, such as 2:1 or 3:1, but variable block may also occur.

A Wenckebach rhythm is usually well-tolerated and rarely requires treatment. It may be observed during the immediate postoperative period following cardiac surgery and should be monitored for progression to more advanced AV block. Mobitz II AV block tends to occur distal to the bundle of His, often because of injury at the time of surgery. This more serious type of AV block usually results in a slow ventricular rate and may require cardiac pacing to support cardiac output. Mobitz II AV block often progresses to complete AV block.

Third-degree AV block is defined as complete failure of the atrial impulses to be conducted to the ventricles. On the ECG, AV dissociation is seen in which the atrial rate is faster than the ventricular rate (see Fig. 8-26, D). Although the atrial rhythm is driven by the sinus node, the ventricular rhythm originates from a site distal to the block. If the block occurs within the AV node or bundle of His, a junctional escape rhythm with a narrow QRS complex may be seen. If the level of block is below the bifurcation of the His bundle, an idioventricular escape rhythm with a wide QRS complex will be observed.[931] The farther down the conduction system this block occurs, the slower will be the escape rhythm.

AV block may be congenital or acquired. Congenital complete AV block (CCAVB) is usually discovered prenatally or shortly after birth and is strongly linked to maternal SSA/Ro and SSA/La autoantibodies,[125] which are associated with collagen vascular diseases, such as systemic lupus erythematosus and Sjögren's syndrome. Congenital AV block may also occur in children with certain structural heart defects, most notably L-transposition of the great arteries (L-TGA, also called congenitally corrected transposition of the great arteries).

AV block in the neonate without structural heart disease may be well tolerated provided the ventricular rate is adequate to maintain effective perfusion. If ventricular rates fall below 65 to 75/min, the neonate often becomes lethargic and demonstrates signs of CHF, such as tachypnea and poor feeding. The fetus may present with hydrops fetalis, necessitating immediate intervention.[433]

Most cases of acquired AV block in children result from injury to the AV node or His bundle at the time of cardiac surgery. Procedures, such as closure of an AV septal defect or ventricular septal defect, tetralogy of Fallot repair, subaortic resection, or aortic or mitral valve replacement, carry a higher risk for surgical AV block, though the incidence of permanent AV block for these repairs is less than 5%.[185,282,387,433] Patients with L-TGA have a much higher incidence of postoperative AV block. Many children will have transient AV block following cardiac surgery, likely caused by edema localized around the nodal region.[185] If the heart block persists beyond 7 to 14 days postoperatively, permanent pacing is recommended.[254]

Acquired AV block may also be a manifestation of other diseases, such as muscular dystrophies, cardiomyopathy, or Kearns-Sayre syndrome. Infections attacking the heart may also lead to AV block. AV block has been reported following bacterial endocarditis, viral myocarditis, rheumatic fever, Lyme disease, Chagas disease, and Rocky Mountain spotted fever.[433,931]

Although AV block increases ventricular diastolic and coronary artery perfusion times, the slow ventricular rate may be inadequate to maintain cardiac output and systemic perfusion, particularly if ventricular function is impaired. In addition, the AV dyssynchrony may further reduce cardiac output by 20% to 30%. Symptoms caused by AV block vary depending on the ventricular rate and presence of associated structural heart disease. Some children with structurally normal hearts and a good ventricular escape rate may do well. Those with structural heart disease and/or a slow escape rate may develop fatigue, dizziness, or syncope. Other symptoms resulting from congestive heart failure may also accompany AV block. Sudden death may occur if the escape rate abruptly falls.[749]

Nursing Assessment and Cardiac Monitoring. Continuous electrocardiographic monitoring is a standard part of critical care. The nurse should ensure that the ECG monitoring system is functioning properly at all times and that alarms are activated and set appropriately. Artifacts may be introduced by dry or loose electrodes, damaged electrode cables, or interference from electrical equipment, resulting in an inaccurate display of the heart rate and poor ECG recording. Monitoring the pulse rate from an arterial pressure wave form or pulse oximetry serves as a good back up to ECG monitoring. A baseline ECG strip taken at the beginning of each shift may be used for comparison in the event of a change in rhythm (Fig. 8-27).

If an arrhythmia is present, the nurse should immediately determine its effects on the child's systemic perfusion. Appropriate assessment includes vital sign measurement, particularly pulse rate and blood pressure, observation of the skin temperature and color, capillary refill time in the extremities, and comparison of apical heart rate with peripheral pulses. The quality of the peripheral pulses also should be determined. If ventricular systole is associated with decreased stroke volume, corresponding peripheral pulses are usually weaker, and an arterial pressure tracing may demonstrate such pulse variations.

If a collapse rhythm, such as pulseless ventricular tachycardia or ventricular fibrillation is present, pulses will not

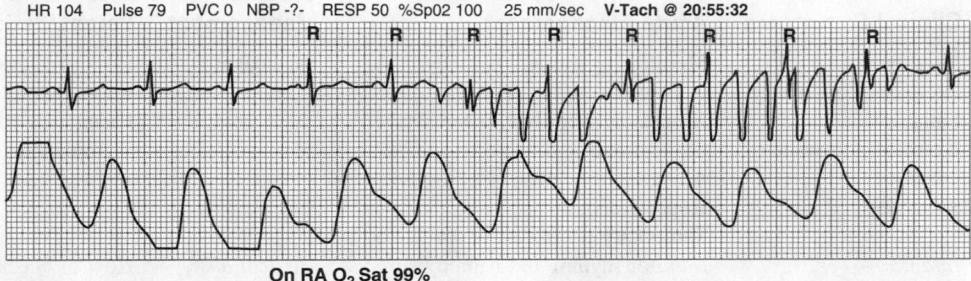

HR 104   Pulse 79   PVC 0   NBP -?-   RESP 50   %SpO2 100   25 mm/sec   **V-Tach @ 20:55:32**

On RA O₂ Sat 99%

FIG. 8-27 Arrhythmia or artifact? A nurse identified this rhythm as ventricular tachycardia. Was the nurse correct? Note that you can "march out" the R-waves (R) throughout this strip and the pulse oximeter waveform corresponds to the R-waves. Artifact from chest physiotherapy, burping a baby, or even shaking the ECG cable can appear similar to ventricular tachycardia. Be sure to assess your patient carefully and use other clues to help with your differential diagnosis.

be palpable. If peripheral pulses are absent and the child's perfusion appears severely compromised, shock resuscitation must commence immediately. If the child has no central pulses (or extreme bradycardia despite effective support of oxygenation and ventilation), cardiopulmonary resuscitation should begin immediately. If possible, someone from the resuscitation team should obtain a rhythm strip to document the event.

If the arrhythmia does not produce a life-threatening compromise in systemic perfusion, further assessment and analysis of the patient's rhythm is possible. A representative rhythm strip should be obtained, and a physician or the on-call provider should be notified. If PVCs are present it is often advisable to record a 2-min rhythm strip so that the frequency of the PVCs can be documented. If time (and patient condition) allows, a 3- or 12-lead ECG should be obtained.

Further evaluation of the arrhythmia will require documentation of precipitating or alleviating factors (e.g., suctioning or administration of medications) and associated changes in the child's clinical condition. Signs of congestive heart failure, alteration in responsiveness, or poor feeding may be indications of compromised systemic perfusion. The nurse should be prepared to report the timing and dosages of any medications the child is receiving and the child's current blood gases, noting any electrolyte and acid-base imbalances.

Acute Management of Arrhythmias

Nursing care of the child with arrhythmias is summarized in Table 8-14.

Bradycardia. The most common cause of bradycardia in infants and children is respiratory compromise. The pediatric nurse caring for a child who suddenly becomes bradycardic must ensure that the airway is patent and provide adequate oxygenation and ventilation. These maneuvers alone will often reverse bradycardia caused by sinus node dysfunction or hypoxemia.

If the bradycardia is vagally mediated, an anticholinergic agent, atropine (0.02 mg/kg), should be given intravenously. In one series, a small atropine dose (per kg) caused mild

slowing of the heart rate,[220] but the need for a minimum atropine dose (0.1 mg) has recently been questioned.[59a] Epinephrine (0.01 mg/kg) may be administered as well. If the heart rate fails to respond adequately to these interventions, isoproterenol, a beta-adrenergic agonist, may be administered as an infusion.[970] In the postoperative cardiac surgery patient, atrial pacing using temporary epicardial pacing wires is the preferred treatment for sinus node dysfunction.

For bradycardic patients with AV block, epinephrine or isoproterenol can be administered to try to support the heart rate acutely. Temporary pacing with transcutaneous or transvenous pacing leads should be instituted as soon as possible. Because of the discomfort associated with transcutaneous pacing, it should be employed for only short periods of time and adequate analgesia must be provided. In the postoperative cardiac surgery patient, temporary epicardial pacing wires can be used. Dual-chamber pacing, when possible, is preferred to provide AV synchrony.

Tachycardia. The most common tachycardia in the critical care unit is sinus tachycardia, which develops in response to the body's demand for increased cardiac output or oxygen delivery. As this acceleration in heart rate is a compensatory mechanism rather than a true rhythm disturbance, treatment is aimed at addressing the underlying cause. Careful assessment of the patient should be performed to discover the reason for the sinus tachycardia. Common causes include hypoxia, hypovolemia (caused by hemorrhage, dehydration, or fluid shifts), anemia, fever, pain, anxiety, stress, or drugs, poisons or toxins. Other less common conditions that lead to sinus tachycardia are cardiac tamponade, pneumothorax, or thromboembolism.[722]

The most common pathologic tachyarrhythmia in infants and children is SVT. Treatment of SVT must consider the degree of hemodynamic compromise because that dictates the urgency of intervention. Treatment may vary depending on the tachycardia mechanism as well. Acute treatment of reentry SVT is generally easier than treatment of automatic SVTs.

Vagal maneuvers are used when the patient with SVT is hemodynamically stable. These are maneuvers that parents can be taught to perform at home in the event their child

Table 8-14 Nursing Care of the Pediatric Patient with Arrhythmias

Arrhythmia	Clinical Symptoms	Acute Management	Chronic Management	Parent/Patient Education
Sinus Node Dysfunction	Slow heart rate Irregular heart beat Fatigue Exercise intolerance Dizziness Syncope	Monitor rhythm and hemodynamic status If unstable, ventilate, oxygenate Epinephrine Atropine Isoproterenolol Temporary pacing	Pacemaker	How to check pulse rate Report symptoms to cardiologist Pacemaker education if device is implanted
Supraventricular Tachycardia	*Infant:* Irritability, lethargy Poor feeding Pallor Sweating CHF *Older child:* Palpitations Fast heart rate Chest discomfort Dizziness	Monitor rhythm and hemodynamic status If stable, vagal maneuvers Overdrive pacing Adenosine—may be diagnostic and/or therapeutic (0.1-0.2 mg rapid IV bolus) If unstable, synchronized cardioversion (0.5-1.0 J/kg) For JET, IV amiodarone or dexmedetomidine plus overdrive pacing	*Medications:* Digoxin for non-WPW only Propranolol Atenolol Flecainide Sotalol Amiodarone RF or cryo ablation	How to check pulse rate Report symptoms to cardiologist How to perform vagal maneuvers (check with cardiologist first) If symptomatic, go to emergency room Medication teaching as needed Procedural teaching if electrophysiology study with ablation is planned
Ventricular Tachycardia	Cardiac arrest or Poor perfusion *Infant:* Lethargy Tachypnea Pallor Poor feeding *Older child:* Palpitations Chest discomfort Dizziness Nausea Syncope	If pulseless: CPR and defibrillation (2-4 J/kg and higher) If pulses: monitor rhythm and hemodynamic status; synchronized cardioversion (0.5-1.0 J/kg) *IV medications:* Amiodarone Lidocaine, Procainamide Correct electrolyte imbalance ECMO or VAD for uncontrolled incessant VT	*Medications:* Amiodarone Beta-blockers Verapamil (in Verapamil-sensitive VT) RF ablation ICD	How to check pulse rate How to perform CPR Call 911 in the event of syncope or arrest Medication teaching as needed Avoid medications that cause QT prolongation Procedural teaching if ICD is planned Activity restrictions as prescribed by cardiologist
Long QT Syndrome	Syncope/presyncope often associated with exercise, noise or stress Palpitations Seizures Cardiac arrest	Monitor rhythm and hemodynamic status For Torsades de pointes, initiate CPR Synchronized cardioversion Administer IV beta blocker (Esmolol) Temporary overdrive pacing to suppress VT	*Medications:* Beta blockers Propranolol Atenolol Possible Alpha blockers Possible Na^+ or Ca^{+2} ion-channel blockers Pacemaker ICD	How to check pulse rate How to perform CPR Call 911 in the event of syncope or arrest Family members need ECGs to evaluate QT (hereditary); consider genetic testing Medication teaching Procedural teaching if pacemaker or ICD is planned *Avoid triggers:* Competitive athletics Loud noises (LQT2) Hypokalemia Medications that cause QT prolongation
AV Block (2° or 3°)	CHF Fatigue Exercise intolerance Dizziness Syncope	Temporary pacemaker	Pacemaker	How to check pulse rate How to perform CPR if pacemaker dependent Call 911 in the event of syncope or arrest Procedural teaching for pacemaker implant Pacemaker education, emphasize no contact or collision-type sports

develops SVT. Vagal maneuvers slow conduction through the AV node and are therefore effective in breaking SVTs in which the AV node is part of the reentry circuit. Specifically, vagal maneuvers can be used for AVRT (including WPW), AVNRT, and PJRT, but they will not work for atrial flutter, IART, or the automatic tachycardias, such as AET or JET.

For infants, eliciting the diving reflex by applying ice to the face works well to increase vagal tone. Ice and water is placed in a plastic bag and applied over the forehead, eyes, and bridge of the nose, with care taken not to obstruct the nares. The tachycardia is successfully converted within 5 to 10 seconds in 33% to 62% of the cases.[639] Also, for infants, stimulation with a rectal thermometer may work as a vagal maneuver as well.

Older children may be instructed in the Valsalva maneuver. This consists of forced expiration against a closed glottis. The basic instruction to "bear down," as if having a bowel movement, may not be well-received by young patients. Asking the child to blow on his thumb like a trumpet or blow into an obstructed straw may be more acceptable ways to elicit the Valsalva maneuver. Gagging, coughing, or performing a head stand may also be effective. Unilateral carotid massage may be used by someone trained in the technique. Ocular pressure should be avoided in children because of the risk of causing retinal detachment.[563]

Adenosine is the drug of choice for acute termination of SVT. Adenosine works by transiently blocking AV nodal conduction. As with vagal maneuvers, adenosine is only effective for those SVTs propagated by a reentry circuit that includes the AV node (AVRT, AVNRT, and PJRT). These circuits are found in 90% of pediatric SVTs. Adenosine is not effective in atrial flutter or IART, but may be diagnostic by slowing the ventricular rate to the point where the underlying atrial tachycardia can be more clearly appreciated.

In order to produce AV block, adenosine must be administered rapidly. A well-functioning IV should be in place, preferably one located more central (e.g., antecubital) rather than distal (e.g., hand). A rhythm strip should be obtained while the drug is administered. Two syringes, one with adenosine (0.1 mg/kg) and the other with an adequate flush, should be attached to a 3-way stopcock near the site of catheter entry into the body. The adenosine should be given IV push, followed immediately by rapid injection of the flush solution (Fig. 8-28). The effects of adenosine are very short, usually less than 10 s, but because it causes AV block, a transcutaneous pacemaker for temporary back-up pacing should be readily available in case bradycardia persists following conversion. Careful ECG and blood pressure monitoring is paramount before, during, and following adenosine administration. If parents are at the bedside, they should be warned about the transient asystole they may see on the cardiac monitor when the drug is given.

If the patient with SVT is hemodynamically unstable, immediate DC cardioversion should be performed using a dose of 0.5-1 Joule/kg. It is important that the "sync" operation is activated to avoid delivering a shock into the T-wave

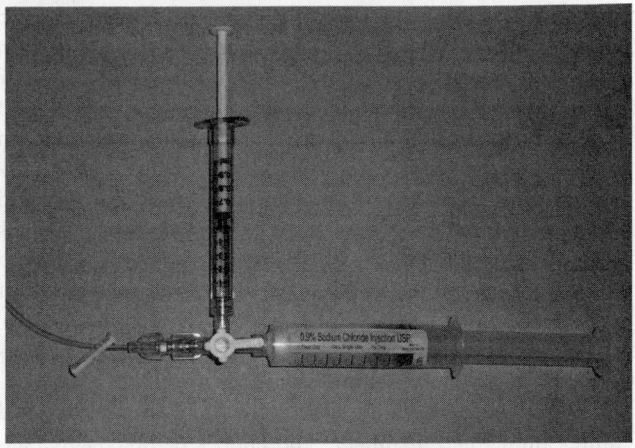

FIG. 8-28 "Two syringe" and stopcock arrangement for rapid administration of adenosine.

and inducing ventricular fibrillation. If the child is conscious, appropriate sedation should be given prior to cardioversion. If the first attempt fails, increase the energy to 2 J/kg and again select "synch" and try again.[479a] If this fails, reevaluate the patient's rhythm to determine if the rhythm could be sinus tachycardia or an automatic tachycardia (AET or JET). These latter rhythms do not respond to DC cardioversion.

Intravenous antiarrhythmic agents may be given for SVTs that are difficult to control or nonresponsive to the above measures. Amiodarone or procainamide are the medications most commonly used (see Tables 8-14 and 8-15). The patient receiving either of these drugs should be monitored closely for hypotension, bradycardia, AV block, or any proarrhythmic effects. Because both amiodarone and procainamide prolong the QT interval, they are usually not used together and expert consultation is advisable.

The use of a beta-adrenergic blocker, either esmolol or propranolol, may be another option in the acute management of SVT. With beta-blocking agents, the patient should be observed closely for adverse effects, especially bradycardia, hypotension, bronchospasm, or hypoglycemia.[3,486,954]

Overdrive atrial pacing may also be attempted to convert SVT to sinus rhythm. In the postoperative cardiac surgery patient, temporary atrial epicardial pacing wires can be used. Alternatively, a transesophageal pacing catheter can be positioned with the electrodes situated in the esophagus behind the left atrium. An atrial electrogram from these leads can confirm atrial positioning and help with identification of the rhythm by isolating the atrial activity from the ventricular rhythm. Multichannel ECG recording should be performed during this procedure to document the arrhythmia and subsequent conversion. Atrial pacing at a rate 10 to 30/min faster than the atrial tachycardia is then performed for approximately 10 to 30 s to overdrive and suppress the tachycardia and interrupt the reentry circuit.

The management of postoperative JET, as discussed earlier, is aimed at slowing the junctional rate and establishing AV synchrony. This is usually accomplished by infusing an antiarrhythmic agent, typically amiodarone, but procainamide, propafenone, and more recently, dexmedetomidine have been used successfully.[177] Atrial pacing at a rate faster than the JET rate restores AV synchrony (atrial "kick"). Other measures, such as maintaining normothermia or even mild hypothermia, and limiting use of catecholamines, help to decrease junctional automaticity.

In rare instances, an incessant atrial tachycardia with rapid conduction to the ventricles or JET refractory to therapies mentioned above may develop. These conditions pose a high risk for cardiovascular collapse. Radiofrequency ablation of the AV node may be required to intentionally create AV block.[103,898] Permanent ventricular pacing would then be necessary to support an adequate ventricular rhythm.

Ventricular tachycardia is often life-threatening and requires immediate treatment. The child's hemodynamic status and, in particular, the presence or absence of a pulse, helps to determine the course of action. In the event of sustained, wide-complex tachycardia in a hemodynamically unstable patient, if a pulse is palpable, synchronized cardioversion is the treatment of choice, starting at 0.5 to 1 J/kg.[722] Sedation should be given whenever possible to conscious patients prior to shock delivery. Intravenous medications that may help to terminate the tachycardia or prevent recurrence of the tachycardia include amiodarone, procainamide, or lidocaine. If the rhythm appears to be torsades de pointes, or if the baseline ECG shows a prolonged QT interval, amiodarone or procainamide should *not* be given, because these drugs are known to cause QT prolongation.[270,970] Lidocaine and magnesium sulfate are appropriate to use in these patients. Esmolol may also be useful in patients with long QT syndrome.[51]

Pulseless ventricular tachycardia is managed the same as ventricular fibrillation. Both are forms of cardiac arrest and require immediate treatment, starting with basic CPR and oxygen administration. Defibrillation should be performed as quickly as possible, using 2 J/kg initially, followed by 4 J/kg or more if subsequent shocks are necessary.[479a] Epinephrine may given, followed by amiodarone or lidocaine.[722] Magnesium should be given for torsades de pointes or if hypomagnesemia is suspected.

For nonshockable rhythms, namely asystole or pulseless electrical activity (PEA), CPR, oxygen, and epinephrine (every 3 to 5 mins) are recommended.[722] In PEA, possible causes should be explored and addressed.

Antiarrhythmic Drug Therapy. Antiarrhythmic medications are used in acute situations to chemically convert tachycardias, suppress automaticity, and/or control the ventricular rate. Chronically, antiarrhythmic drug therapy is reserved for young infants who may be too small to safely undergo ablation or when an SVT is unlikely to resolve spontaneously. Long-term pharmacologic treatment may also be prescribed for children who are not candidates for ablation, have had failed ablation attempts, or in cases where the rhythm disturbance is not amenable to ablation. Drugs may be used in combination with device therapy to control tachyarrhythmias and reduce the risk of sudden cardiac death. Table 8-15 lists the antiarrhythmic agents used commonly in pediatrics. For each drug the indications, dose, serum level and drug interactions are listed.

The Vaughan Williams classification of antiarrhythmic agents is used to group drugs based on their effect. Class I agents comprise the sodium channel blockers. These drugs slow conduction through the heart and vary in their effect on repolarization. They are used to treat reentrant and automatic tachycardias. Class I agents may prolong the QT interval, so close monitoring is required. Class II agents are beta-adrenergic blockers that slow sinus node and AV node conduction, resulting in decreased heart rates and prolongation of the PR interval. They are prescribed for automatic tachycardias, reentrant tachycardias using the AV node, and long QT syndrome. Beta-blockers may cause hypoglycemia in susceptible children or exacerbate bronchospasm in asthmatic patients. Symptoms of fatigue, inattentiveness in school, and depression have been reported as well. Class III agents are potassium channel blockers that decrease automaticity, slow AV conduction, and prolong cardiac repolarization. They are effective in controlling both reentrant and automatic tachycardias. However, the resulting QT interval prolongation and the potential to trigger torsades de pointes warrant careful monitoring of patients receiving sotalol or amiodarone. Class IV agents are calcium channel blockers. These act by slowing SA and AV node conduction and are useful in treating reentrant SVTs but should not be used in WPW. Intravenous administration of verapamil is contraindicated in infants because severe hypotension and cardiovascular collapse may result.[255]

In-hospital monitoring is recommended when initiating therapy with antiarrhythmic drugs that have a higher risk for proarrhythmic effects. These medications include quinidine, procainamide, disopyramide, flecainide, propafenone, sotalol, and amiodarone.

When antiarrhythmic therapy is initiated the nurse should constantly monitor the effects of the medication on the child's ECG. Rhythm strips should be obtained and recorded in the patient's chart at regular intervals (usually at the beginning of each shift). Recording the absence of arrhythmia is just as important as documenting its occurrence. The nurse should also be vigilant about assessing the patient for side effects from antiarrhythmic drugs.

Long-Term Arrhythmia Management
Long-term arrhythmia management requires intervention beyond the critical care environment.

Device Therapy. Pacemakers are used to treat bradycardia and/or restore AV synchrony. Indications for chronic pacing therapy include sinus node dysfunction with symptomatic bradycardia or heart rates less than 40/min. Pacing is also indicated for congenital AV block with a wide QRS escape rhythm, congenital complete AV block with heart rates less than 55/min in the infant with a structurally normal heart or less than 70/min in the infant with coexisting congenital heart disease, or any child with advanced second- or third-degree AV block that persists at least 7 days after cardiac surgery.[254]

Pacemakers function by sending out an imperceptible electrical impulse to stimulate the heart whenever a pause in the rhythm is detected. The device functions within programmed

Table 8-15 Pediatric Antiarrhythmic Therapy

Drug	Indications	Route/Dose	Serum Concentration, Peak and Half-life	Side Effects/Comments	Drug Interactions
Class I: Sodium Channel Blockers					
A: Moderate Sodium Channel Blocker; Prolongs Repolarization					
Quinidine	AET, post-op AFL	PO: 15-60 mg/kg per day Sulfate q 6 h Gluconate q 8-12 h	2-7 g/mL Peak: 1-2 h (QS) Half-life: 6-8 h (QG)	Hypotension, syncope, headache, tinnitus, nausea, vomiting, diarrhea, rash, thrombocytopenia; monitor QT interval	Digoxin, phenytoin, amiodarone, propranolol, coumadin, rifampin
Procainamide	AVRT, AVNRT, postop AFL/AF, AET, JET, ventricular ectopy	IV: Load: 3-7 mg/kg over 30 to 60 min Maint: 20-60 g/kg per minute PO: 15-100 mg/kg per day q 6 h	4-10 g/mL Peak: 1-2 h Half-life: 3-4 h	Negative inotropy, nausea, vomiting, diarrhea, rash, drug-induced SLE; Contraindicated in myasthenia gravis; monitor QT interval	Amiodarone, digoxin, propranolol, trimethoprim
Disopyramide	Postop AFL, VT	PO: <2 yr: 20-33 mg/kg per day 2-10 yr: 10-24 mg/kg per day >10 yr: 6-14 mg/kg per day q 6-8 h; SR q 12 h	2-5 g/mL Peak: 2 h Half-life: 4-10 h	Negative inotropy, AV block, dry mouth, blurred vision, constipation, urinary retention	Atenolol, phenytoin
B: Weak Sodium Channel Blocker; Shortens Repolarization					
Lidocaine	PVC, VT, VF	IV: Load: 1-3 mg/kg Maint: 10-50 g/kg per minute	1-5 g/mL Half-life: 1.8 h in children; 3.2 h in neonates	Dizziness, drowsiness, tinnitus, paresthesia, slurred speech, visual disturbances, seizures	Propranolol, phenytoin, isoproterenol, Ca channel blockers, cyclosporine, tacrolimus, benzodiazepines
Mexiletine	Ventricular ectopy; LQT3	PO: 4.2-15 mg/kg per day q 8 h	Peak: 1-4 h Half-life: 6-12 h	Nausea, vomiting, headache, tremors, dizziness, drowsiness, paresthesia, rash, hepatitis	Phenytoin, rifampin
Tocainide	Ventricular ectopy	PO: 20-40 mg/kg per day q 8 h	3-7 g/mL Peak: 4 h Half-life: 11 h	Tremors, dizziness, nausea, ataxia, confusion, paresthesia, blood dyscrasias, hepatitis	Metoprolol, propranolol
Phenytoin	Digoxin-induced arrhythmias, postop PVC, VT	IV: Load: 10-15 mg/kg PO: Day 1, 15 mg/kg q 6 h Day 2, 7.2 mg/kg q 6 h Maint: 4-8 mg/kg per day q 8-12 h	10-20 g/mL Peak: 1.5-3 h Half-life: 7-40 h (75 h in premies)	Gingival hyperplasia, ataxia, hypotension, drowsiness, nystagmus, drug-induced SLE; Teratogenic	Coumadin, verapamil, amiodarone, phenytoin, phenobarbital
C: Strong Sodium Channel Blocker					
Flecainide	Newborn SVT, AVRT, AVNRT, JET, PJRT, AET, MAT, VT	PO: 3-6 mg/kg per day q 8-12 h (100-225 mg/m² per day)	0.2-1 g/mL Peak: 1.5-3 h Half-life: 7-12 h	Negative inotropy, worsens CHF, nausea,vomiting, headache, blurred vision, irritability, hyperactivity, dry mouth; Proarrhythmia; Increases pacing thresholds	Digoxin, amiodarone, propranolol, verapamil, disopyramide; Dairy products interfere with absorption
Propafenone	Newborn SVT, AVRT, AVNRT, JET, PJRT, AET, MAT	IV: Load: 0.2 mg/kg q 10 min (Maximum 2 mg) Maint: 4-7 g/kg per minute PO: 8-15 mg/kg per day q 6 h (200-600 mg/m² per day)	0.2-1 g/ML Peak: 2-3 h Half-life: 5-17 h	Worsens CHF, hypotension, headache, blurred vision, paresthesia, bitter taste, constipation, nausea, fatigue, drug-induced SLE; Proarrhythmia	Digoxin, beta-blockers, amiodarone
Class II: Beta-Adrenergic Blockers					
Propranolol	Newborn SVT, AVNRT, JET, PJRT, AET, MAT, VT, long QT	IV: Load: 0.01-0.15 mg/kg PO: 1-4 mg/kg per day q 6 h		Hypotension, bradycardia, worsens CHF, fatigue, insomnia, depression, hypoglycemia, bronchospasm; Contraindicated in asthma	Verapamil, propafenone, quinidine, lidocaine, furosemide
Atenolol	AVRT, AVNRT, JET, PJRT, AET, MAT, VT, long QT	PO: 1-2 mg/kg per day q 12-24 h	Peak: 2-3 h Half-life: 5-9 h (16 h in neonates)	Less bronchoconstriction, hypoglycemia than propranolol; Bradycardia	Verapamil
Nadolol	Long QT	PO: 1-2 mg/kg per day q 24 h	Peak: 3-4 h Half-life: 12-24 h	Bronchoconstriction in asthmatics, headache, sleep disturbances, abdominal pain	

Continued

Table 8-15 Pediatric Antiarrhythmic Therapy—cont'd

Drug	Indications	Route/Dose	Serum Concentration, Peak and Half-life	Side Effects/Comments	Drug Interactions
Esmolol	Acute reduction of ventricular rate in AFL, AF	IV: Load: 500 g/kg Maint: 50 g/kg per minute (up to 200 g/kg per minute)	Half-life: 9 min	Hypotension, somnolence, headache, dizziness, nausea, vomiting	Digoxin, coumadin, morphine
Sotalol	Newborn SVT, AVRT, AVNRT, PJRT, AET, MAT, postop AFL/AF, postop PVC, VT, long QT	PO: 2-8 mg/kg per day q 12 h (40-350 mg/m² per day)	Half-life: 12 h	Bradycardia, hypotension Proarrhythmic	Verapamil
Class III: Potassium Channel Blockers					
Amiodarone	Newborn SVT, AVRT, JET, PJRT, AET, CAT, postop AFL/AF, PVC, VT	IV: 5 mg/kg >15-30 min Repeat in 15 min if needed Maint: 10-20 mg/kg per day PO: Load: 10 mg/kg per day q 12 h × 1-2 weeks (max. 1.2 Gm/day) Maint: 5-10 mg/kg per day q 24 h	0.5-2.5 mg/mL Peak: 5-6 h (PO) Half-life: 8-107 days (average 1 mo)	Bradycardia, hypotension, corneal microdeposits, nausea, ataxia, rash, photosensitivity, skin discoloration, thyroid and liver dysfunction, constipation; Side effects less common in children than adults	Digoxin, quinidine, procainamide, phenytoin, flecainide, coumadin, cyclosporine
Class IV: Calcium Channel Blockers					
Verapamil	IV: SVT if >1 y PO: Newborn SVT (not WPW), AVRT, AVNRT	IV: Load: 75-150 g/kg Maint: 5 g/kg per minute PO: 4-17 mg/kg per day q 8 h	0.1-0.3 g/mL Half-life: 12 h	*IV administration is not recommended in infants* Hypotension, bradycardia, atrioventricular block, asystole, CHF, flushing, constipation	Beta-blockers, digoxin, quinidine, disopyramide, coumadin, midazolam
Diltiazem	Postop AFL/AF	IV: Load: 0.25 mg/kg over 2 min Maint: 2 g/kg per minute PO: 120-360 mg/d (adult dose)		Hypotension	Digoxin, propranolol, cyclosporine, carbamazepine
Class V: Digitalis Glycoside					
Digoxin	Newborn SVT (not WPW), AVRT, AVNRT, PJRT, AET, MAT	PO: TDD* Premature infant: 20 g/kg Full-term newborn: 30 g/kg Infant <2 years: 40-50 g/kg Children >2 years: 30-40 g/kg Maint: 25% of TDD daily q 12 h IV: Reduce PO dose by 20% to 25%	1-2 ng/mL up to 3.5 ng/mL in infants Half-life: Premie: 61 h Newborn: 35 h Infant: 18 h Children: 37 h	Digoxin toxicity: anorexia, nausea, vomiting, lethargy, visual changes, headache, seizures, gynecomastia, atrioventricular block, SVT, PVCs, VT, VF (treat digoxin-induced arrhythmias with phenytoin)	Quinidine, amiodarone, verapamil, phenytoin, coumadin, erythromycin, spironolactone
Class VI: Purinergic Agent					
Adenosine	Acute treatment of AVRT, AVNRT, PJRT	IV: 0.1-0.2 mg/kg rapid bolus Double every several minutes up to 4.4 mg/kg	Half-life: <10 s	Transient sinus bradycardia, arrest, atrial ectopy, atrial fibrillation, PVCs, hypotension, flushing, irritability, nausea, chest pain, headache, bronchoconstriction in asthmatics	Quinidine, digoxin, verapamil

Data from: Bink-Boelkens MT: Pharmacologic management of arrhythmias. *Pediatr Cardiol* 21(6):508-515, 2000; Hanisch DG, Van Hare GF: Long-term antiarrhythmic drug therapy. In Zeigler VL, Gillette PC, editors: *Practical management of pediatric cardiac arrhythmias*, Armonk, NY, 2001, Futura, pp. 231-265; Kannankeril PJ, Fish FA: Disorders of cardiac rhythm and conduction. In Allen HD, Driscoll DJ, Shaddy RE, Feltes TF, editors: *Moss and Adams' heart disease in infants, children, and adolescents*, ed 7, Philadelphia, 2008, Lippincott Williams & Wilkins, pp. 293-342.

*TDD: total digitalizing dose: Initially give half of TDD; then in 8 h, give one fourth of TDD; 8 h later, give last one fourth of TDD.

AET, Atrial ectopic tachycardia; *AF*, atrial fibrillation; *AFL*, atrial flutter; *AVRT*, atrioventricular reentry tachycardia; *CHF*, congestive heart failure; *JET*, junctional ectopic tachycardia; *Load*, loading dose; *Maint.*, maintenance dose; *MAT*, multifocal atrial tachycardia; *AVNRT*, atrioventricular nodal reentry tachycardia; *PJRT*, permanent junctional reciprocating tachycardia; *PVC*, premature ventricular contractions; *SLE*, systemic lupus erythematosus; *SVT*, supraventricular tachycardia; *VF*, ventricular fibrillation; *VT*, ventricular tachycardia; *WPW*, Wolff-Parkinson-White syndrome.

timing parameters including a base pacing rate, upper tracking rate, and programmed AV delay (see Chapter 21).

Implantable cardioverter-defibrillators (ICDs) are used to treat ventricular tachyarrhythmias and prevent sudden cardiac death in patients deemed to be at high risk. The ICD analyzes heart rates above a set tachycardia detection zone to identify VT or ventricular fibrillation. Various algorithms may be programmed according to the patient's diagnosis or type of tachycardia. The ICD may first attempt overdrive pacing maneuvers to try to convert VT. Ultimately, the ICD will charge and then deliver a shock to the heart to eliminate VT or VF. ICDs can function as pacemakers as well if rate support is needed.

Ablation Procedures. Many tachyarrhythmias are amenable to ablation procedures. Catheter ablations are performed in the catheterization laboratory by an electrophysiologist. An electrophysiology study is first performed to "map" the arrhythmia using three to five electrode catheters strategically positioned within the heart to produce multiple intracardiac electrograms. Once the electrical pathway or arrhythmogenic focus responsible for a tachycardia is located, an ablation catheter is positioned at that site. Radiofrequency (RF) energy heats the catheter tip to 50 to 60° C, creating a localized "burn" to abolish the tissue's ability to conduct impulses. When the electrical pathway is situated near the AV node, as in AVNRT, cryoablation, using liquid nitrous oxide at temperatures of −70 to −80° C, "freezes" the site.[192,193] Cryoablation results in a smaller, more discrete lesion with less depth than RF ablation.

Success rates for RF ablation procedures in pediatric patients have been quite good: 97% for AVNRT, 94% for AVRT, 92% for AET, 85% for IART, and 78% for VT.[896,897] The overall complication rate is 3% with a tachyarrhythmia recurrence rate around 10%.[897]

Surgical ablation may be performed in the operating room in conjunction with congenital heart surgery.[586,587] A variety of atrial tachycardias, especially IART, and some ventricular tachycardias may be amenable to ablative techniques performed during open heart surgery. In addition to cryoablation and radiofrequency ablation, the surgeon may make multiple incision lines within the heart to block reentrant tachycardias. Young adult patients undergoing Fontan conversions from an atriopulmonary connection to a total cavopulmonary extracardiac Fontan to improve hemodynamics have had successful treatment of IART and other atrial tachyarrhythmias with the Cox-maze procedure.[586]

HYPOXEMIA CAUSED BY CYANOTIC CONGENITAL HEART DISEASE

Mary Fran Hazinski

Pearls

- To have visible cyanosis, there must be about 3 to 5 gm of desaturated hemoglobin present per dL of blood. This means that the anemic child may not be visibly cyanotic despite the presence of significant hypoxemia; conversely, the polycythemic child may appear very cyanotic despite near-normal arterial oxygen content.

- When cyanotic heart disease is present, systemic venous blood is entering the systemic arterial circulation. Therefore, *no air can be allowed to enter any intravenous line*—it can enter the cerebral arterial circulation and cause a stroke.
- Polycythemia may help the child with cyanotic heart disease maintain near-normal arterial oxygen content despite arterial oxygen desaturation. However, if the child becomes anemic or develops a compromise in cardiac output, systemic oxygen delivery may fall and tissue hypoxia may quickly develop.
- Systemic consequences of polycythemia include thrombocytopenia and thrombocytopathia. In addition, patients may develop hyperviscosity syndrome.

Etiology

Cyanosis is the blue color that may be observed in the mucous membranes, nail beds, skin, and/or sclera of the child with arterial oxygen desaturation. Cyanosis usually is not visible until there are about 3 to 5 gm of reduced hemoglobin (hemoglobin not bound with oxygen) per 100 mL of blood (i.e., per deciliter of blood). This usually correlates to an arterial oxygen saturation of 75% to 85%. Because the degree of cyanosis that is visible is dependent on both the total amount of hemoglobin present and its saturation, cyanosis itself is not a reliable indicator of the degree of hypoxemia present. An anemic patient may be profoundly hypoxemic before cyanosis is observed, and a polycythemic patient may appear extremely cyanotic at only modest levels of arterial oxygen desaturation. In addition, the detection of cyanosis depends on the experience of the observer and the ambient lighting conditions. Mildly cyanotic children can appear extremely cyanotic when they are surrounded by blue linen and acyanotic when surrounded by pink linen.

Acrocyanosis, or peripheral cyanosis, is observed in the extremities and around the mouth of the newborn but does not involve the mucous membranes or nailbeds. Acrocyanosis is normal in the newborn and is considered the result of vasomotor instability. It generally disappears when the child is swaddled (to produce increased warmth) or becomes more active.

Causes of Hypoxemia in Children. Because arterial oxygen desaturation can be caused by either cardiac or respiratory disease it is important for the nurse to carefully document the distribution and degree of cyanosis as well as any precipitating or alleviating factors. Cyanosis that *decreases* with cry generally is thought to be *respiratory* in origin and is relieved by the increase in tidal volume during vigorous cry. Cyanosis that *increases* with cry is usually *cardiac* in origin because the expiratory phase of crying tends to increase resistance to pulmonary blood flow and enhance right-to-left intracardiac shunting in the presence of cyanotic heart disease. Cyanosis that is respiratory in origin usually improves with oxygen administration; cyanosis that is cardiac in origin does not (because the intracardiac shunt allows blood to pass into the systemic circulation without ever entering the lungs). The child with cyanosis resulting from respiratory disease often will demonstrate other signs of respiratory distress, including tachypnea and increased respiratory effort (retractions, nasal flaring, and grunting). The child with cyanosis resulting from heart disease also may be tachypneic but usually will not demonstrate signs of increased respiratory effort (i.e., "quiet tachypnea" is present) unless congestive heart failure or acidosis is also present.

To aid in differentiation of respiratory versus cardiac causes of cyanosis, physicians may obtain an arterial blood gas specimen when the child is breathing room air and then obtain an arterial blood gas specimen when the child is receiving 100% oxygen (Box 8-11). If the child's arterial oxygen tension increases by more than 20 torr or rises above 200 torr while breathing 100% oxygen, the cyanosis is probably respiratory in origin. If the child's oxygen tension does *not* increase appreciably with the administration of oxygen, and particularly if the arterial oxygen tension remains below 50 mm Hg, the cyanosis is probably cardiac in origin. Because the child with cyanotic congenital heart disease has intracardiac shunts, some systemic venous blood bypasses the lungs and that shunted blood is never exposed to the increased alveolar (inspired) oxygen concentration.

When cyanotic heart disease is present, systemic venous blood is entering the systemic (arterial) circulation. This can result from:

- Severe obstruction to right heart or pulmonary flow and shunting of blood from the right to the left side of the heart (or from pulmonary artery to aorta);
- Mixing of arterial and venous blood within the heart or great vessels; or
- Transposition of the great vessels

The specific cardiac defects that cause cyanosis are discussed in the fourth section of this chapter. The following discussion summarizes the potential systemic consequences of arterial oxygen desaturation and medical and nursing interventions.

Pathophysiology

The two major compensatory responses to chronic hypoxemia are the development of polycythemia (increase in hemoglobin concentration to increase oxygen carrying capacity of the

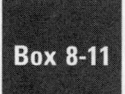

Box 8-11 **Hyperoxia Test for Newborns with Suspected Cyanotic Heart Disease (to distinguish intrapulmonary from intracardiac shunt)[364]**

(1) Administer room air to the newborn (10–15 min, if tolerated)
(2) Obtain baseline arterial PO_2 from right radial artery (via arterial puncture or transcutaneous oxygen monitor—pulse oximetry oxyhemoglobin saturation cannot be used)
(3) Administer 100% oxygen (via mask, oxygen hood or endotracheal tube, if intubated) for 10–15 min
(4) Obtain arterial PO_2 from right radial artery (via arterial puncture or transcutaneous oxygen monitor—pulse oximetry oxyhemoglobin saturation cannot be used)

Results:

- PaO_2 <50 mm Hg despite administration of 100% oxygen: cyanotic heart disease likely
- PaO_2 50–250 mm Hg: cyanotic heart disease possible
- PaO_2 >250 mm Hg: cyanotic heart disease unlikely

blood) and an increase in the oxygen release to the tissues (related to increased erythrocyte levels of 2,3 diphosphoglycerate or 2,3 DPG). Each of these compensatory mechanisms may produce complications.

Systemic Consequences of Polycythemia. Chronic arterial oxygen desaturation stimulates erythropoietin secretion by the kidney, producing erythropoiesis (red blood cell production) and polycythemia. Perinatal polycythemia is normal, and the neonate may have a hematocrit as high as 65% within the first hours of life (particularly if the umbilical cord is "milked" toward the infant before it is cut). Within the first weeks of life, however, if the hematocrit does not fall, polycythemia is present.

Polycythemia increases the viscosity of the blood; this can lead to systemic complications including thromboembolic events, brain abscess, and coagulopathies. The development of microcytic anemia further increases the viscosity of the blood and red blood cells;[540] this produces a high risk of spontaneous thromboembolic events. The incidence of spontaneous cerebrovascular accidents among children with uncorrected cyanotic congenital heart disease was approximately 1.6%/year in the 1970s before corrective procedures were available.[698] The risk is highest among those patients with a mean hematocrit above 60%, a mean hemoglobin concentration of 20 g/dL or higher, and microcytic anemia (a low mean corpuscular hemoglobin concentration and/or mean corpuscular volume).

Children with uncorrected cyanotic congenital heart disease can develop brain abscesses. Although this complication is becoming rare because corrective procedures are performed at a young age, it should be suspected in the child with cyanotic heart disease who develops fever, headaches, or signs and symptoms of increased intracranial pressure. Based on natural history of cyanotic congenital heart disease again from the 1970s, the incidence of brain abscess is highest in children greater than 2 years of age and in those children with tetralogy of Fallot or transposition of the great vessels.[269] The pathophysiology of brain abscess formation is not understood completely, but it seems to be related to an episode of bacteremia and some compromise in cerebral microcirculation.

Children with polycythemia and chronic hypoxemia often develop a hemorrhagic diathesis (a coagulopathy), which may produce severe postoperative bleeding. They often demonstrate thrombocytopathia with or without thrombocytopenia because platelet survival time is shortened and platelet aggregation is reduced.[202] The severity of the thrombocytopenia and thrombocytopathia is directly related to the severity of hypoxemia and to the severity of the polycythemia (i.e., the lower the oxygen saturation and the higher the hemoglobin, the more significant the effect on the platelet number and function). Synthesis of vitamin K-dependent clotting factors in the liver also is impaired, but does not improve with administration of vitamin K.

Polycythemia can cause a hyperviscosity state.[202] Vascular shear stresses are increased when blood viscosity increases. As a result, pulmonary vascular resistance increases as the hematocrit rises, especially when pulmonary blood flow is reduced. Children with cyanotic heart disease may develop pulmonary vascular disease within 1 year even if pulmonary blood flow is normal. It is thought that these vascular changes are related to the shear stresses and the development of pulmonary microemboli.

Children may develop systemic complications of hyperviscosity. These may produce headache, increased cyanosis, decreased exercise tolerance and spontaneous cerebral thromboembolism (stroke).

Digital clubbing (rounding and enlargement of the tips of fingers and toes) occurs after several months of chronic hypoxemia. The etiology of clubbing is understood poorly, but it is thought to be related to abnormal peripheral circulation secondary to the hypoxemia and polycythemia.

Increased Levels of 2,3 DPG. Children with chronic hypoxemia have high levels of erythrocyte 2,3 diphosphoglycerate. This shifts the oxyhemoglobin dissociation curve to the *right* so that at a given arterial oxygen tension (PaO_2) the hemoglobin is less well saturated. As a result, cyanosis will be apparent at a PaO_2 that normally would not be associated with cyanosis; for this reason, cyanosis is detected readily in the child with cyanotic heart disease at relatively mild levels of hypoxemia. However, the rise in 2,3 DPG also facilitates oxygen release to the tissues so that tissue oxygenation is not as severe as it otherwise would be for the level of hypoxemia.

Hypercyanotic Spells. Children with unrepaired cyanotic heart disease may demonstrate paroxysmal hypercyanotic episodes; they occur most commonly in children with tetralogy of Fallot, but are seen in children with other cyanotic defects as well. The development of these spells is not correlated with the degree of cyanosis or hypoxemia present or with the child's hematocrit. They occur most commonly during the first year of life. These episodes can be very frightening to observe because the child suddenly becomes deeply cyanotic, hypoxemic with tissue hypoxia, and hyperpneic and may lose consciousness or develop seizures.

Hypercyanotic spells are incompletely understood, but seem to be related to an acute reduction in pulmonary blood flow or an acute increase in oxygen requirement in the presence of fixed pulmonary blood flow and relatively fixed oxygen delivery. Hyperpnea also has been proposed as a possible contributing factor. Blood gas analysis of children during hypercyanotic episodes documented arterial oxygen saturations as low as 15% to 33% and arterial oxygen tensions as low as 20 mm Hg.[631]

The development of hypercyanotic spells is considered an indication for urgent surgical intervention to improve systemic arterial oxygenation. These spells are dangerous because they are associated with the development of profound hypoxemia and probable cerebral hypoxia; death and cerebrovascular accidents may occur during these episodes.

Clinical Signs and Symptoms

Because polycythemia increases the oxygen-carrying capacity of the blood the child's arterial *oxygen content* may be normal or near-normal despite the presence of hypoxemia (a low arterial oxygen tension), provided the hemoglobin concentration remains elevated and cardiac output is adequate. Therefore the presence of *hypoxemia* does not mean that tissue *hypoxia*

is present (For an example of calculation of oxygen content in a patient with cyanotic heart disease, see Evolve Box 8-4 in the Chapter 8 Supplement on the Evolve Website).

The signs of deterioration in the child with cyanotic heart disease include deterioration in systemic perfusion (development of pallor, increased respiratory distress, gasping respirations, lethargy, cool extremities, and oliguria), development of metabolic/lactic acidosis, or a significant fall in the child's arterial oxygen tension (less than the child's normal or less than 30 to 35 mm Hg). These findings should be reported to a physician or on-call provider immediately.

The child's hemoglobin and hematocrit levels should be monitored often because anemia will significantly reduce the child's arterial oxygen-carrying capacity and oxygen content, and anemia or worsening polycythemia can increase the child's risk of thromboembolic events. Signs of cerebral vascular accident include sudden onset of paralysis, paresthesia, altered speech, seizure, extreme irritability or lethargy, pupil dilation with decreased response to light, or a full fontanelle.

Signs and symptoms of brain abscess formation can be extremely nonspecific. Therefore it is necessary for all members of the healthcare team to be aware of the risk of brain abscess in these children, particularly during episodes of bacteremia. Signs of brain abscess include seizures, focal neurologic abnormalities, fever, nausea, vomiting, headache, or signs of increased intracranial pressure.

If significant polycythemia is present the child's coagulation profile will be abnormal; the clotting time will be prolonged, fibrinogen may be reduced, and vitamin K dependent clotting factors will be reduced. The platelet count may be reduced, but even when the platelet count is normal, platelet function is probably reduced.

Nursing staff must recognize hypercyanotic spells when they occur and must notify a physician immediately if they are observed. These spells are most likely to occur in the morning and most frequently are precipitated by crying, defecation, or feeding. The child may become deeply cyanotic following feeding, bowel movements, or vigorous crying. Often the child is diaphoretic, irritable, and hyperpneic before and during the spell and may lose consciousness as the spell progresses. Many children sleep deeply following the spells. Characteristics of hypercyanotic spells are summarized in Box 8-12, and treatment of the spells is reviewed below.

When cyanotic heart disease is suspected in the neonate a chest x-ray, echocardiogram, and 12-lead ECG are performed. Careful physical examination often will reveal a characteristic murmur (refer to Tables 8-25 and 8-26 later in this chapter).

Management

The following information focuses on supportive measures that maximize the child's arterial oxygen content and minimize the child's risk of systemic consequences of chronic hypoxemia and polycythemia. Specific management of individual defects is reviewed later in this chapter (see Specific Diseases, Cyanotic Heart Defects).

The nurse must be able to recognize changes in the child's clinical condition as soon as they occur. Signs of deterioration in the child with cyanotic heart disease include increased

Box 8-12   Recognition and Management of Hypercyanotic Spells

Description

Most often observed during infancy

Usually occur in morning, typically following episode of crying or vagal stimulation

Characterized by progressive irritability, diaphoresis, cyanosis, hypoxemia, hyperpnea

Child may become profoundly hypoxic and lose consciousness

Stroke, death may occur

Medical and Nursing Management

Comfort child and place in knee–chest position

Administer oxygen

Notify physician or on-call provider

Per physician order or protocol, administer:

Morphine sulfate (sedative): 0.1 mg/kg IV or IM

Propranolol (beta-adrenergic blocking agent): 0.15-0.25 mg/kg per dose slow IV push

Phenylephrine (alpha agonist to constrict systemic arteries): 5 to 20 mcg/kg per dose IV bolus (infusion: 0.1-0.5 mcg/kg per minute, titrated to effect) infusion)

Ketamine (anesthetic) may be used: 0.25-0.5 mg/kg IV

Absolutely no air can enter any intravenous line

Administer isotonic fluid bolus (10 mL/kg).

Treat documented acidosis with sodium bicarbonate.

Intubate and support oxygenation and ventilation, if needed.

Schedule surgical intervention (physician).

saturation and rise in pH), the dose can be titrated to approximately 0.01 to 0.05 mcg/kg per minute.

PGE_1 infusion can produce hypotension and can precipitate congestive heart failure. Additional potential side effects include vasodilation or cutaneous flush, bradycardia, pyrexia, seizure-like activity, respiratory depression, and infection. The incidence of these complications increases as the duration of infusion increases (beyond 48 h) and as long ago as the 1970s was found to be highest in neonates weighing less than 2.0 kg.[370]

Fluid administration may be required if hypotension develops during PGE_1 therapy. If apnea occurs the infant usually resumes breathing when stimulated, although respiratory support may be indicated if apnea recurs. The seizure-like activity that occasionally is observed does not seem to indicate actual seizures, although abnormalities in EEGs have been noted; this activity disappears when the PGE_1 infusion is discontinued.

Because the child with cyanotic congenital heart disease has an *intracardiac* (rather than an intrapulmonary) shunt, increased inspired oxygen concentrations usually will not improve systemic arterial oxygenation. However, if the child is profoundly cyanotic, dissolved oxygen (that will be increased during supplementary oxygen therapy) can become a relatively important method of increasing tissue oxygen delivery. In addition, increased inspired oxygen concentrations may reduce pulmonary vascular resistance and result in increased pulmonary blood flow.

When cyanotic heart disease is present, some systemic venous blood is entering the systemic arterial circulation and bypassing the lungs. Therefore *absolutely no air can be allowed to enter any intravenous line* because it may enter the cerebral circulation, producing a cerebral air embolus (stroke). The entire length of the IV tubing and system should be checked routinely, and all tubing connections must be taped securely. Any air in stopcocks or injection ports must be removed. Infusion pump "air in line" alarms will not reliably detect small amounts of air, and are not reliable to identify air in the IV administration system.

Dehydration must be prevented when cyanosis and polycythemia are present because it may result in hemoconcentration and increased blood viscosity, and a greater risk of spontaneous thromboembolic events. The child's level of hydration must be evaluated frequently. The infant's fontanelle should not be sunken, mucous membranes should be moist, and tearing should be present with cry in the infant older than approximately 6 to 8 weeks. Skin turgor should be good, and the eyes should not appear sunken. If orders for "nothing by mouth" (NPO) are required before catheterization or surgery an intravenous catheter should be inserted to enable maintenance of hydration.

When hypercyanotic spells develop, the child should be placed in the knee-chest position immediately. This position often improves pulmonary blood flow and may increase systemic oxygenation. Oxygen is administered during these episodes to promote pulmonary vasodilation, improve pulmonary blood flow, to increase dissolved oxygen, and slightly increase systemic arterial oxygen transport (refer to Box 8-12). Intravenous morphine sulfate (0.1 mg/kg per dose),

severity of cyanosis, increased respiratory rate and effort, irritability or lethargy, poor systemic perfusion, and the development of metabolic acidosis. These changes must be brought to the attention of the on-call provider immediately.

If the neonate has a ductal-dependent cyanotic congenital heart defect (so that most or all of the child's pulmonary blood flow is supplied through the ductus arteriosus), an acute deterioration will be observed during the first days of life when the ductus begins to close. At this point, prostaglandin E_1 will be administered intravenously to maintain ductal patency. Because approximately 80% of the administered prostaglandin E_1 is metabolized in one pass through the infant's lungs, the drug must be administered continuously.

Prostaglandins are endogenous lipids with a variety of systemic effects. Prostaglandin E_1 has been found to produce vasodilation and smooth muscle relaxation, particularly in the wall of the ductus arteriosus. Pulmonary and systemic vasodilation also will occur. As a result, pulmonary blood flow through the ductus is enhanced and the neonate's arterial oxygen tension and oxyhemoglobin saturation usually improve significantly.

The initial IV dose of prostaglandin is 0.05 to 0.1 mcg/kg per minute. Some institutions recommend administration of an initial bolus of 0.1 mcg/kg when the infusion is begun.

Peripheral intravenous administration appears to be as effective as central venous administration of PGE_1. Once the infant has demonstrated improvement in response to the PGE_1 infusion (i.e., increased PaO_2 and oxyhemoglobin

propranolol (0.15-0.25 mg/kg per dose, given slowly), or continuous infusion of phenylephrine (5-20 mcg/kg bolus or infusion of 0.1-0.5 mcg/kg per minute) will be administered. Ketamine may also be used. The physician or on-call provider should be notified immediately and urgent surgical intervention is typically scheduled. Propranolol administration often is continued until surgery is performed.

Because anemia reduces the child's arterial oxygen-carrying capacity the child's hemoglobin and hematocrit levels should be monitored closely and supported. The mean corpuscular volume and mean corpuscular hemoglobin concentration also should be checked frequently, and iron supplementation ordered as needed.

When the child with cyanotic congenital heart disease and polycythemia undergoes surgical repair, postoperative bleeding should be anticipated. Fresh frozen plasma and platelets usually are ordered for postoperative administration. In some cardiovascular surgical centers, fresh, unrefrigerated whole blood is made available for use in the immediate postoperative period to provide the most active clotting factors and platelets. This blood usually is donated by family members and friends on the day of surgery (donors are typed and blood is screened for infection before surgery) and designated for use by a specific patient.

If the older child with inoperable cyanotic heart disease becomes symptomatic from profound polycythemia (hematocrit exceeding 60% to 70%), periodic phlebotomies may be performed as a palliative measure to reduce respiratory distress and improve exercise tolerance.[202] The child is admitted to the hospital for the phlebotomy because the risk of cerebrovascular accident is significant.

A central venous catheter is inserted, blood is withdrawn in small increments, and the volume is replaced with saline, half-normal saline, or a glucose crystalloid solution. Although the child's red blood cell production will replace the withdrawn blood quickly, the periodic phlebotomy may provide temporary relief of symptoms such as dyspnea, poor exercise tolerance, headache, and malaise. Phlebotomy has been shown to reduce peripheral vascular resistance, improve ventricular stroke volume, increase systemic blood flow, and improve systemic oxygen transport.

PULMONARY HYPERTENSION

Jo Ann Nieves

Pearls
- Term neonates have a very reactive pulmonary vascular bed with elevated pulmonary vascular resistance for the first weeks of life.
- The effects of cardiopulmonary bypass can lead to elevated pulmonary vascular resistance.
- Patients at risk for postoperative pulmonary hypertension may be kept sedated with neuromuscular blockade and mechanical ventilation support for at least the first 24 hours after surgery to minimize the incidence of pulmonary hypertensive episodes.
- Effective pulmonary vasodilators: Oxygen administration, alkalotic pH, sedation with pain control

- Inhaled nitric oxide is a selective pulmonary vasodilator with a half life of 3 to 6 seconds, and must be administered continuously.
- Rebound pulmonary hypertension can occur during the final weaning of nitric oxide to less than 5 parts per million.
- Endotracheal suctioning is a frequent trigger for acute pulmonary vasoconstriction.

Etiology
Pulmonary hypertension is a potentially lethal condition that may be encountered anytime in patients with congenital or acquired heart disease. Many conditions can lead to the development of the elevated pulmonary vascular pressure and resistance found in pulmonary hypertension, including pulmonary, metabolic, hematologic, or immunologic problems (Table 8-16).[810] Congenital heart lesions that may cause pulmonary hypertension include lesions causing increased pulmonary blood flow or elevated pulmonary venous pressure. Pulmonary hypertension often occurs in the postoperative cardiac surgical period and is common in infants who have had elevated pulmonary vascular resistance for weeks or months.[935] Approximately 5% to 10% of adults with congenital heart disease develop pulmonary hypertension.[240]

All patients with pulmonary hypertension require *anticipatory* care interventions geared to *prevent* severe exacerbations of the pulmonary hypertensive condition.[652]

Pathophysiology
The pulmonary arteries evolve during fetal life and continue to develop after birth. At term the pulmonary arteries have muscular, thick walls and narrow lumens. Pulmonary vascular resistance (PVR) and pulmonary artery pressure (PAP) are normally higher at birth than later in life.

The thick medial muscle layer of the pulmonary arteries begins to thin immediately after birth and continues to regress during the first days of life. Within 24 hours after birth, mean pulmonary artery pressure has fallen to approximately one half of mean systemic pressure, if the ductus arteriosus has constricted normally. Normal pulmonary vascular resistance index (normalized to body surface area) is approximately 8 to 10 Wood units $\times$ m^2 body surface area during the first week of life, but falls to adult levels (1-3 Wood units $\times$ m^2 body surface area) within a few weeks in patients at sea level. This fall in PVR results in a parallel fall in the pulmonary artery and right ventricular systolic and end-diastolic pressures. Term neonates will have elevated pulmonary vascular resistance for the first 2 to 6 weeks of life.[267] Pulmonary vascular hemodynamics are summarized in Table 8-17.

During the neonatal period the muscular pulmonary arteries remain very reactive. In the patient with pulmonary hypertension many conditions can lead to pulmonary *vasoconstriction,* including alveolar hypoxia, acidosis, hyperexpansion (overdistention) of the alveoli, endotracheal suctioning, atelectasis, cardiopulmonary bypass, hypoventilation, high hematocrit, agitation, pain, and sympathetic stimulation.[935,938] It should be noted that *alveolar hypoxia is the most potent and consistent stimulus for pulmonary vasoconstriction,* so it must be avoided in infants and children with pulmonary hypertension.[745]

Pulmonary hypertension is present when mean PAP is greater than 25 mm Hg at rest, or greater than 30 mm Hg with exercise,[613,745] with pulmonary artery occlusion pressure less

Table 8-16   Risk Factors for Development of Pulmonary Hypertension

Risk Factor	Condition
Congenital or acquired heart disease:	
Acyanotic systemic to pulmonary artery shunts under high pressure	AVSD, large VSD, large PDA
Increased pulmonary venous pressure	TAPVR, LV failure, severe MS, pulmonary vein stenosis
Cyanotic congenital heart disease	Truncus arteriosus, TGA with large VSD, univentricular heart with high pulmonary blood flow
Adult with congenital heart disease and left to right shunt	ASD
Eisenmenger's syndrome	Patient who has developed irreversible pulmonary vascular damage with PVR higher than SVR; cyanosis is present
Presence of longstanding surgical systemic to pulmonary artery shunt	Waterston shunt, Potts shunt, central shunt
Pretransplant recipient with longstanding cardiac dysfunction	LV failure, dilated cardiomyopathy
Cardiac surgery	Cardiopulmonary bypass and hypothermia may result in endothelial cell injury, release of vasoconstrictors agents, impaired nitric oxide production, formation/exposure to microemboli, and atelectasis
Age	Neonates have highly reactive pulmonary vascular beds
Chromosomal abnormality	Down syndrome: Potential development of accelerated progression and severity of pulmonary vascular disease

ASD, Atrial septal defect; *AVSD*, atrioventricular septal defect; *LV*, left ventricle; *MS*, mitral stenosis; *PDA*, patent ductus arteriosus; *TAPVR*, total anomalous pulmonary venous return; *TGA*, transposition of the great arteries; *VSD*, ventricular septal defect.

Table 8-17   Assessment of Pulmonary Hypertension

Parameter	Sea Level at Rest	Altitude (~15,000 feet) at Rest (mm Hg)
Normal Pulmonary Artery Pressure (PAP)	20/10 mm Hg	38/14
Mean PAP	15 mm Hg	26
Hypertension Mean PAP	• >25 mm Hg at rest • >30 mm Hg with exercise	
Pulmonary vascular resistance, index units		
Normal	1 to 3 (infant to adult)	
Elevated	>3 units	
Newborns, term	8 to 10	

Modified from Rosensweig EB, Barst RJ: Clinical management of patients with pulmonary hypertension. In Allen HD, Driscoll DJ, Feltes TF, Shaddy RE, editors: *Moss & Adams heart disease in infants, children, and adolescents including the fetus and young adult*, ed 7, Philadelphia, 2008, Lippincott Williams & Wilkins.
See Table 8-3 for Calculation of Pulmonary Vascular Resistance.

than 15 mm Hg and a pulmonary vascular resistance index greater than 3 Wood units.[637] Severe elevation of PAP is present when the PAP equals or exceeds the systemic arterial pressure.

The precise mechanism for development of pulmonary hypertension in congenital heart disease is unknown.[938]

Congenital heart defects that markedly increase pulmonary blood flow under high pressure (such as a large ventricular septal defect) stimulate pulmonary vasoconstriction and result in persistence of the pulmonary artery medial muscle layer, so it does not thin normally immediately after birth. The normal fall in pulmonary vascular resistance occurs over weeks instead of days. As a result, symptoms attributable to congenital heart disease with increased pulmonary blood flow from an uncomplicated left-to-right shunt usually are not apparent until the full-term infant is about 4 to 12 weeks of age.

The increased pulmonary blood flow can cause progressive pulmonary arterial wall muscular thickening so the muscle layer extends into more terminal vessels. If the pulmonary hypertension continues, vessel walls hypertrophy and the lumens narrow with progressive obstruction and increased pulmonary vascular resistance.

In general, if the increased pulmonary blood flow is under high pressure, the pulmonary hypertension may develop within months or years, particularly in children with a large patent ductus arteriosus (PDA) or large septal defects such as atrioventricular septal defect (AVSD), truncus arteriosus or large VSD. If the increased pulmonary blood flow occurs under low pressure, the pulmonary hypertension may never develop or may take decades to develop, such as may be diagnosed in an adult with atrial septal defect.[734]

Severely increased pulmonary venous pressures also produce pulmonary hypertension, in conditions such as chronic left ventricular failure, pulmonary vein stenosis or severe mitral valve disease. Newborns with hypoplastic left heart syndrome and a restrictive atrial septal defect or intact atrial septum have severe, life threatening elevations of pulmonary artery pressures (see section, Specific Diseases, Single Functioning Ventricle).[514] The risk of development of pulmonary hypertension is high among all infants with total anomalous pulmonary venous connection (TAPVC), whether pulmonary drainage is obstructed or not. Pulmonary hypertension will be severe in TAPVC with obstruction and urgent surgical intervention is required. In these conditions, pulmonary venous pressure increases. The pulmonary veins undergo similar changes and become arterialized with progressive muscular thickening.[938] Children with any of these lesions should be suspected to have pulmonary hypertension and they require implementation of perioperative pulmonary hypertensive precautions during nursing care.

Children with cyanotic heart disease may develop pulmonary vascular disease within 1 year, particularly in transposition of the great arteries with ventricular septal defect. It is thought that these changes are related to the shear stresses and the development of pulmonary microemboli, which can narrow the lumina of small pulmonary arterioles. These complications are most likely when the hematocrit is 60% to 70%. Patients with a surgically created Potts (descending aorta to left pulmonary artery) or Waterston shunt (ascending aorta to right pulmonary artery) can develop pulmonary hypertension in a short period of time after shunt creation[403]; for this reason, these shunts are rarely performed today.

Several factors, including alveolar hypoxia, prematurity, lung disease, and congenital heart disease may affect normal postnatal pulmonary vascular development. If the infant is born prematurely the medial muscle layer of the pulmonary arteries may develop incompletely, so the muscle layer may regress in a shorter period of time. In addition, the pulmonary arteries of the extremely premature infant may demonstrate less constrictive response to hypoxia and to increased flow. For these reasons the very premature neonate may demonstrate a fall in pulmonary vascular resistance, and resultant shunting of blood from the aorta to pulmonary artery through a patent ductus arteriosus, or congenital heart lesion within a few hours after birth.

Patients living at high altitudes also characteristically demonstrate delayed postnatal fall in pulmonary vascular resistance, because their inspired oxygen tension is relatively low, creating a mild alveolar hypoxia.[745] The presence of alveolar hypoxia during the first days of life may delay or prevent the normal fall in pulmonary vascular resistance, because the hypoxia stimulates pulmonary vasoconstriction. Alveolar hypoxia is present in premature neonates with severe respiratory distress syndrome; this may delay the perinatal fall in pulmonary vascular resistance. As a result, when the premature infant has lung disease and congenital heart disease (CHD), symptoms of the left to right shunt from the defect may not develop until the lung disease begins to resolve and PVR falls. In a premature infant with single ventricle, this impacts the presentation of symptoms, as well as the ratio of systemic versus pulmonary blood flows.

Patients with Down syndrome and congenital heart disease with increased pulmonary blood flow are at higher risk of developing pulmonary hypertension at an accelerated rate and greater severity than patients with the same congenital heart defect but without Down syndrome.[613,926] Pulmonary hypertension can be aggravated by presence of acute or chronic respiratory illness, including respiratory syncytial virus (RSV), bronchopulmonary dysplasia (BPD), asthma, or chronic airway obstruction.[96,403,717] Preoperative screening to detect RSV infection is performed prior to surgical intervention to minimize the potential for perioperative exacerbation of pulmonary hypertension by active RSV infection.

Pulmonary vascular disease results when a congenital heart defect producing increased pulmonary blood flow or pulmonary venous obstruction is left uncorrected. The pulmonary vascular bed, persistently exposed to increased blood flow and increased pressure, remodels and the changes progress into permanent obstructive vessel damage, with progressive vessel narrowing and loss of the smallest pulmonary arteries.[613] Children with TGA and VSD, large PDA, or truncus arteriosus can develop pulmonary vascular disease in the first 6 months of life, if untreated.[613] Children with unrepaired AVSD can develop pulmonary vascular disease by 2 years of life, particularly if Down syndrome is also present.[613]

If the child develops pulmonary vascular disease, left-to-right shunting of blood is reduced because the pulmonary and systemic circulations offer approximately equal resistance to flow. The child's symptoms actually may improve during this period. As pulmonary vascular resistance increases further, it exceeds systemic vascular resistance and a *right-to-left* shunt develops with cyanosis. The pulmonary vascular bed no longer vasodilates in response to inhaled oxygen, nitric oxide, or oral or intravenous pulmonary vasodilators. This reversal of the direction of the shunt as a result of elevated pulmonary vascular resistance is called *Eisenmenger syndrome*.[810] Once this develops, the patient will have central cyanosis, the pulmonary vascular disease is irreversible, the disease is usually progressive, and the cardiac lesion is inoperable.[613]

Patients with *Eisenmenger syndrome* demonstrate breathlessness, central cyanosis, syncope, and right-sided heart failure.[296] The patient requires ongoing medical therapy (oxygen, pulmonary vasodilators, diuretics) to maximize RV function, exercise capacity, and comfort.[296,745] All patients with pulmonary vascular disease and Eisenmenger syndrome are at highest risk during anesthesia, intubation, or respiratory illnesses, because these stimuli can cause extreme elevations in pulmonary resistance and RV failure, with resultant critical drop in systemic arterial oxygen saturation, and pulmonary hypertensive crisis. Lung transplantation with correction of the congenital heart lesion or heart lung transplantation may be considered.[296,395]

Diagnosis and Clinical Signs and Symptoms of Pulmonary Hypertension

Diagnosis. The diagnosis of pulmonary hypertension is established primarily by echocardiography, which provides the definitive diagnosis of any underlying structural heart defects, and, in most cases estimates of the pulmonary artery pressure (PAP), the right atrial pressure, any tricuspid or pulmonary regurgitation, and evaluation of RV function. Presence of ventricular septal bowing into the LV during late systole to early diastole is an indicator of pulmonary hypertension.[967] The echocardiogram guides the patient care team to identify the new development of pulmonary hypertension, and RV status, and enables close ongoing monitoring of the response to therapeutic interventions. Echocardiography quickly identifies if pulmonary hypertension develops in conditions not typically at risk for exacerbation of pulmonary hypertension, such as a post cardiac catheterization newborn following intervention for aortic valve stenosis or a child with postoperative elective atrial septal defect repair.

All of the information related to the pulmonary vascular hemodynamics is obtained through direct measurements made during cardiac catheterization to determine severity and reversibility of the pulmonary hypertension and, thus, potential for surgical intervention for the underlying defect.[321] Such assessment is performed prior to cardiac transplantation to minimize the risk of RV dysfunction post transplant[321] (see Chapter 17). It may also be performed for patients undergoing the Glenn or Fontan procedures for single ventricle circulation, because they require low pulmonary vascular resistance for optimal postoperative cardiac output and recovery.[321] Even mild elevations in PVR may result in severe impairment of cardiac output in Fontan circulation.[717]

As noted above, in addition to baseline hemodynamics, the reversibility or reactivity of the pulmonary vascular resistance to vasodilator drugs can be evaluated during cardiac catheterization. Administration of 100% oxygen, inhaled nitric oxide, intravenous prostacyclin or adenosine should produce pulmonary vasodilation,[638] indicating a "reactive" pulmonary vascular bed. Pulmonary vasodilation should be associated with increased pulmonary blood flow, decreased pulmonary artery pressure and increased cardiac output. A decrease in mean PAP by 10 mm Hg to reach a mean PAP < 40 mm Hg with a normal or high cardiac output is defined as a response to vasodilator therapy.[637] The lowest achievable PVR can be identified. Patients may respond to pulmonary vasodilator therapies without a return to normal pulmonary vascular resistance, and therefore will be identified with elevated perioperative risk for residual pulmonary hypertension,[321] so appropriate anticipatory care can be planned.

Failure to respond to administration of pulmonary vasodilators identifies *irreversible* pulmonary arterial damage and is termed a "fixed" pulmonary vascular bed with inoperable congenital heart disease. This is *Eisenmenger syndrome,* and usually corresponds to a pulmonary vascular resistance above 12 Wood units.[613]

The patient with pulmonary hypertension requires careful observation and support following cardiac catheterization to avoid hypoventilation and other causes of alveolar hypoxia, acidosis or any other factors that may contribute to further pulmonary vasoconstriction.[638,804] Patients with suprasystemic PAP before noncardiac surgery or cardiac catheterization were found to have significant risk of major perioperative complications, including pulmonary hypertensive crisis and cardiac arrest.[140] Common factors promoting pulmonary vasodilation will need to be supported, with avoidance of the clinical situations that cause further pulmonary vasoconstriction. (See section, Management of Pulmonary Hypertension).

Evaluation of actual histologic (structural) changes in pulmonary arteries requires a biopsy, which may be accomplished through a thoracotomy or thoracocscopy.[717] However, these biopsies are rarely performed[613] and are associated with a 30% in-hospital mortality.[408]

Clinical Signs. Despite optimal care, patients with pulmonary hypertension can experience exacerbations that can lead to hemodynamic instability, and, if not successfully treated, can be fatal. Anticipation and early detection is crucial to management and avoidance of progression. An acute pulmonary hypertensive event can be triggered by pulmonary vasoconstriction with resultant rise in pulmonary vascular resistance and pressures. The right ventricle is stressed but may not immediately fail, and systemic arterial blood pressure is stable initially. Signs and symptoms of a pulmonary hypertensive event include an acute rise of pulmonary artery pressure. Clinical signs can include tachycardia, and signs of poor perfusion, but a stable arterial blood pressure. Acute increases in afterload, such as reactive pulmonary vasoconstriction, are poorly tolerated during the neonatal period,[935] and are poorly tolerated by a dysfunctional postoperative RV, so may rapidly progress to a hypertensive crisis. (See Table 8-18.)

A pulmonary hypertensive event can quickly deteriorate to a pulmonary hypertensive "crisis." These crises seem to be associated with severe pulmonary vasoconstriction, an acute rise in right ventricular afterload, right ventricular failure, decreased left ventricular filling and sudden deterioration in cardiac output and systemic perfusion with a sudden fall in arterial pressure. Most of the "crises" occur with weaning of mechanical ventilation[717] or suctioning, but they can occur at any time. The pulmonary artery systolic pressure rises to or exceeds systemic pressure. The signs of a pulmonary hypertensive event versus crisis are summarized in Table 8-18. Once these events develop, they often cluster and must be avoided by promoting factors that produce pulmonary vasodilation and avoiding conditions that contribute to pulmonary vasoconstriction. Rapid recognition of a pulmonary hypertensive event is critical to avoid deterioration to a crisis. A crisis left untreated quickly progresses to cardiovascular collapse, arrest, and death.

Clinical signs of RV failure in the patient with pulmonary hypertension can include tachycardia, a loud pulmonic component of the second heart sound, palpable right ventricular heave, hepatomegaly, ascites, peripheral edema, and signs of inadequate perfusion. Patients older than 1 year of age may demonstrate elevated jugular venous pressure. A holosystolic blowing murmur of tricuspid regurgitation can be heard over the lower left sternal border.[967] Signs of inadequate cardiac output will quickly produce a metabolic acidosis, drop in mixed venous oxygen saturation, and a rise in serum lactate (greater than 2.2 mmol/L). For further information, see Chapter 6 and the Postoperative Care section in this chapter (and Table 8-35 later in this chapter).

Management of Pulmonary Hypertension

Prevention. Neonates, infants, and children with many forms of heart disease are at risk for developing elevated pulmonary vascular resistance. Since it is difficult to predict if or when pulmonary hypertension will develop, surgical correction is scheduled to eliminate the possibility. Medical management of congenital heart patients at risk for developing pulmonary hypertension includes close monitoring of status to optimize the timing for interventions in each child. Almost all congenital heart lesions corrected in a timely manner have resolution of the pulmonary hypertensive structural changes with a return of normal hemodynamics.[717] Lesions such as atrioventricular septal defect, large patent ductus arteriosus,

Table 8-18 Clinical Signs and Symptoms of Pulmonary Hypertension Events and Crises

Condition	Pulmonary Hypertension Event	Pulmonary Hypertension Crisis
Definition	Acute rise in PAP with stable arterial blood pressure	Paroxysmal event in which PAP systolic pressures match or exceed systemic pressures, resulting in RV failure and immediate fall in left atrial preload and systemic hypotension
Focus on *early detection* of *these signs*:		
Heart rate	Elevated	Elevated-late bradycardia
Arterial blood pressure	Stable	Decreased
O_2 saturation	Stable or decreased	Decreased, cyanosis
Central venous/right atrial pressure	Stable or elevated	Elevated
Left atrial pressure	Stable	Decreased to elevated as LV end diastolic pressure rises
Cardiac output/SVO$_2$	Decreased	*Severely* decreased
Serum lactate	Normal	Increased (>2.2)
Systemic perfusion	Decreased	*Severely* decreased

From Nieves J, Kohr L: Nursing considerations in the care of patients with pulmonary hypertension. *Pediatr Crit Care Med* 11(2 Suppl):S74-S78, 2010.

and truncus arteriosus are typically repaired during the first months of life to prevent permanent pulmonary hypertension and optimize the potential for controllable pulmonary vascular resistance perioperatively. Critical pulmonary hypertensive conditions in the newborn are emergencies and are treated immediately after birth (i.e., obstructed total anomalous pulmonary venous return or hypoplastic left heart syndrome with intact atrial septum).[514]

Children undergoing single ventricle staged palliations require low pulmonary vascular resistance for survival.[926,935] Moderate increases in PVR or PAP can lead to critical alterations or failure of Fontan or Glenn circulations. In two-ventricle circulations, elevated pulmonary vascular resistance increases right ventricular afterload and work, forcing the right ventricle to generate higher pressure to maintain normal cardiac output through the pulmonary vascular bed.

In the postoperative period if right ventricular (myocardial) dysfunction is present (particularly in the presence of a right ventriculotomy), an increase in pulmonary vascular resistance can trigger progressive right ventricular failure and low cardiac output. Children with right ventricular dysfunction, particularly postoperative newborns with a right ventriculotomy following repair of tetralogy of Fallot, truncus arteriosus, or neonatal Ross procedure, often require pulmonary hypertension precautions during care to minimize such elevations in pulmonary vascular resistance, while optimizing cardiac output.

General Treatment Approaches. A significant increase in PVR impedes blood flow and causes right ventricular strain that impairs right ventricular filling, producing right ventricular volume and pressure overload. Tricuspid regurgitation develops, and right atrial pressure rises as the right ventricle continues to fail.[967]

If the right ventricle is not able to increase pressure sufficient to maintain normal flow into the pulmonary circulation, left atrial filling decreases. As the right ventricular volume and pressure increase, the ventricular septum bows toward the left, into the LV outflow tract. The LV compliance will decrease, with an increased LV end diastolic and LA pressure. The pulmonary venous return will decrease, with further fall

in cardiac output and coronary perfusion (a pulmonary hypertensive crisis).[845] Treatment strategies for pulmonary hypertension management may be initiated when the systolic PAP is more than half the systemic systolic blood pressure.[845]

As noted, there are many neonates, infants and children at risk for the development of postoperative pulmonary hypertension. Neonates are particularly sensitive to changes in afterload and poorly tolerate sudden increases in pulmonary or systemic vascular resistance.[938] In addition, some patients with apparently normal pulmonary vascular resistance may develop reactive pulmonary vasoconstriction.

Common critical care procedures that can increase pulmonary vascular resistance include hypoxia, sympathetic stimulation, acidosis, endotracheal suctioning, hypoventilation, and alveolar hyperinflation.[935] Alveolar hypoxia is the most potent trigger for pulmonary vasoconstriction.[745] Nurses must remain vigilant during noncardiac surgical procedures such as sedated echocardiograms, cardiac catheterization, endotracheal intubation, sedation, or exposure to anesthesia, which may lead to exacerbation of pulmonary hypertension.

In the preoperative setting caution is necessary in using additional oxygen and other pulmonary vasodilators in children with uncorrected left to right shunting lesions and identified pulmonary hypertension. Use of pulmonary vasodilators, such as oxygen, increase the volume of left-to-right shunts, increasing pulmonary blood flow, but this can also lead to worsening symptoms of congestive heart failure, pulmonary congestion and left heart overload. Excessive increases in pulmonary flow may also lead to a decrease in systemic perfusion in these children.

Postoperative Care. The nurse caring for the child postoperatively should be aware of the child's preoperative health status, intraoperative cardiovascular function, intraoperative echo findings and particular postsurgical complications, including anticipating the risk for pulmonary hypertension. Pulmonary hypertension and pulmonary vascular resistance can be elevated following cardiopulmonary bypass. Factors such as pulmonary vascular endothelial cell dysfunction, atelectasis, microemboli, hypoxic pulmonary vasoconstriction and release of potent vasoconstrictive substances can contribute to postoperative pulmonary vasoconstriction.[845,935,938] The length of cardiopulmonary bypass has also been implicated in the development of postoperative pulmonary vascular reactivity.[935]

Treatment of any patient at risk for pulmonary hypertension requires anticipatory care with elimination of factors that cause pulmonary vasoconstriction and administration of oxygen and other therapies that promote pulmonary vasodilation. The goals of care will include avoiding severe exacerbations in pulmonary vascular resistance and providing therapies to decrease pulmonary vascular resistance, with subsequent improvement of right ventricular function and cardiac output. Nurses will need to monitor continually for risks and signs of pulmonary hypertension. Therapies to avoid triggering pulmonary vasoconstriction will focus on optimizing oxygenation, ventilation, pain control, pulmonary vasodilating medications and sedation; these are summarized in Table 8-19.

If a child's calculated PVR is high, or if the child is known to have increased PVR from preoperative studies or perioperative echocardiographic studies, meticulous attention to ventilation management and respiratory care are required. Precise management of ventilation in children with congenital heart disease is crucial and may have a significant effect on pulmonary vascular resistance; PVR can be controlled by manipulating aspects of ventilation.[935]

The child may be kept sedated with neuromuscular blockade for at least the first 24 hours after surgery to minimize the incidence of pulmonary hypertensive episodes, hemodynamic instability, and crisis.[42,935] Use of oxygen and controlled ventilation promotes pulmonary vasodilation and assists with stabilizing pulmonary artery pressure.[632,876] During mechanical ventilation, the tidal volume must be appropriate and barotrauma prevented. A normal functional residual capacity is optimal because it promotes lower PVR.[935]

Hypoventilation is avoided because it will increase PVR with the associated acidosis and hypercapnia. Hypoventilation may result from weaning ventilation, sedation, premature extubation, a significant leak around the endotracheal tube (can lead to variable tidal volume), or endotracheal tube obstruction or displacement. Pleural effusion, lobar collapse, and pulmonary infections are avoided or promptly treated; these can lead to alveolar hypoxia, hypercapnia, and acidosis

Table 8-19	Strategies to Minimize Pulmonary Vasoconstriction[267,938]
Avoid	**Encourage**
Factors that RAISE PVR by pulmonary vasoconstriction	Factors that LOWER PVR by pulmonary vasodilation
• Hypoxia	• Oxygen
• Acidosis/hypercarbia	• Alkalosis/hypocarbia
• Agitation/pain	• Sedation/anesthesia
• Excessive hematocrit	• Normal to low hematocrit
• Hyperinflation	• Normal functional residual capacity
• Atelectasis, hypoventilation	• Nitric oxide

From Nieves J, Kohr L: Nursing considerations in the care of patients with pulmonary hypertension. *Pediatr Crit Care Med* 11(2 Suppl):S74-S78, 2010.

with resultant increased pulmonary vasoconstriction. Low lung volumes (because of risk for atelectasis), excessive lung volumes, hyperinflation, and high PEEP are also to be avoided because they may provoke pulmonary vasoconstriction and increased pulmonary vascular resistance.[935,938]

Blood gases will require close monitoring to prevent and treat the patient with pulmonary hypertension. Acidosis with a blood pH below normal is avoided as it can provoke pulmonary vasoconstriction. Alveolar hypoxia must be avoided; an alveolar PaO_2 below 50 to 60 mm Hg provokes pulmonary vasoconstriction. Prompt detection and treatment of acidemia and hypoxemia are required. An arterial PaO_2 of greater than 100 mm Hg is expected in children with a biventricular cardiac repair who receive supplementary oxygen.

Oxygen is a potent pulmonary vasodilator.[935] In infants, high levels of inspired oxygen, especially 100% oxygen (FiO_2 of 1.0), decrease pulmonary vascular resistance.[935]

Oxygen therapy is used with caution in the patient with unrepaired single ventricle physiology (e.g., truncus arteriosus or hypoplastic left heart syndrome) because pulmonary vasodilation can cause pulmonary over-circulation with systemic hypoperfusion (see section, Specific Diseases, Single Functioning Ventricle). In single ventricle physiology the balance between systemic and pulmonary blood flow must be carefully controlled through manipulation of PVR. Cyanotic heart disease is present (no air can be allowed to enter any IV line), and a "balanced" shunt is generally present if systemic hemoglobin saturation is maintained near 80% with a PaO_2 of near 40 mm Hg.[935] The patient care team should develop individualized target parameters (such as pH, $PaCO_2$, PaO_2, central venous pressure) for each patient with or at risk for pulmonary hypertension that require notification of the cardiac care team and prompt intervention.

Alkalosis is a pulmonary vasodilator. Serum pH is the dominant factor causing pulmonary vascular tone changes, not the $PaCO_2$.[784] A mild alkalosis (pH approximately 7.5) can be created with mechanical hyperventilation to reliably decrease PVR in infants.[935] However, hypocarbia will decrease cerebral perfusion, so should be used with caution. Alkalosis can also be achieved by adding a continuous infusion of sodium bicarbonate.[784] A $PaCO_2$ less than 25 mm Hg should be avoided because of the risk of compromise in cerebral oxygenation and perfusion.

Endotracheal suctioning has been identified as a strong stimulus provoking acute pulmonary vasoconstriction.[935] Premedication with IV fentanyl can help to block the stress response.[371] Hyperventilation with the delivery of 100% inspired oxygen should be provided before and after each suction pass. Hyperoxygenation has been shown to reduce suction-induced hypoxia[669] and can promote pulmonary vasodilation, so additional manual ventilator breaths with higher oxygen flow should be provided before and after every suction pass. Inline, closed suctioning systems allow suctioning while maintaining a continuous gas flow and PEEP as well as lung volume.[788] However, the nurse must be adept with the use of such a system. If the intubated child has an open suctioning system, two people should be available to suction the patient. One person provides hand or mechanical ventilation and ensures that oxygenation is maintained. The second provides skilled, sterile, gentle suctioning,[788] while monitoring heart rate, end tidal CO_2, systemic arterial oxygen saturation, and hemodynamics.

A pulmonary hypertensive event must be detected promptly to avoid the rapid deterioration to a pulmonary hypertensive crisis. If the patient deteriorates during suctioning, the suctioning is stopped and support of optimal airway, oxygenation, and ventilation provided. Hand ventilation with 100% oxygen is provided until the child's heart rate, color, and cardiovascular function are stable. During a pulmonary hypertension crisis, therapies include: administration of 100% oxygen, intravenous fentanyl bolus, additional sedation, neuromuscular blockade, alkalinization, and efforts to precisely control ventilation and improve cardiac output. The bedside nurse should also verify that infusions of vasodilator therapies (inhaled and intravenous) continue without interruption. Inotropic support, if used, may further escalate PVR. Initiation of inhaled nitric oxide may be required.

During weaning of mechanical ventilation the child's pulmonary pressure and systemic perfusion should be monitored carefully because hypoventilation will produce alveolar hypoxia, hypercapnia, and acidosis, and can result in pulmonary vasoconstriction with decreased RV function. Prevention or prompt correction of acidosis will be required. An arterial PaO_2 of greater than 100 mm Hg is expected in the child with a biventricular repair receiving supplementary oxygen therapy. During the weaning of oxygen therapy, the arterial blood gas and pulse oximetry is monitored for decreasing PaO_2 and arterial oxyhemoglobin desaturation. The care team should be notified if the PaO_2 is less than 90 mm Hg, the arterial oxyhemoglobin saturation is less than 94%, or if a previously identified critical parameter develops. A planned, controlled extubation process is needed with continuous monitoring of systemic perfusion and staff ready to manage in the event of decompensation.[845] Following extubation, supplementary oxygen and adequate analgesia (to maximize efforts for pulmonary toilet and minimize excessive oxygen consumption) are used.

Sedation and pain control are provided to minimize exacerbation of pulmonary vasoconstriction. Agitation and pain can cause stimulation of the sympathetic nervous system with subsequent pulmonary vasoconstriction.[935] Continuous infusions of sedation with intermittent bolus doses are required while mechanical ventilation is provided. Narcotic bolus doses of fentanyl have been shown to blunt the stress response[371] associated with endotracheal suctioning. Pain resulting from chest tube removals, suctioning, venipuncture, intravenous catheter changes or infiltration, or large dressing or tape removals can lead to agitation and pain, with additional risk for pulmonary hypertension; fentanyl premedication should be considered, particularly in labile patients. Continuous infusion of fentanyl (5 mcg/kg per hour) with doses as high as 10 to 15 mcg/kg per hour have been used to treat patients with labile pulmonary hypertension.[935] Neuromuscular blockade with intravenous muscle relaxants may be required.

Normothermia is maintained to minimize additional oxygen consumption. Bathing, discomfort, and excessive stimulation are avoided until the risk for pulmonary hypertensive episodes has passed.

When a pulmonary artery (PA) catheter is present, the pulmonary artery pressure (PAP) can be monitored continuously with rapid detection of alterations. The effect of interventions on the PAP can be monitored, including the addition or weaning of therapies.[935,938] PVR can be calculated and mixed venous oxygen saturation measured.[132] Guidelines for PA line management and removal have been published.[132]

Fluid volume status requires ongoing assessment. Right ventricular dysfunction may require a high right atrial pressure and CVP to optimize RV preload, thus maintaining adequate cardiac output. Both hypovolemia and hypervolemia can alter right ventricular preload, leading to decreased cardiac output. Presence of a sinus rhythm is essential. In the patient with severe RV dysfunction and pulmonary hypertension, tachyarrhythmias with loss of atrioventricular synchrony further critically impair preload and stroke volume, decrease cardiac output, and require immediate treatment (see section, Arrhythmias).[967] Development of bradycardia is ominous and may result from development of profound myocardial hypoperfusion and ischemia.[804]

Nurses should anticipate higher risk of pulmonary hypertensive events or crises developing with extubation, intubation, weaning oxygen, weaning ventilator support (caused by rise in $PaCO_2$, fall in PaO_2, and development of alveolar hypoxia), weaning of sedation or analgesia, discontinuing of neuromuscular blockade, weaning pulmonary vasodilators (nitric oxide), and with painful procedures, in particular suctioning. Continuous monitoring is essential.

Nurses can provide care within a set of individualized parameters identified by the care team for each patient. These may include monitoring for identified specified therapeutic limits, including the highest acceptable pressure (e.g., for right atrial and pulmonary artery pressure), the lowest acceptable invasive or noninvasive oxygenation and carbon dioxide parameters (e.g., lowest PaO_2 or arterial oxyhemoglobin saturation allowed, highest end tidal CO_2), blood gas limits (e.g., for target pH, $PaCO_2$), mixed venous oxygen saturation, or serum lactate limits. These limits will be valuable during the weaning process, when pulmonary hypertensive events and hemodynamic instability may develop.

Selected patients may have a residual atrial communication ("atrial pop-off") in place postoperatively to allow some right-to-left shunting of blood when either right ventricular end-diastolic pressure or right atrial pressure increase.[938] This atrial communication may be present following newborn truncus arteriosus repair, when RV function and pulmonary hypertension are anticipated or with fenestrated Fontan procedures. This right-to-left shunt can optimize left ventricular preload, preserve cardiac output, and cause transient systemic arterial desaturation.[845] Because this shunt allows systemic venous blood to enter the systemic arterial circulation, no air can be allowed to enter any IV line due to risk of systemic emboli. As the RV function improves and elevated pulmonary vascular resistance resolves, the patient will show improved arterial oxygen saturations because of less right-to-left shunting.[938]

Drug Therapy. The causes for pulmonary hypertension in the critical care unit are frequently multifactorial; therefore, multiple approaches to therapies are required for the best care.[938]

Combinations of inotropic support and vasodilator therapy may be used to treat pulmonary hypertension by the inhaled, intravenous, or oral routes of delivery. The optimal medications produce pulmonary vasodilation, decreased PVR, lower PAP, and resultant ease of RV workload without systemic arterial hypotension. Ultimately this will increase pulmonary blood flow and improve cardiac output. Inhaled nitric oxide therapy is common. Unfortunately, most parenteral and oral vasodilators dilate both arteries and veins; thus, this therapy may produce complications such as profound systemic hypotension and critical lowering of coronary perfusion pressure.[938] If vasodilators are administered continuously, it is important that the child's fluid volume status be assessed, because hypotension is more likely to occur during therapy if hypovolemia is present.

Inotropes and Vasodilators. Inotropic support in combination with vasodilators are used to support RV function, improve cardiac output and resolve systemic hypotension. However, pulmonary hypertension can also be exacerbated by an increase in catecholamine agents.[876,938]

Dobutamine maintained at less than 5 mcg/kg per minute in combination with other pulmonary vasodilators may be useful therapy. Inotropic support by use of dobutamine above 5 mcg/kg per minute, norepinephrine, dopamine, isuprel, vasopressin, epinephrine, and phenylephrine are limited by the potential for further progression of pulmonary vasoconstriction and tachycardia.[967]

Milrinone (Primacor) has both vasodilatory and positive inotropic effects. It has been shown to produce selective and additive pulmonary vasodilation when used in combination with inhaled nitric oxide for children after congenital heart disease surgery.[471]

In the immediate postoperative period, Milrinone (Primacor) is a frequently used pulmonary vasodilator, which has been shown to additionally provide positive inotropic support and increase cardiac index.[151]

Other agents that decrease pulmonary vascular resistance include dobutamine and isuprel, but development of tachycardia can limit use.[935] Additional intravenous vasodilators include nitroglycerin or sodium nitroprusside. Prostaglandin E_1 also may promote pulmonary vasodilation in the newborn. These vasodilators usually are administered in conjunction with a sympathomimetic inotropic agent (see Chapter 6).

Nitric Oxide. Nitric oxide (NO) is an endothelium-derived relaxing factor. It is produced in the lung capillary cells, and it acts in vascular smooth muscle cells to promote pulmonary vasodilation. When administered by inhalation, it produces selective pulmonary vasodilation at the best ventilated alveoli, improving the match of ventilation and perfusion.[267] Nitric oxide is FDA approved for treatment of pulmonary hypertension in term and near term newborns.[86] Nitric oxide is rapidly inactivated by hemoglobin; thus, it does not cause systemic hypotension.[938]

Signs of effective therapy include improved signs of systemic perfusion status, lower pulmonary artery pressure and pulmonary vascular resistance, and improved arterial oxygen saturation and PaO_2.[298,619] Nitric oxide is effective at low doses (2-20 parts per million) and dilates constricted pulmonary arteries when vasoconstriction is not caused by hypoxia.[617,736]

The onset of effect is 1 to 3 minutes,[736] with a half-life of only 3 to 6 seconds.[488] The delivery of nitric oxide must be continuous—it cannot be interrupted for suctioning or transports. Most patients will have an in-line suction device (Ballard) for continual gas flow while suctioning. Toxicity is rare.

Nitric oxide administration may be a most helpful therapy for treatment of pulmonary hypertensive crisis[424] and NO use may decrease time of mechanical ventilation.[619] Use after a Fontan-type procedure has been described.[298,935] Patients with pulmonary venous hypertensive disorders (TAPVC, congenital mitral stenosis) and low cardiac output are described as being highly responsive to NO.[938] These children tend to have muscularized pulmonary veins, as well as pulmonary arteries. Both of these sites respond to the NO.[938] Inhaled nitric oxide therapy can be used prophylactically for patients at risk of pulmonary hypertensive crisis.

As noted, use of nitric oxide with milrinone results in greater decreases in pulmonary artery pressure than use of milrinone alone.[471] Patients with severe LV failure or left-sided obstructive lesions (as in obstructed TAPVR) treated with NO can develop increased left ventricular end-diastolic and left atrial pressures with increased pulmonary capillary wedge pressure, pulmonary edema, and poor tolerance of NO therapy.[845] Cautious monitoring for effects of therapy are necessary.[86]

Methemoglobinemia may develop as a complication of nitric oxide inhalation; thus, the methemoglobin concentration is evaluated in the arterial blood gas several times each day and should be kept below 3%.[488] Toxic methemoglobin levels are most commonly associated with nitric oxide therapy at high concentrations over prolonged time periods.[929] Elevated methemoglobin levels usually respond to reduction of the inhaled concentration or discontinuation of NO.[86] Nitrogen dioxide is monitored and maintained less than 3 parts per million.

Rebound pulmonary hypertension may develop during the final weaning of NO to less than 5 ppm and is associated with higher pulmonary artery pressure,[37] difficult ventilation,[785] systemic arterial oxygen desaturation, and cardiovascular instability.[705] Thus, nitric oxide must be weaned gradually with careful attention to initiation of therapies promoting pulmonary vasodilation and avoiding stimuli that provoke pulmonary vasoconstriction. Initial therapy for the rebound pulmonary hypertension includes increased inspired oxygen, sedation, and if persistent, the reinstitution of NO. Pretreatment with Sildenafil (Viagra) or Revatio 1 hour before discontinuing NO has been shown to effectively prevent rebound pulmonary hypertension,[37,643] and reduce the length of mechanical ventilation.[643]

If the postoperative infant does not improve with the administration of NO, an anatomic cause for elevated pulmonary vascular resistance must be considered.[938] The abnormality may require surgical or cardiac catheterization intervention. Despite aggressive perioperative interventions, the severity of pulmonary hypertension and cardiovascular dysfunction may finally require initiation of mechanical support of the circulation until resolution (see Chapter 7).

New and Evolving Therapies. Additional therapies are under investigation for the treatment of pulmonary hypertension.[6,274,404] Major pathways at the cellular level have been discovered to contribute to pulmonary hypertension, including the vasodilating nitric oxide pathway and the prostaglandin pathway. The vasoconstrictor pathway effects are produced by endothelins. Pulmonary hypertension is thought to be a result of an imbalance of vasodilation or vasoconstriction. Therapeutic drug therapies are under investigation that will help, individually or used in combination, to improve the balance between pulmonary vasodilation and pulmonary vasoconstriction.[967] The medications and treatment pathways are reviewed in detail by Humbert et al[397] and Barst et al.[60]

Sildenafil (Viagra) is used for treatment of pulmonary hypertension by promoting pulmonary vasodilation. This drug is approved by the FDA for treatment of adult pulmonary hypertension. Sildenafil has a somewhat selective pulmonary vasodilating effect.[935] An oral/nasogastric dose 0.5 mg/kg every 4 hours was found to be as effective as 2.0 mg/kg.[720] To reduce development of rebound pulmonary hypertension with weaning of NO, the dose is given 1 to 1.5 hours before the NO is discontinued. Peak drug effect occurs in 30 to 60 minutes,[967] with a half-life of 4 hours. Sildenafil is contraindicated in patients receiving oral or intravenous nitrates because of the risk of refractory hypotension.[38] In children, the optimal dose for sildenafil is likely to be 0.3 to 1.0 mg/kg three times/day, but is yet to be determined.[274] Pediatric congenital heart disease clinical trials in the United States are in progress.

Bosentan (Tracleer) is used as chronic oral therapy for pulmonary hypertension in adults.[6] It blocks pulmonary vasoconstriction by endothelin, a potent pulmonary vasoconstrictor, endogenously secreted by the vascular endothelium. Bosentan was first found to be successful in adults in the Breathe 2006 study,[295] in which patients with Eisenmenger syndrome showed significant improvement in exercise capacity and hemodynamics, fewer symptoms, but no change in pulmonary vascular disease. Bosentan is administered under monthly surveillance of hepatic function studies because it can alter hepatic function. Pregnancy is contraindicated.

Letairis (Ambrisentan and Sitaxsentan), are additional orally administered endothelin blocker medications.[6] Letairis was approved by the FDA for use in adults in June 2007. Pediatric studies for endothelin blocking agents are in progress.

Epoprostenol (Flolan) is a prostacyclin producing pulmonary vasodilation, approved by the FDA for treatment of chronic severe pulmonary hypertension.[404] This intravenous drug is used most often for chronic outpatient therapy.[938] In the immediate postoperative unstable patient it can precipitate a systemic hypotension. Flolan is costly, has specific guidelines for initiation with dose titration, and must be administered by continuous IV infusion because it has such a short half life (2 to 3 min).[404,613,967]

Additional prostacyclin analogues have been shown to be effective when studied in adult patients. These include subcutaneous Treprostinil (Remodulin), a subcutaneous infusion with a longer half-life (3 to 4 hours).[967] Remodulin was approved for use by the FDA in 2002. An inhaled prostaglandin drug, Iloprost (Ventavis), can be given by nebulizer

---

Box 8-13	**Advanced Concepts: Pulmonary Hypertension**

- Bosentan (Tracleer) blocks vasoconstriction at the pulmonary vascular endothelial level.
- Alkalotic pH can be maintained by manipulation of mechanical ventilation support and infusion of alkalotic solutions.
- Pulmonary hypertensive crises result in severe, life-threatening impairment of RV function, systemic hypoperfusion, and hypotension.
- Sildenafil administration before weaning inhaled nitric oxide has increased successful discontinuation.
- Fentanyl IV bolus blunts the stress response associated with endotracheal suctioning and painful procedures, thus decreasing incidence of acute pulmonary vasoconstriction.

---

treatments 6 to 9 times/day, lasting 10 to 15 minutes each.[404] Iloprost was FDA approved for adults in 2004, and limited studies are available in children. Each of these medications is currently used as an "off label" therapy in children.

Transition and Advanced Care. Patients with pulmonary hypertension may be admitted to the critical care unit for postoperative care, after cardiac catheterization, following noncardiac surgery procedures, for respiratory illness, or when pulmonary hypertensive drugs are initiated or changed, necessitating nurses to closely monitor for responses to therapy. Communication and collaboration of current status, response to treatments, and plan of care involving all team members is imperative to avoid exacerbation of pulmonary hypertension, which can become life-threatening. Some advanced concepts in the management of these patients are listed in Box 8-13.

Children with severe pulmonary hypertension often receive medications in the home setting, including continuous oxygen and intravenous infusions, to promote pulmonary vasodilation.[745] Nurses must ensure that home medications for pulmonary hypertension are not interrupted upon hospital admission, particularly those medications with a short half-life, such as IV Flolan. Families require comprehensive nursing education focusing on their child's PHTN management.

CONGENITAL HEART DISEASE IN ADULTS

Jo Ann Nieves and Susan M. Fernandes

Pearls

- An estimated 90% of patients born with congenital heart disease today are expected to reach adulthood.
- Adult survivors with congenital heart lesions outnumber affected children.
- Few congenital heart lesions are "cured." Most patients have ongoing risk of sequelae or complications unique to each type of congenital heart defect. These patients require lifelong follow-up by specialists in congenital heart disease.
- Transition of the adolescent into adult clinic requires a planned, progressive change resulting in an adult who can manage all aspects of care.

- Most adults with congenital heart disease are "lost to follow-up" care. Reasons include insufficient patient and family instruction regarding lifelong follow-up needs and loss of insurance coverage.

Etiology/Epidemiology

Improved surgical techniques and medical therapies for pediatric patients with congenital heart disease have made survival into adulthood an expectation, but lifelong medical surveillance is necessary to maintain optimal health. Adults with congenital heart disease (ACHD) now outnumber the population of children with congenital heart disease, with greater than 1 million adult survivors.[946] An estimated 90% of patients with congenital heart disease who receive treatment are expected to reach adulthood.[215] The population of ACHD patients is increasing at a rate of 5%/year.[107] The patients who survived complex neonatal interventions (arterial switch, Ross, Norwood, tetralogy of Fallot repairs) from the 1980s are now adults with emerging issues. An estimated half of these survivors have moderate to complex disease, requiring lifelong, continuous care from ACHD specialists for optimal management.[383,926] The most complex ACHD patients will need lifelong followup at a minimum of every 6 to 12 months at a regional ACHD program with expertise in adult CHD care.[926]

Unfortunately, noncompliance in follow-up may be an issue for many adolescents and adults. Many patients present after gaps in care (often >10 years) during late adolescence and early adulthood; such gaps are associated with increased morbidity and mortality.[402,728,915,945] The inability to achieve continuity of care is likely multifactorial, with forces including limitations in the patient's and family's understanding of the illness and care required, limitations in health insurance, and adolescent rebellion.[131,625,943] Access to adult congenital heart clinics remains limited; families report difficulty finding specialists to care for the adult patient with congenital heart disease.

Many ACHD patients "feel well" and seek follow-up only after they become ill. They can mistakenly believe they are "cured" and may not understand their lesion or potential consequences such as a ventricular dysfunction, thrombosis, arrhythmias, or pulmonary hypertension. The patient may seek medical care only when symptoms of significant sequelae have developed.

Transitioning (self-care management) programs, even when limited in scope, are thought to improve patient knowledge and compliance with medical management and follow-up.[953] Given the significant risk of morbidity and mortality in patients with complex congenital heart disease without adequate follow-up, some form of transitioning (self-care management) education is imperative to improve patient outcomes.

Transitioning and Transfer

Transitioning is defined by Blum and colleagues as, "the purposeful, planned movement of adolescents and young adults with chronic physical and medical conditions from child-centered to adult-oriented healthcare systems."[87] This notion has been publicly and academically discussed since 1984 (with the national Minnesota "Youth with Disability: The Transition Years" conference), with recommendations from several related conferences and publications.[87,744]

The patient with congenital heart disease shares many of the same general issues as other patients with chronic diseases (struggle for independence, personal risk-taking, noncompliance with medical therapy, participation in unprotected sexual behavior, and increased personal emotional exposure and tendency for depression).[66,110,834]

Patients with congenital heart disease do have many things in common with other patients with chronic disease, yet each patient with congenital heart disease is unique, given the wide spectrum of disease and variable physical, medical, and intellectual impact on any given patient. In addition, the management of the adult with congenital heart disease requires specialized training that few providers can offer. In light of these observations, Knauth and colleagues[482] specified that transitioning should exclude transferring of care. They defined transitioning as a process by which adolescents and young adults with chronic childhood illnesses are prepared to take charge of their lives and their health in adulthood. It is an individualized educational process that ideally begins before children reach adolescence and continues until they are capable of assuming full responsibility for their care[485] and is recommended to begin by age 12 years.[926]

In the ideal environment, once a patient successfully transitioned he or she would be transferred to an adult-oriented healthcare system able to care for the cardiac, other medical, and psychosocial issues. Until resources are available to supply this level of care, we must provide all patients with the necessary skills to take responsibility for their health regardless of where or by whom care is provided.

To address specific needs in congenital heart disease, the American College of Cardiology, 32nd Bethesda Conference outlined recommendations for transition and transfer of care.[171,273,513,925]

Although the optimal approach to provide transitioning (self-care management) education to adult patients with congenital heart disease has not yet been established, experts in the field proposed a life span model that focused on developmental issues faced by these patients. The areas of concentration included physical development, social and family relations, emotional health, medical issues, health behaviors, screening and prevention, and treatment issues. Using this information, many centers have developed checklists covering several of these areas to ensure that the patient has acquired the necessary skills before transfer of care. An example of such a checklist is provided in Table 8-20. In addition, either electronic or paper complete medical healthcare passports should be carried by patients with details of current and past history specifics, as well as contact information for immediate access to their ACHD healthcare providers.[926]

Patients who have undergone early childhood total surgical correction for patent ductus arteriosus, atrial septal defect, small ventricular defect, and mild pulmonary stenosis typically have few if any hemodynamic residua and therefore require infrequent evaluation and treatment.[215] Most other patients have some form of residua or sequelae of their disease or the treatment and will require lifelong care by ACHD specialists.[926]

Table 8-20 Sample Checklist for Transitioning of Care

NAME _____

MR# _____ DATE TRANSITION INITIATION ___/ ___/ _____

DATE OF BIRTH ___/ ___/ _____ DATE OF SKILL REVIEW ___/ ___/ _____

	STATUS		
Completed	Practice	Initiate	Skill
			Patient can ask questions independently
			Patient can answer questions independently
			Patient is able to make follow-up appointments without support
			Patient is able to call for prescription refills or send mail order independently
			Patient can describe medical condition using appropriate terminology
			Patient can describe the long-term potential complications associated with his or her condition.
			Patient can describe symptoms that require immediate and semiurgent attention
			Patient can name his or her medications
			Patient understands the purpose of his or her medications and the side effects
			Patient understands the impact of medication mismanagement
			Patient has a healthcare passport
			Patient has a primary care physician (planned adult internist)
			Patient has a life/career plan for after high school/college
			Patient has a plan to pay for medical coverage after discontinuation of parent's health plan
			Patient understands impact of smoking
			Patient understands the impact of alcohol use
			Patient understands the risks of illicit drug use
			Patient understands the risk of pregnancy, sexually transmitted diseases, and contraception
			Patient understands the risk of congenital heart disease/anomalies in offspring (availability of genetic counseling for further information)
			Patient knows how to contact the hospital and outside support resources

Developed for clinical use by Susan M. Fernandes, MHP, PA-C, for Adult Congenital Heart Program, Children's Hospital, Boston.

Most patients with ACHD are *palliated,* not "repaired" or "fixed," and they require lifelong care.[196] Complications of the defect or treatment can include arrhythmias, thrombosis, sudden death, ventricular or valvular dysfunction, pulmonary hypertension, and endocarditis.[946] Additional problems can result from residual shunts, valvar disease, ventricular dysfunction, and arterial pathology. These issues may require further surgical or cardiac catheter-based interventions.[215] Approximately 50% of adult patients with CHD face additional surgery, arrhythmias, complications, heart failure or, if inappropriately managed, premature death.[301,304,305] Late complications increase in frequency over time, typically developing in the second, third, or fourth decade of life; they can be irreversible and potentially fatal.

Occasionally, a congenital heart defect is not diagnosed until adult years; this may be the result of widespread availability of echocardiography.[510] A new diagnosis in the adult can include simple lesions, such as an atrial septal defect or a bicuspid aortic valve, to complex lesions, such as L-transposition of the great arteries diagnosed at the age 60 to 70 years,[331] with the new development of symptoms, cardiac rhythm disturbances, or congestive heart failure. In some lesions, late diagnosis is complicated by the presence of pulmonary hypertension.

Cardiac catheterization based interventional procedures can be used to treat a variety of adult lesions. Interventions can include balloon dilation, stent placement, occlusion by devices, valve replacement (pulmonary or aortic), valve intervention, and therapeutic arrhythmia procedures (see Cardiac Catheterization).

ACHD survivors require appropriate testing and follow-up for likely residuae and sequelae. Echocardiograms are used but may not be optimal because of poor echocardiographic "windows" (sites to enable visualization of specific cardiac structures). Cardiac MRI (magnetic resonance imaging) is an increasingly important tool for the complete evaluation of complex congenital anatomy and surgical interventions in the adolescent and adult.[197] The MRI studies can identify and follow important residual problems, and enable calculation of chamber volumes, quantify valve regurgitation, and enable evaluation of ventricular function, baffle leaks, patency of Fontan pathways, aortic arch status, residual lesions, and flow characteristics. (For additional information, see the MRI section at the end of this chapter.).[197,215,314] Cardiac catheterization is used most frequently for interventions.[215]

Residuae and Sequelae of Congenital Heart Disease
Anticipatory management and ongoing care are critically important and must take place in a center with expertise in complex ACHD care. These patients require expert care for the complications associated with congenital heart interventions and aging. The goal is to monitor for and detect sequelae and provide timely treatment with regular follow-up care. Required management can include simple to complex imaging, cardiac catheter interventions, medications, cardiac pacing or defibrillator implantation, surgery, or cardiac

| Box 8-14 | **Adult Congenital Heart Disease: Symptoms to Report**[215] |

- Palpitations
- Syncope, near syncope
- Edema
- Decreased energy
- Fatigue
- Focal neurologic symptoms
- Chest pain/back pain
- Diarrhea, abdominal distension (Fontan patients)
- Symptoms of heart failure
- Increasing cyanosis

If cyanotic, also report hemoptysis, joint pain, headache, epistaxis, or myalgia.

transplantation. Development or progression of symptoms to report is summarized in Box 8-14.[215]

Lesion-specific guidelines and recommendations for the management of adults with congenital heart disease were published in December, 2008, by the American College of Cardiology and the American Heart Association.[927] Lesion-specific pathways have also been developed for testing and follow-up of congenital heart lesions in the adult; these are covered extensively by Daniels,[215,216] Gatzoulis and Webb,[304] and Deanfield et al,[227] It is important to note that each patient requires a unique plan for lifelong management; patients with identical original defects may have vastly different presentations in adult years. For example, patients with coarctation may have different ages at intervention, unique forms of surgery or catheterization intervention, specific associated lesions, and unique aortic arch anatomy.[215] Each patient also has unique risk factors for acquired coronary artery disease, such as potential obesity, tobacco use, hypertension, diabetes mellitus, hyperlipidemia, or family history of coronary artery disease.[215] Many patients do not report the symptoms that they are experiencing that might suggest an increased risk of heart failure and arrhythmias.[215] Protocols for routine diagnostic testing can monitor for the development of known lesion-specific significant long-term complications and may enable prevention of serious, potentially irreversible disability.

Heart failure can be right- or left-sided, and related to systolic or diastolic dysfunction or pulmonary hypertension. Structurally significant lesions (whether unoperated or residual lesions) may be treated in selected cases by cardiac catheter interventional procedure or, when applicable, surgery.[510] Ventricular dysfunction and heart failure are treated primarily with drug therapy, and treatment of pulmonary hypertension as needed (see section, Pulmonary Hypertension).

The details of a patient's surgical history is important, given the wide variation of surgical technique and the clinical implications. As an example, a Fontan procedure may have been performed with a right atrium to pulmonary artery anastomosis, a lateral tunnel, an extracardiac conduit, or a modification of any one of those. Even less complex lesions such as a coarctation repair can have numerous variations including

an end-to-end anastomosis, an interposition graft or a left subclavian flap plasty, which interrupts normal arterial flow to the arm. This along with original versions of the Blalock Taussig shunt may lead to future *inaccurate* upper extremity blood pressures, which could have significant implications if not noted.

Arrhythmias. Arrhythmias are the most common cause of sudden cardiac death in ACHD,[352] and affect up to 50% of adults with congenital heart disease.[946] Patients with uncorrected and corrected congenital heart disease may present with arrhythmias. For example, patients with uncorrected atrial septal defect may develop atrial fibrillation or flutter. Ninety percent of patients with late sudden cardiac death related to arrhythmias have tetralogy of Fallot, D-transposition of the great arteries, coarctation of the aorta, or aortic stenosis.[352] Antiarrhythmic therapy can be used to treat specific rhythms, but proarrhythmic effects must be monitored. Therapies are detailed by Harris.[352] Treatments can include medications, cardiac pacing, implantation of cardiac defibrillators, or surgical interventions such as the Maze procedure[46] in the management of patients' status post right atria to pulmonary artery Fontan procedure with subsequent development of atrial re-entry tachycardia or atrial fibrillation.[864] The Maze procedure or Cox-Maze III procedure involves cryoablation ($-160\,^{\circ}C$) as well as surgical atrial incisions of the abnormal conduction pathways during open heart surgery.[864]

Cyanosis. Cyanosis can affect patients with uncorrected cyanotic lesions, those with uncorrected shunt lesions and Eisenmenger syndrome, those with cyanotic heart defects and palliative procedures (e.g., systemic artery to pulmonary artery shunts, systemic vein to pulmonary artery shunts, central aorta to pulmonary artery shunts [e.g., Waterston, Potts shunt]), Fontan-type procedures with fenestrations, or complex surgical repairs where atrial fenestration remains.

Polycythemia with hematocrit rising to 60% or above may produce symptoms of headache, dizziness, dyspnea, fatigue, and neurologic changes.[215] Dehydration must be avoided because of hyperviscosity and risk for stroke or emboli. All intravenous systems require meticulous removal of any air or clots because of risk of paradoxic emboli to the brain, kidney, or heart.[215] Thrombocytopenia and coagulopathies are common (see Hypoxemia Caused by Congenital Heart Disease).

Phlebotomy is not routinely performed unless the patient becomes symptomatic. An equal volume of whole blood may be removed and replaced with saline or albumin. Potential complications of phlebotomy include stroke, seizures, and death.[864]

If the cyanosis is associated with pulmonary hypertension (e.g., Eisenmenger syndrome), the patient requires pulmonary hypertensive care precautions. In addition, medical management is required (see the following).

Cyanotic adults may also develop hyperuricemia, gouty arthritis, and altered renal function requiring treatment with allopurinol or colchicines.[864] Hypoperfusion and chronic hypoxia also lead to renal disease.[215]

Pulmonary Hypertension. Pulmonary hypertension can develop as a consequence of congenital heart disease in 15% to 30% of patients,[511] those repaired at a later age, or those with significant unrepaired left-to-right shunts.[215] Patients with single ventricle with Glenn and Fontan palliations or staged correction require the lowest possible pulmonary resistance for survival.[511] Evaluation of the status of the pulmonary vascular bed may include cardiac catheterization with measurement of the reactivity to pulmonary vasodilator therapy (see Common Diagnostic Tests, Cardiac Catheterization).

Patients may demonstrate hypoxemia as a result of pulmonary hypertension and progression to *Eisenmenger* syndrome with reversal of the intracardiac shunt. This pulmonary hypertension is typically unresponsive to oxygen.[926] Pulmonary vasodilator treatments include oxygen therapy to treat hypoxemia (particularly at night),[215] inhaled nitric oxide or epoprostenol,[511] prostacyclines, endothelin receptor antagonists (Bosentan),[912] and phosphodiesterase five inhibitors (Sildenafil).[511]

Pulmonary hypertensive precautions are vital during periods of illness or procedures requiring anesthesia because these situations include risk for conditions such as acidosis, alveolar hypoxia, pain, agitation, and hypoventilation that may provoke pulmonary vasoconstriction. Goals of care will include lowering PAP, decreasing PVR and RV afterload while maximizing RV function, ultimately improving cardiac output. Nursing care will focus on optimizing ventilation, improving RV function, providing adequate sedation, treating pain, avoiding metabolic and respiratory acidosis, avoiding atelectasis, avoiding anemia, and minimizing energy expenditure needs.[511] In the immediate cardiac surgery postoperative period, reactivity of the pulmonary vascular bed is heightened.[511] Support of systemic blood pressure may be required with use of agents such as norepinephrine to maintain coronary perfusion.[511]

Adequate hydration is essential, and hypotension must be avoided.[215] Strategies for care attempt to decrease pulmonary artery pressure, enhance right ventricular function, and avoid development of pulmonary hypertensive events or crises with subsequent right ventricular failure (see Sectons "Pulmonary Hypertension" and "Management").

Selected Eisenmenger syndrome patients may require phlebotomy because of symptomatic hyperviscosity, with specific guidelines to avoid acute adverse reactions and even death. For further information, see Daniels[215] and Warnes et al.[926]

Conduit Obstruction. Extracardiac conduits and baffles can develop obstruction over time, requiring reintervention. The conduits connect the subpulmonary ventricle to the pulmonary arteries in tetralogy of Fallot and other complex congenital heart disease.[398] Treatments include cardiac catheterization intervention (balloon angioplasty or stent implantation).

Conduit replacement is possible with early low mortality; of patients reoperated at a mean age of 9.6 years, 55% were free from conduit reoperation at 10 years, and 31.9% at 20 years.[228] Developments in percutaneous pulmonary valve replacement have resulted in avoiding surgical revisions in many of the cases treated[550] and are FDA approved since 2009.[598] Patients with conduits require lifelong periodic reevaluation[526] in adult CHD clinics.[215,926]

Adult Cardiovascular Problems

Additional impacts on cardiac health related to adult lifestyle and hereditary issues include smoking, obesity, hypertension, hypercholesterolemia, and coronary artery disease. Healthy adults (18 to 65 years old) should ideally complete at least 30 minutes of regular physical activity per day, 5 days a week,[354] yet many adult patients with congenital heart disease are uncertain of their specific goals and limits, requiring additional assessment from their cardiology team and education about the benefits of exercise.[246] (See http://www.heart.org/HEARTORG/Conditions/CongenitalHeartDefects/CareTreatmentfor CongenitalHeartDefects/Congenital-Heart-Defects-and-Physical-Activity_UCM_307738_Article.jsp). Aerobic functional capacity compared with healthy adults has been found to be diminished in patients with congenital heart disease, and significantly lower than normal.[280] Typical low-intensity exercises such as walking, casual swimming, and dancing are encouraged. Individualized instructions are recommended (see http://www.americanheart.org/presenter.jhtml?identifier=11081).

Atherosclerotic heart disease is a major cause of morbidity and mortality in adults in the United States and many countries.[369] Atherosclerotic heart disease begins to develop in early childhood, even in the patient with congenital heart disease,[578] and guidelines for primary prevention in children have been identified.[369]

Lifestyle choices and modifiable risk factors can have a major impact on morbidity and mortality of patients with congenital heart disease. Minimizing cardiovascular risk factors, and following a healthy lifestyle can minimize the risks of complications related to coronary artery disease. Strategies include management of diet, regular exercise, and avoiding cigarette smoking.[186] Obesity is a common finding in children with congenital heart disease.[703] A known independent risk factor for type 2 diabetes and heart disease is obesity,[683] which should be avoided. (See http://www.heart.org/HEARTORG/Conditions/CongenitalHeartDefects/CareTreatmentforCongenitalHeartDefects/Recommendations-for-Heart-Health_UCM_307739_Article.jsp).

Long-Term Outcomes of Specific Defects

As patients age following surgical intervention for congenital heart disease, information is accumulating regarding long-term outcomes.

Bicuspid Aortic Valve. Bicuspid aortic valve is the most common congenital lesion, present in about 1% to 2% of the population.[215,926] The lesion can progress over time, requiring patients to be monitored for potential development of aortic valve calcification, regurgitation, and stenosis. Aortic root dilation and dissection may also develop.[926]

When indicated, therapeutic interventions may include interventional catheterization balloon valvuloplasty, or surgery for aortic valve intervention or replacement, or a Ross procedure (see section, Specific Diseases, Aortic Stenosis).

Coarctation of the Aorta. Coarctation of the aorta may be diagnosed late in life, and the patient may present with upper extremity hypertension with decreased lower extremity pulses and blood pressures. Late complications of repair include recoarctation, aortic aneurysm or dissection, and sudden death. Systemic hypertension has been reported in up to 70% of patients after coarctation repair,[427] and must be differentiated from hypertension caused by recoarctation through use of physical exam (arm and leg blood pressure gradients) and diagnostic studies. Systemic hypertension may occur during rest or activity, and may require medical therapy.[215,926] Blood pressures may be decreased in the left arm if a left subclavian artery flap was used in the original repair. The cause of the high risk of hypertension and aortic dissection is unknown.[215]

Recoarctation incidence is 8% to 54% and in selected cases may be treated with transcatheter therapy (stent, angioplasty).[215] An aortic aneurysm may form in the left subclavian flap or patch aortoplasty repair site.[197] Bicuspid aortic valve is present in about half of patients with coarctation of the aorta.[527a] These bicuspid valves can develop significant stenosis or regurgitation.[196]

Atrial Septal Defect. The adult with an undiagnosed atrial septal defect may present with a cerebrovascular accident or transient ischemic attack following a paradoxic embolism across the atrial septal defect.[215] Factors leading to arrhythmia development include chronic right heart volume overload, ventricular dysfunction,[926] late date at operation, or the presence of pulmonary hypertension.[352] About 50% of those patients with preoperative atrial arrhythmias have postoperative arrhythmias, particularly if they are 40 years old or older at the time of surgery. The presence of atrial arrhythmias can result in need for anticoagulation.[352] Transcatheter device closure is possible for many with secundum type lesions (see Specific Defects, Atrial Septal Defect).

Adult patients presenting with sinus venosus or primum defects require surgical repair.[802] Pulmonary hypertension may be present in the unrepaired adult. Atrial septal defects repaired early in life are typically symptom free, but atrial arrhythmias (fibrillation or flutter) may develop in the operated[608,926] and the unoperated patient.[352,926]

Tetralogy of Fallot. Tetralogy of Fallot is the most common complex defect with the longest survival history.[946] Most adult patients have undergone surgical repair in childhood or even adolescence,[352] and some have undergone initial palliative shunt procedure. Some patients may have a right ventriculotomy with a patch or a valved conduit between the right ventricle and pulmonary artery, whereas others have surgical removal of the pulmonary valve with a transannular patch and resultant free pulmonary regurgitation.

If the pulmonary valve is present, it may become insufficient or stenotic and the distal pulmonary arteries obstructed. Postoperative patients may develop arrhythmias. Atrial arrhythmias (flutter, fibrillation or supraventricular tachycardia) develop in up to one third of patients.[743] Ventricular tachycardia and sudden cardiac death are known complications.[215,926] By 35 years after surgery, the estimated risk for sustained ventricular tachycardia is 11.9%, and for sudden death is 8.3%.[302]

RV size correlates with QRS duration. The combination of older age at correction and QRS duration of 180 ms or longer, as well as older age at initial repair[352] predict risk of sustained ventricular arrhythmias and sudden cardiac death.[303] Right bundle branch block (RBBB) is a common finding in patients who had surgical correction many years ago, but in itself is not predictive of a worse prognosis (although RBBB with QRS 180 ms or higher is).[352]

The most common problem following surgical correction of tetralogy of Fallot is pulmonary regurgitation, which causes chronic right ventricular volume overload and may progress to right ventricular enlargement and systolic dysfunction.[215,926] Severe right ventricular dilation and mild global right ventricular systolic dysfunction are associated with higher risk for adverse clinical outcomes in patients with repaired tetralogy of Fallot.[482] Progressive aortic root dilation and potential for aortic dissection may also develop.[215] Pulmonary regurgitation is the most common reason for late reoperation.[946]

Tetralogy of Fallot survivors require lifelong monitoring, including regular evaluation with MRI,[482,926] for each of these potential complications and to avoid progression of decreased cardiac function. Surveillance for potential arrhythmias is required. Treatment for arrhythmias includes cardiac pacing, use of implantable cardioverter/defibrillators, antiarrhythmic therapy or radiofrequency ablation, or arrhythmia intervention during reoperation[352] for pulmonary valve replacement. Selected cases may undergo transcatheter pulmonary valve replacement via cardiac catheterization.[598] Long-term survival at 32 years is 86%.[641] Tetralogy of Fallot is the most common diagnosis for patients with implantable cardioverter defibrillators.[467]

Transposition of the Great Arteries. Atrial switch for d-transposition of the great artery (Mustard or Senning procedure) requires extensive atrial incisions and suture lines.[352] As a result, patients who undergo these procedures require lifelong regular monitoring[215,926] for development of arrhythmias (atrial tachycardia, sick sinus syndrome) and are at risk for sudden cardiac death. Loss of sinus rhythm is common, with only 18%[950] to 40%[310] of survivors in sinus rhythm 15 to 20 years after surgery. Pacemaker implantation is anticipated in about one-fifth of adults with long-term followup after a Mustard procedure.[352]

Pacemakers can be used to treat bradyarrhythmias or tachyarrhythmias,[352] and radiofrequency ablation or medications can be used to treat tachyarrhythmias.[215] Despite close followup, about 7% of patients have sudden cardiac death after atrial switch.[950]

After an atrial switch procedure for d-transposition of the great arteries, the right ventricle is the systemic ventricle (pump) for life and progressive dysfunction develops by the second or third decade of life in about 15% of postoperative patients,[950] with progression to ventricular arrhythmias in the failing ventricle.[352] The tricuspid valve, exposed to systemic pressures, can become dysfunctional. Narrowing in the left ventricular outflow area can also develop.

Reconstruction of the atrial flow pathways can rarely result in the serious complication of baffle obstruction of pulmonic or systemic venous return.[215] Baffle leaks causing atrial shunting are common but they are often small.[215] If despite optimal medical management the ventricular dysfunction becomes severe, either staged surgical anatomic correction (arterial switch procedure) or cardiac transplant may be planned. Patients with d-TGA, VSD, and pulmonary stenosis repair will have undergone a Rastelli procedure with a conduit between the right ventricle and pulmonary artery, that will require continued surveillance.

Arterial switch became the treatment of choice for transposition of the great arteries in the 1980s. Follow-up shows good systemic ventricular function and sinus rhythm,[946] although the patients having additional VSD repair are reported at higher risk for arrhythmias.[359] Potential long-term issues include the need for serial assessment of ventricular function and surveillance for the development of arrhythmias, stenosis at the great vessel suture sites,[946] neo-aortic root dilation, and development of valvar regurgitation.[186]

Coronary artery lesions, found in 5% of patients following the arterial switch operation, are progressive and can be treated by coronary angioplasty or surgery.[719] Coronary atherosclerosis remains a concern and requires careful followup.[692] The progression of coronary artery disease after the arterial switch procedure is unknown. The most common cause for reoperation is pulmonic stenosis.[547] Survival at 15 years after the initial operation is 88%,[547] but long-term outcome is unknown.[186,215,926]

Single Ventricle. Although it is a rare condition, patients with a single ventricle account for a disproportionate share of the morbidity and mortality found in adults with congenital heart disease.[946] Single ventricle includes diagnoses of tricuspid atresia, mitral atresia, double inlet LV, hypoplastic right or left ventricle, or single ventricle. These patients will remain cyanotic until they undergo Fontan-type correction. The first patients with a Fontan-type staged palliation and correction are now in their fourth decade of followup.[466] Young adults with a univentricular heart who are unrepaired have a poor prognosis.[215]

The original Fontan procedures (1970s) connected the right atrium directly to the pulmonary arteries, or connected the right atrium to the right ventricle, exposing the right atrium to high systemic venous pressure.[352] Over time elevated right atrial pressure can lead to right atrial enlargement, hypertrophy, and slowed atrial conduction.[352] A severely enlarged right atrium is often seen in patients with a classic Fontan procedure and a failing Fontan circuit, which contributes to development of medically resistant complex atrial arrhythmias.[926] Atrial distension and surgical incisions with subsequent scarring also contribute to arrhythmia formation.[352] Atrial tachycardia and sick sinus syndrome may be observed, particularly in those patients with the right atrium included within the Fontan pathway.[352] Atrial tachycardia can develop in up to 50% of adults with Fontan procedure,[226,926] and sinus bradycardia or junctional escape rhythm has been reported in up to 15% of patients.[352] Sustained atrial arrhythmias may cause patients to present with congestive heart failure, low cardiac output, and can lead to development of atrial thrombi.[352] Anticoagulation therapy is often required in the presence of sustained atrial arrhythmias.[352] Therapy for arrhythmias can include antiarrhythmic therapy, pacemaker (typically

epicardial if ventricular), radiofrequency ablation, or arrhythmia intervention during reoperation.[352]

Many long-term complications have been reported following single ventricle palliations. Outcomes have improved, but systemic ventricle dysfunction may develop, particularly with a right ventricular systemic pump.[311] The less efficient right atrium to pulmonary artery Fontan type surgical procedure has become obsolete,[311] replaced by the total cavopulmonary artery connections (superior vena cava to pulmonary artery shunt plus intraatrial lateral tunnel or extracardiac conduit).[467] The use of external conduits from the inferior vena cava to the pulmonary artery results in a sutureless right atrium, and potentially may decrease incidence of postoperative atrial arrhythmias.[311] Some patients may have a lateral tunnel connecting the inferior vena cava to an intraatrial tunnel, then the pulmonary arteries. Long-term data are not yet available to define long-term outcomes of these two procedures.[311]

Pulmonary vein compression, pulmonary artery stenosis, Fontan pathway obstruction, atrioventricular valve insufficiency, arrhythmias, hepatic dysfunction, hepatic fibrosis, and cirrhosis may each develop after the Fontan procedure.[47,215,926] Protein losing enteropathy is reported in 3.7% of patients following Fontan-type correction and is associated with a poor clinical course,[311] with a 50% 5-year mortality after the diagnosis.[612,926]

The function of the single systemic ventricle and atrioventricular valve can deteriorate, and must be monitored closely, particularly in those patients with a right ventricle performing a lifetime of systemic work. Heart failure risk in Fontan patients is reported to be higher in those patients with the (single) morphologic right ventricle functioning as the systemic ventricle.[944] Currently, many patients with the Fontan operation have hypoplastic left heart syndrome, with a resultant systemic right ventricle, creating concerns regarding long-term right ventricle status.[311]

Arterial oxygen saturations will be monitored for the potential late development of cyanosis caused by fenestration of the Fontan or the development of pulmonary arteriovenous malformations (AVM), systemic venous collaterals, or baffle leaks.[215] Patients developing cyanosis[215] or residual stenosis may require diagnostic or therapeutic cardiac catheterization. Cardiac magnetic resonance imaging (MRI) cannot be completed if the patient has a cardiac pacemaker.

The failing Fontan circuit may require surgical revision with conversion to an extracardiac Fontan and a form of the Maze procedure for treatment of intractable atrial tachycardia.[926] Recent reported perioperative mortality is 1%,[46,226] and late mortality is 5%.[46]

Survival at 25 years after Fontan-type correction has been reported at 70%.[467] The most frequent causes of late death in Fontan patients are sudden death (9.2%), thromboembolism (7.9%), and heart failure (6.7%), with an arrhythmic origin presumed for the sudden deaths.[467] Absence of aspirin or warfarin therapy is a predictor of death caused by thromboembolic event.[467] The risk for thromboembolic death increases sharply 15 years after Fontan surgery.[467] All single ventricle patients require continuous lifelong care in a center with expertise in ACHD care. In the presence of single ventricle dysfunction or protein-losing enteropathy, a heart transplant may be beneficial.[926] More information is needed regarding long-term outcome of these patients.

Reproductive Health in Women with Congenital Heart Disease

Women with congenital heart disease appear to have similar sexual activity and fertility rates as their healthy peers.[137,245,609,729] Pregnancy planning in this patient population is required to reduce maternal and/or fetal morbidity. Yet, few patients seek advice regarding birth control and family planning.[428,738,835] It is imperative, therefore, that the healthcare team caring for these patients maximize opportunities to discuss pregnancy prevention and planning. Detailed information regarding pregnancy, contraception, and delivery for patients with congenital heart disease is included in the Chapter 8 Supplement, section, Adults with Congenital Heart Disease, on the Evolve Website.

Medical and surgical advances have made survival into adulthood an expectation for patients with congenital heart disease. With these advances have come an influx of women with moderate and complex congenital heart disease who desire pregnancy. Although pregnancy and delivery are associated with significant hemodynamic changes such as increased blood volume, increased stroke volume, increased cardiac output, and decreased systemic vascular resistance, most women with repaired congenital heart disease appear to tolerate pregnancy and delivery with only minimal risk.[809]

The majority of women with congenital heart disease tolerate pregnancy and delivery without significant risk, although there are many obstetric, cardiac, anesthesia, genetic, and psychosocial factors to consider. In patients with more than simple disease, a multidisciplinary approach in a regional center is essential to optimize maternal and fetal outcomes.

Perioperative Care for the Patient with Adult CHD

Perioperative care for the patient with ACHD for minor (elective noncardiac procedures) and major procedures, as well as emergency admissions[426] requires comprehensive medical, surgical, and nursing management. The team must be knowledgeable about the cardiac anesthesia requirements, the potentially complex hemodynamics, any residual structural abnormalities, anticoagulation needs, and physiologic abnormalities related to each congenital heart lesion. Adults with important co-morbidities such as coronary artery disease or renal failure may require postprocedure recovery in an adult cardiac critical care unit with the consultation of the required adult subspecialists. Adults without significant comorbidities may be treated in a section of the pediatric cardiac critical care unit. Communication among the congenital surgical, interventional cardiology, and adult medical subspecialists is essential to provide optimal care, involving nursing education regarding the defect pathophysiology, hemodynamics, surgical intervention, and likely postoperative complications. The healthcare team must continue to monitor for and document long-term outcomes.

Procedures. Cardiac catheterization may be required in adults with CHD for hemodynamic assessments. Interventions are commonly performed for complex pulmonary artery stenosis, baffle stenosis, or residual aortic narrowing. Shunting defects, including fenestrations, may be sealed with devices (see Common Diagnostic Tests, Cardiac Catheterization). Pulmonary valves and aortic valves are now replaced by transcatheter interventions in selected cases. Pediatric electrophysiology studies to detect and treat atrial or ventricular arrhythmias may include implantation of a cardiac pacemaker with possible cardioverter defibrillator.[388]

Postoperative Care. Comprehensive guidelines are available for the perioperative assessment and management of patients with adult congenital heart disease undergoing noncardiac surgery.[196] When cardiovascular surgery is required, reoperations are the most common type of surgery needed.[802] High-risk patients require close postoperative surveillance in a critical care or coronary care unit, particularly patients with cyanosis, pulmonary hypertension, ventricular dysfunction, or single ventricle.[196]

The most common reported complication in the postoperative cardiac surgery adult (occurring in 10.8% of patients) is atrial arrhythmias.[1] The postoperative team must carefully monitor the patient's volume status, hemodynamics, and electrolyte balance, and be observant for evidence of hypoxemic pulmonary hypertensive episodes or crisis and be aware of all drug therapies required. Each cardiac lesion carries risks of particular rhythm disturbances, and unexpected arrhythmias may occur at any time.

Conduction anomalies are common in adults with uncorrected cyanotic CHD,[802] including ventricular or supraventricular ectopy. Perioperative development of arrhythmias can lead to sudden, severe low cardiac output. Immediate evaluation and prompt treatment are required.[802] Monitoring for development of cardiac ischemia includes monitoring for ST segment changes and ventricular ectopy. Atrial and ventricular pacing wires can assist in management (see Arrhythmia Detection and Management).

Bleeding is a potential risk following reoperation, particularly in the patient with longstanding cyanosis.[802] Reoperation requires incisions through vascular scar tissue and chronic hypoxemia is associated with thrombocytopenia and thrombocytopathia. In addition, patients with chronic hypoxemia may demonstrate a decrease in vitamin K-dependent clotting factors. For these reasons, bleeding should be anticipated and plenty of blood should be available for postoperative blood replacement.

Cardiac reserve may be limited in many cyanotic patients, and excessive blood loss can rapidly cause hemodynamic instability. Target hemoglobin values and plans for coagulation factor replacement are individualized based on the specific congenital lesion, operative interventions, and associated risk factors. A patient with expected residual cyanosis cannot tolerate anemia, because it decreases oxygen-carrying capacity and reduces oxygen content and likely oxygen delivery.

The risk of perioperative low cardiac output is increased in the presence of chronic hypoxemia, ventricular hypertrophy, chronic volume or pressure overload, ventricular dysfunction, and arrhythmias. In the postoperative period, reactivity of the pulmonary vascular bed is heightened,[511] so pulmonary hypertension precautions are vital (see section, Pulmonary Hypertension).

Pulmonary hemorrhage may develop with interventions that increase pulmonary blood flow, particularly after interventional cardiac catheterization. Mechanical ventilation and pulmonary support are required. Development of pneumonia, infection, fever, thrombosis, or pulmonary edema can seriously destabilize the patient with ACHD, even after a minor procedure. Supplementary oxygen can help to decrease the pulmonary vascular resistance, although if cyanotic heart disease is present it may not increase the arterial oxygen saturation.[196] Parameters for acceptable and expected oxygen saturation levels and PaO_2 are required.

Smoking can compromise pulmonary function preoperatively and postoperatively. Encourage pulmonary toilet hourly while awake with incentive spirometry, and encourage the patient to get out of bed and walk or at least sit in a chair as soon as possible. Intermittent pneumatic compression or the use of antiembolism stockings should be used to reduce the risk of deep vein thrombosis (DVT).[196]

Risk of DVT is increased with prolonged bedrest, neuromuscular blockade, and limited range of motion. Early ambulation is optimal. Monitor for signs of DVT, including redness or pain in the leg calves. Signs of pulmonary embolus include sudden dyspnea, tachypnea, increased oxygen requirement, and rales. An arterial blood gas will not establish the diagnosis. Massive pulmonary embolism can result in acute right ventricular failure, low cardiac output, and myocardial ischemia with ST segment changes. Diagnosis is confirmed by lung perfusion scan or pulmonary angiogram. Treatment includes immediate, heparinization, and hemodynamic supportive care. In acute situations, fibrinolytics (recombinant tissue plasminogen activator or rTPA) are administered. Cardiopulmonary bypass may be employed to remove the embolus (pulmonary embolectomy).

Renal dysfunction is a known risk in patients with chronical cyanotic hypoxemia.[802] Cardiopulmonary bypass can further exacerbate renal dysfunction. Perioperative care includes maintaining optimal cardiac output with careful fluid balance and support of systemic perfusion. Volume replacement requires normal saline infusions typically of 500 cc or more (10 cc/kg), administered as a bolus to optimize cardiac filling pressures. Infusion by syringe injections (often used for pediatric patients) does not allow administration of sufficiently large volumes when resuscitation is required.

Relative hypovolemia can result from rewarming and vasodilation, fever, increased capillary permeability, and use of vasodilators. Signs can include sinus tachycardia, decreased central venous or intracardiac pressures, and signs of decreased perfusion.

Standard medication doses for adults are used, including doses for resuscitation drugs, antiarrhythmic therapy, and antibiotics. Intravenous drug infusions in the adult can be specifically concentrated by the clinical pharmacist to avoid excessive fluid volume administration. Doses must be titrated individually with consideration of any renal or hepatic dysfunction.

Cyanotic patients are at greater risk of postural hypotension because of a greater right-to-left shunt.[196] Changes in movement should be gradual.

Effective pain management is essential to minimize catecholamine surges.[196] The patient with ACHD may have sensitization to and greater fear of painful procedures because of a previous history of inadequately managed pain during prior surgeries or hospitalization.[707] Discussion of plans for pain control and patient-controlled analgesia help to control potential anxiety. Patients with preoperative history of illegal drug use or preoperative prescription narcotics typically require higher doses of analgesia postoperatively. Inadequate analgesia can lead to decreased chest physiotherapy and ambulation.

Many adult survivors of congenital heart disease have unique alterations in neurologic status related to the presence of genetic syndromes (Down, DiGeorge, Williams) or previous neurologic alterations leading to developmental delays and increased dependence on family involvement in care. Rest and privacy are essential. The adult's bedtime ritual can be assessed. Some may use prescriptions, rituals, or over-the-counter medications to promote sleep.

Unique developmental needs and degree of family involvement may be present in the patient with ACHD. Some may rely heavily on a parent and/or significant other for making decisions and daily activities. Survivors require guidance in terms of educational and vocation choices. Some of the survivors of complex congenital heart disease management are at risk for inattention, hyperactivity, and developmental disabilities, and require remedial school services.[798]

Issues with independence and interdependence may exist, as well as other psychological challenges found in patients with chronic illness, as detailed in Claessens et al[180] and Tong et al.[867] Providers should assess the patient's knowledge and independence in areas of self-care.

Transitioning to Adult Specialist Care

The transitioning process from pediatric to adult-focused CHD care is life-altering for patients, parents, and staff. The act of transfer may be a substantial source of stress for the patient, parent, and longtime caregiver. Therefore all involved parties should be involved in the transitioning process. The concept of transitioning should be discussed early, around age 12 if the patient is emotionally and intellectually ready, and should continue until the patient demonstrates the ability to take responsibility for self-care. It is essential to provide adequate resources for support of the family at this time, including both in-hospital resources and outside patient support resources. The Adult Congenital Heart Association (ACHA) and American College of Cardiology developed a "Passport" document to allow patients to concisely identify their specific cardiac health needs and endocarditis prophylaxis requirements. The healthcare team can provide lesion specific identification of patient conditions, therapies, and the suggested guidelines for ACHD care. A clinic resource list now identifies ACHD clinics nationwide, and is available on the ACHA web site (www.achaheart.org).

Education with respect to employment, insurance needs, and social service resources are also required by many. Continued monitoring and instruction regarding management of noncardiac surgical procedure care and required collaboration with the adult CHD team are essential to optimize care and safety, and minimize morbidity and mortality risks.

Ultimate goals are to optimize ACHD survival and maximize quality of life. It is clear that all patients with congenital heart disease require lifelong collaborative care from pediatric and adult specialists who will provide ongoing screening for known complications and potentially unexpected sequelae of the defect and therapies. These complex patients face potential long-term and possible life-threatening complications. Transition from the pediatric into the ACHD clinic is a vital priority.

Resources for Healthcare Professionals and Families

- Adult Congenital Heart Association (ACHA): www.achaheart.org
  - "Passports" for CHD, extensive patient education materials, pamphlets available
- American Heart Association: http://www.heart.org/HEARTORG
- International Society of Adult Congenital Cardiac Disease (ISAACD): http://www.isaccd.org/

POSTOPERATIVE CARE AND ANTICOAGULATION FOR THE CHILD WITH CONGENITAL HEART DISEASE

Mary Rummell, Patricia Ann E. Schlosser, Sandra Staveski, Winnie Yung

This section provides an overview of postoperative care of the child after cardiovascular surgery. For information about common problems such as congestive heart failure or pulmonary hypertension, please refer to the information in the previous major section of this chapter, Common Clinical Problems. For specific postoperative complications associated with each congenital heart defect, please refer to the information about the defects in the section Specific Diseases.

ADMISSION TO THE CRITICAL CARE UNIT

The transfer (handoff) of patients from the surgical team to the critical care team can result in technical errors (i.e., delivery of inappropriate infusions, incorrect ventilator settings) and errors of omission. In the past several years, the development of standard handoff procedures and checklists, some of which were learned from consultation with managers of Formula One racing teams and aviation models, have been shown to reduce such errors.[146,147]

Before the patient arrives in the critical care unit, (PCCU), all equipment necessary for the child's care should be set up in working order with appropriate alarm limits established. Whenever possible, the equipment should be transferred with the patient, to avoid the need to change intravenous pumps or monitoring equipment. PCCU personnel should document errors associated with the transfer and standardize this transfer to reduce such errors.

To improve efficiency of patient admission to the critical care unit, each member of the receiving team should be in an assigned position with specific assigned responsibilities (Fig. 8-29). Patient transfers should include a transfer checklist or form, equipment and technology transfer, information transmission, and finally, discussion and plan for the patient.[146]

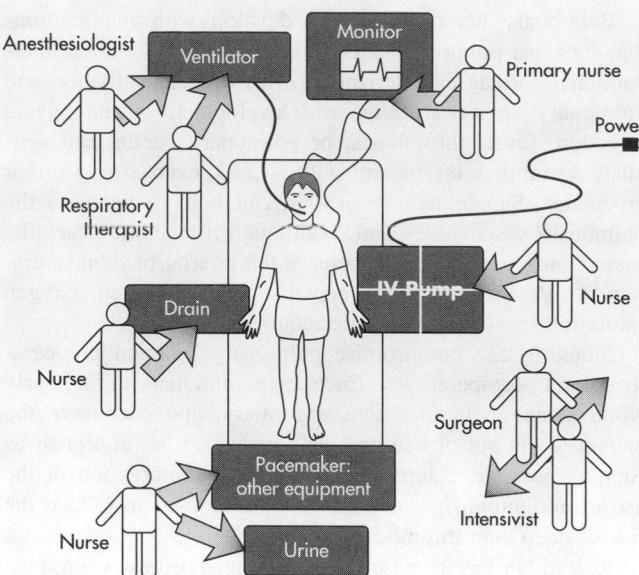

FIG. 8-29 Organization of team for transfer of care from surgical to postoperative critical care team. (Based on Catchpole KR, de Leval MR, Mcewan A, et al: Patient handover from surgery to intensive care: using Formula 1 pit-stop and aviation models to improve safety and quality. *Pediatr Anesth* 17:470-478, 2007.)

CARDIOVASCULAR FUNCTION

Nursing management after cardiac surgery requires understanding of the child's preoperative and postoperative anatomy and physiology, the surgical intervention itself, intraoperative events, the effects of cardiopulmonary bypass (in many cases), the child's baseline condition, and any co-morbidities. Nurses are in a unique position to optimize care delivery and coordinate care for these complex children by virtue of their knowledge, skills, and extended presence at the bedside. The child's cardiovascular function requires close observation through physical examination, hemodynamic monitoring, and laboratory analysis.

Cardiac Output

Cardiac output is the amount of blood ejected from the systemic ventricle in one minute. Cardiac output is a product of heart rate and stroke volume. Stroke volume is affected by preload, afterload, and contractility. Cardiac output may be indexed to body surface area, reported as a cardiac index (CI); normal CI is 3.5 to 4.5 L/min per m² body surface area.

At various stages during the life cycle, there are important developmental components to consider when caring for a patient after cardiac surgery. The infant and child are very dependent on an adequate heart rate to maintain effective cardiac output; bradycardia often is associated with a fall in cardiac output. Children can increase stroke volume in response to volume administration, but the response is limited, particularly during the neonatal period when diastolic ventricular compliance is low with less response to volume loading than in the older infant or adult. It is important to keep these and other developmental considerations in mind as you care for the child after cardiac surgical intervention.

Careful assessment of cardiac output is particularly important during the postoperative period. Adequate postoperative systemic perfusion requires a heart rate appropriate for the child's age and clinical condition, sufficient cardiac preload and intravascular volume, adequate myocardial function, and appropriate ventricular afterload (resistance to ventricular ejection). If cardiac preload or myocardial function is inadequate or if ventricular afterload is excessive, cardiac output may fall. Assessment of cardiac output is accomplished through monitoring heart rate, blood pressure, intracardiac pressures, peripheral perfusion, acid-base status, serum lactate, temperature, urine output, and mixed venous oxygen saturation.[73] The moment the child returns from surgery the nurse should form an opinion of the child's systemic perfusion and cardiovascular function. The nurse also should be aware of the "filling" (central venous, atrial) pressures at which systemic perfusion is best and inform the interdisciplinary team of the findings.

Hemodynamic Monitoring

Postoperative patients will have one or more invasive monitoring catheters depending on the defect, surgical intervention, and anticipated hemodynamic monitoring requirements. Invasive catheters are used for hemodynamic monitoring and blood sampling, as well as for administration of vasoactive infusions, nutrition, and volume expanders. On admission to the pediatric critical care unit (PCCU), the team should check the chest radiograph to verify appropriate placement of the catheters.

It is imperative that all monitoring catheters be zeroed and calibrated and transducers set at the phlebostatic reference point (level of the right atrium) or as established by unit protocol. Transducers placed at a level (relative to the right atrium) different from the level at which they were zeroed and calibrated will provide inaccurate measurements (see Chapter 21). Transthoracic and intracardiac catheters have been shown to be safe to use, but carry associated risks such as thrombus formation, malfunction, and infection.[272]

Left atrial catheters are typically used only for monitoring because administration of anything into these catheters may cause the potentially devastating complication of embolization of air, particulate matter, or thrombus into the cerebral or coronary circulation. It is important to note that children with mixing physiology (i.e., systemic venous blood entering the systemic arterial circulation) are at increased risk for embolic events from all intravenous catheters and therefore should have absolutely no air, thrombus, or particulate matter in their intravenous lines. For more information on hemodynamic monitoring, see Chapter 21.

Preload

The pressure in a ventricle at the end of diastole (i.e., the end-diastolic pressure) provides the preload to stretch of the child's ventricular fibers. It is affected by the child's intravascular volume as well as ventricular compliance. Inadequate intravascular volume can result from hemorrhage, vasodilatation during rewarming, third spacing of fluids related to systemic inflammatory response following cardiopulmonary bypass (CPB), aggressive diuresis, or inadequate fluid administration (Table 8-21).[73]

Ventricular compliance (change in volume divided by change in pressure) is the distensibility of the ventricle; it is

Table 8-21	Potential Causes of Elevated or Reduced Right or Left Atrial Pressure	
Invasive Catheter	**Elevated Pressures**	**Reduced Pressures**
Right atrial or central venous	Volume overload; decreased right ventricular function; tamponade; artifact; catheter malfunction	Hypovolemia; artifact
Left atrial	Volume overload; decreased left ventricular function; tamponade; arrhythmia; artifact	Hypovolemia; artifact; decreased left atrial pressure in combination with high RA and/or CVP can develop with PHTN

typically low immediately after cardiovascular surgery, particularly if a ventriculotomy incision was performed or the ventricle is hypertrophied and the surgery resulted in significant alteration of flow patterns.

Preload is evaluated through examination of "filling" pressures (atrial pressures and central venous pressure) and assessment of liver distension, peripheral and pulmonary edema, and fontanelle fullness. The optimal preload is determined at the bedside and varies from patient to patient and in the same patient over the course of postoperative care. A higher preload is likely to be required early in the postoperative period than as the heart recovers. The bedside nurse should note the "filling" pressure (CVP or right or left atrial pressure) at which systemic perfusion is best.

Preload is manipulated through volume administration and diuresis. Fluid boluses and volume resuscitation should be managed by using the appropriate volume expander based on the clinical situation. For example, hypovolemia not related to bleeding is managed by administration of isotonic crystalloid or colloid. By comparison, hypovolemia related to significant bleeding is managed by correction of abnormal coagulation factors and administration of packed red blood cells.

The child's circulating blood volume should be calculated before the child returns from surgery and all blood losses should be considered as a proportion of the child's circulating blood volume:
- Neonates: 80 to 85 mL/kg
- Infants: 75 to 80 mL/kg
- Children: 70 to 75 mL/kg
- Adolescents/Adults: 65 to 70 mL/kg

Please refer to Chapter 6 for fluid administration guidelines in the treatment of shock.

If the child's chest tube output averages 3 mL/kg per hour, these losses will total 10% to 15% of the child's circulating blood volume within 3 hours. If this blood loss is not replaced, significant cardiovascular compromise and shock can result. It is advisable to replace chest tube output once it totals 5% to 10% of the child's circulating blood volume. Replacement should occur as quickly as the output is draining; use atrial filling pressures and other hemodynamic monitoring pressures to guide your fluid management. Chest tube output of 3 to 5 mL/kg per hour constitutes significant hemorrhage, and the source of the bleeding must be identified. If excessive chest tube output continues despite normal clotting function the child typically requires re-exploration, which may occur in the operating room or at the bedside.

Contractility

Impaired contractility or myocardial dysfunction may influence cardiac output. Drugs, anesthesia, hypoxia, acidosis, ischemia, electrolyte imbalance, extensive ventriculotomy, residual lesions, myocardial resection, and tamponade all affect contractility.[73] Hypercapnia and alveolar hypoxia can increase pulmonary vascular resistance and can contribute to left ventricular dysfunction; therefore if they develop, mechanical ventilatory support generally must be instituted or adjusted. Note that if the child has a single functioning ventricle with a bidirectional Glenn, hemi-Fontan, or Fontan-type physiology, support of spontaneous ventilation is preferred to positive pressure ventilation, when possible. Mild hypercapnia may actually improve cardiac output in these patients.[935]

Acidosis should be treated promptly because it can depress ventricular contractility, leading to decreased perfusion, decreased systemic arterial pressure, and/or increased filling pressures. Treatment (except in tamponade) includes correction of metabolic abnormalities and, if necessary, use of inotropic and afterload reducing agents (see the following).

Afterload

Afterload is impedance or resistance to ventricular ejection. Increased afterload can result from increased pulmonary or systemic vasoconstriction or residual outflow tract obstruction.

Systemic Vascular Resistance. Systemic vasoconstriction may be a compensatory mechanism in a low cardiac output state or from administration of vasoconstrictors. Treatment of increased afterload involves avoidance of precipitating factors, intravenous nonspecific vasodilating agents (SVR and PVR), inhaled vasodilators (PVR), and mechanical ventilator manipulation to optimize cardiopulmonary interactions (e.g., intubation and supporting ventilation for reducing left ventricular afterload).

If systemic vascular resistance (SVR) is high or even normal in the presence of ventricular dysfunction, or the child demonstrates significant peripheral vasoconstriction with poor systemic perfusion, treatment with vasodilators usually is indicated. These agents are nonspecific and may cause dilatory effects in both the systemic and pulmonary beds. When intravenous vasodilators are administered, the child's fluid volume status must be adequate because hypotension may develop, especially during initiation of therapy.

Vasodilators can reduce ventricular preload and afterload because they produce venous and arterial dilation (see Chapter 6). During vasodilator therapy, assess the warmth of the child's extremities, capillary refill, serum lactate, urine output, and blood pressure to determine the effectiveness of therapy. If multiple agents are used, it is also important that the dose of only one medication be changed at any one time so that the patient's response to each change can be determined.

Pulmonary Vascular Resistance. Pulmonary vasoconstriction can result from alveolar hypoxia, acidosis, hyperinflation of the lung, and hypothermia. In addition, cardiopulmonary bypass can affect vascular tone and permeability. Pain may also affect vascular tone.[73] Elevated pulmonary vascular resistance (PVR) may be a developmental, acute, or chronic condition. For example, newborns have reactive pulmonary vascular bed and are susceptible elevated PVR. Additionally, some children have a genetic predisposition for pulmonary hypertension, such as children with trisomy 21.[652] For further information, see Box 8-1 and Table 8-16.

The effects of cardiopulmonary (CPB), pulmonary leukosequestration, microemboli, and hypothermia have been implicated in pulmonary vascular endothelium dysfunction, and elevated PVR with increased pulmonary vasoreactivity in the postoperative period.[73,206,667] Excessive pulmonary blood flow and left-to-right intracardiac shunts before and after CPB, elevated pulmonary venous pressure, lung pathology, blood products, and Protamine are several of the other risk factors associated with postoperative elevation in PVR.[73,667,845] Post-CPB pulmonary endothelium dysfunction may be responsible for increased generation of pulmonary vasoconstricting mediators and decreased endogenous nitric oxide (NO) production associated with vasodilatation.[71,73]

An increase in the child's pulmonary vascular resistance also may be an acute cause of inadequate systemic perfusion postoperatively. An acute rise in PVR with resulting decreased cardiac output, acidosis, hypoxemia, and increased right ventricular (RV) afterload can worsen any preexisting RV dysfunction.[4,7,73,206]

Pulmonary hypertension (PHTN) is characterized by an elevation in pulmonary artery pressure and PVR. It is defined as a systolic pulmonary artery pressure (PAP) greater than 35 mm Hg or a mean PAP greater than 25 mm Hg at rest. Often in the clinical setting, the severity of PHTN is discussed in relation to systemic arterial pressures. Treatment for PHTN typically begins at approximately half systemic pressures. In the absence of a pulmonary artery catheter, it is possible to assess for effects of PVR by monitoring the systemic venous atrial or central venous filling pressures. A child experiencing PTHN will have a rising right atrial or central venous pressure, falling left atrial (or pulmonary venous atrial) pressure, and falling blood pressure.

PHTN can lead to RV failure, low cardiac output state, impaired oxygen delivery, and shock. The goals of care are to decrease PVR and maximize RV function, and optimize cardiac output.[652] Support of right ventricular function and output is important. Milrinone, dopamine, or epinephrine may be used to support cardiac output. Optimizing right ventricular preload can improve cardiac output, because elevated right atrial pressures are required to maintain adequate ventricular filling.[845]

The child with perioperative pulmonary hypertension requires precise postoperative ventilator management and must remain well oxygenated and ventilated, as well as warm. Providers should make an effort to treat pain and agitation and minimize stimulation (see section, Common Clinical Conditions, Pulmonary Hypertension). Respiratory mechanisms to lower PVR include ensuring adequate gas exchange, maintaining functional residual capacity, and avoiding hypoinflation or hyperinflation. Alveolar hypoxia, such as may be produced by hypoventilation, pneumothorax, airway obstruction, suctioning, and atelectasis, must be avoided. A mild alkalosis will promote pulmonary vasodilation. These children usually require mechanical ventilator support for several days, and then *gradual* weaning is attempted. During weaning the child's pulmonary pressure (if available) and systemic perfusion should be monitored carefully because hypoventilation produces alveolar hypoxia and can result in pulmonary vasoconstriction.

These children may also require blunting of stress responses with opioid or benzodiazepines, and ventilation with sedation and neuromuscular blockade may be needed. There may be benefit to premedicating the child with an opioid and/or benzodiazepine before suctioning or noxious stimuli to blunt responses to the stimulus. Clustering care to prevent excessive stimulation may reduce the potential for PHTN crisis as well.

Prevention or prompt correction of acidosis is required with either respiratory or metabolic maneuvers to achieve a pH of approximately 7.5.[652] Pulmonary vasodilatation with specific and nonspecific agents is frequently accomplished through administration of inhaled nitric oxide (specific) and/or milrinone (nonspecific). If inhaled nitric oxide is administered it should be weaned slowly to avoid rebound effect. Weaning from any PVR therapy should be accomplished in a stepwise, methodical fashion.[845]

Endotracheal suctioning is a well-known noxious stimulus that can provoke PHTN. Hyperventilation and hyperoxygenation have been shown to reduce suctioning induced hypoxia.[669] The use of in-line suctioning catheters may be beneficial as well.[442] If open suctioning is required, two nurses should perform the procedure. The first nurse provides hand or mechanical ventilation and maintains oxygenation. If inhaled nitric oxide is being used, ensure that there is delivery of the drug into the hand ventilation circuit. The second nurse provides skilled, gentle suctioning. Children with extremely labile pulmonary vascular beds should have a physician or advanced practice nurse present during suctioning. Please refer to Common Clinical Conditions, Pulmonary Hypertension for further information.

Heart Rate and Arrhythmias

An abnormal heart rate or rhythm can compromise cardiac output postoperatively.

The incidence of arrhythmia after pediatric cardiac surgery has been reported to be as low as 8.8% to as high as 48%; arrhythmias can be a major cause of morbidity.[807,961]

The most common arrhythmias after cardiac surgery involve rate or conduction abnormalities. The heart rate must always be evaluated in light of age and clinical condition. For example, in neonates a sinus tachycardia to 210/min may be tolerated if needed to increase cardiac output. By comparison, the same heart rate in an older child may curtail diastolic filling and significantly compromise cardiac output.

Preprocedural and procedural factors can contribute to postoperative arrhythmias, and include young age, small size, exposure to anesthesia, CPB, hypothermia, surgical incisions,

increased circulating catecholamines, surgical cardiac incisions and suture lines, and hemodynamic lability.[807,816]

Therapeutic treatment of arrhythmias includes medication (e.g., propranolol, procainamide, amiodarone), pacing (e.g., pacemaker therapy, overdrive pacemaker therapy), and nonpharmacologic interventions (e.g., thermoregulation, sedation, vagal stimulation, cardioversion, defibrillation). Prompt recognition and treatment of arrhythmias can reduce morbidity and mortality (see section, Common Clinical Conditions, Arrhythmias).

Postoperative rhythm disturbances can be characterized by bradyarrhythmias and tachyarrhythmias. Bradyarrhythmias include sinus node dysfunction and atrioventricular block. Tachyarrhythmias include atrial tachycardias, junctional tachycardia, and ventricular tachycardia. The most common arrhythmias after pediatric cardiovascular surgery include supraventricular tachycardia, junctional ectopic tachycardia, and various forms of heart block.[807] Loss of atrioventricular synchrony accounts for an approximate 20% to 30% reduction in cardiac output and causes inadequate tissue perfusion.[43]

Maintaining normal electrolyte balance is very important in the prevention and treatment of many rhythm disturbances. Such balance can be challenging to achieve during aggressive diuretic management (see Chapter 12).

Significant ventricular arrhythmias such as ventricular tachycardia or ventricular fibrillation are relatively uncommon in children after cardiovascular surgery, and the appearance of such arrhythmias usually indicates serious deterioration in the child's acid-base or electrolyte balance, oxygenation, or cardiovascular function (see section, Common Clinical Conditions, Arrhythmias).

Accurate diagnosis and immediate intervention are essential to successful management of arrhythmias. Poor heart rate variability in light of clinical changes is an important finding in the identification of arrhythmias. Additionally, cannon "a" waves visible on atrial tracings can provide clues in detection of rhythm disturbances.[73,750] Definitive diagnosis is made by 12-lead electrocardiogram.

Pacemaker wires can also be used to diagnose arrhythmias. An atrial wire tracing performed using the pacemaker wires may be a useful tool in the diagnosis of tachyarrhythmias when the P wave is not easily identified or is obscured by the QRS complex. Please refer to section, Common Clinical Conditions, Arrhythmias for more information.

Temporary pacemaker therapy is common in the postoperative period. Therefore, many children receiving surgical repair involving manipulation near the conduction system have temporary epicardial pacing leads placed during their surgical repair. The leads (or wires) are brought through the child's chest wall. They may be unipolar or bipolar (two terminals in contact with and separated from each other by myocardium). The advantages of bipolar over unipolar leads are: (1) less between-chamber interference, (2) less electrical interference, (3) lower pacing thresholds, and (4) better sensing of local electrograms.[815] Each of the pacemaker leads can be attached to an external pacemaker via a cable.

When pacing is provided or available on "standby," the child's cardiac threshold should be determined and recorded in the nursing records. If heart block is present it is important that the appropriate pacemaker demand rate is set so that the child will receive appropriate pacing support when needed (see Chapter 21). If the child is pacemaker-dependent, the child's pacing threshold should be checked once daily (as opposed to multiple times). In addition, a back-up pacemaker must be readily available with settings programmed and new batteries in place, and the nurse must be able to quickly access transcutaneous pacemaker pads and the device. Assessment of ventricular capture is aided by the presence of a functioning arterial catheter.

If pacing is required and the child does not regain his or her native rhythm within 10 to 14 days, consideration is given to placement of a permanent pacemaker. Pacemakers and defibrillators are now commonly used with children. The diversity and complexity of pediatric patients and those with congenital heart disease makes device management a highly individualized art.[178,815] For further information, see Chapter 21.

Low Cardiac Output Syndrome (LCOS)

Cardiac output/index may progressively decrease in the initial postoperative period and nadirs at 9 to 12 h after CPB.[937] The progressive decline in cardiac index can be associated with elevations in SVR and PVR. A postoperative cardiac index of less than 2.0 to 2.5 L/min per m^2 body surface area indicates the presence of low cardiac output; this is associated with poor systemic perfusion and shock. Early signs of postoperative shock may include tachycardia, decreased intensity of peripheral pulses, cool and pale (or mottled) extremities, prolonged capillary refill time, decreased urine output, and extreme irritability or lethargy. Later signs of shock include hypotension, bradycardia, hypoxemia, and metabolic acidosis. Anticipation, proactive management, and vigilance are important to maintaining stability in the postoperative child.

Potential sources of LCOS include: (1) residual lesion; (2) myocardial ischemia secondary to circulatory arrest, hypothermia, aortic crossclamp and reperfusion injury; (3) insufficient intraoperative myocardial protection and cardioplegia; (4) inflammatory response to CPB; (5) changes in SVR and PVR; (6) arrhythmias; (7) cardiac tamponade; (8) continuation of preoperative ventricular dysfunction, (9) complications of surgery; and (10) infections.[43,73,386,939] Cardiac catheterization and echocardiography may be required to explore potential causes of LCOS because residual lesions are unlikely to improve with medical therapies. Surgical or catheterization interventions may be required. Measures to assess and treat LCOS are important in reducing time on mechanical ventilation, hospitalization, and overall mortality and morbidity.[73,667] Pharmacologic treatment of LCOS is presented in more detail in Chapter 6.

Extracorporeal membrane oxygenation (ECMO) may be considered for refractory LCOS states or cardiac arrest. Cardiac ECMO can be used as a short-term bridge to recovery, or a bridge to long-term mechanical support or transplantation. A system for rapid deployment ECMO requires a skilled team and resource availability to ensure expeditious initiation of ECMO support. Effective use of rapid deployment ECMO has been associated with decreased mortality in children with heart disease with reversible decompensated states and after cardiac arrest.[73,516,940] Please see Chapter 7 for further information about ECMO and ventricular assist devices.

Tamponade

Tamponade is a rare but life-threatening complication and can be a sudden cause of decreased systemic perfusion in the postoperative cardiovascular patient. The pericardial sac surrounding the heart is composed of nonelastic, fibrous tissue. The sac contains a small volume of fluid to cushion and protect the myocardium. Although a slow accumulation of fluid in a relatively noncompliant pericardial sac initially may be tolerated at the expense of ventricular filling,[418] the sudden accumulation of pericardial fluid will not be tolerated and generally produces rapid deterioration.

Cardiac tamponade can be associated with the removal of intracardiac catheters in the PCCU.[418] Flori and colleagues[272] studied the use and associated morbidities of intracardiac catheters and found them to be safe. However, young infants and children with thrombocytopenia or catheters in the left atria or pulmonary artery position had greater need for intervention after catheter removal, so added precautions are warranted in this age group.[272] Careful evaluation of hematologic status, patency of chest tubes, blood product availability, pain and agitation status, and the patient's hemodynamics before catheter removal may minimize complications.[73] Please refer to Box 8-15 before removing transthoracic and intracardiac catheters.

Signs of Tamponade

Signs of tamponade may be similar to those of shock, and may include hypotension and tachycardia, a narrowing of the child's pulse pressure, and a high central venous and left atrial

---

Box 8-15	**Considerations for Transthoracic and Intracardiac Catheter Removal**

1. Check the child's most recent coagulation studies (such as: PT, PTT, INR, Platelets)
2. Verify that platelets are at least 70,000/mm^3 and INR less than 1.5. If child does not meet or exceed these criteria, obtain order for transfusion, and transfuse with appropriate blood product prior to line removal.
3. Blood products should be double-checked with another nurse. Keep tubing at bedside in case of emergent need for administration.
4. Continuous arterial hemodynamic monitoring should be utilized during the removal procedure and for at least one hour after.
5. Ensure the child has adequate IV access prior to intracardiac catheter removal.
6. Ensure chest tube patency prior to removal.
7. Evaluate the child's need for sedation/analgesia; an active child may elevate pressures and increase the potential for bleeding.
8. Check the child's hematocrit one hour post line removal or sooner if bleeding is suspected.
9. Assess the child for signs of tamponade (such as: tachycardia, narrow pulse pressure and high atrial pressures) and bleeding (presence of blood in chest tubes, decreased blood pressure, pallor, altered mental status)
10. If there is a sudden arterial waveform dampening, assume the child is experiencing cardiac tamponade and initiate resuscitation.
11. Document vital signs appropriately.

pressure. The child's heart sounds may become muffled, or the QRS complexes on the child's ECG may become smaller, but these are inconsistent and often late findings. Signs of tamponade may be indistinguishable from those of low cardiac output. If clots have formed around the right or left side of the heart alone, signs of isolated right or left heart tamponade (and isolated systemic or pulmonary venous hypertension, respectively) may be noted occasionally.

Significant pericardial effusion or tamponade can be visualized quickly using echocardiography. A chest radiograph is often not helpful and may be normal in appearance or may show increased heart size and pulmonary vascular congestion, although these findings may be difficult to differentiate from those caused by congestive heart failure. In children with delayed sternal closure, fluid accumulation is easily diagnosed by assessing the impermeable membrane (e.g., silastic patch) for bulging and fluid retention.

Tamponade should be suspected if the child's systemic perfusion deteriorates and right and left atrial or central venous pressures rise simultaneously and equally. The child may also demonstrate *pulsus paradoxus* (a fall in systolic blood pressure by 8 to 10 mm Hg during inspiration), but this finding is difficult to appreciate in the tachypneic or hypotensive infant or child. Clotting of the chest tube and resultant tamponade should be suspected if the child has excessive chest tube output that decreases abruptly as the child's systemic perfusion worsens and right and/or left atrial pressures rise.

Management

The child with tamponade requires immediate evacuation of pericardial fluid, and an emergency mediastinal exploration may have to be performed in the PCCU. Open-chest massage also may be required.

Emergent Mediastinal Exploration in the PCCU

Excessive bleeding and acute tamponade are life-threatening emergencies in the PCCU and may require emergent mediastinal exploration. This may be a low-volume, high-risk procedure in a PCCU and requires all team members to understand roles and specific duties, sterile technique, proper skin preparation, special equipment, and the importance of sequencing.[874] Checklists have been shown to be effective in establishing consistent protocols for opening and closing the chest in places such as the PCCU.[811] Please refer to Table 8-22 for an example of a checklist for Preparation for Elective Chest Closure.

Postoperative Heart Failure

Heart failure is present when cardiac function is incapable of providing sufficient oxygenated blood to meet metabolic demands. Ventricular dysfunction leading to heart failure can be caused by arrhythmias, increased afterload (e.g., aortic stenosis or hypertension), increased preload (e.g., mitral regurgitation or left-to-right shunts), or intrinsic muscle impairment (e.g., ischemia) or a combination of these factors.[529] The term *congestive heart failure* relates to heart failure that is associated with pulmonary congestion and edema that develop because of fluid retention. Heart failure can be present postoperatively, particularly if the child demonstrated it preoperatively, has residual lesions, or if repair of complex heart disease was performed.

Signs of Heart Failure

Signs of heart failure may include signs of systemic and/or pulmonary venous congestion. Isolated right or left ventricular failure may initially produce signs of systemic or pulmonary venous congestion, although biventricular failure will eventually develop.

Signs of systemic venous congestion in the postoperative patient include a high central venous or right atrial pressure, hepatomegaly, and periorbital edema. Ascites also may be present if systemic venous pressures are high.

Signs of pulmonary venous congestion include a high pulmonary arterial wedge or left atrial pressure. If the child is mechanically ventilated, high-peak inspiratory pressures and decreased lung compliance may be noted. If the child is breathing spontaneously, tachypnea and increased respiratory effort will be present.

The size of the heart on the chest radiograph is usually large, and pulmonary vascular markings will be prominent if pulmonary venous congestion is present.

Management

Management includes maximizing cardiac output while minimizing oxygen demand. The targets of treatment are improving cardiac function (improving cardiac contractility), and reducing cardiac work (decreasing afterload) and diuresis. Therapy includes administration of an inodilator, milrinone, or other vasodilators (e.g., nitroprusside) and diuretics. It may also include administration of digoxin, beta-blockers, and nesiritide, a natriuretic peptide.[308,553] Management of congestive heart failure is summarized in Common Clinical Conditions, Congestive Heart Failure.

Postcardiotomy Syndrome

Postcardiotomy (or postpericardiotomy) syndrome is defined as pericardial inflammation secondary to a surgical cardiotomy, producing pain, a friction rub and occasionally with ECG changes suggestive of ischemia. Other findings include fever (greater than 38.5° C), leukocytosis, pericardial and/or pleural effusion, malaise and arthralgia. The pain typically appears 3 to 6 weeks after a pericardiotomy.[199] Because many patients with the syndrome have an elevated C reactive protein (CRP), erythrocyte sedimentation rate, and antiheart antibodies, an autoimmune process has been implicated. In addition, a rise in viral titers also has been documented in many of the patients, suggesting that a viral illness also may be involved.

Treatment of postcardiotomy syndrome involves administration of antiinflammatory agents, observation for and treatment of pleural or pericardial effusion, and general supportive care. Aspirin or indomethacin is typically administered to reduce pericardial inflammation. The nurse should monitor for evidence of fluid retention and should be alert for signs of pleural and pericardial effusion, including signs of cardiac tamponade. The aspirin or indomethacin therapy usually reduces the chest pain and arthralgia, and bedrest may be recommended until the symptoms of pericarditis subside.

Steroids have been implicated in hastening recovery but should be reserved for refractory cases that do not respond to conventional therapies. Surgical intervention may be required for pericardiocentesis or a pericardial window for very difficult cases.[199]

Table 8-22   **Preparation for Elective Chest Closure—PCCU/CVCCU RN Checklist**

Communication

Verify OR team is notified and is coming to assist

Verify if anesthesia is coming; if not, notify PCCU/CVCCU team immediately

Notify charge nurse

Labs and Meds

Pt NPO (4-6 h pre-procedure)

Meds	Emergency medications (pre-drawn and ready for use)
	D/C Heparin drip 4-6 h before procedure (req MD order); after procedure, follow up to see if plan to restart heparin (usually restart 4 h after if no s/s bleeding).
	Antibiotic (cefazolin or vancomycin) ordered by MD
Labs	Recent coags, Hct, and platelet count (within 6 h of procedure; notify MD immediately if abnormal)
	Lab slip for specimen culture: per protocol to indicate "wound culture" and specify "mediastinal"
Blood	*Blood ordered—PRBCs to bedside* and placed in ice cooler; perform 2 RN check and have blood filter tubing and administration line ready.

Patient Setup

Bedside Monitor	ECG electrodes on patient extremities, i.e., away from surgical site
	ECG-QRS tone volume is audible
	Pulse-oximeter securely on and accurate
Chest Tubes	Mark level of chest tube drainage so can account for fluid accumulated during procedure
Pacer	Patient externally paced? Physician may consider asynchronous pacing during cautery
	Pacing wires to pacing cables; pacer at bedside and turned on—ensure recent battery change
Patient	Take down chest tube and sternal wound dressings
	Position patient's head to left (away from surgeon's side); small roll under patient's shoulders
	Place Bovie pad on patient and connect to Bovie machine
IV and Arterial Catheters	Medication administration set with extension tubing and stopcock
	Volume administration set with extension tubing and stopcock
	Situate arterial line to ensure accessibility during procedure
Airway with Respiratory Therapist	Confirm ETT is secure and confirm pt's ETT placement with RT (check morning chest x-ray)
	Anesthesia bag and appropriate size mask at bedside
	Secure ETT if necessary and suction pt before procedure if necessary

Room and Bedside Setup

Signs on doors "sterile procedure/do not enter"; minimize entry of nonessential personnel during procedure

Hats/masks—ready to distribute to those in room during procedure

Clear patient bedside area of all unnecessary equipment and furniture

Defibrillator, including internal handles and paddles

Additional wall suction set up × 2; and set up the large portable suction as back-up

Culture tube with pt's lab label, warm saline to be placed in warmer

Right Side of Patient (Surgeon side)	*Left Side of Patient*
Light source; with a back-up headlight available	All pleurovacs (preferred at foot of bed, if possible)
	Urometer (preferred at foot of bed, if possible)
Bovie/Bovie pad attached to patient	All IV and arterial catheters, pumps, tubing, and transducers (or, head or foot of bed)
	Pacing cables and pacer
Enough suction tubing to reach surgeon	Ventilator tubing and ventilator (or, able to suction w/o contaminating surgical field)
	Large portable suction (foot of bed, if possible)

Personnel	Sedation performed by:
	• Anesthesiologist (will bring medication and flowsheet) or
	• Sedation-qualified provider from PCCU/CVCCU team (will need to organize medication, administration set, sedation flowsheet, and "time out" before procedure)
	OR Team to assist in procedure
	RT notified and at bedside during procedure; safety checks done and ensure ETT secure
	RN to remain at patient bedside to coordinate care and assist as needed
	2nd RN in addition to patient's nurse

Chest Closure Checklist. Modified from a checklist developed by Winnie Yung, MN, RN, CCRN, for Lucile Packard Children's Hospital at Stanford, Palo Alto, California.

THERMOREGULATION AFTER CARDIAC SURGERY

The general goal of thermoregulation after cardiac surgery is maintenance of normothermia with minimal oxygen consumption. However, there are specific arrhythmias that are blunted with the use of systemic cooling such as junctional ectopic tachycardia (JET). It is important to recognize that children who have not received neuromuscular blockade (with sedation) during systemic cooling may start to shiver in an attempt to raise their core temperature. Continuous temperature monitoring is important if systemic cooling therapies are initiated.

The neonate is unable to shiver to generate heat when exposed to cold stress. Instead, the infant breaks down brown fat to generate heat; this is an energy-requiring process. As a result, cold stress increases the infant's oxygen consumption and must be prevented to minimize the infant's oxygen requirements. Additionally, neonates have a larger body surface area to mass ratio and decreased temperature regulation mechanisms and so can quickly become hypothermic. Cold stress also results in hypoglycemia, hypoxia, and acidosis that are detrimental to the postoperative patient.[73]

It is important that environmental temperatures be maintained through the use of a radiant warming device. It is important to note that any heating device with a servo control usually is designed with a skin probe in the feedback loop. The heat output of the unit is then increased when the child's skin temperature falls and decreased when the child's skin temperature rises. If the child has decreased skin perfusion resulting from low cardiac output state, the warmer may continue to generate heat whether the infant's core temperature is high or low. Therefore, the nurse should monitor the servo control setting, skin, and patient temperatures whenever the warmers are used in the presence of cardiovascular compromise.

Older children are able to shiver to generate heat. However, they also may require warming if hypothermic bypass was used during cardiovascular surgery. If the child is hypothermic and peripherally vasoconstricted after surgery, fluid administration should be carefully regulated as the child is warmed. While the child is peripherally vasoconstricted, little fluid administration may be required to maintain adequate cardiac filling pressures. Once the child's temperature increases, peripheral vasodilatation results in expansion of the intravascular space, and the child may require additional fluid administration to maintain adequate cardiac filling pressures.

Hyperthermia in the postoperative period can result from activation of inflammatory biomarkers produced by CPB, overzealous warming, and/or low cardiac output state. Elevated body temperature increases metabolic demand and oxygen consumption, exacerbates tachyarrhythmias, and may potentiate neurologic injury risk.[73] Treatment includes surface cooling and antipyretics.

REPERFUSION INJURY

Reperfusion-induced pulmonary dysfunction is an important clinical problem in some patients after cardiovascular surgery. There are several blood supply networks in the lungs with extensive connections to support lung tissue oxygenation.[922] Postoperative lung dysfunction is observed in some patients after correction of tetralogy of Fallot with pulmonary atresia and major aortopulmonary collaterals or extensive pulmonary artery reconstruction to provide improved pulmonary blood flow.

A phenomenon of "reperfusion pulmonary edema" has also been reported after catheter dilation or surgical intervention to enlarge stenotic blood vessels. The phenomenon is likely associated with insufficient capillary density or arterial smooth muscle to accommodate a sudden elevation in blood flow or hydrostatic pressure.[740]

Patients with pulmonary reperfusion injury typically develop pulmonary edema with a marked mismatch between ventilation and perfusion. Depending on the extent of the mismatch and reperfusion injury, patients may require sedation and mechanical ventilation for several days. If the patient is profoundly hypoxemic, extracorporeal membrane oxygenation (ECMO) may be required (see Chapter 7).

RESPIRATORY FUNCTION

Most children with congenital cardiac defects should not have baseline parenchymal lung disease. However, several common respiratory problems are associated with congenital cardiac defects, including bronchopulmonary dysplasia, tracheal and/ or bronchial malacia, and in some rare cases lung agenesis.

Cardiopulmonary bypass has a profound impact on respiratory mechanics in the postoperative period and may result in excessive pulmonary fluid, decreased lung compliance, or pulmonary hypertension. Respiratory issues presenting in the postoperative period can also be caused by changes with pulmonary blood flow such as reperfusion injury or may include pleural effusion, chylothorax, phrenic nerve injury, airway injury or obstruction (e.g., compression of bronchus), poor nutrition, or weakness associated with prolonged intubation or steroid use. Finally, residual lesions may complicate respiratory mechanics and should be considered when there are several failed attempts to wean and extubate from mechanical ventilation.

The complex relationship between the cardiac and pulmonary system can be especially exaggerated in a patient with a congenital cardiac defect. The mechanics of inhalation and exhalation work in tandem with cardiac filling and output; therefore alterations in intrathoracic pressure associated with respiratory variation and positive pressure ventilation can influence myocardial function.[73] Moreover, carbon dioxide and oxygen play an important role in the balancing the pulmonary and systemic circulations and hence, hemodynamic stability in children with mixing physiology. The goal of respiratory management is to optimize gas exchange and tissue oxygenation based on the child's physiology and surgical repair. Cardiopulmonary interactions are presented in detail in Chapter 9.

Respiratory Assessment

Careful and continuous assessment and support of the child's airway, oxygenation, and ventilation are required throughout the postoperative period. Assessment should include clinical examination, continuous evaluation of arterial oxyhemoglobin saturation (via pulse oximetry), arterial blood gas analysis as needed, capnometry and capnography (monitoring of end-tidal carbon dioxide pressure), and hemodynamic monitoring.

The postoperative recovery period can be variable; the child may be extubated soon after surgery or remain intubated for days or even months until stable. If an advanced airway is anticipated for more than 48 h postoperatively, consideration should be given to placement of an arterial line for blood gas sampling and continuous hemodynamic monitoring.

General assessment of an intubated patient should be performed on an hourly basis, and more frequently as needed. Once the patient arrives in the PCCU, assessment and support of the child's airway and breathing should be the top priority. Clinical examination of the child for secure placement of endotracheal tube (ETT), symmetric chest rise, equal aeration of all lung fields, and appropriate oxygen saturation should be quickly completed on admission to establish a baseline assessment.

A chest radiograph is performed as soon as patient is settled in the PCCU to confirm ETT depth of insertion and evaluate location of intracardiac catheter(s), central venous catheter(s), and chest tube(s). As part of the multidisciplinary PCCU admission team, the respiratory therapist will connect the patient to the mechanical ventilator and set parameters based on orders from the anesthesia and PCCU teams (per hospital protocol). Further changes in ventilator settings will be based on the initial arterial blood gas result and the child's physiology.

An end-tidal carbon dioxide ($PetCO_2$) sensor is commonly attached to the ventilator circuit to provide a continuous recording of exhaled carbon dioxide. The end-tidal CO_2 should be noted during arterial blood gas sampling for tracking its association with $PaCO_2$. By doing so, future ventilator changes may be performed without the need for blood sampling that can lead to iatrogenic blood loss.

Pain and sedation management is ordered based on the projected length of intubation and the child's clinical status. The nurse should understand the overall postoperative plan of care before administrating opioid and benzodiazepines to avoid prolonged intubation. Postoperative physiology dictates the appropriate level of oxygen saturation. Patients with cardiac diseases require detailed investigation for the cause of any compromising respiratory sign or symptom, as respiratory compromise can quickly lead to unstable hemodynamics. Observation of the patient's level of consciousness and color, auscultation of the lung and heart sounds, and palpation of peripheral pulses and temperature of distal extremities should be performed to differentiate the respiratory or cardiac origin of respiratory distress. The child's color may not be the most reliable tool for determining the level of oxygenation because cyanosis is not apparent until severe hypoxemia is present and it may not be observed if the child is anemic.

The Intubated Postoperative Cardiac Patient

Patients with complete cardiac repair should have normal oxygen saturation (greater than 95%). Patients with mixing physiology or with residual shunts may have optimal oxygen saturation between 75% and 85%. The fraction of inspired oxygen on the ventilator is set based on postoperative physiology so as to avoid hypoxia or pulmonary overcirculation. Depending on the size of the patient and other known respiratory co-morbidity, physicians may choose to use either volume controlled or pressure controlled mode of ventilation.

Although oxygen plays a very important role in pulmonary overcirculation, a child in distress should never have oxygen withheld.

Weaning from mechanical ventilation can be straightforward or complex based on the patient's physiology. In straightforward patients, the sequence of planned extubation is to minimize sedation, observe for respiratory drive, maintain clear lung sounds by suctioning as needed, and employ a trial of constant positive airway pressure (CPAP), with an arterial blood gas result confirming readiness for extubation. However, special precautions must be made for patients with pulmonary hypertension and other complex respiratory issues. Postoperative pulmonary hypertension is anticipated with cardiac defects such as truncus arteriosus, atrioventricular septal defect, multiple or large ventricular septal defect, and obstructed total anomalous pulmonary venous return (see section, Pulmonary Hypertension for specific recommendations). Additionally, suctioning can cause changes in the balance of systemic and pulmonary circulations in single ventricular physiology patients, and therefore should be performed with care, and in the initial postoperative period may require a physician or allied healthcare provider presence.

Administered Specialty Gases

Nitric oxide, nitrogen hypoxic gas, and carbon dioxide mixtures are specialty gases commonly used to treat congenital cardiac defects. Inhaled nitric oxide is used to treat pulmonary hypertension. Nitric oxide is synthesized endogenously as a signaling compound responsible for vasodilatation. Inhaled nitric oxide localizes vasodilatation in the pulmonary circulation. Daily methemoglobin blood test should be monitored in patients receiving nitric oxide. Methemoglobinemia (methemoglobin greater than 1% to 3%) may cause tissue hypoxia because methemoglobin cannot bind with oxygen to form oxyhemoglobin. See the section on Pulmonary Hypertension for more information.

Inhaled nitrogen hypoxic gas mixture is a specialty gas with increased nitrogen content to provide less than normal fraction of inspired oxygen (FiO_2 less than 0.21). Nitrogen increases pulmonary vascular resistance by providing a lower alveolar PO_2 for patients with single ventricle physiology who have pulmonary overcirculation. The effect of this hypoxic gas mixture is over an extended period of time; therefore it is not the treatment for acute decompensation. The nurse must also monitor these patients for hypoxemia. Inhaled carbon dioxide may also be used in the treatment of overcirculation.

The Extubated Postoperative Cardiac Child

The child should not be extubated until stability is ensured and so ventilatory support should be continued if hemorrhage, severe heart failure, significant arrhythmias, or shock are present. If right ventricular function is poor, hypoventilation, acidosis, and hypothermia can produce pulmonary vasoconstriction; this will increase right ventricular afterload and can result in right ventricular failure. Therefore, after surgical repair of defects such as severe tetralogy of Fallot, truncus arteriosus, or in the presence of pulmonary hypertension, prolonged mechanical ventilatory support is planned until the child's cardiac function is stable. Weaning is then performed gradually, with careful attention given to both cardiac and respiratory response to weaning. If needed, noninvasive respiratory support, such as noninvasive positive pressure ventilation (e.g., noninvasive pressure support ventilation with CPAP), heated humidified high-flow nasal cannula, and supplementary oxygen through nasal cannula may be provided to bridge respiratory rehabilitation. Chest physiotherapy should not be administered unless the child's cardiovascular function is stable. Chest physiotherapy is not indicated for pulmonary edema. Postural drainage, percussion, vibration, and combinations of hand ventilation and vibration may be helpful for treating atelectasis or consolidation.

Common Pulmonary Complications

Atelectasis

Postoperative right upper lobe atelectasis develops frequently in infants, although this complication can also be related to right mainstem bronchus endotracheal (ETT) tube migration. Left lung atelectasis also can develop from inadvertent right mainstem bronchus intubation during mechanical ventilation. After extubation, left lower lobe atelectasis may develop if significant cardiomegaly causes compression of this lobe or the left main bronchus.

Signs of atelectasis include altered pitch or decreased intensity of breath sounds over the involved area, although these may be difficult to appreciate because breath sounds are transmitted easily from other lung areas. Chest expansion may be decreased on the involved side. The involved lung areas are dull to percussion, and atelectasis produces opacity on the chest radiograph. Treatment includes vigorous chest physiotherapy. If a mucous plug is thought to be the cause of persistent atelectasis, bronchoscopy and bronchial lavage may be performed by a physician in the critical care unit.

Pneumothorax

A pneumothorax can develop postoperatively if the pleural spaces were entered during surgery and if the air is drained inadequately by the pleural chest drainage system. Pneumothorax also can develop spontaneously or during pleural chest tube removal. Signs of pneumothorax include decreased intensity and/or change in pitch of breath sounds over the involved area. If the child with a pneumothorax is receiving mechanical ventilatory support, peak inspiratory pressures often are elevated and the nurse may note increased resistance to hand ventilation. If the child is breathing spontaneously, tachypnea and increased respiratory effort may be noted, and chest expansion may be decreased on the involved side. If the child develops a tension pneumothorax, agitation, hypotension, a shift in the mediastinum, extreme cardiorespiratory distress, and severe hypoxemia will develop.

If the pneumothorax is small, treatment may include administration of supplementary oxygen and frequent assessment to ensure that air accumulation has not increased. If a significant pneumothorax is present, a thoracentesis will be performed or a chest tube will be inserted. The development of a tension pneumothorax constitutes a medical emergency and requires prompt aspiration of the air by thoracentesis or chest tube. With the development of a tension pneumothorax a shift in heart sounds toward the uninvolved side (resulting from a mediastinal shift) may be detected, and pulsus paradoxus (a drop in systolic blood pressure by 10 mm Hg or more during inspiration) may be noted. The hemoglobin saturation will fall if the pneumothorax is significant. This should trigger an alarm if pulse oximetry is used. If a large pneumothorax develops suddenly in the infant, the most significant clinical finding may be the development of hypotension and bradycardia resulting from severe hypoxemia.

Hemothorax

A hemothorax can develop from bleeding in the mediastinum (if the pleural spaces are entered and communicate with the mediastinum) or from bleeding from the great vessels. Hemothorax also can result from erosion of the aorta by the tip of a thoracic chest tube. If a chest tube is in place, hemothorax is apparent when a large quantity of blood enters the chest drainage system. If a chest tube is not in place, a hemothorax will cause a decrease in intensity or a change in quality (pitch) of breath sounds over the involved area. If blood accumulation is significant and the child is mechanically ventilated, peak inspiratory pressures may rise and there may be resistance to hand ventilation. If the child is breathing spontaneously, tachypnea and increased respiratory effort usually are noted. Chest expansion on the involved side usually is decreased.

If a significant hemothorax develops acutely, hypotension and signs of hypovolemia will develop. The presence of fluid in the chest will create opacity on the chest radiograph. Treatment requires evacuation of the fluid by means of thoracentesis or chest tube insertion. Surgical exploration of the bleeding site also may be indicated, and administration of packed red blood cells may be required.

Pleural Effusions

Pleural effusions may develop as a result of congestive heart failure or postcardiotomy syndrome. They also may develop in patients with high pulmonary venous pressure such as the Fontan physiology without a fenestration. Accumulation of thoracic fluid can cause tachypnea, increased respiratory effort, and a change in the pitch of breath sounds. Treatment requires thoracentesis or chest tube insertion. The child usually will receive diuretics to minimize accumulation of fluid. If postcardiotomy syndrome is suspected, aspirin or steroids may be ordered (see section Postcardiotomy Syndrome earlier in this section).

Chylothorax

Chylothorax is the accumulation of lymph fluid in the chest. It occurs as the result of injury to or obstruction of the thoracic duct or a large lymphatic vessel during cardiac surgery. Surgeries around the aortic arch, such as repair of coarctation of the aorta, or interrupted aortic arch, creation of a subclavian-pulmonary arterial shunt, or ligation of patent ductus arteriosus, are associated with higher incidence of chylothorax. Chylothorax has been reported less frequently after open-heart surgery using a median sternotomy approach. It also may develop in children with high central venous pressure, such as children with tricuspid atresia (especially after a Fontan procedure) or those children who develop vena caval obstruction. However, chylothorax also may also be congenital in origin.

If the surgeon observes lymph in the child's chest at the time of surgery, the healthcare team should be notified so that the chest tubes will be left in place until the presence of chylothorax is confirmed or ruled out. Because the child does not eat for several hours before and after surgery there is often very little fat apparent in lymph drainage during the immediate postoperative period; as a result it may not be apparent that there is lymph fluid in the chest drainage. If the chest tubes are left in place until after the child resumes eating a regular oral diet (one that contains fat), the presence of white or creamy lymphatic drainage from the chest tube will confirm the presence of a chylothorax. If a chest tube is not in place and significant lymphatic drainage is present in the chest, the child can develop severe respiratory distress.

Treatment of chylothorax requires drainage of the lymph fluid by a chest tube or repeat thoracentesis. Many physicians recommend that the child be placed on a medium-chain triglyceride diet because these triglycerides can be absorbed directly in the intestines and passed into portal venous blood, so that they do not enter the lymphatic system and will not contribute to the chylothorax. Administration of these triglycerides and avoidance of long-chain fatty acids is thought to reduce thoracic duct lymph flow and promote healing of the chylothorax. During this conservative management, the child still requires maintenance fluids and calories, and supplementary administration of fat-soluble vitamins (A, D, and E). Parenteral alimentation may be used to provide supplementary caloric intake. If the chylothorax fails to heal after a prolonged period of chest drainage and medium-chain triglyceride diet, octreotide infusion may be used, and finally surgical ligation of the thoracic duct or sclerosis of the chylothorax (with injection of hypertonic fluid or antibiotics into the chest) may be attempted. The child should resume a regular oral diet before discharge so that recurrence or persistence of the chylothorax can be detected promptly and treated.

Diaphragm Paralysis

Temporary or permanent diaphragm paralysis may be a cause of respiratory failure postoperatively. Diaphragm paralysis occurs because of injury to the phrenic nerve during surgery. It is usually temporary in duration, but is likely to produce respiratory failure in young children. Diaphragm paralysis should be suspected in the child who does not tolerate spontaneous ventilation or extubation. The paralyzed hemidiaphragm tends to be drawn up into the ipsilateral chest during spontaneous ventilation, resulting in decreased tidal volume and increased work of breathing. The child's spontaneous ventilation may be improved if the child is placed in a lateral decubitus position, with the paralyzed hemidiaphragm in a dependent position.[419] If positioning fails to assist ventilation adequately, nasal continuous positive airway pressure (CPAP) or intubation and positive pressure ventilation usually is required until diaphragm function recovers. If diaphragm paralysis persists for several weeks, surgical plication if the diaphragm may become necessary to prevent billowing of the hemidiaphragm into the ipsilateral chest during inspiration.

NEUROLOGIC FUNCTION

The child's neurologic system plays many important roles in the postoperative period, such as the sympathetic nervous system exerting a fight-or-flight response in the cardiac system. Endogenous epinephrine and norepinephrine production increases when body senses the need to increase cardiac output, whereas vagal nerves stimulation can induce bradycardia that may be helpful in the management of tachyarrhythmia. Additionally, the patient's neurologic function plays a crucial role in the child's quality of life after cardiac surgery. Cyanosis, congenital cardiac shunts, surgical shunts, arrhythmias, anticoagulation therapy, poor cardiac output, and other cardiac anatomic defects may increase the risk of thromboembolism, intracranial hemorrhage, and hypoxic insult to the brain.[167] Intraoperative and postoperative events associated with cardiac surgery can cause potential neurologic issues. These factors include anesthesia, acidosis, hypoxia, embolic events, CPB, ischemia, and deep hypothermic circulatory arrest.[73] Therefore, neurologic assessment in a postoperative cardiac patient is a high priority.

Neurologic Assessment and Potential Complications

Assess the child's neurologic function as soon as the child returns from surgery. The child's pupils should constrict in response to light and the child's movements should be appropriate for age unless neuromuscular blockers were administered. The child's level of consciousness will vary based on opioid and benzodiazepine use.

Seizure activity may be a sign of brain injury (e.g., perioperative neurologic insult) or may result from fever, hypoglycemia, or electrolyte imbalance. It is very difficult to evaluate the presence of seizures in the child receiving neuromuscular blockade. Nystagmus, sluggish pupil response, unexplained, or wide fluctuation in blood pressure and oxygen saturation may be the only clinical signs of seizures in these patients. In this case, an electroencephalogram may be required to determine if seizure is present. Because status epilepticus causes increased cerebral blood flow and oxygen requirements it must be promptly recognized and treated (see Chapter 11).

Hemiplegia or coma may result from hypoxia, acidosis, shock, or a thromboembolic event. Thrombus, particulate matter, or air bubbles from intravenous therapy entering the circulatory system can be extremely detrimental in mixing physiology and can cause stroke in these children. Paraplegia may result from local injury to spinal cord circulation during crossclamping for coarctation of the aorta repair. It is imperative to evaluate lower as well as upper limb movement bilaterally.

Hypoxic insult to the brain in patients with low cardiac output state or after cardiac arrest is a major concern for this vulnerable population. Avoidance and treatment of hypoxia and acidosis is important in maintaining neurologic integrity. Near infrared spectroscopy technology for continuous regional monitoring of oxygen saturation (rSO_2) in the brain and/or the kidneys is commonly used in the operating room. Many PCCUs have adopted the technology by the bedside to improve cerebral protection strategies and for early detection of shock. A probe is placed on the forehead for cerebral rSO_2, another probe is placed on the flank area for renal

rSO_2 monitoring. Interpretation of rSO_2 is in the context of pulse oximetry. Trending of rSO_2 may provide early warning signs of low cardiac output leading to regional insults. Renal rSO_2 is typically higher than cerebral rSO_2 because of high blood flow to the kidneys. More research is needed to show the predictability of continuous monitoring of regional oxygen saturation on neurologic outcomes of postoperative children.[376]

Hypoxic encephalopathy may develop 48 to 72 hours after a significant or prolonged fall in cardiac output. Many studies in the adult and newborn populations have demonstrated the benefit of therapeutic hypothermia for 24 to 48 hours after cardiac arrest (or, in neonates, after hypoxia and ischemia). More research is needed on the benefits of neurologic protection with regional or systemic hypothermia in children.

Careful assessment is needed in neonatal cardiac patients to detect neurologic injury. Routine head ultrasound should be considered for premature infants with neurologic insults, because this population has significant risk of associated intraventricular hemorrhage. Effort must be made on a daily basis to wean FiO_2 delivered by mechanical ventilation for the neonatal population so as to minimize the risk of oxygen toxicity in infants.

Horner syndrome may develop after any surgery that requires dissection around the aortic arch and the sympathetic cervical ganglia. The symptoms of Horner syndrome include ipsilateral ptosis of the upper eyelid, pupil constriction, narrowing of the palpebral fissure, and decreased perspiration. These signs appear on the same side as the injury and the ipsilateral pupil constriction may make the contralateral pupil appear to be dilated. When Horner syndrome is present, however, both pupils should still constrict briskly in response to light. Although the signs of Horner syndrome do not disappear, they often become less obvious over a period of months.

If abnormalities in postoperative neurologic function are suspected, a neurologic evaluation usually is ordered so that a specialist can evaluate the extent and severity of the child's injury. If the neurologic dysfunction is temporary and minimal, the parents often are reassured when a neurologist verifies such a conclusion. However, if the child has suffered significant neurologic injury, the early involvement of the neurologist can be very helpful.

RENAL FUNCTION AND FLUID/BLOOD COMPONENT THERAPY

The kidneys are very sensitive indicators of cardiac output and intravascular fluid status. Therefore, urine output is monitored as an indicator for renal perfusion and cardiac output. Renal function is also monitored by serum blood urea nitrogen level and serum creatinine level. Renal failure is categorized as pre-renal, renal, and postrenal types. Acute pre-renal failure is the most common type of renal failure in postoperative cardiac patients. The causes of pre-renal failure are decreased cardiac output, dehydration, sepsis, and critical hemorrhage.

Fluid Balance

Fluid balance is an important aspect of care, and the nurse must be diligent with calculating fluid intake and output and identifying imbalance before it becomes severe. The effects of CPB and osmotic diuresis resulting from elevated glucose levels in the CPB prime may cause generous diuresis in the initial postoperative period. However, if hypothermia is used, renal perfusion may be compromised, causing low urine output. Within several hours after surgery as the cardiac index and serum glucose concentration fall, urine output typically falls as well. Antidiuretic hormone is secreted in response to stress such as surgery, and may cause fluid retention. At any point in the postoperative period, a decrease in renal perfusion can compromise renal function and result in decreased urine output. For these reasons, if perfusion is adequate, fluid administration often is restricted during the immediate postoperative period to 50% to 75% of maintenance fluids. Diuretic therapy is usually started within the first 24 to 48 hours after surgical intervention to reduce volume overload, improve lung compliance, and reduce the workload of the heart.

Early in the child's postoperative period, the nurse should help the healthcare team identify the parameters for central venous pressure, right atrial pressure, and/or left atrial pressure at which the child's systemic perfusion is best. This pressure may be maintained through infusion of packed red blood cells, fresh-frozen plasma, 5% albumin, or any isotonic crystalloid solutions. The type of solution is determined by the child's hematocrit, recent blood loss, presence of coagulopathies, electrolyte balance, acid-base status, urine output, and cardiac physiology. For example, if the child's hematocrit is low or he or she is bleeding, packed red blood cells are administered. Additionally, children with mixing physiology are usually supported with a higher hematocrit level for optimal oxygen transport. If the child's serum albumin is low, 25% albumin may be administered to increase intravascular oncotic pressure and optimize diuretic therapy. The nurse should be aware of fluid replacement strategies in patients with ventricular dysfunction because quick infusion of a large amount of fluid to these patients may exacerbate their dysfunction.

Hemorrhage

As noted, chest tube output equal to or greater than 3 mL/kg body weight per hour for 3 hours or more is significant. This blood loss must be replaced to prevent hypovolemic shock. In addition, the cause of the bleeding must be identified and corrected. A coagulation panel is usually obtained immediately after arrival in the PCCU to determine if there has been complete reversal of anticoagulation used in CPB, and whenever there is bleeding or possibility of liver dysfunction. Protamine sulfate may need to be administered to patients not completely reversed from their anticoagulation after CPB.

If clotting factors or fibrinogen are low, they are replaced with cryoprecipitate or fresh-frozen plasma as needed. Platelet transfusion may be necessary if thrombocytopenia is present. If platelet count remains low despite repeated platelet transfusion, heparin induced thrombocytopenia should be considered. The presence of ecchymotic lesions, petechiae, or diffuse bleeding from puncture sites also would reinforce the diagnosis of coagulopathy. The use of protamine and platelet replacement should be judicious in shunt-dependent physiology patients.

Children with cyanotic heart disease are likely to demonstrate postoperative bleeding because they may develop a coagulopathy related to their hypoxemia. Any child who requires repeat operations also may demonstrate postoperative bleeding because scar tissue, which is highly vascular, must be dissected to gain cardiac exposure. Cold agglutinins can be triggered by hypothermic surgery or even administration of cold blood (i.e., blood that is not warmed adequately before administration), producing hemolysis and bleeding.

Bleeding that requires reoperation is called a "surgical bleed" and may be caused by oozing from a suture line, a residual atrial or great vessel opening, or a divided collateral vessel. Surgical bleeding should be suspected when the child's chest tube output is sanguineous and totals 3 mL/kg per hour for 3 hours or 5 mL/kg for 1 hour, despite evidence of good clot formation in the chest tubes. Persistent surgical bleeding requires re-operation so that the site of bleeding can be sutured or cauterized and the possibility of tamponade eliminated.

Electrolyte Balance

Electrolytes are measured on admission to the PCCU and routinely thereafter depending on the child's condition. Proper electrolyte balance is important to support optimal cardiac contractility, suppress arrhythmias, and reduce the potential for seizure activity in the postoperative period. Infants and young children have a limited ability to maintain normal blood glucose levels and are susceptible to the effects of hypoglycemia. Hypoglycemia can profoundly influence the child's hemodynamics or be the cause of postoperative seizures. Hyperglycemia may also develop as part of a stress response and as the result of glucose used in the bypass prime. Insulin may be administered to keep the blood glucose less than 150 mg/dL (or per unit policy), but careful monitoring is required to avoid hypoglycemia.

Diuretic therapy can cause significant electrolyte imbalances and hyponatremia or a rapid fall in serum sodium concentration may additionally place patients at risk for seizures. Calcium acts as a positive inotrope, increases contractility, and is involved in myocardial depolarization, therefore calcium imbalances may compromise cardiac function and contribute to arrhythmias. Potassium and magnesium derangements may also contribute to arrhythmias. Therefore, meticulous management of electrolytes is important in postoperative cardiac surgical patients. For a complete discussion of electrolyte management, see Chapter 12.

Urine Output

Urine output should remain at least 0.5 mL/kg per hour for the first 24 hours after surgery and then should be maintained at least 1 mL/kg per hour. Neonates and infants should demonstrate a urine volume of approximately 2 mL/kg per hour.

If urine output is inadequate, it is important to separate *pre-renal* from *renal* causes. Pre-renal failure occurs when renal perfusion is compromised secondary to heart failure, shock, or inadequate circulating blood volume. Treatment of heart failure or shock may require elimination of excessive intravascular water (diuresis) or inotropic therapy, whereas the treatment of inadequate circulating blood volume requires fluid administration.

The nurse should assess the child's hydration and check for evidence of systemic venous congestion (increased liver span, high central venous pressure, and periorbital edema) or pulmonary venous congestion (tachypnea, decreased lung compliance, increased respiratory effort, high left atrial or pulmonary artery wedge pressure, rales, and pulmonary edema).

Occasionally, children develop significant intravascular hemolysis during or immediately after cardiopulmonary bypass. Signs of hemolysis include excretion of rusty-colored urine that contains cell casts and hemoglobin. In addition, the child may demonstrate bleeding from the gastrointestinal tract, chest tubes, or endotracheal tube because of damage to platelets and erythrocytes. If the child demonstrates hemoglobinuria, it is essential that renal blood flow and urine volume be kept at satisfactory levels so that the hemoglobin can be "flushed out" of the kidneys. In addition, the kidneys should not be required to concentrate urine maximally until cell fragments and hemoglobin have been excreted.

If the child's urine output is inadequate despite the presence of adequate systemic perfusion, adequate hydration, and the administration of diuretics, renal failure should be suspected. Too often, the assumption is made that the child with decreased urine output requires further fluid administration. It is only after several large boluses of fluid are administered without result that the diagnosis of renal failure is made; at this point, the child may be hypervolemic. If renal failure is thought to be present, fluid intake should be restricted and potassium administration should be curtailed. Serum samples usually are sent for analysis of blood urea nitrogen (BUN), creatinine, and potassium. Unless the child is anuric, simultaneous urine sampling for creatinine also is accomplished so that some estimation of urine creatinine clearance can be made. Administration of sodium polystyrene sulfonate, glucose, insulin, or calcium gluconate also may be required to reduce serum potassium concentrations. Peritoneal dialysis may be required to eliminate excess intravascular fluid and control the child's serum potassium concentration; however, this is not a very aggressive modality. If the patient is hemodynamically stable and can tolerate a large fluid volume shift, hemodialysis is the therapy of choice. For patients who are critically ill, continuous renal replacement therapy is the most effective and safe form of therapy.

NUTRITION

Nutrition is crucial to the recovery process, especially in the cardiac postoperative period when resting energy expenditure is substantially increased.[128] For example, the nutritional needs of an infant with congenital heart disease are typically between 120 and 150 kcal/kg per day.[658] Moreover, weight gain is a crucial factor in determining readiness for second-stage palliation in infants with single ventricle physiology.[677] Therefore, the importance of adequate nutrition should not be underestimated. A nurse-driven algorithm to advance enteral feeds has been shown to be beneficial for optimizing nutrition without increased risk in a high-risk population.[102] Nutritional assessment in these children is done by recording daily weight, tracking daily caloric intake, monitoring albumin and prealbumin level, or performing an indirect calorimetry test.

Trophic enteral feeding (continuous feeds at a rate of 1-5 mL/hour) should be considered as soon as the patient is stabilized, to reduce the risk of translocation of gut flora. Contraindications to enteral feeding include hemodynamic instability, necrotizing enterocolitis (NEC), and/or other gastrointestinal emergencies, and patients with these conditions should have total parental nutrition initiated. Children with congenital heart disease are at increased risk for NEC and should be monitored for symptoms. These symptoms may include temperature instability, lethargy, acidosis, abdominal distension, vomiting, bloody stools, and/or pneumatosis intestinalis.[73] Treatment includes nasogastric suction, intravenous fluids, and broad-spectrum antibiotics. Historically, umbilical catheterization has been considered another contraindication to enteral feeding; however, recent research has shown the judicious use of trophic feeds to be acceptable and potentially beneficial.[357] When patients have aortic arch abnormalities, feeding should be advanced with careful monitoring of tolerance and monitoring for abdominal distension or bleeding.

Consultation with an occupational therapist should be considered for trialing high-risk infants during their first oral feeding. High-risk infants include those who have never fed before surgery, or have focal cord paralysis, prolonged intubation, or a weak cry. If gastroesophageal reflux or aspiration is suspected, further studies are warranted to determine a safe feeding plan. A nasogastric tube may be left in place to supplement oral feeding and support weight gain in fragile infants. These infants may be limited to several oral feedings daily or to a time limit such as 15 minutes to minimize caloric consumption and promote weight gain. Nasojejunal tube feeding may be used if patients have feeding intolerance with gastric feeds or when aspiration is suspected or confirmed. Approaches to feeding are reviewed in Chapter 14.

ANALGESIA AND SEDATION

Assessment and management of pain and anxiety in children are challenging, particularly in preverbal children. Assessment is further complicated if neuromuscular blockade with sedation is needed. The nurse can use physiologic parameters to support comfort management plans. Hypertension, tachycardia, diaphoresis, and pupil responses can be helpful indicators in measuring discomfort, but it may be difficult to separate signs of cardiovascular compromise from those of anxiety and those produced by pain. If the child is responsive, developmentally appropriate pain and sedation scales should be used consistently (see Chapter 5).

Opioids are used to provide pain control and benzodiazepines are used for anxiolysis. Care should be used when administering opioids such as morphine because they may cause a histamine release with resultant vasodilation and elevation in PVR. Shorter-acting, synthetic opioids such as Fentanyl do not stimulate a histamine response and may be preferable. Acetaminophen and nonsteroidal antiinflammatory drugs may be effective in pain control as well.[73] Nonsteroidal drugs may potentate bleeding and nephrotoxicity, so they should be used with care. Insufficient and excessive pain control and sedation should be avoided.

When the child requires long-term mechanical ventilation and sedative and narcotic use, gradual tapering of the dose is required and careful observation for signs of withdrawal is needed. Please refer to Chapter 5 for further discussion.

INFECTION

In any cardiovascular surgical patient, infection is a leading cause of morbidity and mortality. Consider the typical child admitted to the PCCU after cardiac surgery. There could be several invasive hemodynamic monitoring catheters, an endotracheal tube, a sternal incision, chest tubes, and a urinary catheter so as to effectively manage the child in the postoperative period. Surgical site infections (SSIs), catheter-associated bloodstream infections (CA-BSIs), sepsis, ventilator-associated pneumonias (VAP), endocarditis, and urinary tract infections (UTIs) all lead to prolonged hospitalization, and potential mortality risk. Additional factors thought to increase the child's risk of postoperative infection include noncardiac co-morbidities, young age, poor nutritional status, high complexity cardiac operation, long preoperative length-of-stay, preoperative ventilation, genetic abnormalities, multiple blood transfusions, re-operation for bleeding, prolonged stay in the PCCU, and extended device use.[203] Implementation of evidenced-based care bundles developed by the Institute of Healthcare Improvement (IHI) has been shown to be effective in reducing hospital-associated infections (HAIs).[204] Additionally, establishment of unit-based infection elimination programs, checklists, intensive team education, team vigilance with procedures such as line insertion and management, and an assessment tool identifying and targeting patients at greatest risk have been associated with a reduction in HAIs as well (see Chapter 22).[204,603]

Handwashing is the single most important factor in the prevention of HAIs and should be performed by all hospital personnel before and after patient contact. Because studies have documented inconsistent handwashing practices in PCCUs, it is imperative that critical care nurses ensure good handwashing technique by every member of the healthcare team.[600,776] The PCCU nurse caring for the child with heart disease is that patient's personal safety officer and can have a profound effect on patient outcome.

Compliance with prophylactic administration of broad-spectrum staphylocidal antibiotics in the operating room *before the incision is made* has been found to decrease the postoperative incidence of deep and superficial wound infections after thoracic operations.[755] Often these prophylactic antibiotics are administered for three doses and up to 5 days postoperatively in an attempt to prevent postoperative bacteremia.

Many children may demonstrate a low-grade fever on the night after surgery; however, the child who develops a high fever or a fever beyond the first 48 hours postoperatively should be examined carefully for evidence of infection. Blood cultures usually are drawn any time the fever exceeds 38.5° C, and cultures of urine and tracheal aspirate also may be ordered. When prosthetic material is used during surgical or catheter intervention it is especially important to prevent or treat postprocedural bacteremia promptly, because the prosthetic material is particularly susceptible to bacterial aggregation (see Bacterial Endocarditis in Specific Diseases).

The nurse should assess the appearance of the child's wound and catheter insertion sites daily and report any evidence of infection (erythema, drainage, etc.) to a physician. Wound drainage should be cultured immediately. Surgical site infection reduction bundles have been effective in reducing SSIs in pediatric cardiac patients.[297,755] Deep wound infections usually require incision and drainage and may require frequent or continuous irrigation. Timely diagnosis, aggressive sternal débridement, and appropriate antibiotics have been associated with a reduction in morbidity and mortality.[869] Mediastinitis can cause endocarditis in the child with a cardiac prosthetic valve, patch, or conduit. Reduction in hospital-associated infections is an open area for critical care nurses to positively influence their patients, please refer to Chapter 22.

NURSING CARE PLAN

For a summary of postoperative care, see Box 8-16. Special considerations in neonates are addressed in Box 8-17, and care of the adult with congenital heart disease is summarized in Box 8-18.

PSYCHOSOCIAL ASPECTS OF CARDIOVASCULAR CARE OF THE CHILD AND FAMILY

Erin L. Marriott

Preprocedural Preparation

Adequate preparation of the child and family is essential for a planned cardiovascular procedure, such as cardiac catheterization or surgery. The American Heart Association has developed "Recommendations for Preparing Children and Adolescents for Invasive Cardiac Procedures" outlining methods of assessment, planning, and preparation of children who are to undergo cardiac procedures.[526] The American Family Children's Hospital has developed an online video that can be viewed by children and their parents before a cardiac catheterization or EP study (http://www.uwhealth.org/video/pediatric-cardiace-catehterization-procedures/26816).

Preparation of each child and family for cardiovascular surgery requires careful planning that considers the child's cognitive and social level of development and the child's and family's perception of the child's health. A child who perceives herself or himself to be well should not be told that the surgeon will "make him or her better" because the child actually will feel worse immediately after surgery. Conversely a child who is acutely conscious of cyanosis may find the prospect of looking at (pink) lips and fingernails after surgery to be reassuring and exciting. In some children pre-procedural preparation may increase anxiety, so this must be taken into consideration.

Preoperative teaching is provided at a level appropriate to the child's cognitive abilities and anxiety level. Much information can be obtained from the child during play. For preschool and school-age children it is helpful to make a suitcase including hospital equipment (dressings, tape, syringes, monitor "pasties," IV equipment) and dolls for use by the child in *nonstructured but monitored* play. The nurse will ensure that the child will not enter unsupervised into

physically or emotionally traumatic activity while monitoring the child's comments about and use of particular hospital equipment. Because dolls are also present the child may choose to use the equipment during doll play, or ignore threatening hospital equipment completely and pursue doll play only. In either case, valuable information is obtained about the child's coping style.

The same suitcase and equipment may be used later in a *structured* session to prepare the child for the upcoming surgery. During this structured session the nurse can tell a story about a doll having a noisy (or squeaky) heart fixed; then the child is free to draw personal comparisons. This structured play session also provides an opportunity for the nurse to clarify significant misconceptions the child may have regarding medical or surgical therapy.

Older children may benefit from coping skills training. This includes guided imagery, positive self-talk, conscious breathing, muscle relaxation, biofeedback, and refocusing.[526] Children who receive coping skills training in preparation for heart surgery have better in-hospital and postdischarge adjustment than children who only receive routinely provided information.[136]

If possible preoperatively, the child and family should have the opportunity to meet the nurses and physicians who will be caring for the child postoperatively. If the same nursing staff is involved throughout the child's hospitalization, continuity of care is fostered. If an entirely new staff will be involved in the child's care immediately after surgery the family should have the opportunity to meet the new staff before surgery.

The child's preoperative visit to the PCCU must be planned and supervised carefully. The sight of a critically ill patient unclothed and covered with tubes may be overwhelming and frightening, but the child may be unable to verbalize fears or clarify misconceptions. Such a sight can *increase* rather than decrease the child's anxiety. Another option is to have the child visit a mock PCCU or operating room that is set up similar to what he or she would see without the risk of seeing an actual patient. Computer programs may be used to familiarize patients and family members with the postoperative equipment and plan.

The staff should be careful in the choice of words used to describe postoperative monitoring equipment. "Chest tubes" may be better called "drains," and monitoring leads can be called "special band-aids." It is best to familiarize the child with only that equipment that the child definitely will *see* or *feel* postoperatively because much of the equipment will be removed or out of sight by the time the child is awake enough to look beyond the horizon of the bed. Parents often are best able to cope with specific definitions of particular tubes once they see their child safely returned from surgery (see Chapter 2).

Postoperative Psychosocial Care

Cardiovascular surgery is extremely stressful for the child and family. Throughout the child's hospitalization, every member of the healthcare team should interact with the child at a level appropriate for the child's psychosocial and cognitive development (see Chapter 2). In addition, the child's specific fears and concerns should always be identified and discussed.

The main features of psychosocial care of a child and family after cardiac surgery are similar to that of any child in the PCCU

Box 8-16 Postoperative Care of the Child After Cardiovascular Surgery

Potential for Postoperative Bleeding

Expected Outcomes:

Patient bleeding will not exceed 3 mL/kg per hour of blood for the first 3 hours or 5 mL/kg per hour for 1 hour without replacement.

Nursing Interventions:

- Obtain postoperative complete blood count and coagulation study results on admission to PCCU; correct abnormal results (per physician orders).
- Ensure proper function and patency of all drainage tubes.
- Ensure adequate intravenous access.
- Monitor quality and quantity of surgical drainage and notify physician or on-call provider of excessive drainage; advocate for early medical intervention.
- Ensure proper pain management and sedation to prevent aggravation of postoperative bleeding.
- Investigate sudden cessation of chest tube output for potential tamponade. Tamponade physiology will be recognized and promptly addressed.

Potential of Inadequate Cardiac Output Related to Decreased Intravascular Volume, Postoperative Ventricular Dysfunction, Increased or Decreased SVR or PVR, Arrhythmias, Tamponade

Expected Outcome:

Patient will maintain adequate cardiac output and/or have their cardiac output supported.

Nursing Interventions:

- Closely monitor central venous pressure (or right atrial pressure if available) and advocate for fluid bolus to maintain preload as needed.
- Closely monitor fluid balance every hour to detect early signs of volume depletion. Fluid overload is also to be avoided so as to prevent increased cardiac workload.
- Closely monitor all hemodynamic monitoring systems and titrate vasoactive infusions as needed to optimize cardiac output.
- Ensure adequate oxygenation and ventilation to avoid increase myocardial oxygen demand.
- Oxygen consumption will be minimized through judicious use of opioids, benzodiazepines, and/or chemical relaxation.
- Systemic and pulmonary afterload will be optimized through ventilation maneuvers.
- Electrolytes will be monitored and replaced to avoid arrhythmias.
- Rhythm disturbances will be promptly recognized and medical team notified.

Potential for End-Organ Dysfunction Related to Inadequate Cardiac Output

Expected Outcome:

Patient will have optimal hepatic, renal, and gastrointestinal function on discharge.

Nursing Interventions:

- Support systemic perfusion.
- Monitor evidence of hepatic, renal, and gastrointestinal function and notify physician or on-call provider of abnormalities. Support function as needed (see Chapters 13 and 14).
- Discuss medication profile with medical team or clinical pharmacist about dosing per hepatic and renal function status.

Potential Impairment of Gas Exchange Related to Pleural Effusion, Chylothorax, Ventilator-Associated Pneumonia, Atelectasis, Diaphragmatic Paresis or Paralysis, Pulmonary Edema

Expected Outcome:

Patient will maintain optimal respiratory function with adequate oxygenation, carbon dioxide elimination, and serum pH.

Nursing Interventions:

- Maintain fluid balance prescribed by medical team. Use diuretics judiciously.
- Reposition patient frequently until ambulatory.
- Provide pulmonary toilet strategies as needed (e.g., chest physiotherapy).
- Ensure appropriate functioning of chest tube drainage systems.
- Provide endotracheal tube (ETT) suctioning as needed. Instill sterile normal saline (NS) for ETT suctioning only when secretions are too thick. Limit volume of NS instillation to 0.5 mL for infant and 1 mL for children to prevent dislocation of colonized bacteria from ETT to lungs.
- Follow Institute for Healthcare Improvement (IHI) VAP bundle to prevent ventilator-associated pneumonia (see Chapters 9 and 22).
- Strive for early extubation.
- Optimize sedation and analgesia (see Chapter 5).
- Encourage use of early ambulation, incentive spirometer, coughing, and blowing bubbles after extubation.

Potential Alteration in Cerebral Perfusion and Function Related to Decreased Lung Compliance, Hypoxemia, Inadequate Perfusion, Thromboembolism, Cerebral Hemorrhage, Seizure Activity/Status Epilepticus

Expected Outcome:

Patient will demonstrate baseline (preoperative) neurologic function on discharge.

Nursing Interventions:

- Document patient's baseline neurologic function.
- Correct hypotension, hypoxemia, and acidosis as quickly as possible.
- Monitor near-infrared spectroscopy (NIRS) cerebral tissue oxygenation (normal range >50%). Notify provider of decreased oxygenation.
- Perform frequent neurologic assessments (e.g., level of consciousness, orientation, and pupil shape, size, and reactivity), especially for patients receiving heparin therapy.
- Perform frequent assessment of muscular tone and bilateral symmetry to detect early signs of stroke.
- Support cardiac output and systemic perfusion.
- Assess appropriateness of sedation and analgesia to allow for neurologic assessments.

Potential for Infection Related to Surgical Site Infection/ Mediastinitis, Central Line Associated Blood Stream Infection, Urinary Tract Infection, Ventilator-Associated Pneumonia, Sepsis, Endocarditis

Expected Outcome:

Patient will not demonstrate signs or symptoms of infection such as fever or hypothermia, leukocytosis, or leukopenia, localized infection or inflammation, positive wound or blood

Continued

Box 8-16 **Postoperative Care of the Child After Cardiovascular Surgery—cont'd**

culture, or elevated C-reactive protein (CRP). If the child does demonstrate symptoms, prompt identification and reporting will occur.

Nursing Interventions:

- Ensure that all providers wash hands before and after patient contact.
- Educate and ensure family and other visitors wash hands before and after patient contact.
- Strictly adhere to hospital infection control policy.
- Follow IHI SSI bundle (see section on infection) to prevent surgical site infection.
- Follow IHI CABSI insertion and maintenance bundle (see section on infection) to prevent catheter-associated bloodstream infection.
- Follow IHI VAP bundle.
- Follow IHI UTI bundle.
- Monitor patient for signs and symptoms of infection and notify medical team immediately if there is a positive sign or symptom.
- Administer antibiotics as ordered.
- If infection is present, monitor for evidence of sepsis (tachycardia, BP instability, thrombocytopenia, temperature instability).

Potential for Pain and Discomfort Related to Delayed Sternal Closure, Surgical Incision, Multiple Invasive Catheters or Procedures, Prolonged Immobilization

Expected Outcome:

Patient will be comfortable with no evidence of significant pain during postoperative period (see Chapter 5).

Nursing Interventions:

- Assess pain when vital signs are assessed by using validated developmentally appropriate pain assessment tool.
- Assess level of sedation by using validated sedation assessment tool.
- Perform reassessment of pain and/or sedation 30-60 min after intervention.
- Avoid overmedication in an effort to prevent iatrogenic complications such as delayed extubation, ventilator-associated pneumonia, and delayed physical rehabilitation.

Potential Compromise in Nutrition Related to Inadequate Caloric Intake to Meet Demand, Impaired Gastrointestinal Absorption, Necrotizing Enterocolitis, Volume Overload, Increased Resting Energy Expenditure

Expected Outcome:

Patient will receive adequate caloric and nutritional intake to support recovery.

Nursing Interventions:

- Occupational therapist to assess oral feeding and swallow study as needed.
- Registered dietitian to assess nutritional needs routinely during hospitalization.
- Advocate for early enteral feeding to promote intestinal endothelium health.
- Closely monitor feeding tolerance and adjust feeding appropriately.
- Total parenteral nutrition is generally used only when enteral feeding is contraindicated or insufficient to provide nutrition needed.

- May need to limit oral feeding time and supplement with nasogastric feeds.
- Obtain daily weight with graphic record at bedside before morning rounds.

Impairment in Physical Mobility Related to Critical Care Stay and/or Prolonged Hospitalization

Expected Outcome:

Patient will resume baseline level of mobility on discharge.

Nursing Interventions:

- Reposition while patient is bedridden.
- Provide range of motion exercise while patient is bedridden.
- Maintain neutral joint positions while patient is sedated and/or receiving neuromuscular blockade.
- Provide adequate analgesia for early ambulation.
- Incorporate physical therapy early in postoperative period.

Potential Child and Family Knowledge Deficit Related to Child's Cardiovascular Disease, Hospitalization, Prognosis

Expected Outcome:

Patient and family will demonstrate appropriate and accurate knowledge through discussion of child's disease, postoperative and followup care.

Nursing Interventions:

- Ascertain what patient/family understands about disease, therapy, and prognosis.
- Consult with child life specialist to assist patient (as age-appropriate) with proper preparation for surgery and procedures.
- Consult with child life specialist and/or clinical psychologist to assist patient and/or siblings with coping.
- Assess and document child and family's learning needs and barriers to learning.
- Encourage child and family to ask questions and participate in care when appropriate.
- Record specific teaching information (including terminology used) so healthcare team can use consistent terms and reinforce identical information.

Potential Child/Family Anxiety Related to Child's Life-Threatening Condition, Long-Term Prognosis, Unknown Aspects of Surgery, and Hospitalization

Expected Outcome:

Patient/family will demonstrate manageable levels of anxiety as evidenced by absence of behavior that interferes with patient's medical care and will access resources appropriately during hospitalization.

Nursing Interventions:

- Maintain open communication with patient and family.
- Answer all questions honestly at the appropriate level for patient/family understanding.
- Prepare patient (as age appropriate) and family for procedures. Include child life specialist as appropriate for child's age and clinical condition.
- Encourage family participation in patient care as appropriate.
- Encourage child's expression of feelings and emphasize acceptability of expression.
- Assess family's resources and refer to appropriate hospital support services, such as social work and chaplaincy.

Box 8-17   Special Considerations for Nursing Care of the Neonatal Cardiac Surgical Patient

Potential Alteration in Cerebral Perfusion and Function of Central Nervous System Related to Oxygen Toxicity, Cerebral Hemorrhage, Prolonged Undetected Seizures
Expected Outcome:
Patient will maintain optimal progress with appropriate neurologic development on discharge.
Nursing Interventions:
- Encourage kangaroo care (skin-to-skin contact when infant held by mother) for all preterm infants as soon as infant is sufficiently stable.[344]
- Titrate FiO_2 to the minimal level needed to prevent hypoxemia. (The goal is to prevent oxygen toxicity to the developing brain.)
- Premature infants are more prone to intraventricular hemorrhage (IVH); routine head ultrasound should be considered to detect and monitor IVH.
- Nurses must learn to recognize seizures in newborns (signs may be very subtle) and notify the physician or on-call provider if seizure is suspected.

Risk of Disorganized Infant Behavior
Expected Outcome:
Infant and parents will have a strong bond and attachment on discharge.

Nursing Interventions:
- Encourage kangaroo care (skin-to-skin contact when mother holds infant) for preterm infants and other infants as soon as infant is sufficiently stable.[344]
- Practice family-centered care to involve parents/caregivers with as much care during hospitalization as possible.

Risk of Ineffective Thermoregulation
Expected Outcomes:
Infant will not experience cold stress and will maintain normothermia during hospitalization.
Nursing Interventions:
- Place infant under overhead warmer during the immediate postoperative period to maximize visibility of the infant while supporting infant's temperature.
- Cover infant's head (if there is no scalp peripheral IV) to prevent heat loss.
- Once cardiovascular function is stable, enclosed infant bed (e.g., isolette) may be used for infants less than 1500 g to prevent draft and fluctuation of temperature.

Box 8-18   Potential Postoperative Challenges when Caring for Adults with Congenital Heart Disease

1. Bleeding/coagulation
Patients with longstanding hypoxemia, cyanosis, and compensatory polycythemia often develop postoperative bleeding that may be related to:
- Extensive collaterals, which can be friable and difficult to find and ligate or cauterize
- Complex repairs that typically require extensive suture lines
- Decreased platelet count, platelet activity, and numbers and consumption of coagulation factors

Adults with congenital heart disease may require counseling regarding postoperative anticoagulation, menses, and possibly contraception. (Oral contraceptives can be associated with thromboembolic events or may exacerbate pulmonary hypertension and deep vein thrombosis.)

2. Cardiac output
The risk of perioperative myocardial injury is high for many reasons, including chronic volume overload and pressure leading to ventricular dysfunction and poor ventricular compliance, arrhythmias, heart failure, and multiple surgical interventions.

3. End-organ perfusion
Cyanotic patients are prone to renal dysfunction. Hyperuricemia or gouty arthritis can be markers of abnormal renal function.

4. Gas exchange
Chronic polycythemia, plastic bronchitis (single ventricle) can impair gas exchange.

5. Cerebral perfusion
Patients with mixing of systemic and pulmonary venous blood are at risk for thromboembolic events. Severely hypoxemic patients have polycythemia (hyperviscosity) and may require phlebotomy. Complications can include stroke, seizures, and even death.

6. Infection
Infective endocarditis can develop from dental procedures, poor oral hygiene, nail biting/picking, acne, tattoos, body piercing, or in males, genitourinary procedures.

7. Nutrition
Protein-losing enteropathy may occur in single ventricle patients after Fontan procedure. Adults may benefit from tight glycemic control.

8. Physical mobility
The patient may be physically limited by heart disease.

9. Pain/discomfort
The adult with congenital heart disease may have a previous experience with inadequate analgesia postoperatively, and may need education about advances in pain management. Preoperative abuse of drugs or alcohol may predispose to the patient to delirium and withdrawal.

10. Knowledge deficit
The patient may be very knowledgeable or have a very limited knowledge base.

11. Anxiety
Cumulative hospitalization experiences (fear, effects of financial impact, preexisting emotional disorders), anxiety about being in a PCCU versus adult unit, privacy, and dependence versus independence issues may all manifest.

From Gatzoulis MA, Webb GD, Daubeney PEF. *Diagnosis and management of adult congenital heart disease.* New York, 2003, Churchill Livingstone.

setting. There are specific aspects to be addressed in dealing with families affected by congenital heart disease (CHD).

Children with CHD report a significantly impaired psychosocial quality of life.[890] This is true even if their CHD is mild or corrected. There is also significantly lower school functioning in children with CHD; this is thought to result from neurodevelopmental problems that have been reported in children with CHD. Early referral for psychological counseling or other interventions is necessary.[890] Children may benefit from group settings such as camps that provide an opportunity for children with CHD to relate to peers in similar situations. One example is Camp Odayin (http://www.campodayin.com) in Minnesota.

Parents may feel in some part responsible for their child's cardiac defect. Mothers report psychosocial problems more often than fathers.[519] The nurse may help parents by providing opportunities to discuss fears and concerns and reduce the parents' guilt by reinforcing information provided by the cardiovascular team. Interestingly, the severity of the child's heart disease does not determine the amount of parenting stress.[889]

Members of the healthcare team should avoid the tendency to underestimate the stress that the family is likely to demonstrate when a child has a "simple" cardiac defect or procedure, and particularly avoid comparison with other patients cared for by the team. Positively, families who have a child with CHD reported they felt closer because of their experience and also had a sense of competence as they are able to manage their child's chronic illness.[114]

The family's financial situation has a great effect on psychosocial morbidity.[519] Consultation with a pediatric social worker may help the family to find community resources that may reduce financial stress. Home care nursing may alleviate family stress by relieving the parents from some of the stress of caring for their child.[519]

Group therapy may be helpful for some parents so as to identify with other parents who have children with CHD.[519] A good social network helps to foster resiliency in families dealing with CHD.[837,911] Mended Little Hearts (http://www.mendedlittlehearts.org) is a national program that provides support for parents of children with CHD. Their web site provides educational information, networking, and information about local chapters.

Many medical centers care for a large number of pediatric cardiovascular surgical patients. This large volume of patients usually results in a reduced risk of death or complications because the entire healthcare team is accustomed to caring for children perioperatively and is prepared to deal with anticipated complications. Although the child's care will be "routine" for the nursing and medical staff, the hospitalization experience will be far from routine for the child and family. A sensitive and compassionate nurse treats every patient as unique and demonstrates concern and warmth for each child and family. For more comprehensive information refer to Chapter 2 and, as applicable, Chapter 3.

Sources of Stress with Hospitalization

Parents report a feeling of helplessness and a loss of control. This loss of control can be exacerbated if the parents are not updated periodically. During preoperative clinic visits, parents should receive instructions on how to prepare for surgery,

estimated length of stay, and resources available during hospitalization. At this time, the parents should have an understanding of the proposed surgery. During the preoperative clinic visit, patients and parents are given sufficient amount of time to have their questions answered to achieve full informed consent. During surgery, parents should receive information about their child's condition and the progress of the surgery (direct from the operating room, with the approval and direction of the cardiovascular surgeon) at regular intervals, and they should be able to see their child in the PCCU as quickly as possible after the child's return from surgery. Many parents are so relieved to see that their child has survived the surgical procedure that they fail to notice most of the monitoring equipment surrounding the bedside until later.

It is essential that the parents be allowed to visit their child as frequently as they desire, barring medical emergency in the unit. In addition, the parents should be allowed to participate in care of their child to a limited extent (e.g., a parent may wish to assist with the child's bath or help rub lotion on the child's legs). This opportunity to nurture the child helps parents regain some control of the situation and feel useful in their child's care.

Posttraumatic Stress in the PCCU

The environment of the PCCU can cause a tremendous amount of traumatic stress to children and families. The most common sources of stress for parents in the PCCU have been identified and include sights and sounds in the PCCU (alarms, ventilators), the child's appearance, the child's behaviors and emotional reactions, procedures performed on the child, staff communication, staff behavior, the sight of other critically ill children in the unit, and the witnessed stress of other families.[112] Parents are more likely to be extremely stressed if the critical care hospitalization was unexpected or it resulted from unanticipated deterioration in the child's condition.[112] Some children are found to have posttraumatic stress disorder (PTSD) after a PCCU stay.[727] Proper preparation before surgery and procedures may decrease the likelihood of PTSD. The service of a child life specialist should be introduced to the family during preoperative care and offered throughout the hospitalization. PTSD is also found to be more prevalent in children with multiple hospitalizations.[727] Signs and symptoms of PTSD in children related to hospitalization are indicated in Table 8-23.

Chronic Disease

A child with complex heart disease is likely to survive a series of medical and surgical interventions, and confront a variety of psychological, social, and medical stressors.[396] Living with complex heart disease can include long stays in the PCCU. These long stays require nurses to provide psychosocial and educational supports to optimize care of this fragile patient population that may not be routine in standard care delivery. The syndrome of the chronically, critically ill (CCI) patient is emerging as life-sustaining technologies advance care delivery. During any hospitalization, these children can face multiple episodes of instability and prolonged interventions to save their lives. Many children with CCI have resulting comorbidities from these periods of instability that require management by numerous providers.

Table 8-23	Potential Signs of Posttraumatic Stress Disorder in Children After Critical Care	

Children	Adolescents
• Broad range of moods	• Flashbacks
• Anxiety, irritability, hyperalertness	• Physiologic arousal (e.g., easily startled, tachycardia)
• Behavioral problems	• Emotion-focused coping strategies, such as avoidance
• Agitation	• Distraction
• Disorganized behavior	• Denial
• Repetitive play	
• Avoidance or emotional numbing	
• Dissociation	
• Sleep disruptions	
• Altered relationships with family and friends	

McDowell B. When children experience PTSD in the CCU. *American Association of Critical Care Nurse*, available at www.aacn.org/wd/nti2009/nti_cd/data/papers/main/28330.pdf. Accessed 03/28/2010.

Multiple psychosocial responses and mood alterations accompany the physical issues associated with long stays in the PCCU. CCI symptom identification and management are an essential aspect of nursing care. Noxious symptoms can include communication difficulties, thirst, pain, fatigue, worry, posttraumatic stress disorder, dyspnea, inability to sleep, and general discomfort.[135] Interventions to standardize care, ameliorate symptoms, and improve communication with the patient and his or her family have been shown in the adult literature to be effective in improving patient and family satisfaction with care.[135]

The syndrome of CCI has well-documented social, emotional, and financial burdens to individuals, their parents, caregivers, and the healthcare system.[372] Primary nursing teams and advanced practice nurses (APNs) are in an excellent position to manage and coordinate care to reduce care fragmentation, enhance communication, and minimize morbidity and mortality for these complex patients.

In an adult study, the use of experienced critical care nurses as liaisons between the family and critical care team was well received and provided opportunities for nurses to establish trust early during the hospitalization.[372] Lily et al[536] implemented a structured process for proactive communication with a family meeting within 72 hours of admission. Early ongoing meetings provide a structured process for communication and enable families and clinicians to tailor interventions to meet the needs of the child. Relationship-focused care is an important aspect of providing holistic care. Additionally, complementary and adjunct therapies have been shown to be effective in enhancing the experiences of these patients as well and include physical activity, therapeutic beds, spiritual care, music therapy, massage therapy, pet visitation, and re-engagement with school.[521]

A large cardiac center performed a study aimed at developing criteria for predicting extended hospital stays in infants with congenital heart disease and found that preoperative organ dysfunction, need for nasogastric feeds, and total support time were indicators for long stays in the PCCU.[322]

This is an important consideration for some of the most complex neonates after surgical repair. Nurses and APNs are in a good position to minimize morbidity by focusing on the feeding practices of neonates.

ANTICOAGULATION

Mary Rummell

Pearls

• Antithrombotic therapy has increased in the pediatric population.
• Infants and children with congenital heart disease are anticoagulated for prosthetic heart valves, systemic to pulmonary shunts, abnormal intracardiac blood flow, and devices implanted to open or close blood vessels.
• Medications used for anticoagulation therapy in children are the same as those used in adults; however, little research has been done to study therapy in children.
• Consistency is the key to antithrombotic therapy in children—consistent daily dose of medication, consistent time of daily dose, consistent monitoring, and consistent diet.

Overview

Anticoagulation (antithrombotic) therapy is used both to prevent a thromboembolism and treat a thromboembolism once one has occurred. The choice of therapy depends on the medical/surgical disease of the patient. The use of antithrombotic therapy has increased significantly in pediatric patients over the past decade. Four groups of pediatric patients account for this increase: critically ill neonates, children with cancer who require long-term vascular access, children with genetic or acquired coagulation abnormalities, and children with specific congenital and acquired heart disease.[25,731] This section addresses antithrombotic therapy used for neonates, infants, and children with congenital and acquired heart disease.

Antithrombotic therapy in the group of children with congenital heart disease includes therapy for patients with prosthetic heart valves, systemic to pulmonary shunts, abnormal patterns of intracardiac blood flow (single ventricle), and devices to open or enlarge blood vessels or close vessels and/or septal defects. Children with acquired heart disease receive anticoagulants to prevent a thromboembolic event in an inflamed or enlarged coronary artery (Kawasaki disease) or decreased myocardial function from myocarditis.[25,622,731] Therapy is most frequently initiated with heparin administered intravenously in the pediatric critical care unit. A continuous heparin infusion is started when hemostasis is obtained after cardiac surgery that results in a shunt-dependent blood flow to the pulmonary circulation or the placement of prosthetic heart valves; during and after interventional catheterization; or at the time of the initial diagnosis of the acquired heart disease.

The challenge of antithrombotic therapy for the group of children with congenital and acquired heart disease is compounded by the operative or medical factors encountered by the infant or child before the initiation of antithrombotic therapy. Disruption of essential clotting factors during cardiopulmonary bypass, administration of heparin during interventional cardiac

Table 8-24	Management of Alterations in Hemostasis Before Initiation of Anticoagulation
Tests of Hemostasis	**Management Guidelines**
Hematocrit	<30%: give red blood cells
Platelet count	<50-75,000 mm^3 and bleeding: give platelets
Prothrombin time (PT-INR)	>2.0: give FFP
Activated partial thromboplastin time (aPTT)	>1.5-2 × normal: give FFP
Fibrinogen level	<100 mg/dL: give cryoprecipitate

From DeLoughery TG: Critical care clotting catastrophes. *Crit Care Clin* 21:3, 2005.

catheterization procedures (see Common Diagnostic Studies, Cardiac Catheterization), and any sepsis or low cardiac output must be controlled before anticoagulation is initiated. Clotting factors should be assessed and abnormalities corrected (Table 8-24). Blood products needed to correct the abnormality must be administered slowly with careful monitoring to prevent inadvertent clot formation.[230]

Adult antithrombotic therapy is based on well-designed clinical studies. Although the same antithrombotic agents are used for both adults and children, the results of adult studies cannot be extrapolated to infants and children. The hemostatic system of the neonate is immature. The neonate's capacity to generate thrombin is both delayed and decreased. This capacity remains consistently low (about 25% less than adults) throughout childhood.[742] Vitamin K deficiency in the neonate affects the vitamin K-dependent clotting factors II, VII, IX, X, protein C, and protein S. These factors are also significantly reduced during the first 6 months of life because the liver is immature.[742] Plasma concentrations of antithrombin are low at birth, increasing to adult levels by about 3 months of age.

In addition to the varied maturation of the hemostatic system, many factors make the use and monitoring of antithrombotic therapy in the pediatric patient a challenge. These factors include difficulty in obtaining and maintaining venous access, unpredictable pharmacokinetics that necessitate more frequent monitoring, substantial risk from changing diets, and medical conditions that require the addition or discontinuation of medications that affect both the hemostatic system and the response of the patient to the anticoagulant. Current guidelines for pediatric anticoagulation are based on small studies or case reports.[731] Well-designed large studies are needed to guide pediatric anticoagulation therapy.

Anticoagulant agents act by inhibiting coagulation factors that act together in a complex cascade to form fibrin strands as part of the process of hemostasis (see Chapter 15 and an illustration of the coagulation cascade in the Chapter 15 Supplement on the Evolve Website). Factors II (prothrombin) and X are two of the most important factors targeted by anticoagulants; the effect of all anticoagulants is determined by their reduction of the activity of these factors.

The pharmacology, monitoring, and pediatric concerns for the most common parenteral and oral agents are summarized

in the following. Note that the major side effect of all of these medications is bleeding.

Parenteral Agents Used for Pediatric Antithrombotic Therapy

Heparin, Unfractionated

Heparin is a complex mucopolysaccharide that effects anticoagulation by activating antithrombin III. Antithrombin III inactivates thrombin and the factors IX, X, XI, XII, plasmin, and kallikrein, and thereby prevents the conversion of fibrinogen to fibrin. The heparin is cleared primarily by the reticuloendothelial system and is not affected by decreased renal and hepatic function.

Heparin is administered by both intravenous and subcutaneous routes. Intramuscular administration causes large hematomas. Intravenous administration is initiated in the immediate postoperative period for newborns who have shunt-dependent pulmonary blood flow and infants and children who have prosthetic heart valves. When heparin is administered intravenously, it provides almost instant anticoagulation and has a half-life of about 90 minutes. Therefore, it is critical that hemostasis is established in the postoperative period before heparin therapy is initiated.

Subcutaneous heparin is used infrequently in children because of erratic absorption. It is used when an oral agent is contraindicated. The most frequent subcutaneous use occurs when a young woman with a prosthetic heart valve is pregnant or anticipating pregnancy. In these patients the oral agent, warfarin, is not used because of potential teratogenic effect.[731] Anticoagulation effects are monitored using the activated partial thromboplastin time (aPPT).

The dose for systemic heparinization may vary by cardiac surgeon, institution, or indication for anticoagulation. General guidelines include an initial loading doses range from 50 to 100 U/kg administered over 10 minutes, followed by a maintenance dose of 10 to 20 U/kg per hour. Infusion rates are titrated to maintain a desired aPTT level (usually 60-75 seconds). Heparin is neutralized by protamine. Long-term use can cause osteoporosis.[731,742,839]

Low Molecular Weight Heparin (LMWH). Enoxaparin is a heparin derivative that affects anticoagulation by activating antithrombin III and inactivating coagulation factor Xa with a lesser effect on thrombin. Enoxaparin is administered subcutaneously in both treatment and prophylactic doses. The treatment dose, primarily used for an intracardiac thrombus, is 1 mg/kg twice a day for infants greater than 2 months of age to adult. The prophylactic dose for this age range is 0.5 mg/kg twice daily. Children less than 2 months old require a higher dose per kg.[731,742,839] The subcutaneous dose must be consistently given in the same site: abdomen, buttocks, or thighs. In general, do not use the abdomen for injection in infants less than 2 months of age with single ventricle. Liver hematomas have been reported in infants with enlarged livers who received subcutaneous doses of LMWH in the abdomen.

Anti-factor Xa levels may be monitored. Levels are drawn on initiation of treatment doses and then as needed or with an increase in weight of 1 kg (see Box 8-19 for sample guidelines). Protamine is used for intentional overdose, but has only partial effect.[731,742,839]

Box 8-19	Sample Guidelines for Use of Subcutaneous Low Molecular Weight Heparin in Children

Treatment Dose: Enoxaparin
- <2 months of age = 1.5 mg/kg bid SQ*
- >2 months of age = 1 mg/kg bid SQ*
- Hematology consultation recommended for all patients with new clots

Prophylactic Dose: Enoxaparin
- <2 months of age = 0.75 mg/kg bid SQ*
- >2 months of age = 0.5 mg/kg bid SQ
- *For patients less than 2 months of age with single ventricle, SQ enoxaparin should not be administered in the abdomen; use thighs or buttocks (site must be consistent).*

Monitoring
- Draw LMW Heparin levels 3 to 4 hours after third or fourth SQ dose *(Correct timing of blood sampling is essential.)*
- Treatment dose target level (Anti Xa): 0.5-1 u/mL
- Prophylactic dose target level (Anti Xa): 0.54-0.1 u/mL

Note: all SQ doses must be consistently given in same site—abdomen *or* thighs *or* buttocks.

Oral Agents Used for Pediatric Antithrombotic Therapy

Transition from heparin to warfarin typically occurs in the pediatric critical care unit.

Warfarin

Warfarin is a vitamin K antagonist that has been used for 50 years and continues to be the most common oral anticoagulant used for the prophylaxis and treatment of thromboembolic disorders.[702,731] A coumarin derivative, warfarin acts by interfering with the hepatic synthesis of the vitamin K-dependent clotting factors, II, VII, IX, X, protein C, protein S, and protein Z. These factors decrease gradually depending on their half-life. Factor VII has a half-life of 6 hours, and factor II, prothrombin, has a half-life of 92 hours. Thus, the anticoagulation effect of warfarin is first seen around 8 to 12 hours and may persist for 1 to 5 days after the drug is stopped. A relatively steady state is reached 72 hours after the initial dose.

Warfarin may have a more antithrombotic effect (rather than a simple anticoagulant effect) by the reduction in prothrombin and factor X levels. This decreases the ability to generate thrombin, the main modulator of clot formation. Warfarin is readily absorbed orally with a peak concentration 90 minutes after ingestion. Food slightly slows the absorption.[731,742,839]

Ninety percent of warfarin is bound to albumin. It is accumulated in the liver and then is metabolized and transformed by different pathways.

The suggested initial dose of warfarin for infants greater than 2 months of age and children is 0.2 mg/kg daily for 2 to 4 days and 0.1 mg/kg for those with liver disease. Older children and adults initially receive 5 to 15 mg daily for 2 to 4 days.[839] Many factors influence this initial dose and subsequent doses in addition to liver disease. These factors include cardiac and renal output, especially perioperative cardiac function; nutritional status before surgery, which may be reflected in low serum albumin; acute and chronic disease; concurrent medications; and current diet, including type and amount of food and/or formula ingested.[25,407,564,731,839]

Children are vulnerable to genetic and developmental factors that affect the hemostatic system and response to warfarin. Genetic factors may influence the response requiring as much as a 20-fold higher dose to achieve an anticoagulant effect.[742] At birth, the vitamin K clotting factors are approximately 50% of the adult levels.[742] Because of the immature hemostatic system of the neonate, warfarin is not used during the first 2 months of life.

Children frequently have acute bacterial or viral illnesses that require the initiation of medications or influence their dietary intake. Medication interactions with warfarin are listed in Box 8-20, A and B.

Different forms of dietary intake of vitamin K further influence warfarin effects. The two forms of vitamin K include vitamin K_1 (phylloquinones) and vitamin K_2 (menaquinones). Most of the vitamin K stores in the liver are menaquinones and are thought to originate from the diet rather than intestinal flora. Vitamin K_1 is found in green leafy vegetables, and vitamin K_2 occurs in various foods such as yogurt and organ meats, but is also produced by the bacterial flora of the colon

Box 8-20	Medications That Alter the Anticoagulation Effect of Warfarin[407,564,731,839]

A. Medications That Enhance the Anticoagulation Effect of Warfarin
Antibiotics: Acetaminophen
Cephalosporins (High-dose, long-term use)
Alcohol (intermittent use): Ciprofloxacin
Antiarrhythmics: Erythromycin
Antidepressants: Metronidazole
Antiviral agents: Neomycin
Aspirin, Penicillin
Dipyridamole, Sulfonamides
Cimetidine, Sulfamethoxazole, and Corticosteroids:
    Trimethoprim (Bactrim)
Fluconazole, Tetracycline
Iloprost
Bosentan
Nonsteroidal antiinflammatory drugs
Thyroid hormones
Tricyclics
Vitamin E

B. Medications That Decrease the Activity of Warfarin
Alcohol (chronic use)
Antacids
Antibiotics (Ampicillin*, Augmentin*, Nafcillin, Rifampin)
Antihistamines
Barbiturates
Phenytoin
Estrogens, Progestogens
Tegretol
Vitamin K
Retinoids

*If diarrhea develops, there may be an increased effect.

and small intestine. Children with acute bacterial and viral illness do not eat in typical patterns and have frequent gastroenteritis. This significantly decreases the intake of vitamin K and production by bacterial flora, resulting in an increase in the prothrombin time-international normalized ratio (PT-INR).[702,731]

Healthy infants and children often have significant changes in the vitamin K in their diets. Breastfed babies receive little dietary vitamin K, whereas formula-fed infants receive increasing doses of vitamin K as their daily intake of formula increases.[39,702,742]

The risks of warfarin administration include serious and potentially fatal hemorrhage or necrosis and/or gangrene of the skin and other tissues. Warfarin is a known teratogen that causes midline defects in the fetus. A cardiologist and high-risk perinatologist must carefully follow women who are taking warfarin and become pregnant or plan to become pregnant. The best plan is to change the anticoagulation therapy to subcutaneous heparin.

Anticoagulation therapy using warfarin is monitored by the prothrombin time adjusted with the international normalization ratio (PT-INR). The target PT-INR is determined by the reason for anticoagulation. The frequency of monitoring is based on the time from the initiation of therapy, the PT-INR, concurrent illnesses, initiation of new medications or changes in doses of current medications, pending surgical or dental procedures, or changes in diet. Lifetime monitoring must continue at least monthly.

Increased PT-INR with symptomatic bleeding is treated with the administration of intravenous vitamin K and/or intravenous fresh-frozen plasma. Nonsymptomatic levels of PT-INR may be decreased by lowering the dose or by giving oral vitamin K. In the infant, several ounces of infant formula may be used.[731,742,839]

Warfarin is available as a tablet in many strengths, from 1 mg to 10 mg. The daily dose of warfarin will change as a result of the PT-INR monitoring. Combining tablets as doses change helps to provide a consistent daily dose.

Patient and Parent Education and Monitoring

Patient and parent education needs to start with the initiation of oral antithrombotic therapy. Ideally, it should start with the initial planning of the surgical procedure. Education should include:

- Why the medication is ordered and how it works
- When to call the primary provider monitoring the anticoagulation
- Desired effects and side effects
- How and why to monitor the PT-INR
- Food and drug interactions
- Safety measures directed at the age of the infant or child

Outpatient monitoring of the anticoagulation therapy is frequent and necessary to provide safe care. Home monitoring with a whole blood monitor is safe. The PT-INR is obtained by a fingerstick point of care test.[175] These monitors are expensive and only a few states have Medicaid approval and financial support. Private insurance companies are more reluctant to cover the costs of the monitor and test strips. The process to obtain a home monitor should start as soon as the need

for long-term anticoagulation therapy is known. The process is long and may require documentation of need from a cardiologist.

Helping parents provide appropriate safety guidelines for anticoagulated children is very important. Bleeding, especially into the child's head or a joint, is the major risk of anticoagulation. The risk of bleeding will be affected by the developmental level and activity of the child. A helmet and padded joint protection should be used during any activity in which there is a risk of joint or head injury. Helmets should even be encouraged for infants learning to walk. Participation in sports should be directed to low-impact activities, such as swimming, golf, and tennis.

Parents should be supported to plan the activities in collaboration with their child. They should also provide information on anticoagulation to the school and any activity in which the child is involved. The child should wear a Medi-Alert ID bracelet to identify the use of an anticoagulant.

With all of the variability inherent in anticoagulation with warfarin, emphasis should be placed on consistency. It is important to take the prescribed warfarin dose daily and at the same time. Even though the diet affects the patient response to the medication, it is better to allow the child to eat those foods that he or she prefers and adjust the dose of warfarin to the child's diet. It is also important to communicate any change in health or in medications to the caregiver monitoring the child's anticoagulation. The dose of warfarin can be adjusted to prevent large fluctuations in the PT-INR when the child has a viral illness or a new antibiotic is initiated.

Antiplatelet Therapy
Aspirin

The effect of aspirin is mediated through inhibition of prostaglandin synthetase action. This prevents formation of the platelet-aggregating substance thromboxane A2. Therapy includes both low and high doses.[622,731,742,839] Although the dose of aspirin is stated in the mg/kg format, it is generally dosed in fractions of the 81-mg chewable tablet.

Antiplatelet regimes differ at different pediatric cardiac centers. At Boston Children's Hospital, the dose is 40 mg/day for patients less than 10 kg and 81 mg/day for those greater than 10 kg. Patients less than 2.5 kg would take 40 mg every other day. At Miami Children's Hospital, all babies receive 21 mg/day (one quarter of an 81 mg tablet). Infants with bidirectional Glenn shunts generally take 40 mg/day. Children take 40 to 81 mg/day after Fontan surgery. The tablet should be chewed or crushed and taken with food or after eating to prevent direct irritation from the tablet on the gastric mucosa.

Dipyridamole

Dipyridamole inhibits platelet aggregation by inhibiting the activity of adenosine deaminase and phosphodiesterase. This may cause vasodilation, especially in coronary arteries. It may also stimulate release of prostacyclin. Dipyridamole is used in conjunction with warfarin to allow a lower PT-INR in higher-risk patients with thromboembolic disease. Patients with prosthetic heart valves are included in this

Box 8-21
Advanced Concepts in Anticoagulation Therapy in Children

Box 8-21

- Anticoagulation in the neonate is affected by the immaturity of the hemostatic system. The newborn's ability to generate thrombin and vitamin K deficiency affects both medications available for use in the neonatal period and the newborn's response to these medications.
- Anticoagulation therapy is difficult to monitor in infants and children because of the variations in the development and maturation of the hemostatic system, the ability to maintain and obtain venous access, unpredictable pharmacokinetics, changing diets, and frequent bacterial and viral illnesses.
- Patient and parental education are very important in the success and safety of both short- and long-term anticoagulation therapy.

category.[622,731,742,839] The dose of dipyridamole is 3 to 6 mg/kg per day for children and 25 to 100 mg for adults. It is administered three to four times a day, making compliance more difficult.

Clopidogrel (Plavix)

Clopidogrel inhibits platelet aggregation by irreversibly modifying the platelet ADP receptor. The benefit of the addition of clopidogrel to conventional therapy following systemic to pulmonary shunts was recently evaluated in a multicenter, randomized, double-blind, placebo-controlled study.[941] The primary objective of the study was to determine if clopidogrel reduced the all-cause mortality and shunt-related morbidity in neonates or infants (less than 3 months of age) with cyanotic congenital heart disease palliated with a systemic-to-pulmonary artery shunt. A clopidogrel dose of 0.2 mg/kg per day was given once daily.[941] In this study, the addition of clopidogrel to aspirin therapy did not reduce all-cause mortality or shunt-related morbidity.[941]

Advanced Concepts

Anticoagulation therapy in children requires a thorough understanding of the therapeutic and side effects of the drugs used and developmental aspects of hemostatic/coagulation function. In addition, influence of the child's diet and other drug therapy must be considered. Advanced concepts in anticoagulation therapy are listed in Box 8-21.

SPECIFIC DISEASES

Information in this section summarizes the etiology, pathophysiology, clinical signs and symptoms and management of children with common congenital and acquired (inflammatory) heart diseases. When common clinical conditions such as congestive heart failure or hypoxemia are mentioned in this section, the reader is asked to refer to the detailed discussion of these conditions in the Common Clinical Conditions section of this chapter. When postoperative care is summarized it is presumed that the nurse will monitor for signs of shock, cardiopulmonary arrest, congestive heart failure, bleeding, arrhythmias, and respiratory distress; these

potential complications and other details about postoperative care are addressed in the third (preceding) section of this chapter, Postoperative Care and Anticoagulation for the Child with Congenital Heart Disease. In this section, the postoperative complications listed for each defect include those *most likely* to occur following the specific procedure discussed; the nurse should still assess the patient for signs of other common postoperative complications.

This section is divided into subsections, beginning with information about acyanotic defects. The acyanotic defects include those with left-to-right shunts and those with right and left heart obstructive defects. The left-to-right shunt defects include patent ductus arteriosus, aortopulmonary window, atrial septal defects, ventricular septal defects, and atrioventricular septal defects (also called atrioventricular canal or endocardial cushion defects). The acyanotic obstructive defects include pulmonary valve stenosis and aortic valve stenosis, coarctation of the aorta, interrupted aortic arch and mitral valve dysfunction. The next subsection summarizes cyanotic defects that produce increased or decreased pulmonary blood flow; these include some obstructive lesions. This subsection contains information about tetralogy of Fallot and double-outlet ventricles including double-outlet right and left ventricles and transpositions. The subsection on single functioning ventricles includes tricuspid atresia, pulmonary atresia with intact ventricular septum, and hypoplastic left heart syndrome. The next subsection includes information about vascular rings, coronary artery and vascular anomalies, and the final subsection includes common infection and inflammatory diseases of the heart, including endocarditis, myocarditis, and cardiomyopathy, and tumors.

Of course, division of congenital heart defects into categories is somewhat artificial and some defects will present in or progress to different categories, based on severity or combination of defects. For example, severe pulmonary valve stenosis may present as a cyanotic rather than an acyanotic defect. As a result, the bedside nurse must apply and adapt the information contained in this section to each patient, as appropriate.

Congenital heart defects and the palliative or corrective procedures to treat them result in areas of turbulent blood flow within the heart that provide potential foci for endocardial infection if bacteremia develops. Because a potential focus for endocarditis exists, children with some congenital heart defects should receive antibiotic prophylaxis during periods of increased risk of bacteremia; such prophylaxis is detailed in Bacterial Endocarditis later in this part of the chapter. Appropriate antibiotic prophylaxis is important when procedures are performed during hospitalization, and parents must be taught the importance of antibiotic prophylaxis and prompt treatment of infection.

ACYANOTIC DEFECTS: LEFT-TO-RIGHT SHUNTS

A common feature of left-to-right shunt defects is increased pulmonary blood flow. The magnitude of the shunt and the resulting volume and pressure of the increased pulmonary blood flow is affected by pulmonary vascular resistance (PVR). PVR, in turn, is affected by a variety of factors including alveolar oxygenation, and by the maturation of the pulmonary vasculature, the response of the pulmonary vasculature to increased blood flow, and the anatomic features (e.g., size, location) of the defect.[628]

When a left-to-right shunt is present, the increased pulmonary blood flow is the basis for most resulting symptoms, particularly tachypnea. Tachypnea is frequently associated with mild respiratory distress. Greater respiratory effort further increases metabolic demand. Because a significant volume of blood recirculates through the pulmonary vascular bed, venous return to the left heart is increased and combined ventricular output is increased. Heart failure in these patients is referred to as "high-output" failure rather than "low-output" failure or shock. When heart failure develops, ventricular end-diastolic pressures increase, leading to increased systemic and pulmonary venous pressures. Hepatomegaly develops because the compliant hepatic veins dilate to accommodate the increase in circulating blood volume and pressure.[30] Hypertrophy of the ventricular myocardium will develop if the increased volume load persists.[628]

The increase in work of breathing can substantially increase oxygen consumption and caloric requirements, and so may result in failure to thrive. The tachypneic infant will likely not feed well, compounding nutritional compromise. Heart failure also results in increased catecholamine secretion modulated by neural and hormonal mechanisms ("fight or flight" response). As a result, the infant/child with high-output heart failure is also tachycardiac and diaphoretic. To maintain physical growth, the patient with high-output failure must increase caloric intake.[30] For further information, see Congestive Heart Failure and Altered Nutrition in the Common Clinical Conditions section of this chapter.

Patent Ductus Arteriosus (PDA)

Mary Rummell

Pearls

- The maturity of the pulmonary vascular bed, the anatomic features of the ductus arteriosus and the relative difference between pulmonary and systemic vascular resistances affect the degree of left-to-right shunt.
- The gestational age of the infant determines the response of the ductus arteriosus to oxygen and prostaglandins.

Etiology

A patent ductus arteriosus (PDA) is persistence of the fetal structure, the ductus arteriosus, after birth (Fig. 8-30). The ductus arteriosus is derived from the left sixth embryologic aortic arch and connects the main pulmonary trunk (at the origin of the left pulmonary artery) to the descending aorta just below the left subclavian artery. When a right aortic arch is present, the ductus typically connects the right pulmonary artery with the right aortic arch. The ductus varies in length and is as large as or larger in diameter than the descending aorta in the fetus.[449,628]

During fetal life the ductus arteriosus diverts blood away from the (high-resistance) pulmonary circulation to the

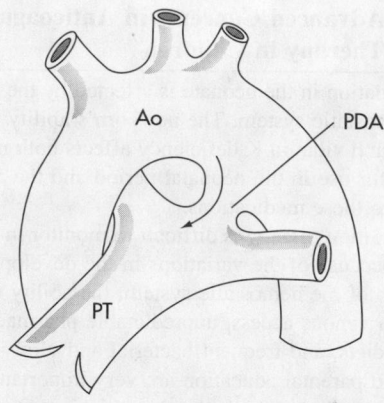

FIG. 8-30 Patent ductus arteriosus (PDA). The PDA extends from the bifurcation of the pulmonary trunk (PT) to the aorta (Ao), joining the aorta just beyond the origin of the left subclavian artery. (From Perloff M: *Clinical recognition of congenital heart disease*, ed 5, Philadelphia, 2003, Saunders. Fig. 20-1.)

descending aorta and toward the low-resistance placental circulation. The ductus carries 55% to 60% of the combined ventricular output.[628]

The intimal layer of the ductus arteriosus is thicker and more mucoid than the intimal layer of the pulmonary artery and the aorta. The smooth muscle in the medial layer of the ductus is arranged in both leftward and rightward patterns with an increased amount of hyaluronic acid; this facilitates constriction and closure of the ductus after birth. By comparison, the medial layer of the wall of the pulmonary artery and aorta consists of circumferential layers of muscle fibers.

The precise mechanisms of ductal closure are not fully understood. Functional closure occurs in two phases. In the first phase, immediately after birth, contraction and cellular migration of the medial smooth muscle produce shortening and thickening of this layer and protrusion of the media into the ductal lumen with thickening of the intimal layer. These thickened cushions or mounds result in functional closure of the ductus within about 12 hours of birth. Infolding of the endothelium; disruption and fragmentation of the elastic fibers; and cellular proliferation, hemorrhage, and necrosis in the subintimal layers result in replacement of the muscle fibers with fibrotic connective tissue to form the ligamentum arteriosum within about 2 to 3 weeks after birth.[628]

The increase in the partial pressure of oxygen (PaO_2) that normally occurs after birth stimulates constriction of the ductus arteriosus. However in preterm infants the ductus is not constricted at even high levels of oxygen tension. Prostaglandins play an important role in ductal patency or constriction. Prostaglandins dilate the ductus, and a normal fall in endogenous prostaglandins after birth contributes to constriction of the ductus. Administered prostaglandin inhibitors (e.g., indomethacin) can cause ductal constriction.[449,628] Other vasoactive substances (bradykinin, acetylcholine, and endogenous catecholamines) also contribute to ductal constriction and closure.

The PDA accounts for about 5% to 10% of all congenital heart defects in full-term infants.[686] The incidence is much higher in premature infants (8 of 1000 premature infants have a PDA), particularly those with pulmonary disease and varies inversely with birthweight. Hemodynamically significant PDA is noted in almost 80% of infants with a birthweight of less than 1000 g, because ductal constrictive response to oxygen is related to gestational age.[628]

Ductus closure may be delayed if the neonate's arterial oxygen tension does not rise normally after birth. For example, the incidence of PDA is about 30% higher at high altitudes (i.e., 4500-5000 m [about 14,700-16,000 feet] above sea level), and neonates with cyanotic congenital heart disease characteristically demonstrate delayed closure of the ductus. A PDA also may be present as part of the rubella syndrome, and it may be seen occasionally in otherwise healthy, normal full-term infants.

A functionally closed ductus may reopen if the arterial oxygen tension falls, such as occurs with asphyxia, meconium aspiration, or pneumonia. It may also reopen in response to administered prostaglandin (e.g., for infants with cyanotic congenital heart disease or lesions with ductal-dependent systemic perfusion).[628]

Pathophysiology

With a PDA, several factors impact the magnitude of the left-to-right shunt: the diameter and length of the ductus, the pressure difference between the aorta and pulmonary artery, and the relative resistances in the systemic and pulmonary circulations.[628] With the first breaths after birth, alveolar oxygenation improves and pulmonary vascular resistance begins to fall; as a result, the pulmonary to systemic flow through the ductus decreases dramatically.[449] Once the umbilical cord is clamped, the systemic vascular resistance becomes slightly greater than the pulmonary vascular resistance, so any flow through the ductus initially becomes bidirectional and then ultimately reverses so it flows from the aorta into the pulmonary circulation.

As noted, the diameter and length of the ductus influences the magnitude of the left-to-right shunt. If the ductus is long and narrow the small diameter and the length add to the resistance to flow. By comparison, a short, wide ductus will offer little resistance to blood flow and allow a large shunt that will increase pulmonary blood flow. In addition, a short, wide ductus allows the blood to flow from the aorta into the pulmonary artery under relatively high pressure. The magnitude and pressure of the pulmonary blood flow through a PDA is likely to increase as pulmonary vascular resistance continues to fall over the first 2 months of life.[628]

There are several compensatory mechanisms, including the Frank-Starling law, adrenergic response, and myocardial hypertrophy that all help maintain cardiac output and systemic perfusion despite high-output heart failure. However, these mechanisms may not be as well developed or expressed in the neonate and particularly the premature neonate as they are in the older infant or child.[628] Even at term the newborn's myocardial structure has higher water content and fewer contractile elements than the myocardium of adults.[30] Neonatal myocardium—especially the myocardium of the preterm neonate—has a more modest response to stretch, so there is limited ability to increase stroke volume in response to volume administration and increased ventricular end-diastolic

pressure. All result in decreased ability to compensate for increased ventricular end-diastolic volume and pressure. In addition, sympathetic nervous innervation of the left ventricle is not complete until term or just after birth.

Myocardial perfusion is also affected by a large PDA. Higher left ventricular diastolic pressure, faster heart rates with shorter diastolic filling time, and lower aortic pressures from ductal flow (runoff) all can compromise coronary artery blood flow. Physiologic anemia also affects myocardial function. Lower hemoglobin concentrations in newborns (even lower in premature newborns) and fetal hemoglobin affect oxygen delivery to the myocardial tissue.[628] In addition to decreased myocardial perfusion, the decrease in systemic blood flow may compromise other organ systems, with resulting renal insufficiency, necrotizing enterocolitis, and intraventricular hemorrhage.[30]

Increased pulmonary blood flow through the PDA is associated with a variety of pulmonary complications, including increased pulmonary interstitial water, increased work of breathing, and decreased diaphragm blood flow. Reduced diaphragm blood flow probably substantially reduces the effectiveness of ventilation. Pulmonary edema may be observed in neonates with only a moderate ductal shunt because capillary permeability is higher in neonates than in older infants.[628]

The high pressure, high volume pulmonary blood flow that can result from a PDA (particularly a short, wide PDA) creates a risk of pulmonary vascular disease. The systemic and pulmonary arterial pressures can become equal. This high pulmonary vascular pressure can prevent the normal postnatal regression of medial smooth muscle in the pulmonary arteries. If the ductus remains open, true pulmonary vascular disease may develop with increased medial smooth muscle, intimal damage with cellular proliferation and hyalinization, and ultimately thrombosis and fibrosis of the small pulmonary arteries.[628]

With some congenital heart defects, flow through the ductus arteriosus is required for pulmonary or systemic blood flow; these defects are called *ductal-dependent* defects. Defects such as pulmonary atresia have ductal-dependent pulmonary blood flow. This means that blood flow from the aorta to the pulmonary artery provides the only source of pulmonary blood flow. When the ductus begins to constrict after birth, the newborn develops profound hypoxemia. Defects such as hypoplastic left heart syndrome have ductal-dependent systemic blood flow. With such defects, blood flow from the ductus into the aorta supports systemic blood flow. When the ductus begins to constrict after birth, systemic perfusion is compromised and shock develops.

Clinical Signs and Symptoms

Clinical features vary depending on the volume and pressure of the left-to-right shunt and the age of the patient. In the preterm infant with no lung disease a systolic murmur may be heard at 24 hours of age. The widespread use of surfactant has reduced severe respiratory disease, so the symptoms of a PDA appear earlier than when severe disease is present. As lung disease resolves and oxygenation improves, vasodilation causes pulmonary vascular resistance to fall, increasing the left-to-right shunt.[30] As the magnitude of the left-to-right shunt increases, the systolic murmur becomes louder and extends into early diastole. A middiastolic flow rumble may be heard at the apex.

If the shunt is small, a murmur may be the only sign of a PDA.[30,628,686] The classic continuous so-called "machinery murmur" heard in an older infant or child with a moderate PDA is not initially heard in the premature or term infant. With an increasing shunt the murmur is louder in all affected patients and may be accompanied by a suprasternal thrill. The pulmonic component of the second heart sound may be increased, especially in the infant with pulmonary disease. The precordium will be active, and the peripheral pulses bounding (because aortic flow runs off into the pulmonary artery).

The preterm, term infant, and child with a significant left-to-right shunt is dyspneic, tachypneic, and tachycardic. (For further information regarding auscultatory findings, see Table 8-25.)

Table 8-25   Clinical, Radiographic and Electrocardiographic Characteristics of Acyanotic Congenital Heart Defects

Defect	Clinical	Chest x-ray	ECG
Patent ductus arteriosus (PDA) (large L →R shunt)	±CHF Bounding pulses (low diastolic BP) if large shunt	±Cardiomegaly (LA, LV enlargement) ↑ PA, pulmonary vascular markings	±LVH (combined LVH and RVH if pulmonary hypertension develops)
Atrial septal defect (ASD)	Often asymptomatic during childhood (CHF rare) Fixed splitting of second heart sound Adults may develop atrial arrhythmias and CHF	Right atrium, right ventricle may be enlarged ↑ PA, pulmonary vascular markings	Mild RVH
Ventricular septal defect (VSD)	CHF present if shunt large	*Large shunt:* Cardiomegaly (RV, LA, LV enlargement) ↑ PA, pulmonary vascular markings *Pulmonary hypertension:* ↓ peripheral pulmonary vascular markings ↑ RV, main PA	*Large shunt:* LAE, LVH Possible RVH *Pulmonary hypertension:* RAE, RVH
Atrioventricular Septal Defect (AVSD)	CHF present if shunt large	*Partial AVSD* (see ASD) *Complete AVSD:* cardiomegaly (all chambers) ↑ PA, pulmonary vascular markings	*Partial AVSD:* left axis deviation, RAE, RVH *Complete AVSD:* LAE, RAE, LVH, RVH, left axis deviation
Double-outlet right ventricle (DORV)	*With subaortic VSD without PS:* CHF	*With subaortic VSD without PS:* ↑ PA, pulmonary vascular markings cardiomegaly (RV, LV, LA enlargement)	*With subaortic VSD without PS:* RVH, LVH, LAE
Tetralogy of Fallot	Cyanosis (proportional to severity of pulmonary obstruction), Pulmonary murmur S₂ often single	Narrow mediastinum, decreased pulmonary vascular markings. RVH causes cardiac silhouette to tilt up (likened to the upturned toe of a boot) Right aortic arch present in some (about 25%)	RVH
Pulmonary stenosis	Asymptomatic (cyanosis, CHF may be present if PS critical in infants)	May be normal ± ↑ RV size ↑ PA (poststenotic dilatation) if vascular stenosis	RVH, ± RAE look for RV "strain" (ECG reliably reflects severity)
Coarctation of the aorta (CoA)	CHF during infancy if severe ↓ lower extremity pulses, B/P ± differential cyanosis if preductal (rarely appreciable)	LV, ascending aorta enlargement (RV, PA enlargement if preductal CoA) Aortic silhouette may resemble "E" or "3" "Rib-notching" created by intercostal arteries if CoA present in older child	±LVH (RVH if preductal CoA) ±LAE
Aortic stenosis (AS)	May be asymptomatic CHF if AS severe during infancy	May be normal Ascending aorta dilated (if valvular AS)	±LVH, ±LAE (ECG *not* reflective of severity)
Hypoplastic left heart syndrome (HLHS)	CHF, cyanosis, shock	Cardiomegaly (RA, RV enlargement) ↑ PA, pulmonary vascular markings	RVH, right axis

If the neonate is receiving mechanical ventilator support for lung disease, increased support requirements (including increased inspiratory pressure or increased supplementary oxygen requirements) may indicate the development of a shunt through the PDA. The murmur may only be heard between breaths or when the neonate is briefly removed from ventilator support (e.g., for suctioning).[628]

Evidence of left ventricular hypertrophy often is noted on clinical examination and by electrocardiographic criteria in the older infant and child (Table 8-26). The echocardiogram usually documents evidence of a large shunt, and an increase in the ratio of left atrial size/aortic size. The chest radiograph may be normal in asymptomatic patients with a small shunt, but cardiomegaly and increased pulmonary vascular markings are generally identified if a large shunt and congestive heart failure are present. Pulmonary interstitial edema also may be apparent. The main pulmonary artery may be prominent (for further information, see, also, Table 8-25).

If the clinical presentation is typical and if no additional abnormality is suspected, the diagnosis is made on the basis of clinical examination, chest radiograph, and echocardiogram. Cardiac catheterization is commonly used as an intervention to close the duct, using one of several devices. If the clinical presentation is atypical or if the presence of other cardiac anomalies is suspected, a cardiac catheterization may be performed. The catheterization will reveal an increase in oxygen saturation in the pulmonary artery. Right ventricular and pulmonary artery pressures will be elevated if pulmonary hypertension is present. Aortic contrast injection will demonstrate the shunt into the pulmonary artery.

If pulmonary hypertension develops, the patent ductus arteriosus murmur may decrease in intensity or be absent. The pulmonary component of the second heart sound will be increased.

If pulmonary vascular resistance is approximately equal to systemic vascular resistance, the child may develop bidirectional shunting through the PDA. This causes arterial oxygen desaturation; the child may demonstrate cyanosis, particularly of the lower extremities and when the infant cries.

Table 8-26 Characteristic 12-Lead Electrocardiographic (ECG) Patterns in Congenital Heart Disease

CHD Category/Defect	Axis	P Wave	QRS	Other
Left-to-Right Shunts				
PDA				Left precordial ST/T abnormalities
ASD	+90 to 150		rSR' in right precordium	
VSD or DORV		LAE	LVH	With high flow
		RAE	RVH	With high pulmonary vascular resistance or PS
AVSD (AV Canal, Endocardial Cushion Defect)	−20 to −150	(P and QRS as with VSD above)		Counterclockwise vector loop
Obstructive Lesions				
PS	+90 to 280	±RAE	RVH	ECG sensitive index of severity
AS		±LAE	±LVH	ECG *not* a sensitive index of severity
Aortic coarctation				
In newborn	Rt. axis	±RAE	RVH	
After 6-12 mo	Lt axis	±LAE	±LVH	
Anomalous drainage of pulmonary veins with obstruction	+90 to 210	RAE	RVH	qR pattern in right precordium
Cyanotic Defects				
Tetralogy of Fallot	+90 to 180	RAE	RVH	Early transition from right-to-left precordial pattern
Tricuspid atresia	−30 to −150*	RAE	LVH	*If great vessels transposed, QRS axis may be +
Pulmonary atresia	Right	RAE	**	**RV forces depend on RV size
Ebstein anomaly of tricuspid valve	Right	RAE	WPW pattern common	
Transposition	Right			Normal for newborn
Truncus arteriosus	Most often normal as newborn			
Miscellaneous				
Anomalous origin of left coronary artery				Ischemia or myocardial infarction pattern
Asplenia/Polysplenia syndrome				Atrial axis anomalies +RVH

From Berman WJ: *Pediatric electrocardiographic interpretation.* St Louis, 1991, Mosby-Year Book.
WPW, Wolff-Parkinson-White syndrome.

If the neonate has ductal-dependent pulmonary blood flow (i.e., cyanotic congenital heart disease with pulmonary blood flow occurring only through the ductus arteriosus), profound hypoxemia and cyanosis will develop when the ductus begins to constrict. The hypoxemia is not relieved with oxygen administration (refer to Hypoxemia in the second section of this chapter and Cyanotic Defects later in this section of the chapter).

If the neonate has ductal dependent systemic blood flow, signs of poor systemic perfusion will develop when the ductus begins to constrict. Without treatment, these signs will progress to circulatory collapse (see section, Obstructive Lesions, Single Functioning Ventricle).

Management

Treatment of a PDA is aimed at closing the ductus. In the asymptomatic older child and adult with a PDA presenting only with a murmur, the need for PDA closure remains controversial.[399,628] Before echocardiography was available, the natural history of the PDA included some spontaneous closure, but also included high infant mortality, and risk of bacterial endocarditis, heart failure, and pulmonary vascular disease with a mortality rate of 60% before 60 years of age. However, the widespread use of echocardiography enables early identification and evaluation of the ductal shunt.

With current therapy and closure at the time of diagnosis the complications of the ductal shunt are eliminated.[449] The PDA may be closed pharmacologically, it may be closed surgically, and it can be closed using a device in older infants and young children. The timing and method of ductal closure in the premature infant remain open to debate. Before the ductus is closed in the preterm infant, medical management includes the maintenance of adequate hemoglobin concentration and hematocrit, normal serum electrolytes, adequate blood glucose, and nutritional support. To provide peripheral oxygenation and improve cardiac output, the hematocrit should be maintained greater than 45%. Management of congestive heart failure includes careful management of intravascular volume, diuretic administration, fluid restriction, and possible sodium restriction. Digitalis is not administered in the preterm infant because complications are high and therapeutic effect is minimal.[628] For further information, see Common Clinical Conditions, Congestive Heart Failure.

Pharmacologic Closure. In the premature neonate, the use of a prostaglandin synthetase inhibitor, indomethacin, to promote ductal closure has until recently replaced surgical intervention as the first-line therapy for the management of symptomatic PDA in this patient population.[628] Indomethacin therapy is most effective when it is administered before 10 days of age. The initial dose is 0.2 mg/kg either intravenously or by nasogastric tube. The intravenous dose is preferred because of the unpredictable absorption of the nasogastric dose. Subsequent doses depend on the age of the neonate at the time of the initial dose. For neonates less than 48 hours of age at initial dose, the next two doses are 0.1 mg/kg; if the neonate is 2 to 7 days of age at initial dose, the next two doses are 0.2 mg/kg; and if the neonate is greater than 7 days of age at initial dose, the next two doses are 0.25 mg/kg. The three doses are given 12 to 24 hours apart. If the urine output decreases, the number of doses may be reduced or the time

between doses increased. Renal side effects are more severe if fluid intake is restricted before indomethacin therapy.[628] If the symptoms of the left-to-right shunt remain, and renal and platelet function remain within normal limits (or adequate), additional doses of indomethacin may be administered (in some cases, consideration is given to repeating the course).

Indomethacin should not be administered to neonates with decreased renal function (serum creatinine greater than 1.6 mg/dL or blood urea nitrogen greater than 20 mg/dL), overt bleeding, shock, necrotizing enterocolitis, or echocardiographic evidence of myocardial ischemia.[628] In recent series, indomethacin therapy failed in more than one fourth of the premature infants who received it, with either the ductus failing to constrict or reopening following initial closure.[173,184,778] The risk factors associated with indomethacin failure included extreme prematurity (all failures occurred in neonates less than 27 weeks' gestation) and lack of exposure to antenatal betamethasone.

Indomethacin has been administered prophylactically during the first 24 hours of life to prevent symptomatic deterioration from a ductal shunt in extremely premature neonates (birthweight less than 1000 g). Although this practice often prevents the cardiorespiratory deterioration associated with the development of a large ductal shunt, it has not been demonstrated to reduce morbidity or mortality from the PDA. The current practice is to initiate therapy immediately on diagnosis of a PDA, usually before 72 h of age.[628] Indomethacin is not effective beyond the neonatal period.[30]

Ibuprofen has been used as an alternative to indomethacin. Early studies indicated that ibuprofen had less negative effect on renal function and urine output. Ibuprofen also has less effect on cerebral vasculature and cerebral blood flow, but does not reduce risk of intraventricular hemorrhage. A recent trial of ibuprofen prophylaxis was ended because an increased incidence of pulmonary hypertension was detected in study patients.[628]

If medical therapy has failed to close the PDA, surgical intervention should be performed 1 to 2 days after failed medical therapy.

Device Closure. For infants and children, the goal of treatment is to interrupt the left-to-right shunt. If the ductus in a term infant is abnormal, the failure to constrict is related to a structural abnormality.[628] Heart failure may be seen in infants less than 6 months of age but rarely develops later. Closure of the PDA in the catheterization laboratory may be delayed until the child is large enough to have a device placed in the ductus. But if congestive heart failure or failure to thrive is present, surgical intervention is indicated.[449]

At the present time the majority of PDAs in children and adults are closed during cardiac catheterization. The exceptions are the premature infant and when the infant's PDA is very large and short.[545] The most common devices used are Gianturco embolization coils (more than one may be used), each consisting of a stainless steel wire with Dacron fibers twisted in the wire, and Amplatzer Vascular Plug, a plug constructed of nitinol wire mesh. The Dacron in a Gianturco embolization coil adds thrombogenicity to the wire, but Dacron is not included in the Amplatzer Vascular plug.[628]

The coil is placed through a catheter that is advanced retrograde through the aorta to the site of the junction of the ductus and the aorta. The catheter delivering the coil crosses the ductus and enters the pulmonary artery. The coil is advanced beyond the tip of the catheter, and one loop is placed in the pulmonary artery. The catheter is then pulled back through the narrowest part of the ductus to the ampulla at the attachment of the ductus to the aorta. The rest of the coil is then advanced out of the catheter.

If a left-to-right shunt is detected after the first coil is placed, one or more additional coils may be deployed. The greatest risk of this procedure is coil migration (4%) into the pulmonary arteries. More than half of these embolized coils were successfully retrieved; the rest remained in place with no adverse effects.[545,628] The greatest risk of coil migration occurs when a patent ductus arteriosus is greater than 4 mm in diameter.

The Amplatzer Vascular Plug (AVP) is used for moderate to large ducts. The AVP is delivered in an antegrade fashion through a central venous catheter that is threaded through the right ventricle and then into the pulmonary artery and through the ductus to the junction of the aorta. The device is positioned in the aorta and pulled back into the aortic ampulla. The rest of the body of the plug is deployed in the body of the ductus with a small part of the plug at the pulmonary artery end of the ductus. The plug is not recommended for infants less than or equal to 5 kg.

With current use of the coil and the plug, the PDA is closed successfully in greater than 97% of the procedures with the overall risk of inadvertent embolizations at less than 1%.[545,580,628,910] After therapeutic catheter intervention, antiplatelet prophylaxis is usually prescribed for 3 to 6 months. Antibiotic prophylaxis for subacute bacterial endocarditis is recommended for 12 months or longer if a persistent shunt remains.[399]

If the neonate has a ductal-dependent cyanotic congenital heart defect, prostaglandin E$_1$ will be administered to *maintain* ductal patency. For further information the reader is referred to Hypoxemia in the second section of this chapter and to Cyanotic Defects later in this section of the chapter.

Surgical Intervention. Early surgical ligation of a PDA in premature neonates was shown to reduce the duration of mechanical ventilatory support and the length of the hospital stay.[628] Therefore prompt surgical PDA ligation is recommended if pharmacologic ductal closure fails.

Closed-heart surgery may be performed thorascopically or through a left, lateral thoracotomy. Although there is risk of recannulation, ligation (tying of the ductus) is favored over division (cutting and oversewing) for the smallest premature neonates (less than 1000 g) because it minimizes the dissection required and shortens the time required for lung retraction and anesthesia. Most surgeons clip the ductus to minimize the need for dissection and the risk of vocal cord dysfunction associated with dissection.[628,757] For all others the ductus is divided and oversewn. If the ductus is calcified, hypertensive, and fragile (generally this occurs only in elderly patients) the procedure is performed with cardiopulmonary bypass on standby.

Morbidity and mortality for surgical elimination of the ductus are typically extremely low (less than 1% mortality).

The neonatal myocardium is very sensitive to afterload, and the change in afterload with ligation of the ductus arteriosus will affect the myocardial performance index and cardiac output of the premature neonate. To maintain cardiac output, inotropic support, usually with dopamine, is required for approximately 24 hour postoperatively.[656]

The highest surgical risk is observed in children and adults with PDA who have developed pulmonary hypertension and Eisenmenger syndrome (a left-to-right shunt becomes a right-to-left shunt as the result of the development of pulmonary hypertension). These patients require careful evaluation and diagnostic studies preoperatively.[275] PDAs have been successfully closed using devices in adult patients with pulmonary hypertension.

Postoperative complications of PDA surgical repair (see Table 8-27)[851–853] include those of a thoracotomy (bleeding, atelectasis, hemothorax, and pneumothorax). In addition, phrenic or recurrent laryngeal nerve injury may occur.[851–853] Vocal cord paralysis may be associated with recurrent laryngeal nerve injury; this complication is relatively uncommon and is observed almost exclusively in very small neonates.

Advanced concepts regarding the care of the child with a PDA are presented in Box 8-22.

Table 8-27	**Summary of Surgical Repair of PDA, 2009-2010**[851–853]		
Age Group	**Total Number PDA Closures**	**Rank: Top 25 Surgeries in Age Group**	**Discharge Mortality (%)**
Neonate (0-30 days)	4701	First	6.4
Infant (31 days to 1 year)	2011	Fourth	2.7
All patients (all ages)	6968	First	3.1

Box 8-22	**Advanced Concepts: Patent Ductus Arteriosus**

- Heart failure from a left-to-right shunt is "high output" failure.
- Patent ductus arteriosus appears earlier in the preterm infant when surfactant is used to prevent pulmonary disease.
- The preterm infant has less compensatory mechanisms to handle the increased volume load from the left-to-right shunt.
- The symptoms of a PDA in a neonate during mechanical ventilation for lung disease may include requirement for increased pressure and/or oxygen support.
- Abrupt closure of the PDA with surgical ligation in the preterm infant will decrease myocardial performance and require inotropic support.

Aortopulmonary Window (Aortopulmonary Septal Defect)

Mary Rummell

Etiology

An aortopulmonary window is a defect between the ascending aorta and the pulmonary artery. With this defect, there must be two distinct semilunar valves.[445]

Septation of the fetal truncus arteriosus is influenced by neural crest cells. However, embryologic studies demonstrate that the neural crest cells do not affect the development of an aortopulmonary window. Studies also demonstrate that the aortopulmonary window is not associated with DiGeorge syndrome or any other chromosomal deletions in 22Q11.[30]

Aortopulmonary window accounts for 0.2% to 0.6% of all congenital heart defects. Nearly half of these patients have associated anomalies; the most common include interrupted aortic arch, anomalous origin of the coronary arteries, and anomalous origin of right pulmonary artery. Although these associated anomalies are found in the same area in the heart, they appear to be embryologically unrelated.[628]

Pathophysiology

The physiologic effects of an aortopulmonary window are similar to the left-to-right shunt of a large patent ductus arteriosus (PDA) or a ventricular septal defect. Once the pulmonary vascular resistance falls in the first days to weeks of life, blood is shunted from the aorta across the defect into the pulmonary circulation. These defects are discrete, most commonly large and unrestrictive, and are positioned between the semilunar valves and the bifurcation of the pulmonary artery as illustrated in Fig. 8-31.

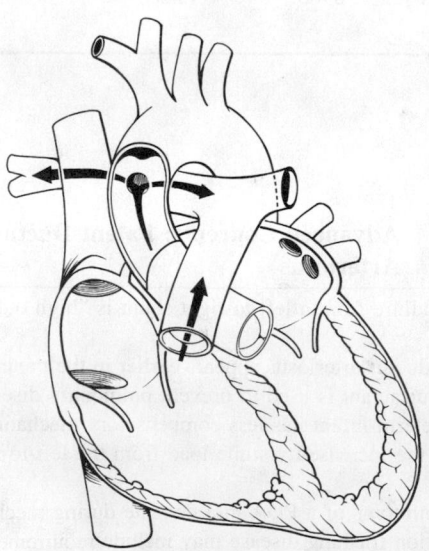

FIG. 8-31 Aortopulmonary window. The defect between the aorta and pulmonary artery produces a left-to-right shunt from the aorta into the pulmonary circulation. Shunting of blood occurs during both systole and diastole. If the defect is large, the volume of the shunt will be large and under high pressure.

These defects typically produce early congestive heart failure. Without repair, pulmonary vascular disease often develops, perhaps as early as 1 year of age.[445] This defect does not close spontaneously. Prompt surgical repair is indicated when the diagnosis is made.[30,686]

Clinical Signs and Symptoms

Clinical signs and symptoms of an aortopulmonary window vary with the size of the defect and the associated anomalies. A very small defect may not produce signs or symptoms other than a systolic ejection murmur.

The defect characteristically produces a loud, systolic murmur at the upper left sternal boarder or a machinery murmur, similar to that produced by a patent ductus arteriosus. Additionally, there may be a mid-diastolic murmur at the apex caused by the flow of the large volume of pulmonary venous return across the mitral valve. The second sound may have a louder pulmonary component from pulmonary hypertension. An ejection click may also be heard in the pulmonary area.[445,628] A right ventricular impulse may be felt along the left sternal boarder, and a thrill may be present at the upper left sternal border. Pulses may be bounding, or if the defect is associated with an interrupted aortic arch, femoral pulses may be markedly decreased when the patent ductus arteriosus closes.

Signs of congestive heart failure often are present, and left ventricular hypertrophy may be apparent on the clinical examination, the chest radiograph, and the ECG. Signs of right ventricular hypertrophy will be present if pulmonary vascular disease develops.

Echocardiography can accurately diagnose an aortopulmonary window and associated anomalies. The defect can also be identified by a fetal echocardiogram.[628] Cardiomegaly and increased pulmonary vascular markings are typically apparent on chest radiograph, unless the defect is very small.

Cardiac catheterization is usually not necessary but will document elevated pulmonary pressures, usually equal to systemic pressures. Contrast injection into the aorta will reveal the shunt into the pulmonary artery. Small defects have been successfully closed with a device during catheterization.[445,628]

Management

Closure of the defect is indicated in virtually all cases. Surgical closure is usually planned as soon as the diagnosis is made. If signs and symptoms of heart failure are severe, preoperative treatment of congestive heart failure (e.g., diuretics) is helpful to reduce pulmonary congestion. Newborns with an aortopulmonary septal defect and interrupted aortic arch may require prostaglandin E_1 to maintain ductal patency to support systemic blood flow preoperatively.

Recommended surgical treatment of an aortopulmonary window requires a median sternotomy with hypothermic cardiopulmonary bypass. Best outcomes are achieved with patch closure through an aortic incision under direct visualization.[275] Postoperative complications include bleeding, low cardiac output, pulmonary hypertension, and congestive heart failure.[156]

Atrial Septal Defect (ASD)

Mary Rummell

Pearls

- Atrial septal defects are present in 1 in 1000 live births.
- Most atrial septal defect in infants close spontaneously.
- Secundum defects may be closed by a septal occluder device.
- Some atrial septal defects require surgical closure. These include sinus venosus atrial septal defect, coronary sinus atrial septal defects, and primum atrial septal defects.

Etiology

An atrial septal defect is any opening in the atrial septum other than a competent foramen ovale.[708] Atrial septal defects result from improper septal formation early in fetal cardiac development. Most occur sporadically. However, some occur with genetic syndromes, most commonly Holt-Oram syndrome, Down syndrome, and Noonan syndrome. The incidence of atrial septal defects is 1 per 1000 live births,[458] but ASDs are found in about 30% to 50% of children with other forms of congenital heart disease.[686]

ASDs are classified into three major types, according to their location relative to the fossa ovalis (Fig. 8-32 illustrates the three types of ASDs: the ostium secundum, ostium primum, and sinus venosus).

The *ostium secundum* is the most common type of ASD, accounting for 50% to 70% of all ASDs. It is located in the region of the fossa ovalis (the foramen ovale). Historically, a patent foramen ovale has not been included in this category unless atrial dilation occurs from increased volume, and the flap closing the foramen ovale becomes incompetent, allowing a left-to-right or a right-to left shunt.[708] Although functional closure of the fetal foramen ovale may occur at birth, anatomic closure of the foramen ovale does not occur in 25% to 30% of the population. This failure is thought to be responsible for paradoxic emboli (from a right-to-left shunt across the foramen ovale) associated with cryptogenic stroke and decompression illness.[169] Migraine headaches have also been linked to patent foramen ovale.

The *ostium primum* defect accounts for about 30% of ASDs. This defect is located anterior to the fossa ovalis where the atrial septum originates from the endocardial cushion. It usually is associated with a defect in ventricular septal tissue as well as with anomalies of one or both atrioventricular valves. (See section, Atrioventricular Septal Defects/Endocardial Cushion Defects.)

The *sinus venosus* ASD is located posterior and superior to the fossa ovalis, typically near the junction of the superior vena cava and the right atrium. This defect can also occur at the junction of the inferior vena cava and right atrium. It often is associated with partial anomalous pulmonary venous return (PAPVR). With PAPVR, some of the pulmonary veins empty directly into the right atrium or superior vena cava instead of into the left atrium.

Anomalies of the atrioventricular valves may be associated with ASDs. As noted, ostium primum ASDs are often associated with anomalies of one or both atrioventricular valves. Mitral valve prolapse is present in about 20% of patients with either a secundum or sinus venosus ASD.[458,686]

Less common forms of ASDs include Chiari network, characterized by multiple fenestrations in the atrial septum that allow a left-to-right shunt (from left-to-right atrium), and a coronary sinus septal defect at the expected site of the coronary sinus as an "unroofed" coronary sinus. When the coronary sinus is unroofed, coronary sinus (i.e., venous) blood flows into the left atrium (a form of right-to-left shunt). Thus, this defect results in bidirectional shunting of blood at the

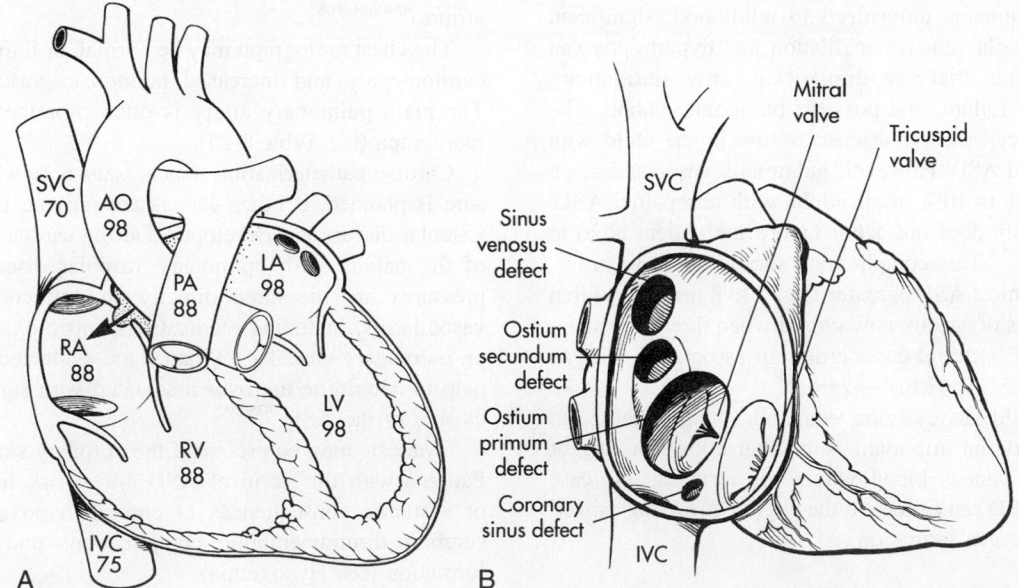

FIG. 8-32 Atrial septal defect (ASD). **A,** Typical oxyhemoglobin saturations observed in the cardiac chambers and great vessels when an ASD is present. **B,** Common types of ASD, and their relationship to the superior vena cava (SVC), the inferior vena cava (IVC) and the mitral and tricuspid valves. (From Kambam J: Patent ductus arteriosus. In Kambam J, editors: *Cardiac anesthesia for infants and children*. St Louis, 1994, Mosby.)

atrial level, with resulting hypoxemia and cyanosis. This unusual form of ASD typically is associated with persistent left superior vena cava.[458]

A common atrium is the most severe form of ASD. The septum primum, septum secundum, and the atrioventricular canal septum are all absent. A common atrium is usually associated with heterotaxy syndrome[458] (for further information, see section, Essential Anatomy and Physiology, Fetal Development of the Heart and Great Vessels).

A patent foramen ovale may serve as a necessary channel for shunting of blood between the right and left atria. This is most commonly observed in patients with obstruction to right atrial flow (tricuspid atresia), obstruction to right ventricular flow (pulmonary atresia), transposition of the great arteries, or obstruction of left ventricular flow (hypoplastic left heart syndrome).[362]

Pathophysiology

The resistance (and compliance) of the ventricles and the ventricular outflow tracts determine the magnitude and direction of shunt across an ASD.[458,708] At birth, the right ventricle is thicker and less compliant than the left ventricle. Pulmonary vascular resistance begins to fall with the first few breaths following birth, but the right ventricle takes weeks to remodel and for resistance to decrease.[30] Therefore, a significant shunt does not typically develop for the first weeks of life.

This defect usually is tolerated well and often produces no symptoms during childhood. An occasional neonate with ASD will develop symptoms of heart failure. Such newborns typically have extracardiac anomalies and developmental delay but do not have hemodynamic changes that are different from newborns without heart failure.[708] Heart failure may also develop in neonates with ASD and additional cardiac defects, such as ventricular septal defect, patent ductus arteriosus, coarctation of the aorta, or those with myocardial dysfunction, an anatomically small left ventricle and systemic hypertension.[458]

If an ASD remains unrepaired to adulthood, significant right atrial and right ventricular dilation and hypertrophy can develop, producing atrial arrhythmias (e.g., atrial fibrillation), congestive heart failure, and possible paradoxic emboli. The risk of pulmonary vascular disease is low in the child with an uncomplicated ASD. However, pulmonary vascular disease is reported in 5% to 10% of all adults with unrepaired ASD, although it usually does not occur before the patient is 20 to 30 years of age.[458] This complication should decrease in frequency because most ASDs greater than 7 to 8 mm in children more than 6 years of age are now closed when they are discovered. The risk of bacterial endocarditis in association with an uncomplicated ASD is virtually zero.[708]

When the child has cyanotic congenital heart disease, an ASD may provide an important shunt that allows mixing of oxygenated and venous blood within the atria. In this case the size of the ASD can influence the degree of mixing as well as the arterial oxygen saturation.

Clinical Signs and Symptoms

Most children with secundum or sinus venosus ASD are asymptomatic. (See Atrioventricular Septal Defects for information about ostium primum atrial septal defects.)

The characteristic heart murmur associated with an ASD is a soft systolic ejection murmur heard over the left second intercostal space and an early to mid-diastolic murmur at the lower left sternal border. This systolic murmur results from increased blood flow across an otherwise normal pulmonary valve; this causes a "relative stenosis" because when a larger than normal volume passes through a normal (not larger than normal) valve orifice, turbulence results. The diastolic murmur results from increased flow from the right atrium across the tricuspid valve into the right ventricle.

The first heart sound is louder at the left lower sternal boarder, and the second heart sound is heard best at the left upper sternal border. The pathognomonic auscultatory finding of an ASD is the presence of fixed splitting of the second heart sound. This split does not vary with respirations and it results from prolonged right ventricular ejection, caused by the increased blood flow into the right atrium, right ventricle and the pulmonary circulation (see Table 8-25). If pulmonary hypertension develops, the split narrows and the pulmonary component of the second heart sound increases.

Right ventricular hypertrophy may produce a sternal lift on clinical examination and right ventricular hypertrophy may be apparent on the ECG (see Table 8-26). A two-dimensional echocardiogram will demonstrate the position as well as the size of the atrial septal defect. It will also demonstrate the effects of the left-to-right shunt, including right ventricular and right atrial enlargement as well as a dilated pulmonary artery. Color-flow Doppler studies will enhance the evaluation of the shunt.

In adolescents and children who are overweight, the transthoracic echo may not provide clear visualization, and a transesophageal echocardiogram is needed. Echocardiographic studies may be augmented by "bubble" studies. During this study agitated normal saline is injected into a peripheral vein, and contrast bubbles are visualized in the left atrium.[458,686,708]

The chest radiograph may be normal, or it may demonstrate cardiomegaly and increased pulmonary vascular markings. The main pulmonary artery is often prominent on the chest radiograph (see Table 8-25).

Cardiac catheterization is necessary only when device closure is planned, if other defects are present, or if pulmonary vascular disease has developed. During cardiac catheterization of the patient with pulmonary vascular disease, pulmonary pressures are measured directly and effects of pulmonary vasodilators, including medications, nitric oxide, and oxygen on pulmonary vascular resistance are evaluated. These studies help to determine the risks associated with surgical or device closure of the ASD.[708,892]

Cyanosis may be present if the coronary sinus is unroofed. Patients with this form of ASD are at risk for development of systemic consequences of chronic hypoxemia, including cerebral thromboembolic complications and brain abscess formation (see Hypoxemia).

Management

Management of an atrial septal defect is determined by the type of defect and presence of symptoms.

Nonsurgical Treatment. Most children with secundum ASDs are asymptomatic. Because of the frequency of echocardiograms, ASDs have been identified in as many as 24% of newborns. The average age at diagnosis is 5 months. Most infants with ASDs (estimated as greater than 90%) have spontaneous closure of this defect by 1 year. Defects 8 mm or larger in diameter are the defects that commonly cause a significant left-to-right shunt and most likely will not close spontaneously. These defects should be surgically closed.[351,458,708]

Device closure has also been successfully performed in infants, even premature newborns. Placement involves hybrid techniques with hepatic and periatrial access.[235,537]

Spontaneous ASD closure can occur in infants with congestive heart failure.[351,708] Children diagnosed with secundum ASD after infancy usually have large defects. These children are followed until they are 4 to 6 years old before elective closure of the secundum ASD. Spontaneous closure of the smaller defects occurs in 34% of children, with 77% showing regression in the size of the defect. Unfortunately, some ASDs can become larger; typically this occurs in children who were diagnosed at an older age, and they require device or surgical closure.

The primary reason to close an atrial septal defect is to prevent pulmonary vascular disease[458] and adult complications such as atrial fibrillation and congestive heart failure. The presence and severity of functional limitations increases with age, with 5% to 10% of patients with ASDs developing pulmonary vascular disease if the defect is not closed. Although pulmonary vascular disease may develop in childhood, it usually does not develop before 20 years of age.[708]

Catheter Intervention. Transcatheter closure of ASDs has been performed with increasing success during the past several years. Criteria for device placement include evidence of right ventricular overload and appropriate septal anatomy. The secundum ASD must have a surrounding rim that is sufficient to anchor the device, and the stretch diameter must not exceed that specific to the device.

Several devices have been evaluated and the Amplatzer Septal Occluder (ASO) was the first to receive FDA approval in 2001.[708] (See Evolve Fig. 8-3 for illustrations of Amplatzer Occluders in the Chapter 8 Supplement on the Evolve Website.) The ASO is a double-disc device of nitinol mesh. The two discs are linked to each other with a central waist. Dacron fabric is incorporated into each disc and the waist. The ASO device is the most effective for closing large defects; stretch diameter must not be larger than 36 to 38 mm.[892] The Helex septal occluder is currently being evaluated to close small or moderate defects with a stretch diameter less than 20 mm (see illustration of Helex septal occluder in Evolve Fig. 8-4 in the Chapter 8 Supplement on the Evolve Website).[422,515,910]

Closure devices are placed in the catheterization laboratory with either transthoracic or transesophageal echocardiographic guidance. Complete closure rates have been satisfactory, with the ASO achieving 98% to 100% closure with few complications. Complications include device malposition, device embolization, thrombus formation, infection, and erosion of adjacent structures. Transient atrioventricular heart block has also been reported.[27,708] These devices become endothelialized in a few weeks. Aspirin is prescribed for 3 to 6 months after placement to minimize the risk of thrombus formation. Both the Amplatzer Septal Occluder and the Helex septal occluder can safely be used in the magnetic resonance imaging (MRI) scanner. The artifact created by the occluder is small enough to allow anatomic and functional MRI even in the immediate vicinity of the device.[545]

Although device closure has been attempted in sinus venosus ASDs, surgical closure is preferred. Because these defects are almost always associated with anomalous pulmonary venous return, the surgical procedure involves patch placement to close the defect and direct the pulmonary venous return to the left atrium.

Coronary sinus atrial septal defects also require surgical closure. Surgical repair depends on the anatomy.[275,458]

Surgical Intervention. Surgical closure of the ASD most frequently is completed through a median sternotomy incision on cardiopulmonary bypass. To reduce visible scarring, other surgical approaches can be used. The most frequent alternative approach is a "mini-sternotomy" through an incision on the lower half of the sternum.[458] Other approaches include a limited right lateral thoracotomy with the incision starting below the scapula and ending at the mid axial line.[11,800] Thorascopic approaches have also been used.

A secundum ASD is closed directly with sutures (primary closure) or with autologous pericardium or prosthetic patch material (patch closure). Mortality is virtually zero, and hospital stay is normally less than 3 days. Complications include bleeding, arrhythmias, and post-pericardiotomy syndrome.[458]

Surgical repair of a sinus venosus defect is more complicated, especially if anomalous pulmonary veins are present. An intracardiac patch may be required as a baffle or the superior vena cava may be translocated to direct pulmonary venous return to the left atrium. If the defect is an inferior sinus venosus defect, the procedure becomes more complex to direct hepatic venous return or anomalous pulmonary venous return to the appropriate atrium.

Repair of a coronary sinus ASD is tailored to the anatomy. If a left superior vena cava (SVC) is present, it may be ligated if a bridging vein to the right superior vena cava exists, or flow from the left SVC will be baffled (directed under a patch) to the right atrium. Postoperative mortality is less than 4%.

Complications following repair of a sinus venosus or coronary sinus ASD include arrhythmias, such as heart block, and postoperative obstruction to venous return. If cyanosis is noted in the postoperative period, reevaluation of pulmonary or systemic drainage is required.

Long term followup from surgical closure of ASDs in children with low pulmonary artery pressures shows excellent results (Table 8-28),[851–853] with a 95% survival rate compared with a matched population survival rate of 98%.[708] Surgical closure usually alleviates symptoms, and residual defects are rare. Occasional patients demonstrate persistent arrhythmias or develop late arrhythmias. Cardiomegaly as evident on a preoperative chest radiograph or ECG may be evident for months or years postoperatively.[458]

Advanced concepts regarding atrial septal defects are listed in Box 8-23.

Table 8-28   Summary of Surgical Repair of ASD, 2006-2010[851–853]

Age Group	Total Number of ASD Surgical Procedures*	Rank: Top 25 Surgeries in Age Group	Discharge Mortality
Neonate (0-30 days)	–	No ASD or Partial Anomalous Pulmonary Venous Connection (PAPVC)	–
Infant (31 days to 1 year)	–	ASD and PAPVC: not listed in top 25 most common procedures	–
Child (>1 year to <18 years)	3455 (for ASD patch and direct closure, and for PAPVC)	ASD: Patch closure is most common surgical procedure	0%
		ASD: Primary closure is 14th	0.3%
		PAPVC: 23rd	0.3%

*Primary closure of ASD may be completed with other surgery for congenital heart disease.

Box 8-23   Advanced Concepts: Atrial Septal Defect

- The direction of blood flow across an atrial septal defect is determined by the resistance or compliance of the ventricles.
- A significant shunt from an atrial septal defect usually does not develop in the newborn because it takes the right ventricle weeks to months to remodel and resistance to decrease.
- Because the defect is well tolerated and a significant number of secundum atrial septal defects close spontaneously, closure can wait until the child is 4 to 6 years of age.
- The primary reason to close an atrial septal defect is to prevent pulmonary vascular disease and other complications (e.g., atrial arrhythmias). Such complications usually do not develop until the second decade of life or later.

Ventricular Septal Defect (VSD)

Mary Rummell

Pearls

- A VSD is the most common congenital heart defect.
- VSDs may cause early congestive heart failure.
- Many VSDs close spontaneously or do not require surgical or device closure.
- Some VSDs require surgical repair.
- The risk of surgical closure of VSDs is low, even in the neonatal period.

Etiology

A ventricular septal defect is the most common congenital heart defect, accounting for 15% to 20% of all congenital heart defects.[686] It occurs as frequently as 2.5 in 1000 live births, although only about one in five or fewer of the defects require closure, either during catheterization or surgery.[457]

A VSD results when the interventricular septum fails to close after the first 7 weeks of fetal life. The reasons for this failure are not clear and are felt to be multifactorial. Although these defects are the most common present in many genetic and chromosomal syndromes, including trisomy 13, 18, and 21, Holt-Orem and Cornelia de Lange syndromes, the vast majority of VSDs are not associated with any defects.[457,597,686] They are, however, more common in premature and low-birthweight neonates.

VSDs can occur as a single defect, as multiple defects, in association with another defect, or as a component of more complex congenital heart disease. Physiologic consequences range from trivial to severe. VSDs are classified by location in the ventricular septum.[597]

Although many terms have been used to classify VSD location, the current terms for the four major locations are: perimembranous, outlet, inlet, and muscular. A summary of the four classifications is presented in Table 8-29, and locations are illustrated in Fig. 8-33.

Perimembranous VSDs, also called membranous conoventricular and infracristal defects, are the most common type of VSD, accounting for 70% to 80% of all VSDs.[597,686] The membranous septum is a small area just below the aortic valve. Defects in this area include the muscular tissue adjacent to the membranous septum. The membranous septum overlaps a small segment of the right atrium, and defects occasionally occur in this area.

Outlet (conal) VSDs account for 5% to 7% of all VSDs with several-fold higher incidence in Far Eastern countries. Outlet VSDs have also been called supracristal, conal, subpulmonary, or subarterial VSDs.[457,686] The outlet defect is located in the conal septum just below the pulmonary valve. Because of its location, a cusp of the aortic valve can prolapse into this defect, causing aortic valve insufficiency.

The third type of ventricular septal defect, an inlet defect, occurs in 5% to 8% of all VSDs. It is located posterior and inferior to the membranous septum below the septal leaflet of the tricuspid valve. This form of a VSD may also be referred to as an endocardial cushion defect or AV canal defect, but unlike the atrioventricular septal defects, it usually does not involve either of the atrioventricular valves.[597]

The fourth type of VSD is the muscular defect, located in the muscular septum. Muscular VSDs constitute 5% to 20% of all VSDs. The defect may be single when viewed from the left side but appears to be multiple when viewed from the right ventricle because the shunted blood flows around trabeculations (criss-crossing muscular and fibrous tissue strands) that form the right ventricular walls. Muscular defects are found in the apex, in the central or mid-muscular region, or in the anterior or marginal region of the septum. Multiple defects involving all components of the ventricular septum are usually referred to as a "Swiss cheese" septum.

Table 8-29 **VSD Classification**

Defect	Previous Names	Incident (%)	Description
Perimembranous	Infracristal, membranous, conoventricular	80	Located in membranous septum just below aortic valve. Usually extends into muscular, inlet, and outlet areas.
Outlet	Supracristal, conal, infundibular, subpulmonary, doubly committed subarterial	5-7	Located just beneath the pulmonary valve.
Inlet	Endocardial cushion defect or AV canal defect.	5-8	Posterior and inferior to the membranous septum below the septal leaflet of the tricuspid valve.
Muscular		5-20	Located in the muscular septum.
1. Central			Midmuscular, may appear to have many defects on RV side, but have only a single defect on the LV side.
2. Apical			Apex of ventricular septum, RV may appear to have multiple defects, but only one on LV side.
3. Marginal			Occurs along RV septal junction
4. "Swiss cheese" septum			Multiple defects throughout muscular septum.

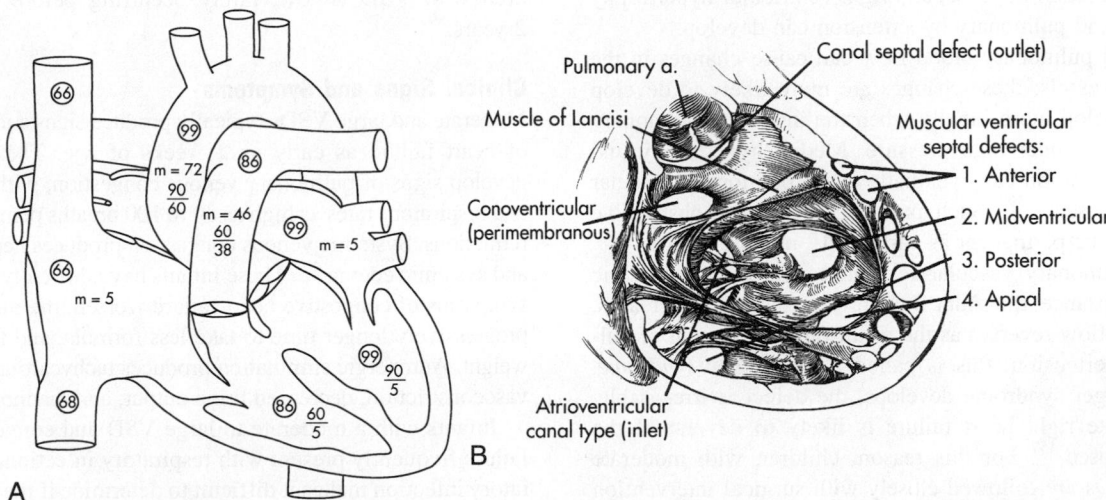

FIG. 8-33 Ventricular septal defect (VSD). **A,** Typical intracardiac pressures (systolic, diastolic and mean [m]) and oxyhemoglobin saturations (in circles). Note step-up in oxyhemoglobin saturation from the right atrium (66%) to the right ventricle (86%) indicating left-to-right shunt at the ventricular level. Right ventricular pressure (60/5) is elevated compared with the normal right ventricular pressure, but is less than the left ventricular pressure (90/5), indicating that the VSD in this illustration is *restrictive*. The pulmonary artery pressure is elevated as well. (From Nichols DG. *Critical heart disease in infants and children,* ed 2, St Louis, 2006, Mosby (Fig. 24-8). **B,** Classification of ventricular septal defects (VSDs) and potential locations: atrioventricular canal (inlet) type; muscular VSDs (anterior [1], midventricular [2], posterior [3], and apical [4]); conoventricular septal defect, which includes perimembranous and malalignment conoventricular septal defects; and conal septal (outlet) defects. The orifice of the pulmonary artery (pulmonary a.) is indicated. (From Sellke F: *Sabiston and spencer's surgery of the chest,* ed 8, Philadelphia, 2009, Saunders; Fig. 117-4.)

Many (30% to 40%) membranous and muscular VSDs may close spontaneously. Spontaneous closure occurs more frequently in small defects and during the first 6 months of life. Defects do not enlarge with age, so they may become relatively smaller as the infant grows. Inlet and outlet defects do not close spontaneously.

Pathophysiology
The primary variable that determines the hemodynamic consequences of a VSD is the size of the defect. Small to medium defects restrict the volume and the pressure of the

left-to-right shunt. However, large defects (approaching the size of the aortic orifice) do not restrict flow, so the magnitude of the shunt is determined by the difference between pulmonary and systemic vascular resistances.[597]

Immediately after birth, pulmonary vascular resistance normally falls rapidly as the small, muscular pulmonary arteries change from vessels with small lumens and thick medial muscle walls to vessels with larger lumens and thinner walls.[30] When pulmonary vascular resistance falls normally, right ventricular pressure decreases and approaches adult levels by 7 to 10 days of life.[597]

The normal postnatal decline in pulmonary vascular resistance may be delayed if a large VSD is present, and this will, in turn, delay development of symptoms of the shunt. The increase in pulmonary blood flow resulting from a VSD will increase left atrial and pulmonary venous pressure and slow the normal decline in pulmonary vascular resistance, so it may take weeks to fall. When pulmonary vascular resistance eventually falls, the left-to-right shunt through the VSD increases. Increased pulmonary blood flow causes increased pulmonary venous return to the left side of the heart with resultant left atrial and ventricle enlargement and development of congestive heart failure, usually at 2 to 8 weeks of age.[597] If signs of congestive heart failure develop at this age, blood flow to the pulmonary arteries is typically at least twice the systemic blood flow or more.[457]

When the VSD is large, the volume of the shunt into the pulmonary circulation is large. Left ventricular hypertrophy develops rapidly in response to the volume load resulting from increased pulmonary venous return. In addition, when the VSD is large, the pressures in the right ventricle and the pulmonary circulation increase, and right ventricular hypertrophy and failure and pulmonary hypertension can develop.

Increased pulmonary blood flow can cause changes in the pulmonary vessels; these changes are more likely to develop and can develop more rapidly when the increased pulmonary blood flow is under high pressure. Medial hypertrophy and intimal proliferation can eventually cause pulmonary vascular obstructive disease.[597] Such pulmonary vascular obstructive disease may be permanent as early as 12 months of age.

Once pulmonary vascular resistance approaches systemic vascular resistance, the shunt flow through the VSD decreases. If the shunt flow reverses as the result of development of pulmonary hypertension, this is called *Eisenmenger syndrome*. If Eisenmenger syndrome develops, the defect is irreparable, because acute right heart failure is likely to develop if the defect is closed.[457] For this reason, children with moderate to large VSDs are followed closely with surgical intervention planned before the development of pulmonary hypertension.[686] For further information, see Common Clinical Conditions, Pulmonary Hypertension.

Several factors may cause the newborn with a VSD to develop signs of congestive heart failure within the first few days of life rather than at several weeks of age. In a rare form of membranous defect, the left ventricle ejects directly to the right atrium. This defect produces a significant shunt and substantial increase in pulmonary blood flow. Other factors that promote early signs of congestive failure include additional cardiac anomalies (particularly any defect that increases resistance to left ventricular or systemic blood flow), respiratory infection, anemia, other congenital anomalies, and prematurity. Left heart abnormalities, including aortic stenosis, coarctation of the aorta, and interrupted aortic arch, can contribute to left ventricular failure and pulmonary edema, and they also magnify the difference between pulmonary and systemic resistance and increase the magnitude of the left-to-right shunt. Mitral valve stenosis or any pulmonary venous obstruction will substantially increase pulmonary venous congestion and pulmonary hypertension.[597]

Other factors may affect the pulmonary or systemic blood flow in patients with a VSD. In a membranous defect the great arteries may be malaligned, either to the right or left and the malalignment may obstruct right or left ventricular outflow. Such malalignment may affect the direction, volume, and pressure of the shunt flow. Tetralogy of Fallot and double outlet right ventricle with a subaortic VSD and pulmonary stenosis are examples of malaligned VSD associated with obstruction to pulmonary blood flow and a right-to-left shunt through the VSD (see section, Tetralogy of Fallot, Double Outlet Right Ventricle).[457]

In an outlet defect the right coronary cusp of the aortic valve may prolapse into the defect, because the defect in the ventricular septum results in inadequate support for the aortic root. In addition, a venturi effect on the valve leaflets can contribute to development of aortic insuffiency.[361,597] Once aortic insufficiency develops it is likely to increase with age.[597] The right or noncoronary cusp of the aortic valve may also prolapse into a membranous defect; this may reduce flow through the defect but obstruct the right ventricular outflow tract.[686]

The risk of bacterial endocarditis in infants and young children with VSD is low, rarely occurring before the age of 2 years.[597]

Clinical Signs and Symptoms

Moderate and large VSDs typically produce signs and symptoms of heart failure as early as 2 weeks of age. The infant will develop signs of pulmonary venous congestion, with tachypnea and respiratory rates as high as 80 to 100 breaths per minute with retractions. Systemic venous congestion produces hepatomegaly and systemic edema.[457] These infants have difficulty feeding; as symptoms of congestive heart failure worsen, the infant takes a progressively longer time to take less formula, and fails to gain weight. Adrenergic stimulation produces tachycardia, peripheral vasoconstriction, decreased urine output, and diaphoresis.

Infants with a moderate to large VSD and congestive heart failure frequently present with respiratory infection. The respiratory infection makes it difficult to determine if the respiratory distress is caused by the left-to-right shunt or the infection.[597]

The murmur of a moderate VSD is harsh and holosystolic, and is usually associated with a thrill. When pulmonary blood flow is twice systemic blood flow, a third heart sound may be heard, with a mid-diastolic rumble. This sound is best heard at the apex and results from increased flow of pulmonary venous return across the mitral valve. The second heart sound is split with the pulmonary component at normal intensity.[457,597,686]

With large shunts, increased precordial activity is apparent over both the right ventricular (parasternal) and left ventricular (apical) areas. The high volume of pulmonary blood flow and pulmonary venous return increase left ventricular volume, resulting in a hyperdynamic precordium. The systolic murmur is S1 coincident and is heard best along the left sternal border; it may end before the second heart sound. The second heart sound is narrowly split and has a loud pulmonary component. Some patients with VSDs have an early diastolic murmur indicating mild pulmonary or aortic valve insufficiency. Either condition indicates increased pathology: the pulmonary valve insufficiency indicates increased pulmonary artery pressure and the aortic valve insufficiency indicates prolapse of the aortic valve cusp. There is also a third heart sound, and a diastolic rumble can be heard at the apex.[457,597]

Infants with infundibular pulmonary stenosis may develop cyanosis from a right-to-left shunt pathology similar to tetralogy of Fallot. Cyanosis may also be seen in the older child with a large VSD and pulmonary hypertension (i.e., pulmonary vascular disease with Eisenmenger syndrome—see section, Common Clinical Conditions, Pulmonary Hypertension).

The chest x-ray and electrocardiogram also vary with the size of the ventricular septal defect (see Tables 8-25 and 8-26). If the VSD is small the ECG and chest x-ray may be normal.[686] With a moderate VSD there is increased pulmonary venous return to the left ventricle, resulting in left ventricular hypertrophy (LVH) on the ECG. Cardiomegaly, increased pulmonary vascular markings, and an enlarged main pulmonary artery segment will be visible on the chest radiograph.[597] In young infants with large VSDs, right ventricular hypertrophy may not be as marked on the ECG as in older infants who have pulmonary hypertension. When the right ventricular pressure equals the left ventricular pressure, biventricular hypertrophy is apparent on ECG and the left atrial enlargement may produce a biphasic P wave.

Cardiomegaly will be present on chest radiograph and results from enlargement of both ventricles and the left atrium. Increased pulmonary vascular markings (increased pulmonary blood flow) will also be present.[597,686]

Two-dimensional echocardiography accurately identifies the defect anatomy and any associated anomalies, including overriding atrioventricular valves, prolapse of the aortic valve cusp, aortic valve regurgitation, and ventricular outflow tract obstruction. Color-flow Doppler studies provide information regarding restriction of flow through the defect and allow assessment of pulmonary and right ventricular pressures. Measurement of left atrial and ventricular diameters provides information about shunt volume.

Transesophageal echocardiography is used preoperatively to further define the defect. It may also be used intraoperatively to evaluate closure of the defect(s).[457,597]

Because echocardiography provides precise details of the anatomy and allows assessment of pulmonary and ventricular pressures and shunts, cardiac catheterization is rarely necessary unless device closure is anticipated. Cardiac catheterization is used to evaluate pulmonary vascular disease (see section, Common Clinical Conditions, Pulmonary Hypertension).

Management

Medical Management. Because most VSDs are small, the infant who is asymptomatic (i.e., without signs of congestive heart failure or pulmonary hypertension) by 6 months of age can be followed conservatively. A large number of these defects close spontaneously; 75% to 80% close within the first 2 years. Children with small defects should be followed every 3 years to monitor for aortic valve prolapse or regurgitation.[457,597,686,759] Prophylaxis for bacterial endocarditis is recommended for VSDs associated with complex heart disease (see Bacterial Endocarditis).

Infants with moderate and large defects and early (i.e., within the first few weeks of life) signs and symptoms of congestive heart failure and failure to thrive are treated medically with nutritional supplementation. A high-calorie formula is generally needed to maximize caloric intake while limiting fluid intake (see section, Common Clinical Conditions, Nutritional Compromise). Medical treatment usually includes diuretics and medications to reduce systemic afterload (see section, Common Clinical Conditions, Congestive Heart Failure).[597] Infants who do not respond to medical therapy, especially those with signs and symptoms of pulmonary hypertension, require device (during catheterization) or surgical closure of the defect.[481,597]

A large number of infants with moderate defects and early signs and symptoms of congestive heart failure improve with medical management. In these infants the defect either decreases in size or becomes relatively smaller as the infant grows. When the defect becomes relatively smaller, it restricts the volume and pressure of the left-to-right shunt, which in turn results in decreased signs and symptoms of heart failure and decreased risk of pulmonary vascular disease.[481]

VSD closure has been recommended to prevent bacterial endocarditis, decrease the risk of aortic valve regurgitation, and prevent ventricular outflow obstruction and pulmonary vascular disease. However, as many as 94% of patients with small to moderate VSDs who were medically managed are in New York Heart Association Class I at 15 years after their diagnosis. In addition, both surgical repair and device closure have been associated with late rhythm disturbances, aortic valve regurgitation, and bacterial endocarditis.[67,481,597] The medical and surgical team must always monitor outcomes and weigh the potential risks and benefits of medical management versus defect closure.

Device Closure. Experience with percutaneous device closure of muscular and membranous VSDs is more limited than device closure of patent ductus arteriosus or atrial septal defects. The initial experience with device closure of VSDs included mid-muscular defects, postoperative residual defects, VSDs that were difficult to reach surgically, or fenestrated defects.[484] Devices can be placed percutaneously, intraoperatively, and periventricularly through an open sternotomy,[27,40,389,545] and they have evolved rapidly over the past several years.

The Amplatzer septal occluder is currently the most frequently used ventricular closure device, with FDA approval since December 2001. The Amplatzer device is a double-disc device of nitinol mesh. The two discs are linked to each other with a central waist. Dacron fabric is incorporated into each disc and the waist. Modifications of this device, still in investigational use, include the Amplatzer muscular VSD occluder and the Amplatzer membranous VSD occluder. The Amplatzer membranous VSD occluder, the newest member and the first with an asymmetric design, was first used clinically in 2002. The Amplatzer family of devices is illustrated in Evolve Fig. 8-3 in the Chapter 8 Supplement on the Evolve Website.

Percutaneous transcatheter VSD closure is more difficult than that of atrial septal defects. Multicenter studies report successful closure in 95.3% of cases using several types of devices. Postcatheter complications include vascular complications, hemolysis, infection, device embolization, arrhythmias, valve regurgitation, and residual shunt. Mortality averages 0.2%.

The most significant complicating arrhythmia is complete atrioventricular block, occurring in 2.8% of patients at various intervals after device placement.[139,285] Aspirin is usually given for 3-6 months after device implantation until the device becomes endothelialized.[27]

Surgical Closure. Palliative surgery using a pulmonary artery band is no longer used, even for small infants with significant left-to-right shunts. Indications for early surgery include uncontrolled congestive heart failure with failure to thrive. Surgical repair is successfully performed within the first few months of life in infants as small as 2 kg. Additional indications for closure include large defects even without symptoms, defects with elevated pulmonary pressures, defects producing a pulmonary-to-systemic shunt ratio greater than 2:1, and defects with associated aortic cusp prolapse. Defects associated with elevated pulmonary pressure and signs of pulmonary hypertension are repaired as soon as signs of pulmonary hypertension are noted or before 2 years of age to prevent pulmonary vascular disease.[457,597]

VSDs are closed surgically through a median sternotomy on hypothermic, cardiopulmonary bypass. Muscular, perimembranous, and inlet defects are closed from the right atrium through the tricuspid valve (i.e., without a ventriculotomy). Subpulmonary defects are closed through the pulmonary valve (so the incision is made in the pulmonary artery). Outlet and perimembranous defects that involve prolapse of the aortic valve cusps require careful attention to support of the aortic valve cusp and avoiding injury to the conduction system.[275,457] Multiple defects, especially near the ventricular apex, may require a small apical ventriculotomy or device closure. The device may be placed intraoperatively.[457]

A variety of materials are used to close VSDs, including autologous pericardium, woven Dacron, or homograft material, and selection is determined by surgeon preference.[275] Intraoperative echocardiography and color flow Doppler are used to determine residual shunts or additional defects before the patient is removed from cardiopulmonary bypass or before the patient leaves the operating room.

Postoperative complications include congestive heart failure and arrhythmias. Right bundle branch block is usually present postoperatively if surgery is performed in patients less than 6 months of age. If closure of an apical ventricular septal defect required a ventriculotomy, postoperative myocardial dysfunction is likely.[457] Postoperative complications are likely in infants with respiratory infections before surgical repair.[597]

Long-term survival of patients with VSD is good. Spontaneous closure of small defects is almost 80%. Ninety-four percent of symptomatic infants with moderate defects who respond to medical treatment and do not require surgical or catheter intervention continue to do well 15 years after initial diagnosis. Most infants with large, symptomatic VSDs who require surgery within the first year have excellent results with normal growth, development, and activity. Limited longitudinal studies show that pulmonary hypertension is rare; sinus node dysfunction is also rare; but progressive aortic valve insufficiency is more common. Children repaired after 2 years of age may demonstrate increased postoperative pulmonary resistance that may be progressive.[597,759]

Table 8-30	Summary of Surgical Repair of VSD, 2006-2010[851–853]		
Age Group	Total Number of VSD Surgical Procedures	Rank: Top 25 Surgeries in Age Group	Discharge Mortality
Neonate (0-30 days)	181	22nd—patch repair	3.3%
Infant (31 days to 1 year)	3884	1st—patch repair	0.6%
Child (>1 year to <18 years)	1440	2nd—patch repair	0.1%

Box 8-24	Advanced Concepts: Ventricle Septal Defect (VSD)

- The primary determinant of a left-to-right shunt and the pulmonary artery pressure is the size of the defect; once it is approximately half the size of the aortic outflow tract, it allows a relatively unrestricted shunt. Location of the defect also influences shunt volume and pressure.
- If the defect is large, the relative difference between pulmonary and systemic outflow tract resistance (including any subvalvular or valvular stenosis or pulmonary artery or aortic narrowing and resistances in the vascular bed) determines the volume of a left-to-right shunt.
- The presence of a loud murmur and a thrill does not indicate a significant left- to-right shunt.
- Closure of a ventricular septal defect is indicated for
  - Uncontrolled congestive heart failure and failure to thrive
  - Signs and symptoms of increased pulmonary resistance
  - Signs and symptoms of aortic valve prolapse

In the discharge mortality data (Table 8-30) from the STS Congenital Heart Surgery Data Summary,[851–853] mortality for surgical closure of VSD is highest in neonates. Infant discharge mortality is twice that of the child, but is just slightly greater than 1%. Therefore it appears that repairing symptomatic infants in the first year of life is the best management of large symptomatic ventricular septal defects.

Advanced concepts for the nurse caring for the infant or child with VSD are provided in Box 8-24.

Atrioventricular Septal Defect (AVSD)/AV Canal Defect

Mary Rummell

Pearls

- Atrioventricular septal defects are a group of abnormalities with a common finding—absence of atrioventricular septum. There are two forms of AVSDs—partial and complete.

○ With partial AVSD the mitral annulus and the tricuspid valve annulus are separate and complete

○ With complete AVSD, the mitral and tricuspid valve share some tissue—there is a single atrioventricular valve annulus.

• AVSDs do NOT close spontaneously. All require surgical repair.

Etiology

Atrioventricular septal defects (AVSD) are a group of abnormalities of the atrioventricular septum and atrioventricular valves.[150] The one common finding in this group of abnormalities is the absence of the atrioventricular septum; therefore the term atrioventricular septal defect is used for this group of defects.[30] AVSDs are mainly derived from faulty fetal development of the atrioventricular septum and the embryologic endocardial cushion tissue; thus, they are also called endocardial cushion defects.

Atrioventricular septal defects occur in 4% to 5% of all congenital heart defects. The estimated incidence is 0.19 in 1000 live births. An AVSD is the most common defect identified on fetal echocardiography,[150,686] and the most common congenital heart defect in children with Down syndrome (see section, Essential Anatomy and Physiology, Etiologies of CHD: Noninherited and Genetic Factors). Patients with Down syndrome and AVSD rarely have associated cardiac defects. Children with AVSD but no Down syndrome may also have heterotaxy syndrome with asplenia and polysplenia.[575] A common atrium is associated with Ellis-van Creveld syndrome.[150]

The AVSDs are divided into two forms: partial and complete (Fig. 8-34). In the partial form there are two distinct atrioventricular valve annuli: the tricuspid valve (with possible cleft) and a cleft mitral valve. In the complete form of AVSD there is a common atrioventricular valve annulus.

A typical partial AVSD includes a primum atrial septal defect (ASD) with a cleft in the anterior leaflet of the mitral valve. The tricuspid valve may also have a cleft in the septal leaflet.

The complete form of AVSD includes a persistent fetal common atrioventricular canal. It is composed of a primum atrial septal defect that is contiguous with an inlet ventricular septal defect (VSD). When the common atrioventricular valve is open, the valve and the septal defects form a "canal" in the center of the heart, hence the name atrioventricular canal defect.[150,575,686]

In both partial and complete forms of AVSD there is downward displacement of the left atrioventricular valve so that both valves are on the same plane. This creates a deficiency in the length of the ventricular septum from the inlet portion to the apex and increases the length from the apex to the aortic valve. The result is an elongated and narrowed left ventricular outflow tract, commonly called a "gooseneck" deformity as illustrated in Fig. 8-35.

There is wide variability among AVSDs with many variations of the atrial and ventricular septal defects and of atrioventricular valve anomalies. These variations provided the basis for complex terminology used in previous classifications. The current trend is to use the generic term *AVSD* and then describe the anatomy and shunting present.[150,575]

Pathophysiology

The physiology seen in this group of defects may be similar to that observed with an atrial septal defect (ASD), ventricular septal defect (VSD), or both, with the possibility of atrioventricular valve regurgitation (refer to Atrial Septal Defect and Ventricular Septal Defect, above). Every possible variation is seen with anatomic differences in both the size of the defect(s) and/or the degree of atrioventricular valve incompetence.[575]

Partial AVSD. In the partial form of AVSD, the primum ASD is usually large. A tongue of connective tissue (it is different from endocardial cushion tissue) separates the tricuspid valve annulus from the mitral valve annulus. This tissue displaces the right and left atrioventricular valves toward the ventricular septum where they may be firmly attached.[686] A small, restrictive inlet ventricular septal defect may also be present; it is typically referred to as an intermediate or transitional AVSD.[275]

Patients with primum ASDs usually demonstrate symptoms of left-to-right shunts earlier that those with

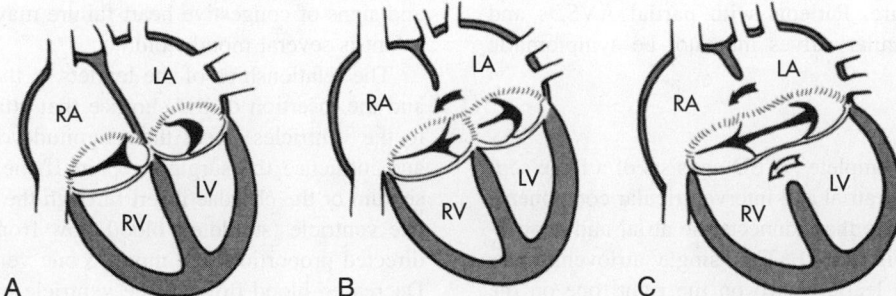

FIG. 8-34 Diagram of the atrioventricular (AV) valve(s) and cardiac septa in partial and complete atrioventricular septal defects (AVSDs). **A,** Normal AV valve anatomy with no septal defect. **B,** Partial AVSD with an ostium primum atrial septal defect (ASD) (*solid arrow showing left to right atrial shunt*) *and* clefts in the mitral and tricuspid valves. **C,** Complete AVSD. An ostium primum ASD (*solid arrow indicates resulting atrial shunt*) and an inlet ventricular septal defect (*open arrow indicates ventricular shunt*) are present. There is a common AV valve with large anterior and posterior bridging leaflets. LA, left atrium; LV, left ventricle; RA, right atrium; RV, right ventricle. (From Park MK. *Pediatric cardiology for practitioners,* ed 5, Philadelphia, 2008, Elsevier, Fig. 12-15.)

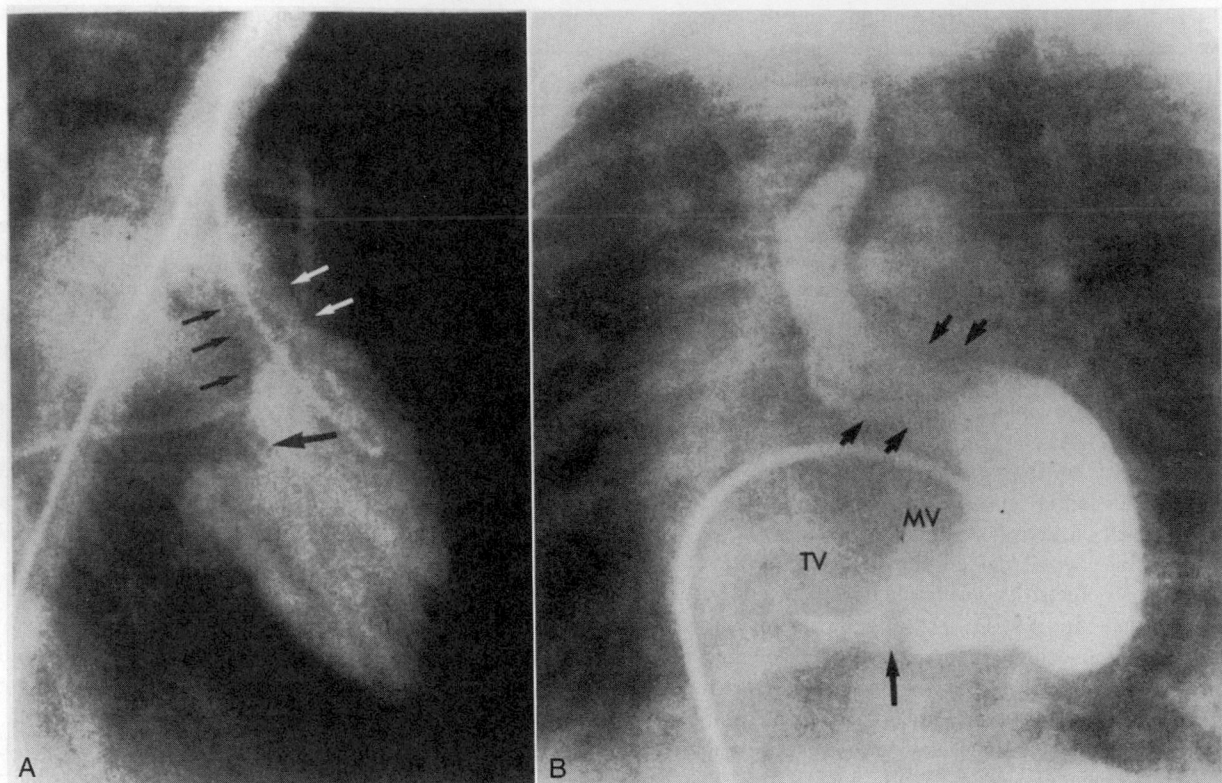

FIG. 8-35 Left ventricular angiograms depicting characteristic features of atrioventricular septal defects (AVSDs). **A,** The injection of contrast into the left ventricle creates a silhouette of the large cleft in the mitral valve (*large black arrow*). During systole, contrast material can be seen flowing back into the left atrium through the insufficient mitral valve. The downward displacement of the mitral valve creates a characteristic elongation of the left ventricular outflow tract (the "gooseneck" deformity), which is outlined by five small (black and white) arrows. **B,** This complete atrioventricular canal defect can be identified, because injection of contrast material into the left ventricle outlines both the mitral and tricuspid valve orifices (TV and MV); these valve rings are not separate and complete. A small indentation in the contrast material (*single large arrow*) is created by some ventricular septal tissue, but the contrast material reveals the ventricular level shunt. The elongation ("gooseneck" deformity) of the left ventricular outflow tract (four *small arrows*) is apparent.

secundum ASDs. The cleft in the anterior leaflet of the mitral valve may allow for left ventricle to right atrial shunting; the degree of shunting depends on the competence of the valve. Infants with significant mitral regurgitation may develop early (i.e., within the first weeks of life) symptoms of congestive heart failure. Patients with partial AVSDs and competent atrioventricular valves may not be symptomatic until adulthood.[150]

Complete AVSD. A complete AVSD consists of a large septal defect with both interatrial and interventricular components and a single valve orifice that connects the atrial and ventricular chambers (see Fig. 8-34). This single atrioventricular valve usually has five leaflets: two on the right, one on the left, plus an anterior and a posterior leaflet that bridge the ventricular septum. Although the valve is very abnormal, it may be competent. The resulting pathophysiology is that of a large ventricular septal defect: Increased pulmonary blood flow and signs of congestive heart failure typically develop in the first months of life. The risk of pulmonary vascular disease is high. Left-to-right shunting and resultant symptoms and risk of

pulmonary vascular disease are enhanced if the common atrioventricular valve is regurgitant.

In patients with Down syndrome, pulmonary vascular resistance may remain elevated during the first weeks of life. In these patients, development of a significant left-to-right shunt and signs of congestive heart failure may be delayed until the infant is several months old.[575]

The relationships of the leaflets to the crest of the septum and the insertion of the chordae that attach the valve leaflets to the ventricles affect the magnitude of the resulting shunt and influence the surgical repair. If the leaflets override the septum or the chordae insert through the defect into the opposite ventricle (straddle), blood flow from the atrium may be directed proportionately more to one ventricle than the other. Decreased blood flow to one ventricle may cause that ventricle to become hypoplastic, creating an "unbalanced" defect with either right or left ventricular dominance. Marked ventricular hypoplasia may prevent a two-ventricular repair. Ventricular hypoplasia is uncommon in patients with Down syndrome and AVSDs.[575,686]

When an AVSD is present, the location of the conduction system is abnormal. The septal defect results in posterior displacement of the atrioventricular (AV) node, so it is closer to the coronary sinus. In addition, the bundle of His is displaced inferiorly so it courses along the lower rim of the ventricular septal defect. On the electrocardiogram the posterior displacement of the AV node produces a prolonged PR interval (first-degree AV block), and "superior" QRS axis (left axis deviation). The abnormal location of the conduction system must be considered during the surgical correction.[150,275]

Children with unrepaired AVSDs require antibiotic prophylaxis against subacute bacterial endocarditis (SBE), although SBE is rare during in infancy. Postoperatively SBE prophylaxis is typically required for patients with valvular insufficiency, because that will cause turbulence near the septal defect patch (refer to Bacterial Endocarditis later in this section of the chapter).[686]

Clinical Signs and Symptoms

Partial AVSD. Children with a partial AVSD are usually asymptomatic. When this defect is associated with moderate or severe mitral valve regurgitation, symptoms of excessive pulmonary blood flow and congestive heart failure may develop during early infancy. These children are tachypneic, tire easily, and have recurrent respiratory infections and poor weight gain.[150,686]

The left-to-right shunt and resulting symptoms will be more severe in the presence of associated left heart abnormalities, such as subaortic stenosis, left atrioventricular valve disease, or aortic arch abnormalities.[575] Symptoms may also be more severe if a common atrium is present.

The typical murmur of a partial AVSD is a systolic ejection murmur heard best at the upper left sternal border, radiating to the lung fields. The second heart sound is widely split and fixed during inspiration (because ejection of the increased volume of blood flow through the pulmonary valve takes longer than ejection of blood flow through the aortic valve). If mitral valve regurgitation is present, the murmur is holosystolic. A mid-diastolic murmur may be present at the apex if the left-to-right shunt is large.

Many children with AVSD have only left-to-right shunting of blood unless or until pulmonary vascular disease develops. However, the child may be mildly cyanotic if a common atrium allows mixing of systemic and pulmonary venous blood.[150,686]

On electrocardiogram about half of patients with AVSD demonstrate left axis deviation and a prolonged PR interval (first-degree AV block). Many patients demonstrate right ventricular hypertrophy with increased right ventricular volume load.[686]

The primary imaging technique for a partial AVSD is two-dimensional echocardiography. The defect in the lower atrial septum is clearly visualized, as is the cleft in the mitral valve. As with all forms of AVSD the deficiency of the inlet portion of the ventricular septum, the inferior displacement of the atrioventricular valves, and the attachment of the AV valves to the ventricular septum are visible. In a partial AVSD the two separate atrioventricular valve orifices are equidistant from the cardiac apex. Color-flow Doppler demonstrates the left-to-right shunt and enables estimation of the right ventricular systolic pressure.[150]

Cardiac catheterization is rarely necessary but if performed, angiography will demonstrate the characteristic "gooseneck" deformity. Chest radiography may demonstrate cardiomegaly and increased pulmonary vascular markings. Right atrial enlargement may result from the jet of blood flow through the cleft mitral valve.[150]

Complete AVSD. In the complete form of AVSD, excessive pulmonary blood flow results in tachypnea, frequent respiratory infections, and failure to thrive within 1 to 2 months after birth (see section, Congestive Heart Failure). If the infant does not develop early symptoms, persistence of increased pulmonary resistance or early onset of pulmonary vascular obstructive disease should be suspected.

Atrioventricular valve regurgitation increases the symptoms of congestive heart failure and complicates management preoperatively and postoperatively. Patients with AV valve regurgitation are at increased risk for reoperation.

Preoperatively, the murmur resembles that of a large ventricular septal defect with a holosystolic murmur heard best at the lower left sternal boarder; it is usually accompanied by a thrill. There is also a holosystolic apical murmur from left AV valve regurgitation that may radiate toward the left axilla. The second heart sound is narrowly split with a louder pulmonary component. The precordium is usually hyperactive, and the liver is enlarged.[686]

Characteristic left axis deviation with a prolonged PR interval is present on electrocardiogram (see Table 8-26). Right ventricular hypertrophy is always evident, and most patients also have left ventricular hypertrophy.[150]

As noted, two-dimensional echocardiography is the primary diagnostic tool for identifying complete AVSDs. It provides complete imaging of all components and allows evaluation of the severity of abnormalities. Additional defects, including secundum atrial septal defects and additional ventricular septal defects, can be visualized and important information about the size and position of the atrioventricular valves, the anatomy of the leaflets, and the locations of the attachment of the papillary muscles in the left ventricle and the septal wall can be demonstrated with this technology. The relative size of both ventricles is also assessed.[150,686] This information is essential for the surgical repair.

The chest radiograph of a child with a complete AVSD demonstrates cardiomegaly with a prominent pulmonary artery and increased pulmonary vascular markings. Cardiac catheterization is rarely needed to define the anatomy, but the characteristic "gooseneck" deformity will be demonstrated on the left ventricular angiogram. In an older child cardiac catheterization is necessary to evaluate pulmonary vascular resistance and rule out pulmonary vascular obstructive disease before complete repair.[150] For further information, please refer to section, Common Clinical Conditions, Pulmonary Hypertension.

Frequently children with Down syndrome and AVSD have higher pulmonary vascular resistance than systemic vascular resistance, and their pulmonary vascular resistance is higher than that of children with AVSD without Down syndrome. Although some histologic studies show no difference in lung tissue between children with and without Down syndrome, other studies have demonstrated that children with Down syndrome have relative pulmonary parenchymal hypoplasia.[150] However, when 100% oxygen is administered to children with Down syndrome and AVSD in the cardiac catheterization lab, pulmonary vascular resistance decreases and the difference between the pulmonary and systemic resistances is eliminated or reversed. This supports the belief that the cause of the high pulmonary vascular resistance in children with AVSD and Down syndrome is related to chronic nasopharyngeal obstruction, relative hypoventilation, and alveolar hypoxia. In addition, sleep apnea seen in children with Down syndrome produces hypoventilation, hypercarbia, and increased pulmonary vascular resistance.[150] Hemodynamic studies of patients with AVSD and Down syndrome have documented a fixed and elevated pulmonary vascular resistance in 11% of patients less than 1 year of age.[150]

Management

The management of the child with AVSD is determined by the child's symptoms, anatomy, and presence of pulmonary vascular disease. Surgical intervention is ultimately required because the defects do not close spontaneously and are not amenable to catheter closure.

Repair of Partial AVSD. Because the partial AVSD rarely causes congestive heart failure, management consists of surgical closure between 6 and 12 months of age. If the diagnosis is not made until the infant is older, surgical repair is performed when the diagnosis is made.[575]

If significant mitral valve regurgitation is present, repair should not be delayed. Regurgitant flow thickens the leaflets around the cleft. Although some surgeons feel that this is beneficial to provide more secure sutures, most feel that the distortion and foreshortening of the valve leaflets prevent the surgical achievement of a competent valve.[145]

Repair of an AVSD is preformed through a median sternotomy incision and uses hypothermic cardiopulmonary bypass. The defect is approached through the right atrium. If there is a small, restrictive inlet ventricular septal defect, this defect will be closed first. Careful placement of sutures in this area is necessary to avoid surgically induced atrioventricular block.[275] The cleft in the mitral valve is then sutured to prevent regurgitation and the primum ASD is closed with autologous pericardium. Synthetic patch material is avoided because it can contribute to hemolysis if there is persistent mitral valve regurgitation postoperatively. At the time of surgery, the surgeon verifies that the mitral valve is competent. Surgical results are excellent with an operative mortality of 2%.[575]

The most frequent postoperative complication is arrhythmia. Supraventricular tachycardia is the most common rhythm disturbance, occurring in about 16% of children following correction of AVSD. Complete heart block is seen in 3%.[575]

Reoperation may be needed in 10% to 15% of patients after repair of AVSD. The most common indication for reoperation is mitral valve regurgitation, although some patients may require reoperation for subaortic stenosis. The goal for reoperation of the mitral valve is to repair the valve, but some require replacement. Surgery may be delayed with little added risk if valve replacement seems likely.[575,686]

Repair of Complete AVSD. For the child with complete atrioventricular septal defect preoperative management includes medical therapy for congestive heart failure using diuretics and afterload reduction (see section, Common Clinical Conditions, Congestive Heart Failure). Medical management also includes nutritional support to minimize failure to thrive (see section, Common Clinical Conditions, Altered Nutrition and Potential Gastrointestinal Complications).

To prevent permanent development of pulmonary vascular obstructive disease and to treat congestive heart failure, surgical repair for uncomplicated complete AVSDs is typically performed in early infancy (at about 2 to 4 months).[575]

The goals of surgical repair of an infant with a balanced, complete AVSD include complete closure of the atrial and ventricular septal defects and effective use of the available atrioventricular septal valve tissue to create two competent atrioventricular valves. In an uncomplicated complete AVSD this may be accomplished in infants in the neonatal period, including those weighing as little as 3 kg.[45,492] The critical component of this repair is the repair of the valve, particularly the left atrioventricular or mitral valve. Dysfunction of the right-sided atrioventricular (tricuspid) valve is much better tolerated than dysfunction of the left atrioventricular valve.[275,575]

A pulmonary artery banding is a palliative procedure performed through a left thoracotomy, without cardiopulmonary bypass. A "band" of synthetic material is placed around the pulmonary artery in an attempt to reduce pulmonary blood flow, decrease the severity of congestive heart failure, and reduce the risk of pulmonary vascular disease. This band on the pulmonary artery may cause distortion of the pulmonary valve or artery.[153]

Only in extreme cases—including complex anatomy, sepsis or respiratory illnesses such as respiratory syncytial virus or pneumonia—is palliative surgery with placement of pulmonary artery band considered.[145,150,153] Some centers report successful outcomes with pulmonary artery banding for infants less than 1 month of age and less than 5 kg who exhibit significant congestive heart failure unresponsive to medical treatment. Successful banding has also been reported for infants with significant associated anomalies. However, the combined reported mortality rate (for banding and later debanding with complete repair) is as high as 15%.[150,686]

For complete correction of AVSD the defect is approached through a median sternotomy incision and repaired during hypothermic, cardiopulmonary bypass. The repair is performed through an incision in the right atrium. Based on the preference of the surgeon, either a single patch or double patch technique is used to close the atrial septal defect and ventricular septal defect and reconstruct the atrioventricular valve (Fig. 8-36).[41,145,150,275,575,623]

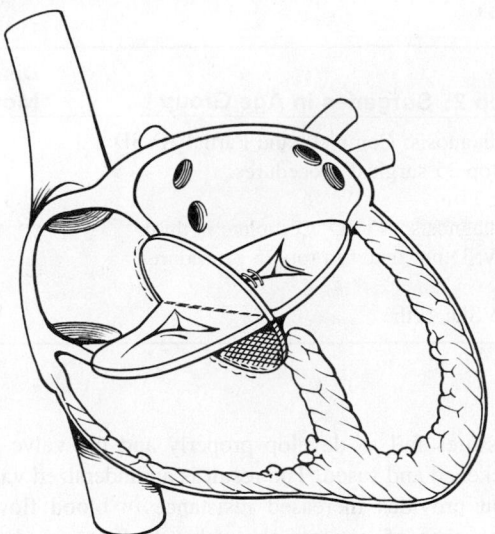

FIG. 8-36 Surgical correction of atrioventricular septal defect. A patch is used to close the atrial septal defect (pericardium is usually used). When a complete AVSD is present (as shown), a second woven patch (usually Dacron) can be used to close the ventricular septal defect. The patches are placed to divide common atrioventricular valve tissue, particularly the bridging anterior leaflet. Clefts in the mitral valve are sutured to prevent significant postoperative mitral insufficiency while avoiding the creation of mitral stenosis. (From Bender HW, et al: Repair of atrioventricular canal malformation in the first year of life. *J Thorac and Cardiovasc Surg* 84:518, 1982.)

In the single patch technique repair of AVSD, autologous pericardium is used to close the defects. In the double patch procedure, a Dacron patch is used to close the VSD and autologous pericardium is used to close the ASD. Usually the cleft in the left atrioventricular valve is sutured to form a bi-leaflet valve. Chordal attachments of the atrioventricular valve must be identified preoperatively with a surface echocardiogram or in the operating room with a transesophageal echocardiogram. The surgeon visually confirms the anatomy and makes the appropriate adjustments in patch placement. The abnormal location of the conduction system makes it critically important that the surgeon place the sutures to avoid the conduction tissue. Direct injury to the conduction tissue or edema around the sutures can cause postoperative heart block, including complete atrioventricular block.[275]

Postoperative complications following repair of complete AVSDs include persistent mitral valve regurgitation, low cardiac output, pulmonary hypertension, elevated left atrial pressures, and arrhythmias such as heart block and junctional atrial tachycardia. Because the atrioventricular valve has been reconstructed and risk of persistent AV valve regurgitation remains, volume loading to increase cardiac output should be avoided if at all possible for the first 24 postoperative hours. Volume loading may put tension on the site of valve sutures and can increase AV valve regurgitation. Atrial filling pressures should be maintained at lower values with inotropic support used to increase cardiac output, as needed. If either a residual ventricular septal defect or significant AV valve regurgitation is thought to be present, aggressive afterload reduction is needed.[153]

Postoperative mortality is related to pulmonary hypertension. It is important to recognize any anatomic causes of pulmonary hypertension, such as severe left atrioventricular valve stenosis or regurgitation, or a residual ventricular septal defect.[153] The trend toward earlier age of repair has decreased the risk of pulmonary hypertension. When correction is performed at less than 3 months of age, fixed elevated pulmonary vascular resistance is rare and outcomes are good. If surgical repair occurs at 6 months of age or older, pulmonary vascular resistance may be elevated and postoperative pulmonary arterial hypertensive crises may be observed postoperatively.[575] (For additional information, please refer to Common Clinical Conditions, Low Cardiac Output and Common Clinical Conditions, Pulmonary Hypertension, as well as the third section of this chapter, Postoperative Care and Anticoagulation.)

Postoperative arrhythmias may be problematic following repair of complete AVSD. As noted, the conduction tissue is in an abnormal position at the rim of the septal defect. Sinoatrial dysfunction may be present preoperatively, and complete heart block may be present postoperatively. When dysfunction of the sinoatrial node is present, cardiac output may be improved with atrial pacing. The preferred treatment of complete heart block is AV sequential pacing. Atrioventricular valve regurgitation may increase if ventricular (ventricular sensing, pacing inbited, or VVI) pacing is provided, rather than atrioventricular pacing.[153]

The mortality rate following repair of AVSD averages 3% to 10%. The surgical mortality is the same for patients with and without Down syndrome. Increased mortality risk for complete repair of an AVSD is associated with very young age at operation, severity of preoperative atrioventricular valve regurgitation, hypoplasia of the left ventricle, increased or fixed pulmonary vascular resistance, and severity of preoperative symptoms.[150,686]

If additional defects are present they can increase the operative risk. Patients with complex forms of atrioventricular septal defects include unbalanced AVSD (surgical risk is highest for right ventricular dominant defect; this means left ventricular hypoplasia is present) and when the defect is present in combination with tetralogy of Fallot, transposition of the great arteries, and double outlet ventricles. Please refer to those associated defects discussed in the following sections.

Surgical repair of AVSDs is one of the great success stories in the past several decades of congenital cardiac surgery.[150] In the STS Congenital Heart Surgery Data Summary, partial AVSD repairs in children have a postoperative mortality of 0%, and infant repairs of complete AVSD repairs has a mortality of 2% (Table 8-31).[851-853] Long-term survival is excellent. Reoperation is required for 2.5% of patients, most often indicated for progressive left atrioventricular valve regurgitation or for relief of left ventricular outflow tract obstruction.[150] Endocarditis remains a long-term postoperative risk for most patients, so antibiotic prophylaxis is recommended for periods of increased risk of bacteremia (see section, Bacterial Endocarditis).

Care of the infant or child with AVSD is both challenging and rewarding. Advanced concepts regarding atrioventricular septal defects are listed in Box 8-25.

Table 8-31   Summary of Surgical Repair of AVSD 2006-2010[851-853]

Age Group	Total Number of AVSD Surgical Procedures	Rank: Top 25 Surgeries in Age Group	Discharge Mortality
Neonate (0-30 days)	–	Primary diagnosis: Complete and Partial AVSD not in top 25 surgical procedures.	–
	696	PA Band: 11th	12.8%
Infant (31 days to 1 year)	2241	Primary diagnosis: AVSD, Complete is third;	2.2%
	–	Partial AVSD not listed in top 25 procedures	–
	564	PA Band	5.5%
Child (>1 year to <18 years)	526	Partial AVSD: 19th	0.0%

Box 8-25   Advanced Concepts: Atrioventricular Septal Defect (AVSD)

- Atrioventricular septal defects are the most common defects in patients with Down syndrome.
- The degree of atrioventricular valve regurgitation determines the onset of symptoms in both forms of AVSDs.
- A delay in the onset of symptoms past 2 months may indicate persistent pulmonary hypertension.
- Surgical repair of complete AVSD is performed before 6 months of age to prevent pulmonary vascular obstructive disease.
- Abnormal development of the conduction system is an important risk factor for postoperative arrhythmias, especially complete heart block.

ACYANOTIC DEFECTS: OBSTRUCTIVE LESIONS

Pulmonary Stenosis

Nancy A. Rudd

Pearls

- Pulmonary stenosis can present as critical stenosis in the newborn period, requiring urgent valvuloplasty.
- Pulmonary stenosis presenting in the older infant or child may be mild, moderate, or severe; mild stenosis is unlikely to progress in severity but moderate and severe stenosis typically will progress in severity.
- Diagnosis is made by echocardiography. The treatment of choice for most pulmonary stenosis is a valvuloplasty performed during cardiac catheterization.
- Surgical intervention is typically indicated when critical pulmonary stenosis is not responsive to valvuloplasty, when valve leaflets are dysplastic or when there are multiple areas of obstruction in the pulmonary outflow tract.

Etiology

Pulmonary Valve Stenosis. Pulmonary valve stenosis results from abnormal formation of pulmonary valve leaflets during fetal cardiac development. The normal pulmonary valve has three leaflets and is situated between the distal right ventricular outflow tract and the proximal main pulmonary artery. Pulmonary valve stenosis most commonly occurs when valve

commissures fail to develop properly and the valve leaflets are thickened and fused. The result is an undersized valve orifice that provides increased resistance to blood flow. In a small number of patients the valve leaflets are dysplastic (abnormally shaped), and the pulmonary valve annulus is small. Either defect impedes flow from the right ventricle to the pulmonary artery.

The error in pulmonary valve formation likely occurs late in embryologic development. If the error occurred early in fetal life, the outcome would be complete underdevelopment of the pulmonary outflow tract. Familial cases of pulmonary valve stenosis have been reported, and siblings of patients with pulmonary stenosis have an increased incidence of congenital heart disease.[711]

Pulmonary stenosis is responsible for 8% to 12% of all congenital heart defects and may manifest with varying degrees of severity and at any age. Isolated pulmonary valve stenosis with an intact ventricular septum accounts for 80% to 90% of right ventricular outflow tract obstructive lesions and is one of the most common congenital heart defects.[711] Isolated pulmonary valve stenosis is not commonly associated with other cardiac lesions.

The morphology of isolated pulmonary valve stenosis can be categorized into anatomic subgroups including descriptive terms such as domed, tricuspid, bicuspid, unicommissural, hypoplastic, and dysplastic. Thickened leaflets and commissural fusion are typically present in all subgroups except the dysplastic subgroup. Dysplastic stenosis accounts for approximately 10% to 20% of all cases of isolated pulmonary valve stenosis,[620] and is the most common type of pulmonary stenosis associated with chromosomal anomalies and syndromes such as Noonan's syndrome.

Supravalvular and Infundibular Stenosis. Less common but additional forms of right ventricular outflow tract obstruction include supravalvular and infundibular pulmonary stenosis (also referred to as subvalvular stenosis). Supravalvular pulmonary stenosis is a rare lesion that occurs with Noonan's syndrome and occasionally with William's syndrome.[451]

Primary infundibular stenosis accounts for approximately 5% of all cases of right ventricular outflow tract obstruction. There are two types of isolated infundibular stenosis. The first type results from fibromuscular thickening in the wall of the right ventricular infundibulum. The other form is characterized by an obstructive muscle band at the junction of the right ventricle cavity and the proximal infundibulum.[620] More commonly, infundibular pulmonary stenosis occurs in combination with three other lesions to create tetralogy of Fallot (see Tetralogy of Fallot later in this section of the chapter).

Pathophysiology

Pathophysiology and management strategies for all forms of isolated right ventricular outflow obstruction vary with the location and severity of the stenosis and the presentation of symptoms. Most patients have either critical pulmonary stenosis, which presents in the newborn period, or valvular pulmonary stenosis, which presents in older infants and children.[620]

With any pulmonary stenosis, the radius of the valve orifice is reduced and resistance to flow through the pulmonary valve is increased. To maintain normal flow across the small outflow tract, the right ventricle must generate a higher pressure proportional to the severity of the pulmonary stenosis. The resulting right ventricular hypertension and the obstruction of blood flow through the right ventricular outflow tract produces a quantifiable pressure gradient between the right ventricle and the main pulmonary artery that is directly related to the degree of stenosis. If the right ventricle cannot increase pressure proportionate to the severity of the pulmonary stenosis, blood flow (right ventricular output and pulmonary blood flow) will decrease.

The calculated gradient across the stenotic valve is categorized as mild (less than 40 mm Hg), moderate (40-80 mm Hg), or severe (greater than 80 mm Hg) based on the pressure gradient between the right ventricle and pulmonary artery. These severity classifications are shown in Box 8-26.

Critical pulmonary stenosis of the newborn, if untreated, can lead to hemodynamic instability soon after birth. Severely limited right ventricular output and the presence of right ventricular hypertrophy at birth causes decreased diastolic compliance, elevated right ventricular pressure, and corresponding elevation in right atrial pressure. Typically newborns with critical pulmonary stenosis have an associated atrial shunt (through an atrial septal defect [ASD] or a patent foramen ovale [PFO]). The tricuspid valve and right ventricular size are usually normal, although some hypoplasia may be present. Because right atrial pressure substantially exceeds left atrial pressure, a right-to-left atrial level shunt develops, resulting in cyanosis. This shunt increases left ventricular output.

Myocardial oxygen supply may be compromised by hypoxemia and lower diastolic coronary perfusion pressure resulting from low-resistance runoff into the pulmonary circulation

from the patent ductus arteriosus (PDA). If the defect is not detected early after birth, closure of the ductus arterious results in decreased pulmonary blood flow, worsening hypoxemia, acidosis, and cardiovascular collapse.[620]

When valvular pulmonary stenosis is present in older infants and children, the main hemodynamic effect is a rise in right ventricular pressure proportionate to the severity of valve obstruction. Chronic elevation of this pressure results in the development of right ventricular hypertrophy and decreased right ventricular compliance. Over time, this right ventricle may dilate and fail. Tricuspid regurgitation may develop and worsen right ventricular failure.[451] Other associated right-heart findings include poststenotic dilation of the main pulmonary artery caused by the jet of blood flowing through the narrowed valve oriface.

When pulmonary stenosis is mild, it does not usually progress in severity. However, with moderate or severe forms of pulmonary stenosis, the severity typically increases with age because the size of stenotic orifice remains fixed as the patient grows.

Clinical Signs and Symptoms

This cardiac defect is often discovered because a murmur is detected during routine auscultation at birth. Auscultatory findings in valvular pulmonary stenosis reveal a normal first heart sound followed by a pulmonary ejection click in patients with mild or moderate stenosis. With severe stenosis the click occurs so early in systole that it merges with the first heart sound and becomes inaudible.[711] A systolic ejection murmur is also present, loudest at the upper left sternal border with radiation over the entire precordium, axillae, and back. The intensity of the murmur generally increases with the degree of obstruction, and severe stenosis typically produces a grade IV murmur and a palpable thrill.

Neonates with critical pulmonary stenosis are cyanotic at birth for hemodynamic reasons discussed earlier. Initially cardiac output is maintained if an adequate atrial shunt is present, but cyanosis is apparent. With ductal closure, cyanosis worsens and hemodynamic deterioration is associated with tachycardia, tachypnea, and respiratory distress.[620] Of note, patients with severe stenosis and right heart failure may have an unusually soft murmur because cardiac output is low, so blood flow through the stenotic pulmonary valve is limited.

Most infants and children with mild pulmonary valve stenosis are asymptomatic and have normal growth and development. Even with moderate pulmonary stenosis, symptoms often do not present until late infancy or childhood. Fatigue or exertional dyspnea may result because cardiac output is limited by the fixed obstruction. Severe, longstanding obstruction may cause symptoms of congestive heart failure. Less common findings include chest pain, syncope, or ventricular arrhythmias.[620]

Cardiac catheterization is no longer needed for the diagnosis of pulmonary stenosis but is indicated for therapeutic intervention. The ECG can be somewhat helpful in diagnosing pulmonary stenosis. About half of patients with mild pulmonary stenosis have a normal ECG and half demonstrate a right ventricular conduction delay.[711] With moderate to severe pulmonary stenosis, the ECG is almost always abnormal with

---

Box 8-26 | **Classification of Pulmonary Stenosis Based on Severity of Pressure Gradient Between Right Ventricle and Pulmonary Artery**

Mild stenosis: <40 mm Hg gradient
Moderate stenosis: 40-80 mm Hg gradient
Severe stenosis: >80 mm Hg gradient

right axis deviation and right ventricular hypertrophy proportional to the severity of obstruction (see Table 8-26 as needed).

The definitive diagnostic technique for pulmonary stenosis is two-dimensional echocardiography with color Doppler. Echocardiography delineates the size of the pulmonary annulus, the level of obstruction, and valve leaflet mobility, shape, number, and thickness. Echocardiographic calculation of the pressure gradient across the pulmonary outflow tract has been shown to correlate well with direct measurements and is about 10% greater than peak-to-peak pressure gradients obtained in the cardiac catheterization laboratory.[288] The degree of obstruction is classified as mild, moderate or severe based on pressure ranges detailed in Box 8-26.

Reports of the natural history for children with pulmonary valve stenosis are mixed. Several reports have documented that the degree of obstruction present at initial diagnosis correlates with progression of the obstruction over the child's lifetime[751] and that children presenting at a younger age are more likely to have progression to severe obstruction.[360] However, one study using serial echocardiograms documented a diminishing degree of stenosis in children with initial mild to moderate levels of obstruction.[320] Therefore because it not currently possible to predict with certainty which subset of children will have significant progression of obstruction, all patients diagnosed with even mild stenosis require close followup with a pediatric cardiologist.

Management

Medical Management. Catheter intervention is the accepted first line treatment for symptomatic pulmonary valve stenosis. When relief of obstruction is indicated, balloon dilation has become the treatment of choice, and surgical intervention is rarely undertaken. A continuous infusion of prostaglandin E_1 is required to maintain ductal patency in newborns with critical pulmonary stenosis as they await catheter intervention.

Pulmonary Valvuloplasty. Currently catheter intervention is the accepted initial treatment for pulmonary valve stenosis at any age and for all valve morphologies. Advances in equipment and technique allow even small neonates with critical pulmonary valve stenosis to undergo immediate valvuloplasty in the neonatal period.

Any symptomatic older infant or child requires catheter intervention as soon as the diagnosis of pulmonary stenosis is made. Even asymptomatic patients with severe obstruction should undergo semielective valvuloplasty.

The technique of percutaneous pulmonary balloon valvuloplasty was first described in early 1980s.[430] Typically a balloon is chosen that is 20% to 40% larger than the pulmonary valve annulus measured angiographically. The balloon is positioned and inflated at the midpoint of the anatomic narrowing. Relief of obstruction results as the valve tears along fused commissures. In patients with a large pulmonary annulus, simultaneous inflation of two balloons may be necessary. The neonate or young infant with an extremely small pulmonary valve orifice may require initial dilation with a small coronary angioplasty balloon to enlarge the orifice enough to allow subsequent dilations with larger balloons.[711]

Any neonate with unsuccessful pulmonary balloon valvuloplasty should undergo immediate surgical valvotomy.

Results with percutaneous balloon valvuloplasty to treat isolated pulmonary valve stenosis have been very good.[594] A successful outcome is defined as a postprocedure Doppler gradient less than 36 mm Hg without the need for repeat valvuloplasty or valvotomy. The Valvuloplasty and Angioplasty of Congenital Anomalies Registry reported followup data for 533 patients up to 8 years after initial catheter intervention. Eighty-four percent were noted to be free from further catheter or surgical procedures and 75% had gradients less than 36 mm Hg. Of those with an initial gradient greater than 36 mm Hg, just over half showed spontaneous regression of gradients to less than 36 mm Hg. Of the remaining 62 patients, 25 underwent subsequent surgery, 23 had repeat balloon valvuloplasty, and 14 remained with gradient greater than 36 mm Hg. Restenosis following initial intervention was also assessed. For patients with optimal immediate results only 12% had a significant gradient at followup or required reintervention for progressive stenosis.[594]

Patients with lower balloon valvuloplasty success rates are those with dysplastic pulmonary valves. Although balloon dilatation effectively splits fused commissures of typical stenotic valves, the thickened leaflets of a dysplastic valve do not respond as predictably to balloon dilation. Reported valvuloplasty associated complications (although uncommon) include vein tears, vein thrombosis, arrhythmia, perforation of the right ventricular outflow tract, tamponade, seizures, and stroke.[828]

Most patients treated with pulmonary valvuloplasty have some degree of pulmonary insufficiency following dilation. In a large follow-up study looking at degree of pulmonary regurgitation, 26% of patients had no regurgitation, 22% had trivial regurgitation, 45% had mild regurgitation, 7% had moderate regurgitation, and no patients demonstrated severe regurgitation.[594] Some speculate that use of excessively large balloons corresponds with more severe insufficiency. Some residual postprocedure stenosis with little or no insufficiency is thought to be preferable to aggressive dilation that eliminates any gradient but is more likely to produce significant pulmonary regurgitation. Any degree of insufficiency must be monitored over time for possible progression and need for intervention. Overall, results of balloon dilation of pulmonary valve stenosis as long as 20 years ago are favorable.[640]

Despite successful relief of obstruction, a small percentage of infants with critical pulmonary stenosis may have persistent cyanosis after catheter intervention. Their right-to-left shunt probably results from low compliance of the right ventricle that is likely to be temporary. Typically the cyanosis resolves over a few weeks as right ventricular compliance improves, right atrial pressure decreases and the right-to-left shunt decreases. Temporary prostaglandin therapy can be used to augment insufficient forward flow across the pulmonary valve and into the pulmonary circulation.

If ductal dependency persists following valvuloplasty, one of two treatment strategies is undertaken.[711] One available strategy is temporary placement of an aortopulmonary shunt that remains in place until the right heart grows sufficiently and right ventricular compliance improves. A second strategy is stenting (open) of the ductus in the interventional catheterization laboratory using an intravascular stent.[640] At a later time when hemodynamically acceptable, these temporary shunts can be closed surgically or by interventional catheterization methods.

Patients who initially have mild hypoplasia of right heart structures at birth usually have sufficient growth of these underdeveloped areas over a period of months following relief of pulmonary outflow obstruction. However, in a small population of neonates with critical pulmonary stenosis, persistent right ventricular hypoplasia may necessitate staged single ventricle palliation (see section, Single Functioning Ventricle).

Surgical Management: Valvotomy. Isolated pulmonary stenosis is no longer a defect that is treated surgically. With the introduction of pulmonary balloon valvuloplasty, surgical pulmonary valvotomy is reserved for those patients with dysplastic valves resistant to dilation or when the pulmonary outflow tract has multiple areas of obstruction not conducive to valvuloplasty alone.[451] As noted, any neonate with critical pulmonary valve stenosis not responsive to balloon dilation requires immediate surgical valvotomy.

When surgery is indicated to address isolated pulmonary valve stenosis, open commissurotomy is the most common surgical procedure performed. Via median sternotomy and using cardiopulmonary bypass, the main pulmonary artery is opened transversely or longitudinally to expose the valve. The valve commissures are incised to the annulus. If annular enlargement (enlargement of the valve orifice) is required, a transannular patch made of autologous pericardium or prosthetic material is inserted. In the case of dysplastic valves, a simple valvotomy may not be effective in relieving obstruction, and partial or even total removal of the valve may be required.

The degree of pulmonary insufficiency present following surgical intervention varies from patient to patient. Mild pulmonary insufficiency is usually well tolerated. However, patients requiring patch augmentation or valve removal are frequently left with moderate or severe pulmonary insufficiency. If the insufficiency is progressive and pulmonary regurgitation becomes severe, a valve replacement may be necessary.

Surgical Management of Supravalvular Pulmonary Artery Stenosis and Primary Infundibular Stenosis. Surgical management mirrors that for isolated pulmonary valve stenosis. However, unlike isolated pulmonary valve stenosis, the primary mode of management for these two lesions is surgical.[620] In most cases of supravalvular stenosis, patch enlargement is all that is required. If infundibular obstruction is present, an extremely small incision is made in the pulmonary outflow tract to allow resection of the infundibular muscle under direct visualization. The infundibular stenosis may also be resected via transatrial route through the tricuspid valve. Recent surgical outcomes reported for this lesion are not available because balloon valvuloplasty has replaced surgery as the primary treatment strategy for this lesion.

Surgical Management: Pulmonary Valve Replacement. The presence of induced pulmonary insufficiency following surgical pulmonary valvotomy or pulmonary balloon valvuloplasty may necessitate the insertion of a competent valve in the pulmonary position. Controversy exists regarding the precise indications for intervention. At present, reported intervention criteria usually include echocardiographic evidence of progressive right ventricular dilation and associated enlargement of the pulmonary valve annulus leading to increasing tricuspid insufficiency. Clinical indications include progressive decrease in exercise tolerance, signs of right heart failure, or the presence of atrial or ventricular arrhythmias.[250]

A variety of prosthetic valves can be surgically placed in the pulmonary position, including homograft valves, xenograft valves, pericardial valves, and mechanical valves. Valve replacement requires open heart surgery using cardiopulmonary bypass. If a mechanical valve is placed, long-term anticoagulation is indicated (see Postoperative Care and Anticoagulation).

Ideally, pulmonary valve replacement should occur when the child is sufficiently grown to receive a valve that will last to adult years, but it should be performed before irreversible damage to the right ventricle and tricuspid valve has occurred. The concern is that implanted valves have limited longevity because calcifications and intimal thickening can develop over time, resulting in pulmonary stenosis or insufficiency. Most children requiring a prosthetic valve placement during infancy or early childhood will require subsequent valve replacement(s).

Since 2000, successful percutaneous pulmonary valve replacement has been performed using a bovine jugular venous valve sutured inside a stent.[91] The possible benefit of eliminating the need for repeat thoracotomy and cardiopulmonary bypass makes this a potentially appealing option, and although long-term followup regarding effectiveness and safety of this intervention is not yet available, research in this area of interventional cardiac catheterization is ongoing.[470]

Antibiotic prophylaxis against endocarditis is no longer recommended postoperatively, with the exception of prosthetic pulmonary valves and for a 6-month period after placement of prosthetic material to augment the pulmonary outflow tract or repair the pulmonary valve.[951]

Advanced concepts regarding pulmonary stenosis are listed in Box 8-27.

Box 8-27	**Advanced Concepts: Pulmonary Valve Stenosis**

The intensity of a murmur of pulmonary stenosis often increases in proportion to the degree of obstruction of flow across the stenotic area. However, patients with severe pulmonary stenosis may have an unusually soft murmur because right heart failure and low cardiac output can limit blood flow across the right ventricular outflow tract.

Aortic Stenosis (AS)

Nancy A. Rudd

Pearls

- Aortic stenosis may be valvular, subvalvular (subaortic), or supravalvular (supraaortic).
- The severity of aortic stenosis may be estimated by Doppler or during cardiac catheterization.
- Estimates of the severity of aortic stenosis will be falsely low if cardiac output is low.
- Percutaneous balloon aortic valvuloplasty has replaced surgical valvotomy as the therapy of choice for valvular aortic stenosis in infants and children requiring intervention.
- Subvalvular and supravalvular aortic stenosis require surgical intervention.

Etiology

The term *aortic stenosis* is used to indicate any obstruction of outflow from the left ventricle to the ascending aorta in the region of the aortic valve. Embryologically, the aortic valve develops from three ridges of subendocardial tissue that form when the aortopulmonary septum divides into the aortic and pulmonary trunks. A normal aortic valve is trileaflet and functions without obstruction. Abnormal development of either the number or morphology of the valve cusps and commissures results in varying forms and degrees of aortic stenosis.

The degree of abnormal development of the aortic outflow tract results in a clinical continuum of congenital aortic stenosis. This continuum can range from a normally functioning, but malformed bicuspid aortic valve, to severe aortic stenosis in the fetus resulting in hypoplastic left heart syndrome (HLHS; detailed elsewhere—see section, Single Functioning Ventricle). In general, obstructive lesions are categorized based on the location of the obstruction: valvular stenosis, subvalvular stenosis, or supravalvular stenosis.

Valvular aortic stenosis is the most common form, occurring in about 75% of all patients with aortic outflow obstruction. Stenosis of the valve is caused by decreased orifice size resulting from thickening and rigidity of valve leaflets. Males with valvular aortic stenosis outnumber females 4:1; however, subvalvular and supravalvular stenosis are only slightly more common in males that females. The most common abnormality of the aortic valve is a bicuspid aortic valve and occurs in about two thirds of patients with valvular aortic stenosis. An estimated 1% to 5% of all infants are born with a bicuspid aortic valve, although only a small percentage develops stenosis from fusion of the two abnormal leaflets.

Subvalvular aortic stenosis or *subaortic* stenosis is the second most common form of aortic obstruction and accounts for about 20% of patients with left ventricular outflow tract obstruction. Subaortic stenosis can occur as an isolated lesion or in association with other congenital heart defects. Three types of subaortic stenosis are described. The discrete membranous type is a fibromuscular ring with a central orifice that is located below the aortic valve. A second type is the hypertrophic type. This form results from hypertrophy of the interventricular septum and anterior leaflet of the mitral valve and leads to dynamic outflow tract obstruction that is often called *hypertrophic cardiomyopathy* (HCM). The least common type of subaortic stenosis is the fibromuscular tunnel type, which consists of a long segment of narrowing beneath the aortic valve.[444]

Supravalvular aortic stenosis, or *supraaortic* stenosis, the least common form of aortic obstruction, is caused by either localized or diffuse fibromembranous narrowing of the aorta above the aortic valve and coronary arteries. The aortic valve leaflets may also be thickened and abnormal and in some cases, the coronary artery ostia can be obstructed by membranous tissue.[780]

Aortic stenosis is believed to result from a complex interaction of genetic and environmental factors. Proposed causes include abnormal formation of the valve cusps during embryologic development and environmental influences such as prenatal infection or metabolic disturbances causing damage to the valve resulting in stenosis. Familial patterns of left ventricular outflow tract obstruction have been reported ranging from bicuspid aortic valve, to valvular AS, to coarctation of the aorta, to hypoplastic left heart syndrome (HLHS) and suggest a hereditary link as well. Recent genetic research has linked abnormalities in the chromosomal regions 5q, 13q, 18q,[572] and the occurrence of aortic stenosis. Genetic defects associated with aortic stenosis include Turner syndrome and Jacobsen syndrome. Supravalvular aortic stenosis is associated with William's syndrome.[780]

Aortic stenosis is one of the more common forms of congenital heart disease (CHD), occurring in 4% to 8% of all infants born with CHD. It is now appreciated that congenital aortic stenosis is more common than previously recognized because many adults diagnosed with "acquired" aortic stenosis actually have congenitally bicuspid aortic valve. Additional or associated congenital heart defects occur in 20% of patients with congenital aortic valve stenosis. The most common are VSD, PDA, coarctation of the aorta, and mitral valve anomalies. Aortic insufficiency is often associated with aortic stenosis.

Pathophysiology

All forms of aortic stenosis produce obstruction of left ventricular outflow resulting in impedance to left ventricular ejection. Whenever there is obstruction to left ventricular outflow the left ventricle must generate higher pressure to maintain normal flow beyond the area of resistance. As a result, left ventricular hypertension develops that is proportional to the degree of aortic obstruction. This pressure overload leads to the development of left ventricular hypertrophy and can lead to left ventricular failure, resulting in elevated left ventricular end-diastolic and left atrial pressures and pulmonary edema.

Aortic stenosis can compromise blood flow to the coronary arteries, because the stenosis can reduce coronary perfusion pressure (difference between aortic end-diastolic pressure and right atrial pressure) and results in prolonged ejection (systole) and shortened diastole (the predominant time that the left coronary artery perfuses the left ventricle). The mismatch between coronary artery perfusion (oxygen delivery) and oxygen demand can be magnified during periods of stress or exercise when oxygen demand is increased; during these periods tachycardia further reduces ventricular diastolic filling and coronary perfusion time and the gradient across the aortic stenosis increases.[531] If hypertrophy is severe, blood supply to the subendocardial tissue may be inadequate, resulting in subendocardial ischemia, arrhythmias, and even myocardial infarction.

When supravalvular aortic stenosis is present, left ventricular hypertrophy still occurs. However, coronary artery perfusion is usually adequate because the coronary artery ostia are located proximal to the aortic obstruction.

The degree of obstruction in AS is typically expressed in terms of catheter-derived peak-to-peak gradient, peak instantaneous echo Doppler gradient, mean systolic pressure gradient calculated from Doppler measurements, or mean pressure gradients derived from simultaneous catheter recordings. The pressure measurement necessary to quantify aortic stenosis as mild, moderate or severe is based on the measurement technique used and often varies from one institution to another.

Clinical Signs and Symptoms

Valvular Stenosis. Neonates, infants and children present with varying degrees of valvular aortic stenosis. Those with mild to even moderate stenosis are relatively asymptomatic. Some neonates have such left heart hypoplasia that they are incapable of sustaining systemic circulation; these infants require single ventricle palliation (see section, Single Functioning Ventricle).

Neonates with adequate left ventricular size but critical aortic valve obstruction may initially tolerate even moderate obstruction; however, gradients may increase substantially during the first days or weeks of life when left ventricular function becomes hyperdynamic, the ductus arteriosus closes, or associated defects such as muscular ventricular septal defects (VSD) close spontaneously. When the ductus arteriosus closes, pulmonary vascular resistance falls, and pulmonary blood flow and venous return to the left atrium increase. If the left ventricle cannot generate the high pressure required to maintain this blood flow through the stenotic outflow tract, signs and symptoms of heart failure or even cardiogenic shock develop and can be fatal without appropriate intervention.

Neonates with critical aortic stenosis are pale, dyspneic, and tachycardic. Physical examination reveals a hyperactive precordium, poor distal pulses, poor peripheral perfusion, and cyanosis. A cardiac murmur is frequently absent when low cardiac output is present. Although a gallop rhythm may be appreciated, an ejection click is rarely heard.[780]

Infants with severe but not critical AS typically present in infancy with signs and symptoms of heart failure, including poor feeding, tachypnea, and growth failure. Physical examination reveals a hyperactive precordium and a thrill is palpated in the suprasternal notch. A precordial thrill is often present with mild to moderate stenosis. On auscultation a characteristic ejection murmur is often heard along the left upper sternal border, radiating to the neck. A systolic ejection murmur may not be present if LV function is significantly reduced and blood flow across the aortic valve (cardiac output) is limited. The presence of a systolic ejection click points to valvular rather than supravalvular or subvalvular

obstruction. In addition, patients may develop right ventricular failure and hepatomegaly.

Older children with valvular aortic stenosis can be relatively asymptomatic with appropriate growth and development. Some report easy fatigability, which appears to be unrelated to the severity of AS. Those who develop severe obstruction are at greatest risk for exercise intolerance, anginal pain, syncopal events, and even sudden death. Older children typically have normal vital signs, including blood pressure. Auscultation may reveal a systolic ejection murmur with intensity proportional to the extent of stenosis. Approximately one third of patients also have a diastolic murmur resulting from aortic regurgitation. More than half of children with valvular aortic stenosis have an ejection click heard best at the apex or lower left sternal border. Visible apical activity and an increased left ventricular impulse on palpation are found with severe aortic stenosis.

The diagnosis of aortic stenosis is almost always made by physical examination and echocardiography. Two-dimensional echocardiography with color Doppler analysis is used to estimate the level and severity of obstruction, evaluate valve and left ventricular outflow tract morphology, and estimate left ventricular function and the degree of aortic regurgitation. Doppler-derived peak instantaneous pressure gradients are calculated across the stenotic aortic valve. Traditionally, catheter-derived peak-to-peak pressure gradients recorded during cardiac catheterization were used to estimate the severity of stenosis and direct management. It is important to note that the Doppler-derived peak instantaneous pressure gradient represents a different physiologic parameter (i.e., calculated from blood flow velocities) than the catheter-derived peak-to-peak pressure gradient, and the two are not interchangeable. The Doppler peak instantaneous gradient is higher than peak-to-peak gradients obtained during catheterization.[780] A mean systolic pressure gradient can be calculated from the Doppler measurements, and this echocardiographic assessment of severity of obstruction is shown to correlate well with mean pressure gradients derived from simultaneous catheter recordings in the catheterization laboratory.[972] Many centers currently favor using mean pressure gradients to guide clinical management of aortic stenosis.

The ECG is of limited use in diagnosing children with AS and has limited utility in distinguishing mild from severe obstruction. A 24-hour ambulatory ECG (Holter) monitor in asymptomatic patients may detect ventricular arrhythmias. A strong relationship has been reported between arrhythmias and sudden death in patients with AS.[780]

The chest radiograph in newborns with critical aortic stenosis and CHF reveals cardiomegaly with venous congestion. A dilated ascending aorta may be seen in older patients with valvular aortic stenosis and results from post-stenotic dilatation. Exercise testing may be of value in evaluating children who want to participate in sports. The development of ST-segment or T-wave changes consistent with myocardial ischemia may indicate significant obstruction in an otherwise asymptomatic patient.

Cardiac catheterization is no longer used for routine diagnosis and is reserved for patients with associated defects that cannot be completely evaluated noninvasively, or if therapeutic intervention is indicated. Cardiac magnetic resonance imaging (MRI) is becoming a useful noninvasive mode for assessing ventricular mass and function as well as defining the morphology of the valve, annulus size, and coronary artery anatomy.

Subvalvular Aortic Stenosis. Subvalvular stenosis that occurs as an isolated lesion is rarely clinically significant in newborns and infants.[544] Patients with mild or moderate obstruction are typically asymptomatic. The lesion is often discovered during evaluation of associated cardiac defects.

Frequently subvalvular aortic stenosis is identified when echocardiography is performed for evaluation of a murmur. More than one-half of affected patients have a characteristic harsh systolic ejection murmur and a high frequency diastolic murmur of AR is heard in some patients.

The physical examination can help distinguish fixed from dynamic subaortic stenosis as seen in hypertrophic cardiomyopathy. In patients able to perform a Valsalva maneuver, the intensity of the murmur typically decreases in fixed subvalvular AS and increases in hypertrophic cardiomyopathy (HCM). Subvalvular AS often progresses rapidly during infancy and early childhood; however, the disorder may remain stable for years as some adults have only mild obstruction.[76] Diagnosis is confirmed by echocardiography, which enables determination of the location and extent of the obstruction and evaluation of left ventricular function and the integrity of the aortic and mitral valves.

Supravalvular Aortic Stenosis. Supravalvular AS is often suspected based on auscultatory findings. Affected children typically have a loud systolic ejection murmur. Unlike in valvular AS, there is no associated ejection click or diastolic murmur of aortic regurgitation. Other possible findings include a thrill in the suprasternal notch and a higher blood pressure in the right arm compared to the left arm caused by a jet of high-pressure flow in the ascending aorta (the Coanda effect). A blood pressure difference between the two arms of more than 10 mm Hg has been noted in approximately two thirds of patients.[544]

The diagnosis of supravalvular AS is confirmed by echocardiography and enables assessment of the severity of obstruction, left ventricular function, and the degree of left ventricular hypertrophy. Magnetic resonance imaging with angiography can be used when physical examination or other findings suggest associated defects of the vascular tree as MRI provides excellent anatomic detail of supravalvular aortic obstruction and associated aortic branch vessel disease.

Management

The American College of Cardiology and American Heart Association have developed joint ACC/AHA guidelines for the management of patients with aortic stenosis that consider age, clinical status and gradient across the stenosis.[780] It is important to note that the gradient across the obstructed area will be falsely lowered when cardiac output is low. Conversely, conditions that increase cardiac output (e.g., anemia, fever, exercise) will result in an increase in the gradient across the obstructed area. Asymptomatic children with Doppler peak instantaneous gradients of greater than 70 mm Hg should be considered for cardiac catheterization with possible balloon valvuloplasty. If the catheter measured peak-to-peak gradient is greater than 60 mm Hg, balloon valvuloplasty is indicated.

Children with symptoms such as dyspnea on exertion, syncope, angina, or ischemic changes on a resting or exercise ECG should have valvuloplasty if the peak-to-peak gradient in greater than 50 mm Hg. If the gradient is less than 50 mm Hg other causes of these symptoms and ECG changes should be investigated.

Valvuloplasty is not recommended for asymptomatic children with peak-to-peak gradients less than 50 mm Hg unless there is a concern that low cardiac output is contributing to underestimation of the severity of obstruction. Even children with mild degrees of aortic stenosis are at risk for progression over time and require periodic echocardiographic assessment.[62] If clinical findings do not appear to correlate with Doppler evaluation, cardiac catheterization may be indicated for direct measurement of peak-to-peak gradient.

Problematic aortic stenosis of all types requires treatment with either valvuloplasty or surgery. The goal of these interventions will be to relieve the aortic obstruction without creating significant aortic insufficiency. The management of each form of aortic stenosis, whether valvular, subvalvular, or supravalvular, is somewhat different and is summarized in the following pages.

Valvular Aortic Stenosis. The management approach is determined by the degree of obstruction present and is independent of the age of the patient. Medical therapy for neonates with critical AS includes intravenous administration of prostaglandin E_1 to open or maintain the ductus arteriosus, thus providing a means of right-to-left shunting (from pulmonary artery to aorta) and adequate antegrade systemic perfusion and retrograde aortic and coronary artery perfusion.

Medical therapy in children and adolescents consist of periodic evaluation to monitor for potential progression of valve dysfunction and need for exercise restrictions. These children are managed according to ACC/AHA recommendations.[780]

Percutaneous balloon aortic valvuloplasty has replaced surgical valvotomy as the therapy of choice for valvular aortic stenosis in infants and children requiring intervention. The aortic valve leaflets in children are typically pliable and easy to dilate and/or tear. By comparison, adult AS is not as amenable to balloon dilation because calcification of valve leaflets in the adult makes them less amenable to successful dilation. The major risk of balloon valvuloplasty is the development of significant aortic regurgitation.

Valvuloplasty is accomplished through the retrograde insertion of a balloon catheter from the femoral artery to the aorta and then beyond the aortic valve. The balloon is inflated to tear and separate the valve leaflets. Excessive valve dilation is avoided to prevent the development of aortic insufficiency that may lead to left ventricular dilation and dysfunction. Repeat balloon dilation is often effective in patients who develop recurrent obstruction, with gradient reduction of at least 50% in most patients. Repeat intervention is required more often in newborns than in older children.[771] Aortic wall injury has been reported as a procedure-related complication in neonates undergoing balloon aortic valvuloplasty is, but it has not resulted in significant mortality.[117]

The long-term outcome of balloon aortic valvuloplasty has been reported in two large series.[593,629] In children undergoing intervention at ages 1 month to 20 years, the average reduction in peak transvalvular gradient was 56 to 60 mm Hg and procedural mortality was 0.7%. Moderate to severe aortic regurgitation was found in 13% of patients immediately after balloon dilatation and in 38% 3.5 years after intervention.[593,629]

Data regarding the outcome of neonatal balloon aortic valvuloplasty is available from retrospective reviews undertaken at two centers.[346,599] In one study, early mortality fell significantly in recent years, from 22% (1985-1993) to 4% (1994-2002). The initial gradient reduction was 54% and significant AR developed in 15%.[599] The second study evaluated neonates who underwent balloon aortic valvuloplasty between 1 and 30 days of age from 1994 to 2004.[346] During the 3.5-year follow-up period, there were 31 reinterventions. Patients with a small aortic annulus were more likely to require aortic valve replacement. Catch-up growth of the left heart structures was reported but the size of the mitral valve remained below normal range for body surface area.[599]

In the treatment of valvular aortic stenosis, the alternative to balloon aortic valvuloplasty is surgical valvotomy performed via median sternotomy under cardiopulmonary bypass. An incision is made in the aorta, just above the coronary arteries, and the fused commissures are incised carefully under direct visualization. The goal of surgical intervention for valvular aortic stenosis is relief of the aortic obstruction without creation of significant aortic insufficiency. Incision is performed only for those commissures with adequate leaflet attachment; otherwise aortic insufficiency is likely to result. An alternative option is closed aortic valvotomy, performed without cardiopulmonary bypass, using calibrated dilators or balloon catheters. Currently this option is rarely used.

Children who develop severe aortic regurgitation following balloon dilation require surgical intervention. In such patients, valve repair can be effective and usually preferred to valve replacement. Surgical repair of residual aortic valve stenosis and aortic regurgitation is influenced by the size of the aortic annulus. If there is no significant annular hypoplasia, a surgical valve-sparing procedure can be performed. Repair techniques include commissurotomies, cusp extensions with pericardial patches, tightening of commissural edges, and shaving of fibrous material from valve cusps.

Aortic valve replacement is reserved for those patients with progressive aortic regurgitation not amenable to surgical intervention or those with recurrent stenosis refractory to balloon valvuloplasty. Options for aortic valve replacement during childhood include bioprosthetic or mechanical valves. Bioprosthetic valves, either homograft or heterograft, avoid the need for anticoagulation, but longevity of these valves and their lack of growth potential are limiting factors. In the early years of replacement, bioprosthetic valves had a failure rate in children as high as 20%. Failure resulted from progressive calcification in as little as 6 years.[917] Replacement with a mechanical prosthesis is the most durable alternative; however, the valve has no growth potential and lifelong anticoagulation is required because of the risk of thromboembolic events. Anticoagulation introduces a risk of hemorrhagic complications. The child and parents require careful instruction about the importance of the anticoagulation, medical followup, and the signs of thromboembolic or hemorrhagic complications (see Postoperative Care and Anticoagulation).

An alternative to valve replacement in infants and small children with aortic stenosis is the Ross procedure (pulmonary autograft). The child's pulmonary valve (with a cuff of tissue) is transplanted to the aortic position, and a pulmonary homograft is placed in the pulmonary valve position. The coronary arteries are reimplanted into the cuff of tissue so they are located immediately above the transplanted pulmonary valve (Fig. 8-37). This procedure avoids the need for anticoagulation, and the neoaortic valve (pulmonary autograft) has potential for growth. The major disadvantage of the Ross procedure in infants and children is that pulmonary homograft dysfunction is inevitable and can occur soon after initial operation. Fortunately, recent modifications to the Ross procedure have reduced the frequency of pulmonary autograft dysfunction and in some reports the function of the neoaorta remains stable for many years. Long-term survival after the Ross procedure is greater than 95%.[780]

When aortic valve stenosis is complicated by obstruction from a hypoplastic aortic annulus or diffuse subaortic stenosis, a Konno procedure (aortoventriculoplasty) is performed to enlarge the annulus. Through a median sternotomy approach and under cardiopulmonary bypass, a longitudinal incision is made in the aorta. By way of a right ventriculotomy, the aortic annulus is entered and an incision is made into the ventricular septum. A prosthetic patch is used to enlarge the left ventricular outflow tract and a prosthetic aortic valve is placed. A pericardial patch is then used to close the right ventriculotomy (Fig. 8-38). Potential problems after the Konno procedure include complete heart block, right ventricular outflow tract obstruction and residual VSD.

An evolving alternative to surgical valve placement is the percutaneous aortic valve implantation. The technique required for catheter delivery of a prosthetic aortic valve is progressing but not currently an option for children with aortic stenosis.[780]

There is limited comparative data between surgical valvotomy and balloon aortic valvuloplasty. In one series of 110 newborns with critical valvular aortic stenosis, surgical valvotomy was performed as the initial procedure in 28 and balloon aortic valvuloplasty was the initial procedure in 82, and survival and freedom from reintervention at 5 years were similar in both groups. Balloon aortic valvuloplasty resulted in a greater reduction in the systolic gradient (65% vs. 41%) and a lower mean residual postoperative gradient (20 vs. 36 mm Hg), but more frequent clinically significant aortic regurgitation (18% vs. 3%).[595]

Subvalvular Aortic Stenosis. Management of the asymptomatic infant or child with discrete *subvalvular* aortic stenosis is very similar to that of the child with valvular aortic stenosis. Children with a left ventricular outflow tract gradient less than 30 mm Hg and no significant left ventricular

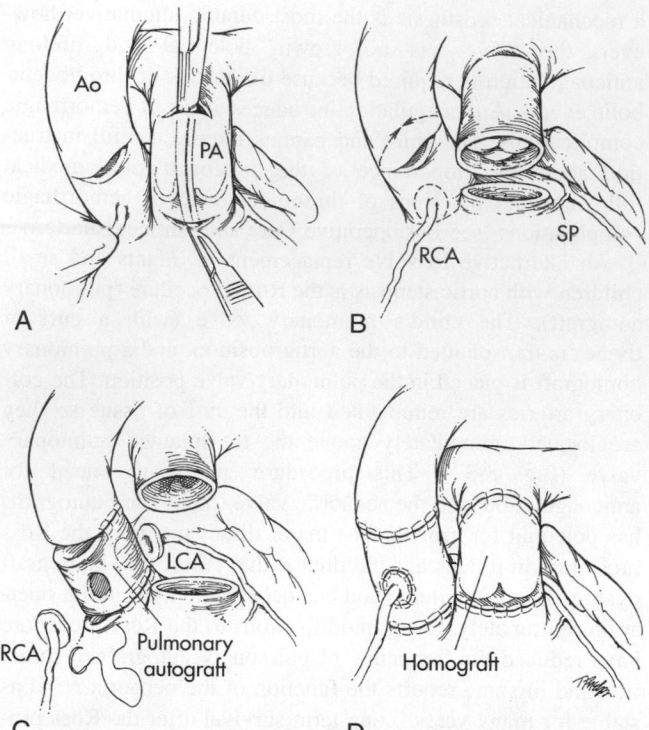

FIG. 8-37 Surgical correction of critical aortic stenosis with pulmonary autograft: Ross procedure. **A,** After the patient has been placed on cardiopulmonary bypass with cardioplegia solution, the pulmonary autograft procedure is performed by making a small incision in the aorta (Ao). If the aortic valve requires replacement, an incision is made in the main pulmonary artery (PA) adjacent to the origin of the right pulmonary artery, and a right-angle clamp is placed across the pulmonary artery and used to identify the right ventricular surface proximal to the pulmonary valve. An incision is then made in the right ventricle (RV); and **B,** the proximal pulmonary valve is removed with a cuff of muscle tissue. The posterior division of the valve from the right ventricle should follow a horizontal plane to prevent injury to the first septal perforator (SP) branch of the left anterior descending coronary artery. After the proximal portion of the pulmonary valve has been removed, the pulmonary artery is transected at the level of the bifurcation through the initial incision made in the pulmonary artery. **C,** With the autograft removed, the previously performed incision in the aorta is extended so that the aorta is transected above the level of the valve. The coronary arteries (right coronary artery [RCA] and left coronary artery [LCA] are then removed with large buttons of surrounding sinus tissue. The aortic valve and all remaining aortic tissue is removed from the base of the heart. The pulmonary autograft is then sewn to the base of the heart. The left coronary artery (LCA) and the right coronary artery (RCA) are implanted into the autograft. **D,** The procedure is completed by placing a cryopreserved homograft in the right ventricular outflow tract to reestablish right ventricle-to-pulmonary artery continuity. (From Ungerleider RJ: Congenital aortic stenosis. In Nichols DG, et al, editors: *Critical heart disease in infants and children.* St Louis, 1995, Mosby.)

hypertrophy are monitored closely for progression, especially during the first several years of life. Echocardiographic evaluation is warranted for any change in symptoms or clinical examination.

Because obstruction is very likely to recur, recommendations for appropriate timing of surgical intervention range from soon after diagnosis to longer periods of observation. Surgery is typically deferred in the first decade of life if the obstruction is moderate or less and aortic regurgitation is trivial. The presence of significant aortic regurgitation is considered an indication for surgery even if the obstruction is moderate or less.

In contrast to valvular aortic stenosis, subvalvular aortic stenosis does not respond to balloon dilation, so surgical correction of the obstruction is the definitive therapy. The surgery is performed through a median sternotomy incision with use of cardiopulmonary bypass. An incision is made in the aorta above the aortic valve and resection of the subvalvular discrete membrane or fibromuscular ring is performed. If subaortic obstruction is the result of a tunnel-like narrowing of the left ventricular outflow tract and a small aortic valve annulus, a patch may be required to enlarge the entire left ventricular outflow tract and annulus also known as the Konno procedure (described earlier for aortic valvular stenosis). Modifications of this intervention are used if subvalvular obstruction is severe but the aortic annulus is adequate, including a modified patch enlargement of the left ventricular outflow tract alone.

Surgical outcomes have improved in recent years and operative mortality rates are very low. Reported postoperative complications include recurrent obstruction in addition to those previously associated with the Konno procedure. Recurrence of subaortic stenosis was evaluated in a recent report of 111 patients who underwent successful surgical resection of discrete subaortic stenosis between 1984 and 2001. Rate of re-operation was 14% at a median followup of 8.2 years. Factors associated with reoperation included a lesion in closer proximity to the aortic valve and a peak Doppler gradient of greater than or equal to 60 mm Hg. Age at initial operation was not a factor, but severity of disease at initial operation was associated with greater likelihood of reoperation.[313]

Supravalvular Aortic Stenosis. Infants and children with mild *supravalvular* aortic stenosis are followed at regular intervals to detect any increase in obstruction. Congestive heart failure and other signs of severe aortic outflow obstruction do not commonly occur in infants with supravalvular aortic stenosis. The risk of sudden death is approximately the same as that reported with valvular aortic stenosis.

Definitive therapy for supravalvular aortic stenosis, whether discrete or diffuse, consists of surgical correction of the obstruction. The indications for surgery vary based on type and degree of stenosis. Surgery for the discrete form of supravalvular AS is usually successful in alleviating the stenosis. Techniques range from single patch enlargement just above the aortic root to bifurcated patch placement extending into two sinuses, and even three sinus patch enlargements.[144]

Treatment of diffuse obstruction is more complex and surgical options include extensive endarterectomy with patch aortoplasty or resection of the stenotic segment with end-to-end anastomosis to the distal ascending aorta. Late complications of surgery include residual stenosis and valvular dysfunction requiring aortic valve replacement. Transcatheter stent placement has been undertaken at a few centers with varying results as an alternative therapy in children with associated involvement of aortic branch vessels.

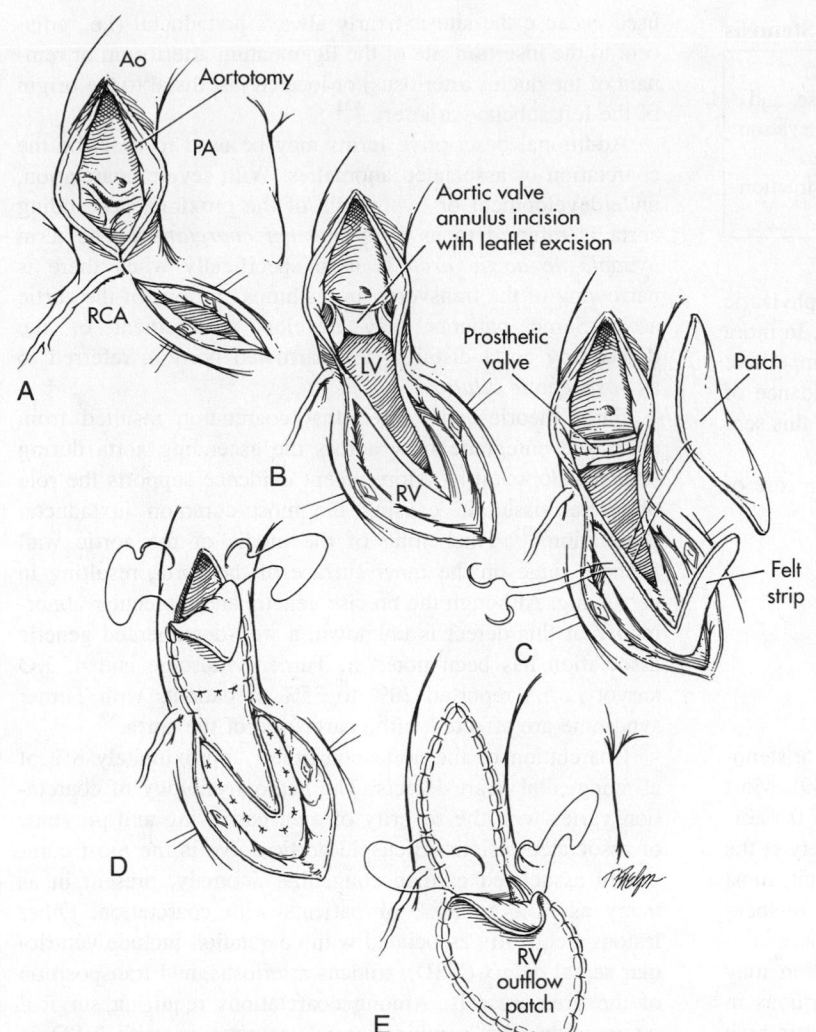

FIG. 8-38 Surgical correction of critical aortic stenosis: Konno procedure. An aortoventriculoplasty is performed with the patient on cardiopulmonary bypass, the aorta cross-clamped, and the heart protected with cardioplegia solution. **A,** A vertical aortotomy is extended just to the left side of the right coronary artery (RCA) and connected to a right ventriculotomy. The right ventriculotomy is performed below the pulmonary valve, and extended (see dotted line) toward the vertical aortotomy. Once these incisions are joined, another incision can be made across the aortic valve annulus **B,** and into the interventricular septum, so the incision is open from the right ventricle (RV) to the left ventricle (LV). The aortic valve leaflets are removed. **C,** A prosthetic valve is then sewn in the valve annulus, using interrupted (or continuous) sutures for the posterior portion of the valve ring. A prosthetic patch is placed and the valve ring sutures are brought through the patch, then through the interventricular septum, and then through a Teflon felt strip. This reconstructs and enlarges the left ventricular (LV) outflow tract and places the patch on the LV surface so the LV pressure will help to hold the patch in place. This patch is then secured. **D,** to the anterior portion of the prosthetic valve ring, and the suture line for the patch is continued around the aortotomy. **E,** Finally, the right ventricular (RV) outflow tract is repaired with an additional patch of either Gore-Tex or pericardium. AO, aorta; PA, pulmonary artery. (From Ungerleider RM: Congenital aortic stenosis. In Nichols DG, et al, editors: *Critical heart disease in infants and children.* St Louis, 1995, Mosby.)

Outcomes after surgical correction of supravalvular aortic stenosis include operative mortality rates ranging 1% to 9% with variability likely owing to nature of the stenosis and the presence of associated lesions. Main predictors of worse survival and more frequent reoperation were the presence of diffuse versus discrete stenosis and the presence of associated aortic valve disease.[854-856] Operative risk is also higher in patients with diffuse arteriopathy as seen in William's syndrome.

The clinical course and natural history for patients with aortic stenosis is not completely known as diagnostic techniques and the evolution of treatment options have simultaneously progressed. It is generally accepted that aortic stenosis presenting in infancy is more severe and carries a higher mortality rate with or without treatment than cases presenting in childhood.

The long-term outcome of congenital aortic stenosis was evaluated in the Second Natural History Study of Congenital Heart Defects.[443] This report included 371 patients with AS, mostly children, who had undergone diagnostic cardiac catheterization between 1958 and 1969. This report provides some useful information about the natural history of this defect, despite the fact that many of the patients did receive therapy. Patients with gradients less than 50 mm Hg were treated

medically, those with intermediate gradients had either medical or surgical therapy, and a surgical valvotomy was performed for gradients across the aortic valve of greater than or equal to 80 mm Hg. A total of 92.3% of all participants were in New York Heart Association functional class I. The 25-year survival was 92.4% for patients with initial peak systolic ejection gradients less than 50 mm Hg and 81% for those greater than or equal to 50 mm Hg. The likelihood of requiring surgery in 25 years was 20%, 40%, and 60% for patients with initial gradients of less than 25, 25 to 49, and 50 to 79 mm Hg, respectively. Sudden death occurred in 5% of the patients and accounted for more than one-half of all cardiac deaths. The patients succumbing to sudden death were almost all older than 10 years of age and had significant obstruction and/or aortic regurgitation; 19 had prior surgery.

According to the 2007 American Heart Association endocarditis prophylaxis guidelines,[951] antibiotic prophylaxis to prevent bacterial endocarditis is no longer recommended in patients with valvular aortic stenosis, supravalvular aortic stenosis, or subvalvular aortic stenosis except in those with a prior history of endocarditis or a repair that required prosthetic material or device. In the latter, antibiotic prophylaxis is recommended for the first 6 months after repair unless a residual defect is present in which case prophylactic antibiotics are continued beyond the 6-month period. In more severe cases of aortic obstruction, participation in competitive sports should probably be restricted along with avoidance of strenuous activity (see Bacterial Endocarditis later in this section of the chapter).

Please refer to Box 8-28 for advanced concepts in care of the patient with aortic stenosis

Coarctation of the Aorta

Nancy A. Rudd

Etiology

Coarctation of the aorta is a constriction (narrowing) or stenosis of a portion of the aorta or aortic arch (Fig. 8-39). Most commonly there is a discrete congenital narrowing of the aortic arch occurring just distal to the left subclavian artery at the level of insertion of the ductus arteriosus. As a result, most coarctations are accurately described as juxtaductal in location. This description can be too simplistic, however, as coarctation anatomy can vary considerably. The coarctation may include stenosis of a long segment or it may be tortuous in presentation; it may be associated with transverse aortic arch hypoplasia or rarely the coarctation may be located in the abdominal aorta.

Past classifications of simple coarctation included either preductal (infantile type) or postductal (adult type). This terminology, although accurate for some patients, is no longer used because the site is nearly always juxtaductal (i.e., adjacent to the insertion site of the ligamentum arteriosum or remnant of the ductus arteriosus) or located just distal to the origin of the left subclavian artery.[421]

Additional descriptive terms may be used to describe the coarctation or associated anomalies. With severe coarctation, underdevelopment or hypoplasia of the proximal descending aorta is referred to as *long segment coarctation*. The term *hypoplastic aortic arch* is used specifically when there is narrowing of the transverse and isthmus portions of the aortic arch. Some patients may develop enlargement of the descending aorta distal to the narrowed portion, referred to as *poststenotic dilation*.

Early theories speculated that coarctation resulted from decreased antegrade flow across the ascending aorta during fetal development.[753] More recent evidence supports the role of ductal tissue in causing the most common juxtaductal coarctation.[905] Thickening of the media of the aortic wall forms a ridge on the inner surface of the aorta, resulting in narrowing. Although the precise genetic and molecular abnormality of this defect is unknown, a well-documented genetic association has been noted in Turner syndrome and 45,XO karyotype. A reported 20% to 35% of patients with Turner syndrome are affected with coarctation of the aorta.[68]

Coarctation of the aorta constitutes approximately 8% of all congenital heart defects. The pathophysiology of coarctation varies with the severity of arch narrowing and presence of associated lesions. Bicuspid aortic valve is the most commonly associated cardiac congenital anomaly, present in as many as 50% to 80% of patients with coarctation. Other lesions frequently associated with coarctation include ventricular septal defect (VSD), truncus arteriosus, and transposition of the great vessels. Among coarctations requiring surgical intervention, the combination of coarctation with VSD is almost as common as coarctation alone.[421] Coarctation is frequently associated with other left heart obstructive lesions, including aortic stenosis, subaortic narrowing, mitral stenosis, left ventricular and left ventricular outflow tract hypoplasia. Coarctation that occurs as one part of a constellation of left

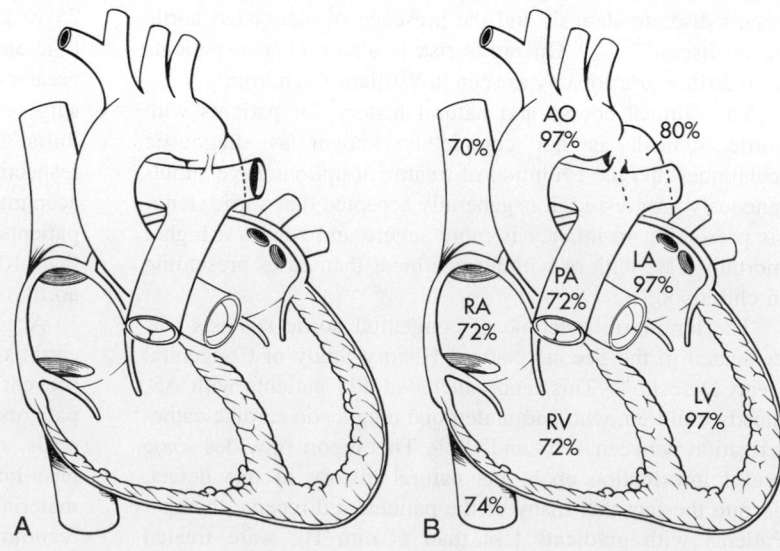

FIG. 8-39 Coarctation of the aorta. **A,** Postductal coarctation. This coarctation is in the region of the ductus arteriosus. **B,** Preductal coarctation. Typical oxyhemoglobin saturations in cardiac chambers and great vessels are depicted. When the ductus arteriosus is patent, the descending aorta is perfused largely with systemic venous blood from the right ventricle through the ductus. AO, aorta; LA, left atrium; LV, left ventricle; PA, pulmonary artery; RA, right atrium; RV, right ventricle.

sided obstructive lesions is called *Shone's complex* (see section, Essential Anatomy and Physiology, Etiologies of CHD: Noninherited and Genetic Factors). The most severe form of this constellation of left heart lesions results in hypoplastic left heart syndrome (see later section, Single Functioning Ventricle).[159]

Pathophysiology

Following birth when the ductus arteriosus constricts, the medial layer of a portion of the aorta also constricts, creating a narrowing in the aorta. The area of stenosis can vary from a mild degree of narrowing producing only a small pressure gradient to severe obstruction causing near interruption of systemic blood flow to the lower body. Therefore, depending on the severity of coarctation and the presence of additional lesions, hemodynamic effects may range from mild upper extremity hypertension to congestive heart failure or even shock.

When there is obstruction to aortic flow, the left ventricle must generate higher pressure to maintain normal flow through the narrowed area, so hypertension will be present in the aorta and in the arteries branching from the aorta proximal to the obstruction. In addition, hypotension will be present in the aorta and arteries branching from the aorta distal to the stenotic area. The decreased flow and hypotension to the lower extremities and abdominal organs may result in ischemia of the organs perfused by the part of the aorta that is distal to the coarctation site. The head and neck vessels and coronary arteries are perfused from the part of the aorta that is proximal to the level of obstruction so they receive hypertensive blood flow.

Because the left ventricle must generate high pressure to maintain blood flow through the narrowed aorta, significant left ventricular hypertrophy may be present. Left ventricular failure may develop. If the coarctation is severe, ductal closure can result in acute development of left ventricular failure, including decreased stroke volume, elevated left ventricular end-diastolic and left atrial pressures, and pulmonary venous congestion. Low cardiac output can cause impaired myocardial perfusion, leading to cardiogenic shock.[68] Inadequate systemic perfusion may produce severe acidosis and renal and gastrointestinal ischemia.

Some cases of significant coarctation result in development of arterial collateral vessels flowing from the aorta and arterial branches that are proximal to the level of obstruction to vessels that will carry blood flow back into the aorta distal to the level of obstruction. These vessels provide a source of low-pressure flow to the descending aorta and the tissues perfused by the descending aorta.

Clinical Signs and Symptoms

Clinical presentation for this cardiac defect can vary from cardiovascular collapse in neonates following ductal closure to asymptomatic hypertension in older infants and children. The pattern of clinical signs and symptoms can be divided into two categories: coarctation of the aorta presenting in the neonatal period and coarctation presenting in later infancy or during childhood.

Neonatal Coarctation of the Aorta. Neonatal coarctation of the aorta typically presents during the first week to 10 days of life and is typically associated with severe signs of shock. At birth, a newborn with severe coarctation may appear asymptomatic while the ductus arteriosus remains patent. Because pulmonary vascular resistance is high during the first hours of life, the presence of a patent ductus arteriosus (PDA) allows right-to-left shunting of blood from the main pulmonary artery to the descending aorta. Before spontaneous ductal closure the only symptom of coarctation may be mild cyanosis of the lower extremities (with a differential oxygen saturation noted with pulse oximetry). Following ductal closure, left ventricular failure and poor systemic perfusion develop and progressive signs and symptoms of deterioration include poor feeding or vomiting secondary to decreased bowel perfusion, tachypnea, pallor, listlessness and acidosis. Pulses in the lower extremities are weak or absent and severe hypotension is present in the lower extremities. Signs of multisystem organ failure can develop, including renal failure, seizures, necrotizing enterocolitis, and possible death.[421]

Coarctation of the Aorta Presenting During Infancy or Childhood. If coarctation of the aorta does not produce signs and symptoms during the first days and weeks of life, and if the degree of narrowing is mild or moderate in severity, the infant or child with coarctation often remains asymptomatic. Some patients may report headaches resulting from upper body hypertension or exercise intolerance and leg pain with activity, because it is impossible to increase cardiac output to tissues perfused by the distal aorta.[421] Patients with severe coarctation can be asymptomatic if arterial collateral blood supply produces near normal blood flow into the descending aorta (beyond the coarctation) and into the femoral arteries, but this is uncommon.

Physical examination reveals diminished, delayed, or absent lower extremity pulses. In fact, the pathognomonic clinical findings of coarctation of the aorta include discrepant arterial pulses and systolic blood pressures between the upper and lower extremities.[68] The upper extremity blood pressure is often elevated for age. Comparative upper and lower extremity measurements usually reveal a pressure gradient of 15 mm Hg or greater. In rare cases the presence of an aberrant right subclavian from the descending aorta (beyond the coarctation) will result in no blood pressure differential between upper and lower extremities.

To identify coarctation, the blood pressure in the right arm should be compared to the blood pressure in either lower extremity. The left arm blood pressure should not be compared to lower extremity blood pressures to identify a blood pressure gradient because the origin of the left subclavian artery is near the coarctation, and this location may result in lower blood pressure in the left arm than in the right arm.

Auscultation may reveal several different murmurs based on the location and severity of the coarctation and the presence of any arterial collateral vessels. A systolic ejection click may indicate the presence of a bicuspid aortic valve. A systolic ejection murmur produced by flow through the coarctation site is best heard at the upper left sternal border or over the left interscapular area of the back. A continuous murmur may also be produced from collateral vessels when present. Neonates with diminished cardiac output may have faint murmurs, and the presence of a gallop rhythm may be the most notable auscultatory finding.[68]

A plain chest radiograph in older patients presenting with coarctation of the aorta demonstrates a normal to mildly enlarged heart. Neonates or young infants with severe coarctation and congestive heart failure may demonstrate moderate to severe cardiomegaly and increased pulmonary vascular markings.

Erosion of the undersurface of the ribs (rib-notching) visible in an anterior-posterior (AP) chest radiograph results from dilation of intercostal vessels that provide arterial collateral blood supply. Rib-notching is not seen in infants because the collateral vessels must enlarge and it will take time to erode the lower surface of the ribs; typically rib-notching is found only in children older than 5 years with uncorrected coarctation.

A "figure 3 sign" may be identified on the AP chest radiograph, caused by the contour (silhouette) of the aortic arch. This contour includes a prominent aortic bulge proximal to the coarctation, a discrete indentation of the aorta at the coarctation site, and post-stenotic dilatation in the aorta immediately beyond the coarctation.[68]

The ECG is usually normal in neonates and infants with coarctation. The ECG of children and adolescents with coarctation may show increased left-sided voltages indicating left ventricular hypertrophy.

Magnetic resonance imaging (MRI) is a useful imaging tool for evaluating coarctation. It provides detailed imaging of head and neck vessels as well as the imaging of the immediate site of the coarctation, the entire aortic arch including the abdominal aorta, and it enables identification of collateral vessels if present. In addition, MRI studies can be used to estimate pressure gradients and aortic blood flow.

High-quality echocardiographic studies frequently provide sufficient physiologic and anatomic detail to accurately diagnose coarctation of the aorta. Images are readily obtainable in infants but can be more difficult to obtain in older children and adults because imaging windows are poor. Doppler imaging may be helpful: a high velocity signal in the area of the coarctation site and the presence of an altered waveform and diastolic runoff in the descending aorta is diagnostic of coarctation. Associated lesions can also be visualized via echocardiography, including bicuspid aortic valve and VSD. Left ventricular hypertrophy or dysfunction can be identified.

Diagnostic cardiac catheterization is only indicated if there are associated cardiac lesions. In the past, angiography was used to identify collateral blood flow or define arch anatomy poorly visualized by echocardiography; MRI is now diagnostic. Currently cardiac catheterization serves a therapeutic role in the management of some patients with coarctation of the aorta.

If left untreated, the natural history for patients with coarctation of the aorta is dismal. Severe coarctation in the neonate would likely be fatal, and mild or moderate coarctation and hypertension can eventually produce complications such as congestive heart failure, aortic rupture, and bacterial endocarditis. One large natural history study reported a mean age at death for patients with untreated coarctation of 34 years.[134]

Intervention is currently recommended for all patients diagnosed with coarctation of the aorta. The appropriate therapy is dictated by the presentation of the patient.

Management

Medical Management. Medical management is required to stabilize neonates and young infants with severe coarctation. Prostaglandin E_1 (PGE_1) infusion is provided to maintain patency of the ductus arteriosus or to reopen a closed ductus. The ductus provides a route of blood flow from the main pulmonary artery to the descending aorta, to maintain perfusion to the vital organs below the area of coarctation. Preoperative management with PGE_1 improves organ perfusion, allowing correction of shock, acidosis and ischemia. After adequate medical stabilization, early surgical intervention is indicated.

Additional medical management during and beyond the neonatal period may include diuretic therapy for the infant with congestive heart failure. Support of organ function (e.g., renal replacement therapies) may be needed.

Surgical Therapy. Surgical therapy is the primary intervention for coarctation of the aorta in neonates, infants, and small children. Catheter intervention strategies such as balloon dilation and stent placement are alternative therapies for management of native coarctation in older patients. Surgical correction of coarctation of the aorta is usually a closed-heart procedure (i.e., without cardiopulmonary bypass) performed via a left thoracotomy. If other cardiac defects such as VSD require simultaneous repair, a sternotomy may be performed; cardiopulmonary bypass is used for the intracardiac repair.

A variety of surgical repairs have been used over the years to treat coarctation (Fig. 8-40). Presently the most frequently used approach is the end-to-end anastomosis and the second most common approach is the subclavian flap repair.

During the procedure, once the aorta is dissected, clamps are placed above and below the narrowed area. During dissection care is taken to avoid injury to lymphatic vessels as well as to the vagus, phrenic, and recurrent laryngeal nerves. If collateral vessels are present, they are generally ligated and divided to prevent intraoperative and postoperative bleeding.[44]

With the end-to-end approach the stenotic area of the aortic arch and ductal tissue are resected, and then the two ends of the aorta are anastomosed (sewn) together. Advantages to this technique include removal of ductal tissue and lack of prosthetic material (that can act as a site for infection). Disadvantages include a circumferential suture line and the resulting potential for recoarctation (narrowing) at that repair site.

A variation of this end-to-end anastomosis technique is used in cases of hypoplasia of the isthmus or transverse arch. The incision extends onto the transverse arch and under the left common carotid and the length of the incision is used to widen or extend the end-to-end anastomosis.

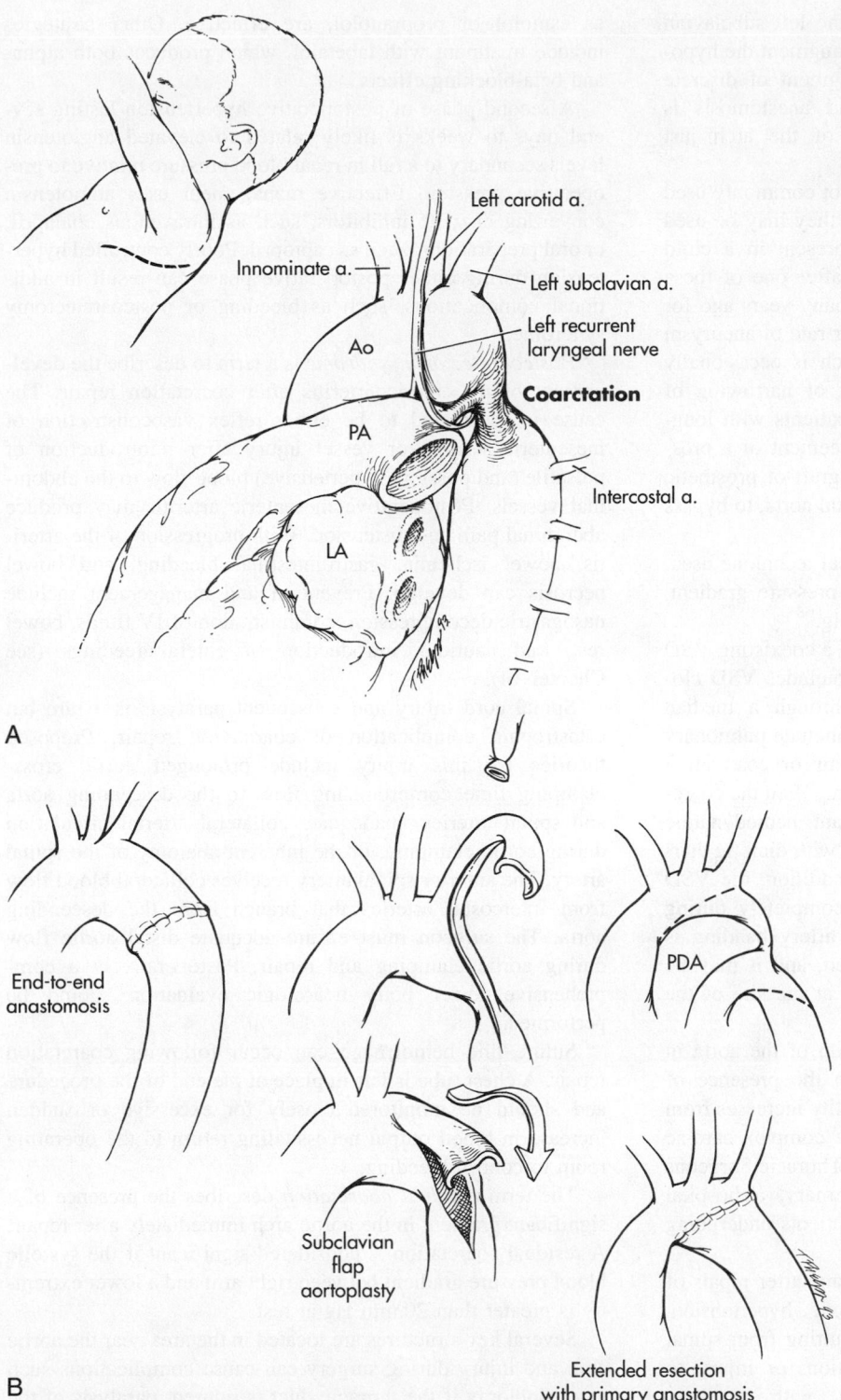

FIG. 8-40 Surgical approach to coarctation of the aorta (CoA). **A,** Typical surgical incision and surgical anatomy. **B,** Three operative procedures commonly used in repair of CoA: resection of the stenotic segment and end-to-end aortic anastomosis, subclavian flap aortoplasty, and extended resection with primary anastomosis. **A,** artery; Ao, aorta; LA, left atrium; PA, pulmonary artery; PDA, patent ductus arteriosus. (From Schwengel DA, Nichols DG, Cameron DE: Coarctation of the aorta and interrupted aortic arch. In Nichols DG, et al, editors: *Critical heart disease in infants and children,* ed 2, St Louis, 2006, Mosby, Fig. 27-10.)

The subclavian flap procedure requires that the left subclavian artery be ligated (tied off) and divided (cut). A longitudinal incision is made through the proximal segment of the subclavian artery and down the aorta to the area just beyond the coarctation. The subclavian stump is then opened and turned down and stitched to the aorta, resulting in a patch of autologous tissue enlarging the area of coarctation. Potential advantages of this technique include avoidance of prosthetic material (that would act as a potential site for infection) and the potential for growth of the patch site as the child grows. In addition a circumferential suture line is avoided. The major disadvantage is the required sacrificing of the left subclavian artery.

More recently some centers have used a reverse left subclavian flap approach to repair discrete coarctation accompanied by distal arch hypoplasia. The left subclavian artery is mobilized as described. In this variation, the left subclavian flap is turned back in a reverse direction to augment the hypoplastic portion of the aortic arch. The segment of discrete narrowing is removed and an end-to-end anastomosis is performed, extending under the portion of the arch just enlarged by the reverse flap.[421]

Several techniques used in the past are not commonly used at present, but are mentioned here because they may be used for unique situations, and they may be present in a child who develops recoarctation several years after one of these procedures. Prosthetic patches were used many years ago for the aortoplasty, but they resulted in a higher rate of aneurysm formation than expected. A prosthetic patch is occasionally used in a small child with long segment of narrowing of the aortic arch. Another option for older patients with long-segment coarctation or recoarctation is placement of a prosthetic interposition graft. Rarely, a bypass graft or prosthetic tube is placed between the proximal and distal aorta, to bypass the stenotic area of the aorta.

Initially after repair, regardless of surgical technique used, most patients have a mild residual blood pressure gradient. Most gradients are less than 10 to 20 mm Hg.[68]

Optimal management of coarctation with a coexisting VSD remains controversial. A one stage repair includes VSD closure at the time of coarctation repair through a median sternotomy approach. Additional strategies include pulmonary artery banding at time of coarctation repair or coarctation repair alone with no initial VSD intervention. Often the coarctation repair alone will produce significant hemodynamic improvement, and the patient can be treated with diuretic therapy if the VSD remains symptomatic. In addition, the VSD may become relatively smaller or close completely during the next several months. If a pulmonary artery banding is performed, later debanding will be required, and it may be necessary to enlarge the pulmonary artery at the site of the band constriction.[159]

Surgical mortality for isolated coarctation of the aorta in infants and older children is near 0%. In the presence of associated lesions such as large VSD, mortality increases from 2% to 10% and is even higher when more complex cardiac defects are also present.[68] In the Society of Thoracic Surgeons Congenital Heart Surgery Executive Summary, a hospital mortality rate of 1.5% is reported for all patients undergoing coarctation repair from 2006 to 2010.[820]

Potential early postoperative complications after repair of coarctation of the aorta include paradoxic hypertension, postcoarctectomy syndrome, paraplegia resulting from spinal cord ischemia, bleeding, residual coarctation, or injury to nearby structures such as lymphatics with resultant chylothorax.[159] Late hypertension and recurrent coarctation may also develop.

Paradoxic hypertension is common postoperatively and appears to have multiple etiologies. In the first 24 to 48 hours after surgery, hypertension is likely related to elevated catecholamine levels from the stress of surgery and resetting of the baroreceptors in the aortic arch and carotid arteries. Medical management must include adequate sedation and analgesia (see Chapter 5). In addition, vasodilators, such as nitroprusside or hydralazine, used in conjunction with a beta-blocker such

as esmolol or propranolol, are effective. Other strategies include treatment with labetalol, which produces both alpha- and beta-blocking effects.

A second phase of postoperative hypertension lasting several days to weeks is likely related to elevated angiotensin levels secondary to a fall in renal blood pressure relative to preoperative pressure. Effective management uses angiotensin converting enzyme inhibitors, such as intravenous enalapril, or oral preparations, such as captopril. Poorly controlled hypertension during either postoperative phase can result in additional complications, such as bleeding or postcoarctectomy syndrome.

Postcoarctectomy syndrome is a term to describe the development of mesenteric arteritis after coarctation repair. The cause is speculated to be either reflex vasoconstriction of mesenteric vessels or vessel injury after reintroduction of pulsatile (and possibly hypertensive) blood flow to the abdominal vessels. Postoperative mesenteric arteritis may produce abdominal pain and distension. With progression of the arteritis, bowel ischemia, gastrointestinal bleeding, and bowel necrosis can develop. Prevention and management include nasogastric decompression, administration of IV fluids, bowel rest, and cautious introduction of enteral feedings (see Chapter 14).

Spinal cord injury and subsequent paralysis is a rare but catastrophic complication of coarctation repair. Proposed theories for this injury include prolonged aortic cross-clamping time compromising flow to the descending aorta and spinal arteries, inadequate collateral arterial circulation during aortic clamping, or the inherent anatomy of the spinal artery. The anterior spinal artery receives collateral blood flow from intercostal arteries that branch from the descending aorta. The surgeon must ensure adequate distal aortic flow during aortic clamping and repair. Postoperatively a comprehensive lower body neurologic evaluation should be performed.

Suture line hemorrhage can occur following coarctation repair. A chest tube is left in place at the end of the procedure and should be monitored closely for excessive or sudden increase in blood output necessitating return to the operating room to control bleeding.

The term *residual coarctation* describes the presence of a significant gradient in the aortic arch immediately after repair. A residual coarctation is considered significant if the systolic blood pressure gradient between right arm and a lower extremity is greater than 20 mm Hg at rest.

Several key structures are located in the area near the aortic arch and injury during surgery can cause complications such as chylothorax if the thoracic duct is injured, paralysis of the hemi-diaphragm in the case of phrenic nerve damage, and vocal cord paralysis with recurrent laryngeal nerve injury.[159] A chylothorax is likely present if milky chest tube drainage is observed; the volume of drainage will increase with resumption of enteral feeding postoperatively.

If a subclavian flap is utilized for the repair, the subclavian artery is sacrificed, so it will not be possible to obtain a cuff pressure or arterial sample from the left arm. In addition, venipunctures should not be performed on that arm. The arm may feel cool and appear mottled for several hours or even days after surgery until collateral vessels improve perfusion to the arm. Minor growth retardation of the left arm has been reported after use of the subclavian artery for arterioplasty.[44]

Careful and regular followup is required following repair of coarctation. Late complications after surgical repair of coarctation include the development of recurrent coarctation, hypertension not associated with residual coarctation, and aneurysm formation.

Recurrent coarctation implies the development of restenosis after an initially successful repair and has been reported after every type of coarctation repair.[44] Restenosis is thought to be related to scar tissue formation at the site of aortic anastomosis or to inadequate resection of ductal tissue at the time of initial repair. Balloon angioplasty is currently the initial therapy of choice to address recoarctation.

Persistent systolic hypertension not caused by recurrent coarctation is more common when the initial coarctation repair is performed after 5 years of age. These patients require pharmacologic therapy, such as angiotensin converting enzyme (ACE) inhibitors (captopril or enalapril) to prevent secondary cardiovascular complications of hypertension.

Aneurysm formation in the aortic arch at the repair site can occur following any surgical approach although the highest incidence has been reported following prosthetic patch aortoplasty.[111] If aneurysms are present, they must be monitored closely for signs of progression as rupture can cause sudden death.

Interventional Therapy. Interventional therapy for treatment of coarctation of the aorta includes percutaneous balloon angioplasty and intravascular stenting. These less invasive alternative therapies can be used to treat both native (never operated) and recurrent (after surgical repair) coarctation. Balloon dilation angioplasty was first undertaken to treat restenosis of surgically resected coarctation. Later the technique was expanded to include dilation of native coarctation. Balloon angioplasty has been successful in the treatment of discrete native coarctation,[258] and some centers routinely manage coarctation in the interventional catheterization laboratory. This approach is not universal, however, chiefly because of concerns regarding residual stenosis and aneurysm formation. Documented significant (greater than 20 mm Hg) residual gradients have been reported in 14% to 27% of patients, and aneurysm formation in 5% to 10% of patients after angioplasty.[611]

The treatment of recurrent coarctation with balloon dilation has become the first-line intervention at most centers. The reported incidence of residual stenosis and of aneurysm formation following balloon dilation for recurrent coarctation are similar to those reported following treatment of native coarctation although the theoretical advantage of dilating a fibrous postsurgical scar is thought to reduce the likelihood of aneurysm development.

Complications from balloon dilation of recurrent and native coarctation are rare but can occur. Acute tears in the aortic wall are rare but serious complications. Aneurysms of the aortic wall can develop early following dilation or may appear years after the dilation. Arterial vessel injury was more frequently reported early in the balloon angioplasty experience;

Box 8-29	**Advanced Concepts: Coarctation of the Aorta**

In cases of infant coarctation, a blood pressure gradient may not initially be detected if a patent ductus arteriosus is present. Because pulmonary vascular resistance may still be elevated in the first hours and days after birth, blood can flow to the descending aorta via the ductus arteriosus, resulting in adequate lower extremity perfusion and relatively equal upper and lower limb blood pressures. Blood flowing to the descending aorta is desaturated, so lower extremity oxyhemoglobin saturation is decreased.

however, advances such as smaller balloon profiles and the use of indwelling sheaths has greatly reduced vessel injury.[640]

Coarctation stenting has been shown to be effective in treating discrete native and recurrent coarctation. The use of intravascular stents for primary treatment of coarctation in larger adolescents and adults has become the treatment of choice at some centers. General practice requires placement of a stent into the aorta only if it is expandable to the adult diameter of the aorta.[640] Currently this prevents the use of stents in treatment of coarctation in infants and children because the large femoral sheath size necessary to deliver adult-size stents is too large for small patients. Balloon-expandable stents have the reported benefit of providing endovascular stability and may diminish the incidence of late aneurysm formation.[417]

Antibiotic prophylaxis against bacterial endocarditis in patients with coarctation of the aorta is recommended for 6 months after surgical repair using prosthetic material and indefinitely if a significant residual coarctation gradient is present. The presence of a bicuspid aortic valve alone no longer necessitates antibiotic prophylaxis; however, adherence to current American Heart Association guidelines for endocarditis prophylaxis is recommended (see Bacterial Endocarditis later in this section of the chapter).[951]

Advanced concepts in the management of the infant with severe coarctation of the aorta are listed in Box 8-29.

Interrupted Aortic Arch

Nancy A. Rudd

Etiology

Interrupted aortic arch (IAA) is defined as the congenital absence or atresia of a segment of the aortic arch resulting in complete separation between the ascending and descending aorta. Interrupted aortic arch is classified into three types is based on the site of interruption (Fig. 8-41). In *Type A*, the interruption occurs just distal to the left subclavian artery at the level of the isthmus. This subtype may be a variant of severe coarctation of the aorta and accounts for approximately 30% of patients with interrupted aortic arch. In *Type B* the aorta is interrupted between the left carotid and the left subclavian artery; the left subclavian artery arises from the descending aortic segment. This form of interrupted aortic arch is the most common, responsible for about 70% of all interrupted aortic arch. In *Type C* the interruption is between the right innominate artery and the left carotid artery. This type is very rare and accounts for only 1% of cases of interrupted aortic arch.

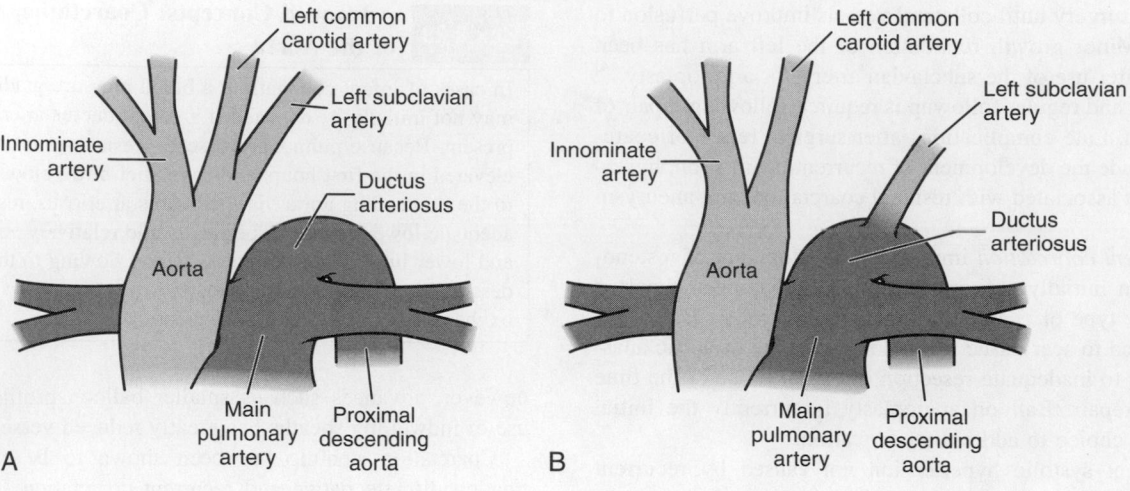

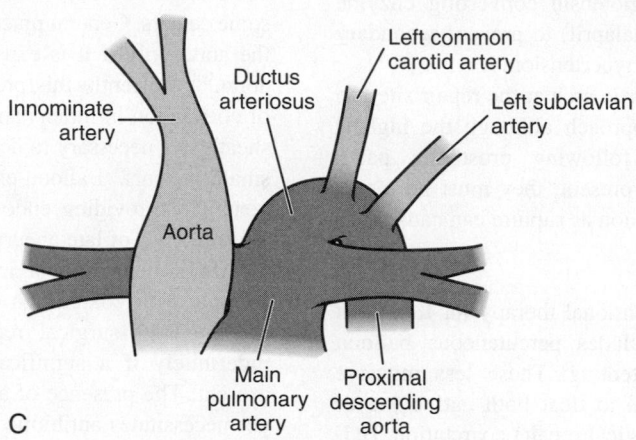

FIG. 8-41 Anatomic types of interrupted aortic arch. **A,** Type A, interruption just distal to the left subclavian artery. **B,** Type B, interruption between the left subclavian and left common carotid arteries. **C,** Type C, interruption between the left common carotid and innominate arteries. (Redrawn from Mavroudis C, Backer CL, editors: *Pediatric cardiac surgery,* ed 3, Philadelphia, 2003, Mosby.)

This defect is thought to result from faulty formation of the aortic arch system during fetal development (see Evolve Fig. 8-1 in the Chapter 8 Supplement on the Evolve Website). Abnormalities in development of the left fourth arch in the embryo are felt to play a role in the occurrence of all three subtypes of IAA.[930] There is also a strong link between chromosomal deletion of 22q11 (DiGeorge syndrome), and interrupted aortic arch, specifically Type B, so this syndrome should be ruled out in newborns with Type B IAA.

Interrupted aortic arch accounts for approximately 1.5% of all congenital heart defects. Interrupted aortic arch is rarely present as an isolated defect; most infants have additional congenital heart defects. The most commonly associated lesion is an isolated VSD. Other accompanying defects include ASD, truncus arteriosus, aortopulmonary window, transposition of the great arteries, double outlet right ventricle, and single ventricle.[421] Type A interruption has been noted in a markedly large subgroup of patients with transposition of the great arteries, whereas Type B interruptions are more commonly associated conotruncal anomalies, malalignment-type VSD, and subaortic obstruction.[930]

Pathophysiology

Presentation of these patients typically is similar to presentation for other ductal-dependent left heart and aortic obstructive lesions, such as critical coarctation of the aorta. The neonate becomes acutely ill with signs of heart failure in the first days of life. After spontaneous closure of the ductus arteriosus, acute cardiovascular collapse ensues, because perfusion of the descending aorta and lower body occurs only through arterial collateral flow. If untreated, ischemic injury to the gut, liver, and kidneys will occur. Soon severe acidosis will develop resulting in injury to all body systems, including the heart and brain.[420]

Clinical Signs and Symptoms

Clinical signs and symptoms of interrupted aortic arch are the same as those described for critical coarctation of the aorta in the neonate. The neonate is tachypneic with evidence of decreased systemic perfusion, severe metabolic acidosis, and oliguria or anuria. The discrepancy in peripheral pulses will be affected by the anatomic subtype of interrupted aortic arch and the presence of an open or closed ductus arteriosus.

For example, a neonate with Type B interruption and a closed ductus should have a palpable pulse in the right arm but absent left arm and femoral pulses.

Cyanosis is not a common clinical finding, particularly when the ductus closes, because the head and right arm are perfused with oxygenated blood from the left ventricle, and the left arm and lower body are perfused only with blood flow delivered to the descending aorta via collateral circulation.

In rare instances, patients with interrupted aortic arch have survived to adulthood without symptoms. These patients usually have extensive collateral circulation that maintains adequate descending aortic blood flow.

Prenatal diagnosis of many cardiac defects, including interrupted aortic arch, allows early intervention to maintain patency of the ductus arteriosus, preventing ductal constriction and the resulting period of low cardiac output. For those patients not identified prenatally, the diagnosis of interrupted aortic arch is suspected by the clinical presentation. It must be differentiated from coarctation of the aorta, aortic atresia, and hypoplastic left heart syndrome.

Two-dimensional (2D) echocardiography is the most important diagnostic tool in identifying this defect. Images pinpoint the site of interruption, the length of discontinuity, the diameter of the aortic annulus, and the diameter of the ascending aorta. All of these anatomic details influence the surgical management of this cardiac lesion. Angiography is still used in some centers to confirm the diagnosis and further delineate arch anatomy. However, accurate diagnosis can be made using echocardiography alone, eliminating the need for invasive cardiac catheterization in a neonate who is often in shock. Recently three-dimensional cardiac magnetic resonance imaging (3D cardiac MRI) has been used to identify the arterial branching pattern and area of separation between the proximal and distal aorta.

Management

Initial medical management includes maintenance or restoration of ductal patency with infusion of prostaglandin E_1, fluid resuscitation, correction of acid-base and electrolyte imbalances, and inotropic support as necessary to optimize systemic perfusion (see Shock, Chapter 6). Once the neonate is stabilized, surgical correction is undertaken as soon as possible.

The surgical approach is via a median sternotomy. Typically all types of interrupted aortic arch can be reconstructed by direct anastomosis of the upper and lower segments of the arch after liberal dissection of each component. If indicated, homograft augmentation of the resected area can be performed to achieve an adequate arch diameter. Prosthetic tube grafts are generally not used for initial neonatal repair because they are rapidly outgrown and may complicate reintervention at a later date.

Whenever possible, simultaneous correction of coexisting cardiac defects such as VSD, transposition of the great arteries, and aortic stenosis is performed. Palliative operations used in the past are not often employed because primary one-stage repair in the neonatal period is considered optimal management.

Postoperative complications include those discussed after repair of severe coarctation of the aorta during infancy. In addition, pulmonary hypertension may be present in the early postoperative period (see section, Common Clinical Conditions, Pulmonary Hypertension) and residual obstruction within the arch or subaortic area may require surgical reintervention.[158]

The natural history of unrepaired interrupted aortic arch is death within days of birth, and surgical mortality as recently as the 1990s was high.[673] With advances in surgical intervention and postoperative care, survival for interrupted aortic arch with VSD is 92% at 1 month.[820]

Antibiotic prophylaxis against bacterial endocarditis is recommended for a 6-month period after surgical repair if prosthetic material was used. Also, if a significant residual aortic arch gradient is present following repair, adherence to current American Heart Association guidelines for endocarditis prophylaxis is recommended (for further information, see Bacterial Endocarditis later in this section of the chapter).[951]

Mitral Valve Dysfunction
Nancy A. Rudd

Etiology

A normal mitral valve is made up of five parts: the valve leaflets, valve annulus, papillary muscles, chordae tendineae, and left ventricular wall (Fig. 8-42). The valve has a smaller anterior or aortic leaflet and a larger posterior or mural leaflet. Congenital mitral valve abnormalities are relatively rare but include isolated mitral stenosis and mitral regurgitation.

Congenital mitral valve abnormalities are commonly associated with additional congenital heart defects. Congenital mitral stenosis frequently occurs in association with other left heart obstructive lesions, such as coarctation of the aorta or aortic stenosis. Congenital mitral regurgitation is more commonly associated with atrioventricular septal defect (particularly complete AV canal), isolated mitral valve cleft, or mitral valve prolapse.

Most mitral valve disease in the pediatric population is acquired. Causes of acquired mitral stenosis and mitral regurgitation are listed in Box 8-30 and detailed in the sections immediately following.

Mitral Valve Stenosis. Mitral stenosis is defined as a narrowing of the mitral valve orifice that can involve the leaflets, the annulus, or both. Isolated mitral stenosis is a rare form of congenital heart disease and accounts for less than 0.5% of congenital heart defects.

Stenosis of the mitral valve results in obstruction of flow to the left ventricle from the left atria. It can be caused by pathology in the supravalvular, valvular, or subvalvular regions. Congenitally stenotic valves frequently produce obstruction at more than one level.

A variety of terms are used to describe abnormal stenotic mitral valves. The term *mitral arcade* valve implies the presence of thickened leaflets, absent or abnormal chordal insertions, and fused commissures. A "parachute" mitral valve takes the form of a funnel or the dome of a parachute with

FIG. 8-42 Mitral valve anatomy, shown in relationship to tricuspid valve (TV), pulmonary valve (PV) and aortic valve. Ao/RCC, aortic valve, right coronary cusp; Ao/NCC, aortic valve, noncoronary cusp; Ao/LCC, aortic valve, left coronary cusp, RCA, right coronary artery; LCA, left coronary artery; LAD, left anterior descending branch of LCA; LCir, left circumflex branch of LCA. (From Nichols DG, et al, editors: *Critical heart disease in infants and children*, ed 2, St Louis, 2006, Mosby, Fig. 28-1.)

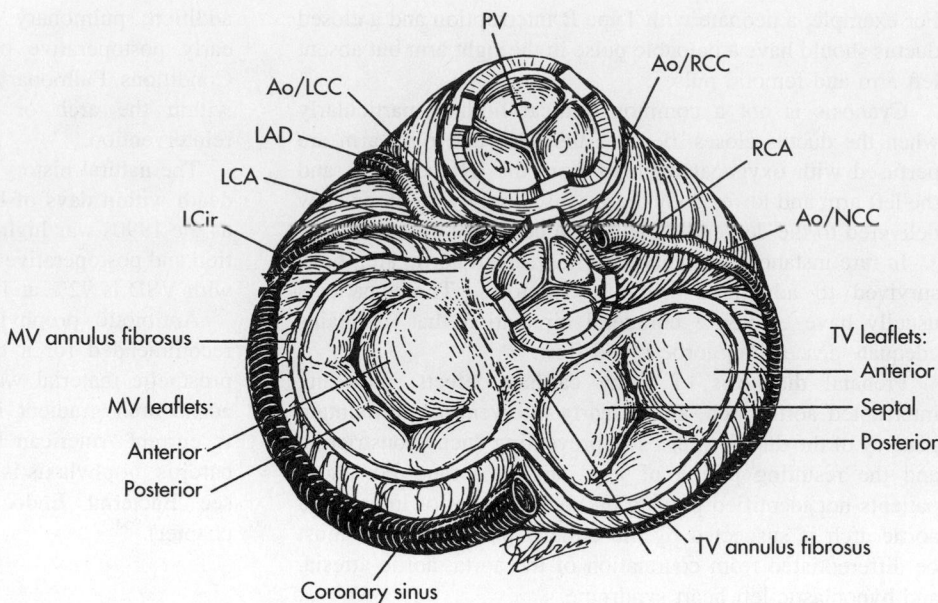

Mitral Stenosis
- Rheumatic fever
- Endocarditis
- Collagen vascular disease (e.g., lupus erythematosus)
- Infiltration disorders (e.g., glycogen storage disease)
- Cardiac tumors in area of mitral valve apparatus
- Surgical intervention (e.g., AVSD repair)

Mitral Regurgitation
- Rheumatic fever
- Myocarditis
- Endocarditis
- Kawasaki disease related coronary abnormality resulting in ischemia
- Dilated cardiomyopathy
- Papillary muscle infarction resulting from ischemic injury
- Postoperative, following surgical repair

---

multiple small holes in the sides of the tissue and no true central orifice; it is considered the most severe form of congenital mitral stenosis.[309] Lastly, the mitral valve can be entirely normal from a structural perspective but hypoplastic. This small size makes the valve functionally stenotic as is often the case in hypoplastic left heart syndrome (see section, Single Functioning Ventricle).

Mitral Valve Regurgitation. Mitral regurgitation, also referred to as mitral insufficiency, is far more common than mitral stenosis. Causes include dilation of the valve annulus to a point where leaflets no longer appose each other, resulting in central regurgitation. Mitral regurgitation can also result from structural abnormalities similar to those causing mitral

stenosis such as dysplastic leaflets, isolated leaflet cleft, leaflet prolapse, or abnormal chords and papillary muscles.

Mitral Valve Prolapse. Mitral valve prolapse is present when the mitral valve leaflets move back across or prolapse across the mitral valve annulus into the left atrium during ventricular systole. In the past mitral valve prolapse was often over diagnosed in children using echocardiographic criteria. However, more recent studies using consistent diagnostic criteria found rates of occurrence in the general population between 0.6% and 2.4%.[271,279]

Mitral valve prolapse occurs both as a primary lesion and in association with a variety of other disorders. It is strongly associated with connective tissue disorders such as Ehlers-Danlos syndrome and is almost always present in patients with Marfan syndrome. Mitral valve prolapse is also associated with congenital heart defects such as ASD, Ebstein anomaly, and corrected transposition.

Pathophysiology

Mitral Valve Stenosis. When there is obstruction to blood flow from the left atrium to the left ventricle, the left atrium dilates and left atrial pressure increases. This left atrial hypertension causes elevation in pulmonary venous pressure and pulmonary congestion. The increased pulmonary venous pressure will cause elevated pulmonary arterial pressure, requiring increased right ventricular systolic pressure. In addition, severe obstruction of blood flow from the left atrium to the left ventricle can produce decreased cardiac output, although left ventricular function is usually maintained. Extreme mitral stenosis, as seen in Shone syndrome or hypoplastic left heart syndrome may prevent the left heart from supporting systemic circulation and the child may be dependent on flow from the right ventricle through the pulmonary artery and ductus arteriosus to maintain adequate systemic blood flow.[421]

Mitral Valve Regurgitation. As with mitral stenosis, mitral regurgitation increases left atrial and pulmonary venous pressures and ultimately increases pulmonary artery pressure. However, mitral regurgitation also results in left ventricular volume overload and may produce left ventricular dysfunction. Once mitral regurgitation of any origin is present, it is likely to progress because the regurgitation itself results in left ventricular dilation and further mitral valve annulus dilation and insufficiency.

Mitral Valve Prolapse. The consequences of mitral valve prolapse are determined by the degree of mitral regurgitation, which in turn is directly proportional to the amount of prolapse and the extent of annular dilation. The hemodynamic consequences of mitral regurgitation apply to infants and children with mitral valve prolapse.

Clinical Signs and Symptoms

The clinical presentation of mitral stenosis and mitral regurgitation is multifactorial and depends on the severity of obstruction or regurgitation and potential compounding effects if both lesions are present. Mild mitral stenosis or regurgitation is usually not associated with symptoms. In the setting of moderate mitral stenosis, infants present with symptoms typical of congestive heart failure, including tachypnea, diaphoresis, poor feeding, and failure to thrive. The presence of pulmonary venous congestion increases risk of respiratory infections. Older children may present with orthopnea, dyspnea on exertion, and exercise intolerance. Symptoms of moderate to severe mitral insufficiency are often identical to those of mitral stenosis.

Arrhythmias, including atrial flutter and atrial fibrillation can develop in patients with significant atrial enlargement caused by either mitral stenosis or insufficiency. These arrhythmias can be detected by Holter or event monitor. Echocardiography is the diagnostic tool of choice in patients with mitral stenosis and mitral regurgitation.

Mitral Valve Stenosis. Auscultatory findings in mitral stenosis include an opening snap, which is a sharp high-pitched sound occurring after the second heart sound (S2), corresponding to the mitral valve opening. The murmur associated with mitral stenosis is heard at the apex and is a low-frequency, mid-to-late diastolic murmur. The pulmonary component of the second heart sound is increased if pulmonary hypertension is present.

Increased right heart forces and right-axis deviation are present on the ECG for both mitral stenosis and regurgitation. The chest x-ray of patients with moderate to severe mitral stenosis demonstrates prominent pulmonary vasculature and cardiomegaly with left atrial enlargement.

In assessing mitral stenosis, 2D echocardiographic images can identify structural abnormalities at the valvular, subvalvular, and supravalvular levels. Doppler flow studies across the mitral valve enable calculation of the flow gradient from the left atrium to the left ventricle. Mild stenosis results in a mean gradient of 4 to 5 mm Hg, a moderate gradient is 6 to 12 mm Hg, and a gradient greater than 13 mm Hg indicates

severe stenosis. Severe stenosis is often associated with systemic right heart pressures. It is important to remember, however, that the estimated gradient is affected by flow through the mitral valve and the presence of a left-to-right atrial level shunt can decrease the estimated gradient (because flow across the valve is decreased) and a left-to-right ventricular level shunt may increase the gradient (because pulmonary blood flow and the flow of pulmonary venous return across the mitral valve is increased).

A second echocardiographic method of evaluating the severity of mitral stenosis is to measure functional size of the mitral valve orifice. Normal values have been identified for children and relate to body surface area, allowing calculation of Z scores. A Z score of -2.5 to -3.0 indicates a low likelihood that the mitral valve is functional.[421]

Cardiac catheterization may be helpful in some cases of mitral stenosis if echocardiography alone is unable to determine Doppler gradients or right heart pressures. Ideally, left atrial and left ventricular pressures are measured simultaneously to definitively calculate the pressure gradient. The left atrial pressure can be estimated via pulmonary artery wedge pressure: after a balloon-tipped catheter is inserted through the right heart and into the pulmonary artery, inflation of the balloon occludes the antegrade flow through the pulmonary artery so the pressure distal to the balloon can reflect left atrial pressure. However there are several caveats to this estimation of left atrial pressure (see Pulmonary Artery Catheters in Chapter 21).

Mitral Regurgitation. Physical examination findings with mitral regurgitation include a hyperactive precordium and a high frequency holosystolic blowing murmur heard at the apex with radiation to the left axillae. If mitral insufficiency is severe, a diastolic rumble can be heard secondary to increased blood flow crossing the mitral valve. The pulmonary component of the second heart sound may be increased if pulmonary hypertension has developed.

Patients with mitral regurgitation have an enlarged left ventricle. Increased right heart forces and right-axis deviation are seen on the ECG for both mitral stenosis and regurgitation, but patients with mitral regurgitation also demonstrate increased left heart forces.

Echocardiography can very effectively diagnose mitral regurgitation, often identifying even very trivial regurgitation. Mitral regurgitation is usually graded as mild, moderate, or severe. Echocardiography is also able to localize the regurgitation as either central or through a cleft and can identify the presence or progression of left atrial and left ventricular enlargement. Cardiac catheterization is not necessary or specifically useful in identifying the source or severity of insufficiency.

Mitral Valve Prolapse. Current diagnostic criteria for mitral valve prolapse include both auscultatory and echocardiographic findings. A mid-to-late systolic click with or without a murmur of mitral regurgitation is present on physical examination. Two-dimensional echocardiography to confirm the diagnosis of mitral valve prolapse requires visualization of the mitral valve apparatus falling back into the left atrium across the plane of the mitral valve in systole.

Patients with mitral valve prolapse can be asymptomatic. Presenting complaints may include palpitations, atypical or nonspecific chest pain, decreased exercise tolerance or fatigue, and syncopal or near syncopal episodes. The palpitations are attributed to premature atrial contractions or premature ventricular contractions. Supraventricular tachycardia and ventricular arrhythmias are common in those patients with moderate to severe mitral regurgitation resulting in left atrial and left ventricular enlargement. The type of chest pain reported is of variable severity and not reproducible during an exercise stress test.

Management

Mitral Valve Stenosis. Management of mitral stenosis is determined by the severity of the obstruction. Patients with mild mitral stenosis are often followed clinically with serial echocardiograms performed to evaluate any left atrial enlargement and the progression of the gradient across the mitral valve. These patients are often asymptomatic and the stenosis may or may not progress.

Moderate degrees of mitral stenosis produce pulmonary venous obstruction and pulmonary venous congestion that can often be successfully managed medically while closely monitoring for signs of deteriorating left or right ventricular function or worsening pulmonary hypertension. Patients with severe mitral stenosis require early intervention.

Medical Therapy. Treatment targets relief of symptoms of congestive heart failure. Pulmonary edema is treated with diuretic therapy. Patients with poor weight gain, frequent respiratory infections, or echocardiographic signs of worsening ventricular function require further intervention.

Pulmonary venous congestion from mitral stenosis increases the risk of severe respiratory illnesses including respiratory syncytial virus (RSV). The administration of palivizumab (Synagis), a humanized monoclonal antibody against the RSV is recommended in infants and children younger than 24 months with hemodynamically significant heart disease such as mitral stenosis. Palivizumab is administered monthly during RSV season and timing varies by geographic region.

Interventional Therapy. The low incidence of congenital mitral stenosis has limited the experience with balloon mitral valvuloplasty in smaller children. As a result, mitral valve balloon valvuloplasty is primarily performed in patients with rheumatic mitral stenosis. Balloon dilation should not be attempted for treatment of mitral stenosis if the valve leaflets are poorly defined or there is parachute-like anatomy.

Successful balloon dilation reduces the degree of stenosis and delays the need for surgical intervention until the child is larger. Unfortunately, the unwanted tradeoff for relief of stenosis is mitral insufficiency. Currently percutaneous balloon valvuloplasty of the mitral valve should be contemplated only in select patients at centers with established experience and skill.[92]

Surgical Therapy. Surgical intervention for mitral stenosis involves repair or replacement of the mitral valve. Typically much effort is made to avoid mitral valve surgery in infants and children because results are variable, morbidity can be high, and often there is need for valve replacement. The surgical approach for each patient must consider valve anatomy and the presence of any associated lesions. Closure of an associated PDA or VSD may sufficiently reduce the pulmonary venous return and blood flow through the mitral valve that the mitral valve gradient is reduced and need for mitral valve surgery is eliminated or postponed. Approaches to repairing a stenotic mitral valve include resection of a supravalvular mitral ring, commissurotomy, splitting of fused cords or papillary muscles, muscle resection, or enlargement of the mitral annulus.

When mitral valve repair is not possible, replacement becomes necessary. Most commonly the valve is replaced with a prosthetic (mechanical) valve although placement of a bioprosthetic valve (homograft or heterograft) in the mitral position is an option. Unfortunately, bioprosthetic valves exposed to left ventricular (systemic) pressures deteriorate quickly, requiring early reintervention.[164]

Mitral valve replacement in small patients requires careful consideration of valve size because a prosthetic or bioprosthetic mitral valve placed during childhood is eventually outgrown and will require another valve replacement. Alternately, placing too large a prosthesis into the native valve annulus can result in complete heart block.

Placement of a mechanical mitral valve results in the need for long-term anticoagulation and its associated risks in infants and children (see Postoperative Care and Anticoagulation). In adolescent females the use of bioprosthetic valves is preferred because the warfarin required for anticoagulation of mechanical valves has teratogenic potential.[65] The preferred valve for smaller children is a low-profile bileaflet valve. For infants with a valve annulus smaller than the smallest prosthetic valve available, supra-annular mitral valve replacement is a surgical option.[421]

Mitral Valve Regurgitation. Therapy to treat mitral regurgitation varies with the severity of the insufficiency. Mild to moderate regurgitation can be palliated temporarily with medical anticongestive therapy (diuretics) and close monitoring of left ventricular function. Progression to moderate insufficiency or the acute development of severe regurgitation necessitates surgical intervention.

Medical Therapy. Medical management of mild to moderate mitral regurgitation includes standard pharmacologic therapy for congestive heart failure. Specifically, afterload reduction with use of angiotensin converting enzyme inhibitors is beneficial in treating mitral insufficiency and should be maximized.

Interventional Therapy. Currently there are no interventional catheter techniques that are effective in the management of mitral regurgitation.

Surgical therapy. The criteria for surgical intervention to treat mitral regurgitation are less stringent than for repair of mitral stenosis because surgical intervention generally substantially improves the degree of insufficiency regardless of the anatomic cause. Delay in repair can worsen the chance of successful repair if left ventricular dysfunction develops or secondary changes to the valve occur.

The initial surgical attempt is almost always valve repair with valve replacement reserved as a final option. Surgical intervention for a regurgitant valve consists of assessment of annulus size, ensuring that leaflets are mobilized, leaflet repair if necessary, and closure of any clefts.[509]

Operative techniques for addressing the mitral regurgitation include cleft closure, chordal shortening, and annuloplasty for central regurgitation.[421] The placement of an annuloplasty ring to aid in reduction of annulus size is typically avoided in infants and children because it may restrict the growth of the annulus. The procedure for mitral valve replacement for mitral regurgitation is the same as for mitral stenosis; however, the presence of annulus dilation eliminates the need for supra-annular valve placement.

Postoperative Care. Postoperative care after mitral valve surgery requires close assessment for changes in left ventricular compliance, and monitoring for elevated left atrial pressure and pulmonary hypertension. The placement of a left atrial pressure catheter intraoperatively facilitates this postoperative management.[155]

In addition to monitoring for possible development of complete heart block mentioned earlier, other potential postoperative complications following valve implantation include thrombus formation on the surface of the mechanical valve and hemolysis. The absence of a mechanical click raises concern regarding possible thrombus formation on the mechanical valve leaflets. The development of a perivalvular leak can result in a shearing force that lyses red blood cells.

Results for surgical management of mitral valve disease vary by complexity of the repair needed and the presence of associated cardiac defects. Straightforward repair of mitral regurgitation carries the lowest surgical risk with documented hospital mortality of 1.1% to 3.3%. However, for surgical repair of complex mitral anomalies with concurrent intracardiac disease, mortality prior to discharge as high as 26.6% has been reported.[337,955] Unfortunately, patients undergoing surgical repair of the mitral valve often require reoperation and possible valve replacement.

In general, mitral valve replacement carries a higher mortality rate and less favorable prognosis than mitral valve repair. For children requiring valve replacement, early series reported operative mortality as high as 33%; however, recent advances in perioperative management have decreased hospital mortality to 5.8% for isolated mitral valve replacement.[337]

Mitral Valve Prolapse. The natural history of mild mitral valve prolapse with mild mitral regurgitation is generally excellent. Surgical repair or replacement of the mitral valve is needed for those patients with moderate to severe mitral regurgitation, and should be undertaken before the development of significant left atrial or left ventricular enlargement.

Box 8-31	**Advanced Concepts: Mitral Valve Dysfunction**

- The ausculatory exam findings alone can often diagnose mitral valve prolapse. Patients with mitral valve prolapse have a mid-systolic click and late systolic murmur. The most important feature of the murmur and click in mitral valve prolapse is its variability with maneuvers designed to increase or decrease the left ventricular systolic volume.
  - With maneuvers such as moving from a squat to a standing position, which decrease left ventricular systolic function and thus decrease venous return, the click and murmur occur earlier in systole.
  - With maneuvers that increase left ventricular systolic volume, such as moving from a standing to a squatting position, the click and murmur occur later in systole.
- The timing of the click can also vary with the severity of the prolapse and regurgitation. A later click and murmur are usually associated with milder prolapse, whereas more significant prolapse and regurgitation cause the click to move earlier into systole.

Operative techniques include those reviewed in the discussion of surgical management of mitral stenosis and mitral regurgitation.

Patients with mitral valve prolapse may require endocarditis prophylaxis. For those with mitral valve prolapse without valvular regurgitation, endocarditis prophylaxis is not recommended. If there is valvular dysfunction and associated insufficiency, the patient falls into the moderate risk category and endocarditis prophylaxis is recommended. And finally, those with mitral valve prolapse resulting in a bioprosthetic or prosthetic cardiac valve placement are considered to be high-risk for endocarditis and endocarditis prophylaxis is recommended (see Bacterial Endocarditis later in this section of the chapter).[952]

Advanced concepts for the care of the child with mitral valve dysfunction are listed in Box 8-31.

CYANOTIC DEFECTS

General principles in the care of the child with cyanotic heart disease are summarized in the section, Common Clinical Conditions, Hypoxemia. When the newborn demonstrates cyanosis it is important to determine if the cyanosis is cardiac (i.e., caused by congenital heart disease) or pulmonary in origin. The hyperoxia test is often performed (Box 8-32).[364]

If cyanotic heart disease is likely or possible and pulmonary or systemic blood flow is dependent on the ductus arteriosus, prostaglandin E_1 is administered to reopen and keep the ductus patent. The administration of PGE_1 is summarized in Box 8-33. Further evaluation and management is described for each congenital defect.

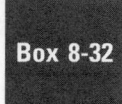

Box 8-32

Hyperoxia Test for Newborns with Suspected Cyanotic Heart Disease (to distinguish intrapulmonary from intracardiac shunt)[364]

1. Administer room air to the newborn (10-15 min, if tolerated)
2. Obtain baseline arterial PO_2 from right radial artery (via arterial puncture or transcutaneous oxygen monitor—pulse oximetry oxyhemoglobin saturation cannot be used)
3. Administer 100% oxygen (via mask, oxygen hood, or endotracheal tube, if intubated) for 10–15 min
4. Obtain arterial PO_2 from right radial artery (via arterial puncture or transcutaneous oxygen monitor—pulse oximetry oxyhemoglobin saturation cannot be used)

Results:

- PaO_2 is <50 mm Hg despite administration of 100% oxygen: cyanotic heart disease likely
- PaO_2 is 50–250 mm Hg: Cyanotic heart disease possible
- PaO_2 >250 mm Hg: Cyanotic heart disease unlikely

Box 8-33   Prostaglandin E-1 Administration

- Initial dose: 0.05-0.1 mcg/kg per minute IV/IO
- Maintenance infusion: 0.01-0.05 mcg/kg per minute IV/IO infusion
- May produce vasodilation, hypotension, apnea, fever, agitation, and seizures
- May also produce hypoglycemia and hypocalcemia

Tetralogy of Fallot and Pulmonary Atresia with Ventricular Septal Defect

Lisa M. Kohr

Pearls

- The degree of cyanosis is determined by the severity of right ventricular outflow tract obstruction.
- Neonates with tetralogy of Fallot (TOF) with severe pulmonary stenosis have ductal-dependent pulmonary blood flow, requiring PGE_1 and surgical intervention.
- Hypoxemic spells can occur during activities that increase oxygen demand such as crying and feeding. Note that blood flow to the lungs is limited by the right ventricular outflow tract obstruction. Conditions that may contribute to hypoxemic spells:
  - Dehydration
  - Anemia
  - Acidosis

Etiology

Tetralogy of Fallot refers to the association of four cardiac abnormalities described in detail in 1888 by French physician Etienne Fallot. The four cardiac anomalies include a ventricular septal defect, right ventricular outflow tract obstruction, overriding aorta (it arises above the ventricular septal defect) and right ventricular hypertrophy (Fig. 8-43). If an atrial septal

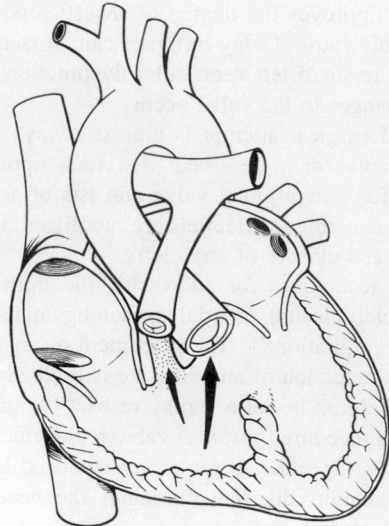

FIG. 8-43 Tetralogy of Fallot. This defect is defined as the association of four anomalies: a ventricular septal defect, pulmonary infundibular stenosis (often the pulmonary valve and main pulmonary artery are small), dextroposition of the aorta (the aorta shifts to the right and overrides the VSD), and right ventricular hypertrophy. Pentalogy of Fallot includes these four defects plus an atrial septal defect; this association of anomalies often occurs with a small left ventricle. The arrows show direction of the blood flow from the right ventricle into the pulmonary artery and aorta. The more severe the obstruction, the smaller the pulmonary blood flow and the larger the shunt from the right ventricle into the aorta.

defect is also present, the defect is known as *pentalogy of Fallot*. In the classic form of pentalogy of Fallot, the left ventricle is small, because much of pulmonary venous return is diverted to the right side of the heart through the ASD.

Tetralogy of Fallot is thought to result from inadequate development of the subpulmonary conus during fetal life. This not only produces pulmonary infundibular stenosis, but also causes malalignment of the conal septum during fetal cardiac development, resulting in a large unrestrictive ventricular septal defect that is approximately equal to the size of the aorta. The bundle of His is generally located at the posteroinferior edge of the defect, placing the infant at risk for arrhythmias during the postoperative phase.

In addition to infundibular stenosis, valvular and supravalvular pulmonary stenosis may be present in varying degrees. The pulmonary valve is almost always involved in the obstruction. A bicuspid pulmonary valve is present in nearly two-thirds of patients with TOF and the pulmonary annulus is typically smaller than normal for age.[886]

The aorta is displaced to the right (toward the right ventricle) because the subpulmonary conus and pulmonary outflow tract have not developed normally. As a result, the aorta sits directly over the ventricular septal defect; this also may be referred to as an *overriding aorta*. Right ventricular hypertrophy is merely a compensatory response to the obstruction to right ventricular outflow.

Tetralogy of Fallot is the most common cyanotic congenital heart lesion and is responsible for approximately 9% of all congenital heart defects.[886] It may be associated with additional intracardiac anomalies that are likely to alter the clinical presentation or management. Common combinations include pulmonary atresia with ventricular septal defect, tetralogy of Fallot with absent pulmonary valve, and tetralogy of Fallot with atrioventricular canal defect. Patients with tetralogy of Fallot often have a right aortic arch, multiple ventricular septal defects, or persistent left superior vena cava.

When the pulmonary stenosis is extreme, there is no anatomic connection between the right ventricle and the pulmonary artery. This severe form of tetralogy of Fallot may be referred to as *pulmonary atresia with ventricular septal defect,* or pseudotruncus arteriosus. It is discussed briefly here and again in the Truncus Arteriosus section.

Rarely, tetralogy of Fallot is associated with a rudimentary or absent pulmonary valve. This occurs in 5% of children with tetralogy of Fallot, and produces valvular insufficiency during the neonatal period.[886] As a result, aneurysmal dilation of the main pulmonary artery as well as the right and left branch pulmonary arteries develops. The dilated pulmonary artery and branch arteries compress the trachea and right and left main bronchii and may result in significant respiratory compromise.

Tetralogy of Fallot may be associated with an atrioventricular septal defect (see Atrioventricular Septal Defect earlier in this chapter). This combination occurs in less than 2% of infants with tetralogy of Fallot and is associated with trisomy 21. As part of the atrioventricular canal portion of the defect, an atrial septal defect is present in addition to an anterior valve leaflet that is common to both the tricuspid and mitral valves. Moderate or severe atrioventricular valve insufficiency is present.

Pathophysiology

Tetralogy of Fallot. The hemodynamic changes that develop with uncomplicated tetralogy of Fallot are determined by the severity of obstruction to pulmonary blood flow. When pulmonary infundibular and valvular stenosis is mild, the right ventricular pressure is only mildly increased; there is minimal shunting of blood through the ventricular septal defect because pulmonary vascular resistance is approximately equal to systemic vascular resistance. The result is a balanced shunt and balanced pulmonary and systemic circulations. The pulmonary stenosis is protective; it prevents development of a significant pulmonary shunt once pulmonary vascular resistance falls. This form of tetralogy is often referred to as "pink" (acyanotic) tetralogy of Fallot. It does not require treatment in the newborn period and patients are typically discharged home from the newborn nursery to feed and grow, on no medications. Hypoxemia and cyanosis will typically develop with progression of right ventricular outflow tract obstruction. As right ventricular obstruction increases, more blood shunts from the right ventricle across the ventricular septal defect into the aorta, causing systemic arterial oxygen desaturation. Initially, oxygen desaturation is only noted during exertion (e.g., during vigorous cry); however, when significant pulmonary stenosis is present, cyanosis is present even at rest. The increased right ventricular obstruction results in right ventricular hypertrophy.

Suprasystemic right ventricular hypertension does not develop in patients with tetralogy of Fallot because the ventricular septal defect serves to "vent" the right ventricle.

The greater the resistance to pulmonary blood flow, the greater is the volume of the right-to-left shunt through the ventricular septal defect into the aorta.[886]

Approximately 8% of children with tetralogy of Fallot have abnormalities in coronary artery anatomy.[886] The most common abnormalities include a single coronary artery arising from the aorta (with later branching into the right and left coronary arteries), or a left anterior descending coronary artery arising from the right coronary artery. One result of these anomalies is that the left anterior descending coronary artery may cross over the right ventricular outflow tract. It is extremely important that this anomalous coronary artery distribution be identified preoperatively so that surgical repair can be planned to avoid coronary artery injury.[886] This may necessitate cardiac catheterization to delineate coronary anatomy if the coronary arteries are not clearly visualized with echocardiography. In addition, it is important to identify the presence of multiple ventricular septal defects, aortopulmonary collaterals, and the extent of right ventricular outflow tract obstruction before surgical repair.

Pulmonary Atresia with VSD. When pulmonary blood flow is significantly compromised such as in the neonate with tetralogy of Fallot with severe pulmonary stenosis or pulmonary atresia with VSD, pulmonary blood flow is dependent on the ductus arteriosus. As a result, severe hypoxemia develops when the ductus begins to close. Rarely, older children with unrepaired tetralogy of Fallot are seen for evaluation. These children generally develop collateral vessels from the descending aorta to the bronchial arteries to supply pulmonary arteries with additional blood flow.

Tetralogy of Fallot with Absent Pulmonary Valve. If an infant has tetralogy with absent pulmonary valve, pulmonary insufficiency is present from birth and produces right ventricular dysfunction. There is aneurysmal dilation of the main pulmonary artery that may involve the branch pulmonary arteries. The dilated pulmonary artery compresses the tracheobronchial tree, producing airway obstruction and air trapping with possible emphysema. These infants also have right-to-left shunting of blood through the ventricular septal defect, with resultant arterial oxygen desaturation.

Tetralogy of Fallot with Atrioventricular Septal Defect. The combination of tetralogy of Fallot with atrioventricular septal defect produces a left-to-right shunt at the atrial level. Mitral insufficiency is present and if significant, will increase left atrial pressure and increase the magnitude of left-to-right shunting through the atrial septal defect. If a ventricular component is present, right-to-left shunting will occur through the AVSD, with resulting hypoxemia.

Clinical Signs and Symptoms

Tetralogy of Fallot. The hallmark symptom of tetralogy of Fallot is cyanosis that is directly proportional to the degree of pulmonary stenosis. The infant with mild pulmonary stenosis may not demonstrate any symptoms because there is minimal shunt through the ventricular septal defect. If the pulmonary stenosis is severe or pulmonary atresia is present, the right-to left shunt through the ventricular septal defect will be significant and the infant will demonstrate severe cyanosis even at rest. (See Hypoxemia in the second section of this chapter for a discussion of the potential systemic consequences of polycythemia.)

Neonates with tetralogy of Fallot and mild pulmonary stenosis generally are monitored in the hospital until the patent ductus arteriosus closes to ensure there is a sufficient amount of antegrade blood flow across pulmonary valve. After the ductus constricts, the neonate may demonstrate cyanosis with exertion, but should generally maintain an oxyhemoglobin saturation greater than 75%. As the infant grows and becomes more active, the right ventricular outflow tract obstruction usually becomes more severe because it does not grow proportionate to the child's growth. The fixed obstruction caused by the pulmonary stenosis prevents an increase in pulmonary blood flow and oxygen delivery during periods of increased oxygen requirement. The infant usually begins to demonstrate progressive cyanosis and decreased exercise tolerance at 4 months of age.

If a newborn presents with cyanosis of unknown origin at birth, a hyperoxia test is performed. One hundred percent oxygen is administered to the infant in an attempt to determine whether the etiology of the cyanosis is cardiac or pulmonary related (see Box 8-32). If the arterial oxygen tension (PaO_2) remains less than 50 mm Hg after administration of 100% oxygen, the cyanosis is likely caused by cyanotic congenital heart disease.

The neonate with tetralogy of Fallot and severe pulmonary stenosis or small branch pulmonary arteries generally presents with cyanosis at birth. In these infants, most pulmonary blood flow is provided through the ductus arteriosus. If the infant has been diagnosed in utero, a prostaglandin E_1 infusion is initiated at birth to prevent constriction of the ductus arteriosus (see Box 8-33). If prostaglandin E_1 is not administered, the neonate will likely become profoundly hypoxemic and acidotic as the duct closes. These neonates will also require surgical correction or a palliative intervention to improve pulmonary blood flow.

Unrepaired infants with tetralogy of Fallot may begin to develop hypoxemic spells as early as the first months of life depending on the severity and progression of pulmonary stenosis. Hypoxemic spells are thought to be caused by a transient increase in right ventricular outflow tract obstruction and a fall in systemic vascular resistance; these changes decrease pulmonary blood flow and promote right-to-left shunting across the ventricular septal defect, resulting in progressive hypoxemia. The spells typically occur in the morning, particularly during activities that increase oxygen demand such as during crying, defecation, or feeding. Infants who are dehydrated, anemic, acidotic, or have increased circulating catecholamines are at particular risk for developing hypoxemic spells.

With the onset of hypoxemic spells (also called "tet" spells or hypercyanotic spells), the infant becomes acutely cyanotic, hyperpneic, irritable, and diaphoretic and arterial oxyhemoglobin saturation falls. Late in the spell the infant may become limp and lose consciousness. If an arterial blood gas is obtained during the spell, hypercapnia, hypoxemia, and acidosis will be noted. Hypercyanotic spells can result in stroke, seizures, or death, so the development of hypoxemic spells is typically considered an indication for surgery. Administration of a beta-blocker such as propranolol may be indicated if a delay in surgery is warranted. Beta-blockade acts to relax the right ventricular infundibulum, decrease right ventricular response to agitation, and decrease the incidence and severity of hypoxemic spells.

Children with tetralogy of Fallot who are not repaired in infancy develop polycythemia caused by chronic hypoxemia. When the hematocrit approaches 60%, the infant may demonstrate a more rapid respiratory rate and increased work of breathing because polycythemia increases blood viscosity, which decreases the velocity of pulmonary blood flow. Infants with unrepaired tetralogy and chronic hypoxemia demonstrate clubbing of the tips of the fingers and toes.

If the iron intake of the infant with chronic hypoxemia is inadequate, a microcytic anemia will develop that will not only decrease arterial oxygen content but will increase risk of cerebrovascular accident (stroke). The infant may have a normal hemoglobin concentration for age but may demonstrate a relative anemia because polycythemia is present. The mean corpuscular hemoglobin concentration (MCHC) and mean corpuscular volume (MCV) should be followed to identify and treat microcytic anemia.

On physical examination, a systolic ejection murmur can be heard best at the second intercostal space along the left sternal border. This murmur is caused by flow through the narrowed pulmonary outflow tract. The murmur disappears during hypoxemic episodes because blood flow across the narrowed pulmonary outflow tract decreases substantially. Bruits may be heard over the child's back if the child has developed extensive collateral circulation to the lungs.

If moderate or severe pulmonary stenosis is present, the presence of a sternal lift indicates right ventricular hypertrophy. Right ventricular hypertrophy in addition to right axis deviation will be evident on the electrocardiogram. Echocardiography can fully delineate the intracardiac and extracardiac anatomy (including size and position of the ventricular septal defect, appearance of the right ventricular outflow tract, aortic position, and size of main and branch pulmonary arteries) and can enable estimation of right ventricular pressure and the gradient across the pulmonary valve.

Cardiac catheterization is rarely performed because of the advanced imaging capabilities of echocardiography. Indications for cardiac catheterization include the presence of multiple ventricular septal defects or the need to further delineate the pulmonary vascular and coronary artery anatomy. These children can develop a hypoxemic episode during the procedure. As a result, noninvasive diagnostic modalities such as computed tomography-angiography or magnetic resonance-angiography provide safer diagnostic options.

On chest radiograph, a narrow mediastinum is observed because the main pulmonary artery segment is small. The classic radiographic cardiac contour in the infant with tetralogy of Fallot resembles the shape of a boot. The apex of the heart is elevated because right ventricular hypertrophy is present; as a result, the apex resembles the upturned toe of a boot. Pulmonary vascular markings are decreased when pulmonary stenosis is severe, unless collateral vessels to the lungs have developed. Approximately one-fourth of patients with tetralogy of Fallot have a right aortic arch (see Table 8-25).

Pulmonary Atresia with VSD and Collateral Pulmonary Blood Flow. Prenatal diagnosis assists in the management of this group of patients. Postnatal diagnosis may be delayed if aorta to pulmonary artery collateral flow provides sufficient pulmonary blood flow. In many instances, the collaterals become stenotic, at which time the child will develop cyanosis. If collateral flow is significant, signs and symptoms of congestive heart failure and failure to thrive develop by about 3 to 6 months of age. Other significant findings include a continuous murmur due to collateral flow, and a single S_2.

The chest radiograph reveals mild to moderate cardiomegaly with no main pulmonary artery segment and increased pulmonary vascular markings. Cardiac catheterization is routine to assist with delineation of the branch pulmonary artery anatomy, which may be small and nonconfluent.

Tetralogy of Fallot with Absent Pulmonary Valve. Infants with tetralogy of Fallot and absent pulmonary valve often have mild cyanosis, congestive heart failure, and significant respiratory distress. These infants have a muffled, single second heart sound because only the aortic valve closure is heard. A harsh, systolic ejection murmur (caused by pulmonary infundibular stenosis) and a prominent, low-frequency diastolic murmur (resulting from pulmonary insufficiency) may be present and accompanied by a thrill.

Right ventricular hypertrophy is evident on clinical examination and on the ECG. The chest radiograph typically reveals an enlarged heart, increased pulmonary vascular markings and a large pulmonary artery silhouette. Echocardiography reveals right ventricular dilation as well as dilation of main, right and left pulmonary arteries. The pulmonary valve is absent. Cardiac catheterization is rarely needed for diagnosis.

Tetralogy of Fallot with Atrioventricular Canal Defect. This combination of lesions often tempers the symptoms that normally would be produced by either lesion alone. The pulmonary stenosis associated with tetralogy of Fallot prevents excessive pulmonary blood flow that normally would result from the atrioventricular septal defect, so that signs of severe congestive heart failure are not observed. If pulmonary stenosis is mild or moderate, pulmonary blood flow is decreased, and cyanosis may be readily apparent. Atrioventricular valve regurgitation is usually present.

The child with tetralogy of Fallot and atrioventricular septal defect demonstrates a pulmonary systolic murmur as well as a systolic murmur heard over the left lower sternal border (VSD murmur). An apical systolic murmur produced by mitral insufficiency is also present.

The ECG confirms the presence of right ventricular hypertrophy, but a superior axis deviation consistent with atrioventricular septal defect is also noted. Findings on chest radiograph are dependent on the severity of the combined lesions. Echocardiography reveals features consistent with tetralogy of Fallot as well as the presence of a common

atrioventricular valve leaflet. Cardiac catheterization is rarely performed in these children because echocardiography provides adequate preoperative information.

Management

Tetralogy of Fallot. With the expanded use of fetal ultrasound, a diagnosis of congenital heart disease is often established before birth. This allows the medical team to prepare for the immediate initiation of PGE_1 and transfer to a cardiac center for medical and surgical management at birth. Many of these neonates have umbilical lines placed and they may be intubated as a precautionary measure for transport to a tertiary care center.

Medical Management of Tetralogy of Fallot. If the neonate is diagnosed postnatally, the infant will present with cyanosis shortly after birth. A hyperoxia test is typically administered to assist in differentiating the cause of the hypoxia. Failure to respond to 100% oxygen (i.e., PaO_2 less than 50 mm Hg) is most likely caused by a cyanotic cardiac lesion, and initiation of prostaglandin E_1, and an echocardiogram is warranted.

Initial medical management in the newborn period is directed at maintaining adequate oxygenation and preventing hypoxemic spells until surgical correction is performed. If mild pulmonary stenosis is present, the infant will generally be monitored in the hospital while the patent ductus closes and then follow-up care is provided to prevent complications until surgical care is performed. Clinicians should consider chromosomal analysis and fluorescent in situ hybridization (FISH) testing as part of routine newborn care before discharge. Ten percent of infants with conotruncal defects have an associated chromosomal abnormality. The most common genetic disorder is 22q11 microdeletion, which places the infant at risk for vascular anomalies in addition to the cardiac lesion (see Section, Essential Anatomy and Physiology, Etiologies of CHD: Noninherited and Genetic Factors).

The infant should be kept well hydrated to prevent hemoconcentration, and microcytic anemia should be avoided because it decreases oxygen content and increases the child's risk of cerebral thromboembolic events. Parents should be taught when to notify a physician or nurse practitioner if the infant develops diarrhea, nausea, vomiting, or fever, so that dehydration can be prevented or promptly treated and antibiotic prophylaxis can be prescribed if needed. The parents should be taught to monitor for signs of hypoxemic episodes. Instruction should include potential triggers and should include alleviating maneuvers such as calming the child and placement in the knee-chest position. If a hypoxemic spell does develop, surgery should be scheduled.

Whenever the infant or child with uncorrected tetralogy of Fallot is admitted to the hospital, it is essential that no air be allowed to enter any IV line because systemic venous blood may shunt directly into the aorta and any IV air may cause a cerebral air embolus. All staff members should be aware that infants with tetralogy of Fallot may develop hypoxemic spells.

Hypoxemic spells are treated by calming the infant, placing the child in the knee-chest position and administering oxygen, a potent pulmonary vasodilator. The on-call physician or nurse practitioner should be notified immediately if any spells

Box 8-34 Management of Hypercyanotic Spells

- Calm the child
- Administer oxygen
- Place child in knee chest position
- Administer morphine (0.1 mg/kg IV or IM) to improve pulmonary blood flow
- Administer intravenous fluids (bolus isotonic crystalloids or packed red blood cells if needed to maintain adequate hemoglobin and hematocrit)
- Administer propranolol (beta-adrenergic blocking agent)
  - reduces dynamic obstruction to pulmonary blood flow
  - IV dose: 0.15-0.25 mg/kg per dose, slow IV push
- Administer IV phenylephrine (alpha-agonist)
  - produces arterial and venous constriction. This should increase venous return to the right ventricle, and reduce right-to-left shunt and hypoxemia.
  - IV bolus: 5-20 mcg/kg per dose
  - IV infusion: 0.1-0.5 mcg/kg per minute, titrate to effect
  - IM dose: 0.1 mg/kg per dose
- Ketamine (anesthetic) may be considered because it increases systemic vascular resistance (and therefore reduces the right-to-left shunt and hypoxemia and should improve pulmonary blood flow). A sedative IV dose is 0.25-0.5 mg/kg.

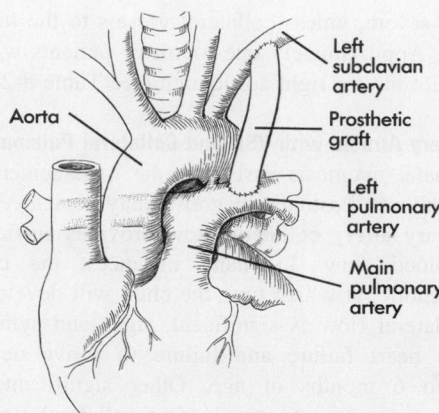

FIG. 8-44 Modified (Prosthetic) Blalock-Taussig shunt. A prosthetic shunt, usually made of polytetrafluoroethylene (Gore-Tex or Impra) is sewn between the patient's subclavian artery and the pulmonary artery to provide a systemic-to-pulmonary artery shunt.

develop, and the bedside nurse should anticipate administering a weight-appropriate dose of intravenous morphine sulfate (0.1 mg/kg). If these maneuvers do not alleviate the spell, propranolol, phenylephrine or ketamine may be given. Sodium bicarbonate may be administered to correct acidosis. In addition, volume in the form of packed red blood cells may be ordered to maintain the hematocrit greater than or equal to 45% and alpha-agonists may be administered to increase systemic vascular resistance (and reduce the right-to-left shunt, thereby increasing pulmonary blood flow). A beta-blocking agent may be given to relax the RV infundibulum and decrease RV outflow tract obstruction (Box 8-34).

Complete corrective surgery is typically performed for the symptomatic full-term neonate with tetralogy of Fallot. The optimal age for elective correction of tetralogy of Fallot remains controversial. Surgery is generally recommended when the child's oxyhemoglobin saturation decreases to less than 70% to 80%.

Palliation of Tetralogy of Fallot. Many centers use a staged approach for premature or small-for-gestational-age infants. A staged surgical approach involves the placement of a Blalock-Taussig or modified Blalock-Taussig systemic to pulmonary artery shunt. The modified Blalock-Taussig shunt procedure involves placement of a 3.5- to 4.0-mm Gore-Tex tube between the innominate artery and ipsilateral pulmonary artery (Fig. 8-44). Additional palliative shunts for cyanotic heart disease are illustrated in the Evolve Fig. 8-5 and described in Evolve Table 8-2 in the Chapter 8 Supplement on the Evolve Website. Creation of a systemic to pulmonary artery shunt can be performed through a thoracotomy; however, a median sternotomy approach may be considered to enable initiation of cardiopulmonary bypass to support oxygenation in infants

considered to be at high risk for hypoxemic spells during anesthesia induction. Placement of the Blalock-Taussig shunt can result in scarring and branch pulmonary artery distortion at the distal anastomosis; such scarring and distortion must be addressed at the time of complete repair.

There are technical challenges to the placement of an optimal shunt: too large a shunt can result in excessive pulmonary blood flow with symptoms of congestive heart failure, a wide pulse pressure and bounding pulses resulting from aortic runoff. Too small a shunt results in continued hypoxemia. Rarely, reoperation is required to revise the size of the shunt.

The expected range of oxyhemoglobin saturation after the placement of a systemic to pulmonary artery shunt is 75% to 85%. During the immediate postoperative period, the nurse should monitor for signs of hypovolemia caused by osmotic diuresis, especially if the infant was placed on cardiopulmonary bypass for the procedure. This places the infant at risk for hemoconcentration, clot formation, and shunt occlusion. Arterial punctures and cuff blood pressure measurement should be avoided on the arm and artery used for the shunt.

Immediate postoperative complications also include bleeding and shunt occlusion. When a polytetrafluoroethylene shunt is used for the creation of the systemic-to-pulmonary artery shunt, the infant's platelet count will likely fall in the first day after surgery because platelets adhere to the shunt material until it endothelializes. The infant's platelet count should be monitored and it should gradually return to normal. To prevent clot formation, a heparin infusion may be ordered until the infant is tolerating enteral feedings and aspirin therapy (10 mg/kg every other day, or per protocol) can be started (see Antiplatelet Therapy in section, Postoperative Care and Anticoagulation for the Child with Heart Disease).

Signs of inadequate pulmonary blood flow or possible shunt occlusion include a change in the intensity of the continuous shunt murmur, a drop in baseline oxyhemoglobin saturation, increased cyanosis or acidosis. If shunt occlusion is suspected based on physical exam and echocardiographic findings, the nurse should prepare the infant for cardiac catheterization and/or surgery. In some cases, the nurse may administer a bolus of heparin and begin a heparin drip (if one is not present) in the hopes of maintaining shunt patency.

Occasionally, injury to the phrenic nerve, thoracic duct, or recurrent laryngeal nerve may occur when the surgical approach is via left thoracotomy. Phrenic nerve injury causes diaphragm paralysis, which may not be apparent while the child receives positive pressure ventilation, but should be suspected if the infant has difficulty weaning from ventilator support. A chest radiograph obtained while the infant is removed briefly from positive pressure ventilator support will reveal elevation of the hemidiaphragm on the involved side. If the diagnosis still remains unclear, observation of spontaneous breathing under fluoroscopy can confirm the diagnosis. Diaphragm paralysis is generally temporary and function returns within several weeks. If the condition prevents effective spontaneous ventilation, the team may consider diaphragm plication.

Injury to the thoracic duct can result in chylothorax that is not apparent until the infant begins taking oral or enteral nutrition containing long chain triglycerides. If the thoracic duct has been injured, the chest tube drainage will turn to a milky white. If a chest tube in not in place, the infant may develop a pleural effusion on the left side. (See Postoperative section, Chylothorax, for management strategies.)

Injury to the recurrent laryngeal nerve can lead to vocal cord paralysis. This condition is usually temporary and unilateral. Diagnosis of this condition typically begins when a weak or absent cry is noted after extubation. If persistent, the infant may be at risk for aspiration; therefore, a speech evaluation should take place to assess whether the infant can safely take oral feedings. If vocal cord paralysis is suspected, an otolaryngology specialist should be consulted to confirm the diagnosis.

Nonsurgical palliation has been reported for a select subgroup of infants with tetralogy of Fallot. These procedures include a balloon valvuloplasty to open the stenotic pulmonary valve and improve antegrade flow through the native pulmonary artery. In addition, a stent may be inserted to open the narrow right ventricular outflow tract. Both procedures are performed in the cardiac catheterization laboratory in high-risk infants and can only be done if the branch pulmonary arteries are contiguous. Both procedures attempt to provide a secure source of pulmonary blood flow until corrective surgery is performed; they may prove to be a viable alternative in the staging process.

Surgical Correction of Tetralogy of Fallot. Corrective surgery is electively performed at approximately 3 to 6 months of age; however, some centers delay elective repair until 1 year of age. The goals for surgical repair include closure of the ventricular septal defect and reconstruction of the right ventricular outflow tract.

Whenever possible a ventriculotomy is avoided and the repair is usually accomplished via a transatrial and transpulmonary approach. An incision is made in the right atrium and the surgeon gains access to the right ventricle through the tricuspid valve and closes the VSD from this approach (Fig. 8-45). Through this approach, the VSD is closed using a Dacron patch, directing LV flow to the aorta. Resection of the pulmonary stenosis is accomplished through

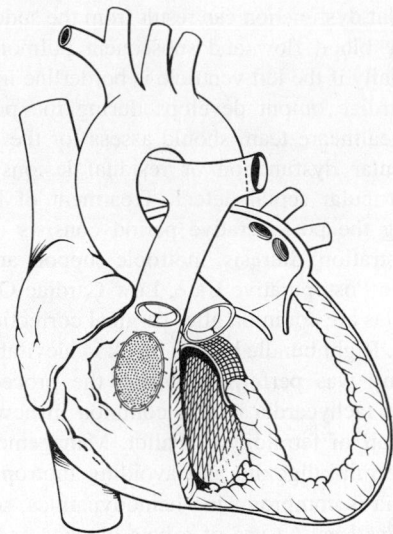

FIG. 8-45 Surgical correction of tetralogy of Fallot. Pulmonary infundibular stenosis is resected, and the ventricular septal defect (VSD) is closed with a patch. The pulmonary outflow tract is enlarged with one or two patches if necessary (one is depicted here). When possible, to avoid a right ventriculotomy incision, an atriotomy incision is performed, and the surgeon enters the right ventricle through the open tricuspid valve. The VSD is identified and closed from this approach. An incision is also made in the main pulmonary artery above the pulmonary valve, the pulmonary valve is opened and subpulmonary stenosis is resected.

the pulmonary artery. The surgeon makes an incision in the pulmonary artery, opens the pulmonary valve, and resects the subvalvular stenosis. The hypertrophic right ventricular infundibular muscle is resected and a pulmonary valvotomy is performed if needed. A right ventriculotomy is occasionally needed. Any existing systemic to pulmonary artery shunt is taken down at the time of repair.

If the pulmonary outflow tract and main pulmonary artery are small, a patch may be placed across the pulmonary outflow tract and if necessary, in the main pulmonary artery with extension onto the branch pulmonary arteries. Use of a transannular patch to enlarge the pulmonary valve annulus can reduce resistance to right ventricular ejection but can create valvular insufficiency. If pulmonary insufficiency is severe, the volume load produced by the insufficiency may cause severe postoperative right ventricular dysfunction.

Reoperation late in adolescence may be required to correct the valvular insufficiency. Reoperation may also be required if residual pulmonary branch stenosis is present because this increases resistance to pulmonary flow and magnifies pulmonary insufficiency.

Immediate postoperative complications include bleeding, low cardiac output, right ventricular dysfunction, and arrhythmias, especially junctional ectopic tachycardia. Additional complications include heart block, residual pulmonary stenosis, right ventricular outflow tract obstruction, and/or ventricular septal defect, pulmonary insufficiency, or damage to the aortic valve. Right heart failure may result from right ventricular dysfunction and is more likely to occur in neonates with pulmonary hypertension or those with residual pulmonary stenosis or significant pulmonary insufficiency.

Left ventricular dysfunction can result from the sudden increase in pulmonary blood flow and subsequent pulmonary venous return, especially if the left ventricle is borderline in size.

If low cardiac output develops during the postoperative period, the healthcare team should assess for the presence of right ventricular dysfunction or residual lesions such as a residual ventricular septal defect. Treatment of low cardiac output during the postoperative period consists of judicious fluid administration, diuresis, inotropic support and afterload reduction (see Postoperative Care, Low Cardiac Output).

Arrhythmias are common after surgical correction of tetralogy of Fallot. Right bundle branch block is inevitable if a right ventriculotomy was performed during the procedure. Junctional ectopic tachycardia is also common in newborns after complete repair of tetralogy of Fallot. Management includes mild hypothermia, digoxin, and avoiding inotropic drugs. If the arrhythmia is compromising hemodynamics, sedation and paralysis as well as the use of a beta-blocker or amiodarone may be used. If the junctional rate is slowed with beta-blockade and the patient has temporary pacing wires in place, overdrive pacing may allow for capture and conversion to sinus rhythm. Other arrhythmias seen during the postoperative period include heart block, supraventricular tachycardia, and premature ventricular contractions.

Abnormal neurodevelopmental outcomes have been found on follow-up and may be related to the exposure of the neonatal brain to cardiopulmonary bypass and prolonged hospitalizations. Studies comparing neurodevelopmental outcomes and the timing of the complete repair using cardiopulmonary bypass have found lower intelligence scores in the children who underwent complete repair as a neonate.[257,538,618]

Early mortality after complete repair has been reported at 5%. The incidence of sudden death late after tetralogy of Fallot repair is reported to be approximately 2% to 7%.[886] This risk of sudden death is extremely low among those patients with an excellent operative result, but is significant among patients with persistent severe right ventricular hypertension and a history of ventricular tachycardia. Life-long follow-up is required by this population for the management of residual pulmonary stenosis, chronic pulmonary regurgitation, and ventricular arrhythmias. Late reoperation may be necessary to preserve right ventricular function and exercise tolerance.[49] Endocarditis is a lifelong risk because there is typically some residual defect (e.g., mild pulmonary stenosis or insufficiency) adjacent to the VSD patch (and any other patches placed during the repair).

Pulmonary Atresia with VSD. The neonate will require administration of prostaglandin E_1 to maintain ductal patency. Surgical intervention will be required.

Surgical Correction of Pulmonary Atresia with VSD. Eligible children generally present in congestive heart failure with adequate arterial oxygen saturations and adequate pulmonary artery segments with a left-to-right (aorta to pulmonary) shunt. Surgical repair often consists of several steps: first, the pulmonary arteries are unifocalized; second, a right ventricular to pulmonary artery conduit is placed to promote growth of the proximal and distal pulmonary arteries. The ventricular septal defect is completely closed in children who have forward flow through the right ventricular outflow tract and adequately sized pulmonary arteries.

A postoperative right ventricular-to-left ventricular pressure ratio of less than two-thirds to three-fourths to one on direct measurement in the operating room is associated with good long-term results. Postoperative complications include right ventricular dysfunction, residual ventricular septal defect, pulmonary artery stenosis, right ventricular hypertension, aortic regurgitation, and arrhythmias, including heart block. Subsequent cardiac catheterizations may be necessary to assess the pulmonary arteries and need for balloon angioplasty or stenting. Reoperation will be required for conduit replacement if significant conduit stenosis or regurgitation develop. Endocarditis is a lifelong risk (see Bacterial Endocarditis later in this section).

Tetralogy of Fallot with Absent Pulmonary Valve. If the neonate with tetralogy of Fallot with absent pulmonary valve is symptomatic, generally with respiratory compromise, then severe dilation of the pulmonary artery and compression of the tracheobronchial tree is probably present. This condition produces signs of airway obstruction and air trapping necessitating the use of mechanical ventilation with positive end-expiratory pressure. Surgical repair requires cardiopulmonary bypass. The aneurysmal main and branch pulmonary arteries are plicated to relieve compression on the distal trachea and bronchus; the ventricular septal defect is closed and a right ventricle to pulmonary conduit is inserted.

Early mortality is significant, especially among symptomatic neonates with airway compromise. Postoperative complications include persistent respiratory failure, congestive heart failure, shock, and arrhythmias. Aggressive pulmonary toilet must be provided to these neonates to prevent further complications. Some infants require a tracheostomy.

Tetralogy of Fallot with Atrioventricular Canal. Definitive repair for this complex heart defect is typically performed between 6 and 12 months of age when the infant becomes symptomatic and is refractory to medical therapy. Cardiopulmonary bypass is instituted to perform a two-patch repair of the atrioventricular canal. An atriotomy is used to place a Dacron patch to close the ventricular septal defect and a pericardial patch is used to close the atrial septal defect. The common leaflet is sandwiched between the two patches, and this prevents the need for the surgeon to incise the common leaflet. The cleft in the mitral valve is closed with sutures and an incision is made in the pulmonary artery to facilitate resection of the pulmonary infundibular stenosis. Patch enlargement of the pulmonary outflow tract or insertion of a valved conduit is occasionally necessary. Postoperative complications include atrioventricular valve regurgitation, low cardiac output, congestive heart failure, arrhythmias, heart block, and bleeding. Right ventricular outflow tract obstruction may result from suboptimal placement of the intraventricular patch.

Advanced Concepts

Because many patients with tetralogy of Fallot have associated defects that affect the clinical presentation and medical and

Box 8-35   **Advanced Concepts: Tetralogy of Fallot (TOF)**

- TOF with mild PS produces a balanced shunt: the pulmonary stenosis prevents a large left-to-right shunt through the VSD, but it is not so severe as to produce a right-to-left shunt.
- TOF with severe PS presents with cyanosis and pulmonary blood flow is decreased substantially.
- Hypoxemic spells can be triggered by events that increase myocardial oxygen consumption. However, because of the obstruction to pulmonary blood flow is fixed, pulmonary blood flow cannot increase. This causes tissue hypoxia, acidosis, and further decrease in pulmonary blood flow. If the cycle is not broken, the infant will become severely cyanotic and acidotic. Shock can develop.

surgical management, it can be challenging to anticipate the clinical course and management (see Box 8-35). Skilled nursing assessment and care are required.

Ebstein Malformation

Mary Fran Hazinski

Etiology

Ebstein malformation is a congenital anomaly of the tricuspid valve that was first described by Wilhelm Ebstein in 1866. In this rare defect the tricuspid valve leaflets do not attach normally to the tricuspid valve annulus. The valve leaflets are dysplastic, and two of the leaflets (the medial or septal leaflet and the posterior leaflet) are displaced inferiorly, adhering to the right ventricular wall (Fig. 8-46).[61]

The cause of Ebstein malformation is unknown. The defect results when the tricuspid valve leaflets fail to develop normally from the interior aspect of the embryonic right ventricular myocardium during the fifth week of fetal cardiac development.

The anatomy of this defect varies widely, and additional associated intracardiac abnormalities are common. Atrial or ventricular septal defects and L-transposition ("corrected transposition" or ventricular inversion) are often present. When L-transposition is present, the anomalous tricuspid valve is on the *left* side, receiving pulmonary venous return.

Pathophysiology

Hemodynamic alterations resulting from Ebstein anomaly are related to the effects of this anomaly on right atrial size and pressure, tricuspid valve function, and right ventricular size and function. The inferior displacement of the tricuspid valve leaflets effectively incorporates a variable portion of the right ventricle into the right atrium, so a portion of the ventricle is "atrialized." As a result, the right atrium is dilated and right ventricular size is compromised. The atrialized portion of the right ventricle may *appear* to be relatively normal, or may be extremely thin with little ability to contract.[61]

The function of the tricuspid valve varies widely in Ebstein. The function is affected by the chordal attachments of the valve leaflets. Frequently the leaflets are attached

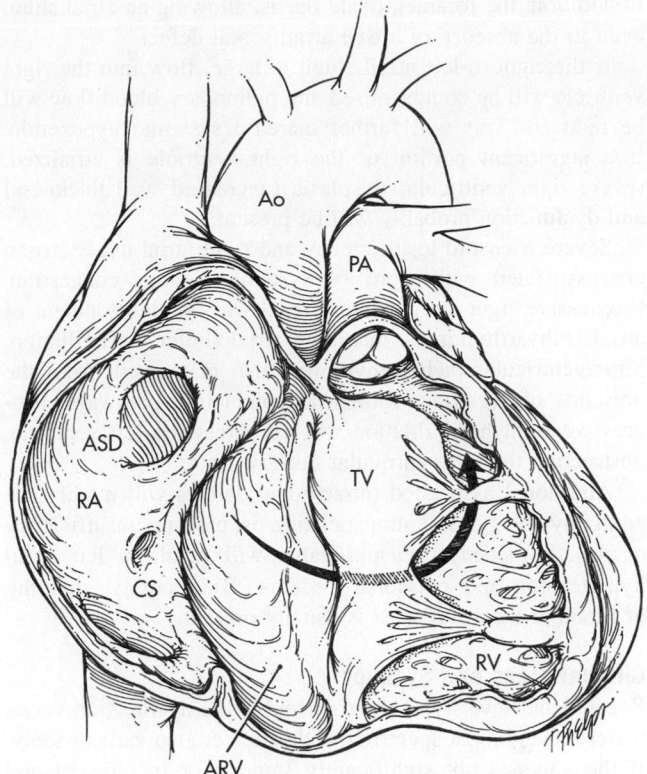

FIG. 8-46 Native anatomy of Ebstein anomaly. The tricuspid valve (TV) is displaced into the right ventricle (RV), leaving an atrialized portion of the RV (ARV) above the level of the displaced TV leaflets but below the level of what should be the tricuspid annulus. The anterior leaflet of the TV is large and sail-like and may obstruct the RV outflow tract. The posterior and septal TV leaflets are small, and a large ostium secundum defect (ASD) is seen. Ao, aorta; CS, coronary sinus; PA, pulmonary artery; RA, right atrium. (From Davidson DL, Bando K, Haelnaer M, Cameron DE: Ebstein anomaly. In Nichols DG, editor: *Critical heart disease in infants and children*, ed 2, Philadelphia, 2005, Elsevier, p. 908, Fig. 37-1.)

abnormally (tethered) to the right ventricular wall; this restricts leaflet motion and results in valvular insufficiency and stenosis. If the valve is minimally displaced and minimally tethered and is relatively competent, hemodynamic effects may be minimal.

Significant displacement and tethering of the tricuspid valve leaflets results in tricuspid insufficiency and stenosis. Right atrial pressure rises and right-to-left shunting of blood occurs through a foramen ovale or (less commonly) through a true atrial septal defect, resulting in hypoxemia.

During atrial systole, blood is propelled from the right atrium into the atrialized portion of the right ventricle, as well as into the true remaining right ventricle. During ventricular systole any contraction of the atrialized right ventricle results in regurgitation of blood into the true right atrium.

Right-to-left shunting of blood at the atrial level is typically greatest during the neonatal period. Until pulmonary vascular resistance falls, right ventricular systolic and end-diastolic pressures will be high; this increases tricuspid insufficiency.

In addition, the foramen ovale opens, allowing an atrial shunt even in the absence of a true atrial septal defect.

If the right-to-left atrial shunt is large, flow into the right ventricle will be compromised and pulmonary blood flow will be reduced. This will further increase systemic hypoxemia. If a significant portion of the right ventricle is atrialized, severe right ventricular dysplasia (decreased wall thickness) and dysfunction probably will be present.

Severe tricuspid insufficiency and right atrial hypertension are associated with signs of systemic venous congestion. Progressive right atrial dilation results in the development of atrial tachyarrhythmias, including atrial flutter or fibrillation. Supraventricular tachyarrhythmias also may result from the presence of accessory intraatrial conduction pathways. Progressive right heart dilation will compress the left ventricle, obstructing the left ventricular outflow tract.

Additional associated intracardiac defects will modify the pathophysiology. If L-transposition is present, insufficiency of the (left-sided) tricuspid valve will result in left atrial hypertension and pulmonary edema. Bidirectional shunting of blood at the atrial level is usually present.

Clinical Signs and Symptoms

Because the severity of the tricuspid valve dysfunction varies widely, the clinical spectrum of this defect also varies widely. If the valve is not significantly stenotic or insufficient and displacement is minimal, the patient may be asymptomatic during infancy and early childhood. Cyanosis may be present during the neonatal period, but disappears when pulmonary vascular resistance falls. Older infants may demonstrate cyanosis only during exercise. Late development of atrial arrhythmias is also common.[61]

Although Ebstein anomaly is a relatively rare congenital heart defect, it is one of the most common congenital heart defects diagnosed in utero. If the tricuspid valve is severely dysfunctional, significant right atrial dilation and systemic edema will be present in utero, producing hydrops, fetal pleural and pericardial effusions, and cardiomegaly, which are detected readily by fetal echocardiogram. Those defects diagnosed in utero are usually of the most severe form and carry the worst prognosis.

After birth, tricuspid valve dysfunction and right atrial hypertension result in a large right-to-left atrial shunt (through a foramen ovale), so that severe cyanosis is observed during the first days of life. In addition, signs of congestive heart failure also are observed. Cyanosis and congestive heart failure may be severe until pulmonary vascular resistance falls (when the neonate is several weeks old); at that point the infant's condition often improves.

Right ventricular dysplasia and dysfunction contribute further to the signs of tricuspid insufficiency, congestive heart failure, and cyanosis. Severe right heart dilation produces bulging of the ventricular septum toward the left ventricle, with resultant obstruction of the left ventricular outflow tract. Right atrial dilation also may be associated with stasis of systemic venous blood and paradoxic emboli to the left atrium; these may embolize to the systemic arterial circulation.

The hypoxemic child with Ebstein anomaly will develop compensatory polycythemia and is at risk for the development of systemic complications of this polycythemia. For further information, see Common Clinical Conditions, Hypoxemia in the second section of this chapter.

A systolic murmur of tricuspid insufficiency often is heard best at the left lower sternal border. Note that this location is unusual for tricuspid valve sounds but occurs because the valve leaflets are displaced inferiorly. The first heart sound may be normal or diminished in intensity, and tricuspid closure may produce a click. A diastolic murmur may be present, although its origins are unclear.[899]

Radiographic appearance of the heart and pulmonary vasculature vary widely among patients with Ebstein anomaly. The heart size and pulmonary vascular markings may be normal if the tricuspid valve is affected mildly; these findings most commonly are observed in older children. In the symptomatic infant the heart often is massively enlarged, with decreased pulmonary vascular markings (this distinguishes Ebstein anomaly from many other cyanotic heart lesions). Marked convexity of the right heart shadow (indicative of right atrial enlargement) is usually apparent. Massive right atrial enlargement produces a cardiac silhouette that resembles an inverted funnel; the mediastinum with small pulmonary artery silhouette creates a narrow top of the funnel, and the widened cardiac silhouette produced by right atrial enlargement creates the widened bottom of the funnel.

The electrocardiogram is always abnormal; right bundle branch block and right atrial enlargement are the most consistent features. Wolff-Parkinson-White syndrome (supraventricular tachycardia resulting from accelerated intraatrial conduction pathways) or other supraventricular atrial tachyarrhythmias are also common. The P-R interval usually is prolonged, and right axis deviation is common (see Table 8-26 and Common Clinical Conditions, Arrhythmias).

The echocardiogram enables thorough evaluation of the location and chordal attachments of the tricuspid valve leaflets, the size and wall thickness of the right ventricle, and the function of the heart in general. Those echocardiographic features associated with a severe form of Ebstein malformation and poor prognosis include: tethered distal attachments of the anterosuperior tricuspid leaflet, right ventricular dysplasia, left ventricular outflow tract obstruction (resulting from right heart dilation and septal deviation), and total combined area of the right atrium and atrialized right ventricle that is greater than the total combined area of the functional right ventricle, left atrium, and left ventricle. These risk factors are similar for patients of all ages with Ebstein malformation.

Cardiac catheterization is rarely necessary because the anatomy of Ebstein anomaly can be documented clearly by echocardiography. In fact the risk of fatal arrhythmias is so high that catheterization is avoided in many institutions. If catheterization and angiocardiography are performed, the child's heart rate and rhythm must be monitored closely and antiarrhythmic drugs must be prepared at the bedside.

The child with Ebstein anomaly is at risk for all of the systemic consequences of hypoxemia and polycythemia. Intracardiac conduction defects, including the presence of intraatrial conduction pathways, may also be present, and supraventricular tachycardia often develops. The PR interval is usually prolonged.

Management

Nonsurgical support of the patient with Ebstein anomaly requires treatment of congestive heart failure and management of arrhythmias. Diuresis cannot be too aggressive because hemoconcentration increases the risk of thromboembolic phenomena. Throughout therapy, until final surgical correction is performed, it is imperative that absolutely *no air be allowed to enter any intravenous line* because it may be shunted into the systemic arterial circulation, producing a cerebral air embolus (stroke). These children should not be allowed to become dehydrated; that may result in hemoconcentration and increased risk of thromboembolic events (see section, Common Clinical Conditions, Hypoxemia).

If pulmonary blood flow is severely compromised and hypoxemia is severe, the neonate should receive prostaglandin E_1 to maintain ductal patency (see Box 8-33). Indications for surgical intervention in any patient with Ebstein malformation include severe cyanosis and increasing polycythemia (including neonates dependent on ductal pulmonary blood flow), congestive heart failure refractory to medical management, tachyarrhythmias secondary to an accessory intraatrial conduction pathway, paradoxic emboli, or progressive disability.

Any surgical intervention for Ebstein anomaly will be palliative in nature. Classical palliative procedures for cyanotic heart disease, including systemic to pulmonary shunts, are generally not associated with relief of symptoms and clinical improvement. "Corrective" surgical procedures for Ebstein anomaly are still being refined, but if two ventricles are to be maintained, either tricuspid valve replacement or reconstruction is performed.

Although valve replacement can be performed, complications are higher than for other valve replacements. In addition, the child will outgrow the valve and subsequent re-replacement will be needed.

Reconstruction of the tricuspid valve requires plication of the atrialized portion of the right ventricle and repair of the tricuspid valve, freeing it from abnormal right ventricular attachments. Plication of the atrialized right ventricle is performed through insertion of mattress sutures passed through pledgets of Teflon cloth from the normal valve ring through folds created in the atrialized portion of the right ventricle to the rim of the displaced valve leaflets; the sutures are pulled together to pull the valve leaflets toward their normal position (Fig. 8-47). Sutures through the atrialized wall must

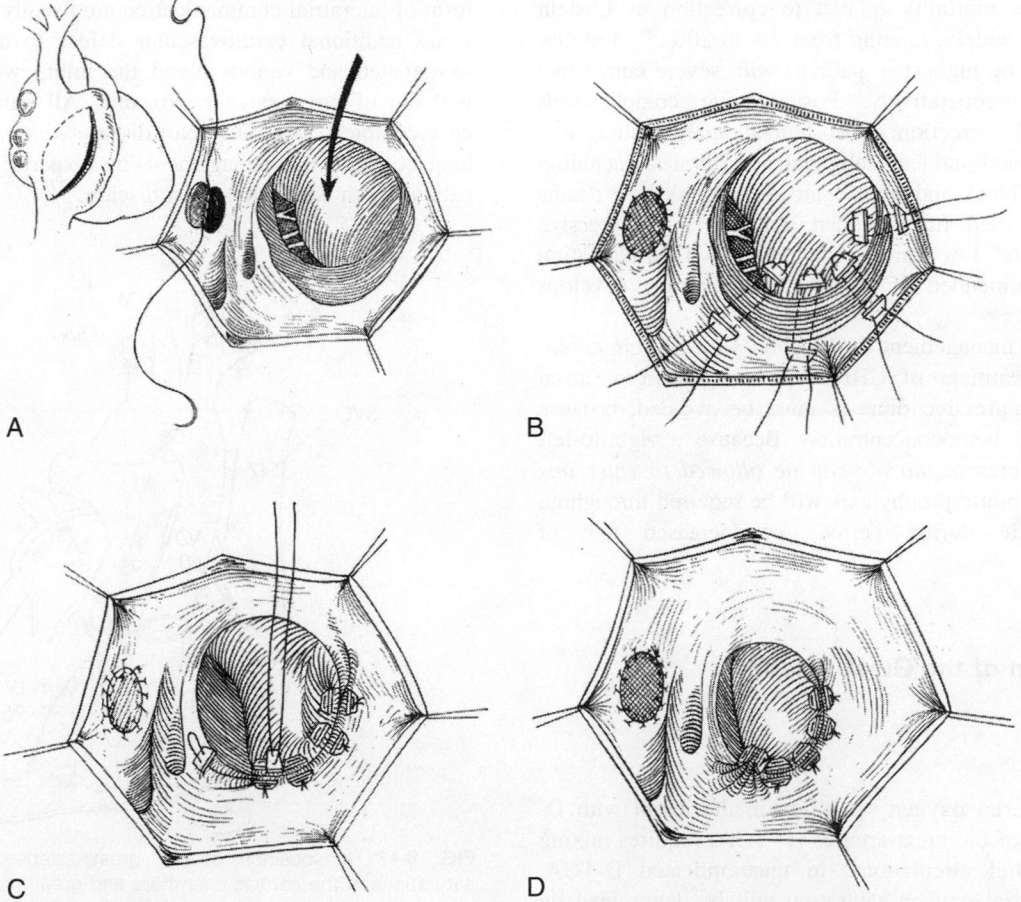

FIG. 8-47 Danielson repair of Ebstein anomaly, view from right atrial incision (atriotomy). **A,** Atrial septal defect is closed with a patch. Displaced tricuspid valve is indicated by arrow. **B and C,** Mattress sutures are passed through pledgets of woven material; they appear as rectangles above the valve annulus (in this figure they are depicted near the lower edge of the atrial incision at the bottom of each figure). The mattress sutures are used to pull folds of the atrialized ventricle and the displaced valve ring into the normal tricuspid valve position. **D,** A tricuspid annuloplasty is performed to reduce the size of the annulus. (Reproduced with permission from Perloff M: *Congenital heart disease in adults,* ed 3, Philadelphia, 2008, Saunders, Fig. 15-17.)

be carefully placed to avoid injuring coronary artery branches and the surgeon assesses the effects of suture placement. An annuloplasty is performed to reduce the size of the tricuspid valve orifice and ensure satisfactory tricuspid valve function. The associated atrial septal defect or patent foramen ovale is closed with a patch.[163] Successful tricuspid valvuloplasty is dependent on an intact anterior valve leaflet. If the anterior leaflet is abnormal or the surgeon is unable to fashion a functioning valve from existing tissue, a prosthetic valve is inserted. If accessory intraatrial conduction pathways are producing supraventricular arrhythmias, these are interrupted at the time of surgery.

The child may be managed as a patient with tricuspid atresia, in effect ignoring the right ventricle. Palliation and correction will be as for tricuspid atresia (see Tricuspid Atresia later in this section).

Children with Ebstein anomaly may be referred for cardiac transplantation rather than corrective surgery. Long-term results of transplantation for children with complex heart disease have not yet been determined, although it is hoped that these children will have better functional outcome immediately after transplantation than has been reported after surgical correction of the Ebstein anomaly.[693]

Perioperative mortality related to correction of Ebstein anomaly varies widely, ranging from 7% to 20%.[36] Mortality rates appear to be highest in patients with severe congestive heart failure preoperatively. Postoperative complications after traditional correction of Ebstein anomaly include low cardiac output and sudden malignant arrhythmias (including complete heart block and ventricular fibrillation). Late deaths have been reported from sudden arrhythmias, progressive heart failure and low cardiac output.[36,693] Transplantation may be recommended if clinical deterioration develops postoperatively.

Nonsurgical management of the child with Ebstein anomaly requires treatment of CHF and management of atrial arrhythmias. Aggressive diuresis must be avoided, because it may lead to hemoconcentration. Because a right-to-left shunt is often present, *no air can be allowed to enter any IV system.* Antibiotic prophylaxis will be required throughout the child's life during periods of increased risk of bacteremia.

Transposition of the Great Arteries

Jo Ann Nieves

Pearls

- Adequate arterial oxygen saturation in the infant with D-transposition of the great arteries (D-TGA) requires mixing of two parallel circulations. In uncomplicated D-TGA, systemic arterial oxygen saturation will be determined by the mixing of systemic and pulmonary venous blood and by the volume of effective pulmonary blood flow (i.e., systemic venous blood that enters the pulmonary circulation).
- Prostaglandin E_1 dilates the ductus arteriosus, enhancing intercirculatory mixing in the newborn with hypoxemia and D-TGA.

- A balloon atrial septostomy is performed to increase intercirculatory mixing at the atrial level, with resultant improved oxygen saturation.
- An arterial switch procedure is typically performed in the first weeks of life before pulmonary vascular resistance falls and the left ventricle accommodates to the lower resistance.

Etiology

When isolated D-TGA is present the aorta arises from the anatomic right ventricle and the pulmonary artery arises from the anatomic left ventricle. With this dextro-transposition (D-transposition of the great arteries, or D-TGA) the aorta lies anterior and to the right of the pulmonary artery (Fig. 8-48). D-TGA is the focus of this section and is abbreviated as TGA. L-transposition of the great arteries is addressed in the following section, and is referred to as congenitally corrected transposition of the great arteries (CCTGA).

D-transposition is often associated with additional congenital heart defects. A ventricular septal defect (VSD) is present in nearly half of patients with TGA, and a VSD with left ventricular outflow tract obstruction in 10%.[933] Coarctation of the aorta or aortic arch anomaly is present in about 5% of patients with TGA.[933] A patent ductus arteriosus and some form of interatrial communication are usually present. If there is no additional cardiovascular defect to allow mixing of oxygenated and venous blood the infant with transposition will die of progressive hypoxemia. All patients with TGA have complex congenital heart disease which will require life-long, continuous management by experts in the care of patients with congenital heart disease.[927]

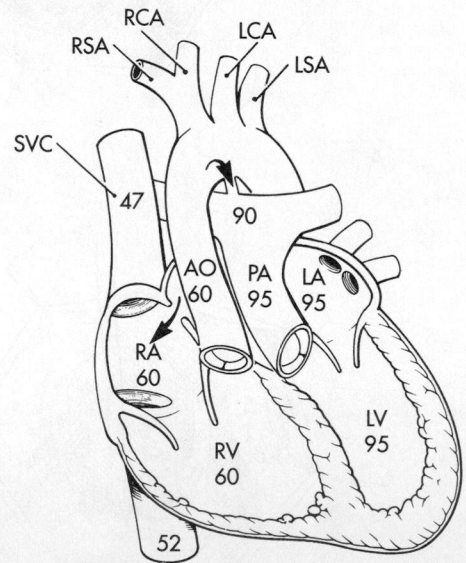

FIG. 8-48 Transposition of the great arteries. Typical oxygen saturations in the cardiac chambers and great vessels when some shunting (mixing) of blood occurs at the atrial level and through a patent ductus arteriosus. AO, aorta; LA, left atrium; LCA, left carotid artery; LSA, left subclavian artery; LV, left ventricle; PA, pulmonary artery; RCA, Right common carotid artery; RSA, right subclavian artery; RV, right ventricle; SVC, superior vena cava. (From Kambam J: Transposition of the great arteries. In Kambam J, editor: *Cardiac anesthesia for infants and children.* St Louis, 1994, Mosby.)

Pathophysiology

In TGA, the systemic and pulmonary venous circulations are completely separated, existing as two parallel circulations. Hypoxemic systemic venous blood enters the right atrium, the morphologic right ventricle, and is then recirculated into the systemic circulation through the aorta. Fully saturated pulmonary venous blood from the lungs enters the left atrium, flows into the morphologic left ventricle, and is recirculated back into the lungs via the pulmonary artery. As a result the body receives only recirculated, hypoxemic blood, which is incompatible with survival.[686]

Arterial oxygen desaturation is present at birth. The degree of hypoxemia/arterial oxygen desaturation present is determined by the amount of mixing between systemic and pulmonary venous blood. Survival in TGA depends on adequate mixing of blood between the two parallel circulations (Fig. 8-49).[287] Mixing of the two circulations can occur at a patent foramen ovale or other atrial communication, a ventricular septal defect and across a patent ductus arteriosus. The more mixing between the systemic and pulmonary venous blood that occurs in the heart or great vessels, the more saturated is the systemic arterial blood; if there is little mixing of systemic and pulmonary venous blood, arterial oxygen saturation is low (hypoxemia is severe). Higher concentrations of inspired oxygen do not improve the hypoxemia.[686,933]

Because hypoxemia is always present until surgical correction, the child is at risk for the development of complications of hypoxemia and polycythemia. Pulmonary vascular disease may also develop during infancy, whether or not pulmonary blood flow is increased.[933]

The degree of arterial oxygen desaturation is also determined by the effective pulmonary blood flow. This refers to the amount of desaturated systemic venous blood that enters the pulmonary circulation. It is not helpful if only oxygenated pulmonary venous blood returns to the pulmonary circulation; some desaturated systemic venous blood must also enter the pulmonary circulation.

If an intact ventricular septum is present the neonate is dependent on the mixing of blood through an interatrial communication and the patent ductus arteriosus. The most common form of interatrial communication in infants with TGA is a patent foramen ovale, although a true atrial septal defect is present in a small number of patients (5%).[933] If the foramen ovale is competent, very little shunting and mixing of blood occurs at the atrial level and the newborn will be profoundly hypoxemic and cyanotic, with a PaO₂ of 15 to 25 mm Hg.[933]

If the foramen ovale is moderately dilated, bidirectional interatrial shunting of blood occurs. In TGA with intact ventricular septum, right-to-left atrial shunting occurs during ventricular diastole because the left ventricle and pulmonary circulation offer less resistance to flow than the right ventricle and systemic circulation (particularly once pulmonary vascular resistance begins to fall). This right-to-left (systemic to pulmonary) shunting is enhanced during patient inspiration.[933] Left-to-right shunting of blood occurs during ventricular systole because the left atrium is less distensible than the right atrium, and the left atrial pressure rises more than right atrial pressure during ventricular systole.[933] If the foramen ovale is dilated significantly, bidirectional shunting of blood will occur freely, resulting in interatrial mixing of systemic and pulmonary venous blood and improvement in systemic arterial oxygen saturation. If adequate mixing of blood is present at the atrial level, and through the ductus arteriosus the neonate may demonstrate an arterial oxygen tension of approximately 30 to 45 mm Hg. A potential source of increasing cyanosis can result if a previously open interatrial communication begins to narrow and becomes restrictive.[933]

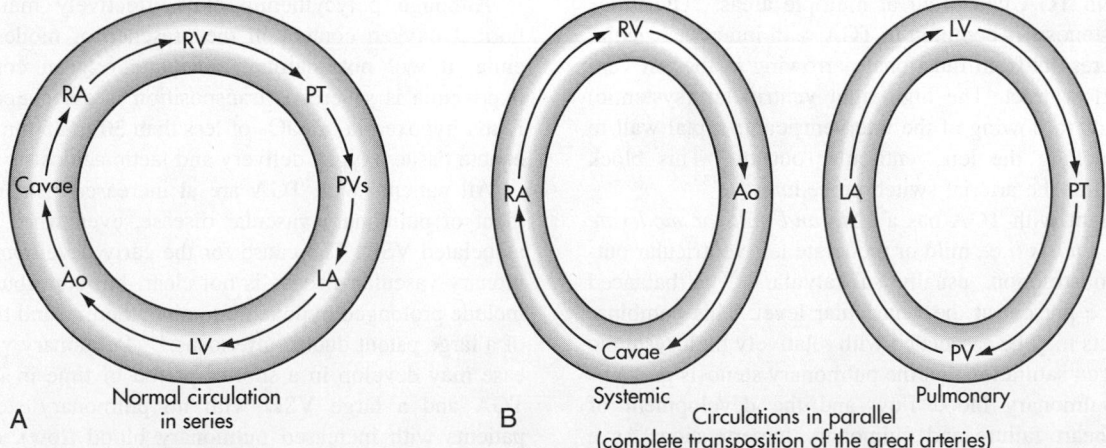

FIG. 8-49 Illustrations of the normal (series) pulmonary and systemic circulations and the distinctive parallel circulations in transposition of the great arteries. **A,** In the normal heart, there is a single circulation in series, with flow from the right ventricle (RV) into the pulmonary trunk (PT), through the pulmonary circulation into the pulmonary veins (PVs), left atrium (LA), left ventricle (LV), aorta (Ao), to the systemic circulation, then back to the heart via the venae cavae (cavae), into the right atrium (RA), and back to the right ventricle. **B,** In complete D-transposition of the great arteries, there are two circulations in parallel. The systemic circulation is characterized by flow from the right ventricle into the aorta and systemic circulation, returning through inferior and superior venae cavae to the right atrium, and back to the right ventricle. The pulmonary circulation is characterized by flow from left ventricle into pulmonary trunk and the pulmonary arteries, returning via the pulmonary veins to the left atrium, and back to the left ventricle. (From Perloff M: *Clinical recognition of congenital heart disease,* ed 5, Philadelphia, 2003, Saunders, Fig. 27-5.)

Because the ductus arteriosus provides some mixing of pulmonary and systemic venous blood, when the ductus arteriosus begins to constrict the neonate with TGA and an intact ventricular septum usually develops profound cyanosis, hypoxemia, and acidosis. Severe arterial hypoxemia can lead to anaerobic metabolism, lactate production, metabolic acidosis, hypoglycemia, hypothermia, and death will result if the intracardiac mixing does not improve.[933]

If a *ventricular septal defect (VSD)* is present, the size can range from small to large and it can be located anywhere in the septum. One-third of the defects are small, creating only small hemodynamic changes, and many of the muscular defects decrease in size or close.[933] The direction and magnitude of shunting are determined in part by the location and size of the VSD. A VSD located just under the pulmonary valve increases blood flow to the pulmonary circulation. The magnitude of the shunt is also determined by the presence of any left ventricular outflow tract obstruction. When the VSD is large with no left ventricular outflow tract obstruction, pulmonary blood flow is substantial, and the magnitude of pulmonary venous return favors a left-to-right shunt at the atrial and ventricular level during ventricular diastole.[933] During ventricular systole a right-to-left shunt occurs; some systemic venous blood from the right ventricle shunts to the pulmonary circulation (through the VSD) because the pulmonary circulation offers the path of less resistance.[933] The combination of a large VSD without pulmonic stenosis and with low pulmonary vascular resistance results in high pulmonary blood flow with development of CHF, and mild cyanosis (relatively high—but not normal—oxygen saturation).[933] The patient with TGA and VSD often has additional associated anomalies, including coarctation of the aorta, pulmonic stenosis or atresia, interrupted aortic arch, or atrioventricular valve anomalies.[287,686]

Pulmonary stenosis or left ventricular outflow tract obstruction in TGA can occur at multiple areas. "Dynamic" pulmonary stenosis is common in TGA with intact ventricular septum and results from functional narrowing in the left ventricular outflow tract. The high right ventricular (systemic) pressure leads to bowing of the interventricular septal wall to the left, blocking the left ventricular outflow. This block disappears after the arterial switch procedure.[287,933]

If the infant with TGA has a *VSD and mild or moderate pulmonary stenosis* (i.e., mild or moderate left ventricular outflow tract obstruction, usually subvalvular),[287] a balanced shunt may be present at the ventricular level. This combination of defects may be associated with relatively high systemic arterial oxygen saturation, yet the pulmonary stenosis prevents excessive pulmonary blood flow and the development of congestive heart failure and pulmonary hypertension. As a result, the infant may have few symptoms and may demonstrate adequate growth initially during infancy.[287] Systemic venous blood also may shunt into the left heart through a patent foramen ovale or the ventricular septal defect. As a result, adequate mixing of systemic and pulmonary venous blood occurs, and a higher systemic arterial oxygen saturation is present than that observed with isolated TGA.

If transposition is associated with a *VSD and severe subvalvular pulmonary stenosis* (i.e., severe left ventricular outflow tract obstruction) the total amount of pulmonary blood flow is reduced. Although the pulmonary stenosis does enhance the shunting of oxygenated blood from the left ventricle into the right ventricle or aorta, the absolute volume of pulmonary venous return (and oxygenated pulmonary venous blood available to mix with desaturated systemic venous blood) is reduced, so systemic arterial oxygen saturation is low. Profound hypoxemia and acidosis usually develop once the ductus arteriosus begins to close because the ductus provides a major source of pulmonary blood flow.

Bronchopulmonary collateral vessels have been found in more than 30% of children with TGA.[933] These vessels join the pulmonary vascular bed potentially providing an additional systemic to pulmonary artery pathway to improve effective pulmonary blood flow. The collateral vessels may contribute to the development of pulmonary vascular disease,[933] and typically need to be closed via interventional cardiac catheterization procedures if they persist after surgical repair.

In another variant of TGA, both great vessels exit from the right ventricle. This defect is also known as *double outlet right ventricle or the Taussig-Bing anomaly*. This lesion is discussed in a later section on double outlet right ventricle.

Unrepaired TGA produces chronic arterial oxygen desaturation.[287,686,927,933,935] Compensatory polycythemia develops to maintain effective oxygen delivery to the tissues. This polycythemia increases blood viscosity and introduces the risk of cerebral thromboembolism,[287] particularly during episodes of bacteremia, microcytic anemia, or dehydration. For these reasons the patient with cyanotic heart disease should not be allowed to become dehydrated, and an intravenous catheter should be inserted to enable administration of intravenous fluids whenever the child is placed NPO for cardiac catheterization or surgery (see section, Common Clinical Conditions, Hypoxemia).

Although polycythemia may effectively maintain near-normal oxygen content in the presence of moderate hypoxemia, it will not maintain adequate oxygen content when hypoxemia is severe. If transposition is associated with profound hypoxemia (a PaO_2 of less than 30 to 35 mm Hg), inadequate tissue oxygen delivery and lactic acidosis will develop.

All patients with TGA are at increased risk for development of pulmonary vascular disease, even when there is no associated VSD. The cause for the early development of pulmonary vascular disease is not clear, but contributing factors include prolonged hypoxemia, polycythemia, and the presence of a large patent ductus arteriosus.[933] Pulmonary vascular disease may develop in a shorter period of time in infants with TGA and a large VSD with no pulmonary stenosis (i.e., patients with increased pulmonary blood flow), even if the VSD narrows or closes.[287] The current approach to TGA includes surgical repair in the first weeks of life, possibly leading to a lower incidence of progressive pulmonary vascular obstructive disease.[933]

Transposition of the great arteries is associated with an increased risk of bacterial endocarditis. As a result the child with uncorrected transposition should receive appropriate antibiotic prophylaxis during episodes of increased risk of bacteremia (see Bacterial Endocarditis later in this section).

Clinical Signs and Symptoms

Transposition of the great arteries produces early and almost universal cyanosis during the neonatal period if there is inadequate mixing of systemic and pulmonary venous blood (e.g., if there is intact ventricular septum, a small ventricular septal defect, and a restrictive foramen ovale). Initially cyanosis may be mild, but it will progress.[933] Often the ductus arteriosus provides the major site of mixing of systemic and pulmonary venous blood, so profound cyanosis and acidosis usually develop when the ductus begins to close.

All neonates with TGA are tachypneic, typically without retractions,[287] and most are hyperpneic. Feeding is prolonged with the infant tiring quickly.[287] This increase in respiratory rate and tidal volume is thought to be stimulated by hypoxemia. The cyanosis does not change directly with administration of oxygen or crying.[287] However, oxygen administration can help decrease pulmonary vascular resistance, so pulmonary blood flow increases; this can lead to improved mixing of systemic and venous blood and some improvement in arterial oxygen saturation.[686]

If a large (unrestrictive) *VSD* is associated with transposition of the great arteries, cyanosis may be minimal during the neonatal period, especially while the ductus arteriosus is patent. However, signs of congestive heart failure usually develop once pulmonary vascular resistance falls (at approximately 2 to 6 weeks of age) and pulmonary blood flow increases. The infant usually demonstrates a progression from tachycardia and mild tachypnea to respiratory distress.[287] Dyspnea and feeding difficulties may develop.[686] Cyanosis is more notable with crying and stress.[933] If the infant has a VSD with coarctation or interrupted aortic arch, heart failure may develop days after birth[287] (see section, Common Clinical Conditions, Congestive Heart Failure).

If a large *PDA* is present, signs of heart failure may develop because the PDA provides a large shunt into the pulmonary circulation. The neonate often demonstrates tachypnea and mild cyanosis. Less than half of these infants will have the characteristic findings of a large PDA, including bounding pulse, continuous murmur, and mid-diastolic rumble.[933]

The combination of TGA, *VSD and mild pulmonary stenosis* often results in a balanced shunt. The pulmonary stenosis enhances mixing of systemic and pulmonary venous blood at the ventricular level and allows adequate pulmonary blood flow. Moderate pulmonary stenosis will prevent excessive pulmonary blood flow, so that congestive heart failure usually does not develop. If transposition of the great arteries is associated with *VSD and severe pulmonary stenosis,* the newborn typically demonstrates severe hypoxemia and cyanosis, particularly once the ductus arteriosus begins to close. Clinical findings are similar to those observed when tetralogy of Fallot or pulmonary atresia with intact ventricular septum is present.[933]

Peripheral pulses are not unusual, and the infant's precordium is usually quiet. Most neonates with TGA and intact ventricular septum have no heart murmur. The S2 is single and loud.[686] A grade 2/6 or softer systolic murmur might be heard along the mid to upper left sternal border, possibly representing a functional murmur produced by the left ventricular outflow tract.[933] A ventricular septal defect produces a holosystolic murmur after several days of age, and the infant may show signs of congestive heart failure and mild cyanosis.[686]

Right ventricular hypertrophy may produce a sternal lift. The ECG may not be helpful during the neonatal period because it normally indicates right ventricular hypertrophy during the first days of life.[287] Persistent signs of right ventricular hypertrophy, including upright T waves in V1 beyond the first days of life, are suggestive of right ventricular hypertrophy.[686] If a large ventricular septal defect or PDA is present, clinical and electrocardiographic evidence of biventricular hypertrophy will be noted (see Table 8-26).[686]

Echocardiography is the chief diagnostic tool used in the preoperative and postoperative evaluation of the infant and child with TGA.[933] The 2D echocardiogram will confirm the diagnosis of transposition of the great arteries and enable identification of any associated intracardiac defects or malposition. Doppler interrogation will estimate gradients along the left ventricular outflow tract.[287] A specialized fetal echocardiogram can diagnose TGA in utero, allowing for the prompt treatment of the newborn with PGE_1 administration before development of clinical deterioration.

Unless a ventricular septal defect is present, the heart size usually appears normal on the chest radiograph. Because the aorta lies in front of the pulmonary artery the mediastinum often appears to be very narrow and the cardiac silhouette is said to resemble the appearance of an "egg-on-side."[686] If a large ventricular septal defect is present, generalized cardiomegaly and increased pulmonary vascular markings are usually apparent once pulmonary vascular resistance falls and pulmonary blood flow increases. If severe pulmonary stenosis is present, pulmonary vascular markings will be decreased.

Cardiac catheterization is no longer required to confirm the diagnosis of D-TGA because this is accomplished by echocardiography. Catheterization may be performed to confirm information about the coronary anatomy, delineate specific aspects of associated defects, or to enable performance of a balloon atrial septostomy.[287] If the newborn has adequate intercirculatory mixing and an arterial switch is planned for the first days of life, an atrial septostomy may not be completed.[933]

If catheterization is performed immediately after birth, a catheter inserted via the umbilical vein or by percutaneous femoral artery entry,[933] will pass through the right atrium into the right ventricle, entering the aorta. If the catheter is passed through the foramen ovale it will enter the left atrium, left ventricle, and pulmonary artery. Arterial oxygen saturation in the aorta will be reduced, and saturation measurements made in the atria and ventricles will reveal the presence and significance of any additional intracardiac shunts. Angiocardiography will demonstrate spatial relationships and the presence of any additional shunts or defects.

Management

Medical Management. If the newborn demonstrates severe cyanosis during the first days of life, transposition of the great vessels should be suspected. Severe hypoxemia (PaO_2 less than 30 mm Hg) or acidosis must be reported immediately to the provider. An IV infusion of prostaglandin E₁ is initiated (see Box 8-33), and an echocardiogram is obtained on an urgent basis. Immediate therapy is directed to creating adequate mixing of systemic and pulmonary venous blood to maximize the arterial oxygen saturation and improve systemic oxygen delivery. In addition, therapy is directed to optimize ventilation in order to maximize pulmonary venous saturation; increased pulmonary venous saturation will, in turn, improve the arterial oxygen saturation. Supportive measures include administration of oxygen, treatment of acidosis, PGE₁ infusion, and respiratory support.

Throughout the diagnostic testing and hospitalization it is important that *no air be allowed to enter any IV system* because it may enter the systemic arterial circulation, producing a cerebral air embolus (see Common Clinical Problems, Hypoxemia).

The prostaglandin E₁ (PGE₁) infusion not only promotes patency of the ductus arteriosus, it also lowers pulmonary and systemic vascular resistance. As a result, effective pulmonary blood flow is increased and the PaO₂ and arterial oxygen saturation usually rises. Side effects of PGE₁ can include hypotension, requiring IV volume administration, and apnea requiring potential elective intubation with mechanical ventilation (see section, Common Clinical Conditions, Hypoxemia). If the neonate has transposition of the great arteries, a VSD, and no pulmonary stenosis, the increased pulmonary blood flow caused by prostaglandin administration can produce congestive heart failure, requiring inotropic support and diuresis.

If the PaO₂ remains very low (15 to 20 mm Hg), with an elevated PaCO₂ (despite adequate ventilation) and metabolic acidosis, this indicates poor mixing of the systemic and pulmonary venous blood and severely decreased effective pulmonary blood flow, most often seen with transposition and an intact ventricular septum. The causes for severe hypoxemia can include a restrictive foramen ovale and pulmonary hypertension.[935]

If the PGE₁ infusion does not lead to improved PaO₂ and a restrictive foramen ovale is present, prompt cardiac catheterization will likely be planned to perform a Rashkind balloon atrial septostomy in order to improve interatrial mixing (see Palliative Procedures). Additional treatment includes measures to decrease pulmonary vascular resistance (including oxygen administration and possible mild hyperventilation or administration of sodium bicarbonate to create alkalosis). These measures will not only increase effective pulmonary blood flow, they will also increase mixing of pulmonary and systemic venous blood at the atrial level (through the septostomy).[935] Provision of higher concentrations of inspired oxygen can promote pulmonary vasodilation with a decrease in pulmonary resistance, but will not greatly affect PaO₂ unless it reduces PVR and increases effective pulmonary blood flow.[287,933,935]

In the severely hypoxemic newborn, maximizing the oxygen delivery status will include improving mixed venous oxygen saturation, optimizing ventilation, and minimizing oxygen consumption. Because most systemic venous blood is recirculated to the body, the mixed venous oxygen saturation

has a major effect on the arterial oxygen saturation.[935] Providing sedation, mechanical ventilation, maintaining normothermia and neuromuscular blockade can each decrease oxygen consumption. Treat anemia to maximize oxygen content and delivery, although the ideal hemoglobin concentration threshold for transfusion has not been established in infants with cyanotic heart disease. Correct hypocalcemia and hypoglycemia.[686] Infants with TGA and a large VSD will require the usual therapies for congestive heart failure, including diuretics and possible digoxin (see section, Common Clinical Conditions, Congestive Heart Failure).[686] Cardiac output can be increased with inotropic support and vasodilation.

The management plan for the patient with TGA must be determined by the cardiology and cardiovascular surgical teams. No one surgical procedure or sequence provides optimal results for every patient. Therefore the cardiovascular team will recommend the procedure that should provide the best early and late results for each patient, in light of that patient's unique anatomy. Because infants with TGA are at risk for the development of complications of chronic hypoxemia and polycythemia, including cerebrovascular accident and pulmonary hypertension, early correction (during the neonatal period or early infancy) currently is favored if the anatomy is suitable. If early correction cannot be accomplished the infant should be monitored closely for complications of polycythemia (see section, Common Clinical Conditions, Hypoxemia).

Palliative Procedures. Several palliative procedures may be performed to improve systemic arterial oxygenation, increase interatrial mixing, and improve oxygen delivery.

Rashkind Septostomy. Before the recent success of the arterial switch corrective procedures, the Rashkind balloon septostomy was performed as the standard neonatal palliative procedure. Currently the septostomy may be performed to improve interatrial mixing of blood when neonatal hypoxemia is severe (particularly in neonates with simple D-TGA). However, the septostomy may not be performed if the TGA is associated with a large ventricular septal defect or surgical correction during the neonatal period is anticipated. If atrial (venous) correction of transposition is planned, the surgeon may wish to preserve atrial septal tissue to be used in the correction.

The Rashkind balloon septostomy can be performed at the bedside with echocardiographic guidance or it may be performed during cardiac catheterization. A balloon-tipped catheter is inserted in the umbilical or femoral vein and advanced through the inferior vena cava to the right atrium. It is passed through the foramen ovale into the left atrium, guided by echocardiography or fluoroscopy. The balloon is inflated and pulled back sharply into the right atrium, tearing and enlarging the septum primum flap of the fossa ovalis. If an adequate septostomy is achieved, the neonate's arterial oxygen saturation should rise by 10% or more and any interatrial pressure gradient should be minimal.[686] If the neonate fails to improve after the septostomy, it may have been inadequate; however, additional factors are likely to contribute to inadequate intracardiac mixing of blood, and repeat septostomies are rarely helpful.[933] It is postulated that those neonates with an unsatisfactory response to the septostomy despite adequate size of the interatrial defect (5 to 6 mm) may demonstrate a delayed fall in pulmonary vascular resistance with a resultant low pulmonary blood flow and decreased left atrial volume and pressure that decreases the interatrial mixing of pulmonary venous blood with systemic venous blood.[933] For these infants, surgical correction is probably necessary.

The balloon septostomy may not be successful in infants older than 2 months of age. These infants may require use of an atrial septal needle puncture followed by balloon dilation of the atrial opening, and potential placement of a stent in the atrial opening to maintain patency.[287] A catheter with an extendable blade tip may also be used to open the atrial septum.[933]

The PGE_1 infusion can usually be discontinued after a successful atrial septostomy.[933] The neonate must be monitored closely after the septostomy because arrhythmias, tamponade, and cerebrovascular accident have been reported after this procedure. Rare complications include perforation of the atrial wall, inferior vena caval injury, or damage to the atrioventricular valve.[933] Any blood loss during the catheterization should be quantified, and blood replacement is occasionally necessary.

Some infants demonstrate gradual worsening of hypoxemia after catheterization, and PGE_1 infusion may need to be restarted. Redevelopment of severe hypoxemia (demonstrated by a fall in PaO_2 and arterial oxygen saturation), worsening tachypnea, increased respiratory effort, irritability, or lethargy should be reported to a physician immediately. The neonate should be maintained in a neutral thermal environment (to reduce oxygen consumption), and ventilatory support should be available. Neurologic function should be evaluated frequently because cerebrovascular accidents (stroke), or ischemia may result from profound hypoxemia, or in the interval between palliation and corrective surgery. If deterioration occurs, urgent surgical intervention is often necessary.

Septectomy. The Blalock-Hanlon septectomy is rarely performed because early neonatal arterial repair is now provided, and if more interatrial mixing is required similar results usually can be obtained nonsurgically with the Rashkind procedure.[933] The procedure was, however, widely used in the past, so older patients may have had this procedure. The Blalock-Hanlon septectomy procedure does not require cardiopulmonary bypass. An atrial septal defect is made by clamping the posterior aspect of the interatrial septum and accessing and incising the septum within the clamped area. Following the atrial septectomy the systemic and pulmonary venous blood should mix better at the atrial level, producing an increase in arterial oxygen saturation.[933]

Systemic to Pulmonary Anastomosis. The infant born with TGA, VSD, and severe pulmonary stenosis will have severe cyanosis. An arterial switch cannot be performed, because the severe pulmonary stenosis is left ventricular outflow tract obstruction that would become severe aortic stenosis. Some infants will undergo a neonatal Rastelli procedure. If the Rastelli procedure will not be performed in the neonatal period, a palliative aortopulmonary shunt (see Fig. 8-44,

Modified Blalock-Taussig shunt; and Evolve Fig. 8-5 and Evolve Table 8-2 in the Chapter 8 Supplement on the Evolve Website) will be created to improve pulmonary blood flow until future physiologic correction by a Rastelli procedure. Operative mortality can be as low as 5%.[933]

Surgical Correction: Arterial Switch (Jatene) Procedure. The arterial switch operation is now established as the corrective procedure of choice for D-TGA with and without a VSD.[287,686,933] This procedure produces both anatomic and physiologic correction of TGA by restoring the normal anatomic relationships of the great vessels and the coronary arteries to the ventricles. The procedure was attempted initially in the early 1960s with no success because coronary artery relocation could not be accomplished. Following extensive advancements in pediatric cardiac surgery, Dr. Jatene and his colleagues reported the first survivor from the arterial switch procedure in 1975.[411]

The arterial switch procedure is accomplished using cardiopulmonary bypass and hypothermia, with a brief period of circulatory arrest or low-flow bypass.[583] Any existing intracardiac defects are corrected, and then the great vessels are transected approximately 1 to 2 mm above the semilunar valves. (The aorta is transected distal to the coronary artery ostia.) The coronary arteries, each surrounded by a cuff of adjacent aortic wall, are removed from the original aortic trunk, and these arteries are transplanted into the former pulmonary artery stump, because that stump (arising from the left ventricle) is now the neoaortic root. The great vessels are then sewn into their new locations so that the aorta arises from the left ventricle and the pulmonary artery arises from the right ventricle (Fig. 8-50). The Lecompte maneuver will pass the anterior aorta back to the posterior position, behind the bifurcation of the pulmonary artery.[583] Pericardial patches can be used to close the defects created by the removal of the coronary arteries from the former aorta (now the new pulmonary artery). An interposed prosthetic tubular conduit or direct connection joins the pulmonary artery connections.[933]

After the arterial switch, the left ventricle must be able to immediately support the systemic circulation. Following birth, the left ventricle in D-TGA with intact ventricular septum will eject blood into the pulmonary circulation. Although the pulmonary vascular resistance (PVR) is elevated for the first hours and days after birth, it soon begins to fall; as PVR falls, the left ventricle is able to maintain pulmonary blood flow by ejecting blood at lower and lower pressures. Most centers recommend surgical correction for newborns with TGA with intact ventricular septum during the first week or two of life, while the left ventricle is accustomed to generating high pressures to eject into a pulmonary circulation with relatively high resistance. Successful arterial switch for TGA with intact ventricular septum beyond 3 weeks to 2 months of age has been reported with no increase in mortality, but it may require preparation of the left ventricle to generate high pressure.[432] Planned postoperative circulatory support has been used successfully when the arterial switch is performed beyond 6 weeks of age. The planned circulatory support can allow the LV time to adapt to performing systemic work.[84]

FIG. 8-50 Surgical correction of transposition of the great arteries: "arterial switch" (Jatene) procedure. The aorta and pulmonary arteries are transected **A**, and the coronary arteries are removed from the original proximal aorta **B**. The great vessels are "switched" so that they will arise from the correct ventricles **C and D**, and the coronary arteries are moved to the new aorta, also called the neoaorta **C**. (From Kambam J: Transposition of the great arteries. In Kambam J, editor: *Cardiac anesthesia for infants and children.* St Louis, 1994, Mosby.)

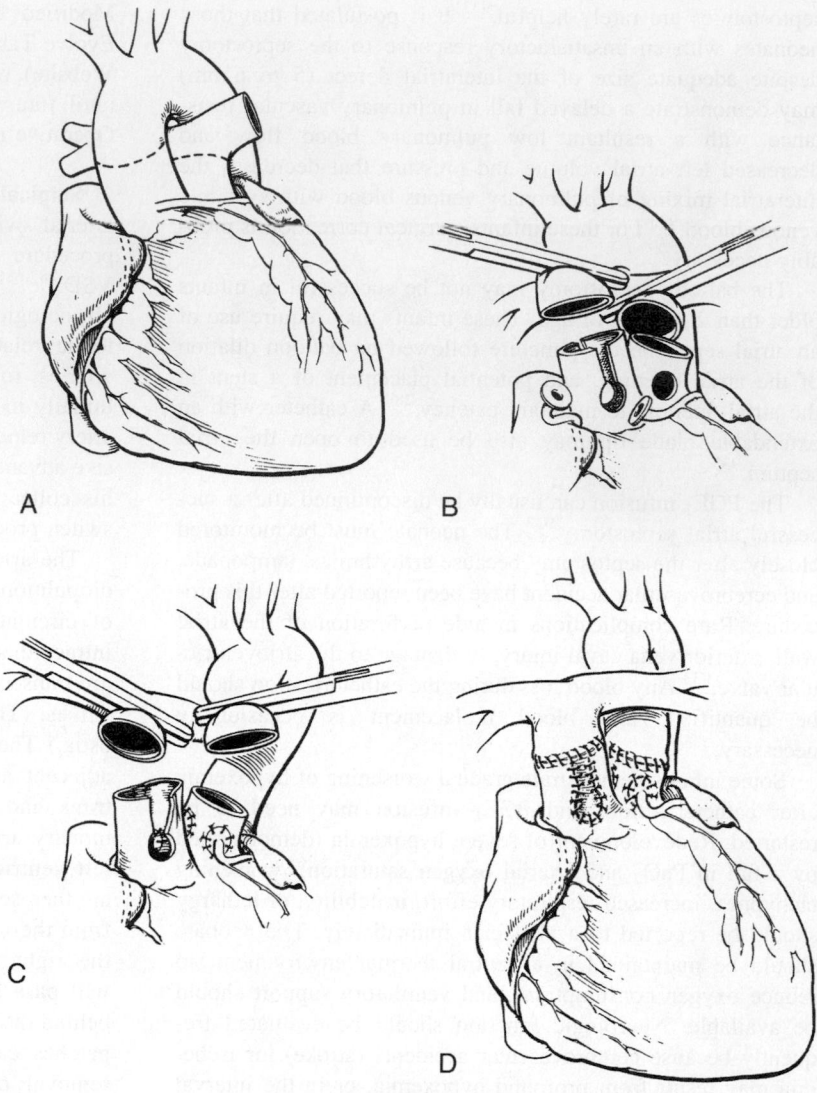

Surgical correction of D-TGA with a small or moderate VSD is also typically scheduled within the first weeks of life. When a large VSD is present, both the left and right ventricle will maintain high pressure. As a result, the arterial switch procedure can be scheduled beyond the first weeks of life without further preparation of the LV.[287]

When "dynamic" subpulmonary stenosis is caused by bowing of the ventricular septum into the pulmonary outflow tract, the stenosis is typically eliminated when the arterial switch procedure is performed, so it will not produce postoperative left ventricular outflow tract obstruction.[287] If an area of discrete fibromuscular narrowing is present along the left ventricular outflow tract, this can be resected during arterial switch surgery.

As noted, the arterial switch is now widely recognized as the corrective procedure of choice for TGA with VSD and the Taussig-Bing anomaly (TGA with double-outlet right ventricle and subpulmonic VSD).[933] Correction of TGA with VSD is generally accomplished during the first months of life.[583] The arterial switch procedure cannot be performed in the child with TGA and subvalvular pulmonary stenosis or a small left ventricle because the stenosis would become subaortic stenosis after arterial switch.

Postoperative mortality following the arterial switch procedure is reported in the neonate at 2.5% by the 2006-2010 Society of Thoracic Surgeons data centers, 7.3% if a VSD is also closed (http://sts.org/sites/default/files/documents/STSCONG-NeonatesSummary_Fall2010.pdf).[821] Mortality in patients weighing less than 2.5 kg is higher than in larger infants.[211,714] Factors associated with an increase in perioperative risk include multiple VSDs, intramural coronary arteries, aortic arch abnormalities, and atrioventricular valves that straddle the VSD. Factors leading to early postoperative mortality include coronary artery kinking or obstruction, hemorrhage from the multiple suture lines, and a left ventricle which is unprepared to sustain systemic function.[933]

Arterial oxygen saturation should be normal after the arterial switch procedure. Postoperative complications include low cardiac output related to LV dysfunction. This complication occurs when the LV cannot immediately support the systemic circulation after surgery. This complication is uncommon in infants after the arterial switch procedure in the first several weeks of life, but may occur in the older infant with an unprepared left ventricle. However, low cardiac output should be anticipated after any corrective procedure. CHF may be severe if a right ventriculotomy was performed. Many issues can lead to low cardiac output syndrome in the first 6 to 18 hours after complex cardiac surgery.[935]

The left atrial pressure is often elevated in LV failure, and volume administration may lead to further elevation in left atrial pressure because left ventricular compliance is likely to be low. The extremely elevated LA pressure can lead to pulmonary edema and low cardiac output. Treatment includes inotropic support, slow volume administration with close monitoring of hemodynamic tolerance, and initiation of afterload reduction. If the LV failure remains unresponsive to medical management, mechanical circulatory support may be required until improvement (see Postoperative Nursing Care and Anticoagulation in the third section of this chapter).[935]

Coronary artery kinking, stretching, occlusion, or compression by the neopulmonary artery can produce myocardial ischemia, leading to LV dysfunction, arrhythmias, and failure to wean from cardiopulmonary bypass.[583,933] Signs may range from symptoms of chronic low cardiac output to acute cardiogenic shock. Bedside monitoring and serial 12-lead ECG can assess the progression of ST segment changes and arrhythmias caused by myocardial ischemia.[935] Some patients with obstruction in the coronary arteries may show no immediate signs, but the occlusions can be found at later cardiac catheterization.[844] Neurologic complications are possible after arterial switch (see Postoperative Nursing Care and Anticoagulation).

The presence of residual lesions (residual VSD, subaortic stenosis) after an arterial switch procedure can contribute to a low cardiac output state. Such lesions can be detected by assessment for abnormal hemodynamics or murmurs, and can be diagnosed by echocardiography.

Postoperative pulmonary hypertension can develop, with risk for RV failure. It is more likely to develop in the infant with transposition of the great arteries and a VSD who is several weeks old because this infant has experienced several weeks of high pulmonary artery pressure and high pulmonary blood flow. Extensive suture lines under high pressure during systole and diastole may be potential sites of bleeding, so hypertension should be avoided and systemic blood pressure controlled. Delayed sternal closure may be necessary.

All patients with transposition of the great arteries have extremely complex congenital heart disease and require lifelong, continuous monitoring by a cardiologist with expertise in management of adults with congenital heart disease.[186,924,927]

In contrast to results from atrial switch (intra-atrial repair) procedures, infants undergoing arterial switch procedures have a low incidence of rhythm disturbances and most patients have a normal sinus rhythm postoperatively.[933] Closure of an associated VSD during an arterial switch procedure is a risk factor for development of arrhythmias.[359]

Left ventricular function has been assessed as normal at 10 years.[229] A high incidence of aortic insufficiency has been reported, but is rarely more than trivial to mild.[933] Neo-aortic (anatomic pulmonary) root dilation has been reported in 70% of patients with no patients having severe aortic regurgitation.[229] The etiology and long-term effects of the aortic root dilation are not known, but are of concern.[933]

Late coronary ischemia or infarction has been reported in up to 8% of patients after arterial switch operation,[927,933]

and fatal infarctions have been reported in 1% to 2% of patients.[933] Coronary lesions can be treated with restoration of normal myocardial perfusion through interventional cardiac catheterization or surgery.[719]

Pulmonary artery stenosis has been reported as the most frequent cause for reintervention,[933] requiring cardiac catheterization intervention or reoperation in 5% to 30% of cases. Bronchial arteries can lead to systemic to pulmonary shunt and potential development of pulmonary vascular disease.[766] Neurodevelopmental abnormalities and learning disabilities have been reported in patients with D-TGA[647]; therefore ongoing developmental assessment and therapeutic interventions are important.

Follow-up studies are in progress and the true long-term outcomes are unknown. Potential postoperative complications are being monitored and may not be clear until several decades in the future.

Maintenance of Left Ventricular Mass: Pulmonary Artery Banding. If repair cannot be accomplished during the neonatal period and arterial switch correction is planned, it is imperative that the left ventricle be capable of generating systemic pressure and ejecting into a high resistance circulation. When pulmonary vascular resistance falls normally in the presence of TGA, left ventricular muscle mass will regress. This may render the left ventricle incapable of performing later as the systemic ventricle. Therefore to maintain or improve left ventricular muscle mass and function for a future arterial switch correction, a pulmonary artery banding may be performed as the first-stage palliative procedure, without use of cardiopulmonary bypass. The LV muscle retraining can occur within 7 to 10 days in most cases, so that the arterial switch operation can take place during the same hospitalization ("rapid two-stage arterial switch").[95,933] A systemic-to-pulmonary artery shunt is often created simultaneously to ensure adequate pulmonary blood flow.[933] The mortality after newborn pulmonary artery banding should be less than 5%.[933]

Low cardiac output syndrome is often seen after the first stage pulmonary artery banding,[933] so the team should plan to treat this complication. When the left ventricle is ready for the arterial switch, the surgery will be completed in the standard manner with removal of the pulmonary artery banding and closure of the systemic to pulmonary shunt.

Intraatrial Correction (Venous Switch or Atrial Repair). The Mustard and the Senning procedures result in a physiologic (rather than an anatomic) correction of TGA, using pericardium or portions of the patient's atrial septum and (for the Senning) the external atrial wall to redirect pulmonary and systemic venous flow within the atria. The Mustard procedure (illustrated in Evolve Fig. 8-6 in the Chapter 8 Supplement on the Evolve Website) uses autologous pericardium or synthetic material for creation of the atrial baffle, while the Senning procedure uses portions of the atrial tissue to create the intracardiac baffle.

In the atrial switch repair for TGA, desaturated systemic venous blood is diverted ultimately to the mitral valve and into the left ventricle, so that it is ejected into the pulmonary artery. Oxygenated pulmonary venous blood is diverted into the tricuspid valve and into the right ventricle, and is ejected into the aorta. Timing for the atrial switch procedure differs from the newborn timing for an arterial switch operation. The atrial switch procedure can be delayed for weeks to months after birth, once the balloon atrial septostomy is performed.[933]

Because the right ventricle continues to function as the systemic ventricle for life, long-term results are often suboptimal. Reported survival at 30 years ranges from 79.3%[626] to 80% at 28 years.[950] Early mortality after the Mustard and Senning operations is similar and low, less than 5% at most centers.[878] Immediate postoperative problems include bleeding, neurologic complications, including thromboembolic events, arrhythmias, and low cardiac output related to inadequate right ventricular (systemic pump) function or loss of sinus rhythm. Obstruction of systemic venous blood flow (producing hepatomegaly, upper body edema) or pulmonary venous blood flow (producing pulmonary venous congestion and pulmonary edema on chest radiograph) may develop and can be confirmed by echocardiography. Superior vena caval (SVC) obstruction is more common after the Mustard procedure and pulmonary venous obstruction is more common after the Senning procedure.[935]

Continuous ECG monitoring can detect bradyarrhythmias or tachyarrhythmias resulting from edema surrounding sutures or interruption of the conduction pathways; such arrhythmias can further compromise cardiac output. Temporary epicardial pacing wires may be used for pacing or diagnostic atrial electrocardiograms. At discharge, only 80% of patients with an atrial switch remain in sinus rhythm.[935]

An atrial switch procedure may occasionally be performed if the child's anatomy is unsuited to the arterial switch. This procedure is not typically used for correction of TGA with VSD because VSD closure through the tricuspid valve is difficult and may damage the valve, and both initial and late mortality are high. Postoperative complications are the same as those described for TGA.

Both the Mustard and the Senning procedures are associated with significant, progressive late complications.[933] For many reasons, the morphologic right ventricle may not be capable of functioning as the systemic ventricle on a long-term basis.[933] In addition, arrhythmias are problematic.

Baffle obstruction affects about 10% of patients after atrial switch. Baffle obstruction of flow from the superior vena cava into the heart produces a form of superior vena caval syndrome, including edema of the face and head, hydrocephalus, and chylothorax.[217,287,933] Less commonly (in about 1% of patients) the baffle obstructs the flow of blood from the inferior vena cava to the heart,[933] producing hepatomegaly and ascites. Signs of inferior vena caval obstruction will be difficult to distinguish from signs of congestive heart failure. Baffle obstruction of pulmonary venous return to the heart affects about 2% of patients as either an early or late postoperative complication. Signs include pulmonary venous congestion and unexplained arterial oxygen desaturation.[933] Treatment for these complications may include interventional cardiac catheterization or re-operation.

Leaks within the baffle can cause shunting of blood at the atrial level, leading to risk of paradoxical emboli, particularly if atrial arrhythmias are also present.[927] Trivial leaks are found in 10% to 20% of patients and significant leaks, requiring reintervention in 1% to 2%.[933] Cardiac MRI is an excellent tool for serial assessment of the RV function, baffle status,[217] and cardiac status following atrial switch procedures. Cardiac CT is an important diagnostic modality for atrial switch patients who have cardiac arrhythmias requiring implantation of a cardiac pacemaker or an automatic implanted cardioverter-defibrillator (AICD).[197]

The overall incidence of postoperative arrhythmias following intraatrial repair of transposition of the great arteries is not known.[217] A range of 18%[950] to 40%[310] of patients are reported to be in sinus rhythm 15 to 20 years after atrial switch. Arrhythmias include symptomatic bradycardia-tachycardia syndromes ("sick sinus syndrome") that can produce palpitations, dizziness, or even syncope and risk of sudden death,[927] and may require pacemaker implantation.[933] Atrial flutter or tachycardia occurs in 5% to 15% of long-term survivors. Use of antiarrhythmics alone may cause additional bradycardia.[287] Potential injury to the sinus node or sinus artery, extensive atrial incisions, and late longstanding atrial enlargement can each contribute to the arrhythmias.[287] There is also a disturbing 2% to 10% incidence of sudden death, but it is not known if the risk is specifically related to atrial or ventricular arrhythmias.[933]

The tricuspid valve may not function well as the systemic atrioventricular valve.[287] Moderate to severe tricuspid (systemic) valve regurgitation develops in 5% to 10% of patients following atrial switch repair of TGA with VSD, potentially related to tricuspid valve damage during the surgical repair. Significant tricuspid regurgitation in TGA with intact ventricular septum after atrial switch is rare (1% to 2%).[933]

Right ventricular dysfunction often develops after the Senning or Mustard repair of TGA, although it is often asymptomatic. In the adult with an atrial baffle surgery, the development of RV (systemic) or tricuspid valve failure is the most important complication.[927] Although exercise performance is universally decreased,[933] 76% of patients surviving 28 years after atrial switch were reported to be in New York Heart Association class I, with minimal symptoms.[950] If the child develops right ventricular dysfunction or significant tricuspid valve insufficiency, pulmonary venous congestion, and respiratory distress can develop quickly. For the severely symptomatic patient, cardiac transplant or surgical conversion to an anatomic correction (arterial switch) may be considered. If staged surgical correction is planned, a pulmonary artery band must first be placed, to retrain the left ventricle for systemic performance.

Damus-Stansel-Kaye Procedure for TGA. An alternative to arterial switch (which requires coronary artery relocation) or intraatrial correction for TGA is the Damus-Stansel-Kaye procedure (1975). This procedure avoids the need for coronary artery relocation. In this procedure the pulmonary artery is transected before the bifurcation (i.e., the main trunk is separated from the branches). The end of the main pulmonary trunk is sewn into the side of the ascending aorta. This enables left ventricular outflow to enter the original pulmonary artery trunk and then flow into the aorta. If a VSD is present, it is closed in the typical manner, to direct left ventricular blood flow to the neoaortic (native pulmonary) valve.[583] The aortic valve (the semilunar valve from the right ventricle) remains closed because pressure in the aorta remains higher than the pressure in the right ventricle.[583] A pulmonary homograft is placed to connect the right ventricle to the pulmonary artery bifurcation. Future cardiac catheterization intervention or surgery will be required for the valved conduit, because it will require later replacement. This procedure may be extremely useful in the neonate with TGA and coronary artery patterns unsuitable for arterial switch and those with double outlet right ventricle and subpulmonic VSD (see Double Outlet Right Ventricle later in this section) or children with single ventricle and severe subaortic stenosis.[933]

Rastelli Procedure for TGA with VSD and Pulmonary Stenosis. Rastelli initially described this procedure for the intraventricular repair of TGA with large VSD and significant preoperative pulmonary stenosis (left ventricular outflow tract obstruction). The procedure also may be modified for the correction of truncus arteriosus.

A median sternotomy incision is performed and cardiopulmonary bypass is required; hypothermia may be used during infancy. A right ventriculotomy incision is made and the VSD is closed with a patch ("baffle") to divert left ventricular outflow through the VSD into the aorta. The pulmonary valve orifice is closed. Then a valved extracardiac conduit is placed to connect the right ventricle to the main pulmonary artery. The goal is to provide anatomic correction of the TGA pathology (so the left ventricle is the systemic ventricle) while bypassing what would become left ventricular outflow obstruction.[933] This surgical correction is accomplished before 2 years of age, and mortality is approximately about 5%.[933]

Postoperative complications include low cardiac output, congestive heart failure, bleeding, arrhythmias, and neurologic complications. Low cardiac output should be anticipated after any corrective procedure. CHF may be severe because a right ventriculotomy is required. Future interventions will be required to treat conduit stenosis by interventional cardiac catheterization[598] or surgical replacement of the valved extracardiac conduit.[933]

REV Procedure for TGA with VSD and Pulmonary Stenosis. The REV procedure was developed by Lecompte for repair of D-TGA with VSD and severe pulmonic stenosis. Left ventricular flow is directed into the aorta by an intraventricular baffle. The pulmonary artery is directly connected to the right ventricle using an anterior patch.[583,686] No valved conduit is used in the pulmonary outflow tract and no valve is present between the right ventricle and the pulmonary artery. The procedure allows complete repair in infancy, but requires lifelong monitoring to determine the impact of pulmonary regurgitation.[933]

Nikaidoh Procedure for TGA with VSD and Pulmonary Stenosis. The Nikaidoh procedure provides another surgical option for correction of D-TGA with VSD and severe pulmonary stenosis. The aortic root (with the coronary arteries) is mobilized and translocated to the original pulmonary artery position. The left ventricular outflow tract is reconstructed relieving the obstruction and an intraventricular baffle is placed to tunnel left ventricular flow into the aorta. The Lecompte maneuver places the ascending aorta behind the pulmonary artery. The right ventricular to pulmonary artery connection is reconstructed with a pericardial patch or homograft.[583,686]

Long-Term Follow-Up and Advanced Concepts in Care

Care of the patient with transposition requires an individual approach. As a result, it can be challenging to understand the child's anatomy, the surgical procedure performed, the resulting blood flow pathways, and likely postoperative complications. As the child grows, readmission may be needed for the management of any potential sequelae of any interventions performed. Each patient with TGA has extremely complex congenital heart disease, requiring lifelong, continual care by cardiologists with expertise in the management of adults with congenital heart disease.[927] Some advanced concepts in the care of the patient with D-TGA are highlighted in Box 8-36.

Box 8-36   Advanced Concepts: Transposition of the Great Arteries

- Management of TGA with a large ventricular septal defect (VSD) is challenging because aggressive diuresis causes hemoconcentration and increases risks of thromboembolic events.
- To improve systemic arterial oxygenation in the newborn with TGA and severe cyanosis requires improvement in mixing of systemic and pulmonary venous blood and increased effective pulmonary blood flow. Although an intervention such as a balloon septostomy or corrective surgery may be necessary, provide optimal bedside support:
  - Ensure that airway is patent and support of ventilation is optimal.
  - Verify correct administration of the prostaglandin E_1 infusion.
  - Monitor arterial blood gas values and maintain PaO_2 above 30 mm Hg.
  - Support factors that promote pulmonary vasodilation and eliminate factors that can contribute to pulmonary vasoconstriction:
    - Prevent alveolar hypoxia that develops with pulmonary edema, atelectasis, and hypoventilation.

  - Titrate supplementary oxygen to promote pulmonary vasodilation.
  - Consider administration of sodium bicarbonate or short-term hyperventilation to raise serum pH and reduce pulmonary vascular resistance.
  - Optimize oxygen supply-demand relationship to maximize systemic venous saturation.
    - Maximize cardiac output (consider fluid bolus administration, inotropic support).
    - Maximize arterial oxygen content (evaluate hemoglobin concentration, avoid anemia, titrate inspired oxygen concentration and positive end-expiratory pressure).
    - Minimize oxygen consumption (treat fever, pain, and anxiety; prevent shivering; consider sedatives, analgesics, and possible neuromuscular blockade with sedation during ventilation to reduce work of breathing).
  - Patients with D-TGA plus coarctation of the aorta or interrupted aortic arch can present with reverse differential cyanosis: they demonstrate more cyanosis of the upper body than the cyanosis of the lower body. Coarctation of the aorta is found in 5% of patients with D-TGA.[933]

Congenitally Corrected Transposition (CCTGA, or L-transposition)

Jo Ann Nieves

Pearls

- The sequence of blood flow is normal with CCTGA (systemic venous blood is ejected into the pulmonary circulation and pulmonary venous blood is ejected into the systemic circulation), but the ventricle supporting the systemic circulation is a morphologic right ventricle with a tricuspid atrioventricular valve. This can create complications for long-term function.
- Patients with CCTGA are at high risk for development of postoperative complete heart block.
- Anatomic correction for CCTGA involves the complex "double switch" procedure.

Etiology

Congenitally corrected transposition of the great arteries (CCTGA, also known as L-transposition) is present when the atria are in the normal position and receive the correct venous return, but they are connected to right and left ventricles that are inverted in right-to-left position (i.e., they are discordant). The right atrium connects to the mitral valve and the morphologic (anatomic) left ventricle and the left atrium connects to the tricuspid valve and the morphologic (anatomic) right ventricle. The ventricles are connected to the "wrong" great vessels, because the morphologic left ventricle is located on the right and ejects into the pulmonary artery and the morphologic right ventricle is located on the left and ejects into the aorta. The aorta is in a leftward (levo-) position relative to the pulmonary artery.[332]

This defect results from embryologic left or L-looping of the ventricle (instead of right or dextral [D] looping), so the aorta is located to the left of the pulmonary artery, with the ascending aorta *anterior* and arising from the anatomic or morphologic right ventricle (see section, Essential Anatomy and Physiology, Fetal Development of the Heart and Great Vessels). This lesion may also be called L-TGA or corrected transposition. The defect is considered "corrected" because systemic venous blood is ejected into the pulmonary artery and pulmonary venous blood is ejected into the aorta. Transposition of the great arteries is present because the aorta is in a leftward position relative to the pulmonary artery. This lesion is referred to here as CCTGA. CCTGA is rare, responsible for approximately 0.5% of congenital heart disease. Patients with CCTGA do not often have extracardiac anomalies.[332]

CCTGA frequently occurs in association with other congenital heart defects, including VSD (70%), pulmonary or subpulmonary stenosis (40%), and systemic (tricuspid) valve abnormalities (90%).[217] The ventricular septum is malaligned, which frequently results in an associated VSD and also can contribute to abnormalities in the AV node. The conduction system is abnormal and may be unstable in most patients with CCTGA; the incidence of complete heart block increases at 2% per year of age,[217] until by adult life

30% have complete heart block.[437] If a VSD is present, the AV bundle courses along the anterior rim of the defect and may be injured during surgical closure of the VSD. Coronary anatomy may also be abnormal; main coronary artery branches may course along the front of the pulmonary artery and right ventricular outflow tract and single coronary artery may be present.

Rare patients with no associated cardiac lesions can maintain normal or near normal right heart function into their sixties and seventies,[332] with survival to 84 years of age reported.[959] Continual, lifelong care by experts in congenital heart disease is required.

Pathophysiology

The blood flow pathways are not altered in isolated CCTGA; systemic venous return ultimately enters the right atrium and is ejected into the pulmonary circulation, and pulmonary venous return enters the left atrium and is ejected into the systemic circulation. However, the systemic venous return enters the right atrium, flows through a *mitral* valve into a morphologic (structural) left ventricle, and is then ejected into a posterior pulmonary artery. The pulmonary venous return flows into the left atrium, then through a *tricuspid* valve into a structural right ventricle and is then ejected into an anterior aorta.

The hemodynamics with CCTGA vary as the result of associated anatomic lesions. For example, a large VSD with no pulmonary stenosis will produce congestive heart failure in the first weeks of life. If there are no additional anatomic lesions, the patient has a normal oxygen saturation and intracardiac pressures during infancy and childhood.

Complete heart block can be present at birth and develops spontaneously in many patients.[447] Unless surgical intervention occurs, the RV must perform as the systemic pump for life. The tricuspid valve (on the systemic side of the heart) may become insufficient when it functions as the atrioventricular valve that is exposed to high pressure. The incidence of systemic tricuspid valve insufficiency is high and increases with increasing age; the insufficiency is also progressive.[332] Systemic ventricular (right ventricular) dysfunction is common. Patients with CCTGA and no associated lesions have a 25% incidence of congestive heart failure by 45 years of age, and two thirds of patients with associated defects develop CHF by adult years.[333] Sudden death is rare.[332]

Clinical Signs and Symptoms

The clinical features are directly related to the associated cardiac lesions.[447] If a large VSD (with no pulmonary stenosis) or severe tricuspid regurgitation is present early signs of congestive heart failure will be present,[332] requiring management (see section, Common Clinical Conditions, Congestive Heart Failure). If moderate to severe subpulmonic stenosis with VSD is present, the patient will present with systemic arterial oxygen desaturation and cyanosis (see section, Common Clinical Conditions, Hypoxemia).

The ECG will reveal varying degrees of heart block,[447] and conduction defects can develop at any time.[437] In the chest radiograph, an anterior and leftward ascending aorta can be identified.[447] Dextrocardia or mesocardia is found in 25% of patients with CCTGA.[332]

A systolic murmur at the left sternal border or separate apical systolic murmur (i.e., separate from tricuspid regurgitation) may be heard.[437] Diagnosis is confirmed by echocardiography. Cardiac catheterization is needed specifically for interventions, including treatment of pulmonic stenosis, device closure of ventricular septal defect, or for measuring and evaluating pulmonary arterial pressure.[447]

Management

The surgical intervention required is extremely variable and depends on the type and severity of associated lesions. A palliative shunt to increase pulmonary blood flow may be completed for patients with pulmonary stenosis and hypoxemia (see Fig. 8-44; and Evolve Fig. 8-5 and Evolve Table 8-2 in the Chapter 8 Supplement on the Evolve Website).[447] Repair of a VSD commonly leads to postoperative complete heart block, and complete heart block may complicate any procedure, so temporary pacing wires will typically be placed.[437] Tricuspid valve repair is rarely successful; most patients require replacement with a mechanical valve and subsequent lifelong anticoagulation (see Postoperative Care and Anticoagulation).[332] In all other respects, postoperative care is similar to the care required for all cardiovascular surgical patients.

The current surgical approach to CCTGA targets anatomic repair to attempt to avoid progressive, long-term problems including early mortality, right ventricular (systemic pump) failure, and tricuspid regurgitation.[447] Development of right ventricle (systemic pump) dysfunction or dilation is typically an early indication for surgical intervention.[924]

Anatomic correction for CCTGA was first reported in 1989[958] and results in the morphologic left ventricle becoming the systemic ventricle. CCTGA with intact ventricular septum may be corrected anatomically using a combination of an atrial switch (Senning) together with an arterial switch procedure (see TGA). This is termed a *double switch* (Fig. 8-51). A staged conversion for a double switch procedure can include initial banding of the pulmonary artery to prepare the morphologic LV for systemic work. A Senning plus Rastelli operation may be completed for the patient with CCTGA, VSD, and left ventricular outflow obstruction.[447] Survival is improving, with hospital mortality ranging from 0% to 8.9%.[249] Ten-year survival ranges from 77.6%[249] to 80% at 16 years for the intraventricular rerouting group.[799] Reoperations are required for conduit replacement after a Rastelli operation. Other patients may require conversion to single ventricle staged interventions or cardiac transplantation. (Perioperative Care is detailed in Transposition of the Great Arteries.)

Lifelong care by expert congenital heart disease specialists is required for patients with CCTGA and involves ongoing monitoring for rhythm disturbances and signs of systemic (right) ventricular and tricuspid valve dysfunction. MRI and CT exams (for those patients with a pacemaker) provide valuable information during followup. Management of the symptomatic patient can involve aggressive management of heart failure, a double switch operation, or cardiac transplantation.[217]

It is challenging to understand the combined hemodynamic consequences of CCTGA and associated cardiac defects. Some advanced concepts for the care of patients with CCTGA are presented in Box 8-37.

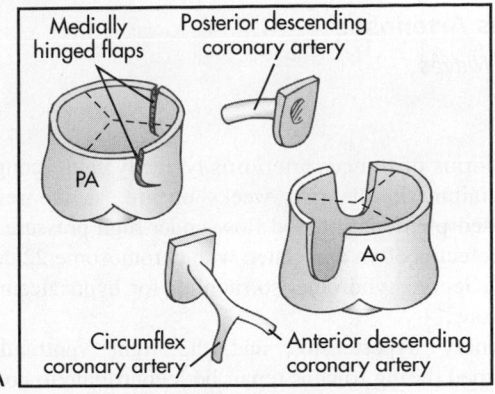

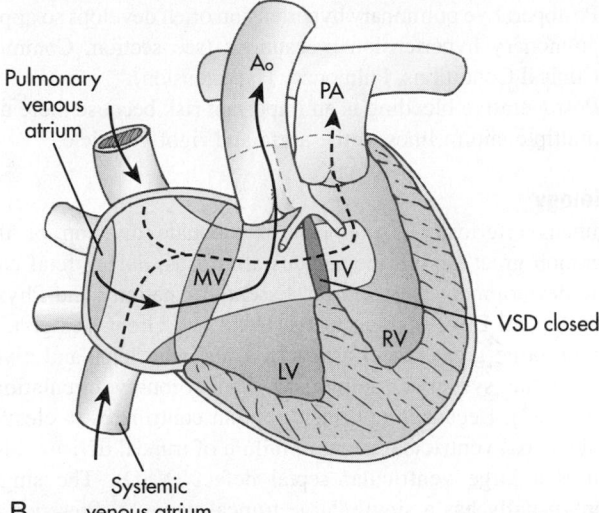

FIG. 8-51 Atrial-arterial switch ("double switch") for congenitally corrected transposition of the great arteries (CCTGA). **A,** The great vessels are switched with relocation of the coronary arteries to the neoaorta. **B,** A baffle is placed within the atria to divert systemic venous blood to the left side of the heart, where it will pass through the tricuspid valve and morphologic (structural) right ventricle and then into the new pulmonary artery and pulmonary circulation. The baffle also diverts pulmonary venous blood to the right side of the heart where it will pass through the mitral valve and into the morphologic left ventricle, the new aorta, and then to the systemic circulation. (From Selke WA. *Sebastian and Spencer's surgery of the chest*, ed 8, St Louis, 2010, Elsevier, Fig. 126-6.)

Box 8-37	**Advanced Concepts: Congenitally Corrected Transposition (CCTGA, also called L-transposition)**

- Complete heart block may be present at birth in CCTGA and develops spontaneously in 2% of patients per year.
- CCTGA patients with no associated lesions may present as adults with initial bradycardia caused by complete heart block or congestive heart failure related to right ventricular or tricuspid valve dysfunction.
- It can be confusing to understand the effects of associated lesions with CCTGA. It is helpful to draw a cartoon of the heart, noting the positions of the mitral (right side) and tricuspid (left side) valves, and note the presence of an infundibulum in the systemic ventricle (because it is a morphologic right ventricle). This may allow better insight into the hemodynamic consequences of associated defects.

Truncus Arteriosus

Jo Ann Nieves

Pearls

- Most forms of truncus arteriosus typically cause congestive heart failure in the first weeks of life, as the result of increased pulmonary blood flow under high pressure.
- This defect is often associated with chromosome 22 deletion and DiGeorge syndrome, so monitor for hypocalcemia and infections.
- Pulmonary hypertension and the right ventriculotomy performed during truncus repair both contribute to postoperative right ventricular dysfunction.
- Postoperative pulmonary hypertension often develops so apply pulmonary hypertension precautions (see section, Common Clinical Conditions, Pulmonary Hypertension).
- Postoperative bleeding is an important risk because there are multiple suture lines in the aorta and right ventricle.

Etiology

Truncus arteriosus results from inadequate division of the common great vessel, the truncus arteriosus, during fetal cardiac development (see section, Essential Anatomy and Physiology, Fetal Development of the Heart and Great Vessels). A single, large great vessel arises from the ventricles and gives rise to the systemic, pulmonary, and coronary circulations (Fig. 8-52). Because the truncal septum contributes to closure of the conal ventricular septum, failure of truncal division also causes a large ventricular septal defect (VSD). The single trunk usually has a single, large truncal valve.[127] Presence of the single semilunar valve differentiates truncus arteriosus from aortic and pulmonary valve atresia because although

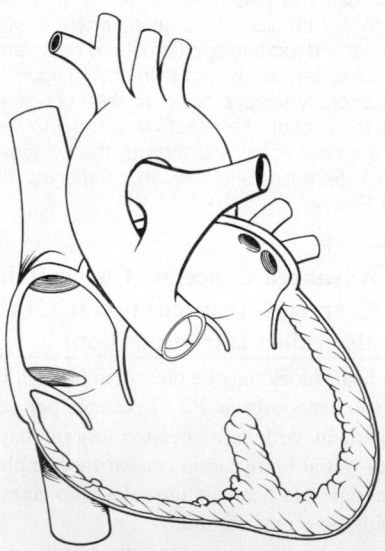

FIG. 8-52 Truncus arteriosus, Type I. In all forms of truncus, a large trunk arises from the ventricles, straddling a ventricular septal defect (VSD). This trunk receives the outflow from both ventricles and supplies the systemic, pulmonary, and coronary circulations. In truncus I, the main pulmonary artery branches directly from the trunk. Pulmonary stenosis may be present, although pulmonary blood flow is typically increased. The truncal valve may be stenotic or insufficient.

there is a single arterial trunk arising from the heart in all of these lesions, in aortic and pulmonary valve atresia, there is a second atretic semilunar valve present.[127]

Truncus arteriosus is frequently associated with DiGeorge syndrome (see section, Essential Anatomy and Physiology, Etiologies of CHD: Noninherited and Genetic Factors).[127] Truncus arteriosus is a rare condition with reported 0.006 to 0.0.43 incidence per 1000 live births.[291,694] Lifelong, continual care will be required by experts in the care of patients with congenital heart disease.

The major forms of truncus arteriosus are distinguished by the anatomic origin of the pulmonary arteries (Fig. 8-53). Collett and Edwards[191] described *Type I* truncus arteriosus with a short main pulmonary artery rising from the trunk, just above the large truncal valve and giving rise to both pulmonary arteries. In *Type II* truncus arteriosus there is no main pulmonary artery segment, and the right and left pulmonary arteries originate near each other from the back of the truncus at the same level. In *Type III* truncus arteriosus the right and left pulmonary arteries arise separately from the lateral aspect of the truncus, and there is no main pulmonary artery segment.[127] Any one of these three forms of truncus arteriosus may be associated with stenosis of the pulmonary artery or arteries. Van Praagh and van Praagh[904] presented a truncus arteriosus classification system that includes commonly associated lesions, absence of a pulmonary artery or aortic arch underdevelopment, including complete interruption of the aortic arch. The Collett and Edwards classification of the major forms of truncus[82,191] is summarized in Table 8-32.

The Collett and Edwards *Type IV* truncus arteriosus is now recognized as a form of pulmonary atresia with ventricular septal defect,[127] so the reader is referred to the section on pulmonary atresia with VSD presented earlier in this section.

Pathophysiology

Because the single great vessel straddles the large ventricular septal defect, it receives the output of both ventricles. The large ventricular septal defect causes equalization of ventricular pressures, and both ventricles share a common outflow tract; as a result both right and left ventricular pressures will be high. The pulmonary vascular bed receives blood flow under high (systemic arterial) pressure,[127] during both systole and diastole, because blood flow runs off from the aorta into the pulmonary artery during diastole. The volume of the pulmonary blood flow will be determined by the degree of pulmonary stenosis and the pulmonary vascular resistance.[455]

At birth, blood flow to both the systemic and pulmonary circulations is approximately equal because both circulations offer approximately equal resistance to flow. Once the pulmonary vascular resistance falls the pulmonary circulation provides less resistance to flow, so there will be a greater tendency for blood from the common great vessel to flow into the pulmonary circulation (i.e., a large left-to-right shunt develops into the pulmonary circulation). Patients with truncus arteriosus can develop pulmonary vascular obstructive disease as early as 6 months of age if the lesion is not surgically treated.[455]

Both pulmonary venous (oxygenated) and systemic venous blood from the left and right ventricles is ejected into the common trunk, so the systemic and pulmonary circulations receive

Collett and Edwards

Van Praagh

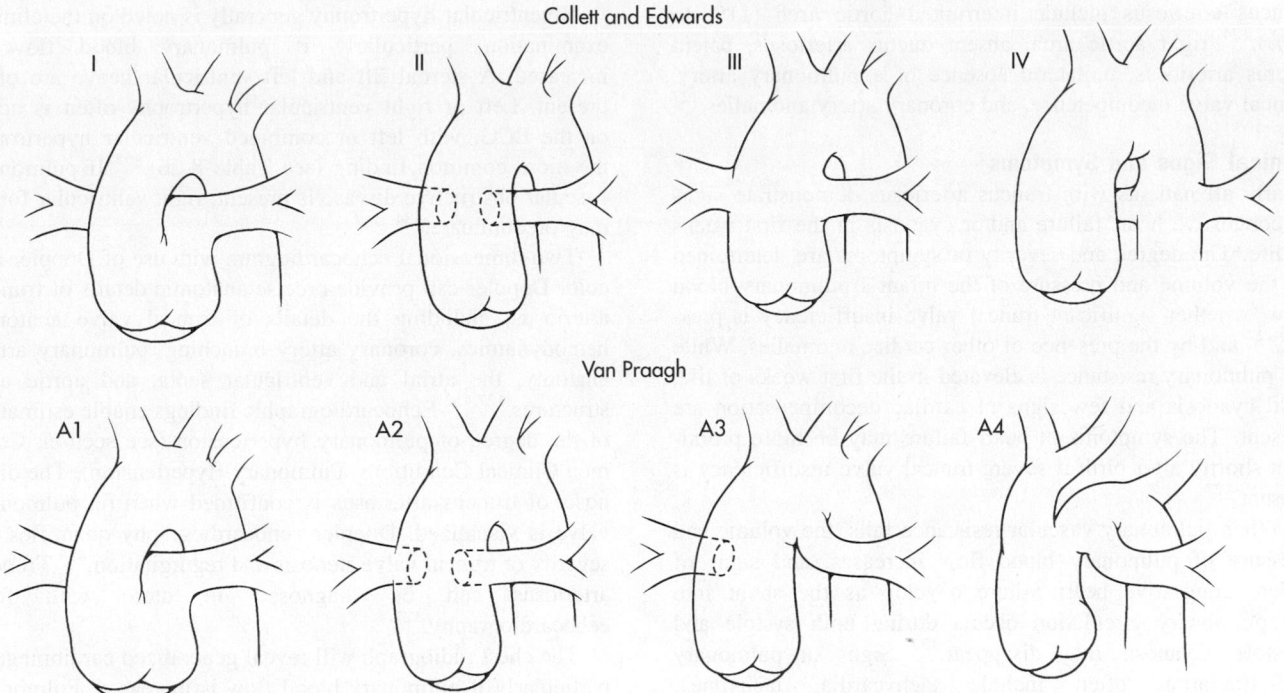

FIG. 8-53 The Collett and Edwards and the Van Praagh classifications of truncus arteriosus. (From Selke WA. *Sebastian and Spencer's surgery of the chest*, ed 8, St Louis, 2010, Elsevier, Fig. 121-1).

Table 8-32 Classification of Truncus Arteriosus[82,191]

Type	Description[191]	Occurrence (%)
I	Short main pulmonary artery branches from trunk, giving rise to right and left pulmonary arteries.	48-68
II	Right and left pulmonary artery branches arise close together from the posterior surface of the trunk (so there is no main pulmonary artery).	29-48
III	The right and left pulmonary arteries branch from the lateral aspects of the trunk, and may be at some distance from each other at different levels of the trunk (so there is no main pulmonary artery).	6-10
IV	There are no main, right, or left pulmonary arteries; currently classified as pulmonary atresia with ventricular septal defect.	

mixed venous blood. The level of systemic arterial oxygen saturation usually corresponds to the volume of pulmonary blood flow; the greater the pulmonary blood flow, the larger the proportion of oxygenated pulmonary venous blood that enters the common great vessel from the left ventricle, and the higher will be the arterial oxygen saturation.

Pulmonary artery or pulmonary artery ostia stenosis is uncommon.[127] In rare cases the deformed truncal valve tissue may obstruct the ostia of the pulmonary artery during ventricular systole.[127] If *mild pulmonary stenosis* is present, pulmonary blood flow may be sufficient to prevent profound hypoxemia, and the pulmonary stenosis may prevent excessive pulmonary blood flow and development of congestive heart failure. If *severe pulmonary stenosis or atresia* of a pulmonary artery is present, pulmonary blood flow may be severely reduced, so that little oxygenated blood is returning to the left ventricle and entering the systemic circulation; therefore hypoxemia can be severe from birth. In these neonates the patent ductus arteriosus provides an important source of pulmonary

blood flow during the first days of life, and hypoxemia is likely to worsen when the ductus begins to close (see section, Common Clinical Conditions, Hypoxemia).

If there is an absence of one pulmonary artery branch, the lung on the involved side is usually small until collateral circulation develops to that lung. If a pulmonary artery is absent, it is more common for the artery to be absent on the same side as the aortic arch. This is in contrast to tetralogy of Fallot; if a pulmonary artery is absent with tetralogy, the pulmonary artery that is absent is more often on the side opposite side the aortic arch.[127]

The truncal valve is rarely normal and leaflets are commonly thickened or deformed.[124] The truncal valve leaflet anatomy can be tricuspid (69%), bicuspid (9%), quadricuspid (22%), pentacuspid (0.3%), or unicommissural (0.3%).[286] Most patients have some degree of truncal valve regurgitation.[455] If severe truncal valve insufficiency is present, severe congestive heart failure and cardiac decompensation can result. Commonly associated defects among patients with truncus arteriosus include interrupted aortic arch (11% to 14%),[124] right aortic arch, absent ductus arteriosus, patent ductus arteriosus, unilateral absence of a pulmonary artery, truncal valve incompetence, and coronary artery anomalies.[127]

Clinical Signs and Symptoms

Nearly all patients with truncus arteriosus demonstrate signs of congestive heart failure and/or cyanosis in the first weeks of life. The degree and severity of symptoms are determined by the volume and pressure of the infant's pulmonary blood flow, whether significant truncal valve insufficiency is present,[127] and by the presence of other cardiac anomalies. While the pulmonary resistance is elevated in the first weeks of life, mild cyanosis and few signs of cardiac decompensation are present. The symptoms of heart failure may be more prominent shortly after birth if severe truncal valve insufficiency is present.[127]

When pulmonary vascular resistance falls, the volume and pressure of pulmonary blood flow increases, and signs of severe congestive heart failure develop as the shunt into the pulmonary circulation occurs during both systole and diastole. Cyanosis may disappear.[127] Signs of pulmonary overcirculation often include tachycardia, tachypnea, retractions, sweating, poor feeding,[127] and hepatomegaly with failure to thrive.[584] The patient with a large shunt into the pulmonary circulation may demonstrate bounding pulses and a widened pulse pressure. These signs indicate a "runoff" of blood from the systemic circulation into the pulmonary circulation during diastole.[127] Severe pulmonary vascular obstructive disease is likely to develop at an early age.[559] Little or no cyanosis is present in patients with increased pulmonary blood flow.[127] A precordial bulge on the left may be seen,[127] caused by ventricular hypertrophy. These signs and symptoms may develop earlier or be more severe if the truncal valve is grossly insufficient because the insufficiency will contribute an additional volume load to the ventricles.[127]

If *pulmonary stenosis is mild,* congestive heart failure may not develop unless significant truncal valve insufficiency is present. The infant with mild pulmonary stenosis may be protected from the development of pulmonary vascular disease, yet have sufficient pulmonary blood flow so that cyanosis is only mild or moderate. The cyanosis may worsen with increasing age.[127] If *pulmonary stenosis is severe* or one pulmonary artery branch is absent, severe cyanosis is usually present at birth and worsens once the ductus arteriosus begins to close (see section, Common Clinical Conditions, Hypoxemia).

Truncus arteriosus produces a normal first heart sound followed by an ejection click related to maximal opening of the truncal valve.[127] The second heart sound is typically loud and single.[127] A loud, pansystolic murmur is heard along the lower left sternal border and radiates to the entire precordium, accompanied by a thrill.[127] A diastolic high-pitched murmur may be heard along the left lower sternal border if the truncal valve is insufficient.[127] If pulmonary blood flow is increased a diastolic low-pitched rumble can be heard at the apex, resulting from the large flow of the pulmonary venous return from the left atrium, across the mitral valve, and into the left ventricle.[127]

Biventricular hypertrophy generally is noted on the clinical examination, particularly if pulmonary blood flow is increased. A sternal lift and left ventricular heave are often present. Left or right ventricular hypertrophy often is noted on the ECG, with left or combined ventricular hypertrophy the more common finding (see Table 8-26).[455] If pulmonary vascular obstructive disease is present, right ventricular forces may predominate.[584]

Two-dimensional echocardiogram with use of Doppler and color Doppler can provide precise anatomic details of truncus arteriosus, including the details of truncal valve anatomy, hemodynamics, coronary artery branching, pulmonary artery anatomy, the atrial and ventricular septa, and aortic arch structures.[127,455] Echocardiographic findings enable estimation of the degree of pulmonary hypertension (see section, Common Clinical Conditions, Pulmonary Hypertension). The diagnosis of truncus arteriosus is confirmed when no pulmonary valve is visualized. Doppler echocardiography quantifies the severity of truncal valve stenosis and regurgitation.[455] Truncus arteriosus can be diagnosed in utero with fetal echocardiography.[127]

The chest radiograph will reveal generalized cardiomegaly, particularly if pulmonary blood flow is increased. Pulmonary vascular markings will be increased and the pulmonary artery segment will be absent.[584] Approximately one third of patients with truncus arteriosus have a right aortic arch, and the combination of a right aortic arch and increased pulmonary blood flow is strongly suggestive of truncus arteriosus.[127] The ascending aorta may appear dilated, and the hilus of either lung (most commonly the left hilus) may be displaced upward if the corresponding pulmonary artery rises from a point high on the ascending aorta. If longstanding pulmonary vascular obstructive disease is present, pulmonary vascular markings will be decreased.[584]

Cardiac catheterization is infrequently required before surgical correction in early infancy, but is indicated preoperatively to delineate uncertain anatomy, evaluate the status of pulmonary vascular disease, and evaluate the response to pulmonary vasodilator therapy (100% oxygen, nitric oxide) when elevated pulmonary vascular resistance is present[127,455] (see section, Common Clinical Conditions, Pulmonary Hypertension). Patients presenting with truncus arteriosus beyond infancy undergo cardiac catheterization to assess the pulmonary vascular resistance,[559] in order to determine the feasibility of surgical intervention. The perioperative risk is higher in patients with truncus arteriosus and pulmonary arterial resistance greater than 8 U/m^2 body surface area (see Table 8-3 in Essential Anatomy and Physiology section of this chapter).[559]

If the cardiac catheterization is performed, an increase in oxygen saturation in the right ventricle will be observed, resulting from the left-to-right shunt through the ventricular septal defect. In most patients the systemic arterial oxygen saturation will be higher than the pulmonary arterial oxygen saturation because systemic venous blood streams preferentially into the pulmonary circulation and pulmonary venous blood streams preferentially into the systemic circulation.[129] Right ventricular hypertension is present in all patients. A pressure gradient may be measured across the truncal valve if valvular stenosis is present. Pulmonary stenosis also may be noted; it occurs most commonly at the origin of the pulmonary artery (or arteries) from the trunk, although peripheral pulmonary artery stenosis also has been observed.

Pulmonary vascular resistance will be calculated carefully from measurements of pulmonary blood flow and pressure because these infants are at risk for the development of pulmonary vascular disease. Reactivity of the pulmonary vascular bed to pulmonary vasodilator therapy will be tested[127] (see section, Common Clinical Conditions, Pulmonary Hypertension).

The angiocardiogram delineates a single great vessel (the truncus) and helps differentiate between truncus arteriosus and pulmonary atresia. Both right and left ventricular angiography will demonstrate the location of the ventricular septal defect, the trunk, and the anatomy of the pulmonary arterial circulation. A contrast injection in the common great vessel will identify coronary artery anatomy and may demonstrate the presence of truncal valve insufficiency.

Without surgical intervention, patients with truncus arteriosus have a 75% 1-year mortality rate.[191] As a result the risk of endocarditis in the nonoperated infant is not known; all patients with truncus arteriosus should receive antibiotic prophylaxis for periods of increased risk of development of bacteremia (see Bacterial Endocarditis in this section of the chapter) preoperatively and postoperatively (they will have a prosthetic cardiac valve).[952]

Management

Medical Management. Nonsurgical treatment of the infant with truncus arteriosus is aimed at reducing the signs and symptoms of congestive heart failure and preventing complications of polycythemia, arterial hypoxemia, and pulmonary hypertension. Because all patients with truncus arteriosus have some systemic venous blood entering the systemic arterial circulation, *no air can be allowed to enter any IV system* until corrective surgery has been performed. If the infant has congestive heart failure, treatment with digoxin and diuretics and possible vasodilators is necessary while optimizing nutritional status (see section, Common Clinical Conditions, Congestive Heart Failure).

Single ventricle care guidelines must be followed, including use of room air, avoiding hypocarbia, avoiding anemia (maintain hematocrit near 40 percent), and close monitoring for signs of systemic hypoperfusion (see section, Single Functioning Ventricle). However, excessive diuresis and the resulting hemoconcentration it can produce must be avoided because the infant's hematocrit can rise sharply, increasing the risk of thromboembolic events (see section, Common Clinical Conditions, Hypoxemia).

Surgical Management. Because infants with truncus arteriosus and high pulmonary blood flow can develop pulmonary vascular disease within a short period of time, Doppler echocardiography is performed as soon as the diagnosis is suspected. If the child is diagnosed beyond infancy, a cardiac catheterization is required to calculate the pulmonary vascular resistance and further delineate the anatomy.

In general, surgical repair of truncus arteriosus is performed during the first 2 to 6 weeks of infancy, before the development of decompensated congestive heart failure, increased pulmonary vascular resistance, or cardiac cachexia.[584] Early correction also eliminates the risk of complications such as pulmonary vascular disease or thromboembolic events. Delays in operation can produce chronic ischemia of the hypertrophied ventricle, which is perfused by desaturated blood at low aortic diastolic pressure (and therefore, low coronary perfusion pressure).[127] Occasionally the infant's anatomy is unsuitable for total correction, and palliative surgical procedures are then performed.

When the neonate with truncus arteriosus and pulmonary stenosis or absence of a pulmonary artery branch has severe cyanosis at birth, prostaglandin E_1 should be administered intravenously to prevent closure of the ductus arteriosus (or reopen it), because the ductus is providing an important route for pulmonary blood flow. After an echocardiogram, a cardiac catheterization may be performed, and surgical intervention is necessary. During prostaglandin therapy and diagnostic studies, absolutely *no air can be allowed in the IV systems* because air may enter the systemic circulation, producing a cerebral air embolus (see section, Common Clinical Conditions, Hypoxemia).

Palliative Surgical Intervention. Pulmonary artery banding may be performed if excessive pulmonary blood flow produces congestive heart failure unresponsive to medical management. However, this procedure is associated with a very high mortality rate, and the banding may not prevent the development of pulmonary vascular disease. For these reasons, complete correction usually is preferred to pulmonary artery banding in infancy.[127] Pulmonary artery banding is contraindicated if significant truncal valve incompetence is present because it will worsen the vavular insufficiency.

Surgical Correction. As noted, surgical correction of the symptomatic newborn is accomplished during the first weeks of life.[127] There are three goals of surgical correction: establishment of continuity between the RV and the pulmonary artery, closure of the VSD, and correction of any associated lesions.

Surgical correction of truncus arteriosus uses a modification of the Rastelli procedure; a median sternotomy incision is performed and cardiopulmonary bypass is used with periods of deep hypothermia and circulatory arrest employed for infants. The pulmonary artery or arteries are separated from the trunk, and any remaining defect in the aorta is patched or primarily closed. The trunk then becomes the aorta. If the pulmonary arteries have been removed as separate vessels they are joined together, and a patch may be used to enlarge the common pulmonary artery confluence. An interrupted aortic arch is repaired under circulatory arrest.[584]

A right ventriculotomy incision is made to close the ventricular septal defect. The VSD patch is placed so left ventricular outflow is directed to the truncal valve; this temporarily isolates the right ventricle and completes the conversion of the common trunk into the aorta. A conduit is then placed between the right ventricle and the pulmonary artery or arteries (Fig. 8-54).

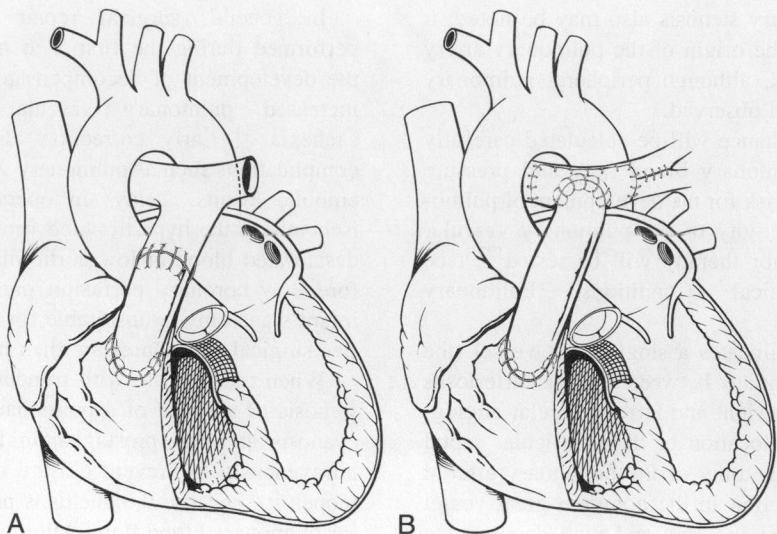

FIG. 8-54 Surgical correction of truncus arteriosus. **A,** Correction of truncus Type I. Correction of all forms of truncus requires separation of the pulmonary circulation from the trunk, patch closure of the ventricular septal defect (VSD) to direct left ventricular outflow into the trunk, and joining of the right ventricle to the pulmonary circulation. A valved pulmonary artery homograft is typically used for the correction. **B,** Surgical correction of truncus arteriosus with unifocalization of the pulmonary artery supply. When the right and left pulmonary arteries are separated from the descending aorta they must be joined together to form a single vessel (this is called *unifocalization*). A patch may be used to create a pulmonary artery of sufficient size. As with all forms of truncus correction, the ventricular septal defect (VSD) is closed with a patch that diverts left ventricular outflow into the trunk. The right ventricle is joined with new pulmonary artery. A valved pulmonary artery homograft is typically used.

In the past woven conduits containing porcine valves (Hancock conduits) were used in the repair; however, the porcine valves tended to calcify rapidly, they developed neointimal hyperplasia with a narrowed lumen, and they degenerated in children.[584] The valves also became relatively stenotic as the child grew. For this reason, antibiotic-treated, cryopreserved valved aortic or pulmonary artery homografts from cadaver donors are now preferred as conduits because they have greater longevity in children.[127,584] and may be used without anticoagulation. Valved bovine jugular vein conduits have been used successfully in neonates without early fibrocalcification.[176] All patients with valved conduits require long-term followup and are at risk for development of valve obstruction or regurgitation that may require reintervention by cardiac catheterization or reoperation for replacement.[221]

Nonvalved conduits or direct anastomosis of the right ventricle to the pulmonary arteries with anterior patch angioplasty can also be performed[119] provided the pulmonary vascular resistance is low. Note that even moderate elevation in pulmonary vascular resistance produces significant pulmonary valve insufficiency. Continued life-long management will be required by experts in the care of complex congenital heart disease. This management will include echocardiographic evaluation of cardiac function and evaluation of the conduit.

The conduits used in truncus correction must be small when definitive surgery is performed during infancy. The conduit size selection is important; too small a conduit will produce obstruction to pulmonary blood flow, and too large a conduit will be compressed when the chest is closed. The major problem with extracardiac conduits is that replacement will be needed as the child grows, and progressive conduit calcification or degeneration can occur.[127]

Somatic growth is now the primary factor that determines the need for conduit replacement.[584] Patients with smaller (less than 19 mm) RV to pulmonary artery homograft conduits and younger age require earlier conduit intervention or replacement.[88] Reoperations for conduit replacement have a low risk.[127] Limited homograft availability, particularly in small sizes, has prompted the search for additional conduits, including the use of bovine valved jugular vein (Contegra) conduits.[176] Pulmonary valve replacement via cardiac catheterization procedure will be possible in selected patients.[598] The search for the ideal extracardiac pulmonary valve conduit is ongoing.

Occasionally, repair or (rarely) replacement of the truncal valve is required during correction of truncus arteriosus with severe truncal valve insufficiency. Truncal valve repair techniques have produced excellent results.[584] The severely dysfunctional truncal valve may later be replaced at the time of reoperation for conduit replacement,[127] with a low risk.[367] Truncal valve replacement is avoided during infancy because the problems of valvular stenosis and anticoagulation during childhood are significant.

Despite the selection of an ideal conduit, it may not be possible to close the sternum at the end of surgery. If this occurs, the skin, subcutaneous tissues and sternum may be left separated, covered with a silastic patch for several days and then closed as tolerated. Conduit insertion can cause crowding of the thorax that can produce tamponade and compression of the coronary arteries (see Postoperative Care and Anticoagulation in the third section of this chapter). Any postoperative bleeding can contribute to tamponade, because there is little room in the mediastinum. Tamponade must be ruled out whenever signs of low cardiac output develop.

An intraoperative transesophageal echocardiogram (TEE) can help evaluate the repair (including identification of any residual VSD or truncal valve incompetence). In addition, the TEE is used to evaluate RV function and severity of pulmonary hypertension.

Potential postoperative complications include low cardiac output, congestive heart failure, bleeding, arrhythmias, and neurologic complications such as thromboembolic events and seizures.[935] The child is at risk for complications of cyanotic heart disease, including thromboembolism and bleeding. Sutures lines are under high pressure in the aorta and RV outflow. Systemic hypertension should be avoided to minimize excessive bleeding.

Right bundle branch block is an inevitable result of the right ventriculotomy incision.[935] Loss of sinus rhythm, development of complete heart block, and slow heart rate for clinical condition all compromise cardiac output, necessitating temporary external cardiac pacing. The systemic arterial oxygen saturation should be normal postoperatively unless a persistent atrial or ventricular septal defect is present and causes a right to left shunt.

Low cardiac output is relatively common after correction of truncus arteriosus. The right ventriculotomy incision and conduit insertion contribute to right ventricular dysfunction, which is exacerbated if pulmonary hypertension is present. Fluid administration is typically titrated to keep the CVP/right atrial (RA) pressure 12 to 15 mm Hg in the immediate postoperative period to optimize preload and cardiac output.[157]

Surgeons may elect to establish a small atrial defect or patent foramen ovale intraoperatively for patients expected to have RV dysfunction or pulmonary hypertension postoperatively. Such an atrial opening (or "pop-off") allows a right-to-left atrial shunt when RA pressure (also right ventricular end-diastolic pressure) rises; such a shunt decompresses the right atrium and ventricle and improves cardiac output, but causes transient systemic arterial oxygen desaturation during periods of elevated right atrial pressure.[942] During these periods the bedside nurse will note the arterial oxygen saturation in the 80% to 90% range, depending on the magnitude of right-to-left atrial shunt present. If no atrial communication is left patent in these patients, right ventricular dysfunction can progress and cause decreased right ventricular output, reduced left ventricular filling, leading to left ventricular dysfunction and poor systemic perfusion.[942]

If preoperative pulmonary hypertension is present, postoperative pulmonary hypertensive crises should be anticipated. Meticulous management of mechanical ventilatory support with use of pulmonary hypertensive patient care guidelines should be planned for the first several days postoperatively. Pulmonary hypertensive events in the postoperative period are more common in patients who have experienced weeks or months of elevated pulmonary artery blood flow and pressure, particularly older patients (greater than 3 months of age).[935] Care guidelines to promote pulmonary vasodilation will be used, including maintenance of adequate alveolar oxygenation (avoid or promptly treat atelectasis, pneumothorax, hypoventilation, or pulmonary edema) and maintenance of alkalosis, normothermia, and normal hematocrit. Sedation, continuous analgesia (and possible neuromuscular blockade)

should be provided to minimize oxygen delivery demands and avoid agitation, and pain (see Chapter 5).

Interventions that are likely to create pulmonary vasoconstriction will be avoided. Alveolar hypoxia is a primary cause of acute pulmonary vasoconstriction, and must be prevented or promptly treated. Suctioning can often trigger pulmonary hypertensive episodes and should be performed very carefully with close monitoring of heart rate, oxyhemoglobin saturation and blood pressure. Acidosis, alveolar hyperdistention, pain, agitation, and hypothermia should be prevented because they may stimulate pulmonary arterial vasoconstriction and worsen pulmonary hypertension. A mild alkalosis usually is maintained. Weaning from ventilatory support should be accomplished gradually to avoid hypoventilation. Vasodilator therapies may include milrinone or inhaled nitric oxide (see section, Common Clinical Conditions, Pulmonary Hypertension for guidelines for care).[935]

Left ventricular dysfunction is likely to develop if pulmonary stenosis was present preoperatively because the left ventricle is then unaccustomed to a normal volume of pulmonary venous return. Low cardiac output is managed with judicious fluid administration and inotropic support. Vasodilator therapy also improves ventricular performance and systemic perfusion (see Shock in Chapter 6).

Often the chromosome evaluations are not yet confirmed at the time of surgery. Patients with truncus arteriosus require close monitoring for development of hypocalcemia that often develops in patients with DiGeorge syndrome.[935]

Patients with a right ventriculotomy and transient right ventricular dysfunction often develop pleural effusions and possibly ascites. Particularly in young patients, the pleural effusions and increased interstitial lung water can be a sign of right heart failure and increased systemic venous pressure that impedes lymphatic return to the venous circulation.[942] The effusion will be cleared with chest tube insertion and drainage and diuretic therapies.

If there are continued signs of postoperative low cardiac output despite medical management, prompt evaluation by echocardiogram is indicated to assess for the presence of residual conditions, including pulmonary hypertension, ventricular dysfunction, or the presence of an anatomic problem. A significant residual ventricular septal defect, truncal (neoaortic) valve insufficiency, pulmonary arterial stenosis, residual right ventricular outflow tract obstruction or homograft valve compression may require surgical or cardiac catheterization intervention.[935]

Replacement of the truncal valve with a mechanical valve requires long-term anticoagulation with close monitoring to maintain therapeutic International Normalized Ratio (INR) values. Patient and family education is needed so they are aware of risks associated with anticoagulation in children (see Postoperative Care and Anticoagulation). Patients with mechanical valves or homographs require lifelong antibiotic prophylaxis before dental procedures and at other times of risk of bacteremia.[952]

Postoperative hospital mortality before discharge after neonatal correction of truncus arteriosus is reported at 10.9% by the Society of Thoracic Surgeons (http://sts.org/sites/default/files/documents/STSCONG-NeonatesSummary_Fall2010.pdf)

reporting centers (2006-2010), and has also been reported at 3.4% by Kalavrouziotis, in infants with a mean age at surgery of 28 days.[429] Operative risk is highest in severely symptomatic infants, in the presence of interrupted aortic arch,[494] in those requiring initial truncal valve replacement,[935] and those with preoperative pulmonary hypertension. Children with truncus arteriosus and chromosomal microdeletion 22q11.2 have higher morbidity and mortality.[504]

Whenever a prosthetic valve (or any implanted prosthetic material) is placed, prevention of bacterial endocarditis is extremely important because bacteria can lodge in the prosthetic material and be extremely difficult to eliminate. A prosthetic patch will likely be endothelialized within 6 months, unless a residual defect is present near the patch. However, because a prosthetic valve and prosthetic material is used for the conduit, the child is considered at high risk for adverse outcome from endocarditis. Strict perioperative asepsis is required with all invasive procedures. Antibiotic prophylaxis should be administered during periods of increased risk of bacteremia, especially during dental work or wound infections (see Bacterial Endocarditis later in this section of the chapter). The child's family should be taught to consult a provider whenever the child develops a fever or other signs of infection, and antibiotics usually are administered. Blood cultures should be drawn before initiation of antibiotics whenever the child develops high fever and elevation in white blood cell count, with or without localized signs of infection.

Chronic anticoagulation may not be necessary after placement of a heterograft valved conduit. Patients with truncus arteriosus repair require lifelong congenital heart care. Late mortality following surgical repair of truncus arteriosus is approximately 9% to 12%.[238,565] This late mortality results from valve or conduit failure or obstruction, progression of pulmonary vascular disease, persistent heart failure or low cardiac output, arrhythmias, or reoperation for conduit replacement. If a porcine valve is present in the conduit it may calcify, producing pulmonary valvular stenosis as early as 2 years after placement. When any porcine valve is placed during childhood it tends to develop obstruction to some degree within 2 to 8 years after initial surgery; 6% to 30% of the conduits fail within 5 years.[244] For this reason, porcine valves are now rarely used. If the conduit is placed during infancy, replacement with a larger conduit is planned 1 to 3 years later. Conduit replacement surgery has thus far been associated with a relatively low mortality.

Dilation of a stenotic conduit during cardiac catheterization can delay inevitable conduit replacement.[429,661] Nonsurgical pulmonary valve conduit replacement, begun in 2000 by Bonhoeffer, uses a bovine jugular venous valve mounted on a stent to replace the patient's dysfunctional pulmonary valve. It is placed during an interventional cardiac catheterization.[469] In 2009, this method of pulmonary valve conduit replacement was approved by the FDA for use in the United States. The pulmonary valve implantation procedure has been shown to increase exercise capacity.[551]

Postoperative dysfunction can be caused by the development of central pulmonary artery stenosis and aortic obstruction. Both can be improved by cardiac catheterization interventional balloon dilation and possible stent implantation.[455]

Box 8-38   Advanced Concepts: Truncus Arteriosus

- RV dysfunction is common postoperatively and typically requires maintenance of an elevated RA pressure/CVP to optimize right ventricular preload and cardiac output.
- A "pop-off" small atrial defect may be established intraoperatively to allow for a right-to-left atrial shunt when right atrial (and right ventricular end-diastolic) pressure is high. This "pop-off" often decompresses the right atrium and ventricle and improves cardiac output, but it causes cyanosis.
- Lifelong followup is required, and future surgical replacement of RV to pulmonary artery conduit or pulmonary valve replacement by cardiac catheterization will be needed.

Adults with surgically repaired truncus arteriosus can develop progressive dilation of the aorta (the original truncal artery), and are at risk for development of ascending aortic aneurysm, dissection, rupture or new aortic (truncal valve) regurgitation.[127] Ongoing monitoring by experts in the management of adult congenital heart disease will include assessment for development of truncal valve stenosis or insufficiency and ventricular dysfunction (both systolic and diastolic) and evaluation of pulmonary homograft/conduit status,[127] using echocardiography and MRI/MRA studies.

Patients with repaired truncus arteriosus are expected to undergo at least two additional open heart procedures or interventional cardiac catheterizations for replacement of a failed right ventricle to pulmonary artery conduit. Results of surgical conduit replacement have been excellent.[584] Future advances and clinical research for the conduits will focus on providing improved longevity and growth with the potential for fewer complications and for longer intervals between operations.[584]

Care of the patient with truncus arteriosus requires careful monitoring and prompt treatment of congestive heart failure, arrhythmias, and pulmonary hypertension. Some advanced concepts regarding the care of the patient with truncus arteriosus are listed in Box 8-38.

Anomalous Pulmonary Venous Connection/Total Anomalous Pulmonary Venous Connection (TAPVC)

Gwen Paxson Fosse

Etiology

Anomalies of the pulmonary veins and their connections result from failure of the pulmonary veins to join normally to the left atrium during fetal cardiopulmonary development. In the first weeks of pregnancy the venous channels of the primitive gut (splanchnic plexus) and the early lung buds are a common system. As the development progresses, there are stages in which communication between pulmonary veins and the right atrium, superior vena cava, ductus arteriosus, and portal venous system is normal. If these connections persist, anomalous pulmonary venous return occurs at various points in the systemic venous channels.[453,900,948]

The Society of Thoracic Surgeons—Congenital Heart Surgery Database Committee and representatives from the European Association for Cardiothoracic Surgery reviewed the classifications of anomalous pulmonary venous return based on errors of embryology of pulmonary venous channels and described the following major categories: partial anomalous pulmonary venous connection, total anomalous pulmonary venous connection, atresia of the common pulmonary vein, cor triatriatum, and stenosis or abnormal number of pulmonary veins.[368,857–860] This section focuses on total anomalous pulmonary venous connection with a brief description of related lesions.

Partial Anomalous Pulmonary Venous Connection (PAPVC).

With PAPVC one to three of the four pulmonary veins drain anomalously to systemic venous channels or to the right atrium. The resulting physiology is similar to that of an atrial septal defect with left-to-right shunt. For further information see Atrial Septal Defect.

Scimitar Syndrome. When *scimitar syndrome* (a form of PAPVC) is present, either all or some of the right pulmonary veins drain anomalously to the inferior vena cava.[152] Most commonly the right upper lobe drains normally; however, right middle and lower lobes drain into the inferior vena cava near the level of the right leaf of the diaphragm. The anomalous vein coursing to the inferior vena cava creates a crescent-shaped opacification on chest radiographs, hence the name scimitar syndrome. The right lung is usually hypoplastic and one or more lobes may be missing (usually the right upper lobe). Abnormalities of right lung bronchial branching are also present. The right pulmonary artery is usually small in size, and one or more arteries often arise from the aorta to supply the lower portion of the right lung.

These vascular and bronchial anomalies result in sequestration (isolation of the area from normal air and blood supplies) of the right lower lobe and progressive signs and symptoms of respiratory distress. Chronic pulmonary infections and air trapping are likely to develop. The child with *scimitar syndrome* may be asymptomatic, but usually is referred for cardiopulmonary evaluation after repeated pulmonary infections.

Management may include repair of venous drainage and the sequestration may be treated by lobectomy of the involved lobes of the lung and ligation of anomalous arteries and veins. In a small case series, coil embolization of the anomalous vessels has been reported to be effective in eliminating symptoms of chronic pulmonary infections.[888]

Atresia of the Common Pulmonary Vein.

In this rare and severe anomaly the common pulmonary vein ends in a blind pouch. The characteristics and management are similar to that of TAPVC. However, without immediate diagnosis and intervention, this lesion is incompatible with life.[527]

Cor Triatriatum.

Another embryologic aberration of the pulmonary veins is cor triatriatum. In this defect, the common pulmonary vein is incompletely merged with the left atrium, causing a membranous division of the left atrium into an inflow portion and an outflow portion with a resulting obstruction of pulmonary venous flow. The pathophysiology is similar to that of mitral stenosis.

Stenosis or Abnormal Number of Pulmonary Veins.

Characteristics and management of other abnormalities of the pulmonary veins is determined by the specific anatomy.

Total Anomalous Pulmonary Venous Connection.

TAPVC, also known as total anomalous pulmonary venous drainage or total anomalous pulmonary venous return, is the focus of the remainder of this section. When all four pulmonary veins drain into the systemic venous circulation and/or right atrium, there is total anomalous pulmonary venous connection. Often there is persistence of the embryologic common pulmonary vein where the four pulmonary veins converge. In TAPVC, all systemic and pulmonary venous return mixes in the right atrium, increasing right heart and pulmonary arterial flow (unless there is increased pulmonary vascular resistance). With this anatomy, there is not a normal inflow of blood into the left atrium, but some of the mixed venous blood passes from the right atrium through a patent foramen ovale or atrial septal defect to the left side of the heart. Because the inflow to the left side of the heart is altered, there may be some degree of underdevelopment of the left atrium and ventricle that may impact cardiac output.

With any type of TAPVC, pulmonary venous obstruction may be present, leading to pulmonary venous congestion, pulmonary hypertension, and congestive heart failure. The site of obstruction can include the point at which the pulmonary veins enter the systemic venous circulation, in the common vein itself, a restrictive atrial septal defect, or a small and noncompliant left atrium.[948]

There are four major types of total anomalous pulmonary venous connection; these types are labeled according to the location of the pulmonary venous connection to the systemic venous circulation (Fig. 8-55). In Type I, *supracardiac* TAPVC (45% of cases)[500] the pulmonary veins join systemic veins that ultimately enter the superior vena cava or a they join a persistent left superior vena cava. Approximately half of the patients with this type have some pulmonary venous obstruction.[948] Type II, *cardiac* TAPVC (25% of cases)[500] is the second most common form of the defect; in this defect the pulmonary venous blood drains into the right atrium directly or through the coronary sinus to the right atrium. Pulmonary venous obstruction is rare in this type.[948] When Type III, *infradiaphragmatic* TAPVC (25% of cases)[500] is present, the pulmonary veins join to form a common pulmonary vein that descends below the diaphragm and drains into the ductus venosus or portal vein so pulmonary venous blood passes through the liver before entering the hepatic vein and returning through the inferior vena cava to the right atrium. This type of TAPVC is virtually always associated with some degree of pulmonary venous obstruction.[948] When Type IV, or *mixed* TAPVC (5% of cases)[500] is present, some pulmonary veins join the systemic circulation at one site, and other pulmonary veins enter the systemic circulation at a second site. Mixed TAPVC is the least common form of anomalous pulmonary venous connection.

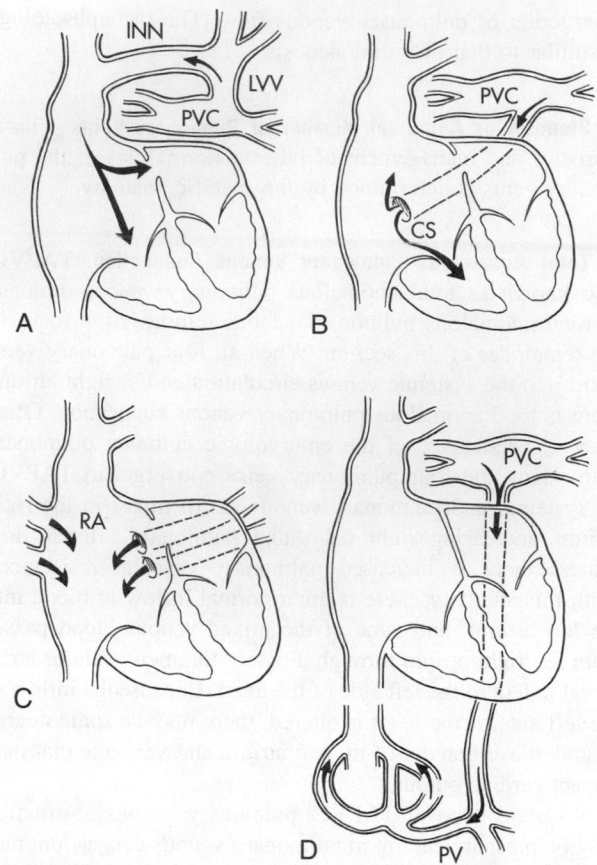

FIG. 8-55 The four most common anatomic defects in total anomalous pulmonary venous connection (TAPVC). **A,** TAPVC with the pulmonary venous confluence (PVC) draining to the innominate vein (INN) via a left vertical vein (LVV). **B,** TAPVC with the common PVC draining into the coronary sinus (CS). **C,** TAPVC with pulmonary veins joined directly to the right atrium (RA). **D,** Infradiaphragmatic TAPVC, with the common PVC draining into the portal vein (PV). (From Murphy AM, Greeley WJ. Total anomalous pulmonary venous connection. In Nichols DG, et al, editors. *Critical heart disease in infants and children.* St Louis, 1995, Mosby.)

The incidence of total anomalous pulmonary venous connection is reported as less than 1% to 3% of all congenital heart defects, but constitutes 2.6% of the heart defects of critically ill infants.[80,453] TAPVC may be seen with asplenia or polysplenia and the incidence of TAPVC is high in infants with asplenia or polysplenia.[453] TAPVC has a 3:1 male preponderance and newborns with TAPVC have higher rates of birth weight less than 2.5 kg, gestational age less than 38 weeks, and are more likely to be small for gestational age than infants without TAPVC.[201] There may be a genetic predisposition to the anomalous progress of pulmonary vein growth that results in pulmonary venous anomalies and some exposure histories have indicated a possible association between TAPVC and parental exposure to lead or pesticide exposure.[405,948] Extracardiac anomalies have been reported with pulmonary venous anomalies, including heterotaxy syndromes (asplenia and polysplenia), congenital diaphragmatic hernia, chromosome 12 abnormalities, and Turner syndrome.[334,353,378] Approximately half of infants with TAPVC have an associated patent ductus arteriosus, and associated major cardiac anomalies are present in about one third, including double

outlet right ventricle, single ventricle anatomies, ventricular septal defect, transposition of the great arteries, and complex malformations.[400,718,948] Those with asplenia or polysplenia (heterotaxy patients) typically have other cardiac defects which substantially alter the pathophysiology. Pulmonary vein stenosis is a more prevalent complication in asplenia patients (occurring in greater than 30% of patients).[453] Heterotaxy patients appear to have a comparable survival rate overall compared with nonheterotaxy patients with TAPVC, despite their higher incidence of other cardiac malformations and pulmonary vein reoperation rate.[630] Patients with single ventricle physiology have a worse prognosis and techniques to improve survival continue to be explored.[347,546]

Pathophysiology

With all forms of total anomalous pulmonary venous connection, pulmonary and systemic venous blood mix, and this mixed venous blood ultimately returns to the right atrium. Some mixed venous blood enters the left atrium through a patent foramen ovale or a true atrial septal defect. As a result, the oxygen saturation of the blood in both the right side and left side of the heart (and ultimately the systemic arterial circulation) are the same. Additional pathophysiology is determined by the presence or absence of obstruction to pulmonary flow.

With *unobstructed* pulmonary venous channels, in most cases of total anomalous pulmonary vein connection, once pulmonary vascular resistance falls, a large portion of the mixed venous blood returning to the right atrium flows preferentially into the right ventricle and ultimately into the pulmonary circulation. This produces increased pulmonary blood flow under low pressure, similar to that produced as a result of a large atrial septal defect. When pulmonary blood flow is large, the volume of pulmonary venous return is large. If this large volume of pulmonary venous return passes unobstructed into the systemic venous circulation, the mixed venous blood returning to the heart will have relatively high oxygen saturation. Some of this highly saturated venous blood ultimately passes from the right to the left atrium, into the left ventricle, and into the aorta and systemic circulation. As a result the greater the quantity of the pulmonary blood flow, the higher the arterial oxygen saturation. With this physiology there may also be compromised cardiac output resulting from the decreased volume in the left heart and potentially smaller size and compliance of the left ventricle.[152]

Obstruction to pulmonary venous drainage is present in approximately one third of all patients with total anomalous pulmonary venous connection; it can occur with any form of the defect, although it is most common with infradiaphragmatic TAPVC. When pulmonary venous return is obstructed, pulmonary venous pressure rises and pulmonary interstitial edema develops. The high pulmonary venous pressure produces an increase in pulmonary vascular resistance and pulmonary arterial pressure. These changes in pulmonary resistance and pressure develop within the first months of life. Pulmonary vascular resistance is increased in all patients with obstruction to pulmonary venous return, and histologic evidence of pulmonary arterial hypertension has been observed in infants as young as 1 to 3 months old. It is important to note, however, that the risk of pulmonary hypertension is high among all patients with this defect, whether pulmonary drainage is obstructed or not.

Clinical Signs and Symptoms

Fetal diagnosis of partial and total anomalous pulmonary venous connection is possible with advanced sonographic equipment and careful checking of pulmonary venous anatomy. Fetal diagnosis enables expedited newborn intervention.[168,416,893] The natural history of TAPVC is that 80% of involved and untreated infants die during the first year of life.[460]

More than half of all infants with total anomalous pulmonary venous connection are cyanotic during the first month of life. Nearly two thirds have developed congestive heart failure by 3 months of age, and more than 90% of infants with this defect have congestive heart failure and/or cyanosis during the first year of life. Cyanosis usually increases significantly with exercise or vigorous cry. The signs and symptoms of TAPVC primarily depend on the absence or presence (and degree) of pulmonary venous obstruction (Table 8-33).[152,160,268,453,479,948,957,962]

Table 8-33 Signs and Symptoms of TAPVC[152,160,268,453,479,948,957,962]

Assessment	Unobstructed Pulmonary Veins	Obstructed Pulmonary Veins
Physical exam	Infant typically does not appear so ill—may be asymptomatic for years. Symptoms can be similar to those of a large ASD and may include: failure to thrive, tachypnea, recurrent respiratory infections, minimal or no cyanosis, hepatomegaly, and prominence of left side of chest.[957]	With severe obstruction: seriously ill infant with respiratory distress, cyanosis, and hepatomegaly. Symptoms may mimic those of persistent pulmonary hypertension of the newborn. Progressive pulmonary hypertension and cyanosis.
Auscultation	Gallop rhythm possible. Systolic ejection murmur at LUSB, diastolic rumble at lower sternal border.	Usually there is no murmur but a systolic murmur may be present. Loud 2nd heart sound. May have a gallop.
Pulse oximetry	Minimally reduced.	Variable oxygen saturation but may be very low.
Electrocardiography	RV hypertrophy, P pulmonale	RV hypertrophy, P pulmonale
Chest x-ray	Enlarged heart, excessive pulmonary blood flow but not pulmonary edema. In supracardiac TAPVC to the left innominate vein a bilateral bulge in the superior mediastinum may be noted, giving the mediastinum the appearance of a figure eight or a snowman.	Heart normal size or slightly enlarged, evidence of pulmonary edema.
Echocardiography—with TAPVC attempts are made to see all four pulmonary veins to identify multiple drainage sites if present. Transesophageal only after sternotomy or in bigger patients because it may cause compression of pulmonary veins[160]	Common and individual veins visualized. Assessment of PA and RV pressure is possible if there is tricuspid regurgitation.	Can be difficult with critically ill infant. Visualization of a common vein and its connection to systemic venous circulation (which are typically dilated with low-velocity flow when obstruction is present), right-to-left flow at PFO/ASD, small left atrium. If PDA is present, you will see right-to-left shunt, site(s) of obstruction, enlarged and hypertensive RV, and possible bowing of the ventricular septum and tricuspid regurgitation. Absence of pulsatile pulmonary venous blood flow by Doppler suggests obstruction.
Magnetic Resonance Imaging and Angiography	Anatomic details	Anatomic details
Cardiac Catheterization	Typically not necessary in infants. In older patients it may be indicated to evaluate pulmonary hypertension or vascular obstruction.	Risky in this population. Typically is not necessary for this lesion unless there are associated cardiac defects. May be employed to enlarge a restrictive atrial septal communication or dilate a pulmonary venous obstruction in a critically ill patient to delay surgery until patient is more stable.

TAPVC Without Pulmonary Venous Obstruction. If pulmonary venous obstruction and hypertension are absent the infant usually develops signs of failure to thrive or congestive heart failure in the first year of life, although occasional patients with supracardiac or cardiac total anomalous pulmonary venous connection have survived to adulthood without development of significant symptoms.

Approximately half of infants with TAPVC have a cardiac murmur. It is usually a soft systolic murmur heard best at the lower left sternal border. This systolic murmur also may be heard when scimitar syndrome is present. If pulmonary blood flow is significantly increased, the volume of mixed venous return to the right atrium is large, and a tricuspid diastolic rumble may be heard at the lower right and left sternal border. Fixed splitting of the second heart sound is often caused by increased pulmonary blood flow.

If there is no obstruction to pulmonary venous return, cyanosis may be minimal and physical and electrocardiographic findings will be similar to those observed when a large atrial septal defect is present. Signs of congestive heart failure may not be present. Right ventricular hypertrophy causes a sternal lift, and right ventricular hypertrophy and right axis deviation are apparent on the ECG in all patients. Right atrial hypertrophy also is noted beyond 1 month of age. The echocardiogram documents the presence of right atrial and ventricular enlargement. A two-dimensional echocardiogram usually reveals the presence of a patent foramen ovale; inability to demonstrate continuity between the pulmonary veins and the left atrium helps confirm the diagnosis.

When the infant has total anomalous pulmonary venous connection without obstruction, cardiomegaly is usually apparent on the chest radiograph. In addition, pulmonary vascular markings are increased. If supracardiac total anomalous pulmonary venous connection to the left innominate vein is present, a characteristic bilateral bulge may be visible in the superior mediastinum, giving the entire mediastinum the appearance of a figure eight or a snowman.

TAPVC with Pulmonary Venous Obstruction. If pulmonary venous obstruction is present, the infant usually becomes critically ill during the first days to months of life. The infant is very cyanotic. Once pulmonary edema develops signs of respiratory distress and congestive heart failure are observed.

There may be no heart murmur noted. If pulmonary hypertension is present, a loud second heart sound is heard, and if congestive heart failure is present a gallop may be noted.

Because there is obstruction to pulmonary venous drainage into the systemic circulation, the amount of mixed venous return to the right atrium is not excessive. Right ventricular hypertrophy develops once pulmonary vascular resistance is increased so that a sternal lift may be noted, and right ventricular hypertrophy and right axis deviation will be noted on the ECG. Right atrial hypertrophy may or may not be noted. The echocardiogram will reveal right ventricular hypertrophy, and 2D echocardiography often demonstrates the presence of the patent foramen ovale and no visible continuity between the left atrium and pulmonary veins.

The heart size is usually normal on chest radiograph. Pulmonary interstitial edema gives the lung fields a "ground glass" appearance of passive pulmonary congestion.

Management

With any form of partial or total anomalous pulmonary venous connection, the site of pulmonary venous connection must be established. Echocardiography, doppler studies, and other imaging modalities and surgical visualization may be utilized. Repair of PAPVC is discussed under the section, Atrial Septal Defect, earlier in the chapter.

Critically ill patients with TAPVC with obstructed pulmonary venous flow and hemodynamic compromise require emergent intervention. Mechanical ventilation to enable oxygenation, mild hyperventilation and reduction of pulmonary vascular resistance are necessary to maximize oxygen delivery.

Prostaglandin E_1 administration may be helpful to preserve flow to the systemic circulation. Inotropic support and correction of metabolic acidosis may be necessary. The newborn may be emergently taken to surgery or extracorporeal membrane oxygenation (ECMO) may be employed to stabilize the patient before surgery. Some symptomatic infants with TAPVC may be scheduled for urgent surgery because the risk of mortality is high in this population.

For patients with no or minimal symptoms, surgery is typically recommended as soon after diagnosis as is feasible based on the patient's status.[268,479] Until surgery is performed the patient requires vigorous management of congestive heart failure and the prevention of pulmonary vascular disease, endocarditis, and systemic consequences of cyanotic heart disease and polycythemia (see Common Clinical Conditions, Congestive Heart Failure and Common Clinical Conditions, Hypoxemia).

Interventional cardiac catheterization may be employed to enlarge a restrictive atrial septal communication or dilate a pulmonary venous obstruction in a critically ill patient to delay surgery until the patient is more stable. This is a controversial approach because the mortality risk is substantial and the risks of immediate surgery versus interventional cardiac catheterization must be carefully weighed.[500]

Preoperatively and throughout patient management the family must be informed of patient risk factors depending on the specific condition. It is critical that families understand the potential for postoperative development of pulmonary venous stenosis.[787]

Surgical techniques vary depending on the preferences of the surgeon. The focus in all techniques is providing unrestricted flow between the pulmonary veins and the left atrium, directing all pulmonary venous blood to the left atrium, eliminating the anomalous pulmonary venous connection, and closing any inter-atrial communication. Repair of total anomalous pulmonary venous return is performed through a median sternotomy with use of cardiopulmonary bypass and profound hypothermia. Vascular cannulation and cardiopulmonary bypass are initiated and the patient is cooled to 18° C to 20° C. If a patent ductus is present it is ligated. Then cardiopulmonary bypass flow is reduced for low-flow hypothermic bypass or, if the surgeon prefers, cardiopulmonary bypass is discontinued for deep hypothermic circulatory arrest to complete the repair (this is typically necessary in neonates).[479,500]

Because patients with TAPVC typically have decreased flow to the left ventricle preoperatively, they may have low cardiac output and poor coronary circulation. This can make intraoperative management very difficult. Aggressive support of left ventricular function, coronary flow and systemic perfusion is warranted.[500]

Repair of *supracardiac total anomalous pulmonary venous connection* to a common vein is accomplished by anastomosis of the common pulmonary venous sinus (where the right and left pulmonary veins join) to the back of the left atrium. The atrial septal defect is closed with a pericardial or woven patch. For supracardiac TAPVC to the superior vena cava a baffle may be used to redirect the pulmonary venous flow through the atrial septum to the left atrium.

As an alternative, the surgeon may divide the superior vena cava above the point of the pulmonary venous entry. The upper portion of the superior vena cava is then anastomosed to the right atrial appendage. Then the area containing the junction of the pulmonary veins and superior vena cava as it enters the right atrium is diverted to the left atrium using a baffle.[923]

When the infant has *cardiac total anomalous pulmonary venous connection to the coronary sinus,* the surgeon joins the ostium of the coronary sinus to the foramen ovale (an incision in the atrial septum is made to join the coronary sinus and foramen ovale and create one large atrial septal defect). A woven patch is then placed over the common orifice so that pulmonary venous return remains on the left atrial side of the patch. If the TAPVC is directly to the right atrium a baffle can be used or the atrial septal patch can be placed in such a way that all pulmonary venous return is directed to the left atrium.

When *infradiaphragmatic total anomalous pulmonary venous connection* is present the confluence of pulmonary veins behind the left atrium leads to a descending vertical vein. The descending common vertical pulmonary vein is ligated at the level of the diaphragm and the confluence of the pulmonary veins is joined to the left atrium. The atrial septal communication is closed.[479]

Repair of the *mixed type of total anomalous pulmonary venous connection* incorporates the previously described techniques as necessary to accomplish the repair.

Postoperative care for patients with TAPVC must include all the usual measures after cardiac surgery with cardiopulmonary bypass. Because these infants often have hypoplastic pulmonary arteries and/or pulmonary hypertension at the time of surgery and because the effects of cardiopulmonary bypass may exacerbate pulmonary vascular reactivity, pulmonary artery pressure is usually high during the immediate postoperative period.[787] Controlled mechanical ventilatory support is then required, and weaning must be performed slowly and carefully while monitoring the infant's pulmonary pressure.

These infants may have a hyperreactive pulmonary vascular bed and are at risk for life-threatening pulmonary hypertensive crises, so agitation, acidosis, hypothermia, and alveolar hypoventilation (all of which can produce pulmonary arterial constriction) must be prevented and great caution must be employed with endotracheal suctioning. Pulmonary vasodilator agents may be helpful in the postoperative period. Agents that may be used are inhaled nitric oxide, tolazoline hydrochloride, prostacyclin (PGI_2), dobutamine, milrinone, magnesium sulfate, and alprostadil (Prostin VR). Systemic blood pressure must be monitored for undesirable systemic hypotension during administration of these vasodilators (for further information see Common Clinical Conditions, Pulmonary Hypertension).

Ventilation problems are exacerbated if phrenic nerve injury occurs during the dissection necessary for the repair. If a small left atrium is present or if there is some stenosis at the junction of the pulmonary veins and the left atrium, pulmonary interstitial edema may complicate the infant's postoperative course. Meticulous respiratory care is essential and pulmonary edema may necessitate use of diuretics and assisted ventilation with oxygen and positive end-expiratory pressure (PEEP).[500,948] For further information see Respiratory Failure in Chapter 9.

In severe cases it may be determined at the end of the operation that ECMO and/or delayed sternal closure is necessary for the immediate postoperative period. If the infant demonstrates severe congestive heart failure preoperatively or a small left noncompliant ventricle, severe congestive heart failure or low cardiac output may develop postoperatively. Optimizing heart rate and cardiac output are warranted. The reduced compliance of the left ventricle can result in poor tolerance of rapid fluid boluses, so cautious monitoring is advised during fluid administration.[152] Arrhythmias (particularly supraventricular tachyarrhythmias or heart block) must be treated promptly because they may cause rapid deterioration in cardiac output.

Discharge mortality has been reported for all patients with surgical repair of TAPVC at 10.1% (compared with 3.7% for all congenital heart surgeries) for the 4 years from 2006 to 2010 by the Society of Thoracic Surgeons Congenital Heart Surgery Database Report.[857] In further detail the reported hospital mortality was: 15.5% for neonates and 2.1% for infants (correction of only partial anomalous pulmonary venous return is reported for children, with mortality of 0.3%).[858–860]

A significantly higher mortality is reported for the repair of infradiaphragmatic total anomalous pulmonary venous connection, particularly if the infant is acidotic with profound pulmonary edema at the time of surgery. Mortality also remains highest in the youngest patients and those with cardiac connection type and/or pulmonary venous obstruction.[436]

Late outcomes are typically good without cardiovascular problems. Late mortality varies after the repair of total anomalous pulmonary venous connection, but it is significant. The late mortality most often results from progressive pulmonary vascular disease and possible pulmonary venous obstruction at the site of anastomosis to the left atrium.[787]

Changes in surgical techniques with use of absorbable sutures or sutureless methods have resulted in a decreased postoperative pulmonary vein stenosis.[233,505] Late recurrence of pulmonary venous obstruction develops in 5% to 10% of patients, and is typically evident within the first 6 months postoperatively. If the obstruction is discrete at the pulmonary venous confluence or at the site of the anastomosis, reoperation or interventional cardiac catheterization for balloon angioplasty and/or endovascular stent placement may be helpful. In some instances the obstruction is caused by intimal fibrotic hyperplasia in the pulmonary venous walls that may not be amenable to surgical intervention.[479,500,948] Neurodevelopmental difficulties with fine motor function, visual-motor integration, and attention deficit have also been reported.[17,478,948]

TAPVC repair survivors appear to have a greater incidence of sinus node dysfunction long term, but significant arrhythmias are uncommon.[843] Long-term followup has documented that exercise performance may be mildly compromised, possibly related to common residual pulmonary abnormalities.[592]

DOUBLE OUTLET VENTRICLES AND MALPOSITIONS
Gwen Paxson Fosse

Etiology of Double-Outlet Ventricles
When both great arteries arise entirely or predominantly (greater than 50%) from one ventricle the condition is called double outlet ventricle; this may occur with either the right or the left ventricle and the great arteries may arise from a normal or a hypoplastic ventricle.[342] Double outlet right ventricle (DORV) occurs in 0.03 to 0.2/1000 live births,[448] representing 1% to 1.5% of patients with congenital heart disease.[341] Double outlet left ventricle (DOLV) is a rare anomaly and occurs much less frequently than DORV.[341]

During embryology the truncus arteriosus is divided by the formation of a spiral septum into the pulmonary artery and aorta. As this conotruncal septum forms to divide the outflow area of the right and left ventricles, it shifts to the left. This processes can be disrupted by genetic, pharmacologic, and other triggers.[605] If the conotruncal septum fails to shift, both great arteries arise from the right ventricle. This explains why DORV is far more common than DOLV.[826]

Other processes of embryology may result in double outlet ventricles. The conus or primitive ventricular outlet normally evolves into the RV outlet but when the conus is bilateral the result is DORV. In the rare situation when the conus is entirely or almost completely absent, DOLV results. Abnormal cardiac looping may also result in double outlet right or left ventricle with normally related or transposed great arteries and with or without ventricular inversion.[901] With double outlet ventricles there can be normal or opposite atrial to ventricular connection.[341] Normal embryologic development is presented in more detail in Essential Anatomy and Physiology, Fetal Development of the Heart and Great Vessels in this chapter.

In a normal heart the aortic valve is located to the right and anterior to the pulmonic valve; the pulmonary valve is higher than the aortic valve and has a conus below it. When DORV is present the great vessels frequently are side-by-side in the same (anteroposterior) plane, and the aortic and pulmonic

valves lie at the same level. Because the aorta in DORV arises from the right ventricle and has a conus, the normal aortic-mitral valve continuity is absent. There is usually a conus below both the aorta and the pulmonary artery; subpulmonary stenosis is present in nearly one third of the involved patients, and subaortic stenosis also may be present. A ventricular septal defect nearly always is associated with DORV. The great vessels may be normally related or transposed. Additional cardiovascular anomalies, including anomalous coronary arteries, occur in approximately half of the patients with double outlet right ventricle.

In DOLV both great arteries arise predominantly from the left ventricle and neither of them has a significant conus (infundibular muscle). The pathology can be similar to DORV in that it may be varied and can include a ventricular septal defect, tetralogy of Fallot anatomy, features of transposition of the great arteries, and other cardiac malformations.[341]

Double Outlet Right Ventricle (DORV)
Pathophysiology
Because both vessels rise from the right ventricle, there must be a ventricular septal defect present as an outlet for the left ventricle. There are many forms of DORV; the hemodynamic consequences of each form are determined by the location of the ventricular septal defect, its relationship to the great vessels, the presence and severity of subpulmonic stenosis, and the degree of mixing between systemic and pulmonary venous blood within the right ventricle. In all forms of DORV, right ventricular hypertension and hypertrophy are present because the right ventricle ejects into both the pulmonary artery and aorta.

Five classifications of double outlet right ventricle are described as the minimal dataset for the Congenital Heart Surgeons Society's nomenclature database, and these classifications determine surgical management. The five classifications are[498,920]:

1. VSD Type: with subaortic or doubly committed ventricular septal defect *without* pulmonary outflow tract obstruction (simple DORV)
2. Tetralogy of Fallot Type: with subaortic or doubly committed ventricular septal defect *with* pulmonary outflow tract obstruction
3. Transposition of Great Arteries Type: with subpulmonic ventricular septal defect, Taussig-Bing malformation
4. Remote VSD Type: noncommitted ventricular septal defect *with or without* pulmonary outflow tract obstruction
5. DORV with intact ventricular septum

DORV with Subaortic VSD and Without Pulmonary Outflow Tract Obstruction (VSD or "Simple DORV" Type). In nearly half of the patients with DORV the great vessels lie side-by-side, there is a subaortic ventricular septal defect (the VSD is located just below the aorta), and pulmonary stenosis is absent. As a result, most pulmonary venous blood from the left ventricle will flow through the ventricular septal defect, directly into the aorta. As long as pulmonary vascular resistance is high during the neonatal period, pulmonary blood flow is not increased. Aortic blood flow comes primarily from the pulmonary venous blood in the left ventricle through the ventricular septal defect; therefore cyanosis usually is *not* present.

Once pulmonary vascular resistance falls, at approximately 4 to 12 weeks of age, there is increased blood flow into the pulmonary artery and pulmonary circulation because the pulmonary circulation provides less resistance to flow. Blood flow into the pulmonary artery comes from both the right and left ventricles (through the ventricular septal defect) and is under high pressure because both the right and left ventricles generate equal pressure. This high-pressure pulmonary blood flow usually produces congestive heart failure and increases the patient's risk of development of pulmonary vascular disease. As a result the hemodynamic effects of this form of double outlet right ventricle are similar to those seen with a simple large ventricular septal defect.

DORV with Subaortic or Doubly Committed VSD with Pulmonary Outflow Tract Obstruction (Tetralogy of Fallot Type). The hemodynamic effects of this form of DORV are similar to those of tetralogy of Fallot. If the stenosis is mild, most of the right ventricular output enters the pulmonary artery, and left ventricular output enters the aorta (through the ventricular septal defect). Congestive heart failure is unlikely because the pulmonary stenosis prevents a large shunt into the pulmonary circulation. If the stenosis is moderate or severe, however, pulmonary blood flow is reduced and systemic venous blood from the right ventricle enters the aorta in an amount proportional to the degree of pulmonary stenosis: the greater the stenosis, the greater the effective right-to-left shunt of blood into the aorta. As with tetralogy of Fallot, the child will be hypoxemic and cyanotic in a degree proportional to the pulmonary stenosis and the magnitude of the right-to-left shunt.

DORV with Subpulmonic VSD (Transposition of the Great Arteries Type; Taussig-Bing Malformation). When a subpulmonic VSD is present without pulmonic stenosis in the patient with DORV, systemic venous blood from the right ventricle flows preferentially into the aorta, and pulmonary venous blood from the left ventricle flows preferentially into the pulmonary artery through the ventricular septal defect. A rare form of this type of DORV is a Taussig-Bing malformation. This defect is characterized by a subpulmonic VSD *without* pulmonary stenosis. In addition, the aorta and pulmonary artery assume a relationship that is similar to that observed with D-transposition of the great vessels. Typically, the aorta and pulmonary artery are side by side, but occasionally the pulmonary artery is posterior and to the left of the aorta. The hemodynamic effects of these anomalies are similar to those seen with transposition of the great arteries.

As long as pulmonary vascular resistance is high during the neonatal period, cyanosis is present with no signs of congestive heart failure. Once pulmonary vascular resistance falls, at approximately 4 to 12 weeks of age, blood from the right and left ventricles will flow preferentially into the pulmonary artery because the pulmonary circulation offers less resistance to flow. Cyanosis is still present and congestive heart failure typically develops. An additional intracardiac shunt (e.g., an atrial septal defect or a patent ductus arteriosus) must be present to allow oxygenated pulmonary venous blood from the left heart to be diverted to the aorta and systemic circulation.

DORV with Remote VSD Type (Noncommitted Ventricular Septal Defect) With or Without Pulmonary Outflow Tract Obstruction. In this form of DORV, the VSD is not near either great vessel.[498] This type of DORV may be seen with a common atrioventricular septal defect (atrioventricular canal).[920] The pathophysiology is determined by the volume of pulmonary blood flow. If pulmonary blood flow is decreased the pathophysiology is similar to tetralogy of Fallot; if pulmonary blood flow is increased, VSD pathophysiology prevails.

DORV with Intact Ventricular Septum. Rarely, there is no VSD associated with DORV; this form of DORV usually is associated with a hypoplastic left ventricle.

Associated Anomalies. Each of the preceding types can be further described in terms of great artery relationships, absence or presence of aortic outflow obstruction, absence or presence of a conus (muscle under the pulmonary and/or aortic outflow), and coronary artery anatomy.[920] Other anomalies that may be associated with DORV are patent ductus arteriosus, pulmonary artery anomalies, atrioventricular valve abnormalities (stenosis, atresia, straddling, and complete AV canal defect), coarctation of the aorta, coronary artery anomalies, ventricular hypoplasia, unroofed coronary sinus syndrome, systemic venous anomalies (persistent left SVC, azygous continuation of IVC), ASD, atrioventricular discordance, juxtaposed atrial appendages, superior-inferior ventricles, situs inversus totalis, double chambered right ventricle, and dextrocardia.[342,498]

Clinical Signs and Symptoms

As noted, DORV can cause a wide variety of clinical signs and symptoms. The clinical presentation is determined by the location of the ventricular septal defect, its relationship to the great vessels, and the presence and severity of any pulmonic stenosis. Each of these affects the streaming of blood flow, so there may be balanced pulmonary and systemic arterial flow or preferential flow to one of the great vessels, resulting in either decreased or increased pulmonary blood flow. In turn, arterial oxygen saturation and the volume load of the heart are affected.

In most DORV the ECG shows right ventricular hypertrophy and the chest radiograph is not diagnostic.[448] Clinical features of the five types of DORV are described in the following. Echocardiography provides the details about the VSD, valves, great arteries, and coronary arteries.[498] DORV may be diagnosed prenatally with fetal echocardiography but is challenging.[472]

Because echocardiography is accurate in determining the diagnosis, cardiac catheterization is not routinely used to diagnose DORV, although hemodynamic assessment by catheterization may be needed in childhood or later.[498] Typical catheterization findings of the native anatomy are described in the following.

The natural history of this lesion depends on the type of DORV found—it may be similar to the natural history for a VSD, tetralogy of Fallot, or transposition of the great arteries. In some cases the associated cardiac anomalies and/or the early development of pulmonary vascular disease leads to a less favorable prognosis.[498]

DORV with Subaortic VSD and without Pulmonary Outflow Tract Obstruction (VSD or "Simple DORV" Type). Signs and symptoms are similar to those of infants with large ventricular septal defects. The neonate is usually asymptomatic while pulmonary vascular resistance is high. Once pulmonary vascular resistance falls, pulmonary blood flow increases, pulmonary hypertension is present, and signs of congestive heart failure develop.

A harsh, holosystolic murmur is present at the left lower sternal border as a result of the ventricular septal defect. A systolic pulmonic murmur is noted, and a gallop rhythm may be present with congestive heart failure. If the volume of pulmonary blood flow is large, a mitral diastolic rumble may be heard at the apex, resulting from the large flow of pulmonary venous blood from the left atrium to the left ventricle. Because both ventricles are large, a sternal lift and a left ventricular heave may be noted on clinical examination. Biventricular hypertrophy is noted on the ECG and echocardiogram.

The origin of both great vessels from the right ventricle will be apparent on the echocardiogram; the lack of continuity between the aorta and the mitral valve and the abnormal relationship of the great vessels also will be apparent. The relationship of the ventricular septal defect to the aorta may not be visualized on the echocardiogram. The chest radiograph will reveal cardiomegaly with biventricular hypertrophy and increased pulmonary vascular markings.

Cardiac catheterization will reveal an increase in oxygen saturation in the right ventricle and pulmonary artery as a result of the left-to-right shunt through the ventricular septal defect. Right ventricular pressure will equal left ventricular pressure. The right and left ventricular angiocardiograms will reveal the origin of both great vessels from the right ventricle; the relationship of the aorta and aortic valve to the pulmonary artery and pulmonic valve and the relationship of the ventricular septal defect to the great vessels will be visualized, and aortic-mitral valve discontinuity will be observed. Pulmonary pressure and flow and pulmonary vascular resistance must be calculated carefully because the risk of pulmonary hypertension is high in these patients.

DORV with Subaortic or Doubly Committed VSD and Pulmonary Outflow Tract Obstruction (Tetralogy of Fallot Type). Clinical signs and symptoms are similar to those produced by tetralogy of Fallot. Cyanosis may be minimal at birth. However, as the pulmonic stenosis becomes relatively more severe, more systemic venous blood shunts into the aorta, and the infant becomes progressively more cyanotic. Hypercyanotic spells may be noted (see Common Clinical Problems, Hypoxemia).

These infants have a harsh systolic murmur heard over the left lower sternal border caused by the ventricular septal defect, and a systolic pulmonic murmur resulting from the pulmonic stenosis. Congestive heart failure does not occur. Biventricular hypertrophy is apparent on the clinical examination, ECG, and chest radiograph. This is one way this form of DORV can be distinguished from tetralogy of Fallot. The chest radiograph depicts decreased pulmonary vascular markings.

The ECG most commonly demonstrates biventricular hypertrophy. In addition, first-degree AV block (prolonged P-R interval) and complete right bundle branch block also may be noted. A superior axis usually is present.

Cardiac catheterization reveals an increase in oxygen saturation in the right ventricle just at the level of the ventricular septal defect, because pulmonary venous blood from the left ventricle must flow through the ventricular septal defect to the right ventricle before passing into the aorta. Arterial oxygen desaturation also will be noted. Right and left ventricular pressures are usually equal, and measurement of a pressure gradient between the right ventricle and pulmonary artery will confirm the presence of pulmonic stenosis. Right and left ventricular angiograms will confirm the location and relationship of the great vessels and the location of the ventricular septal defect. In addition, the location and severity of pulmonic stenosis will be documented.

DORV with Subpulmonic VSD (Transposition of the Great Arteries Type; Taussig Bing Malformation). Signs and symptoms are similar to those produced by transposition and a ventricular septal defect. Mild to moderate cyanosis is present from birth, and congestive heart failure develops once pulmonary vascular resistance falls at approximately 4 to 12 weeks of age. The Taussig-Bing malformation is one of the few congenital heart defects in which high pulmonary blood flow and congestive heart failure can be associated with severe cyanosis.

A harsh systolic ejection murmur is present at the left lower sternal border, resulting from the ventricular septal defect. A gallop may be noted when congestive heart failure develops. Signs of right ventricular hypertrophy are present on clinical examination and on the ECG and chest radiograph. Signs of left ventricular hypertrophy are usually also noted. Conduction abnormalities are rare.

The echocardiogram reveals the dextroposition (rightward displacement) of the aorta and the position of the pulmonary artery, overriding the ventricular septal defect. Some forms of this defect (so-called left-sided Taussig-Bing anomaly) may be difficult to differentiate with certainty from transposition of the great vessels with a ventricular septal defect.

The chest radiograph reveals generalized cardiomegaly with right (and often left) ventricular hypertrophy. Pulmonary vascular markings are increased.

Cardiac catheterization reveals equal right and left ventricular pressures. An increase in arterial oxygen saturation is noted in the right ventricle (and often in the pulmonary artery) as a result of the flow of oxygenated blood from the left ventricle through the ventricular septal defect, into the right ventricle, and into the pulmonary artery. Blood in the aorta is desaturated because this blood comes primarily from the right ventricle. A right ventricular angiogram reveals the emergence of the pulmonary artery and the aorta from the right ventricle.

The aorta is usually located to the right of the pulmonary artery, and the aortic valve is at the same level as the pulmonic valve. A left ventricular angiogram reveals the location of the ventricular septal defect and the preferential streaming of left ventricular blood into the pulmonary artery. Pulmonary pressure will be high, and pulmonary vascular resistance should be calculated carefully because the risk of pulmonary vascular disease is high.

DORV with Remote VSD Type (Noncommitted Ventricular Septal Defect) With or Without Pulmonary Outflow Tract Obstruction. Clinical manifestations are determined by the volume of pulmonary blood flow. If pulmonary blood flow is decreased the manifestations will be similar to those described in the DORV-Tetralogy of Fallot Type (see the preceding). If the pulmonary blood flow is increased, the symptomatology will be similar to the DORV-VSD Type (see the preceding).

DORV with Intact Ventricular Septum. Clinical signs and symptoms in this anatomy are those that are seen with single ventricle physiology (see section, Single Functioning Ventricle).

Management

The interventions for DORV may involve palliative procedures (systemic to pulmonary artery shunt, pulmonary artery banding, interventional catheterization procedures to improve pulmonary flow, or others). Repair procedures can be similar to those used for conventional VSDs, those used for tetralogy of Fallot, those used for transposition of the great arteries, and those used for truncus arteriosus with pulmonary stenosis (see relevant defects elsewhere in this section of the chapter). These include using a patch to redirect flow from one ventricle through the VSD to one of the great arteries (simultaneously eliminating mixing of systemic and pulmonary venous blood and closing the VSD), the arterial switch operation, the "atrial switch" procedure (i.e., the Mustard or Senning procedures redirect systemic venous return to the left ventricle so it is ejected into the pulmonary circulation and redirects pulmonary venous return to the right ventricle so it is ejected into the systemic circulation), the Damus-Kaye-Stansel procedure, the Rastelli procedure (patching of the VSD to divert left ventricular flow into what will be the aorta, and insertion of a valved conduit to join the right ventricle to the main pulmonary artery), and repairs for associated anomalies. The intraventricular tunneling procedures may require surgical enlargement of the ventricular septal defect; this must be accomplished carefully to avoid damage to conduction tissue.

Additional surgical techniques that have not been described for the preceding may be required for complex anatomies.

• The Kawashima procedure is similar to a bidirectional Glenn procedure (creation of a superior vena cava to pulmonary artery fistula) but it directs a greater proportion of the systemic venous return to the pulmonary arteries. This procedure is done when the patient has an interrupted inferior vena cava, so all but the hepatic venous return is diverted away from the heart and to the pulmonary artery.[440]

• *Reparation l'etage ventriculaire* (REV procedure or Lecompte maneuver) is used when the ventriculoarterial relationships are not normal. It involves creating left ventricle to aortic flow and right ventricle to pulmonary flow without using an extracardiac conduit. A tunnel patch from the VSD to the aortic root is placed. Then the aorta is positioned posterior to the pulmonary artery and the main pulmonary artery is moved anteriorly where a patch is placed as a roof over the incised right ventricular outflow tract into the pulmonary artery (the pulmonary valve is not preserved).[498]

• The Nikaidoh procedure involves translocation of the right-sided aortic root into a position within the incised VSD and pulmonary artery (when the pulmonary artery is the great vessel closer to the left ventricle). After this translocation is accomplished a patch is used to establish left ventricle to aorta flow. Right ventricle to pulmonary artery flow is then achieved in a way similar to that described in the REV procedure.[653] The Nikaidoh procedure avoids creation of aortic insufficiency and aortic outflow obstruction.[960]

In the past, DORV repair has been associated with relatively high mortality. In recent years the outlook has improved for biventricular repairs of some types of DORV, with reported ranges of hospital mortality from 0% to 32%. In univentricular palliations of DORV in earlier years, hospital mortality neared 50%, but in the current era is approximately 5% to 10%.[498] Some of the biventricular repairs, the Rastelli type repair in particular, is associated with worse late outcomes than the Fontan (single ventricle correction) procedure, so this should be considered when there is a borderline case for biventricular repair.[100]

With selected anatomies such as DORV with noncommitted VSD and DORV with atrioventricular septal defects and heterotaxy, biventricular repairs can have acceptable outcomes.[31] Factors associated with greater mortality include atrioventricular valve regurgitation, pulmonary venous obstruction, and neonatal presentation.[840] In complex DORV with discordant atrioventricular and ventriculoarterial connections the challenging approach of combining the Senning or Mustard procedure with the Rastelli procedure has been associated with acceptable outcomes.[391] The hospital mortality rate reported in the Society of Thoracic Surgeons—Duke Clinical Research Institute 2010 Congenital Report Executive Summary was 4.1% in infants who underwent tunnel repairs for DORV.[822]

If pulmonary vascular disease is present preoperatively, postoperative ventilatory support must be excellent. Weaning from ventilatory support must be performed very gradually because alveolar hypoxia, acidosis, or hypothermia can produce pulmonary arterial constriction and increased pulmonary vascular resistance. This increases right ventricular afterload and can precipitate deterioration in pulmonary blood flow and systemic perfusion.[100,472]

Late complications after surgical repair of double outlet right ventricle include progression of pulmonary vascular disease, persistent arrhythmias, conduit failure, recurrent ventricular septal defect, and development of left ventricular outflow tract obstruction. A significant incidence of late sudden death has been reported and is probably the result of arrhythmias (including progressive heart block). The need for reoperation to address complications of surgically created tunnels is more likely with complex tunnels.[498]

If prosthetic material is used for the surgical repair the child will require antibiotic prophylaxis in the early postoperative period. Preoperatively and postoperatively, adherence to current American Heart Association recommendations for endocarditis prophylaxis is required (see Bacterial Endocarditis later in this section).

DORV With Subaortic VSD Without Pulmonary Outflow Tract Obstruction (VSD or "Simple DORV" Type). When congestive heart failure develops, aggressive medical management will be required. Although pulmonary artery banding may be performed initially as a palliative measure, many surgeons prefer early total correction of this defect unless additional cardiac anomalies are present.

Surgical correction requires a median sternotomy incision and use of cardiopulmonary bypass. Hypothermia also is used in small infants. A right ventriculotomy cardiac incision is made, avoiding any anomalous coronary arteries. The ventricular septal defect is closed with placement of a prosthetic patch that diverts left ventricular outflow into the aorta; this creates an intraventricular tunnel from the left ventricle through the VSD to the aorta, while closing the VSD. Postoperative complications include congestive heart failure, low cardiac output, and arrhythmias. Operative risk is especially high if pulmonary hypertension or severe symptoms were present preoperatively.

DORV with Subaortic or Doubly Committed VSD with Pulmonary Outflow Tract Obstruction (Tetralogy of Fallot Type). Surgical management is similar to that for tetralogy of Fallot (refer to discussion of this defect earlier in this chapter). During IV therapy, *no air should be allowed in IV systems* because air may flow into the systemic arterial circulation, producing a cerebral air embolus.

Nurses caring infants with this form of DORV should be alert for the development of hypercyanotic episodes. If these develop the infant should be placed in a knee-chest position, and oxygen should be administered. Morphine sulfate or propranolol may be administered in an attempt to improve pulmonary blood flow and arterial oxygen saturation. A phenylephrine infusion (0.1 to 0.5 mcg/kg per minute) may also be provided to improve systemic oxygenation and perfusion (refer to Box 8-34).

These infants should be kept well hydrated to avoid hemoconcentration and resultant increase in the serum hematocrit and blood viscosity that will decrease pulmonary blood flow. The parents should be taught the importance of prevention of dehydration and contacting a healthcare provider whenever vomiting, diarrhea, or other potential causes of dehydration develop (see section, Common Clinical Conditions, Hypoxemia).

If the infant with double outlet right ventricle of the tetralogy type is extremely hypoxemic or develops hypercyanotic episodes, interventional catheterization for a pulmonary valvotomy or surgical creation of a systemic-to-pulmonary artery shunt may be recommended. This palliative surgery does not require use of cardiopulmonary bypass and should reduce the infant's hypoxemia (refer to Tetralogy of Fallot). Postoperatively and until surgical correction, it is still imperative that air be eliminated from IV administration systems because systemic venous blood is still entering the systemic arterial circulation, and IV air can produce a cerebral air embolus.

Corrective surgery for DORV of the tetralogy type is similar to that performed for repair of tetralogy of Fallot. A median sternotomy incision is used, and cardiopulmonary bypass is required. Hypothermia also may be used in small infants. The surgical repair usually is performed through a right ventriculotomy. The pulmonic stenosis is relieved by excision of the muscular stenotic pulmonary infundibulum, and a pulmonary valvotomy also may be performed. The ventricular septal defect is closed with a prosthetic patch so that left ventricular outflow enters the aorta—the ventricular septal defect patch helps to divert this blood into the aorta. One or two patches may be used to enlarge the right ventricular outflow tract, minimizing residual pulmonic stenosis.

If an anomalous coronary artery crosses the right ventricular outflow tract where the surgical incision or patch placement is planned, or if it is difficult to patch the ventricular septal defect without obstructing the flow of blood from right ventricle to pulmonary artery, a valved conduit may be placed between the right ventricle and the pulmonary artery. Postoperative complications after repair of DORV of the tetralogy type include congestive heart failure, low cardiac output, bleeding, arrhythmias, infection, and neurologic complications.

DORV with Subpulmonic VSD (Transposition of the Great Arteries Type; Taussig Bing Malformation). Medical and nursing management for this form of DORV is challenging. If the infant develops severe symptoms of congestive heart failure at approximately 1 to 3 months of age, treatment with digoxin and diuretics is indicated (see section, Common Clinical Conditions, Congestive Heart Failure). However, aggressive diuresis should be avoided because it may produce hemoconcentration, causing a rise in the infant's hematocrit to unacceptable levels that increase the risk of thromboembolic events (see section, Common Clinical Conditions, Hypoxemia). Therefore a balance between adequate treatment of congestive heart failure and prevention of hemoconcentration must be achieved. Whenever the infant is hospitalized (until the corrective surgery is performed), *no air can be allowed in any IV system* because some systemic venous blood is passing into the systemic arterial circulation, and IV air may cause a cerebral air embolus (stroke).

If congestive heart failure is refractory to medical management, pulmonary artery banding may be recommended to reduce the quantity and pressure of pulmonary blood flow. Banding should relieve the symptoms of congestive heart failure and reduce the risk of pulmonary vascular disease. However, because the reduction in pulmonary blood flow by banding may worsen the infant's hypoxemia, it may be necessary to create a systemic-to-pulmonary artery shunt at the same time. The typical results of the combined procedures have led many surgeons to prefer correction to palliation.

Surgical correction of the double outlet right ventricle with subpulmonic ventricular septal defect without pulmonic stenosis requires a median sternotomy and use of cardiopulmonary bypass. Hypothermia is also often used for repair during infancy. Surgery may be performed through a right atriotomy or ventriculotomy incision. Whenever feasible, VSD closure is performed in conjunction with an arterial switch procedure. If the arterial switch procedure is not feasible (e.g., the coronary arteries are not transferable), a Damus-Stansel-Kaye procedure is performed. Both the arterial switch and the Damus-Stansel-Kaye procedures are reviewed in detail with Transposition of the Great Arteries earlier in this section of the chapter. Operative risk is highest for these repairs. Postoperative complications include congestive heart failure, low cardiac output, bleeding, arrhythmias, and neurologic complications.

DORV with Remote VSD Type (Noncommitted Ventricular Septal Defect) With or Without Pulmonary Outflow Tract Obstruction. The management is determined by the anatomy and is either that described for tetralogy of Fallot or similar to that for a VSD. In some cases there are not two adequate atrioventricular valve and ventricle combinations; this anatomy necessitates a single ventricle surgical approach (see section, Single Functioning Ventricle).

DORV with Intact Ventricular Septum. Typically the single ventricle approach, with stages of surgery culminating with a Fontan procedure, is needed for this type of DORV (see section, Single Functioning Ventricle).

Double Outlet Left Ventricle (DOLV)
Pathophysiology
Double outlet left ventricle is a rare anomaly in which both great arteries (aorta and pulmonary artery) arise from the left ventricle. At one point this lesion was thought to be embryologically impossible, but the diagnostic findings were clearly reported by Paul et al.[688] The pathophysiology can resemble that of DORV and is determined by the precise anatomy of a VSD, the position of the great vessels in relation to each other and the VSD, whether normal or discordant atrioventricular relationships are present, the presence of single or two ventricles, and the presence or absence of pulmonary and/or aortic outflow tract obstruction.[846]

A number of additional associated anomalies have been reported with DOLV, including coronary artery anomalies, patent ductus arteriosus, coarctation of the aorta, interrupted aortic arch, juxtaposed atrial appendages, anomalous pulmonary and systemic venous connections, situs inversus, Ebstein malformation of the tricuspid valve, atrioventricular valve atresia, subaortic stenosis, double inlet left ventricle, and many others.[342,846]

Clinical Signs and Symptoms
Findings are dependent on the specific anatomy, especially the presence or absence of pulmonary outflow tract obstruction. Signs and complications of increased pulmonary blood flow (congestive heart failure, pulmonary vascular disease) similar to those produced by a large VSD may be present when there is no obstruction to pulmonary flow. In about one third of patients, there is significant obstruction to pulmonary flow resulting in cyanosis and findings similar to those described with tetralogy of Fallot.[448,498]

With the infrequency and variability of DOLV, diagnostic features are difficult to generalize. Physical findings, chest radiograph, and electrocardiogram can provide clues about physiology, but they do not provide conclusive diagnostic information. The diagnosis may be made with echocardiography and cardiac catheterization, but may also be made intraoperatively.[498]

Management
Surgical techniques described for DORV (discussed in the preceding pages) are used for DOLV and the surgical procedure is affected by the presence or absence of pulmonary stenosis.[498] For DOLV *with* pulmonary outflow obstruction, surgical intervention may include intraventricular tunnel repairs, pulmonary artery translocation, the REV procedure, or the Rastelli procedure.[921] The REV procedure has been an effective treatment for DOLV in infants that avoids use of an extracardiac conduit that would necessitate reoperation for replacement when the patient outgrows the conduit.[498] For DOLV *without* pulmonary stenosis, surgical interventions would be the same as those for DORV without pulmonary stenosis. Surgical intervention for DOLV with right ventricular hypoplasia employs a single ventricle surgical approach (see section, Single Functioning Ventricle).[921]

Outcomes are difficult to ascertain because of the small numbers and the variable anatomy, but are thought to be similar to the outcomes seen with DORV.[498]

If prosthetic material is used for the surgical repair the child will require antibiotic prophylaxis in the early postoperative period. Preoperatively and postoperatively, adherence to current American Heart Association recommendations for endocarditis prophylaxis is encouraged.

SINGLE FUNCTIONING VENTRICLE

Overview of Single Functioning Ventricle
Jo Ann Nieves

Pearls
- Optimal circulation in patients with palliated single ventricle is associated with signs of adequate systemic perfusion and a systemic arterial oxygen saturation of 75% to 85%.
  - Systemic arterial oxygen saturation greater than 85% with signs of decreased systemic perfusion suggest pulmonary overcirculation (and inadequate systemic blood flow). Ongoing assessment is critical to verify adequate oxygen delivery and stable systemic perfusion.
  - Systemic arterial oxygen saturation less than 75% requires further evaluation and can lead to inadequate oxygen delivery. Interventions or therapies are needed to promote adequate pulmonary blood flow and pulmonary vasodilation and prevent pulmonary vasoconstriction.
- A hematocrit greater than 40% is necessary to optimize oxygen carrying capacity in the child with single ventricle physiology.

- All patients undergoing Glenn, Fontan, or Kawashima procedures must have normal pulmonary vascular resistance.
- Caution is required when the patient with single ventricle patient receives nothing by mouth (i.e., is NPO) or has inadequate fluid intake, because the patient can rapidly become dehydrated with resulting inadequate systemic perfusion and decreased oxygen saturation. Hemoconcentration can increase risk of thromboembolic events.

Overview of Etiology

Single ventricle refers to any congenital cardiac malformation where one ventricle is hypoplastic or absent. The heart may have significant hypoplasia of an AV valve or the apical portion of either ventricle.[591] The etiology of each defect producing single ventricle physiology is described separately in the following sections.

Overview of Pathophysiology

The physiology and hemodynamics resulting from a univentricular heart are determined by individual variations such as obstruction to flow within the heart, status of flow across the atrial septum, the volume and mixing of systemic and pulmonary venous return, the pulmonary vascular resistance and the status of the AV valve regurgitation.[468] In all defects with single ventricle physiology, the systemic and pulmonary venous return will mix in the single ventricle with resulting systemic arterial oxygen desaturation.[591]

The volume and ratio of systemic and pulmonary blood flows are determined by the vascular resistances in the pulmonary and systemic outflow tracts and pulmonary and systemic circulations.[468] The presence or absence of obstruction to pulmonary blood flow helps to determine the presenting clinical signs, including congestive heart failure and cyanosis.[342] If no obstruction to pulmonary (artery) blood flow exists, pulmonary hypertension will be present early and, if untreated, can progress to severe pulmonary vascular obstructive disease by the age of 2 years.[342] Obstruction to pulmonary venous return can also lead to pulmonary hypertension.

The patient with single ventricle physiology may have varying degrees of obstruction to systemic outflow (see Hypoplastic Left Heart Syndrome [HLHS] and also Aortic stenosis elsewhere in this section of the chapter) and heterotaxy. Such obstruction can contribute to pulmonary overcirculation and, once the ductus begins to close, to poor systemic perfusion.

The goal for single ventricle patients is a Fontan circulation where all systemic venous return is directed passively into the pulmonary arteries, without the assist of a ventricular pumping chamber.[591] Patients with single ventricle lesions requiring Glenn- and Fontan-type palliations require the lowest possible pulmonary vascular resistance for survival.[512] These procedures create nonpulsatile pulmonary blood flow that is passive so flow is dependent on a gradient between the systemic venous (right atrial) pressure and left atrial pressure.[589]

If a single ventricle is present *without significant obstruction to pulmonary blood flow*, hypoxemia will be present from birth because pulmonary and systemic venous blood will mix in the ventricle. If there is good mixing of pulmonary and systemic venous blood, hypoxemia may be mild. Once pulmonary vascular resistance falls, pulmonary blood flow increases and signs of congestive heart failure develop.

If the single ventricle is associated *with significant obstruction to pulmonary blood flow*, hypoxemia will be present and may be severe from birth. If pulmonary atresia is present, pulmonary blood flow is dependent on the ductus arteriosus, and severe hypoxemia will develop when the ductus begins to close.

Unrepaired patients with univentricular anatomy have a poor prognosis. About 70% of those with left ventricular anatomy die by age 16 years. If the right ventricle is the systemic ventricle, about 50% die within 4 years after diagnosis.[624] Patients with double inlet left ventricle have survived to the seventh decade of life with unoperated, well-balanced circulations.[22] Survival is very poor (23% at 5 years) if the patient has associated total anomalous pulmonary venous return.[307] All patients with single ventricle have very complex lesions and many potential complications, so require continuous, lifelong cardiac care by experts in the care of patients with congenital heart disease.[927]

Overview of Clinical Signs and Symptoms

If there is *no significant obstruction to pulmonary blood flow*, cyanosis may be mild during the neonatal period. Once pulmonary vascular resistance falls in the first 2 to 6 weeks of life, pulmonary blood flow increases significantly, and signs of congestive heart failure develop. If signs of congestive heart failure develop earlier (during the first 2 weeks of life), associated lesions can be present, including AV valve abnormalities, coarctation or other lesions. The signs of congestive heart failure include tachypnea, tachycardia, hepatomegaly, failure to thrive, and diaphoresis.[342] The risk of pulmonary hypertension is significant. Arterial oxygen saturation may near 90%, reflecting excessive pulmonary blood flow.

A grade 3-4 over 6 systolic murmur is heard over the left sternal border. A diastolic murmur of pulmonary regurgitation may be heard at the upper left sternal border.[686] The chest radiograph will reveal increased heart size and pulmonary vascular markings.[686]

The ECG can be highly variable because the anatomy of the univentricular heart may vary widely.[468] The electrocardiogram is suggestive of a single ventricle if Q waves are abnormal and Q waves may be absent in right precordial leads or noted only with right precordial leads. First or second degree heart block may be present.[686] The ECG in patients with a common-inlet atrioventricular (AV) connection and a common AV valve typically demonstrates moderate to severe left axis deviation.[342] The risk of complete heart block is high when the single ventricle is associated with congenitally corrected transposition (CCTGA or levo-transposition of the great arteries [L-TGA]).[81]

The two-dimensional echocardiogram is the most useful noninvasive tool for the diagnosis, and typically reveals two atrioventricular valves opening into the single ventricle. Echocardiography enables classification of the single ventricle, identification of any rudimentary chamber, and other anatomic details. Magnetic resonance imaging (MRI) is extremely valuable in detailing anatomy, extracardiac abnormalities, volumes, and function.[342]

Cardiac catheterization will demonstrate specific details of cardiac anatomy and function, AV valve function, and the status of the pulmonary vascular bed.[342] Initial palliative treatment may involve interventional cardiac catheterization.

Overview of Management (Including Surgical Procedures)

The management of the child with a single ventricle is individualized based on the child's symptomatology and anatomy. Nonsurgical management is determined by the magnitude of pulmonary blood flow and the severity of hypoxemia. The ultimate goal for a single functioning ventricle is a staged Fontan circulation. The management from birth is directed toward making each patient an optimal candidate for the Fontan procedure.

The Fontan circulation is typically achieved in two stages, beginning at approximately 4 to 6 months of age with surgery to create a superior vena cava (SVC) to pulmonary artery shunt (bidirectional Glenn). Timing for the Fontan surgery is individualized for each patient,[589] but is typically performed at about 1 to 2 years of age.[591] The Fontan redirects the IVC blood flow into the pulmonary arteries, resulting in total separation of systemic and pulmonary venous blood.[591] Until the single ventricle is corrected it is imperative that *no air be allowed to enter any intravenous system,* because this air may be shunted into the systemic arterial circulation, producing a cerebral air embolus (stroke).

Children with single ventricle will require ongoing assessment of oxygen delivery and systemic perfusion to ensure that both are adequate. Careful assessment is required even when the arterial oxygen saturation is within the expected ranges for condition.

Beginning in the newborn period, most patients require palliative procedures to relieve cyanosis or prevent congestive heart failure (Box 8-39).[589] The corrective procedures must also consider the presence of any associated defects; thus the particular surgical approach will be individualized. Cardiac transplantation may also be performed.

If *significant obstruction to pulmonary blood flow* is present, prostaglandin E_1 administration is required during the first days of life to maintain ductal patency; a palliative procedure is then performed to stabilize pulmonary blood flow. A surgical pulmonary-to-systemic shunt can be created (see Fig. 8-44), and the ductus can then be ligated (Additional palliative shunts are illustrated in Evolve Fig. 8-5, and are described in Evolve Table 8-2 in the Chapter 8 Supplement on the Evolve Website). Depending on the interventions required for associated conditions (e.g., pulmonary artery arterioplasty), cardiopulmonary bypass may be required for the surgery. In selected cases the patient may instead undergo interventional cardiac catheterization as the initial palliation, for placement of a stent in the ductus arteriosus to maintain ductal patency and adequate pulmonary blood flow.[18,93,614]

If *significant obstruction to systemic blood flow* is present, such as variants of hypoplastic left heart syndrome, management during the first days of life will include administration of prostaglandin E_1 to maintain ductal patency and systemic flow. A palliative Norwood, Damus-Kaye-Stansel procedure or hybrid stage I palliation is then performed (see Hypoplastic Left Heart Syndrome later in this section of the chapter).

General Nursing Care. General nursing assessment and anticipatory interventions for single ventricle circulation involve support of adequate tissue oxygen delivery. In true single ventricle defects, the systemic arterial oxygen saturation is almost directly related to the volume of pulmonary blood flow. The greater the volume of pulmonary blood flow, the higher the volume of oxygenated pulmonary venous blood returning to the left atrium to mix with the (desaturated) systemic venous return, and the higher will be the resulting (mixed) systemic arterial oxygen saturation.[514] An arterial oxygen saturation of 80% indicates a pulmonary to systemic

---

Box 8-39 Surgical Approach to Single Functioning Ventricle

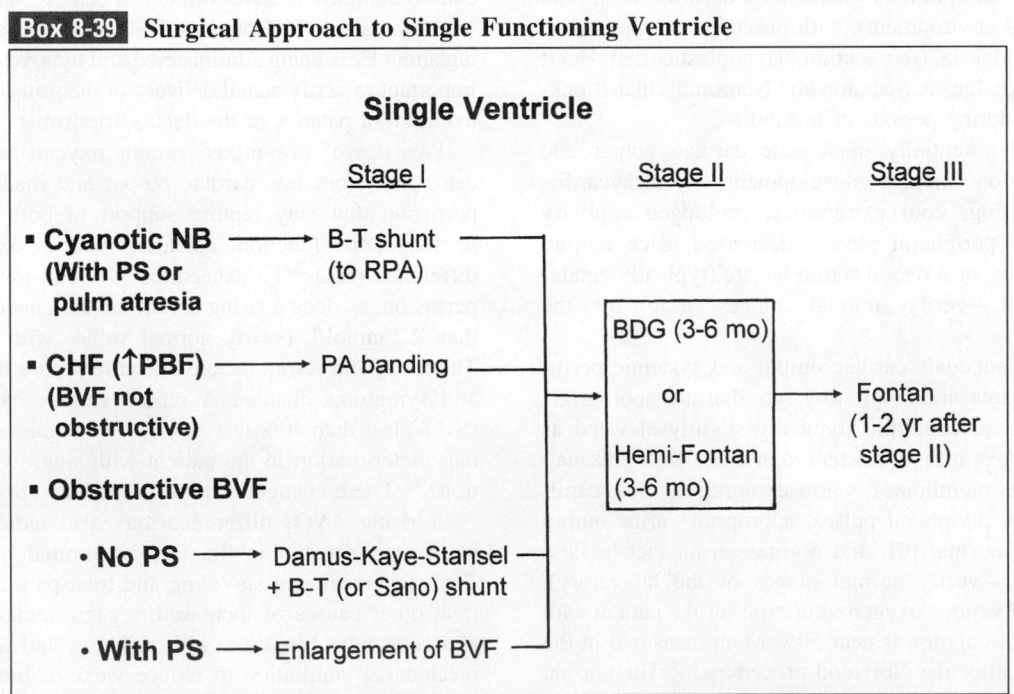

From Park MK. *Pediatr cardiol for practitioners,* ed 5, Philadelphia, 2008, Elsevier (Fig. 14-63).
BDG, Bidirectional Glenn; *B-T* Blalock-Taussig; *BVF,* bulboventricular foramen; *CHF,* congestive heart failure;
NB, newborn; *PBF,* pulmonary blood flow; *PS,* pulmonic stenosis; *RPA,* right pulmonary artery.

blood flow ratio (QP/QS ratio) of nearly 1:1, assuming 95% to 100% pulmonary venous saturation and a 65% mixed venous saturation.[935]

Nursing care practices and therapies must promote a balance between systemic and pulmonary blood flow so both are optimized. Even when the arterial oxygen saturation is adequate (i.e., near 80%), typical clinical signs used to evaluate systemic perfusion do not reliably indicate actual tissue oxygen delivery.[384] The arterial blood gas is, however, an excellent indicator of hemodynamic stability in the patient with single ventricle physiology.[935] Adequate peripheral perfusion is indicated by a normal pH and an arterial oxygen saturation near 80% with a Qp:Qs ratio near 1:1.[935] The arterial oxygen tension (PaO_2) must remain greater than 30 mm Hg. Even when the arterial oxygen saturation is as expected, children with single ventricle physiology require ongoing assessment to verify adequate oxygen delivery and stable systemic perfusion. The arterial oxygen saturation may be within the acceptable or targeted range despite profound circulatory derangements.[881]

Care is generally provided in room air, because oxygen is a potent pulmonary vasodilator that will increase pulmonary blood flow. A high inspired oxygen concentration can lead to excessive pulmonary blood flow (indicated by an arterial oxygen saturation greater than 85% to 88%) and resultant systemic hypoperfusion and development of lactic acidosis.[935] The inspired oxygen concentration and ventilation support is tailored to maintain the PaO_2 near 40 mm Hg, the $PaCO_2$ near 40 mm Hg, and the pH near 7.40. Hypocarbia and creation of alkalosis result in pulmonary vasodilation, and so are avoided unless there is a need to increase pulmonary blood flow.

The hematocrit is maintained at least at 40% to optimize oxygen carrying capacity in these patients with cyanosis and chronic arterial oxygen desaturation. Efforts are made to minimize oxygen consumption by maintaining normothermia (and a neutral thermal environment), with provision of appropriate sedation and analgesia (see section, Hypoplastic Left Heart and Chapter 5, Analgesia, Sedation and Neuromuscular Blockade), especially during periods of instability.

Indicators of potentially inadequate cardiac output and systemic perfusion include development of tachycardia, tachypnea, mottling, cool extremities, prolonged capillary refill, decreased peripheral pulses, decreased urine output, metabolic acidosis, or a rise in serum lactate (typically greater than 2.2 mmol/L—verify normal ranges used by the laboratory).

Indicators of adequate cardiac output and systemic perfusion are a heart rate and respiratory rate that are appropriate for age and clinical condition (typically slightly elevated as the result of hypoxemia), consistent skin color with pink nail beds and mucous membranes, warm extremities, brisk capillary refill, strong peripheral pulses, appropriate urine output for fluid intake, normal pH, and normal serum lactate (less than 2.2 mmol/L—verify normal ranges of the laboratory). The target mixed venous oxygen saturation for the patient with single ventricle circulation is near 50% when measured in the SVC of patients after the Norwood procedure.[881] The normal target arteriovenous oxygen saturation difference (systemic arterial saturation [SaO_2] minus mixed venous oxygen saturation, or $\Delta Sa\text{-}vO_2$) is near 25%.

General care for patients with unrepaired single ventricle circulation will avoid factors that can lead to inadequate systemic perfusion. Hyperventilation with excessive use of oxygen is avoided, as are hypocarbia and alkalosis because they promote pulmonary vasodilation. Such pulmonary vasodilation can result in pulmonary overcirculation, with subsequent systemic hypoperfusion and development or worsening of congestive heart failure and myocardial dysfunction. This combination will produce acidosis despite an arterial oxygen saturation in excess of 90%,[935] and requires rapid recognition and intervention.

Sinus tachycardia remains the most efficient way to increase cardiac output in newborns and infants. When any arrhythmias develop it is important to assess the impact of the arrhythmia on systemic perfusion; the greater the effect of the arrhythmia on perfusion, the more urgent the treatment needed. Excessive tachycardia, loss of AV synchrony and bradycardia are not well tolerated and may produce a fall in coronary as well as systemic perfusion, leading to rapid patient deterioration.

Systolic hypertension and high systemic vascular resistance may contribute to excessive pulmonary blood flow, increased myocardial work and increased oxygen consumption,[520,602] requiring initiation of afterload reduction (vasodilator) therapy. No air can be allowed in any IV system because it may flow into the systemic arterial circulation causing a cerebral embolic event (e.g., stroke).

An arterial saturation less than 70% or PaO_2 of less than 30 mm Hg is undesirable, as it indicates inadequate pulmonary blood flow, and eventually leads to the development of tissue hypoxia and acidosis. Management involves assessment and support of adequate airway and ventilation *first*. Pulmonary venous desaturation may be caused by hypoventilation, endotracheal tube obstruction or displacement, atelectasis, pleural effusion, infection and pneumothorax. Supplementary oxygen can be administered and titrated to achieve an arterial oxygen saturation above 75% but less than 85%. Preoperatively, if prostaglandin E_1 is being administered and hypoxemia worsens, it is important to verify actual delivery of the infusion and assess for evidence of patency of the ductus arteriosus.

Presence of low mixed venous oxygen saturation (SvO_2) can result from low cardiac output and inadequate systemic perfusion that may require support of both respiratory and hemodynamic function. An arteriovenous oxygen saturation difference ($\Delta Sa\text{-}vO_2$) exceeding 30% can indicate worsening perfusion, as does a rising serum lactate concentration greater than 2.2 mmol/L (verify normal values with the laboratory). The SvO_2 and serum lactate decrease *before* the clinical signs and symptoms change. A mixed venous oxygen saturation (SvO_2) less than 40% is a *very early* indicator of cardiopulmonary deterioration in the patient with single ventricle circulation.[384] These changes require immediate attention.

A rising AVO_2 difference may also indicate an increase in oxygen demand in the face of limited oxygen delivery. Treat fever, prevent shivering and treat pain and identify and treat other causes of increased oxygen demand and consider neuromuscular blockade with sedation and analgesia during mechanical ventilation to reduce work of breathing. Anemia with subsequent impaired oxygen delivery can decrease arterial saturation and oxygen delivery, and requires transfusion to raise the hematocrit greater than 40%.

Hypotension may lead to decreased pulmonary blood flow and decreased arterial oxygen saturation, requiring IV volume administration or vasoactive therapy, and adjustment of vasodilator therapy. A diastolic blood pressure of less than 30 mm Hg is avoided because it will reduce coronary artery perfusion pressure (aortic end-diastolic pressure—right atrial pressure).[591]

An echocardiogram may be required to identify potential causes of arterial oxygen desaturation. Evaluation includes assessment of any existing shunt, examination of the ductus arteriosus (if present) and assessment of the size of the pulmonary artery and pulmonary veins (to identify any obstruction to pulmonary arterial or pulmonary venous flow), and assessment of diaphragm and cardiac function.

Caution is required to avoid excessive diuresis and avoid, identify, and promptly treat any dehydration. Dehydration with decreased intravascular volume can lead to lower cardiac output and systemic arterial oxygen saturation and can also produce hemoconcentration with subsequent risk of thromboemboli.

Treatment for elevated arterial oxygen saturation (greater than 85%), with pulmonary overcirculation and poor systemic perfusion includes measures to *increase* pulmonary vascular resistance. Inspired oxygen concentration is decreased to room air, to avoid the vasodilatory effects of increased alveolar oxygenation. If the child is receiving mechanical ventilation, interventions to increase pulmonary vascular resistance include changes in support to produce an increase in $PaCO_2$ with intentional hypercarbia to 45 mm Hg or above. If the patient is tachypneic on the ventilator, sedation and neuromuscular blockade may be initiated. An arterial PaO_2 of at least 30 mm Hg is desired,[514] with a pH of 7.35 to 7.40. Sedation can be used to suppress the infant's intrinsic respiratory drive, allowing the $PaCO_2$ to rise. PEEP can contribute to increased pulmonary vascular resistance.[881]

Alveolar hypoxia can be created with use of inhaled nitrogen to reduce the inspired oxygen concentration to 14% to 20% to create pulmonary vasoconstriction and thus *limit* pulmonary blood flow.[935] Inhaled carbon dioxide (2% to 5%) can cause pulmonary vasoconstriction.[935] When the arterial oxygen saturation is elevated, it may be appropriate to decrease systemic vascular resistance using intravenous vasodilators (e.g., Primacor up to 1 mcg/kg per minute, Phenoxybenzamine, or Nipride) or oral vasodilators (e.g., Enalapril, Captopril).

Despite the presence of an elevated arterial oxygen saturation, some infants may be minimally symptomatic, tolerating oral feedings with signs of adequate perfusion. Ongoing surveillance is still needed to evaluate adequacy of oxygen delivery and systemic perfusion. Echocardiogram may be completed to assess potential causes for elevated saturation, including extra sources of pulmonary blood flow from aortopulmonary collaterals or the development of an aortic arch obstruction with subsequent excessive flow through a prosthetic shunt or stented patent ductus arteriosus.

Throughout the care of patients with single ventricle, optimizing nutrition is critical for growth. Interventions are required to maximize caloric intake, monitor weight gain and minimize excessive metabolic demand. Infants with hypoplastic left heart palliation are expected to consume 110 to 130 cal/kg per day with fortified breast milk or formula prepared to deliver 24 to 27 calories per ounce.[881] It is also common for the patient with single ventricle to have difficulty with oral intake, GE reflux, and altered feeding (see section, Common Clinical Conditions, Altered Nutrition). Normal rate of weight gains in infants following Norwood Stage I surgery have been achieved using calorie enhanced formulas with home surveillance of nutrition and weight gains.[891]

Palliative Surgery for Univentricular Heart with Excessive Pulmonary Blood Flow: Pulmonary Artery Banding. Palliative surgery for univentricular heart with uncontrolled increase in pulmonary blood flow can include pulmonary artery banding during early infancy. Banding can be performed via a midsternal incision, without cardiopulmonary bypass. The pulmonary artery banding can help prevent development of pulmonary vascular obstructive disease[342]; it will decrease the volume and pressure of pulmonary blood flow and decrease symptoms of congestive heart failure (CHF). Postoperative care includes titration of vasoactive support and intravascular volume and all aspects of typical perioperative cardiovascular care. The sudden application of new afterload by the pulmonary artery band may not be well tolerated, so myocardial dysfunction may be present postoperatively.

The systemic oxygen saturation following pulmonary artery banding should remain 75% to 80%. Following banding signs of an excessively tight band include signs of decreased pulmonary blood flow with excessive cyanosis, an arterial oxygen saturation less than 70%, poor perfusion, and acidosis. If the band is too loose, signs of pulmonary overcirculation with high arterial oxygen saturation (greater than 80%) and congestive heart failure may persist, and continued treatment for CHF will be required.

The Society of Thoracic Surgery 4-year database (2006-2010) reports hospital mortality for pulmonary artery banding is high at 12.8% in neonates and 5.5% in infants (compared to an overall pediatric surgical hospital mortality of 3.2%).[823] The use of percutaneously adjustable pulmonary artery bands have improved survival and decreased the need for reoperation.[842]

Palliative Surgery for Univentricular Heart with Systemic Outflow Tract Obstruction: The Damus-Kaye-Stansel Procedure. This procedure requires cardiopulmonary bypass with aortic cross-clamping. In this procedure the pulmonary artery is transected before the bifurcation (i.e., the main trunk is separated from the branches). The end of the main pulmonary trunk is sewn into the side of the ascending aorta. This enables ventricular outflow to enter the original pulmonary artery trunk (bypassing the subaortic stenosis) and then flow into the aorta[591] (Fig. 8-56). A modified Blalock-Taussig shunt is created to provide pulmonary blood flow. A patch is placed to close the opening in the distal main pulmonary artery.

Postoperative care for the Damus-Kaye-Stansel procedure is similar to that required after the Norwood procedure with a modified Blalock-Taussig shunt. Because the child has single ventricle hemodynamics, the desired arterial oxygen saturation is near 80%. Bleeding is a potential complication because the child has extensive aortic suture lines exposed to arterial pressure.[591]

Ongoing interstage mortality in patients with palliated single ventricle have led to establishment of specialized

FIG. 8-56 The Damus-Kaye-Stansel procedure in a patient with double-inlet left ventricle and subaortic stenosis. A, Blood flow pathways before the surgical procedure. The aorta (AO) arises from a hypoplastic right ventricular outflow tract (RVOT) chamber that receives blood flow from the left ventricle through the bulboventricular foramen (BVF). The small outflow tract produces subaortic stenosis. The main pulmonary artery (MPA) arises from the left ventricle, and supplies blood flow to the pulmonary circulation, and, via the patent ductus arteriosus, to the aorta and systemic circulations. B, Blood flow pathways after the procedureThe MPA is transected and the trunk is sewn end-to-side to the ascending AO, providing unobstructed blood flow from the left ventricle into the aorta. A systemic shunt, such as a Blalock-Taussig shunt, is created (not shown) to provide pulmonary blood flow. LA, left atrium; LV, left ventricle; PDA, patent ductus arteriosus. (From Nichols DG. *Critical heart disease in infants and children*, ed 2, Philadelphia, 1995, Elsevier, Fig. 38-3.)

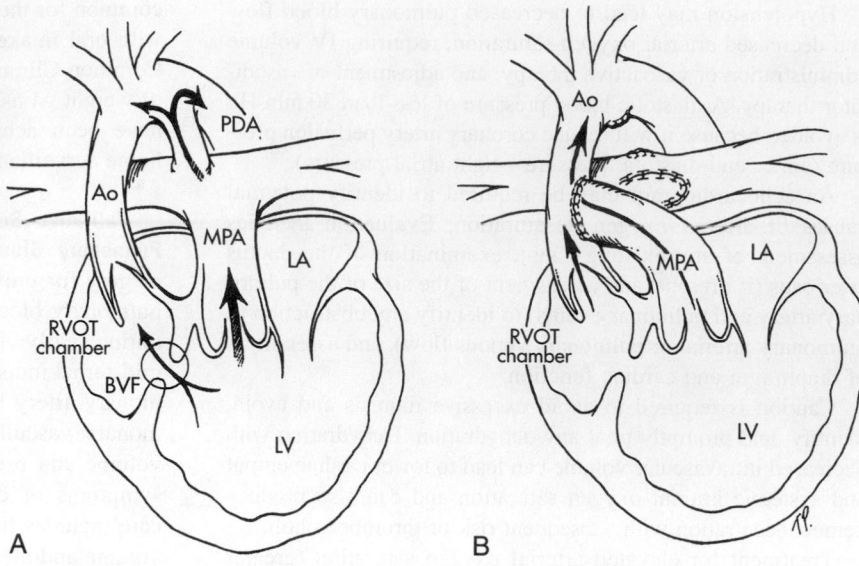

interstage home monitoring programs. These programs have improved survival of patients following the Norwood procedure and include monitoring of oxygen saturation and daily weight, and establishing parameters for additional repeat followup.[318] National, multicenter quality improvement collaboratives by the Joint Council on Congenital Heart Disease are underway to reduce clinical practice variations and improve outcomes for children with HLHS.[502] Risks for interstage death after the Norwood procedure and before the second stage Glenn procedure range from 5% to 15%[881] (see Hypoplastic Left Heart Syndrome). Infants with palliative shunts are at risk for sudden interstage death.[262]

Family education and extensive preparation for optimal home management and follow-up care are required. Prophylaxis for risk of infective endocarditis is required because of the presence of prosthetic materials and presence of palliated cyanotic heart disease (see Bacterial Endocarditis later in this section of the chapter).

Palliative Surgery for Univentricular Heart with Inadequate Pulmonary Blood Flow: Systemic-to-Pulmonary Shunt. Pulmonary blood flow may be increased through the creation of a surgical systemic-to-pulmonary shunt. Alternatively, a stent may be placed in the ductus arteriosus to keep it open.

After surgery for a systemic to pulmonary artery shunt or placement of a stent within the ductus arteriosus to maintain ductal patency, titration of volume administration, inotropic support, and ventilatory management are required to balance systemic and pulmonary blood flow and prevent ventricular overload. Postoperatively, monitor for signs that the shunt is patent: an arterial oxygen saturation consistently greater than 70%, adequate systemic perfusion, low diastolic blood pressure with a wide pulse pressure (because the shunt creates a runoff of aortic blood flow into the pulmonary artery), and a continuous murmur. Clinical signs of a narrowing or closing shunt include a falling arterial oxygen saturation (a fall of greater than 10% from baseline or to less than 75%), rising diastolic blood pressure, a change in or disappearance of the shunt murmur, signs of poor perfusion,

metabolic acidosis, or rising serum lactate greater than 2.2 mmol/L (verify threshold for lactic acidosis with the laboratory).

Shunt thrombosis is an emergency when the shunt is the only source of pulmonary blood flow. Immediate care can include administration of intravenous heparin, drugs to raise arterial blood pressure, and intravenous volume administration. Emergent echocardiogram is needed and urgent shunt revision may be needed.

The Society of Thoracic Surgery 4-year database (2006-2009) documents a relatively high mortality for prosthetic shunt surgery. Hospital mortality among neonates with single ventricle following creation of a modified Blalock-Taussig shunt is 6.9%, and 10% for a central shunt, while a 8.9% mortality is reported for a modified Blalock-Taussig shunt in infants without single ventricle physiology.[823]

Use of oral aspirin in children with prosthetic shunts appears to lower the risk of death and the occurrence of shunt thrombosis.[533] Anticoagulation can initially include IV heparin (once the risk of postoperative bleeding is resolved), transitioning to oral aspirin therapy, but may include other anticoagulants such as Coumadin or Lovenox (a low molecular weight heparin) if the shunt or stent are judged to be at higher risk for thrombus occlusion.

Some patients continue to have antegrade pulmonary blood flow from the heart through the stenotic pulmonary outflow tract. When antegrade pulmonary blood flow from the heart is present, the arterial oxygen saturation is expected to trend higher than when a shunt alone provides all pulmonary blood flow.

Palliative Surgery for Univentricular Heart: The Bidirectional Glenn and Hemi-Fontan Procedure (Cavopulmonary Anastomosis). The bidirectional Glenn and hemi-Fontan procedures may be performed as second-stage palliative procedures for hypoplastic left heart syndrome or as palliative procedures for other single functioning ventricle defects, such as tricuspid atresia. Both involve creation of a connection between the superior vena cava and the main pulmonary artery to divert all SVC blood to the pulmonary circulation. SVC flow is equal to about half of the total systemic venous return, and is slightly more than half of the systemic venous return in the infant.[935]

The bidirectional Glenn and the hemi-Fontan improve effective pulmonary blood flow and increase systemic arterial oxygen saturation by reducing the volume of systemic venous blood that enters the heart to mix with pulmonary venous blood. Both procedures also decompress the single ventricle because they reduce the total venous volume that the ventricle must eject, reducing the risk of ventricular dysfunction and atrioventricular valve insufficiency.[935] As a result, both procedures improve survival and outcome from the later corrective procedure (the Fontan or variant of Fontan procedure).

The Glenn anastomosis can be performed with or without cardiopulmonary bypass. The hemi-Fontan is more extensive and requires cardiopulmonary bypass but facilitates later completion of the corrective Fontan (or modified Fontan) procedure.[589,881] Typically, when either procedure is performed, previous palliative procedures (e.g., a systemic to pulmonary artery shunt or ductal stent) are taken down.

The bidirectional Glenn or hemi-Fontan and ultimate Fontan procedures require the presence of low pulmonary vascular resistance and low pulmonary venous pressures (which are related to the compliance of the single ventricle),[298] and both require central pulmonary arteries that are undistorted and of adequate size.[589] If pulmonary vascular resistance is elevated, these palliative procedures and ultimate correction cannot be performed. Therefore close collaboration between the cardiologist and cardiovascular surgeon is required to determine the ideal procedure and optimal time for surgical intervention.

Preoperative evaluation before second-stage palliation with the bidirectional Glenn or hemi-Fontan procedure includes echocardiogram with possible cardiac catheterization or cardiac MRI. The cardiac catheterization evaluates anatomy, hemodynamics, and suitability for the procedure. Interventional procedures during the preoperative catheterization may also include closure of aortopulmonary or venovenous collateral vessels and angioplasty dilation of the pulmonary arteries with possible stenting of any narrowed structures.

Cardiac MRI may be performed after first-stage palliations to evaluate for potential complications or sequelae. These can include aortic arch obstruction, pulmonary artery branch deformities and pulmonary vein compression or stenosis. The shunt status is also evaluated.[314]

The MRI before[118] and after the Glenn procedure provides extensive information and in an increasing number of cases may substitute for diagnostic catheterization.[314] Successful bidirectional Glenn procedures are achievable with calculated pulmonary vascular resistance up to 3-4 wood units (indexed to body surface area) or pulmonary artery mean pressure up to 20 mm Hg.[589] For further information see Common Clinical Conditions, Pulmonary Hypertension.

The Hemi-Fontan Procedure. The hemi-Fontan procedure is so named because it diverts roughly half of systemic venous blood flow into the pulmonary circulation. The procedure requires cardiopulmonary bypass. It involves creation of an anastomosis between the side of the SVC and the main pulmonary artery (Fig. 8-57, A). The SVC is not disconnected from

the right atrium, but a patch is placed at the SVC inlet to the right atrium to prevent SVC blood flow from entering the heart. The connection may alternatively include arteriotomies in the superior and inferior surfaces of the right pulmonary artery to allow for the connection to the superior vena cava (SVC).[589]

The Glenn Anastomosis. The Glenn anastomosis is performed with or without cardiopulmonary bypass. It involves division of the superior vena cava above the heart. The top portion (bringing venous blood from the head and upper extremities) is sewn directly into the top of the main pulmonary artery (on the patient's right side) and the cut end of the SVC that leads to the right atrium is oversewn. If a right and left SVC are present, a bilateral bidirectional Glenn is performed to join each SVC to the corresponding pulmonary artery.[935] Occasionally, bilateral SVC's are present and the much smaller SVC can be ligated.[935]

The Glenn results in the diversion of all superior vena caval venous blood away from the heart and directly into the pulmonary arteries. The bidirectional Glenn immediately relieves overload of the functioning single ventricle, increases ventricular function, and improves the function of the AV valves.[935] By directing a significant portion of desaturated systemic venous blood directly into the pulmonary circulation, effective pulmonary blood flow and systemic oxygenation is improved, particularly in young children.

In most centers, the Glenn procedure is performed as a stage 2 palliation technique for hypoplastic left heart syndrome. It follows an initial Norwood palliation, and is performed when the infant is about 4 to 6 months of age. This delayed timing for the second stage has followed reports that earlier performance of cavopulmonary anastomoses (i.e., at less than 4 months of age) resulted in lower arterial oxygen saturation in the early postoperative period and longer length of hospital stay.[410]

Postoperative Care After the Glenn or Hemi-Fontan. Potential early postoperative complications of the Glenn and the hemi-Fontan procedures include bleeding, chylothorax, pleural effusion, and superior vena caval obstruction. Arterial oxygen saturation should be near 80% to 85% for infants in room air.[589,935] In the older patient, the arterial oxygen saturation may be lower after the Glenn because the volume of systemic venous return from the upper body that is diverted to the lungs is a smaller portion of total systemic venous return in older than in younger patients.[935] Repair of additional lesions, such as pulmonary artery or aortic reconstruction, can add to the complexity of the postoperative course.

Oxygen therapy can be used without restriction following the Glenn procedure. During the immediate postoperative period, the head of the bed should be elevated with the head in a midline position, to enhance blood flow from the superior vena cava into the pulmonary arteries. The face and upper extremities are often edematous and plethoric in appearance during the immediate postoperative period (parents should be informed about this potential change in appearance in advance), but the child's appearance should return to normal within several days.

Small increases in pulmonary vascular resistance can lead to systemic venous hypertension with low cardiac output despite a technically successful procedure.[476] Pulmonary hypertension can be present and pulmonary vascular resistance can be elevated after cardiopulmonary bypass.[935,942]

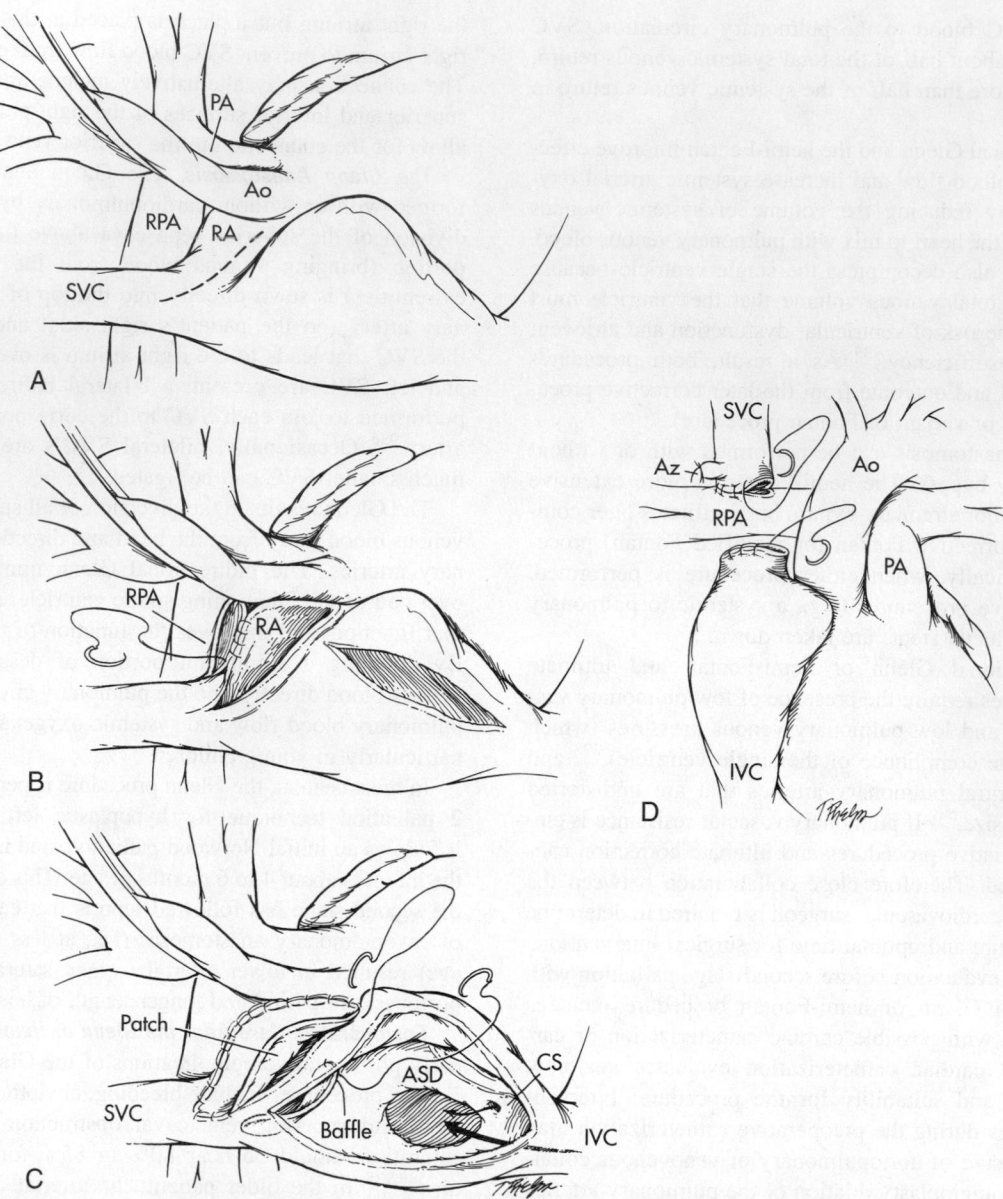

FIG. 8-57 The hemi-Fontan/Bi-Directional Glenn operations. **A,** The hemi-Fontan operation from the surgeon's point of view (this view is rotated 90 degrees counterclockwise from other figures of congenital heart defects and surgical repairs included in this chapter). A right atrial spiral incision is made, extending from the superior vena cava (SVC) to the surface of the right atrium (RA). **B,** After incision in the right pulmonary artery (RPA), a vascular confluence is created incorporating the cardiac end of the SVC, the cephalad portion of the RA (the portion nearest the head), and the RPA. **C,** The confluence is roofed with a patch of polytetrafluoroethylene (PTFE). A second PTFE baffle forms the floor of this confluence and separates the inferior vena cava (IVC) and coronary sinus (CS) blood from the SVC blood, thus diverting IVC and coronary sinus venous return through the atrial septal defect (ASD) to the left atrium. AO, aorta. **D,** The bidirectional Glenn operation. After transection of the superior vena cava (SVC), the cephalad end (i.e., bringing venous return from the head and upper extremities) is anastomosed to the right pulmonary artery (RPA). The cardiac end of the SVC is oversewn. The azygous (Az) vein is ligated (tied off). Blood flow from the inferior vena cava (IVC) passes through the atrial septal defect (ASD) to the left atrium, and thus contributes to left ventricular preload. AO, aorta. (From Nichols DG. *Critical heart disease in infants and children,* ed 2, Philadelphia, 1995, Elsevier, Figs. 39-8 and 39-9.)

Treatment for elevated pulmonary vascular resistance can include the use of oxygen, vasodilators, and milrinone. Inhaled nitric oxide has been shown to be beneficial[8,298] in the early postoperative period after Fontan and Glenn procedures.

Patients with elevated pulmonary vascular resistance (greater than 3.5 Wood units) or elevated mean pulmonary artery pressures (greater than 18 mm Hg) have been found to have higher risk for postoperative superior vena caval syndrome, low oxygen saturation (less than 70% to 75%), and death.[174] High SVC pressure with high arterial oxygen saturation may indicate the presence of a large aortopulmonary collateral vessel producing an effective left-to-right shunt.[591]

Marked elevations in the SVC pressure result in decreased systemic perfusion.[8]

Initial postoperative SVC pressure may exceed 15 mm Hg, but should fall to 12 mm Hg or less within 2 days.[591] For flow to occur through the Glenn, pulmonary vascular resistance must be low, so anything that causes pulmonary vasoconstriction will reduce blood flow through the Glenn and increase SVC pressure.

A superior vena caval syndrome may develop when SVC pressure is elevated; this syndrome produces upper body edema and plethora.[935] Possible causes of superior vena caval syndrome include obstruction at the anastomosis, elevated pulmonary resistance or distortions of the pulmonary arteries with obstruction to flow.[935] The elevated SVC pressure can be associated with an elevated transpulmonary gradient (SVC pressure minus intraatrial pressure).[591] Identification of the cause for persistent SVC pressure elevation despite treatment requires a search for anatomic causes[8] that can generally be treated during cardiac catheterization.

The Glenn anastomosis places cerebral blood flow and cardiopulmonary blood flow in a series, and autoregulatory mechanisms in these two tissue beds respond to changes in acid-base status and carbon dioxide tension in opposite ways.[393,935] Increased alveolar oxygenation will produce pulmonary vasodilation. Factors known to produce pulmonary vasoconstriction (e.g., hypoventilation, acidosis, and reducing alveolar oxygenation) will cause cerebral vasodilation. Recent studies have shown that hypercarbia (maintaining the $PaCO_2$ approximately 55 mm Hg) after a bidirectional Glenn will increase cardiac output by increasing cerebral blood flow, pulmonary blood flow and systemic arterial oxygenation, without significant elevation in pulmonary vascular resistance.[98,99,393,935]

Elevated atrial pressures may result from ventricular dysfunction, presence of arrhythmias with loss of AV synchrony, and atrioventricular valve regurgitation. The elevated atrial pressures can cause elevation in the SVC pressure.[591] Heart rhythm disturbances may include sinus node dysfunction, treated with chronotropic medication therapy or temporary pacing.[935]

Pulmonary management includes weaning positive pressure ventilation to allow spontaneous ventilation as soon as possible. Early extubation is optimal to promote pulmonary blood flow. The arterial PaO_2 should remain greater than 30 mm Hg. Hypercapnia with the $PaCO_2$ approximately 55 mm Hg (range, 45-55 mm Hg) can increase cardiac output, systemic oxygenation, and pulmonary and cerebral blood flow.

After the bidirectional Glenn procedure the patient does not usually improve in response to inhaled nitric oxide,[5] but cases of impaired pulmonary circulation after bidirectional Glenn have been treated successfully with inhaled nitric oxide[298] and sildenafil[646] to promote pulmonary vasodilation. Improved pulmonary blood flow results in improved systemic arterial oxygenation and systemic blood flow and decreases the transpulmonary gradient. If there is difficulty in weaning mechanical ventilation, rule out a diaphragm paralysis.

Systemic arterial hypertension is often present postoperatively. Causes can include pain, intracranial hypertension, or catecholamine secretion.[935] Treatment may include administration of vasodilators. Caution is required to avoid aggressive lowering of the blood pressure, because it may have a negative affect on cerebral perfusion pressure.[935] Irritability is a common postoperative finding and requires provision of comfort measures, analgesics and sedation (see Chapter 5, Sedatives, Analgesics, and Neuromuscular Blockade).

Severe hypoxemia and cyanosis, with low arterial oxygen saturation (less than 70% to 75%), or an arterial PaO_2 of less than 30 mm Hg requires prompt identification and intervention. Such hypoxemia can be caused by pulmonary venous desaturation resulting from pulmonary problems such as atelectasis, elevated diaphragm, pleural effusion, tube obstruction, or pulmonary edema. Increased pulmonary vascular resistance and resulting decrease in pulmonary blood flow can also cause lower arterial oxygen saturation, because less pulmonary venous blood returns to the heart to mix with the systemic venous return from the inferior vena cava.

Persistent low cardiac output with low mixed venous oxygen saturation can lead to worsening hypoxemia and cyanosis, so treatment must focus on improving cardiac output. A hematocrit of at least 40% is maintained to optimize oxygen carrying capacity. A cardiac catheterization procedure may be required for complete assessment, definitive diagnosis, and intervention to treat the cause of the severe hypoxemia and cyanosis. Interventions may include sealing decompressing collateral venous vessels, angioplasty, and possible stenting of a stenotic anastomosis or pulmonary vessel.

Deterioration in arterial oxygen saturation in the weeks to months postoperatively can be caused by opening of venovenous collaterals (from the superior vena cava into the right atrium or inferior vena cava). Such collaterals will decompress (reduce) the elevated SVC pressure,[686] but will increase cyanosis. The venous collaterals can be identified by echocardiography with a "bubble study," injecting agitated saline into an upper extremity and watching for the movement of the saline into the heart. An echocardiogram may also reveal a previously undiagnosed left superior vena cava or a baffle leak (in the intracardiac SVC patch for the hemi-Fontan).[935]

Persistent elevation of SVC pressure can lead to persistent pleural effusions and interstitial infiltrates if the pulmonary lymphatic vessels cannot drain into the hypertensive central veins.[591] Pleural effusions are managed with diuresis and control of intravascular volume. Drainage is monitored for the development of chylous effusion, a whitish, opaque fluid. The chyle volume is increased, particularly with oral feedings containing fats (see Postoperative Care after Fontan Procedure, Pleural and Pericardial Effusions). Untreated pleural effusions further decrease pulmonary blood flow and arterial oxygen saturation, leading to worsening cyanosis.[591]

The bidirectional Glenn for infants has a hospital mortality of 1.8% in the 4-year (2006-2010) report from the Society of Thoracic Surgeons (STS) database, and 2.5% in infants undergoing bilateral bidirectional Glenn. Reported STS mortality for the hemi-Fontan procedure is 3.2%. Survival at 1 year was 96%, and at 5 years was 89% in a recent 10-year analysis,[777] with preoperative atrioventricular valve regurgitation identified as a risk factor for death or transplant.

Patients undergoing the Glenn procedure in the past may have undergone the original Glenn connection (first reported in 1958), joining the SVC exclusively to the right pulmonary artery. This method is no longer used because it was associated with a high rate of complications, including the development of pulmonary arteriovenous fistulae, pulmonary artery or superior vena caval distortion, loss of continuity between right and left pulmonary arteries, and failure of normal right pulmonary artery development.[342] The bidirectional Glenn procedure is not associated with significant occurrence of pulmonary arteriovenous fistulae.[726]

When pulmonic stenosis or a pulmonary band is present the bidirectional Glenn may be created and an existing systemic-to-pulmonary artery shunt may be left intact to provide additional antegrade pulmonary blood flow. The bidirectional Glenn with additional antegrade pulmonary blood flow may produce a resting arterial oxygen saturation of approximately 90%. This combination may serve as the final surgery if the patient is found to be a suboptimal Fontan candidate.[133]

If pulmonary *arteriovenous malformations* develop, desaturated venous blood within the lungs bypasses the pulmonary capillary bed and returns into the pulmonary veins without gas exchange, so hypoxemia and cyanosis worsen.[881] The possible cause for the formation of these vessels is the lack of a "hepatic factor."[489] Hepatic factor is a postulated (but not yet identified) substance in hepatic venous blood; if hepatic venous blood does not traverse the pulmonary circulation (i.e., if it bypasses the lungs), patients are more likely to develop pulmonary arteriovenous malformations or fistulae. Completion of the Fontan procedure restores the "hepatic factor" flow through the pulmonary circulation, with potential resolution of pulmonary arteriovenous malformations.[881]

With time and growth the relative quantity of systemic venous return from the upper body diminishes, causing the child to become increasingly hypoxemic, cyanotic, and polycythemic.[342] As the child grows, oxygen consumption increases and the growth of the lower body results in an increase in the volume of desaturated systemic venous returning to the heart via the inferior vena cava.[881] Once this growth in the lower body occurs, the Glenn anastomosis will not provide sufficient pulmonary blood flow,[241] and an additional surgical procedure will be needed to improve pulmonary blood flow. Typically, a Fontan-type correction is anticipated. In selected cases, an additional systemic to pulmonary artery shunt will be placed with no progression to the Fontan.

Selected patients will be eligible to have a "one-and-a-half" ventricle repair, with surgical correction of blood flow at the ventricular level and maintenance of the bidirectional Glenn.[522] Alternatively, a bi-ventricular repair can be accomplished with takedown of the previously completed Glenn and Fontan procedures.[379] Selected patients with unmanageable, severely decreased ventricular function may be referred for cardiac transplantation.

Corrective Surgery: The Completion Fontan Procedure (and Variations of the Fontan). The correction of a single functioning ventricle is a variant of the original procedure described by Fontan in 1971. The procedure diverts all systemic venous blood flow into the pulmonary circulation. When accomplished after a bidirectional Glenn or hemi-Fontan (procedures that divert superior vena caval blood flow into the pulmonary circulation), the procedure diverts the inferior vena caval flow under a baffle or through an extracardiac conduit into the pulmonary circulation[591] (Fig. 8-58). The Fontan is typically completed with use of cardiopulmonary bypass,[591] although extracardiac Fontan completion without cardiopulmonary bypass is reported.[797] Following the Fontan procedure the coronary sinus venous return will drain into the heart, resulting in a small right to left shunt with a decrease in systemic arterial oxygen saturation by one to two percent (Fig. 8-58).[591]

Preoperative Evaluation. Before the Fontan procedure, evaluation includes echocardiogram and cardiac catheterization to assess hemodynamics and suitability for Fontan procedure. Interventional procedures during the catheterization may include closure of aortopulmonary collateral vessels and dilation and possible stenting of narrowed structures including the pulmonary arteries or aorta.

"Ideal" hemodynamic criteria for a Fontan procedure include: low pulmonary vascular resistance (less than 2 Wood units, indexed to body surface area), pulmonary artery mean pressure less than 15 mm Hg, central pulmonary arteries that are large and without distortion, good ventricular function and low pulmonary venous atrial pressure (less than 5 mm Hg).[589] Mild elevation in pulmonary vascular resistance (greater than 3 Wood units) can prevent a successful Fontan procedure.[342] A 24-hour Holter monitor can detect loss of AV synchrony or bradycardia. After cardiac catheterization, patients may have transient complete heart block related to catheter manipulation.[452]

Fenestrated Fontan. The Fontan procedure produces passive flow of systemic venous blood through the pulmonary circulation. Because no ventricle ejects the flow forward into the lungs,[942] blood flow requires that pulmonary venous and left atrial pressures and pulmonary vascular resistance remain low. Patients with increased risk factors, including elevated pulmonary pressure or elevated pulmonary vascular resistance or less than optimal ventricular function, may have restricted forward flow through a conventional Fontan, with decreased pulmonary venous return and low cardiac output. These patients may undergo a *fenestrated* Fontan, first described in 1990.[108] In the fenestrated Fontan, there is a hole (fenestration) placed in the Fontan baffle to allow some inferior vena caval blood flow to enter the pulmonary venous atrium. This creates a right-to-left shunt whenever pressure in the Fontan baffle is elevated. The fenestration allows maintenance of cardiac output despite elevated pulmonary vascular resistance, although the systemic oxygen saturation will be lower than normal (as the result of the right-to-left shunt through the fenestration).

Use of the fenestrated Fontan and use of modified ultrafiltration to control intravascular volume have been shown to decrease the duration and severity of pleural effusions after the Fontan.[306] Children with a fenestrated Fontan have been shown to have fewer complications, with less chest tube drainage and shorter length of hospital stay, and they are less likely to need additional postoperative procedures.[523] With a right-to-left shunt, risk for systemic embolization exists. No air can be allowed to enter any intravenous device (see section, Common Clinical Conditions, Hypoxemia) as long as the fenestration is present.

Fenestrations are expected to cause systemic oxygen *desaturation,* so it is essential that the bedside nurse and

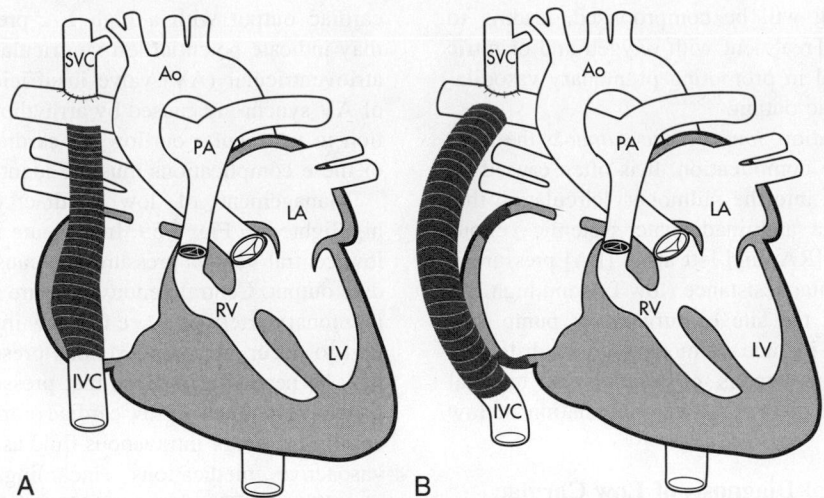

FIG. 8-58 Fontan correction for single ventricle. **A,** Lateral tunnel Fontan procedure for tricuspid atresia with normally related great arteries. Systemic venous return is channeled into the pulmonary circulation by direct anastomosis of the superior vena cava to the right pulmonary artery and insertion of an intraatrial baffle to divert the blood flow from inferior vena cava to the right pulmonary artery. If there is residual blood flow through the pulmonary valve, the main pulmonary artery is ligated (tied off) at the time of surgery. **B,** Extracardiac Fontan procedure for tricuspid atresia with normally related great arteries. This procedure is similar to the lateral tunnel Fontan procedure, except that the systemic venous return from the inferior vena cava is directed to the right pulmonary artery through an extraatrial conduit. AO, aorta; IVC, inferior vena cava; LA, left atrium; LV, left ventricle; PA, pulmonary artery; RV, right ventricle; SVC, superior vena cava. (From Sidebotham D, McKee A, Gillham M, et al: *Cardiothoracic critical care.* Philadelphia, 2007, Butterworth Heinemann/Elsevier, Figs. 15-6 and 15-7.)

receiving team know if such fenestrations were created, so the team will know to expect arterial oxygen desaturation. If the oxygen saturation rises or is higher than postoperative baseline values, the fenestration may have closed or become occluded; this must be promptly reported to the surgical team. Spontaneous fenestration closure may occur immediately after or days after surgery, causing acute deterioration with hypotension, renal failure, and excessive edema, in the presence of normally (fully) saturated blood.[589] Echocardiographic evaluation for fenestration patency and prompt interventional venous cardiac catheterization may involve balloon dilation or placement of a stent[55] or an ASD dilation device to reopen the fenestration. Cardiac catheter intervention perforation of the extracardiac conduit with implantation of a covered stent into the Fontan fenestration has been successful for the patient with a failing Fontan caused by closure of the fenestration.[616]

Outcomes have improved for both the standard and high-risk Fontan patient with fenestrated Fontan.[621] By 1 year after surgery, 20% to 40% of fenestrations close spontaneously.[686] Elective, future fenestration closure is completed with interventional cardiac catheterization and implantation of the Amplatzer device (see Atrial Septal Defect, and Evolve Fig. 8-2 in the Chapter 8 Supplement on the Evolve Website),[389,621] or occlusion device. After fenestration closure, the arterial oxygen saturation is expected to rise.

If there is no fenestration in the Fontan circuit, all IVC blood flow will enter the pulmonary artery and systemic arterial blood should be near fully saturated (i.e., arterial oxygen saturation above 95% and near 100%) following surgery. Excellent outcomes with this procedure have been reported.[758]

Patients with heterotaxy variants may have complex venous anatomy including an interrupted IVC that does not

enter the right atrium. Instead, the IVC joins to the azygous venous system and eventually enters the SVC; this anatomy is particularly likely in patients with polysplenia and bilateral left-sidedness.[591] In these patients completion of a bilateral bidirectional Glenn is equivalent to near completion of a Fontan procedure because both the SVC and IVC blood flow will then enter the pulmonary arterial system. The only lower body venous flow not entering the pulmonary circulation is the hepatic blood.[591] This bilateral cavopulmonary anastomosis procedure has been called the Kawashima procedure.

Postoperative Care After Fontan Procedure. Extubation with spontaneous ventilation should be allowed as soon as it is feasible after Fontan surgery because it may improve hemodynamics.[935] Systemic venous return is facilitated by the subatmospheric pleural and intrathoracic pressures generated by spontaneous inspiration.[942] If positive pressure ventilation must be provided, extremely high levels of positive end-expiratory pressure (PEEP) should be avoided because they can impede pulmonary blood flow and contribute to a fall in cardiac output.[942] A PEEP of 3 to 5 cm H_2O can be used without causing hemodynamic compromise,[942] and can help improve ventilation-perfusion matching by reducing areas of microatelectasis.[935] Positive pressure ventilation can decrease preload to the right and left atria and increase afterload to the pulmonary circulation.[942] Ventilation goals, however, include extubation with spontaneous ventilation as soon as possible. Non-fenestrated Fontan patients should have arterial saturations above 95%.

Pulmonary pressure and pulmonary vascular resistance can be elevated following cardiopulmonary bypass.[935,942] With even small increases in pulmonary resistance or any impediment to forward flow through the pulmonary vascular bed, the left heart filling will be compromised, leading to lower cardiac output.[253] Treatment with oxygen and or nitric oxide has been successful in promoting pulmonary vasodilation and improving cardiac output.[298,327]

After the Fontan operation, *low cardiac output* is the most common and most severe complication. It is often caused by inadequate flow of blood into the pulmonary circulation that results from hypovolemia and inadequate systemic venous pressure (low right atrial [RA] and left atrial [LA] pressures), elevated pulmonary vascular resistance (low LA and high RA pressures), obstruction at the site of surgery, or pump failure.[935] Additional causes include pulmonary artery distortion or hypoplasia, pulmonary venous obstruction, or residual left-to-right shunts (Table 8-34).[342] The combination of low

cardiac output with a high LA pressure is worrisome and may indicate potential left ventricular dysfunction, significant atrioventricular (AV) valve insufficiency or obstruction, loss of AV synchrony caused by arrhythmias, presence of obstruction to ventricular outflow, or cardiac tamponade.[934,935] Any of these complications must be identified and treated.

Management of low cardiac output after Fontan is highlighted in Fig. 8-59. Inadequate intravascular volume and low central venous pressure can cause postoperative low cardiac output. Central venous pressure must equal or exceed the pulmonary artery pressure for flow into the pulmonary circulation to occur. A central venous pressure of 12 to 15 mm Hg may be needed to provide that pressure gradient and forward flow.[750] Treatment of low cardiac output requires both judicious administration of intravenous fluid as well as administration of vasoactive medications (including inotropic agents and vasodilators). Therapy should be modified based on evaluation of the child's systemic perfusion, including assessment of mixed venous oxygen saturation, serum lactate and urine output. Avoid relative hypovolemia, with low central venous pressure and resultant low left atrial pressure.

Diuretics, including Lasix and Aldactone (an aldosterone antagonist) are used to treat congestive heart failure,[881] but aggressive diuresis is avoided. Afterload reduction is used to improve cardiac output and decrease single ventricle end-diastolic (filling) pressure,[384] as well as decrease elevated systemic vascular resistance.[589]

Management of low cardiac output includes efforts to reduce pulmonary vascular resistance (see section, Common Clinical Conditions, Pulmonary Hypertension). These efforts include administration of supplementary oxygen even if arterial oxygen saturation is adequate.[591] Avoid acidosis, hypoventilation,

Table 8-34	**Differential Diagnosis of Low Cardiac Output After Fontan**	
RA pressure	**LA pressure**	**Cause(s)**
Low	Low	Hypovolemia
High	Low	High pulmonary vascular resistance, baffle obstruction, pulmonary artery hypoplasia or stenosis
High	High	Ventricular dysfunction, atrioventricular valve stenosis or regurgitation, arrhythmia, outflow obstruction, tamponade

Reproduced with permission from Wernovsky G, Bove EL: Early bidirectional cavopulmonary shunt in young infants. In Chang AC, Hanley F, Wernovsky G, Wessel DL, editors: *Pediatric cardiac intensive care.* Baltimore, 2008, Williams & Wilkins, p. 283.

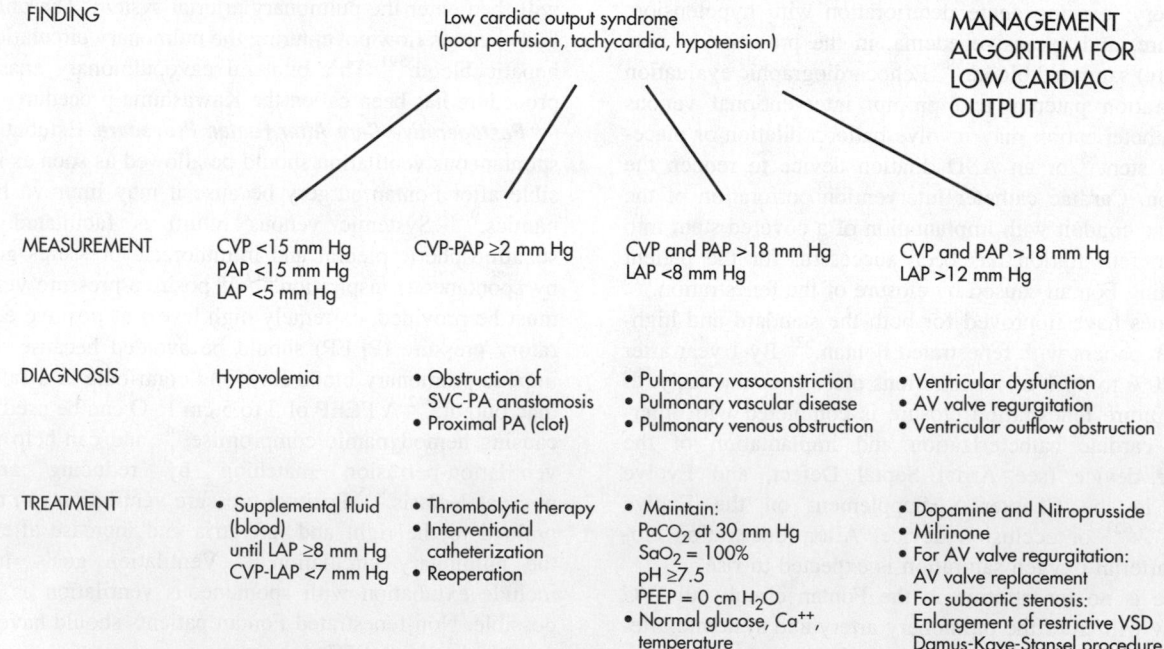

FINDING	Low cardiac output syndrome (poor perfusion, tachycardia, hypotension)			MANAGEMENT ALGORITHM FOR LOW CARDIAC OUTPUT
MEASUREMENT	CVP <15 mm Hg PAP <15 mm Hg LAP <5 mm Hg	CVP-PAP ≥2 mm Hg	CVP and PAP >18 mm Hg LAP <8 mm Hg	CVP and PAP >18 mm Hg LAP >12 mm Hg
DIAGNOSIS	Hypovolemia	• Obstruction of SVC-PA anastomosis • Proximal PA (clot)	• Pulmonary vasoconstriction • Pulmonary vascular disease • Pulmonary venous obstruction	• Ventricular dysfunction • AV valve regurgitation • Ventricular outflow obstruction
TREATMENT	• Supplemental fluid (blood) until LAP ≥8 mm Hg CVP-LAP <7 mm Hg	• Thrombolytic therapy • Interventional catheterization • Reoperation	• Maintain: PaCO$_2$ at 30 mm Hg SaO$_2$ = 100% pH ≥7.5 PEEP = 0 cm H$_2$O • Normal glucose, Ca^{++}, temperature	• Dopamine and Nitroprusside • Milrinone • For AV valve regurgitation: AV valve replacement • For subaortic stenosis: Enlargement of restrictive VSD Damus-Kaye-Stansel procedure

FIG. 8-59 Management algorithm for low cardiac output after Fontan-type correction of tricuspid atresia or single ventricle. *AV,* Atrioventricular; *CVP,* central venous pressure; *LAP,* left atrial pressure; *PA,* pulmonary artery; *PAP,* pulmonary artery pressure; *PEEP,* positive and expiratory pressure; *SVC,* superior vena cava; *VSD,* ventricular septal defect. (Modified from Okanlami O, et al: Tricuspid atresia and the Fontan operation. In Nichols DG, et al, editors. *Critical heart disease in infants and children.* St Louis, 1995, Mosby.)

atelectasis (or other causes of alveolar hypoxia), hypothermia, and agitation. Anemia is treated to support adequate oxygen-carrying capacity and arterial oxygen content. Factors that increase oxygen consumption (fever, pain, agitation, and infection) should be avoided or promptly treated. When cardiac output is optimized and there is a good balance between oxygen delivery and oxygen demand, the mixed venous oxygen saturation will rise. In addition to monitoring and support of the arterial oxyhemoglobin saturation, the PaO_2 must be monitored and maintained above 30 mm Hg (Table 8-35).

A CVP greater than 15 to 18 mm Hg suggests difficulty with passive Fontan flow into the pulmonary capillary bed.[591] *Anatomic obstruction* in the Fontan systemic venous pathway leads to elevated transpulmonary gradient (CVP minus LAP) with a value above 10 mm Hg suggesting difficulty with passive Fontan flow into the pulmonary circulation.[591] Clinical signs include hepatomegaly, ascites, edema of the head and neck, anasarca, and signs of low cardiac output. The left atrial pressure is derived from the common atrial pressure with typical desired pressure slightly greater than 5 mm Hg (but not a lot higher).

Bleeding is most likely to occur if a coagulopathy existed preoperatively (related to chronic hypoxemia and polycythemia—see section, Common Clinical Conditions, Hypoxemia) or a significant amount of scar tissue (from previous palliative surgical procedures) was dissected. If synthetic polytetrafluoroethylene is used for the surgical correction, platelet adherence to the surface of this material will produce a fall in the child's platelet count immediately after surgery.

Continued cyanosis/hypoxemia may result from pulmonary venous desaturation related to atelectasis, elevated diaphragm, pleural effusions, pneumothorax, hypoventilation, or pulmonary edema (Table 8-36). Excessive cyanosis may be caused by a leak in the intracardiac baffle (or an intentional fenestration). If a fenestration is present within the Fontan circuit, right-to-left shunting with systemic desaturation is expected. Cyanosis may also result from decreased mixed venous oxygen saturation.

Veno-venous collaterals may develop (from the SVC to the pulmonary venous atrium), but typically take weeks or months to develop after bidirectional Glenn or Fontan procedures. These collaterals increase cyanosis and require assessment and device closure during cardiac catheterization. It is uncommon for current bidirectional Glenn patients to develop pulmonary arteriovenous malformation (AVM) fistulae, which shunt blood flow away from the pulmonary capillaries and produce cyanosis. If these are present preoperatively in the Fontan patients, they will cause persistent cyanosis in the postoperative period. Pulmonary AVMs cannot be closed with coils or devices during cardiac catheterization, and must resolve over time. The cause for development of pulmonary AVMs is suspected to be lack of flow of a "hepatic factor" into the pulmonary circulation; when hepatic venous blood flows through the pulmonary circulation following the Fontan procedure, the problem resolves. Cyanosis and inability to wean from mechanical ventilation can also be related to diaphragm paralysis, with resultant risk for hypoventilation, atelectasis and increased pulmonary resistance.

Chronically cyanotic patients often develop collateral vessels from the systemic to the pulmonary arteries, resulting in increased pulmonary blood flow.[434] The collateral vessels can cause ventricular volume overload,[434] requiring transcatheter occlusion either before or after the Fontan procedure. Echocardiography with agitated saline contrast can be used to diagnose a right-to-left intrapulmonary or intracardiac

Table 8-35 Optimizing Pulmonary and Systemic Blood Flow in Patients with Single Ventricle

Support Goals	Avoid and Correct
ARTERIAL oxygen saturation: *75%-85%*	*Arterial oxygen saturation >85%*: May indicate excessive pulmonary blood flow, and cause CHF, respiratory distress, pulmonary edema *Arterial oxygen saturation <70%*: Indicates decreased pulmonary blood flow, intrapulmonary shunt or reduced systemic venous oxygen saturation; will likely lead to development of acidosis. Verify patent airway and appropriate inspired oxygen and ventilation.
Signs of adequate systemic perfusion	*Inadequate systemic perfusion*, metabolic acidosis *AIR in any IV system* (risk of right-to-left shunt, embolus to systemic circulation)
Mixed venous saturation near 50% (or within 10% of baseline)	*Mixed venous saturation <40%* indicates inadequate oxygen delivery-demand/consumption balance
Serum lactate <2.2 mmol/L	*Serum lactate >2.2 mmol/L*
OXYGEN: *Carefully titrate* use of oxygen to achieve desired oxygen saturation. Oxygen is a potent pulmonary vasodilator that typically *increases* pulmonary blood flow.	
ARTERIAL BLOOD GAS: *Aim for "40-40-40"* (PaO_2: 40 mm Hg, $PaCO_2$: 40 mm Hg, pH 7.40)	*HYPERVENTILATION*: Decreases cerebral blood flow and may contribute to reduced cardiac output and arterial oxygen saturation after cavopulmonary anastomosis. *ACIDOSIS* increases pulmonary vascular resistance; metabolic acidosis indicates inadequate tissue oxygenation
Keep *Hematocrit* at least 40%	*Anemia*

Table 8-36	Differential Diagnosis of Cyanosis After the Superior Cavopulmonary Anastomosis and the Fontan Completion	
	Bidirectional Glenn/Hemi-Fontan	**Fontan Completion**
Pulmonary venous desaturation	Ventilation/perfusion mismatch • Pleural effusion • Pneumothorax • Hemothorax • Chylothorax • Pulmonary edema • Atelectasis • Bacterial pneumonia/viral pneumonitis • Arteriovenous malformation	Ventilation/perfusion mismatch • Pleural effusion • Pneumothorax • Hemothorax • Chylothorax • Pulmonary edema • Atelectasis • Bacterial pneumonia/viral pneumonitis • Arteriovenous malformation
Systemic venous desaturation	Decreased oxygen delivery • Anemia • Low cardiac output • Decreased ventricular function • Severe atrioventricular valve regurgitation • Pericardial tamponade Increased oxygen consumption • Sepsis Decompressing vein • Venovenous collateral from superior cavopulmonary circuit via the systemic venous circuit to the systemic ventricle Baffle leak (only for hemi-Fontan)	Decreased oxygen delivery • Anemia • Low cardiac output • Decreased ventricular function • Severe atrioventricular valve regurgitation • Pericardial tamponade Increased oxygen consumption • Sepsis Decompressing vein • Venovenous collateral from superior cavopulmonary circuit to the systemic ventricle Baffle leak (only for lateral tunnel Fontan completion) Fenestration that is too large
Decreased pulmonary blood flow	Increased pulmonary vascular resistance Pulmonary venous hypertension Restrictive atrial communication Decompressing vein Baffle leak	Increased pulmonary vascular resistance Pulmonary venous hypertension Restrictive atrial communication Decompressing vein Baffle leak Pulmonary artery obstruction

From Marino BS, Spray TL, Greeley WJ. Separating the circulations: cavopulmonary connections (Bidirectional Glenn, hemi-Fontan) and the modified Fontan operation. In Nicholls DG, editor in chief. *Critical heart disease in infants, children and adolescents*, ed 2, Philadelphia, 2006, Saunders. Table 41-2.

shunt in the patient with unexplained cyanosis following a Glenn or Fontan operation.[162,474] The agitated saline can help to detect location of a Fontan leak.[474]

Pleural and pericardial effusions are common postoperative problems requiring prolonged hospitalization.[935] The causes are multifactorial.[577] Elevated systemic venous pressure impedes lymphatic return into the venous circulation.[591] Treatment by evacuation is needed because large fluid collections compress the lung, raising pulmonary vascular resistance,[589] and significant pericardial effusions can cause tamponade.

An effusion is a *chylothorax* when milky appearing lymph fluid drains into the chest. Insertion of chest tubes may be necessary if pleural fluid accumulation compromises ventilation and oxygenation. Chylothorax can require initiation of and long-term management with a diet low in long-chain triglycerides,[138] with Portagen as the infant formula. Because this fluid represents fluid loss from the body the total amount of fluid drained must be considered when evaluating the child's fluid balance. In addition, fat-soluble vitamins may be lost in the lymph fluid so replacement of vitamins A, D,

K, and E is often required.[138] Some children lose large proteins, including coagulation factors and fibrinogen, in this fluid; monitoring of the coagulation panel is advisable. Replacement of intravascular volume may be required with protein, electrolytes, and immunoglobulins.[935] Octreotide IV infusion has been used with improvement.[161] Thoracic duct ligation may be required for persistent drainage.

Recent factors associated with decreased incidence of effusions include use of fenestrations in the Fontan circuit, use of modified ultrafiltration, and the use of an "adjustable atrial septal defect."[935] Systemic venous congestion can lead to additional complications, including pericardial effusion, ascites, and liver congestion, which may produce liver dysfunction.

After the Fontan procedure, anticoagulation is typically initiated with aspirin, dipyridamole, or Coumadin (once intracardiac catheters and temporary pacing wires are removed). Slower venous blood flow occurs through the Fontan circuit, with passage through prosthetic materials, making patients susceptible to thrombus formation.[591,881] Choice of therapy remains a matter of debate[571] The persistent right-to-left fenestration shunt may also increase risk for thrombus formation and systemic embolization.

Rare complications include the development of plastic bronchitis with the formation of thick, tenacious protein casts within the bronchus.[325,949] These casts cause life threatening obstruction of the airway and can result in pulmonary failure. Management is complex and involves repeated bronchoscopies.[709]

Arrhythmias can be problematic postoperatively. The presence of a normal sinus rhythm is not required for successful function of the Fontan, although the presence of chronic atrial fibrillation is worrisome because it often is associated with severe right atrial dilation and may indicate the presence of a severely restrictive atrial septal defect or left ventricular failure. Temporary or permanent cardiac pacing wires can be used postoperatively to control the cardiac rhythm.

Heart block or junctional tachyarrhythmias (loss of AV synchrony) raise intracardiac pressures, causing increased resistance to atrial filling and resulting in lower ventricular filling volume, additional pulmonary venous congestion, and low cardiac output as effective atrial contractility is lost or the atria contract against a closed AV valve.[695] Loss of sinus rhythm, with escape rhythms such as junctional ectopic tachycardia, are poorly tolerated.[589,935]

Potential arrhythmias, including atrial flutter or fibrillation, primary atrial tachycardia, or accelerated junctional tachycardia, may develop postoperatively.[342] Sinus node dysfunction is common after Fontan completion,[591] possibly related to sinus node injury or interruption of sinus node blood supply.[591] Sinus node dysfunction may result from an atrial septal defect; if an atrial septal defect is restrictive preoperatively, it leads to right atrial dilation.[342] The atrial arrhythmias may reappear if significant right atrial hypertension develops postoperatively.

Preoperative Holter monitoring to establish baseline rhythm alterations can indicate the need for placement of permanent epicardial wires and a pacemaker generator during the Fontan procedure. Treatment can include temporary or permanent pacing and use of antiarrhythmic drugs. Atrial pacing wires allow for accurate rhythm diagnosis (see section, Common Clinical Conditions, Arrhythmias).[589]

Early perioperative Fontan failure may be related to multiple factors, including myocardial injury or elevated pulmonary vascular resistance.[394,935] If elevated systemic venous pressure and low cardiac output persist despite maximal support, patients are brought to the cardiac catheterization laboratory for evaluation of their hemodynamics and anatomy. Transcatheter interventions have been completed safely in the early postoperative period after the Fontan procedure, including balloon angioplasty, occlusion of residual antegrade pulmonary flow or insertion of stents in narrowed Fontan or arterial structures.[83] During interventional cardiac catheterization, an emergent fenestration may be created in the extracardiac Fontan circuit to improve cardiac output.[616] A Fontan "takedown" to a bidirectional cavopulmonary shunt is uncommon, but may be a life-saving measure in the face of severe low cardiac output.[589]

Neurologic and developmental monitoring is required in patients with a single ventricle because risk for unfavorable developmental sequelae is high.[648] Poor neurologic outcome is particularly likely in children with hypoplastic left heart syndrome who can have cognitive, motor, and neurologic deficits.[554,767] Developmental evaluations are essential, with initiation of an early intervention programs, ongoing assessment and other interventions as needed.

Multiple factors create higher risks for developmental delay, including prolonged hypoxemia, unstable hemodynamics, multiple cardiac catheterizations, congestive heart failure, and a series of surgical procedures.[648] An increased incidence of preoperative and postoperative periventricular leukomalacia, a nonspecific sign of cerebral white matter injury, has been found among patients who have undergone neonatal open-heart surgery.[557]

Physical activity level is reduced after Fontan procedures.[596] Single ventricle patients with a Fontan procedure have been reported to have reduced exercise capacity.[682,966] Obesity has the potential to increase pulmonary vascular resistance, as well as lead to other morbidities, and should be prevented in patients after the Fontan procedure.[596] Ongoing care requires attention to promoting physical activity and healthy heart living.

After the Fontan procedure, most children demonstrate significant symptomatic improvement, although most also demonstrate abnormalities in exercise tolerance. In general the child demonstrates a high heart rate, high ventilation for oxygen consumption, and oxygen desaturation with exercise. Most children have an increase in physiologic dead space and a ventilation/perfusion mismatch, whether or not a Glenn anastomosis was performed before the Fontan procedure.[934] Left ventricular ejection fraction often is reduced after the Fontan procedure, and the capacity to increase cardiac output in response to exercise varies from patient to patient. If left ventricular function is extremely poor, cardiac transplantation ultimately may be performed.[934]

Development of protein losing enteropathy (PLE) after a Fontan is associated with a poor clinical course.[311] The incidence is 4% to 13%.[756] Elevated systemic venous pressures are thought to contribute to protein-losing enteropathy, a loss of proteins throughout the GI tract,[217] but the precise cause unknown.[756] Symptoms include diarrhea, ascites, fatigue, abdominal pain, pleural effusions, shortness of breath, emesis, and peripheral edema.[756] Fecal alpha$_1$-antitrypsin is increased (greater than 200 mg/dL) and serum albumin is chronically low (less than 3.9 g/dL).[756]

Interventions include heparin administration, a high protein/low-fat diet, diuretic therapy, medications to improve cardiovascular function (afterload reduction, inotropic support), albumin infusions,[612,756] prednisone,[612,862] octreotide, budesonide,[849] sildenafil[730] and creation of atrial fenestration.[612] After the onset of PLE, survival is 46% to 59%,[756] with 50% mortality in 5 years.[612]

Monitoring of calcium, serum albumin, and total protein is required for patients with PLE, with intermittent infusions of these substances if needed. Subcutaneous heparin therapy has been shown to provide subjective symptomatic improvement in most patients, but it does not increase the clinical remission or decrease the need for albumin administration.[756] No cure is known.[217]

The outcomes of the Fontan procedure with the evolving modalities of management require ongoing evaluation. Transcatheter fenestration with creation of an interatrial communication for the Fontan circuit has not prevented protein-losing enteropathy.[914]

Postoperative mortality associated with the Fontan procedure reported by centers in the Society of Thoracic Surgeons (2006-2010)[823] database is 1.3% for the extracardiac fenestrated Fontan and 1.2% for the nonfenestrated procedure. The STS database reports postoperative hospital mortality of 1.0% for the fenestrated lateral tunnel.[823] Adults (greater than 18 years old) presenting for Fontan revision/conversion have 8% mortality prior to discharge. Mortality for children with Down syndrome is higher following both the Glenn and Fontan surgery, and the procedures are rarely performed in these children.[339]

Results of the Fontan palliation continue to improve. Survival at 20 years after Fontan procedure ranges from 82.6%[466] to 87%.[672] The leading causes of death after Fontan are related to thromboembolism, sudden death, and heart failure.[466] For double inlet left ventricle patients, 78% are reported to be alive at 12 years.[468] Ten percent of the patients with single left ventricle develop complete heart block.[452] A 15-year followup of extracardiac Fontan patients had 85% survival at 15 years (including operative deaths), with 92% of long-term survivors free from late heart failure. Three percent of the patients developed extracardiac conduit obstruction, and 3% experienced ventricular failure.[319] Extracardiac conduit total cavopulmonary connection 10-year survival is reported at 93.6% with low morbidity, no restenosis, and 115/126 in normal sinus rhythm.[642]

Risk factors for adverse early and late outcomes include preoperative impaired ventricular function and elevated pulmonary vascular resistance.[392] Late complications of the Fontan procedure include the development of conduit obstruction; this may cause sudden death if a Glenn anastomosis is not in place. Late arrhythmias, including atrial arrhythmias and complete heart block, also have been reported, requiring antiarrhythmic therapy and potential pacemaker insertion. Although many patients are able to resume normal daily activities without difficulty, others demonstrate persistent signs of systemic venous congestion and low cardiac output.

Late Fontan failure symptoms include those of congestive heart failure, as well as the development of protein losing enteropathy.[394] Maintenance of low pulmonary artery pressure and vascular resistance with adequate unobstructed pulmonary blood flow and pulmonary venous return are important for optimal long-term Fontan hemodynamics.[676] Cardiac catheter intervention dilation of Fontan pathway stenosis can improve hemodynamics, as well as improve or relieve chronic ascites.[676] For those patients who develop intractable atrial arrhythmias requiring Fontan conversion, the procedure is completed with low mortality and is effective.[582]

Orthotopic cardiac transplantation remains an option for the patients with single functioning ventricule and may be an option for patients with severe ventricular dysfunction. The long-term morbidity and mortality related to transplant have prevented it from becoming a primary option for surgical management.[342]

Transcatheter Fontan Procedure. A transcatheter Fontan procedure has been developed as an interventional cardiac catheterization procedure using a covered stent.[207,292,294,761] During the bidirectional Glenn, the patient undergoes placement of an aperture at the cardiac end of the SVC to pulmonary artery anastomosis. This aperture is perforated at the time of the transcatheter Fontan with placement of a stent. This procedure has resulted in improved outcomes compared with surgical Fontans, including shorter length of stay, postprocedural extubation, no arrhythmias, and no plural effusions. Successful Fontan stent dilation to accommodate for growth has been reported.[761]

Future Challenges and Advanced Concepts

Future issues for the young adult and adult with single ventricle palliations are numerous and reviewed by Khairy et al.[468] Late medical, adult issues can include chronic low cardiac output, hypoxemia, protein-losing enteropathy, arrhythmias, ventricular dysfunction, thromboembolism, and Fontan pathway obstruction. Development of venous collaterals to the left atrium or development of pulmonary arteriovenous malformation may cause increased cyanosis.

Regular evaluation of the hepatic function is mandatory because late cirrhosis and hepatic dysfunction may develop and has been correlated with the duration of the Fontan circulation.[48] Employment may be hindered because many patients have documented limitations in exercise capacity, as well as potential neurodevelopmental limitations. Lifelong care in an expert adult CHD clinic is critical to provide comprehensive, continuous, lifelong anticipatory management[927] (see section, Common Clinical Conditions, Adult Congenital Heart Disease).

For advanced concepts in the care of the child with single functioning ventricle, see Box 8-40.

Box 8-40 | Advanced Concepts: Single Functioning Ventricle

- Oxygen is a potent pulmonary vasodilator, and use of supplementary oxygen in patients with single ventricle is unnecessary if systemic arterial oxygen saturation is above 85% or the PaO_2 is greater than 40 mm Hg.
- A fenestrated Fontan baffle will be created in patients with single ventricle who have less than optimal preoperative hemodynamics. The fenestration allows for right-to-left atrial shunting in the presence of elevated Fontan circuit pressures. This relieves venous congestion and helps to maintain cardiac output and oxygen delivery.
- Patients with a fenestrated Fontan are expected to have variable arterial oxygen saturation, with oxygen saturation inversely related to the magnitude of right-to-left shunting across the fenestration. Increasing saturation to near normal levels (>90%) may be a sign of a closing fenestration and must be evaluated immediately.
- New or increasing hepatomegaly or ascites is worrisome in patients after Fontan-type procedures, and suggests elevated Fontan circuit pressures.

Tricuspid Atresia

Jo Ann Nieves

Pearls

- Type IB is the most common form of tricuspid atresia, and includes a ventricular septal defect and pulmonic stenosis. This defect presents with cyanosis in the first days of life.
- The infant with tricuspid atresia with large VSD and no pulmonic stenosis will develop heart failure in the first weeks of life as the result of excessive pulmonary blood flow.
- Single ventricle physiology care is required for all patients with tricuspid atresia before second-stage bidirectional Glenn (or hemi-Fontan).
- Staged palliations are required, concluding with Fontan-type hemodynamics.

Etiology

Tricuspid atresia results from a complete lack of formation of the tricuspid valve during fetal cardiac development. There is no blood flow between the right atrium and right ventricle. Tricuspid atresia is associated with a hypoplastic (very small) right ventricle (Fig. 8-60).

In all forms of tricuspid atresia the systemic venous blood returns to the right atrium and must pass through an atrial septal defect or widely patent foramen ovale into the left atrium.[253] The mitral valve (the only atrioventricular valve) connects the left atrium to the dominant left ventricle. A ventricular septal defect is often present.[865]

There are several forms of tricuspid atresia (Table 8-37). Normally related great arteries (Type I) are present in approximately 70% to 80%,[253] but tricuspid atresia may also be associated with transposition of the great arteries (Type II)

Table 8-37	Classification of Tricuspid Atresia and Frequency of Occurrence	
Type I	**Tricuspid atresia: normally related great arteries**	**70%-80%**
Ia	No VSD and pulmonary atresia	
Ib	Small VSD and pulmonary stenosis	
Ic	Large VSD without pulmonary stenosis	
Type II	**Tricuspid atresia: D-transposition of the great arteries**	**12%-25%**
IIa	VSD with pulmonary atresia	
IIb	VSD with pulmonary stenosis	
IIc	VSD without pulmonary stenosis	
Type III	**Tricuspid atresia: with L-transposition of the great arteries**	**3%-6%**

From Epstein ML. Tricuspid atresia, stenosis and regurgitation. In Allen HD, Driscoll DJ, Feltes TF, Shaddy RE, editors. *Moss and Adams' heart disease in infants, children, and adolescents, including the fetus and young adult,* ed 7, Philadelphia, 2008, Lippincott Williams & Wilkins.

or other complex anomalies (Type III). Subcategories of tricuspid atresia have been named according to the degree of obstruction to pulmonary blood flow.[406]

Tricuspid atresia was found in less than 3% of patients with congenital heart disease from the New England Regional Infant Cardiac Registry.[330,724] Multiple cardiac anomalies are reported in less than 20% of cases.[253] Coarctation of the aorta occurs most often, in about one third of patients with tricuspid atresia and transposition of the great arteries.[253,454] Aortic arch obstruction was found in 25% of newborns with fetal diagnosis of tricuspid atresia.[916] The 1-year survival rate for patients with tricuspid atresia without surgical intervention is as low as 10%, and is affected by the anatomy and associated defects.[236] Survival into the sixth decade of life with no surgery has been reported in the presence of a balanced circulation.[865] Continuous, lifelong care by congenital heart disease experts is required.

Pathophysiology

Tricuspid Atresia with Normally Related Great Arteries. The only outlet for the right atrium is an atrial septal defect, so systemic venous blood enters the right atrium and passes through the interatrial communication to the left atrium. Systemic and pulmonary venous blood completely mix in the left atrium and left ventricle, with the resulting saturation dependent on the relative volume of systemic and pulmonary venous blood. The left atrium is dilated but usually morphologically normal.[406] The mixed venous blood passes through the mitral valve, into a large, well-developed left ventricle. From the left ventricle, some of the mixed venous blood can pass into the hypoplastic right ventricle though the ventricular septal defect (VSD), then into the pulmonary outflow tract and pulmonary artery. The volume of pulmonary blood flow depends on the size of the VSD and the degree of any pulmonary stenosis.[253]

The most common form of tricuspid atresia, present in about half of all patients with tricuspid atresia, is Type IB,

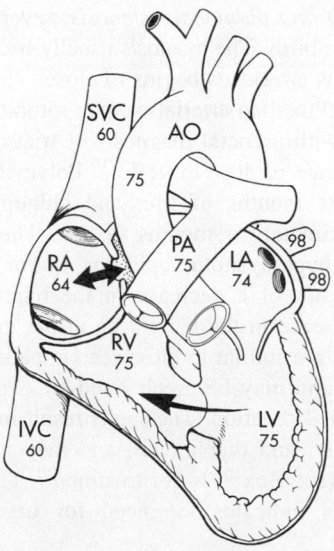

FIG. 8-60 Tricuspid atresia with normally related great arteries, ventricular septal defect and pulmonary stenosis (Type IB). Typical oxygen saturations within the cardiac chambers and great vessels are depicted. Tricuspid atresia may also be associated with transposition of the great arteries and without pulmonary stenosis. (From Striepe V. Tricuspid atresia. In Kambam J, editor. *Cardiac anesthesia for infants and children.* St Louis, 1994, Mosby.)

tricuspid atresia with a *small VSD and pulmonary stenosis*.[236,454] With this combination of defects, blood flow to the pulmonary circulation (and oxygenated pulmonary venous return to the left atrium) will be limited, so cyanosis will be present at birth. Pulmonary overcirculation will not develop when the pulmonary vascular resistance drops in the first weeks of life.[253] In fact, pulmonary blood flow is decreased, and cyanosis can be significant, but no heart failure is present. The patients are at risk for the development of systemic consequences of chronic hypoxemia and resultant polycythemia (see section, Common Clinical Conditions, Hypoxemia). The infundibular stenosis can create a dynamic obstruction that can become severe.

The atrial septal defect is often a widely stretched patent foramen ovale or an ostium secundum atrial septal defect.[253] If the interatrial communication is restrictive (too small), right atrial hypertension and systemic venous congestion with hepatomegaly will be present. In addition, signs of decreased cardiac output and hypoxemia are observed.[253]

As the infant with Type IB tricuspid atresia grows, the ventricular septal defect often becomes relatively smaller. In addition, the pulmonary infundibular stenosis may increase. For these reasons, pulmonary blood flow is typically further reduced, and the infant becomes progressively more cyanotic. Regular medical examinations are necessary to detect changes in the clinical presentation, and avoid the development of severe hypoxemia.

If the tricuspid atresia is present with *no VSD and normally related great vessels* (Type IA), there is no shunt from left to right at the ventricular level, so no intracardiac path for pulmonary blood flow, and the neonate usually demonstrates profound cyanosis from birth. This cyanosis worsens when the ductus arteriosus begins to close, because the ductus provides the only source of pulmonary blood flow. The right ventricle may be absent and the pulmonary valve atretic.[253]

Tricuspid Atresia with Transposition of the Great Arteries. If transposition of the great vessels is present, the pulmonary artery arises from the left ventricle and the aorta arises from the right ventricle. If no pulmonic stenosis is present (Type IIC), pulmonary blood flow will be increased once pulmonary vascular resistance falls at approximately 4 to 12 weeks of age. The excessive pulmonary blood flow under high pressure results in symptoms of congestive heart failure.[253] The greater the volume of pulmonary blood flow, the greater the proportion of oxygenated blood returning to the left ventricle and the higher the systemic arterial oxygen saturation. As a result cyanosis usually decreases as pulmonary blood flow increases. However, the price of this increase in pulmonary blood flow is severe CHF, pulmonary hypertension, and the risk of pulmonary vascular disease. Increased pulmonary venous return contributes to the development of left ventricular volume overload and left ventricular dysfunction.

In tricuspid atresia with transposition of the great arteries, the right ventricle forms a subaortic chamber from which the aorta arises. Subaortic stenosis can result from a restrictive VSD, which minimizes shunting of blood from the left ventricle into the small right ventricle (the systemic outflow chamber),[454] obstructing systemic blood flow. Subaortic stenosis

can also result from a narrow infundibular area.[253] Severe narrowing will decrease systemic circulation, which can produce shock, hypotension, or metabolic acidosis.[253] When this combination of defects is present, systemic perfusion will deteriorate substantially as the ductus arteriosus begins to constrict after birth.

Coarctation of the aorta may be present with tricuspid atresia. The clinical findings of aortic coarctation will also be found, producing upper extremity hypertension with decreased blood pressure and pulses to the lower extremities, gastrointestinal tract, and kidneys.[253] A bicuspid aortic valve may also be present.

The risk of bacterial endocarditis is significant in children with tricuspid atresia before and after palliative surgery. As a result, it is extremely important that antibiotic prophylaxis be administered during periods of increased risk of bacteremia preoperatively and after palliative surgery with prosthetic shunts and corrective surgery (see Bacterial Endocarditis later in this section of the chapter). Patients with tricuspid atresia and increased pulmonary blood flow who survive infancy are at risk for the development of pulmonary vascular disease.

Clinical Signs and Symptoms

All newborns with tricuspid atresia have systemic arterial desaturation resulting from the complete mixing of systemic and pulmonary venous return at the atrial level. By 1 week of age, most patients are noted to be cyanotic. The timing of onset and degree of cyanosis are determined by the source and volume of pulmonary blood flow.[253] In an analysis of 225 patients presenting with tricuspid atresia, the most common presenting symptom was cyanosis (88%), followed by congestive heart failure (25%) and circulatory collapse/acidosis (6.2%).[813]

When *normally related great vessels are present with a restrictive VSD and pulmonary stenosis,* severe cyanosis will be present from birth. The cyanosis usually becomes profound when the ductus arteriosus begins to close.

The reported median arterial oxygen saturation in room air for newborns with prenatal diagnosis of tricuspid atresia was 79%, with a range of 40% to 91%.[916] Polycythemia develops during the first months of life, and clubbing is observed beyond approximately 4 months of age. These infants also may develop hypercyanotic episodes (paroxysmal hypoxic spells) as a result of a decrease in the relative size of the VSD or an increase in the narrowing at the infundibulum.[253] These episodes are similar to those seen in patients with tetralogy of Fallot, and may be precipitated by exertion, vigorous cry, feeding, or defecation. The spells result in profound cyanosis, irritability, and diaphoresis, and may result in loss of consciousness (see Box 8-34 for treatment). The development of these spells indicates the need for urgent therapeutic intervention.

When *tricuspid atresia is present with a large VSD (with or without transposition) and no significant pulmonic stenosis* cyanosis may be mild or may not be present at birth.[253] However, signs of congestive heart failure and pulmonary overcirculation develop once pulmonary vascular resistance falls at approximately 4 to 12 weeks of age.[253] Symptoms can include tachypnea, minimal cyanosis and hepatomegaly (see section, Common Clinical Conditions, Congestive Heart Failure).[454]

Murmurs are almost always present (described by Epstein[253]). If the pulmonary valve is patent a systolic pulmonary murmur may be heard at the second intercostal space along the left sternal border. The first heart sound is single because it is produced by mitral valve closure alone (no tricuspid valve closure). The second heart sound is usually also single. Flow through the VSD can produce a holosystolic murmur, and obstruction through the right ventricular outflow tract can produce an ejection murmur. A third heart sound and mid-diastolic rumble may be heard at the apex, caused by increased pulmonary blood flow. A restrictive VSD can produce a palpable thrill. The precordium is usually quiet. A left ventricular impulse is more likely to be appreciated than a right ventricular impulse.

Hepatomegaly may be present, particularly if the atrial septum is obstructing the right-to-left atrial shunt or CHF is present. The pulses are easily palpable in all extremities unless a coarctation is present and produces decreased lower extremity pulses.

ECG characteristics have been described by Epstein.[253] Left axis deviation is present in 85% of patients with Type I tricuspid atresia. Right atrial enlargement often develops in older infants and children, but may not be seen at birth. When increased pulmonary blood flow is present, combined atrial enlargement may be noted. The precordial leads show reduced right ventricular forces. The P-R interval is normal in most patients. A sinus rhythm is typical, but older patients may have atrial tachycardias, including atrial flutter or fibrillation, particularly in the presence of a restrictive atrial septum or a dilated, hypertensive right atrium.

On chest radiograph, the heart size in tricuspid atresia is directly related to the volume of the pulmonary blood flow.[454] The cardiac silhouette is often globular in appearance, with a normal heart size.[253] The right heart border may be prominent when the right atrium is dilated.[253] If pulmonary blood flow is increased (Types IC and IIC), cardiomegaly (caused by increased pulmonary venous return and left ventricular volume load) and increased pulmonary vascular markings develop once pulmonary vascular resistance falls and pulmonary blood flow increases.[253] If pulmonary blood flow is obstructed, heart size will be normal and pulmonary vascular markings will be normal or decreased.[253]

The echocardiogram will confirm the presence of tricuspid atresia and is the diagnostic procedure of choice.[253] The tricuspid valve will not be visible in the expected location; instead an imperforate linear echo density is present. Anatomic details, shunting, estimated pulmonary artery pressure, and ventricular function are identified by echocardiography. Associated defects, including coarctation of the aorta are identified.[253] The degree of obstruction at the VSD, the size and location of the interatrial communication, and the size of the right ventricular outflow tract are quantified by the Doppler echocardiogram.[454] Diagnosis of tricuspid atresia is well established by fetal echocardiography.[916]

Ongoing serial echocardiograms are used to monitor patients who undergo initial first-stage palliation, to monitor for the development of potential deterioration caused by problems such as pulmonary artery stenosis, ventricular dysfunction, evolution of atrial septal obstruction, or mitral valve regurgitation. If atrial fibrillation develops, the echocardiogram is performed to check for the development of atrial thrombi.[253]

Cardiac catheterization is often not required for diagnostic purposes because echocardiography provides detailed information, and advances in CT and MRI imaging yield clear and reliable images. Cardiac catheterization is used to measure the pulmonary vascular resistance, which is a critical factor for successful management, and must be determined before planning the next palliative surgery. Diagnostic studies may be needed to define the source(s) of pulmonary arterial flow, the impact of VSD obstruction, or evaluate other associated lesions, such as truncus arteriosus. Cardiac catheterization will also be required for interventional procedures, such as in selected cases requiring balloon atrial septostomy relief of a restrictive atrial septum, dilation of narrowed pulmonary arteries, or closure of collateral vessels.[388]

Angiocardiograms can evaluate the presence, location, and severity of any pulmonary stenosis or distortion. Initial surgical palliation with a systemic to pulmonary artery shunt or placement of a pulmonary artery band can lead to distortion of the pulmonary arteries. Angiography can also define any associated cardiac lesions. The precise size and location of collateral arteries (from the descending aorta to the lungs) or collateral venous vessels (creating a right-to-left shunt) are demonstrated by angiography.

Management

Medical Management. Greater than half of all newborns with tricuspid atresia demonstrate cyanosis in the first days of life. The cyanosis often progresses when the ductus arteriosus closes, the VSD becomes relatively smaller or closes, or there is progression in severity of the pulmonary stenosis. When significant cyanosis is present at birth, a substantial portion of pulmonary blood flow is probably dependent on the ductus arteriosus. If cyanosis is severe at birth, prostaglandin E_1 (0.05 to 0.1 mcg/kg per minute initial infusion, titrated to 0.01 to 0.05 mcg/kg per minute infusion as tolerated) is administered to maintain ductal patency during the diagnostic studies and possibly until surgery can be performed (see section, Common Clinical Conditions, Hypoxemia, and Box 8-33).

Patients with tricuspid atresia typically undergo a series of procedures that eventually result in diversion of systemic venous return directly into the pulmonary arterial circulation. This eliminates the right-to-left atrial level shunt, and results in normal systemic arterial oxygenation and decompression of the left ventricle.[253]

Initial interventions are therapies to promote a balanced circulation, with sufficient pulmonary blood flow and adequate systemic oxygen delivery, while promoting growth and minimizing congestive heart failure and risk of pulmonary vascular disease. The goals of intervention for the newborn include: (1) establishing/maintaining a sufficient source of pulmonary blood flow to avoid extreme hypoxemia;

(2) preventing excessive pulmonary blood flow, pulmonary hypertension, and the risk of pulmonary vascular disease; (3) maintaining a stable pulmonary artery anatomy for future surgical procedures.[253] A balanced systemic and pulmonary circulation is indicated by signs of adequate systemic perfusion, normal pH and systemic arterial oxygen saturation near 80%.[935] Activities to maintain effective pulmonary and systemic flow are listed in Table 8-35 (located earlier in the chapter).

If the echocardiogram identifies potential obstruction at the interatrial septum, a cardiac catheterization for a Rashkind balloon atrial septostomy (use of a balloon to tear a hole in the atrial septum) is performed. This septostomy usually is not required, however, because the foramen ovale typically is dilated.

If congestive heart failure is caused by *increased* pulmonary blood flow under high pressure (as occurs when a large ventricular septal defect is present without pulmonary stenosis), judicious medical management with diuretics and digoxin is indicated (see section, Common Clinical Conditions, Congestive Heart Failure). It is important to avoid aggressive diuresis, because hemoconcentration increases the risk of thromboembolic events, including cerebrovascular accident. The infant should be kept well hydrated to prevent hemoconcentration, although aggressive fluid administration should be avoided because it may precipitate or worsen congestive heart failure. Pulmonary artery banding may be performed if congestive heart failure is refractory to medical management.

Hypercyanotic spells occur in approximately 16% to 45% of infants with tricuspid atresia. If hypercyanotic episodes are observed, place the infant in the knee-chest position and administer 100% oxygen by nonrebreather face mask. Morphine sulfate (0.1 mg/kg IV or IM) provides sedation. The deeply cyanotic patient may require IV fluids and a vasopressor drug to increase the systemic vascular resistance (e.g., phenylephrine).[935] This medication should be kept at the bedside of any infant known to have a history of such spells (for further information, refer to Box 8-34). Anything producing a fall in systemic vascular resistance should be avoided, because it will contribute to further reduction in pulmonary blood flow (i.e., blood is diverted to the systemic circulation) and worsening cyanosis.[935] *No air can be allowed to enter any IV system* (may cause systemic/cerebral embolus).

Children with single ventricle physiology often are delayed in growth and may demonstrate difficulty feeding. Promoting adequate nutrition and growth is a critical component of care. Typically a concentrated formula (providing at least 24 calories per ounce) is provided with a goal of delivering more than 120 cal/kg per day. In the patient with single ventricle, when the arterial oxygen saturation is elevated (indicating excessive pulmonary blood flow that is likely associated with decreased systemic arterial flow) and during any low cardiac output state, mesenteric hypoperfusion is likely to be present. It is important to monitor for signs of necrotizing enterocolitis in the newborn including gastric distension, vomiting, and heme-positive stools. When enteral feedings are provided, monitor for increased volume of gastric residuals (see section, Common Clinical Conditions, Altered Nutrition).

Palliative Surgery. All surgical approaches are staged and palliative for tricuspid atresia; no biventricular repair is available. All staged procedures target a Fontan-type final procedure, so ultimately all systemic venous blood is directed into the pulmonary circulation. Palliative procedures are designed to divert some systemic venous (i.e., superior vena caval) blood to the pulmonary circulation and provide sufficient pulmonary blood flow to ensure adequate oxygenation while protecting the pulmonary vascular bed from developing elevated resistance. A low pulmonary vascular resistance is critical for a successful Fontan-type procedure.

The newborn with tricuspid atresia typically requires surgical intervention. If *subpulmonic stenosis is present,* a prostaglandin E_1 infusion is provided and surgical or interventional catheterization is needed to increase pulmonary blood flow. A subclavian-to-pulmonary artery shunt, such as a Blalock-Taussig or modified prosthetic shunt (see Fig. 8-44; and Evolve Fig. 8-5 and Evolve Table 8-2 in the Chapter 8 Supplement on the Evolve Website) is often performed to provide adequate pulmonary blood flow under controlled pressure and stimulate growth of the pulmonary arteries. When the shunt is created, the prostaglandin E_1 infusion will be discontinued. Some forms of palliative surgery are performed without cardiopulmonary bypass, while others require bypass. If the main pulmonary artery is small, a central prosthetic graft may be inserted between the aorta and the main pulmonary artery. These shunt procedures and perioperative care are discussed in Tetralogy of Fallot, Management, earlier in this chapter.

In selected cases, an alternative palliative procedure to increase pulmonary blood flow in the child with ductal-dependent circulation involves placement of a stent within the ductus arterious during cardiac catheterization.[18,149] This avoids the need to create a surgical shunt in selected newborns. A balloon atrial septostomy is performed if a restrictive ASD is present.

In the presence of *excessive pulmonary blood flow,* pulmonary artery banding may be performed. Pulmonary artery banding can decrease the pulmonary blood flow and alleviate symptoms of congestive heart failure, but may not prevent development of pulmonary vascular disease. If the banding is too tight, the patient may develop severe hypoxemia, with systemic arterial oxygen saturation less than 75%, leading to metabolic acidosis. If the band is too loose, the symptoms of congestive heart failure will continue. Care after pulmonary artery banding is briefly reviewed in the Single Functioning Ventricle, Overview of Management section.

Alternatively, the main pulmonary artery may be detached from the heart and an aortopulmonary shunt can be created, to provide pulmonary blood flow through a path that has a controlled diameter to restrict the volume and the pressure of the pulmonary blood flow. A surgical atrial septectomy is also completed if the interatrial septum is restrictive or has the potential to be restrictive.

If *D-transposition of the great arteries is present with obstruction to systemic flow* through the VSD into the transposed aorta, surgery will be performed to provide unobstructed systemic flow. The Damus-Kaye-Stansel procedure may be performed: the pulmonary artery is transected before the bifurcation (i.e., the main trunk is separated from the branches). The end of the main pulmonary trunk is then sewn into the side of the ascending aorta. This procedure enables ventricular outflow to enter the original pulmonary artery trunk (bypassing the subaortic stenosis) and then flow into the aorta (see section, Single Functioning Ventricle, Overview of Management). An additional aortopulmonary shunt is created to provide pulmonary blood flow. A target arterial oxygen saturation for these patients with single ventricle hemodynamics is near 80%. Bleeding is a potential concern because of the extensive suture lines under systolic pressure[591] (see section, Single Ventricle, Overview of Management). Following the surgery, flow into the aorta arises through both the pulmonary valve (from the left ventricle) and through the restrictive VSD and into the right ventricle and the aorta.[253]

Cavopulmonary Anastomosis. Either the bidirectional Glenn or the hemi-Fontan procedure is typically performed as the second stage surgery to improve effective pulmonary blood flow and arterial oxygen saturation and to decompress the left ventricle. These procedures and postoperative care are presented in detail in Single Functioning Ventricle, Overview of Management (see Box 8-39).

Completion Fontan-Type Procedure. The completion surgery for tricuspid atresia leads to total separation of the systemic and pulmonary venous blood by redirection of all systemic venous blood directly into the pulmonary arteries. The procedure is typically performed at 2 to 4 years of age.[253,454] The bidirectional Glenn and Fontan procedures require low pulmonary artery pressure and vascular resistance.[253] A cardiac catheterization is done before the surgery to determine the ideal procedure and the optimal time for surgical correction for each child.

This final stage Fontan-type procedure redirects inferior vena caval blood flow to the pulmonary arteries by means of an extracardiac conduit or with an intracardiac baffle.[591] These procedures are illustrated and described in detail in Single Functioning Ventricle, Overview of Management, in previous pages. Pulmonary blood flow is provided without a ventricular pumping chamber.[311] Cardiopulmonary bypass is required for most surgical Fontan-type procedures, but occasional cases have been reported of Fontan completion without use of bypass.[123]

The arterial oxygen saturation following the Fontan is typically in the high 80% to low 90% because the coronary sinus venous blood continues to drain into the right atrium, so it mixes with the pulmonary venous return, and then enters the systemic arterial circulation.[591] This continued mixing of coronary sinus venous blood creates, in effect, a small right-to-left shunt. Arterial oxygen desaturation will also be present if a fenestrated Fontan is created to allow for right-to-left shunt flow and relief of potentially high pressure within the Fontan circuit. For details regarding postoperative care and complications, please see Single Functioning Ventricle, Overview of Management.

Several forms of cardiac catheterization based, nonsurgical Fontan completion have been successful and are under continued refinement.[207,292,761]

Variations of the Fontan procedure have been completed since 1971. The current mortality reported after a fenestrated Fontan procedure is 2.4%, and a bidirectional Glenn 1.4%.[823] Interstage deaths caused by shunt thrombosis and unexplained deaths can also occur.[813]

Patients with tricuspid atresia who are not eligible for Fontan-type surgery may be eligible for cardiac transplantation. Factors that may prevent eligibility for the Fontan in tricuspid atresia include severe pulmonary artery distortion, pulmonary hypertension or elevated pulmonary vascular resistance, ventricular dysfunction, and progressive subaortic stenosis.

The survival of patients continues to improve with the wide use of Fontan-type interventions. Before use of the Fontan modifications, expected survival to young adulthood was about 50%.[253] The outcomes vary widely with reported 10-year survival at 82% for tricuspid atresia patients with a Fontan procedure, whether diagnosis occurred during fetal life or after birth.[813,916] The current goal is to achieve a Fontan circulation whenever possible.

Long-term complications are common and can include development of ventricular failure, atrial arrhythmias (particularly if the right atrium is included as part of the Fontan circuit), protein-losing enteropathy, Fontan pathway obstruction, increasing hypoxemia, collateral vessel malformations (venous and arterial), thromboembolism, recurrent pulmonary effusions, diminished exercise capacity, cirrhosis of the liver, and endocarditis.[253,865] These potential complications and required care are detailed by Thorne,[865] and are summarized in the Postoperative Care section of Single Functioning Ventricle, Overview of Management.

Advanced Concepts

Care of the patient with tricuspid atresia requires excellence in cardiopulmonary support. Continuous lifelong care by experts in congenital heart disease is required. Details regarding care after palliation are provided in the Overview of Single Functioning Ventricle, Overview of Management section and advanced concepts are listed in Box 8-41.

Box 8-41 **Advanced Concepts: Tricuspid Atresia**

- Approximately one third of patients with tricuspid atresia and transposition of the great arteries (Type II) have coarctation of the aorta.
- Patients with tricuspid atresia often have profound cyanosis at birth, and most require intervention during the neonatal period.
- In tricuspid atresia with a large VSD (with or without transposition) and no significant pulmonic stenosis, cyanosis may be mild or may not be present at birth. Signs of congestive heart failure and pulmonary overcirculation develop once pulmonary vascular resistance falls at approximately 4-12 weeks of age.
- The child with tricuspid atresia requires careful balance of systemic and pulmonary blood flow to maintain adequate systemic oxygenation and perfusion while minimizing risk of pulmonary vascular disease and ventricular dysfunction.

Pulmonary Atresia with Intact Ventricular Septum (IVS)

Jo Ann Nieves

Pearls

- The newborn with pulmonary atresia and intact ventricular septum (IVS) is dependent on the presence of an atrial septal defect for right-to-left shunt, to allow exit of systemic venous blood flow from the right heart, and is also dependent on a patent ductus arteriosus to provide pulmonary blood flow.
- Right ventricular to coronary artery connections (sinusoids) develop with extreme RV hypertension; they develop most commonly in patients with small tricuspid valves and small, hypertrophied right ventricles. These sinusoids contribute to ischemia of both the right and left ventricles.
- Single ventricle physiology care is required.
- Staged palliations can lead to biventricular repair.
- After pulmonary valve perforation and dilation the newborn may not achieve sufficient arterial oxygen saturation for days or weeks and often requires continued observation and continuation of prostaglandin E_1 therapy until that time.

Etiology

In pulmonary atresia there is complete obstruction to right ventricular outflow. When pulmonary atresia is present *without* a ventricular septal defect, this defect is called pulmonary atresia with *intact ventricular septum (IVS)*. It results from failure of appropriate septation of the truncus arteriosus into both a pulmonary artery and aorta, with failure of pulmonary valve development. This form of the defect may also be called "hypoplastic right heart syndrome."[936]

Right heart underdevelopment associated with pulmonary atresia can range from mild to severe, so the right ventricle size ranges from near normal to markedly hypertrophied with an underdeveloped chamber. The tricuspid valve, which is often dysplastic and stenotic, can be severely regurgitant with features of Ebstein anomaly.[662] Typically the pulmonary valve is atretic, with fused valve leaflets,[936] and there is a well-developed main pulmonary artery, with normally developed right and left pulmonary arteries. An atrial septal defect is present with either a patent foramen ovale or a secundum atrial septal defect; this allows the obligatory right-to-left atrial shunt (Fig. 8-61, A).[662]

Coronary artery anomalies are common, including the development of *coronary sinusoids*. These sinusoids are fistulae between the right ventricular cavity and the coronary arteries, producing retrograde flow of systemic venous blood from the right ventricular chamber through the coronary circulation.

Fetal studies suggest pulmonary atresia with intact ventricular septum is related to acquired progressive, altered hemodynamics in utero leading to lack of right heart ejection with subsequent fusion of the pulmonary valve leaflets.[454] It is a rare lesion with an estimated incidence of 0.083 per 1000 live births.[264] The New England Regional Infant Cardiac Program data reports that this defect represents 3.1% of all congenital heart defects. Extracardiac anomalies are rare.[454] All patients with pulmonary atresia and intact ventricular septum have extremely complex congenital heart disease requiring lifelong, continuous care by a cardiologist with expertise in management of adult patients with congenital heart disease.[927]

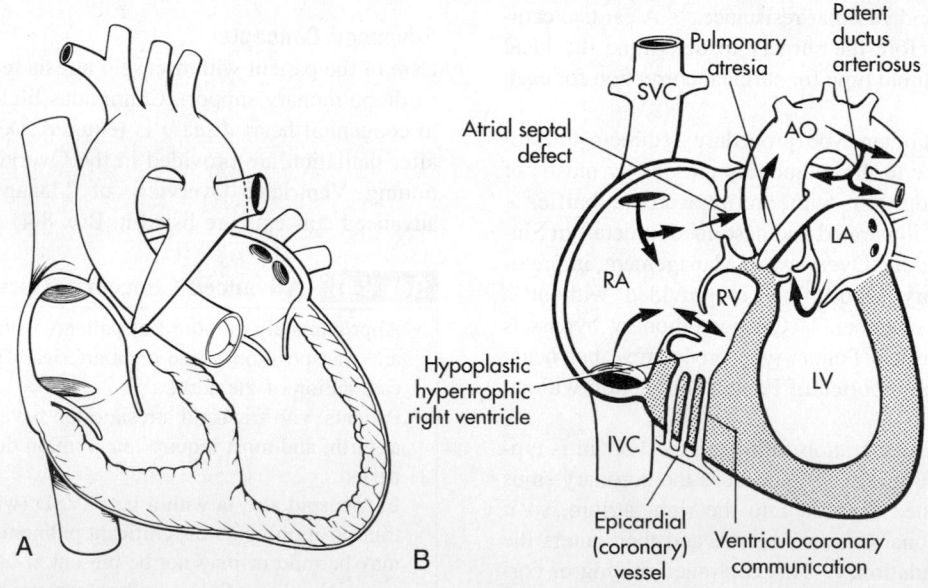

FIG. 8-61 Pulmonary atresia with intact ventricular septum. **A,** There is no outflow from the right ventricle, and the ventricle is small and extremely hypertensive and hypertrophied. There must be a source of pulmonary blood flow, such as the patent ductus arteriosus (PDA) depicted here. **B,** Right ventricular sinusoids may develop between the coronary arteries and the hypertensive right ventricular cavity. Desaturated systemic venous blood flows from the right ventricle through the sinusoids into the coronary arteries (particularly the left anterior descending branch). This results in perfusion of the myocardium with desaturated blood. (From Striepe V. Pulmonary atresia with intact ventricular septum. In Kambam J, editor. *Cardiac anesthesia for infants and children.* St Louis, 1994, Mosby.)

Pathophysiology

The hemodynamics of pulmonary atresia with intact ventricular septum are similar to those resulting from other forms of single ventricle (including tricuspid atresia), with pulmonary blood flow dependent on patency of the ductus arteriosus (see Overview of Single Ventricle earlier in this section).[936] When there is lack of anatomic continuity between the right ventricle and pulmonary artery, blood must enter the pulmonary circulation through another shunt or the newborn will develop profound and progressive hypoxemia when the ductus arteriosus begins to close; without intervention, this hypoxemia will lead to death.

Because there is no outflow from the right ventricle, an obligatory right-to-left shunt at the atrial level leads to complete mixing of the systemic and pulmonary venous return in the left heart. The right atrium is always dilated, and an interatrial communication is always present; this communication usually occurs through a patent foramen ovale or secundum atrial septal defect. The interatrial communication is rarely restrictive in size.[662] The pulmonary valve is atretic with fused leaflets.[450]

Systemic venous blood enters the right heart and quickly fills the right ventricle, but has no outflow path. Right ventricular end-diastolic and right atrial pressures rise, and tricuspid insufficiency often results. The increase in right atrial pressure opens the foramen ovale, so that systemic venous blood flows from the right to the left atrium and mixes with pulmonary venous blood. The mixed venous blood enters the left ventricle and is ejected into the aorta. A patent ductus arteriosus or some other form of systemic-to-pulmonary artery shunt must be present to provide flow from the systemic circulation into the pulmonary arterial circulation. The systemic arterial oxygen saturation varies directly with the volume of pulmonary blood flow; the greater the volume of pulmonary blood flow, the higher will be the systemic arterial oxygen saturation.[662]

The lack of a right ventricular outflow tract results in constant and extraordinarily high right ventricular afterload, severe right ventricular hypertrophy and extreme right ventricular hypertension; the RV systolic pressure may rise to 200 mm Hg.[450] The hypertrophy and hypertension are responsible for many of the pathophysiologic changes that are associated with pulmonary atresia and intact ventricular septum.

The size of the right ventricle varies widely from a hypertrophied, tiny, hypertensive cavity to a hugely dilated, thin-walled cavity with low pressure, and can even include a normal-sized ventricle.[219] The tricuspid valve is rarely normal, the annulus size is variable, and the valve is often hypoplastic, dysplastic, stenotic, or regurgitant.[662] In some cases the tricuspid valve has features of Ebstein anomaly (see Ebstein Anomaly).[662] The tricuspid valve diameter is presented as a "Z score" (the number of standard deviations by which the patient's tricuspid valve measurement deviates from the population mean).[219] The size of the right ventricular cavity correlates well with the size of the tricuspid valve.[349] In most (90%) patients with pulmonary atresia and IVS, the RV cavity size is small; it is severely reduced in 54% of the cases.[349] Typically, the cavity size is severely compromised by massive right ventricular hypertrophy. Endocardial fibroelastosis can be present.[662]

Coronary artery abnormalities are common, and are found in as many as 70% of patients with this defect.[770] Anomalies include coronary artery atresia at the origin, obstruction or occlusion of the coronary arteries, and sinusoids/fistulae between the right ventricle and coronary arteries.[454] Newborns can demonstrate evidence of coronary artery abnormalities at birth, including stenoses and interruptions that can produce myocardial ischemia.[662]

The most common coronary abnormalities are the fistulae between the right ventricle and coronary artery. When these fistulae are present, endothelium-lined channels within the RV muscle mass, known as *sinusoids,* connect the RV cavity to the coronary artery tree.[620] These sinusoids allow systemic venous blood from the hypertensive right ventricle to flow retrograde into the left anterior descending artery and/or the right coronary artery (see Fig. 8-61, B). This retrograde flow of desaturated blood into the coronary circulation results in ischemia of both the right and left ventricles. The involved coronary arteries may be dilated and tortuous, stenotic, or interrupted, with thick walls and small lumens. The coronary artery sinusoids are most likely to develop in patients with the smallest, most hypertensive right ventricles, the lowest "Z score" for the tricuspid valve (i.e., the most negative "Z score" value, indicating that the size of the tricuspid valve is much smaller than present in the population).[662] Patients with a normal or near-normal right ventricle are unlikely to develop coronary sinusoids.[770]

The coronary sinusoids are thought to develop during fetal life because there is no outflow from the right ventricle and extreme RV hypertension is present. After birth, a variety of factors compromise coronary perfusion pressure and flow (coronary perfusion pressure = aortic end-diastolic pressure − right atrial pressure). Tachycardia, use of prostaglandin E_1, creation of systemic to pulmonary shunts (by surgery or via stent within the ductus arteriosus) and use of vasodilator therapy can all decrease aortic end-diastolic pressure, and right atrial pressure is consistently elevated. These factors can reduce coronary artery perfusion pressure, enhance blood flow through the coronary sinusoids and compromise myocardial perfusion, causing myocardial ischemia and possible infarction.[662]

Coronary stenosis or atresia can develop proximal to the coronary fistulae, making the myocardium dependent on retrograde perfusion with desaturated blood from the RV through the fistulae into the coronary arteries. This combination is referred to as *RV dependent coronary circulation* (RVDCC).[338] In these cases the RV pressure will need to remain high for any type of coronary perfusion to occur, because the aortic end-diastolic pressure may not be sufficient to provide antegrade coronary blood flow through the stenosed or atretic coronary vessels.[662]

The sinusoids can be minor or extensive and their development correlates directly with the degree of RV hypoplasia and resulting RV hypertension.[936] When RVDCC is present, decompression of the RV (by a pulmonary valvotomy or an RV transannular patch), or other therapeutic interventions, which reduce RV hypertension can lead to coronary hypoperfusion, with resulting myocardial ischemia, infarction, ventricular dysfunction, malignant ventricular arrhythmias, and even death.[662,936] RVDCC is reviewed by Guleserian et al[338] and is reported in 3% to 34% of patients with pulmonary atresia and IVS.

The main pulmonary artery trunk is typically somewhat smaller than normal.[450] The normal size of the pulmonary artery with this defect is in sharp contrast to the diminutive size of the pulmonary arteries observed in patients with pulmonary atresia *with* a ventricular septal defect (see Tetralogy of Fallot).[450] Occasionally, hypoplasia of either the right or the left pulmonary artery is present.

The pulmonary venous return occurs through pulmonary veins that are typically joined normally to the left atrium. The left ventricular has variable degrees of hypertrophy.[662] The left ventricle receives both systemic and pulmonary venous return, so left ventricular dilation and dysfunction may develop. This dysfunction is exacerbated by the development of right ventricular-coronary artery sinusoids and consequent compromise in oxygen delivery to the myocardium.

Successful fetal percutaneous pulmonary balloon valvuloplasty intervention has been initiated to alter the development of pulmonary atresia with intact ventricular septum *in utero* to enable ultimate biventricular management.[33,877,883] Echocardiographic criteria have been established to identify potential candidates for fetal pulmonary valve intervention with the goal of preventing progressive RV hypoplasia.[739,762] The risk of pulmonary hypertension is low.

Clinical Signs and Symptoms

Significant cyanosis and hypoxemia are present at birth. Profound cyanosis usually is observed once the ductus arteriosus begins to close, and will progress rapidly if untreated, causing metabolic acidosis and hemodynamic collapse. The hypoxemia is not responsive to oxygen administration.[662]

Once the ductus is reopened with prostaglandin E$_1$ therapy, the desired arterial oxygen saturation is near 80%, with a normal pH. An arterial oxygen saturation greater than 90% suggests pulmonary overcirculation and will likely be associated with systemic hypoperfusion.[935]

A pansystolic murmur caused by tricuspid insufficiency can be heard along the left sternal border.[662] A patent ductus arteriosus murmur can be heard at the second or third intercostal space, particularly once prostaglandin E$_1$ therapy has begun.[662] There may be no murmur.[450]

The pulse pressure is wide with a low diastolic pressure caused by the runoff of aortic blood flow into the ductus arteriosus, then into the pulmonary vascular circulation.[620] The aortic diastolic pressure in a patient with a patent ductus arteriosus or a systemic to pulmonary shunt may be very low, leading to decreased coronary artery perfusion.[620] The pulses are often normal, unless a large patent ductus produces bounding pulses or low cardiac output produces diminished pulses.[662]

The liver may become enlarged if the atrial septum is severely restrictive or the tricuspid valve is severely regurgitant.[662] Tachycardia, and other signs of congestive heart failure also may be noted, and a left ventricular heave may be palpated.

Classic ECG findings include sinus rhythm, with left ventricular hypertrophy or dominance, decreased right ventricular forces, and right atrial enlargement.[662] ECG evidence of left ventricular hypertrophy is in contrast to the typical dominant right ventricular forces normally observed in the neonate.[620] Malignant ventricular arrhythmias may be observed. ST-segment abnormalities (depression or elevation) are frequently seen, indicating subendocardial ischemia[662] (depression when the QRS is positive) or infarction (indicated by ST-segment elevation when the QRS is positive).

The cardiothoracic ratio on the chest radiograph ranges from mildly to substantially enlarged.[662] Massive cardiomegaly will be seen in pulmonary atresia with Ebstein anomaly,[662] or with significant tricuspid regurgitation.[454] Pulmonary vascular markings will be diminished. The upper left heart border will be concave because the normal main pulmonary artery shadow is absent.

The echocardiogram is the primary mode of diagnosis and demonstrates absence of the right ventricular outflow tract. The echocardiogram enables evaluation of RV cavity size and function, tricuspid valve annulus size (including Z score) and function, the size and location of the atrial defect, the volume of the atrial shunting, the patency of the ductus arteriosus, and pulmonary artery branch anatomy. A tricuspid valve Z score of less than or equal to 2.5 has been shown to predict significant coronary artery abnormalities and the presence of right ventricular-dependent coronary circulation.[770]

Cardiac catheterization is often required for complete evaluation and to allow potential interventional therapies. Cardiac catheterization will conclusively demonstrate the anatomy needed to establish a treatment plan, including the distribution of the coronary arteries; identification of any atresia, stenosis, or interruption in the coronary arteries; the identification of right ventricle to coronary artery fistulae; and the status of right ventricular-dependent coronary circulation.[662,935] Cardiac catheterization documents the absence of anatomic continuity between the pulmonary artery and aorta, and it the source, magnitude, and distribution of pulmonary arterial blood flow. In addition, the size of the common pulmonary artery or right and left pulmonary artery branches is visualized during angiography in order to determine the appropriate surgical intervention.

As part of the treatment during cardiac catheterization, a balloon atrial septostomy may be performed to treat a restrictive atrial septum. In selected cases, the plan will include perforation of the pulmonary valve or insertion of a PDA stent (see Palliative Procedures in the Management section, below).

Management

Medical Management. Initial management for pulmonary atresia with intact atrial septum involves establishment of vascular access and immediate administration of PGE$_1$ (initial infusion: 0.05-0.1 mcg/kg per minute, then titrated to 0.01-0.05 mcg/kg per minute) to maintain ductal patency (see Box 8-33). Metabolic acidosis will require treatment. The infant is at risk for the development of complications of hypoxemia and polycythemia. *No air can be allowed to enter any IV system* because it can enter the systemic arterial circulation, producing an air embolus.

Single ventricle guidelines for care are followed, with goals including an arterial oxygen saturation of 75% to 85%, and signs of adequate oxygen delivery and systemic perfusion (see Overview of Single Functioning Ventricle, Overview of Management earlier in this section). A high arterial oxygen saturation (90% or above) with signs of poor perfusion can indicate excessive pulmonary blood flow with subsequent systemic hypoperfusion; this development requires intervention to improve the systemic blood flow, including changes in mechanical ventilation support, reduction in inspired oxygen concentration or inhaled nitrogen (to reduce inspired oxygen concentration and alveolar oxygenation). Excessively high systemic vascular resistance or very low pulmonary vascular resistance can result in increased pulmonary blood flow and higher arterial oxygen saturation, but may result in inadequate systemic and coronary artery perfusion and decreased tissue oxygen delivery with acidosis, myocardial ischemia, and compromised splanchnic and renal flow.

Inotropic support may be necessary if signs of inadequate perfusion are present. CHF requires careful management of intravascular volume while avoiding hemoconcentration. Severe tachycardia (which shortens diastolic filling time and coronary artery perfusion time) or further lowering of the aortic diastolic pressure must be avoided in patients with right ventricular-dependent coronary circulation because either condition will exacerbate coronary ischemia.[662] Antibiotic prophylaxis is required before selected invasive procedures (see Bacterial Endocarditis).

The anatomy of pulmonary atresia with intact ventricular septum can be complex with wide variability in tricuspid, right ventricular, and coronary artery anatomy. Each patient requires an individualized approach in selection of surgical or interventional cardiac catheterization therapy, or a combination of these ("hybrid" procedure). No single procedure is appropriate for all patients.

Palliative Procedures. The initial palliative procedure provides some form of pulmonary blood flow.[454] Interventions include creation of a systemic to pulmonary shunt, or right ventricular (RV) decompression (with a valvotomy or transannular patch), or a combination of RV decompression and a shunt.[620] The goal of any palliative treatment is to establish adequate systemic arterial oxygenation with balanced pulmonary and systemic blood flow. The long-term goal is to maximize RV growth to enable a biventricular repair whenever possible, with separation of the systemic and pulmonary venous circulations, and RV to pulmonary artery continuity.[219]

Ultimately the degree of RV development will determine the strategy for biventricular repair, intermediate repair, or univentricular repair.[620] A univentricular palliation treatment path is used when most or all of the coronary circulation is dependent on the RV, or when extensive RV-coronary fistulae are present.[662] Options for management of the patient with pulmonary atresia with intact ventricular septum are summarized in Table 8-38.

Interventional Catheterization. Perforation of the pulmonary valve during cardiac catheterization allows some blood flow across the right ventricular outflow tract. Since the 1990s radiofrequency energy has been used in the cardiac catheterization lab to perforate the pulmonary valve and establish antegrade pulmonary blood flow, with anticipation that the flow will stimulate RV growth and allow acute RV decompression. Laser-guided techniques also can be used. After pulmonary valve perforation, balloon dilation is performed. Perforation can be accomplished in 80% of patients with pulmonary atresia and intact ventricular septum.[662] Complications occur in nearly 15% of patients, however, and can include perforation and tamponade. Mortality is approximately 8%.[389]

Another intervention that can be performed during cardiac catheterization to improve pulmonary blood flow is placement of a stent within the ductus arteriosus to maintain ductal patency.[783] Future potential coarctation (i.e., stenosis or narrowing) of the left pulmonary artery associated with the

Table 8-38	**Newborn Interventions for Pulmonary Atresia with Intact Ventricular Septum by Anatomic Considerations**[315,620,662,936]	

Anatomy Type	Intervention
RV and tricuspid valve—adequate size, no sinusoids	Surgery: Neonatal complete surgical repair with RV outflow reconstruction[936] *Biventricular repair*
Mild RV hypoplasia, without RVDCC; tricuspid valve Z score of: 0 to −2[620]	Surgery: Transannular patch along the right ventricle outflow tract Cardiac catheterization: Pulmonary valvotomy[620] Goal: *Biventricular repair*
Moderate RV hypoplasia, tricuspid valve Z score is: −2 to −3; the coronary artery perfusion is not dependent on the RV[620]	Surgery: Pulmonary outflow tract procedure with a Blalock-Taussig shunt[620] Goal: *Biventricular repair*
Severe RV hypoplasia, the tricuspid valve Z value is less than or equal to: −3[620] Likely to have sinusoids[620]	Surgery: Blalock-Taussig shunt Cardiac catheterization: Stent in PDA. *Univentricular repair*
RV dependent coronary artery circulation, sinusoids[662]	Surgery: Blalock-Taussig shunt Cardiac catheterization: Stent in PDA *Univentricular repair*[662]
Severe tricuspid regurgitation	Surgery: Blalock-Taussig shunt[662] with potential creation of tricuspid atresia[662] Consider cardiac transplantation[662] *Univentricular repair*

PDA, Patent ductus arteriosus; *RV,* right ventricle; *RVDCC,* right ventricular-dependent coronary circulation.

site of ductus arteriosus stent insertion requires ongoing assessment.[18]

The atrial right-to-left shunt often persists despite relief of the RV outflow obstruction because of the combined effects of tricuspid stenosis, annular hypoplasia, and a small, noncompliant RV. The prostaglandin E_1 infusion may be continued for days to weeks to ensure sufficient pulmonary blood flow, arterial oxygen saturation, and oxygen delivery. Postprocedure care includes the guidelines for single ventricle care presented in the section, Single Functioning Ventricle, Overview of Management earlier in this section of the chapter, and Cardiac Catheterization in the last section of this chapter.

If hypoxemia persists, an additional source of pulmonary blood flow can be created with a surgical Blalock-Taussig shunt or a stent placed within the ductus during a cardiac catheterization. A source of additional pulmonary blood flow is required in 33% to 70% of patients.[350,662] Throughout the hospitalization, IV tubing must be kept free of air, because any air entering the systemic venous circulation may ultimately be shunted into the systemic arterial circulation, and may produce a cerebral air embolus.

When successful, these interventional therapies avoid the use of cardiopulmonary bypass in the newborn, and can facilitate later biventricular repair or "one-and-a-half ventricle" repair.[350] The long-term results of this approach continue to be analyzed.[662]

Surgical Palliation to Increase Pulmonary Outflow and Blood Flow. Improved pulmonary blood flow can be achieved by a surgical pulmonary valvotomy. A closed transventricular pulmonary valvotomy does not require use of cardiopulmonary bypass. A curved blade is inserted through a small stab wound in the right ventricular outflow tract; the stab wound is surrounded by purse-string sutures (to prevent bleeding). A similar procedure may be performed using inflow occlusion and a small incision in the pulmonary artery. The valvotomy improves pulmonary blood flow and decompresses the right ventricle. In addition, it enables right ventricular ejection of blood, and so may stimulate growth of the hypoplastic right ventricle.[620] Postoperatively, management as for single ventricle physiology is needed (as detailed in the Single Functioning Ventricle, Overview of Management).

Open-heart procedures performed in the newborn include an open pulmonary valvotomy followed by insertion of a patch in the pulmonary outflow tract. The ductus arteriosus can be ligated if systemic arterial saturation is adequate.[620] If pulmonary blood flow (and systemic arterial saturation) remains inadequate after the valvotomy, a systemic-to-pulmonary artery shunt is also created. Postoperative complications include progressive right ventricular dysfunction, low cardiac output, and malignant ventricular arrhythmias. Congestive heart failure also may be present, with signs of systemic venous congestion. After any palliative procedure, *absolutely no air can be allowed to enter any intravenous system* because systemic venous blood continues to be shunted into the systemic arterial circulation.

Patients who have RV outflow reconstruction with creation of a Blalock-Taussig shunt can present with signs of low cardiac output if previously undiagnosed RV coronary sinusoids produce myocardial ischemia. Such low cardiac output is particularly likely if the right ventricular outflow reconstruction produced decompression of the right ventricle in patients with right ventricular-dependent coronary circulation. Signs of myocardial ischemia include ventricular arrhythmias and ECG changes (ST segment depression or elevation and T wave changes) immediately after surgery. An echocardiogram will confirm areas of myocardial dyskinesis or akinesis.[936]

If pulmonary insufficiency and tricuspid insufficiency are both present postoperatively, an ineffective *"circular shunt"* can develop. This shunt can develop after pulmonary valvotomy or RV outflow reconstruction that produces pulmonary insufficiency and creation of a systemic to pulmonary shunt. The systemic to pulmonary shunt delivers blood flow from the aorta to the pulmonary circulation; because pulmonary insufficiency is present, some of the shunted blood flows retrograde into the RV. If tricuspid valve regurgitation is also present, some of the blood from the RV is ejected back into the right atrium and then shunts right-to-left into the left atrium, ultimately flowing into the aorta and systemic circulation. This blood can then flow back through the systemic to pulmonary shunt, into the pulmonary artery, and back into the RV to the right atrium, left atrium, and aorta. The net result of this circular shunt is inadequate *systemic* blood flow. Signs of poor perfusion, including oliguria, metabolic acidosis, and systemic hypotension may develop several days after surgery.[662] Therapies to decrease this postoperative physiology include increasing pulmonary vascular resistance and lowering systemic vascular resistance. The patient may require narrowing of the shunt or repair of the tricuspid valve.[936]

Surgical Correction. Following the initial procedure for pulmonary atresia with intact ventricular septum, the patient must be monitored to determine the timing and procedure appropriate for the second intervention. In children with mild RV hypoplasia who have successful RV outflow decompression (by balloon valvotomy, surgical valvotomy, or transannular patch), the RV hypertrophy can regress, RV compliance can improve, and the RV can grow, increasing the volume of pulmonary blood flow.

A lung perfusion scan may be performed to determine blood flow distribution and identify branch pulmonary artery narrowing. An echocardiogram and cardiac catheterization are typically performed when the infant is 3 to 6 months of age to determine if the RV will be capable of supporting normal pulmonary blood flow. If the RV has grown sufficiently, the existing aorta to pulmonary shunt will be closed in the cardiac catheterization laboratory with devices[454] or via surgery. Some patients may only need an additional pulmonary balloon valvuloplasty and device closure of the atrial septal defect as the final intervention to complete biventricular repair.

More commonly an additional surgical procedure is needed to relieve RV outflow obstruction, including infundibular resection, pulmonary valvotomy, or placement of a transannular patch. The atrial septal defect may be closed, or the surgeon may choose to leave an atrial septal defect to allow a postoperative right-to-left shunt in case right ventricular function is borderline. The atrial defect can also be closed by cardiac catheterization device at a time in the future, when RV compliance and function improve.[620]

"One-and-a-half Ventricle" Repair. If RV development continues to be borderline, and the tricuspid valve is small, a "one-and-a-half ventricle" repair can be completed.[620] This consists of a bidirectional Glenn (SVC to right pulmonary artery shunt) anastamosis[936] to direct SVC flow directly into the pulmonary circulation. The IVC flow continues to enter the right atrium, and flows through the tricuspid valve, and is ejected by the right ventricle into the pulmonary circulation. A right ventricular outflow enlargement is performed to relieve residual pulmonary stenosis. When the atrial septal defect is closed, total separation of the systemic and pulmonary venous blood and separation of the systemic and pulmonary circulations is achieved.[620] If atrial septal defect closure is not tolerated, a restrictive atrial opening may be left with plans for future closure via an interventional cardiac catheterization procedure. Immediately after surgery the atrial defect allows for right-to-left atrial shunting, and systemic arterial desaturation is present (see Single Functioning Ventricle, Overview of Management, Palliative Surgery for Univentricular Heart: The Bidirectional Glenn and Hemi-Fontan Procedure [Cavopulmonary Anastomosis] in this section, and the section, Postoperative Care and Anticoagulation).

Patients treated with an RV outflow tract enlargement procedure combined with a systemic to pulmonary artery shunt for mild to moderate RV hypoplasia require ongoing echocardiographic assessment of RV and tricuspid valve growth. If adequate growth is observed, a cardiac catheterization is performed and the shunt is temporarily occluded to evaluate adequacy of systemic arterial saturation (a sign of adequate pulmonary blood flow and adequate RV output). A temporary balloon may also be inserted to occlude the atrial septal defect to assess the ability of the RV to maintain adequate cardiac output. If the arterial oxygen saturation is maintained during catheterization testing, the shunt may be permanently closed. The catheterization may show need for additional surgery to enlarge the RV outflow tract as the next procedure.[620]

Biventricular Repair. When the right ventricle and both pulmonary arteries are of adequate size, total correction of the pulmonary atresia can be performed using a median sternotomy incision, cardiopulmonary bypass, and hypothermia in the newborn or after successful staged palliation during infancy. A transannular patch (with or without a cusp) or a conduit is inserted between the right ventricle and pulmonary artery; the use of antibiotic-treated cryopreserved valved pulmonary or aortic homografts currently is preferred over the use of prosthetic conduits. After biventricular repair, the atrial septal defect may be closed, or an atrial defect may be allowed to remain open temporarily to decompress the right heart in the immediate postoperative period; this will produce varying degrees of right-to-left shunting of blood and varying degrees of systemic arterial oxygen desaturation and cyanosis. Later, when flow patterns are established, the ASD may be closed during cardiac catheterization or additional surgery.

Postoperative complications after biventricular repair or "one-and-a-half ventricle" repair include low cardiac output, congestive heart failure, arrhythmias, bleeding, and neurologic complications. Severe congestive heart failure and right ventricular dysfunction (with signs of severe systemic venous congestion, including tachycardia, hepatomegaly, ascites, and pleural effusions) may develop after right ventricular outflow reconstruction. As noted, a small atrial defect may be left in place after any of these procedures, to allow for a right-to-left shunt when residual RV dysfunction is present. It is important to know if a residual ASD is present, because this will cause systemic arterial oxygen desaturation. In addition, if a residual ASD and right-to-left shunt is present, no air can be allowed to enter any intravenous catheter, because it may be shunted into the systemic arterial circulation and may produce a cerebral air embolus.

Ventricular dysfunction and signs of myocardial ischemia, ventricular arrhythmias, or ventricular infarction can develop in patients with RV sinusoids. It is important to monitor for ST-segment changes postoperatively.

Univentricular Repair. If the tricuspid valve and RV continue to be severely hypoplastic, they will be too small to support adequate pulmonary blood flow, and biventricular repair will not be possible. A staged univentricular pathway is planned and a bidirectional cavopulmonary anastomosis is performed with closure of the systemic to pulmonary artery shunt as the second stage. Postoperative evaluation will monitor RV and tricuspid valve status to determine future suitability for RV outflow tract enlargement with a "one-and-a-half-ventricle" repair, or completion of a Fontan procedure (see Single Functioning Ventricle, Overview of Management, Corrective Surgery: The Completion Fontan Procedure).

If the patient has an initial systemic to pulmonary artery palliation (shunt or stenting of the ductus arteriosus) and a univentricular heart pathway is anticipated, cardiac catheterization is performed at 3 to 6 months of age in preparation for the second-stage bidirectional Glenn with takedown of the systemic to pulmonary artery shunt. A total cavopulmonary connection (Fontan procedure) will then be completed.

For children with RV-dependent coronary circulation the Fontan pathway is planned to maintain elevated RV pressure, directing oxygenated (pulmonary venous) blood into the RV then into the coronary arteries via retrograde flow. This may include a lateral tunnel or extracardiac Fontan. The surgical procedure is planned to avoid even temporary RV decompression during cardiopulmonary bypass, because RV decompression can lead to lethal myocardial ischemia.[620] The Fontan procedure (with or without a fenestration) joins the inferior vena caval flow to the pulmonary artery, so that systemic venous blood is diverted into the pulmonary arteries; oxygenated pulmonary venous blood must be able to flow through the tricuspid valve and into the RV and then into the coronary circulation (see Single Functioning Ventricle, Overview of Management, Corrective Surgery: The Completion Fontan Procedure).

Perioperative mortality varies widely and by specific procedure. The Society of Thoracic Surgeons, reporting 2006-2010 data, identify 7.1% (modified shunt) to 11.9% (central shunt) overall hospital mortality in neonates undergoing systemic to pulmonary artery shunts.[823] Biventricular repair management strategies and outcomes have been reported, but broad application is limited due to the variability in intracardiac and great vessel anatomy.[183] The Congenital Heart Surgeon Society database for 408 neonates with pulmonary atresia and intact ventricular septum reports 77% survival at 1 month, 60% survival at 5 years, and 58% survival at 15 years of age. A biventricular repair was reported in 33%, a Fontan in 20%, and a "one-and-a-half ventricle" repair in 5%. Outcomes continue to improve.[34]

The survivors of pulmonary atresia with intact ventricular septum are now beginning to reach adulthood and they will require lifelong care. Long-term results are affected by the patient's unique hemodynamics and the subsequent interventions. Late survivors can develop arrhythmias, residual right ventricular outflow obstruction, right atrial dilation, tricuspid regurgitation, and pulmonary regurgitation. Some may continue to have cyanosis from residual atrial septal defects or other shunts. The specific potential problems are varied because of the unique forms of palliation performed, possible progression of coronary artery abnormalities, and—for those with the univentricular interventions—all of the potential complications related to the Fontan procedure. These late complications, assessments, and late management options are detailed by Daubeney.[219] Lifelong, continuous care is required into adulthood by experts in the management of adults with congenital heart disease.[927]

Some advanced concepts in the care of the child with pulmonary atresia and intact ventricular septum are listed in Box 8-42.

Hypoplastic Left Heart Syndrome (HLHS)
Jo Ann Nieves

Pearls

- As the PDA closes in the newborn with HLHS, inadequate systemic perfusion will result in shock.
- The optimal circulation in patients with single ventricle physiology produces an arterial oxygen saturation of 75% to 85% with signs of adequate systemic perfusion.
- In the patient with single ventricle physiology:
  - An arterial oxygen saturation greater than 85% with signs of decreased perfusion suggests pulmonary overcirculation (excessive pulmonary blood flow) that can lead to systemic hypoperfusion and inadequate systemic oxygen delivery.
  - An arterial oxygen saturation less than 70% indicates inadequate pulmonary blood flow or low cardiac output that can result in tissue hypoxia and lactic (metabolic) acidosis.
- A hematocrit greater than 40% is necessary to optimize oxygen carrying capacity when single ventricle physiology is present.
- It is important to monitor upper versus lower extremity pulses and blood pressures after the Norwood procedure. A pressure differential of greater than 10 mm Hg with elevation in upper extremity blood pressure may indicate recoarctation of the aorta after the Norwood procedure.

Box 8-42   Advanced Concepts: Pulmonary Atresia with Intact Ventricular Septum (IVS)

- A "circular shunt" can develop after creation of a systemic to pulmonary artery shunt if severe pulmonary and tricuspid insufficiency develop.
  - Pulmonary insufficiency can result from RV outflow tract reconstruction with a transannular patch or from a percutaneous pulmonary valvotomy. Tricuspid insufficiency can result from right ventricular dysfunction and dilation.
  - In the presence of both pulmonary and tricuspid regurgitation, blood from the aorta flows through the systemic to pulmonary artery shunt into the pulmonary artery, then flows retrograde (through the insufficient pulmonary valve) into the right ventricle. The blood can then flow retrograde (through the insufficient tricuspid valve) into the right atrium. Blood from the right atrium can flow through the atrial septal defect to the left atrium and into the ventricle and can be ejected into the aorta, to again flow through the systemic to pulmonary shunt.
    - A circular shunt produces low cardiac output.
- Decreased aortic diastolic pressure, tachycardia, and hypovolemia in the presence of RV sinusoids or RV-dependent coronary circulation will reduce myocardial oxygen delivery and produce myocardial ischemia. Such

ischemia can produce ventricular arrhythmias and low cardiac output.
  - Reduced aortic diastolic pressure decreases coronary perfusion pressure in general. In patients with RV sinusoids it will also increase retrograde flow of systemic venous blood from the right ventricle through the sinusoids.
  - Tachycardia decreases coronary perfusion time.
  - Hypovolemia reduces right ventricular end-diastolic pressure and decreases retrograde perfusion through the sinusoids. Patients with RV-dependent coronary circulation have limited antegrade flow from the coronary artery, so anything that reduces RV pressure will reduce the major source of blood flow to the coronary circulation. Decreased aortic diastolic pressure will also reduce what little antegrade flow is present through the coronary circulation
- Signs of myocardial ischemia include ST-segment depression (in leads with upright QRS complex) and T-wave abnormalities. Myocardial infarction can produce ST-segment elevation (in leads with upright QRS complex). These changes require immediate recognition and therapy.

Etiology

Hypoplastic left heart syndrome (HLHS) consists of a small, often tiny left ventricle, aortic and/or mitral valve stenosis or atresia, normally related great vessels, and an intact ventricular septum (Fig. 8-62). The ascending aorta supplies the coronary circulation with retrograde flow (from the patent ductus into the aorta), but the aorta is hypoplastic; approximately half of patients with HLHS have an aortic diameter less than 2 mm.[879] The left atrium is small because it receives limited blood flow during fetal development and the atrial septum is thick, with a foramen ovale that can be small or closed.[514] Eighty percent of patients have localized coarctation of the aorta.[358] The most serious form of the defect includes aortic atresia. The fetus with severe aortic valve disease has decreased or reversed blood flow through the patent foramen ovale in utero; the decreased flow results in less stimulus for development of left heart structures.[561,881]

Hypoplastic left heart syndrome is responsible for between 1.4% and 3.8% of all congenital heart defects.[881] Patients with HLHS can have extracardiac anomalies, including congenital diaphragmatic hernia, malrotation, and biliary atresia.[881] A genetic basis for HLHS has been identified, with sibling recurrence risk at 8% and the presence of HLHS-associated cardiovascular malformation in one fifth of siblings.[375] Before 1979 there was no intervention for HLHS, so mortality was 100%.[514] Rapidly evolving treatment strategies for HLHS have dramatically improved survival in the last decade and include fetal echocardiographic diagnosis, prenatal

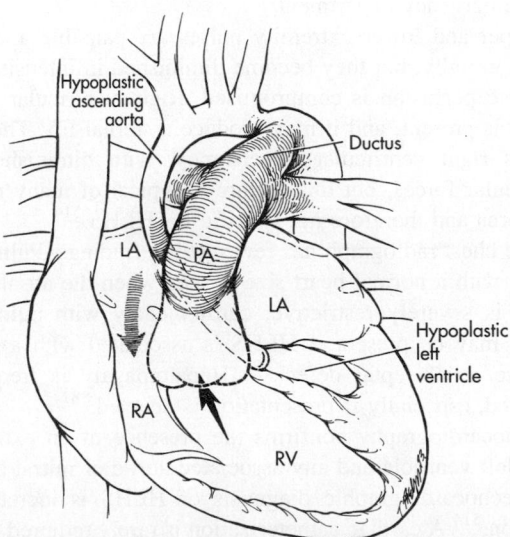

FIG. 8-62 Hypoplastic left heart syndrome: native anatomy. The syndrome includes a hypoplastic left ventricle, aortic valve atresia, and a diminutive ascending aorta. Systemic blood flow is generated by the right ventricle. Systemic venous blood flows from the right ventricle into the pulmonary artery (PA), through a patent ductus arteriosus (ductus) into the aorta. Pulmonary venous return enters the left atrium and flows through the foramen ovale or an atrial septal defect to the right ventricle. The amount of right ventricular output that flows into the pulmonary versus systemic circulations is determined by the relative resistances in the pulmonary and systemic circulations. LA, Left atrium; RA, right atrium; RV, right ventricle. (From Nichols SC, Steven JM, Jobes AB. Hypoplastic left heart syndrome. In Nichols GD, et al, editors. *Critical heart disease in infants and children*, St Louis, 1995, Mosby.)

transcatheter cardiac interventions, newborn staged surgical reconstruction, heart transplantation, and collaborative hybrid (cardiac catheter interventional and surgical) newborn palliation procedures. However, HLHS remains a leading cause of infant mortality and childhood morbidity among children with congenital heart disease.[375]

Pathophysiology

In HLHS systemic and pulmonary venous blood mix at the atrial level. Because there is a small left ventricular chamber with or without aortic or mitral valve obstruction, there is resistance to flow into the aorta and there is inadequate systemic perfusion. Survival after birth is dependent on the flow of blood from the right ventricle into the pulmonary artery and then through a patent ductus arteriosus to supply the systemic and coronary circulations. This flow from the ductus arteriosus supplies the descending aorta with antegrade flow; the ascending aorta (including the brain) and coronary arteries are perfused with retrograde flow. Thus, the right ventricle must supply the pulmonary, systemic, and coronary circulations. The left heart is too small to support the systemic and coronary circulations.

In HLHS, a parallel circulation exists, so the total ventricular output is divided between the pulmonary and systemic circulations and the volume of flow to each circulation is determined by the relative vascular resistance in each circuit.[514,935] When the ductus arteriosus is widely patent and pulmonary vascular resistance is high at birth, there may be balanced flow to the systemic and pulmonary circulations with adequate arterial oxygen saturation and systemic perfusion.

An optimal balance of blood flow to the pulmonary and systemic circulations produces adequate systemic oxygen delivery without excessive volume load to the single, systemic right ventricle. This corresponds to a pulmonary to systemic flow ratio (Qp/Qs) of 1:1, an arterial oxygen saturation of near 80%, a pulmonary venous saturation about 95%, a mixed venous oxygen saturation about 65%, and cardiac output approximately normal.[935] The systemic arterial oxygen saturation is almost directly related to the amount of pulmonary blood flow; the greater the amount of pulmonary blood flow, the higher is the amount of oxygenated pulmonary venous blood returning to the left atrium to mix with the (desaturated) systemic venous return, and the higher is the oxygen saturation ejected by the right ventricle into the pulmonary, coronary, and systemic circulations.[514]

Pulmonary vascular resistance decreases immediately after birth, leading to increased pulmonary blood flow.[935] When the pulmonary vascular resistance is less than the systemic vascular resistance, blood flows preferentially into the pulmonary vascular bed, and the arterial oxygen saturation rises. The normal postnatal rise in systemic vascular resistance also enhances blood flow into the pulmonary vascular bed. Signs of congestive heart failure typically develop. Pulmonary congestion is likely to be significant because the increased volume of pulmonary venous return to the left atrium cannot flow freely into the left heart; obstruction to flow through the left heart increases pulmonary venous pressure with resultant pulmonary edema and work of breathing. The increased pulmonary blood flow may potentially cause systemic hypoperfusion because blood is diverted into the pulmonary circulation and away from the systemic circulation.

When the arterial oxygen saturation approaches 90%, pulmonary blood flow is very high and systemic flow is significantly compromised. If the oxygen tension in the alveoli is high, pulmonary vasodilation occurs, resulting in further increase in pulmonary blood flow. The single right ventricle has excessive volume load, so dysfunction will rapidly develop with dilation, elevated end-diastolic pressure, and progressive tricuspid regurgitation. Signs of heart failure include tachycardia, poor perfusion, and metabolic acidosis.[935] The right ventricle exceeds maximal performance volume when the volume overload is four to five times normal, or the pulmonary to systemic flow ratio (Qp/QS) is 4:1.[514]

Progressive deterioration of systemic perfusion is associated with compromised coronary artery perfusion. Factors associated with progressive right ventricular dysfunction include excessive volume load (resulting from increased pulmonary blood flow and increased pulmonary venous return), increased right ventricular afterload (caused by the constricting ductus arteriosus and any pulmonary vasoconstriction that results from pulmonary edema and alveolar hypoxia), and poor coronary perfusion. As right ventricular dysfunction worsens, the ventricle will dilate and tricuspid regurgitation will develop. This leads to an increase in right and left atrial pressures and worsening of pulmonary venous hypertension and pulmonary edema.

An important determinant of symptoms from HLHS is the size of the interatrial communication. When severe mitral or aortic obstruction is present, blood will shunt from the left to the right atrium through a stretched foramen ovale. A nonrestrictive atrial septal defect allows an unrestricted left-to-right atrial shunt.[514] If the interatrial communication is restrictive, the left atrial pressure will rise, increasing pulmonary venous pressure and ultimately increasing total pulmonary vascular resistance.[514] This can eventually help to limit pulmonary blood flow.[514] However, the left atrial hypertension will impair gas exchange.[514] Pulmonary edema, respiratory distress, and progressive severe hypoxemia/cyanosis develop if a severely restrictive atrial septal defect or an intact atrial septum is present. Elevated pulmonary vascular resistance or a drop in systemic vascular resistance reduce pulmonary blood flow and increase cyanosis.

Clinical Signs and Symptoms

At birth the neonate may appear to be normal, but symptoms generally develop within 48 hours.[2] There is no specific murmur associated with this defect.[881] A third heart sound may be heard if ventricular dysfunction is present, and tricuspid regurgitation may produce a loud S1.[881] If an unrestricted atrial septal defect is present, systemic perfusion and the systemic arterial oxygen saturation may initially be adequate while the ductus arteriosus is patent. As pulmonary vascular resistance begins to fall, pulmonary blood flow is increased, producing elevation in systemic arterial oxygen saturation and the development of signs of congestive heart failure, including tachycardia, tachypnea, and dyspnea. Because the infant is unable to breathe and suck at the same time, severe tachypnea is associated with poor feeding.

As the ductus arteriosus begins to spontaneously close, pulmonary blood flow increases and aortic blood flow and systemic perfusion decrease generally independent of the pulmonary vascular resistance.[935] Cyanosis or pallor and signs of poor systemic perfusion develop rapidly, with signs including tachycardia, weak peripheral pulses, a narrowed pulse pressure, and peripheral vasoconstriction with possible lethargy.[514] Continued ductal closure combined with the normal postnatal fall in pulmonary vascular resistance leads to progressive deterioration in systemic blood flow. Decreased coronary perfusion can lead to further myocardial dysfunction. The newborn may suddenly develop symptoms of circulatory collapse, including absence of palpable peripheral pulses, ashen color, gasping respirations, and severe cyanosis. Profound metabolic acidosis develops despite a high PaO_2 (70 to 100 mm Hg).[935]

The development of pulmonary edema, respiratory distress, and progressive, severe cyanosis will be seen if a severely restrictive atrial septal defect or intact atrial septum is present.[686] Respiratory support with elective intubation and assisted ventilation will be required. The patients with severely restrictive atrial septal defect or an intact septum are often unresponsive to conventional medical intervention and require urgent interventional catheterization.[881]

Newborns who are discharged home before the development of obvious symptoms may present at 2 to 3 days of age, with the parents reporting difficulty feeding or "funny breathing." Gasping respirations with profound low cardiac output, acidosis, and renal failure may be seen on presentation to an emergency department.

Upper and lower extremity pulses are palpable and symmetric initially, but they become diminished in intensity once systemic perfusion is compromised. Right ventricular hypertrophy is present, and it may produce a sternal lift. The ECG reveals right ventricular hypertrophy, with diminished left ventricular forces, but this feature is typical of many normal newborns and therefore not specific for HLHS.[514]

The chest radiograph has few specific findings. Pulmonary edema with a normal heart size is seen when the atrial septal defect is severely restrictive; cardiomegaly with pulmonary edema may be present if HLHS is associated with a nonrestrictive atrial septal defect.[881] Hepatomegaly is frequently observed, especially if presentation is delayed.[881]

Echocardiography confirms the presence of an extremely small left ventricle and any associated aortic or mitral atresia. Fetal echocardiographic diagnosis of HLHS is increasingly common.[514] A cardiac catheterization is rarely required except in newborns with a severely restrictive atrial septal defect or intact atrial septum; catheterization allows interventional atrial septostomy for these newborns. These infants typically demonstrate severe pulmonary hypertension, pulmonary edema, low cardiac output, and cyanosis.

Management

Medical Management. Newborns with hypoplastic left heart syndrome can die at any time before institution of therapy. A *prostaglandin E₁ infusion* must be provided immediately (initial infusion, 0.05 to 0.1 mcg/kg per minute) to keep the ductus arteriosus open until the diagnosis is confirmed (see Box 8-33). IV Prostaglandin E$_1$ almost invariably reopens the ductus arteriosus, but may produce apnea, so providers should be prepared to perform intubation and provide mechanical ventilation.[514]

The PGE$_1$ dose can be decreased to the lowest effective dose (0.01-0.05 mcg/kg per minute) once ductal patency is confirmed.[881] Because all circulations are perfused by the right ventricle, until complete correction and separation of systemic and pulmonary venous blood is accomplished surgically, *no air can be allowed to enter any IV system* because it may be shunted into the cerebral arterial circulation, causing a cerebral air embolus (stroke). The patient is at risk for all complications associated with hypoxemia and polycythemia until that time (see section, Common Clinical Conditions, Hypoxemia).

Support of adequate systemic perfusion and oxygen delivery are critical throughout care in the patient with single ventricle circulation. The arterial blood gas is an excellent indicator of hemodynamic stability in these patients.[935] Adequate peripheral perfusion is indicated by a normal pH and an arterial oxygen saturation near 80%; these findings are associated with a pulmonary to systemic flow ratio (Qp:Qs) near 1:1.[935] Inadequate systemic perfusion and oxygen delivery, excessive pulmonary blood flow, and likely myocardial dysfunction are indicated by metabolic acidosis with arterial oxygen saturation in excess of 90%.[935] Early detection and treatment of altered oxygen delivery is important to minimize end organ ischemia and improve survival. Note that arterial oxygen saturation may be within the acceptable range despite profound circulatory derangements, so continuous monitoring and careful assessment are needed.[881]

Development of signs of systemic hypoperfusion must be reported immediately to the healthcare provider responsible for managing the infant's care. Signs of systemic hypoperfusion include worsening tachycardia, diminished quality of peripheral pulses, decreased urine output, and pulmonary congestion. Serial serum lactate measurements help evaluate adequacy of oxygen delivery; a rising or persistently high lactate indicates acidosis that is not responding to therapy.

Near infrared spectroscopy (NIRS) sensors over the forehead and kidney area on the lower back have been used to identify real-time trends in oxygenation of the brain and somatic tissue, and to monitor response to interventions.[315] After palliation for HLHS, cerebral saturations greater than 50% and somatic values greater than 60% have predicted better outcomes.[590]

After the reopening of the ductus, therapies to support right ventricular function may include inotropic support. If severe signs of low cardiac output develop, the right ventricle must be supported to recover from insults and stressors, including probable ischemia caused by poor coronary perfusion, volume overload, increased afterload, and acidosis.[514] Hypoglycemia and hypocalcemia require correction.

Profoundly low cardiac output can lead to gastrointestinal dysfunction, hepatic dysfunction or failure, renal failure, fluid overload, and hyperkalemia; these complications require supportive therapies. Vasoactive therapy must be carefully titrated to prevent excessive vasoconstriction and further reduction in organ blood flow. Doses of all drugs should be evaluated

and adjusted as needed if new renal or hepatic dysfunction develops.[514]

High doses of inotropic support are undesirable because they cause excessive vasoconstriction that will contribute to a further increase in pulmonary blood flow and will divert even more blood flow from the systemic to the pulmonary circulation. As a result, arterial oxygen saturation and mean arterial blood pressure require careful monitoring.[935]

Oxygen administration is necessary if the arterial oxygen saturation is less than 70%. The arterial blood gas must be closely monitored for development of acidosis or an oxygen tension below 30 mm Hg; these findings must be immediately reported to the on-call provider because they may be associated with inadequate oxygen delivery.

If the atrial septal defect is severely restrictive or the atrial septum is intact, obstruction to pulmonary blood venous return to the left atrium can contribute to pulmonary edema, and produce poor oxygenation and profound hypoxemia, with PaO$_2$ of 20 mm Hg. When the atrial septal defect is restrictive, medical therapy to increase pulmonary blood flow, including oxygen administration and mechanical ventilation will not increase the PaO$_2$.[514] If the atrial septum is intact or the atrial septal defect is restrictive, urgent interventional cardiac catheterization or surgery is indicated to open the atrial septal defect and decompress the left atrium. This condition remains highly lethal despite prenatal diagnosis,[323] but has shown improving outcomes with fetal atrial septostomy intervention.[908]

Cardiac catheterization intervention should improve systemic arterial oxygenation and relieve left atrial and pulmonary hypertension and pulmonary edema.[329] Room air should be used to avoid the pulmonary vasodilation resulting from high alveolar oxygen tension that is produced by oxygen therapy. If high arterial oxygen saturation is associated with poor perfusion, metabolic acidosis, or other signs of inadequate tissue oxygen delivery, interventions are needed to increase pulmonary vascular resistance and reduce excessive pulmonary blood flow; this will improve systemic perfusion. Such measures include decreasing the inspired oxygen concentration, elective intubation, mechanical ventilation support, sedation, and possible neuromuscular blockade (see Chapter 5). Controlled hypoventilation is used to increase arterial carbon dioxide levels and create a mild respiratory acidosis. Alkalosis creates pulmonary vasodilation, and is therefore avoided. As a result, mild alveolar hypoxia and mild hypercarbia are maintained preoperatively and can improve systemic circulation.[935]

Sedation can be used to suppress the infant's intrinsic respiratory drive, because a rapid spontaneous respiratory rate will likely further decrease the PaCO$_2$. Positive and-expiratory pressure (PEEP) can result in increased pulmonary resistance.[881] Inspired gases can be manipulated to reduce excessive pulmonary blood flow and improve systemic hypoperfusion.[935] Alveolar hypoxia can be created with addition of inhaled nitrogen to reduce the inspired oxygen concentration to 14% to 20%; such interventions will produce pulmonary vasoconstriction and thus limit pulmonary blood flow.[935] Inhaled carbon dioxide (2% to 5%) can be used to promote pulmonary vasoconstriction.[935]

Afterload reduction can further decrease the systemic vascular resistance,[881,935] but the diastolic blood pressure should not fall below 30 mm Hg to avoid compromising coronary blood flow.[590] As pulmonary blood flow is controlled, the arterial oxygen saturation should decline to the acceptable range with signs of improved systemic perfusion. The right ventricular function will typically improve when the pulmonary to systemic flow ratio (QP/QS) falls from 4:1 to 2:1 or lower because the decrease in pulmonary venous return will reduce right ventricular volume overload.[514]

Inotropic support with milrinone can aid right ventricular contractility and reduce systemic vascular resistance.[514] Hypertension and a rise in systemic vascular resistance are avoided because they will again increase pulmonary blood flow, with the potential return of poor systemic perfusion.

If at all possible the neonate should be allowed to continue to breathe spontaneously in room air. If mechanical ventilation is required, room air is often used to prevent excessive pulmonary vasodilation. Supplementary oxygen therapy may be required for severe hypoxia, lung pathology, or a restrictive atrial septal defect.[881]

Surgical Intervention. Since the late 1970s the Norwood procedure (Fig. 8-63, A) has become increasingly successful when performed as a first-stage palliation for hypoplastic left heart syndrome.[315,659,881] Staged surgical intervention, completed by a Fontan-like procedure, ultimately results in separation of single ventricle circulations. Cardiac transplantation during the neonatal period may also be offered, particularly if right ventricular or tricuspid valve dysfunction remains severe despite medical management.

A modification of the Norwood procedure, the Sano operation (see Fig. 8-63, B), was developed in the 1990s. Most recently a staged "hybrid" intervention combining interventional cardiac catheterization and surgery without cardiopulmonary bypass has become available.[293] (See Hybrid Procedures in Cardiac Catheterization and Interventions.)

It is important to note that some parents may decline surgical intervention for the newborn with HLHS. In selected cases when unrecoverable decompensation occurs at presentation or multiple congenital anomalies are present, compassionate care is offered to the family. In these cases, comfort measures only are provided, with no surgical intervention, and the parents are supported until the infant dies (see Chapter 3).

The goal of each first stage intervention for HLHS is to provide unobstructed systemic blood flow from the right ventricle into the aorta. A source of controlled pulmonary blood flow is needed with care taken to protect the pulmonary artery architecture from development of distortions, and the pulmonary vascular bed from development of hypertension and vascular disease. Obstruction to pulmonary venous return is eliminated by establishing an adequate interatrial communication to ensure an unrestricted flow from the left to the right atrium. The final staged procedure for HLHS uses a modification of the Fontan procedure to separate pulmonary and systemic blood flow within the heart.

The Norwood Procedure. This operation establishes permanent, unobstructed systemic blood flow from the right ventricle into a reconstructed neo-aorta. This procedure requires cardiopulmonary bypass, altered perfusion (circulatory arrest or regional perfusion), and deep hypothermia.[881] Pulmonary blood flow is provided by a prosthetic shunt from an aortic branch to a pulmonary artery. To eliminate obstruction to pulmonary venous return, the interatrial septum is resected.

The distal main pulmonary artery is transected. The aorta is incised longitudinally from the left subclavian artery, across the arch to the ascending aorta. An anastomosis is created between the trunk of the proximal main pulmonary artery and the ascending aorta and aortic arch. A portion of pulmonary homograft can be used to complete aortic reconstruction and prevent development of stenosis. Pulmonary blood flow

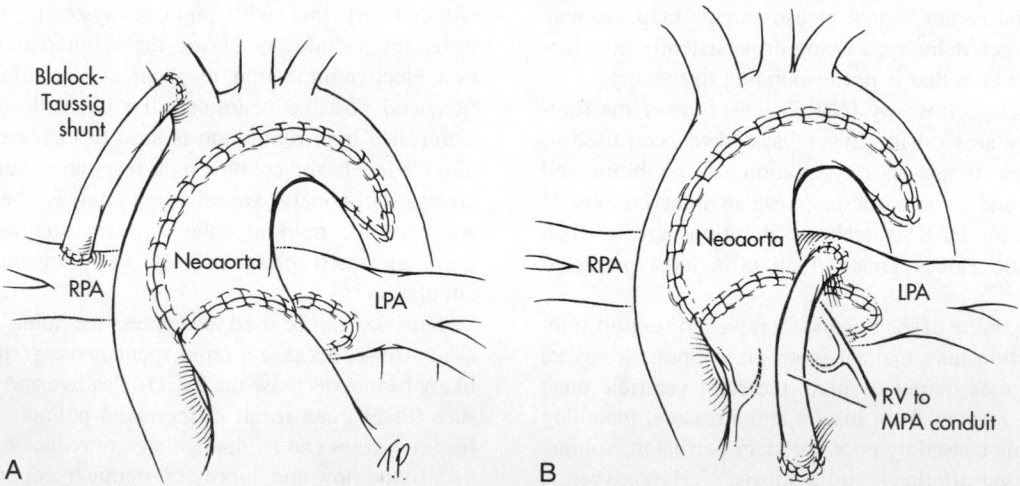

FIG. 8-63 Stage I Norwood procedure for hypoplastic left heart syndrome. **A,** Stage I Norwood procedure with pulmonary blood flow provided by a modified right Blalock-Taussig shunt. The main pulmonary artery is transected right before it branches into the right pulmonary artery (RPA) and left pulmonary artery (LPA). The new aorta (neoaorta) is created by joining the main pulmonary artery trunk to the original aorta. Pulmonary blood flow is provided by a Blalock-Taussig (subclavian to pulmonary artery) prosthetic shunt. **B,** In the Sano modification, a 5-mm conduit is inserted between the right ventricle (RV) and the main pulmonary artery (MPA) to provide pulmonary blood flow. (From Nichols GD. *Critical heart disease in infants and children.* St Louis, 1995, Mosby, Fig. 40-7, A and B.)

is created by insertion of a 3- to 4-mm Gore-Tex systemic-to-pulmonary artery shunt between the innominate artery (or the aorta) and the pulmonary artery. The existing atrial septal defect or patent foramen ovale is enlarged (see Fig. 8-63, A and B).

After the completion of the stage 1 procedure, parallel circulations exist. The right ventricle receives systemic and pulmonary venous blood and ejects that mixed venous blood into the new aorta that was fashioned from the aorta and original pulmonary artery trunk. Pulmonary blood flow occurs through the systemic-to-pulmonary artery shunt. Pulmonary venous return enters the left atrium and flows chiefly into the right atrium, and is mixed with systemic venous blood in the right ventricle.

Several postoperative complications can develop after the Norwood procedure. The same single ventricle circulation guidelines for care are to be followed as during the preoperative period, with targeted arterial oxygen saturation near 80%.

Optimizing systemic oxygen delivery remains crucial. Low cardiac output syndrome is common during the first 24 to 48 postoperative hours,[935] and inotropic medications are required. There are many causes of low cardiac output syndrome after intervention for complex neonatal congenital heart disease using cardiopulmonary bypass. Causes of low cardiac output after the Norwood procedure can include residual anatomic lesions such as residual aortic arch obstruction.[935] In addition, metabolic demands are increased postoperatively. It is important to note that neonates can develop shock despite the presence of an adequate arterial blood pressure, so close observation is needed to detect signs of poor perfusion (see Shock in Chapter 6).[568]

Inotropic medications are titrated carefully to support cardiac output and systemic perfusion while avoiding a significant increase in systemic vascular resistance that can lead to increased pulmonary blood flow with systemic hypoperfusion and the potential for decreased systemic oxygen delivery. Cardiovascular surgical centers have reported improved survival and neurologic outcome with the routine initiation of mechanical circulatory assistance in the operating room, at the conclusion of the Norwood procedure (see Chapter 7). This practice enables support of cardiovascular function to meet the increased postoperative oxygen requirements.[887]

Continuous close monitoring for adequacy of oxygen delivery versus consumption (demand) is needed and includes the typical monitoring for the complex postoperative patient with additional measurements. Oxygen delivery status can be continually or intermittently evaluated with the use of a catheter in the superior vena cava to measure central venous oxygen saturation ($ScvO_2$). Goal directed therapy targeting an $ScvO_2$ of 75% as an indicator of adequate systemic oxygen delivery versus demand has resulted in improved survival after HLHS palliation.[590,880] Continuous $ScvO_2$ monitoring has also decreased the incidence of sudden circulatory collapse in the postoperative period.[882] An $ScvO_2$ saturation below 45% may be associated with ischemic brain injury.[590] The difference between the arterial and central venous oxygen saturation should also be assessed. A rising arterial venous oxygen saturation difference is a strong indicator of inadequate oxygen delivery, and a difference of 40% to 50% or more indicates severely low cardiac output.[384,935] A rising serum lactate also indicates inadequate systemic oxygen delivery.

Near infrared spectroscopy (NIRS) sensors over the forehead and kidney area on the lower back have been used to identify real-time trends in oxygenation of the brain and somatic tissue. After palliation for HLHS, cerebral saturations greater than 50% and somatic values greater than 60% have predicted better outcomes.[590] Trends can be continually monitored and response to therapies assessed with good correlation between $ScvO_2$ saturations and NIRS saturations[590] for additional details of postoperative care.

Postoperatively, excessive pulmonary blood flow is present if the arterial oxygen saturation is greater than 85% to 88%.[935] Although both pulmonary and systemic vascular resistance should be evaluated and optimized, the primary determinant of the pulmonary to systemic flow ratio is the systemic vascular resistance. Successful treatment methods to improve systemic perfusion involve therapies to decrease systemic vascular resistance.

Afterload reduction enhances systemic blood flow and improves systemic oxygen delivery as more blood flows to the systemic circulation (and less to the pulmonary circulation). Milrinone is often used as both a vasodilator and positive inotropic agent (it is an inodilator).

Phenoxybenzamine has been used successfully for prolonged afterload reduction through alpha-adrenergic blockade both post cardiopulmonary bypass and in the postoperative period. Decreasing the systemic vascular resistance can lead to a more balanced single ventricle circulation with a more stable postoperative course and higher systemic oxygen delivery.[382] However, use of phenoxybenzamine can lead to sustained, excessive vasodilation and systemic hypoperfusion, requiring the initiation of catecholamines, including norepinephrine to optimize the systemic vascular resistance.[591] When inotropic support is required during the use of phenoxybenzamine with low mixed venous saturation and elevated systemic vascular resistance, epinephrine may be useful.[591] The arterial diastolic pressure should be maintained at greater than 30 mm Hg[590] to maintain adequate coronary perfusion pressure.

Elevated systemic resistance and arterial blood pressure can result from a residual aortic arch obstruction. Clinical exam and echocardiography can be used to evaluate the reconstruction and detect any obstruction.

Monitor for bleeding. Bleeding may occur at any of the extensive suture lines along the aorta, because these suture lines are exposed to systemic pressure. Post-bypass coagulopathy can also contribute to bleeding. Anemia must be avoided and the hematocrit maintained at least 40% to support adequate oxygen-carrying capacity.

Titrate preload (with volume therapy) to maintain right atrial and right ventricular end-diastolic pressure, and support optimal cardiac output. Typically an initial CVP of 12 to 14 mm Hg is maintained.[881]

Monitor for arrhythmias. Sinus tachycardia is the newborn's most efficient mechanism to raise cardiac output, and it is a nonspecific sign of distress. As a result, development of tachycardia should prompt careful assessment of the newborn's airway, oxygenation, ventilation, and perfusion.

Malignant arrhythmias including bradycardia, loss of sinus rhythm, or supraventricular tachycardia are not well tolerated and can lead to severe low cardiac output.

Monitor for neurologic complications, including seizures. Closely monitor the neonate's serum ionized calcium and provide supplementation as needed. *Absolutely no air can be allowed to enter any intravenous system* because it may be shunted into the cerebral circulation, producing a cerebral air embolus (stroke).

Additional support. Elective delayed sternal closure may be used. Methods to minimize oxygen consumption include providing narcotics and sedation and maintenance of normothermia and a neutral thermal environment. For further information about management, see Single Functioning Ventricle, Overview of Management.

Monitor for signs of deterioration. A decrease in pulmonary blood flow may result from hypotension or low systemic vascular resistance. A narrowed shunt can produce increasing cyanosis and development of metabolic acidosis at any time postoperatively. The shunt murmur may change and the diastolic blood pressure may increase. If shunt occlusion is suspected, immediate therapy is indicated, including heparinization to minimize clot progression, elevation of the arterial blood pressure with epinephrine (to enhance shunt flow), and rapid echocardiogram. Elective heparinization to decrease the possibility of prosthetic shunt occlusion may begin after the risk of postoperative bleeding has passed, with eventual transition to anticoagulation with aspirin or low molecular weight heparin. Hypoxemia unresponsive to therapy requires initiation of cardiopulmonary support or ECMO.

The atrial septal defect may become obstructive, leading to pulmonary venous hypertension; this is particularly likely in those patients undergoing the hybrid stage 1 intervention. Signs may develop gradually and include increasing tachypnea, decreasing arterial oxygen saturation, cyanosis, oxygen dependence, poor feeding, and signs of pulmonary venous congestion on chest radiograph. The shunt murmur intensity may decrease.[514] The diagnosis can be made by echocardiography and treatment can include interventional cardiac catheterization to dilate the atrial septum, with possible stent implantation.

Right ventricular dysfunction and tricuspid regurgitation can develop requiring additional inotropic support and initiation of afterload reduction to reduce systemic vascular resistance (ventricular afterload). If treatment does not improve ventricular function, the infant may require an early second-stage bidirectional Glenn procedure, with tricuspid valve plication. Some infants are referred directly for cardiac transplantation.

Nutrition is initially provided parenterally. As the risk for systemic hypoperfusion subsides, enteral feeding begins, increasing gradually to 110 to 130 kcal/kg per day using fortified formula or breast milk.[881] Optimal nutrition is critical for growth after palliation, but may be complicated by the development of poor oral feeding, impaired circulation with mesenteric hypoperfusion, necrotizing enterocolitis, or presence of postoperative recurrent laryngeal nerve injury.[591,935] Necrotizing enterocolitis increases the risk for death.[412] Malnutrition is common,[461] with formula intolerance and prolonged feedings associated with impaired somatic growth until after the second stage surgical procedure.[645,825]

Nasogastric or gastrostomy tube feedings may be required. Normal rate of weight gain in infants following Norwood Stage I surgery have been achieved using calorie enhanced formulas with home surveillance monitoring of nutrition and weight gains.[891] Management of these potential challenges is reviewed in the section, Common Clinical Conditions, Altered Nutrition and Potential Gastrointestinal Complications.

Re-coarctations in the aorta are reported in 11% to 37%[170] of patients, and reintervention is most commonly required in the first 6 months after the Norwood procedure.[35] Clinical symptoms include decreased femoral pulses and hypertension in the upper extremities. A gradient of 10 mm Hg or more between the blood pressures in the upper and lower extremities (with the higher pressure in the upper extremities) requires assessment by echocardiography. Re-coarctation also leads to high arterial saturation because the obstruction in the aorta increases systemic vascular resistance, so it increases pulmonary blood flow.[935] The increased pulmonary blood flow can lead to even further pressure and volume load for the right ventricle, resulting in poor ventricular function and signs of heart failure. Re-coarctation is treated successfully by balloon dilation during interventional cardiac catheterization and possible aortic stent implantation or re-operation.[170]

Late complications include progressive congestive heart failure, pulmonary artery distortion, pulmonary vein stenosis and sudden death. The systemic to pulmonary artery shunt (Blalock-Taussig or other) or RV to PA conduit provide the only source for pulmonary blood flow and can progressively narrow at any time, causing increased cyanosis and hypoxemia.

Approximately 5% to 16%[502,812] of immediate survivors of stage 1 Norwood die in the interval between stage 1 and the stage 2 procedures. Multiple risk factors for interstage death include postoperative arrhythmias, decreased ventricular function at discharge,[502,812] and residual or recurrent lesions.

The limited cardiac reserve and chronic hypoxemia and cyanosis in patients with palliated HLHS reduce their tolerance of dehydration, fever, increased metabolic demands, serious respiratory illness, or advancing heart failure. Use of home monitoring protocols have improved interstage survival for surgical[316–318,502] and hybrid stage I[293] palliated HLHS by providing extensive parental education and combinations of home oxygen saturation monitoring, daily weights with digital scales, surveillance for intercurrent illness, and monitoring of oral intake.[318,881,891] National, multicenter quality improvement collaboratives are underway by the Joint Council on Congenital Heart Disease to reduce clinical practice variations and improve long-term outcomes for children with HLHS.[502]

The Sano Procedure. This first stage intervention for HLHS is identical to the Norwood procedure except that the source for pulmonary blood flow is a 5- to 6-mm graft sewn between the right ventricle and the main pulmonary artery.[881] Insertion of this graft requires a small right ventriculotomy (Fig. 8-63, B).

The described potential advantage of the Sano procedure includes the fact that the right ventricle to pulmonary artery connection avoids the low diastolic pressure that results from the aortic runoff with a systemic to pulmonary artery shunt.[514] The aortic diastolic blood pressure has been found to be higher after the Sano procedure, but there is more variability in pulmonary blood flow.[208,316]

Potential postoperative complications include the development of conduit stenosis that produces cyanosis and hypoxemia and requires intervention.[496] Oxygen therapy should be used for these infants with cyanosis because their shunt to the pulmonary system only occurs during systole, rather than during systole and diastole as following a systemic to pulmonary artery shunt.

Reports have not documented any difference between the Norwood and the Sano procedure when freedom from cardiac transplantation after 12 months[670] and survival are evaluated.[53,54,316,317] It may take years to determine the effects of the ventriculotomy and right ventricular to pulmonary artery shunt on right ventricular function and the pulmonary vascular bed.[53]

Long-Term Survival Following Palliation. Survival for infants undergoing the initial palliation for HLHS has dramatically improved in the last decade, with survival to hospital discharge as high as 93%[209,880] to 95%.[315] A 39% 15-year survival rate was reported for patients undergoing a Norwood procedure from 1984 to 1999.[556] Mortality remains high for the Norwood procedure, with the Society of Thoracic Surgeons data centers reporting 18.2% mortality prior to hospital discharge (compared to the 3.2% overall mortality in the Society for Thoracic Surgeons congenital heart disease surgical registry).[823]

The long-term results of this procedure are unknown. There is concern that the right ventricle may not function indefinitely as a systemic ventricle, and that progressive right ventricular dysfunction will develop in a significant number of patients. Life-long continuous followup by experts in congenital heart disease care is mandatory.

Neurodevelopmental disabilities have been reported,[326,554,798,836] include delays in visual-motor integration, motor development, executive function, and behavioral abnormalities. All patients with hypoplastic left heart syndrome require close, ongoing developmental screening for potential complications requiring therapeutic intervention, with a focus on maximizing the neurocognitive outcomes.[115] The risks for developmental delay are summarized by Tweddell et al.[881]

Exercise performance has been shown to decline with age in children undergoing staged interventions for complex congenital heart disease.[413] HLHS is an extremely complex congenital heart defect with multiple variations. To minimize morbidity and maximize quality of life, every child with HLHS requires continual, lifelong care by experts in management of adult congenital heart disease. Guidelines for management of adults with congenital heart disease are published by Warnes et al.[927] Case reports have documented successful pregnancies following the Nowood procedure and later Fontan procedures.[674,910]

Fetal Intervention. Fetal aortic valvuloplasty has been performed to treat aortic stenosis with a goal of preventing the progression to HLHS in the fetus.[562] Growth of the aorta and left ventricle with biventricular circulation has been documented postnatally following the fetal surgery.[562]

Stage 2 and Stage 3 Procedures. A bidirectional Glenn or hemi-Fontan procedure (SVC to pulmonary artery) may be performed at 4 to 6 months of age.[514] A Fontan-type procedure (IVC to the pulmonary artery) anastomosis is the final stage for correction of hypoplastic left heart syndrome and is typically completed near the age of 2 to 4 years.

The Fontan operation separates the pulmonary and systemic circulations. The desaturated systemic venous blood is diverted directly into the pulmonary circulation. Fully saturated pulmonary venous blood is ejected into the systemic circulation by the right ventricle (see section, Single Ventricle, Overview of Management [Including Surgical Procedures]). Before these staged procedures, catheter-based interventions may be completed to treat residual lesions. The goal is to prepare the myocardium and pulmonary vascular bed, avoiding pulmonary vessel distortion and maintaining normal pulmonary vascular resistance.

Advanced Concepts

Advanced concepts in the care of the patient with hypoplastic left heart syndrome are listed in Box 8-43.

Box 8-43 **Advanced Concepts: Hypoplastic Left Heart Syndrome**

- Following stage I palliation, targeted oxygen saturation is approximately 80%. An elevated arterial oxygen saturation (above 85% to 88%) can indicate pulmonary overcirculation that can compromise systemic blood flow and perfusion.
- An elevated arterial oxygen saturation following creation of a systemic to pulmonary artery shunt can be caused by development of aortic re-coarctation distal to the placement of the Blalock-Taussig (or systemic to pulmonary artery) shunt. Assess for difference between upper versus lower extremity pulses and blood pressures.
- A restrictive atrial septal defect may develop following stage I palliation, particularly after a hybrid stage I procedure. A restrictive atrial septal defect limits the left to right atrial shunt and produces elevated left atrial and pulmonary venous pressures, pulmonary edema, increasing hypoxemia, cyanosis, and respiratory distress.
- Oxygen is a potent pulmonary vasodilator and use in single ventricle patients is unnecessary if the systemic arterial oxygen saturation is above 75% or the PaO_2 is greater than 30 mm Hg.
- Interstage morbidity and mortality remain significant after palliation for HLHS. Changes in feeding, increased respiratory effort, tachycardia, lack of weight gain, and irritability may signal adverse hemodynamic changes requiring intervention.

CORONARY ARTERY AND VASCULAR ANOMALIES

Coronary Artery Anomalies

Gwen Paxson Fosse

Etiology

For many years, the coronary arteries were thought to originate from sinuses that formed in the trabeculations of the developing myocardial cells in the embryo. More recently, it has been discovered that the embryonic epicardial cells invade the surface and develop the coronary vascularity. This process is dependent on growth factors, adhesion molecules, and chemotactic factors, which contribute to the formation of the coronary vessels. The coronary arteries grow from the peritruncal area into the aorta. Abnormalities of the signaling pathways or factors that direct this development can result in congenital anomalies of the coronary arteries.[497,581] The anomalies may be described in terms of abnormal origin, course, orifices, number, or connections of the coronary arteries.[283]

Coronary artery anomalies occur in 0.2% to 1.2% of the population, and rarely occur as isolated congenital defects.[242] Coronary fistulae are rare, but with advances in echocardiography there is increasing recognition of this anomaly.[456] Anomalies of the origin of a coronary artery from the pulmonary artery were also thought to be rare but they, too, have been recognized with greater frequency as the result of advances in echocardiography. The most common of these, anomalous origin of the left coronary artery from the pulmonary artery, occurs in only 0.25% to 0.5% of live births.[588]

There are normally two coronary arteries that carry oxygenated blood from the aorta: the left coronary artery, which branches into the left anterior descending and left circumflex arteries, and the right coronary artery. After the cardiac tissue is perfused (from epicardium, through the myocardium to the endocardium) with substrate and oxygen,[283] the coronary venous blood drains into the anterior cardiac veins or the coronary sinus and then into the right atrium.

There are minor, major, and secondary coronary artery anomalies in terms of their anatomic significance. Certainly, many congenital cardiac malformations have secondary abnormalities of coronary artery origin or route but such secondary abnormalities are not the subject of this section. Secondary abnormalities are described with the primary congenital heart defects elsewhere in this Specific Diseases section of this chapter.

Isolated coronary anomalies include the coronary variations such as anomalous aortic origins (origin from the wrong sinus of Valsalva in the aortic valve, which in some cases can be clinically significant), high take-off, multiple ostia, single ostium, abnormal branching, stenoses, and others. Another coronary anomaly is coronary aneurysm; in children it is most often associated with Kawasaki disease. An abnormal intramyocardial course of coronary arteries (known as bridging), typically does not require intervention.

The anomalies addressed here include anomalous coronary artery origins from the pulmonary artery instead of from the aorta; some anomalous aortic origins of coronary arteries;

fistulas of a coronary arteries; and congenital atresia of the left main coronary artery.[242,446,456,588]

Pathophysiology

Anomalous Coronary Artery Origins from the Pulmonary Artery. Anomalous left coronary artery originating from the pulmonary artery (ALCAPA, Bland White Garland syndrome) is the most common of these anomalies. When the left coronary artery arises from the pulmonary artery, it is likely that no changes occur during fetal life when pressures in the aorta and pulmonary artery are approximately equal. After birth, the left ventricle is perfused with desaturated blood flow from the pulmonary artery, under low pressure; this leads to left ventricular ischemia and often causes heart failure. Soon, collateral vessels develop from branches of the *right* coronary artery to branches of the anomalous left coronary artery. Once the collateral vessels develop, blood flow from the right coronary artery travels retrograde through the branches of the left coronary artery into the low resistance pulmonary artery, instead of perfusing the high resistance coronary vasculature. The effect is a "steal" of right coronary blood flow, causing angina and ischemia.[242]

Other anomalous coronary artery origins from the pulmonary artery are rarer: anomalous origin of the right coronary artery from the pulmonary artery (ARCAPA), anomalous origin of the circumflex coronary artery from the pulmonary artery (ACxPA), and anomalous right and left coronaries from the pulmonary artery.[242]

Anomalous Aortic Origins of Coronary Arteries. Some of these variations are not clinically significant, whereas others can be fatal. When there is aberrant origin of the left main coronary artery (LMCA) from the right aortic sinus of Valsalva (RASV) or aberrant origin of the right coronary artery (RCA) from the left aortic sinus of Valsalva (LASV) there can be cardiac symptoms and sudden death caused by episodes of ischemia.[242] When the LMCA originates from the RASV, the right coronary artery provides the majority of coronary circulation; the risk of ischemia and sudden death is particularly high if the path of the left main coronary artery courses between the great arteries, because it can be compressed.[242]

Coronary Artery Fistulas. Fistulas are the most common type of hemodynamically significant coronary anomalies; they can be congenital or acquired. Fistulas can be isolated or can occur in combination with other heart defects.[242] They can involve the right (most common), left, or both coronary arteries.[497] The fistulous connection can involve a coronary vein, a vena cava, a chamber of the heart, a great artery, pulmonary vessels, or an aorto-left ventricular tunnel.[242,446,456,497]

A fistula produces shunting of flow from the higher pressure to the lower pressure end of the fistula. The most common type of fistula is a coronary artery to right-heart structure (arteriovenous) fistula, which results in a left-to-right shunt.[497] When the fistula connects to a left heart structure (arterioarterial fistula) there may be runoff from the aorta during low pressure phases of the cardiac cycle; this runoff can increase left ventricular volume load.[497]

Congenital Atresia of the Left Main Coronary Artery (CALM). In this very rare anomaly, the right coronary artery perfuses the entire heart. It does this in a retrograde fashion via collaterals to the left anterior descending and the circumflex coronary arteries. This lesion is associated with supravalvular aortic stenosis particularly with Williams-Beuren syndrome.[588]

Clinical Signs and Symptoms

Anomalous Coronary Artery Origins from the Pulmonary Artery. Anomalous left coronary artery from the pulmonary artery (ALCAPA) often produces ischemia and symptoms in early infancy with evidence of pain (presumably caused by angina), failure to thrive, signs of heart failure, and in some cases, signs of low cardiac output (shock). The symptoms may mimic those of cardiomyopathy or endocardial fibroelastosis.

In cases of adequate collateral circulation, symptoms may not develop until later childhood and even into adult years. Signs may include a nonspecific systolic murmur at the base or an apical pansystolic murmur caused by mitral regurgitation secondary to left ventricular failure. Cardiomegaly, hepatomegaly, and rales may be present.

A hoarse cry in infancy has been reported as the presenting symptom of ALCAPA, and it has been theorized that dilation of the pulmonary artery impinges on the recurrent laryngeal nerve.[16] ARCAPA is rarely associated with sudden death.[947]

On electrocardiogram there is often evidence of left ventricular hypertrophy and there may be ST-segment changes related to ischemia or infarction. Cardiomegaly and pulmonary edema are often visible on chest radiograph. Echocardiography shows the dilated left ventricle with changes in function, possibly mitral valve changes, and the anomalous coronary artery may be evident. Definitive diagnosis can be made with cardiac catheterization and cineangiography delineating the coronary anatomy.[431,497]

Anomalous Aortic Origins of Coronary Arteries. There may be no distinct clinical or ECG findings with this anomaly. Angina may be described with or without exertion. Diagnosis can be made by angiography, echocardiography, magnetic resonance imaging,[497] and computed tomography.[283] If the anomalous coronary artery courses between the aorta and the right ventricular infundibulum (pulmonary root), there may be compression of the coronary artery, particularly with strenuous exertion. Such compression can lead to sudden ischemia and sudden death that may be the first indication of the anomaly. Some patients do have a history of syncope or prolonged chest pain.[581]

Anomalous coronary artery origin (left main coronary artery from the RASV, with the artery coursing between the aorta and the right ventricular outflow tract) was found in 35% of the victims in the U.S. military recruit sudden death autopsy data; some had a history of syncope and/or exertional chest pain.[251]

Coronary Artery Fistulas. Patients with coronary artery fistulas typically present later in life with a continuous murmur, mild cardiomegaly, increased pulmonary vascular markings on chest radiograph, or infective endocarditis; the fistula may be an incidental finding when angiography is performed for other reasons. Symptoms are rare unless there is an exceptionally large fistula but can include symptoms of heart failure caused by a left-to-right shunt, angina, or myocardial infarction.

The ECG and chest radiograph may be normal or may provide suggestive but nonspecific evidence. Echocardiography may establish the diagnosis, particularly if the fistula is large. Cardiac catheterization can provide the definitive diagnosis with aortography and selective coronary angiograms.[336,497] Endocarditis and aneurysm with rupture have been reported with this lesion.[456]

Congenital Atresia of the Left Main Coronary Artery (CALM). Clinical findings are virtually the same as with ALCAPA. Definitive diagnosis is made during catheterization and angiography, which allows differentiation of these lesions.[588]

Management

Anomalous Coronary Artery Origin from the Pulmonary Artery. Diagnosis of anomalous left coronary artery originating from the pulmonary artery (ALCAPA) is an indication for surgery. A median sternotomy incision, cardiopulmonary bypass, hypothermia, and cardioplegia are typically used for this surgery. Careful management is necessary in patients with symptoms of poor myocardial perfusion, to avoid ventricular fibrillation before establishing cardiopulmonary bypass.

Surgical strategies are aimed at constructing a system of two coronary arteries perfused with aortic blood flow. Surgical approaches vary depending on the position of the coronary artery in relation to the aorta. If possible the left coronary artery is transferred from the pulmonary artery to the aorta. A Takeuchi procedure (tunnel repair) may be required if the coronary artery is not near the aorta. An aortopulmonary connection (window) is created and blood from the aorta is tunneled through the window to the coronary origin in the pulmonary trunk.

In older patients when other alternatives are not possible, a connection from a subclavian artery to the coronary artery (Meyer procedure) may be created to provide coronary arterial flow. Coronary bypass grafting techniques may be used in some cases. Another option is ligation of the coronary artery to eliminate the steal phenomenon, but this is associated with higher mortality.

Death in the first year of life occurs in about 65% of patients with ALCAPA if there is no surgery. Surgical intervention is associated with high early and late survival, especially if there is no significant left ventricular dysfunction or mitral regurgitation preoperatively.[154,497,588]

When the right or both coronary arteries originate from the pulmonary artery the surgical approach is similar to that described above.[497] ARCAPA has a lower surgical risk than ALCAPA.[947]

Anomalous Aortic Origins of Coronary Arteries. Surgical approaches to these defects are aimed at restoring the normal anatomy and avoiding proximal obstruction of the coronary ostia. Strategies may include coronary artery bypass grafting, opening the origin of the coronary artery within the aorta to create unobstructed coronary flow, an unroofing procedure to open the origin of the artery, or reimplantation of the coronary artery.

When the coronary artery courses between the great arteries, the pulmonary artery trunk may be separated from the aorta to prevent coronary compression. Because the frequency of this defect is low and the anatomy varies widely, the outcomes with and without surgery are difficult to ascertain.[497,588] Ischemia may develop even after surgical creation of a new ostia. Such ischemia may create persistent risk of sudden death.[116]

Coronary Artery Fistulas. In rare cases, spontaneous closure of a fistula has been reported. Intervention is recommended only if symptoms are present. In some cases coil occlusion of the fistula is possible during cardiac catheterization. Otherwise, surgery is performed through a median sternotomy incision and usually requires cardiopulmonary bypass. The fistula is identified, approached through the vessel or chamber, and sutures are used to close the connection. Without treatment the natural history of these defects has not been clearly determined, but surgical and hospital mortality, rate of complications, and late mortality are all very low.[497]

Congenital Atresia of the Left Main Coronary Artery (CALM). Surgery is recommended upon diagnosis. Open-heart surgery coronary artery bypass techniques are employed to establish left anterior descending coronary artery flow. Without treatment the prognosis is poor and surgery is associated with low mortality.[588]

Preoperative and Postoperative Care. For all coronary artery anomalies, nursing care involves managing congestive heart failure and low cardiac output (including symptomatic arrhythmias) as needed. It is important to identify any signs of ST-segment or T-wave changes indicative of ischemia or infarction (see Arrhythmias).

The postoperative period may be complicated by low cardiac output and ventricular arrhythmias.[154] For this reason, it is advisable to avoid excessive volume resuscitation or excessive catecholamine administration in the postoperative period. Extracorporeal membrane oxygenation may be employed as needed in the early postoperative period to improve survival (see Chapter 7).[154,588]

Vascular Rings
Etiology
Vascular rings are created by abnormal branches of the aorta and systemic arteries that form a ring of vessels that encircle and potentially compress the trachea and esophagus. The most common vascular rings are created by a double aortic arch, a right aortic arch with left ligamentum arteriosus (the ligament formed after constriction of the ductus arteriosus or aberrant left subclavian artery), an anomalous innominate or left common carotid artery, or a pulmonary artery sling.[930] These forms of vascular rings are illustrated and described in Table 8-39.[459]

During fetal life, six pairs of aortic arches are initially formed. These arches reform and involute, and they contribute to the formation of the aortic arch, the innominate and left subclavian arteries, and the right and left pulmonary arteries (see Evolve Fig. 8-1 in the Chapter 8 Supplement on the Evolve Website). If this process is disrupted, anomalies of the aortic arch and its major branches can result in the formation of a vascular ring. Anomalies of aortic arch formation have been found in patients with chromosome 22q-11 deletion.[930]

Pathophysiology
The specific complications resulting from a vascular ring will be determined, in part, by the location of the anomalous vessels. However, if compression of the trachea and esophagus is significant, it will cause upper airway obstruction. This compression often is exacerbated during feeding when the esophagus further compresses the trachea. A prolonged expiratory time may be present, and air trapping may develop.

Vascular rings often are associated with additional cardiovascular malformations. Common associated lesions include atrial septal defect, ventricular septal defect, and tetralogy of Fallot. Abnormalities of the tracheobronchial tree may be present.

Clinical Signs and Symptoms
The most striking signs of vascular ring are those of respiratory distress. The infant may appear normal at birth, but usually demonstrates progression of symptoms during the first months of life. The infant may develop recurrent respiratory infections and frequently demonstrates wheezing or stridor. Congestion often is present and is not cleared by coughing. Esophageal compression (most commonly associated with an aberrant right subclavian artery) is associated with the development of dysphagia.

Typically the signs of respiratory distress worsen during feeding and when the infant is placed in a reclining position. Cyanotic episodes or the development of apnea are ominous signs and indicate the presence of severe obstruction and risk of respiratory arrest; these children require urgent surgical intervention.

The infant often lies with the neck hyperextended and prefers the upright position. A crowing stridor often is observed.[930]

A plain lateral chest film may demonstrate compression of the trachea and esophagus. In addition, the presence of a right aortic arch or double aortic arch often is detected by plain chest radiograph or echocardiography. An echocardiogram also allows identification of the vessels involved in the compression.

Computed tomography (CT) angiography (with contrast injection into a peripheral vein) allows visualization of the ring in multiple planes. When a vascular ring is present but not all vessels are patent, one of "three Ds" can typically be identified by computed tomography, on the side opposite the side of the aortic arch: **d**iverticulum (a large vessel arising from the descending aorta that gives rise to a smaller vessel that suddenly tapers), **d**imple (a tapered outpouching of the aorta that has a blind ending), and the **d**escending aorta that is opposite the side of the aortic arch. A ligamentum arteriosus will not be visible on an angiogram. Additional studies such as a barium swallow (contrast esophagram) may be required to

Table 8-39 Vascular Rings

Lesion	Symptoms	Plain Film (Chest x-ray)	Barium Swallow	Bronchoscopy	Angiography	Treatment
Double arch	Stridor; Respiratory distress; Swallowing dysfunction; Reflex apnea	AP—Wider base of heart; Lat.—Narrowed trachea displaced forward at C3-C4	Bilateral indentation of esophagus	Bilateral tracheal compression—both pulsatile	Diagnostic but often unnecessary	Ligate and divide smaller arch (usually left)
Right arch and ligamentum/ductus	Respiratory distress; Swallowing dysfunction	AP—Tracheal deviation to left (right arch)	Bilateral indentation of esophagus R > L	Bilateral tracheal compression—R. pulsatile	Usually unnecessary	Ligate ligamentum or ductus
Aberrant right subclavian	Occasional swallowing dysfunction	Normal	AP—Oblique defect upward to right; Lat.—Small defect on right posterior wall	Usually normal	Diagnostic but often unnecessary	Ligate artery
Anomalous innominate	Cough; Stridor; Reflex apnea	AP—Normal; Lat.—Anterior tracheal compression	Normal	Pulsatile anterior tracheal compression	Unnecessary	Conservative. If apnea, suspend artery
Pulmonary sling	Expiratory stridor; Respiratory distress	AP—Low left hilum, right emphysema/atelectasis; Lat.—Anterior bowing of right bronchus and trachea	±Anterior indentation above carina between esophagus and trachea	Tracheal displacement to left; Compression of right main bronchus	Diagnostic	Detach and reanastomose to main pulmonary artery in front of trachea

From Keith HM: Vascular rings and tracheobronchial compression in infants. *Pediatr Ann* 6(8):542-543, 1977.

determine the location and severity of tracheoesophageal compression.

A bronchoscopy can be performed to confirm the presence of tracheal compression, particularly if an anomalous innominate artery is present. Typically, when compression of the trachea by an anomalous innominate artery is observed during bronchoscopy, bronchoscopic pressure against the site of compression will result in obliteration of the pulse in the ipsilateral arm.

Management

The child with vascular ring and respiratory distress must be monitored closely because apnea and respiratory arrest may develop. Surgical intervention is planned during infancy to remove the tracheal compression so the trachea can grow.

Surgical intervention is accomplished through a thoracotomy incision. If a double aortic arch is present, the smaller (remnant or diminutive) arch is tied and divided, and the ligamentum arteriosus also is divided. If an anomalous innominate artery is contributing to tracheal compression, it often is pulled away from the trachea and suspended by sutures from the posterior portion of the sternum. If a pulmonary artery sling is present the anomalous pulmonary vessel usually is ligated, and an anastomosis is performed anterior to the trachea between the anomalous pulmonary vessel and the left pulmonary artery.

Respiratory secretions are often copious postoperatively because the child is able to mobilize and clear the secretions. For this reason, pulmonary hygiene must be excellent.

CARDIAC INFECTION, INFLAMMATION AND TUMORS

Infective Endocarditis

Gwen Paxson Fosse

Etiology

Infective endocarditis is an infection and inflammation of a structure of the heart that results from attachment of a microorganism (usually bacteria) to damaged cardiac endothelial tissue. Infective endocarditis can cause cardiac and extracardiac complications. This disease was previously known as "bacterial endocarditis" but the name was changed to reflect the fact that causative organisms in addition to bacteria have been implicated.

Although most endocarditis is caused by bacteria, less commonly, endocarditis results from fungal, viral, or rickettsial organisms. Organisms most frequently found are *Staphylococcus, Streptococcus viridans,* and *Enterococcus*; all have adherent factors that allow them to attach to tissue.[499]

Infective endocarditis causes significant mortality and morbidity. The brain is the most common site of endocarditis emboli, and cerebrovascular complications of endocarditis carry a mortality rate of 80% to 90%.[247,499] In pediatrics, endocarditis caused by staphylococci has the highest mortality rate.[573] Factors that impact prognosis include age, etiologic event, presence of congestive heart failure, extent of cardiac involvement, and presence of complications.

Endocarditis is most likely to affect children with underlying cardiovascular disease (congenital or acquired), which provides an abnormal endocardial surface to which microorganisms can adhere. This is especially true in children who have areas of high-velocity turbulent flow (e.g., associated with aortic stenosis, ventricular septal defect, and other high-velocity shunting lesions) where shunting blood can damage endothelium (see also Box 8-44). Other children at risk are those who have undergone surgical intervention for congenital heart disease, particularly procedures involving placement of prosthetic materials (valves, grafts, etc.).[737] Nearly 20% of involved patients, however, have no known cardiovascular disease.

Other risk factors in the neonatal and pediatric critical care population include the use of invasive technology and intracardiac catheters (these account for 8% to 10% of pediatric endocarditis), immunocompromise, presence of ventriculoatrial shunts for hydrocephalus,[266] intravenous drug abuse (especially associated with right heart endocarditis),[234] and body art (piercings, especially of colonized mucosal surfaces, and tattoos), particularly if there is also a cardiac risk factor.[69,172,214,348,956] Historically the purposes of body art have included marking rights of passage, religious celebrations, utilitarian reasons, military and prisoner marking, and cosmetic purposes.[172,956] Popularity of body art was rekindled in the Punk era at the end of the 1970s and has increased in recent years, especially among adolescents and young adults.[741]

Box 8-44   **Endocarditis Risk Factors in Pediatrics**

Relatively High Risk Factors
- Previous infective endocarditis
- Prosthetic heart valves
- Cyanotic congenital heart disease
- Patent ductus arteriosus
- Aortic regurgitation
- Aortis stenosis
- Mitral regurgitation
- Mitral stenosis with regurgitation
- Ventricular septal defect
- Coarctation of aorta
- Surgically repaired intracardiac lesion with residual hemodynamic abnormality

Intermediate Risk Factors
- Mitral valve prolapse with regurgitation
- Pure mitral stenosis
- Tricuspid valve disease
- Pulmonary stenosis
- Asymmetrical septal hypertrophy (hypertrophic cardiomyopathy)
- Bicuspid aortic valve disease
- Calcific aortic sclerosis with minimal hemodynamic abnormality
- Degenerative valve disease in elderly patients
- Surgically repaired intracardiac lesion with minimal hemodynamic abnormality less than six months after surgery

From Sharan L, Kamlesh M. Managing infective endocarditis. *Fed Pract* 18 (11):48, 2001.

Although endocarditis occurs in children of all ages, nearly half of the patients involved are older than 10 years of age. Because this form of infection can result in progressive cardiovascular dysfunction, thromboembolic events, and possible death, preventive measures are essential and prompt detection and treatment are needed.

Gram positive cocci are most commonly responsible for pediatric endocarditis, and *streptococcus* (primarily *S. viridans*) and *staphylococcus* (primarily *S. aureus*) are identified in approximately 80% of all cases of pediatric endocarditis.[573] Enterococcus can also cause endocarditis and is associated with concurrent urinary tract infections.[573]

Fungal organisms, although rare, are particularly virulent and are most likely to be identified in neonates or other immunologically compromised patients. A small number (5% to 7%)[573] of patients with endocarditis remain culture negative primarily because antibiotics are often administered before cultures are obtained.

Pathophysiology

Infective endocarditis requires the presence of an invading organism as well as predisposing host factors (Fig. 8-64). As noted, most affected children have underlying valvular or other structural heart disease that create pressure gradients and turbulent blood flow.

Microorganisms gain entry to the cardiovascular system in a variety of ways. Typically, endocarditis results from an extracardiac infection or an organism that originates in a colonized mucosal surface or infected tissue and gains entry via the oral cavity, the vascular system, the genitourinary or gastrointestinal tract, or with an injury (including trauma from dental, surgical, or other procedures) to colonized or infected tissues. Activities of daily life such as chewing, brushing teeth, and bowel movements routinely result in bacteremias, which are typically low grade, and the normally functioning immune system prevents consequent infection.

The most common congenital heart defects found among patients with bacterial endocarditis are ventricular septal defect and aortic stenosis. Tetralogy of Fallot, coarctation of the aorta, patent ductus arteriosus, and transposition of the great vessels are also relatively common associated defects.

Turbulent blood flow results in mural tissue damage with deposition of platelets and fibrin and thrombus formation. Circulating microorganisms become trapped in this thrombus, becoming the focus of the endocarditis. These foci were described by Lazare Riviere in 1646, "In the left ventricle of the heart, round caruncles were found like the substance of the lungs,... resembled a cluster of hazelnuts and filled up the opening of the aorta." These colonies of microorganisms and the resulting deposition of fibrin and platelets form lesions, commonly called vegetations, which usually become encased in a fibrin network. The fibrin network makes phagocytosis by circulating leukocytes and elimination by circulating antibiotics difficult. In addition, the lesions may contribute to valvular insufficiency or portions of the lesions may embolize to other organs. The potential manifestations and consequences of endocarditis are numerous (Box 8-45) and are associated with significant mortality and morbidity.

The pathophysiology of bacterial endocarditis is not limited to the immediate effects of the bacterial lesions and any hemodynamic or embolic consequences they produce. The infectious process also results in complement activation and activation of portions of the inflammatory response that may contribute to the development of renal dysfunction.

Box 8-45 **Potential Manifestations and Consequences of Endocarditis**

Cardiovascular
- Damaged or destroyed valves
- Damage of the aorta
- Endocardial changes
- Pericarditis
- Myocarditis
- Myocardial infarction due to emboli
- Fistula formation
- Abscess formation
- Rhythm disturbances
- Hemorrhage of eroded vessels

Neurologic
- Cerebral infarction caused by emboli
- Acute hemiplegia
- Seizure, ataxia
- Aphasia
- Change in mental status
- Abscess formation
- Mycotic aneurysm
- Meningitis

Other
- Immunologic
  ◦ Hypergammaglobulinemic state
  ◦ Increased circulating immune complexes
  ◦ Splenomegaly
- Renal
  ◦ Glomerulonephritis
  ◦ Renal failure
- Emboli of infected debris with ischemia or infarcts—lungs, liver, spleen, kidneys, and skin.
- Sepsis and multisystem organ failure

From Korkola SJ, Tchervenkov CI, Mavroudis C. Infective endocarditis. In Mavroudis C, Backer CL, editors. *Pediatric cardiac surgery*, ed 3, Philadelphia, 2003, Mosby/Elsevier, p. 769.

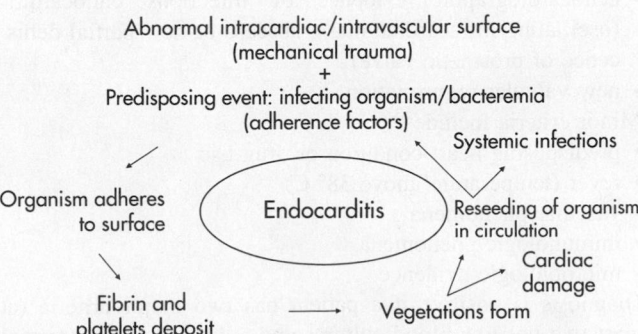

FIG. 8-64 Pathophysiology of endocarditis.

The lesions eventually heal after successful antimicrobial therapy, but weeks of intravenous therapy usually are required to ensure destruction of the organism. There may be significant sequelae (as listed in Box 8-45), necessitating a variety of medical or surgical interventions.

Clinical Signs and Symptoms

The onset of endocarditis can be acute and fulminant, potentially resulting in death within weeks, or slow and insidious with low-grade fever, malaise, and night sweats recurring over months. A high index of suspicion for endocarditis is needed when caring for a patient with a cardiac lesion. Findings are often subtle and early detection and treatment are imperative to limit endocardial damage and reduce mortality and morbidity. Any indication that a patient may have endocarditis warrants investigation: obtain blood cultures promptly.

Some of the symptoms of endocarditis can mimic those seen with active rheumatic fever but positive blood cultures will distinguish between the two. Acute rheumatic fever and endocarditis do not happen simultaneously.[289]

If endocarditis is present on the left side of the heart, systemic emboli often produce extremity ischemia with pain and compromise of perfusion, renal dysfunction, arthralgia, or focal neurologic signs; specific signs are determined by the location of the embolus. Additional signs of endocarditis include the development of new or changing murmurs, fever, and subtle signs of illness, including malaise, headache, or arthralgia. The list of possible signs and symptoms is extensive (Table 8-40).[104]

The presence of endocarditis is suggested by a positive blood culture. Blood cultures are positive in 85% to 95% of cases of infective endocarditis.[248] If a child has received antibiotics before the identification of the infecting organism, special techniques may allow isolation of the organism from subsequent blood cultures. Repeat blood cultures (up to three sets in 24 h) are often necessary to isolate an organism, and a small number of children with endocarditis never have a positive blood culture.

Additional nonspecific laboratory tests suggestive of endocarditis include positive acute phase reactants. The erythrocyte sedimentation rate is typically elevated, as is the C-reactive protein. Some laboratories are able to perform complex antigen or antibody studies or isolate peripheral reticuloendothelial cells; these studies are not used widely.

Although the ECG may not be helpful in the diagnosis of endocarditis (other than possible onset of new conduction disturbances), the echocardiogram often enables visualization of vegetations and is considered an essential tool in diagnosis. A negative echocardiogram, however, will not rule out the presence of endocarditis. The chest radiograph may show evidence of congestive heart failure and/or changes indicative of pulmonary embolic lesions or abscess.

Diagnosis often is based on the Duke Criteria for the Diagnosis of Infective Endocarditis.[248,532] Major criteria include[532]:

- positive blood culture for microorganisms typical for endocarditis (two positive cultures typically required, drawn more than 12 h apart although single positive culture for

Table 8-40 Signs and Symptoms of Endocarditis

Sign/Symptom	Incidence in Endocarditis Population (%)
Fever*	95-100
Onset of murmur	80-85
New or changing murmur	10-40
Chills	42-75
Sweating	25
Anorexia and weight loss	25-55
Malaise	25-40
Dyspnea	20-40
Cough	25
Stroke	13-20
Headache	15-40
Nausea, vomiting	15-20
Myalgia/arthralgia	15-30
Chest pain	8-35
Abdominal pain	5-15
Back pain	7-10
Confusion	10-20
Neurological abnormalities	30-40
Embolic event	20-40
Splenomegaly	15-50
Clubbing	10-20
Peripheral manifestations*	
Osler's nodes (painful lesions on finger and toes)	7-10
Splinter hemorrhages (seen in nail beds)	5-15
Petechiae	10-40
Janeway lesions (nontender lesions on palms/soles)	6-10
Retinal lesions/Roth spots (retinal hemorrhage with pale center)	4-10
Evidence of vascular phenomena (emboli, infarcts, hemorrhage, aneurysm)*	Variable depending on location

From Braunwald E, Zipes DP, Libby P. *Heart disease*, ed 6, Philadelphia, 2001, Saunders, p. 1730, lexi.com/web/news.isp?id=100025.
*Duke Minor Criteria for diagnosis of endocarditis. Durack DT, Lukes AS, Bright DK. The Duke Endocarditis Service. New criteria for diagnosis of infective endocarditis: utilization of specific echocardiographic findings. *Am J Med* 96:200-209, 1994.

Coxiella burnetii or antiphase 1 IgG antibody titer greater than 1:800 acceptable)
- evidence of endocardial involvement
- echocardiographic evidence of infectious endocarditis (oscillating intracardiac mass, abscess or new partial dehiscence of prosthetic valve)
- new valvular regurgitation.

Minor criteria include[532]:
- predisposing heart condition or drug use
- fever (temperature above 38° C)
- vascular phenomena
- immunologic phenomena
- microbiologic evidence.

Diagnosis is positive if a patient has two major criteria (at least two positive blood cultures and evidence of endocardial involvement typically determined by transthoracic or transesophageal echocardiographic evidence), one major plus three minor criteria, or five minor criteria.[248,532]

Prevention and Management

Prevention. Prevention rather than need to treat endocarditis is the goal. However, several aspects of endocarditis prophylaxis remain controversial. For many years the American Heart Association (AHA) has published extensive recommendations regarding antibiotic prophylaxis for the prevention of endocarditis under a variety of circumstances; these recommendations have been revised over the years based on review of published evidence. These guidelines address the administration of specified antibiotics before an event that is likely to cause entry of causative organisms into the circulation of an individual with risk factors. It is always prudent to obtain and follow the most current guidelines published by the AHA.[951]

In 2007 significant revisions were made in the AHA Guidelines for Endocarditis Prophylaxis because of the absence of high-level evidence that the prophylaxis decreases costs, reduces the risk for allergic reactions (including anaphylaxis) by reducing exposure to antibiotics, and reduces antibiotic overuse that can promote development of resistant organisms.

The 2007 Guidelines noted:

The major changes in the updated recommendations include the following: (1) The Committee concluded that only an extremely small number of cases of infective endocarditis might be prevented by antibiotic prophylaxis for dental procedures even if such prophylactic therapy were 100% effective. (2) Infective endocarditis prophylaxis for dental procedures is reasonable only for patients with underlying cardiac conditions associated with the highest risk of adverse outcome from infective endocarditis. (3) For patients with these underlying cardiac conditions, prophylaxis is reasonable for all dental procedures that involve manipulation of gingival tissue or the periapical region of teeth or perforation of the oral mucosa. (4) Prophylaxis is not recommended based solely on an increased lifetime risk of acquisition of infective endocarditis. (5) Administration of antibiotics solely to prevent endocarditis is not recommended for patients who undergo a genitourinary or gastrointestinal tract procedure. These changes are intended to define more clearly when infective endocarditis prophylaxis is or is not recommended and to provide more uniform and consistent global recommendations."[951]

Table 8-41 highlights the AHA guidelines for prevention of infective endocarditis, published in October 2007.[951]

The 2007 AHA Endocarditis Prevention guidelines produced some controversy. Concerns have been expressed regarding confusion over changes, medical and dental legal considerations, and no recommended prophylaxis for some lesions that were previously considered at higher risk for endocarditis, such as ventricular septal defect, patent ductus arteriosus, and aortic stenosis. Apprehension is natural following major guidelines changes because antibiotic prophylaxis was recommended in past guidelines for more types of congenital heart defects, and was recommended preoperatively

and postoperatively (without a 6-month limitation) and in some cases was recommended even if postoperatively the child had no residual defect.

Currently, in many cases the recommendation for prophylaxis is based on the presence of residua.[951] Because the heart is a dynamic organ in dynamic individuals the absence of residua at one moment may not be so later. Also, residua may be difficult to rule out when diagnostic techniques may be hindered by lack of cooperation in young children. Practitioners are advised to use judgment to make appropriate decisions in each individual case.

Nonpharmacologic endocarditis prevention measures are those which educate patients and parents and can reduce events that cause bacteremia (Box 8-46). These precautions should always be followed and included in published and online information for patients and parents. It is the duty of nurses and the entire healthcare team to teach patients and parents about these precautions, which include appropriate antibiotic treatment of infections, good dental hygiene and care, timing of dental care to avoid dental procedures close to the time of cardiac interventions, good skin care, and education about risky behaviors and risk factors.

Treatment. Effective treatment of endocarditis requires several weeks of intravenous antibiotic therapy. Delay of effective antibiotic therapy is associated with greater incidence of complications. The choice of antibiotics is determined by the organism and its sensitivity to antibiotics, as well as the site(s) of associated infection. During therapy the serum peak bactericidal titer will be monitored to evaluate the effectiveness of the antibiotic regimen and the likelihood of cure.

If a prosthetic valve is infected, 6 weeks of intravenous antibiotic therapy will be required. If cardiovascular deterioration, systemic embolic events, obstruction, regurgitation, or staphylococcal endocarditis with heart failure are present with prosthetic valve endocarditis, valve replacement will be required under urgent conditions.[499]

Surgery may be necessary to remove infected tissue and restore better hemodynamics. For endocarditis without a prosthetic valve, surgical indications may include refractory congestive heart failure, uncontrolled infection, repeated serious embolic episodes, fungal or other difficult-to-treat endocarditis, the presence of prosthetic material, progressive renal failure, severe valve dysfunction, the presence of an echocardiographically identifiable intracardiac vegetation (although this is controversial), and invasion of cardiac tissue leading to conduction disturbances, abscesses, or cardiac fistulae.[495,499] Surgery may be indicated after the acute endocarditis is resolved if there are significant hemodynamic sequelae amenable to repair. Before surgical intervention the child's neurologic status must be monitored closely to detect any evidence of cerebral emboli.

Postoperative care includes all typical interventions after cardiac surgery, with emphasis on care likely to be required in light of the valve or tissue involved. Additional considerations are hemodynamic consequences associated with sepsis (see Chapter 6), treatment of other affected organs, anticoagulation implications if a mechanical valve is used and the patient has experienced hemorrhagic complications,

Table 8-41 Prevention of Infective Endocarditis: 2007 Guidelines from the American Heart Association

A. Cardiac Conditions Associated with the Highest Risk of Adverse Outcome from Endocarditis for Which Prophylaxis with Dental Procedures is Reasonable

Prosthetic cardiac valve or prosthetic material used for cardiac valve repair

Previous Infective Endocarditis (IE)

Congenital heart disease (CHD)*

- Unrepaired cyanotic CHD, including palliative shunts and conduits
- Completely repaired congenital heart defect with prosthetic material or device, whether placed by surgery or by catheter intervention, during the first 6 months after the procedure[†]
- Repaired CHD with residual defects at the site or adjacent to the site of a prosthetic patch or prosthetic device (which inhibit endothelialization)

Cardiac transplantation recipients who develop cardiac valvulopathy

B. Dental Procedures for Which Endocarditis Prophylaxis Is Reasonable for Patients Identified in Part A

All *dental procedures* that involve manipulation of gingival tissue or the periapical region of teeth or perforation of the oral mucosa[‡]

C. Regimens for a Dental Procedure

Situation	Agent	REGIMEN: SINGLE DOSE 30-60 MIN BEFORE PROCEDURE	
		Adults	Children
Oral	Amoxicillin	2 g	50 mg/kg
Unable to take oral medication	Ampicillin	2 g IM or IV	50 mg/kg IM or IV
	OR		
	Cefazolin or ceftriaxone	1 g IM or IV	50 mg/kg IM or IV
Allergic to penicillins or ampicillin-oral	Cephalexin[§,‖]	2 g	50 mg/kg
	OR		
	Clindamycin	600 mg	20 mg/kg
	OR		
	Azithromycin or clarithromycin	500 mg	15 mg/kg
Allergic to penicillins or ampicillin and unable to take oral medication	Cefazolin or ceftriaxone[‖]	1 g IM or IV	50 mg/kg IM or IV
	OR		
	Clindamycin	600 mg IM or IV	20 mg/kg IM or IV

D. Summary of Major Changes in 2007 Guidelines

We concluded that bacteremia resulting from daily activities is much more likely to cause IE than bacteremia associated with a dental procedure.

We concluded that only an extremely small number of cases of IE might be prevented by antibiotic prophylaxis even if prophylaxis is 100% effective.

Antibiotic prophylaxis is not recommended based solely on an increased lifetime risk of acquisition of IE.

Limit recommendations for IE prophylaxis only to those conditions listed in part A of this table.

Antibiotic prophylaxis is no longer recommended for any other form of CHD, except for the conditions listed in part A of this table.

Antibiotic prophylaxis is reasonable for all dental procedures that involve manipulation of gingival tissues or periapical region of teeth or perforation of oral mucosa only for patients with underlying cardiac conditions associated with the highest risk of adverse outcome from IE (see part A).

Antibiotic prophylaxis is reasonable for procedures on respiratory tract or infected skin, skin structures, or musculoskeletal tissue only for patients with underlying cardiac conditions associated with the highest risk of adverse outcome from IE (see part A).

Antibiotic prophylaxis solely to prevent IE is not recommended for GU or GI tract procedures. If enterococcal colonization is present in the urinary tract, elective urinary tract procedures should be deferred until it is eradicated.

Although these guidelines recommend changes in indications for IE prophylaxis with regard to selected dental procedures (see text), the writing group reaffirms that those medical procedures listed as not requiring IE prophylaxis in the 1997 statement remain unchanged and extends this view to vaginal delivery, hysterectomy, and tattooing. Additionally, the committee advises against body piercing for patients with conditions listed in part A because of the possibility of bacteremia, while recognizing that there are minimal published data regarding the risk of bacteremia or endocarditis associated with body piercing.

The Council on Scientific Affairs of the American Dental Association has approved the guideline as it relates to dentistry. In addition, this guideline has been endorsed by the American Academy of Pediatrics, Infectious Diseases Society of America, the International Society of Chemotherapy for Infection and Cancer, and the Pediatric Infectious Diseases Society.[¶]

Wilson W, Taubert KA, Gewitz M, et al: Prevention of infective endocarditis. Guidelines from the American Heart Association: A Guideline from the American Heart Association Rheumatic Fever, Endocarditis, and Kawasaki Disease Committee, Council on Cardiovascular Disease in the Young, and the Council on Clinical Cardiology, Council on Cardiovascular Surgery and Anesthesia, and the Quality of Care and Outcomes Research Interdisciplinary Working Group. *Circulation* 116:1736-1754, 2007. Copyright 2007 American Heart Association, Inc.

*Except for the conditions listed above, antibiotic prophylaxis is no longer recommended for any other form of CHD.

[†]Prophylaxis is reasonable because endothelialization of prosthetic material occurs within 6 months after the procedure.

[‡]The following procedures and events do not need prophylaxis: routine anesthetic injections through noninfected tissue, taking dental radiographs, placement of removable prosthodontic or orthodontic appliances, adjustment of orthodontic appliances, placement of orthodontic brackets, shedding of deciduous teeth, and bleeding from trauma to the lips or oral mucosa.

[§]Or other first- or second-generation oral cephalosporin in equivalent adult or pediatric dosage.

[‖]Cephalosporins should not be used in an individual with a history of anaphylaxis, angioedema, or urticaria with penicillins or ampicillin.

[¶]If these guidelines are applied outside of the United States of America, adaptation of the recommended antibiotic agents may be considered with respect to the regional situation.

IM, Intramuscular; *IV*, intravenous.

Box 8-46	Nonpharmacologic Endocarditis Prevention Measures

- Provide patient/family with a current AHA Prevention of Bacterial Endocarditis wallet card, which is available in English and Spanish at www.americanheart.org.
- Teach the child and family that they should seek appropriate antibiotic treatment for infections.
- Encourage good dental hygiene and regular dental care.
- Elective dental treatment should be performed at least 1-2 months before or 4-6 months after cardiac surgery to try to avoid a potentially significant bacteremic episode in temporal proximity to cardiac surgery.[818]
- Counsel patients and families regarding potentially greater risks of complications from intravenous drug abuse, piercings, and tattooing for individuals with many types of cardiac disease.[706]
- Encourage good skin care—cleaning wounds, avoiding nail biting, and refraining from manipulation of acne lesions. Treatment of chronic acne should be discussed with a physician.[706]
- Educate patients and families about:
  - Risks and pathophysiology
  - Their responsibility to be advocates for the child and to inform care providers of risks
  - Signs of endocarditis with emphasis on fever and the need to inform physicians of any symptoms that might warrant obtaining blood cultures

continued antibiotic therapy, and observation for recurrent infection.[499]

Throughout therapy, support of cardiovascular function is required. Valvular endocarditis often results in congestive heart failure, so limitation of fluid intake and diuretic therapy are frequently required (see Common Clinical Problems, Congestive Heart Failure).

Treatment of lesions of other organs must occur simultaneous with treatment of the endocarditis. Outcomes have improved with the advent of interventional radiology and catheterization techniques such as device occlusion of vessels that have become hemorrhagic as the result of erosion from infection.

Myocarditis

Gail L. Stendahl

Etiology

Myocarditis is an inflammatory process that involves the cardiac muscle; most result from viral infection (Box 8-47). Each decade there has been a shift in viral demographics of myocarditis. In the 1970s and 1980s, coxsackievirus was most common, but in the 1990s and 2000s viral causes included adenovirus and a broader range of enteroviruses. Most recently, parvovirus B19 has become a commonly identified pathogen in patients with suspected myocarditis.[873]

Nonviral causes of myocarditis include infectious agents such as rickettsiae, fungi, bacteria, protozoa, and other parasites (Box 8-48). Noninfectious etiologies include drug toxicity, as with some antimicrobial medications, along with

Box 8-47	Viral Causes of Myocarditis

Enterovirus	Varicella
Coxsackie A	Mumps
Coxsackie B	Measles
Echovirus	Rabies
Poliovirus	Hepatitis B, C
Adenovirus	Rubella
Parvovirus B19	Rubeola
Cytomegalovirus	Respiratory syncytial virus
Herpesvirus	Human immunodeficiency virus
Influenza A	Epstein-Barr virus

From Towbin, JA. Myocarditis. In Allen HD, Shaddy RE, Driscoll DJ, Feltes TF, editors. *Moss and Adams' heart disease in infants, children, and adolescents, including the fetus and young adult*, ed 7. Philadelphia, 2008, Lippincott Williams & Wilkins, p. 1208, Table 58-1.

hypersensitivity, autoimmune, collagen-vascular diseases, or other disorders such as Kawasaki disease and sarcoidosis (Box 8-49).[873]

In most cases, myocarditis remains idiopathic.[873] The incidence of myocarditis is difficult to determine because of the varied presentation; patients may be asymptomatic or may develop cardiogenic shock and die. Estimated prevalence frequently ranges from 1 to 10 per 100,000 persons. Viral RNA has been detected in myocardial tissue in pediatric patients with sudden death.[179] Infants and young children may be more prone to the development of myocarditis because of a higher overall rate of enteroviral and adenoviral infections.[528]

Box 8-48	Nonviral Causes of Myocarditis

Rickettsial	Protozoal	Fungi and Yeasts
Rickettsia rickettsii	*Trypanosoma cruzi*	*Actinomycosis*
Rickettsia tsutsugamushi	Toxoplasmosis	Coccidioidomycosis
	Amebiasis	Histoplasmosis
		Candida
Bacterial	**Other Parasites**	
Meningococcus	*Toxocara canis*	
Klebsiella	Schistosomiasis	
Leptospira	Heterophyiasis	
Mycoplasma	Cysticercosis	
Salmonella	*Echinococcus*	
Clostridia	Visceral larva migrans	
Tuberculosis	Trichinosis	
Brucella		
Legionella pneumophila		
Streptococcus		
Smallpox		

From Towbin, JA. Myocarditis. In Allen HD, Shaddy RE, Driscoll DJ, Feltes TF, eds. *Moss and Adams' heart disease in infants, children, and adolescents, including the fetus and young adult*, ed 7. Philadelphia, 2008, Lippincott Williams & Wilkins, p. 1208, Table 58-2.

Box 8-49	Causes Of Myocarditis: Noninfectious Etiologic Agents

Toxic	Hypersensitivity/Autoimmune
Scorpion	Rheumatoid arthritis
Diphtheria	Rheumatic fever
	Ulcerative colitis
	Systemic lupus erythematosus
	Mixed connective tissue disease
	Scleroderma
	Whipple disease
Drugs	**Other**
Sulfonamides	Sarcoidosis
Phenylbutazone	Kawasaki disease
Cyclophosphamide	Cornstarch
Neomercazole	
Acetazolamide	
Amphotericin B	
Indomethacin	
Tetracycline	
Isoniazid	
Methyldopa	
Phenytoin	
Penicillin	

From Towbin, JA. Myocarditis. In Allen HD, Shaddy RE, Driscoll DJ, Feltes TF, eds. *Moss and Adams' heart disease in infants, children, and adolescents, including the fetus and young adult*, ed 7. Philadelphia, Lippincott Williams & Wilkins, 2008, p. 1208, Table 58-3.

Pathophysiology

Three related mechanisms result in myocardial injury from infectious agents, including invasion of the myocardial cells, production of a myocardial toxin, and immune-mediated myocardial damage.[528] The process can be divided into three phases: infection and proliferation, autoimmunity, and progression to dilated cardiomyopathy. The immune-mediated changes led by T-lymphocytes and macrophages are the predominant mechanisms that result in myocardial injury. The increased effect of T cells, activation of cytokines, and synthesis of nitric oxide destroys the myocytes, causing ventricular remodeling and progression to dilated cardiomyopathy.[528]

Several changes result in the pathophysiologic response in patients with myocarditis. First, the sympathetic nervous system may preserve blood pressure and systemic blood flow through vasoconstriction. This adrenergic response is associated with tachycardia and an increase in ventricular afterload. Congestive heart failure develops with disease progression. The increase in ventricular end-diastolic volume and pressure results in increased left atrial pressure, which, in turn, increases pulmonary venous pressure and leads to pulmonary edema.

Eventually, all cardiac chambers dilate, particularly the left ventricle. This dilation, in addition to causing poor ventricular function, creates worsening pulmonary edema and symptoms of congestive heart failure. The ventricular dilation may also cause mitral regurgitation, further increasing left atrial volume and pressure.

During the healing stages of myocarditis, fibroblasts replace normal cells, resulting in scar formation. Reduced elasticity and ventricular performance can produce persistent heart failure. In addition, ventricular arrhythmias commonly accompany fibrosis.[528]

There are subtypes of myocarditis based on presenting symptoms, clinical course, outcome, and histology.[528] Fulminant myocarditis is characterized by a distinct, sudden onset of cardiac failure, severe left ventricular dysfunction, and cardiogenic shock. Acute myocarditis represents the largest group of patients. The onset of symptoms is often indistinct, and patients seem to develop a more gradual deterioration in ventricular function. Chronic myocarditis is characterized by an unclear onset of congestive heart failure with a slow progressive deterioration in ventricular function.[528]

Clinical Signs and Symptoms

The clinical presentation depends on the age of the child. Nonspecific flulike illness or episodes of gastroenteritis may precede symptoms of congestive heart failure. Newborns and infants present with poor appetite, fever, irritability or listlessness, pallor, and diaphoresis. Older children and adolescents commonly have a recent history of viral disease before presentation.[873]

Typically the child has fever, tachycardia disproportionate to the degree of fever present, arrhythmias, and signs of congestive heart failure, including a gallop rhythm, tachypnea, and signs of systemic and pulmonary edema (see section, Common Clinical Conditions, Congestive Heart Failure). The parents may note lethargy, and the child may complain of chest pain, weakness, myalgia, or constant fatigue. A history of asthma or congenital heart disease can skew the clinical picture.[885]

If significant myocardial dysfunction is present the child may have signs of poor systemic perfusion or shock (see Shock in Chapter 6). A systolic tricuspid or mitral murmur may be noted that is consistent with the development of atrioventricular valve insufficiency resulting from progressive ventricular dilation. Often, a third heart sound (gallop rhythm) develops as the result of rapid filling of a noncompliant, poorly contractile left ventricle.[885] Pulsus alternans may result from decreased ventricular contractility, and a pericardial or pleural friction rub also may be present.

The initial evaluation of a child with suspected myocarditis includes evaluation of the chest radiograph, electrocardiogram (ECG), and cardiac biomarkers. An echocardiogram should be performed to evaluate ventricular function and the degree of any mitral regurgitation.[870]

The chest radiograph may reveal cardiomegaly, pulmonary venous engorgement, and pulmonary edema. It may be difficult to distinguish any increase in the size of the cardiac silhouette produced by a pericardial effusion from the cardiomegaly associated with a poorly functioning myocardium. Pleural effusions also may be noted.

Blood tests (e.g., complete blood count, erythrocyte sedimentation rate, C-reactive protein, and other chemistry profiles) usually are not helpful to confirm the diagnosis of myocarditis. Cardiac biomarkers showing myocardial injury often are elevated, including creatinine phosphokinase myocardial band (CPK-MB) fraction, Troponin I and/or Troponin T. These can be followed serially to assess ongoing inflammation and injury.[528]

The B-Type natriuretic peptide (BNP) blood test is a measurement of cardiac hormone produced by the ventricular myocardium in response to volume expansion and pressure overload. It is a hormonal marker of ventricular dysfunction and a surrogate quantifiable marker of the degree of congestive heart failure; BNP can also be useful when monitored serially. Viral serologic tests and polymerase chain reaction (PCR) assays of blood, stool, urine, and nasopharyngeal specimens can be adjunctive methods in diagnosing myocarditis; however, they are often negative.[873]

The echocardiogram is required to rule out the presence of structural heart disease, and it will enable evaluation of heart size, ventricular contractility, and atrioventricular (AV) valve function. The echocardiogram also will confirm the presence of any significant pericardial effusion.

Cardiac magnetic resonance imaging (MRI) is an emerging field that is capable of showing delayed enhancement of the affected myocardium. The cardiac MRI can show nodular and patchy areas of inflammation, often seen first in the lateral and inferior wall of the heart; these can be used later to guide biopsy.

A cardiac catheterization may be performed if there is any question about the presence of structural heart disease, pulmonary hypertension, coronary artery anatomy, or severe ventricular dysfunction with AV valve disease. The cardiac catheterization typically shows depressed cardiac index, elevated left ventricular end-diastolic pressure, and elevated mean atrial pressure. Angiography shows decreased left ventricular function with or without mitral regurgitation although the utility of angiography to evaluate ventricular and valve function has recently decreased because the quality of available noninvasive imaging is extremely high.

During catheterization an endomyocardial biopsy (EMB) may be obtained to allow histologic grading of the myocarditis and possible explanation of the causative organism. Right ventricle EMB using the Dallas Criteria for classification continues to be the "gold standard" for the diagnosis of myocarditis.[528] Improvement in diagnostic accuracy can be achieved by using immunohistochemical markers for lymphocytes and applying polymerase chain reaction (PCR) techniques to detect the presence of virus in a biopsy specimen.[189] This is often extremely valuable in the establishment of the cause and in some cases to guide therapy.

Management

Treatment of the child with myocarditis includes managing the underlying infection or disease (if identified), maximization of ventricular function, and cardiovascular support (optimize heart rate, preload and contractility, and reduce afterload). Because the symptomatic child with myocarditis is at risk for development of serious arrhythmias and sudden cardiac arrest (sudden death), admission to the critical care unit and continuous electrocardiographic monitoring and observation are required.

If an infectious agent is found the child may require isolation or treatment with antimicrobial agents. The physician may recommend that the child be maintained on bedrest to reduce cardiac output requirements. Fever should be treated with antipyretics, because fever will increase oxygen consumption and myocardial work.

Assisted ventilation along with continuous positive airway pressure relieves the excessive work of breathing, improves pulmonary edema and oxygenation, and may have a beneficial effect in reducing left ventricular afterload. In the setting of low cardiac output, severe ventricular dysfunction, and absence of cardiac reserve, endotracheal intubation should be carefully planned with contingency plans ready to enact if the child decompensates. Risk of decompensation is high during intubation because the sedation needed may lead to hypotension, cardiovascular collapse, and even cardiac arrest.[528]

Patients with fulminant myocarditis and cardiogenic shock require aggressive intervention to support circulation. Treatment of shock requires maintenance of adequate intravascular volume, correction of electrolyte or acid-base imbalances and use of inotropic and vasodilator therapy. Intravenous inotropic agents should be used judiciously and may be more helpful for short-term stabilization than for longer-term support. When low cardiac output and elevated systemic vascular resistance are present, milrinone therapy should be considered. The major advantages of milrinone are that it does not increase heart rate and it improves relaxation of the heart.[528]

Mechanical circulatory support with extracorporeal membrane oxygenation (ECMO) or ventricular assist devices may be life-saving in patients with fulminant myocarditis when inotropic agents are ineffective in maintaining adequate cardiac output (see Chapter 7). The use of ventricular assist devices versus transplantation in acute and fulminant myocarditis as a bridge to recovery remains controversial; assist devices are thought to be underused as a therapy.[528]

Transplantation may be the only option for children with significant cardiac failure resulting from myocarditis. Preferably, children are not listed for transplant until they have progressed to the chronic phase of the disease, because recovery is possible even in the most severe cases.[64]

Treatment of arrhythmias requires administration of antiarrhythmic drugs, although these medications should be used with caution because many of them also depress myocardial contractility. If antiarrhythmic therapy is prescribed the nurse must assess the child carefully for signs of decreased systemic perfusion and notify a physician or other on-call provider immediately if these develop. If arrhythmias remain unresponsive to pharmacologic therapy, pacing wires may be inserted to allow overdrive pacing (see section, Common Clinical Conditions, Arrhythmias).

If a significant pericardial effusion is present the nurse must monitor for signs of cardiac tamponade, including a rise in central venous pressure, poor systemic perfusion, progressive unremitting tachycardia, and pulsus paradoxus. Pericardiocentesis may be required to decompress the pericardium (see Evolve Fig. 19-2 in the Pediatric Trauma information in the Chapter 19 Supplement on the Evolve Website).

Patients with mild-to-moderate cardiac failure should be treated with conventional pharmacologic agents, including diuretics (e.g., furosemide, spironolactone), angiotensin-converting enzyme inhibitors or angiotensin receptor blockers, and possibly digoxin.[528] Digoxin, if employed, should be used judiciously in low dose and without a loading dose, to reduce risk of toxicity. Anticoagulation with aspirin, warfarin, or intravenous heparin may be used to prevent thrombus formation when the left ventricle is dilated and function is severely depressed.

After stabilization, beta-adrenergic antagonists, such as carvedilol, may be introduced cautiously and the dose slowly titrated up over time. Beta blockers are effective in improving systolic function in adults with heart failure, although data remain limited regarding effectiveness in children.[793] Beta-blockers are currently being used in pediatrics in hopes to reduce mortality and improve left ventricular ejection fraction in chronic heart failure.[528]

Use of corticosteroids in the treatment of myocarditis is controversial, because steroids may suppress the child's immune response, and result in progression of the initial infectious process. Occasionally, if myocarditis produces severe complications, including arrhythmias unresponsive to medical management, corticosteroids may be administered in an attempt to reduce myocardial inflammation. Overall survival in children has not differed in patients who received steroids in addition to conventional therapy versus those who received conventional therapy alone.[252]

Immunosuppression for the treatment of myocarditis remains controversial.[873] Immunosuppressive agents that are administered early in the course of myocarditis increase viral replication, damage heart cells, and increase mortality. If immunosuppression is used it should be initiated only during the autoimmune phase of the disease process. Treatment with intravenous immunoglobulin (IVIG) can alter the immune response and may improve outcomes by reducing ongoing myocardial cell damage.[189] The IVIG may also neutralize the antibodies that form against the causative virus and lead to ongoing damage via an autoimmune mechanism.

Monitoring the critically ill child with myocarditis in the critical care unit can be very challenging. The nurse must be able to recognize early clinical signs of deterioration. The most common assessment techniques used for children at risk for cardiovascular compromise or collapse include invasive hemodynamic monitoring, frequent careful clinical evaluation by experienced providers, and laboratory assessment of end-organ function, blood gases, and serum lactate, along with routine continuous noninvasive measures of vital signs, pulse oximetry and the use of near infrared spectroscopy (NIRS) to detect trends in oxygen delivery or consumption.

These critically ill patients are often treated with a myriad of agents to manage afterload, prevent arrhythmias, and support oxygenation, ventilation and nutrition and to optimize cardiac output. When the child is unresponsive to these management strategies, the timely use of ECMO and/or ventricular assist devices are additional modalities available as supportive therapy for myocarditis (see Chapter 7).

Potential novel therapies for future treatment of myocarditis include vaccinations, virus specific drugs, and protease inhibitors. Vaccination has been used successfully to prevent diseases.[873] The efficacy of vaccines has led to the suggestion that a broadly specific enteroviral vaccine would be beneficial for reducing the incidence of myocarditis. The use of antiviral medications requires further investigation. In addition, because viruses release proteases that can lead to myocardial damage, protease inhibitors may be reasonable agents to consider for clinical investigation. Continued improvements in alternatives for myocardial support along with ongoing research into genetic markers that may identify patients at risk hold promise for the future.

Throughout the management of the child with myocarditis, the patient and the family will require emotional support and clear, concise, and consistent information. If the child is admitted with signs of cardiopulmonary compromise that require critical care support and monitoring, the possibility of mortality is real and heightens the importance of effective communication with the family.

The parents should be allowed to remain with the child as often as is feasible in hopes of reducing their anxiety and that of the child. It is only through careful coordination of care, a shared understanding of the pathophysiology and clinical issues, and thoughtful open communication between healthcare providers and the family that we can maximize the opportunities for these children to have the best possible outcome.

Cardiomyopathy

Gail L. Stendahl

Etiology

Cardiomyopathy is defined as a disease of the myocardium with cardiac dysfunction. It is usually associated with mechanical and/or electrical problems, and the patient may exhibit ventricular hypertrophy or dilation. Cardiomyopathies can be confined to the heart or may be related to a systemic disorder, often leading to death or a progressive heart failure-related disability.[570]

The term *primary cardiomyopathy* is used to indicate myocardial disease unrelated to congenital heart disease, pulmonary or systemic hypertension, or coronary artery or valvular heart disease. Cardiomyopathy also may develop as a secondary complication of systemic disease, viral infection, or exposure to chemicals or drugs. Some forms of congenital heart disease produce secondary ventricular dysfunction with effects similar to cardiomyopathy. For example, the child with transposition may develop severe right ventricular dysfunction after intraatrial (atrial—not arterial) correction. In most patients, however, the cause of cardiomyopathy is unknown.

Cardiomyopathy is uncommon, accounting for only 1% of all pediatric cardiac disease.[524] Risk factors for the development of pediatric cardiomyopathy include the infant or adolescent age group, gender (3:2 male predominance), African-American race, and, most importantly, the presence of an affected family member. More than 50% of pediatric cardiomyopathy cases develop before 1 year of age. This early incidence may represent a genetic component. The incidence peaks again in adolescence. Lower socioeconomic status is associated with higher incidence of cardiomyopathy. These data suggest that genetic and environmental factors are interrelated and contribute to the risk of cardiomyopathy. The presence of a family member with cardiomyopathy increases the incidence for all first-degree relatives: 9% to 20% of all cardiomyopathies are inherited.[212]

Pathophysiology

Three forms of cardiomyopathy are commonly identified: (1) dilated cardiomyopathy, (2) hypertrophic cardiomyopathy, and (3) restrictive cardiomyopathy. A discussion of each of these follows. All forms of cardiomyopathy are associated with ventricular dysfunction, decreased ventricular ejection fraction, and an increase in myocardial mass.

Dilated Cardiomyopathy. Dilated cardiomyopathy (DCM) is the most common form of the cardiomyopathies; it accounts for at least half of all cases, with a population incidence of 0.58 per 100,000 children.[189] Most cases of DCM are idiopathic in origin. Severe infections and overwhelming systemic inflammation may cause severe systolic dysfunction that may look like DCM. Myocarditis is a relatively common cause of DCM, accounting for 2% to 15% (diagnosed by endomyocardial biopsy) of DCM cases; the percentage is slightly higher in children less than 2 years of age.

There are multiple patterns of inheritance in familial DCM. Neuromuscular diseases may result from genetic mutations and may be autosomal or related to abnormalities of mitochondrial DNA (maternal inheritance). Duchenne's and Becker's muscular dystrophy (both X-linked disorders located in the dystrophin gene locus) have cardiomyopathy as a prominent feature. Barth syndrome, another X-linked disorder, is caused by a genetic mutation for the tafazzin gene. It is characterized by both cardiac and skeletal involvement and can present with DCM, with or without ventricular noncompaction.[524]

Regardless of the etiology, depressed cardiac function is the common feature in all forms of DCM. Some patients with cardiomyopathy, particularly those with restrictive or hypertrophic variants, may present initially with predominantly diastolic dysfunction. Systolic function may initially be preserved; however, the systolic function can deteriorate over time. Furthermore, the various forms of cardiomyopathy can have overlapping phenotypes (e.g., dilated cardiomyopathy with restrictive physiology).

Initially, cardiac output is often maintained despite decreased contractility by increased end-systolic function and end-diastolic volume creating increased wall tension. This increased tension stimulates myocyte hypertrophy and normalizes cardiac output. Over time, these compensatory changes result in unfavorable remodeling and progressive ventricular dilation with alteration in the normal ventricular geometry. As the function declines, the dilation and wall tension continue to increase, causing pooling of blood in the heart chambers. At this point, the elevated wall tension decreases myocardial efficiency and increases myocardial oxygen consumption. Eventually, these compensatory mechanisms are not sufficient to maintain adequate cardiac output. Additional stress, such as a febrile illness or exercise, may exacerbate symptoms.

Diminished cardiac output results in hypoperfusion of organs and may cause end-organ damage. Decreased renal blood flow activates the renin-angiotensin system to help maintain perfusion pressure by promoting fluid retention and vasoconstriction, and potentiating catecholamines. The sympathetic nervous system is stimulated, producing an increase in heart rate and contractility. At the expense of increased afterload, vasoconstriction maintains perfusion to vital organs. In short, the compensatory physiologic changes caused by the failing heart produce additional myocardial strain, ventricular dilation, and dysfunction.

The failing ventricle continues to dilate; the stretch on the cardiac myocytes distorts the conduction system, there is increased myocardial work and decreased cardiac output, and the patient is susceptible to arrhythmias, end organ dysfunction, and ischemia. Current medical therapies largely serve to neutralize this counterproductive physiology.

Microscopic examination of the cells shows hypertrophy of the myocytes. The progression of symptoms is dependent on the acuity of the decompensation.[524]

Hypertrophic Cardiomyopathy. Hypertrophic cardiomyopathy (HCM) is the second most common form of cardiomyopathy[524]; it accounts for 42% of childhood cardiomyopathy with an incidence of 0.47/100,000 children.[189] HCM is one of the most common inherited cardiac disorders, with a prevalence in young adults of 1 in 500. Many children with this form of cardiomyopathy have first-degree relatives with similar heart disease, and sudden death is frequently reported in family members.

As is the case with dilated cardiomyopathy, metabolic and mitochondrial abnormalities may cause HCM.[212] In addition, Wolff-Parkinson-White syndrome has been associated with HCM. Although this disease generally appears in the second or third decade of life, occasionally symptoms develop during childhood and may be progressive, with significant morbidity and mortality.[524]

The characteristic feature of HCM is the progressive and asymmetric thickening of the myocardium, especially in the area of the ventricular septum. The thickened myocardium invades the ventricular cavity, dramatically decreasing the cavity size. Left ventricular outflow tract obstruction is often present and may be associated with systolic anterior motion (SAM) of the mitral valve with secondary mitral insufficiency.

Intracellular calcium is known to regulate contractile function and relaxation. As the cardiac myocytes begin to hypertrophy, there is an increase in the release of intracellular calcium during diastole, which leads to diastolic dysfunction. Histologic examination reveals myocyte hypertrophy, myofiber disarray, and patchy fibrosis.[872]

Hypertrophic cardiomyopathy usually produces a decrease in ventricular compliance and ejection fraction, and it can result in the development of mitral regurgitation, arrhythmias, congestive heart failure, and/or low cardiac output.

Restrictive Cardiomyopathy. Restrictive cardiomyopathy is the least common form of cardiomyopathy; among children it is quite rare, accounting for fewer than 3% of pediatric cardiomyopathy cases.[189] Restrictive cardiomyopathy presents with normal or near-normal systolic function but impaired ventricular filling resulting from increased stiffness and reduced diastolic volume of either or both ventricles.[189] Primary types of restrictive cardiomyopathy include endomyocardial fibrosis, hypereosinophilic syndrome, familial, and most commonly idiopathic cardiomyopathy. Secondary types are related to multisystem disorders, including infiltrative and storage disease.

Pediatric cases are generally idiopathic or related to cardiotoxicity or endocardial fibroelastosis (EFE), with up to one third occurring in a familial pattern. Differentiation from many of the secondary causes relies on morphologic criteria. Tissue analysis is often pursued given the dismal prognosis of the disease and the desire to exclude any potentially treatable disorder.[189]

The characteristic feature of restrictive cardiomyopathy is a marked increase in the stiffness of the myocardium or endomyocardium, resulting in a reduced ventricular size. The consequence is impaired ventricular filling, leading to elevated diastolic pressures and marked atrial dilation. Pulmonary hypertension secondary to left atrial hypertension is present from the early stages of this disease.

If endomyocardial fibrosis is present, it may be noted as a distinct disease or in association with bacterial endocarditis or eosinophilic leukemia. As endocardial or myocardial lesions progress, ventricular expansion during diastole is restricted so ventricular end-diastolic pressure increases and stoke volume declines.[231] Eventually the ventricular lumen may be obstructed by fibrotic tissue and thrombus formation. These ventricular thrombi can embolize to the pulmonary or systemic circulations.

Clinical Signs and Symptoms

Children with cardiomyopathy may be asymptomatic or show signs of severe congestive heart failure (CHF). The rate of symptom progression varies and depends on the nature of the disease and the body's ability to increase cardiac output to meet the demands of the body. As ventricular dysfunction worsens, the child shows symptoms of left- and/or right-heart failure.

The findings of CHF vary with the age of the patient. Infants usually present with feeding intolerance. Symptoms include tachypnea, increased respiratory effort with retractions, diaphoresis during feeding, prolonged periods of irritability, and failure to thrive. Children and adolescents initially present with exercise intolerance or dyspnea with exertion, fatigue, orthopnea, tachypnea, dyspnea, and edema. Sympathetic nervous system redistribution of blood flow away from skin, gut, and kidney can lead to gastrointestinal symptoms, including abdominal pain after meals, nausea, vomiting, and anorexia. Additional symptoms may include new onset palpitations and syncope. Occasionally, patients are asymptomatic except when arrhythmias are present; sudden cardiac arrest (sudden death) may be the first sign of the disease.

Vital signs reveal an elevated heart rate (for age) with decreased heart rate variability. Tachycardia initially compensates for the decreased stroke volume. Pulses may be weak with a narrow pulse pressure, as systemic vascular resistance increases and cardiac output decreases. The blood pressure is low to normal and may be maintained until just before cardiovascular collapse. The respiratory rate is elevated. Cyanosis is uncommon but pallor or mottling may be present.[212] The patient may also be febrile as the result of an acute infectious process that may be exacerbating symptoms that otherwise would be subtle.[671]

Cardiac examination may reveal cardiomegaly, increased precordial impulse or lateral displacement of the apical impulse. The heart sounds may be distant or muffled. Although murmurs are not always present, a systolic murmur often is noted along the left sternal border. The murmur may be caused by progressive left ventricular outflow tract obstruction (in the child with hypertrophic cardiomyopathy) or by mitral regurgitation. An extra heart sound, secondary to elevated ventricular filling pressure, may be auscultated as a gallop rhythm. Jugular venous distension may be present, but is difficult to appreciate in young children.[671]

Abdominal examination can reveal hepatomegaly and ascites. Nonspecific generalized abdominal pain also may be present, resulting from mesenteric ischemia. Dependent edema is common and can be seen in the eyelids and the scrotum of infants or in the legs of children and adolescents.[212] Vasoconstriction can cause extremities to be cool and poorly perfused. Capillary refill time is increased.

The chest radiograph classically reveals cardiomegaly, typically from left atrial and left ventricular enlargement. The left atrial enlargement may elevate the left main stem bronchus and cause airway obstruction or left lung atelectasis. In younger children, lung fields often appear hyperexpanded with flattening of the diaphragm. Elevated pulmonary venous pressure leads to pulmonary congestion. Pleural effusions may also be present.[212]

The echocardiogram demonstrates ventricular dilation, disproportionate ventricular septal thickening, or possible obstruction of the left and/or right ventricular outflow tracts. Echocardiographic findings show globally decreased contractility without regional wall motion abnormalities. Color and pulse-wave Doppler can determine the presence and degree of valve regurgitation, assess cardiac output by aortic flow velocities, determine the degree of diastolic dysfunction by atrioventricular (AV) valve inflow pattern, and estimate pulmonary artery and right ventricular pressures. Echocardiography is beneficial for monitoring patients longitudinally as well as for detecting changes in ventricular function, thrombus formation, wall stress, pulmonary vascular disease, and valvular regurgitation.[212]

The electrocardiogram (ECG) is usually abnormal, although no specific criteria are diagnostic for cardiomyopathy. Usually, evidence of left (and possible right) ventricular hypertrophy, arrhythmias and ST segment changes consistent with myocardial injury may be noted (see section, Common Clinical Conditions, Arrhythmias, ST-Segment Deviation), T-wave inversion, abnormal Q waves, and diminished R waves also may be present on lateral precordial leads.

Evidence of atrial hypertrophy may be present. A Holter monitor allows for determination of chronotropic (heart rate) variability, identification of ST segment changes, and assessment of T-wave alternans.

Acute myocardial injury or inflammation can be detected with serum biomarkers, such as cardiac troponins I and T. These biomarkers are intracellular proteins that are sensitive and specific for acute myocyte injury. Elevation of troponin should alert clinicians to look for ischemia, myocarditis, or an acute inflammatory process as the cause of the cardiomyopathy. Patients with infectious causes for cardiomyopathy may have an elevated white blood cell count with a lymphocytosis, and trends in inflammatory markers (e.g., C-reactive protein [CRP] and erythrocyte sedimentation rate [ESR]) should be monitored. Providers must closely monitor end-organ function. Blood and nasopharyngeal cultures for viruses are usually not diagnostic.

In patients presenting with CHF, progression of heart failure can be monitored with B-type natriuretic peptide levels. These hormones are secreted from the ventricles in response to dilation and wall stress. Monitoring of BNP levels may be useful in managing cardiomyopathy in children. Depending on the age and presentation of the cardiomyopathy, a metabolic evaluation with blood and urine analysis should be considered. In addition, molecular testing is available to screen for genetic defects that led to cardiomyopathy.[212]

Cardiac catheterization is performed to evaluate left ventricular filling, pulmonary capillary wedge pressure, and pulmonary artery and central venous pressures; these measurements and evaluation can help guide therapy. Endomyocardial biopsy remains the gold standard to exclude myocarditis and may be useful in the diagnosis of metabolic abnormalities, mitochondrial defects, and infiltrative disease. Biopsy results are often nonspecific, showing myocyte hypertrophy and fibrosis. Polymerase chain reaction (PCR) analysis and electron microscopy may provide a more definitive diagnosis that can affect prognosis and treatment.[212]

Cardiac magnetic resonance imaging (MRI) is a useful tool for the measurement of myocardial mass and thickness, particularly when echocardiography is inadequate. Three-dimensional reconstruction of data enables quantification of the disorder. Recent work using delayed enhancement after gadolinium administration has demonstrated the capacity to identify areas of myocardial fibrosis, a finding with prognostic importance.[189]

Management

Management of a child diagnosed with cardiomyopathy should begin by ruling out treatable causes, minimizing the risks of complications from the cardiomyopathy and providing supportive care for the heart failure symptoms.[212] The clinical picture of a child with cardiomyopathy includes low cardiac output, fluid retention and peripheral vasoconstriction. Therapy is aimed at increasing cardiac output, enhancing tissue oxygen delivery, and sustaining vital organ function. If a treatable metabolic abnormality (e.g., carnitine deficiency) is present, appropriate treatment should be started without delay. Confirmatory diagnostic testing from urine and plasma sampling can still be performed with concurrent treatment of the presumed deficiency.

The short-term management of patients with heart failure consists of supportive care. Acute symptoms of CHF may be improved with administration of inotropes, such as dopamine or epinephrine, but these strategies are rarely useful as longer-term therapies. At low doses, dopamine increases renal blood flow. At higher doses, it increases cardiac output but can also increase peripheral vascular resistance and cause arrhythmias.[671] Therefore, inotropes should be used judiciously and may serve as a bridge to alternative therapies such as mechanical support, biventricular pacing, or cardiac transplantation. Incremental titration should be used as the clinical situation dictates. Milrinone, an inodilator (inotrope and vasodilator), may decrease left ventricular work by promoting relaxation and increasing ventricular compliance.

Diuresis is essential to control signs and symptoms of CHF. Intravenous diuretic therapy is used during acute decompensation and can be transitioned to oral therapy once the systemic or venous congestion improves. It is critical to monitor electrolytes during initial or escalation of diuretic therapy because electrolyte imbalances can lead to life-threatening arrhythmias.[524]

When the acute decompensation has been controlled, patients are often converted to an oral regimen of afterload reduction with angiotensin-converting enzyme (ACE) inhibitors such as enalapril or captopril, diuretic therapy with spironolactone, and a loop diuretic such as furosemide or hydrochlorothiazide, and a beta-receptor antagonist, usually carvedilol or metoprolol.[524]

Beta-adrenergic agents may be effective in the treatment of both dilated and hypertrophic cardiomyopathy in adults, but their utility in pediatrics remains controversial and unproven. Approximately one third of symptomatic adults improve after administration of a beta-blocker. Although the predominant mechanism by which improvement occurs is unclear, it is thought that carvedilol reduces myocardial oxygen requirements and may decrease apoptosis (programmed cell death).[671] Carvedilol does not usually produce immediate improvement in the short term and has not been shown to reduce the risk of sudden fatal arrhythmias among patients with cardiomyopathy.

Calcium channel blockers, such as amlodipine, have also been effective in the treatment of hypertrophic cardiomyopathy, although experience in children is limited. Sudden death is a risk factor for children receiving calcium channel blockers, so they require close monitoring with initiation of this therapy.

Digoxin should be used with caution in acutely ill children. Use of digoxin in patients with inflamed myocardium may promote ventricular arrhythmias. Digoxin is not recommended for children with hypertrophic cardiomyopathy and adequate ventricular systolic function because digoxin may worsen the left ventricular outflow tract obstruction. Digoxin, however, may be beneficial in low doses for symptomatic patients with dilated cardiomyopathy.[671]

If the child has developed intraventricular or intraatrial thrombi, anticoagulant therapy will be initiated. Careful monitoring of systemic perfusion and pulmonary function is required to detect evidence of systemic or pulmonary emboli. Thrombus formation can occur when there is stasis of blood in enlarged chambers of the heart. If a clot is detected, it should be aggressively treated with heparin and eventually switched to warfarin or Lovenox. Patients with global ventricular dilation and dysfunction may benefit from low dose aspirin as an antiplatelet agent or prophylactic anticoagulation with Coumadin even in the absence of identified thrombus formation.[212]

Prevention or treatment of secondary arrhythmias (particularly malignant ones) can be challenging because antiarrhythmic drugs often produce myocardial depression. Despite this, many patients with chronic arrhythmias benefit from antiarrhythmic therapy. Depending on the nature of the arrhythmia, treatment may include beta-blockade, amiodarone, or class 1 agents such as lidocaine or mexiletine. Antiarrhythmic drugs and/or radiofrequency ablation are used when the diagnosis of tachycardia-induced cardiomyopathy is established.[671] The therapy of choice depends on the nature of the tachycardia, but establishing sinus rhythm with rate control is imperative and usually leads to marked improvement in ventricular function. Many effective antiarrhythmics, such as procainamide, have negative inotropic effects, may not produce rapid cardioversion, and should be used with caution in this group. Ultimately, these patients should often be considered for ablative therapy as a potential cure (see section, Common Clinical Conditions, Arrhythmias).

Cardiac resynchronization therapy has been used in adult patients with left bundle branch block and decreased ventricular function. This therapy has been shown to be helpful in improving symptoms and decreasing hospitalizations. Experience with this therapy is limited in pediatric patients, although early reports suggest that this is a promising therapy for selected patients. Further studies are needed in the pediatric population.[671]

Children that are not responsive to medical management for CHF may benefit from surgical palliative therapies before heart transplantation. Surgical palliation with bridging techniques, such as ventricular assist devices, intraaortic balloon pumps, and extracorporeal membrane oxygenation, have allowed some patients who normally would not have survived to live long enough to receive a heart transplant (see Chapter 7).[212]

Cardiac transplantation should be considered if short-term survival is unlikely or when severe symptoms are unresponsive to conventional therapy. Patients with heart failure symptoms who cannot be weaned from intravenous inotropic support fall into this category. In addition, patients managed on diuretics, angiotensin-converting enzyme inhibitors, and beta-blockers who have persistent New York Heart Association class III or IV heart failure symptoms, ongoing failure to thrive, or severely depressed ventricular function after 6 months of appropriate therapy should be considered candidates for cardiac transplantation (see Chapter 17).[679]

The natural history of cardiomyopathy is affected by the cause (primary versus secondary) and any coexisting risk factors. Primary cardiomyopathies are usually progressive, despite aggressive anticongestive medical therapy, whereas secondary causes may or may not be progressive. Although many children with secondary cardiomyopathy recover ventricular function, children with marked myocardial injury in early childhood should be followed closely.[212]

The prognosis of children with cardiomyopathy is dependent on the cause of the disease and the age at presentation. Traditionally, approximately one third of children with cardiomyopathy were expected to recover completely, another one third were expected to improve but with some residual dysfunction, and the remaining one third were predicted to die or require transplantation. However, these results have improved in recent years. Sudden death may occur at any stage regardless of ventricular function and may be precipitated by comorbidities, such as progressive ventricular dysfunction, CHF, arrhythmias, conduction disturbances, and/or thromboembolic events.[212]

Children with ventricular dysfunction benefit from reducing modifiable cardiovascular risk factors, such as hypertension, diabetes, hypercholesterolemia, and obesity. Secondary prevention strategies can limit the ongoing myocardial injury after the initial insult. Children should be encouraged to eat a well-balanced diet and participate in a regular physical activity or a cardiac rehabilitation program whenever possible. In addition, routine screening for some high-risk groups is recommended.[212]

Cardiac Tumors
Gwen Paxson Fosse

Etiology
The incidence of primary cardiac tumors is reported to be 0.027% to 0.32% in children.[199,576] Primary myocardial, intracardiac, or epicardial masses/tumors are rare but do occur in infants and children, and are most commonly benign. However, they may produce hemodynamic compromise, hemolysis, or embolic phenomena, so they must be identified and treated. The incidence of benign primary cardiac tumors in children is increasing, but these tumors are also more frequently detected and diagnosed, particularly with echocardiographic techniques.[574] Primary cardiac malignant tumors represent less than 10% of the primary cardiac tumors in children.[199,576]

Pathophysiology
Cardiac tumors in pediatrics may cause no significant pathophysiology, but they may have very significant effects depending on the type, number, location, and size of the tumor(s). Right heart tumors can cause right heart failure and left heart tumors can cause or mimic mitral or aortic valve dysfunction. Tumors can result in cardiac inflow and/or outflow obstruction, they may compress vessels and chambers, interfere with valve function, cause coronary artery changes with potential ischemia, infiltrate the myocardium, and cause arrhythmias, embolization, and sudden death.[199,574] There are both benign and malignant cardiac tumors in children (described in the following).

Benign Masses and Tumors. Benign masses and tumors include rhabdomyomas, fibromas, myxomas, teratomas, hemangiomas, angiomas, hamartomas, thrombi, and other uncommon tumors. These are presented briefly in the following.

Rhabdomyoma. The rhabdomyoma is the most common cardiac tumor seen in children, and is typically diagnosed in infants less than 1 year of age. These benign tumors, composed of cardiac myocytes, often (in 78% to 90% of patients) occur as a result of tuberous sclerosis (an autosomal dominant disorder involving tumors of many organ systems and developmental delay) and may be diagnosed prenatally.[574] The rhabdomyoma is usually multiple and is located within the walls of the ventricles, particularly within the septum. Cardiovascular effects occur when the tumor obstructs a coronary artery or a valve or the outflow tract of a ventricle. Arrhythmias also may develop.

These tumors can be removed successfully, resulting in resolution of all symptoms (including all arrhythmias). In more than half of the cases these tumors spontaneously regress or completely disappear.[574]

Fibroma. A fibroma is the second most common cardiac tumor seen during childhood. It, too, is benign, and is diagnosed most frequently during the first year of life. This tumor is firmer than a rhabdomyoma, and is usually a solitary tumor that compresses surrounding structures as it grows. These tumors appear to invade the myocardium and can cause inflow and/or outflow tract obstruction, distortion and changes to atrioventricular valve apparatus, and coronary artery changes.[574] Arrhythmias are reported in approximately one third of affected patients, and sudden death may occur.

In approximately half of involved patients the fibroma cannot be excised completely, although it can be debulked. Long-term survival after complete excision is excellent, but must be more guarded after partial resection.

Myxomas. Myxomas are common in adults but rare in the pediatric population. They most often are found in the left atrium but can occur in other chambers. There is typically a stalk that connects the myxoma, which allows it to be mobile, so embolization can occur. Some myxomas are a familial form and they can be associated with Carney complex, an autosomal dominant disorder.[574]

Teratomas. Teratomas are usually single and intrapericardial but in rare cases have been reported to involve cardiac chambers. They are composed of embryonic germinal layers and may be diagnosed in the fetus. They are often large and cystic, causing compression of vessels and chambers and pericardial effusion. Surgical removal is typically possible without recurrence. On rare occasions teratomas may be malignant.[574]

Hemangiomas/angiomas. Hemangiomas/angiomas consist of large blood vessels and vascular channels involving the myocardium. They are usually single. If symptoms develop, surgical removal may be warranted. Many hemangiomas/angiomas have been successfully treated with steroids or interferon resulting in regression.[574]

Hamartomas. Hamartomas typically involve the left ventricle and present early with ventricular tachycardia necessitating electrophysiologic studies and surgery with inspection and excision of the tumor (typically very small) and cryoablation of the margins. The outcome using this approach is reported to be good.[199]

Thrombi. Thrombi have increased in incidence and there is also increased detection through the use of improved imaging techniques including echocardiography. The growth in the population of critically ill infants and children has resulted in conditions amenable to the formation of thromboemboli. The use of indwelling catheters also has added to this phenomenon. Survival of children with single ventricle physiology, Fontan operations, cardiomyopathies, and those who have had Kawasaki disease contribute to the population at risk for thrombi.[574] With an intracardiac mass in the presence of an indwelling catheter, a blood culture can be obtained from the site to determine if the mass is infected or is an endocarditis vegetation.[401]

Other Masses. Other tumors including lipomas, papillary tumors, accessory endocardial cushion tissue, and fibroelastoma can be associated with pathophysiology similar to that mentioned for other tumors.[576]

Malignant Cardiac Tumors. Malignant cardiac tumors are extremely rare in children.[574] The most common malignant types found in pediatric patients are rhabdomyosarcomas, angiosarcomas, fibrosarcomas, lymphosarcoma, giant cell sarcoma, fibromyxosarcoma, neurogenic sarcoma, leiomyosarcomas, and undifferentiated sarcoma.[199,576] They are associated with right heart chamber involvement, local invasion of the heart, and hemorrhagic pericardial effusions.[199] Stroke and myocardial infarction have been reported complications of pediatric cardiac tumors.[636] Metastases to lung, brain, and liver are not unusual.

Without treatment survival is typically less than 1 year. With surgery and chemotherapy reported survival has improved.[199]

Secondary Cardiac Tumors. Secondary cardiac tumors, aggressive local tumors, or metastatic malignancies are more common than primary cardiac neoplasms in children and can cause the same pathophysiology as that seen with primary malignant tumors. Lymphomas, leukemias, neuroblastomas, and extracardiac sarcomas are associated with secondary cardiac involvement in children.[199,576] Orthopnea and abnormal echocardiography should raise the suspicion of cardiac infiltration, which might not otherwise be appreciated promptly enough for meaningful intervention.[786] Renal and hepatic malignancies, including Wilms tumors, may have direct extension of tumor into the inferior vena cava and right atrium requiring chemotherapy with possible surgery.[199,576] Life-threatening embolic phenomena have been reported with extracardiac malignancies resulting in myocardial infarction and pulmonary emboli.[28,423]

Clinical Signs and Symptoms

The size, location and number of tumors have a major effect on presenting symptoms. Some tumors are small and asymptomatic and may remain undetected. The tumor location may be indicative of tumor type and composition. Diagnosis may be made in the fetus, neonate, child, and adolescent.

Signs and symptoms may be related to myocardial dysfunction and obstruction of blood flow. Clinical features may resemble congenital heart defects with congestive heart failure and include low cardiac output, murmurs, cyanosis, and arrhythmias. Additional findings in the child and adolescent may include fever, malaise, weight loss, arthralgias, myalgias, emboli, exercise intolerance, chest pain, and syncope.[199,574]

Electrocardiography will certainly reveal arrhythmias, but also may be suggestive of chamber enlargement and myocardial ischemia.[574] Ventricular preexcitation or supraventricular tachycardia can be presenting symptoms in infants with some cardiac tumors.[607]

The chest radiograph may show the contours of a mass as well as areas of calcification if they are present in the tumor. Echocardiography can be invaluable in evaluating the hemodynamics and deciphering details about the tumor to aid in diagnosis of the tumor type. Other imaging modalities, including magnetic resonance imaging, computed tomography, and cardiac catheterization, can provide additional information.[199,574]

Management

Diagnosis of the type of tumor and knowledge of the specific characteristics can be paramount in determining the management approach. Medical management with serial surveillance may be the only recommendation.

Management of thrombi can be very challenging. For a thrombus mass, antibiotic therapy may be employed if infection is present. Assessment for a hypercoagulable state or collagen vascular disease may be helpful in determining etiology and management of a thrombus. Thrombolysis may be warranted and is most effective with freshly clotted material, but the risk of emboli must be considered. Intracardiac thrombi can pose a risk of emboli or obstruction to flow, in which case surgical resection may be recommended. Thrombi in a child with underlying cardiac anomalies, foreign surfaces, stagnant areas of flow, or abnormal flow through a baffle or tunnel may warrant surgical intervention.[401] Decision-making must involve consideration of the risk/benefit ratio for both thrombolysis and surgical intervention.[199,574]

In cases of hemodynamic compromise with the presenting symptoms of a tumor, medical interventions to stabilize the child must be the first priority. In newborns this may involve the use of prostaglandin E$_1$ (PGE$_1$) to maintain ductal patency (initial dose: 0.05-0.1 mcg/kg per minute, refer to Box 8-33).[576]

Surgical resection can be successful and life-saving for tumors such as myxomas, teratomas, and others that are causing embolic phenomena, hemodynamic compromise, or arrhythmias. Surgical management may or may not require cardiopulmonary bypass. The approach depends on the location of the tumor(s), but if at all possible, incisions are made in the atria or great vessels, avoiding ventriculotomy. Ideally, complete resection occurs, but in some cases the involvement of critical structures may prevent total resection.

If complete resection is not possible the child will require serial evaluation to detect changes in the tumor. In rare cases cardiac transplantation has been performed for massive fibromas. Radiofrequency or other ablation techniques may be employed successfully to treat tumor-associated arrhythmias.[199,574]

Malignant tumors, both primary and secondary, raise issues of both a medical and surgical nature. The cardiology, cardiovascular surgery, and hematology/oncology teams must work closely together to determine the treatment plan. Surgical cavectomy has been reported with success for children with Wilms tumor and intravascular thrombus into the right atrium.[733] Individualized treatment plans are necessary to address the specific medical needs in children with primary cardiac malignant tumors to avoid potential complications.[636]

Outcomes for those with benign tumors are usually quite good. Those with underlying congenital heart disease, systemic conditions, or malignancy have varied outcomes depending on the nature of their associated disorders.

Kawasaki Disease (Mucocutaneous Lymph Node Syndrome)

Caroline A. Rich

Etiology and Epidemiology

Kawasaki disease (KD) is an immune-mediated, multisystem vasculitis of infancy and early childhood with self-limited clinical course and unknown etiology. It was formerly called mucocutaneous lymph node syndrome.

Most cases of KD occur in children between 1 and 8 years of age with 85% of children affected under the age of 5 years. The disease is more common in the Japanese-American population. The male to female ratio is 1.5:1.[684,838]

Pathophysiology and Clinical Signs and Symptoms

Kawasaki disease is characterized by systemic inflammation manifested by fever for at least 5 days (usually greater than 39° C and remittent) and four of five clinical criteria (Box 8-50).[684,838]

Other associated features include irritability, abdominal pain, diarrhea, vomiting, elevated platelet count (by second week of illness), C-reactive protein and erythrocyte sedimentation rate, hyponatremia, and leukocytosis with bandemia (high percentage of band forms). Other findings include urethritis with sterile pyuria, anterior uveitis, mild hepatic dysfunction, arthralgia, aseptic meningitis, pericardial effusion, gallbladder hydrops, and myocarditis manifested by congestive heart failure (CHF).

Box 8-50   Clinical Criteria for Kawasaki Disease[684,838]

- Bilateral bulbar conjunctival infection without exudate
- Oral mucous membrane changes, including erythema of mouth and pharynx, strawberry tongue, and red cracked lips
- Erythema and edema of palms of hands and soles of feet, and periungual desquamation (after acute phase of illness)
- Polymorphous rash
- Cervical lymphadenopathy (at least one lymph node >1.5 cm in diameter)

Supporting Laboratory Findings in Kawasaki Disease
- Albumin less than 3 g/dL
- Anemia for age
- Elevated alanine aminotransferase
- Platelet count greater than 450,000/mm^3 after 7 days
- White blood cell count greater than 15,000/mm^3
- Elevated C-Reactive Protein
- Erythrocyte sedimentation rate greater than 40 mm/h
- Sterile pyuria

There is no diagnostic test available to confirm KD. The diagnosis is established by fulfillment of the clinical criteria and exclusion of other possible illnesses, such as measles, parvovirus B19 infection, adenovirus, enterovirus, scarlet fever, drug reactions (Stevens-Johnson syndrome), staphylococcal scalded skin syndrome, toxic shock syndrome, and juvenile rheumatoid arthritis.[684,838]

Children with fever and two or three of the typical clinical criteria for 5 days or more, with three or more supporting laboratory findings are said to have incomplete KD. These children should have an echocardiogram and receive treatment. If there are less than three supporting laboratory findings, an echocardiogram is suggested; treatment is warranted if the echocardiogram is positive for coronary artery aneurysms or dilation.

The major complication of KD, especially in infants younger than 1 year of age, is coronary artery aneurysms. These aneurysms occur in 20% to 25% of untreated children with KD, but develop in only 4% of those who receive adequate therapy. Other cardiac sequelae may include myocarditis, decreased myocardial contractility, coronary arteritis without aneurysms, mild mitral valvular regurgitation, and pericardial effusion.[684,838]

Clinical findings at presentation that have been associated with an increased incidence of coronary artery aneurysms include treatment delay beyond 10 days; age less than 1 year or greater than 8 years; male gender; fever greater than 14 days; or fever persisting after IVIG administration.[684,838]

Coronary artery aneurysms have been visualized with echocardiogram as soon as a few days after onset of illness, but more typically occur between 1 and 4 weeks after onset of illness; later than 6 weeks is uncommon. Giant coronary artery aneurysms (greater than 8 mm in diameter) are likely to be associated with long-term complications, such as myocardial infarction.

Acute myocardial infarction (AMI) may develop during the acute phase of illness. This diagnosis can be difficult to make in children because it is so rare. The infarction often occurs at night during sleep or rest and is accompanied by pallor, inconsolable crying, abdominal pain, and vomiting.

Management

Management of KD during the acute phase is directed at decreasing inflammation of the myocardium and coronary artery wall. Once the acute phase has passed, therapy is directed at prevention of coronary artery thrombosis.

Intravenous immune globulin (IVIG) and aspirin initiated within 10 days of the onset of the fever substantially decreases progression to coronary artery dilation and aneurysms.[20] The recommended IVIG dose is 2 g/kg as a single dose given over 10 to 12 hours. Aspirin is administered in doses of 80 to 100 mg/kg per day in four divided doses during the acute phase. The dose of aspirin is decreased to 3 mg/kg per day, 48 hours after the resolution of fever. Aspirin is discontinued if no coronary artery abnormalities have been detected by 6 to 8 weeks after the onset of illness.[684,838]

An echocardiogram should be obtained early in the acute phase of illness and 6 to 8 weeks after onset. Children diagnosed with KD should be assessed during the first 2 months for arrhythmias, CHF, and valvular regurgitation.

Approximately 10% of patients with KD fail to defervesce with initial IVIG treatment. Failure to respond is usually defined as persistent or recrudescent fever more than 36 h after completion of initial IVIG infusion. Retreatment with IVIG (dose: 2 g/kg) is recommended.[918] Although corticosteroids are the treatment of choice in other forms of vasculitis, their use has been limited in children with KD.[805]

Early detection of KD and prompt initiation of therapy with IVIG and aspirin have reduced mortality to less than 0.1% to 0.2% and the prevalence of coronary artery aneurysm to approximately 5%. The principal cause of death is AMI resulting from coronary artery occlusion attributable to thrombosis or progressive stenosis.[684,838]

Measles and varicella immunizations should be deferred 11 months after IVIG administration.

COMMON DIAGNOSTIC TESTS

Punkaj Gupta and Stephen M. Schexnayder

The field of pediatric critical care has undergone a fundamental transition over the past few years with recent advances in medical technology. The major imaging modalities for structural and functional evaluation of most organ systems in the body are ultrasonography (including echocardiography), computed tomography, magnetic resonance imaging, and nuclear medicine techniques. This section includes description of these imaging modalities, potential complications, and nursing interventions needed for these procedures.

ECHOCARDIOGRAPHY

Description

Sonography has evolved to become one of the most versatile modalities for diagnosing and guiding treatment in critically ill children. It consists of both cardiac (echocardiography) and noncardiac (head, lung, abdominal, and vascular) ultrasound. Echocardiographic examination provides extensive noninvasive anatomic and hemodynamic information in real time. This painless procedure involves the transmission of high-frequency, pulsed-sound waves from piezoelectric crystals located within the ultrasound transducer. The pulse-sound waves are transmitted into the chest and then are reflected back, received, and recorded by the same transducer.

All tissues in the body impede or absorb high-frequency sound waves in a different way, so that the sound waves reflected back to the receiver are of differing strengths. The distance of a reflecting surface from the transducer is calculated on the basis of the time it takes the energy to reach the structure and return to the transducer. This information then determines the location of dots representing that structure on a display screen. This process is repeated approximately 1000 times/s (1000 Hz) to create an image.[259,312,675,808,819]

Echocardiography can be a rapid, noninvasive, objective tool in the assessment of ventricular function and preload during resuscitation of a critically ill child. Echocardiography can also be used to evaluate the dimensions of the cardiac chambers and great vessels, the location and motion of cardiac valves, and the size and location of septal and other defects. In

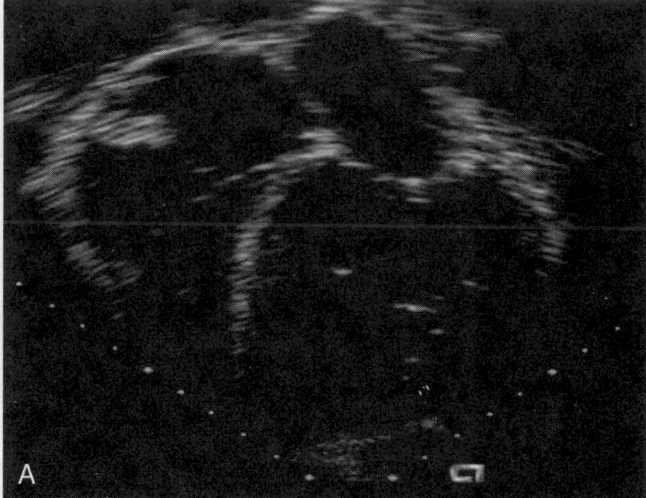

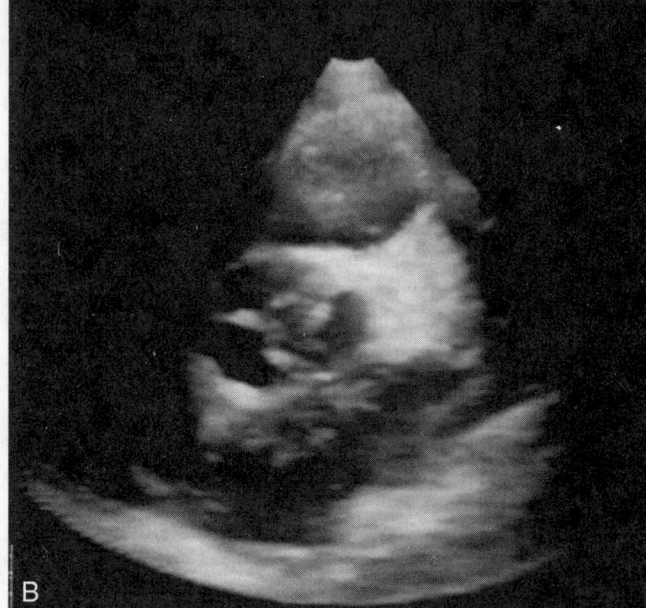

Box 8-51	**Common Indications for Echocardiography in Critically Ill Children**

Assessment of hemodynamics

Assess myocardial contractility and regional wall abnormalities

Assess volume status

Assess noninvasive cardiac output

Estimate filling pressures and predict volume responsiveness

Assess right heart function

Detect pericardial effusion/tamponade

Detect pulmonary embolus

Diagnose diastolic ventricular dysfunction

Resuscitation

Differentiate fine ventricular fibrillation from true asystole

Assess cardiac standstill for prognostication purposes

Perform focused evaluation in resuscitation (FEER) to look for potentially reversible causes of PEA or asystole, such as pericardial effusion/tamponade, hypovolemia, pulmonary embolism, or tension pneumothorax

Other Diagnostic Uses

Congenital heart disease

Primary or secondary cardiomyopathy

Primary pulmonary hypertension

Cerebrovascular infarct (embolic)

Rhythm and conduction abnormalities

Cardiac and pericardiac tumors

Arteriovenous malformations

Rheumatic heart disease

Kawasaki disease

Chest pain

Syncope

Suspected endocarditis

Deep vein thrombosis

Procedural Guidance in PCCU

Balloon atrial septostomy

Pericardiocentesis

Line displacement or dislodgement

FIG. 8-65 A, Four chambered view of the heart in a normal two-dimensional echocardiogram. B, Three-dimensional echocardiographic image. This is a short axis view of a tricuspid aortic valve leaflet. (Images courtesy of Dr. Ritu Sachdeva, Division of Pediatric Cardiology, Arkansas Children's Hospital.)

addition, bedside echocardiography can be used to differentiate fine ventricular fibrillation from true asystole during resuscitation.[105,106,710] Box 8-51 summarizes some of the common indications for echocardiography in critically ill children.

The ability to assess myocardial function, volume status, and cardiac output noninvasively is very useful in the management of complicated or mixed shock states.[166,716,779] Although the culture is changing, echocardiography still remains a forte of cardiologists in the majority of tertiary care centers in United States.

Three forms of echocardiography currently are used, namely *M-mode* (or motion-mode) echocardiography, 2D echocardiography, and 3D echocardiography.[259,675] M-mode (or motion-mode) echocardiography uses a single crystal to obtain an image of the heart at one point. The only axis that is evaluated is depth, so only structures located directly under the transducer are visualized. Spatial orientation of objects can

only be achieved by moving or angling the transducer. M-mode is now used primarily for evaluation of left ventricular dimensions and function; it has largely been replaced with 2D echo imaging. In rare cases, 2D-directed M-mode may be useful for assessing certain structures, such as native and prosthetic valve leaflets.

Two-dimensional or *cross-sectional* echocardiography uses many crystals to pass a planar beam of ultrasound through the heart to obtain an image of a cardiac plane (Fig. 8-65, A). The ultrasound beam is swept rapidly in an arc, creating multiple M-mode images, which are then aligned to create a cross-sectional image of the heart. Because this form of echocardiography can provide a spatially correct image of the heart and great vessels, it is more useful for the determination of anatomic relationships of structures within the heart. The three basic elements of any 2D echocardiogram include imaging sweeps for anatomic delineation, Doppler interrogation for blood flow velocity and direction, and measurement of systolic and diastolic function.

Three-dimensional echocardiography is one of the significant advances in this field because it provides realistic visualization of cardiac valves and congenital abnormalities as well as accurate assessment of cardiac chamber volumes (Fig. 8-65, B). Real-time 3D echocardiography allows fast acquisition of pyramidal datasets during a single breath-hold without the need for off-line reconstruction, thus eliminating motion artifacts known to have adversely affected the earlier multiplane acquisition and reconstruction methodology.[715,801]

Color Doppler echocardiography yields color-coded Doppler signals overlaid on an echocardiographic image of the heart. With such Doppler studies, blood flow of differing speeds (e.g., shunting blood) is identified by different colors. Directionality of blood flow is determined by whether the frequency shift is higher (i.e., the flow is toward the probe) or lower (the flow is away from the probe). Various color maps are used to encode this information, but a commonly used map displays blood flow toward the transducer in red and flow away in blue (see Evolve Fig. 8-7 in the Chapter 8 Supplement on the Evolve Website). The use of color enables rapid and obvious visualization of small or multiple shunts or small amounts of valvular regurgitation and may enable identification of small vascular pathways (e.g., sources of pulmonary blood flow in patients with pulmonary atresia) that are not detected by standard echocardiography. In addition, Doppler derived calculations provide quantitative and semiquantitative estimation of valvular regurgitation, intracardiac and extracardiac shunts, and myocardial motion.[324]

Transesophageal echocardiography (TEE) is another modality of echocardiography, most frequently used in the operating room or during the perioperative period, where the acoustic windows are limited by dressings over the incision (Fig. 8-66).[690] The transesophageal approach does not compromise the operative field and images are not obscured by

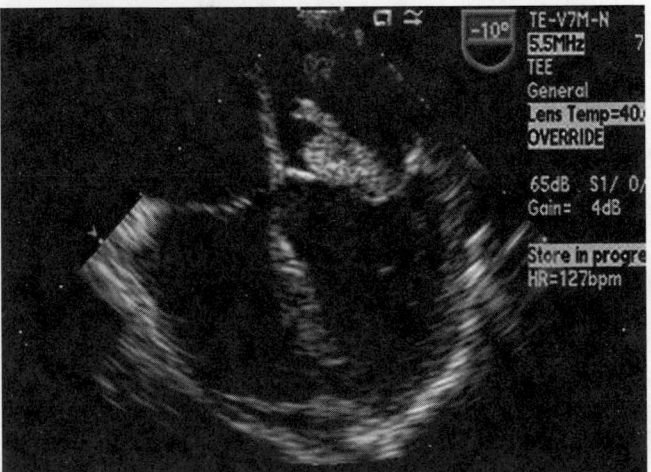

FIG. 8-66 Transesophageal echocardiogram (TEE) image showing mitral valve vegetation in a 3-year-old girl. (Courtesy of Dr. Ritu Sachdeva, Division of Pediatric Cardiology, Arkansas Children's Hospital.)

chest tubes and dressings as with transthoracic imaging. Occasionally the image quality with transesophageal echocardiography can be compromised by adjacent nasogastric tubes.

TEE offers high-quality imaging of patients who otherwise pose a challenge to the echocardiographer. Structures that are particularly well suited to TEE examination are those located closest to the esophagus, including the atrial septum, pulmonary veins, superior vena cava, AV valves, left ventricular outflow tract, aortic valve, and coronary artery origins. With the advancement in technology, transesophageal probes are available for patients as small as 2 to 2.5 kg.

Procedure

Echocardiography can be performed at the bedside or in the echocardiography laboratory. It does not require any specific preparation. The infant or child is placed in a reclining or semireclining position at the start of the procedure and it may be necessary to turn the patient occasionally during the procedure.

A single, flat-tipped transducer that is approximately 6 inches in length is used to obtain the surface echocardiogram; this transducer sends and receives the sound waves. To minimize artifact and maximize sound transmission, small amounts of electrocardiographic gel or paste are applied to the child's chest, where the transducer is placed. During the procedure the infant or child merely feels the touch of the transducer and gel. TEE is obtained through a transducer inserted into the esophagus.

Because the images produced during the echocardiogram will be blurred by motion artifact, it is very important that the infant and/or child be motionless during the procedure. Usually the infant and/or child will be quieted by the use of a pacifier or feeding with a bottle. Parent presence, the use of pacifiers or favorite objects, a quiet environment, and the therapeutic use of music or videos can all be provided in a hospital environment. If all attempts at holding and quieting fail, the physician may elect to prescribe a mild sedative for the infant. Oral chloral hydrate provides deep sedation usually lasting 60 to 120 min, which should be adequate for a complete study in a child with complex congenital heart disease.[542,644] Intravenous midazolam or narcotics may be preferable in some situations, particularly in critical care settings. Institutional guidelines for procedural sedation should be followed, and qualified medical personnel not involved in performing the echocardiography should be responsible for monitoring the child's cardiorespiratory status.[19]

Potential Complications

Although a relatively safe procedure, it has been our experience that a child with marginal hemodynamic status has the potential to decompensate during echocardiography. Therefore, the bedside nurse should monitor the hemodynamic status of the child very closely throughout the procedure. Procedural sedation may produce complications. Because managing procedural sedation is the responsibility of pediatric cardiovascular nurses, the bedside nurse should be well versed with these complications. Adequate care must be taken to keep the critically ill infant or child warm and comfortable during the procedure.

A transesophageal echocardiogram (TEE) may produce complications such as oropharyngeal and esophageal injury and compression of airways and vascular structures. Contraindications to TEE include unrepaired tracheoesophageal fistula, significant esophageal stricture, active gastrointestinal bleeding, and an uncontrolled airway in a patient with significant cardiorespiratory compromise.[690]

Nursing Interventions

There is no specific nursing care required before, during, or after echocardiography. It is important that the nurse observe the patient carefully throughout the procedure, and ensure that the patient is kept warm. Unstable children must be monitored closely. The study will progress more quickly if the nurse is able to help keep the infant or child quiet, content, and motionless. Often this requires creativity and a lot of patience. The nurse should keep a bottle (unless the infant can have nothing by mouth) and pacifier nearby during echocardiography of the infant and several toys available during echocardiography of the child. Children often enjoy watching their heart "on TV."

COMPUTED TOMOGRAPHY (CT)

Description

A computed tomography (CT) scan combines a series of x-ray views taken from many different angles to produce cross-sectional images of the bones and soft tissues inside the patient's body. The data are digitized and converted to cross-sectional images with the help of powerful array processors. These devices record, digitize, store, and tomographically reconstruct hundreds of projection images acquired at many angles about the patient, using special mathematical algorithms. One major advantage in favor of CT scan is quick image acquisition time. Helical (spiral) scanners have so substantially shortened the acquisition times required for high-quality images that sedation for CT is unnecessary in the vast majority of infants and children who can refrain from moving briefly or can be restrained appropriately. Box 8-52 summarizes some of the common indications of CT scan in critically ill children.[52,57,58,223,335]

Procedure

A CT scan is a quick, painless procedure that requires positioning the child on the CT examination table. The patient is typically scanned while lying supine, although lateral and prone positions are occasionally used. A CT machine resembles a large, square doughnut. A flat "patient couch" is situated in the circular opening, which is about 24 to 28 inches in diameter. The patient lies on the couch, which can be moved up, down, forward, and backward to position the patient for imaging. Straps and pillows may be needed to maintain the correct position and hold the patient still during the exam. Motion will degrade the quality of the examination. If contrast material is used, it will be swallowed, injected through an intravenous line (IV), or administered by enema, depending on the type of examination.

Box 8-52	Common Indications for Computed Tomography in Critically Ill Children

Acute trauma
Nonaccidental trauma
Increased intracranial pressure
Acute neurologic deficit
Encephalopathy
Suspected CNS infection
Intractable headaches
Shunted hydrocephalus with a suspected shunt obstruction
Head and neck masses
Mediastinal pathology such as lymphoma, tumor, or great vessel disease (aortic aneurysm or dissection)
Cardiac or pericardial disease, such as tumor, inflammation, or pericardial effusion
Suspected pulmonary embolus
Abnormal collection in any body cavity as abscess, empyema, or pneumocephalus
Evaluation of spinal cord abnormality
Detection and confirmation of calcification in any body part

Potential Complications

Although the scanning itself causes no pain, there may be some discomfort because the child must remain still for several minutes. The CT scan can be particularly stressful for children with claustrophobia or chronic pain. Because the child must remain in a closed chamber and there is limited visibility of and access to the child during the procedure, it has the potential for short-term complications such as unintentional extubation and hemodynamic collapse during the process.

If contrast is used, complications may include reaction to iodinated contrast, contrast infiltration at the injection site, and long-term complications such as contrast-induced nephropathy. Contraindications to CT in children are unusual and include syndromes in which radiation could induce chromosome breaks and increase the genetic predisposition to tumors (e.g., ataxia telangiectasia, Nijmegen breakage syndrome).[335]

Nursing Interventions

The bedside nurse should remove any metal jewelry or clothing accessories to prevent artifacts from decreasing the diagnostic quality of the images. If IV contrast is to be used the patient should remain NPO (not given anything by mouth) for at least 4 hours before the procedure. The critical care team taking care of the patient should determine the need for oral contrast before moving the patient to the radiology suite. The child requires close monitoring throughout the procedure. For children who cannot hold still for the examination, procedural sedation may be needed.

If the patient is in the critical care unit, the bedside nurse accompanies the child to and remains with the child at the CT scanner. (The nurse remains in the observation room rather than at the side of the scanner.) Any medications the child requires should accompany him or her to the scanner, and resuscitation drugs and equipment must be readily available. If the patient is intubated, both the bedside nurse and a respiratory therapist or a provider capable of re-intubation as well as re-intubation equipment typically accompany the child. Tube position must be verified when the child is transferred into and out of the scanner or repositioned in the scanner.

Although the intravenous contrast agent is typically administered by the radiology technicians or physician in the radiology suite, the bedside nurse is typically responsible for maintaining vascular access and monitoring the injection site for evidence of infiltration or inflammation. If the patient has a known allergy to iodine, then premedication will be necessary to prevent a histamine reaction. The reaction can be mild, such as hives, to life-threatening, including upper airway obstruction with laryngospasm. With newer and safer nonionic contrast, reactions have become less common.

NUCLEAR MAGNETIC RESONANCE IMAGING (NMRI OR MRI)

Description

Clinical magnetic resonance imaging (MRI) uses the magnetic properties of hydrogen and its interaction with both a large external magnetic field and radio waves to produce highly detailed images of the human body. In its early days, MRI was known as NMR, or nuclear magnetic resonance. Although the name has changed, the basic principles are the same. MR images are generated by analysis of signals produced by hydrogen nuclei of molecules in varying tissues as the spins of the nuclei are aligned in a strong external magnetic field and then perturbed by radiofrequency pulses. In an MRI machine, a radio frequency transmitter is briefly turned on, producing an electromagnetic field. The photons of this field have just the right energy, known as the resonance frequency, to flip the spin of the aligned protons in the body. As the intensity and duration of application of the field increase, more aligned spins are affected. After the field is turned off, the protons decay to the original spin-down state and the difference in energy between the two states is released as a photon. It is these photons that produce the electromagnetic signal that the scanner detects. An image can be constructed because the protons in different tissues return to their equilibrium state at different rates, a difference that can be detected.

MRI is used to image every part of the body, and is particularly useful for tissues with many hydrogen nuclei and little density contrast, such as the brain, muscle (including myocardium), connective tissue, and most tumors. MRI often provides more sensitive and specific imaging information about pediatric CNS abnormalities than does ultrasound or computed tomography technology. MRI also has redefined the role of invasive procedures such as myelography, ventriculography, cisternography, and angiography. Box 8-53 summarizes some of the common indications of MRI in critically ill children.[24,52,57–59,635]

All personnel and monitoring and support equipment must be safe for the magnet. The American Society for Testing and Material (ASTM) International developed the following terminology for labeling of implanted devices[21,796]:

Box 8-53 | **Common Indications for Magnetic Resonance Imaging in Critically Ill Children**

Acute trauma
Nonaccidental trauma
Hypoxic ischemic injury
Meningitis or meningoencephalitis
Intracranial or spinal fluid collections and/or Infections
Intractable seizure activity
Evaluation of spinal column and spinal neuraxis
Unexplained and intractable headaches
Unexplained hydrocephalus
Investigation of orbital pathology
Toxic metabolic injury
Vascular disease and hemorrhage
Muscular and vascular anomalies in any body part
Postinfectious encephalomyelitis

- **MR safe:** An item that poses no known hazards in any MR environment
- **MR conditional:** An item that has been demonstrated to pose no known hazards in a specified MR imaging environment with specified conditions of use
- **MR unsafe:** An item that is known to pose hazards in all MR environments

Procedure

The MRI scanner is normally located well away from critical care units. The patient is positioned on the moveable examination table. The patient lies inside a large, cylinder-shaped magnet. Radio waves 10,000 to 30,000 times stronger than the magnetic field of the earth are then sent through the body. These radio waves and the magnet affect the body's atoms, forcing the nuclei into a different position. As they move back into place, they send out radio waves of their own. The scanner picks up these signals and a computer turns them into a picture. These pictures are based on the location and strength of the incoming signals. If a contrast material is used during the examination, it is injected into the intravenous (IV) catheter after an initial series of scans. Additional series of images are taken during or after the injection.

Straps and bolsters may be used to keep the child still and maintain the correct position during imaging. An audiovisual system within the scanner greatly reduces the need for sedation in children greater than 3 years of age.

Potential Complications

There are no known complications to MRI scanning. The principal drawback of MR imaging is the long acquisition time, which frequently necessitates procedural sedation for children less than 8 years old and for some who are older. As noted, the use of audiovisual systems may distract or calm the child and reduce need for sedation.

Another drawback of MRI is the incompatibility of ferromagnetic materials within the imaging suite. In critically ill ventilator-dependent children, plastic and aluminium

MR-compatible monitors and ventilators are available, but children with metallic bullet fragments or implants, including cardiac pacemakers and neurostimulators, may not be able to undergo MRI.

Although the scanning itself causes no pain, there may be some discomfort for some children from having to remain still for several minutes to a few hours. The MRI machine produces loud thumping and humming noises; therefore earplugs are typically provided during the scan. The MRI scan is particularly stressful for children with claustrophobia and/or chronic pain.

Because the child must remain in a closed chamber with limited access during the procedure, this procedure has the potential for short-term complications such as inadvertent extubation, hemodynamic collapse, contrast infiltration at the injection site, anaphylactoid reactions from the gadolinium contrast agents, and/or long-term complications from gadolinium contrast as nephrogenic systemic fibrosis (NSF). MR contrast agents are generally safer than iodinated contrast agents in patients who are unstable or have impaired renal function or a prior history of anaphylactoid reaction to iodinated contrast agents.

Nursing Interventions

Before entering the MRI suite, the bedside nurse should remove any MRI-incompatible metal jewelry or clothing accessories. A detailed list of MR-compatible medical devices is available on the web site maintained by Frank Shellock at http://www.mrisafety.com. In addition to magnet issues, metallic devices can also create artifacts and distortions in the surrounding tissues.

Given the long acquisition time of the procedure, all devices and catheters must be secured before the start of the procedure. Careful cardiorespiratory monitoring is required throughout the procedure, often performed via a camera in the scanner and a screen in the observation area. For children who cannot hold still for the examination, procedural sedation may be needed. If the patient is in the critical care unit, the bedside nurse should accompany the child throughout transportation to and from and during the procedure in the MRI suite. (The nurse will observe the child in the observation room during the actual procedure.)

To continue sedation or vasopressor infusions during the MRI, the bedside nurse should attach and flush long tubing extensions before the transport to allow continuation of all infusions during the MRI. Because most infusion pumps are incompatible with the MRI, they must remain outside of the MRI suite. The long tubing allows use of these infusion pumps; the tubing stretches from the patient through a hole in the wall of the MRI suite to the pumps. If the patient is intubated, both the bedside nurse and the respiratory therapist are responsible for ensuring that the endotracheal tube is well secured and remains in place throughout the procedure.

Although intravenous contrast is generally administered by the radiology technicians or a physician in the radiology suite, the bedside nurse is responsible for maintaining the intravenous catheter and monitoring the injection site. Infiltration of the contrast material can result in a painful tissue injury around the site.

NUCLEAR CARDIOLOGY

Definition

Radionuclide imaging is an extremely reliable method of evaluating ventricular function and myocardial perfusion. These studies use an injected radionuclide (such as technetium or thallium) and record its movement through the cardiac chambers, vascular space, or myocardial muscle. The advantages of this highly sensitive and specific technique are the ability to detect and prognosticate coronary disease, reproduce similar results, and assess myocardial viability.

Radionuclide methods often lack sufficient resolution to precisely characterize complex morphology in congenital heart lesions. However, these methods provide an accurate and reproducible quantitative assessment of the physiologic consequences of structural heart disease. The radionuclide method most often is used to assess the size of left-to-right shunts in four major congenital lesions: atrial septal defect, ventricular septal defect (VSD), patent ductus arteriosus, and partial anomalous pulmonary venous return. These tests expose the patient to radiation and are associated with increased cost.[50,213,493,696,875]

Procedure

The scintigraphic technique involves the rapid injection of a bolus of radionuclide (usually 99m Tc-DTPA), into the circulation while monitoring the transit through the heart and lungs with the gamma camera. For small infants (i.e., premature newborn infants), a butterfly needle can be used in a temporal scalp vein to deliver a compact bolus of radionuclide to the central circulation. In older children and adults, either a butterfly needle or a small plastic catheter can be inserted, preferably into an external jugular vein, although an antecubital vein can also be used. The delivery of a compact nonfragmented bolus of radionuclide is critical to allow accurate determination of the size of the shunt. With good injection technique, the success rate should be greater than 90%.

The study is done in the anterior projection using a converging collimator (which provides magnification) in infants and ideally a high sensitivity parallel collimator in older children and adults. A dynamic acquisition with a sampling rate of two to four frames per second is adequate for evaluation of shunts.[213]

Potential Complications

The only potential complication related to this study is extravasation of the radionuclide. Extravasation at the peripheral site may cause local tissue burns and extravasation from a central venous line into the thoracic space or pericardium may produce cardiorespiratory compromise.

Nursing Interventions

Because these studies require injection of a radionuclide, reliable intravenous access must be established. The radionuclide is injected by laboratory personnel, and the bedside nurse is responsible for monitoring the injection site and the patient's condition during the study.

CARDIAC CATHETERIZATION AND INTERVENTION

Jo Ann Nieves and Ruby L. Whalen

Pearls

- Pediatric cardiac catheterization procedures are primarily for interventional purposes.
- Cardiac catheterization interventional procedures alter cardiac hemodynamics. Each patient must be monitored for potential complications, including decreased systemic perfusion, arrhythmias, bleeding, tamponade, and compromised limb perfusion.
- Interventional procedures are typically performed under general anesthesia.
- Anemia may develop from blood loss during the procedure. A hematocrit less than 40% is undesirable in the child with single ventricle physiology or cyanotic heart disease and will lead to inadequate oxygen carrying capacity and delivery. Transfusion therapy may be required.
- Increasingly complex interventions: About 70% of cardiac catheterizations are now interventional, and many delay or eliminate the need for surgical intervention. Patient acuity is often high.
- When patients have short length of stay (admitted and discharged within 24 hours) the teaching provided by the bedside nurse is crucial.
- Care is anticipatory; to anticipate complications the bedside nurse requires knowledge of the child's diagnosis, intervention, and change in anatomy/and physiology caused by the catheterization.

Cardiac catheterization involves insertion of a radiopaque catheter through an artery and/or vein into the heart. This procedure is performed under fluoroscopy so the location and movement of the catheter can be visualized. Throughout catheterization, pressure measurements are made and oxygen saturations are recorded to provide complete hemodynamic and anatomic data about blood flow patterns (including shunts) within the heart. Structures such as cardiac chambers, valves, or great vessels can be visualized through injection of a radiopaque contrast agent. Rapid sequential radiographs, called angiograms, are made to record the flow of contrast through the heart. References that provide excellent reviews of the technique of cardiac catheterization and analysis of the data include Grifka[336] and Lock[545].

Assessment of the pulmonary vascular bed is required in patients with elevated pulmonary vascular resistance to determine operability or before transplant. Response to vasodilator therapy will be evaluated, including response to oxygen and medications such as nitric oxide, prostacyclin, and sildenafil. Fontan and Glenn procedures require low pulmonary vascular resistance. Pulmonary hypertensive precautions in care are required to avoid exacerbation of the pulmonary vascular hypertension. (See section, Common Clinical Conditions, Pulmonary Hypertension, and Specific Diseases, Single Functioning Ventricle.)

Since the 1980s advances in echocardiography and magnetic resonance imaging have progressively improved the precision of noninvasive diagnosis of congenital heart defects, decreasing the need for diagnostic cardiac catheterization.[336]

Diagnostic cardiac catheterization is still required when complete diagnosis or hemodynamic information is not possible with noninvasive methods. Diagnostic catheterization may also take place when the patient's clinical signs and symptoms are not consistent with the diagnosis, or when the clinical course is not progressing as expected.[336]

The assessment of pulmonary vascular resistance is one of the most common indications for diagnostic catheterization,[336] particularly in those patients who will undergo creation of a complete systemic venous to pulmonary arterial connection.[253] Selected patients undergo MRI study and, therefore, no longer require routine preoperative diagnostic cardiac catheterization prior to bidirectional Glenn procedure.[118]

Therapeutic interventions have rapidly evolved as the primary reason for cardiac catheterization. The interventional cardiologist uses devices to dilate stenotic structures, close defects, and create vascular connections in patients with congenital heart disease of all ages, from the unborn fetus to the adult. In many cases patients no longer require surgical intervention, and in selected cases surgery is delayed. Many procedures take place as a day procedure or require overnight admission, have a relatively painless and rapid recovery, and are safe and effective.[660] Many lesions previously classified as inoperable can be managed at cardiac catheterization.[545] In selected patients a hybrid procedure will combine the simultaneous skills of the surgeon with the interventional cardiology team to optimize patient management.

Critically ill patients requiring cardiac catheterization postoperatively may be moved to the catheterization suite on mechanical cardiopulmonary support circuits for diagnostic catheterization and catheter intervention. Electrophysiologic studies are used to identify and eliminate intracardiac conduction pathways and sources of arrhythmias.

The most common percutaneous interventional procedures in the adult patient with congenital heart disease include lesion closures by devices or coils, balloon valvuloplasty, balloon angioplasty with or without stent placement to treat native, recurrent or prosthetic conduit lesions, and arrhythmia assessment or therapies. Adult interventions are detailed in Inglessis and Landzberg[399] and Holzer and Cheatham.[388]

Procedure

Cardiac catheterization is performed in a catheterization laboratory where appropriate catheters, devices, anesthesia, and radiographic equipment are located. The infant or child usually receives nothing by mouth before the catheterization to minimize the possibility of vomiting and aspiration during the procedure. Oral sedation is prescribed before the catheterization in patients presenting for outpatient, elective catheterization, and additional sedation is administered as needed during the procedure. General anesthesia is often used for interventional procedures.[664] Vascular access is typically placed in patients with cyanotic heart disease and/or polycythemia before the catheterization to ensure adequate hydration and sedation.[336]

The patient's right femoral artery and vein often are used for the procedure; the umbilical vessels may be used in the neonate. In the older child the femoral artery and vein or vessels in the antecubital fossa or axilla, jugular, or subclavian veins may be used for the catheterization. Percutaneous puncture, usually via the Seldinger technique, is performed most often to gain access to the artery or vein. Transhepatic access may be required if femoral access is not possible. Surgical access via a cutdown in the neck may be used as access for interventional procedures treating the aortic valve in newborns or the descending aorta to optimize access during hybrid intervention.[663]

Right heart catheterization is accomplished through insertion of a catheter into a vein; for purposes of simplicity, the remaining description assumes normally related atria, ventricles, and great vessels. The catheter is passed into the superior or inferior vena cava and into the right atrium and then the right ventricle and pulmonary artery. Pressure measurements and oxygen saturation analyses are made in each location to detect the presence and location of abnormal chamber hypertension or intracardiac shunts.

The left heart often can be entered by passage of the catheter from the right atrium through a probe-patent foramen ovale to the left atrium. If the cardiologist is not able to enter the left atrium from the right atrium, a catheter can be inserted into a systemic artery, retrograde into the aorta and then into the left ventricle, or the atrial septum can be punctured to allow access into the left heart.

When all necessary pressure and oxygen saturation measurements have been recorded, angiograms are performed. Angiograms depict any shunting that occurs as the result of congenital heart defects or valvular dysfunction, and document areas of narrowing or dilation in blood flow pathways.

Associated procedures may be accomplished during cardiac catheterization. As noted, defects may be created or closed, and valves and vessels may be dilated. Specific information regarding therapeutic catheterization is comprehensively covered by Nykanen and Zahn,[663] Lock,[545] and Holzer and Cheatham.[388,389]

Conduction system mapping can be performed along with therapeutic management of refractory arrhythmias (comprehensive information in Saul[772]). Transvenous intracardiac pacing wires also may be inserted during catheterization and fluoroscopy

Sedation and analgesia are continued during the procedure with a variety of agents, including morphine, fentanyl, ketamine, midazolam, and propofol (see Chapter 5).[336,664] Agents that produce systemic vasodilation, such as propofol, are avoided in patients with right-to-left shunts, because they enhance the right-to-left shunt and can worsen hypoxemia.[336]

Medication may be administered during the catheterization to allow detailed assessment of the patient's hemodynamic response. Continual monitoring of all hemodynamic and respiratory responses occurs throughout the procedure, observing for variations in heart rate, oxygen saturation, blood pressure, and ventilatory status.

At the end of the catheterization procedure the catheters are removed and pressure is applied to the puncture site. Products that apply pressure over the access sites may be secured in place with specific removal guidelines (i.e., they are removed several hours later). The infant or child is returned to the unit for close observation. If a catheter was

passed through a surgical systemic to pulmonary artery shunt, anticoagulation therapy may be ordered to minimize the risk of thrombus within the shunt (see Postoperative Care, Anticoagulation).

If the child is normally ambulatory, the physician typically requests that he or she remain in bed for several hours after the catheterization. After percutaneous cardiac device placement a chest radiograph or echocardiogram is typically obtained to evaluate device position before discharge home.[664] Nursing care is reviewed in the following sections.

If cardiac catheterization is performed electively on a stable child the mortality rate is low, reported at 0.2%,[143] with 2.4% serious complications. If, however, the procedure is performed on an emergency basis on a critically ill patient, the morbidity and mortality will be higher. The risks of catheterization also are increased for infants and children with elevated pulmonary vascular resistance, arrhythmias, or hypoxemia, and for those children with tetralogy of Fallot or other cyanotic defect who have a history of hypercyanotic episodes (see section, Common Clinical Conditions, Hypoxemia).

Therapeutic Cardiac Catheterization

Cardiac catheterization interventions in congenital heart disease are often guided by transesophageal echocardiogram (TEE), intravascular ultrasound (IVUS) or intracardiac echocardiogram (ICE). *Hybrid procedures* combine the simultaneous skills of the surgeon with the interventional cardiology team. Interventions can be completed intraoperatively, including implantation of stents in the pulmonary or systemic vasculature under direct vision or cardioscopic imaging.[663] Surgeons can assist planned catheter interventions by providing alternative open surgical vessel access for interventions via the carotid artery or direct access to the aortic valve or descending aorta.[663] Improved outcomes are reported with early (less than 24 hours) cardiac catheterization and catheter based intervention in children who cannot be separated from cardiopulmonary bypass at the end of a surgical procedure.[663,965]

Occlusion of Lesions

Atrial septal defect (ASD) transcatheter device closure began in 1975.[781] Secundum ASDs are most frequently closed by the Amplatzer septal occluder device, approved by the FDA in 2001 (see Evolve Figs. 8-3 through 8-5 in the Chapter 8 Supplement on the Evolve Website). The Amplatzer is a double-disk of nitinol wire mesh and fibers, available up to 38 mm in diameter.[389] The Helex (up to a 35 mm device) has a long nitinol wire with polytetrafluoroethylene fabric that allows tissue in-growth to seal the defect.[649] ASD occluders have also included the Sideris, CardioSEAL, and STARFlex devices.[389]

Rhythm disturbances are common within the first 24 hours after ASD device closure,[374] but typically resolve quickly.[389] Patients with ASDs are at increased risk for paradoxic emboli if they develop deep vein thrombosis.[26] Device embolization is rare, but can occur into the pulmonary, left heart, or systemic circulation.[664] Adults with large ASD with deficient rims are at highest risk for embolization.[389]

Adults with large unrepaired ASDs can develop atrial arrhythmias and heart failure. They may have left ventricular diastolic dysfunction, with development of elevated left atrial pressure, pulmonary edema, and ventilator dependence after closure of the ASD, when the "pop off" flow across the atrial septum is sealed.[256] Closure of large ASDs may precipitate headaches in patients with a previous history.

Ventricular septal defects (VSDs) in the muscular septum may be closed by percutaneous placement of the FDA approved muscular VSD Amplatzer occluder device, available up to 18 mm (see Evolve Fig. 8-3 in the Chapter 8 Supplement on the Evolve Website).[139,389] A transcatheter approach or periventricular (midsternal chest incision with the heart beating, no cardiopulmonary bypass) closure may be used.[389] Complications include potential embolization, arrhythmias (most frequently heart block), and blood loss requiring transfusion.[664] The transcatheter device closure of perimembranous VSD is under investigation with potential concerns including development of heart block in 1%[579] to 5%,[389] within days to months after the procedure. New or increased valve regurgitation (aortic or tricuspid) has been reported in up to 9%, with most improving or resolving by 6 months after the procedure.[390]

Vascular structure occlusions include sealing of aortopulmonary collateral vessels, pulmonary arteriovenous fistulae producing cyanosis, residual shunts, Blalock-Taussig shunts, venous malformations and coronary AV fistulae.[545] Devices used to occlude these vessels include Gianturco embolization coils and stainless steel coils with synthetic Dacron fibers.[389] The Gianturco-Grifka vascular occlusion device consists of a nylon bag filled with long stainless steel wires. It may be used to occlude vascular tubular structures.[389]

Closure of a patent ductus arteriosus (PDA) can use coils or the Amplatzer duct occluder device made of nitinol wire mesh (FDA approved). The Nit-Occlud PDA occlusion system (nitinol wire device wound into a helix-type loop) is also available.[389] Complications can include dislodgement and migration of coils into the systemic or pulmonary circulations.[664]

Fontan fenestrations may be closed with septal closure devices in patients with transcutaneous oxygen saturations of 90% or less after Fontan completion.[389] The Amplatzer septal occluder is the most common device used after balloon test occlusion of the fenestration to assure favorable hemodynamics.[389]

Implanted devices can embolize. When monitoring for device embolization assess for signs of altered perfusion status or development of arrhythmias or ECG changes. Auscultation may reveal a change in the cardiac murmur. Changes in peripheral perfusion can occur with migration into the aorta or branches. Some embolizations may be completely asymptomatic. CXR and echo are monitored for status of device location before the patient's discharge home. Dislodged devices may be retrieved with cardiac catheterization or surgery.

Structure Enlargement

Obstructive congenital heart lesions can be treated with percutaneous cardiac catheterization procedures that use balloon angioplasty and cutting balloons and may include placement of endovascular stents.[389] Balloon angioplasty is performed to stretch a vessel to its maximum diameter.[545] The angioplasty results in stretching or vessel tear of the intima, media,

and rarely the adventitia.[389,664] The vessel will then heal in an open position.[545] Because vessels recoil to a smaller size after angioplasty, a stent may be placed to increase the diameter to a larger size than would result from an angioplasty alone.[545] Stent implantation is most commonly used to enlarge branch pulmonary artery stenosis, for treatment of coarctation (see Fig. 8-67),[389] and to enlarge narrowed modified Blalock-Taussig or Sano Gore-Tex grafts.[725]

All stents used for congenital cardiovascular lesions in the United States are used in an "off-label" basis, because they were not designed and have not been approved for the specific intervention.[389] Covered stents are used to treat ruptured vessels or aortic aneurysms.[389] Stent implantation in infants is safe with re-dilations scheduled to keep pace with somatic growth.[827] Hybrid procedures may be completed with placement of stents planned in the operating suite, along with the cardiac surgical procedure.[389]

Balloon angioplasty of all types of pulmonary arteries is a widely accepted procedure,[389] and is one of the most common interventions performed in the developed world.[26] Repeated, staged interventions may be needed to treat distal pulmonary artery stenosis[389] or long segment stenosis (also called hypoplastic pulmonary arteries),[545] particularly to decrease RV strain before replacement of the pulmonary valve or in the presence of RV dysfunction.[388]

Vessels treated by angioplasty or stenting may develop aneurysm or dissection, or they may rupture.[664] Patients with diseases involving arteriopathies, such as William syndrome, are at increased risk of vessel rupture with dilation. The pulmonary vessels are the most likely to rupture after angioplasty, with presenting signs including acute hemoptysis, pulmonary hemorrhage, hemothorax, and pleural or pericardial effusions with tamponade.[664] Progression of bleeding must be monitored and ventilation supported. Pulmonary edema may develop because of increased blood flow after angioplasties, particularly in patients with multiple peripheral pulmonary artery stenoses (as in William or Alagille syndrome).[664] Surgical intervention may be required.

All bioprosthetic conduits placed for surgical palliation of tetralogy of Fallot, truncus arteriosus, or other complex repairs develop obstruction because of calcification, shrinkage, or compression,[545] and they do not grow as the child grows. Right ventricle to pulmonary artery conduit stenosis can be treated with angioplasty and stents to delay reoperations for conduit change.[545]

In newborns to adults, valvar pulmonic stenosis requiring intervention is treated by percutaneous balloon dilation as the standard therapeutic intervention.[389] For the first several days after balloon valvuloplasty for treatment of critical pulmonary valve stenosis of the newborn, decreased right ventricular compliance and residual elevation of right ventricular pressure may initially prevent sufficient antegrade flow across the valve, with resultant cyanosis and continued requirement for prostaglandin E1 infusion. Once right ventricular compliance improves, pulmonary blood flow and arterial oxygen saturation rise days later.[664] Restenosis of the pulmonary valve may occur in 25% to 50% of neonates.[545] Beyond the neonatal period, a single valvotomy will likely produce sufficient pulmonary blood flow for decades, with restenosis rare.

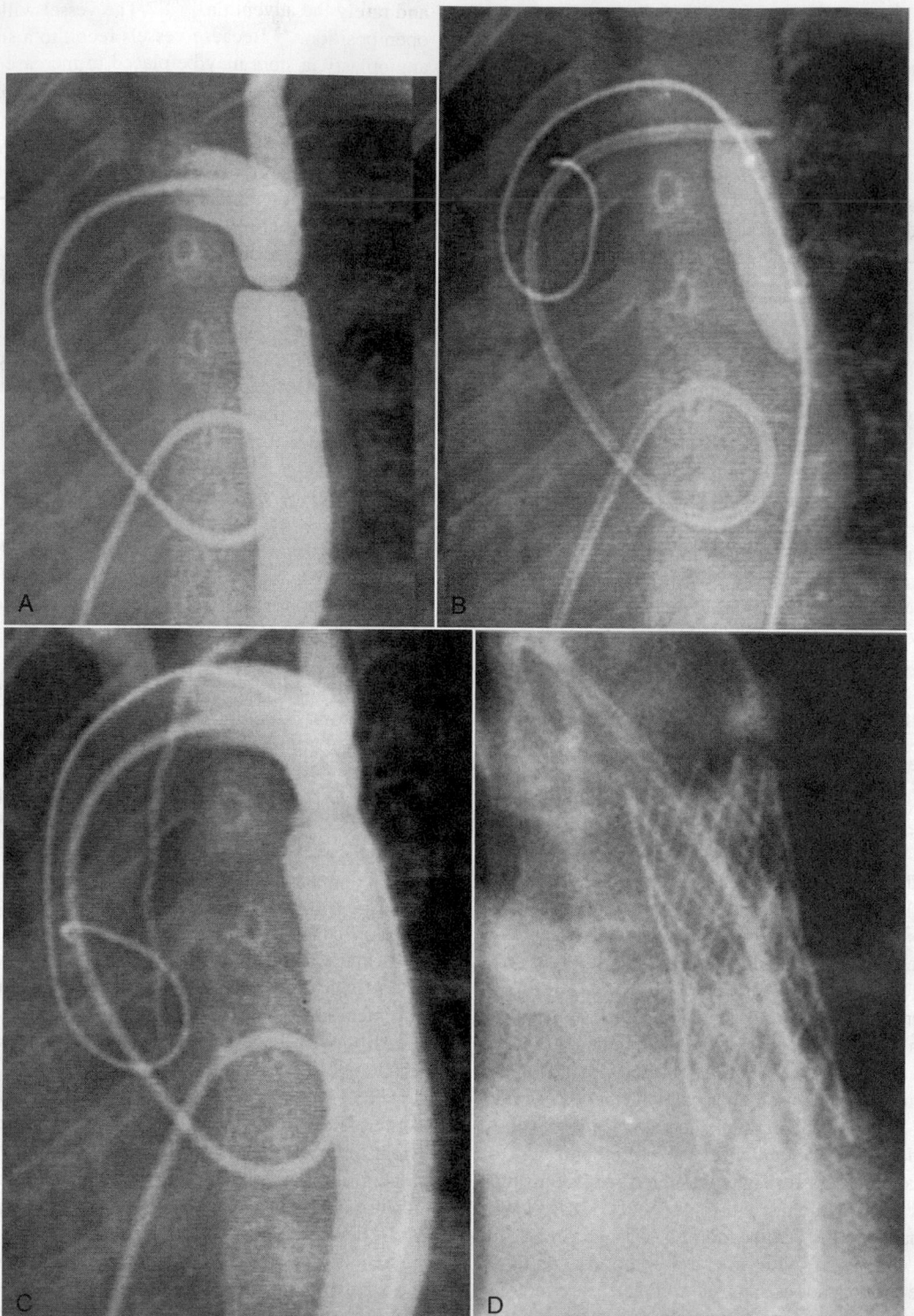

FIG. 8-67 Balloon angioplasty and stent placement during cardiac catheterization for coarctation of the aorta. **A,** Contrast injection depicts coarctation of the aorta. **B,** Balloon is inflated to dilate coarctation area. **C,** Contrast injection shows relief of coarctation. **D,** Stent is placed to support continued aortic enlargement.

Atretic pulmonary valves may be perforated with radio-frequency energy during cardiac catheterization, then balloon dilation is used to increase forward blood flow.[26] An estimated 50% of these infants require infusion of prostaglandin E_1 to provide additional pulmonary blood flow for several hours or days after cardiac catheterization. If severe hypoxemia and cyanosis persist, the infant may require future surgical aortopulmonary shunt or ductal stenting.[389] The major risk of radiofrequency valve perforation is perforation of the heart with resultant pericardial effusion and potential tamponade.[26]

In patients with pulmonary atresia/intact ventricular septum, radiofrequency valve perforation can facilitate pulmonary artery growth and provide the potential for eventual biventricular repair.

Aortic valve stenosis treated by balloon valvotomy increases valve diameter and decreases the gradient across the valve. It is important to note that neonates with critical aortic obstruction may have a falsely low transvalvular gradient at the beginning of the procedure because cardiac output is low.[545]

An aortic valvotomy may produce aortic regurgitation if excessive dilation or torn leaflets result. Severe aortic regurgitation produces symptoms including low diastolic pressure, tachycardia, diastolic murmur, signs of coronary ischemia, hypotension, and poor systemic perfusion. Surgical intervention may be required.

Critically ill neonates may continue to require hemodynamic support after successful aortic valvotomy because of pre-existing poor left ventricular function. Aortic valve balloon valvuloplasty is usually considered palliative versus curative,[389] although as many as two thirds of patients are free from surgery in the long term.[276] Percutaneous placement of a stent can relieve tunnel subaortic stenosis.[545] In the neonate with critical aortic stenosis, surgical access to the carotid artery permits safe and effective access to the valve for intervention.

Mitral valve balloon valvotomy may be performed for congenital or acquired (rheumatic) stenosis. In most patients with mitral stenosis caused by rheumatic heart disease, mitral balloon valvotomy is the initial intervention of choice.[545] These patients require careful assessment and care, particularly if they have pulmonary hypertension before intervention.[664] Mitral regurgitation may be present postprocedure and require surgical intervention.

Aortic coarctation balloon angioplasty is less common in small children and infants because of the high risk of recoarctation (near 66%).[389] The goal of the procedure is to reduce the gradient to less than 10 mm Hg, or effect a 90% relief of the obstruction.[389] Adults and school-aged children with primary coarctation or recoarctation are often treated with placement of an aortic stent (Fig. 8-67).[388,545] After angioplasty, vessel dissection is uncommon, but if it occurs it can be treated by placement of a covered stent. An aneurysm may be seen early and late after coarctation dilation.[389] Persistent, severe chest pain can indicate extension of the aortic tear; therefore this should be reported to a physician immediately.[664] Hypertension is present before intervention because of the aortic coarctation, and severe elevations must be controlled after the treatment to avoid the risk of vessel rupture.[664]

An unrestrictive atrial shunt is required for patients with simple transposition of the great arteries and other complex lesions to improve mixing of systemic and pulmonary venous blood and optimize arterial oxygen saturation. In hypoplastic left heart syndrome (HLHS), adequate cardiac output requires an adequate interatrial communication. The balloon atrial septostomy is a life-saving procedure for infants with simple transposition of the great arteries and acidosis related to a restrictive atrial shunt.[389] Percutaneous access through umbilical or femoral vein is typical with echocardiographic guidance in the PCCU. A deflated balloon is passed through the venous system, into the right atrium, across the atrial septum. The balloon is inflated with dilute contrast and pulled rapidly across the atrial opening, into the right atrium, to force a perforation in the septum. After adequate septostomy, the atrial pressures should immediately equalize, and hemodynamic status should improve.[389] Above the age of 1 month, the atrial septum may be too thick or tough for adequate septostomy requiring additional use of a blade atrial septostomy or cutting balloon atrial septostomy.[389]

A highly restrictive atrial shunt or intact atrial septum in HLHS has been managed by emergent balloon atrial septostomy in the effort to stabilize hemodynamics before first-stage palliation or cardiac transplantation.[908] Fetal intervention has been performed for this condition with reports of improving hospital survival after first-stage palliation.[908] Placement of an intraatrial stent may be required to maintain nonrestrictive atrial communication,[525] and cutting balloons or radiofrequency perforation may be used.[389,691] Before catheterization, infants with HLHS and severely restrictive atrial shunt or intact atrial septum are typically gravely ill, with severe cyanosis and pulmonary hypertension.[685] After atrial septostomy or stent implantation, the interatrial communication can progressively restenose.[691] Despite atrial septostomy, mortality in patients born with severely restrictive atrial shunt or intact atrial septum remains high.[323]

After an atrial switch procedure (Mustard or Senning operation for transposition of the great arteries) residual anatomic lesions can emerge.[388] Systemic or pulmonary venous baffle obstruction can be treated by percutaneous catheter dilation and stent implantation. Leaks within the atrial baffles may be sealed with a septal device occluder.[388] Electrophysiology therapy may be required for recurrent arrhythmias.

Pulmonary vein stenosis has a poor long-term outcome, despite surgical and therapeutic cardiac catheterization intervention.[232] Complications frequently develop after placement of pulmonary vein stents, and include stent embolization into the systemic circulation.[389]

Fontan fenestrations can be created with percutaneous catheterization by perforation of the extracardiac conduit and a covered stent may be inserted to maintain fenestration patency. Such fenestrations can result in improved cardiac output, pleural effusions, and ascites.[615] A Fontan procedure can be completed during cardiac catheterization with percutaneous placement of a large covered stent extending from the inferior vena cava into the superior vena cava and pulmonary arteries.[292]

Significant pulmonary insufficiency leads to RV dilation with subsequent risk for RV dysfunction and arrhythmias. Such insufficiency may develop in patients after tetralogy of Fallot repair,[483] and some patients ultimately require reoperation for insertion of a valved right ventricle to pulmonary artery conduit. Surgically placed valved conduits have limited life spans.[550] Since 2000, successful percutaneous valve replacement has been accomplished within a stent placed in the pulmonary position to treat both pulmonary stenosis and regurgitation.[91] A bovine jugular venous valve is used within a platinum stent that can be expanded to a maximum of 22 mm in diameter (Fig. 8-68, A).[389,598] Potential complications can include homograft rupture, device migration, coronary

FIG. 8-68 Pulmonary valve replacement by cardiac catheterization. **A,** Melody Transcatheter Pulmonary Valve (TPV, Medtronic Incorporated), a natural tri-leaflet bovine jugular vein valve sewn into metal frame. **B,** Melody TPV is sewn into a metal frame (stent). **C,** The transcatheter pulmonary valve has been placed during cardiac catheterization into proper location, restoring pulmonary valve function and adequate blood flow to the lungs. (A and B, Copyright 2010 Medtronic, Inc. Melody TPV is a Humanitarian Use Device. Authorized by federal law (USA) for use in patients with regurgitant or stenotic Right Ventricular Outflow Tract (RVOT) conduit (≥ 16 mm in diameter when originally implanted). The effectiveness of this system for this use has not been demonstrated. C courtesy of Dr. Evan Zahn, Miami Children's Hospital.)

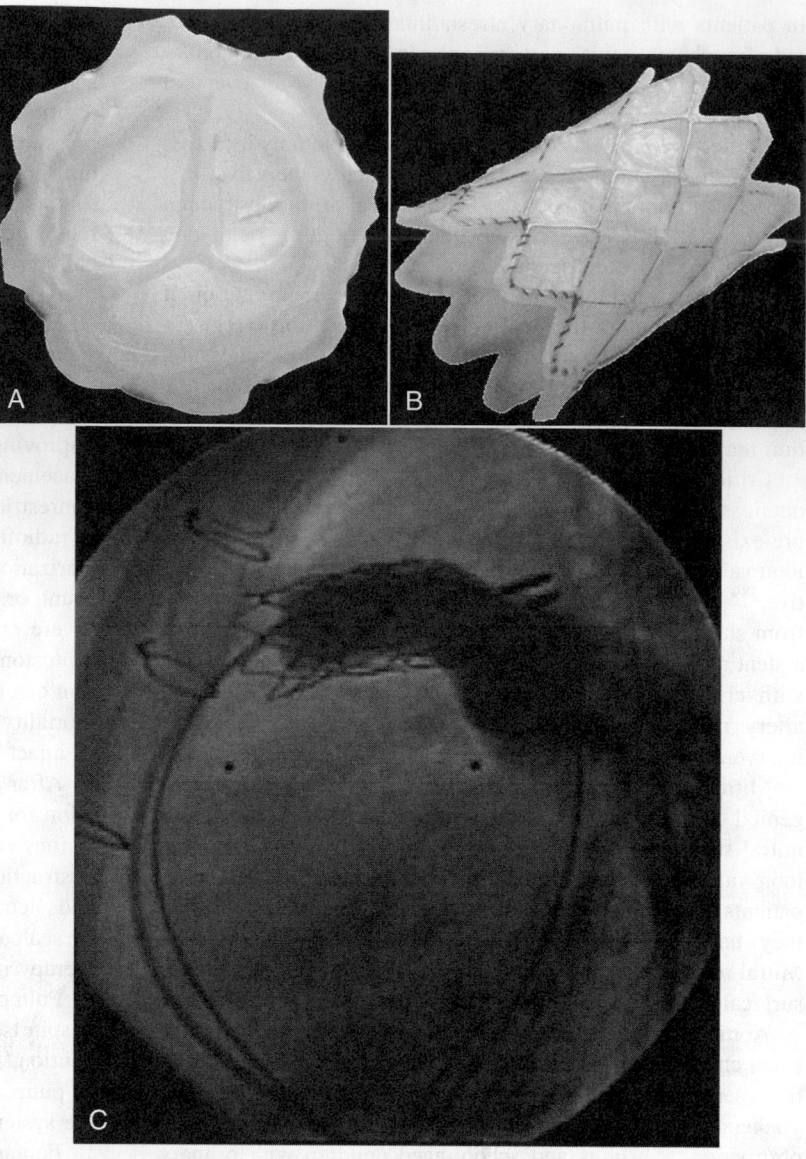

compression, and later stent fracture.[550] Surgical intervention for valved conduit replacement is delayed,[550] but evaluation and long-term outcome analysis continue. Percutaneous aortic valve implantations and mitral valve repairs have begun in adults, with increasing success.[260,389]

Coils may be used to close PDAs (Fig. 8-69). Stents may be used to keep the PDA open in patients awaiting cardiac transplant for HLHS,[94] and as an alternative to initial palliative surgical shunt, to maintain pulmonary blood flow in ductal-dependent pulmonary circulation (Fig. 8-70).[18,93,614] Stents may also be placed to widen a narrowed Gore-Tex shunt. Potential complications include progressive narrowing of the stent with cyanosis requiring re-intervention, stent migration, intravascular hemolysis, and worsening of pulmonary artery stenosis.[18,614]

Other Cardiac Catheterization Procedures

Endomyocardial biopsy by cardiac catheterization remains the mainstay in the diagnosis of rejection both early and late after heart transplantation.[545] The biopsies can produce

complications; myocardial perforation is the most common (see the section on Endomyocardial Biopsy).

Electrophysiology studies are performed to identify cardiac rhythm abnormalities and definitively treat them by elimination of abnormal atrial or ventricular arrhythmia pathways. The procedures are similar to cardiac catheterization with various potential access sites at the antecubital veins, jugular, and femoral vessels. Radiofrequency energy applies heat to burn lesions and interrupt arrhythmia pathways. Cryoablation applies extreme cold at the catheters tip to ultimately burst the cells responsible for arrhythmias.[772] These procedures are reviewed in detail by Saul.[772]

General anesthesia is often used to ensure that the patient remains motionless during critical points in the procedure, and to keep the patient comfortable during a potentially long procedure.[772] Radiofrequency energy can cause AV block in children[775] and coronary artery injury.[85] Cryoablation is safer,[772] having minimal effect on the adjacent coronary arteries[814] and a lower incidence of thrombus formation.[465] Additional potential complications include vascular injury,

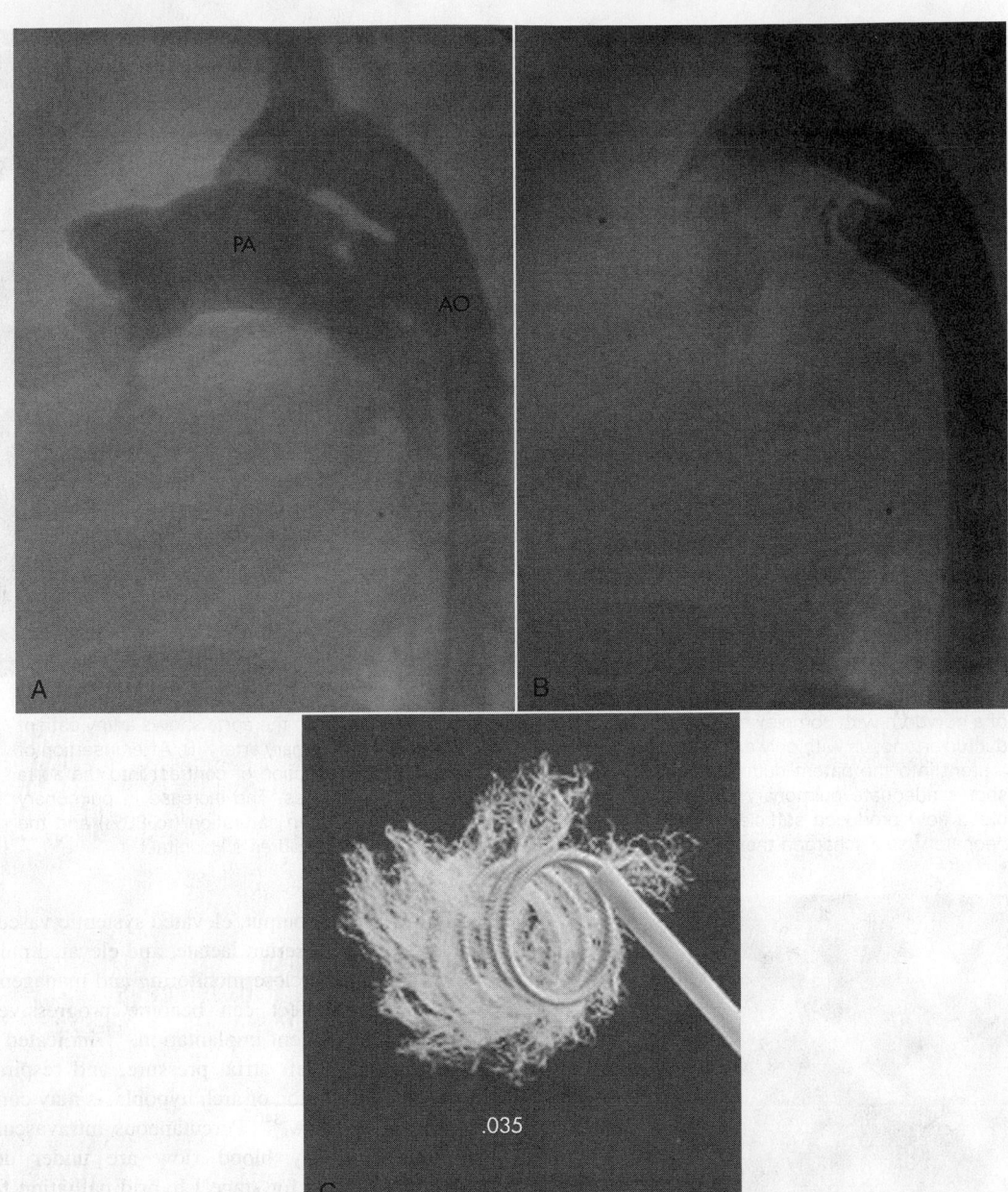

FIG. 8-69 Closure of patent ductus arteriosus (PDA) with coil. **A,** Angiogram with contrast, lateral view, shows blood flow into the arch of the aorta (Ao), through the PDA and into the main pulmonary artery (PA) and then into the right and left pulmonary arteries and pulmonary circulation. **B,** Angiogram with contrast in the same view after insertion of coil. This image confirms that blood flows into the aorta and no longer enters the pulmonary artery. The PDA has been closed. **C,** Gianturco coil. (A and B courtesy of Dr. Evan Zahn, Miami Children's Hospital; C permission for use granted by Cook Medical Incorporated, Bloomington, Indiana.)

embolic injury, valvular regurgitation, and minor skin irritations or burns at electrode skin sites.[503] Mortality is low for ablation procedures, reported at 0.097%,[503] but up to 0.89% in patients with structural heart disease.[774]

Hybrid Procedures

Hybrid procedures combine the interventional cardiac catheterization procedure with a surgical procedure. Hybrid procedures include periventricular closure of the ventricular septal defect,[40] as well as intraoperative placement of stents in the pulmonary arteries or the aorta.

Newborns with hypoplastic left heart syndrome (HLHS) may undergo a hybrid first-stage intervention to extend the waiting time for cardiac transplant, allow time for left ventricular growth,[12] and minimize the newborn's exposure to cardiopulmonary bypass, cardioplegic arrest, and circulatory arrest.[534] The stage I hybrid procedure for HLHS includes surgical bilateral pulmonary artery banding with cardiac catheterization placement of a stent within the ductus arteriosus (Fig. 8-71), possibly followed by enlargement of the interatrial communication via septostomy.[130,340,783] Postcatheterization hemodynamics in stage I hybrid HLHS patients can include

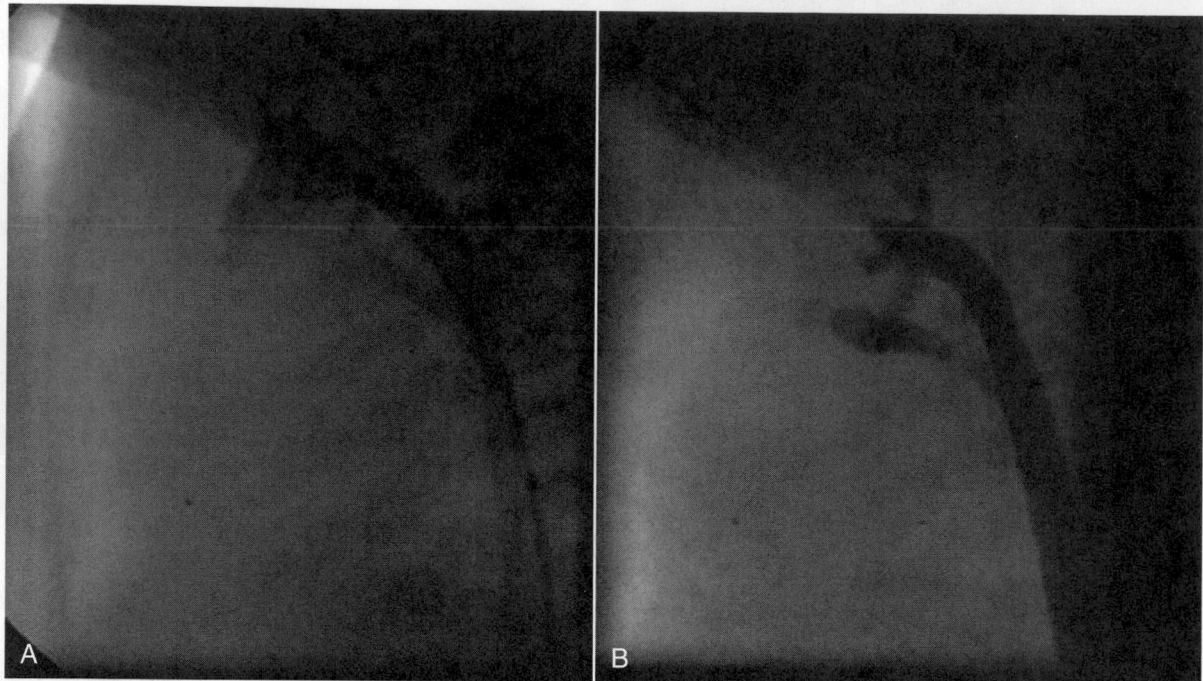

FIG. 8-70 Patent ductus arteriosus (PDA) stent placed by cardiac catheterization. These are two lateral views of a newborn with complex single ventricle physiology. **A,** Contrast injection in the aorta shows a tiny patent ductus arteriosus with only a small amount of contrast entering the left pulmonary artery. **B,** After insertion of a stent into the patent ductus arteriosus during cardiac catheterization, injection of contrast into the aorta shows adequate pulmonary blood flow with filling of the pulmonary arteries. The increase in pulmonary blood flow produced sufficient improvement in the neonate's arterial oxygen saturation (to 80%) and the neonate was discharged the next day. (Courtesy of Dr. Evan Zahn, Miami Children's Hospital.)

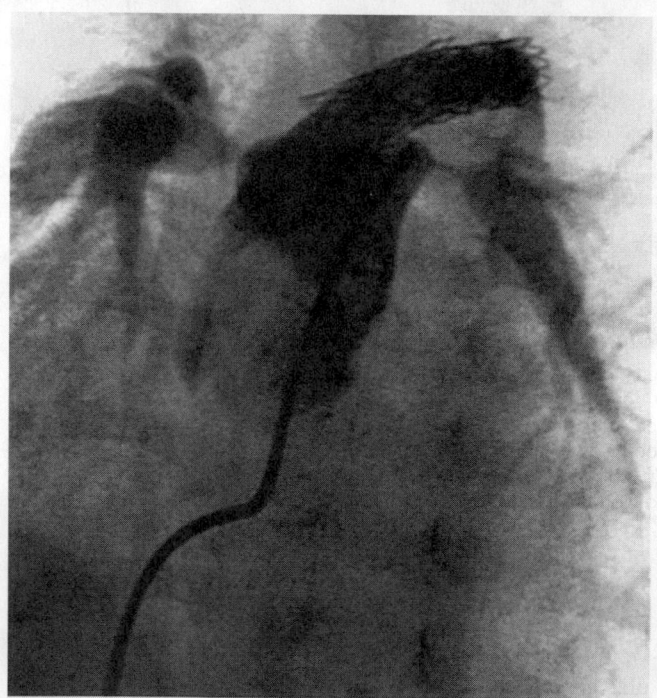

FIG. 8-71 Hybrid procedure stage I for hypoplastic left heart syndrome. Contrast injection into the aorta allows visualization of the patent ductus arteriosus and the right and left pulmonary arteries. A stent has been placed in the patent ductus arteriosus by cardiac catheterization (the wire mesh is visible above the pulmonary arteries). Pulmonary artery bands have been surgically placed around the right and left pulmonary artery to reduce/control pulmonary blood flow. (Courtesy of Dr. Evan Zahn, Miami Children's Hospital.)

early low cardiac output, elevated systemic vascular resistance, acidosis and high serum lactate, and elevated pulmonary blood flow,[534] requiring close monitoring and management.

The atrial defect can become progressively restrictive even after atrial stent implantation,[691] indicated by increasing cyanosis, rising left atrial pressure, and respiratory distress. Preductal coarctation or arch hypoplasia may compromise pulmonary blood flow.[340] Percutaneous intravascular devices to control pulmonary blood flow are under development.[94] Long-term results for stage I hybrid palliation for HLHS and Fontan completion with a covered stent are unknown.

Fetal Intervention

Fetal in utero interventional valvuloplasty is performed at select programs for cases of critical aortic valvar obstruction, with the aim of preventing fetal progression to hypoplastic left heart syndrome.[791,884] Intact or highly restrictive interatrial communication,[908] and pulmonary atresia with intact ventricular septum[689] have also been treated by fetal in utero dilation. Fetal aortic valve intervention has led to biventricular repairs.[545] Long-term outcomes must be analyzed.

Clinical Trials

The development of transcatheter devices to treat congenital heart lesions have rapidly progressed over the past decade. Septal occluder devices, intravascular stents, and transcatheter valves have become more readily available. This has led to the expansion of clinical research trials into the domain of interventional congenital cardiology. Clinical trials exist for ASD and VSD closure devices, stent procedures, and transcatheter pulmonary valves. When caring for a child who is enrolled in a clinical trial, the nurse must be aware of the responsibilities of each member of the research team. Adherence to the trial's protocol is imperative if access to devices is to continue and grow. Byers[126] reported that 75% of families enrolled in clinical research trials thought that the treatment provided was the standard of care.

Potential Complications of Cardiac Catheterization

Potential complications of any cardiac catheterization include arrhythmias, particularly atrial or ventricular irritability (and resultant supraventricular or ventricular arrhythmias), or the development of atrioventricular (AV) block. Bleeding, cardiac perforation, tamponade, cerebrovascular accident, stroke, pulmonary hemorrhage, pulmonary edema, contrast agent reactions, brachial plexus injury, skin pressure lesions, or hypothermia may also occur. Arterial or venous vascular injury may occur as well.[336]

Interventional catheterization often involves anticoagulation and insertion of large sheaths, and may require long procedure times. This can increase the risk of bleeding from the access site, hematoma formation, vessel spasm, and thrombus. Frequent assessment of the extremity is vital for early detection and treatment to avoid limb ischemia and permanent complications.

Hypoventilation may result because of the effects of sedation or prostaglandin infusions, or in patients with Down syndrome because of the risk of airway obstruction.[336] Emboli into the systemic or venous circulations can be caused by air, thrombus, or broken catheters or wires.[336] Patients with infundibular pulmonic stenosis (including tetralogy of Fallot) may experience hypercyanotic episodes during or after the catheterization despite careful maintenance of hydration and sedation and careful catheter manipulation (see section, Common Clinical Conditions, Cyanotic Heart Disease).[336] Air or thrombus embolization to cerebral vessels is a known complication. This risk increases in the cyanotic or iron-deficient patient, or if multiple catheter exchanges occurred during the catheterization.[660,663] Devices placed during interventional procedures may embolize within the heart or distal vascular sites. Aortic stents can migrate distally. Although complications are rare, the nurse should exercise a high index of suspicion with focus on anticipation of potential problems.[336,660,663]

Nursing Management

Any patient who returns from the cardiac catheterization procedure with hemodynamic instability or new, sudden arrhythmias after a device placement must be assessed for suspected device displacement. A device placed to occlude an atrial septal defect can migrate into the mitral valve or aorta. A device placed to close a patent ductus arteriosus can migrate into the pulmonary arteries or the aorta, particularly if the patient has pulmonary hypertension. Initial efforts focus on maintaining adequate oxygenation, ventilation, and hemodynamic stability. An immediate echocardiogram can assist in evaluating the position of the device within the heart. A chest radiograph also provides a general idea of device location, but interpretation may be complicated by unusual anatomy.

Patients with elevated pulmonary vascular resistance may develop acute elevations in pulmonary resistance with right heart failure. If a pulmonary hypertension event occurs after cardiac catheterization, management focuses on optimizing airway, ventilation, and oxygenation; treatment of pain and anxiety; optimizing carbon dioxide tension, and correction of hypothermia (see section, Common Clinical Conditions, Pulmonary Hypertension, Management).

Alternative routes of vascular access (ARVA) have grown with the increasing complexity of patients and interventional procedures. Alternative access routes involve, but are not limited to, access for catheterization via carotid, brachial, hepatic, and open chest/direct cardiac puncture.[222] Two common ARVA sites are carotid and hepatic access. Carotid access is often used emergently to treat critical aortic stenosis, or for PDA stent placement. Hepatic venous access is used in the setting of femoral vein occlusion. The nurse must be aware of the access route used for the procedure and assess the patient accordingly.

When caring for a child who is part of a clinical research study, the bedside nurse must ensure that the family understands they are part of a clinical trial. Family support and education are paramount. Compliance with the treatment protocol, prompt notification of adverse events to the clinical research team, and reporting of conflicts of interest are the responsibility of the nursing team.

The past decade has witnessed significant changes in cardiac catheterization therapy. Although the volume of diagnostic procedures has decreased, an increase in interventional treatment of congenital heart disease has been associated with higher acuity and complexity of cases.[660] Improved noninvasive diagnostic methods have brought about earlier diagnosis and treatment. This, in turn, has had a significant effect on required postcatheterization nursing care.

Anesthesia is used for many interventional cases, patients are younger, undergoing corrective treatment in the cath lab, and with short LOS as most are day procedures with patient admitted day of the procedure and discharged within 24 h. In addition, more patients undergoing cardiac catheterization are unstable, with problems such as early postoperative low cardiac output or pulmonary hypertension,[336] and they require critical care.

Most cardiac catheterizations are performed percutaneously, and therefore do not include an incision that requires sutures. However, pressure is applied to the vascular access site, and the nurse should monitor for evidence of bleeding or hematoma formation and for evidence of obstruction of the venous or arterial catheterization site.

Patients may return to the nursing unit with only intravenous fluids and oxygen for recovery. However, interventional catheterizations create significant changes in physiology. This necessitates need for nursing care centered on a high index of suspicion for potential complications.

General nursing management of the patient before and after cardiac catheterization is summarized in Box 8-54. Intervention-specific care after interventional cardiac catheterization is summarized in Box 8-55. Finally, advanced concepts related to care of the child undergoing cardiac catheterization are summarized in Box 8-56.

Text continues on p. 461

Box 8-54   Nursing Care for the Child Undergoing Cardiac Catheterization

Precardiac Catheterization
Potential Problems
Anxiety (patient/family) and knowledge deficit related to patient's health status, anticipated catheterization

Expected Patient Outcomes
- Patient/family demonstrates comprehension of preparation for procedure, catheterization itself, and postcatheterization care
- Patient/family's anxiety does not interfere with appropriate activity

Nursing Interventions
- Orient child/family to nursing care unit, policies, personnel, catheterization lab (as age appropriate)
- Orient child/family to preparation for catheterization, including tests, medications (including holding anticoagulants, premedication, and effects and planned sedation or anesthesia), need for nothing by mouth before catheterization
  - Instruct patient (as appropriate to age) and family regarding procedure itself
  - Discuss postcatheterization care with patient (if appropriate to age) and family
  - If child is greater than 2 years old, toys or puppets may be used to demonstrate experiences the child will remember
- During and after catheterization procedure, provide support and simple explanations of catheterization results; orient patient to time and place frequently while patient is recovering from sedation. Involve child life therapist.
- Provide written information on procedure and child's condition
- Provide online teaching web sites to reinforce teaching

Postcardiac Catheterization
General Care for All Patients
- Continuous cardiorespiratory monitoring, including monitoring of oxyhemoglobin saturation by pulse oximetry
- Assessment and support of airway, oxygenation, and ventilation as needed
- Frequent assessment of perfusion of affected extremity
- Exposure of pressure dressing, monitoring for bleeding, hematoma
- Bedrest/immobilization
- Administration of intravenous fluids
- Frequent neurologic checks
- Strict recording of fluid intake and output
- Discharge planning and teaching

Initial Evaluation at Admission after Catheterization ("Quick look" assessment)
- Evaluate general appearance, color, perfusion
- Evaluate airway, oxygenation, ventilation including color, oxyhemoglobin saturation, respiratory effort
- Evaluate systemic perfusion: heart rate and rhythm, four extremity pulses, blood pressure, skin color, skin temperature, capillary refill
- Check catheterization site(s)
- Evaluate and monitor temperature (core and peripheral)
- Evaluate hydration
- Evaluate neurologic function, responsiveness, and movement
- Check all infusion sites

1. Potential Arrhythmias, Decreased Cardiac Output
- Related to injury to conduction system, physiology stress of catheterization, underlying cardiac disease, reaction to sedation/anesthesia or contrast agent, hypothermia. Arrhythmias may be more common in patients with single ventricle anatomy, or severe/critical aortic stenosis.[336]
- Common arrhythmias include: tachycardia/supraventricular tachycardia (SVT), bradycardia, heart block (particularly with AV discordance, d-transposition of the great arteries [d-TGA], and tetralogy of Fallot [TOF]),[336] or severe right ventricular outflow tract obstruction. Ventricular fibrillation may develop in patients with aortic stenosis or pulmonary atresia with intact ventricular septum.[664]

Expected Patient Outcomes
Stable cardiac output as measured by adequate BP, good peripheral perfusion, regular/appropriate cardiac rate and rhythm, intimal bleeding from catheterization site, adequate urine output (average, approximately 1-2 mL/kg per hour), absence of systemic or pulmonary venous congestion, normal body temperature

Nursing Interventions
- Obtain baseline ECG on arrival to unit and continuously (or per unit routine). If arrhythmia develops:
  - Monitor for changes in ECG, ECG axis, or ST-segment changes, palpitations, chest pain, and shortness of breath
  - Note effect on systemic perfusion (note if BP drops with aberrant beat)
  - Note any precipitating or alleviating factors, and response to medications
  - Notify provider
  - Treat as needed (see also, Common Clinical Conditions, Arrhythmias)
  - Administer oxygen and support perfusion as needed
  - SVT/tachycardia: Anticipate adenosine or cardioversion
  - Bradycardia/heart block
    - Ensure adequate oxygenation and ventilation
    - Determine if it is a first-, second-, or third-degree heart block.
    - Anticipate the administration of medications, and initiate pacemaker therapy.
- Assess heart rate: Ascertain if it is adequate for clinical condition (see Table 8-12 earlier in this chapter and pages inside front cover); notify physician and on-call provider if heart rate is excessive or insufficient
- Assess vital signs, including body temperature
- Assess apical and peripheral pulses for strength, regular rate, and rhythm. If any irregularities or pulse discrepancies exist, notify physician, assess perfusion, and obtain rhythm strip. Be prepared to provide CPR.
- Assess central and peripheral perfusion and blood pressure every 15 min initially, then every 1-2 h as appropriate or per unit routine. Notify on-call provider of evidence of poor perfusion or hypotension and treat
- Assess level of consciousness

2. Potential Bleeding/Cardiac Tamponade
Related to vessel rupture or cardiac perforation, embolization of an implanted device and subsequent heart or vessel damage. When caring for a child who has undergone placement of a device such as ASD/VSD/transcatheter valve implant/endovascular stent, device migration and internal bleeding must be considered if the patient develops signs of hemodynamic compromise or decreased perfusion.

Box 8-54 **Nursing Care for the Child Undergoing Cardiac Catheterization—cont'd**

Expected Patient Outcomes

Stable cardiac output as measured by adequate blood pressure, normal heart rate and rhythm, normal peripheral pulses and perfusion, normal hemoglobin/hematocrit, absence of signs of cardiac tamponade, absence of hemoptysis, or hematuria (consider retroperitoneal bleed)

Nursing Interventions

- Monitor hemoglobin and hematocrit as ordered
- Closely monitor systemic perfusion and blood pressure for evidence of low cardiac output—tachycardia; cool, clammy extremities; decreased urine output; change in behavior or responsiveness; cyanosis, mottling, or pallor; evidence of pulmonary edema; decreasing blood pressure. Notify physician/on-call provider immediately if they develop.
- Monitor for signs of cardiac tamponade—pallor, tachycardia, decreased blood pressure or decreased pulse pressure, decreased heart sounds, restlessness, cool extremities, tachypnea, neck vein distension, hypotension not responsive to fluid administration. Notify physician/on-call provider immediately if they occur and be prepared for emergency measures if necessary.

Note: Signs of tamponade may be virtually identical to the signs of shock. Pulsus paradoxus may be impossible to appreciate if child is tachypneic or hypotensive.

3. Potential Alteration in Body Temperature

Related to cool temperatures in catheterization suite and flushing of catheters with cold fluids during the procedure.[664]

Expected Outcomes

Patient will be kept warm during and after cardiac catheterization, and core and peripheral temperature will be normal.

Nursing Interventions

- Assess temperature with vital signs. Keep patient warm but avoid hyperthermia.
- Monitor for signs of hypothermia, including, bradycardia/hypotension, hemodynamic compromise because of vasoconstriction, lethargy/CNS depression, prolonged recovery from sedation or anesthesia, peripheral cyanosis, metabolic acidosis

4. Potential Site Complications: Bleeding/Compromised Perfusion to Extremity

- Related to anticoagulation, arterial access, larger sheath size, especially for device implantation such as aortic/pulmonary stents, device closures, or transcatheter valve implantation.
- Treatment of coarctation requires a larger sheath in the aorta/femoral artery.
- Bleeding from catheterization site may cause hematomas, weakened pulse, or venous/arterial congestion. Arterial compromise can lead to long-term issues with growth of the affected extremity and significant ischemia; may ultimately require amputation of extremity if allowed to progress. Vigilant monitoring and prompt treatment are important.
- The incidence of arterial spasm and vessel thrombosis increases with smaller children (<5 kg) larger sheaths, and longer vessel access times.

Expected Patient Outcomes

Perfusion of catheterized extremity remains adequate as indicated by: warmth, brisk capillary refill, pink color, strong pulses, appropriate movement and sensation (use opposite limb for comparison)

Nursing Interventions

- Monitor catheterization site and dressing for evidence of bleeding. If bleeding is excessive and does not stop with application of pressure, notify physician/on-call provider immediately.
- If bleeding occurs, apply pressure one to two fingers cephalad to (above) catheterization site, remove the dressing to inspect the site while maintaining pressure, hold pressure until hemostasis is achieved, while assessing peripheral pulses frequently during this time to ensure adequate perfusion to extremity. If pressure device is present (i.e., Safeguard), inflate device to apply pressure while palpating distal pulse to the extremity.

Note: Many institutions have protocols for management of pressure devices.

- Maintain bedrest for 4 to 8 hours as ordered. Head of bed can be elevated 30-45 degrees as per institution protocol.
- *Monitor for arterial compromise*: Often results in cool, pale, mottled extremity. If any of these symptoms occur, notify physician/on-call provider immediately.
  - Monitor pulses of extremity distal to catheterization site; notify physician immediately of any decrease in pulses (if spasm or thrombus occurs in artery, distal artery can rapidly become thrombosed, and ischemia of extremity will result)
  - Assess color and warmth of extremity
  - Application of heat to contralateral extremity may help maintain circulation to catheterized extremity (by producing reflex vasodilation), but heat should never be applied to involved extremity because it merely increases O_2 consumption of already compromised tissue
  - If thrombus develops in artery, surgical removal may be required
  - Anticipate anticoagulation therapy such as Heparin infusion, Lovenox injections. If administered early may prevent thrombus formation. Streptokinase or tPA may be used if pulse does not return.[336]
  - Attempt to prevent flexion of catheterized extremity at catheterization site for 6 hours or as ordered
  - Maintain bed rest for 6 to 12 hours after catheterization (or as ordered)
  - Administer pain medication as ordered (and needed); monitor patient's response and systemic perfusion
  - Monitor for evidence of excessive edema or bleeding at catheterization site; notify physician if bleeding is not stopped by application of pressure
  - Apply ice to catheterization site as needed and ordered
- *Monitor for venous compromise*: Often results in signs of venous congestion, such as edema, extremity discoloration (extremity becomes dusky), increase in size of extremity.

Note: When venous cutdown is performed, vein used for the catheterization is often tied off at end of procedure, especially in small infants. In this case, extremity distal to catheterization site is likely to become edematous and slightly cyanotic as venous blood is trapped in extremity; collateral veins will quickly provide venous drainage, but initial discomfort should be expected.

Continued

Box 8-54   Nursing Care for the Child Undergoing Cardiac Catheterization—cont'd

- Monitor pulses of extremity distal to catheterization site
- If edema is present, elevate extremity to facilitate venous return; notify physician immediately if edema causes decrease in arterial pulses (indicates compromise of arterial circulation)
- Monitor for evidence of bleeding at catheterization site and notify physician if it is not relieved by pressure
- Maintain bed rest for 4 to 6 hours after catheterization (as ordered)
- Monitor for evidence of arteriovenous fistula: AV fistulas are rare but can develop after cardiac catheterization, particularly in older children. Smaller AV fistulas are usually asymptomatic, but larger communications may cause symptoms and may require treatment.
  - Monitor for pain, development of large hematoma/bruise, presence of visible veins on surface of leg, leg swelling, palpation of a bruit, or auscultation of shunt at the catheterization site
  - Monitor perfusion to extremity
  - Provide pain management
  - Anticipate further treatment involving coil embolization or surgical ligation

5. Potential Respiratory Compromise

Related to sedation or general anesthesia, precatheterization respiratory compromise or upper airway obstruction (e.g., Down syndrome, velocardiofacial syndrome), postextubation upper airway edema, or pulmonary edema associated with reperfusion syndrome (e.g., with tetralogy of Fallot, pulmonary atresia, and other diagnoses after pulmonary artery angioplasty or stent implantation to increase pulmonary blood flow)

Expected Patient Outcomes

Adequate respiratory function as demonstrated by appropriate rate and effort, equal and adequate lung aeration bilaterally, appropriate oxyhemoglobin saturation and heart rate for patient

Nursing Interventions

- Monitor respiratory rate (see pages inside front cover) and effort. Notify physician/on-call provider if rate or effort is insufficient or excessive; respiratory support (oxygen therapy, ventilation) may be necessary
- Monitor for airway obstruction: Snoring, nasal flaring, retractions, gasping for breath, use of accessory muscles. Reposition head (head tilt/jaw thrust), consider need for oxygen
- Monitor for laryngospasm: Agitation, stridor, hypoxia, diminished/absence of breath sounds. Provide positive-pressure ventilation via bag/mask and notify physician/on-call provider immediately
- Monitor oxyhemoglobin saturation: Notify physician/on-call provider of inadequate/inappropriate oxyhemoglobin saturation. Consider assessments compared to the baseline status prior to catheterization procedure and potential presence of single ventricle circulation.
- Auscultate lungs: Notify physician/on-call provider of inadequate aeration, ventilation
- Monitor CXR for atelectasis, symptoms of pulmonary congestion
- If reperfusion syndrome is suspected, anticipate administration of oxygen, diuretics, aggressive pulmonary toilet, or mechanical ventilation

6. Potential Dehydration/ Potential Compromise in Renal Function

Related to inadequate fluid intake before and during procedure, diuresis, or nephrotoxicity caused by contrast agents. Patients with cyanotic heart disease are at increased risk for development of hemoconcentration if dehydrated.

Expected Patient Outcome

Patient will demonstrate adequate urine output (1-2 mL/kg per hour)

Nursing Interventions

- Monitor urine output; notify physician if urine output is inadequate despite sufficient fluid intake

  Note: A small child may rapidly become dehydrated when kept NPO for hours while awaiting catheterization; ensure adequate parenteral and/or oral fluid intake before, during, and after catheterization.
- Typically, generous fluid administration is provided (if tolerated) to facilitate urinary excretion of contrast agent. If patient is oliguric despite sufficient intake, restriction of fluid intake may be needed to prevent overload.
- If the patient has a persistent right to left intracardiac shunt, no air can be allowed into any IV system due to the risk for cerebral or systemic embolization.
- Assess fluid balance; notify physician or on-call provider of imbalance
- Test urine for hematuria; notify physician if blood is present and monitor urine output closely

6. Potential Allergic Reaction

Related to contrast agent, catheters, medications, equipment. Most occur during or in the early postcatheterization period. Latex allergies should be considered in some patients. Many pediatric catheterization suites now use low osmolality/nonionic agents, yet contrast agents can still result in pulmonary compromise/edema.

Expected Patient Outcomes

Patient will remain free of symptoms of allergic reaction

Nursing Interventions

Monitor for signs of allergic reaction: changes in skin color, rash, hives, itching, low-grade fever, diaphoresis, respiratory difficulty, vasodilation, and hypotension. If allergic reaction is suspected, notify physician/on-call provider immediately, administer oxygen if necessary, anticipate administration of antihistamines, treat specific symptoms (i.e., support airway, oxygenation, ventilation, perfusion)

7. Potential Neurologic Compromise

Related to embolization of thrombus, air or device, cyanotic heart disease, and polycythemia. Potential for neurologic event increases with multiple catheter exchanges, use of large sheaths, polycythemia with iron deficiency anemia, and procedures involving left heart, head and neck vessels, aorta, and right-to-left intracardiac shunts.

Expected Patient Outcomes

Patient will respond in age-appropriate and developmentally appropriate manner

Nursing Interventions

- Document baseline neurologic status
- Immediately report failure to progress to baseline movement, speech, activity

Box 8-54 Nursing Care for the Child Undergoing Cardiac Catheterization—cont'd

- Frequently assess neurologic function: Notify physician/on-call provider if changes. Note that increased somnolence may indicate neurologic compromise.
- Monitor for seizure activity; notify physician/on-call provider immediately if present

8. Potential Knowledge Deficit/Comfort/Anxiety

Many cardiac catheterization patients are admitted and discharged within 24 h. Extensive teaching is necessary in a short time period. Postprocedure patients are often awake but with enforced limited mobility, which can be challenging for the nurse, patient, and family. Pain may be present.

Expected Patient Outcome

Patient/family possesses adequate information to comply with postcatheterization care regimen and general health maintenance

Nursing Interventions

- Assess level of pain and provide medication as ordered
- Offer child services where available
- Assess family's understanding of diagnosis, procedure and necessary care. Provide additional teaching if necessary, consult with support services such as social work where applicable
- Provide child/family with appropriate instruction regarding wound care, physician and other follow-up appointments and emergency telephone numbers, signs of infection, activity restrictions (if any), and medications

- Discuss implications of catheterization results with patient/family to obtain their perceptions of physician's recommendations and clarify any misconceptions they may have
- Review appropriate diet with child/family as indicated

9. Potential for Infection Caused by Invasive Procedure, Wound

Expected Patient Outcome

Patient will remain free of symptoms of infection, including fever or temperature instability, leukocytosis, erythema or drainage at catheterization site, evidence of endocarditis or pericarditis

Nursing Interventions

- Monitor catheterization site for edema, erythema, heat, or discharge; notify physician if present
- Monitor patient's temperature; blood cultures are usually recommended if fever higher than 101.3° F (38.5° C)
- Inform family that a low-grade fever is not uncommon 24 to 48 hours after cardiac catheterization. Notify physician if fever persists or temperature is higher than 100.4° F (or accepted parameters per institution).
- Monitor white blood cell (WBC) count and platelet count if infection is suspected
- Monitor for evidence of endocarditis (high fever, appearance of new heart murmur, hematuria) and pericarditis (cardiac friction rub, loss of heart tones, ECG changes)

Box 8-55 Intervention-Specific Nursing Management Following Cardiac Catheterization*

I. Device Implantation

This includes ASD/VSD occluders, PDA closure devices, coils, intravascular stents, and implantable valves.

General Nursing Interventions

- Monitor for symptoms of infection. Most patients receive a course of antibiotics during hospitalization and observe SBE prophylaxis as per American Heart Association Guidelines for up to 6 months after implantation (see section, Specific Diseases, Endocarditis, and Table 8-41).
- Patients with septal occluder devices, stents to the pulmonary artery circulation or venous system, or implantable heart valves often are discharged home on antiplatelet/anticoagulation therapy for up to 6 months (see Postoperative Care, Anticoagulation).
- A chest radiograph, echocardiogram, and CBC are often obtained and reviewed by the physician before patient discharge. Lung perfusion scans are often ordered after pulmonary artery stents are placed.
- Review discharge medications and necessary endocarditis prophylaxis (see Table 8-41). Include potential side effects of medications (i.e., increased incidence of bruising with anticoagulation), when to call provider (i.e., development of frequent nosebleeds, multiple bruises, bleeding with teeth brushing).

Nursing Interventions After ASD Device Closure

- Monitor for symptoms of device migration: Palpitations, ECG changes, chest pain, dyspnea, bleeding/low cardiac output, systemic or venous obstruction: venous congestion, jugular distension

- Monitor for aortic perforation, bleeding, device interference with AV valves, low cardiac output
- Patients may develop headaches after ASD closure. Include in discharge teaching

Nursing Interventions After VSD Device Closure

- Will likely require longer procedure times, and use of large sheaths, and may be associated with significant blood loss during procedure
- Obtain baseline hemoglobin/hematocrit, assess for hypovolemia, hypotension, hypothermia
- Monitor for arrhythmias: ventricular tachycardia, fibrillation, heart block
- Assess for loss of pedal pulses indicating possible vasospasm or thrombus
- Anticipate need for ventilatory support, inotropes, vasopressors, pacing, cardioversion[660]

Nursing Interventions After PDA Device Closure

- Monitor patient for symptoms of device migration
- If patient develops abdominal/flank pain/distension, chest pain, shortness of breath, hematuria, decreased lower extremity pulses, or signs of decreased cardiac output and perfusion, consider device migration into the aorta. Notify physician immediately and anticipate immediate return to catheterization suite or surgery for removal
- If patient develops hemoptysis, shortness of breath, arrhythmias, or decrease in oxygen saturation, consider device migration into pulmonary circulation or heart. Treat symptoms and notify physician immediately
- Coarctation and left pulmonary artery stenosis are known complications of PDA closure.

Continued

Nursing Care After Aortic Stent Implantation

These patients are considered at high risk of bleeding from catheterization site because of the use of a large arterial sheath and required anticoagulation.

- Perform frequent and vigilant assessment of entry site and extremity pulses (per order/routine)
- Maintain strict bed rest for 4-6 h as per orders/routine
- Monitor for device migration (see Symptoms in PDA Device closure section)
- Monitor neurologic status: Catheters in close proximity to head and neck vessels increase the risk of thrombus
- Patients may be discharged with beta-blocker or antihypertensive therapy

Nursing Care After Pulmonary Artery/Conduit Stent Implantation

Signs of stent migration dependent on location (pulmonary artery versus right ventricle)

- Monitor for signs of potential stent migration into the right heart: Congestive heart failure, jugular distension, hepatomegaly, dyspnea, ventricular arrhythmias, palpitations, tachycardia, cyanosis, and symptoms of low cardiac output.
- Monitor for evidence of coronary artery ischemia (can develop if device compresses the coronary arteries), specifically ST segment changes in ECG. Notify physician immediately, administer oxygen, obtain CXR, anticipate blood/fluid administration and emergent return to catheterization suite or surgery.
- Large sheath size: Monitor patient for retroperitoneal bleeding and symptoms of decreased cardiac output/shock
- Assess for reperfusion injury in patients with complex pulmonary artery disease/severe pulmonary artery stenosis as discussed under Respiratory Compromise.

II. Balloon Dilation/Valvuloplasty

Angioplasty and valvuloplasty is performed for stenotic vessels and valves. The narrowed area is stretched or may be torn. Severity of symptoms is dependent on the degree of stenosis before and after intervention (moderate, severe, or critical). With severe or critical valvular stenosis, the patient may be labile after catheterization and require support of ventilation and diuretic therapy.

General Nursing Interventions

- Monitor for bleeding, arrhythmias, signs of valvar insufficiency, and heart perforation/tamponade (low cardiac output)
- Monitor neurologic status: Balloon rupture during the procedure may cause air embolism or thrombus formation
- Assess and support systemic perfusion
- Anticipate postcatheterization chest radiograph, echocardiogram, and ECG before discharge
- Patient will require endocarditis prophylaxis for 6 months (see section, Specific Diseases, Endocarditis, and Table 8-41)

Nursing Interventions After Pulmonary Valvuloplasty

Manipulation of the right ventricular outflow tract may cause a hypercyanotic episode (see section, Common Clinical Conditions, Cyanotic Heart Disease).

- Monitor oxyhemoglobin saturation, color, heart rate and rhythm, respiratory effort, and serum pH and serum lactate for evidence of progressive hypoxemia.[336]
- Anticipate need for volume administration and support of oxygenation and ventilation
- Assess for symptoms of right heart failure

Nursing Interventions After Pulmonary Angioplasty

- Assess for reperfusion syndrome, support airway, oxygenation and ventilation
- Monitor patient for vessel rupture: Symptoms of low cardiac output

Nursing Interventions After Aortic Valvuloplasty

- Monitor arterial access site for bleeding
- Monitor for signs of neurologic impairment
- Monitor for symptoms of aortic insufficiency—widening pulse pressure, weak/thready pulse, hyperdynamic precordium, ventricular arrhythmias

III. Radiofrequency Ablation
General Nursing Interventions
- Monitor access sites, including neck.

Monitor for bleeding/infection

- Monitor ECG for arrhythmias especially heart block or recurrent SVT
- Monitor for evidence of pericardial effusion/tamponade
- After left-sided pathway ablations patients are often discharged home on antiplatelet therapy. Review during discharge teaching.

IV. Special Considerations
A. Intervention/Access through Surgical Shunts to Pulmonary Arteries: Nursing Interventions
- Monitor for symptoms of shunt stenosis/occlusion:
  ○ Increasing cyanosis, increasing O_2 requirements, decreased respiratory and cardiac function
- Anticipate aggressive anticoagulation therapy, intubation, possible emergent return to cath lab/OR

B. Hybrid Procedure for HLHS: Nursing Interventions
These procedures will alter hemodynamics significantly. Patients are often labile in the postcatheterization period. Monitor for:
- Potential excessive cyanosis
- Restriction to pulmonary blood flow caused by excessively tight pulmonary artery band or ductal stent narrowing
- Restrictive atrial shunt, limiting pulmonary venous return; symptoms of heart failure
- Low cardiac output, excessively low mixed venous saturations
- Anemia, hematocrit <40%
- Heart failure, pulmonary edema caused by excessive pulmonary flow (indicated by arterial oxyhemoglobin saturation >85%)—typically the result of insufficient pulmonary banding

C. Patients Critically Ill Before Procedure: Nursing Interventions
Monitor for and be prepared to treat pulmonary hypertensive crises, severe hypoxemia, arrhythmias (see appropriate sections in Common Clinical Conditions)

D. Early Postoperative Intervention: High-Risk Patients: Nursing Interventions
- Monitor for internal bleeding caused by catheter crossing new suture lines
- Anticipate that patient may be hemodynamically unstable after procedure and will likely require support of circulation (e.g., inotropic or vasoactive support) and support of oxygenation and ventilation
- Monitor for cardiorespiratory instability, renal intolerance of contrast, infection

*Information in this box is intended to supplement that contained in Box 8-54. It highlights potential complications associated with specific catheterization interventions.

Box 8-56	Advanced Concepts: Care of the Child Undergoing Cardiac Catheterization

- Cardiac catheterization procedures in shunted patients may involve catheter manipulation through the surgical shunt with resultant elevated risk for shunt thrombosis. Systemic anticoagulation to avoid shunt thrombus is prescribed. Close monitoring for signs of altered shunt flow with increasing cyanosis is required.
- Hybrid Stage I procedures for hypoplastic left heart syndrome result in single ventricle physiology postcatheterization. Bilateral pulmonary artery bands and a stent within the ductus arteriosus are placed.
- Hybrid Stage I procedures for HLHS may develop restrictive atrial septum with elevated left atrial pressures, pulmonary hypertension, cyanosis, and inadequate cardiac output, requiring re-intervention.
- Distal pulmonary artery intervention provides treatment for stenosis inaccessible to surgical treatment.

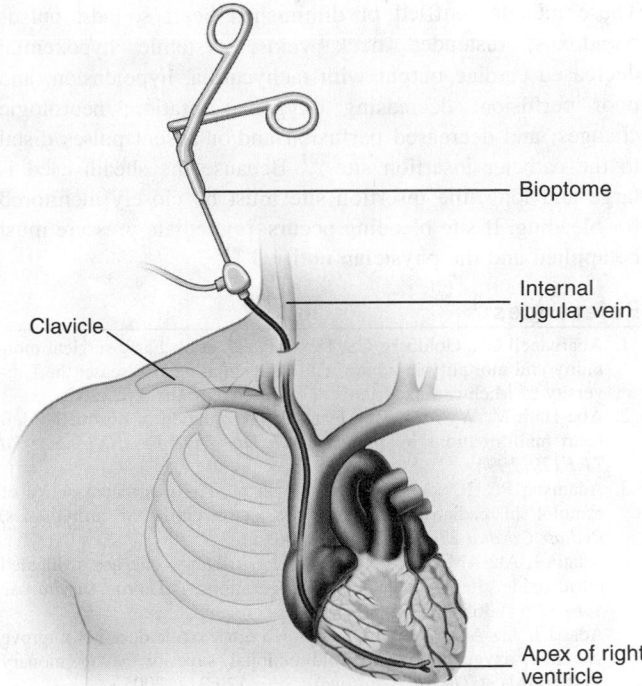

FIG. 8-72 Endomyocardial biopsy technique showing the bioptome in place in the right ventricle. (Redrawn from Copeland JG, Stinson EB. *Curr Probl Cardiol* 4:1-5, 1979.)

ENDOMYOCARDIAL BIOPSY

Definition

An endomyocardial biopsy is a diagnostic procedure that removes a small piece of the heart muscle for laboratory analysis. This procedure aids in making the diagnosis of specific myocardial disorders that are seldom diagnosed by noninvasive tests.[198] Diagnosis of these myocardial disorders guides treatment.

Endomyocardial biopsy remains the standard for diagnosing acute viral myocarditis and for diagnosing myocardial disease seen in hyperplastic obstructive cardiomyopathy, mitochondrial disorders, and storage diseases.[165,188] (Please refer to the section, Myocarditis and the section, Cardiomypathy.)

Endomyocardial biopsy is also used to obtain tissue for rejection surveillance after cardiac transplantation (see Chapter 17).[475]

Because patients with myocardial disorders often present with new-onset heart failure and cardiogenic shock, early diagnosis is vital to guide treatment.[198]

Procedure

Endomyocardial biopsy is usually performed in the cardiac catheterization suite under fluoroscopic guidance. Fluoroscopy is preferred over two-dimensional echocardiography because it provides detailed information about the course of the catheter and the biopsy sites.[198] Hemodynamic data are often obtained with the myocardial samples.

Specimens of heart endocardium and myocardium are obtained using a flexible bioptome. A bioptome is a solid catheter that has sharpened cusps that are opened and closed by the cardiologist to pinch off a piece of heart tissue. The bioptome is introduced through a long sheath directing the bioptome cusps to the biopsy site in the ventricular wall, as illustrated in Fig. 8-72. A variety of sizes of bioptomes and sheaths allow access even in small infants. Percutaneous access is obtained through right and left jugular or subclavian veins, right and left femoral veins, and right and left femoral arteries. The right

internal jugular vein is the most common site used for posttransplant surveillance biopsies.[198]

Potential Complications

Acute complications of endomyocardial biopsy include perforation and resultant pericardial tamponade, ventricular or supraventricular arrhythmias, heart block, pneumothorax, puncture of central arteries, pulmonary embolization, nerve paresis, venous hematoma, damage to the tricuspid valve, and creation of an arteriovenous fistula.[198] The risk of complications varies with the skill and experience of the operator and the clinical condition of the patient. The use of the long sheath has reduced the risk of damage to the tricuspid valve.

Delayed complications include those seen with cardiac catheterization. These involve bleeding at the access site, pericardial tamponade, and deep vein thrombosis. The overall complication rate is less than 1% in greater than 4000 biopsies, with the major complications resulting from sheath insertion and biopsy procedure. Reported deaths have resulted from perforation and pericardial tamponade.[198]

Nursing Interventions

The nurse must monitor the child's appearance, electrocardiographic rhythm, blood pressure, and pulse oximetry throughout the procedure and during the postprocedure period. Signs of poor systemic perfusion, respiratory distress, bleeding, or arrhythmias must be immediately reported to the physician.

The nurse must have a high sensitivity to signs of cardiac tamponade and venous and arterial thrombosis and/or emboli.

These include muffled or diminished heart sounds; pulsus paradoxus; distended neck veins; systemic hypoxemia; decreased cardiac output with tachycardia, hypotension, and poor perfusion; decreasing oxygen saturation; neurologic changes; and decreased perfusion and/or absent pulses distal to the catheter insertion site.[721] Because the sheath used is large and long, the insertion site must be closely monitored for bleeding. If site bleeding occurs, immediate pressure must be applied and the physician notified.[806]

References

1. Abarbanell GL, Goldberg CS, Devaney EJ, et al: Early surgical morbidity and mortality in adults with congenital heart disease: the University of Michigan experience. *Congen Heart Dis* 3:82, 2008.
2. Abu-Harb M, Wyllie J, Hey E, et al: Presentation of obstructive left heart malformations in infancy. *Arch Dis Child Fetal Neonatal Ed* 71:F179, 1994.
3. Adamson PC, Rhodes LA, Saul JP, et al: The pharmacokinetics of esmolol in pediatric subjects with supraventricular arrhythmias. *Pediatr Cardiol* 27(4):420–427, 2006.
4. Adatia I, Atz AM, Jonas RA, Wessel DL: Diagnostic use of inhaled nitric oxide after neonatal cardiac operations. *J Thorac Cardiovasc Surg* 112(5):365–392, 1996.
5. Adatia I, Atz AM, Wessel DL: Inhaled nitric oxide does not improve systemic oxygenation after bidirectional superior cavopulmonary anastomosis. *J Thorac Cardiovasc Surg* 129:217, 2005.
6. Adatia I, Shekerdemian L: The role of calcium channel blockers, steroids, anticoagulation, antiplatelet drugs, and endothelin receptor antagonists. *Pediatr Crit Care Med* 11(2 Suppl):S46–S51, 2010.
7. Adatia I, Wessel DL: Diagnostic and therapeutic uses of inhaled nitric oxide in congenital heart disease. In Zapol WM, Bloch KD, editors: *Nitric Oxide and the Lung*, New York, 1997, Marcel Dekker.
8. Agarwal HS: Inhaled nitric oxide use in bidirectional Glenn anastomosis for elevated Glenn pressures. *Ann Thorac Surg* 81:1429, 2006.
9. Agarwala B: Failure to thrive. In Koenig P, Hijazi ZM, Zimmerman F, editors: *Essential pediatric cardiology*, New York, 2004, McGraw-Hill.
10. Aguinaga L, Primo J, Anguera I, et al: Long-term follow-up in patients with the permanent form of junctional reciprocating tachycardia treated with radiofrequency ablation. *Pacing Clin Electrophysiol* 21(11 Pt 1):2073–2078, 1998.
11. Ak K, Aybek T, Wimmer-Greinecker G, Ozaslan F, et al: Evolution of surgical techniques for atrial septal defect repair in adults: a 10-year single-institution experience. *J Thoras Cadiovas Surg* 134 (3):757–764, 2007.
12. Akinturk H, Michel-Behnke I, Valeske K, et al: Hybrid transcatheter-surgical palliation: basis for univentricular or biventricular repair: the Giessen experience. *Pediatr Cardiol* 28:79, 2007.
13. Alexander ME: Ventricular arrhythmias in children and young adults. In Walsh EP, Saul JP, Triedman JK, editors: *Cardiac arrhythmias in children and young adults with congenital heart disease*, Philadelphia, 2001, Lippincott Williams & Wilkins, pp. 201–234.
14. Alexander ME, Cecchin F, Walsh EP, et al: Implications of implantable cardioverter defibrillator therapy in congenital heart disease and pediatrics. *J Cardiovasc Electrophysiol* 15(1):72–76, 2004.
15. Allanson JE, Hall G, Van Allen MI: Noonan phenotype associated with neurofibromatosis. *Am J Med Genet* 21:457–462, 1985.
16. Allen DR, Schieken RM, Donofrio MT: Hoarseness as the initial clinical presentation of anomalous left coronary artery from the pulmonary artery. *Pediatr Cardiol* 26(5):668–671, 2005.
17. Alton GY, Robertson CM, Sauve R, et al: Early childhood health, growth, and neurodevelopmental outcomes after complete repair of total anomalous pulmonary venous connection at 6 weeks or younger. *J Thorac Cardiovasc Surg* 133(4):905–911, 2007.
18. Alwi M, Choo KK, Latiff HA, et al: Initial results and medium-term follow-up of stent implantation of patent ductus arteriosus in duct-dependent pulmonary circulation. *J Am Coll Cardiol* 44(2):438–445, 2004.
19. American Academy of Pediatrics Committee on Drugs: Guidelines for monitoring and management of pediatric patients during and after sedation for diagnostic and therapeutic procedures. *Pediatrics* 89:1110, 1992.
20. American Academy of Pediatrics Committee on Infectious Diseases: Intravenous gamma-globulin use in children with Kawasaki disease. *Pediatrics* 82:112, 1988.
21. American Society for Testing and Materials (ASTM) International: *ASTM F2503-05: standard practice for marking medical devices and other times for safety in the magnetic resonance environment, 2005:* West Conshohocken, PA, 2005, ASTM International. Available from http://www.astm.org.
22. Ammash NM, Warnes CA: Survival into adulthood of patients with unoperated single ventricle. *Am J Cardiol* 77:542–544, 1996.
23. Andreasen JB, Johnsen SP, Ravn HB: Junctional ectopic tachycardia after surgery for congenital heart disease in children. *Int Care Med* 34(5):895–902, 2008.
24. Andrew ER: Nuclear magnetic resonance and the brain. *Brain Topogr* 5:129, 1992.
25. Andrew M, Michelson A, Bovill E, et al: Guidelines for antithrombotic therapy in pediatric patients. *J Pediatr* 132(4):575–588, 1998.
26. Andrews RE, Tulloh RMR: Interventional cardiac catheterization in congenital heart disease. *Archiv Dis Child* 89:1168, 2004.
27. Andrews RE, Tullah RMR: Interventional cardiac catheterization in congenital heart disease. *Arch Dis Child* 89:1170–1171, 2004.
28. Aragon J: A rare noncardiac cause for acute myocardial infarction in a 13-year-old patient. *Cardiol Rev* 12(1):31–36, 2004.
29. Arensman FW, et al: Early medical and surgical intervention for congenital cyanotic heart defects. *J Thorac Cardiovasc Surg* 84:88, 1982.
30. Artman M, Mahony L, Teitel DF: *Neonatal cardiology.* New York, 2002, McGraw-Hill.
31. Artrip JH, Sauer H, Campbell DN, et al: Biventricular repair in double outlet right ventricle: surgical results based on the STS-EACTS International Nomenclature classification. *Eur J Cardiothorac Surg* 29(4): 545–550, 2006.
32. Arumanayagam M, Chan S, Tong S, Sanderson JE: Antioxidant properties of carvedilol and metoprolol in heart failure: a double-blind randomized controlled trial. *Cardiovasc Pharmacol* 37:48–54, 2001.
33. Arzt W, Tulzer G, Aigner M, et al: Invasive intrauterine treatment of pulmonary atresia/intact ventricular septum with heart failure. *Ultrasound Obstet Gynecol* 2(2):186, 2003.
34. Ashburn DA, Blackstone EH, Wells WJ, et al: Determinants of mortality and type of repair in neonates with pulmonary atresia and intact ventricular septum. *J Thoracic Cardiovasc Surg* 127: 1000, 2004.
35. Ashcraft TM, Jones K, Border WL, et al: Factors affecting long-term risk of aortic arch recoarctation after the Norwood procedure. *Ann Thorac Surg* 85:1397, 2008.
36. Attenhofer Jost CH, Connolly HM, Edwards WD, et al: Ebstein anomaly: review of a multifaceted congenital cardiac condition. *Swiss Med Wkly* 135:269–281, 2005.
37. Atz AM, Adatia I, Wessel DL: Rebound pulmonary hypertension after inhalation of nitric oxide. *Ann Thorac Surg* 62(6):1759, 1996.
38. Atz AM, Wessel DL: Sildenafil ameliorates effects of inhaled nitric oxide withdrawal. *Anesthesiology* 91(1):307–310, 1999.
39. Babu K, McCormick M, Bird S: Pediatric dietary supplement use. An update. *Clin Pediatr Emerg Med* 6:2, 2005.
40. Bacha EA, Cao QL, Galantowicz ME, et al: Multicenter experience with preventricular device closure of muscular ventricular septal defects. *Pediatr Cardiol* 26(2):169–175, 2005.
41. Backer CL: Complete atrioventricular canal: comparison of modified single-patch technique with two-patch technique. *Ann Thorac Surg* 84 (6):2038–2046, 2007.
42. Backer CL, Badden HP, Costello JM, Mavroudis C: Perioperative care. In Mavroudis C, Backer CL, editors: *Pediatric cardiac surgery*, ed 3, Philadelphia, 2003, Mosby.
43. Backer CL, Baden HP, Costello JM, Mavroudis CM: Perioperative care. In Mavroudis CM, Backer CL, editors: *Pediatric cardiac surgery*, ed 3, St Louis, 2003, Mosby, pp. 119–142.
44. Backer CL, Mavroudis C: Coarctation of the aorta. In Mavroudis C, Backer CL, editors: *Pediatric cardiac surgery*, ed 3, Philadelphia, 2003, Mosby/Elsevier.
45. Backer CL, Stewart RD, Mavroudis C: Overview: history, anatomy, timing, and results of complete atrioventricular canal. *Semin Thorac Cardiovasc Surg Pediatr Card Surg Annu* Jan 3-10, 2007.
46. Backer CL, Tsao S, Deal BJ, Mavroudis C: Maze procedure in single ventricle patients. *Semin Thorac Cardiovasc Surg Pediatr Card Surg Annu* 44–48, 2008.

47. Baek JS, Bae EJ, Ko JS, Kim GB, et al: Late hepatic complications after Fontan operation; non-invasive markers of hepatic fibrosis and risk factors. *Heart* 96(21):1750–1755, 2010.

48. Baek JS, Bae EJ, Ko JS, et al: Late hepatic complications after Fontan operation; non-invasive markers of hepatic fibrosis and risk factors. *Heart* 96(21):1750–1755, 2010.

49. Bailliard F, Anderson RH: Tetralogy of Fallot. *Orphanet Journal of Rare Diseases* 4(2):1–10, 2009.

50. Baker E, Ellam S, Lorber A, et al: Superiority of radionuclide over oximetric measurement of left to right shunts. *Br Heart J* 53:535, 1985.

51. Balcells J, Rodriguez M, Pujol M, Iglesias J: Successful treatment of long QT syndrome-induced ventricular tachycardia with esmolol. *Pediatr Cardiol* 25(2):160–162, 2004.

52. Ball W Jr: *Pediatric neuroradiology.* Philadelphia, 1997, Lippincott-Raven.

53. Ballweg JA, Dominguez TE, Ravishankar C, et al: A contemporary comparison of the effect of shunt type in hypoplastic left heart syndrome on the hemodynamics and outcome at stage 2 reconstruction. *J Thorac Cardiovasc Surg* 134:297, 2007.

54. Ballweg JA, Dominguez TE, Ravishankar C, et al: A contemporary comparison of the effect of shunt type in hypoplastic left heart syndrome on the hemodynamics and outcome at Fontan completion. *J Thorac Cardiovasc Surg* 140:537, 2010.

55. Bar-Cohen Y, Perry SB, Keane JF, Lock JE: Use of stents to maintain atrial defects and Fontan fenestration in congenital heart disease. *J Interv Cardiol* 18:111, 2005.

56. Bar-Cohen Y, Silka MJ: Congenital long QT syndrome: diagnosis and management in pediatric patients. *Curr Treat Options Cardiovasc Med* 8(5):387–395, 2006.

57. Barkovich A: *Pediatric neuroimaging.* Philadelphia, 2000, Lippincott-Raven.

58. Barkovich AJ, Naidich TP, editors: *Pediatric neuroradiology, neuroimaging clinics of North America,* Philadelphia, 1994, Saunders.

59. Barnes PD: Editorial: imaging in the pediatric patient with headache. *Int Pediatr* 17(2):67, 2002.

60. Barst RJ, Gibbs SR, Ghofrani HA, et al: Updated evidence-based treatment algorithm in pulmonary arterial hypertension. *J Am Coll Cardiol* 54:78–84, 2009.

61. Bart RD, Bremner RM, Starnes VA: Ebstein anomaly. In Nicholls DG, editor in chief. *Critical heart disease in infants and children,* ed 2, Philadelphia, 2006, Saunders.

62. Bartz PJ, Driscoll DJ, Keane JF, et al: Management strategy for very mild aortic valve stenosis. *Pediatr Cardiol* 27:259, 2006.

63. Basson CT, Huang T, Lin RC, et al: Different TBX5 interactions in heart and limb defined by Holt-Oram syndrome mutations. *Proc Natl Acad Sci USA* 96:2919–2924, 1999.

64. Batra AS, Lewis AB: Acute myocarditis. *Curr Opin Pediatr* 13(3):234–239, 2001.

65. Baylen BG, Atkinson DE: Congenital mitral insufficiency. In Allen HD, Shaddy RE, Driscoll DJ, Feltes TF, editors: *Moss and Adams' heart disease in infants, children, and adolescents, including the fetus and young adult,* ed 7, Philadelphia, 2008, Lippincott Williams & Wilkins.

66. Beasley PJ, D'Angelo EJ, Landzberg M, DeMaso DR: Depression and anxiety in adults with congenital heart disease: a pilot study. *Heart Lung* 32(2):105–110, 2003.

67. Beekman RH: Commentary to Most patients with a moderate ventricular septal defect will not require intervention. *J Pediatr* 151(5):554, 2007.

68. Beekman RH: Coarctation of the aorta. In Allen HD, Shaddy RE, Driscoll DJ, Feltes TF, editors: *Moss and Adams' heart disease in infants, children, and adolescents, including the fetus and young adult,* ed 7, Philadelphia, 2008, Lippincott Williams & Wilkins.

69. Beerman HL, Lane RA: A survey of scientific literature on the medical complications of tattoos. *Am J Med Sci* 227:444–465, 1954.

70. Beery TA, Shooner KA, Benson DW: Neonatal long QT syndrome due to a de novo dominant negative hERG mutation. *Am J Crit Care* 16:412–415, 2007.

71. Beghetti M, Silkoff PE, Caramori M, et al: Decreased exhaled nitric oxide may be a marker of cardiopulmonary bypass-induced injury. *Ann Thorac Surg* 66:532–534, 1998.

72. Behrman RE, Kliegman RM, Jenson HB, editors: *Nelson textbook of pediatrics,* ed 17, Philadelphia, 2004, Saunders Elsevier.

73. Beke DM, Braudis NJ, Lincoln P: Management of pediatric postoperative cardiac surgery patient. *Crit Care Nurs Clin North Am* 17(4):405–416, 2005.

74. Benditt DG: Sinus node dysfunction: pathophysiology, clinical features, evaluation and treatment. In Zipes DP, Jalife J, editors: *Cardiac electrophysiology: from cell to bedside,* Philadelphia, 1990, Saunders, pp. 713–714.

75. Benson DW Jr, Gallagher JJ, Sterba R, et al: Catecholamine induced double tachycardia: case report in a child. *Pacing Clin Electrophysiol* 3(1):96–103, 1980.

76. Beppu S, Suzuki S, Matsuda H, et al: Rapidity of progression of aortic stenosis in patients with congenital bicuspid aortic valves. *Am J Cardiol* 71:322, 1993.

77. Berne RM, Levy MN. *Cardiovascular physiology.* ed 5, St Louis, 1986, Mosby.

78. Berne RM, Levy MN. *Cardiovascular physiology.* ed 8, St Louis, 2001, Mosby.

79. Bernstein D: Developmental biology and the cardiovascular system. In Behrman RE, Kliegman RM, Jenson HB, editors: *Nelson textbook of pediatrics,* ed 17, Philadelphia, 2004, Saunders Elsevier.

80. Bharati S, Lev M: Congenital anomalies of the pulmonary veins. *Cardiovasc Clin* 5:23, 1973.

81. Bharati S, Lev M: The course of the conduction system in single ventricle with inverted (L-) loop and inverted (L-) transposition. *Circulation* 51:723–730, 1975.

82. Bharati S, McAllister H, Rosenquist G: The surgical anatomy of truncus arteriosus communis. *J Thorac Cardiovasc Surg* 67:501, 1974.

83. Bhole V, Wright JG, De Giovanni JV, et al: Transcatheter interventions in the early postoperative period after the Fontan procedure. *Catheter Cardiovasc Interv* 77:92, 2011.

84. Bisoi AK, Sharma P, Chauhan S, Reddy SM, et al: Primary arterial switch operation in children presenting late with d-transposition of great arteries and intact ventricular septum. When is it too late for a primary arterial switch operation? *Eur J Cardiothorac Surg* 38(6):707–713, 2010.

85. Blaufox AD, Saul JP: Acute coronary artery stenosis during slow pathway ablation for atrioventricular nodal reentrant tachycardia in a child. *Cardiovasc Elctrophysiol* 15:97, 2004.

86. Bloch KD, Fumito I, Roberts JD, Zapol WM: Inhaled NO as a therapeutic agent. *Cardiovasc Res* 75(2):339, 2007.

87. Blum RW, Garell D, Hodgman CH, et al: Transition from child-centered to adult health-care systems for adolescents with chronic conditions. A position paper of the Society for Adolescent Medicine. *J Adolesc Health* 14(7):570–576, 1993.

88. Boethig D, Goerler H, Westhoff-Bleck M, et al: Evaluation of 188 consecutive homografts implanted in pulmonary position after 20 years. *Eur J Cardiothorac Surg* 32(1):133, 2007.

89. Boineau JP: The early repolarization variant: an electrocardiographic enigma with both QRS and J-STT anomalies. *J Electrocardiololgy* 40:3e1–e10, 2007.

90. Boineau JP: The early repolarization variant: normal or a marker of heart disease in certain subjects. *J Electrocardiololgy* 40: 3e11–e16, 2007.

91. Bonhoffer P, Oudjemline Y, Qureshi SA, et al: Percutaneous replacement of pulmonary valve in a right-ventricle to pulmonary-artery prosthetic conduit with valve dysfunction. *Lancet* 356:1403–1405, 2000.

92. Bonow RO, Carabello BA, Chatterjee K, et al: ACC/AHA 2006 guidelines for the management of patients with valvular heart disease. A report of the American College of Cardiology/American Heart Association Task Force on Practice Guidelines (Writing committee to revise the 1998 guidelines for the management of patients with valvular heart disease). *J Am Coll Cardiol* 48:1, 2006.

93. Boshoff DE, Michel-Behnke I, Schranz D, Gewillig M: Stenting the neonatal arterial duct. *Expert Rev Cardiovasc Ther* 5(5):893–901, 2007.

94. Boucek MM, Chan KC, Bright JM: Percutaneous selective pulmonary artery bands (Joeys) in a pulmonary overcirculation model. *Catheter Cardiovasc Intern* 70:98, 2007.

95. Boutin C, Jonas RA, Sanders SP, et al: Rapid two-stage arterial switch operation: acquisition of left ventricular mass following pulmonary artery banding in infants with transposition of the great arteries. *Circulation* 90:1304, 1994.

96. Boyer KM: RSV and the timing of surgery for congenital heart disease. *Crit Care Med* 27(9):2065, 1999.

97. Bradley DJ, Fischbach PS, Law IH, et al: The clinical course of multifocal atrial tachycardia in infants and children. *J Am Coll Cardiol* 38(2):401–408, 2001.

98. Bradley SM, Simsic JM, Mulvihill DM: Hyperventilation impairs oxygenation after bidirectional superior cavopulmonary connection. *Circulation* 98:II372–II377, 1998.

99. Bradley SM, Simsic JM, Mulvihill DM: Hypoventilation improves oxygenation after bidirectional superior cavopulmonary connection. *J Thorac Cardiovasc Surg* 126:1033–1039, 2003.

100. Bradley TJ, Karamlou T, Kulik A, et al: Determinants of repair type, reintervention and mortality in 393 children with double-outlet right ventricle. *J Thorac Cardiovasc Surg* 134(4):967–973, 2007.

101. Brashers VL, McCance K: Structure and function of the cardiovascular and lymphatic systems. In McCance K, Huethers S, Brashers VL, Rote NS, editors: *Pathophysiology: the biologic basis for disease in adults and children*, ed 6, Philadelphia, 2010, Mosby.

102. Braudis NJ, Curley MAQ, Beaupre K, et al: Enteral feeding algorithm for infants with hypoplastic left heart syndrome post stage I palliation. *Pediatr Crit Care Med* 10(4):460–466, 2010.

103. Braunstein PW Jr, Sade RM, Gillette PC: Life-threatening postoperative junctional ectopic tachycardia. *Ann Thorac Surg* 53(4): 726–728, 1992.

104. Braunwald E, Zipes DP, Libby P: Endocarditis. In *Heart disease*, ed 6, Philadelphia, 2001, Saunders, p. 1730.

105. Breitkreutz R, Price S, Steiger HV, et al: Focused echocardiographic evaluation in life support and peri-resuscitation of emergency patients: a prospective trial. *Resuscitation* Aug 27. [Epub ahead of print], 2010.

106. Breitkreutz R, Walcher F, Seeger FH: Focused echocardiographic evaluation in resuscitation management: concept of an advanced life support-conformed algorithm. *Crit Care Med* 35(5 Suppl): S150–S161, 2007.

107. Brickner ME, Hillis LD, Lange RA: Congenital heart disease in adults. First of two parts. *N Engl J Med* 342:256, 2000.

108. Bridges ND, Lock JE, Castaneda AR: Baffle fenestration with subsequent transcatheter closure: modification of the Fontan operation for patients at increased risk. *Circulation* 82:1681–1689, 1990.

109. Bristow MR: Mechanism of action of beta-blocking agents in heart failure. *Am J Cardiol* 80:26L–40L, 1997.

110. Britto MT, Garrett JM, Dugliss MA, et al: Risky behavior in teens with cystic fibrosis or sickle cell disease: a multicenter study. *Pediatrics* 101(2):250–256, 1998.

111. Bromberg BI, Beekman RH, Rocchini AP, et al: Aortic aneurysm after patch aortoplasty repair of coarctation. *J Am Coll Cardiol* 14:734–741, 1989.

112. Bronner MB, Peek N, Knoester H, et al: Course and predicators of posttraumatic stress disorder in parents after pediatric intensive care treatment of their child. *J Pediatr Psychol* Advance access published online on February 11, 2010.

113. Brooke BS, Habashi JP, Judge DP, et al: Angiotensin II blockade and aortic-root dilation in Marfan's syndrome. *N Engl J Med* 358:2787–2795, 2006.

114. Brosig CL, Mussatto KA, Kuhn EM, et al: Psychosocial outcomes for preschool children and families after surgery for complex congenital heart disease. *Pediatr Cardiol* 28(4):255–262, 2007.

115. Brosig CL, Mussatto KA, Kuhn EM, Tweddelll JS: Neurodevelopmental outcome in preschool survivors of complex congenital heart disease: implications for clinical practice. *J Pediatr Healthcare* 21:3, 2007.

116. Brothers JA, McBride MG, Seliem MA, et al: Evaluation of myocardial ischemia after surgical repair of anomalous aortic origin of a coronary artery in a series of pediatric patients. *J Am Coll Cardiol* 50(21):2978–2982, 2007.

117. Brown DW, Chong EC, Gauvreau K, et al: Aortic wall injury as a complication of neonatal aortic valvuloplasty: incidence and risk factors. *Circ Cardiovasc Intervent* 1:53, 2008.

118. Brown DW, Gauvreau K, Powell AJ, et al: Cardiac magnetic resonance versus routine cardiac catheterization before bidirectional Glenn anastomosis in infants with functional single ventricle: a prospective randomized trial. *Circulation* 116:2718, 2007.

119. Brown JW, Ruzmetov M, Okada Y, et al: Truncus arteriosus repair: outcomes, risk factors, reoperation and management. *Eur J Cardiothorac Surg* 20(2):221–227, 2001.

120. Brugada P, Brugada J: Right bundle branch block, persistent ST segment elevation and sudden cardiac death: a distinct clinical and electrocardiographic syndrome. A multicenter report. *J Am Coll Cardiol* 20(6):1391–1396, 1992.

121. Buchhorn R, Bartmus D, Siekmeyer W, et al: Beta-blocker therapy of severe congestive heart failure in infants with left to right shunts. *Am J Cardiol* 81:1366–1368, 1997.

122. Bulbul ZR, Rosenthal D, Brueckner M: Genetic aspects of heart disease in the newborn. *Semin Perinatol* 17(2):61–75, 1993.

123. Burke RP, Jacobs JP, Ashraf MH, et al: Extracardiac Fontan operation without cardiopulmonary bypass. *Ann Thorac Surg* 63:1175, 1997.

124. Butto F, Lucas RV, Edwards JE: Persistent truncus arteriosus: pathologic anatomy in 54 cases. *Pediatr Cardiol* 7:95, 1986.

125. Buyon JP, Hiebert R, Copel J, et al: Autoimmune-associated congenital heart block: demographics, mortality, morbidity and recurrence rates obtained from a national neonatal lupus registry. *J Am Coll Cardiol* 31(7):1658–1666, 1998.

126. Byers J: Protecting patients during clinical research. *Crit Care Nurse* 24(1):53–59, 2004.

127. Cabalka AK, Edwards WD, Dearani JA: Truncus arteriosus. In Allen HD, Driscoll DJ, Feltes TF, Shaddy RE, editors: *Moss and Adams' heart disease in infants, children, and adolescents, including the fetus and young adult*, ed 7, Philadelphia, 2008, Lippincott Williams & Wilkins.

128. Cabreraa AG, Prodhanb P, Bhuttab AT: Nutritional challenges and outcomes after surgery for congenital heart disease. *Curr Op Cardiol* 25:88, 2010.

129. Calder L, Van Praagh R, Sears WP, et al: Truncus arteriosus communis: clinical, angiocardiographic, and pathologic findings in 100 patients. *Am Heart J* 92:23, 1976.

130. Calderone CA, Benson L, Holtby H, et al: Initial experience with hybrid palliation for neonates with single-ventricle physiology. *Ann Thorac Surg* 84:1294, 2007.

131. Callahan ST, Winitzer RF, Keenan P: Transition from pediatric to adult-oriented healthcare: a challenge for patients with chronic disease. *Curr Opin Pediatr* 13(4):310–316, 2001.

132. Callow L: Pulmonary artery intracardiac line: care and management. In Verger JT, Lebet RM, editors: *AACN procedural manual for pediatric acute & critical care*, Philadelphia, 2008, Elsevier Saunders.

133. Calvaruso DF, Rubino A, Ocello S, et al: Bidirectional Glenn and antegrade pulmonary blood flow: temporary or definitive palliation? *Ann Thorac Surg* 85:1389, 2008.

134. Campbell M: Natural history of coarctation of the aorta. *Br Heart J* 32:633–640, 1970.

135. Campbell GB, Happ MB: Symptom identification in the chronically, critically ill. *AACN* 21(1):64–79, 2010.

136. Campbell LA, Kirkpatrick SE, Berry CC, Lamberti JJ: Preparing children with congenital heart disease for cardiac surgery. *J Pediatr Psychol* 20(3):313–328, 1995.

137. Canobbio MM, Perloff JK, Rapkin AJ: Gynecological health of females with congenital heart disease. *Int J Cardiol* 98(3):379–387, 2005.

138. Cardillo K: Nutrition interventions for chylous effusions. *Support Line* 6:18, 2001.

139. Carminati M, Butera G, Chessa M, et al: Transcatheter closure of congenital ventricular septal defects: results of the European Registry. *Eur Heart J* 28:2361–2368, 2007.

140. Carmosino MJ, Friesen RH, Doran A, Ivy DD: Perioperative complications in children with pulmonary hypertension undergoing noncardiac surgery or cardiac catheterization. *Anesth Analg* 104(3): 521, 2007.

141. Casella ES, et al: Developmental physiology of the cardiovascular system. In Rogers MC, editor: *Textbook of pediatric intensive care*, Baltimore, 1987, Williams & Wilkins.

142. Casey FA, McCrindle BW, Hamilton RM, Gow RM: Neonatal atrial flutter: significant early morbidity and excellent long-term prognosis. *Am Heart J* 133(3):302–306, 1997.

143. Cassidy SC, Schmidt KG, van Hare GF, et al: Complications of pediatric cardiac catheterization: a three-year study. *J Am Coll Cardiol* 19:1285, 1992.

144. Castanada AR, Jonas RA, Mayer JE, Hanley FL, editors: Obstruction of the left ventricular outflow tract. *Cardiac surgery of the neonate and infant*, Philadelphia, 1994, Saunders, p. 315.

145. Castaneda AR, Jonas RA, Mayer JEN, Hanley FL: Atrioventricular canal. In *Cardiac surgery of the neonate and infant*. Philadelphia, 1994, Saunders.

146. Catchpole KR, de Leval MR, Mcewan A, et al: Patient handover from surgery to intensive care: using Formula 1 pit-stop and aviation models to improve safety and quality. *Pediatr Anesth* 17:470–478, 2007.

147. Catchpole K, Sellers R, Goldman A, et al: Patient handovers within the hospital: translating knowledge from motor racing to healthcare. *Qual Sat Healthcare* 19:318–322, 2010.

148. Cecchin F, Johnsrude CL, Perry JC, Friedman RA: Effect of age and surgical technique on symptomatic arrhythmias after the Fontan procedure. *Am J Cardiol* 76(5):386–391, 1995.

149. Celebi A, Yalcin Y, Erdem A, et al: Stent implantation into the patent ductus arteriosus in cyanotic congenial heart disease with duct dependent or diminished pulmonary circulation. *Turk J Pediatr* 49 (4):413, 2007.

150. Cetta F, Minich L, Edwards WD, et al: Atrioventricular septal defects. In Allen HD, Driscoll DJ, Shaddy RE, Feltes TF, editors: *Moss and Adams' heart disease in infants, children, and adolescents, including the fetus and young adult*, ed 7, Philadelphia, 2008, Lippincott Williams & Wilkins.

151. Chang AC, Atz AM, Wernovsky G, et al: Milrinone: systemic and pulmonary hemodynamic effects in neonates after cardiac surgery. *Crit Care Med* 23:1907, 1995.

152. Chang AC, Burke RP: Anomalous pulmonary venous connection. In Chang AC, Hanley FL, Wernovsky G, Wessel DL, editors: *Pediatric cardiac intensive care*, Toronto, 1998, Williams & Wilkins, p. 227.

153. Chang AC, Burke RP: Common atrioventricular canal. In Chang AC, Hanldey FL, Wernovsky G, et al., editors: *Pediatric cardiac intensive care*, Baltimore, 1998, Williams & Wilkins.

154. Chang AC, Hanley FL: Anomalous origin of the left coronary artery from the pulmonary artery. In Chang AC, Hanley FL, Wernovsky G, Wessel DL, editors: *Pediatric cardiac intensive care*, Baltimore, 1998, Williams & Wilkins, pp. 312–316.

155. Chang AC, Jacobs J: Mitral valve disease. In Chang AC, Hanley FL, Wernovsky G, Wessel DL, editors: *Pediatric cardiac intensive care*, Canada, 1998, Williams & Wilkins.

156. Chang AC, Jacobs J: Aorticopulmonary window. In Chang AC, Hanley FL, Wernovsky G, Wessel DL, editors: *Pediatric cardiac intensive care*, Baltimore, 1998, Williams & Wilkins.

157. Chang AC, Reddy M: Truncus arteriosus. In Chang AC, Hanley F, Wernovsky G, Wessel DL, editors: *Pediatric cardiac intensive care*, Baltimore, 1998, Williams & Wilkins.

158. Chang AC, Starnes VA: Interrupted Aortic Arch. In Chang AC, Hanley FL, Wernovsky G, Wessel DL, editors: *Pediatric cardiac intensive care*, Canada, 1998, Williams & Wilkins.

159. Chang AC, Starnes VA: Coarctation of the aorta. In Chang AC, Hanley FL, Wernovsky G, Wessel DL, editors: *Pediatric cardiac intensive care*, Baltimore, 1998, Williams & Wilkins.

160. Chang YY, Chang CI, Wang MF, et al: The safe use of intraoperative transesophageal echocardiography in the management of total anomalous pulmonary venous connection in newborns and infants: a case series. *Paediatr Anaesth* 15(11):939–943, 2005.

161. Chan SY, Lau W, Wong WH, et al: Chylothorax in children after congenital heart surgery. *Ann Thorac Surg* 82:1656, 2006.

162. Chang RK, et al: Bubble contrast echocardiography in detecting pulmonary arteriovenous shunting in children with univentricular heart after cavopulmonary anastomosis. *J Am Coll Cardiol* 33:2052, 1999.

163. Chauvaud S, Berrebi A, d'Attellis N, et al: Ebstein anomaly: repair based on functional analysis. *Eur J Cardiothorac Surg* 23:525–531, 2003.

164. Chauvaud S, Waldmann T, d'Attellis N, et al: Homograft replacement of the mitral valve in young patients: mid-term results. *Eur J Cardiothorac Surg* 23:560–566, 2003.

165. Checchia PA, Kulik TJ: Acute viral myocarditis: diagnosis. *Pediatr Crit Care Med* 7(6 Suppl.):S8–S11, 2006.

166. Cheitlin MD, Armstrong WF, Aurigemma GP, et al: ACC/AHA/ASE 2003 guideline update for the clinical application of echocardiography: summary article: a report of the American College of Cardiology/American Heart Association Task Force on Practice Guidelines (ACC/AHA/ASE Committee to Update the 1997 Guidelines for the Clinical Application of Echocardiography). *Circulation* 108:1146, 2003.

167. Chen J, Zimmerman R, Javik GP, et al: Perioperative stroke in infants undergoing open heart operations for congenital heart disease. *Ann Thorac Surg* 88:823, 2009.

168. Chen YY, Hsu CY: Prenatal diagnosis and antenatal history of total anomalous pulmonary venous return. *Taiwanese J Obstet Gynecol* 45(3):283–285, 2006.

169. Cheng TO: Is patent foramen ovale the culprit in women with migraine and cardiovascular disease. *Int J Cardiol* 113(3):442, 2006.

170. Chessa M, Dindar A, Vettukattil JJ, et al: Balloon antioplasty in infants with aortic obstruction after the modified stage I Norwood procedure. *Am Heart J* 40:227, 2000.

171. Child JS, Collins-Nakai RL, Alpert JS, et al: Task force 3: workforce description and educational requirements for the care of adults with congenital heart disease. *J Am Coll Cardiol* 37(5):1183–1187, 2001.

172. Chivers L: Body adornment: piercings and tattoos. *Nurs Stand* 16 (34):41–45, 2002.

173. Chorne N, Jegatheesan P, Lin E, et al: Risk factors for persistent ductus arteriosus patency during indomethacin treatment. *J Pediatr* 151(6):629–634, 2007.

174. Chowdhury UK, Airan B, Kothari SS, et al: Surgical outcomes of staged univentricular-type repairs for patients with univentricular physiology and pulmonary hypertension. *Indian Heart J* 56:320, 2004.

175. Christensen TD, Andersen NT, Maegaard M, et al: Oral anticoagulation therapy in children: successfully controlled by self-management. *Heart Surg Forum* 7(4), 2004, doi:10-1532/HSF98.20041000.

176. Christenson JT, Sierra J, Colina Manzano NE, Jolou J, et al: Homografts and xenografts for right ventricular outflow tract reconstruction: long-term results. *Ann Thorac Surg* 90:1287–1293, 2010.

177. Chrysostomou C, Beerman L, Shiderly D, et al: Dexmedetomidine: a novel drug for the treatment of atrial and junctional tachyarrhythmias during the perioperative period for congenital cardiac surgery: a preliminary study. *Anesth Analg* 107(5):1514–1522, 2008.

178. Chun T: Pacemaker and defibrillator therapy in pediatrics and congenital heart disease. *Future Cardiol* 4(5):469–479, 2008.

179. Cioc AM, Nuovo GJ: Histologic and in situ viral findings in the myocardium in cases of sudden unexpected death. *Mod Pathol* 15:914, 2002.

180. Claessens P, Moons P, Dierckx de Casterle B, et al: What does it mean to live with congenital heart disease? A qualitative study on the lived experiences of adult patients. *Eur J Cardiovasc Nurs* 4:3, 2005.

181. Clark EB: Pathogenetic mechanisms of congenital cardiovascular malformations revisited. *Semin perinatol* 20:465, 1996.

182. Clark EB: Growth, morphogenesis, and function: the dynamics of cardiovascular development. In Moller JM, Neal WA, editors: *Fetal, neonatal, and infant heart disease*, New York, 1989, Appleton-Century-Crofts, pp. 1–22.

183. Cleuziou J, Schreiber C, Eicken A, Hörer J, et al: Predictors for biventricular repair in pulmonary atresia with intact ventricular septum. *Thorac Cardiovasc Surg* 58(6):339–344, 2010.

184. Clyman RI, Chorne N: Patent ductus arteriosus: evidence for and against treatment (editorial). *J Pediatr* 150:216–219, 2007.

185. Cohen MI, Vetter VL: Postoperative atrioventricular conduction defects. In Balaji S, Gillette PC, Case CL, editors: *Cardiac arrhythmias after surgery for congenital heart disease*, New York, 2001, Arnold Publishers, pp. 85–118.

186. Cohen M, Wernovsky G: Is the arterial switch operation as good over the long term as we thought it would be? *Cardiol Young* 16 (Suppl 3):117, 2006.

187. Cohen S, Springer C, Avital A, et al: Amino-terminal pro-brain type natriuretic peptide: heart or lung disease in pediatric respiratory distress? *Pediatrics* 115:1347–1350, 2005.

188. Colan SD: Cardiomyopathies. In Keane JF, Lock JE, Fyler DC, editors: *Nadas' pediatric cardiology*, ed 2, Philadelphia, 2006, Elsevier.

189. Colan SD: Cardiomyopathies. In Keane JF, Lock JE, Fyler DC, editors: *Nadas' pediatric cardiology*, ed 2, Philadelphia, 2006, Elsevier, pp. 421–422.

190. Coleman KB: Genetic counseling in congenital heart disease. *Crit Care Nurs Q* 25(3):8–16, 2002.

191. Collett R, Edwards J: Persistent truncus arteriosus: a classification according to anatomic types. *Surg Clin North Am* 29:1245–1270, 1949.

192. Collins KK, Dubin AM, Chiesa NA, et al: Cryoablation versus radiofrequency ablation for treatment of pediatric atrioventricular nodal reentrant tachycardia: initial experience with 4-mm cryocatheter. *Heart Rhythm* 3(5):564–570, 2006.

193. Collins KK, Dubin AM, Chiesa NA, et al: Cryoablation in pediatric atrioventricular nodal reentry: electrophysiologic effects on atrioventricular nodal conduction. *Heart Rhythm* 3(5):557–563, 2006.

194. Collins KK, Rhee EK, Delucca JM, et al: Modification to the Fontan procedure for the prophylaxis of intra-atrial reentrant tachycardia: short-term results of a prospective randomized blinded trial. *J Thorac Cardiovasc Surg* 127(3):721–729, 2004.

195. Collins KK, Van Hare GF, Kertesz NJ, et al: Pediatric nonpostoperative junctional ectopic tachycardia medical management and interventional therapies. *J Am Coll Cardiol* 53(8):690–697, 2009.

196. Colman JM: Noncardiac surgery in adult congenital heart disease. In Gatzoulis MA, Webb GA, Daubeney PEF, editors: *Diagnosis and management of adult congenital heart disease*, Edinburgh, 2003, Churchill Livingstone.

197. Cook SC, Raman SV: Imaging modalities for adolescents and adults with congenital heart disease. In Allen HD, Driscoll DJ, Feltes TF, Shaddy RE, editors: *Moss and Adams' heart disease in infants, children, and adolescent including the fetus and young adult*, ed 7, Philadelphia, 2008, Lippincott Williams & Wilkins.

198. Cooper LT, Baughman KL, Feldman AM, et al: The role of endomyocardial biopsy in the management of cardiovascular disease. A scientific statement from the American Heart Association, the American College of Cardiology, and the European society of Cardiology. Endorsed by the Heart Failure Society of America and the Heart Failure Association of the European Society of Cardiology. *Eur Heart J* 28:3076–3093, 2007.

199. Cope JT, Lindsey JH, Irving LK: Cardiac tumors. In Mavroudis C, Backer CL, editors: *Pediatric cardiac surgery*, ed 3, Philadelphia, 2003, Mosby/Elsevier.

200. Copeland JG, Sinson EB: Human heart transplantation. *Curr Probl Cardiol* 8(4):1–5, 1979.

201. Correa-Villasenor A, Ferencz C, Boughman JA, Neill CA: Total anomalous pulmonary venous return: familial and environmental factors. The Baltimore-Washington Infant Study Group. *Teratology* 44(4):415–428, 1991.

202. Corrigan JJ. Hematologic aspects of pediatric cardiology. In Allen HD, Driscoll DJ, Feltes TF, Shaddy RE, editors: *Moss & Adams heart disease in infants, children, and adolescents including the fetus and young adult*, ed 7, Philadelphia, 2008, Lippincott Williams & Wilkins.

203. Costello JM, Graham DA, Morrow DF, et al: Risk factors for central line-associated bloodstream infection in a pediatric cardiac intensive care unit. *Pediatr Crit Care Med* 10(4):453–459, 2009.

204. Costello JM, Morrow DF, Graham DA, et al: Systematic intervention to reduce central line associated bloodstream infection rates in a pediatric cardiac intensive care unit. *Pediatrics* 121:915–923, 2008.

205. Cowrie MR, Jourdain P, Maisel AS, et al: Clinical applications of B-type natriuretic peptide (BNP) testing. *Eur Heart J* 24:1710–1718, 2003.

206. Craig J, Fineman LD, Moynihan P, Baker AL: Cardiovascular critical care problems. In Curley MAQ, Moloney-Harmon P, editors: *Critical care nursing of infants and children*, ed 2, Philadelphia, 2001, Saunders.

207. Crystal MA, Yoo SH, Mikailian H, Benson LN: Catheter-based completion of the Fontan circuit: a nonsurgical approach. *Circulation* 114:e5, 2006.

208. Cua CL, Galantowicz ME, Turner DR, et al: Palliation via hybrid procedure of a 1.4 kg patient with a hypoplastic left heart. *Congenit Heart Dis* 2:191, 2007.

209. Cua CL, Thiagarajan RR, Gauvreau K, et al: Early postoperative outcomes in a series of infants with hypoplastic left heart syndrome undergoing stage I palliation operation with either modified Blalock-Taussig shunt or right ventricle to pulmonary artery conduit. *Pediatr Crit Care Med* 7:286, 2006.

210. Cummings RM, Mahle WT, Strieper MJ, et al: Outcomes following electroanatomic mapping and ablation for the treatment of ectopic atrial tachycardia in the pediatric population. *Pediatr Cardiol* 29(2): 393–397, 2008.

211. Curzon CL, Milford-Beland S, Li JS, et al: Cardiac surgery in infants with low birth weight is associated with increased mortality: analysis of the Society of Thoracic Surgeons Congenital Heart Database. *J Thorac Cardiovasc Surg* 135(3):546, 2008.

212. Dadlani G, Harmon W, Liphultz S: Dilated cardiomyopathy. In Chang AC, Towbin JA, editors: *Heart failure in children and young adults*, Philadelphia, 2006, Elsevier, pp. 248–263.

213. Dae MW: Pediatric nuclear cardiology. *Semin Nucl Med* 37(5): 382–390, 2007.

214. Dahnert I, Schneider P, Handrick W: Piercing and tattoos in patients with congenital heart disease: is it a problem? *Z Kardio* 93(8): 618–623, 2004.

214a. Dallman PR, Shannon K, Pearson HA: Developmental changes in red blood cell production and function. In Rudolph CD, Rudolph AM, Hostetter MK, Lister G, Siegel NH, editors: *Rudolph's Pediatrics*, ed 21, New York, 2003, McGraw-Hill.

215. Daniels CJ: Adult congenital heart disease: lesion specific pathways. In Allen HD, Driscoll DJ, Feltes TF, Shaddy RE, editors: *Moss and Adams' heart disease in infants, children, and adolescent including the fetus and young adult*, ed 7, Philadelphia, 2008, Lippincott Williams & Wilkins.

216. Daniels CJ: The young with congenital heart disease. In Allen HD, Driscoll DJ, Feltes TF, Shaddy RE, editors: *Moss and Adams' heart disease in infants, children, and adolescent including the fetus and young adult*, ed 7, Philadelphia, 2008, Lippincott Williams & Wilkins.

217. Daniels CJ: The adolescent and adult with congenital heart disease. In Allen HD, Driscoll DJ, Feltes TF, Shaddy RE, editors: *Moss and Adams' heart disease in infants, children, and adolescents, including the fetus and young adult*, ed 7, Philadelphia, 2008, Lippincott Williams & Wilkins.

218. Danner E, Joeckel R, Phillips S, Goday P: Weight velocity in infants and children. *Nutr Clin Pract* 24:76–79, 2009.

219. Daubeney PEF: Pulmonary atresia with intact ventricular septum. In Gatzoulis MA, Webb GA, Daubeney PEF, editors: *Diagnosis and management of adult congenital heart disease*, Edinburgh, 2003, Churchill Livingstone.

220. Dauchot P, Gravenstein JS: Effects of atropine on the electrocardiogram in different age groups. *Clin Pharmacol Ther* 12:274–280, 1971.

221. Dave H, Mueggler O, Comber M, et al: Risk factor analysis of 170 single-institution contegra implantations in pulmonary position. *Ann Thorac Surgery* 91:195, 2011.

222. Davenport JJ, Lam L, Whalen-Glass R, et al: The successful use of alternative routes of vascular access for performing pediatric interventional cardiac catheterization. *Catheter Cardiovasc Interv* 72(3): 392–398, 2008.

223. Davis PC, Hopkins KL: Imaging of the pediatric orbit and visual pathways: computed tomography and magnetic resonance imaging. *Neuroimaging Clin North Am* 9:93, 1999.

224. Deal BJ: Supraventricular tachycardia mechanisms and natural history. In Deal BJ, Wolff GS, Gelband H, editors: *Current concepts in diagnosis and management of arrhythmias in infants and children*, New York, 1998, Futura, pp. 117–143.

225. Deal BJ, Keane JF, Gillette PC, Garson A Jr, : Wolff-Parkinson-White syndrome and supraventricular tachycardia during infancy: management and follow-up. *J Am Coll Cardiol* 5(1):130–135, 1985.

226. Deal BJ, Mavroudis C, Backer CL: Arrhythmia management in the Fontan patient. *Pediatr Cardiol* 28:448, 2007.

227. Deanfield J, Thaulow E, Warnes C, et al: Management of grown up congenital heart disease. *Eur Heart J* 24:1035, 2003.

228. Dearani JA, Danielson GK, Puga FJ, et al: Late follow-up of 1095 patients undergoing operation for complex congenital heart disease utilizing pulmonary ventricle to pulmonary artery conduits. *Ann Thorac Surg* 75:399, 2003.

229. de Koning WB, van Osch-Gevers M, Harkel AD, et al: Followup outcomes 10 years after arterial switch operation for transposition of the great arteries: comparison of cardiologic health status and health-related quality of life to those of a normal reference population. *Eur J Pediatr* 167(9):994–1004, 2007.

230. DeLoughery TG: Critical care clotting catastrophes. *Crit Care Clin* 21:3, 2005.

231. Denfield S: Restrictive cardiomyopathy and constrictive pericarditis. In Chang AC, Towbin JA, editors: *Heart failure in children and young adults*, Philadelphia, 2006, Elsevier, pp. 264–277.

232. Devaney EJ, Chang AC, Ohye RG, et al: Management of congenital and acquired pulmonary vein stenosis. *Ann Thorac Surg* 81:992, 2006.

233. Devaney EJ, Ohye RG, Bove EL: Pulmonary vein stenosis following repair of total anomalous pulmonary venous connection. Semin Thorac Cardiovasc Surg. *Pediatr Cardiol Surg Annu* 9:51–55, 2006.

234. DeWitt DE, Pauuw DS: Endocarditis in injection drug users. *Am Fam Physician* 53:2045–2409, 1996.

235. Diab KA: Device closure of atrial septal defects with the Amplatzer septal occluder: safety and outcome in infants. *J Thoras Cadiovasc Surg* 134(4):960–966, 2007.

236. Dick M, Fyler DC, Nadas AS: Tricuspid atresia: clinical course in 101 patients. *Am J Cardiol* 36:327, 1975.

237. Dick M 2nd, Russell MW: Ventricular tachycardia. In Deal BJ, Wolff GS, Gelband H, editors: *Current concepts in diagnosis and management of arrhythmias in infants and children. armonk*, Futura, 1998, NY, pp. 181–222.

238. DiDonato RM, Fyfe DA, Puga FJ, et al: Fifteen year experience with surgical repair of truncus arteriosus. *J Thorac Cardiovasc Surg* 89:414, 1985.

239. Diercks DB, Shumaik GM, Harrigan RA, et al: Electrocardiographic manifestations: electrolyte abnormalities. *J Emerg Med* 27(2): 153–160, 2004.

240. Diller GP, Gatzoulis MA: Pulmonary vascular disease in adults with congenital heart disease. *Circulation* 115(8):1039, 2007.

241. Diller GP, Uebing A, Willson K, et al: Analytical identification of ideal pulmonary-systemic flow balance in patients with bidirectional cavopulmonary shunt and univentricular circulation: oxygen delivery or tissue oxygenation? *Circulation* 114(12):1243–1250, 2006.

242. Dodge-Khatami A, Mavroudis C, Backer CL: The Society of Thoracic Surgeons Congenital Heart Surgery Nomenclature and Database Project: Coronary Arteries. *Ann Thorac Surg* 69(suppl): S270–S297, 2000.

243. Dorostkar PC, Silka MJ, Morady F, Dick M 2nd: Clinical course of persistent junctional reciprocating tachycardia. *J Am Coll Cardiol* 33 (2):366–375, 1999.

244. Downing TP, Danielson GK, Schaff HV, et al: Replacement of obstructed right ventricular-pulmonary arterial conduits with nonvalved conduits in children. *Circulation* 72(Suppl II):II–84, 1985.

245. Drenthen W, Pieper PG, van der Tuuk K, et al: Fertility, pregnancy and delivery in women after biventricular repair for double outlet right ventricle. *Cardiology* 109(2):105–109, 2008.

246. Dua JS, Cooper AR, Fox KR, Graham Suart A: Physical activity levels in adults with congenital heart disease. *Eur J Cardiovasc Prev Rehabil* 14:287, 2007.

247. Du Plessis AJ: Neurologic conditions. In Chang AC, Hanley FL, Wernovsky G, Wessel DL, editors: *Pediatric cardiac intensive care*, Toronto, 1998, Williams & Wilkins.

248. Durack DT, Lukes AS, Bright DK: The Duke Endocarditis Service. New criteria for diagnosis of infective endocarditis: utilization of specific echocardiographic findings. *Am J Med* 96:200–209, 1994.

249. Dyck JD, Atallah J: Congenitally corrected transposition of the great arteries. In Allen HD, Driscoll DJ, Feltes TF, Shaddy RE, editors: *Moss and Adams' heart disease in infants, children, and adolescents, including the fetus and young adult*, ed 7, Philadelphia, 2008, Lippincott Williams & Wilkins.

250. Earing MG, Connolly HM, Dearani JA, et al: Long-term followup of patients after surgical treatment for isolated pulmonary valve stenosis. *Mayo Clin Proc* 80:871, 2005.

251. Eckart RE, Jones SO 4th, Shry EA, et al: Sudden death associated with anomalous coronary origin and obstructive coronary disease in the young. *Cardiol Rev* 14(4):161–163, 2006.

252. English RF, Janosky JE, Ettedgui JA, Webber SA: Outcomes for children with acute myocarditis. *Cardiol Young* 14:488, 2004.

253. Epstein ML: Tricuspid atresia, stenosis and regurgitation. In Allen HD, Driscoll DJ, Feltes TF, Shaddy RE, editors: *Moss and Adams' heart disease in infants, children, and adolescents, including the fetus and young adult*, ed 7, Philadelphia, 2008, Lippincott Williams & Wilkins.

254. Epstein AE, DiMarco JP, Ellenbogen KA, et al: ACC/AHA/HRS 2008 Guidelines for Device-Based Therapy of Cardiac Rhythm Abnormalities: a report of the American College of Cardiology/ American Heart Association Task Force on Practice Guidelines (Writing Committee to Revise the ACC/AHA/NASPE 2002 Guideline Update for Implantation of Cardiac Pacemakers and Antiarrhythmia Devices) developed in collaboration with the American Association for Thoracic Surgery and Society of Thoracic Surgeons. *J Am Coll Cardiol* 51(21):e1–62, 2008.

255. Epstein ML, Kiel EA, Victorica BE: Cardiac decompensation following verapamil therapy in infants with supraventricular tachycardia. *Pediatrics* 75:737–740, 1985.

256. Ewert P, Berger F, Nagdyman N, et al: Masked left ventricular restriction in elderly patients with atrial septal defects: a contraindication for closure? *Cathet Cardiovasc Interv* 52:177, 2001.

257. Fallon P, Aparício JM, Elliott MJ, Kirkham FJ: Incidence of neurological complications of surgery for congenital heart disease. *Arch Dis Child* 72:418–422, 1995.

258. Fawzy ME, Awad M, Hassam W, et al: Long-term outcome (up to 15 years) of balloon angioplasty of discrete native coarctation of the aorta in adolescents and adults. *J Am Coll Cardiol* 43:1062–1067, 2004.

259. Feigenbaum H: *Echocardiography.* Philadelphia, 1994, Lea & Febiger.

260. Feldman T, Leon MB: Prospects for percutaneous valve therapies. *Circulation* 116:2866, 2007.

261. Fenton M, Burch M: Understanding heart failure. *Arch Dis Child* 92:812–816, 2007.

262. Fenton KN, et al: Interim mortality in infants with systemic to pulmonary artery shunts. *Ann Thorac Surg* 76:152–157, 2003.

263. Ferencz C, Neill CA, Boughman JA, et al: Congenital cardiovascular malformations associated with chromosome abnormalities: an epidemiologic study. *J Pediatr* 114(1):79–86, 1989.

264. Ferencz C, Rubin JD, McCarter RJ, et al: Congenital heart disease: prevalence at livebirth. The Baltimore-Washington Infant Study. *Am J Epidemiol* 121:31, 1985.

265. Ferencz C, Villasenor AC: Epidemiology of cardiovascular malformation: the state of the art. *Cardiol Young* 1(4):264, 1991.

266. Ferrieri P, Gewitz MH, Gerber MA, et al: AHA scientific statement: unique features of infective endocarditis in childhood. *Circulation* 105:2115, 2002.

267. Fineman JR, Heymann MA, Morin FC III: Fetal and postnatal circulations: pulmonary and persistent pulmonary hypertension of the Newborn. In Allen HD, Clark EB, Gutgesell HP, Driscoll DJ, editors: *Moss & Adams heart disease in infants, children, and adolescents including the fetus and young adult*, ed 6, Philadelphia, 2001, Lippincott Williams & Wilkins.

268. Fink BW: *Congenital heart disease.* ed 2, Chicago, 1985, Year Book.

269. Fischbein CA, et al: Risk factors for brain abscess in patients with congenital heart disease. *Am J Cardiol* 34:97, 1974.

270. Fishberger SB, Hannan RL, Welch EM, Rossi AF: Amiodarone for pediatric resuscitation: a word of caution. *Pediatr Cardiol* 30(7): 1006–1008, 2009.

271. Flack JM, Kvasnicka JH, Gardin JM, et al: Anthropometric and physiologic correlates of mitral valve prolapse in a bethink cohort of young adults: the CARDIA study. *Am Heart J* 138:486, 1999.

272. Flori H, Johnson LD, Hanley FL, Fineman JR: Transthoracic intracardiac catheters in pediatric patients recovering from congenital heart defect surgery: associated complications and outcomes. *Crit Care Med* 28:8, 2997–3001, 2000.

273. Foster E, Graham TP Jr, Driscoll DJ, et al: Task force 2: special healthcare needs of adults with congenital heart disease. *J Am Coll Cardiol* 37(5):1176–1183, 2001.

274. Fraisse A, Wessel DL: Acute pulmonary hypertension in infants and children: cGMP-realted drugs. *Pediatr Crit Care Med* 11(2 Suppl): S37–S40, 2010.

275. Fraser CD, Carberyy KE: Congenital heart disease. In Townsend CM, Beauchamp RD, Evers BM, Mattox KL, editors: *Sabiston textbook of surgery*, ed 18, Philadelphia, 2008, Elsevier, Available electronically on MD Consult.

276. Fratz S, Gildein HP, Balling G, Sebening W, et al: Aortic valvuloplasty in pediatric patients substantially postpones the need for aortic valve surgery: a single-center experience of 188 patients after up to 17.5 years of follow-up. *Circulation* 177:1201, 2008.

277. Frazier L, Johnson RL, Sparks E: Genomics and cardiovascular disease. *J Nurs Scholarship* 37(4):315–321, 2005.

278. Freed MD: Fetal and transitional circulation. In Keane JF, Lock JE, Fyler DC, editors: *Nadas' pediatric cardiology*, ed 2, Philadelphia, 2006, Saunders Elsevier.

279. Freed LA, Levy D, Levine RA, et al: Prevalence and clinical outcome of mitral-valve prolapse. *NEJM* 341:1, 1999.

280. Freiedriksen PM, Therrien J, Veldtman G, et al: Lung function and aerobic capacity in adult patients following modified Fontan procedure. *Heart* 85:295, 2001.

281. Fried I, Bar-Oz B, Perles Z, et al: N-terminal pro-B-type natriuretic peptide levels in acute versus chronic left ventricular dysfunction. *J Pediatr* 149:28–31, 2006.

282. Friedman RA: Sinus and atrioventricular conduction disorders. In Deal BJ, Wolff GS, Gelband H, editors: *Current concepts in diagnosis and management of arrhythmias in infants and children*, Armonk, NY, 1998, Futura, pp. 89–116.

283. Friedman AH, Fogel MA, Stephens P Jr, et al: Identification, imaging, functional assessment and management of congenital coronary arterial abnormalities in children. *Cardiol Young* 17(Suppl 2): 56–67, 2007.

284. Friedman WF, George BL: Treatment of congestive heart failure by altering loading conditions of the heart. *J Pediatr* 106:697, 1985.

285. Fu Y, Bass J, Amin Z, et al: Transcatheter closure of perimembranous ventricular septal defects using the new Amplatzer membranous VSD occluder. *J Am Coll Cardiol* 47(2):319–325, 2006.

286. Fuglestad SJ, Puga FJ, Danielson GK, Edwards WD: Surgical pathology of the truncal valve: a study of 12 cases. *Am J Cardiovasc Pathol* 2:39, 1988.

287. Fulton DR, Fyler DC: D-Transposition of the great arteries. In Keane JF, Lock JE, Fyler DC, editors: *Nadas' pediatric cardiology*, ed 2, Philadelphia, 2006, Elsevier.

288. Fyler DC: Pulmonary Stenosis. In Fyler DC, editor: *Nadas' pediatric cardiology*, Philadelphia, 1992, Hanley.

289. Fyler DC: Rheumatic fever. In Keane JF, Lock JE, Fyler DC, editors: *Nadas' pediatiatric cardiology*, ed 2, Philadelphia, 2006, Elsevier.

290. Fyler DC, Buckley LP, Hellenbrand WE, Cohn HE: Report of the New England regional infant cardiac program. *Pediatrics* 65(suppl 2):375–461, 1980.

291. Fyler DC, Buckley LP, Hellenbrand WE, et al: Report of the New England Regional Infant Cardiac Program. *Pediatrics* 65(Suppl 2): 387, 1980.

292. Galantowicz M, Cheatham JP: Fontan completion without surgery. *Semin Thorac Cardiovasc Surg Pediatr Card Surg Annu* 7:48, 2004.

293. Galanowitz M, Cheatham JP: Lessons learned from the development of a new hybrid strategy for the management of hypoplastic left heart syndrome. *Pediatr Cardiol* 26:190, 2005.

294. Galantowicz M, Cheatham JP, Phillips A, et al: Hybrid approach for hypoplastic left heart syndrome: intermediate results after the learning curve. *Ann Thorac Surg* 2063:85, 2008.

295. Galie N, Geghetti M, Gatzoulis MD, et al: Bosentan therapy in patients with Eisenmenger syndrome: a multi-center, double-blind, randomized, placebo-controlled study. *Circulation* 114(1):48, 2006.

296. Galie N, Manes A, Palazzini M, et al: Management of pulmonary arterial hypertension associated with congenial systemic-to-pulmonary shunts and Eisenmenger syndrome. *Drugs* 68(8):1049, 2008.

297. Galvin P: Reducing surgical site infections in children undergoing cardiac surgery. *AJN* 19(12):49–55, 2009.

298. Gamillscheg A, Zobel G, Urlesberger B, et al: Inhaled nitric oxide in patients with critical pulmonary perfusion after Fontan-type procedure and bidirectional Glenn anastomosis. *J Thorac Cardiovas Surg* 113(3):435, 1997.

299. Garson A Jr: *The electrocardiogram in infants and children: a systematic approach*. Philadelphia, 1983, Lea & Febiger.

300. Garson A Jr: Ventricular arrhythmias. In Gillette PC, Garson A Jr, editors: *Pediatric arrhythmias: electrophysiology and pacing*, Philadelphia, 1990, Saunders, pp. 427–500.

301. Gatzoulis MA: Adult congenital heart disease: education, education, education. *Nat Cln Pract* 3(1):2, 2006.

302. Gatzoulis MA, Balaji S, Webber SA, et al: Risk factors for arrhythmia and sudden cardiac death late after repair of tetralogy of Fallot: a multicentre study. *Lancet* 356:975, 2000.

303. Gatzoulis MA, Till JA, Sommerville J, et al: Mechanoelectrical interaction in tetralogy of Fallot. QRS prolongation related to right ventricular size and predicts malignant ventricular arrhythmias and sudden death. *Circulation* 92:231, 1995.

304. Gatzoulis MA, Webb GD: Adults with congenital heart disease: a growing population. In Gatzoulis MA, Webb GA, Daubeney PEF, editors: *Diagnosis and management of adult congenital heart disease*, Edinburgh, 2003, Churchill Livingstone.

305. Gatzoulis MA, Webb GD, Daubeney PEF: *Diagnosis and management of adult congenital heart disease*. New York, 2003, Churchill Livingstone.

306. Gaynor JW, Bridges ND, Cohen MI, et al: Predictors of outcome after the Fontan operation: is hypoplastic left heart still a risk factor? *J Thorac Cardiovasc Surg* 123:237, 2002.

307. Gaynor JW, Collins MH, Rychik J, et al: Long-term outcome of infants with single ventricle and total anomalous pulmonary venous connection. *J Thorac Cardiovasc Surg* 117:506, 1999.

308. Gazit AZ, Oren PP: Pharmaceutical management of decompensated heart failure syndrome in children: current state of the art and a new approach. *Curr Treat Opt Cardiovasc Med* 11:403–409, 2009.

309. Geggel RL, Flyer DC: Mitral valve and left atrial lesions. In Keane JF, Lock JE, Fyler DC, editors: *Nadas' pediatric cardiology*, ed 2, Philadelphia, 2006, Elsevier.

310. Gelatt M, Hamilton RM, McCrindle BW, et al: Arrhythmia and mortality after the Mustard procedure: a 30-year single-center experience. *J Am Coll Cardiol* 29(1):194–201, 1997.

311. Gersony WM: Fontan operation after 3 decades. What we have learned? *Circulation* 117:13, 2008.

312. Geva T: Echocardiography and Doppler ultrasound. In Garson A, Bricker JT, Fisher DJ, Neish SR, editors: *The science and practice of pediatric cardiology*, Baltimore, 1997, Williams & Wilkins.

313. Geva A, McMahon CJ, Gauvreau K, et al: Risk factors for reoperation after repair of discrete subaortic stenosis in children. *J Am Coll Cardiol* 50(15):1498–1504, 2007.

314. Geva T, Powell AJ: Magnetic resonance imaging. In Allen HD, Driscoll DJ, Feltes TF, Shaddy RE, editors: *Moss and Adams' heart disease in infants, children, and adolescent including the fetus and young adult*, ed 7, Philadelphia, 2008, Lippincott Williams & Wilkins.

315. Ghanayem NS, Hoffman GM, Mussatto KA, et al: Perioperative monitoring in high-risk infants after stage 1 palliation of univentricular congenital heart disease. *JThorac Cardiovasc Surg* 140:857, 2010.

316. Ghanayem NS, Jacquiss RD, Cava JR, et al: Right ventricle-to-pulmonary artery conduit versus Blaclock-Taussig shunt: a hemodynamic comparison. *Ann Thorac Surg* 82:1603, 2006.

317. Ghanayem NS, Tweddell JS, Hoffman G, et al: Optimal timing of the second stage of palliation for hypoplastic left heart syndrome facilitated through home monitoring, and the results of early cavopulmonary anastomosis. *Cardiol Young* 16(Suppl 1):61, 2006.

318. Ghanayem NS, et al: Home surveillance program prevents interstage mortality after the Norwood procedure. *J Thorac Cardiovasc Surg* 126(5):1367–1377, 2003.

319. Giannico S, Hammad F, Amodeo A, et al: Clinical outcome of 193 extracardiac Fontan patients: the first 15 years. *J Am Coll Cardiol* 47:2065, 2006.

320. Gielen H, Daniels O, van Lier H: Natural history of congenital pulmonary valvular stenosis: an echo and cardiographic assessment. *Cardiol Young* 9:129, 1999.

321. Giglia TM, Humpl T: Preoperative pulmonary hemodynamics and assessment of operability: is there a pulmonary vascular resistance that precludes cardiac operation? *Pediatr Crit Care Med* 11(2 Suppl):S57–S66, 2010.

322. Gillespie M, Kuipers M, Van Rossem M, et al: Determinants of critical care unit length of stay for infants undergoing cardiac surgery. *Congenit Heart Dis* 1:152–160, 2006.

323. Glatz JA, Tabbutt S, Gaynor JW, et al: Hypoplastic left heart syndrome with atrial level restriction in the era of prenatal diagnosis. *Ann Thorac Surg* 84:1633, 2007.

324. Goldberg SJ, Allen HD, Marx GR, Flinn CJ: Clinical application of Doppler Echocardiography to flow measurements. In In Sanders SP, Yeager S, Williams RG, editors: *Doppler Echocardiography*, Philadelphia,, 1985, Lea & Febiger, p. 92.

325. Goldberg DJ, Dodds K, Rychik J: Rare problems associated with the Fontan circulation. *Cardiol Young* 20(Suppl 3):113, 2010.

326. Goldberg CS, Schwartz EM, Brunberg JA, et al: Neurodevelopmental outcome of patients after the Fontan operation: a comparison between children with hypoplastic left heart syndrome and other functional single ventricle lesions. *J Pediatr* 137(5):646, 2000.

327. Goldman AP, Delius RE, Deanfield JE, et al: Pharmacologic control of pulmonary blood flow with inhaled nitric oxide after the fenestrated Fontan operation. *Circulation* (Suppl):II44, 1996.

328. Goldmuntz E, Lin AE: Genetics of congenital heart defects. In Allen HD, Driscoll DJ, Shaddy RE, Feltes TF, editors: *Moss and Adams' heart disease in infants, children, and adolescents*, ed 7, Philadelphia, 2008, Lippincott Williams & Wilkins.

329. Gossett JG, Rocchini AP, Lloyd TR, Graziano JN: Catheter-based decompression of the left atrium in patients with hypoplastic left heart syndrome and restrictive atrial septum is safe and effective. *Catheter Cardiovasc Interv* 67:619, 2006.

330. Grabitz RG, Joffres MR, Collins-Nakai RL: Congenital heart disease: incidence in the first year of life. The Alberta Heritage Pediatric Cardiology Program. *Am J Epidemiol* 128(2):381–388, 1988.

331. Graham TP Jr, Markham L, Parra DA, Bichell D: Congenitally corrected transposition of the great arteries: an update. *Curr Treat Options Cardiovasc Med* 5(9):407–413, 2007.

332. Graham TP: Congenitally corrected transposition. In Gatzoulis MA, Webb GA, Daubeney PEF, editors: *Diagnosis and management of adult congenital heart disease*, Edinburgh, 2003, Churchill Livingstone.

333. Graham TP, Bernard YD, Mellen BG, et al: Long-term outcome in congenitally corrected transposition of the great arteries: a multi-institutional study. *J Am Coll Cardiol* 36:255, 2000.

334. Graziano JN. Congenital Diaphragmatic Hernia Study Group: Cardiac anomalies in patients with congenital diaphragmatic hernia and their prognosis: a report from the Congenital Diaphragmatic Hernia Study Group. *J Pediatr Surg* 40(6):1045–1049, 2005.

335. Griffiths PD, Morrison GD: Computed tomography in children. *BMJ* 329:930, 2004.

336. Grifka RG: Cardiac catheterization and angiography. In Allen HD, Shaddy RE, Driscoll DJ, Feltes TF, editors: *Moss and Adams' heart disease in infants, children, and adolescents, including the fetus and young adult*, ed 7, Philadelphia, 2008, Lippincott Williams & Wilkins.

337. Grossi EA, Galloway AC, LaPietra A, et al: Minimally invasive mitral valve surgery: a 6-year experience with 714 patients. *Ann Thorac Surg* 74:660–663, 2002.

338. Guleserian KJ, Armsby LB, Thaigarajan RR, et al: Natural history of pulmonary atresia with intact ventricular septum and right-ventricle-dependent coronary circulation managed by the single ventricle approach. *Ann Thorac Surg* 81:2250, 2006.

339. Gupta-Malhotra M, Larson VE, Rosengart RM, et al: Mortality after total cavopulmonary connection in children with the down syndrome. *Am J Cardiol* 105(6):865–868, 2010.

340. Gutgesell HP, Lim DS: Hybrid palliation in hypoplastic left heart syndrome. *Curr Opin Cardiol* 22:55, 2007.

341. Hagler DJ: Double outlet right ventricle and double outlet left ventricle; and univentricular atrioventricular connection. In Allen HD, Shaddy RE, Driscoll DJ, Feltes TF, editors: *Moss and Adams' heart disease in infants, children, and adolescents, including the fetus and young adult*, ed 7, Philadelphia, 2008, Lippincott Williams & Wilkins.

342. Hagler DJ, Edwards WD: Univentricular atrioventricular connection. In Allen HD, Shaddy RE, Driscoll DJ, Feltes TF, editors: *Moss and Adams' heart disease in infants, children, and adolescents, including the fetus and young adult*, ed 7, Philadelphia, 2008, Lippincott Williams & Wilkins.

343. Hagler DJ, O'Leary PW: Cardiac malpositions and abnormalities of atrial and visceral situs. In Allen HD, Driscoll DJ, Shaddy RE, Feltes TF, editors: *Moss and Adams' heart disease in infants, children, and adolescents including the fetus and young adult*, ed 7, Philadelphia, 2008, Lippincott Williams & Wilkins.

344. Hall D, Kirsten G: Kangaroo mother care: a review. *Transfusion Med* 18(2):77–82, 2008.

345. Hammerer-Lercher A, Geiger R, Mair J, et al: Utility of N-terminal pro-B-type natriuretic peptide to differentiate cardiac diseases from noncardiac diseases in young pediatric patients. *Clin Chem* 52:1415–1419, 2006.

346. Han RK, Gurofsky RC, Lee KJ, et al: Outcome and growth potential of left heart structures after neonatal intervention for aortic valve stenosis. *J Am Coll Cardiol* 50:2406, 2007.

347. Hancock Friesen CL, Zurakowski D, Thiagarajan RR, et al: Total anomalous pulmonary venous connection: an analysis of current management strategies in a single institution. *Ann Thorac Surg* 79 (2):596–606, 2005.

348. Handrick w, Nenoff P, Muller H, Knofler W: Infections caused by piercing and tattoos—a review. *Wiener Medizinische Wochenschrift* 153(9-10):194–197, 2003.

349. Hanley FL, Dade RM, Blackstone EH, et al: Outcomes in neonatal pulmonary atresia with intact ventricular septum: a multiinstitutional study. *J Thorac Cardiovasc Surg* 105:406, 1993.

350. Hannan RL, Zabinsky JA, Stanfill RM, et al: Experience with PA IVS management. Society of Thoracic Surgeons 44th Annual Meeting, Fort Lauderdale, FL, January, 2008, Abstract, poster.

351. Hanslik A, Pospisil U, Salzer-Muhar U, et al: Predictors of spontaneous closure of isolated secundum atrial septal defects in children: a longitudinal study. *Pediatrics* 118:1560–1665, 2006.

352. Harris L, Balaji S. Arrhythmias in the adult with congenital heart disease. In Gatzoulis MA, Webb GD, Daubeney PEF, editors: *Diagnosis and management of adult congenital heart disease*, Philadelphia, 2003, Churchill Livingstone.

353. Harris DL, Siu BL, Hummel M, et al: Mosaic ring 12p and total anomalous pulmonary venous return. *Am J Med Genet Part A* 131 (1):91–93, 2004.

354. Haskell WL, Lee IL, Pate RR, et al: Physical activity and updated recommendation for adults from the American College of Sports Medicine and the American Heart Association. *Circulation* 116:1081, 2007.

355. Hastreiter AR, van der Horst RL, Chow-Tung E: Digitalis toxicity in infants and children. *Pediatr Cardiol* 5:131, 1984 (review article).

356. Hastreiter AR, van der Horst RL, Voda C, Chow-Tung E: Maintenance digoxin dosage and steady-state plasma concentration in infants and children. *J Pediatr* 107(1):140–146, 1985.

357. Havranek T, Johanboeke P, Madramootoo C, Carver JD: Umbilical artery catheters do not affect intestinal blood flow responses to minimal enteral feedings. *J Perinatol* 6:375–379, 2007.

358. Hawkins JA, Doty DB: Aortic atresia: morphologic characteristics affecting survival and operative palliation. *J Thorac Cardiovasc Surg* 88:620, 1994.

359. Hayashi G, Kurosaki K, Echigo S, et al: Prevalence of arrhythmias and their risk factors mid- and long-term after the arterial switch operation. *Pediatr Cardiol* 27(6):689, 2006.

360. Hayes CJ, Gersony WM, Driscol DJ, et al: Second natural history study of congenital heart defects: results of treatment of patients with pulmonary valvular stenosis. *Circulation* 87:1–28, 1993.

361. Hazinski MF: Cardiovascular problems. In Hazinski MF, editor: *Nursing care of the critically ill child*, ed 2, St Louis, 1992, Mosby.

362. Hazinski MF: Cardiovascular problems. In Hazinski MF, editor: *Manual of pediatric critical care*, St Louis, 1999, Mosby.

363. Hazinski MF: Cardiac anomalies associated with genetic or maternal health factors. In *Manual of pediatric critical care*, St Louis, 1999, Mosby, p. 86.

364. Hazinski MF, Samson R, Schexnayder S, editors: *Considerations for evaluation of the cyanotic neonate*, In 2010 Handbook of Emergency Cardiovascular Care for Healthcare Providers, Dallas, 2010, American Heart Association, p. 79.

365. Heerdt PM: Digitalis pharmacodynamics: considerations in critical illness. In Chernow B, editor: *The pharmacologic approach to the critically ill patient*, ed 2, Baltimore, 1988, Williams & Wilkins.

366. Heimburger DC, Weinsier RL: *Handbook of clinical nutrition*. ed 3, St Louis, 1997, Mosby, p. 235.

367. Henaine R, Azarnoush K, Belli E, et al: Fate of the truncal valve in truncus arteriosus. *Ann Thorac Surg* 85(1):172, 2008.

368. Herlong JR, Jagger JJ, Ungerleider RM: Pulmonary venous anomalies: the Society of Thoracic surgeons Congenital Heart Surgery Nomenclature and Database Project. *Ann Thorac Surg* 69 (Suppl):S56, 2000.

369. Heyman LL, Meininger JC, Danaiels SR, et al: Primary prevention of cardiovascular disease in nursing practice: focus on children and youth. *Circulation* 116:344, 2007.

370. Heymann MA. Pharmacologic use of prostaglandin Ej in infants with congenital heart disease. *Am Heart J* 101:837, 1981.

371. Hickey PR, Hahnsen DD, Wessel D, et al: Blunting of stress responses in the pulmonary circulation of infants by fentanyl. *Anesth Analg* 64:1137, 1985.

372. Hickman RL, Douglas PA: Impact of chronic critical illness on psychological outcomes of family members. *AACN* 21(1):80–91, 2010.

373. Hidaka N, Tsukimori K, Chiba Y, et al: Monochorionic twins in which at least one fetus has a congenital heart disease with or

without twin-twin transfusion syndrome. *J Perinat Med* 35(5): 425–430, 2007.

374. Hill SL, Berul CI, Patel HT, et al: Early ECG abnormalities associated with transcatheter closure of atrial septal defects using the Amplatzer septal defects using the Amplatzer septal occluder. *J Inter Card Electrophysiol* 4:469, 2000.

375. Hinton RB Jr, Martin LJ, Tabangin ME, et al: Hypoplastic left heart syndrome is heritable. *J Amer Coll Cardiol* 50:1590, 2007.

376. Hirsch JC, Charpie JR, Ohye RG, et al: Near-infrared spectroscopy: what we know and what we need to know. A systematic review of the congenital heart disease literature. *J Thorac Cardiovasc Surg* 137:154, 2009.

377. Hjalmarson A, Goldstein S, Fagerberg B, et al: Effects of controlled-release metoprolol on total mortality, hospitalizations, and well-being in patients with heart failure: the Metoprolol CR/XL Randomized Intervention Trial in congestive heart failure (MERIT-HF). *JAMA* 283:1295–1302, 2000.

378. Ho VB, Bakalov VK, Cooley M, et al: Major vascular anomalies in Turner syndrome: prevalence and magnetic resonance angiographic features. *Circulation* 110(12):1694–1700, 2004.

379. Hoashi T, Bove EL, Devaney EJ, et al: Outcomes of 1½- or 2-ventricle conversion for patients initially treated with single-ventricle palliation. *J Thorac Cardiovasc Surg.* 141:419, 2011.

380. Hoffman JIE: Congenital heart disease: incidence and inheritance. In Gillette PC, editor: *Pediatric clinics of North America*, Philadelphia, 1990, Saunders.

381. Hoffman TM, Bush DM, Wernovsky G, et al: Postoperative junctional ectopic tachycardia in children: incidence, risk factors, and treatment. *Ann Thorac Surg* 74(5):1607–1611, 2002.

382. Hoffman GM, Ghanayem NS, Kampine JM, et al: Venous saturation and anaerobic threshold in neonates after the Norwood procedure for hypoplastic left heart syndrome. *Ann Thorac Surg* 70:1515, 2000.

383. Hoffman JI, Kaplan S, Liberthson RR: Prevalence of adult congenital heart disease. *Am Heart J* 147:425, 2004.

384. Hoffman GM, Tweddelll JS, Ghanayem NS, et al: Alteration of the critical arteriovenous oxygen saturation relationship by sustained afterload reduction after the Norwood procedure. *J Thoracic Cardiovasc Surg* 127:738–745, 2004.

385. Hoffman TM, Welty SE: Physiology of the preterm and term infant. In Allen HD, Driscoll DJ, Shaddy RE, Feltes TF, editors: *Moss and Adams' heart disease in infants, children, and adolescents including the fetus and young adult*, ed 7, Philadelphia, 2008, Lippincott Williams & Wilkins.

386. Hoffman TM, Wernovsky G, Atz AM, Kulik TJ, et al: Efficacy and safety of milrinone in preventing low cardiac output syndrome in infants and children after corrective surgery for congenital heart disease. *Circulation* 996–1002, 2003.

387. Hoffman TM, Wernovsky G, Wieand TS, et al: The incidence of arrhythmias in a pediatric cardiac intensive care unit. *Pediatr Cardiol* 23(6):598–604, 2002.

388. Holzer RJ, Cheatham J: Therapeutic cardiac catheterization in adults with congenital heart disease. In Allen HD, Driscoll DJ, Feltes TF, Shaddy RE, editors: *Moss and Adams' heart disease in infants, children, and adolescent including the fetus and young adult*, ed 7, Philadelphia, 2008, Lippincott Williams & Wilkins.

389. Holzer RJ, Cheatham JP: Therapeutic cardiac catheterization. In Allen HD, Driscoll DJ, Shaddy RE, Feltes TF, editors: *Moss and Adams' heart disease in infants, children, and adolescents, including the fetus and young adult*, ed 7, Philadelphia, 2008, Lippincott Williams & Wilkins.

390. Holzer R, de Giovanni J, Walsh KP, et al: Transcatheter closure of perimembranous ventricular septal defects using the Amplatzer membranous VSD occluder: immediate and midterm results of an international registry. *Catheter Cardiovasc Inter* 68:620, 2006.

391. Horer J, Haas F, Cleuziou J, et al: Intermediate-term results of the Senning or Mustard procedures combined with the Rastelli operation for patient with discordant atrioventricular connections associated with discordant ventriculoarterial connections or double outlet right ventricle. *Cardiol Young* 17(2):158–165, 2007.

392. Hosein RB, Clarke J, McGuirk SP, et al: Factors influencing early and late outcome following the Fontan procedure in the current era. The 'Two Commandments'? *Eur J Cardiothorac Surg* 31:344, 2007.

393. Hoskote A, Li J, Hickey C, et al: The effects of carbon dioxide on oxygenation and systemic, cerebral and pulmonary vascular hemodynamics after the bidirectional superior cavopulmonary anastomosis. *J Am Coll Cardiol* 44:1501–1509, 2004.

394. Huddleston CB: The failing Fontan: options for surgical therapy. *Pediatr Cardiol* 28:472, 2007.

395. Huddletson CB: Lung transplantation for pulmonary hypertension in children. *Pediatr Crit Care Med* 11(2 Suppl):S53–S56, 2010.

396. Human DG: Living with complex heart disease. *Pediatr Child Health* 14:161–166, 2009.

397. Humbert M, Sitbon O, Simonneau G: Treatment of pulmonary arterial hypertension. *N Engl J Med* 351:1425, 2004.

398. Inglessis I, Abbara S, de Moor M: Which diagnostic modality for adult congenital heart disease? *J Cardiovasc Comput Tomogr.* 2(1): 23–25, 2008.

399. Inglessis I, Landzberg MJ: Interventional catheterization in adult congenital heart disease. *Circulation* 115(12):1622–1633, 2007.

400. Ishiyama M, Kurosawa H, Shinoka T, Imai Y: Double-outlet right ventricle with left malposition of the great arteries and total anomalous pulmonary venous connection. *Gen Thorac CV Surg* 55(2):57–60, 2007.

401. Issenberg HJ: Miscellaneous topics. In Chang AC, Hanley FL, Wernovsky G, Wessel DL, editors: *Pediatric cardiac intensive care*, Toronto, 1998, Williams & Wilkins.

402. Iversen K, Vejlstrup NG, Sondergaard L, Nielsen OW: Screening of adults with congenital cardiac disease lost for follow-up. *Cardiol Young* 17(6):601–608, 2007.

403. Ivy D: Diagnosis and treatment of severe pediatric pulmonary hypertension. *Cardiol Rev* 9(4):227, 2001.

404. Ivy DD: Prostacyclin in the intensive care setting. *Pediatr Crit Care Med* 11(2 Suppl):S41–S45, 2010.

405. Jackson LW, Correa-Villasenor A, Lees PS, Dominici F, et al: Parental lead exposure and total anomalous pulmonary venous return. *Birth Defects Res* 70(4):185–193, 2004.

406. Jacobs ML: The functional single ventricle and Fontan's operation. In Mavroudis C, Backer CL, editors: *Pediatric cardiac surgery*, ed 3, Philadelphia, 2003, Mosby/Elsevier.

407. Jacobs LG: Warfarin pharmacology, clinical management, and evaluation of hemorrhage risk for the elderly. *Clin Geriatr Med* 22(1), 2006.

408. Jaklitsch MT, Linden BC, Braunlin EA, et al: Open-lung biopsy guides therapy in children. *Ann Thorac Surg* 71:1179–1785, 2001.

409. Janousek J, Paul T, Luhmer I, et al: Atrial baffle procedures for complete transposition of the great arteries: natural course of sinus node dysfunction and risk factors for dysrhythmias and sudden death. *Z Kardiol* 83(12):933–938, 1994.

410. Jaquiss RD, Ghanayem NS, Hoffman GM, et al: Early cavopulmonary anastomosis in very young infants after the Norwood procedure: impact on oxygenation, resource utilization, and mortality. *J Thorac Cardiovasc Surg* 127:982, 2004.

411. Jatene AD, Fontes VF, Paulista PP, et al: Successful anatomic correction of transposition of the great vessels. *J Thorac Cardiovasc Surg* 72:364, 1976.

412. Jeffries HE, Wells WJ, Starnes VA, et al: Gastrointestinal morbidity after Norwood palliation for hypoplastic left heart syndrome. *Ann Thorac Surg* 81:982, 2006.

413. Jenkins PC, Chinnock RE, Jenkin KJ, et al: Decreased exercise performance with age in children with hypoplastic left heart syndrome. *J Pediatr* 152(4):507, 2008.

414. Jenkins KJ, Correa A, Feinstein JA, et al: Noninherited risk factors and congenital cardiovascular defects: current knowledge: a scientific statement from the American heart association council on cardiovascular disease in the young: endorsed by the American academy of pediatrics. *Circulation* 115:2995–3014, 2007.

415. Joey's journey: our life with lissencephaly: Joey's journey: our life with lissencephaly, 2012. http://lfurlotte.tripod.com/.

416. Johnson BA, Ades A: Infants born with TAPVC have a natural history of death in 80% during the first year of life without intervention. *Clin Pernatol* 32(4):921–946, 2005.

417. Johnston TA, Grifka RG, Jones TK: Endovascular stents for treatment of coarctation of the aorta: acute results and followup experience. *Cathet Cardiovasc Interv* 62:499–505, 2004.

418. Johnston LJ, McKinley DF: Cardiac tamponade after removal of atrial intracardiac monitoring catheters in a pediatric patient: case report. *Heart Lung* 256–261, 2000.

419. Joho-Arreola AL, Bauersfeld U, Stauffer UG, et al: Incidence and treatment of diaphragmatic paralysis after cardiac surgery in children. *Eur J Cardiothorac Surg* 27:53, 2005.

420. Jonas RA: Interrupted aortic arch. In Mavroudis C, Backer CL, editors: *Pediatric cardiac surgery*, ed 3, Philadelphia, 2003, Mosby/Elsevier.

421. Jonas RA: *Comprehensive surgical management of congenital heart disease*. New York, 2004, Oxford University Press.

422. Jones TK: Results of the U.S. multicenter pivotal study of the HELEX septal occluder for percutaneous closure of secundum atrial septal defects. *J Coll Cardiol* 49(22):2215–2221, 2007.

423. Jones DH, Schlatter MG, Cornelius AS, Neirottie RN: A massive pulmonary tumor embolism after surgical manipulation and biopsy of a pelvic mass. *Pediatr Anesthes* 90(2):322, 2000.

424. Journois D, Pouard P, Mauriat P, et al: Inhaled nitric oxide as a therapy for pulmonary hypertension after operations for congenital heart defects. *J Thorac Cardiovas Surg* 107:1129, 1994.

425. Jung AD: Gastroesophageal reflux in infants and children. *Am Fam Physician* 64(11):1853–1860, 2001.

426. Kaemmerer H, Bauer U, Pensi U, et al: Management of emergencies in adults with congenital heart disease. *Am J Cardiol* 101:521, 2008.

427. Kaemmerer H, Oelret F, Bahlmann J, et al: Arterial hypertension in adults after surgical treatment of aortic coarctation. *J Thorac Cardiovasc Surg* 46:121, 1998.

428. Kafka H, Johnson MR, Gatzoulis MA: The team approach to pregnancy and congenital heart disease. *Cardiol Clin* 24(4):587–605, 2006.

429. Kalavrouziotis G: Truncus arteriosus communis: early and midterm results of early primary repair. *Ann Thorac Surg* 82(6):2200, 2006.

430. Kan JS, White RI, Mitchell SE, et al: Percutaneous balloon valvuloplasty: a new method for treating pulmonary-valves enosis. *NEJM* 307:540–542, 1982.

431. Kang WC, Chung WJ, Choi CH, et al: A rare case of anomalous left coronary artery from the pulmonary artery (ALCAPA) presenting congestive heart failure in an adult. *Int J Cardiol* 115(2):e63–e67, 2007.

432. Kang N, De Leval MR, Elliot M, et al: Extending the boundary of the primary arterial switch operation in patients with transposition of the great arteries. *Circulation* 110(11, Supp 1):II123, 2004.

433. Kannankeril PJ, Fish FA: Disorders of cardiac rhythm and conduction. In Allen HD, Driscoll DJ, Shaddy RE, Feltes TF, editors: *Moss and Adams' heart disease in infants, children, and adolescents*, ed 7, Philadelphia, 2008, Lippincoll Williams & Wilkins, pp. 293–342.

434. Kanter KR, Vincent RN: Management of aortopulmonary collateral arteries in Fontan patients: occlusion improves clinical outcome. *Semin Thorac Cardiovasc Surg Pediatr Card Surg Annu* 5:48, 2002.

435. Kantor PF, Abraham JR, Pipchand AI, et al: The impact of changing medical therapy on transplantation-free survival in pediatric dilated cardiomyopathy. *J Am Coll Cardiol* 55(13):277–284, 2010.

436. Karamlou T, Gurofsky R, Al Sukhni E, et al: Factors associated with mortality and reoperation in 377 children with total anomalous pulmonary venous connection. *Circulation* 115(12):1591–1598, 2007.

437. Karl TR, Cochrane AD: Congenitally corrected transposition of the great arteries. In Mavroudis C, Backer CL, editors: *Pediatric cardiac surgery*, ed 3, Philadelphia, 2003, Mosby/Elsevier.

438. Katz AM: Cardiomyopathy of overload: a major determinant of prognosis in congestive heart failure. *N Engl J Med* 322:100, 1990.

439. Kaufman ES: Mechanisms and clinical management of inherited channelopathies: long QT syndrome, Brugada syndrome, catecholaminergic polymorphic ventricular tachycardia, and short QT syndrome. *Heart Rhythm* 6(8 Suppl):S51–S55, 2009.

440. Kawashima Y, Ktamura S, Matsuda H, et al: Total cavopulmonary shunt operation in complex cardiac anomalies: a new operation. *J Thoracic Cardiovasc Surg* 87(1):74–81, 1984.

441. Kaye DM, Lefkovits J, Jennings GL, et al: Adverse consequences of high sympathetic nervous activity in the failing heart. *J Am Coll Cardiol* 26:1257–1263, 1995.

442. Kayln A, Blatz S, Fenerstake S, et al: Closed suctioning of intubated neonates maintains better physiologic stability: randomized trial. *J Perinatol* 23:218–222, 2003.

443. Keane JF, Driscoll DJ, Gersony WM, et al: Second natural history study of congenital heart defects: results of treatment of patients with aortic valvular stenosis. *Circulation* 87:I16, 1993.

444. Keane JF, Fyler DC: Aortic outflow abnormalities. In Keane JF, Lock JE, Fyler DC, editors: *Nadas' pediatric cardiology*, ed 2, Philadelphia, 2006, Elsevier.

445. Keane JF, Fyler DC: Aortopulmonary window. In Keane JF, Lock JE, Fyler DC, editors: *Nadas' pediatric cardiology*, ed 2, Philadelphia, 2006, Elsevier.

446. Keane JF, Fyler DC: Coronary artery anomalies. In Keane JF, Lock JE, Fyler DC, editors: *Nadas' pediatric cardiology*, ed 2, Philadelphia, 2006, Elsevier.

447. Keane JF, Fyler DC: Corrected" transposition of the great arteries. In Keane JF, Lock JE, Fyler DC, editors: *Nadas' pediatric cardiology*, ed 2, Philadelphia, 2006, Elsevier.

448. Keane JF, Fyler DC: Double-Outlet Right Ventricle. In Keane JF, Lock JE, Fyler DC, editors: *Nadas' pediatric cardiology*, ed 2, Philadelphia, 2006, Elsevier, p. 735.

449. Keane JF, Fyler DC: Patent ductus arteriosus. In Keane JF, Lock JE, Fyler DC, editors: *Nadas' pediatric cardiology*, ed 2, Philadelphia, 2006, Elsevier.

450. Keane JF, Fyler DC: Pulmonary atresia with intact ventricular septum. In Keane JF, Lock JE, Fyler DC, editors: *Nadas' pediatric cardiology*, ed 2, Philadelphia, 2006, Elsevier, pp. 729–734.

451. Keane JF, Fyler DC: Pulmonary stenosis. In Keane JF, Lock JE, Fyler DC, editors: *Nadas' pediatric cardiology*, ed 2, Philadelphia, 2006, Elsevier.

452. Keane JF, Fyler DC: Single ventricle. In Keane JF, Lock JE, Fyler DC, editors: *Nadas' pediatric cardiology*, ed 2, Philadelphia, 2006, Elsevier.

453. Keane JF, Fyler DC: Total anomalous pulmonary venous return. In Keane JF, Lock JE, Fyler DC, editors: *Nadas' pediatric cardiology*, ed 2, Philadelphia, 2006, Elsevier, p. 773.

454. Keane JF, Fyler DC: Tricuspid atresia. In Keane JF, Lock JE, Fyler DC, editors: *Nadas' pediatric cardiology*, ed 2, Philadelphia, 2006, Elsevier.

455. Keane JF, Fyler DC: Truncus arteriosus. In Keane JF, Lock JE, Fyler DC, editors: *Nadas' pediatric cardiology*, ed 2, Philadelphia, 2006, Elsevier.

456. Keane JF, Fyler DC: Vascular fistula. In Keane JF, Lock JE, Fyler DC, editors: *Nadas' pediatric cardiology*, ed 2, Philadelphia, 2006, Elsevier.

457. Keane JF, Fyler DC: Ventricular septal defect. In Keane JF, Lock JE, Fyler DC, editors: *Nadas' pediatric cardiology*, ed 2, Philadelphia, 2006, Elsevier.

458. Keane JF, Gev T, Fyler DC: Atrial septal defect. In Keane JF, Lock JE, Fyler DC, editors: *Nadas' pediatric cardiology*, ed 2, Philadelphia, 2006, Elsevier.

459. Keith HM: Vascular rings and tracheobronchial compression in infants. *Pediatr Ann* 6(8):542–543, 1977.

460. Keith JD, Rowe RD, Vlad P, O'Hanley JH: Complete anomalous pulmonary venous drainage. *Am J Med* 16:23, 1954.

461. Kelleher DK, Laussen P, Teixeira-Pinto A, Duggan C: Growth and correlates of nutritional status among infants with hypoplastic left heart syndrome after stage 1 Norwood procedure. *Nutrition* 22:237, 2006.

462. Kelley RI: Barth syndrome. Available from www.barthsyndrome.org. Accessed March 20, 2008, Updated 2007.

463. Kenner C, Gallo AM, Bryant KD: Promoting children's health through understanding of genetics and genomics. *J Nurs Scholarship* 37(4):308–314, 2005.

464. Kertesz NJ, Friedman RA, Fenrich AL, Garson A Jr, : The incidence of perioperative arrhythmias. In Balaji S, Gillette PC, Case CL, editors: *Cardiac arrhythmias after surgery for congenital heart disease*, New York, 2001, Arnold, pp. 50–63.

465. Khairy P, Chauvet P, Lehmann J, et al: Lower incidence of thrombus formation with cryoenergy versus radiofrequency catheterization. *Circulation* 107:2045, 2003.

466. Khairy P, Fernandes S, Mayer JE, et al: Long-term survival, modes of death, and predictors if mortality in patients with Fontan surgery. *Circulation* 117:85, 2008.

467. Khairy P, Harris L, Landzberg MJ, et al: Implantable cardioverter-defibrillators in tetralogy of Fallot. *Circulation* 117:363, 2008.

468. Khairy P, Poirier N, Mercier LA: Univentricular heart. *Circulation* 115:800, 2007.

469. Khambadkone S, Bonhoeffer P: Percutaneous pulmonary valve implantation. *Semin Thorac Cardiovascular Surg Pediat Card Surg Annu* 9:23–28, 2006.

470. Khambadkone S, Coats L, Taylor A, et al: Percutaneous pulmonary valve implantation in humans. Results in 59 consecutive patients. *Circulation* 112:1189–1197, 2005.

471. Khazin V, Kaufman Y, Zabeeda D, et al: Milrinone and nitric oxide: combined effect on pulmonary artery pressures after cardiopulmonary bypass in children. *J Cardiothorac Vasc Anesth* 18(2):156, 2004.

472. Kim N, Friedberg MK, Silverman NH: Diagnosis and prognosis of fetuses with double outlet right ventricle. *Prenat Diagn* 26(8): 740–745, 2006.

473. Kimball TR, Daniels SR, Meyer RA, et al: Effect of digoxin on contractility and symptoms in infants with a large ventricular septal defect. *Am J Cardiol* 68:1377–1382, 1991.

474. Kimball TR, Michelfelder EC: Echocardiography. In Allen HD, Driscoll DJ, Feltes TF, Shaddy RE, editors: *Moss and Adams' heart disease in infants, children, and adolescents, including the fetus and young adult*, ed 7, Philadelphia, 2008, Lippincott Williams & Wilkins.

475. Kirklin JK: Is biopsy-proven cellular rejection an important clinical consideration in heart transplantation? *Curr Opin Cardiol* 20(2): 127–131, 2005.

476. Kirklin JK, Brown RN, Bryant AS: Is the "perfect Fontan" operation routinely achievable in the modern era? *Cardiol Young* 18:328, 2008.

477. Kirsh JA, Walsh EP, Triedman JK: Prevalence of and risk factors for atrial fibrillation and intra-atrial reentrant tachycardia among patients with congenital heart disease. *Am J Cardiol* 90(3): 338–340, 2002.

478. Kirshbom PM, Flynn TB, Clancy RR, et al: Late neurodevelopmental outcome after repair of total anomalous pulmonary venous connection. *J Thorac Cardiovasc Surg* 129(5):1091–1097, 2005.

479. Kirshbom PM, Jaggers J, Ungerleider RM: TAPVC. In Mavroudis C, Backer CL, editors: *Pediatric cardiac surgery*, ed 3, Philadelphia, 2003, Mosby/Elsevier, p. 623.

479a. Kleinman ME, Chameides L, Schexnayder SM, et al: Part 14: pediatric advanced life support: 2010 American Heart Association Guidelines for Cardiopulmonary Resuscitation and Emergency Cardiovascular Care. *Circulation* 122(18 Suppl 3):S876–S908, 2010.

480. Kleinman RE: *Pediatric nutrition handbook*. ed 6, Elk Grove, IL, 2009, American Academy of Pediatrics.

481. Kleinman CS, Tabibian M, Starc T, et al: Most patients with a moderate ventricular septal defect will not require intervention. *J Pediatr* 150:583–586, 2007.

482. Knauth A, Verstappen A, Reiss J, Webb GD: Transition and transfer from pediatric to adult care of the young adult with complex congenital heart disease. *Cardiol Clin* 24(4):619–629, vi, 2006.

483. Knauth AL, Gauvreau K, Powell AJ, et al: Ventricular size and function assessed by cardiac MRI predict major adverse clinical outcomes late after tetralogy of Fallot repair. *Heart* 94:211–216, 2008.

484. Knauth AL, Lock JE, Perry SB, et al: Transcatheter device closure of congenital and postoperative residual ventricular septal defects. *Circulation* 110:501–507, 2004.

485. Knauth A, Verstappen A, Reiss J, Webb GD: Transition and transfer from pediatric to adult care of the young adult with complex congenital heart disease. *Cardiol Clin* 24(4):619–629, 2006.

486. Knick BJ, Saul JP: Immediate arrhythmia management. In Zeigler VL, Gillette PC, editors: *Practical management of pediatric cardiac arrhythmias*, Armonk, NY, 2001, Futura, pp. 161–230.

487. Kniffen CL: *Fragile X mental retardation syndrome*. Johns Hopkins University, Mendelian Inheritance in Man. Updated 2007. Available from http://www.ncbi.nlm.nih.gov/omim/300624. Accessed March 16, 2008.

488. Knight D: Newborn drug services: nitric oxide, 2001. Available from http://www.akhealth.co.nz/newborn/DrugProtocols/NitricOxide Pharmacology.htm. Accessed December, 2008.

489. Knight WB, Mee RB: A cure for pulmonary arteriovenous fistulas? *Ann Thorac Surg* 59:999, 1995.

490. Knilans TK: Cardiac arrhythmias in infants and children. In Chou T, Knilans TK, editors: *Electrocardiography in clinical practice: adult and pediatric*, ed 4, Philadelphia, 1996, Saunders, pp. 682–696.

491. Ko JK, Deal BJ, Strasburger JF, Benson DW Jr: Supraventricular tachycardia mechanisms and their age distribution in pediatric patients. *Am J Cardiol* 69(12):1028–1032, 1992.

492. Kogon BE: What is the optimal time to repair atrioventricular septal defect and common atrioventricular valve orifice? *Cardiol Young* 17 (4):356–359, 2007.

493. Kondo C: Myocardial perfusion imaging in pediatric cardiology. *Ann Nucl Med* 18(7):551–561, 2004.

494. Konstantinov IE: Truncus arterious associated with interrupted aortic arch in 50 neonates: a Congenital Heart Surgeons Society study. *Ann Thorac Surg* 81(1):214, 2006.

495. Korkola SJ, Tchervenkov CI, Mavroudis C: Infective endocarditis. In Mavroudis C, Backer CL, editors: *Pediatric cardiac surgery*, ed 3, Philadelphia, 2003, Mosby/Elsevier.

496. Kostolny M, Hoerer J, Eicken A, et al: Impact of placing a conduit from the right ventricle to the pulmonary arteries as the first stage of further palliation in the Norwood sequence for hypoplasia of the left heart. *Cardiol Young* 17:517, 2007.

497. Kouchoukos NT, Blackstone EH, Doty DB, et al: Congenital anomalies of the coronary arteries. In Park M, editor: *Kirklin/Barratt-Boyes cardiac surgery*, ed 3, Philadelphia, 2003, Churchill Livingstone.

498. Kouchoukos NT, Blackstone EH, Doty DB, et al: Double outlet right ventricle. In Park MK, editor: *Kirklin/Barratt-Boyes cardiac surgery*, ed 3, Philadelphia, 2003, Churchill Livingstone-Elsevier.

499. Kouchoukos NT, Blackstone EH, Doty DB et al: editors: *Kirklin/Barrat-Boyes cardiac surgery*, ed 3, Philadelphia, 2003, Churchill Livingstone.

500. Kouchoukos NT, Blackstone EH, Doty DB, et al: Total anomalous pulmonary venous connection. In Kouchoukos NT, Doty DB, editors: *Kirklin/Barratt-Boyes cardiac surgery*, ed 3, Philadelphia, 2003, Churchill Livingstone, pp. 773–775.

501. Kugler JD: Benign arrhythmias: neonate throughout childhood. In Deal BJ, Wolff GS, Gelband H, editors: *Current concepts in diagnosis and management of arrhythmias in infants and children*, Armonk, NY, 1998, Futura, pp. 65–87.

502. Kugler JD, Beekman RH, Rosenthal GL, et al: Development of a pediatric cardiology quality improvement collaborative: from inception to implementation. From the Joint Council on Congenital Heart Disease Quality Improvement Task Force. *Congenit Heart Dis* 4:38, 2009.

503. Kugler JD, Danford DA, Deal BJ, et al: Radiofrequency catheter ablation for tachyarrhythmias in children and adolescents: the Pediatric Electrophysiology Society. *NEJM* 330:1481, 1994.

504. Kyburz A, Bauersfeld U, Schinzel A, et al: The fate of children with microdeletion 22q11.2 syndrome and congenital heart defect: clinical course and cardiac outcomes. *Pediatr Cardiol* 29(1):76, 2008.

505. Lacour-Gayet F: Surgery for pulmonary venous obstruction after repair of total anomalous pulmonary venous return. Semin Thorac Cardiovasc Surg. *Pediatr Cardiol Surg Annu* 9:45–50, 2006.

506. Lacro RV: Dysmorphology. In Keane JF, Lock JE, Fyler DC, editors: *Nadas' pediatric cardiology*, ed 2, Philadelphia, 2006, Elsevier.

507. Lacy CF, Armstrong LL, Goldman MP, Lance LL: *Lexi-comp's drug information handbook*. ed 12, Hudson, OH, 2004.

508. Laird WP, Snyder CS, Kertesz NJ, et al: Use of intravenous amiodarone for postoperative junctional ectopic tachycardia in children. *Pediatr Cardiol* 24(2):133–137, 2003.

509. Lamberti JJ, Mitruka SN: Congenital anomalies of the mitral valve. In Mavroudis C, Backer CL, editors: *Pediatric cardiac surgery*, ed 3, Philadelphia, 2003, Mosby/Elsevier.

510. Landzberg MJ: Adult congenital heart disease. In Keane JF, Lock JE, Fyler DC, editors: *Nadas' pediatric cardiology*, ed 2, Philadelphia, 2006, Elsevier.

511. Landzberg MJ: Congenital heart disease associated pulmonary arterial hypertension. *Clin Chest Med* 28(1):1–13, 2007.

512. Landzberg MJ: Congenital heart disease associated pulmonary arterial hypertension. *Clin Chest Med* 28(1):243–253, 2007.

513. Landzberg MJ, Murphy DJ Jr, Davidson WR Jr, et al: Task force 4: organization of delivery systems for adults with congenital heart disease. *J Am Coll Cardiol* 37(5):1187–1193, 2001.

514. Lang PL, Fyler DC: Hypoplastic left heart syndrome, mitral atresia, and aortic atresia. In Keane JF, Lock JE, Fyler DC, editors: *Nadas' pediatric cardiology*, ed 2, St Louis, 2006, Saunders Elsevier.

515. Latson LA, Jones TK, Jacobson J, et al: Analysis of factors related to successful transcatheter closure of secundum atrial septal defects using the HELEX septal occluder. *Am Heart J* 151(5):1136. e8–1136.e11, 2006.

516. Laussen PC, Roth SJ: Mechanical circulatory support. In Sellke FW, del Nido PJ, Swanson SJ, editors: *Sabiston and spencer: surgery of the chest*, ed 7, vol 2. Philadelphia, 2005, Elsevier.

517. Law IH: Atrioventricular reentry tachycardia. In Dick M, editor: *Clinical cardiac electrophysiology in the young*, New York, 2006, Springer, pp. 51–68.

518. Law YM, Hoyer AM, Reller MD, Silberbach M: Accuracy of plasma B-type natriuretic peptide to diagnose significant cardiovascular disease in children. *J Am Coll Cardiol* 54:1467–1475, 2009.

519. Lawoko S, Soares JJF: Psychosocial morbidity among parents of children with congenital heart disease: a prospective longitudinal study. *Heart Lung: J Acute Crit Care* 35(5):301–314, 2006.

520. Lawrenson J, et al: Manipulating parallel circuits: the perioperative management of patients with complex congenital cardiac disease. *Cardiol Young* 13(4):316–322, 2003.

521. Lee D, Higgins PA: Adjunctive therapies for the chronically, critically ill. *AACN* 21(1):92–106, 2010.

522. Lee YO, Kim YJ, Lee JR, Kim WH: Long-term results of one-and-a-half ventricle repair in complex cardiac anomalies. *Eur J Cardiothorac Surg* .

523. Lemler MS, Scott WA, Leonard SR, et al: Fenestration improves clinical outcome of the Fontan procedure: a prospective, randomized study. *Circulation* 105:207, 2002.

524. Le P, Chrisant M: Cardiomyopathy. In Vetter V, editor: *Pediatric cardiology: the requisites in pediatrics*, St Louis, 2006, Elsevier, pp. 97–109.

525. Leonard GT, Justino H, Carlson KM: Atrial septal stent implant: atrial septal defect creation in the management of complex congenital heart defects in infants. *Congenital Heart Dis* 1:219, 2006.

526. LeRoy S, Elixson EM, O'Brien P, et al: Recommendations for preparing children and adolescents for invasive cardiac procedures. A statement from the American heart association pediatric nursing subcommittee of the council on cardiovascular nursing in collaboration with the council on cardiovascular diseases of the young. *Circulation* 108(20):2550–2564, 2003.

527. Levine MA, Moller JH, Amplatz K, Edwards JE: Atresia of the common pulmonary vein—case report and differential diagnosis. *Am J Roentgenol* 100:322–327, 1967.

527a. Lewin MB, Otto CM: The bicuspid aortic valve: Adverse outcomes from infancy to old age. *Circulation* 111(7):832–834, 2005.

528. Lewis A: Acute myocarditis. In Chang AC, Towbin JA, editors: *Heart failure in children and young adults*, Philadelphia, 2006, Elsevier, pp. 235–247.

529. Lewis AB: The failing myocardium. In Chang AC, Hanley FL, Wernovsky G, Wessel DL, editors: *Pediatric Cardiac Intensive Care*, Philadelphia, 1998, Lippincott Williams & Wilkins.

530. Lewis AB, Chabot M: The effect of treatment with angiotensin-converting enzyme inhibitors on survival of pediatric patients with dilated cardiomyopathy. *Pediatr Cardiol* 14:9–12, 1993.

531. Lewis AB, Heymann MA, Stanger P, et al: Evaluation of subendocardial ischemia in valvular aortic stenosis in children. *Circulation* 49:978, 1974.

532. Li JS, Sexton DJ, Mick N, et al: Proposed modifications to the Duke Criteria for the Diagnosis of Infective Endocarditis. *Clin Inf Dis* 30:633–638, 2000.

533. Li JS, Yow E, Berezny KY, et al: Clinical outcomes of palliative surgery including a systemic to pulmonary artery shunt in infants with cyanotic congenital heart disease: Does aspirin make a difference? *Circulation* 116:236, 2007.

534. Li J, Zhang G, Benson L, et al: Comparison of the profiles of postoperative systemic hemodynamics and oxygen transport in neonates after the hybrid or the Norwood procedure: a pilot study. *Circulation* 116:I179, 2007.

535. Liberthson RR: Sudden death from cardiac causes in children and young adults. *N Engl J Med* 334:1039–1044, 1996.

536. Lily C, De Meo D, Sonna L, et al: An intensive communication intervention for the critically ill. *Am J Med* 109:469–475, 2000.

537. Lim DS: Percutaneous device closure of atrial septal defect in a premature infant with rapid improvement in pulmonary status. *Pediatrics* 119(2):398–400, 2007.

538. Limperopoulos C, Majnemer A, Shevell MI, et al: Predictors of developmental disabilities after open heart surgery in young children with congenital heart defects. *J Pediatr* 141:52–58, 42002.

539. Lin AE: Etiology of congenital heart defects. *Pediatr Pathol* 10:305, 1990.

540. Linderkamp O, et al: Increased blood viscosity in patients with cyanotic congenital heart disease and iron deficiency. *J Pediatr* 95:567, 1979.

541. Lingren V, Rosinsky B, Chin J, Berry-Kravis E: Two patients with overlapping de novo duplications of the long arm of chromosome 9, including one case with DiGeorge sequence. *Am J Med Genet* 49(1):67–73, 1994.

542. Lipshitz M, Marino BL, Sanders ST: Chloral hydrate side effects in young children: causes and management. *Heart Lung* 22(5):408–414, 1993.

543. Lister G: Decreased perfusion and circulatory shock. In Lister GE, First LR, Gershon AA, editors: *Rudolph's textbook of pediatrics*, ed 22, New York, 2011, McGraw-Hill.

544. Liu CW, Hwang B, Lee BC, Lu JH: Aortic stenosis in children: 19-year experience. *Zhonghua Yi Xue Za Zhi (Taipei)* 59:107, 1997.

545. Lock J: Cardiac catheterization. In Keane JF, Lock JE, Fyler DC, editors: *Nadas' pediatric cardiology*, ed 2, Philadelphia, 2006, Elsevier.

546. Lodge AJ, Rychik J, Nicolson SC, et al: Improving outcomes in functional single ventricle and total anomalous pulmonary venous connection. *Ann Thorac Surg* 78(5):1688–1695, 2004.

547. Losay J, Touchot A, Serraf A, et al: Late outcome after arterial switch operation for transposition of the great arteries. *Circulation* 104(Suppl I):1121, 2001.

548. Ludomirsky A, Garson A: Supraventricular tachycardia. In Gillette PC, Garson A, editors: *Pediatric arrhythmias: electrophysiology and pacing*, Philadelphia, 1990, Saunders, pp. 380–425.

549. Lurie IL, et al: *Neurofibromatosis Noonan Syndrome*. Johns Hopkins University, Mendelian Inheritance in Man. 2006, Available from http://www.ncbi.nlm.nih.gov/omim/601321. Accessed March 11, 2008.

550. Lurz P, Coats L, Khambadkone S, et al: Percutaneous pulmonary valve implantation: impact of evolving technology and learning curve on clinical outcome. *Circualtion* 117:1964, 2008.

551. Lurz P, Nordmeyer J, Sachin K, et al: Percutaneous pulmonary valve implantation improves exercise capacity in patients with predominantly stenosis but not predominantly regurgitation. *Circulation* 116(16):(Suppl II):3128A, 2007.

552. Luysman T, Styns-Cailteux M, Tremouroux-Wattiez M, et al: Intravenous enalaprilat and oral enalapril in congestive heart failure secondary to ventricular septal defect in infancy. *Am J Cardiol* 70:959–962, 1992.

553. Madriago E, Silberbach M: Heart failure in infants and children. *Pediatr Rev* 31:4–12, 2010.

554. Mahle WT, Clancy RR, Moss EM, et al: Neurodevelopmental outcome and lifestyle assessment in school-aged and adolescent children with hyoplastic left heart syndrome. *Pediatrics* 105(5):1082, 2000.

555. Mahle WT, Cuadrado AR, Kirshom PM, et al: Nesiritide in infants and children with congestive heart failure. *Pediatr Crit Care Med* 6:543–546, 2005.

556. Mahle WT, Spray RL, Wernovsky G, et al: Survival after reconstructive surgery for hypoplastic left heart syndrome: a 15-year experience from a single institution. *Circulation* 102:III136, 2000.

557. Mahle WT, Tavani F, Zimmerman RA, et al: An MRI study of neurological injury before and after congenital heart surgery. *Circulation* 106(12 Suppl 1):109, 2002.

558. Maillot F, Cook P, Lilburn M, Lee PJ: A practical approach to maternal phenylketonuria management. *J Inherit Metab Dis* 30(2):198–201, 2007.

559. Mair D, Ritter D, Davis G: Selection of patients with truncus arteriosus for surgical correction: anatomic and hemodynamic considerations. *Circulation* 49:144, 1974.

560. Maisel AS, Krishnaswamy P, Nowak RM, et al: Rapid measurement of B-type natriuretic peptide in the emergency diagnosis of heart failure. *N Engl J Med* 347:161–167, 2002.

561. Makikallio K, Levine JC, Marx GR, et al: Fetal aortic valve stenosis and the evolution of hypoplastic left heart syndrome: patient selection for fetal intervention. *Circulation* 110:III690, 2004.

562. Makikallio K, McElhinney DB, Levine JC, et al: Fetal aortic valve stenosis and the evolution of hypoplastic left heart syndrome: patient selection for fetal intervention. *Circulation* 113:1401, 2006.

563. Manole MD, Saladino RA: Emergency department management of the pediatric patient with supraventricular tachycardia. *Pediatr Emerg Care* 23(3):176–185, (quiz: 186-179), 2007.

564. Manzi SF, Shannon M: Drug interactions: a review. *Clin Pediatr Emerg Med* 6(2), 2005.

565. Marcellitti C, McGoon DC, Danielson GK, et al: Early and late results of surgical repair of truncus arteriosus. *Circulation* 55:636, 1977.

566. Marchand V, Baker SS, Baker RD: Enteral nutrition in pediatric population. *Gastrointest Clin North Am* 8(3):669–703, 1998.

567. Marden PM, Smith DW, McDonald MJ: Congenital anomalies in the newborn infant including minor variants. *J Pediatr* 64:357, 1965.

568. Marino BS, Wernovsky G: Preoperative care. In Chang AC, Hanley F, Wernovsky G, Wessel DL, editors: *Pediatric cardiac intensive care*, Baltimore, 1998, Williams & Wilkins.

569. Maron BJ: Sudden death in young athletes. *N Engl J Med* 349:1064–1075, 2003.

570. Maron BJ, Towbin JA, Thiene G, et al: Contemporary definitions and classification of the cardiomyopathies: an American Heart Association Scientific Statement from the Council on Clinical Cardiology, Heart Failure and Transplantation Committee: Quality of Care and Outcomes Research and Functional Genomics and Translational Biology Interdisciplinary Working Groups; and Council on Epidemiology and Prevention. *Circulation* 113:1807, 2006.

571. Marrone C, Galasso G, Piccolo R, et al: Antiplatelet versus anticoagulation therapy after extracardiac conduit fontan: a systematic review and meta-analysis. *Pediatr Cardiol* 32:32, 2011.

572. Martin LJ, Ramachandran V, Cripe LH, et al: Evidence in favor of linkage to human chromosomal regions 18q, 5q and 13q for bicuspid aortic valve ans other associated cardiovascular malformations. *Hum Genet* 121:275, 2007.

573. Marx GR: Infective endocarditis. In Keane JF, Lock JE, Fyler DC, editors: *Nadas' pediatiatric cardiology*, ed 2, Philadelphia, 2006, Elsevier.

574. Marx GR, Fyler DC: Cardiac tumors. In Keane JF, Lock JE, Fyler DC, editors: *Nadas' pediatric cardiology*, ed 2, Philadelphia, 2006, Elsevier.

575. Marx GR, Fyler DC: Endocardial cushion defects. In Keane JF, Lock JE, Fyler DC, editors: *Nadas' pediatric cardiology*, ed 2, Philadelphia, 2006, Elsevier.

576. Marx GR, Moran AM: Cardiac tumors. In Allen HD, Shaddy RE, Driscoll DJ, Feltes TF, editors: *Moss and Adams' heart disease in infants, children, and adolescents, including the fetus and young adult*, ed 7, Philadelphia, 2008, Lippincott Williams & Wilkins.

577. Mascio CE, Austin EH 3rd: Pleural effusions following the Fontan procedure. *Curr Opin Pulm Med* 16:362, 2010.

578. Massin MM, Hovels-Gurich H, Seghavy MC: Atherosclerosis lifestyle risk factors in children with congenital heart disease. *Eur J Cardiovasc Prev* 14:349, 2007.

579. Masura J, Gao W, Gavora P, et al: Percutaneous closure of perimembranous ventricular septal defects with the eccentric Amplatzer device: multicenter follow-up study. *Pediatr Cardiol* 26:216, 2005.

580. Masura J, Tittel P, Gavora P, Podnar T: Long-term outcome of transcatheter patent ductus arteriosus closure using Amplatzer duct occluders. *Am Heart J* 151(3):755.e7–755.e10, 2006.

581. Matherne GP, Lim DS: Congenital anomalies of the coronary vessels and the aortic root. In Allen HD, Shaddy RE, Driscoll DJ, Feltes TF, editors: *Moss and Adams' heart disease in infants, children, and adolescents, including the fetus and young adult*, ed 7, Philadelphia, 2008, Lippincott Williams & Wilkins.

582. Mavroudis C, Deal BJ, Backer CL, et al: 111 Fontan conversions with arrhythmia surgery: surgical lessons and outcomes. *Ann Thorac Surg* 84:1457, 2007.

583. Mavroudis C, Backer CL: Transposition of the great arteries. In Mavroudis C, Backer CL, editors: *Pediatric cardiac surgery*, ed 3, Philadelphia, 2003, Mosby/Elsevier.

584. Mavroudis C, Backer CL: Truncus arteriosus. In Mavroudis C, Backer CL, editors: *Pediatric cardiac surgery*, ed 3, Philadelphia, 2003, Mosby/Elsevier.

585. Mavroudis C, Backer CL, Deal BJ, et al: Evolving anatomic and electrophysiologic considerations associated with Fontan conversion. *Semin Thorac Cardiovasc Surg Pediatr Card Surg Annu* 136–145, 2007.

586. Mavroudis C, Deal BJ, Backer CL, et al: J. Maxwell Chamberlain Memorial Paper for congenital heart surgery. 111 Fontan conversions with arrhythmia surgery: surgical lessons and outcomes. *Ann Thorac Surg* 84(5):1457–1466, 2007.

587. Mavroudis C, Deal BJ, Backer CL, Tsao S: Arrhythmia Surgery in Patients With and Without Congenital Heart Disease. *Ann Thorac Surg* 86(3):857–868, 2008.

588. Mavroudis C, Dodge-Khatami A, Backer CL: Coronary artery anomalies. In Mavroudis C, Backer CL, editors: *Pediatric cardiac surgery*, ed 3, Philadelphia, 2003, Mosby/Elsevier.

589. Mayer JE: Surgical management of the patient with the univentricular heart. In Keane JF, Lock JE, Fyler DC, editors: *Nadas' pediatric cardiology*, ed 2, Philadelphia, 2006, Elsevier.

590. May LE: Somatic and cerebral oximetry aids detection of low cardiac output after stage one palliation of hypoplastic left heart syndrome. *Neonat Int Care* 20:49, 2007.

591. May LE: *Pediatric heart surgery: a ready reference for professionals.* ed 4, Milwaukee, 2008, Maxishare.

592. McBride MG, Kirshbom PM, Gaynor JW, et al: Late cardiopulmonary and musculoskeletal exercise performance after repair for total anomalous pulmonary venous connection during infancy. *J Thorac Cardiovasc Surg* 133(6):1533–1539, 2007.

593. McCrindle BW: Independent predictors of immediate results of percutaneous balloon aortic valvotomy in children. Valvuloplasty and Angioplasty of Congenital Anomalies (VACA) Registry Investigators. *Am J Cardiol* 77:286, 1996.

594. McCrindle BW: Independent predictors of long-term results after balloon pulmonary valvuloplasty. Valvuloplasty and Angioplasty of Congenital Anomalies (VACA) Registry Investigators. *Circulation* 89(4):1751–1759, 1994.

595. McCrindle BW, Blackstone EH, Williams WG, et al: Are outcomes of surgical versus transcatheter balloon valvotomy equivalent in neonatal critical aortic stenosis? *Circulation* 104:I152, 2001.

596. McCrindle BW, Williams RV, Mital S, et al: Physical activity levels in children and adolescents are reduced after the Fontan procedure, independent of exercise capacity, and are associated with lower perceived general health. *Arch Dis Child* 92:509, 2007.

597. McDaniel NL, Gutgesell HP: Ventricular septal defects. In Allen HD, Driscoll DJ, Shaddy RE, Feltes TF, editors: *Moss and Adams' heart disease in infants, children, and adolescents, including the fetus and young adult*, ed 7, Philadelphia, 2008, Lippincott Williams & Wilkins.

598. McElhinney DB, Hellenbrand WE, Zahn EM, Jones TK, et al: Short- and medium-term outcomes after transcatheter pulmonary valve placement in the expanded multicenter US Melody Valve Trial. *Circulation* 122:507–516, 2010.

599. McElhinney DB, Lock JE, Keane JF, et al: Left heart growth, function, and reintervention after balloon aortic valvuloplasty for neonatal aortic stenosis. *Circulation* 111:451, 2005.

600. McGucklin M, Waterman R, Govednik J: Hand hygiene compliance rates in the United States: a one-year multi-center collaboration using product volume usage measurement and feedback. *Am J Med Qual* 24:205–213, 2009.

601. McGuire JK, Kulkarni MS, Baden HP: Fatal hypermagnesemia in a child treated with megavitamin/megamineral therapy. *Pediatrics* 105 (2):e18, 2000.

602. McGuirk SP, Griselli M, Stumper OF, et al: Staged surgical management of hypoplastic left heart syndrome: a single institution 12 year experience. *Heart* 92(3):364–370, 2006.

603. McKee C, Berkowitz I, Cosgrove S, et al: Reduction of catheter-associated bloodstream in pediatric patients: experimentation and reality. *Pediatr Crit Care Med* 9(1):40–46, 2008.

604. McKusick VA, et al: Mendelian inheritance in man. Updated 2006: Available from http://www.ncbi.nlm.nih.gov/omim Accessed March 15, 2008.

605. McQuinn TC, Wessels A: Embryology of the heart and great vessels. In Mavroudis C, Backer CL, editors: *Pediatric cardiac surgery*, ed 3, Philadelphia, 2003, Mosby/Elsevier.

606. Medi C, Kalman JM, Haqqani H, et al: Tachycardia-mediated cardiomyopathy secondary to focal atrial tachycardia: long-term outcome after catheter ablation. *J Am Coll Cardiol* 53(19):1791–1797, 2009.

607. Mehta AV: Rhabdomyoma and ventricular preexcitation syndrome. *Am J Dis Child* 147(6):669–671, 1993.

608. Meijboom F, Hess J, Szatmari A, et al: Long-term, follow-up (9–20 years) after surgical closure of atrial septal defect at a young age. *Am J Cardiol* 72:14431, 1993.

609. Meijer JM, Pieper PG, Drenthen W, et al: Pregnancy, fertility, and recurrence risk in corrected tetralogy of Fallot. *Heart* 91(6):801–805, 2005.

610. Mellion M: Diagnosing Marfan syndrome. *Heart Dis Stroke* Sep/Oct:241–245, 1994.

611. Mendelshon AM, Lloyd TR, Crowley DC, et al: Late followup of balloon angioplasty in children with a native coarctation of the aorta. *Am J Cardiol* 74:696–700, 1994.

612. Mertens L, Hagler DJ, Saure U, et al: Protein-losing enteropathy after the Fontan operation: An international multicenter study. PLE Study Group. *J Thorac Cardiovasc Surg* 115:1063, 1998.

613. Meyers JL: Pulmonary hypertension, Eisenmenger Syndrome, 2007, Available from http://www.emedicine.com/ped/TOPIC2528.HTM, February 8, 2008.

614. Michel-Behnke I, Akintuerk H, Thul J, et al: Stent implantation in the ductus arteriosus for pulmonary blood supply in congenital heart disease. *Catheter Cardiovasc Interv* 61(2):242–252, 2004.

615. Michel-Behnke I, Le TP, Waldecker B, et al: Percutaneous closure of congenital and acquired ventricular septal defects: considerations on selection of the occlusion device. *J Interv Cardiol* 8:89, 2005.

616. Michel-Behnke I, Luedemann M, Bauer J, et al: Fenestration in extracardiac conduits in children after modified Fontan operation by implantation of stent grafts. *Pediatr Cardiol* 26:93, 2005.

617. Miller OI, Celermajer DS, Deanfield JE, Macrae DJ: Very-low-dose inhaled nitric oxide: a selective pulmonary vasodilator after operations for congenital heart disease. *J Thorac Cardiovas Surg* 108:487, 1994.

618. Miller G, Tesman JR, Ramer JC, et al: Outcome after open-heart surgery in infants and children. *J Child Neurol* 11:49–53, 1996.

619. Miller OI, Tang SF, Keech A, et al: Inhaled nitric oxide and prevention of pulmonary hypertension after congenital heart surgery: a randomized double-blind study. *Lancet* 356:1464, 2000.

620. Mitchell MB, Clarke DR: Isolated right ventricular outflow tract obstruction. In Mavroudis C, Backer CL, editors: *Pediatric cardiac surgery*, ed 3, Philadelphia, 2003, Mosby/Elsevier.

621. Momenah TS, Eltayb H, Oakley RE, et al: Effects of transcatheter closure of Fontan fenestration on exercise tolerance. *Pediatr Cardiol* 29:585, 2008.

622. Monagle P, Chan A, Massicotte P, et al: Antithrombotic therapy in children: the seventh ACCP conference on antithrombotic and thrombolytic therapy. *Chest* 126(suppl 3):645S–687S, 2004.

623. Monteiro AJ: Surgical treatment of complete atrioventricular septal defect with the two-patch technique: early-to-mid followup. *Interact Cardiovasc Thorac Surg* 6(6):737–740, 2007.

624. Moodie DS, Ritter DG, Tajik AJ, et al: Long-term followup in the unoperated univentricular heart. *Am J Cardiol* 53:1124, 1984.

625. Moons P, De Volder E, Budts W, et al: What do adult patients with congenital heart disease know about their disease, treatment, and prevention of complications? A call for structured patient education. *Heart* 86(1):74–80, 2001.

626. Moons P, Gewillig M, Sluysmans T, et al: Long term outcome up to 30 years after the Mustard or Senning operation: a nationwide multicentre study in Belgium. *Heart* 90(3):307, 2004.

627. Moore KL, Persaud TVN, Torchia MG: *The cardiovascular system. The developing human: clinically oriented embryology.* ed 8, Philadelphia, 2008, Saunders Elsevier.

628. Moore P, Brook MM, Heymann MA: Patent ductus arteriosus and aortopulmonary window. In Allen HD, Driscoll DJ, Shaddy RE, Feltes TF, editors: *Moss and Adams' heart disease in infants, children, and adolescents, including the fetus and young adult,* ed 7, Philadelphia, 2008, Lippincott Williams & Wilkins.

629. Moore P, Egito E, Mowrey H, Perry SB: Midterm results of balloon dilation of congenital aortic stenosis: predictors of success. *J Am Coll Cardiol* 27:1257, 1996.

630. Morales DL, Braud BE, Booth JH, et al: Heterotaxy patients with total anomalous pulmonary venous return: improving surgical results. *Ann Thorac Surg* 82(5):1621–1627, 2006.

631. Morgan BC, et al: A clinical profile of paroxysmal hyperpnea in cyanotic congenital heart disease. *Circulation* 31:66, 1965.

632. Morris K, Beghetti M, Petros A, et al: Comparison of hyperventilation and inhaled nitric oxide for pulmonary hypertension after repair of congenital heart disease. *Crit Care Med* 28, 2974.2000.

633. Morse RP, Rockenmacher S, Pyeritz RE, et al: Diagnosis and management of infantile Marfan syndrome. *Pediatrics* 86:888–895, 1990.

634. Mueller C, Scholer A, Laule-Kilian K, et al: Use of B-type natriuretic peptide in the evaluation and management of acute dyspnea. *N Engl J Med* 350:647–654, 2004.

635. Mukherji SK, editor: *Pediatric head and neck imaging*, Neuroimaging Clin North Am Philadelphia, 2000, Saunders.

636. Mull CC, Dahdah NS, Scarfone RJ: Cerebral and coronary embolization of a valvular tumor. *Ped Cardiol* 23(1):71–73, 2002.

637. Mullen MP: Diagnostic strategies for acute presentation of pulmonary hypertension in children: Particular focus on use of echocardiography, cardiac catheterization, magnetic resonance imaging, chest computed tomography, and lung biopsy. *Pediatr Crit Care Med* 11(2 Suppl):S23–S26, 2010.

638. Mullen MP: Pulmonary hypertension. In Keane JF, Lock JE, Fyler DC, editors: *Nadas' pediatric cardiology*, ed 2, St Louis, 2006, Saunders Elsevier.

639. Muller G, Deal BJ, Benson DW Jr: "Vagal maneuvers" and adenosine for termination of atrioventricular reentrant tachycardia. *Am J Cardiol* 74:500–503, 1994.

640. Mullins CE: *Cardiac catheterization in congenital heart disease.* ed 1, Malden, MA, 2006, Blackwell.

641. Murphy JG, Gersch BJ, Mair DD, et al: Long-term outcome in patients undergoing surgical repair of tetralogy of Fallot. *N Engd J Med* 329:593, 1993.

642. Nakano T, Kado H, Tachibana T, et al: Excellent midterm outcomes of extradiac conduit total cavopulmonary connection: results of 126 cases. *Ann Thorac Surg* 84:1619, 2007.

643. Namachivayam P, Theilen U, Warwick W, et al: Sildenafil prevents rebound pulmonary hypertension after withdrawal of nitric oxide in children. *Am J Resp Crit Care Med* 174:1042, 2006.

644. Napoli KL, Ingall CG, Martin GR: Safety and efficacy of chloral hydrate sedation in children undergoing echocardiography. *J Pediatr* 129(2):287–291, 1996.

645. Nelson DP: Paying more attention to morbidity in infants with hypoplastic left heart syndrome. *Pediat Crit Care Med* 6:614, 2005.

646. Nemoto S, Umehara E, Ikeda T, et al: Oral sildenafil ameliorates impaired pulmonary circulation early alter bidirectional cavopulmonary shunt. *Ann Thorac Surg* 83:e11, 2007.

647. Newberger J: Neurodevelopmental outcomes after heart surgery in children. In Allen HD, Driscoll DJ, Feltes TF, Shaddy RE, editors: *Moss and Adams' heart disease in infants, children, and adolescents, including the fetus and young adult,* ed 7, Philadelphia, 2008, Lippincott Williams & Wilkins.

648. Newburger JW: Neurodevelopmental outcomes after heart surgery in children. In Allen HD, Shaddy RE, Driscoll DJ, Feltes TF, editors: *Moss and Adams' heart disease in infants, children, and adolescents, including the fetus and young adult,* ed 7, Philadelphia, 2008, Lippincott Williams & Wilkins, pp. 1505–1512.

649. News and Events: FDA approves Gored HELEX septal occluder for treatment of atrial septal defect. *Congenital Cardiology Today* November 22, 2007.

650. Newth J, Hammer J: Pulmonary issues. In Chang AC, Hanley FL, Wernovsky G, Wessel DL, editors: *Pediatric cardiac intensive care*, Baltimore, 1998, Williams & Wilkins.

651. Nielson DE, Robin NH: Advances in the genetics of pediatric heart disease. *Contemp Pediatr* 19(1):85, 86, 88-90, 92, 2002.

652. Nieves J, Kohr L: Nursing considerations in the care of patients with pulmonary hypertension. *Pediatr Crit Care Med* 11(2 Suppl):S74–S78, 2010.

653. Nikaidoh H: Aortic translocation and biventricular outflow tract reconstruction: a new surgical repair for transposition of the great arteries associated with ventricular septal defect and pulmonary stenosis. *J Thorac Cardiovasc Surg* 88:365, 1984.

654. Noe P, Van Driel V, Wittkampf F, Sreeram N: Rapid recovery of cardiac function after catheter ablation of persistent junctional reciprocating tachycardia in children. *Pacing Clin Electrophysiol* 25(2):191–194, 2002.

655. Noonan JA: Noonan syndrome and related disorders: alterations in growth and puberty. *Rev Endocr Metab Disord* 7(4):251–255, 2006.

656. Noori S, Frieduch P, Seri I, Wong P: Changes in myocardial function and hemodynamics after ligation of the ductus arteriosus in preterm infants. *J Pediatr* 150:597–602, 2007.

657. Nora JJ: Causes of congenital heart disease: old and new modes, mechanisms and models. *Am Heart J* 87(2):1–14, 1993.

658. Norris MK, Hill CS: Nutritional issues in infants and children with congenital heart disease. *Crit Care Nurs Clin North Am* 6(1):153–163, 1994.

659. Norwood WI, Kirklin JK, Sanders SP: Hypoplastic left heart syndrome: experience with palliative surgery. *Am J Cardiol* 45:87, 1980.

660. Nykanen DG: Interventional cardiac catheterization procedures: cardiology considerations. In Bissonette B, Dalens B, editors: *Pediatric anesthesia: principles and practice*, New York, 2002, McGraw-Hill.

661. Nykanen D: Interventional cardiac catheterization procedures: cardiology considerations. In Bissonette B, Dalens B, editors: *Principles and practice of pediatric anesthesia*, New York, 2005, McGraw-Hill.

662. Nykanen D: Pulmonary atresia and intact ventricular septum. In Allen HD, Driscoll DJ, Feltes TF, Shaddy RE, editors: *Moss and Adams' heart disease in infants, children, and adolescents, including the fetus and young adult*, ed 7, Philadelphia, 2008, Lippincott Williams & Wilkins.

663. Nykanen D, Zahn EM: Transcatheter techniques in the management of perioperative vascular obstruction. *Cathet Cardiovasc Intervention* 66:573, 2005.

664. O'Hare B, Laussen P: Interventional cardiac catheterization: anesthetic consideration and post procedural management. In Bissonette B, Dalens B, editors: *Pediatric anesthesia: principles and practice*, New York, 2002, McGraw-Hill.

665. O'Neill MJF: *Brugada syndrome*. Johns Hopkins University, Mendelian Inheritance in Man. Updated 2008, Available from http://www.ncbi.nlm.nih.gov/omim/611777, 611875, and 611876 Accessed March 23, 2008.

666. O'Neill MJF: *Long QT syndrome 9*. Johns Hopkins University, Mendelian Inheritance in Man. 2008, Available from www.ncbi.nlm.nih.gov/entrez/dispomim.cgi?id=611818,811819,611820. Accessed March 13, 2008.

667. Odegard KC, Laussen PC: Pediatric anesthesia and critical care. In Sellke FW, del Nido PJ, Swanson SJ, editors: *Sabiston and spencer: surgery of the chest*, ed 7, vol 2. Philadelphia, 2005, Elsevier.

668. Oh MS, Carroll HJ: Electrolyte and acid-base disorders. In Chernow B, editor: *The pharmacologic approach to the critically ill patient*, ed 2, Baltimore, 1988, Williams & Wilkins.

669. Oh H, Seo W: A meta-analysis of the effects of various interventions in preventing endotracheal suction-induced hypoxemia. *J Clin Nur* 12:912–924, 2003.

670. Ohye RG, Sleeper LA, Mahony L, et al: Comparison of shunt types in the Norwood procedure for single-ventricle lesions. *N Engl J Med* 362:1980, 2010.

671. Olson T, Hoffman T, Chan D: Dilated congestive cardiomyopathy. In Allen HD, Shaddy RE, Driscoll DJ, Feltes TF, editors: *Moss and Adams' heart disease in infants, children, and adolescents, including the fetus and young adult*, ed 7, Philadelphia, 2008, Lippincott Williams & Wilkins, pp. 1195–1205.

672. Ono M, Boethig D, Goerler H, et al: Clinical outcome of patients 20 years after Fontan operation: effect of fenestration on late morbidity. *Eur J Cardiothorac Surg* 30:923, 2006.

673. Oosterhof T, Azakie A, Freedom RM, et al: Associated factors and trends in outcomes of interrupted aortic arch. *Ann Thorac Surg* 78:1696–1702, 2004.

674. Opotowsky AR, Shellenberger D, Dharan V, et al: Successful pregnancies in two women with hypoplastic left heart syndrome. *Congenit Heart Dis* 5:476, 2010.

675. Otto CM: *Textbook of clinical echocardiography*. 3rd ed, Philadelphia, 2004, Saunders.

676. Ovroutski S, Ewert P, Alexi-Meskishvili V, et al: Dilatation and stenting of the Fontan pathway: impact of the stenosis treatment on chronic ascites. *J Intevr Cardiol* 21:38, 2008.

677. Owens JL, Musa N: Nutrition support after neonatal cardiac surgery. *Nutr Clin Pract* 24:242, 2009.

678. Packer M, Coats AJ, Fowler MB, et al: Carvedilol Prospective Randomized Cumulative Survival Study Group: Effect of carvedilol on survival in severe chronic heart failure. *N Engl J Med* 344:1651–1658, 2001.

679. Pahl E, Dipchand AI, Burch M: Heart transplantation for heart failure in children. *Heart Fail Clin* 6(4):575–589, 2010.

680. Panagiotopoulos C, McCrindle BW, Hick K, Katzman DK: Electrocardiographic findings in adolescents with eating disorders. *Pediatrics* 105(5):1100–1105, 2000.

681. Pardi G, Cetin I: Human fetal growth and organ development: 50 years of discoveries. *Am J Obstet Gynecol* 194:1088–1099, 2006.

682. Paridon SM, Mitchell PD, Colan SD, et al: A cross-sectional study of exercise performance during the first 2 decades of life after the Fontan operation. *J Am Coll Cardiol* 52:99, 2008.

683. Park MK: Cardiac involvement in systemic diseases. In Park MK, editor: *Pediatric cardiology for practitioners*, ed 5, Philadelphia, 2008, Elsevier.

684. Park MK: Cardiovascular infections. In Park MK, editor: *Pediatric cardiology for practitioners*, ed 5, Philadelphia, 2008, Elsevier.

685. Park M. Hypoplastic left heart syndrome. In Park MK, editor: *Pediatric cardiology for practitioners*, ed 5, St. Louis, 2008, Mosby.

686. Park MK: *Pediatric cardiology for practitioners*. ed 5, Philadelphia, 2008, Mosby Elsevier.

687. Park MK, Guntheroth WG: *How to read pediatric ECGs*. ed 4, Philadelphia, 2006, Mosby Elsevier.

688. Paul MH, Muster AJ, Sinha HN, et al: Double-outlet left ventricle with an intact ventricular septum. Clinical and autopsy diagnosis and developmental implications. *Circulation* 41:129–139, 1970.

689. Pavlovic M, Acharya G, Huhta JC: Controversies of fetal cardiac intervention. *Early Hum Dev* 84:149, 2008.

690. Pearson AC, Castello R, Labovitz AJ: Safety and utility of transesophageal echocardiography in the critically ill patient. *Am Heart J* 119:1083, 1990.

691. Pedra CA, Neves JR, Pedra SR, et al: New transcatheter techniques for creation or enlargement of atrial septal defects in infants with complex congenital heart disease. *Catheter Cardiovasc Interv* 70:731, 2007.

692. Pedra SR, Pedra CA, Abizaid AA, et al: Intracoronary ultrasound assessment late after the arterial switch operation for transposition of the great arteries. *J Am Coll Cardiol* 45:2061, 2005.

693. Perloff JK. Ebstein malformation. In *Congenital heart disease in adults*, ed 3, Philadelphia, 2008, Saunders.

694. Perry LW, Neill CA, Ferencz C, et al: Infants with congenital heart disease: the cases. In Ferencz C, Rubin JD, Loffredo CA, et al., editors: *Perspectives in pediatric cardiology: epidemiology of congenital heart disease, the Baltimore-Washington Infant Study, 1981-1989*, Armonk, NY, 1993, Futura.

695. Perry JC, Walsh EP: Diagnosis and management of cardiac arrhythmias. In Chang AC, Hanley F, Wernovsky G, Wessel DL, editors: *Pediatric cardiac intensive care*, Baltimore, 1998, Williams & Wilkins.

696. Peter C, Armstrong B, Jones R: Radionuclide quantitation of right-to-left shunts in children. *Circulation* 64:572, 1981.

697. Pfeffer MA, Braunwald E, Moye LA, et al: for the SAVE Investigators: Effect of captopril on mortality and morbidity in patients with left ventricular dysfunction after myocardial infarction: results of the Survival and Ventricular Enlargement Trial. *N Engl J Med* 327:669–677, 1992.

698. Phornphutkul C, et al: Cerebrovascular accident in infants and children with cyanotic congenital heart disease. *Am J Cardiol* 32:329, 1973.

699. Piacentini G, Digilio MC, Sarkozy A, et al: Genetics of congenital heart diseases in syndromic and nonsyndromic patients: new advances and clinical implications. *J Cardiovasc Med* 8(1):7–11, 2007.

700. Pierpont ME, Basson CT, Benson DW, et al: Genetic basis for congenital heart defects: current knowledge: a scientific statement from the American Heart Association Congenital Cardiac Defects Committee, Council on CVDY: endorsed by the AAP. *Circulation*. 115 (23):3015–3038, 2007.

701. Pillo-Blocka F: Rapid advancement to more concentrated formula in infants after surgery for congenital heart disease reduces duration of hospital stay: a randomized clinical trial. *J Pediatr* 145:761–766, 2004.

702. Pineo GF, Hull RD: Vitamin K antagonists and direct thrombin inhibitors: present and future. *Hematol Oncol Clin North Am* 19:69–85, 2005.

703. Pinto NM, Marino BS, Wernovsky G, et al: Obesity is a common comorbidity in children with congenital and acquired heart disease. *Pediatrics* 120:e1157, 2007.

704. Pitt B, Zannad F, Remme WJ, et al: for the RALES Investigators: The effect of spironolactone on morbidity and mortality in patients with severe heart failure. Randomized Aldactone Evaluation Study Investigators. *N Engl J Med* 341:709–717, 1999.

705. Poongundran N, Theilen U, Warwick W, et al: Sildenafil prevents rebound pulmonary hypertension after withdrawal of nitric oxide in children. *Am J Respir Crit Care Med* 174:1042–1047, 2006.

706. Popper R: Avoiding endocarditis. *Heart Matters (ACHA)* 9(2):3, 10, 2007.

707. Porter FL, Grunau RE, Anand KJ: Long-term effects of pain in infants. *J Dev Behav Pediatr* 4(20):253–261, 1999.

708. Porter CJ, Edwards WD: Atrial septal defects. In Allen HD, Driscoll DJ, Shaddy RE, Feltes TF, editors: *Moss and Adams' heart disease in infants, children, and adolescents, including the fetus and young adult*, ed 7, Philadelphia, 2008, Lippincott Williams & Wilkins.

709. Preciado D, Verghese S, Choi S: Aggressive bronchoscopic management of plastic bronchitis. *Int J Pediatric Otorhinolaryngol* 74:820, 2010.

710. Price S, Ilper H, Uddin S, et al: Peri-resuscitation echocardiography: Training the novice practitioner. *Resuscitation* Aug 18. [Epub ahead of print], 2010.

711. Prieto LR, Latson LA: Pulmonary stenosis. In Allen HD, Shaddy RE, Driscoll DJ, Feltes TF, editors: *Moss and Adams' heart disease in infants, children, and adolescents, including the fetus and young adult*, ed 7, Philadelphia, 2008, Lippincott Williams & Wilkins.

712. Pryzlepa KA, et al: *Hurler syndrome.* Johns Hopkins University, Mendelian Inheritance in Man. 2008, Available from http://www.ncbi.nlm.nih.gov/omim/607014. Accessed March 15, 2008.

713. Pucci A, Wharton J, Arbustini E, et al: Localization of brain and atrial natriuretic peptide in human and porcine heart. *Int J Cardiol* 92:1558–1664, 1992.

714. Qamar ZA, Goldberg CS, Devaney EJ, et al: Current risk factors and outcomes for the arterial switch operation. *Ann Thorac Surg* 84(3): 871, 2007.

715. Qin JJ, Jones M, Shiota T, et al: New digital measurement methods for left ventricular volume using real-time three-dimensional echocardiography: comparison with electromagnetic flow method and magnetic resonance imaging. *Eur J Echocardiogr* 1:96, 2000.

716. Quinones MA, Douglas PS, Foster E, et al: ACC/AHA clinical competence statement on echocardiography: a report of the American College of Cardiology/American Heart Association/American College of Physicians-American Society of Internal Medicine Task Force on Clinical Competence. *J Am Coll Cardiol* 41:687, 2003.

717. Rabinovitch M: Pathophysiology of pulmonary hypertension. In Allen HD, Driscoll DJ, Feltes TF, Shaddy RE, editors: *Moss & Adams heart disease in infants, children, and adolescents including the fetus and young adult*, ed 7, Philadelphia, 2008, Lippincott Williams & Wilkins.

718. Raff GW, Geiss DM, Shah JJ, et al: Repair of transposition of the great arteries with total anomalous pulmonary venous return. *Ann Thorac Surg* 73(2):655–657, 2002.

719. Raisky O, Bergoend E, Agnoletti G, et al: Late coronary artery lesions after neonatal arterial switch operation: results of surgical coronary revascularization. *Eur J Cardiothorac Surg* 31(5):894, 2007.

720. Raja SG, Danton MD, MacArthur KJ, Pollock JC: Effects of escalating doses of sildenafil on hemodynamics and gas exchange in children with pulmonary hypertension and congenital cardiac defects. *J Cardiothoracic Vasc Anesth* 21(2):203, 2007.

721. Ralston M, Hazinski MF, Zaritsky AL, et al: *PALS provider manual.* Dallas, 2006, American Heart Association.

722. Ralston M, Hazinski MF, Zaritsky AL, et al., editors: *Pediatric advanced life support provider manual*, Dallas, 2006, American Heart Association.

723. Ransom J, Srivastava D: The genetics of cardiac birth defects. *Semin Cell Dev Biol* 18(1):132–139, 2007.

724. Rao PS, editor: *Tricuspid atresia*, Mt Kisco, NY, 1982, Futura, pp. 13–24, 210-229.

725. Rao PS: Role of interventional cardiology in the treatment of neonates, Part III. *Congen Cardiol Today* 6:1, 2008.

726. Reddy VM, Liddicoat JR, Hanley FL: Primary bidirectional superior cavopulmonary shunt in infants between 1 and 4 months of age. *Ann Thorac Surg* 59:1120, 1995.

727. Rees G, Gledhill J, Garralda ME, et al: Psychiatric outcome following pediatric critical care unit (PCCU) admission: a cohort study. *Int Care Med* 30:1607, 2004.

728. Reid GJ, Irvine MJ, McCrindle BW, et al: Prevalence and correlates of successful transfer from pediatric to adult healthcare among a cohort of young adults with complex congenital heart defects. *Pediatrics* 113:e197–2205, 2004.

729. Reid GJ, Siu SC, McCrindle BW, Irvine MJ, Webb GD: Sexual behavior and reproductive concerns among adolescents and young adults with congenital heart disease. *Int J Cardiol* 125(3):332–338, 2008.

730. Reinhardt Z, Uzun O, Bhole V, et al: Sildenafil in the management of the failing Fontan circulation. *Cardiol Young* 20:522, 2010.

731. Reller MD: Congenital heart disease: current indications for antithrombotic therapy in pediatric patients. *Curr Cardiol Rpts* 3 (1):90–95, 2001.

732. Rhodes LA, Wernovsky G, Keane JF, et al: Arrhythmias and intracardiac conduction after the arterial switch operation. *J Thorac Cardiovasc Surg* 109(2):303–310, 1995.

733. Riberio RC, Schettini ST, Abib SDC, et al: Cavectomy for the treatment of Wilm's tumor with vascular extension. *J Urol* 176(1): 279–283, 2006.

734. Rigby ML: Atrial septal defect. In Gatzoulis MA, Webb GD, Daubeney PEF, editors: *Diagnosis and Management of Adult congenital Heart Disease*, Edinburgh, 2003, Churchill Livingstone.

735. Roberts RJ: Cardiovascular drugs. In Roberts RJ, editor: *Drug therapy in infants: pharmacological principles and clinical experience*, Philadelphia, 1984, WB Saunders Co.

736. Roberts JD, Lang P, Bigatello LM, et al: Inhaled nitric oxide in congenial heart disease. *Circulation* 87(2):447, 1993.

737. Rodbard S: Blood velocity and endocarditis. *Circulation* 27:18, 1963.

738. Rogers P, Mansour D, Mattinson A, O'Sullivan JJ: A collaborative clinic between contraception and sexual health services and an adult congenital heart disease clinic. *J Fam Plann Reprod Health Care* 33 (1):17–21, 2007.

739. Roman KS, Fouron JC, Nii M, et al: Determinants of outcome in fetal pulmonary valve stenosis or atresia with intact ventricular septum. *Am J Cardiol* 99(5):699, 2007.

740. Rome JJ, Lock JE: Cardiac catheterization of the critically ill cardiac patient. In Chang AC, Hanley FL, Wernovsky G, Wessel DL, editors: *Pediatric cardiac intensive care*, Philadelphia, 1998, Lippincott Williams & Wilkins.

741. Ronge L: Pediatricians' piercing insight can help teens get the point. *AAP News* 13(1):10–11, 1997.

742. Ronghe MD, Halsey C, Gouldern NJ: Anticoagulation therapy in children. *Pediatr Drugs* 5(12):803–820, 2003.

743. Roos-Hesselink J, Perlroth MG, McGhie J, et al: Atrial arrhythmias in adults after repair of tetralogy of Fallot. Correlation with clinical, exercise, and echocardiographic findings. *Circulation* 91:2214–2219, 1995.

744. Rosen DS, Blum RW, Britto M, et al: Society for Adolescent Medicine: Transition to adult healthcare for adolescents and young adults with chronic conditions: position paper of the Society for Adolescent Medicine. *J Adolesc Health* 33(4):309–311, 2003.

745. Rosensweig EB, Barst RJ: Clinical management of patients with pulmonary hypertension. In Allen HD, Driscoll DJ, Feltes TF, Shaddy RE, editors: *Moss & Adams heart disease in infants, children, and adolescents including the fetus and young adult*, ed 7, Philadelphia, 2008, Lippincott Williams & Wilkins.

746. Rosenthal A: Nutritional considerations in the prognosis and treatment of children with congenital heart disease. In Suskind RM, Lewinter-Suskind L, editors: *Textbook of pediatric nutrition*, ed 2, New York, 1993, Raven.

747. Rose V, Clark E: Etiology of congenital heart disease. In Freedom RM, Benson LN, Smallhorn JF, editors: *Neonatal heart disease*, London, 1992, Springer-Verlag, pp. 3–17.

747a. Ross RD, Bollinger RO, Pinsky WW: Grading the severity of heart failure in infants. *Pediatr Cardiol* 13:72–75, 1992.

748. Ross RD, Daniels SR, Schwartz DC, et al: Plasma norepinephrine levels in infants and children with congestive heart failure. *Am J Cardiol* 59:911–914, 1987.

749. Ross BA, Gillette PC: Atrioventricular block and bundle branch block. In Gillette PC, Garson A Jr, editors: *Clinical pediatric arrhythmias*, Philadelphia, 1999, pp. 63–77.

750. Roth SJ: Postoperative care. In Chang AC, Hanley F, Wernovsky G, Wessel DL, editors: *Pediatric cardiac intensive care*, Baltimore, 1998, Williams & Wilkins.

751. Rowland DG, Hammill WW, Allen HD, et al: Natural course of isolated pulmonary valve stenosis in infants and children utilizing Doppler echocardiography. *Am J Cardiol* 79:344, 1997.

752. Rudolph AM: *Congenital diseases of the heart.* Chicago, 1974, Year Book Medical Publishers.

753. Rudolph AM, Heymann MA, Spitzna U: Hemodynamic consideration in the development of narrowing of the aorta. *Am J Cardiol* 30:514–525, 1972.

754. Ruggiero RJ: Prescription drugs taken during pregnancy, 2008. Available from http://www.visembryo.com/baby/pharmaceuticals.html. Accessed February 17, 2008.

755. Ryckman FC, Schoettker PJ, Hays KR, et al: Reducing surgical site infections at a pediatric academic medical center. *JCJQPS* 35(4):192–198, 2009.

756. Ryerson L, Goldberg C, Rosenthal A, Arrmstrong A: Usefulness of heparin therapy in protein-losing enteropathy associated with single ventricle palliation. *Am J Cardiol* 101:248, 2008.

757. Sachdeva R, Hussain E, Moss M, et al: Vocal cord dysfunction and feeding difficulties after pediatric cardiovascular surgery. *J Pediatr* 151:312–315, 2007.

758. Salazar JD, Zafar F, Siddiqui K, et al: Fenestration during Fontan palliation: now the exception instead of the rule. *J Thorac Cardiovasc Surg* 140:129, 2010.

759. Saleeb SF, Solowiejczyk DE, Glickstein JS, et al: Frequency of development of aortic cuspal prolapse and aortic regurgitation in patients with subaortic ventricular septal defect diagnosed at <1 year of age. *Am J Cardiol* 99:1588–1592, 2007.

760. Salim MA, Case CL, Gillette PC: Chaotic atrial tachycardia in children. *Am Heart J* 129(4):831–833, 1995.

761. Sallehuddin A, Mesned A, Barakati M, et al: Fontan completion without surgery. *Eur J Cardiothoracic Surg* 32:195, 2007.

762. Salvin JW, McElhinney DB, Colan SD, et al: Fetal tricuspid valve size and growth as predictors of outcome in pulmonary atresia with intact ventricular septum. *Pediatrics* 118(2):e415, 2006.

763. Samour PQ, King K: *Handbook of pediatric nutrition.* Boston, 2005, Jones and Bartlett.

764. Sander TL, Klinker DB, Tomita-Mitchell A, Mitchell ME: Molecular and cellular basis of congenital heart disease. *Pediatr Clin North Am* 53:989–1009, 2006.

765. Sanlaville D, Verloes A: CHARGE syndrome: an update. *Eur J Hum Genet* 15(4):389–399, 2007.

766. Santoro G, Carrozza M, Russo MG, Calabro R: Symptomatic aorta pulmonary collaterals early after arterial switch procedure. *Pediatr Cardiol* 29:838–841, 2008.

767. Sarajuuri A: Neurodevelopmental and neuroradiologic outcomes in patients with univentricular heart aged 5 to 7 years: related risk factor analysis. *J Thorac Cardovasc Surg* 133:1524, 2007.

768. Sarubbi B, Musto B, Ducceschi V, et al: Congenital junctional ectopic tachycardia in children and adolescents: a 20 year experience based study. *Heart* 88(2):188–190, 2002.

769. Satiel A, Sanfilippo DJ, Hendler R, Lister G: Oxygen transport during anemia in pigs: effects of digoxin on metabolism. *Am J Physiol* 263(1 pt 2):H208–H217, 1992.

770. Satou GM, Perry SB, Gauvereau K, et al: Echocardiographic predictors of coronary artery pathology in pulmonary atresia with intact ventricular septum. *Am J Cardiol* 85:1319, 2000.

771. Satou GM, Perry SB, Lock JE, et al: Repeat balloon dilation of congenital valvular aortic stenosis: immediate results and midterm outcome. *Catheter Cardiovasc Interv* 47:47, 1999.

772. Saul JP: Electrophysiologic therapeutic catheterization. In Allen HD, Driscoll DJ, Feltes TF, Shaddy RE, editors: *Moss and Adams' heart disease in infants, children, and adolescent including the fetus and young adult,* ed 7, Philadelphia, 2008, Lippincott Williams & Wilkins.

773. Saul JP, Scott WA, Brown S, et al: Intravenous amiodarone for incessant tachyarrhythmias in children: a randomized, double-blind, antiarrhythmic drug trial. *Circulation* 112(22):3470–3477, 2005.

774. Schaffer MS, Gow RM, Moak JP, et al: Mortality following radiofrequency catheter ablation (from the Pediatric Radiofrequency Ablation Registry). Participating members of the Pediatric Electrophysiology Society. *Am J Cardiol* 86:639, 2000.

775. Schaffer MS, Silka MJ, Ross BA, et al: Inadvertent atrioventricular block during radiofrequency catheter ablation. Results of the Pediatric Radiofrequency Ablation Registry. *Pediatric Electrophysiology Society* 94(12):3214–3220, 1996.

776. Scheithauer S, Haefner H, Schwanz T, et al: Compliance with hand hygiene on surgical, medical, and neuralgic intensive care units: direct observation versus calculated disinfectant usage. *Am J Infect Contr* 37(10):835–841, 2009.

777. Scheurer MA, Hill EG, Vasuki N, et al: Survival after bidirectional cavopulmonary anastomosis: analysis of preoperative risk factors. *J Thorac Cardiovasc Surg* 134:82, 2007.

778. Schmidt B, Roberts RS, Fanaroff A, et al: Indomethacin prophylaxis, patent ductus arteriosus, and the risk of bronchopulmonary dysplasia: further analyses from the trial of indomethacin prophylaxis in preterms (TIPP). *J Pediatr* 148:730–734, 2006.

779. Schmidt MA, Ohazama CJ, Agyeman KO, et al: Real-time three-dimensional echocardiography for measurement of left ventricular volumes. *Am J Cardiol* 84:1434, 1999.

780. Schneider DJ, Moore JW: Aortic stenosis. In Allen HD, Shaddy RE, Driscoll DJ, Feltes TF, editors: *Moss and Adams' heart disease in infants, children, and adolescents, including the fetus and young adult,* ed 7, Philadelphia, 2008, Lippincott Williams & Wilkins.

781. Schräder R: Catheter closure of secundum ASD using "other" devices. *Interv Cardiol* 16(5):409–412, 2003.

782. Schranz D, Michel-Behnke IM, Akintuerk H: Letter by Schranz et al. regarding article Comparison of the profiles of postoperative systemic hemodynamics and oxygen transport in neonates after the hybrid or the Norwood procedure: a pilot study. *Circulation* 117:e296, 2008.

783. Schranz D, Michel-Behnke I, Heyer R, Vogel M, Bauer J, et al: Stent Implantation of the Arterial Duct in Newborns with a Truly Duct-Dependent Pulmonary Circulation: A Single-Center Experience with Emphasis on Aspects of the Interventional Technique. *Interv Cardiol* Jul 19: 1–8, 2010.

784. Schreiber MD, Heymann MA, Soifer SJ: Increased arterial pH, not decreased $PaCO_2$ attenuates hypoxia-induced pulmonary vasoconstriction in newborn lambs. *Pediatr Res* 20:113–117, 1986.

785. Schulze-Neick I, Werner H, Penny DJ, et al: Acute ventilatory restriction in children after weaning off inhaled nitric oxide: relation to rebound pulmonary hypertension. *Int Care Med* 25(1):76, 1999.

786. Schulz L, Twite M, Liang X, et al: A case of childhood peripheral T-cell lymphoma with massive cardiac infiltration. *J Ped Hematol/Oncol* 26(1):48–51, 2004.

787. Seale AN, Uemura H, Webber SA, et al: Total anomalous pulmonary venous connection: Morphology and outcome from an international population-based study. *Circulation* 122:2718, 2010.

788. Seckel MA: Ask the experts. *Crit Care Nurse* 28(10):65–66, 2008.

789. Seguchi M, Nakazawa M, Momma K: Further evidence suggesting a limited role of digitalis in infants with circulatory congestion secondary to large ventricular septal defect. *Am J Cardiol* 83:1408–1411, 1999.

790. Seino Y, Ogawa A, Yamashita T, et al: Application of NT-proBNP and BNP measurements in cardiac care: a more discerning marker for the detection and evaluation of heart failure. *Eur J Heart Fail* 6:295–300, 2004.

791. Selamet Tierney ES, Wald RM, McElhinney DB, et al: Changes in left heart hemodynamics after technically successful in-utero aortic valvuloplasty. *Ultrasound Obstet Gynecol* 30:715, 2007.

792. Shaddy R: Beta-adrenergic blockade in the treatment of pediatric heart failure. *Prog Pediatr Cardiol* 12:113–118, 2000.

793. Shaddy RE, Boucek MM, Hsu DT, et al: Pediatric Carvedilol Study Group: Carvedilol for children and adolescents with heart failure: a randomized controlled trial. *JAMA* 298:1171–1179, 2007.

794. Shaddy RE, Tani LY, Gidding SS, et al: Beta-blocker treatment of dilated cardiomyopathy with congestive heart failure in children: a multi-institutional experience. *J Heart Lung Transplant* 18:269–274, 1999.

795. Sheffield JS, Butler-Koster EL, Casey BM, et al: Maternal diabetes mellitus and infant malformations. *Obstet Gynecol* 100(pt 1):925–930, 2002.

796. Shellock FJ, Kanal E: Policies, guidelines, and recommendations for MR imaging safety and patient management. *J Magn Reson Imaging* 1:97, 1991.

797. Shikata F, Yagihara T, Kagisaki K, et al: Does the off-pump Fontan procedure ameliorate the volume and duration of pleural and peritoneal effusions? *Eur J Cardiothorac Surg* 34:570, 2008.

798. Shillingford AJ, Glanzman MM, Ittenbach RF, et al: Inattention, hyperactivity, and school performance in a population of school-age children with complex congenital heart disease. *Pediatircs* 121:759, 2008.

799. Shin'oka T, Kurosawa H, Imai Y, et al: Outcome of definitive surgical repair for congenitally corrected transposition of the great

arteries or double outlet right ventricle with discordant atrioventricular connections: disk analysis in 189 patients. *J Thorac Cardiovasc Surg* 133(5):1318–1328, 2007.

800. Shinkawa T: Atrial septal defect repair through limited lateral thoracotomy in children. *Jpn J Thorac Cardiovasc Surg* 54(11):469–471, 2006.
801. Shiota T, McCarthy PM, White RD, et al: Initial clinical experience of real-time three-dimensional echocardiography in patients with ischemic and idiopathic dilated cardiomyopathy. *Am J Cardiol* 84:1068, 1999.
802. Shore DF: Late repair and reoperations in adults with congenital heart disease. In Gatzoulis MA, Webb GA, Daubeney PEF, editors: *Diagnosis and management of adult congenital heart disease,* Edinburgh, 2003, Churchill Livingstone.
803. Shprintzen RJ: *Shprintzen? DiGeorge? Velo-Cardio-Facial?* 1995, Chaser News Fall.
804. Shukla AV, Almodovar MC: Anesthesia considerations for children with pulmonary hypertension. *Pediatr Crit Care Med* 11(2 Suppl):S70–S73, 2010.
805. Shulman ST: Is there a role for corticosteriods in Kawasaki disease? *J Pediatrics* 142:601–603, 2003.
806. Sievert H, Qureshi SA, Wilson N, Hijazi ZM: *Percutaneous interventions for congenital heart disease.* Andover, Hampshire, 2007, Informa UK Ltd.
807. Silva JN, Van Hare G: Management of postoperative pediatric cardiac arrhythmias: current state of the art. *Curr Treat Opt Cardiovasc Med* 11:410–416, 2009.
808. Silverman NH: *Pediatric echocardiography.* Baltimore, 1993, Williams & Wilkins.
809. Silversides C, Coleman J, Siu S: Physiology and management of pregnancy in the young adult with congenital heart disease. In Allen HD, Driscoll DJ, Feltes TF, Shaddy RE, editors: *Moss and Adams' heart disease in infants, children, and adolescent including the fetus and young adult,* ed 7, Philadelphia, 2008, Lippincott Williams & Wilkins.
810. Simonneau G, Robbins IM, Beghetti M, et al: Updated clinical classification of pulmonary hypertension. *J Am Coll Cardiol* 54(1):s43, 2009.
811. Simpson SQ, Peterson DA, O'Brien-Ladner: Development and implementation of an CCU quality improvement checklist. *AACN Advan Crit Care* 18(2):183–189, 2007.
812. Simsic JM, Bradley SM, Stroud MR, Atz AM: Risk factors for interstage death after the Norwood procedure. *Pediatr Cardiol* 26:400, 2005.
813. Sittiwangkul R, Azakie A, Van Arsdell GS, et al: Outcomes of tricuspid atresia in the Fontan era. *Ann Thorac Surg* 77:889, 2004.
814. Skanes AC, Jones DL, Teefy P, et al: Safety and feasibility of cryothermal ablation within the mid- and distal coronary sinus. *J Cariovascu Electrophysiol* 15:1319, 2004.
815. Skippen P, Sanatani S, Forese N, et al: Pacemaker therapy of postoperative arrhythmias after pediatric cardiac surgery. *Pediatr Crit Care Med* 11(1):133–138, 2010.
816. Skippen P, Sanatani S, Gow RM, Froese N: Diagnosis of postoperative arrhythmias following paediatric cardiac surgery. *Anaesth Int Care* 37(5):705–719, 2009.
817. Sletten LJ, Pierpont MEM: Variation in severity of cardiac disease in Holt-Oram syndrome. *Am J Med Genet* 65:128–132, 1996.
818. Smith P: Primary care in children with congenital heart disease. *J Pediatric Nurs* 16(5):308–319, 2001.
819. Snider AR, Serwer GA, Ritter SB: *Echocardiography in pediatric heart disease.* St Louis, 1997, Mosby.
820. Society of Thoracic Surgeons: *Duke clinical research institute 2010 congenital report executive summary.* Available from: http://sts.org/national-database/database-managers/executive-summaries, 2012.
821. Society of Thoracic Surgeons: *Congenial heart surgery data summary 2006-2010 procedures neonates (0-30 days).* Available from: http://sts.org/national-database/database-managers/executive-summaries, Accessed March 26, 2011, 2012.
822. Society of Thoracic Surgeons: *Duke clinical research institute 2010 congenital report executive summary.* http://sts.org/national-database/database-managers/executive-summaries, 2012.
823. Society of Thoracic Surgeons: Congenial Heart Surgery Data Summary 2006-2010 Procedures http://sts.org/sites/default/files/documents/STSCONG-NeonatesSummary_Fall2010.pdf Accessed March 28, 2011, 2012.

824. Sokoloski MC: Tachyarrhythmas confined to the atrium. In Gillette PC, Garson A Jr, editors: *Clinical pediatric arrhythmias,* ed 2, Philadelphia, 1999, Saunders, pp. 78–96.
825. Srinivasan C, Jaquiss RDB, Morrow R, et al: Impact of staged palliation on somatic growth in patients with hypoplastic left heart syndrome. *Congenit Heart Dis* 5:546, 2010.
826. Srivastava D, Baldwin HS: Molecular determinants of cardiac development and disease. In Allen HD, Shaddy RE, Driscoll DJ, Feltes TF, editors: *Moss and Adams' heart disease in infants, children, and adolescents, including the fetus and young adult,* ed. 7, Philadelphia, 2008, Lippincott Williams & Wilkins, pp. 2510–2523.
827. Stanfill R, Nykanen DG, Osorio S, et al: Stent implantation is effective treatment of vascular stenosis in young infants with congenital heart disease: acute implantation and long-term follow-up results. *Catheter Cardiovasc Interv* 71:831, 2008.
828. Stanger P, Cassidy SC, Girod DA, et al: Balloon pulmonary valvuloplasty: results of the Valvuloplasty and Angioplasty of Congenital Anomalies Registry. *Am J Cardiol* 65:775–783, 1990.
829. Stern H, Weil J, Vogt B: Captopril in dilated cardiomyopathy: acute and long term effects in a prospective study of hemodynamic and hormonal effects. *Pediatr Cardiol* 11:22–28, 1990.
830. Strauss A: *Presentation: the genetic basis of pediatric heart disease. at american heart association 76th scientific sessions.* Orlando, FL. 2003.
831. Stuart AG, Williams A: Marfan's syndrome and the heart. *Arch Dis Child* 92(4):351–356, 2007.
832. Surawicz B, Knilans TK: *Chou's electrocardiography in clinical practice: adult and pediatric.* ed 5, Philadelphia, 2001, W.B. Saunders.
833. Surawicz B, Parikh SR: Prevalence of Male and Female Patterns of Early Ventricular Repolarization in the Normal ECG of Males and Females From Childhood to Old Age. *J Am Coll Cardiol* 40:1870–1876, 2002.
834. Suris JC, Resnick MD, Cassuto N, Blum RW: Sexual behavior of adolescents with chronic disease and disability. *J Adolesc Health* 19(2):124–131, 1996.
835. Swan L, Hillis WS, Cameron A: Family planning requirements of adults with congenital heart disease. *Heart* 78(1):9–11, 1997.
836. Tabbutt S, Nord AS, Jarvik GP, et al: Neurodevelopmental outcomes after staged palliation for hypoplastic left heart syndrome. *Pediatrics* 121(3):476, 2008.
837. Tak YR, McCubbin M: Family stress, perceived social support and coping following the diagnosis of a child's congenital heart disease. *J Adv Nurs* 39(2):190–198, 2002.
838. Takahashi M, Newburger JW: Kawasaki disease (mucocutaneous lymph node syndrome). In Allen HD, Driscol DJ, Shaddy RE, Feltes TF, editors: *Moss and Adams' heart disease in infants, children, and adolescents, including the fetus and young adult,* ed 7, Philadelphia, 2008, Lippincott Williams & Wilkins.
839. Taketomo CK, Hodding JH, Kraus DM: *Pediatric dosage handbook.* ed 13, Hudson, OH, 2006, Lexi-Comp.
840. Takeuchi K, McGowan FX, Bacha EZ, et al: Analysis of surgical outcome in complex double-outlet right ventricle with heterotaxy syndrome or complete atrioventricular canal defect. *Ann Thorac Surg* 82(1):146–152, 2006.
841. Talner NS: Heart failure. In Adams FH, Emmanouil-ides GC, Riemenschneider TA, editors: *Moss' heart disease in infants, children, and adolescents,* ed 4, Baltimore, 1989, Williams & Wilkins.
842. Talwar S, Choudhary SK, Mathur A, et al: Changing outcomes of pulmonary artery banding with the percutaneously adjustable pulmonary artery band. *Ann Thorac Surg* 85:593, 2008.
843. Tanel RE, Kirshbom PM, Paridon SM, et al: Long-term noninvasive arrhythmia assessment after total anomalous pulmonary venous connection repair. *Am Heart J* 153(2):267–274, 2007.
844. Tanel RE, Wernovsky G, Landzberg MJ, et al: Coronary artery abnormalities detected at cardiac catheterization following the arterial switch operation for transposition of the great arteries. *Am J Cardiol* 76:153, 1995.
845. Taylor MB, Laussen PC: Fundamentals of management of acute postoperative pulmonary hypertension. *Pediatr Crit Care Med* 11(2 Suppl):S27–S29, 2010.
846. Tchervenkov CI, Walters HL III, Chu VF: Congenital heart surgery nomenclature and database project: double outlet left ventricle. *Ann Thorac Surg* 69:S264–S269, 2000.

847. Tester DJ, Ackerman MJ: Cardiomyopathic and channelopathic causes of sudden unexplained death in infants and children. *Annu Rev Med* 60:69–84, 2009.

848. Texter KM, Kertesz NJ, Friedman RA, Fenrich AL Jr, : Atrial flutter in infants. *J Am Coll Cardiol* 48(5):1040–1046, 2006.

849. Thacker D, Patel A, Dodds K, et al: Use of oral budesonide in the management of protein-losing enteropathy after the Fontan operation. *Ann Thorac Surg* 89:837, 2010.

850. The CONSENSUS Trial Study Group: Effects of enalapril on mortality in severe congestive heart failure. Results of the Cooperative North Scandinavian Enalapril Survival Study. *N Engl J Med* 316:1429–1435, 1987.

851. The Society of Thoracic Surgeons: *STS Congenital Heart Surgery Data Summary, 2006-2010 Procedures, Infants (31 days-1 year).* Available from: http://sts.org/sites/default/files/documents/STSCONG-InfantsSummary_Fall2010.pdf Accessed March 28, 2011, 2012.

852. The Society of Thoracic Surgeons: *STS Congenital Heart Surgery Data Summary, 2006-2010 Procedures, Neonates (0-30 days).* Available from: http://sts.org/sites/default/files/documents/STSCONG-NeonatesSummary_Fall2010.pdf Accessed March 28, 2012.

853. The Society of Thoracic Surgeons: *STS Congenital Heart Surgery Data Summary, 2003-2006 Procedures, Children (>1 year to <18 years).* Available from: http://sts.org/sites/default/files/documents/STSCONG-ChildrenSummary_Fall2010.pdf Accessed March 28, 2011, 2012.

854. The Society of Thoracic Surgeons: *STS Congenital Heart Surgery Data Summary, 2003-2006 Procedures, Infants (31 days-1 year).* Available from: http://sts.org/sites/default/files/documents/STSCONG-InfantsSummary_Fall2010.pdf Accessed March 28, 2011, 2012.

855. The Society of Thoracic Surgeons: *STS Congenital Heart Surgery Data Summary, 2006-2010 Procedures, Neonates (0-30 days).* Available from: http://sts.org/sites/default/files/documents/STSCONG-NeonatesSummary_Fall2010.pdf Accessed March 28, 2011, 2012.

856. The Society of Thoracic Surgeons: *STS Congenital Heart Surgery Data Summary, 2006-2010 Procedures, Children (>1 year to <18 years).* Available from: http://sts.org/sites/default/files/documents/STSCONG-ChildrenSummary_Fall2010.pdf Accessed March 28, 2011, 2012.

857. The Society of Thoracic Surgeons: *STS congenital heart surgery data summary, 2006-2010 procedures, all patients.* Available from: http://sts.org/sites/default/files/documents/STSCONG-AllPatients-Summary_Fall2010.pdf Accessed March 28, 2011, 2012.

858. The Society of Thoracic Surgeons: *STS congenital heart surgery data summary, 2006-2010 procedures, infants.* Available from: http://sts.org/sites/default/files/documents/STSCONG-InfantsSummary_Fall2010.pdf Accessed March 28, 2011, 2012.

859. The Society of Thoracic Surgeons: *STS congenital heart surgery data summary, 2003-2006 procedures, neonates.* Available from: http://sts.org/sites/default/files/documents/STSCONG-NeonatesSummary_Fall2010.pdf Accessed March 28, 2011, 2012.

860. The Society of Thoracic Surgeons: *STS congenital heart surgery data summary, 2003-2006 procedures, children (>1 year to <18 years).* Available from: http://sts.org/sites/default/files/documents/STSCONG-ChildrenSummary_Fall2010.pdf Accessed March 28, 2011, 2012.

861. The SOLVD Investigators: Effect of enalapril on survival in patients with reduced left ventricular ejection fractions and congestive heart failure. *N Engl J Med* 325:293–302, 1991.

862. Therrien J, Webb GD, Gatzoulis MA: Reversal of protein losing enteropathy with prednisone in adults with modified Fontan operations: long term palliation or bridge to cardiac transplant? *Heart* 82:241, 1999.

863. Thibodeau GA, Patton KT: *Anatomy and physiology.* ed 6, St Louis, 2007, Mosby.

864. Thompson L: Care of the patient with adult congenital heart disease. *Crit Care Nurs Q* 30:3, 2007.

865. Thorne S: Atrioventricular valve atresia. In Gatzoulis MA, Webb GA, Daubeney PEF, editors: *Diagnosis and management of adult congenital heart disease*, Edinburgh, 2003, Churchill Livingstone.

866. Thulstrup AM, Bonde JP: Maternal occupational exposure and risk of specific birth defects. *Occup Med (Lond)* 56(8):532–543, 2006.

867. Tong EM, Sparacino SA, Messias DKH, et al: Growing up with congenital heart disease: the dilemmas of adolescents and young adults. *Cardiol Young* 8:303, 1998.

868. Toriello H: Recent genetic updates. *Spectrum Health XX Files* 6(5):2, 2007.

869. Tororiello TA, Friedman JD, McKenzie D, et al: Mediastinitis after pediatric cardiac surgery: a 15-year experience at a single institution. *Ann Thorac Surg* 76:1655–1660, 2003.

870. Towbin JA: Cardiomyopathies. In Moller JH, editor: *Pediatric cardiovascular medicine*, London, 2000, Churchill Livingstone, p. 758.

871. Towbin JA: Genetics of heart disease. *Pediatr Cardiol Today* 2(8):1–8, 2004.

872. Towbin J: Hypertrophic cardiomyopathy. In Chang AC, Towbin JA, editors: *Heart failure in children and young adults*, Philadelphia, 2006, Elsevier, pp. 278–293.

873. Towbin JA: Myocarditis. In Allen HD, Shaddy RE, Driscoll DJ, Feltes TF, editors: *Moss and Adams' heart disease in infants, children, and adolescents, including the fetus and young adult*, ed 7, Philadelphia, 2008, Lippincott Williams & Wilkins, pp. 1207–1225.

874. Tremper RS: Mediastinal exploration in the surgical intensive care unit. *Dimens Crit Care Nurse* 23(1):24–30, 2004.

875. Treves S, Kuruc A: Radionuclide evaluation of circulatory shunts. *Cardiol Clin* 1:427, 1983.

876. Tulloh R: Management and therapeutic options in pediatric pulmonary hypertension. *Expert Rev Cardiovasc Ther* 4(3):361, 2006.

877. Tulzer F, Arzt W, Franklin RC, et al: Fetal pulmonary valvuloplasty for critical pulmonary stenosis or atresia with intact septum. *Lancet* 360:1567, 2002.

878. Turley K, Hanley FL, Verrier ED, et al: The Mustard procedure in infants (less than 100 days of age). Ten year follow up. *J Thorac Cardiovasc Surg* 96:849, 1988.

879. Tweddell JS: The Norwood procedure with an innominate artery-to-pulmonary artery shunt. *Operative Techniques Thorac Cardiovasc Surg* 10:123, 2005.

880. Tweddell JS, Ghanayem NS, Mussattto KA, et al: Mixed venous oxygen saturation monitoring after stage 1 palliation for hypoplastic left heart syndrome. *Ann Thorac Surg* 84:1301, 2007.

881. Tweddell JS, Hoffman GM, Ghanayem NS, et al: Hypoplastic left heart syndrome. In Allen HD, Driscoll DJ, Feltes TF, Shaddy RE, editors: *Moss and Adams' heart disease in infants, children, and adolescents, including the fetus and young adult*, ed 7, Philadelphia, 2008, Lippincott Williams & Wilkins.

882. Tweddell JS, Hoffman GM, Mussatto KA, et al: Improved survival of patients undergoing palliation of hypoplastic left heart syndrome: lessons learned from 115 consecutive patients. *Circulation* 106 (Suppl 1):182, 2002.

883. Tworetzky W, McElhinney DB, Marx GR, Benson CB, et al: In utero valvuloplasty for pulmonary atresia with hypoplastic right ventricle: techniques and outcomes. *Pediatrics* 124(3):e510–e518, 2009.

884. Tworetzky W, Wilkins-Haug L, Jennings JW, et al: Balloon dilation of severe aortic stenosis in the fetus: potential for prevention of hypoplastic left heart syndrome: candidate selection, technique, and results of successful intervention. *Circulation* 110:2125, 2004.

885. Uhl TL: Viral myocarditis in children. *Crit Care Nurse* 28(1):42–63, 2008.

886. Ungerleider RM: Tetralogy of Fallot. In Nichols DM, editor in chief. *Critical heart disease in infants and children*, ed 2, St Louis, 2002, Elsevier.

887. Ungerleider RM, Shen I, Yeh T, et al: Routine mechanical ventricular assist following the Norwood procedure: improved neurologic outcome and excellent hospital survival. *Ann Thorac Surg* 77:18, 2004.

888. Uthaman B, Ubushaban L, Al-Qbandi M, Rathinasamy J: The impact of interruption of anomalous systemic arterial supply on scimitar syndrome presenting during infancy. *Catheter Cardiovasc Interv* 71(5):671–678, 2008.

889. Uzark K, Jones K: Parenting stress and children with heart disease. *J Pediatr Healthcare* 17(4):163–168, 2003.

890. Uzark K, Jones K, Slusher J, et al: Quality of life in children with heart disease as perceived by children and parents. *Pediatrics* 121 (5):e1060–e1067, 2008.

891. Uzark K, Rudd N, Elixson M, et al: Interstage weight gain in infants following the Norwood operation: Changing the outcome. In *American College of Cardiology Conference*, Poster presentation, April, 2011.

892. Valente AM, Rhodes JF: Current indications and contraindications for transcatheter atrial septal defect and patent foramen ovale device closure. *Am Heart J* 153:581–584, 2007.

893. Valsangiacomo ER, Hornberger LK, Barrea C, et al: Partial and total anomalous pulmonary venous connection in the fetus: two-dimensional and Doppler echocardiographic findings. *Ultrasound Obstet Gynecol* 22(3):257–263, 2003.

894. Van Hare GF: Supraventricular tachycardia. In Gillette PC, Garson A, editors: *Clinical pediatric arrhythmias*, Philadelphia, 1999, Saunders, pp. 97–120.

895. Van Hare GF, Dubin AM: *The normal electrocardiogram*. pp. 253–268, In Allen HD, Driscoll DJ, Shaddy RE, Feltes TF, editors: *Moss and Adams' heart disease in infants, children, and adolescents*, 7th ed, Philadelphia, 2008, Lippincott Williams & Wilkins.

896. Van Hare GF, Javitz H, Carmelli D, et al: Prospective assessment after pediatric cardiac ablation: demographics, medical profiles, and initial outcomes. *J Cardiovasc Electrophysiol* 15(7):759–770, 2004.

897. Van Hare GF, Javitz H, Carmelli D, et al: Prospective assessment after pediatric cardiac ablation: recurrence at 1 year after initially successful ablation of supraventricular tachycardia. *Heart Rhythm* 1 (2):188–196, 2004.

898. Van Hare GF, Velvis H, Langberg JJ: Successful transcatheter ablation of congenital junctional ectopic tachycardia in a ten-month-old infant using radiofrequency energy. *Pacing Clin Electrophysiol* 13 (6):730–735, 1990.

899. Van Mierop LHS, Kutsche LM, Victorica BE: Ebstein anomaly. In Adams FH, Emmanouilides GC, Riemenschneider TA, editors: *Moss' heart disease in infants, children, and adolescents*, ed 4, Baltimore, 1989, Williams & Wilkins.

900. Van Praagh R: Cardiac anatomy. In Chang AC, Hanley FL, Wernovsky G, Wessel DL, editors: *Pediatric cardiac intensive care*, Toronto, 1998, Williams & Wilkins, p. 10.

901. Van Praagh R: Cardiac anatomy. In Chang AC, Hanley FL, Wernovsky G, Wessel DL, editors: *Pediatric cardiac intensive care*, Toronto, 1998, Williams & Wilkins, pp. 3–16.

902. Van Praagh R: Embryology. In Keane JF, Lock JE, Fyler DC, editors: *Nadas' pediatric cardiology*, ed 2, Philadelphia, 2006, Saunders Elsevier.

903. Van Praagh R, et al: Malpositions of the heart. In Adams FH, Emmanouilides GC, Riemenschneider TA, editors: *Moss' heart disease in Infants, children, and adolescents*, ed 4, Baltimore, 1989, Williams & Wilkins.

904. Van Praagh R, Van Praagh S: The anatomy of common aorticopulmonary trunk (truncus arteriosus communis) and its embryologic implications: a study of 57 necropsy cases. *Am J Cardiol* 16:1245, 1965.

905. Van Son JA, Lacquet LK, Smedts F: Patterns of ductal tissue in coarctation of the aorta in early infancy. *J Thorac Cardiovasc Surg* 105:368–369, 1993.

906. Varagich J, Frohlich ED: Local cardiac rennin-angiotensin system: hypertension and cardiac failure. *J Mol Cell Cardiol* 34:1435–1442, 2002.

907. Varan B, Tokel K, Yilmaz G: Malnutrition and growth failure in cyanotic and acyanotic congenital heart disease with and without pulmonary hypertension. *Arch Dis Child* 81:49–52, 1999.

908. Vida VL, Bacha EA, Larrazabal A, et al: Hypoplastic left heart syndrome with intact or highly restrictive atrial septum: surgical experience from a single center. *Ann Thorac Surg* 84:581, 2007.

909. Villain E, Vetter VL, Garcia JM, et al: Evolving concepts in the management of congenital junctional ectopic tachycardia. A multicenter study. *Circulation* 81(5):1544–1549, 1990.

910. Vincent RH, Diehl HJ: Intervention in pediatric cardiac catheterization, CCNQ. *Crit Care Nurs Q* 25(3):37–47, 2002.

911. Visconti KJ, Saudino KJ, Rappaport LA, et al: Influence of parental stress and social support on the behavioral adjustment of children with transposition of the great arteries. *JDBP* 23(5):314–321, 2002.

912. von Loon RLE, Hoendermis ES, Duffels MGJ, et al: Long-term effect of bosentan in adults versus children with pulmonary arterial hypertension associated with systemic-to-pulmonary shunt. Does the beneficial effect persist? *Am Heart J* 154, 2007.

913. Vyas H, Ackerman MJ: Epinephrine QT stress testing in congenital long QT syndrome. *J Electrocardiol* 39(4 Suppl):S107–S113, 2006.

914. Vyas H, Driscoll DF, Cabalka AK, et al: Results of transcatheter Fontan fenestration to treat protein losing enteropathy. *Catheter Cardiovasc Interv* 69:584, 2007.

915. Wacker A, Kaemmerer H, Hollweck R, et al: Outcome of operated and unoperated adults with congenital cardiac disease lost to follow-up for more than five years. *Am J Cardiol* 95(6):776–779, 2005.

916. Wald RM, Tham EB, McCrindle BW, et al: Outcome after prenatal diagnosis of tricuspid atresia: a multicenter experience. *Am Heart J* 5:153, 2009.

917. Walker WE, Duncan JM, Frazier OH Jr, et al: Early experience with the ionescu-shiley pericardial xenograft valve. Accelerated calcification in children. *J Thorac Cardiovasc Surg* 86:570, 1983.

918. Wallace CA, French JW, Kahn SJ, Sherry DD: Initial IVIG treatment failure in kawasaki disease. *Pediatrics* 105:E78, 2000.

919. Walsh EP: Automatic atrial and junctional tachycardias. In Walsh EP, Saul JP, Triedman JK, editors: *Cardiac arrhythmias in children and adults with congenital heart disease*, Philadelphia, 2001, Lippincott Williams & Wilkins, pp. 115–135.

920. Walters HL III, Mavroudis C, Tchervenkov CI, et al: Double outlet right ventricle. The Society of Thoracic Surgeons Congenital Heart Surgery Nomenclature and Database Project. *Ann Thoracic Surg* 69 (Suppl):249, 2000.

921. Walters HL III, Pacifico AD: Double outlet ventricles. In Mavroudis C, Backer CL, editors: *Pediatric cardiac surgery*, ed 3, Philadelphia, 2003, Mosby/Elsevier.

922. Wan NS, Yim AP: Pulmonary ischaemia-reperfusion injury: role of apoptosis. *Eur Respir J* 25:356–363, 2005.

923. Warden HE, Gustafson RA, Tarnay TJ, et al: An alternative method for repair of partial anomalous venous connection to the superior vena cava. *Ann Thorac Surg* 38:601, 1984.

924. Warnes C: Transposition of the great arteries. *Circulation* 114(24): 2699, 2006.

925. Warnes CA, Liberthson R, Danielson GK, et al: Task force 1: the changing profile of congenital heart disease in adult life. *J Am Coll Cardiol* 37(5):1170–1175, 2001.

926. Warnes CA, Williams RG, Bashore TM, et al: ACC/AHA 2008 Guidelines for the Management of Adults with Congenital Heart Disease: a report of the American College of Cardiology/American Heart Association Task Force on Practice Guidelines (writing committee to develop guidelines on the management of adults with congenital heart disease). *Circulation* 118(23): e714–e833, 2008.

927. Warnes CA, Williams RG, Bashore TM, Child JS, Connolly HM, Dearani JA, Del Nido P, Fasules JW, Graham TP Jr, Hijazi ZM, Hunt SA, King ME, Landzberg MJ, Miner PD, Radford MJ, Walsh EP, Webb GD: ACC/AHA 2008 guidelines for the management of adults with congenital heart disease: executive summary: a report of the American College of Cardiology/American Heart Association Task Force on Practice Guidelines (Writing Committee to Develop Guidelines for the Management of Adults with Congenital Heart Disease). *Circulation* 118(23):2395–2451, 2008.

928. Webster G, Berul CI: Congenital long-QT syndromes: a clinical and genetic update from infancy through adulthood. *Trends Cardiovasc Med* 18(6):216–224, 2008.

929. Weinberger B, Laskin DL, Heck DE, et al: The toxicology of inhaled nitric oxide. *Toxicology Sci* 59:5, 2001.

930. Weinberg PM: Aortic arch anomalies. In Allen HD, Shaddy RE, Driscoll DJ, Feltes TF, editors: *Moss and Adams' heart disease in infants, children, and adolescents, including the fetus and young adult*, ed 7, Philadelphia, 2008, Lippincott Williams & Wilkins.

931. Weindling SN: Atrioventricular conduction disturbances. In Walsh EP, Saul JP, Triedman JK, editors: *Cardiac arrhythmias in children and young adults with congenital heart desease*, Philadelphia, 2001, Lippincott Williams & Wilkins, pp. 285–300.

932. Weismann CG, Gelb BD: The genetics of congenital heart disease: a review of recent developments. *Curr Opin Cardiol* 22(3):200–206, 2007.

933. Wernovsky G: Transposition of the great arteries. In Allen HD, Driscoll DJ, Feltes TF, Shaddy RE, editors: *Moss and Adams' heart disease in infants, children, and adolescents, including the fetus and young adult*, ed 7, Philadelphia, 2008, Lippincott Williams & Wilkins.

934. Wernovsky G, Bove EL: Single ventricle lesions. In Chang AC, Hanley F, Wernovsky G, Wessel DL, editors: *Pediatric cardiac intensive care*, Baltimore, 1998, Williams & Wilkins.

935. Wernovsky G, Chang AC, Wessel DL, Ravishankar C: Cardiac intensive care. In Allen HD, Driscoll DJ, Feltes TF, Shaddy RE, editors: *Moss and Adams' heart disease in infants, children, and*

adolescents including the fetus and young adult, ed 7, Philadelphia, 2008, Lippincott Williams & Wilkins.

936. Wernovsky G, Hanley FL: Pulmonary atresia with intact ventricular septum. In Chang AC, Hanley F, Wernovsky G, Wessel DL, editors: *Pediatric cardiac intensive care*, Baltimore, 1998, Williams & Wilkins.

937. Wernovsky G, Wypij D, Jonas RA, Mayer JE, et al: Postoperative course and hemodynamic profile after the arterial switch operation in neonates and infants: a comparison of low-flow cardiopulmonary bypass and circulatory arrest. *Circulation* 92:2226-2235, 1995.

938. Wessel D: Intensive care unit. In Keane JF, Lock JE, Fyler DC, editors: *Nadas' pediatric cardiology*, ed 2, St Louis, 2006, Saunders Elsevier.

939. Wessel DL: Managing low cardiac output syndrome after congenital heart surgery. *Crit Care Med* 29(10):S220-S2230, 2001.

940. Wessel DL, Almodovar MC, Laussen PC: Intensive care management of cardiac patients on extracorporeal membrane oxygenation. In Duncan B, editor: *Mechanical circulatory support for cardiac and respiratory failure in pediatric patients*, New York, 2001, Marcel Dekker.

941. Wessel DL, Berger F, Li JS, Fontecave S, Rakhit A, Newburger JW: for the CLARINET Investigators: A randomized trial of clopidogrel to reduce mortality and shunt-related morbidity in infants palliated with a systemic to pulmonary artery shunt. *Circulation* 122: A19459, 2010.

942. Wessel DL, Laussen PC: Intensive care unit. In Keane JF, Lock JE, Fyler DC, editors: *Nadas' pediatric cardiology*, ed 2, Philadelphia, 2006, Elsevier.

943. White PH: Access to healthcare: health insurance considerations for young adults with special healthcare needs/disabilities. *Pediatrics* 110(6 Pt 2):1328-1335, 2002.

944. Williams I, Atz AM, Cnota JC, et al: Predictors of functional status following Fontan palliation: development of a Fontan functional score. *Circulation* 116(suppl II):II-479 abstract. 2007.

945. Williams RG, Pearson GD, Barst RJ, et al: National Heart, Lung, and Blood Institute Working Group on research in adult congenital heart disease. Report of the National Heart, Lung, and Blood Institute Working Group on research in adult congenital heart disease. *J Am Coll Cardiol* 47(4):701-707, 2006.

946. Williams R, Pearson G, Barst R, et al: Report of the National Heart, Lung, and Blood Institute working group on research in adult congenital heart disease. *J Am Coll Cardiol* 47:701, 2006.

947. Williams IA, Gersony WM, Hellenbrand WE: Anomalous right coronary artery arising from the pulmonary artery: a report of 7 cases and a review of the literature. *Am Heart J* 152(5):1004e9-1004e17, 2006.

948. Wilson AD: *Total anomalous pulmonary venous connection on eMedicine specialties > Pediatrics: cardiac disease and critical care medicine > Cardiology*. Last Updated November 16. 2007.

949. Wilson J, Russell J, Williams W, Benson L: Fenestration of the Fontan circuit as treatment for plastic bronchitis. *Pediatr Cardiol* 26:717, 2005.

950. Wilson NJ, Clarkson PM, Baratt-Boyes BG, et al: Long-term outcome after the Mustard repair for simple transposition of the great arteries: 28-year followup. *J Am Coll Cardiol* 32(3):758, 1998.

951. Wilson W, Taubert KA, Gewitz M, et al: Prevention of Infective Endocarditis Guidelines From the American Heart Association: A Guideline From the American Heart Association Rheumatic Fever, Endocarditis, and Kawasaki Disease Committee, Council on Cardiovascular Disease in the Young, and the Council on Clinical Cardiology, Council on Cardiovascular Surgery and Anesthesia, and the Quality of Care and Outcomes Research Interdisciplinary Working Group. *Circulation* 116:1736-1754, 2007.

952. Wilson W, Taubert KA, Gewitz M, et al: Prevention of infective endocarditis. A guideline from the American Heart Association Rheumatic Fever, Endocarditis, and Kawasaki Disease Committee, Council on Cardiovascular Disease in the Young, and the Council on Clinical Cardiology, Council no Cardiovascular Surgery and Anesthesia, and the Quality of Care and Outcomes Research Interdisciplinary working group. *J Am Dent Assoc* 6(138):739-745, 2007.

953. Wojciechowski EA, Hurtig A, Dorn L: A natural history study of adolescents and young adults with sickle cell disease as they transfer to adult care: a need for case management services. *J Pediatr Nurs* 17(1):18-27, 2002.

954. Wong KK, Potts JE, Etheridge SP, Sanatani S: Medications used to manage supraventricular tachycardia in the infant: a North American survey. *Pediatr Cardiol* 27(2):199-203, 2006.

955. Wood AE, Healy DG, Nolke L, et al: Mitral valve reconstruction in a pediatric population: late clinical results and predictors of long-term outcome. *J Thorac Cardiovasc Surg* 130:66-73, 2005.

956. Wright J: Modifying the body: piercing and tattoos. *Nurs Stand* 10(11):27-30, 1995.

957. Yalta K, Turgut OO, Yilmaz A, et al: Asymptomatic total anomalous pulmonary venous connection with double drainage in a young adult: a case report. *Heart Surg Forum* 10:63, 2007.

958. Yamagishi M, Imai Y, Hoshino S, et al: Anatomic correction of atrioventricular discordance. *J Thorac Cardiovasc Surg* 105:1067, 1993.

959. Yamazaki I, Kondo J, Imoto K, et al: Corrected transposition of the great arteries diagnosed in an 84-year old woman. *J Cardiovasc Surg* 42(2):201, 2001.

960. Yeh T, Ramaciotti C, Leonard SR, et al: The aortic translocation (Nikaidoh) procedure: midterm results superior to the Rastelli procedure. *J Thorac Cardiovasc Surg* 133(2):461-469, 2007.

961. Yildrim SV, Tokel K, Saygili B, Varan B: The incidence and risk factors of arrhythmias in the early period after cardiac surgery in pediatric patients. *Turk J Pediatr* 50(6):549-553, 2008.

962. Yoshioka K, Niinuma H, Kawakami T, et al: Three-dimensional demonstration of total anomalous pulmonary venous return with contrast-enhanced magnetic resonance angiography. *Ann Thorac Surg* 78(6):2186, 2004.

963. Young JB, Abraham WT, Smith AL, et al: Multicenter InSync ICD Randomized Clinical Evaluation (MIRACLE ICD) Trial Investigators: Combined cardiac resynchronization and implantable cardioversion defibrillation in advanced chronic heart failure: the MIRACLE ICD Trial. *JAMA* 289:2685-2694, 2003.

964. Young M, Deal BJ, Wolff GS: Supraventricular tachycardia: electrophysiologic evaluation and treatment. In Deal BJ, Wolff GS, Gelband H, editors: *Current concepts in diagnosis and management of arrhythmias in infants and children*, Armonk, NY, 1998, Futura, pp. 145-180.

965. Zahn EM, Dobrolet NC, Nykanen DG, et al: Interventional catheterization performed in the early postoperative period after congenital heart surgery in children. *J Am Coll Cardiol* 43:1264, 2004.

966. Zajac A, Tomkiewicz L, Podolec P, et al: Cardiorespiratory response to exercise in children after modified fontan operation. *Scand Cardiovasc J* 36:67, 2002.

967. Zamanian RT, Haddad F, Doyle RL, et al: Management strategies for patients with pulmonary hypertension in the intensive care unit. *Crit Care Med* 35(9):2037, 2007.

968. Zaritsky A, Chernow B: Use of catecholamines in pediatrics. *J Pediatr* 105:341, 1984.

969. Zaritsky A, Chernow B: Catecholamines and other inotropes. In Chernow B, editor: *The pharmacologic approach to the critically ill patient*, ed 2, Baltimore, 1988, Williams & Wilkins.

970. Zeigler VL: Pediatric cardiac arrhythmias resulting in hemodynamic compromise. *Crit Care Nurs Clin North Am* 17(1):77-95, xi, 2005.

971. Zeigler VL, Gillette PC, Crawford FA Jr, et al: New approaches to treatment of incessant ventricular tachycardia in the very young. *J Am Coll Cardiol* 16(3):681-685, 1990.

972. Zoghbi WA, Farmer KL, Soto JG, et al: Accurate noninvasive quantification of stenotic aortic valve area by Doppler echocardiography. *Circulation* 73:452, 1986.

Pulmonary Disorders

9

Andrea M. Kline-Tilford • Lauren R. Sorce •
Daniel L. Levin • Nick G. Anas

evolve Be sure to check out the supplementary content available at
http://evolve.elsevier.com/Hazinski.

PEARLS

- Acute disease of the respiratory tract is the most common cause of illness in infancy and childhood.
- Respiratory disease is frequently present in critically ill or injured children; it may be present as a primary clinical problem or as a secondary complication.
- Altered level of consciousness in an infant or child with respiratory disease is often an ominous sign of deterioration.
- Children can have adequate oxygen saturation as documented by pulse oximetry, but they may be hypoxic because of inadequate oxygen delivery.
- Airway resistance increases exponentially as airway lumen size decreases.
- Once the PaO_2 falls below 60 mm Hg, even small additional decreases in PaO_2 are associated with a significant fall in arterial oxygen saturation and therefore in arterial oxygen content.
- Hypercarbia is difficult to detect clinically.

ESSENTIAL ANATOMY AND PHYSIOLOGY

The primary functions of the respiratory system are to move oxygen from the air into the blood and to move carbon dioxide from the blood into the air. This process is known as *gas exchange*. Gas exchange is adequate if arterial oxygen tension (PaO_2) and arterial carbon dioxide tension ($PaCO_2$) are maintained in the normal range. Gas exchange is either inadequate or excessive if these blood gas tensions are abnormal. Ventilation, measured by the elimination or accumulation of $PaCO_2$ is the product of breathing frequency (f) and tidal volume (V_T).

Oxygen and carbon dioxide move between air and blood in the lung by simple diffusion—that is, gases move from an area of high partial pressure to an area of low partial pressure. The respiratory muscles bring oxygen-rich, carbon dioxide-poor air through branching airway tubes to the alveolar air spaces. Oxygen-poor, carbon dioxide-rich systemic venous blood is pumped by the right ventricle through branching pulmonary arteries to lung capillaries, located within the walls of the alveoli. Virtually all cardiac output enters the lungs. Each red blood cell spends approximately 1 second exposed to alveolar air, a brief time that is more than adequate for the complete equilibration of oxygen and carbon dioxide between alveolar gas and capillary blood.

Embryology of the Lung

The respiratory system begins to develop by the fourth week of gestation. A lung bud branches from the primitive esophagus and eventually forms the airways and alveolar spaces. The pulmonary arteries form near the branching airways and their growth matches the growth of the airways. Although virtually all other body systems are physiologically ready for extrauterine life by as early as 25 weeks' gestation, the lungs require more time to mature. Thus lung maturity is the single most important factor that determines whether a premature infant can survive extrauterine life. Table 9-1 summarizes development of the respiratory system. Although the number of airway branches is fixed at birth, airway dimensions increase until the child is approximately 8 years old.[202] Alveoli multiply rapidly from an estimated 20 million alveoli at birth to 200 million by 3 years of age, and the number decreases thereafter. The alveolar surface is lined with type I and type II epithelial cells that are well developed at birth.[99]

Anatomy of the Chest

The thoracic cavity is formed by the ribs, intercostal muscles, and diaphragm, and it contains both lungs and the mediastinal structures. The right lung is composed of three lobes, and the left lung is composed of two lobes.[49] The heart, great vessels, nerves, trachea, and esophagus are located within the mediastinum. Pleural tissue covers each lung and adheres to the surface of the diaphragm and inner surface of the chest wall.

The diaphragm is the principal muscle of inspiration. If the chest wall is sufficiently stiff and expands during inspiratory contraction of the diaphragm, thoracic volume increases in both longitudinal and transverse dimensions, and thoracic cavity pressure decreases.

The diaphragm is innervated on each side of the chest by the phrenic nerve, which is formed by the third, fourth, and fifth cervical spinal nerves. In older children and adults, the chest wall is relatively rigid compared with the chest wall of the neonate and infant. Therefore, when the diaphragm contracts in older patients, intrathoracic pressure falls in proportion to the movement of the diaphragm, and air moves into the lungs (Fig. 9-1).

The ribs angle downward, from back to front, so that contraction of the external intercostal muscles will elevate the rib cage. The chest wall of an infant is compliant, and the external intercostal muscles stabilize the chest wall. When respiratory disease develops, pulmonary compliance is reduced.

483

Table 9-1   **Fetal Respiratory System Development**

Period of Gestation	Development
26 days	Lower respiratory system begins to develop until separation of the respiratory tract from the foregut is achieved
5 weeks	Lung buds form and begin to differentiate into the bronchi
7-10 weeks	Development of the larynx
5-16 weeks	Twenty-four orders of airway branches are formed
13-25 weeks	Canalicular period; bronchi enlarge and lung tissue becomes highly vascular
26-28 weeks	Lungs are capable of gas exchange; type II alveolar cells secrete surfactant
24 weeks to birth	Capillary network proliferates around the alveoli; approximately 8%-10% of cardiac output flows through the lung; pulmonary vascular resistance is high

When the diaphragm contracts and produces a decrease in intrathoracic pressure, intercostal and sternal retractions develop rather than inflation of the lungs (Fig. 9-2). The more the chest wall retracts, the less the lungs inflate.

The diaphragm inserts more horizontally in infants than in older children or adults, and diaphragm contraction can contribute to subcostal retractions, particularly when the infant is supine.[49] The greater the retractions present, the more the diaphragm will need to contract or shorten to generate an adequate V_T. Retractions make ventilation inefficient, with the result that the diaphragm must shorten and move as much as 130% of normal to generate a V_T; this increases the work of breathing and can lead to respiratory muscle fatigue.

The airways distribute gas to all parts of the lung. As air passes through the nose and mouth it is warmed, humidified,

and filtered. The upper airway thus serves as an air filter and an "air conditioner," so air that reaches the trachea has been warmed to body temperature, is fully saturated with water, and is freed of small particles.

The amount of water vapor a volume of gas can contain depends on the temperature of the gas. The higher the temperature of the inspired gas, the greater the amount of water vapor contained in the gas. Heat is transmitted to inspired air by convection, whereas water is added by evaporation from the airway surface. Therefore there is usually a loss of heat and water from the body during breathing. Although a healthy child copes well with this loss, a small infant with lung disease can lose a substantial amount of heat and water when tachypnea develops. When water is lost from the airway surface, ciliary activity and mucociliary clearance are impaired, which can lead to the formation of mucous plugs, atelectasis, air trapping, or infection. When the upper airway is bypassed with an endotracheal tube (ETT) or tracheostomy, inspired gas must be humidified to avoid damage to the airway surface by mucosal drying.

The Upper Airway

The neonate (0-4 weeks of age) breathes predominantly through the nose, so any obstruction in the nose or nasopharynx will increase upper airway resistance and increase the work of breathing. For example, respiratory failure can be exacerbated in neonates by the insertion of a nasogastric tube or obstruction of the nares by secretions.

The airways of infants and children are much smaller than the airways of adults. Resistance to air flow in any airway will increase exponentially if the airway radius is compromised (see Box 9-1 and Fig. 9-3). This means that any decrease in airway radius can significantly compromise effective gas flow or increase the work of breathing. Relatively small amounts of mucus accumulation, airway constriction, or edema can substantially reduce airway radius in the infant or child, resulting in an increase in the resistance to air flow and the work of breathing.

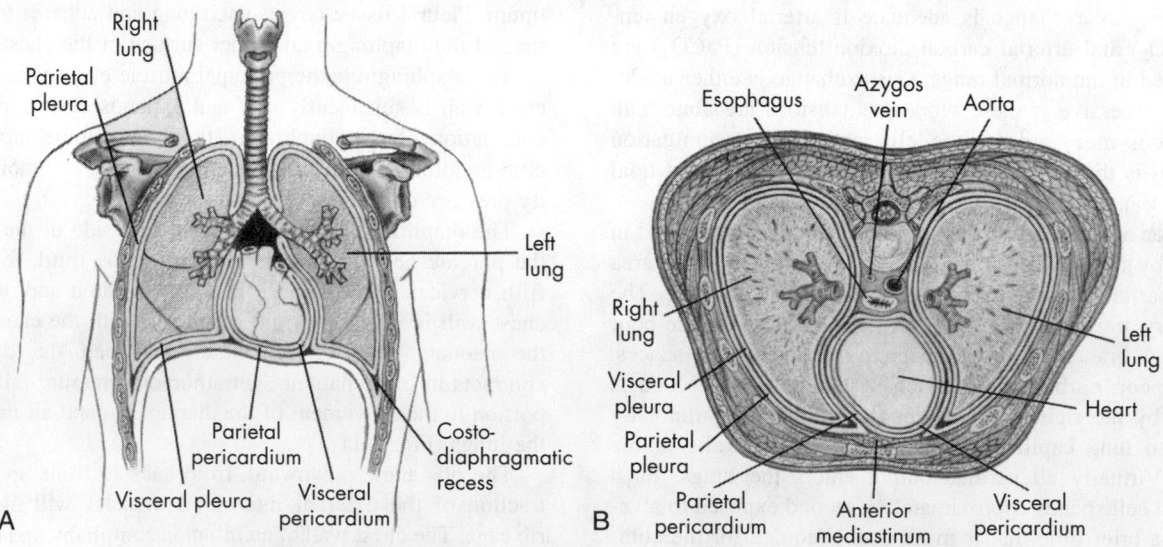

FIG. 9-1 Chest cavity and related structures. **A,** Anterior view. **B,** Cross section. (From Thompson JM, et al: *Mosby's manual of clinical nursing,* ed 2, St Louis, 1989, Mosby.)

Box 9-1   Poiseuille's Law

Resistance to flow increases as radius decreases, and it is increased by length of the tube or vessel.

$R = 8nl/\pi r^4$ when flow is laminar (substitute r^5 power if flow is turbulent)

l, Length of tube; *n*, gas viscosity; *r*, radius of tube.

Upper airway patency is maintained by the active contraction of muscles in the pharynx and larynx. Airway obstruction can develop if these muscles do not function properly or if the neck of an infant is flexed or extended. Airway obstruction can also develop during rapid-eye-movement sleep, when muscle tone is markedly reduced. The upper airway of the infant is fairly pliable and it can narrow during inspiration.

The infant upper airway is shaped like a funnel, whereas the upper airway of the older child and adult is more tubular. The glottis of an infant is located more anteriorly and more cephalad than in an older child, and the epiglottis is longer, making intubation of the trachea more difficult in the small infant, especially when the neck is hyperextended. The narrowest portion of the infant's airway is at the level of the cricoid, whereas the narrowest portion of the airway in the adult is at the level of the vocal cords. Small amounts of edema or obstruction in the cricoid (subglottic) area will produce an increase in airway resistance and can lead to respiratory failure. Postnatally the airways increase in both length and diameter and major changes occur in the terminal respiratory units as the number and size of the alveoli increase.[49,182]

Compliance and Resistance

From the time of the first breath, elastic fibers in the lung tissue create a tendency for the lungs to recoil inward (away from the chest wall). This recoil tendency is balanced by the propensity of the chest wall to spring outward. The net effect of these two opposing forces is to create a subatmospheric pressure in the intrathoracic space at the end of a normal breath (Fig. 9-2). During inspiration, the volume of the thoracic cavity is increased, and intrathoracic pressure becomes more negative with respect to atmospheric pressure. As a result, air moves from the mouth to the alveolar spaces. At the end of inspiration, the elastic recoil of the lungs and chest wall cause alveolar pressure to rise above atmospheric pressure, producing expiratory flow. In a person with normal lungs, expiration is passive and requires no muscular work.[92]

The ratio of lung volume to transpulmonary pressure is called *compliance*. Compliance of the lung (C_L) is a measure

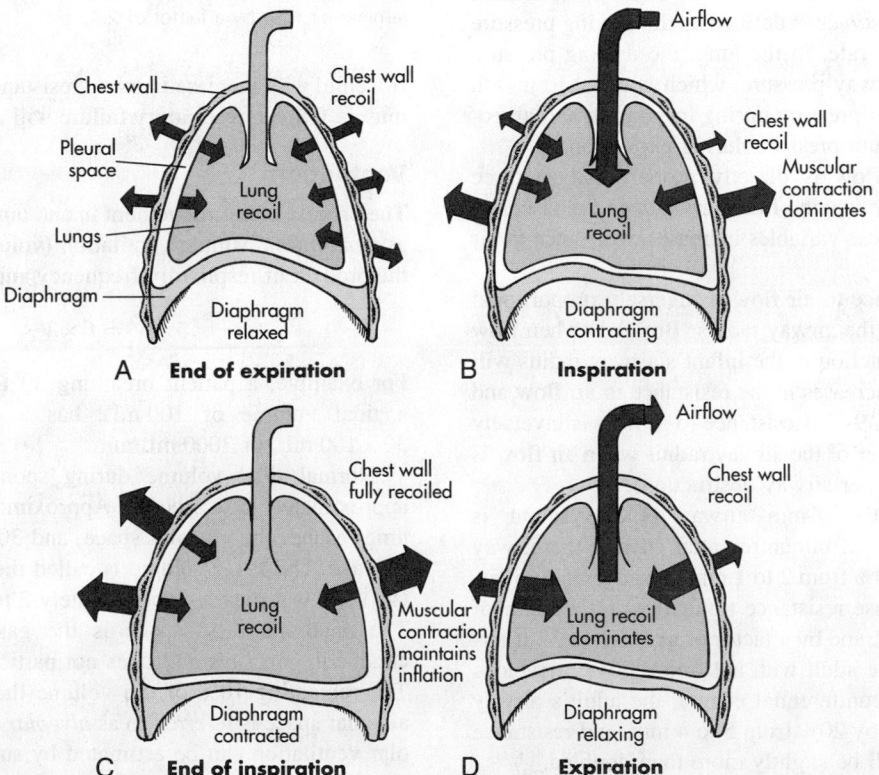

FIG. 9-2 Interaction of forces during inspiration and expiration. Equilibrium between recoil tendencies of lungs (to move inward) and chest wall (to move outward) is reached at the end of each normal expiration (A) and inspiration (C). During inspiration (B), the equilibrium is disrupted, with the chest wall tendency to move outward dominant (*large arrows* indicate chest wall tendencies). During expiration (D), the lung's recoil tendencies are dominant (*large arrows* indicate recoil tendencies). The chest wall and lungs tend to expand and recoil together as the result of the subatmospheric pressure present in the pleural space. (From Brashers VL: Structure and function of the pulmonary system. In McCance KL, Heuther SE: *Pathophysiology: the biologic basis for disease in adults and children*, ed 6, St Louis, 2010, Mosby.)

of the distensibility of the lungs and is defined as the volume change (ΔV) produced by a transpulmonary pressure change (ΔP):

$$C_{\text{L}} = \Delta V / \Delta P.$$

Compliance is high when the volume change produced by a given pressure change is large. Compliant lungs will inflate with very low pressure (i.e., the volume change produced by 1 cm H_2O pressure is large).

If the volume change produced by a given pressure change is small, the lungs are stiff and less compliant. When lung compliance is low, the work of breathing is increased. Compliance is increased in diseases such as emphysema and asthma, and it is decreased by pulmonary edema, pneumothorax, atelectasis, and pulmonary fibrosis. Compliance is difficult to measure, but effective compliance or dynamic compliance of the lung and chest wall can be measured in the intubated child during mechanical ventilation (see sections, Optimal PEEP and Common Diagnostic Tests).

Lung compliance is determined primarily by two factors: surfactant and the elasticity of lung tissue. Surfactant is a lipid material that spreads on the alveolar surface and prevents alveolar collapse as the alveoli get smaller during expiration. Surfactant lowers surface tension at low lung volumes.

Just as compliance is determined by lung tissue factors, resistance is determined primarily by airway size (diameter or radius). *Airway resistance* is defined as the driving pressure divided by the airflow rate. In the lung, the driving pressure for flow is the transairway pressure, which is equal to mouth pressure minus alveolar pressure during inspiration and alveolar pressure minus mouth pressure during expiration.

Resistance to air flow is directly proportional to three variables: flow rate, the length of the airway, and the viscosity of the gas. If any of these variables increases, resistance to air flow will increase.

In addition, resistance to air flow is inversely proportional to the fourth power of the airway radius (Box 9-1) when flow is laminar.[110] Any reduction in the infant's airway radius will result in exponential increases in the resistance to air flow and work of breathing (Fig. 9-3). Resistance to airflow is inversely related to the fifth power of the airway radius when air flow is turbulent (e.g., with upper airway obstruction).

For example, if the 4-mm airway of the infant is compromised by 1 mm of circumferential edema, the airway radius is reduced by 50% from 2 to 1 mm. The decrease in circumference will increase resistance to air flow by a factor of 16 if airflow is laminar, and by a factor of as much as 32 if airflow is turbulent. If the adult with a 10-mm airway develops the same 1 mm of circumferential edema, the adult's airway radius will be reduced by 20% from 5 to 4 mm, and resistance to laminar air flow will be slightly more than doubled.

The small caliber of the pediatric airway increases the potential significance of any disorder that compromises airway size. Airway resistance is highest in the nasopharynx and lowest in the small bronchioles. Airway resistance is substantially increased in diseases such as asthma, cystic fibrosis, chronic lung disease, bronchiolitis, and tracheal stenosis and conditions with increased respiratory secretions. High airway resistance increases the work of breathing and creates respiratory distress.

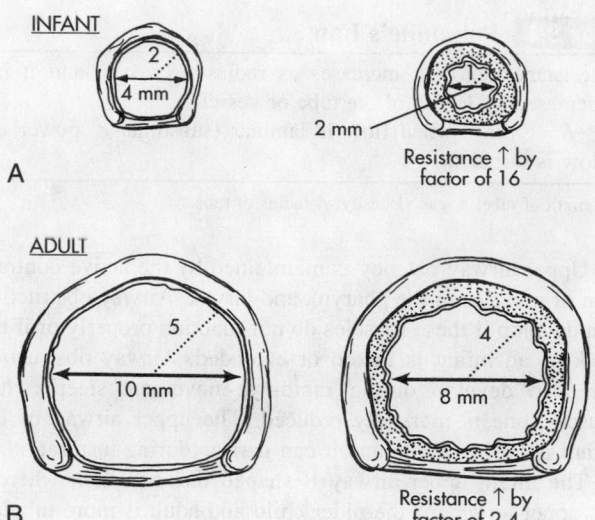

FIG. 9-3 Relative effects of 1 mm of circumferential airway edema in a infant and young adult. A, The infant's larynx is approximately 4 mm diameter, with a 2-mm radius. If 1 mm of circumferential edema develops, it will halve the airway radius and increase resistance to air flow by a factor of 16 if airflow is laminar, and it will increase resistance to turbulent airflow by up to 32 times. B, The young adult possesses a larynx approximately 10 mm in diameter and 5 mm in radius. Development of 1 mm of circumferential edema in the young adult will reduce the radius by approximately 20% (from 5 to 4 mm) and increase resistance to laminar air flow by a factor of 2.4.

If a child with increased airway resistance develops respiratory muscle fatigue, respiratory failure will ensue.

Ventilation

The process of gas movement in and out of the lungs is defined as *ventilation*. Minute ventilation (volume per minute $[\dot{V}]$) is the product of respiratory frequency and tidal volume:

$$\dot{V} = f \times V_{\text{T}}$$

For example, a patient breathing 30 times per minute, with a tidal volume of 100 mL, has a minute ventilation of 30×100 mL, or 3000 mL/min.

Normal tidal volume during spontaneous respiration is approximately 6 to 7 cc/kg. Approximately 70% of tidal volume reaches the alveolar space, and 30% fills the conducting airways. The latter volume is called the *anatomic dead space* (V_{D}) and is typically approximately 2 to 3 cc/kg body weight. The anatomic dead space is the gas that remains in the conducting airways and does not participate in gas exchange. The remaining 70% of the volume that actually reaches the alveolar space is referred to as *alveolar ventilation* (V_{A}). Alveolar ventilation can be estimated by subtracting the anatomic dead space from the tidal volume (V_{T}):

$$V_{\text{A}} = f \times (V_{\text{T}} - V_{\text{D}})$$

For example, if the tidal volume is 100 mL, respiratory rate is 30/min, and the anatomic dead space is 20 mL, then alveolar ventilation would equal $30 \times (100 - 20)$, or 2400 mL/min. Alveolar ventilation is always less than minute ventilation.

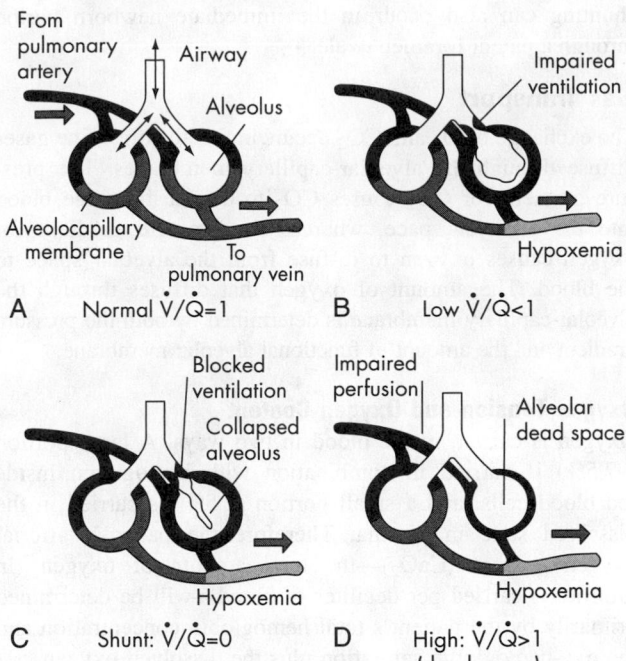

FIG. 9-4 The theoretical respiratory unit with graphic representation of the relationship between ventilation and perfusion in different clinical conditions. **A,** The ideal ventilation-perfusion ratio is $\dot{V}/\dot{Q} = 1$. **B** and **C,** Lung diseases characterized by a loss of alveolar volume (e.g., acute respiratory distress syndrome) create V/Q ratios that are either low $(0 < \dot{V}/\dot{Q} < 1)$—*shown in B*—or zero $(\dot{V}/\dot{Q} = 0$ which is the definition for intrapulmonary shunt)—*shown in C*. Importantly, low $\dot{V}/\dot{Q}$ alveolar units are responsive to oxygen administration (i.e., results in an increase in PaO_2), whereas $\dot{V}/\dot{Q} = 0$ alveolar units (intrapulmonary shunt) are not responsive to oxygen administration. **D,** High $\dot{V}/\dot{Q}$ units (dead space ventilation) are created under any circumstances in which pulmonary perfusion is reduced while alveolar ventilation is maintained. Thus any clinical condition that decreases right ventricular output (e.g., full cardiac arrest) or increases pulmonary vascular resistance (e.g., excessive PEEP) will result in increased dead space ventilation.

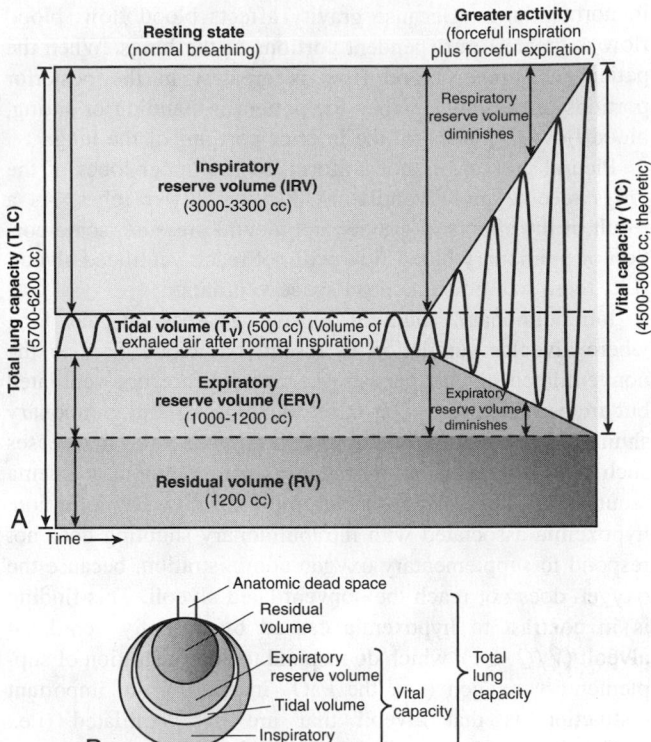

FIG. 9-5 Divisions of total lung capacity. **A** and **B,** Total lung capacity (TLC) is the maximum amount of air contained in the lungs. The total lung capacity is divided into four primary volumes: inspiratory reserve volume (IRV), tidal volume (V_T), expiratory reserve volume (ERV), and residual volume (RV). Capacities are combinations of two or more lung volumes; these include inspiratory capacity (IC), functional residual capacity (FRC), and VC. The IC is the IRV plus the V_T. The FRC is ERV plus the RV. The VC is depicted. Normal adult volumes are shown. (From Patton KT, Thibodeau GA: *Anatomy and physiology,* ed 7, St Louis, 2010, Mosby.)

The rate of removal of carbon dioxide from alveoli and the rate of oxygen delivery to the alveoli are directly related to alveolar ventilation. *Normal alveolar ventilation* is defined as the level of ventilation that results in normal partial pressures of oxygen and carbon dioxide in arterial blood.[103]

Anatomic dead space is just one part of the total dead space ventilation. A more clinically significant portion of dead space is the physiologic dead space. This space represents the volume of ventilation that reaches the alveoli that do not receive any pulmonary blood flow; therefore it is ventilation that does not participate in gas exchange. Ventilation of this portion of the lung is wasted. This concept is illustrated in Fig. 9-4. Normally, physiologic and anatomic dead space volumes are similar, but physiologic dead space can be significant in patients with pulmonary vascular disease or when positive end-expiratory pressure (PEEP) reduces pulmonary blood flow or whenever right ventricular output is reduced.

Lung Volumes

Lung volume measurements require patient effort; therefore accuracy is affected by patient cooperation. Such measurements are difficult or impossible to obtain in children who are uncooperative or who are younger than 5 years.

The total volume of the gas contained in the lung at maximum inspiration is the total lung capacity, Fig. 9-5. The volume that can be expired after a maximal inspiratory effort is the vital capacity (VC). This important and useful measurement of lung function is discussed in detail later in this chapter. VC can be reduced by any acute or chronic lung disease that increases lung stiffness (i.e., reduces lung compliance) or by conditions that limit available intrathoracic space (e.g., scoliosis, pneumonia, pleural effusion).

The volume of gas remaining in the lungs at the end of a normal expiration is the functional residual capacity (FRC). An increase in functional residual capacity usually indicates hyperinflation of the lung, or gas trapping, which is generally found in disorders characterized by decreased expiratory flow, such as chronic lung disease, cystic fibrosis, or asthma. A decrease in FRC may be seen in patients with pulmonary fibrosis or scoliosis.

Ventilation-Perfusion Relationships

As atmospheric air reaches the lungs (ventilation), it is exposed to pulmonary capillary blood perfusing the lungs. The distribution of perfusion and ventilation is not uniform in normal lungs. Because gravity affects blood flow, blood flow is greatest in dependent portions of the lungs. When the patient is supine, blood flow is greatest in the posterior portions of the lungs. When the patient is standing or sitting, blood flow is greatest in the inferior portions of the lung.

Pleural pressure is not uniform, so the upper lobes of the lungs receive more ventilation than the lower lobes. As a result of the effects of gravity and pleural pressure, some portion of pulmonary blood flow will not reach ventilated alveoli (i.e., there will be some dead space ventilation).

Intrapulmonary shunting exists in areas of the lung where alveolar ventilation is absent, but blood flow to the nonventilated alveoli persists (i.e., alveoli are not ventilated but are perfused, so $\dot{V}/\dot{Q}$ is 0; see Fig. 9-4, C). Intrapulmonary shunting is the cause of reduced PaO_2 (hypoxemia) in diseases such as cardiogenic and noncardiogenic pulmonary edema (acute respiratory distress syndrome [ARDS]). By definition, hypoxemia associated with intrapulmonary shunting does not respond to supplementary oxygen administration, because the oxygen does not reach the nonventilated alveoli. This finding is in contrast to hypoxemia caused by partially ventilated alveoli ($\dot{V}/\dot{Q} < 1$), which do respond to administration of supplementary oxygen (i.e., the PaO_2 increases). An important distinction is that alveoli that are not ventilated (i.e., $\dot{V}/\dot{Q} = 0$) must be recruited (opened) for supplementary oxygen to improve oxygenation. With treatment, the $\dot{V}/\dot{Q}$ ratio is converted from zero $\dot{V}/\dot{Q}$ (shunt) to low or normal $\dot{V}/\dot{Q}$ (i.e., to oxygen-responsive hypoxemia).

Intrapulmonary shunt and low $\dot{V}/\dot{Q}$ match are the most common causes of hypoxemia in pediatric lung disorders. These physiologic or abnormal intrapulmonary shunts do not result in hypercapnia (increased $PaCO_2$), because CO_2 is highly soluble in capillary blood and rapidly diffuses into the alveoli, and it is eliminated during expiration (exhalation).

During the first days of life, neonates demonstrate both cardiac and intrapulmonary shunting of blood. The cardiovascular shunt is caused by the patent ductus arteriosus with some desaturated pulmonary arterial blood shunted through the ductus into the arterial circulation (the aorta) without passing through the lungs. This right-to-left shunt occurs because pulmonary vascular resistance is high at birth. Once pulmonary vascular resistance begins to fall, the volume of right-to-left shunt falls. In infants with a patent ductus arteriosus, a PaO_2 of 60 to 80 mm Hg may be normal in the first day of life, but the PaO_2 typically exceeds 80 mm Hg within 2 or 3 days after birth (Table 9-2) as pulmonary vascular resistance falls and the right-to-left shunt ceases. A small amount of right-to-left

Table 9-2	Normal Arterial Blood Gas Values in Children	
	Neonate at Birth	**Child**
pH	7.32-7.42	7.35-7.45
PCO_2	30-40 mm Hg	35-45 mm Hg
HCO_3	20-26 mEq/L	22-28 mEq/L
PO_2	60-80 mm Hg	80-100 mm Hg

The neonatal values represent normal values for neonates during the first days of life. Values for the child are the same as for the adult.

shunting can also occur in the immediate newborn period through a patent foramen ovale.

Gas Transport

The exchange of O_2 and CO_2 occurs in the alveolus. The gases diffuse through the alveolar-capillary membranes. The pressure gradient for CO_2 causes CO_2 to diffuse from the blood into the alveolar space, whereas the pressure gradient for oxygen causes oxygen to diffuse from the alveolar space to the blood. The amount of oxygen that diffuses through the alveolar-capillary membrane is determined by both the pressure gradient and the amount of functional alveolar membrane.

Oxygen Tension and Oxygen Content

Oxygen is carried in the blood in two ways. A large portion (97.5%) is carried in combination with hemoglobin inside red blood cells, and a small portion (2.5%) is carried in the dissolved state in plasma. Therefore the patient's arterial oxygen content (CaO_2)—the total amount of oxygen (in milliliters) carried per deciliter of blood—will be determined primarily by the patient's total hemoglobin concentration and the oxy-hemoglobin saturation plus the dissolved oxygen.

Arterial oxygen content cannot be determined from the PaO_2, which is the partial pressure of oxygen. At sea level, the total pressure of gases in the atmosphere and in the blood must always equal 760 torr. Room air contains 21% oxygen, approximately 79% nitrogen, and a small quantity of inert gases. Therefore the PaO_2 of room air is 21% of 760 torr, or approximately 160 mm Hg, and the partial pressure of nitrogen in room air is 79% of 760 mm Hg, or 600 mm Hg.

In the alveolus at sea level, the total pressure exerted by all gases will still equal 760 mm Hg, but these gases ultimately include both water and CO_2. Water vapor pressure of air that is 100% humidified is 47 mm Hg, so the partial pressure of O_2 in the airways when the patient breathes room air is approximately 150 mm Hg ($0.21 \times [760 - 47]$ mm Hg). Alveolar gas also contains CO_2 with a normal $PaCO_2$ of 40 mm Hg, so the alveolar oxygen tension or partial pressure of oxygen in the alveoli (PAO_2) is approximately 110 mm Hg. When blood passes through the capillary adjacent to the alveolus, CO_2 diffuses from the blood through the alveolar-capillary membrane and into the alveolus, and oxygen diffuses from the alveolus into the blood.

The total pressure of all gases in the blood also totals 760 mm Hg at sea level. The partial pressure of O_2 is approximately 110 mm Hg, and the partial pressure of CO_2 is approximately 40 mm Hg. These numbers reflect the partial pressure of gases (including oxygen) dissolved in the blood.

Approximately 0.003 mL of oxygen is dissolved per deciliter of blood for every mm Hg partial pressure of oxygen present in the blood. For example, if the PaO_2 is 100 mm Hg, 0.3 mL of oxygen is dissolved per deciliter of blood. This dissolved oxygen reflects only a tiny fraction of the oxygen carried in the blood, but this is the number reflected by the PaO_2.

Oxygen is carried most efficiently when it is bound to hemoglobin and each gram of hemoglobin is able to carry 1.34 mL oxygen. The total oxygen content is determined by multiplying the hemoglobin (in g/dL) by 1.34 mL O_2/g of

Box 9-2	Calculation of Total Arterial Oxygen Content

Total oxygen content = O_2 bound to Hgb + dissolved O_2.

The oxygen bound to hemoglobin is calculated by determining the theoretical oxygen-carrying capacity of the blood, or the amount of oxygen carried by the hemoglobin if the hemoglobin is fully saturated:

$$Oxygen\ capacity = Hgb\ concentration(mg/dL)$$
$$\times 1.34mL\ O_2/g\ Hgb$$

Once the patient's arterial oxygen saturation is known, it is multiplied by the theoretical O_2-carrying capacity:

$$O_2\ bound\ to\ Hgb = (O_2\ capacity) \times Arterial\ O_2\ saturation$$

To calculate the amount of dissolved oxygen present in the blood, the child's PaO_2 is multiplied by 0.003 mL O_2 per dL:

$$Dissolved\ oxygen = 0.003mL\ O_2/dL \times PaO_2$$

Finally, the total arterial oxygen content is equal to the sum of the O_2 carried by the hemoglobin and the dissolved O_2:

$$Oxygen\ content(CaO_2) = O_2\ bound\ to\ Hgb$$
$$+ dissolved\ oxygen$$

Hgb, Hemoglobin.

saturated hemoglobin and then multiplying that number by the actual hemoglobin saturation. The small amount of oxygen carried in the dissolved form is then added to the amount of O_2 carried by hemoglobin. The normal arterial O_2 content is approximately 18 to 20 mL O_2 per dL blood (Box 9-2).[271]

To emphasize the difference between PaO_2 and arterial O_2 content, consider the effects of varying hemoglobin concentration in three patients. If the patients all breathe room air, as noted previously, the PaO_2 of all patients will equal approximately 110 mm Hg, regardless of hemoglobin concentration. If the three patients have normal lungs, their hemoglobin will be fully saturated (99%), so their total arterial oxygen content will differ according to their hemoglobin concentration. If the first patient has no hemoglobin at all (concentration of 0 g/dL), the patient's PaO_2 is still 110 mm Hg, but the patient's arterial oxygen content is 0.33 mL/dL (equal to the amount of dissolved oxygen, or $0.003 \times PaO_2$). This example is not realistic, but it makes the point that the PaO_2 is not the same as O_2 content. Consider a second patient with a hemoglobin concentration of 8 g/dL; the second patient's PaO_2 is 110 mm Hg, with a total arterial oxygen content of approximately 11 mL O_2 per dL blood (slightly more than half normal). The third patient has a hemoglobin concentration of 15 g/dL; this patient's PaO_2 is 110 mm Hg, and the patient's arterial oxygen content is approximately 20 mL O_2 per dL blood (normal). Although all three patients have exactly the same PaO_2 and oxygen

saturation, the second patient must almost double cardiac output to maintain the same oxygen delivery as the third patient ($DO_2 = CO \times CaO_2$). These examples illustrate the importance of evaluating hemoglobin concentration, PaO_2, and arterial oxygen saturation when interpreting blood gas results. Additional patient examples are included in Box 9-3.

The Oxyhemoglobin Dissociation Curve

The relationship between the PaO_2 and the hemoglobin saturation is expressed by the oxyhemoglobin dissociation curve, as shown in Fig. 9-6, with the PaO_2 on the horizontal axis and the hemoglobin saturation on the vertical axis. The curve is not linear but S-shaped, with a large plateau at the higher levels of PaO_2. There are several important things to note about the oxyhemoglobin dissociation curve. As noted, the curve flattens when the PaO_2 exceeds 80 to 100 mm Hg; this means that although the PaO_2 continues to rise beyond 100 mm Hg, the hemoglobin cannot become more saturated than 100%, and it cannot carry any more oxygen. Any additional rise in the PaO_2 will result only in increases in the amount of dissolved oxygen in the blood, which contributes only 0.003 mL O_2 per mm Hg rise in PaO_2. Therefore a rise in PaO_2 from 100 to 700 torr does not mean that sevenfold more oxygen is carried in the blood; it is associated with an approximately 10% increase in oxygen content. Because the hemoglobin is fully saturated once the PaO_2 reaches 100 mm Hg, there is usually no advantage to maintaining the patient's PaO_2 any higher than this value.

As shown in Fig. 9-6, the slope of the oxyhemoglobin dissociation curve becomes extremely steep once the PaO_2 is less than 60 mm Hg. Thus when the patient's PaO_2 falls below 60 mm Hg, even small additional decreases in the PaO_2 will be associated with a significant fall in the hemoglobin saturation and arterial oxygen content. Therefore the patient's PaO_2 should be maintained above 60 mm Hg, if possible.

The position of the oxyhemoglobin curve can be altered by several factors (Table 9-3). If the curve is shifted to the right, then hemoglobin has less affinity for oxygen (it is less well saturated) at any partial pressure of oxygen (PaO_2). Conversely, if the curve is shifted to the left, then hemoglobin has a higher affinity for oxygen (the hemoglobin is better saturated) at any given PaO_2.

Factors that shift the curve to the right include acidosis, hypercapnia, and hyperthermia. Under these conditions the oxyhemoglobin saturation and oxygen content is lower at any given PaO_2, but within the normal range the amount of oxygen released to tissues is enhanced, which is an adaptive response that makes oxygen more available in the tissue beds of patients who are likely to need it (e.g., those who are acidotic, hypercapnic, febrile).[271] Factors that shift the oxyhemoglobin dissociation curve to the left include alkalosis, hypocapnia, and hypothermia. Although these factors increase oxyhemoglobin saturation at any given PaO_2, oxygen will not be as readily released to the tissues,[271] because oxygen is more tightly bound to the hemoglobin molecule.

The hemoglobin dissociation curve for fetal hemoglobin is located to the left of the adult hemoglobin curve. Thus at a given PaO_2 and hematocrit, fetal blood contains more oxygen than adult blood. This higher affinity of fetal hemoglobin for

| Box 9-3 | **Calculation of Arterial Oxygen Content from Patient Examples** |

Normal arterial oxygen content is 18-20 mL O_2 per dL blood.

Example 1

Calculate the oxygen content (in mL O_2 per dL) for a child with a hemoglobin concentration of 15 g/dL, a PaO_2 of 100 mm Hg, and an arterial oxygen saturation of 97%.

$$\begin{aligned}
\text{Oxygen content} &= O_2 \text{ carried by Hb} + \text{dissolved } O_2 \\
&= (15\text{g/dL} \times 1.34\text{mL/g} \times 0.97) \\
&\quad + (0.003\text{mL } O_2/\text{mm Hg} \times 100\text{mm Hg}) \\
&= 19.50\text{mL } O_2/\text{dL} + 0.30\text{mL } O_2/\text{dL} \\
&= 19.80\text{mL } O_2/\text{dL}
\end{aligned}$$

Example 2

Calculate the oxygen content (in mL O_2 per dL) for a child with a hemoglobin concentration of 8 g/dL, a PaO_2 of 100 mm Hg, and an arterial oxygen saturation of 97%.

$$\begin{aligned}
\text{Oxygen content} &= O_2 \text{ carried by Hgb} + \text{dissolved } O_2 \\
&= (8\text{g/dL} \times 1.34\text{mL/g} \times 0.97) \\
&\quad + (0.003\text{ml } O_2/\text{mm Hg} \times 100\text{mm Hg}) \\
&= 10.40\text{mL } O_2/\text{dL} + 0.30\text{mL } O_2/\text{dL} \\
&= 10.70\text{mL } O_2/\text{dL}
\end{aligned}$$

Examples 1 and 2 demonstrate the dramatic fall in O_2 content that occurs with a fall in the Hgb concentration. Although both patients have exactly the same PaO_2 and O_2 saturation, the second patient must almost double cardiac output to maintain the same O_2 delivery as the first patient ($DO_2 = CO \times CaO_2$).

Example 3

Calculate the arterial O_2 content (in mL O_2 per dL) for a child with a hemoglobin concentration of 15 g/dL, a PaO_2 of 50 mm Hg, and an arterial O_2 saturation of 85%.

$$\begin{aligned}
\text{Oxygen content} &= O_2 \text{ carried by Hgb} + \text{Dissolved } O_2 \\
&= (15\text{g/dL} \times 1.34\text{mL } O_2/\text{g} \times 0.85) \\
&\quad + (0.003\text{mL } O_2/\text{mm Hg} \times 50\text{mm Hg}) \\
&= 17.09\text{mL } O_2/\text{dL} + 0.15\text{mL } O_2/\text{dL} \\
&= 17.24\text{mL } O_2/\text{dL}
\end{aligned}$$

This example demonstrates the effect of mild hypoxemia on the patient's arterial O_2 content. Most patients tolerate such mild hypoxemia because they are able to maintain O_2 delivery by compensatory increases in cardiac output. The arterial O_2 content of the patient in Example 3 is still significantly higher than the arterial O_2 content of the patient in Example 2, even though the patient in Example 2 has a higher PaO_2 and fully saturated Hgb. This is explained by the higher Hgb concentration of the patient in Example 3.

Hgb, Hemoglobin.

oxygen provides adequate fetal arterial oxygen content and delivery, despite the relatively low PaO_2 in the placenta and fetal circulation. Fetal hemoglobin, however, releases oxygen less readily to the tissues than does adult hemoglobin. Fetal hemoglobin usually disappears within 4 to 6 weeks after birth and is replaced by adult hemoglobin.

Regulation of Carbon Dioxide Tension and Hydrogen Ion Concentration

Carbon dioxide is carried in the blood in several ways. Like oxygen, it can be dissolved in plasma or carried by hemoglobin. In addition, CO_2 can react with water to form carbonic acid (H_2CO_3), or it can combine with other proteins to form carbamino compounds.

Unlike oxygen, the relationship between $PaCO_2$ and the arterial CO_2 content is linear. Furthermore, $PaCO_2$ is directly proportional to the metabolic production of CO_2 and inversely proportional to alveolar ventilation. Thus an increase in alveolar ventilation will result in a decrease in $PaCO_2$. For example, if the patient's $PaCO_2$ falls from 40 to 20 mm Hg, the patient must have doubled alveolar ventilation. Similarly, if the $PaCO_2$ increases from 40 to 60 mm Hg, alveolar ventilation must have decreased by 50%. If the $PaCO_2$ increases, then CO_2 combines with water to form H_2CO_3, and carbonic acid then dissociates into bicarbonate and hydrogen ion:

$$CO_2 + H_2O \leftrightarrow 5H_2CO_3 \leftrightarrow 5H^+ + HCO_3^-$$

The net result of these reactions is a rise in hydrogen ion concentration and a fall in pH, or respiratory acidosis. If this condition persists for several hours, the kidney will respond with the excretion of more hydrogen ions and reabsorption of more bicarbonate. Renal compensation can restore the arterial pH to nearly normal levels (see discussion of renal disorders in Chapter 13).

Alveolar ventilation may either increase or decrease as compensation for primary metabolic disorders. When metabolic acidosis develops, excess hydrogen ions are present, resulting in the formation of more carbonic acid, which then dissociates to CO_2 and water. Total ventilation then increases (e.g., a patient with diabetic acidosis develops hyperpnea), so additional CO_2 is eliminated, and the CO_2 tension falls. The arterial pH will then increase toward normal levels, because hydrogen ions are eliminated as CO_2 is excreted by the lungs.

Alveolar ventilation will decrease when metabolic alkalosis is present. Carbon dioxide may be retained until the $PaCO_2$ is extremely high. Carbon dioxide will combine with water to form carbonic acid, which will dissociate to form hydrogen ions and bicarbonate ions. Hydrogen ions accumulate and the arterial pH decreases. An example of this compensation is a patient who develops hypokalemic, hypochloremic metabolic alkalosis and slows respirations; the $PaCO_2$ rises and the pH falls toward normal. Table 9-4 summarizes changes in the arterial pH, $PaCO_2$, and serum bicarbonate (HCO_3^-) that occur with respiratory and metabolic acidosis and alkalosis.

Regulation of Respiration

Alveolar ventilation is controlled by both neural and chemical factors. Spontaneous respiration requires a rhythmic discharge from the respiratory center in the ventral portion of the brain. The chemical control of breathing is modulated at two

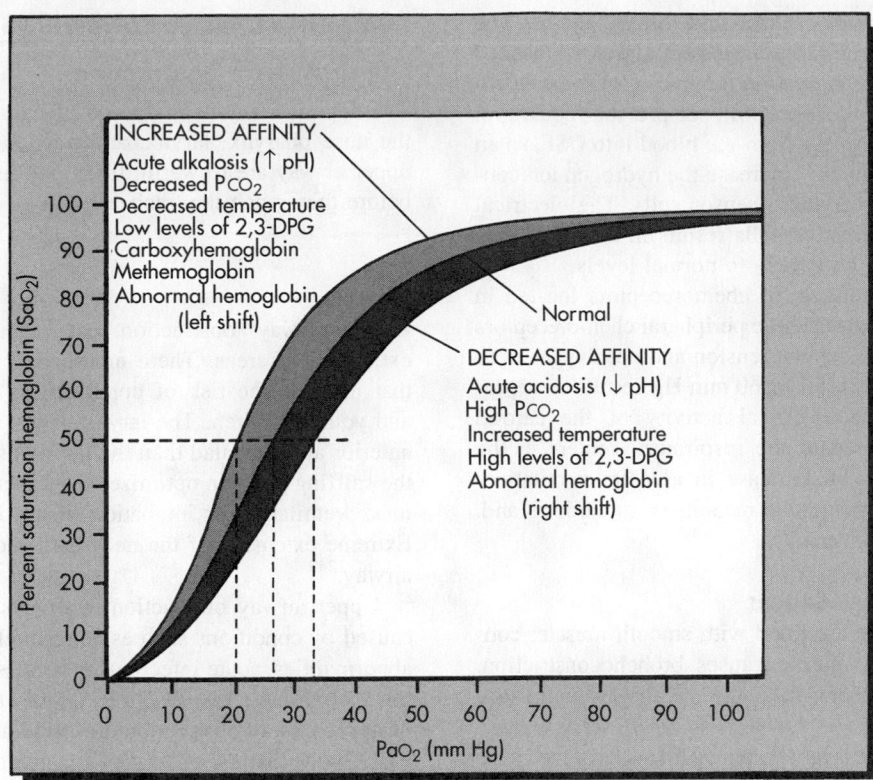

FIG. 9-6 Oxyhemoglobin dissociation curve. The horizontal or flat segment of the curve at the top of the graph is sometimes called the *arterial portion,* or that part of the curve where oxygen is bound to hemoglobin. This portion of the curve is flat because partial pressure changes of oxygen between 60 and 100 mm Hg do not significantly alter the percent saturation of hemoglobin with oxygen. The wide range of partial pressures of oxygen (PaO_2=60-100 mm Hg) represented by the flat part of the curve, allows adequate hemoglobin saturation at a variety of altitudes. For example, a PaO_2 of 100 mm Hg at sea level results in a hemoglobin saturation with oxygen of 98%. The steep part of the oxyhemoglobin dissociation curve occurs after the PaO_2 drops below 60 mm Hg and represents the rapid dissociation of oxygen from hemoglobin. During this phase, oxygen diffuses rapidly from the blood into tissue cells. Conditions associated with altered affinity of hemoglobin for O_2 are listed. P50 is the PaO_2 at which hemoglobin is 50% saturated, normally 26.6 mm Hg. A lower-than-normal P50 represents increased affinity of hemoglobin for O_2, such as is present in conditions such as alkalosis, hypocarbia, hypothermia. The lower P50 means that the hemoglobin will be better saturated at lower PaO_2 (e.g., at normal pH, a 90% oxyhemoglobin saturation is associated with PaO_2 of approximately 60 mm Hg; at an alkalotic pH, a 90% oxyhemoglobin saturation will be associated with a lower PaO_2, probably nearer 50 mm Hg). The increased affinity means that the hemoglobin does not release O_2 to the tissues as readily. A higher P50 is seen with decreased hemoglobin affinity for O_2. With decreased affinity for O_2, the hemoglobin is less saturated at a given PaO_2, but will release the oxygen more readily to the tissues. Note that variation from normal is associated with decreased (low P50) or increased (high P50) availability of O_2 to tissues *(dotted lines).* The *shaded area* shows the entire oxyhemoglobin dissociation curve under the same circumstances. *2,3-DPG,* 2,3-diphosphoglycerate present in higher quantities in children with cyanotic heart disease and in lower quantities in neonates with large amounts of fetal hemoglobin. (From Lane EE, Walker JF: *Clinical arterial blood gas analysis,* St Louis, 1987, Mosby.)

Table 9-3	Shifts in Hemoglobin Dissociation Curve
Shift to Left (Higher oxygen affinity)	**Shift to Right (Lower oxygen affinity)**
Alkalosis	Acidosis
Hypocapnia	Hypercapnia
Hypothermia	Hyperthermia
Fetal hemoglobin (decreased 2,3 DPG)	Increased 2,3 DPG
Methemoglobinemia	Adult hemoglobin

Table 9-4 Changes in Arterial Blood Gases with Acid-Base Imbalances

Arterial Blood Gases	pH	PCO_2	HCO_3^-
Respiratory acidosis	↓	↑	N or ↑*
Respiratory alkalosis	↑	↓	N or ↓*
Metabolic acidosis	↓	N or ↓*	↓
Metabolic alkalosis	↑	N or ↑*	↑

*Complete compensation.
↓, Decreased; ↑, increased; *N,* normal.

respiratory centers: the CO_2 sensor and the O_2 sensor. The sensor for CO_2 is located in the brainstem and is influenced primarily by CO_2-related changes in the hydrogen ion concentration of the cerebrospinal fluid (CSF; see previous equation). Carbon dioxide diffuses freely from the blood into CSF, so an increase in $PaCO_2$ will quickly increase the hydrogen ion concentration in the CSF near these sensor cells. The electrical output of these chemosensitive cells results in an increase in ventilation that restores the $PaCO_2$ to normal levels.

The oxygen sensor consists of chemoreceptors located in the carotid and aortic bodies. These peripheral chemoreceptors detect changes in arterial oxygen tension and not oxygen content. A fall in PaO_2 below 50 to 60 mm Hg results in a progressive increase in the electrical activity of the carotid body, which is transmitted to the respiratory centers in the brainstem and results in an increase in alveolar ventilation. The carotid body sensors are also responsive to acidosis and, to a lesser extent, hypotension.

Neural Control of Airway Caliber

The walls of the airways are lined with smooth muscle; constriction of this smooth muscle causes bronchoconstriction. Relaxation of the smooth muscle lining the airways will cause bronchodilation.

Airway smooth muscle is innervated by branches of the vagus nerve (cholinergic nerves) and to a lesser extent by branches of the sympathetic nervous system (adrenergic nerves). Acetylcholine and related compounds cause bronchoconstriction, whereas acetylcholine antagonists such as atropine cause bronchodilation. Adrenergic stimulation of smooth muscle by epinephrine and related compounds causes bronchodilation. Mucous glands in the lung also have a dual cholinergic and adrenergic innervation. Cholinergic stimulation increases mucus secretion, whereas adrenergic stimulation decreases it.

COMMON CLINICAL CONDITIONS

Upper Airway Obstruction

The upper airway is composed of many structures, including the nose pharynx, larynx, and trachea. The functions of the upper airway are to warm, filter, and humidify inspired gases before they reach the trachea.[92]

Etiology

Upper airway obstruction can occur anywhere in the extrathoracic areas. There are several developmental factors that increase the risk of upper airway obstruction in infants and young children. The larynx of the infant or child is more anterior and cephalad than the larynx of the adult. As a result, the sniffing position optimizes the airway opening during bag-mask ventilation or intubation of the infant or young child. Extreme extension of the neck can lead to obstruction of the airway.[243]

Upper airway obstruction in infants and children may be caused by conditions such as congenital or acquired anatomic abnormalities, acute infectious processes, or compression from other organ systems (Table 9-5). Additional potential causes of upper airway obstruction are listed as follows:

1. Recent history of airway manipulation (e.g., intubation, bronchoscopy, airway surgery)
2. Mucus plugging of an artificial airway (e.g., endotracheal tube or tracheostomy tube)
3. Mechanical obstruction from a foreign body aspiration, with secondary laryngospasm that may result in further airway obstruction
4. Infections associated with acute inflammation and swelling of the upper airway (e.g., croup, epiglottitis, retropharyngeal abscess, peritonsillar abscess)

Table 9-5   **Clinical Diagnosis of Airway Obstruction**

	Croup	Epiglottitis	Bacterial Tracheitis	Foreign Body Aspiration	Retropharyngeal Abscess
Age	3 months to 3 years	1-6 year	3 month to 12 years	Any	Any
Incidence in children presenting with stridor	>80%	5%-10%	About 2%	About 2%	About 2%
Onset	Prodrome, 1-5 days	Rapid, 4-12 h	Prodrome 2-5 days	Acute or chronic	Prodrome variable
Temperature	Low grade	Markedly high	Moderate	None	High
Dysphagia	No	Yes	Rare	No	Yes
Drooling	No	Yes	Rare	No	Yes
Voice	Hoarse	Muffled	Normal	Variable	Muffled occasionally
Cough	Barking	No	Variable	Yes	No
Position	No effect	Erect, leaning (anxious, air hunger)	No effect	No effect	Opisthotonic (meningismus occasionally)
Radiographic findings	Overdistention of hypopharynx and paradoxic narrowing of subglottic portion of trachea	Marked thickening of epiglottis and aryepiglottic folds	"Fuzzy" tracheal walls with narrowing	Soft tissue mass or opaque foreign body in airways	Thickening of retropharyngeal space and anterior displacement of trachea

From Al-Jundi S: Acute upper airway obstruction: croup, epiglottitis, bacterial tracheitis, and retropharyngeal abscess. In Levin DL, Morriss FC, editors: *Essentials of pediatric intensive care*, ed 2, St Louis, 1997, Quality Medical Publishers.

5. Recent history of general anesthesia or sedation, leading to decreased upper airway tone and collapse of upper airway or tongue falling to back of throat
6. Trauma or congenital malformations of the head or neck (e.g., choanal stenosis)
7. Any disease that results in excessive mucus production such as asthma or cystic fibrosis
8. Anaphylactic reaction
9. Adenotonsillar hypertrophy
10. Rapid-eye-movement sleep with decreased pharyngeal muscle tone.

Pathophysiology

Airway obstruction decreases airway diameter and increases the resistance to air flow and work of breathing. The child often can compensate for a mild airway obstruction by increasing the work of breathing, allowing ventilation (air flow) to remain unchanged. When the airway obstruction becomes more severe, the child will no longer be able to compensate and will demonstrate significant increased work of breathing, decreased aeration (ventilation) with eventual hypercarbia, and respiratory failure. When severe, this condition can also lead to hypoxemia and tissue hypoxia.

Clinical Signs and Symptoms

Upper airway obstruction can often be identified from the clinical signs and symptoms. Older children with upper airway obstruction and a normal level of consciousness often assume the position that provides the most relief (i.e., the best air flow). Typically, these children are more comfortable sitting up and leaning forward; this is referred to as the *tripod position*. Signs of respiratory distress are often exacerbated in the supine position or by agitation.

The infant or child will exhibit stridor, a high-pitched sound during inspiration. This sound may be accompanied by a hoarse cough or cry. Inspiratory stridor, hoarseness, and drooling indicate the presence of significant acute upper airway obstruction, which is often associated with airway edema or airway compression. Stertor, or snoring, is often noted in children with upper airway obstruction secondary to adenotonsillar hypertrophy or a tongue that obstructs the posterior pharynx.

The child with mild to moderate airway obstruction may be restless and exhibit tachypnea. The child will often use accessory muscles of respiration, demonstrating nasal flaring and tracheal tugging (supraclavicular retractions). Breath sounds may be adequate, although they may be difficult to assess if the child has concomitant stridor or stertor. Tachycardia may also be noted as a nonspecific sign of distress. Oxygenation usually remains adequate until there is severe obstruction and decompensation. Signs of profound airway obstruction with respiratory failure include slowed respiratory rate, decreased aeration, altered level of consciousness, compromise in systemic perfusion, apnea or gasping, and bradycardia.

Regardless of the site of obstruction, the hallmark of airway obstruction is hypercarbia with a respiratory acidosis. The PaO_2 may initially be normal, although hypoxemia will develop when the patient's condition deteriorates.

Management

Acute upper airway obstruction must be rapidly evaluated and treated. It can sometimes be anticipated and prevented or treated in young children by proper positioning of the head and neck into the sniffing position. Infants with acute respiratory distress who are breathing spontaneously are positioned in the upright or lateral (supported) position, especially after feedings. An infant seat can be used to keep the infant upright. Care must be taken to avoid flexion or hyperextension of the neck, because these positions can cause upper airway obstruction by tracheal compression.

For the older child the side-lying position is preferred immediately after surgery, because the tongue and other upper airway muscles may be hypotonic and occlude the upper airway if the patient is supine. Children with large tonsils or adenoids may manifest signs of airway obstruction, including snoring or stertor if they are allowed to sleep in the supine position.

As noted previously, toddlers and older children with upper airway obstruction often instinctively assume a posture that maximizes airway caliber. It is best to avoid manipulating the child's position until personnel experienced in airway management are present. The young child may be most comfortable when held and supported upright by a parent.

Treatment includes administration of warmed, humidified oxygen by face mask, hood, tent, or blow-by tubing. Minimize noxious stimulation, because agitation can worsen airway obstruction. Inhaled racemic epinephrine is an accepted treatment for upper airway obstruction related to moderate-to-severe croup or postextubation edema. The mechanism of action is thought to be related to α-adrenergic constriction of precapillary arterioles, with resulting fluid reabsorption from the interstitial space and decreased laryngeal mucosal edema. These effects increase airway diameter and ease of gas flow. Doses may be given as often as every 20 minutes. Inhaled l-epinephrine is as effective as racemic epinephrine. These inhaled agents are to be used with caution in patients with tachycardia, arrhythmias, or underlying congenital heart disease, because the agents can potentiate tachycardia.[201]

Inhalation treatment with a helium-oxygen mixture (heliox) provides a lower density gas compared with a nitrogen and oxygen mixture. Helium is an odorless, tasteless inert gas that can be substituted for nitrogen in inhaled gaseous mixtures.[94,167] The benefit of providing inhaled gas with a lower density is that it promotes laminar flow within the upper and lower airways. Laminar gas flow promotes the delivery of oxygen and inhaled medications through the areas of obstruction and facilitates drug deposition (Fig. 9-7). Effects of the helium and oxygen mixture are noted almost immediately; if it is effective, then the patient's work of breathing decreases and aeration improves. If the child is verbal, gas delivery is confirmed if the child speaks in a high-pitched voice. A higher pitched cry may be noted during therapy in preverbal infants.

One limitation to the use of the helium-oxygen mixture is the need for supplementary oxygen. Generally, helium mixtures are delivered at 20% oxygen and 80% helium, 30% oxygen and 70% helium, or 40% oxygen and 60% helium. There is generally no benefit to heliox if the patient needs

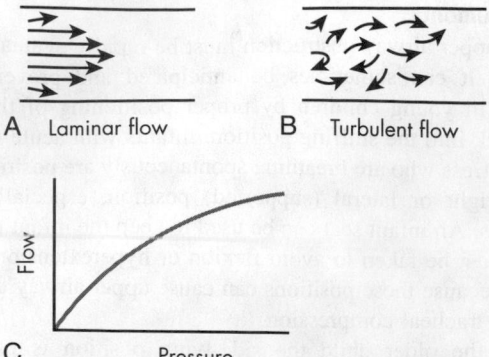

FIG. 9-7 Laminar versus turbulent flow. Schematic depiction of the spatial and velocity profiles of gas molecules within **A,** a laminar and **B,** a turbulent flow regimen. The velocity of the gas molecules is proportional to the length of arrows. During turbulent flow, there is chaotic molecular movement between lamina that results in ever greater pressure being required to achieve incremental flow. **C,** Note the alinear pressure-flow relationship with turbulent flow.

an FiO_2 greater than 0.4 (40% oxygen plus 60% helium), because the gas mixture will have a density similar to that of a standard nitrogen and oxygen mixture. Some children, however, will need less oxygen if the inhaled gas is able to traverse the areas of obstruction to reach the lower airways.

Administration of heliox during mechanical ventilation necessitates close monitoring of the child and the circuit,

because the helium may interfere with the pneumotachometers and ventilator function. Because heliox improves flow through areas of airway obstruction, it can be used to treat disease processes that produce turbulent flow (e.g., asthma). It is often used until therapeutic medications take effect, or it can be used until resolution of the disease process.[94] Most institutions develop specific protocols for management of acute, life-threatening upper airway obstruction to support efficient care (Box 9-4).[6]

When airway obstruction is severe, elective (supportive) intubation is always preferable to emergency intubation (i.e., during resuscitation) of a child with impending respiratory failure. The decision to intubate is based on the patient's clinical appearance. If the child demonstrates severe respiratory distress with significant work of breathing, then consider intubation. Signs of severe airway obstruction include mottling or cyanosis, decreased air movement, altered level of consciousness, stertor, stridor, and compromised systemic perfusion. Apnea or gasping or bradycardia are late signs of severe airway obstruction and should be prevented by timely intubation and respiratory support.

The pulse oximeter is generally not a useful tool in the detection of significant airway obstruction and the need for intubation, because hypoxemia is a late sign of deterioration. However, a downward trend or a sudden substantial decrease in oxyhemoglobin saturation can indicate deterioration, especially when the patient is breathing room air ($FiO_2 = 0.21$).

Box 9-4 Sample Protocol for Management of Epiglottitis

I. Once the diagnosis of epiglottitis is suspected, follow these steps without exception:
  A. Begin continuous observation of the patient. Allow the parents to remain with the patient. Do not place the child in a supine position.
  B. Contact the team designated to secure the airway (i.e., anesthesiologist, intensivist, otolaryngologist).
  C. Place equipment for bag-mask ventilation, intubation, oxygen, suction, tracheostomy, and cardiopulmonary resuscitation at the bedside.
  D. Do not agitate the child with noxious procedures such as oral examination, blood drawing, or intravenous catheter placement.
  E. Begin continuous electrocardiogram, respiratory, and pulse oximetry monitoring.
  F. Obtain lateral neck radiograph only if the child's condition is stable and the diagnosis is uncertain. A physician capable of intubation must accompany the child to the radiology department.
  G. Administer O_2 at 1-2 L/min or at a rate sufficient to maintain O_2 saturation >90% by pulse oximetry.
  H. For worsening airway obstruction consider administering nebulized racemic epinephrine (2.25%): 0.2 mL in 2 mL 0.9% sodium chloride solution.
  I. If complete airway obstruction develops before the arrival of the airway team, begin assisted ventilation with bag and mask with continuous positive pressure during expiration.

II. Once the airway team has arrived, perform the following:
  A. Transport the child to the operating room or critical care unit.
  B. Ask the airway specialist to remain with the child and be prepared for fiberoptic examination, rigid bronchoscopy, or tracheostomy
  C. Induce anesthesia with the patient in a sitting position using an inhalation agent and oxygen. Confirm the diagnosis of epiglottitis. Intubate the child through the oral route with an endotracheal tube one size smaller than estimated from the child's body length and age.
  D. Provide bag-tube ventilation and verify tube position with clinical assessment and an exhaled CO_2 detector. Ensure that the child is well oxygenated.
  E. Obtain a chest radiograph to ensure proper insertion depth of the endotracheal tube and to evaluate for pulmonary abnormalities, including pulmonary edema.
  F. Place an intravenous catheter; obtain blood and epiglottic cultures.
  G. Begin antibiotic therapy with extended-spectrum cephalosporin*, or as indicated based on local and likely pathogens and their susceptibilities.
    1. Cefuroxime: 150 mg/kg/day for 3 days
    2. Ceftriaxone: 80 mg/kg/day for 2 days
    3. Cefotaxime: 200 mg/kg/day for 4 days

Modified from Al-Sundi S: Acute upper airway obstruction: croup, epiglottitis, bacterial tracheitis, and retropharyngeal abrasions. In Levin D, Morriss F, editors: *Essentials of pediatric intensive care,* New York, 1997, Churchill Livingstone.
*Chloramphenicol is no longer recommended because second- and third-generation cephalosporins are effective and far less toxic.

Blood gas analysis or noninvasive CO_2 measurements should be evaluated if hypercarbia is suspected.

The severity and etiology of the upper airway obstruction will determine the treatment needed. Obstruction may be acute, as in cases of infection and tissue inflammation, or it may be chronic, such as with tonsillar and adenoidal hypertrophy. In both categories of airway obstruction, assessment of the effectiveness of gas exchange will help determine appropriate intervention. Some obstruction will resolve with repositioning and suctioning. Significant obstruction, however, may be treated with a nasal trumpet to provide airway stenting, noninvasive positive pressure ventilation, or tracheal intubation and ventilation. Relief of some causes of upper airway obstruction may need surgical intervention.

Lower Airway Obstruction

The lower airways consist of the lungs, conducting airways, and alveoli (i.e., the airways inside the thorax). These airways get progressively smaller, so small changes in airway diameter can have significant effects on airflow and work of breathing.

Etiology

Obstruction in the lower airways can result from airway plugging caused by inflammation with mucosal edema and increased production of thick secretions, or it can result from hyperreactivity of the bronchial smooth muscle that leads to bronchospasm. Some lower airway obstruction results from both causes. Although asthma is the most common cause of lower airways disease and obstruction in pediatric patients, the obstruction can result from other causes, including infections and chronic lung disease.[92]

Pathophysiology

Airflow obstruction results from decreased airway caliber, which causes increased resistance to the flow of both inspired and expired gas. However, exhalation is predominantly affected. Mucus plugging within the small airways results in air trapping and hyperinflation of the lungs, causing the diaphragm to be flattened instead of a typical dome shape at rest[92] (Fig. 9-8).

Clinical Signs and Symptoms

Lower airway obstruction typically produces increased work of breathing, forced or prolonged exhalation, and expiratory wheezing. If the obstruction is severe, verbal children will be unable to speak in complete sentences; they may speak in monosyllables because they need to interrupt speech to breathe. In addition, patients may demonstrate:
- Hypoxemia or cyanosis
- Pulsus paradoxus (a decrease in the amplitude of the pulse oximeter or intraarterial wave form during inspiration)
- Diaphragm fatigue as manifested by paradoxical movement of the abdomen or apnea
- Altered mental status
- Inability to lie supine

Management

A variety of pharmacologic agents is available for management of lower airways obstruction. These medications will be discussed in more detail in the sections on status

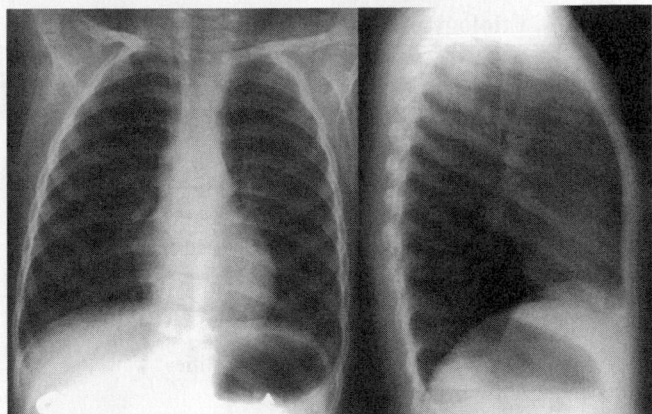

FIG. 9-8 Chest radiographs of a patient with hyperinflation. No infiltrates are noted. The right side is more radiolucent (darker) compared with the left. This is subtle and may be difficult to appreciate unless the chest radiograph is viewed from a distance. The right hemidiaphragm is normally higher than the left hemidiaphragm; they are at about the same level in this patient. These findings suggest hyperinflation of the right lung. The clinical history indicated that the child was jumping on a bed while eating a snack, when she began choking. Since that time, she has experienced respiratory difficulty. Further radiographs revealed bilateral air trapping. Bronchoscopy revealed bilateral bronchial peanut fragment foreign bodies. Impression: Right-sided hyperexpansion and air trapping, which may represent a bronchial foreign body.

asthmaticus and bronchiolitis. In addition to pharmacologic agents, heliox can be used to manage lower airway obstruction. Refer to additional information on heliox in the Upper Airway Obstruction section. Heliox may have additional therapeutic effects, because it may attenuate lung inflammation and reduce mechanical and oxidative stress in the management of acute lung injury.[169] Assisted ventilation, either noninvasive or invasive, is needed in some patients (see section, Status Asthmaticus later in this chapter).

Apnea

Apnea is a common problem in premature infants, and the incidence is inversely related to gestational age. Apnea must not be confused with normal neonatal periodic breathing. Apnea is generally defined as lack of airflow for 20 seconds or longer. Lack of airflow over shorter periods of time is labeled apnea if it is associated with significant bradycardia or cyanosis.[224] More than half of infants younger than 32 weeks postconceptual age will demonstrate some degree of apnea.[224] Apnea in a term infant is never a normal finding and needs further investigation.

Apnea can be either central, when there is no respiratory effort and no airflow, or obstructive, when there is respiratory effort accompanied by paradoxic inward motion of the chest and outward movement of the abdomen, but absence of airflow associated with the effort. Mixed central and obstructive apnea occurs when there is a combination of decreased effort and evidence of obstruction to airflow.

Etiology

The etiology of apnea in the preterm infant may be multifactorial, with delayed maturation of cardiorespiratory control a likely factor. Infants and children with apnea must be

Box 9-5 Etiology of Apnea

Central apnea
- Infection—particularly respiratory syncytial virus (RSV)
- Hypoxia with decreased cardiac output
- Central nervous system pathology, brainstem injuries (infection, stroke, tumor, trauma including inflicted trauma)
- Metabolic disorder—disorders of fatty acid oxidation
- Pharmacologic side effects—especially anesthetics, narcotics
- Cardiac arrhythmias

Obstructive apnea
- Anatomic factors—craniofacial abnormalities, adenotonsillar hypertrophy
- Gastroesophageal reflux

evaluated for a variety of abnormalities (Box 9-5). Apnea in older children may be chronic, as when related to an underlying neurologic condition (e.g., brain tumor, hydrocephalus), or it may be acute as in conditions such as toxic ingestions or traumatic brain injury.

Obstructive apnea is seen in children with structural or mechanical upper airway obstruction (e.g., from adenotonsillar hypertrophy) during sleep. Clinical symptoms are exacerbated with sleep, because the tone in upper airway muscles is reduced in the sleep state. Reduced tone can result in prolapse of structures such as the tongue into the airway, leading to worsening of mechanical obstruction.

Mixed obstructive apnea is frequently documented in children with obstructive apnea syndromes. In these cases, respiratory pauses (central apnea) are present but are rarely physiologically significant. It is presumed that dysfunction in medullary respiratory centers explains both the lack of airway tone associated with obstructed breaths and the absence of effort that defines central apnea.

Management

The management of apnea is determined by the etiology. Patients with central apnea may need to be intubated and mechanically ventilated if it is severe (e.g., respiratory syncytial virus [RSV]-associated apnea, drug overdose, trauma, stroke, hypoxic-ischemic brain injury). Apnea of prematurity generally will resolve by the time the infant reaches 40 weeks postconceptual age. Cardiac and apnea monitoring are indicated for these patients. Some children may need home apnea monitoring.

Treatment includes management of the etiology of the apnea (e.g., underlying cardiac disease, anatomic abnormalities) when possible. If the etiology is not treatable, such as in premature infants, symptom control is the goal. This treatment can include tactile stimulation during events, administration of low-flow oxygen, methylxanthines (e.g., caffeine), or nasal continuous positive airway pressure (CPAP). In older infants and children, a complete evaluation will be needed to identify the etiology of the apnea.

In obstructive sleep apnea (OSA), management focuses on relieving the obstruction. Polysomnography can be used to quantify the respiratory distress index and document the severity of OSA. Surgical management (i.e., tonsillectomy,

adenoidectomy, or both) is often needed for moderate to severe OSA. Nonsurgical management includes positive pressure ventilation, using either CPAP or bilevel positive airway pressure. Patients with severe obstruction may not achieve cure with surgical intervention alone and may need noninvasive positive pressure support after surgical intervention. Commonly, obese children with OSA will achieve improvement in their respiratory distress index and quality of life postoperatively, but OSA does not resolve completely in the majority. In these cases, chronic noninvasive ventilation support may be needed.[160]

If airway obstruction is not resolved and becomes chronic, the chronic alveolar hypoxia can, over time, produce pulmonary hypertension and cor pulmonale (right-sided heart failure caused by pulmonary hypertension). A 12-lead electrocardiogram (ECG) and echocardiogram (Echo) may be indicated to determine whether cor pulmonale is present in children with longstanding OSA. A follow-up polysomnogram is generally indicated 4 to 6 weeks postoperatively or after implementation of noninvasive ventilation to ensure adequate control of obstructive disease. Long-term complications of OSA include cor pulmonale, systemic hypertension, behavioral disturbances, poor school performance, daytime somnolence, and enuresis.

Hypoventilation

Hypoventilation is a result of decreased respiratory effort. It leads to decreased renewal of alveolar gas, so the $PaCO_2$ rises and the PaO_2 falls.[79]

Etiology

True hypoventilation is uncommon. When it occurs, it is most likely to result from central nervous system dysfunction.[79] The condition can be challenging to detect unless the patient is already being monitored or the condition is associated with additional clinical findings such as upper airway obstruction. The differential diagnosis for hypoventilation includes central nervous system injury, use of narcotic or anesthetic agents, neuromuscular disorders, infant botulism, and congenital central hypoventilation syndrome (Ondine's curse).

Head trauma—especially when it is associated with ischemia, an intracranial mass, or infection—can decrease the brainstem response to chemoreceptor stimulation (i.e., hypercarbia or hypoxia). Pharmacologic agents and metabolic toxins can lead to similar clinical findings. In particular, opioid medications decrease the respiratory drive, leading to hypoventilation. This effect may be desirable when using this class of medication to facilitate mechanical ventilation, but it may be a hindrance when working toward extubation or when opioids are administered to children who are not intubated.[80]

Hypoventilation can also be caused by significant muscle weakness. In these clinical situations, the child initiates a breath, but the muscles are so weak that the child is unable to generate adequate tidal volume to achieve CO_2 removal.

Clinical Manifestations

When hypoventilation is present, the rise in $PaCO_2$ approximately equals the fall in PaO_2, so oxyhemoglobin saturation (via pulse oximetry) will fall. Hypercarbia secondary to hypoventilation often produces nonspecific findings. If hypercarbia is severe, somnolence may be noted. Mild hypercapnia is often not associated with any clinical findings, so it is difficult to diagnose in the absence of other findings. Children with reduced respiratory effort associated with hypercarbia and hypoxemia need central nervous system evaluation.[80]

Management

For acute hypoventilation, invasive or noninvasive mechanical ventilatory support is indicated to restore ventilation. Central respiratory stimulants have been successful primarily in neonates, after the child's condition is stabilized. A reversal agent (naloxone) can be administered in cases of pharmacologically induced apnea (i.e., opioids), which can result in increased respiratory effort and temporary reversal of apnea. However, patients need close monitoring for recurrence of bradypnea and apnea, because the duration of action of the narcotic is longer than that of the naloxone. In chronic disease, diaphragm pacing has been provided in an attempt to avoid long-term mechanical ventilation; however, this practice is not widespread.

Airways Malacias

The term *malacia* is derived from a Greek word that means *softness*. Malacia is generally used to describe a weak or insufficiently rigid (i.e., supporting cartilage is insufficiently rigid) portion of the airway that collapses during respiration. The distal third of the trachea is most commonly affected, although any portion of the airway can be involved.[65,152]

The incidence of tracheomalacia is unknown. Although uncommon, it is the most frequent cause of stridor in infants and children. Most children have mild or moderate symptoms that improve with time, as the cartilage becomes more firm. An increased incidence has been described in premature infants.[267]

Etiology

Malacia can be primary or secondary. Primary tracheomalacia occurs when the trachea is unusually collapsible from incomplete hardening of the tracheal cartilage. Secondary malacia occurs in association with conditions that compress the trachea (Table 9-6).

Table 9-6 **Classification of Tracheomalacia**

Primary	Secondary
Congenital absence of tracheal cartilage	Esophageal atresia and tracheoesophageal fistula Vascular rings Tracheal compression from an innominate artery Tetralogy of Fallot with absent pulmonary valve Compression from mediastinal mass Connective tissue disease disorder Prolonged mechanical ventilation

Adapted from McNamara VM, Crabbe DCG: Traceomalacia, *Paediatric Resp Rev* 5:147, 2004.

Pathophysiology

Collapse of the extrathoracic airway (e.g., trachea) during inspiration causes narrowing of the airway lumen, resulting in inspiratory airflow obstruction. This effect can lead to severe respiratory distress and is exaggerated by increased respiratory effort or agitation, particularly during feeding, crying, and coughing, or by the presence of an intercurrent illness.[65,152]

Clinical Signs and Symptoms

Severity of symptoms will be affected by the length, location and severity of the malacia. Most infants with malacia will present with stridor. Stridor and obstruction are exacerbated by agitation and increased respiratory effort, and lessened during sleep and restful breathing. Persistent wheezing with irreversible airway obstruction is another frequent presenting sign. Additional potential symptoms include cough, noisy breathing, hoarseness, dyspnea, and inspiratory retractions.

Management

In cases of primary tracheomalacia, gradual improvement occurs as the tracheal lumen increases in diameter with anatomic growth and firming of supporting cartilage. Most infants demonstrate improvement by 6 to 12 months of age, and signs and symptoms will resolve in most children by 2 years of age.

Symptoms may be alleviated by positioning. Prone positioning will allow gravity to contribute to enlarging or opening of the airway lumen. Conversely, supine positioning can lead to decreased airway lumen diameter and airway collapse.[65] Positioning with the head of the bed elevated may prevent episodes of gastroesophageal reflux, decreasing the risk for gastric contents irritating airways and further compromising airway diameter. Irritating an already collapsing airway can exacerbate symptoms. In addition, proton pump inhibitors, histamine blockers, and prokinetic agents are used often to reduce the effects of gastroesophageal reflux.[267]

Fortunately most cases of malacia are mild. In cases of moderate to severe malacia, conservative measures may not be adequate. Parents should be taught basic life support techniques. These children may also need cardiorespiratory monitoring, oxygen, and noninvasive PPV in the home.[152]

Surgical options for severe tracheomalacia include aortopexy and segmental tracheal resection. The goal of aortopexy is to suspend the aorta in a ventral position to prevent tracheal collapse. Through either a thoracotomy or median sternotomy, the aortic root is exposed and the thymus is resected or retracted.[267] Sutures are placed in the pericardial tissue over the aortic root and in the adventitia of the aortic arch and are tied to the underside of the sternum. As the aorta is pulled forward (i.e., toward the sternum), the front wall of the trachea is also pulled forward by fibrous attachments between the aorta and trachea. Intraoperative bronchoscopy can be used to visualize the trachea and to ensure adequate suspension and reduction of the tracheal compression.[152,267] There are few complications associated with aortopexy surgery. Recurrence (incidence is approximately 10% to 25%) may necessitate additional surgery in some patients. Other less common complications include phrenic nerve palsy, pneumonia, chylopericardium, and wound infections.[267]

If aortopexy does not successfully improve the diameter of the tracheal lumen, another option is to resect the region of malacia. This procedure may cure the malacia, but candidacy for it can be limited by the length of the segment involved, because long segments of malacia cannot be resected.[152]

Additional treatment strategies include placing indwelling endotracheal or endobronchial stents to stabilize the collapsing airway. Expandable metallic airway stents have been used in adults since the 1980s to palliate airway strictures caused by malignancy. Expandable metallic coronary artery stents have been used in children, although experience is limited. In the short term, stents are highly effective in treating malacia. However, because indwelling airway stents do not epithelialize in the same way as endovascular stents, airway stents promote formation of granulation tissue that can contribute to recurrent airway obstruction and bleeding. There is also a risk that the stent may erode into neighboring vessels, causing catastrophic hemorrhage. Newer biodegradable stents are under development.[152]

Vocal Cord Paralysis

The vocal cords are two elastic bands of muscle tissue located just above the trachea in the larynx. Vocalization is normally created when exhaled air passes through closed vocal cords, causing them to vibrate. In the absence of vocalization, the cords remain open to facilitate respiration.

Vocal cord paralysis is the absence of movement of the cords owing to motor nerve dysfunction in the larynx. The paralysis can be unilateral or bilateral. In cases of bilateral paralysis, most cases are abductor palsies, with the cords in close apposition to each other. The cords may not move at all (paralysis), or they may have decreased or abnormal movement (paresis). Although vocal cord paralysis is uncommon, this condition is the second leading cause of stridor in infancy.[58]

Etiology

Vocal cord paralysis may be idiopathic, or it may be associated with surgical procedures or related to a neurologic disorder, birth trauma, or brachial plexus injury. Cardiac procedures such as ligation of a patent ductus arteriosus or manipulation or repair of the aortic arch have been associated with vocal cord dysfunction. The recurrent laryngeal nerve loops around the aortic arch on the left and the subclavian artery on the right before it travels superiorly and enters the larynx. Surgery near these areas can result in manipulation of the nerve, producing vocal cord dysfunction.[250]

Neurologic conditions associated with vocal cord paralysis include midbrain/brainstem dysgenesis, Arnold-Chiari malformation, congenital hydrocephalus, neurofibromatosis, and global hypotonia.[58,162] Neurosurgical procedures near the brainstem also can result in vocal cord paralysis.

Uncommonly, vocal cord injury can be caused by physical trauma during endotracheal intubation. Postoperatively, all children who undergo these surgical procedures need to be monitored for clinical signs of vocal cord paresis.

Clinical Manifestations

Common clinical signs and symptoms include stridor, weak cry or voice, hoarseness, and swallowing dysfunction. In cases of bilateral paresis or paralysis, the stridor is more severe; in fact, children with bilateral paresis will have more significant clinical findings in general.[58] Swallowing dysfunction associated with vocal cord paralysis can lead to aspiration of saliva or food, placing the child at risk for aspiration pneumonitis.[250]

The diagnosis of vocal cord paralysis can be established using either direct bronchoscopy in the operating room or through dynamic assessment of the larynx using flexible fiberoptic laryngoscopy (generally performed at the bedside) to evaluate the motion of the vocal cords. Ultrasonography of the larynx is a useful adjunctive diagnostic technique.[58] The condition is confirmed when the there is no motion or abnormal motion of one or both of the vocal cords.[250]

Management

Spontaneous recovery can occur within approximately 6 months in some children. Intervention of any sort is needed only if the vocal cord injury results in problems with gas exchange or if the child is aspirating food or formula.

Some children will need only thickened foods and positioning with the head of the bed elevated during feeding. In addition, they will need close observation for signs of aspiration. Other children will need alternative enteral nutrition delivery (e.g., gastric tube) to bypass the paretic area. Speech therapy evaluation is crucial to determine the safest method for feeding.[250] Rarely, a tracheostomy is needed to relieve airway obstruction associated with vocal cord paresis and to protect the lungs from soiling.[127]

For children with unilateral vocal cord paresis, surgical intervention is an option, using a CO_2 laser to bring the paralyzed cord into a more medial position (i.e., medialization); this facilitates adduction of the paretic cord with the functional cord. Another method of medialization of the paralyzed vocal cord is to inject it with silicone elastomers. Injection with Teflon (DuPont, Wilmington, DE) is no longer used because it has been associated with granuloma development.[69]

Respiratory Failure

Etiology

Respiratory failure is defined as exchange of O_2 and CO_2 that is insufficient to meet the metabolic demands of the body; this results in hypoxemia, hypercarbia, or both. Virtually any critically ill or injured child is at risk for respiratory failure. Respiratory failure results from hypoventilation, ventilation or perfusion ($\dot{V}/\dot{Q}$) mismatch, diffusion abnormalities, and intrapulmonary shunting.[9,82,243]

Pathophysiology

Respiratory failure can be caused by failure of any component of the respiratory system, including central nervous system control of ventilation, airways, the chest wall, respiratory muscles, or lung tissue including the alveolar-capillary membrane (Box 9-6).

Respiratory failure and hypoxemia result from: hypoventilation, low $\dot{V}/\dot{Q} < 1$ (O_2 responsive), $\dot{V}/\dot{Q} = 0$ (shunt, not O_2 responsive), diffusion disturbances, decreased PaO_2 (decreased SaO_2), and high altitude.[9]

Box 9-6 **Major Components of the Respiratory System and Potential Contribution to Respiratory Failure**

- Brain or central nervous system control of breathing
  - Immaturity
  - Depressed because of narcotics, barbiturates, or anesthetics
  - Impaired in central nervous system disease, insult, or injury
- Airways
  - Bronchospasm
  - Airway obstruction caused by inflammation, edema, or mucus with significant increase in resistance to air flow and work of breathing
  - Airway musculature incompletely developed, so airways are compliant and may be compressed
  - Airway may be compressed by abnormal vascular or other anatomy
  - Artificial airway occlusion or displacement
- Chest wall
  - Extremely compliant in young children, so it may collapse during episodes of respiratory distress, resulting in further compromise in efficiency of respiratory function
  - Excessive inspiratory pressure and volume can be provided inadvertently during positive pressure ventilation.

- Respiratory muscles
  - If any respiratory muscles lack tone, power, or coordination, the upper or lower airway patency may be compromised, reducing inspiratory effort.
  - Diaphragm fatigue or paralysis: Intercostal muscles may be incapable of generating effective tidal volume during early childhood.
  - Phrenic nerve injury
- Lung tissue
  - Cardiogenic or noncardiogenic pulmonary edema
  - Surfactant inactivation
  - Parenchymal lung diseases
  - Anatomic abnormalities can result in lung restriction or compliance problems.
- Alveolar-pulmonary capillary interface (diffusion surface)
  - Pulmonary edema
  - Pulmonary hypertension syndromes
  - Pulmonary emboli
- Excessive positive pressure

The diagnosis of respiratory failure is based on both clinical and physiologic criteria. For example, oxygen criteria alone can be misleading in a child with cyanotic heart disease who is hypoxemic while breathing room air (i.e., intracardiac shunt). Physiologic criteria include hypoxemia while breathing room air and hypercarbia with acidosis. Oxygen therapy may result in a normalization of the PaO_2 in a patient with respiratory failure.[260] The response to oxygen in a patient with lung disease is determined by the percent of alveoli represented by intrapulmonary shunting. If greater than 40% of the lung units are involved in the shunt, positive pressure ventilation and lung recruitment will be needed before oxygen therapy will increase the PaO_2.

Respiratory failure may be present despite oxygen therapy. Hypoxemia can result in inadequate tissue oxygenation and development of lactic acidosis. Cardiac output and pulmonary blood flow increase initially in response to hypoxemia. In addition, the hemoglobin affinity for oxygen is decreased (the oxyhemoglobin dissociation curve shifts to the right; see Fig. 9-6) so that oxygen is released more easily to the tissues.[64] These compensatory mechanisms will help maintain adequate oxygen delivery. With progressive hypoxemia, cardiac output falls and alveolar hypoxia may produce inadequate oxygen delivery.

Clinical Signs and Symptoms of Respiratory Failure

The clinical and physiologic indicators of respiratory failure in children are listed in Box 9-7. These indicators include hypoxemia despite oxygen therapy and hypercarbia with acidosis. The child's baseline oxygenation and respiratory function must also be considered (Box 9-8).

The alveolar-arterial oxygen difference or gradient (A-a DO_2) is an objective calculation used to assess the initial severity and the evolution of lung injury. It is calculated as

follows. A patient breathes a known concentration of oxygen for 15 to 20 min, and then an arterial blood sample is obtained. The inspired oxygen tension (PiO_2) is calculated by multiplying the fractional inspired oxygen concentration (FiO_2) by the difference between the barometric pressure and the water vapor pressure at body temperature (the water vapor pressure at body temperature is 47 mm Hg). The alveolar oxygen tension (PaO_2) is equal to the PiO_2 minus the $PaCO_2$ as shown on the next page:

Box 9-7 **Clinical and Physiologic Indicators of Respiratory Failure**

- Depressed level of consciousness
- Increased respiratory rate and effort, including retractions or grunting, decreased chest wall movement
- Absent or significantly decreased breath sounds
- Cardiovascular signs of distress, including tachycardia, peripheral vasoconstriction, mottled color, and pulsus paradoxus
- Signs of diaphragm muscle fatigue:
  - Paradoxic movement of diaphragm
  - Respiratory alternans
  - Apnea
- Late signs: apnea or gasping, agonal respirations, bradycardia, or hypotension
- Cyanosis and hypoxemia despite supplementary oxygen therapy (e.g., $PaO_2 < 75$ mm Hg despite FiO_2 of 1.00)*
- Hypercarbia ($PaCO_2 > 50$-75 mm Hg)†, especially with acute acidosis
- Rising alveolar-arterial oxygen difference (normal, < 25 mm Hg) or decreasing PaO_2/FiO_2 ratio

*In the absence of intracardiac right-to-left shunt lesion.
†In the absence of chronic lung disease and metabolic alkalosis.

| Box 9-8 | Clinical and Physiologic Criteria for Diagnosis of Respiratory Failure in Children with Chronic Lung Disease, Cyanotic Heart Disease, or Neurologic Disease |

Respiratory failure in the child with chronic lung disease
- Chronic increase in $PaCO_2$ with compensatory metabolic alkalosis
- Acute respiratory acidosis
- Significant increase in work of breathing
- Hypoxemia or hypercarbia exceeding the child's "normal" range
- Compromise in systemic perfusion (cool extremities, mottled color)
- Depressed level of consciousness
- Late signs: apnea, gasping, bradycardia

Respiratory failure in the child with cyanotic congenital heart disease
- Metabolic (lactic) acidosis (increased serum lactate, worsening base deficit)

- Hypoxemia exceeding patient's normal range
- Severe retractions or grunting
- Hypercarbia
- Late signs: apnea or gasping, compromise in systemic perfusion, bradycardia

Respiratory failure in the child with neuromuscular disease
- Decreased respiratory effort
- Weak cough, incompetent swallow or gag
- Use of accessory muscles of respiration
- Decreased tidal volume
- Decreased inspiratory force: cannot generate force more negative than -20 cm H_2O (normal is at least -60 to -100 cm H_2O, and forceful cough is thought to require at least -25 cm H_2O)
- Decreased vital capacity

$$PAO_2 = [FiO_2 \times (760 - 47)] - (PaCO_2/R)$$

$$PAO_2 = PiO_2 - PaCO_2$$

where R = Respiratory exchange quotient, which can be estimated as 1.

Note: If not at sea level, substitute barometric pressure for 760.

The A-a DO_2 is the difference between the calculated PAO_2 and the PaO_2 and is calculated as follows:

$$A - a\ DO_2 = PAO_2 - PaO_2$$

where normal is <25 to 50 mm Hg.

The difference between PiO_2 and the child's arterial oxygen tension increases when perfusion of nonventilated alveoli occurs; this is called an *intrapulmonary shunt*. The severity of intrapulmonary shunting is estimated using a shunt graph (Fig. 9-9). The PaO_2/FiO_2 (*P/F*) ratio is more commonly used in clinical practice to estimate the degree of intrapulmonary shunting (e.g., *P/F* <200 is consistent with ARDS).

Management

The child with respiratory distress and evolving respiratory failure needs continuous monitoring of general appearance and responsiveness, pulse oximetry, and heart rate. The child needs to be kept as comfortable as possible. Position the child for maximal comfort to provide optimal oxygenation, and frequently evaluate the child's airway, oxygenation, ventilation, and perfusion.

If the child's airway is obstructed or if the child appears unable to maintain a patent airway, perform intubation immediately (see section, Intubation below). The goal of therapy for respiratory failure is to maximize O_2 delivery by increasing arterial oxygen content and supporting cardiac output. In addition, reduce oxygen demand by treating fever and pain. Avoid cold stress in young infants through the use of warming devices. A frightened child may be comforted by the presence of the parents. Minimize intrusive examinations and treatments. Monitor fluid intake and

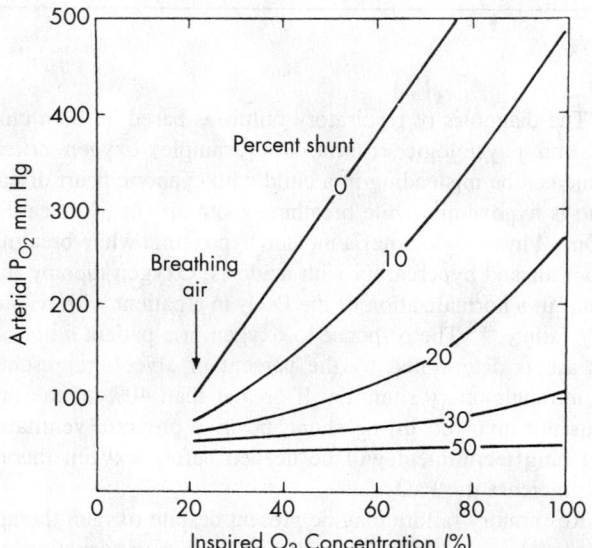

FIG. 9-9 Relationship between inspired O_2 concentration and arterial O_2 tension with changing severity of intrapulmonary shunting. By comparing the patient's FiO_2 to the PaO_2, the percentage of nonfunctioning but perfused alveoli (i.e., the shunt) can be determined. Note that once the intrapulmonary shunt nears 50%, increasing the inspired O_2 concentration will produce little improvement in PaO_2 at this point, treatment must improve alveolar ventilation and the ventilation-perfusion ratio through the use of positive end-expiratory pressure. Changes in cardiac output and O_2 uptake can influence the position of the shunt curves. (From West JB: *Pulmonary pathophysiology: the essentials*, ed 2, Baltimore, 1980, Williams and Wilkins.)

output carefully, because excessive fluid administration can contribute to pulmonary interstitial edema (from capillary leak) and worsening of respiratory failure.

Pulse Oximetry. Pulse oximetry allows continuous evaluation of oxyhemoglobin saturation (SaO_2). To estimate the child's PaO_2 from the SaO_2, consult an illustration of the oxyhemoglobin dissociation curve (see Fig. 9-6). The pulse oximeter uses a photodetector with light-emitting diodes. The photodetector is placed across a pulsatile tissue bed from the diodes. The diodes emit a red light and an infrared light through tissue containing both venous and arterial blood, and a photodetector captures the red and infrared light on the other side of the tissue bed. Oxygenated hemoglobin absorbs little red light, but a large amount of infrared light. A microprocessor determines the difference between the absorption of the red and infrared light and can determine the percentage of the total normal hemoglobin that is oxygenated in the tissue.[206] The pulse oximeter also displays the strength of the pulse and a digital pulse rate.

In order for pulse oximetry to be useful, the signal must be strong and artifact must be minimized. The oximeter is typically placed on the child's finger or toe (the neonate's hand or foot may be used). If movement artifact interferes with pulse oximetry, the disposable sensor and band can be placed on the arm or leg of the neonate. Technology in newer pulse oximeters has reduced motion artifact. Ambient light may also cause artifact, so it may be helpful to wrap the sensor and extremity loosely in gauze. The pulse oximeters are calibrated by the manufacturer, so they do not require calibration by the user.

In addition to light and motion artifact, accuracy of pulse oximetry is limited when tissue perfusion is poor, and it is limited by hemoglobinopathies and by dyes or pigments in the blood and hemoglobin. Poor tissue perfusion decreases the pulsatile flow needed for the detectors and for the calculation. Pulse oximeters calculate only O_2 saturation in normal hemoglobin, so they do not recognize carboxyhemoglobin or methemoglobin. As a result, the oxyhemoglobin saturation displayed by the monitor will overestimate total hemoglobin saturation in patients with these conditions, because it will reflect only the percent of normal hemoglobin that is saturated with oxygen and does not reflect the abnormal hemoglobin compounds. For example, if a child has 15% carboxyhemoglobin, the child's maximum possible oxyhemoglobin saturation is 85%. If the pulse oximeter displays an SaO_2 of 90%, the child's actual oxyhemoglobin saturation is probably 90% of the 85% of hemoglobin that is not bound to carbon monoxide, for an actual saturation of 76% (i.e., $0.85 \times 0.9 = 76.5\%$). If carbon monoxide poisoning or methemoglobinemia are suspected or confirmed, the hemoglobin saturation must be measured by cooximetry in the blood gas laboratory.[206]

Pulse oximeters are generally accurate over a wide range of hemoglobin saturations, although most have a lower limit or threshold hemoglobin concentration below which they are no longer accurate. In addition, clinicians must be aware that a child with severe anemia can have extremely low arterial oxygen content despite a normal oxyhemoglobin saturation, because oxygen-carrying capacity is reduced. In the child with severe anemia, oxygen delivery will fall unless cardiac output increases (see Box 9-2).

The pulse oximeter must have adequate signal strength, and the high and low alarm limits for heart rate and hemoglobin saturation must be set appropriately. Clinicians must be aware of the child's hemoglobin concentration and pH. In general an oxyhemoglobin saturation 94% or higher will be associated with adequate arterial oxygen content (and a PaO_2 greater than 70 mm Hg) unless anemia is present. If the child's pH is maintained in the alkalotic range, an oxyhemoglobin saturation less than 94% may be associated with significant hypoxemia (a PaO_2 less than 60 mm Hg).

An experienced healthcare provider may be able to recognize the presence of pulsus paradoxus (i.e., a fall in systolic blood pressure during spontaneous inspiration) during careful evaluation of the pulse oximetry signal, because the pulse amplitude will decrease during deep spontaneous inspiration. Pulsus paradoxus may be present in children with status asthmaticus when severe air trapping causes hyperinflation of the lungs and flattening of the diaphragm; this places tension on the pericardium. The hyperinflated lungs and the pericardium compress the heart and reduce diastolic filling, and they increase left ventricular afterload. These effects decrease stroke volume and cardiac output, especially during spontaneous inspiration.

Oxygen Administration. Administer warmed, humidified oxygen to the hypoxemic child. This therapy may effectively treat respiratory failure associated with hypoxemia if the child's airway is patent and respiratory effort and ventilation are acceptable (i.e., the child's $PaCO_2$ is normal). Measure and record the concentration of inspired oxygen carefully and assess the response of the child to therapy at frequent intervals.

Nasal cannulae are frequently used to deliver supplementary oxygen to children; they are useful to deliver low levels of oxygen (22%-40%). Flow rates for a standard nasal cannula range from 0.25 to 4 L/min, and they provide limited humidification. Hi-flow nasal cannula are also available.

Face tents are used frequently for older children and adolescents, although they are not made specifically in pediatric sizes. The soft, plastic masklike tent fits around the patient's chin and elastic straps hold it in place around the jaw. A minimum gas flow of 7 L/min is needed to ensure adequate CO_2 removal.

Several kinds of oxygen masks are available for pediatric use. To select a mask of the appropriate size, make certain that the mask is just large enough to cover the child's nose and mouth, because a mask that is too large may cause the patient to rebreathe exhaled gas, and a mask that is too small can prevent adequate gas flow. Most oxygen masks deliver inspired oxygen concentrations up to approximately 55%. A tight-fitting mask with a reservoir bag or special blender can provide inspired O_2 concentrations up to 100%.

Venturi masks are designed to provide more predictable oxygen concentrations, and they are particularly effective at delivering inspired O_2 concentrations between 24% and 50%. The Venturi mask differs from the conventional mask in that it can successfully deliver specific inspired O_2 concentrations, because its total liter flow usually exceeds the patient's inspiratory flow. Therefore all inspired gas contains the same, premeasured O_2 concentration (FiO_2), and no ambient air is entrained. Table 9-7 summarizes the advantages and disadvantages of various oxygen delivery systems (see Chapter 21).

Table 9-7   Advantages and Disadvantages of Typical Oxygen Delivery Systems

System	Advantages	Disadvantages
Oxygen masks	Many sizes available Provides predictable concentration of oxygen (with Venturi mask) whether child breathes through nose or mouth	Skin irritation Fear of suffocation Accumulation of moisture on face Possible aspiration of vomitus Difficulty controlling inspired oxygen concentrations
Nasal cannula	Provides constant oxygen flow even while the child eats and talks Enables more complete observation of child because nose and mouth remain unobstructed	May be uncomfortable or irritating May causing abdominal distension and discomfort or vomiting Difficult to control inspired oxygen concentration if child breathes through mouth Inability to provide mist if desired
Oxygen hood	Provides high concentrations of oxygen (FiO_2 up to 1.00) Enables ready access to patient's chest for assessment	High humidity environment Need to remove patient for feeding and care

Use of Oral or Nasal Airways. Placement of an oropharyngeal or nasopharyngeal airway may be necessary for the control of secretions or the prevention of airway obstruction. These airways are appropriate for short-term use only, and they must be replaced by an endotracheal tube if there is any doubt about the child's ability to maintain a patent airway.

Oropharyngeal airways may prevent occlusion of the pharynx by the tongue of an unconscious patient; they cannot be inserted in a conscious child because they may stimulate vomiting.[194] Occasionally an oral airway is maintained in the obtunded child with an oral endotracheal tube in place to prevent biting on the tube, but a bite block is more appropriate for this purpose.

The size of the oropharyngeal airway is evaluated before insertion by placing the airway on the outside of the child's cheek, with the bite block segment at the lips. The end of the airway should reach the angle of the jaw so that it will reach to the level of the central incisors.[43] Using a tongue blade may be helpful to depress the tongue during insertion.[194] Do not force the airway into the patient, because it can push the tongue back into the pharynx and obstruct the airway.

Nasopharyngeal airways are soft rubber or plastic tubes that provide a conduit for air flow from the nares to the posterior pharyngeal wall and for suctioning of the posterior pharynx.[194] These airways can be used in conscious or unconscious children, and they will maintain airway patency and provide a channel for suctioning the pharynx.

The diameter of the nasopharyngeal airway is sized by comparing the inner circumference of the nare to the outer circumference of the nasopharyngeal airway to be used. The length of the nasopharyngeal airway is equivalent to the distance from the tip of the nose to the tragus of the ear.[194] Lubricate the airway with a water-soluble lubricant before insertion, and do not force it into place if resistance is encountered. If any blanching of the nare is noted after placement, the diameter of the nasopharyngeal airway is too big and a smaller airway is needed. Small or extremely soft airways can become obstructed by mucus, vomitus, or soft tissues, so the airway must be suctioned frequently and its effectiveness needs to be evaluated repeatedly.[194]

Bag-Mask Ventilation. This method of ventilation uses a hand-ventilating bag joined to an oxygen source and a mask. A bag-mask system must be present at every bedside in the critical care unit. Because virtually any patient is at risk for developing respiratory failure, bedside nurses must be prepared to offer support of ventilation whenever necessary. Every healthcare provider must learn good bag-mask ventilation technique. The novice can begin skill acquisition by assisting during the suctioning of an intubated patient. It is important to provide effective ventilation without generating high peak inspiratory pressures, and it is also important to synchronize delivered breaths with the patient's spontaneous ventilatory efforts.

To provide effective bag-mask ventilation, use a self-inflating bag and select a mask to fit properly over the child's nose and mouth. Extend the child's neck slightly, unless cervical spinal injury is suspected in a trauma victim, and lift the jaw. Create a seal between the patient's face and the mask by grasping the mask between the thumb and index fingers of the nondominant hand while lifting the child's lower jaw against the mask using the third, fourth, and fifth fingers; this creates the E-C clamp depicted in Fig. 9-10.

During bag-mask ventilation, the rescuer compresses the bag in synchrony with, or slightly faster than, the child's spontaneous respiratory efforts. Inspiratory volume is administered to produce a visible chest rise. Bag-mask ventilation is effective if the chest expands equally and adequately bilaterally and if equal breath sounds can be auscultated over both sides of the chest during each breath. In addition, if bag-mask ventilation is effective, the child's oxyhemoglobin saturation

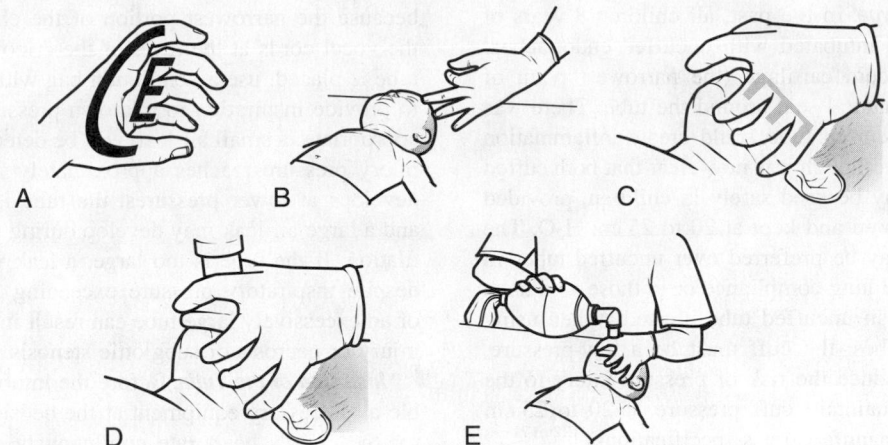

FIG. 9-10 Single rescuer bag-mask ventilation (E-C clamp) technique ("ventilating a baby is as 'E-C' as 1-2-3"). **A,** Hand displaying E-C shape. **B,** The E is formed with the ring, small, and index fingers. The C is formed with the index finger and thumb. **C,** The E fingers rest on the bony ridge of the jaw. **D,** The C fingers are positioned to hold the mask. **E,** Proper E-C clamp for assisted ventilation. (Developed by the New York City EMS project and NYC*EMS! Adapted from the Center for Pediatric Emergency Medicine: Teaching resource for instructors in prehospital pediatrics, ed 2. Available at http://cpem.med.nyu.edu/teaching-materials/tripp-bls. (Modified from Foltin GL, et al: *Teaching resource for instructors in prehospital pediatrics*, New York, 1998, Center for Pediatric Emergency Medicine, Maternal Child Health Bureau, Emergency Medical Services for Children Grant.)

(SaO_2) will rise or remain adequate, and the heart rate will be appropriate for age and clinical condition. Ineffective ventilation produces inadequate breath sounds bilaterally, and the chest fails to rise during ventilation. If the SaO_2 is low or falling and heart rate is decreased, bag-mask ventilation is inadequate.

Bag-mask ventilation can result in the entry of air into the esophagus, producing gastric distension; this can be harmful because the child could vomit and aspirate gastric contents, and gastric dilation can impair diaphragm excursion. If the child is unconscious with no cough or gag reflex, a second person can apply light pressure at the cricoid cartilage during bag-mask ventilation; this will displace the trachea posteriorly and obstruct the esophagus, reducing or preventing further air entry into the esophagus. If this maneuver fails or if gastric distension is significant, insert a nasogastric tube to decompress the stomach (remove it before an intubation attempt).

If prolonged bag-mask ventilation is needed, an endotracheal tube (advanced airway) will be inserted, enabling delivery of mechanical ventilatory support with less potential inflation of the stomach. The endotracheal tube will permit suctioning and application of PEEP to improve oxygenation.

Intubation. The decision to intubate is primarily a clinical decision, based on assessment of gas exchange and respiratory effort. Indications for intubation in the critically ill child include respiratory arrest or apnea, inability to maintain an effective airway (as a result of a depressed level of consciousness), obstructed airway, or edema with stridor, and/or severe hypoxemia or progressive hypercarbia. Intubation will be needed for the child who has multisystem failure or increased intracranial pressure (Box 9-9).

Whenever possible, accomplish intubation on an elective basis (i.e., discuss it during morning and afternoon rounds and plan elective intubation) in anticipation of further deterioration in respiratory function. If nursing and medical assessment and care are skilled, respiratory arrests rarely occur in the hospital, because respiratory deterioration is recognized and appropriate support is provided to prevent the arrest.

Box 9-9 **Indications for Intubation and Mechanical Ventilation**

- Respiratory arrest, gasping, or agonal respirations
- Excessive work of breathing
- Respiratory muscle fatigue
- Upper airway obstruction (anatomic or functional) or potential obstruction (e.g., facial trauma, inhalation injuries)
- Actual or potential decrease in airway protective reflexes (i.e., cough, gag)
- Shock (especially septic shock)
- Anticipated need for mechanical ventilation support (e.g., impending acute respiratory failure, chest trauma, shock, increased intracranial pressure, neuromuscular disease)

- Hypoxemia despite supplementary oxygen ($PaO_2 < 60$ mm Hg with $FiO_2 > 0.6$) in the absence of cyanotic congenital heart disease
- Inadequate ventilation ($PaCO_2 > 60$ mm Hg acutely or unresponsive to other interventions)
- Need for airway and ventilation control for deep sedation or patient transport
- Emergency drug administration
- Altered mental status
- Glasgow Coma Scale score less than 8 (see Chapter 11, Table 11-6)
- Increased intracranial pressure (see Chapter 11)

Selection of Tube Type. In the past, all children 8 years of age and younger were intubated with uncuffed endotracheal tubes, because the cricoid cartilage (the narrowest point of the airway) creates a natural seal around the tube. There was concern that use of a cuffed tube could create inflammation and injury to this area, although it is now clear that both cuffed and uncuffed tubes may be used safely in children, provided cuff pressure is monitored and kept at 20 to 25 cm H_2O. The use of cuffed ETTs may be preferred over uncuffed tubes in children with decreased lung compliance or in those who have a large air leak when an uncuffed tube is used. When using cuffed endotracheal tubes, the cuff must be a low-pressure, high-volume cuff to reduce the risk of pressure injury to the tissues. Monitor and maintain cuff pressure at 20 to 25 cm H_2O pressure (or per manufacturer's specifications).[122a,171]

Selection of Tube Size. When the child is critically ill and is at risk for respiratory failure, intubation equipment should be readily available in a cart at the bedside. Proper ETT size is estimated most accurately from the child's length, and the use of the color-coded Broselow Resuscitation Tape (Vital Signs, Armstrong Medical, Lincolnshire, IL) facilitates determination of proper tube size.[139] If the tape is not available, the uncuffed endotracheal tube size can be estimated roughly from the child's age according to the following formula (accurate in children 1-10 years old)[122a]:

$$\text{Uncuffed ETT size(mm)} = \frac{\text{Age(years)}}{4} + 4$$

The cuffed endotracheal tube can be estimated by the child's age using the following formula[122a]:

$$\text{Cuffed ETT size(mm)} = \frac{\text{Age(years)}}{4} + 3.5$$

The diameter of the ETT is approximately the diameter of the child's small finger. A reference table also can be used to estimate the proper tube size (Table 9-8).

Tube size is evaluated after placement. A tube can be too large yet still pass easily through the child's vocal cords, because the narrowest portion of the child's larynx is below the vocal cords at the level of the cricoid cartilage. Once the tube is placed, use a ventilation bag with pressure manometer to provide inspiration to a known pressure. If the tube size is appropriate, a small air leak will be detectable when the inspiratory pressure reaches approximately 25 cm H_2O. If a leak develops at lower pressures, the tube is probably too small, and a large air leak may develop during positive pressure ventilation. If the tube is too large, a leak will not be detectable despite inspiratory pressure exceeding 25 cm H_2O. The use of an excessively large tube can result in laryngeal or mucosal injury or necrosis or subglottic stenosis.

Insertion of the Tube. Before the intubation attempt, assemble all necessary equipment at the bedside (Box 9-10). Monitor the child's heart rate continuously and make certain the heart rate (QRS tone) is audible.

Oxygen is administered before and between any intubation attempts to ensure that the child is well oxygenated. If a short-acting nondepolarizing or depolarizing neuromuscular blocking agent is administered to facilitate intubation, then atropine may be administered to prevent bradycardia (refer to section, Nursing Care of the Child during Mechanical Ventilation and Chapter 5). Routine administration of atropine before intubation attempts is discouraged, however, because it might prevent or minimize hypoxemic-induced bradycardia and delay the recognition of hypoxemia during intubation.

Intubation of the critically ill child should be attempted only by persons skilled in airway management. The intubation clinician is assisted by one or more team members. Proper positioning before the attempt is essential. Typically, infants and toddlers (without suspected cervical spine trauma) are placed on a flat surface with the chin lifted into a sniffing position. It may be necessary to place the torso on a small pad to achieve proper alignment. Children older than 2 years (without cervical spine trauma) are generally placed with the head on a small pillow, and the chin is lifted into a sniffing position. The child is appropriately positioned for intubation if the opening of the ear canal is above or just level with the front of the shoulder when viewed from the side.

Table 9-8   Endotracheal and Tracheostomy Tube Sizes

Age	Internal Diameter (mm) Cuffed or Uncuffed	Oral Length (cm)	Nasal Length (cm)	Tracheostomy, Internal Diameter (mm)	Suction Catheter (in French Sizes)
Premature	2.5-3.0	8	11	4-5	5½-6
Newborn	3.0-3.5	8.5-10	13	4-5	6-8
6 months	3.5-4.0	10.5-12	15	5.5	8
18 months	3.5-4.5	12-13.5	16	6.0	8-10
24 months	4.5-5.5	13.5-14	17	6-7	10
2-4 year	5.0-6.0	15	18	6-7	10-12
4-7 year	5.5-6.5	16	19	7.0	12
7-10 year	6.0-7.0	17-19.5	21	8.0	12-14
10-12 year	6.5-7.5	20-21	22-25	9.0	14

Formula for estimating of *uncuffed* endotracheal tube:
$\frac{\text{Age(years)}}{4} + 4 = $ mm internal diameter

Formula for estimation of *cuffed* endotracheal tube:
$\frac{\text{Age(years)}}{4} + 3.5 = $ mm internal diameter

Formula for estimation of depth of tube insertion:
Tube internal diameter(in mm) $\times$ 3 $=$ cm insertion at the lip

Box 9-10	Intubation Equipment

- Bag, mask, and oxygen source, cardiac monitor with audible QRS tone
- Endotracheal tube: estimated size for body length and age (see Table 9-8) plus tubes sized 0.5 mm larger and 0.5 mm smaller
- Laryngeal mask airways in a variety of sizes (if available)
- Laryngoscope blade and handle (and extra bulbs and batteries)
  - Infants: 0-1 straight blade
  - Small children: 1 straight blade
  - Children (12-22 kg): 2 straight or curved blade
  - Large children (24-30 kg): 2-3 straight or curved blade
  - Adolescents (32-34 kg): 3 straight or curved blade
- Stylet

- Children 3-17 kg: 6 French
- Children >17 kg: 14 French
- Exhaled CO_2 detector, capnography
- Suction equipment: wall or portable suction
- Appropriate catheter to pass easily through endotracheal tube (usually the next French size above twice the ETT size (in millimeters) will pass readily into any ETT > 3.0 mm)
- Tonsillar suction or 12-14 French suction catheter
- Nasogastric tube
- Tape, liquid adhesive applicators, water-soluble lubricant
- Gloves and goggles
- Neuromuscular blocking agents, sedatives, analgesics, lidocaine
- Magill forceps for nasotracheal intubation

ETT, Endotracheal tube.

One team member holds the ETT (prepared with a stylet if requested) and may provide bag-mask ventilation using 100% oxygen before and after any intubation attempt. That team member may also provide cricoid pressure if requested during the intubation attempt. One team member is responsible for monitoring patient color and heart rate during the intubation attempt and must advise the intubating clinician if the child's heart rate or appearance deteriorates, so that the attempt can be interrupted and hand ventilation can be provided if the child's condition worsens. A respiratory therapist is an important member of the team during this phase of intubation.

It may be necessary to insert a stylet into the tube to pass the tube through the vocal cords. If a stylet is used, insert it only up to the final 1 cm of the tube and bend the proximal end of the stylet over the universal adaptor at the proximal end of the tube, so that the stylet cannot be inadvertently advanced beyond the tip of the tube. It is important to prevent the stylet from extending beyond the end of the tube, because it can perforate the airway. The decision to use a stylet during intubation is made by the intubating clinician. Be prepared to apply pressure to the cricoid cartilage to facilitate intubation.

During intubation, the following materials must be available within reach of the intubating clinician: suction tubing (joined to a suction canister, set to provide approximately -90 cm H_2O suction), a tonsillar suction device, a large suction catheter (used to suction the pharynx, if needed), a suction catheter of appropriate size for suctioning the ETT, liquid adhesive applicator, and tape (torn into strips appropriate for taping the tube), or device to secure the tube.

Suction devices are often needed to remove secretions, vomitus, or blood from the pharynx so that the intubating clinician can visualize the vocal chords. Once the tube is in place, the suction control is set to provide approximately -60 to -150 cm H_2O suction, based on the age of the child (Table 9-9).

Table 9-9	Typical Maximum Negative Pressure for Pediatric Airway Suctioning Based on Age

Age	Typical Negative Pressure (cm H_2O)
Infant	60-80
Child	80-120
Older child	120-150

Orotracheal intubation is typically performed in the critical care unit. It can be achieved rapidly and is associated with few complications. Nasotracheal intubation may be performed if it is difficult to secure the oral tube (e.g., the child has mouth or facial burns or injuries). Nasotracheal intubation has been associated with development of sinusitis, so when it is performed it will be necessary to monitor the patient closely for evidence of sinus infection.

If orotracheal intubation is performed, the laryngoscope blade is inserted into the hypopharynx to control the tongue and lift the lower jaw and tongue upward, so that the vocal cords may be visualized. It may be necessary to suction the area above the vocal cords, with a tonsillar suction or a large suction catheter, to visualize the cords.

If nasotracheal intubation is performed, the tube is lubricated, gently inserted nasally, and advanced until the tip of the tube is visualized in the back of the pharynx. The laryngoscope blade is then used to visualize the cords, and McGill forceps are used to advance the tube from the pharynx through the vocal cords.

Rapid Sequence Intubation. The critically ill or injured infant or child who needs intubation may have a full stomach. In such a child, the goal is to safely insert an airway, without stimulating vomiting. For a patient who needs urgent intubation, rapid sequence intubation (RSI) may be performed (Box 9-11 shows the indications for RSI). RSI is defined as nearly simultaneous delivery of oxygenation, sedation, and neuromuscular blockade for the purpose of intubation.[209] The goal is to provide near immediate intubating conditions.[284]

Preoxygenation is accomplished by providing 100% oxygen to the child while the child is breathing spontaneously. Preoxygenation will typically be effective after 3 to 5 minutes of oxygen administration or four to eight deep breaths, if the child is cooperative. After preoxygenation, an intravenous sedative or anesthetic is administered rapidly, followed almost immediately by a neuromuscular blocker. Cricoid pressure is applied via the Sellick maneuver as soon as the child is deeply sedated (i.e., without cough or gag reflex).[25] During administration of the sedative and neuromuscular blocker, the oxygen mask remains in place on the child's face, but positive-pressure ventilation is not provided, because such ventilation can produce gastric distension and possible regurgitation. The

---

Box 9-11 **Rapid Sequence Intubation**

Indications

- Full stomach or oral intake within the past 4-6 h
- Pharyngeal or upper gastrointestinal bleeding
- Ileus or intestinal obstruction (includes acute onset of illness)
- Tense abdominal distension
- Pregnancy

Relative Contraindications*

- Difficult airway, known or suspected
- Profuse hemorrhage obscuring airway visualization
- Upper airway obstruction
- Increased intracranial pressure*
- Significant facial or laryngeal edema, trauma or distortion

Sequence

1. Brief medical history and focused physical assessment

2. Preparation of patient (positioning), equipment, personnel and medications
3. Establishment of monitoring and IV/IO access
4. Preoxygenation for 3 to 5 min (or four to eight voluntary breaths) with 100% oxygen
5. Administration of IV anesthetic-sedative-analgesic and almost simultaneous delivery of neuromuscular blocker
6. Cricoid pressure (once the patient is deeply sedated)
7. Short period of apnea until the patient has full muscle relaxation
8. Endotracheal intubation
9. Confirmation of tube placement (with clinical exam and device); cricoid pressure is removed once tube position is confirmed and tube cuff (if present) is inflated
10. Postintubation monitoring and observation

Adapted from Ralston M, et al, editors: *PALS provider manual, student CD: respiratory management resources chapter,* Dallas, 2006, American Heart Association; and deCaen A, et al: Airway management. In Nichols DG, editor: *Roger's textbook of pediatric critical care,* ed 4, Philadelphia, 2008, Lippincott Williams and Wilkins.
*Evaluate each patient for the risk/benefit of intubation using RSI.
IO, Intraosseous; *IV,* intravenous.

---

child is apneic for a brief period until full muscle relaxation occurs. As soon as the child is flaccid, intubation is performed by a provider skilled in airway management.[284] Once endotracheal intubation is confirmed and the tube cuff (if used) is inflated, cricoid pressure is removed, the child's lungs are manually ventilated, and proper tube position is confirmed.[243]

The title of the intubating clinician (i.e., resident, fellow, nurse practitioner, respiratory therapist, attending physician) is less important than the level of intubation experience.[198,209] Complications of RSI include hypoxemia, hypotension, and arrhythmia.[198]

Difficult Airway. A difficult airway is present any time the intubating team member has difficulty with bag-mask ventilation or endotracheal intubation. The team may encounter difficult airways in children with a history of challenging intubations or conditions (e.g., obesity, craniofacial abnormalities, facial burns or trauma, macroglossia, open globe, cervical spine injuries, mediastinal mass, musculoskeletal diseases, acute infectious upper airway obstruction) that are likely to make intubation difficult. These difficult airways need to be anticipated and carefully planned.

Every unit caring for seriously ill or injured children must keep a kit readily available with the equipment needed to address a difficult airway, including many types and sizes of laryngoscope blades, ETTs, laryngeal mask airways (LMAs), forceps, stylets, a needle cricothyrotomy-tracheostomy kit, and an intubating bronchoscope.[59]

New techniques that may be helpful for intubating children with difficult airways include a lighted wand stylet or a video laryngoscope (i.e., laryngoscope with video camera). It may be appropriate to consult anesthesia or otolaryngology (ear, nose, and throat) specialists for assistance in managing the difficult airway. In these cases fiberoptic bronchoscopy for intubation is an option.[59]

Laryngeal Mask Airway. The LMA is a supraglottic airway that can be inserted in an unconscious child. It can be inserted blindly, without visualization of the vocal cords (see Evolve

Figure 9-1 in the Chapter 9 Supplement on the Evolve Website). LMAs have been used frequently in the operating room to establish an airway. However, they may also provide an acceptable temporary alternative in a patient with a difficult airway until a more secure airway is achieved (Box 9-12). LMAs are now available in a variety of sizes for pediatric use (Table 9-10). Infants and children who have an LMA placed must be sedated or have significantly depressed level of consciousness to limit airway reflex activity.[243,282]

The LMA is inserted by placing the LMA with the cuff lumen facing upward, so that it opens toward the surface of the tongue. The LMA is advanced into the pharynx until resistance is met. The mask is inflated to seal the hypopharynx, and air flow can then occur through the tube into the trachea (see Evolve Figure 9-1 in the Chapter 9 Supplement on the Evolve Website).[25] Do not exceed recommended cuff inflation volumes (see Table 9-10).

Combitubes. The combitube is a dual-lumen (esophageal-tracheal) tube used to quickly and easily secure an airway.[199] This tube is inserted blindly, without visualization of the glottis (see Evolve Figures 9-2 and 9-3 in the Chapter 9 Supplement on the Evolve Website). When using blind intubation, the tip of the tube can be inserted into either the esophagus or the trachea. The dual lumen allows for ventilation whether the tube is in the esophagus or trachea; however, proper selection of ventilating lumens is needed. Because this tube is available in only large sizes, it can be used only for emergencies in adolescents (older than 12 years).

To insert the Combitube, the intubating clinician performs a jaw thrust and inserts the tube into the middle of the mouth parallel to the pharyngeal wall and advances it gently until the patient's teeth lie between the two black ring markings on the tube. The pharyngeal balloon is inflated, followed by inflation of the esophageal balloon.[199] If the tip of the tube rests in the esophagus, the esophageal blue (distal) lumen and connector are used for ventilation. If the tip of the tube rests in the trachea, the white (tracheal) lumen and connector are used for

Box 9-12 Use of Laryngeal Mask Airway (LMA) in Children

Indications
- Resuscitation of unconscious child when endotracheal intubation is not possible
- Controlling the airway during routine or emergency anesthetic procedures
- Known or suspected difficult airway
- Oropharyngeal trauma with failure of other means in establishing an airway

Contraindications
- Intact gag reflex
- Delayed gastric emptying, unknown oral intake (laryngeal mask airway does not protect from aspiration)
- Low pulmonary compliance requiring high ventilation pressures

Based on information from Binck AC: Intubation: perform, including laryngeal mask airway. In Verger JT, Lebet RM, editors: *AACN procedure manual for pediatric acute and critical care.* St Louis, 2008, Saunders-Elsevier; and Hazinski MF, et al, editors: Airway, ventilation and management of respiratory distress and failure. In: *PALS provider manual,* Dallas, 2002, American Heart Association.

Table 9-10 LMA Sizes and Cuff Inflation Volumes

LMA Airway Size	Patient Size	Maximum Cuff Inflation Volumes (air, mL)*
1	Neonates/infants up to 5 kg	4
1½	Infants 5-10 kg	7
2	Infants/children 10-20 kg	10
2½	Children 20-30 kg	14
3	Children 30-50 kg	20
4	Adults 50-70 kg	30
5	Adults 70-100 kg	40
6	Adults >100 kg	50

Reproduced from LMA Airway management: *Frequently asked questions,* 2008. Available at: http://www.lmana.com/faqs.php#faq03. Accessed June 9, 2011. *These are maximum clinical volumes that should never be exceeded. It is recommended that the cuff be inflated to 60 cm H_2O intracuff pressures.

ventilation (see Evolve Figure 9-2 in the Chapter 9 Supplement on the Evolve Website). To confirm use of the correct (ventilating) lumen, use a CO_2 detection device after delivering 6 to 12 positive pressure breaths. Detection of CO_2 confirms that the lumen used is in communication with the trachea. Reexpansion of the self-inflating bulb will also confirm that the lumen is in communication with the trachea. Although use of the Combitube may be beneficial in an emergency, it is not intended for long-term use.

The EasyTube (Rüsch EasyTube, Teleflex Medical, Durham, NC, www.rusch.com) is another emergency intubation device that can be inserted blindly; it can be used for children longer than 90 cm.[241] The EasyTube is similar to the Combitube, but the lumen is narrower to reduce risk of mucosal damage. Experience with this device is limited.

Evaluating Tube Placement. Once the tube is inserted into the trachea, hand ventilation is provided using a bag with

oxygen, and a team member auscultates both sides of the chest to verify the presence of bilateral breath sounds and auscultates over the stomach to verify that breath sounds are not heard. Chest expansion should be equal and adequate bilaterally. A device is also needed to confirm placement.

If the tube is in the trachea, CO_2 is detected after delivery of six breaths, using a colorimetric CO_2 detector or capnography. A colorimetric CO_2 detector changes color when CO_2 is detected.[194] A capnography waveform is a very reliable indicator of exhaled CO_2 and tracheal tube placement. Because a perfusing cardiac rhythm is needed to deliver CO_2 to the lungs, when cardiac arrest is present, CO_2 may not be detected even when the tube is in the trachea. Excellent chest compressions can produce sufficient cardiac output and pulmonary blood flow, resulting in detection of CO_2 in exhaled air (see Chapter 6). Reexpansion of the bulb of an esophageal detector device indicates tracheal tube placement.

After intubation the appropriateness of the tube size is assessed. If the tube is the appropriate size, an air leak will be detected once an inspiratory pressure of 25 cm H_2O is provided. If a leak is detected at a lower pressure, the tube may be too small, and it may be necessary to replace it with a larger tube once the patient is stable, particularly if the child is mechanically ventilated and has noncompliant lungs. If higher pressures are needed to create a leak, the tube may be too large, and it may be necessary to replace it when the patient's condition is stable.

As long as the advanced airway is in place, the bedside nurse is responsible for verifying tube position and patency on a regular basis and whenever the patient's condition changes. If the tube is in the proper location, both sides of the chest will expand equally and adequately. A unilateral decrease in chest expansion can indicate tube migration or unilateral atelectasis. Right main bronchus intubation, for example, will result in expansion of the right chest, with decreased or absent breath sounds and decreased expansion of the left chest during positive pressure ventilation.

Once the tube is thought to be in proper position, the centimeter number located at the lips is noted, and the tube is taped in position. In general, proper depth of insertion (in centimeters) is estimated for children 1 to 10 years old by tripling the ETT internal diameter (in millimeters). Once the ETT is taped and firmly in place, a chest radiograph is obtained to confirm proper tube insertion depth, and the position of the ETT is adjusted if necessary. If the ETT is properly placed, the tip of the ETT will be no deeper than 1 to 2 cm above the carina and no higher than the first rib (see Figs. 10-20 and 10-21 for examples of the radiographic evaluation of ETT location).

Neither use of the Broselow tape nor the formula to estimate ETT placement can replace clinical assessment. Clinical evaluation and a chest radiograph are needed to confirm appropriate ETT size and depth of insertion.[187] The role of the bedside nurse is critical to this evaluation.

Securing the Endotracheal Tube. The ETT can be secured in a variety of ways to reduce the risk of tube displacement. Unplanned extubations are often preventable occurrences that can affect patient morbidity and mortality.[146] Taping or retaping of the ETT must always be performed by two people. One person is responsible for holding the tube in place and immobilizing the child's head, and the second person is responsible for the taping. Do not attempt this procedure with one person, because movement by the child can result in unplanned extubation.

Commonly, pediatric ETTs are secured with adhesive tape (Fig. 9-11). Taping the ETT typically involves wrapping the tube with pieces of tape that are anchored to each cheek and then split lengthwise and wrapped around the tube and anchored to the skin. Skin integrity is evaluated when the tube is retaped. If skin barrier material is needed before the tape is placed, it is placed on the child's face to protect from skin breakdown. To promote tape adhesion, an adhesive skin preparation can be used over the area to be taped. Breath sounds are assessed immediately before and after retaping to confirm the presence of equal and bilateral breath sounds. Unequal breath sounds, especially with more prominent breath sounds on the right side, may indicate endobronchial intubation resulting from advancement of the tube during retaping. Note the ETT centimeter mark at the child's lips at the start and end of procedure. If there is uncertainty about movement of the tube during retaping, a discrepancy regarding the location of the documented tube measurement, or a change in physical examination results after

tube retaping, notify a provider. A chest radiograph may be ordered to assess the depth of tube insertion.[111]

An umbilical clamp may be used to assist securing the ETT in infants (see Evolve Figure 9-4 in the Chapter 9 Supplement on the Evolve Website). This method allows the ETT to be secured to both the infant's face and the umbilical clamp for tube stabilization. Studies in neonates have documented reduced unplanned extubation rates when using the tape-and-clamp method compared with traditional taping methods.[61,138]

Commercially manufactured devices are available to secure advanced airways, but infant and pediatric sizes are limited. Several studies in adults have evaluated commercially available devices and their effect on unplanned extubations. No single method of securing a tube has been identified as superior for minimizing ETT dislodgement, although there may be some effect on time requirements, patient comfort, incidence of skin breakdown, and cost.[35,84]

Maintaining the Endotracheal Tube. Factors most commonly associated with inadvertent extubation in the critically ill infant or child include lack of recent sedation, patient agitation, lack of restraints, performing bedside procedures, taping

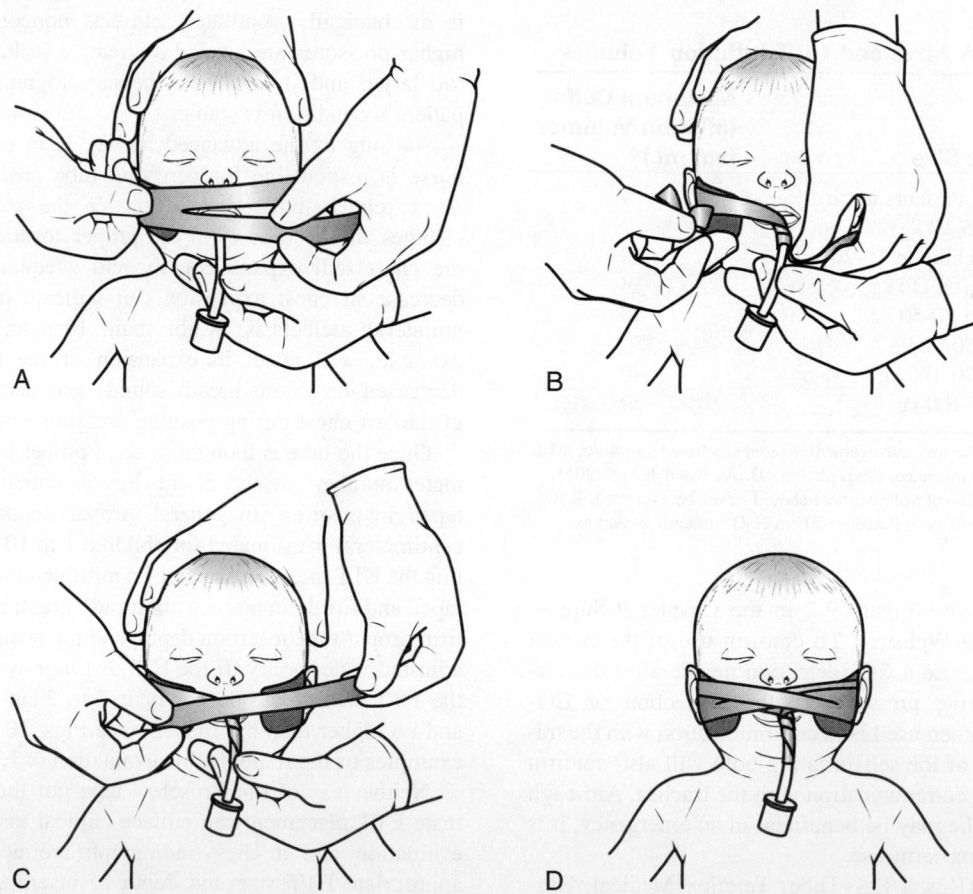

FIG. 9-11 Method of securing an orotracheal tube using split tape. Liquid barrier has been applied to the cheeks and upper lip and the oral endotracheal tube is held in place. **A,** A piece of tape is split lengthwise for half of its length; the solid piece is placed on the right cheek with split portion toward the mouth. **B,** The top half of the split tape is wrapped around the tube in a spiral fashion, beginning across the top of the tube. The tape should be spiraled so that each layer of tape adheres to the tube, rather than to layers of tape. A piece of tape is turned at the end to create a tab that will facilitate later removal. **C,** The bottom split half of the tape is secured across the top lip of the child, extending to the opposite cheek. **D,** The taping has been repeated from the other cheek. (Modified from Jarog DL. *Endotracheal Tube: Taping,* in Verger JT and Lebet RM (Eds). *AACN Procedure Manual for Pediatric Acute and Critical Care,* Philadelphia, 2008, Saunders Elsevier.)

technique, emesis, and coughing.[32,81,134] Not only do patient-specific factors affect the risk of extubation, but nursing staff ratios have been shown to affect the risk of unplanned extubation in the pediatric critical care unit. Higher nurse-to-patient ratios and higher patient acuity-to-nurse ratios have been identified as factors associated with increased incidence of unplanned extubations.[146,197] Experience with intubated patients and the number of pediatric critical care unit beds have not been shown to affect rates of unplanned extubation.[81]

Nurses are uniquely positioned to affect the incidence of unplanned extubation. Attention to the sedation level and judicious administration of analgesia and anxiolytics to intubated children can affect outcomes (see Chapter 5). Daily identification of sedation goals and scores can improve patient safety and reduce frequency of unplanned extubations.[188] Extremity immobilizers may be indicated in active intubated patients.

It is important to use extreme care when moving or repositioning intubated children. The trachea of the infant or child is shorter than that of the adult. Consequently, even small movements of the ETT place the child at risk for inadvertent extubation or endobronchial tube migration. Studies evaluating tracheal tube tip displacement during head-neck manipulation demonstrate that head and neck flexion consistently result in movement of the endotracheal tube tip toward the carina (see Fig. 10-19). Conversely, head and neck extension move the ETT tip away from the carina, increasing risk for extubation.[112,269] Maintain the head in a neutral position throughout the period of intubation. Rotating the head, neck, and torso as a unit can prevent neck torsion and tube displacement. When a chest radiograph is obtained, place the child's head and neck in neutral position with the chest free of extraneous objects that could interfere with radiograph quality.

Causes of Acute Deterioration in the Intubated Child. Whenever a child is intubated, the bedside nurse must ensure that the ETT remains patent and in proper position, and that the child's oxygenation and ventilation are adequate. Causes of acute deterioration in the intubated child include tube displacement or obstruction, pneumothorax, and equipment (i.e., oxygen, ventilator, or bag device) failure and can be recalled using the "DOPE" mnemonic.[122a] Whenever a child with an advanced airway deteriorates acutely, provide hand ventilation with a ventilation bag and attempt to identify or rule out these causes of deterioration (Box 9-13). If hand ventilation cannot move air and expand the chest, the tube is probably displaced out of the trachea or is obstructed. Although bilateral pneumothoraces may be present, they are less common than tube obstruction. Quickly suction the tube in an effort to relieve the obstruction. If the obstruction cannot be eliminated quickly, then remove the tube. Notify a physician or healthcare provider skilled in airway

management and provide ventilation by bag and mask until reintubation can be performed.

Manual ventilator bags. Two types of manual ventilator bags can be used to provide hand ventilation for intubated patients. One type is the self-inflating manual ventilator bag, and the second is the flow-inflating or "anesthesia" bag. Both of these bags come in a variety of sizes to deliver a variety of tidal volumes. However, there are several important differences between these two types of manual ventilator bags.

Self-inflating bags do not require a source of gas flow, so they can be used away from oxygen sources (e.g., during transport when an oxygen tank is empty). Self-inflating bags have a pop-off valve that vents pressure from the bag system when pressure exceeds 35 to 45 mm Hg.[194] Concentrations of delivered oxygen can vary greatly (FiO_2 between 0.30 and 0.60) when this bag is used, because the bag entrains room air when it reexpands after compression. If a reservoir is added to the bag, an FiO_2 of 1.00 (100% oxygen) may be administered. PEEP may also be added to this bag system using a PEEP valve. A disadvantage of this bag is that there is no way to monitor the pressure or volume of inspired air delivered to the patient. In addition, the user tends to lose the "feel" of the lungs while providing hand ventilation. See Chapter 21 for information about self-inflating bags currently being used in the care of critically ill children.

The flow-inflating bag requires continuous gas flow to inflate, but it is able to accurately deliver concentrations of oxygen up to 100%. Flow through the bag is adjusted by changing the oxygen flow and the expiratory or pressure relief valve attached to the bag. In addition, PEEP may be added to this bag by incrementally closing the pressure relief valve until the desired PEEP is achieved. Because this manual ventilator system has no pop-off valve, the inflating or inspiratory pressure provided to the patient is typically measured with a manometer attached to the bag outlet. Because oxygen flow is continuous through this system and no one-way valve is present, the child can receive oxygen flow between manual inflations if breathing is spontaneous.

Because the flow-inflating bag is extremely compliant, the user can develop a good "feel" for the compliance of the child's lungs during manual ventilation. However, if this bag is used by an unskilled person, high inflation pressures may inadvertently develop, causing barotrauma, including pneumothorax.

TYPES OF MECHANICAL VENTILATION

There are many methods of mechanical support of ventilation and oxygenation for a child with diseased lungs. Ventilation support can be intermittent, continuous, short-term, or long-term, and it can use positive or negative pressure, with or without patient effort or cooperation.

Normal Spontaneous Ventilation Cycle

Support of ventilation can be better understood after considering the normal respiratory cycle. Normal mechanics of breathing depend on pressure gradients within the pulmonary system (see Fig. 9-2). Air or gas flows only when a pressure difference exists between two areas, and gas always flows from an area of higher pressure to one of lower pressure. Thus the

Box 9-13	**Causes of Acute Deterioration in the Child with an Advanced Airway "DOPE" Mnemonic**[122a]

- Tube **D**isplacement
- Tube **O**bstruction
- **P**neumothorax
- **E**quipment Failure

intraalveolar pressure must be less than the pressure at the airway opening (atmospheric pressure) for inspiratory flow to occur. As the diaphragm contracts, intrathoracic volume increases and the intrapleural pressure becomes negative with respect to atmospheric pressure. The lung tissue is pulled outward (lung volume increased) and alveolar pressure decreases. This pressure change creates a pressure difference between the atmosphere and the alveolus, and gas flows into the lungs until pressure in the atmosphere is again equal to that within the alveoli. The passive elastic recoil of the lung and thorax tend to return the lung volume to its resting state during expiration. At end expiration, intraalveolar and atmospheric pressures are approximately equal.

Positive Pressure Mechanical Ventilation

Mechanical ventilators provide support in a variety of ways, using different mechanics and microprocessors controlled by the settings prescribed. In general, the mode of ventilation is selected and a series of variables, including the trigger, limit, and cycle, must be adjusted to optimize mechanical ventilation. These adjustable settings are variables of pressure, volume, flow, and time.

With positive pressure ventilation, inspiration is controlled, and exhalation is passive and depends on the elastic recoil of the lungs, relatively low airway resistance, and ETT patency and effective diameter. If airway resistance is high or the ETT is too small or obstructed, exhalation is inhibited and air trapping and hypercarbia may develop

Positive Pressure Ventilation

Positive pressure ventilation delivers a pressure at the airway opening that is greater than the intraalveolar pressure. As a result, pressurized gas is forced from the ventilator unit into the lungs. Pressurized gas will flow preferentially into the areas of the lung that offer the least resistance to air flow.[147] These areas will be the superior and anterior regions of the lung if the patient is supine or semiupright. Positive pressure ventilation results in increased airway pressures and increased intrathoracic pressures. Increased intrathoracic pressure can cause a decrease in both systemic and pulmonary venous return to the heart and a fall in cardiac output that is accentuated if the patient exhibits hypovolemia.

The flow of gas in the pressure mode may be constant, not constant, increasing, or decreasing, depending on the specific ventilator. If the setting is pressure triggered, inspiration starts when a preset pressure is detected. If a ventilator is pressure-cycled, inspiration ceases when the preset inspiratory pressure is reached. If the setting is pressure limited, a peak pressure may be met before the end of inspiration.[259] The tidal volume delivered is determined by the compliance of the patient's lungs, airway resistance, and presence or absence of a leak around the ETT.

Volume

Volume cycled ventilation delivers a preset amount (volume) of gas with each inspiration. If the setting is volume cycled, the inspiration ends when the volume has been reached. If the setting is volume limited, a peak volume may be met before the end of inspiration.[259] The pressure necessary to deliver the volume depends on the compliance of the ventilator circuit, the patient's lung compliance, and airway resistance.

Flow

Flow cycled ventilation delivers a flow of gas. If the setting is flow triggered, inspiration starts when a preset minimum flow is detected. If the setting flow is cycled, the inspiration ends when the inspiration flow meets a preset maximum flow. If the setting is flow limited, the peak flow may be reached before the end of inspiration.[259]

Time

Time cycled ventilation delivers gas based on time. If the setting is time triggered, inspiration starts when a preset time elapses. If the setting is time cycled, inspiration ends when a set inspiratory time has elapsed. There is no time limited setting.[259] As a result, tidal volume is determined by the flow rate of the ventilator.

Negative Pressure Ventilation

Negative pressure ventilators can be used for long-term ventilation of children with neuromuscular disease. The tank ventilator (the so-called iron lung or shell), body suit, and cuirass ventilator are the primary units available. These units create subatmospheric pressure that results in expansion of the chest wall and therefore the lungs, producing inhalation.[60] These devices must cover the child's thorax, and as a result they are cumbersome and limit the activity of and accessibility to the child. The chief advantage of such a system is that an artificial airway is unnecessary if the child's upper airway is patent.

Despite a long history of use in patients with polio and tracheostomies, a recent review of negative pressure ventilation did not identify sufficient research to recommend its use in acute hypoxemic respiratory failure in children.[217] However, there is some evidence to support a growing interest in this ventilation modality for both neonates and adults.[239,247]

Conventional Ventilation Modes

Mechanical ventilation can be delivered in several modes. The appropriate ventilation mode is selected on the basis of factors such as the presence of spontaneous breathing, reason for institution of mechanical ventilation, and severity of the child's cardiopulmonary disease. The two major categories of ventilation support are assist-control, and intermittent mandatory ventilation (IMV).

Assist-Control Mode

Complete mechanical ventilation in the control mode means that the patient cannot contribute any spontaneous breaths during ventilation. Although most children can contribute some effort to the ventilatory cycle, children with impaired central nervous system function (coma, apnea, or neuromuscular weakness) or severe cardiovascular instability may need complete controlled mechanical ventilation. Children who recently have undergone major surgery may conserve energy and stabilize more quickly if they receive mechanical ventilation in the control mode. Children who are able to make adequate breathing efforts and who might fight the ventilator, however, would not be good candidates for the control mode unless they are sufficiently sedated. In this mode there is no additional assistance from the ventilator to support patient-initiated breathing between the controlled breaths. As such, for most children, even the most critically ill, the mode of ventilation typically includes assistance for any additional breaths the child might strive to take.

The assist mode of ventilation provides for facilitated breathing and can be used in addition to controlled ventilation or independent of a mandatory respiratory rate. New ventilatory technology uses pressure support breaths in place of the assist mode. However, children receiving continued ventilatory support may be using ventilators with an active assist mode.

In general, in the assist mode the child initiates a breath and the inspiration occurs with the aid of the ventilator. Inspiratory flow will begin when the patient creates a subatmospheric pressure or, in the case of ventilation with PEEP, reduces pressure to a preset level; this triggers the ventilator and causes it to cycle. The ease of the patient triggering depends on the sensitivity setting on the machine. Once triggered, the machine cycles and delivers a breath.

Children who are extremely weak might not be able to trigger the ventilator to augment a spontaneous breath, and the child will appear distressed and dyssynchronous with the ventilatory cycle. If this occurs, the sensitivity may be adjusted or the mode changed to facilitate spontaneous breathing. An advantage of the assist setting is that the child can augment his or her own breathing and usually feels more comfortable.

Intermittent Mandatory Ventilation (IMV)

During IMV the child receives a preset number of ventilator-generated breaths at mandatory intervals. Between mandatory breaths, however, continuous gas flow is present in the system, so that the child may breathe spontaneously between each IMV breath. The support given to those breaths varies with the type of ventilator in use. Synchronized intermittent mandatory ventilation (SIMV) also provides a preset number of breaths that are synchronized with the child's spontaneous inspiration. With either IMV or SIMV, the patient receives a minimal number of mandatory breaths.

For the IMV or SIMV mode to provide successful ventilation, the mandatory breaths must be provided to complement the patient's spontaneous ventilation. A higher number of mandatory breaths must be provided if the patient's spontaneous ventilatory effort is minimal, and the number of mandatory breaths can be reduced as the patient's spontaneous ventilatory effort increases.

For IMV or SIMV, continuous gas flow must be present through the system so that the patient will receive fresh gas during spontaneous breathing cycles. The demand valve is opened when the patient generates sufficient negative inspiratory pressure or a minimal flow within the central airway, and then gas flow is provided.[147] The opening of the inspiratory valve may create excessive work for small infants and children with small tidal volumes. The ventilator needs to be adjusted to provide continuous flow so that the child is not "locked out" of a supported breath.

Pressure-Support Ventilation

Pressure-support ventilation (PSV) is also known as *inspiratory assist ventilation* and is another method of partial ventilatory support. This mode can be used if the patient demonstrates some effective ventilatory effort; it is often used during weaning, with or without a mandatory respiratory rate. During PSV the patient receives assistance from the ventilator during every patient-initiated breath. The patient initiates a breath by generating a small amount of negative pressure within the system, and pressurized gas is provided to achieve a preset airway pressure. When the patient's inspiration ceases (i.e., inspiratory flow rate declines by a certain percentage or below a certain set volume), pressure support is terminated.[147,260] During PSV the tidal volume delivered with each breath may vary because a maximum pressure, not volume, is set.

An advantage of PSV is that it can reduce the inspiratory effort necessary to overcome the resistance created by an artificial airway or ventilator circuit. In addition, it can provide an additional method of tapering ventilatory support, increasing the patient's spontaneous ventilation, and conditioning respiratory muscles.[30,141,189]

The inspiratory support must be adjusted properly for the resistance created by the ETT and ventilator circuit.[76] If the ventilator is improperly adjusted, with high triggering pressures or low inspiratory flows, the work of breathing is likely to be high. PSV will not successfully ventilate a patient who has a significant air leak around the ETT, and it may be difficult to adjust to support (or wean) an infant with tachypnea.

High-Frequency Ventilation

High-frequency ventilation (HFV) uses rapid respiratory rates (60-3600 cycles/min) at tidal volumes approximating anatomic dead space to achieve adequate oxygenation and ventilation in children with acute lung injury and when conventional ventilation has failed.[115,122,146,259] Two major forms of HFV are currently available: oscillatory ventilation and jet ventilation.

High-Frequency Oscillatory Ventilation. High-frequency oscillatory ventilation (HFOV) moves a small volume of gas into and out of the lungs using a piston that moves at extremely high frequencies to create positive and negative pressure swings (180-1500 cycles/min).[122,147] The effective tidal volume delivered is determined by airway resistance. Carbon dioxide elimination is, in turn, influenced by the effective tidal volume delivered and by vibration frequency. Exhalation is active in HFOV through a change in the pressure from positive to negative. The proposed mechanisms of gas exchange during HFOV include convection, molecular diffusion, pendelluft, asymmetric velocity profiles, direct alveolar ventilation, Taylor dispersion, cardiogenic mixing, accelerated diffusion, and acoustic resonance.[125]

HFOV can improve oxygenation by alveolar recruitment. It does so by opening the lungs using a higher mean airway pressure compared with conventional mechanical ventilation (CMV), then keeping the lungs open during the respiratory cycle. Because HFOV inflates the lungs (alveolar recruitment) and keeps them open using low volume and low or peak pressure, it may reduce barotrauma and volutrauma. Ventilator-induced lung injury (VILI) is believed to be caused by excessive alveolar stretch (volume), especially in patients with low lung volumes. Therefore HFOV may reduce VILI by maintaining an "open" lung while ventilating with extremely low tidal volumes.

Although HFOV has been used effectively for more than 15 years, pediatric data from randomized controlled clinical trials are limited. One well-known clinical trial, published in 1994 by Arnold et al.[10] was a randomized, crossover trial of 70 critically ill children with ARDS. Those treated with HFOV demonstrated improved oxygenation and decreased use of supplementary oxygen 30 days later.[10] Given the limited amount of data both in neonates and children, the current Cochrane reviews on HFOV in acute lung injury found no difference in CMV versus HFOV.[100,281] HFOV is currently being studied by the adult acute respiratory distress syndrome network.[4]

There are special considerations for nursing care of the child receiving HFOV. Respiratory assessment is altered because the child has a chest wiggle instead of standard inspiratory and expiratory phases of ventilation. The chest wiggle reflects the power of ventilation. Depending on the size of the patient, the wiggle will extend down the chest and range between the umbilicus and middle thigh and will be symmetrical.

The sounds in the chest are different when compared with breath sounds heard during CMV. Conventional breath sounds are not present and cannot be described using standard terminology: instead the nurse should describe the pitch, comparing one side of the chest to the other. Monitoring of ventilator settings is similar with HFOV, but the terminology is different (Box 9-14). In addition, monitoring for complications is routine (Box 9-15).

High-Frequency Jet Ventilation. High-frequency jet ventilation (HFJV) uses an injection catheter within the lumen of the central airway to pulse gas under high pressure at a rapid

---

Box 9-14	Definition of High-Frequency Oscillatory Ventilation Terms

- *Frequency (F)*: Rate measure in hertz; 1 Hz = 60 breaths/ min
- *Mean airway pressure (mPaw)*: Mean pressure delivered over time
- *Amplitude (ΔP)*: Change in pressure (in the circuit) above and below the mean airway pressure
- *Power:* Electrical current that controls the movement of the piston[97]

Box 9-15	Potential Complications of High-Frequency Oscillatory Ventilation

- *Hemodynamic Compromise*: Secondary to high mean airway pressure, leading to decreased venous return
- *Barotrauma*: Secondary to hyperinflation and shear force of high gas flow
- *Intraventricular Hemorrhage (neonate)*: Secondary to elevated intrapulmonary pressure that impedes venous return and causes increased venous pressures[97]

---

cycling rate. Tidal volume, usually slightly higher than anatomic dead space, varies with jet driving pressure, frequency, and inspiratory time.[122,147] Exhalation is passive and depends on lung and chest wall recoil. This mode of HFV is specifically helpful in patients with bronchopleural fistula,[259] and it is used much less frequently than HFOV. The most recent Cochrane review for HFJV is for very low-birth weight neonates, and it found no significant difference in those neonates treated with HFJV versus CMV.[114]

Newer Modes of Ventilatory Support

Volume-Support Ventilation

Volume-support ventilation (VSV) is a new mode of ventilation and a mode of partial mechanical ventilation. It is similar to PSV in that it is an assist mode and supports spontaneous breathing. During VSV the patient receives assistance from the ventilator during every patient-initiated breath. With each spontaneous breath, the ventilator delivers a preset tidal volume. The pressure with which this volume is delivered varies depending on the degree of lung injury.[149] This mode has been used as a weaning mode and studied in comparison with PSV.[109,196] Some ventilators will change automatically from VSV to a mandatory ventilation mode if the patient is apneic.[259]

Airway Pressure Release Ventilation

Airway pressure release ventilation (APRV) is a new mode of ventilation. APRV provides CPAP with the aid of an airway release mechanism using a time cycle.[191] The patient breathes spontaneously without a mandatory respiratory rate from the ventilator. Each breath is delivered at two different airway pressures through continuous flow. The main benefit of this method of support is thought to be its application of a lower total airway pressure.[259] In addition, use of a constant expiratory pressure facilitates and maintains alveolar recruitment.[190]

Dual Control Modes

Newer, more sophisticated ventilators have feedback loops that provide information to the ventilator to control pressure, volume, or both. The modes are dual control within a breath or dual control breath-to-breath. In either case, a desired tidal volume is delivered. Dual control within a breath can change from pressure control to volume control within the same breath if the feedback loop is telling the ventilator that the patient is not going to reach the targeted tidal volume. In the breath-to-breath mode, the feedback to the ventilator adjusts the pressure needed to deliver the set tidal volume, so the pressure may vary with each breath.[259]

Pressure Regulated, Volume Control Ventilation

Pressure-regulated volume-control ventilation (PRVCV) is a dual-control breath-to-breath mode. Mandatory breaths are delivered to the patient using a maximal set pressure until a set tidal volume is reached. Using the feedback after the first breath is delivered, the ventilator delivers subsequent breaths at 75% of the pressure to reach the desired tidal volume. Depending on lung compliance, the pressure needed to meet the set tidal volume will vary: it will decrease when compliance improves and increase when compliance deteriorates.[259]

Because PRVCV decreases peak inspiratory pressure (PIP), it may reduce barotrauma. It is considered an advantageous mode when patients have rapidly changing lung compliance and resistance.[149] Some ventilators deliver this mode only in an IMV and not SIMV mode; if that is the case, there is no synchronization with the respiratory effort of the patient, so concomitant sedation and possible neuromuscular blockade is needed.

Positive End-Expiratory Pressure

The use of either PEEP or CPAP is helpful when treating hypoxemia that is unresponsive to supplementary oxygen. The name applied (CPAP or PEEP) is based on method of ventilation. When positive pressure ventilation (PPV) is provided, the end-expiratory pressure is designated as *PEEP*. When a patient is breathing spontaneously (without PPV), positive airway pressure is called *CPAP*. Although the physiologic effects of CPAP and PEEP are identical, the following discussion will refer to the use of PEEP. Effects are the same for CPAP. For further information about cardiopulmonary interactions and potential effects of positive pressure ventilation on cardiac output, see Cardiopulmonary Interactions later in this chapter.

Therapeutic Effects of PEEP

PEEP increases alveolar volume, thereby improving ventilation-perfusion matching. The result is an increase in arterial oxygenation. In addition, PEEP redistributes lung water, moving pulmonary edema fluid into other areas of lung (toward the hilum and away from alveoli) so that the fluid will interfere less with gas exchange. Finally, PEEP therapy can maintain inspiratory muscles in a position of relative mechanical advantage, so it may reduce the work of spontaneous inspiration.[147,222,255]

Studies in adults with cardiac failure have found that positive pressure, including PEEP, improves cardiac output. PEEP decreases left ventricular transmural pressure, and it improves cardiac output by decreasing afterload.[3,173] As a result, it is easier for the left ventricle to eject blood.

Detrimental Effects of PEEP

Potential detrimental effects of PEEP must be considered when initiating or increasing PEEP therapy. PEEP increases intrathoracic pressure and can impede systemic venous return, resulting in a fall in cardiac output, particularly if the patient has hypovolemia. High levels of PEEP may produce alveolar hyperinflation and increase risk of barotrauma and air leak. High levels of PEEP (exceeding 8-12 cm H_2O) can impede cerebral venous return and contribute to increased intracranial pressure. Excessive levels of PEEP also increase pulmonary vascular resistance and decrease pulmonary blood flow, resulting in an increase in dead space ventilation (physiologic dead space).

Determination of Optimal PEEP

The ideal PEEP is the lowest PEEP consistent with maximal oxygen delivery; it is associated frequently with maximal pulmonary compliance. Although high levels of PEEP can increase arterial oxygen content, they can result in a fall in oxygen delivery if cardiac output is compromised relatively more than the oxygen content is improved. Optimal PEEP

Box 9-16 | **Characteristics Associated With Optimal PEEP**

- Optimal PEEP is lowest PEEP consistent with maximal oxygen delivery at the lowest inspired oxygen concentration
- Maintains $PaO_2 > 60$ torr and hemoglobin saturation $>90\%$, with $FiO_2 < 0.5$
- Does not significantly depress cardiac output or compromise systemic perfusion
- Maintains highest mixed venous oxygen tension or saturation (goal: $S\bar{v}O_2 \geq 65\%$ as measured with SVC/PA fiberoptic catheter)
- Reduces intrapulmonary shunting
- Increases lung compliance
- Minimal increase in dead space ventilation
- Optimal PEEP might not correlate with highest PaO_2 or hemoglobin saturation

PA, Posteroanterior; *PEEP,* positive end-expiratory pressure; *SVC,* superior vena cava.

---

will maintain arterial oxygenation (PaO_2 approximately 70-80 mm Hg, hemoglobin saturation approximately 92%) without significantly depressing cardiac output or systemic perfusion, and will reduce the intrapulmonary shunt (Box 9-16).

PEEP therapy often is titrated by evaluating a series of PEEP settings increased by steps of 2 to 4 cm H_2O each time. Because pulmonary artery catheters are rarely used in pediatric patients, monitoring uses physical examination, noninvasive devices, arterial blood gas analysis (including measurements of lactate levels), and arterial and superior vena caval oxyhemoglobin saturation ($S_{cv}O_2$). If excessive levels of PEEP compromise cardiac output, the child's blood pressure, color, perfusion of extremities, SVC oxyhemoglobin saturation, and urine output will deteriorate. In general, titration of PEEP to levels as high as 10 to 12 cm H_2O can be performed using noninvasive assessment of cardiac output. If higher levels of PEEP are thought to be needed, consider monitoring of cardiac output (e.g., use of a pulmonary artery catheter or noninvasive device).

When a thermodilution cardiac output pulmonary artery catheter is in place, the oxygen delivery can be calculated at various levels of PEEP therapy (see Box 9-3). An arterial blood sample is drawn at the same time that a cardiac output calculation is performed. It is important to allow approximately 20 min to elapse each time the PEEP is adjusted before samples are drawn, to provide sufficient time for the maximal therapeutic effects of PEEP to be apparent.[186,234]

In pediatric critical care, the effect of PEEP on $S\bar{v}O_2$ is generally assessed by monitoring trends in the SVC oxyhemoglobin saturation, obtained through a central venous catheter located in the SVC, because such catheters are placed in pediatric patients more frequently than pulmonary artery catheters. If there is no change in patient fever or baseline medical condition—including level of pain, agitation, or sedation—the oxygen consumption is assumed to be stable. A rise in the SVC oxyhemoglobin saturation then suggests improved oxygen delivery, and a fall in the saturation suggests a decrease in oxygen delivery (see, also, chapter 6).

Mild reductions in cardiac output or systemic perfusion during PEEP therapy can be treated effectively by

mechanical ventilation and determining the appropriateness of the ventilator variables

Ensure that the equipment, including the ventilator, tubing, and monitoring devices, are appropriate for the patient. The goals of mechanical ventilation are to maintain adequate gas exchange while avoiding air leaks and oxygen injury, and to maintain oxygen delivery until the lung injury improves sufficiently so that the patient can be liberated from the ventilator. The following are variables to be checked routinely with measurement of vital signs and any time the patient's condition changes.

1. *Respiratory rate.* The appropriate respiratory rate is determined by the child's lung disease, metabolic rate and level of consciousness. The respiratory rate that the nurse counts and records on the flow chart includes the breaths delivered by the ventilator as well as any additional breaths taken by the child. If the ventilator is functioning, the total respiratory rate should never fall below the minimal mandatory rate set on the ventilator.

2. *Tidal volume (V_T).* A tidal volume of 4 to 6 cc/kg body weight is typically used for initial ventilation with a volume ventilator. A higher tidal volume is needed if extremely compliant ventilator tubing is used or if there is a leak around the ETT. In adults with acute lung injury, improved outcomes have been reported when lower tidal volumes (6-8 cc/kg) compared with traditional tidal volumes (10-12 cc/kg) are used.[7,261] Although a similar pediatric study has not been published, most clinicians use a low tidal volume approach.[253] If a pressure-limit ventilator is used, a peak inspiratory pressure of 15 to 30 cm H_2O will deliver the appropriate tidal volume in the patient with normal lung compliance, but this must be confirmed by actual measurement. Higher inspiratory pressure will be needed to ventilate extremely noncompliant lungs. The child's chest must expand during each inspiration provided by a positive pressure mechanical ventilator. If the chest does not move, the tidal volume delivered by the ventilator is inadequate, regardless of the numbers displayed by the ventilator gauges. Monitoring of end-tidal carbon dioxide ($P_{ET}CO_2$) concentration and comparison with the $PaCO_2$ aids in the evaluation of effectiveness of ventilation. If the $P_{ET}CO_2$ and the $PaCO_2$ fall together, the patient's ventilation has improved; if both rise, the patient's ventilation is reduced. If the $P_{ET}CO_2$ falls and the $PaCO_2$ rises, dead space has been added to the system (areas are ventilated that are not perfused). This condition can develop if the lung is overdistended with PEEP. The $P_{ET}CO_2$ can fall without a rise in the $PaCO_2$ when cardiac output falls, and pulmonary blood flow and delivery of CO_2 to the lungs decreases. The $P_{ET}CO_2$ will fall to near zero with spontaneous extubation.

3. *Minute ventilation.* Minute ventilation is the product of V_T and the frequency (*f*) of breaths. Some mechanical ventilators display the minute ventilation, but others do not.

4. *Pressure limit control.* The pressure limit is determined after considering the child's condition and the amount of pressure needed to achieve adequate chest expansion or deliver adequate tidal volume. Pressure limit will be the maximum PIP delivered by either a volume-cycled or a pressure-cycled ventilator. The Acute Respiratory Distress Syndrome Network (ARDSNET) recommends maintaining pressure plateau (P_{PLAT}) $\leq$35 cm H_2O (P_{PLAT} is generally less than PIP), so that children who need PIP >35 cm H_2O need to be evaluated for transition to HFV. The amount of pressure needed to deliver a given tidal volume depends on the compliance of the ventilator tubing and the compliance of the patient's lungs and chest wall (total respiratory compliance). If the child has lung disease and decreased lung compliance, delivery of a given volume will generate higher airway pressures than in a child with normal lung compliance. As the disease and the child's lung compliance improve, the inspiratory pressures usually will decrease. If a volume-cycled ventilator is used, a rise in the peak inspiratory pressure can indicate a decrease in intrinsic lung compliance or an increase in airway resistance. Peak pressure also will increase when secretions form in the child's airways or when a kink or water buildup is present in the tubing. If the child develops a pneumothorax, PIP can increase suddenly. If the patient becomes extubated or disconnected from the ventilator, the PIP will decrease suddenly.

5. *Inspired oxygen concentration.* The amount of oxygen delivered by the ventilator system is the FiO_2. The delivered oxygen concentration is analyzed continuously or at least every hour.

6. *Positive end-expiratory pressure.* If the child is receiving PEEP, the PEEP mode must be maintained at all times. When the child's lungs are ventilated manually with a resuscitation bag, a valve can be added to the manual system to hold the PEEP during manual ventilation. If the child is receiving both PEEP and assist-controlled ventilation, adjustment of the assist trigger is needed so that the child can initiate a breath without having to override the PEEP.

Extracorporeal Membrane Oxygenation

Extracorporeal membrane oxygenation (ECMO) therapy supports cardiac or pulmonary function, or both, using cardiopulmonary bypass with a membrane oxygenator. This system can be used to provide temporary support for the infant or child with reversible cardiac or respiratory failure.

Over the past 30 years, treatment for refractory respiratory failure in neonates has included ECMO with good outcomes and survival. The experience in treating pediatric acute respiratory failure (ARF) with ECMO is less documented. However, more than 7000 children have been treated with ECMO.[213] Two studies demonstrated decreased mortality in children with ARF who were treated with ECMO compared with conventional therapy without ECMO.[235]

Suggested indications for the use of ECMO support include reversible ARF unresponsive to CMV and HFV (for further information, see Box 7-1 and Chapter 7). Several methods of ECMO support can be provided. All forms include removing venous blood from the body, oxygenating and warming the blood in an oxygenator, and returning the blood to the body. Venovenous ECMO diverts patient venous blood to the oxygenator and then returns the oxygenated blood through a large vein to the patient's right atrium. This form of ECMO support may be used in the treatment of respiratory failure, but it requires adequate cardiac function because the patient's heart is still responsible for ejection of normal cardiac output.

Venoarterial ECMO diverts venous blood to the oxygenator and returns the blood to the patient's arterial circulation (the carotid or another large artery). If ECMO support is provided after cardiovascular surgery, the median sternotomy incision will enable cannulation of the aorta. This form of ECMO therapy can provide total cardiac and pulmonary support.

During ECMO therapy, at least one nurse and one perfusionist must remain at the bedside at all times to monitor the patient and the ECMO equipment. The child receives neuromuscular blockers and is totally dependent on the medical team for the provision of adequate oxygenation and perfusion. Adequate analgesia and sedation also must be provided. Mechanical ventilation is provided at minimal settings to prevent atelectasis or complete lung collapse. Providers at the bedside must be able to detect subtle changes in the child's condition and recognize equipment malfunction immediately. Cannula dislodgement or tubing separation can result in immediate fatal hemorrhage, so the cannula must be secured and all tubing must be visible at all times.

Complications of ECMO therapy include bleeding, mechanical or technical problems, infection, and neurologic sequelae (including intracranial hemorrhage). Children may be more likely to demonstrate extracranial hemorrhage than neonates. For further information regarding ECMO therapy, see Chapters 7 and 21.

Weaning from Mechanical Ventilatory Support

Weaning is an organized process of liberating the patient from mechanical ventilation.[259] Weaning can be a smooth process or a long, difficult one. The healthcare team considers weaning when the child's underlying disease process and gas exchange improve, and when the cardiovascular and pulmonary systems stabilize. The child must be ready for weaning (Box 9-17). The following criteria are required for beginning the process of weaning from ventilatory support[259]:

1. Improvement of the condition that necessitated intubation and mechanical support
2. Adequate gas exchange

Box 9-17   Indicators for Initiation of Weaning

1. Achievement of baseline mental status
2. Presence of cough and gag reflexes
3. Absence of fever
4. Spontaneous respiratory effort
5. Normal acid-base balance
6. Oxyhemoglobin saturation $\geq 90\%$ or $PaO_2 \geq 60$ mm Hg (in the absence of cyanotic heart disease)
7. $FiO_2 < 0.5$
8. PEEP < 7 cm H_2O
9. $PaCO_2 < 50$ mm Hg
10. Stable hemodynamics
11. Stable ventilation support for ≥ 24 h
12. No plans that will require significant sedation or operative procedures in the next 12 h

Adapted from Venkataraman ST: Mechanical ventilation and respiratory care. In Fuhrman BP, Zimmerman J, editors: *Pediatric critical care*, ed 3, Philadelphia, 2006, Mosby-Elsevier.
PEEP, Positive end-expiratory pressure.

---

3. Absence of conditions placing an excessive burden on the respiratory system, including cardiac instability or insufficiency, significant malnutrition, multiple system organ failure, or severe hyperinflation
4. Spontaneous ventilation is sustainable by the patient, without excessive energy use when ventilatory support is decreased

It is important to identify and correct any factors that might hinder the weaning process. These factors include cardiac abnormalities such as arrhythmias, myocardial depression, shock, anemia, pain, drug-induced respiratory depression, fever, sleep deprivation, extreme apprehension, abnormal mental status, and depressed airway reflexes. Evaluation of the child's nutritional status and general muscle strength are also important, because poor nutrition or poor muscle strength make weaning a difficult if not impossible task. Recent studies demonstrate that fluid balance has no effect on successful weaning or extubation.[195] In contrast, the use of sedation in the first 24 h of weaning can negatively effect successful extubation.[195]

The type of weaning performed is determined by provider preference and patient needs. Periods without sedation may be useful to observe the patient's respiratory effort, and it may be helpful to avoid continuous infusions of opioids and sedatives. A large study sponsored by the National Institutes of Health is currently evaluating methods to decrease the use of opioids and sedatives and whether such decreased use will reduce total mechanical ventilation time and time to successful extubation.

General Principles of Weaning

Weaning can be performed in a variety of ways, but generally either the child's ventilator support is gradually decreased or the child is weaned using a preset series of steps called a readiness to extubate trial (see spontaneous breathing trials). Regardless of the weaning method selected, the weaning is performed in an organized manner. It is usually inappropriate to make multiple variable changes at the same time. For example, it is not appropriate to expect to decrease the FiO_2, the respiratory rate, and the inspiratory pressure (or tidal volume) simultaneously. The cumulative effect of all these changes may be too great for the child to tolerate, and if he/she does not, the clinicians will not be able to determine which variable was most responsible for the failure.

Frequent evaluation of gas exchange is needed to monitor the success of weaning. Noninvasive devices help reduce the need for frequent blood gasses. If a device is available to analyze the child's end-tidal CO_2, the values may be useful in reflecting trends in the child's arterial CO_2 tension. Pulse oximetry will enable continuous monitoring of the patient's oxygenation, but will not enable the detection of hypercarbia. Transcutaneous O_2 or CO_2 monitoring may also be used (for further information see Common Diagnostic Tests later in this chapter and Chapter 21).

Traditional Weaning of Mechanical Ventilation

Intermittent Mandatory Ventilation Weaning. The traditional method of weaning is a form of IMV. In this mode, continuous fresh gas flow is present in the circuit, and the ventilator provides a preset number of breaths with a predetermined tidal volume. During weaning the mandatory ventilation rate is decreased slowly as the patient's independent respiratory effort increases. Eventually the patient receives only CPAP with supplementary oxygen (for further information about IMV or SIMV, see Conventional Ventilation Modes).

Pressure-Support Ventilation Weaning. During PSV the patient receives assistance from the ventilator during every breath. The patient, however, determines the respiratory rate, tidal volume, and inspiratory time. The medical team determines the inspiratory pressure that will be delivered to assist the patient once spontaneous inspiration begins. The patient initiates a breath, and pressurized gas is provided to achieve a specified airway pressure. As weaning progresses, the preset airway pressure is gradually reduced. A minimal amount of pressure is maintained to overcome the resistance of the ETT during inspiration; the amount varies with the size of the ETT (Table 9-11).[196] If this form of weaning support is inappropriately adjusted, the patient's work of breathing may be excessive, and weaning will not be successful (see section, Conventional Ventilation Modes).

Spontaneous Breathing Trials

Readiness for extubation or spontaneous breathing trials (SBTs) have begun to replace traditional ventilatory weaning practices. Unlike in adults, weaning protocols in children have not yet led to decreased ventilator time.[196] The use of protocols has demonstrated that most children do not need prolonged weaning strategies, and they may be stable for extubation in a short period of time. In addition, there is no one superior SBT method (T-piece, pressure or volume support) that results in more successful extubation and decreased reintubation rates.[73,196]

During SBT the following variables are monitored in each child: respiratory rate, work of breathing, CO_2 levels, oxygenation, heart rate, blood pressure, mental status, and acid-base balance if an arterial catheter is available.[73] The methods used most commonly for SBT are T-piece or PSV/ CPAP weaning. VSV has also been described.

Use of T-piece Weaning. The use of a T-piece is one technique for an SBT. The child is removed from the ventilator circuit and is joined to a T-piece of tubing through which humidified, oxygenated gas flows continuously. The child is joined to the T-piece for up to 2 h and monitored. If the child is stable as monitored (see previous paragraph), the child can be extubated. If the child does not tolerate the trial (see Box 9-18 for indications to halt trial), the child is returned to the previous ventilation support parameters. SBT may be resumed

| Box 9-18 | **Indications to Halt Spontaneous Breathing Trial** |

1. Inability to maintain gas exchange
   - Oxyhemoglobin desaturation with stable FiO_2
   - Need for increased FiO_2
2. Poor effective ventilation: rise in $PaCO_2$ by >10 mm Hg
3. Increased work of breathing beyond baseline: use of accessory muscles
4. Increased respiratory rate: exceeding normal for age
5. Additional signs of distress
   - Change in mental status (anxiety, agitation, lethargy)
   - Increased heart rate exceeding normal range for age
   - Diaphoresis
   - Hypotension

Adapted from Venkataraman ST: Mechanical ventilation and respiratory care. In Fuhrman BP, Zimmerman J, editors: *Pediatric critical care*, ed 3, Philadelphia, 2006, Mosby-Elsevier.

when the child again meets readiness criteria. Very small infants are likely not to tolerate T-piece breathing, because there is no pressure to assist in overcoming the ETT resistance.[259]

Using Pressure-Supported Weaning. PSV and CPAP may also be used for an SBT. As with the T piece trial, the patient is put on either PSV set at a level to overcome resistance of the ETT or CPAP (typically set at the level of PEEP the child is receiving). This setting is maintained for up to 2 h and the child is closely monitored as described previously. If the child is stable, the child can be extubated. If the child does not tolerate the trial (see Box 9-18), the child is returned to the previous ventilation support settings. Additional trials can occur when the child is stable.

Extubation

The decision to perform extubation is made once the child tolerates traditional or modern weaning, which demonstrates readiness for extubation. The overall assessment is based on several factors, including satisfactory gas exchange; acceptable chest radiograph and hematocrit; good cardiac, respiratory, neurologic, and renal function; the ability of the child to cough effectively; and minimal sedation (i.e., sedation has been minimized or eliminated). On occasion, agents used during mechanical ventilation will have to be reversed to ensure that a patient is ready for extubation (see Chapter 5).

Before actual extubation, reintubation equipment is assembled and readily accessible for use if needed urgently. A humidified O_2 device (face tent, face mask, nasal cannula) is prepared and ready for use as soon as the child is extubated. Someone skilled at intubation must be at the bedside before extubation and available for 4 to 6 hours following extubation.

Typically the airway is suctioned immediately before extubation. Deep suctioning is avoided after extubation because it may traumatize glottic and supraglottic tissues, producing edema and upper airway obstruction. The child is monitored for changes in heart rate and apnea during and after the removal of the tube. Some providers recommend that corticosteroids such as dexamethasone be given before and

Table 9-11	**Minimum Pressure Support Settings during Weaning**[195]	
Endotracheal Tube Size	**Pressure Support (cm H_2O)**	
3.0-3.5	10	
4.0-4.5	8	
≥5.0	6	

after extubation in an effort to prevent or reduce the risk of stridor. A typical dose is 0.6 mg/kg given intravenously every 6 h, beginning 24 h before extubation and continuing for four to six doses after extubation. Although dexamethasone has not been proved effective, in a recent study, there was a statistical trend toward benefit.[148]

The inhalation of an aerosol mist containing epinephrine can be used to enhance bronchodilation and to reduce edema immediately after extubation (see section, Upper Airway Obstruction for further information about racemic epinephrine). Persistent stridor may be an indication of inadequate airway patency.

Oral fluids and chest physiotherapy usually are withheld for 4 to 6 hours following extubation to avoid compromising the airway with swallowing maneuvers or coughing. The child receives nothing by mouth if respiratory distress is present. Reintubation can stimulate vomiting, and aspiration of stomach contents can complicate respiratory failure. Monitoring gas exchange is necessary after extubation to assess respiratory function.

The child needs close observation for approximately 24 hours following extubation. Changes in respiratory status such as an increase in hoarseness, wheezing, stridor, chest retractions, or decreased air movement accompanied by tachycardia and anxiety, usually indicate failure of extubation. Such failure may result from upper airway obstruction caused by postextubation edema or from insufficient improvement in the original disease process. In the case of upper airway edema, aerosolized epinephrine therapy may be helpful to avoid reintubation, but reintubation is sometimes necessary.

Predictors of Extubation Failure

Although some variables in intubated children are associated with a higher or lower likelihood of successful extubation, none is 100% predictive. Studied variables include respiratory rate, tidal volume, PIP, oxygenation index, mean airway pressure, and FiO_2.[72,196,258,268] Even after readiness for extubation criteria are met, approximately 15% of children will fail extubation.[72,196] Factors associated with a greater likelihood of extubation failure and longer weaning times include upper airway obstruction, lower respiratory tract problems, apnea, cardiovascular instability, male gender, and higher sedation scores during the first 24 hours of weaning.[196] The length of time the patient has been sedated may also affect ability to wean. Drug "holidays" decrease the length of time on mechanical ventilation (see Chapter 5).

Nursing Care of the Child During Mechanical Ventilation

A nursing care plan is available in Evolve Box 9-1 in the Chapter 9 Supplement on the Evolve Website.

Bedside Assessment

The most important nursing responsibility in the care of the child receiving mechanical ventilation is assessing the adequacy of the ventilatory support. The use of a mechanical ventilator does not ensure that the child's lungs are being ventilated. Nursing assessment is especially important during the first few hours after initiation of mechanical ventilation and whenever a change in ventilation variables is made or the patient is moved (e.g., from bed to gurney or into or out of a computed tomography (CT) scanner).

The primary factors included in this assessment are physical examination, vital signs, oxygenation, airway patency, exhaled or end-tidal CO_2, arterial blood gas analysis, chest radiograph interpretation, and measurement and calculation of pulmonary function variables. The most reliable method of assessment is the physical examination performed by a skilled practitioner. The objective impression that a child "looks good" or "looks bad" is as important, if not more so, than any other assessment the skilled person can make. The vital signs, especially the heart rate and blood pressure, also must be noted. It may be helpful for the nurse to consider the following questions and actions:

1. Is the child fighting the ventilator or does he or she appear agitated or distressed? If so, remove the child from the ventilator, provide manual ventilation (with a bag), and assess air movement and chest expansion for evidence of a malpositioned/displaced ETT, ETT obstruction, pneumothorax or equipment failure (rule out DOPE—see Box 9-13).

2. Is the heart rate too fast or too slow for the child's age and clinical condition? Extreme tachycardia or bradycardia may be an indication of hypoxemia and hypoxia.

3. Is the blood pressure appropriate for the child's age and clinical condition? The hypertensive child may be in pain or may be hypoxic. Hypotension may be caused by hypoxia or acidosis associated with inadequate ventilation, excessive PEEP, or tension pneumothorax.

4. Are the child's color and perfusion acceptable? The child's mucous membranes and nail beds should be pink, extremities warm, and capillary refill time brisk. Normal urine output averages 0.5 to 2 mL/kg body weight per hour if fluid intake is adequate. Deterioration in the child's color or systemic perfusion could be an early sign of hypoxia and respiratory insufficiency.

5. Is the chest rising symmetrically with each positive pressure inspiration? Significant atelectasis or pneumothorax can prevent adequate lung and chest expansion on the involved side.

6. Are the breath sounds equal and adequate bilaterally? If the ETT is in the right bronchus, breath sounds heard over the right chest will be louder and have a different pitch (see item 7) than those heard over the left chest. Because the chest wall of infants and young children is so thin and transmits breath sounds so easily, the child may appear to have adequate breath sounds, even over areas of atelectasis or pneumothorax, until the breath sounds are compared with those heard over normal lung areas.

7. What is the pitch of the breath sounds bilaterally? Because breath sounds can be referred from other areas of the lung, it is important to listen for a change in the pitch of the breath sounds over involved areas. Such a change may be the first sign of atelectasis, pneumothorax, or consolidation.

8. Is the child's level of consciousness appropriate for clinical condition? Extreme irritability or lethargy may be signs of severe hypoxia or hypercarbia.

9. Are the child's oxyhemoglobin saturation (per pulse oximetry) and arterial blood gas values stable? A fall in

oxyhemoglobin saturation or deterioration in blood gas values (reduction in $\dot{V}/\dot{Q}$ matching) may indicate inadequate lung recruitment (needing a possible increase in PEEP), or tube *d*isplacement, tube *o*bstruction, *p*neumothorax, or failure of the *e*quipment, including the ventilator (recall the mnemonic *DOPE*).

10. Is the child's exhaled or end-tidal CO_2 stable and appropriate?

The presence of any abnormalities in these assessments can indicate the presence of hypoxia, abnormal gas exchange, or inadequate ventilatory support.

When the condition of a ventilated patient suddenly worsens, disconnect the child from the ventilator and perform manual ventilation (i.e., with a bag). Quickly assess breath sounds to be certain that the ETT is not displaced or obstructed and assess breath sounds bilaterally for evidence of pneumothorax. Check or ask a colleague to check the ventilator for malfunction. If the tube is patent and the lungs expand bilaterally with hand ventilation and there is no evidence of ventilator malfunction, the patient can be returned to the ventilator and evaluated more thoroughly for other causes of deterioration. The most common causes of sudden deterioration in a child with an advanced airway during mechanical ventilation include tube displacement, tube obstruction, and pneumothorax.

Laboratory Assessment

Laboratory assessment during mechanical ventilation is used only to reinforce the clinical impression. Pulse oximetry provides a continuous display of oxyhemoglobin saturation. Bedside oximeters vary in speed of response, so they might not reflect rapid or severe decreases in oxyhemoglobin saturation.[216,46] As a result, the child's color, perfusion, and clinical appearance must be monitored constantly. For further information, see Pulse Oximetry, under Clinical Signs and Symptoms of Respiratory Failure (earlier in this chapter), and Common Diagnostic Tests (at the end of this chapter) and Chapter 21.

Blood gas analyses often are ordered when mechanical ventilation is initiated or when any change is made in ventilatory variables, but these are now checked less frequently since the development and widespread use of exhaled or end-tidal CO_2 monitoring and pulse oximetry that allow for continuous, noninvasive evaluation of gas exchange. Once an arterial blood gas value is used to confirm end-tidal CO_2 values, the frequency of blood sampling can be reduced. In young infants, frequent blood sampling can lead to phlebotomy-associated anemia, and frequent sampling through the arterial catheter can increase the risk for infection. In children with concomitant acid-base derangements or severe lung disease, checking arterial blood gases may be necessary at regular intervals. Blood gas analyses are useful in the management of children with severe lung disease and may be used to calculate both the A-aO_2 difference and the physiologic shunt. These calculations may be helpful in trending the disease course and response to therapy.

Sedation, Analgesia, and Neuromuscular Blockade

Special care must be provided if the child receives sedation and a neuromuscular blocking agent. These children are completely dependent on the healthcare team for the provision of adequate ventilation and are not able to signal distress or hypoxemia. Loss of muscle tone also places the child at risk for venous pooling and joint hyperextension or dislocation. Whenever the child is turned or moved, the head and extremities must be supported carefully to prevent injury.

The recovery of diaphragm muscle tone after neuromuscular blockade can be gauged by recovery of the rectus muscle, because both recover at approximately the same rate. Neuromuscular blocking agents are not sedatives or analgesics. Sedatives and analgesics must be used with neuromuscular blocking agents (see Chapter 5) to ensure that the child is free of pain and comfortable during treatment. Because the child can still hear, it is necessary to provide frequent, comforting words, explanations (appropriate for age), and reassurances. It may be useful to play a recording of the voices of parents and siblings or familiar music at the child's bedside.

Communication with Intubated Children

Patients, staff members, and family members have all reported challenges and frustrations in communication when patients are intubated. In addition to the advanced airway, barriers to communication include developmental level, fatigue, neurologic disease, and pharmacologic effects.[98] When children are unable to speak and communicate effectively, they can develop feelings of anger and depression, which can ultimately lead to withdrawal.

Low technology tools such as pen and paper and age-appropriate printed pain scores can be used for children who are sufficiently alert. If available, more technologically advanced devices such as computers can be used. In some cases, video conferencing can allow patients to maintain communication with family, friends, and classmates. Members of the healthcare team can increase communication techniques such as attention, touch, and empathy skills. Because continuity of care can facilitate assisted communication, it is important to consider continuity when nursing assignments are made.[98,142]

Positioning

If unilateral lung disease is present, proper positioning of the patient may increase oxygenation. Dependent segments of the lungs are the best perfused segments during positive pressure ventilation. Placing the healthy lung in the dependent position will result in increased perfusion of the good lung and possible improved ventilation of the diseased lung. Some critically ill children will tolerate only small changes in position during the acute phase of their illness. Note that the prone position can improve oxygenation for some patients.[53]

Nonventilatory Methods of Improving Oxygenation

Systemic oxygenation may be improved using anxiolytics, analgesia, and neuromuscular blockade to ensure that mechanical ventilation complements the patient's respiratory effort, position, hemoglobin concentration, and cardiac output.

Anxiolysis, Analgesia, and Neuromuscular Blockade. Mechanical ventilation support must be synchronized with the patient's spontaneous respiratory effort and is accomplished by skilled adjustments to mechanical ventilator settings. If ventilator adjustments alone are unsuccessful, administration of anxiolytics and analgesics and possibly neuromuscular blocking agents is indicated (see Chapter 5).

Minimization of Oxygen Demand. When severe respiratory failure and hypoxemia are present, the goals of treatment are to maximize oxygen delivery and reduce oxygen demand; this includes treatment of fever, pain, and agitation, because all can increase oxygen consumption. If the child is breathing spontaneously with increased work of breathing, providers can consider sedation in the nonintubated patient and sedation with neuromuscular blockade in the intubated patient.

Treatment of Anemia. The optimal hemoglobin concentration for the child with respiratory failure is unknown. Higher levels of hemoglobin will increase blood oxygen carrying capacity and oxygen delivery. An elevated hematocrit, however, will also increase blood viscosity and pulmonary vascular resistance, and both will increase cardiac work. Risks of blood transfusion must also be considered. Recent studies indicate that equally sick, stable patients in the critical care unit, who receive a transfusion may do worse than those who do not. In stable, critically ill children (i.e., with no cardiorespiratory instability), a transfusion threshold of 7 mg/dL decreased transfusions with no increase in adverse events.[126] A similar study has not been performed in unstable critically ill infants and children, particularly those with severe hypoxemia, hemodynamic instability, active blood loss, or cyanotic heart disease. In children with severe respiratory failure, hemoglobin levels are often maintained at approximately 12 mg/dL, although a target hemoglobin concentration needs to be determined for each patient.

Humidification and Pulmonary Hygiene

Humidification

Intubation and mechanical ventilation impair the body's intrinsic mechanisms for removal of respiratory secretions. Specifically, intrinsic mucociliary clearance is lost because most cilia are bypassed by the ETT. In addition, impaired cough effectiveness decreases removal of secretions. Humidification of inspired air is standard of care for secretion management, and warming and humidifying of gases delivered during mechanical ventilation can prevent respiratory tract mucosal injury. Humidification can be achieved in two ways, either through passive heat and moisture exchangers or actively through a heated humidifier. Passive heat and moisture exchangers allow condensation from the patient's exhaled air to be evaporated on inspiration. A heated humidifier passes gas over a heated water bath. Humidifiers that contain a heated wire circuit avoid ventilator circuit condensate, which has been linked with ventilator-associated pneumonia.[223]

There are advantages and disadvantages to each type of humidification system. In patients with copious secretions, heat humidification is more beneficial than a heat and moisture exchanger and may decrease incidence of ventilator-associated pneumonia.[28,223] Heat and moisture exchangers reduce contaminated condensation in the ventilator circuit,

and heated humidifiers preserve mucociliary clearance by containing a higher absolute humidity level.[223]

Suctioning

Airway suctioning is a critical component of secretion removal in intubated patients. The primary goal is to remove secretions in order to prevent airway obstruction and atelectasis while maintaining oxygenation and ventilation.[166] Suctioning has been associated with a variety of adverse consequences, including hypoxemia, bradycardia, pneumothorax, increased intracranial pressure, arrhythmias, mucosal trauma, loss of lung volume, and atelectasis after suctioning.[166,245]

Two methods of ETT suctioning are used commonly in clinical practice. The open suctioning method is performed by removing the child from the mechanical ventilator circuit and suctioning the airway with single-use catheters. This technique has been reported to be associated with loss of PEEP, oxygen desaturation, and cardiac arrhythmias. Loss of lung volume has been documented in infants receiving high-frequency oscillatory ventilation when they are removed from the ventilatory circuit for open suctioning.[245] These detrimental effects are most often noted in patients with cardiovascular instability.[183]

Closed suctioning systems (so-called in-line suction systems) were developed to minimize the adverse effects reported with open suctioning systems. The closed method allows the child to remain attached to the mechanical ventilation system and uses multiuse suction catheters that are encapsulated in a plastic sheath attached to the ventilator circuit. Closed-circuit systems are easy to use, and they result in less adverse physiologic effects when compared with open systems, although correct use requires practice. Decreasing environmental contamination with use of closed-circuit suctioning has been postulated to decrease the risk of ventilator-associated pneumonia, although this finding is not consistently observed.[183,222,232] Disadvantages of closed suctioning systems include increased costs and decreased effectiveness in clearing sections.[183]

If the child has severe lung injury, it may be necessary to provide 100% oxygen for a short time before suctioning. If the open suctioning technique is used with hand ventilation (with a bag), the PIPs provided during manual ventilation need to approximate the proximal airway pressure generated during mechanical ventilation. PIPs measured with a hand ventilator system reflect the true peak pressure at the proximal airway.

Use of normal saline instillation into the artificial airway before suctioning is controversial. The rationale for use is that it may facilitate removal of fixed secretions and prevent the formation of a mucous crust within the artificial airway and the proximal patient airways. However, the saline droplets are too large to travel beyond the area of the carina. Routine saline instillation is not necessary if the inspired gas is warmed and humidified as in standard ventilator circuits. If secretions are observed to be thick, it is important to check the function of the humidification system. Suctioning is performed to clear the ETT of secretions. It is not possible to direct the suction catheter into the patient's right or left main bronchus by turning of the head. Do not attempt bronchial suctioning.

Throughout every suctioning procedure the child's heart rate, blood pressure, and skin color need to be observed closely. Monitor pulse oximetry to assess the effect of suctioning on the patient's oxygenation. In general, make suctioning as brief as possible to prevent vagal stimulation and hypoxemia. If the child develops bradycardia or hypotension or develops cyanosis, mottling, or pallor during suctioning, terminate the suction procedure and provide manual ventilation with a bag, with increased inspired oxygen if needed, until the child is stable.

With open suctioning methods for the intubated patient, manual ventilation is also provided after suctioning. Additional breaths can also be administered after suctioning through the closed system. Doing so will minimize atelectasis and will reverse any hypoxemia or hypercarbia that has developed during suctioning.

Auscultate breath sounds carefully after suctioning to ensure that ventilation is adequate and that secretions have been reduced. The frequency of suctioning required will vary from patient to patient and during the course of the patient's illness. For example, patients with bacterial tracheitis or bronchiolitis may need suctioning every 15 minutes, whereas a comatose patient with healthy lungs may need suctioning only once in several hours. Suctioning is indicated whenever there is evidence of accumulation of secretions or when there is a question of tube obstruction. Suctioning performed unnecessarily or haphazardly will cause mucosal damage and stimulate more mucus production.

Complications of Intubation and Mechanical Ventilation

Intubation and mechanical ventilation are not without risk. Although some patients need these interventions to survive, care is required to minimize associated risks. Traditional intubation involves manipulation of the oral cavity and the posterior pharynx to visualize the vocal cords. After the cords are visualized, the plastic ETT is passed through the child's vocal cords. This is often performed swiftly and efficiently, but a variety of complications can occur during the intubation procedure. In addition, the presence of an ETT itself presents a risk for pediatric patients, and complications may develop during the course of mechanical ventilation (Box 9-19).

Ventilator-Associated Pneumonia
Ventilator-associated pneumonia (VAP) is a hospital-acquired infection that occurs in patients receiving mechanical ventilation. The infection is not present at the time of intubation and develops more than 48 hours after the institution of mechanical ventilation.[279] VAP is the second most common

hospital-acquired infection in children in the critical care unit, after vascular catheter infections.[78] Intubated patients are at risk for VAP because of alterations in first-line host defenses directly related to intubation. The bacterial etiology of VAP is strongly associated with gram-negative bacilli and *Staphylococcus aureus*.[279] Several risk factors for VAP have been identified in the adult population, including aspiration of oropharyngeal secretions or gastric contents and inhalation of aerosolized bacteria and hematogenous spread to the lungs. Risk factors for pediatric patients are similar (Box 9-20), but differ slightly from those in adults.[279]

It may be difficult to establish the diagnosis of VAP in pediatric patients, because a variety of definitions and surveillance mechanisms are used. This results in differences in reported incidence among institutions. Clinical and radiographic criteria have been developed by the National Nosocomial Surveillance System of the Centers for Disease Control and Prevention (Boxes 9-21 and 9-22).[279] Differentiating

---

Box 9-20 Risk Factors for Pediatric Ventilator-Associated Pneumonia

- Prolonged mechanical ventilation
- Neuromuscular blockade
- Altered mental status
- Immunodeficiency or immunosuppression
- Primary blood stream infections
- Severe traumatic brain injury
- Burn injury
- Steroids
- Reintubation
- Congenital neuromuscular weakness

Box 9-21 Criteria for Ventilator-Associated Pneumonia in Children 1-12 Years of Age

- One or more of the following clinical criteria:
  - Fever (body temperature >38° C) without other identified cause
  - Leukopenia (WBC count <4000 per mm^3) or leukocytosis (WBC count >12,000 per mm^3)
- *Plus* radiographic criteria of two or more serial radiographs* with new or worsening and persistent infiltrate, cavitation, or pneumatocele that developed >48 h after initiating mechanical ventilation
- *And* at least two of the following:
  - New-onset purulent sputum, change in character of sputum, or increased respiratory secretions
  - New onset or worsening of tachypnea, dyspnea, or cough
  - Rales or bronchial sounds
  - Worsening oxygenation or ventilation

Adapted from Wright ML and Romano MJ: Ventilator-associated pneumonia in children, *Semin Pediatr Infect Dis* 17:58-64, 2006; and Horan, Andrus, Dudeck, CDC/NHSN surveillance definition of healthcare-associated infection and criteria for specific types of infections in the acute care setting. *Am J Infect Control* 2008;36:309-332. Available at: http://www.cdc.gov/ncidod/dhqp/pdf/nnis/NosInfDefinitions.pdf. Accessed June 26, 2011.
*In children with an absence of underlying pulmonary or cardiac disease, one radiograph is acceptable.
WBC, White blood cell.

Box 9-19 Complications of Intubation and Positive Pressure Ventilation

- Airway trauma, injury
- Ventilator-associated pneumonia
- Aspiration pneumonia
- Oxygen toxicity
- Ventilation-induced lung injury

Box 9-22	Criteria for Ventilator-Associated Pneumonia in Infants Younger than 12 Months

- Worsening gas exchange with at least three of the following clinical criteria
  - Temperature instability without other recognized origin
  - WBC count < 4000 per mm^3 or > 15,000 per mm^3, and more than 10% bandemia on differential
  - Apnea, tachypnea, increased work of breathing, or grunting
  - Rhonchi, rales, wheezing
  - Cough
  - Heart rate < 100/min or > 170/min
  - Plus radiographic criteria of two or more serial radiographs* with new or worsening and persistent infiltrate, cavitation, or pneumatocele that developed > 48 h after initiation of mechanical ventilation

Adapted from Wright ML, Romano, MJ: Ventilator-associated pneumonia in children. *Sem Pediatr Infect Dis* 17:58-64, 2006.
*In infants with an absence of underlying pulmonary or cardiac disease, one radiograph is acceptable
WBC, White blood cell.

between consolidation and atelectasis on a chest radiograph can be challenging in pediatric patients and can complicate the diagnosis of VAP.

Invasive testing can be performed to document the presence of VAP. A few studies have evaluated the sensitivity of sampling lower airway secretions in intubated children to aid in identification of VAP. Either nonbronchoscopic bronchoalveolar lavage or bronchoscopic bronchoalveolar lavage may be used. Nonbronchoscopic alveolar lavage is an alternative to bronchoalveolar lavage with comparable results.[78] It is performed by inserting a suction catheter into the ETT until it meets resistance; saline is then instilled and suctioned.[78] In bronchoscopic lavage, a fiberoptic instrument is used to visualize the airway and obtain a sample of secretions from the lower airways. The nonbronchoscopic technique may be preferred because there is no need for equipment or training in performing bronchoscopy. Both nonbronchoscopic and bronchoscopic bronchoalveolar lavage are relatively safe procedures in infants and children who do not have severe hypoxemia, increased intracranial pressure, hemodynamic instability, or bleeding problems.[78]

Treatment of VAP is determined by the organisms most likely to cause the pneumonia. Empiric antibiotic therapy is initiated while awaiting blood culture results. Pleural fluid can be sampled when an effusion is present. The most commonly identified bacteria include *S. aureus, Pseudomonas aeruginosa,* and other gram-negative organisms.[78] In adults, causative organisms differ between early-onset and late-onset VAP, but this difference has not been documented in children. Antibiotic therapy is tailored to target the causative organism sensitivities when culture results are available; this will limit the risk of developing resistant organisms.

The Centers for Disease Control and Prevention and the Healthcare Infection Control Practices Advisory Committee have recommended strategies for VAP prevention.[78] Suggestions include preferential orotracheal (instead of nasotracheal) intubation and changing of ventilation circuits only when they are visibly contaminated. Other strategies include elevating the head of the bed, routine oral care, meticulous hand washing, and using closed suctioning systems. In adult patients, the use of gastric protective agents that increase gastric pH has been associated with increased incidence of VAP, because the agents may be associated with increased bacterial growth in the stomach[78]; however, similar data are not yet available for pediatric patients. Preventive strategies are most effective if combined with education initiatives for healthcare providers (see Chapter 22, Box 22-7).

Traumatic and Ischemic Complications

Postextubation stridor and tracheal ischemia are potential complications of endotracheal intubation. Postextubation stridor caused by laryngeal edema is relatively common in pediatric patients after endotracheal intubation of any duration. Tracheal ischemia complications are more serious and can result in tracheal stenosis. Laryngeal edema and tracheal ischemia can develop from excessive pressure exerted by the ETT on the tracheal mucosa (cuff-to-tracheal pressure). Although the maximal safe cuff-to-trachea pressure has not been defined, it is generally accepted as 25 mm Hg[96]; however, it can vary slightly based on ETT manufacturer, so the tube manufacturer's recommendation should be used. The low-volume, high-pressure ETT cuffs used in the early days of mechanical ventilation produced excessively high cuff-to-tracheal pressures ($\geq$100 cm Hg) and caused significant tracheal ischemia and necrosis in up to one fifth of patients.[96] High-volume, low-pressure ETT cuffs have substantially decreased the incidence of cuff-induced tracheal ischemic complications. These preformed cuffs expand when inflated to conform to the contours of the trachea, with no pressure generated inside the cuff until the cuff wall comes into contact with the tracheal wall. The cuff inflation pressure is thought to be equal to the cuff-to-tracheal pressure, although it is difficult to quantify this pressure clinically.

Routine measurement of cuff pressures with either manometry or digital palpation is useful in preventing tracheal wall injury and necrosis.[165] In general, recommended cuff inflation pressures are > 18 mm Hg to decrease aspiration and < 20-25 mm Hg to minimize complications of tracheal wall ischemia.[96] Cuff pressure pop-off valves have been specifically designed for pediatric ETTs to avoid cuff pressures greater than 20 cm H_2O (approximately 27 mm Hg). The pop-off valve is a metallic device designed to release any pressure greater than 20 cm H_2O. The proximal luer lock allows connection to a cuff pressure manometer or cuff inflating syringe, and the distal luer lock is connected to the balloon of the tube cuff. The device is reusable. Preliminary information suggests that the pop-off valve limits potentially dangerous manual cuff inflation pressures, although more studies are needed.[68]

The subglottic airway is the narrowest region in the child's trachea, and it is completely surrounded by a cartilage ring. This site is most vulnerable to intubation trauma, including laryngeal lesions or subglottic stenosis.[227] Laryngeal lesions result from trauma to tissues during intubation. Several factors have been linked with laryngotracheal stenosis, including individual susceptibility, movement of the ETT, inappropriately large ETT, excessively high pressures in the ETT cuff, and duration of intubation.[110,150] Children younger than 5 years are at highest risk for airway inflammation and subglottic stenosis, probably related to the small pediatric airway caliber.[150] Pathophysiology includes an ischemic process and ulceration of the respiratory mucosa at the site of contact with the ETT or the ETT cuff. This continuous contact and pressure on the airway tissue can lead to ulceration and inflammation followed by development of granulation tissue. Later, scar tissue forms and the surrounding tissue retracts.[227] In some cases, this can lead to long-term tracheal complications needing surgical intervention.

Subglottic stenosis is a common indication for tracheostomy. Upper airway lesions can be evaluated using flexible fiber-optic laryngoscopy of the upper airway. It is relatively safe and can usually be performed at the bedside with minimal or no sedation.[227] Less commonly, a three-dimensional CT scan can be used to evaluate the level of and severity of the stenosis.[252]

Mild forms of subglottic stenosis often do not need surgical intervention, but moderate to severe cases of subglottic stenosis do. Surgical management can include incision of the airway and placement of a patch (typically pericardial tissue or a rib graft) to enlarge the airway diameter. Surgery for long segment stenosis typically involves resecting a portion of the stenotic trachea and creating anterior and posterior longitudinal incisions in the proximal and distal tracheal segments. The proximal and distal ends are reconnected with the original incisions placed facing each other. The result is a shorter trachea with increased caliber and low incidence of restenosis, because the reconstruction uses existing tracheal tissue.[252] Complications can include granulation tissue at the surgical suture line.[93]

Vocal Cord Paralysis

Although most episodes of postextubation stridor are related to laryngeal edema, some may be caused by vocal cord paresis. This condition is rarely caused by the intubation procedure itself, but it has been described in the literature. Some cases are noted after extubation from a surgical procedure, most often neurosurgical or cardiac. Please see Upper Airway Obstruction in Common Clinical Conditions for more information on vocal cord paralysis.

Postextubation Stridor

Several factors can contribute to postextubation stridor. Large ETT size (relative to the child), lack of an audible leak around the ETT, and lack of an endotracheal leak when checking with a manometer can increase a child's risk for postextubation stridor. At least one study suggests that lack of an audible leak around the ETT is a valid indicator of risk of extubation stridor only in children aged 7 years and older,[157] and no correlation has been found between the absence of a leak and the likelihood of extubation failure.[278]

To decrease airway edema, some clinicians give dexamethasone before and after extubation.[74] A typical dose is 0.6 mg/kg intravenously, given every 6 hours beginning 24 hours before extubation and continuing for four to six doses after extubation. For stridor after extubation, racemic epinephrine may also

be used. Doses differ for patients weighing less than 20 kg (0.25 mL in 3-5 mL NaCl solution is used), 20-40 kg (0.5 mL in 3-5 mL NaCl solution), and more than 40 kg (0.75 mL in 3-5 mL NaCl solution). Some clinicians use a standard unit dose regardless of patient weight. For additional information, see Common Clinical Conditions, Upper Airway Obstruction, earlier in this chapter.

Oxygen Toxicity

Prolonged breathing of high levels of inspired oxygen is known to cause oxidant injuries in airway and lung parenchyma, known as *oxygen toxicity*. Much of the data about oxygen toxicity have been developed in animal models (primarily rat and piglet) and extrapolated to humans.[140] Oxygen toxicity probably results from the formation of high concentrations of oxygen-derived free radicals. A free oxygen radical is an atom or molecule that contains an uneven number of electrons in its outermost orbit; the one unpaired electron makes the atom or molecule highly unstable. Free oxygen radicals either give up an electron or combine with proteins, lipids or carbohydrates and initiate chain reactions that can affect cell membrane stability; these reactions may produce cell injury. Under normal conditions the cell protects itself from the effects of free radicals, and the body can rid itself of some free oxygen radicals. However, in the presence of high levels of inspired oxygen, particularly when combined with lung injury, free oxygen radical production in the lung is accelerated.[136]

It is difficult to separate the pulmonary effects of oxygen toxicity in the patient with respiratory failure from the effects of the patient's underlying disease and from the injury resulting from positive pressure ventilation. Diffuse alveolar damage can develop within a few days of insult, causing increased capillary permeability and interstitial edema. Inflammatory cells then infiltrate the alveoli with proliferation of type 2 pneumocytes and, beyond the first week, with fibroblasts that can lead to intraalveolar fibrosis.[136] The results of these changes are alteration in the diffusion surface, hypoxemia, progressive pulmonary interstitial fibrosis, decreased lung compliance, and increased work of breathing.

The dose and duration of oxygen exposure that causes toxicity is unknown. Postoperative cardiovascular surgical patients have tolerated a short exposure (24-48 hours) to 100% oxygen without oxygen toxicity.[226] However, if underlying lung disease is present or the oxygen is administered at high pressures, tolerance of high inspired oxygen concentration hyperoxia is likely to be drastically reduced.

To reduce the risk of oxygen toxicity, the healthcare team will attempt to identify and provide the minimal inspired oxygen concentration consistent with adequate tissue oxygenation. Frequently, PEEP is increased to levels sufficient to enable reduction of the FiO_2 to less than 0.60. Oxygen is not withheld from a patient with severe hypoxemia because of fear of oxygen toxicity. Risk of oxygen toxicity at that point is a possibility, whereas the consequences of severe systemic hypoxemia and tissue hypoxia are more likely to be realized.[136]

It may be possible to reduce the FiO_2 if the patient's oxygen needs are minimized. Fever and pain must be treated effectively. Neonates and young infants must receive care in a warm environment, because cold stress increases oxygen consumption in young infants. If the patient is demonstrating an increased work of breathing during positive pressure ventilation, it may be necessary to provide controlled ventilatory support with sedation and neuromuscular blockade. The child's systemic arterial oxygenation may increase, and it may be possible to reduce the PIP during mechanical ventilation if sedatives, analgesics, or neuromuscular blocking agents are administered.

No safe levels of inspired oxygen concentration or exposure have been established in critically ill or injured patients. Inspired oxygen concentration is titrated according to patient response and is tapered as soon as possible. Adults with acute lung injury who received pure oxygen during mechanical ventilation can develop atelectasis (loss of lung volume), and the use of higher PEEP and lower FiO_2 can result in maintenance of lung recruitment (lung volume).[2] Therefore ventilation strategies to improve systemic oxygenation need to be more comprehensive than merely increasing inspired oxygen concentration (e.g., they need to include increasing PEEP and PIP). The optimal inspired oxygen concentration for any patient will be the lowest effective amount of oxygen that will support adequate tissue oxygenation as defined by (1) absence of lactic acidosis, (2) normal SvO_2 or SVC oxygen saturation ($\geq 65\%$), and (3) appropriate mental status, systemic oxygen delivery, and end-organ function.

Cardiopulmonary Interactions

Dawn Tucker and Ronald Bronicki

Technology to measure hemodynamic changes during the respiratory cycle has led to better appreciation of the interrelationship between pulmonary and cardiovascular function. The relationship of the heart to the thoracic chamber has been described as a "pressure chamber within a pressure chamber," and changes in intrathoracic pressure associated with spontaneous and mechanical ventilation can affect cardiovascular function. These important interactions between the cardiovascular and pulmonary systems are magnified by cardiopulmonary diseases and by the critical care therapies used.

Volume Pressure Relationships

Cardiopulmonary interaction results from the volume-pressure relationships in the elastic chambers of the thorax and intrathoracic structures. The primary property of an elastic structure is its inherent ability to offer resistance to a distending or collapsing force and to return to its resting or unstressed volume after force has been removed. Change in volume produced by any change in pressure in an elastic structure is determined by the compliance of the structure and the magnitude and direction of the pressure exerted across its wall (i.e., transmural pressure [Ptm]). Compliance is a measure of chamber distensibility, and Ptm is equal to the difference between intra- and extracavitary pressures. A positive Ptm distends the cavity, and a negative Ptm causes the structure to reduce in size (see section, Essential Anatomy and Physiology).

Effects of Ventilation on Right Ventricular Preload

Filling of the right heart is determined primarily by the pressure gradient that exists between the right atrium (RA) and the extrathoracic venous reservoirs (primarily the splanchnic,

splenic, and hepatic tissue beds).[31] The vascular (capillary) pressure within these structures is the upstream pressure responsible for propelling blood back to the heart. This pressure is primarily a function of blood volume and capacitance of the venous circulation.[203]

When RA pressure rises, a compensatory increase in pressure occurs within the venous reservoirs to maintain venous return (otherwise venous return would decrease). These compensatory mechanisms include adrenergic stimulation of venous capacitance vessels and stimulation of the renin-angiotensin-aldosterone system (RAAS).[212] With venoconstriction, the effective compliance of the venous reservoirs immediately decreases. As a result, the pressure within these structures rises, increasing the pressure gradient for venous return, while transferring blood from the periphery. This response is complemented over time by an increase in intravascular volume that results from stimulation of the RAAS. When the upstream driving pressure decreases, venous return invariably decreases. For example, venodilators such as Lasix and nitroglycerin increase venous capacitance and decrease venous return.[95]

Because the RA is an intrathoracic structure, respiratory-induced changes in intrathoracic pressure (ITP) directly affect RA pressure and therefore venous return. During a spontaneous inspiration, ITP falls. As a result, the RA Ptm increases, producing an increase in RA volume. This increase causes the RA pressure to fall and venous return to increase. In contrast, PPV increases ITP, causing a decrease in RA Ptm and a fall in venous return to the heart. If the fall is significant, cardiac output falls and systemic perfusion is compromised.[135]

Effects of Ventilation on Right Ventricular Afterload

The pulmonary system serves as the afterload for the right heart and preload for the left heart. Any abnormal pressure increase in the pulmonary arterial and venous circulations will affect right ventricular (RV) afterload and output as well as left atrial filling. Pulmonary vascular resistance is the main determinant of RV afterload.[236]

Respiration affects pulmonary arterial pressure and RV afterload by altering pulmonary vascular resistance (PVR). Respiration affects PVR by altering lung volumes, blood pH, and alveolar oxygen tension. PVR is lowest at FRC, which is the lung volume from which normal tidal volume breathing occurs (see Fig. 9-5). Pulmonary vascular resistance will increase if lung volumes are less than or greater than FRC. At low lung volumes, atelectasis decreases alveolar oxygenation, causing hypoxic pulmonary vasoconstriction. Hypoxic pulmonary vasoconstriction appears to be mediated by alveolar hypoxia-induced suppression of endogenous nitric oxide production. The use of PEEP recruits (i.e., opens) collapsed lung units, increasing alveolar oxygen tension and thereby releasing hypoxic pulmonary vasoconstriction. If lung volumes rise above the FRC, however, distended alveoli compress blood vessels that reside between adjacent alveoli; this leads to increased PVR.[238]

Alkalosis causes pulmonary vasodilation while acidosis causes vasoconstriction. $PaCO_2$ does not directly affect PVR; rather, the pH affects PVR. In addition, alveolar hypoxia constricts pulmonary arteries. When this occurs, pulmonary blood flow is diverted away from poorly ventilated to well-ventilated alveoli; this matches ventilation to perfusion and improves oxygenation.[23]

Clinical Applications

The extent to which PPV causes venous return to decrease is determined by the pulmonary and cardiac mechanics. First, the degree to which airway pressure is transmitted to intrathoracic vascular structures varies with changes in respiratory mechanics. For a given airway pressure a stiff, noncompliant lung transmits less airway pressure to the heart and therefore has less of an effect on right atrial pressure than when lung compliance is normal. Second, the effects of changes in intrathoracic pressure on venous return are determined by ventricular function (see Chapters 6 and 8, Frank-Starling Law, and Fig. 8-12) and on the adequacy of the compensatory circulatory reflexes described previously. For example, if RV function is characterized by the flat portion of the Frank-Starling (ventricular end-diastolic volume-to-output) curve the patient can tolerate a decrease in venous return with minimal effect on stroke volume and cardiac output. However, if RV function is characterized by the steep upward portion of the Frank-Starling curve, small decreases in systemic venous return can cause a significant fall in stroke volume and cardiac output (see, also, Chapter 6, Fig. 6-2).

A hypovolemic patient will be particularly sensitive to the potential adverse effects of PPV on venous return. This response to PPV can be mitigated by volume replacement before intubation or when systemic perfusion is compromised during PPV. Patients with acute lung injury (ARDS) often need high mean airway pressures to establish adequate oxygenation, and they can benefit from volume administration. Therapies that increase venous capacitance, such as nitroglycerin and other venodilators, typically decrease venous return and may decrease RA filling and cardiac output.

Pathophysiologic states that impair vascular function can significantly compromise venous return. Severe sepsis is characterized by a systemic inflammatory response. Inflammatory mediators, in addition to increasing microvascular permeability, decrease vasomotor tone, which leads to a decrease in systemic vascular resistance and a marked increase in venous capacitance. In addition, some patients may demonstrate a compensatory ventricular dilation to increase ventricular end-diastolic pressure in order to maintain stroke volume despite a fall in ejection fraction. Consequently, these patients require volume resuscitation for many reasons.

Cardiopulmonary interactions need to be considered when interpreting bedside hemodynamics such as central venous pressure (CVP). The interpretation of CVP/RA pressure as an indicator of RV volume will be affected by RV compliance and contractility (i.e., the relationship between a given RV volume and RV end-diastolic pressure). For example, after repair of tetralogy of Fallot, RV compliance is often poor. As a result, these patients often have an elevated CVP-RA pressure, even when the stiff RV is under filled. Another confounding factor in using a CVP-RA pressure as a surrogate for RV volume is the effect that changes in ITP have on right heart size and compliance.[236] As ITP increases with PPV, the Ptm for the RV during diastole decreases. As a result, RV chamber size and filling decrease while the RA pressure increases.[221]

Effects of Ventilation on Left Ventricular Preload

Ventilation primarily influences LV preload through its effects on ITP (and therefore systemic venous return), RV afterload (alterations in gas exchange, blood pH, and lung volume), and LV compliance. As discussed, venous return and RV filling increase as ITP falls. When this occurs, RV volume and pressure rise, causing the pressure gradient across the interventricular septum to decrease during ventricular diastole; this causes the ventricular septum to shift leftward. This septum shift compromises LV diastolic volume and filling and therefore cardiac output, and it is partly responsible for the decrease in systolic blood pressure that occurs during inspiration.[184,185] This phenomenon is known as *pulsus paradoxus,* and the effect of alterations in the position of the septum on cardiovascular function is known as *ventricular interdependence.* The other factor responsible for the decrease in systolic blood pressure with inspiration is the increase in LV afterload that occurs as ITP falls.[208]

The importance of ventricular interdependence is exemplified in patients with pulmonary hypertension and RV failure and in those with isolated RV failure. In these patients, inadequate LV preload results from a decrease in RV ejection, with a resulting decrease in pulmonary blood flow and pulmonary venous return. In addition, the volume- and pressure-loaded RV pushes the intraventricular septum leftward and into the LV cavity. While LV diastolic pressure increases, its surrounding pressure rises to a greater extent as the LV is constrained by the deviated septum and RV pressure and by the pericardium. As a result, LV diastolic Ptm and LV volume are reduced despite the elevated LV diastolic pressure.[31]

Effects of Ventilation on Left Ventricular Afterload

An important determinant of LV afterload is the LV systolic Ptm, which is equal to LV systolic pressure minus ITP.[75] Therefore changes in systolic blood pressure and ITP have a significant effect on LV afterload and function. This fact is particularly important in the setting of LV systolic dysfunction, in which the LV is sensitive to even modest changes in afterload. Increases in LV afterload in these patients will cause stroke volume and cardiac output to fall.

Changes in ITP affect the Ptm of the intrathoracic arteries. In doing so, a pressure gradient is created between intrathoracic and extrathoracic arterial vessels. As ITP increases, the Ptm for the intrathoracic arteries decreases. As a result, the volume of these structures decreases and the pressure within increases. This change creates a waterfall-like effect as a favorable pressure gradient is created between intrathoracic and extrathoracic arterial vessels (Fig. 9-13). If the increase in ITP occurs with LV systole, the LV ejection is assisted. If the increase in ITP occurs during ventricular diastole, the LV ejects into a relatively depleted aorta (akin to an intraaortic balloon pump). The opposite occurs with negative pressure breathing.[31]

Clinical Applications

Stroke volume and cardiac output can be increased by decreasing LV afterload through the use of vasoactive agents that reduce systemic vascular resistance and systolic blood pressure. Stroke volume and cardiac output may also be increased

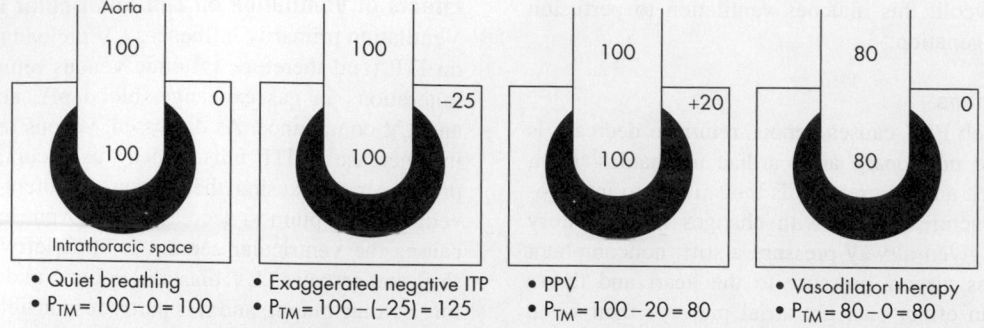

FIG. 9-13 Effects of ventilation on left ventricular afterload. Illustration of the left ventricle, thoracic cavity, and aorta. Similar changes in the left ventricular systolic transmural pressure (P_{tm}) can be generated by manipulating aortic or intrathoracic pressure (ITP). When negative ITPs are exaggerated, as occurs with respiratory disease, the P_{tm} increases significantly. PPV, Positive pressure ventilation. (Reproduced with permission from Bronicki R, Anas N: Cardiopulmonary interaction. *Pediatr Crit Care Med* 10:313-322, 2009.)

by decreasing LV afterload through the use of PPV. It is important to appreciate this concept, because PPV should be considered as a therapeutic strategy to treat LV systolic heart failure.

It is also important to consider the effects of changes in ITP on LV afterload when weaning PPV. Consider the patient with heart failure who has been extubated. The nurse notes stridor from upper airway edema following extubation. In this scenario the patient is no longer receiving LV assistance from PPV and is experiencing a dramatic increase in LV afterload secondary to upper airway obstruction and generation of exaggerated negative ITP. This patient will exhibit pulsus paradoxus that can be demonstrated by monitoring the amplitude of a pulse oximeter waveform and/or arterial catheter waveform.

In contrast to systolic heart failure, diastolic heart failure is characterized by inadequate ventricular filling and low operating volumes. After repair of tetralogy of Fallot, for example, right ventricular diastolic function is often impaired whereas left ventricular systolic function is intact. In this setting, the predominant effect of PPV is on venous return and not on left ventricular ejection. Therefore extubation is beneficial in these patients, because the fall in ITP increases venous return and RV filling as a result of an increase in the RV Ptm during diastole. Other patients at risk for low cardiac output caused by diastolic heart failure who may benefit from extubation include those with the Fontan circulation or hypertrophic cardiomyopathy (see Chapter 8).[221]

Complications During Positive Pressure Ventilation

Impaired Venous Return
See the previous section regarding cardiopulmonary interaction.

Ventilator Induced Lung Injury/Volutrauma
Human lungs can tolerate exposure to extremely high airway pressures without developing injury.[204] For example, Rotta and Steinhorn[204] noted that trumpet players generate extremely high airway pressure, but they also contract muscles to generate high pleural pressure, thus avoiding generation of high transpulmonary pressure. It is now clear that VILI results from lung distension caused by elevated transpulmonary pressures, not from high airway pressures.[204] It remains

unclear how much transpulmonary pressure can be tolerated without causing lung injury.

Mechanical ventilation with high and low tidal volumes will generate different degrees of lung injury, even if peak airway pressures are identical. Studies in animal models have demonstrated that high volumes, whether delivered at high or low pressures, will cause lung injury. Excessive tidal volume produces regional lung overdistention and causes lung injury, known as *volutrauma*.[29,204]

Lung protective strategies for treatment of acute lung injury using conventional ventilation now emphasize reduced tidal volumes, compared with ventilation strategies used in the past, to avoid volutrauma and sufficient PEEP to avoid atelectasis (Fig. 9-14).[4] This strategy is accomplished with

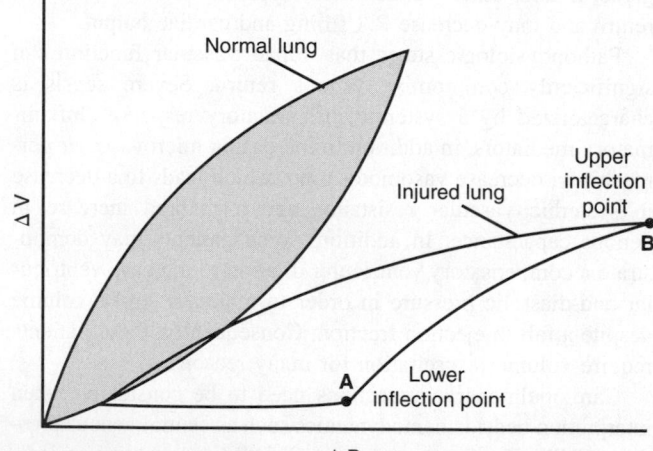

FIG. 9-14 Titration of tidal volume and positive end-expiratory pressure (PEEP) to maintain lung compliance. The compliance curves for a normal lung and an injured lung are depicted here. PEEP is titrated to keep the end expiratory lung volume at a lower inflection point (A) and ventilate at a tidal volume of approximately 6 mL/kg to maintain further changes in pressure below the upper inflection point (B). This ensures ventilation in the most compliant portion of the curve. (From Venegas J, Harris R and Simm B: A comprehensive equation for the pulmonary pressure—volume curve, *J Appl Physiol* 84:389-395, 1998; and Amato M et al.: Beneficial effects of the "open lung approach" with low distending pressures in acute respiratory distress syndrome. *Am J Respir Crit Care Med* 152:1835-1846, 1995.)

the use of low tidal volume and, if needed to improve oxygenation, high PEEP ventilator settings. Such an approach will promote ventilation in a "safe zone."

Permissive hypercarbia (elevated $PaCO_2$) strategies may also be used to reduce the risk of ventilator injury. This approach keeps tidal volume low to avoid volutrauma, even if it allows elevation in arterial CO_2 tension. Hypercarbia is typically well tolerated. Some experimental data suggest that respiratory (hypercarbic) acidosis may contribute to improved outcomes. Permissive hypercapnia can be successful in reducing the complications of mechanical ventilation.[204]

Air Leak Syndromes (Pneumothorax, Pneumopericardium, and Pneumomediastinum)

Mechanical ventilation can result in air leak syndromes. Application of high pressure or large tidal volumes in children with acute severe respiratory disease increases the incidence of air leaking from the respiratory tract. The air can collect around the lung (pneumothorax) restricting lung movement and function, or it can collect in the mediastinum (pneumomediastinum); less commonly, it can collect around the heart (pneumopericardium), causing a tamponade if air accumulates at high pressure.

When mechanical ventilation produces high peak pressures, the risk for air leak syndrome increases. An air leak syndrome may result in sudden clinical deterioration in the patient's color, systemic perfusion, and oxygenation, although the oxyhemoglobin saturation detected by pulse oximetry may not fall immediately. Breath sounds and chest expansion are typically diminished on the side with the pneumothorax, and the heart sounds may be shifted away from the side of the pneumothorax (mediastinal shift). Acute tachycardia and hypotension are often present. If the pneumothorax is small, clinical signs may be more subtle.

A tension pneumothorax must be treated urgently to prevent profound hypoxemia, bradycardia, and hypotension. The diagnosis is made on the basis of clinical examination, and treatment does not wait for confirmation with a chest radiograph. Often a needle decompression (needle thoracostomy) is performed immediately and may be followed by chest tube insertion.

To perform a needle thoracostomy, the needle is inserted in the anterior chest at the second, third, or fourth intercostal space, at the anterior axillary line. When the catheter is inserted successfully into the pleural cavity, a rush of air is often heard or air can be readily aspirated with a syringe. Guidelines for emergency chest tube insertion are provided in detail in Chapter 19. Equal breath sounds and chest expansion, improved oxyhemoglobin saturation, heart rate, blood pressure, and peripheral pulses are all indications of resolution of the tension pneumothorax. A chest radiograph is needed to verify resolution of the pneumothorax.

Other Complications of Mechanical Ventilation

Other complications of mechanical ventilation include complications of immobility (contractures, constipation, and skin breakdown) and psychologic sequelae. These complications, their clinical signs and symptoms, and appropriate nursing interventions are summarized in Table 9-12.

Noninvasive Positive Pressure Ventilation

Whereas some critically ill children need advanced airway and mechanical ventilatory support, others can be managed with noninvasive ventilation. Noninvasive ventilation (NIV) includes a variety of forms of ventilation support that do not involve an advanced or invasive airway (e.g., ETT or tracheostomy). Positive pressure is administered through a mask, nasal prongs, nasal pillows, or helmet interface. The goals are to reduce work of breathing and improve respiratory gas exchange.[237]

Continuous Positive Airway Pressure

Positive pressure can be delivered to maintain a constant minimum positive pressure throughout the respiratory cycle. This form of positive pressure is called *CPAP*. CPAP improves oxygenation by increasing lung volume and improving $(\dot{V}/\dot{Q})$ matching, and it decreases the patient's work of breathing by reducing the work of the respiratory muscles. In addition to improving oxygenation, CPAP increases the child's FRC and prevents both upper airway and alveolar collapse by delivering continuous distending pressure.[137]

Bilevel Positive Airway Pressure

Positive pressure can also be delivered using two levels of pressure during the respiratory cycle. One level of pressure is provided during inspiration (i.e., inspiratory positive airway pressure or IPAP) and a lower level of pressure is maintained between breaths (i.e., expiratory positive airway pressure or EPAP). EPAP is sometimes referred to as CPAP.

Beneficial Effects and Potential Complications

Patients with a variety of disease processes can benefit from NIV. NIV can be effective in children with chronic respiratory and pulmonary disorders as well as in children with neuromuscular weakness and restrictive pulmonary diseases.[237] NIV can also be beneficial for children with acute illnesses such as status asthmaticus, bronchiolitis, pneumonia, and other forms of acute respiratory failure.[20,36] NIV may also be used in patients as adjunct therapy immediately after extubation or when a child demonstrates decompensation after extubation caused by upper airway obstruction, ongoing parenchymal disease, or reduced respiratory effort.[71]

If NIV is effective, tachypnea, work of breathing, oxygenation, and pulmonary index scores will all improve.[36] Early use of NIV and oxygen may be superior to oxygen administration by mask or nasal cannula, and it may decrease the likelihood of intubation and the need for mechanical ventilation.

Contraindications to NIV include absence of a cough or gag, because it can increase the risk of gastric distension, vomiting, and aspiration. Other contraindications are recent craniofacial trauma or surgery, because some of the interface devices (e.g., masks, prongs, nasal pillows, helmet) can exert pressure on or cause contact with these areas. Benefits of NIV, compared with advanced airway insertion and invasive ventilation, include reduced risk of upper airway trauma, less opportunity for deconditioning of respiratory muscles, reduced risk for hospital acquired infection, and reduced need for sedation and analgesia.

Table 9-12 Complications of Intubation and Conventional Positive Pressure Ventilation

Complication	Signs and Symptoms	Intervention
Complications of Intubation		

Postintubation upper airway edema/ injury related to traumatic intubation, inappropriate tube size, tube movement during intubation, accumulation of pulmonary secretions	• Hoarseness, sore throat
	• Signs of upper airway obstruction (stridor, retractions, nasal flaring)
		• Ensure that intubation is performed by skilled personnel and that tube size is appropriate (air leak should be observed when approximately 25 cm H_2O positive pressure ventilation is provided)
		• Provide humidification of inspired air during mechanical ventilation; secretions should be thin; if secretions are thick, check temperature of inspired air
		• Target temperatures:
		  ◦ Neonate: 32° – 34° C
		  ◦ Child: 30° – 32° C
		  ◦ Adolescent: 28° – 30° C
		Check water level and function of humidification system; do not allow inspiratory tubing to rest on cooling mattress (water will precipitate in tubing as inspired air cools)
		• Perform suctioning as needed to keep ETT free of secretions; suction ETT gently—do not attempt deep suctioning of bronchi
		• Tape ETT securely and maintain head in neutral position to prevent tube movement
		• Monitor child closely after extubation to detect early signs of upper airway obstruction
		• Administer inhaled nebulized saline or racemic epinephrine as needed and ordered following extubation, monitor effect
		• Prepare for reintubation as needed

Pneumonia and infection related to invasive tubing and catheters, aspiration, and compromise of nutritional status	• Fever, leukocytosis, leukopenia, increased pulmonary congestion by radiograph and examination	• Ensure good handwashing technique; monitor patient closely for evidence of infection; report signs to physician or provider • Ensure adequate nutritional intake; discuss inadequate nutrition with physician or provider • Monitor for evidence of aspiration; notify physician if observed • Provide oropharyngeal decontamination if ordered • Use aseptic technique during suctioning and dressing changes, keep all wounds dry and provide catheter insertion site care per hospital policy (see Boxes 22-6 and 22-7)
Complications of Oxygen Therapy and Positive Pressure Ventilation		
Oxygen toxicity	• Decreased lung compliance, increased work of breathing, increased ventilation-perfusion mismatch	• Administer lowest possible oxygen concentration consistent with effective oxygen delivery; if high concentrations of inspired oxygen are required, discuss plan with physician or provider for addition and titration of PEEP and other adjustments in mechanical ventilator support • Minimize oxygen requirements; treat fever and pain, keep child comfortable, maintain neutral thermal environment for infants • Administer sedatives and neuromuscular blockers as ordered and needed to reduce work of breathing and facilitate optimal oxygenation and ventilation • Maintain target hemoglobin concentration (discuss plan with physician or provider)
Barotrauma related to positive pressure ventilation	• Pneumothorax: reduced breath sounds or change in pitch of breath sounds and decreased expansion of chest on involved side; if volume	• Monitor peak, mean, and end-expiratory pressures during ventilation; notify physician or provider if these pressures are high (it may be necessary to adjust ventilatory support)

Table 9-12 **Complications of Intubation and Conventional Positive Pressure Ventilation—cont'd**

Complication	Signs and Symptoms	Intervention
	ventilator is used, peak inspiratory pressure will rise with delivery of same volume when pneumothorax develops; tension pneumothorax will result in acute deterioration in systemic perfusion and oxygenation, with bradycardia and hypotension ○ Barotrauma can result in development of chronic lung disease ○ Pneumomediastinum can produce clinical signs similar to cardiac tamponade (including high CVP, hypotension) ○ Subcutaneous emphysema may be observed at high inspiratory pressures	• Maintain emergency thoracentesis and chest tube insertion equipment at bedside • Monitor child continuously for evidence of pneumothorax; notify physician immediately if these signs are observed; prepare for thoracentesis and insertion of chest tube on emergency basis • Monitor for evidence of a compromise in systemic perfusion; suspect pneumomediastinum or tension pneumothorax if cardiac output falls • Be prepared to assist in pericardiocentesis if radiography confirms pneumomediastinum
Decreased cardiac output caused by compromise in systemic venous return and distortion of geometry of left ventricle by high PEEP	• Tachycardia, cool skin, delayed capillary refill, altered level of consciousness, oliguria	• Monitor systemic perfusion closely and notify physician of any deterioration; whenever PEEP is increased, assess the effects on systemic perfusion • Monitor fluid balance, notify physician of any evidence of positive or negative fluid balance • Administer fluid bolus as needed and ordered to support systemic perfusion • Administer inotropic drugs as needed and ordered to support systemic perfusion
Fluid retention resulting from ADH secretion and underlying renal, pulmonary disease	• Weight gain • Positive fluid balance • Hyponatremia, reduced urine specific gravity • Pulmonary edema may develop if significant fluid retention occurs • Significant fluid retention may produce congestive heart failure	• Measure weight daily or twice daily as ordered; notify physician of significant weight gain or loss • Record fluid intake and output carefully; discuss positive fluid balance with physician or provider • Calculate maintenance fluid requirements for patient; discuss fluid administration rate with physician or provider if maintenance or greater than calculated maintenance fluid volume are ordered (and systemic perfusion is adequate) See pages inside front cover. • Auscultate breath sounds and notify physician if pulmonary congestion increases or secretions increase in volume or become frothy • Monitor for signs of CHF; notify physician if these signs are observed • Monitor electrolyte balance and notify physician of development of hyponatremia • Administer diuretics as ordered; monitor effectiveness of therapy
Complications of Critical Illness		
Stress ulcer	• Guaiac-positive gastric drainage • Abdominal pain	• Guaiac test all gastric drainage • Assess conscious patient for any evidence of abdominal pain, tenderness; report any findings to physician • Administer antacids as ordered to maintain pH of gastric secretions >4.0 • Administer histamine (H2) blockers as ordered • Provide nutrition as tolerated and ordered
Compromise in nutritional status	• Weight loss • Reduced serum protein concentration • Poor wound healing	• Weigh patient daily on same scale at same time of day and notify physician of weight loss • Calculate child's maintenance caloric requirements (see pages inside front cover and notify physician if patients fails to receive these

Continued

Nursing Care of the Critically Ill Child

Table 9-12   Complications of Intubation and Conventional Positive Pressure Ventilation—cont'd

Complication	Signs and Symptoms	Intervention
		• Monitor wound healing, skin turgor, notify physician of deterioration • Administer nutritional support as ordered, monitor patient tolerance
Complications of Immobility		
Constipation	• Decreased bowel sounds • Absence of bowel movements	• Monitor bowel function; notify physician of lack of bowel movement • Administer stool softeners as needed and ordered
Diarrhea	• Increased frequency and loose or liquid bowel movements	• Monitor bowel function and volume of stool; notify physician of excessive fluid losses
Corneal, conjunctival damage (if patient unconscious or pharmacologically paralyzed)	• Dry conjunctiva • Corneal abrasions	• If patient is unconscious or receiving neuromuscular blockers, obtain order for lubricating corneal ointment and apply as ordered • If patient is conscious, monitor blink reflex and appearance of conjunctiva; if dryness or redness is noted, notify physician or provider
Paralytic ileus and gastric distension	• Decreased bowel sounds • Increased abdominal girth • Nausea, vomiting	• Monitor bowel sounds twice per shift • Measure abdominal girth once per shift; notify physician of increase • Place NG tube as needed (and with physician order) • Ensure that abdominal distension is relieved before initiation of weaning
Muscle weakness, wasting or contractures	• Decreased range of motion • Limitation of joint movement • Pain with movement	• Provide passive and active range of motion exercises • Change patient position every 1-2 h as tolerated • Position patient with support of joints (e.g., consider use of high-topped shoes to support feet, ankles) • Obtain physical therapy consultation as needed
Atelectasis	• Decreased breath sounds or change in pitch of breath sounds over involved area • Decreased chest expansion on involved side • Radiographic evidence of atelectasis • Hypoxemia	• Provide sighs or hand ventilation at regular intervals during mechanical ventilation • Auscultate breath sounds every hour; notify physician or other on-call provider of change • Change patient position every 1-2 h • Provide chest physiotherapy as needed • Allow patient to sit in chair if tolerated
Skin breakdown, irritation	• Redness, breakdown of skin particularly over bony prominences	• Keep skin dry • Change patient position frequently (every 1-2 hours) • Massage erythematous areas after turning • Notify physician immediately if skin irritation or breakdown is observed

ADH, Antidiuretic hormone; *CHF,* congestive heart failure; *CVP,* central venous pressure; *ETT,* endotracheal tube; *NG,* nasogastric; *PEEP,* positive end-expiratory pressure.

Successful NIV requires optimal mask, nasal prong, or nasal pillow fit. Leaks from ill-fitting masks can allow a significant portion of the positive pressure to escape around the mask or prongs. If the leak is significant, the pressure will escape into the environment, and the positive airway pressure (and its beneficial effects) will not be maintained, rendering the therapy ineffective. Large leaks around the mask or prongs may cause dry eyes or significant eye irritation. Aerophagia, or the swallowing of air, can be associated with NIV and if severe, can result in gastric distension. Insertion of a nasogastric tube may be needed to decompress the air in the abdomen. In rare cases, children may develop air leak syndromes.[137]

Humidified High-Flow Nasal Cannula

Humidified high-flow nasal cannula deliver humidified and warmed respiratory gases via nasal cannula. Historically, nasal cannula flow rates of more than 2 to 4 L/minute have not been supported by the American Association of Respiratory Care, because flow rates at these levels can cause dry nasal passages and may be uncomfortable.[62] If the inspired air is warmed and additional humidity is provided, administration of higher gas flow rates may be better tolerated via nasal cannula. This therapy has been gaining popularity in many pediatric critical care units as an adjunct to the respiratory support options. Although most agree that this therapy delivers some positive pressure, it remains unclear how much pressure is being delivered to patients receiving this therapy at different levels of flow (see Chapter 21).

SPECIFIC DISEASES

Acute Respiratory Distress Syndrome (ARDS)
Etiology

ARDS is respiratory failure secondary to diffuse alveolar-capillary membrane injury resulting in permeability or high protein pulmonary edema.[205] ARDS was first described in 1967 in adult patients with respiratory failure characterized by hypoxemia refractory to oxygen therapy, tachypnea, and poor lung compliance in the absence of elevated left atrial pressure.[11] The name initially given to this disease was *adult respiratory distress syndrome,* to distinguish it from the respiratory failure of premature infants. The term was then changed to *acute respiratory distress syndrome,* because it can be identified in patients of all ages. ARDS results from a direct or indirect insult to the lungs, including but not limited to chest or multisystem trauma, toxin inhalation, metabolic derangements, acute pancreatitis, infection, sepsis, ingestion, or drug overdose. Most frequently, pneumonia, aspiration, and sepsis are the initial events that stimulate lung injury.[77]

The diagnosis of ARDS has been a topic of many consensus conferences. In 1994 the American European Consensus on ARDS defined ARDS (Table 9-13) to clarify the diagnosis and set it apart from the less severe form, acute lung injury.[18]

To identify risk factors associated with mortality for children with ARDS, more than 300 children were studied over several years. In the study, the presence of nonpulmonary organ system dysfunction was associated with a marked increase in mortality. Furthermore, the initial severity of hypoxemia predicted children at high risk for needing prolonged mechanical ventilation and high risk of death. [18]

Pathophysiology

The pathophysiology of ARDS has three stages. Following the acute injury, a *latent period* usually lasts approximately 6 to 48 hours and is followed by acute respiratory failure. Finally, a recuperative period is present that is characterized by severe pulmonary abnormalities, from which the patient either recovers or dies.[205]

Acute Phase. Acute lung injury damages the alveolar-capillary membrane through a variety of known and unknown mechanisms. During the latent period, pulmonary capillary permeability is increased and interstitial edema begins to develop. The alveoli are flooded with proteinaceous and fibrinous fluid, and the transport role of the alveolar membrane is disrupted, contributing to further fluid movement into the alveolus and limited fluid movement out.[155] In an excellent review article, Ware and Matthay[264] provided a schematic illustration of the lung with ARDS (Fig. 9-15).

In ARDS, type II pneumocytes are injured; this causes decreased surfactant production. Surfactant deficiency results in increased alveolar surface tension and an increased tendency toward collapse (atelectasis), contributing to pulmonary dysfunction. Finally, the inflammatory cascade is activated and a variety of mediators are released, leading to further damage. Overall there is an imbalance of proinflammatory and antiinflammatory cytokines (mediators). In addition, in multicenter studies in adult patients with ARDS, decreased levels of activated protein C (an anticoagulant that also acts as a brake on the inflammatory process), and high levels of plasminogen activator inhibitor-1 (a substance that inhibits fibrinolysis) were associated with increased mortality.[263] Although this information is extrapolated from adults, therapies that modulate this inflammatory response may someday be beneficial for children.

Neutrophils and other white blood cells have been implicated in the ongoing damage to the lung. These cells and many proinflammatory mediators lead to cell injury.[265] Multiple confounding variables have been identified as contributing to the alveolar membrane injury, function, repair, and resolution.

The child with ARDS has intrapulmonary shunting ($\dot{V}/\dot{Q} = 0$), increased pulmonary vascular resistance, and thus increased dead space ventilation and increased right ventricular afterload. Hypoxemia is present and is often unresponsive to oxygen administration. The result is decreased lung compliance and substantial increase in the work of breathing.

Late Phase. As the lung begins to heal, fluid is actively transported out of the lungs.[155] This phase of ARDS is also characterized by pneumocyte and fibrin infiltration of the alveoli. The lung begins to heal, but also may become fibrotic in some areas whereas in other areas normal architecture is restored.

Clinical Signs and Symptoms

During the initial lung injury and latent period, the patient often demonstrates only those signs caused by the injurious agent (e.g., drug overdose may be associated with

Table 9-13 **Criteria to Diagnose Acute Lung Injury (ALI) and Acute Respiratory Distress Syndrome (ARDS)**

Criteria	ALI	ARDS
Timing	Acute onset	Acute onset
PaO₂/FiO₂	≤300	≤200
Chest radiograph	Bilateral infiltrates	Bilateral infiltrates
Pulmonary wedge pressure	≤18 mm Hg or absence of clinical evidence of left atrial hypertension	≤18 mm Hg or absence of clinical evidence of left atrial hypertension

From Bernard GR, et al: The American-European consensus conference on ARDS definitions, mechanisms, relevant outcomes and clinical trial coordination, *Am J Respir Crit Care Med* 149:818, 1994.
ALI, Acute lung injury; *ARDS,* acute respiratory distress syndrome.

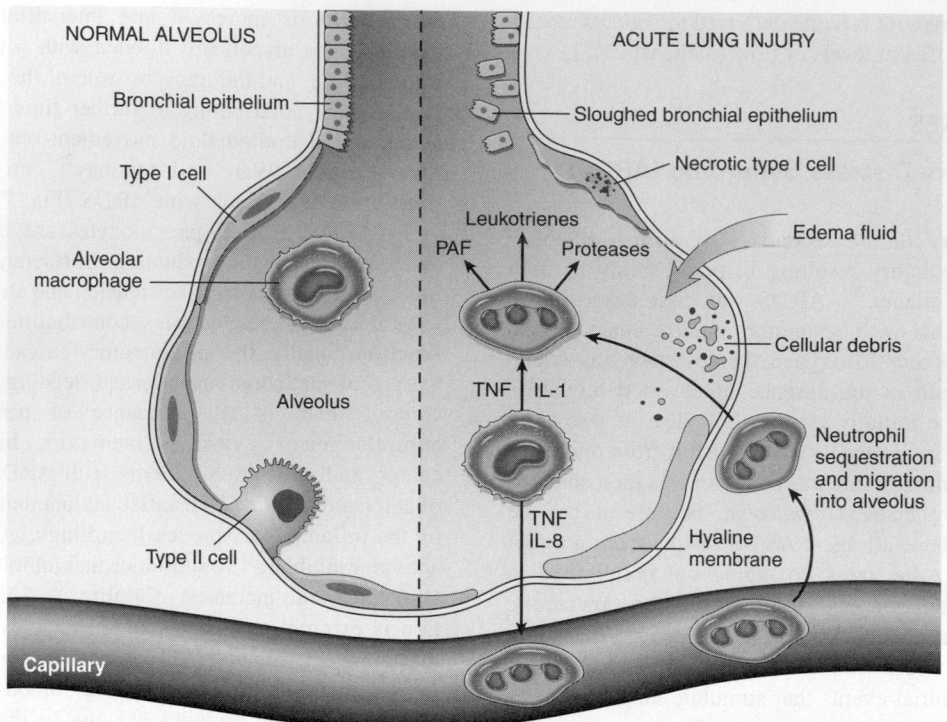

FIG. 9-15 The normal alveolus *(left)* compared with the injured alveolus in the early phase of acute lung injury and the acute respiratory distress syndrome *(right)*. Under the influence of proinflammatory cytokines such as interleukin (IL) 8, IL-1, and tumor necrosis factor (TNF) (released by macrophages), neutrophils initially undergo sequestration in the pulmonary microvasculature, followed by margination and egress into the alveolar space, where they undergo activation. Activated neutrophils release a variety of factors such as leukotrienes, oxidants, proteases, and platelet-activating factor, which contribute to local tissue damage, accumulation of edema fluid in the airspaces, surfactant inactivation, and hyaline membrane formation. Subsequently, the release of macrophage-derived fibrogenic cytokines, such as transforming growth factor β (TGF-β) and platelet-derived growth factor (PGDF), stimulate fibroblast growth and collagen deposition associated with the healing phase of injury. (From Ware LB and Matthay MA: The acute respiratory distress syndrome. *N Engl J Med* 342:1334, 2000.)

cardiovascular instability). Tachypnea, dyspnea, agitation, and hypoxemia are usually the first clinical signs of the acute phase.[155] As the pulmonary edema worsens, respiratory distress increases and evidence of respiratory muscle fatigue may develop. Muscle fatigue may be worsened by shock, hypoxia, and hyperinflation. A chest radiograph at this time likely indicates bilateral pulmonary infiltrates, which is necessary for the diagnosis of ARDS.

Acute respiratory failure is associated with hypoxemia, tachypnea, and increased respiratory effort. Intrapulmonary shunting is typically so severe at this point that hypoxemia is not responsive to oxygen administration. In addition to monitoring arterial blood gases, calculating pressure-to-flow ratios, V_D/V_T ($[PaCO_2 - P_{ET}CO_2]/PaCO_2$), and measuring $S\bar{v}O_2$ may be helpful. Respiratory distress and hypoxemia are severe, necessitating intubation and mechanical ventilation. Hypercarbia is not common at this time, although it may be present in patients with severe ARDS or ARDS complicating chronic lung disease.[230]

Management

Current strategies for mechanical ventilation support in patients with ARDS have evolved from a variety of adult

studies over the past 10 years. However, the pediatric community has embraced these approaches and is routinely instituting them in the care of the critically ill children.

Lung Protective Strategy: High PEEP, Low Tidal Volume. High PEEP with low tidal volume has become routine for treatment of children with lung injury and is especially important in the management of pediatric ARDS. This strategy is derived from studies in adult patients with ARDS that demonstrated a decrease in mortality and increase in ventilator-free days in patients treated with low tidal volumes (6-8 cc/kg) compared with those treated with traditional tidal volumes (10-12 cc/kg).[4] Further study using low tidal volume and high PEEP demonstrated increased survival compared with traditional ventilation strategies.[261] In the study, the PEEP was set 2 cm H_2O above the lower inflection point on the pressure volume curve (P_{flex}), the pressure needed to reexpand the collapsed lung. P_{flex} is identified by evaluating pressure-volume curves on the ventilator (see Figs. 9-12 and 9-13).

The goal of the lung protective strategy is to open the lung and keep it open during ventilation while minimizing additional lung injury. As an additional protective strategy, the plateau pressure is limited to less than 30 cm H_2O. The risk of VILI is associated with the driving pressure or the transpulmonary pressure (P_{ALV} − Ppleural). The lower the P_{ALV} or the higher the Ppleural (PEEP), the lower the driving pressure and the lower the risk of VILI.

PEEP therapy and mechanical ventilation support are adjusted to improve arterial oxygen content without depressing cardiac output. PEEP therapy will increase functional residual capacity, reduce intrapulmonary shunting, and move the edema fluid to less harmful areas of the lung.[220] However, it also may impede systemic venous return, resulting in a compromise of cardiac output, systemic perfusion, and oxygen delivery.

High Frequency Ventilation. Children with ARDS can rapidly escalate to maximal CMV settings and need transition to HFV. The goal is to limit barotrauma and volutrauma and to recruit atelectatic portions of the lung and maintain them in the open position. Please see the previous section on Types of Mechanical Ventilation, High Frequency Ventilation, for additional information.

Permissive Hypercapnia. Mechanical ventilation for ARDS is no longer set to provide normocarbia or achieve a normal blood gas result. Frequently in ARDS patients, high pressures, high tidal volumes, and high overall ventilator settings would be needed to normalize the blood gases.[105] The Hypothermia after Cardiac Arrest Study Group,[106] was the first to report improved outcomes in patients with ARDS who were managed with a low tidal volume, pressure-limited ventilation strategy, tolerating hypercarbia. Over time, it has become clear that an elevated arterial CO_2 tension is not harmful, provided the pH is stable (>7.2). In a reevaluation of the ARDS Network trial[4], Kregenow et al.[124] found that a 12-cc/kg tidal volume strategy was associated with increased mortality, whereas patients receiving ventilation with permissive hypercarbia demonstrated improved survival. Although there are limited data to support this approach in pediatrics, the practice has permeated pediatric critical care.

Surfactant. Surfactant inactivation is part of the pathysiology of ARDS. Although the use of surfactant is not routine in pediatrics, various surfactant preparations (calfactant,[276] bovine,[163] and porcine surfactant[102]) have been evaluated as a treatment modality for ARDS in small studies in children. A metaanalysis of six studies noted overall that surfactant administration improved oxygenation, increased ventilator-free days, and decreased duration of ventilation.[67] Administered surfactant has been successful in reducing mortality from neonatal respiratory distress syndrome (RDS),[50] and it may reduce the severity of and sequelae from RDS.[51]

Other Adjunctive Therapies: Prone Positioning. The prone position can improve oxygenation by producing more homogenous lung inflation, redistributing the inflation gradient redistributed from the dorsal to ventral regions, leading to more regional ventilation in the lung.[181] In large studies of prone positioning, although oxygenation improved, survival and ventilator-free days were not affected.[44,53,54,144] As a result, although not used routinely, prone positioning may be

---

Box 9-23   Prone Positioning Checklist

Patient Selection and Preparation
- Determine patient stability and need for access.
- Secure all tubes and catheters. Retape ETT as needed to the upper lip on the side of the face that will remain superior. Cap nonessential vascular lines and the nasogastric tube. Ensure that all stopcocks are accessible and all connections are secure.
- Provide appropriate sedation, analgesia, and neuromuscular blockade as needed.
- Prepare cushion supports and provide film dressings as needed for the patient's head, chest, pelvis, femur, and lower limbs that will leave the abdomen unrestrained and prevent pressure or friction over bony prominences and toes.
- Move ECG electrodes to the side to ensure accessibility.
- Suction the oropharynx and ETT.
- Inform the child and the family if they are present.
- Free all tubing from any anchoring supports or frames.
- Evaluate the patient. Verify placement of ETT, evaluate oxygenation and perfusion, and check vital signs.

Performing Turn
- Designate responsibilities for handling of the patient and each piece of equipment.
- Turn the patient toward the mechanical ventilator in increments.

Evaluation Immediately After the Turn
- Evaluate the patient (verify placement of ETT, evaluate oxygenation and perfusion, and check vital signs).
- Check all catheters and tubing; reconnect those that were capped.
- Adjust cushions and padding to support the patient, with the head higher than the abdomen and the head of the bed elevated slightly. Check body prominences, abdomen, and toes, and adjust cushions as needed to avoid pressure on these areas.

Adapted from Grant MJC, Curley MAQ: Pulmonary critical care problems. In Curley MAQ, Maloney-Harmon PA, editors: *Critical care nursing of infants and children*, Philadelphia, 2001, WB Saunders.
ECG, Electrocardiogram; *ETT,* endotracheal tube.

---

used to improve oxygenation. Doing so will need organization and planning (Box 9-23).[91]

Other Adjunctive Therapies: Nitric Oxide. Nitric oxide is currently approved by the FDA for use in neonatal RDS, where it has been well demonstrated to improve oxygenation in patients with pulmonary hypertension. In children, however, inhaled nitric oxide has not been demonstrated as an effective therapy for ARDS. Nonetheless, nitric oxide is frequently used because it improves oxygenation as a result of its selective vasodilatory properties, resulting in increased $\dot{V}/\dot{Q}$ matching.

Minimizing of Oxygen Demands. Eliminating fever and pain and maintaining the patient in a thermoneutral environment will decrease oxygen consumption. As noted previously, the use of neuromuscular blockade with sedation may reduce the oxygen consumption by respiratory muscles and will enable better ventilation control of the child with severe respiratory failure. The use of neuromuscular blockade with appropriate sedation (and analgesia, if needed) is particularly important when CMV produces elevated peak inspiratory pressures, because these pressures increase the risk of spontaneous pneumothorax. The use of neuromuscular blockers is not mandatory when children are treated with HFV, although sedation is usually needed (see Chapter 5).

Supportive Care. Careful monitoring and evaluation of fluid administration is necessary in the child with ARDS, because excessive fluid administration may contribute to worsening pulmonary edema and respiratory failure. The goal of fluid therapy is to maintain systemic perfusion and fluid balance using intravenous fluids, feedings, or diuretic therapy. In adults with ARDS, the use of limited fluid administration has been associated with significantly more ventilator-free days, significantly more critical care unit-free days, and slightly reduced mortality when compared with treatment using unrestricted fluid management.[168] Of note, the adult ARDS study did not include patients in shock. Fluid restriction and removal of mediators of lung injury using hemofiltration is not universally practiced, because no randomized trials have evaluated outcomes. Intravascular volume must be maintained at adequate levels, and systemic perfusion must be monitored closely. Urine volume and skin perfusion will serve as reliable indicators of the adequacy of systemic perfusion. If systemic perfusion is compromised by positive pressure ventilation or high levels of PEEP, volume administration or inotropic support usually will restore perfusion to satisfactory levels.

Bronchopulmonary Dysplasia (Chronic Lung Disease of the Premature Infant)
Etiology
Chronic lung disease includes bronchopulmonary dysplasia (BPD), the chronic lung disease occurring in premature infants. It is defined as the need for supplementary oxygen from birth, regardless of the infant's gestational age, for longer than 28 days.[113] BPD was first described by Northway et al.[174] Since that time, estimates of the incidence of BPD have varied widely,[174] as the result of heterogeneity of population risk factors, including antenatal exposures, genetics, and heredity.

BPD is the response of the immature lung to early injury. In the past, high FiO_2 and PPV were both implicated in the development of BPD. The past (i.e., former) BPD was characterized by inflammation and disruption of normal pulmonary structures which lead to heterogeneous airway and parenchymal disease. A "new" BPD has emerged as a developmental disorder characterized by decreased alveolarization, decreased septation, and minimal airway disease. These abnormalities result in less surface area for gas exchange to occur, limited airway injury, inflammation, and fibrosis. Infants with BPD may have only mild respiratory distress, but exposure to multiple contributing factors can result in alterations in normal pulmonary microvascular growth and alveolarization.[13]

Pathophysiology
Infants with BPD demonstrate reduced lung compliance, increased airway resistance, and severe expiratory flow limitation caused by edema and small airway inflammation; these cause both overinflation and atelectasis.[32] Ventilation-perfusion mismatch results in hypercarbia and hypoxemia. Current lung protective ventilation strategies allowing for permissive hypercarbia may limit additional lung injury that had been associated with traditional approaches to ventilation.

The sequelae of chronic hypoxemia include increased pulmonary vascular resistance, pulmonary hypertension, and cor pulmonale. Supplementary oxygen is an essential component of therapy when hypoxemia is present.

Clinical Signs and Symptoms
The chest radiograph of the child with BPD characteristically shows scattered linear infiltrates and patchy areas of hyperinflation (Fig. 9-16). Arterial blood gases usually reveal hypercapnia, mild acidosis (compensated respiratory acidosis), and mild hypoxemia.[228,249] The child may have a barrel chest, tachypnea, retractions, wheezing, crackles, and failure to thrive. In severe forms of old BPD, digital clubbing may be present, which indicates a poor prognosis.

High pulmonary vascular resistance increases right ventricular afterload and may produce right ventricular hypertrophy that may be diagnosed by ECG criteria, even before the patient exhibits overt symptomatology. If right-sided heart failure develops, tachycardia, tachypnea, hepatomegaly, periorbital edema, and a gallop rhythm may be noted.

Management
Once BPD develops, weaning from mechanical ventilation is undertaken gradually, and some patients may need mechanical ventilation at home. As mentioned previously, supplementary oxygen will promote adequate tissue oxygenation and diminish the risk of pulmonary vascular and cardiac complications. Oxygen requirements can vary during activity, sleep, and feeding, so oxygen saturations are monitored by pulse oximetry during a variety of activities and O_2 is titrated accordingly.

Given the role of inflammation in the pathophysiology of BPD, steroids have been used with success. However, long-term outcomes of infants who received dexamethasone therapy demonstrated an increased risk of neurotoxicity. Therefore steroid administration is no longer recommended for routine use in BPD therapy.[8] Intermittent, goal-directed therapy with steroids may still be used with caution in these patients.

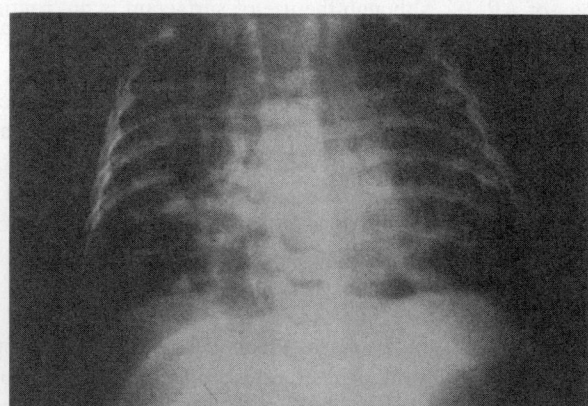

FIG. 9-16 The most common radiographic finding associated with bronchopulmonary dysplasia is the presence of diffuse infiltrates. These infiltrates produce a ground-glass or marbleized appearance in the lung fields. Emphysema may or may not be present. (Courtesy Thomas A Hazinski, Vanderbilt University Medical Center, Nashville, TN.)

Rapid lung growth occurs during the first year of life, and lung function even in patients with chronic lung disease usually improves. Adequate nutrition is essential to the recovery of the infant with BPD, but it may be difficult to achieve. Elevated rates of energy expenditure in chronic lung disease demand a higher caloric intake that is difficult to provide while maintaining fluid restriction.[63] High calorie formulas present an excessive osmotic load to the gastrointestinal tract and may result in diarrhea.

Some infants with BPD suffer from gastroesophageal reflux or may demonstrate poor feeding related to behavioral problems and reduced oral sensitivity following prolonged intubation. Optimization of nutritional support often requires speech therapy, environmental modifications to support eating, and the use of enteral feeding tubes.

Throughout the child's hospitalization, all clinicians must monitor for symptoms of impending respiratory failure, such as increased respiratory effort or worsening hypercapnia or hypoxemia. Acidosis in the child with chronic (compensated) respiratory acidosis may indicate the need for invasive or non-invasive support of ventilation. It is also important to monitor for signs of congestive heart failure, including tachycardia, tachypnea, hepatomegaly, decreased urine output, decreased peripheral perfusion, and rarely periorbital or sacral edema.

Croup (Laryngotracheobronchitis)

Etiology

Croup (laryngotracheobronchitis [LTB]) is a disease of diffuse inflammation that can include the epiglottis, vocal cords, subglottic tissue, trachea, or bronchi, resulting in upper airway obstruction. Infectious LTB is typically viral rather than bacterial in origin. Viral LTB occurs predominantly in children 3 months to 4 years of age; the most common viral pathogens are parainfluenza, RSV, and adenovirus.

Pathophysiology

The subglottic region is the narrowest segment of the upper airway of the infant and young child. It is surrounded by a rigid ring of cricoid cartilage. When infection produces inflammation, secretions and edema in this richly vascularized area, the rigid cartilage limits external extension of the tissue, and the internal airway lumen is narrowed so that airway obstruction develops. In addition, subglottic edema limits vocal cord abduction during inspiration, resulting in increased airway resistance.

Clinical Signs and Symptoms

The child with croup may have a history of rhinitis, mild fever, malaise, and anorexia for 12 to 48 hours before respiratory signs or symptoms appear. The onset of croup is heralded by a barking cough and hoarseness that is typically worse in the evening or at night. The child appears restless and anxious and may have inspiratory stridor. Because airway obstruction increases resistance to airflow, sternal retractions will be present, indicative of increased respiratory effort. On auscultation, diminished breath sounds can be heard and adventitious sounds also may be noted. If airway obstruction is severe, hypercarbia, hypoxemia, tachycardia, and respiratory acidosis may develop.

Severity of croup symptoms can be scored to provide an objective number to monitor for signs of either improvement or disease progression. The most commonly used score is the Westley Croup Score[273] (Table 9-14). However, a number of croup scores are available online, and there is no evidence that one is better than another in determining outcomes in croup. The most important aspect of any scoring system is consistency in application by all members of the healthcare team.

The differential diagnosis of LTB includes epiglottitis, foreign body aspiration, retropharyngeal abscess, diphtheria, trauma, peritonsillar abscess, allergic reaction, angioneurotic edema, or tumor. LTB may be diagnosed by the child's clinical condition.[24] If the clinical condition does not provide enough evidence to support the diagnosis of croup, a lateral radiograph of the neck may be obtained. This test can be expected to show a normal epiglottis and an area of density below the larynx caused by swelling of the tracheal soft tissues.

An anteroposterior view of the neck may show subglottic narrowing manifested by a "steeple effect" or "pencil pointing" in the airway, but this is not diagnostic. The radiograph is obtained to rule out epiglottitis, not to diagnose croup. Direct examination of the oropharynx is performed only by a physician skilled in airway management, ideally in the operating room with another physician present who can perform an emergency tracheostomy.

Management

The treatment for LTB is largely supportive and includes measures that comfort the child and facilitate airflow until the inflammation resolves. Maintenance of a patent airway is vitally important.

Table 9-14 Croup Score

Respiratory Findings	0	1	2
Inspiratory breath sounds	Normal	Harsh with rhonchi (large airway sounds)	Delayed
Stridor	None	Inspiratory	Inspiratory and expiratory
Cough or cry	Normal	Hoarse cry	Bark cough
Retractions and nasal flaring	None	Suprasternal retractions	Suprasternal and intercostal retractions and nasal flaring
Cyanosis (oxyhemoglobin saturation <95%)	None	In room air	With FiO_2 of 0.4

Modified from Al-Jundi S: Acute upper airway obstruction: croup, epiglottitis, bacterial tracheitis, and retropharyngeal abscess. In Levin DL, Morriss FC, editors: *Essentials of pediatric intensive care*, ed 2, 1997, St Louis: Churchill Livingstone and Quality Medical Publishing.

It is also important to minimize the child's anxiety and prevent crying and agitation, which can increase stridor, respiratory distress, and work of breathing. If the child is comforted by the parents or family, they are encouraged to remain at the bedside to decrease the child's agitation. The child is kept as quiet and comfortable as possible. Painful procedures are not performed until a provider experienced in pediatric airway management either confirms or rules out the diagnosis and determines the need for an advanced airway or other support.

Oxygen is administered as needed to treat hypoxemia, titrated based on oxyhemoglobin saturation (pulse oximetry).[164] Because hypoxemia can cause tissue hypoxia that contributes to agitation and worsening of respiratory distress, it must be treated promptly. In the past, the application of mist was thought to moisten secretions and soothe inflamed laryngeal mucosa. Administration of humidified oxygen, however, has not improved outcomes of children with croup in the emergency department.[164]

Heart rate, heart rhythm, and rate, depth, and pattern of respirations need to be monitored, as well as the presence and severity of retractions and nasal flaring. Hoarseness, stridor, cough, and mental status are assessed on a regular basis to detect any signs of deterioration. Tachyarrhythmias may indicate progressive hypoxemia. Arterial blood gas (ABG) analysis can be performed if the child's condition warrants such analysis, although usually this is avoided to prevent agitation. Equipment for intubation and possible tracheostomy must be readily available.

Monitor body temperature and treat fever with antipyretics. Administer intravenous fluids if oral intake is impossible or unsafe because of severe respiratory distress or deterioration. Intravenous fluid administration also may be needed if dehydration is present, but excessive fluid administration is avoided because it can contribute to pulmonary edema. Urine specific gravity is a good indicator of the child's level of hydration.

Inhalation of racemic epinephrine or l-epinephrine can reduce airway edema and has been shown to reduce airway resistance, improve clinical symptoms, and decrease the need for intubation in children with respiratory distress and croup.[24,45] Hourly treatments may occasionally be necessary (see section, Upper Airway Obstruction earlier in this chapter for doses). During and immediately following the racemic epinephrine treatments, monitor for tachycardia or lack of improvement.

A helium-oxygen mixture (heliox) may be beneficial in children with croup, particularly if the child does not need a high inspired oxygen concentration. In one study, when combined with dexamethasone, either heliox or racemic epinephrine improved croup scores.[266] Although there is limited evidence that heliox improves outcomes in croup, it may be beneficial to decrease work of breathing in the short-term care of these children (see the discussion of heliox administration under the section, Upper Airway Obstruction).

Many studies have demonstrated the effectiveness of steroids, including dexamethasone, prednisolone, and budesonide, in relieving symptoms of croup and reducing hospital length of stay.[207] Because steroids improve croup symptoms, few children (less than 1% of children with LTB) will need intubation for the management of respiratory failure.[86]

Epiglottitis
Etiology
Epiglottitis is a medical emergency characterized by inflammation and swelling of the epiglottis, false cords, and aryepiglottic folds, often causing severe upper airway obstruction. Because it involves the structures of the supraglottic region, it can be known as *supraglottitis*. In the past, the primary bacterial agent causing epiglottitis was *Haemophilus influenzae* B. With the introduction of the *Hib* vaccine, the incidence of epiglottitis has decreased overall, and those caused by *H. influenzae B* have been significantly reduced.[218] Other infectious organisms are group A beta streptococcus, *Streptococcus pyogenes, Streptococcus pneumoniae,* and *Staphylococcus aureus,* as well as some fungi and viruses.[90,200] Following widespread use of the *Hib* vaccine, the age of patients with the disease has increased, and it now occurs most commonly in children from 2 years to late school age.[218,274]

Pathophysiology
The epiglottis is a cartilaginous structure covered by mucous membranes; it normally helps to occlude the glottis during swallowing. Edema of the mucous membranes in the area of the epiglottis can obstruct the airway completely in a matter of minutes or hours. Acute and complete occlusion of the airway may be precipitated by stimulating the oropharynx (e.g., examination, manipulation, suctioning) or by any procedure that induces apprehension or anxiety in the child.[110]

Clinical Signs and Symptoms
The clinical course of epiglottitis is characteristically rapid. Unless immediate medical care is provided to maintain airway patency, airway obstruction and death can result. The child with epiglottitis often demonstrates a muffled voice, weak cough, sore throat, drooling, and dysphagia with a high fever (usually >39° C). As the epiglottis increases in size, the child exhibits signs of airway obstruction, including a characteristic inspiratory stridor, sternal retractions, tachycardia, and decreased breath sounds. The child is usually anxious and prefers to sit and lean forward, assuming a tripod position. Late signs of hypoxia include listlessness, cyanosis, and cardiac arrhythmias, including bradycardia and premature ventricular contractions (see Table 9-5).

The definitive diagnosis of epiglottitis is ideally made in the operating room when a physician experienced in airway management examines the upper airway via laryngoscopy and visualizes a cherry-red, swollen epiglottis. The presence of the disease is nearly always an indication for intubation. Typically intubation is performed using an ETT one size smaller than that typically used for the child's age and size. Occasionally intubation is impossible if laryngospasm has occurred; a tracheostomy is then performed.

Management
Once the diagnosis of epiglottitis is suspected, a physician qualified to perform emergency intubation or tracheostomy and all equipment needed for intubation must be readily available. Allow the parents to remain with the child, because their presence may reduce the child's anxiety. If obtained, a lateral radiograph of the neck shows the epiglottis as a large, rounded,

soft-tissue mass at the base of the tongue, and it rules out other pathologies such as retropharyngeal abscess, foreign body, and croup.[219] A radiograph is obtained only when the diagnosis is questioned and care must be taken to prevent agitation.

In the unusual case of a patient with epiglottitis who is not intubated, the goal is to maintain a patent airway while keeping the child quiet and undisturbed. Anxiety and episodes of crying may be minimized by having the child rest in the parent's arms. The parent can deliver oxygen by simple blow-by (a tube or mask with humidified oxygen "blowing by" the child's nose and mouth).

Until intubation is accomplished, it is important to monitor the child's rate and depth of respirations, retractions, and nasal flaring and stridor, as well as the child's color and air movement. Supportive care is provided to minimize the child's energy expenditure and maximize respiratory efficiency. Humidified oxygen (using a facial tent, face mask, or blow-by O_2, as noted previously) is provided.

If cardiorespiratory arrest occurs before insertion of an advanced airway, attempt bag-mask ventilation with 100% oxygen (using a two-person technique to ensure a tight face-to-mask seal and effective jaw lift). Ventilation may not be effective if inflammation is severe or if the child initially struggles. As the child loses consciousness, it may be possible to provide effective bag-mask ventilation. If airway obstruction prevents ventilation by bag-mask technique, a healthcare provider skilled in airway management can insert a large-bore needle (13-15 gauge) into the cricothyroid area to provide oxygenation (it will not provide an effective technique for CO_2 elimination) until an ETT or tracheostomy can be placed.

Typically the ETT can be removed within 24 to 48 hours after antibiotic therapy is started (ceftriaxone or appropriate antibiotic for suspected pathogen). Sedation may be necessary if O_2 and the relief of airway obstruction do not eliminate the patient's agitation, although frequently patients are comfortable as soon as they are intubated. Until swelling of the epiglottis subsides, maintenance of ETT patency and position are critical. Any obstruction or displacement of the tube can produce acute, life-threatening, deterioration. The ETT must be taped securely in place. Secure the child's hands appropriately (as needed) to decrease the risk of spontaneous extubation, which can be a life-threatening event. Reintubation can be extremely difficult in these children, although when the tube is removed early for any reason, even within hours of starting antibiotics, patients are frequently sufficiently improved and reintubation may not be needed.

The child with epiglottitis needs adequate fluid and caloric intake. Before intubation, the child with severe respiratory distress receives nothing by mouth. Intravenous fluids are administered to ensure adequate hydration, although caution is necessary in establishing intravenous access before the advanced airway is placed. Typically, vascular access is achieved in the operating suite after anesthesia is administered and after the airway is placed.

Immediately after extubation, the child receives nothing by mouth for up to 8 hours, until the healthcare team is certain that reintubation will not be needed. If reintubation is needed, the child may have Ludwig's angina (a cellulitis infection of the submandibular space). Once the child is successfully extubated, oral fluids may be provided.

The child and family will need reassurance and support. The acuity of the child's progression of symptoms can be extremely frightening.

Bronchiolitis

Etiology

Bronchiolitis is a lower respiratory tract illness that occurs primarily in young infants. It is characterized by inflammation of the bronchioles, increased mucus production, and bronchoconstriction resulting in airway obstruction and air trapping. Bronchiolitis is caused most frequently by RSV, but other viruses, including adenovirus, influenza, and parainfluenza, also may be isolated. The peak incidence of illness occurs during midwinter and early spring, and the disease typically affects infants of approximately 2 to 4 months of age.[176] Significant symptoms of lower airway obstruction in the child older than 2 years are rare.

Infants with BPD, cyanotic congenital heart disease, prematurity, cystic fibrosis, stem cell or solid organ transplantation (or both), neuromuscular diseases, and immunodeficiency are at increased risk for severe bronchiolitis.[154,178,270] Additional risk factors for severe bronchiolitis include male gender, younger age, birth during RSV season, attendance in day care, and crowded living conditions.[225] Other potential risk factors include exposure to tobacco smoke, asthma in a parent, lower socioeconomic status, time limited breastfeeding and atopic dermatitis.[225,231]

Pathophysiology

The virus responsible for the bronchiolitis replicates in the epithelial cells of the airways, resulting in inflammation, necrosis of the epithelium, and proliferation of nonciliated cells. The lack of bronchial cilia, increased secretions, edema of the submucosal layer, and bronchoconstriction cause obstruction of the small airways. An increase in the functional residual capacity, caused by air trapping, forces the infant to breathe at a higher lung volume; this reduces lung compliance and increases the work of breathing. Scattered areas of atelectasis produce ventilation perfusion mismatching and abnormal gas exchange.

Clinical Signs and Symptoms

Following a 2- to 5-day prodrome of upper respiratory tract infection and fever, the infant develops tachypnea, wheezing, crackles, and retractions. Episodes of apnea and/or cyanosis also may be observed as initial symptoms in small infants. The liver may be palpable secondary to lung hyperinflation. The chest radiograph typically demonstrates hyperinflation, a flattened diaphragm, and atelectasis. Hypoxemia may be detected using pulse oximetry, and both hypoxemia and hypercarbia may be detected with arterial blood gas sampling.

Diagnosis is based primarily on clinical observation and knowledge of epidemiology within the community. A rapid immunofluorescence test for RSV may be used on nasopharyngeal secretions. This test is 70% to 100% sensitive and specific, provided that a good sample of nasopharyngeal secretions is obtained.[101]

Management

The respiratory status of the infant with bronchiolitis must be assessed continuously, with close observation for respiratory fatigue and respiratory failure or apnea. Signs of respiratory failure include a change in respiratory effort (significant increase or decrease in effort), diaphragm fatigue (paradoxic abdominal movement, respiratory alternans, and apnea), cyanosis, hypercarbia, and hypoxemia.

Oxygen is administered to maintain normal arterial oxyhemoglobin saturation. Intubation and ventilation may be necessary if respiratory failure develops or if the infant demonstrates repetitive apnea that is not relieved by nasal suctioning. Administration of nebulized bronchodilators such as beta adrenergic agonists and epinephrine may result in symptomatic improvement in some children. However, there is no evidence that routine administration of bronchodilators improves oxygenation, hospitalization rate, or duration of hospitalization.[119] There is also little benefit from bronchodilators in intubated children with RSV and respiratory failure.[130] For children who have trouble with secretion clearance, administration of nebulized hypertonic 3% saline may facilitate mucociliary clearance.[211] Treatment with corticosteroids is controversial, and there is no evidence of overall effect in decreasing ventilator days in critically ill, children receiving ventilation.[56] Ribavirin is an antiviral agent previously used in the treatment of RSV. More recent data, however, do not support its use in treating RSV. In addition, the routine use of surfactant in children with RSV may show positive trends, but additional rigorous study is needed to determine effectiveness in this disease.[56] Hydration is maintained by the intravenous route when the infant exhibits tachypnea or distress. Contact isolation is recommended for children with bronchiolitis caused by RSV, adenovirus, coronavirus, influenza virus, parainfluenza, and rhinovirus.

Many infants with bronchiolitis, especially small or young infants and those with chronic or congenital diseases, will develop respiratory failure necessitating mechanical ventilation. Although this has traditionally been accomplished with endotracheal intubation, NIV techniques such as face mask CPAP and high-flow nasal cannula may be successful.

Status Asthmaticus

Pathophysiology

Asthma is a diffuse, obstructive pulmonary disease that is characterized by airway inflammation, mucosal edema, increased mucus production, and bronchospasm.[92] Submucosal inflammatory infiltrates in the bronchial tree activate mast cells, epithelial cells, and T lymphocytes that generate proinflammatory cytokines. Inflammatory mediators such as leukotrienes, histamine, and platelet-activating factor are found both locally in the airways and systemically. The inflammatory changes cause epithelial destruction and nerve end exposure, which result in airway hyperreactivity.

Because the airways of the child with asthma are hyperreactive, acute airway obstruction can be triggered by allergens, infections, smoke, exercise, environmental irritants, and stress.[145] Underlying inflammation and bronchospasm lead to impaired gas flow and air trapping, making exhalation difficult.[145] Ventilation-perfusion mismatch results in hypoxemia. Increased work of breathing can lead to respiratory muscle fatigue and hypercarbia.

Increased FRC resulting from air trapping can affect cardiac function. Right ventricular afterload is increased as the result of hypoxic pulmonary vasoconstriction, increased lung volume, and possibly acidosis. If airway obstruction is severe, patients may demonstrate a pulsus paradoxus or an exaggeration in the drop of arterial pressure during inspiration. Severe airway obstruction results in generation of more negative intrapleural pressures. Negative intrapleural pressures increase left ventricular afterload and depressed left ventricular function, and they can lead to cardiogenic pulmonary edema (see section, Cardiopulmonary Interactions earlier in this chapter). Hyperinflation also impairs diaphragm function because the diaphragm is shortened, limiting the tension the muscle fibers can generate.

Clinical Signs and Symptoms

The clinical presentation of status asthmaticus varies by severity of illness and age. Cough, wheezing, prolonged or forced expiration phase and increased work of breathing are typical presenting signs and symptoms. A congested cough may also result from the increased mucus production. Wheezing noted on physical examination indicates obstructed expiratory airflow. Absent or distant breath sounds (or "silent chest") are signs of impending respiratory failure. Other signs indicative of significant respiratory compromise include inability to speak in more than monosyllables, diaphoresis, inability to lie flat, or change in mental status.[145] The presence of pulsus paradoxus correlates with the severity of airway obstruction and may be useful in the assessment of disease progression. Pulsus paradoxus is best illustrated by fluctuations in the wave form from an intraarterial catheter, but may be detected by the reduction in the amplitude of the pulse oximeter waveform during inspiration. Assessment of a child with status asthmaticus is primarily through clinical examination, but some diagnostic tests can be used to augment assessment of severity (Table 9-15).

Chest Radiography. Radiographic studies are not used to diagnose asthma, but will generally demonstrate characteristic air trapping and support clinical examination findings. Flattened diaphragms are typically noted with diseases causing air trapping (see Fig. 9-8). These children are at increased risk for air leak syndromes, and some radiographs may demonstrate a pneumothorax or pneumomediastinum associated with the illness. Often these air leaks are clinically insignificant, but they have the potential to expand and cause clinical deterioration. If the exacerbation of asthma is related to pneumonia, an infiltrate may be noted on a chest radiograph. Frequently, the chest radiograph demonstrates areas of atelectasis that can be confused with true infiltrate.

Carbon Dioxide Monitoring. Blood gas analysis can be used in the assessment of children with status asthmaticus. Generally, however, this method has been replaced by noninvasive oximetry and either transcutaneous CO_2 measurement or capnography. Carbon dioxide monitoring is useful in assessing pulmonary gas exchange. Hypocarbia is noted in the early phases of the exacerbation, and a normalizing CO_2 or hypercarbia in the presence of ongoing symptoms typically indicates deterioration in condition.

Table 9-15 Pediatric Asthma Score

Score	1	2	3
Respiratory rate			
2-3 years	≤ 34	35-39	≥ 40
4-5 years	≤ 30	31-35	≥ 36
6-12 years	≤ 26	27-30	≥ 31
>12 years	≤ 23	24-27	≥ 28
Oxygen Requirement	SpO_2 >95% on room air	SpO_2 >90-95% on room air	SpO_2 <90% on room air or on oxygen
Auscultation	Normal breath sounds or end expiratory wheeze	Expiratory wheeze	Inspiratory and expiratory wheeze or diminished breath sounds
Retractions	None or intercostal	Intercostal and substernal	Severe

Adapted from Kelly CS, et al: Improved outcomes for hospitalized asthmatic children using a clinical pathway. *Ann Allergy Asthma Immunol* 84:509-516, 2000.
Score: mild, 4-6; moderate, 7-9; severe, 10-12, consider admission to pediatric intensive care unit.

Management

The immediate goal of care of the child with status asthmaticus is the relief of airway obstruction and the restoration of effective oxygenation and ventilation. Any child with severe asthma needs careful cardiorespiratory monitoring and a quiet and comfortable environment to alleviate fear and agitation. Supplementary oxygen is administered to maintain the SaO_2 90% to 92% or greater.

Fluid Management. Most children with status asthmaticus will have some level of dehydration at the time of admission. Explanations include increased insensible fluid loss secondary to increased work of breathing, decreased fluid intake during the time of exacerbation, and vomiting related to the underlying cause of the exacerbation. Fluid goals include restoration of euvolemia. Fluid boluses and continuous intravenous fluid therapy may be needed, although care must be taken to avoid overhydration that may contribute to pulmonary edema and worsening of clinical condition.[145]

Pharmacologic Therapy. Treatment with β-receptor agonists is the mainstay of therapy in status asthmaticus (Box 9-24).

Box 9-24 Pharmacologic Management of Status Asthmaticus

Beta 2 agonists
- Albuterol
- Levalbuterol
- Terbutaline

Anticholinergics
- Ipratropium bromide

Corticosteroids
Magnesium Sulfate
Methylxanthine
- Aminophylline
Leukotriene antagonists
- Montelukast
Mucolytics
- Recombinant human deoxyribonuclease
Inhaled anesthetics
- Desflurane
- Isoflurane
- Sevoflurane

These medications bind to the β2-receptors in the smooth muscle lining the airway and will produce smooth muscle relaxation.[145] The most common means of administration of β2-receptor agonists is via nebulization. Intravenous formulations (e.g., terbutaline) may be useful if the child does not tolerate a nebulized formulation or does not exhibit adequate bronchodilation with the inhaled formulation.

β2-Receptor Agonists. The most commonly used inhaled β2-receptor agonist in the United States is albuterol. Other available agents are epinephrine and levalbuterol. Both racemic albuterol and terbutaline are selective for β2-receptor agonists. Levalbuterol is a formulation of R-isomer-albuterol that is thought to have fewer side effects with the same clinical effect as albuterol and terbutaline. S-albuterol (50% of racemic albuterol) was previously thought to be an inert compound, but some studies have demonstrated that this compound may exaggerate airway hyperresponsiveness, trigger a proinflammatory effect in children, and actually cause prolonged bronchoconstriction.[85,114,130,145,170] Terbutaline is the intravenous β2-receptor agonist formulation used in the United States. Other countries use intravenous albuterol.

Side effects related to β2-receptor agonists include tachycardia, arrhythmia, hypertension, and prolongation of the QT interval corrected for heart rate (QTc interval). β2-receptor agonists may also contribute to hypokalemia and hyperkalemia. The most common clinically significant side effects of continuous albuterol or intravenous terbutaline are diastolic hypotension, hypoxemia caused by reversal of hypoxic pulmonary vasoconstriction, tachycardia, and agitation. No studies have demonstrated clinically significant cardiac toxicity related to the administration of terbutaline.[145]

Even when administered under ideal conditions, less than 10% of nebulized medication will reach the lung. Factors affecting drug absorption include the child's tidal volume, breathing pattern, and nebulized gas flow.[145] Some evidence supports the use of metered dose inhalers for medication delivery in children with mild to moderate symptoms. For those needing more frequent or continuous therapy, however, continuous nebulization is used.[145]

Anticholinergics. Anticholinergic medications, most commonly ipratropium bromide, may be used in conjunction with β2-receptor agonists for the treatment of status asthmaticus. These medications are inhaled and are delivered using either nebulization or metered dose inhaler. No systemic absorption occurs, so side effects are minimal. These medications are not considered to be rescue medications and they are used as adjunctive therapy with other bronchodilators. Several studies evaluating the use of ipratropium bromide in ward-hospitalized pediatric patients have failed to demonstrate changes in patient outcomes such as length of stay.[52,88] However, because side effects are minimal and benefits have been reported, ipratropium is used as adjunctive therapy for status asthmaticus.

Corticosteroids. Corticosteroids are central in the management of status asthmaticus. Beneficial effects of steroids include decreased airway inflammation, inhibition of the vascular leak induced by proinflammatory mediators, decreased mucus production, and modification of activation of lymphocytes, eosinophils, mast cells, and macrophages. Oral and intravenous corticosteroids (e.g., methylprednisolone, 0.5-1 mg/kg every 6 hours) are equally effective, although intravenous formulations are often used in critically ill children who may demonstrate tenuous respiratory status or poor tolerance of enteral feedings.[145] The first dose of steroids is administered promptly, because effects will not be noted for 2 to 4 hours.

Magnesium Sulfate. Adjuvant therapy with magnesium sulfate may have a role in the management of status asthmaticus. Magnesium is found in intracellular fluid and is important for cellular electrical activity and many enzymatic reactions.[118] Smooth muscle relaxation secondary to magnesium administration is thought to be secondary to inhibition of calcium uptake.[145]

Magnesium sulfate can be administered intravenously via intermittent infusion dosing, or it can be added to the continuous intravenous fluid formulation. Nebulized magnesium sulfate is also available, but its role in status asthmaticus has not yet been determined.[262] Side effects include flushing, weakness, burning at the infusion site, diarrhea, and hypotension. Several studies have documented the safety of this therapy in pediatric status asthmaticus.[47,48,87]

Leukotrienes. Leukotrienes are naturally occurring mediators that are implicated in the inflammatory process of asthma exacerbations. Leukotriene antagonists are not used in the routine treatment of status asthmaticus,[145] but their role in asthma therapy continues to be explored.

Methylxanthines. Methylaxanthines (e.g., theophylline) were once a mainstay in the management of asthma, but their use has fallen out of favor because of the risk of toxicity. Methylxanthines are phosphodiesterase inhibitors that are thought to stimulate endogenous catecholamine release, stimulate β-adrenergic receptors, augment diaphragmatic contractility, and act as a diuretic.[145] Their role in management of severe pediatric asthma remains unclear, although some studies suggest they may be beneficial.[55,161,275]

Ketamine. Ketamine is a dissociative anesthetic with potent analgesic action. It also possesses bronchodilatory side effects that may be useful in status asthmaticus. Several mechanisms for bronchodilation have been postulated, but the most likely explanation is increasing endogenous catecholamine release. This medication can be considered for procedural use in children with status asthmaticus and for intermediate term sedation for intubated asthmatics.[145]

Mucolytic Agents. Airway obstruction by viscous mucus is one of the pathophysiologic features of an acute asthma exacerbation. The mucous plugs develop after lysis of inflammatory cells, and DNA present in the cell debris contributes to increased adhesiveness and viscosity of secretions. The mucus can be liquefied by administration of recombinant human deoxyribonuclease (dornase alpha) in patients with cystic fibrosis, although addition of single-dose nebulized dornase alpha to the combination of bronchodilator therapy and systemic steroids has not been shown to be beneficial in children with moderate to severe asthma.[26]

Heliox. Heliox can be used to reduce the turbulent airflow associated with asthma. This gas mixture will allow gas and medications to traverse areas of obstruction more easily and allow for improved airflow through the lower airways. To provide the benefits of the lighter weight gas mixture, the ratio of helium to oxygen must be at least 60% helium and 40% oxygen (see Croup [Laryngotracheobronchitis], earlier in this chapter). This gas mixture can be delivered to children who are breathing spontaneously without advanced airways in place and to children receiving either noninvasive or invasive mechanical ventilation. Heliox admixture administration via conventional ventilation appears to be safe, lowers the peak inspiratory pressure, and improves CO_2 removal.[1] Overall, the reported benefits of this gas mixture in status asthmaticus have been mixed.[38,120]

Noninvasive Ventilation. Noninvasive ventilation may be successful for treatment of status asthmaticus. General benefits of NIV are discussed above (see section, Noninvasive Positive Pressure Ventilation earlier in this chapter). Several studies have demonstrated that noninvasive ventilation in status asthmaticus, and lower airways diseases may avoid the need for intubation and mechanical ventilation.[36,242]

Invasive Ventilation. Because the complication rate for invasive ventilation is high for children with status asthmaticus, this method of support needs to be avoided if possible. If intubation is performed, a cuffed ETT is preferred to minimize the air leak associated with the anticipated high pressures needed to provide adequate ventilation. Most complications associated with intubation and ventilation in the child with status asthmaticus occur at the time of intubation or shortly thereafter. The most common complications include hypotension, oxygen desaturation, pneumothorax, subcutaneous emphysema, and cardiac arrest.[37,145] Hypotension related to intrathoracic pressure changes and reduced systemic venous return is usually successfully treated with fluid boluses. If hypotension does not improve with fluid administration, a tension pneumothorax may be present and needs to be ruled out.[145] These children are also at risk for VAP.

Sedation, analgesia, and in many cases neuromuscular blockade will be needed to prevent tachypnea and ventilator dyssynchrony and to decrease the risk of pneumothorax. Optimal ventilator strategies for intubated patients with asthma have not been well described. Shorter inspiratory times allow greater time for the expiratory phase of the respiratory cycle, which is beneficial in obstructive diseases. Pressure control ventilation has been demonstrated to be a safe mode of ventilation for patients with asthma.[210] The use of PEEP remains controversial, although there seems to be good physiologic evidence that PEEP allows for improved expiratory airflow by maintaining airway patency throughout the respiratory cycle. Recent research suggests that intubation and mechanical ventilation itself may increase risk of mortality.[37]

Inhalation Anesthetics. Some inhalation anesthetics are highly potent bronchodilators. These agents have been used in refractory status asthmaticus, although there are significant challenges associated with administration. Safe and proper administration of inhalation agents must be considered before implementation. Administration requires either an anesthesia machine or custom-fitted ventilator with a scavenging circuit and continuous analysis of inspiratory and expiratory gas.[145]

Pneumonia

Etiology

Pneumonia is an inflammation of the lung parenchyma that may be caused by infection, aspiration, chemical inhalation, or toxic agents. The term *pneumonia* covers many disorders that differ widely in causative agents (Box 9-25), disease

---

Box 9-25 | Risk Factors for Pneumonia: Compromised Host Defenses

Bypass of nasal defense
- Tracheostomy
- Endotracheal intubation
- Craniofacial malformations (e.g., cleft palate)

Aspiration
- Bottle propping
- Incompetent cough, gag, or swallow
- Tracheoesophageal fistula (H-type) or cleft
- Gastroesophageal reflux with aspiration

Abnormal cough reflex
- Drugs and anesthetic agents
- Muscular weakness or paralysis
- Pain
- Anatomic defects (e.g., vascular ring, polyps, tracheal web)

Compromise in mucociliary clearance
- Infections (e.g., mycoplasma, pertussis, virus)
- Inhaled toxins
- Abnormal mucus
- Bronchopulmonary dysplasia
- Immotile cilia syndromes

Abnormal airway secretions
- Cystic fibrosis
- Secretory IgA deficiency
- IgG subclass deficiency

Airway obstruction
- Congenital (e.g., pulmonary sequestration, cysts, fistulas)
- Acquired (e.g., retained foreign body, extrinsic airway compression, nodes, masses, bronchiectasis, asthma)

Ig, Immunoglobulin.

---

course, pathology, and prognosis. The likely causative agents vary with the age of the child. The most common bacterial cause of pneumonia in pediatrics is *Streptococcus pneumonia,* followed by *Chlamydia pneumonia* and *Mycoplasma pneumoniae.*[214] In the newborn period, congenital infection caused by cytomegalovirus, herpes simplex, rubella, and toxoplasma must be considered. Acquired newborn infections include group B streptococcus and those caused by gram-negative enterobacillus such as *Escherichia coli* and *Klebsiella* species. *Chlamydia trachomatis* is a common cause of afebrile pneumonia in infants.[214]

In patients with congenital or acquired immunodeficiency, *Pneumocystis carinii, Candida* species, and *Aspergillus* species can cause pneumonia. Approximately 25% of children suffering from bacterial pneumonia can also be co-infected with a virus.[133,158] Respiratory viruses are a common cause of febrile pneumonia, with a peak incidence at 2 to 3 years of age.[214] Pneumonias secondary to parainfluenza virus, adenovirus, metapneumovirus, and rhinovirus are also common in these younger children. Community-acquired methicillin-resistant *Staphylococcus aureus* (CA-MRSA) must be considered as a likely causative agent in areas where it is endemic. Typically CA-MRSA causes local skin and soft-tissue infections, but it can cause pneumonia.[240] CA-MRSA has a susceptibility profile that differs from hospital-acquired *S. aureus.*

Pathophysiology

As noted previously, the term *pneumonia* covers a multitude of disorders that differ widely in causative agents, disease course, pathology, and prognosis. A common feature of all pneumonias is that each involves an inflammatory response. The causative agent is most often infectious, and it is introduced into the lungs through either inhalation or the bloodstream. Depending on the etiologic agent, the pathologic response varies. A virus causes direct injury to the epithelium of the respiratory tract, leading to edema and obstruction, accumulation of debris, and abnormal secretions. Bacteria may also injure the epithelium with the same consequences or cause inhibition of ciliary action, cellular destruction, and an inflammatory reaction in the submucosa.[214]

Pneumonia can be classified as lobar pneumonia (e.g., *Streptococcus pneumoniae),* bronchopneumonia (e.g., *Staphylococcus pneumoniae),* or interstitial pneumonia (e.g., group A streptococcus) on the basis of clinical and radiographic evidence. In lobar pneumonia, one or more lobes are involved. When bronchopneumonia is present, the terminal bronchioles are inflamed. With interstitial pneumonia the inflammatory processes are found within the alveolar walls.

Clinical Signs and Symptoms

Generally, infants and younger children develop more severe symptoms with respiratory infection than do older children. In addition, the natural history of the illness can differ among age groups, because of developmental differences in lung function and respiratory reserve. Although the onset of the disease is typically characterized by rhinitis and cough lasting for several days, the classic presentation throughout childhood is tachypnea.

Infants may demonstrate a period of decreased oral intake followed by development of fever or hypothermia, respiratory distress, apprehension, and restlessness. Respiratory distress is accompanied by increased work of breathing manifested by grunting, use of accessory muscles, nasal flaring, and intercostal, subcostal, and supraclavicular retractions. These infants will likely also have tachycardia and cyanosis. In addition, vomiting, anorexia, and diarrhea may be present with a paralytic ileus causing abdominal distension.

Children and adolescents may demonstrate the characteristic rhinitis and cough followed by rapid onset of fever with chills and chest pain. They may be drowsy and restless, and they can have a dry or productive cough, be anxious, and develop circumoral cyanosis. Pleuritic pain may be present. Gastrointestinal findings may also be present in this age group, and a lower lobe pneumonia frequently presents with signs similar to those of an acute abdomen.

Respiratory findings for pneumonia include diminished breath sounds, crackles, and rhonchi over the affected area of the lung. In small infants, abnormal lung sounds may be heard throughout because the sounds are referred from the involved area through noninvolved tissue. If the child is an infant and is wheezing, the child is more likely to have a viral rather than a bacterial or mixed cause pneumonia.[158] With percussion there is dullness over the affected area. Children with complications of pneumonia including effusion, empyema, or pneumothorax will have more pronounced findings of respiratory distress.

Ideally, a specific pathogen is identified by sputum culture, although this is rarely the case in pediatric patients. Appropriate antibiotic therapy is tailored to culture results. When an expectorated sputum sample cannot be obtained, tracheal aspirate, pleural fluid, or a lung biopsy sample may be obtained and cultured. In children, however, these invasive techniques are usually reserved for immunocompromised patients or those who fail to respond to conventional therapy.

Management

Oxygen and Respiratory Support. Humidified oxygen is administered to children with respiratory distress and hypoxemia. It is important to monitor the child closely throughout hospitalization for evidence of increased respiratory distress. When respiratory distress increases despite oxygen delivery, the child may benefit from the addition of noninvasive respiratory support in the form of a high-flow nasal cannula, bag-mask positive pressure ventilation, or CPAP (see section, Noninvasive Positive Pressure Ventilation earlier in this chapter).

Mechanical Ventilation. Some children with pneumonia will develop respiratory failure and need intubation and mechanical ventilation. Conventional mechanical ventilation (CMV) is typically effective for the treatment of respiratory failure secondary to pneumonia. The goal of ventilatory support is to maximize oxygenation and ventilation. Transitioning to HFV is unusual in children with pneumonia.

Antibiotics. If the child is critically ill, antimicrobial therapy is usually instituted before a pathogen is isolated. Antibiotics are selected based on the age of the child and the likely causative organism. A third-generation cephalosporin generally is recommended for critically ill children. If the child does not improve, additional coverage for atypical agents may be needed. For children living in communities where CA-MRSA is prevalent, consider coverage with vancomycin or clindamycin.[214] For neonates, broad-spectrum antibiotic coverage for possible sepsis is typically provided.

Supportive Care. Children with pneumonia need thorough respiratory assessment and good general supportive care. Respiratory rate, effort, and color are assessed frequently. Auscultation over both lung fields is performed, and the examiner must be alert to the presence of adventitious sounds or alteration in the pitch or intensity of diminished breath sounds, and report deterioration to a provider. Once any area of consolidation or congestion is identified, careful auscultation is needed to identify evidence of clearing or exacerbation.

If the child's cough is ineffective, suctioning may be necessary to remove secretions whether the child is intubated or not. Chest physiotherapy may aid in the mobilization of secretions (see the Chapter 9 Supplement on the Evolve Website for information and illustrations regarding chest physiotherapy). The child with pneumonia may not be able to tolerate a head-down or side-lying position. Pillows may be used to elevate the head of the bed or aid in positioning the patient. The infant may demonstrate improvement when placed in an infant seat, because this position can maximize diaphragm excursion.

Monitor the child's body temperature closely and treat fever with antipyretics to reduce oxygen consumption, improve patient comfort, and decrease the possibility of febrile seizure. Fever in conjunction with tachypnea also increases insensible water loss. Evaluate the child's fluid status frequently and carefully record hourly intake and output and routine weights. Monitor the child's urine volume and specific gravity. Urine output averages 1 mL/kg per hour if fluid intake is adequate. Provide maintenance fluids and titrate them to the child's fluid status. Nutrition can be provided orally or by enteral tube in the child who is not intubated, as tolerated. In the intubated child, enteral tube feedings are begun as soon as possible to support healing.

Some complications of pneumonia (especially staphylococcal pneumonia) are empyema, pleural effusion, pyopneumothorax, and tension pneumothorax. If pleural fluid accumulation is detected by auscultation and a chest radiograph, a thoracentesis can be performed and any fluid obtained is cultured. Continuous chest drainage may be necessary when purulent fluid is aspirated.

Aspiration Pneumonia

Etiology

Aspiration pneumonia is a group of disorders that have in common the contamination of the lower respiratory tract with foreign, nongaseous material. Aspiration events can be asymptomatic, mildly symptomatic, or acute and life-threatening. A variety of substances can be aspirated, including saliva, gastric contents, hydrocarbon, and other materials. Most but not all cases of aspiration pneumonia occur in patients with an impaired level of consciousness or impaired neuromuscular control of swallowing (Box 9-26).

Conditions that Increase Risk of Aspiration

- Altered level of consciousness
- Central nervous system injury or disease (e.g., meningitis, seizures, trauma, poisoning, toxic ingestion)
- Sedation
- General anesthesia
- Dysphagia
- Esophageal dysmotility, neurologic deficit, gastroesophageal reflux
- Mechanical disruption of defensive barriers
- Endotracheal tube, tracheostomy
- Persistent vomiting

Table 9-16 **Classification and Clinical Signs of Aspiration Pneumonia Syndromes**

Type	Aspirated material	Clinical presentation
Chemical pneumonitis	Acid Hydrocarbons	Acute dyspnea, wheezing, cyanosis, pulmonary edema
Reflex airway closure, mechanical obstruction	Inert fluids Oral secretions	Dyspnea, cough, hypoxemia, pulmonary edema
Infection	Oropharyngeal secretions	Cough, sputum changes, fever, infiltrates

Adapted from Bartlett JG: Aspiration pneumonia. *Clin Notes Respir Disease* 18:3, 1980.

Aspiration pneumonia can be classified according to the type of substance aspirated, known as the *inoculum*. The classification and clinical signs of the most common forms of aspiration pneumonias are listed in Table 9-16. Disease secondary to the aspiration of particulate matter is referred to as *foreign body aspiration* in this chapter (see section, Foreign Body Aspiration later in this chapter).

Chemical pneumonitis may result from the aspiration of gastric acid or hydrocarbons. Toxic manifestations of the aspiration of various forms of hydrocarbons are listed in Table 9-17.

Inert fluids that can be aspirated include saline, water, barium, and many nasogastric feeding solutions. They may fail to produce a chemical pneumonitis and do not harbor sufficient bacteria to produce infection. Aspiration of upper airway secretions is a common form of aspiration pneumonia. The oropharynx harbors a variety of flora normal for that portion of the airway, but which can cause infections in the lung. Massive aspiration events can produce direct injury to the mucosal surface of the respiratory tract, resulting in diffuse alveolar damage, hemorrhage, and necrotizing bronchiolitis. In severe forms, the clinical disease closely resembles ARDS, with similar outcomes.[179]

Pathophysiology

The severity of the lung injury is affected by the pH of the aspirated material and the presence of bacteria, and in the case of hydrocarbons, by the volatility and viscosity of aspirated material (see Table 9-16). Pulmonary hemorrhage, necrosis, surfactant impairment, and pulmonary edema may occur, resulting in abnormal compliance and $\dot{V}/\dot{Q}$ mismatching. Intubation and mechanical ventilation may be necessary.

Clinical Signs and Symptoms

Most patients develop respiratory symptoms within 2 hours of the aspiration event. Beyond that time, complications are unlikely unless vegetable matter was aspirated (see next paragraph).[116] Acid aspiration can produce immediate pulmonary symptoms that worsen over the first 24 hours. Coughing, vomiting, tachypnea, dyspnea, wheezing, and cyanosis may be noted as well as pulmonary edema and hemoptysis. Fever usually results from the necrotizing pneumonitis and does not necessarily indicate a superimposed bacterial infection.

Clinical signs of the aspiration of oral secretions may not be distinguishable from other forms of acute bacterial pneumonia. Aspirated vegetable matter (e.g., peanut, carrot, popcorn) may not produce symptoms for several weeks following aspiration. There may be an increase in cough or fever, and sputum will be foul smelling.

Chest radiograph changes may worsen over the first 72 hours following aspiration, and then begin to clear (Fig. 9-17). Abnormalities can persist for 4 to 6 weeks, lagging far behind clinical improvement. Marked perihilar densities are initially visible, followed by progression to consolidation. Air trapping with the possible formation of pneumatoceles and cysts may occur rarely. Infiltrates are most likely to be observed in the right upper lobe of the supine, intubated patient, but they may be present in any lobe. The presence of a normal chest radiograph, normal breath sounds, and lack of pulmonary symptoms does not rule out the possibility of aspiration pneumonia.

Management

Treatment of aspiration pneumonia is primarily supportive and includes frequent monitoring of respiratory status, management of bronchospasm, support of oxygen delivery, and PPV when needed. Airway clearance with oropharyngeal and tracheal suctioning is performed, as clinically indicated.[177] Children with aspiration pneumonia are at a high risk for developing air leaks, so they need close observations for signs and symptoms of pneumothorax, pneumomediastinum, and pneumopericardium. Treatment is similar to that described for ARDS in severe cases (see sections regarding ARDS and Nursing Care of the Child During Mechanical Ventilation earlier in this chapter).

If gastroesophageal reflux is suspected, elevate the head of the bed during and after every feeding. Studies in critically ill patients that have compared small bowel feeding tubes to gastric feeding tubes have failed to demonstrate superiority of one form of feeding over the other to prevent aspiration pneumonia related to gastroesophageal reflux.[66,104,153,256] When nasogastric feedings are administered with an infusion pump, the child must be monitored carefully, because an infusion pump will continue to infuse the feeding even when the child is vomiting. Residual volume is not a valid marker for risk of aspiration in critically ill patients.[151]

Table 9-17   **Clinical Features and Toxic Manifestations Following Aspiration of Common Hydrocarbons**

Classification	Examples	Toxic Manifestations
Aliphatic (low viscosity hydrocarbons)	Petroleum ether Gasoline Naphtha (lighter fluid, cleaning fluid, paint thinner) Kerosene (fuel, lighter fluid, paint thinner) Mineral seal oil (furniture polish)	Most commonly ingested, most likely to cause pulmonary toxicity Chemical pneumonitis CNS depression (caused by hypoxemia) Coma, respiratory arrest Gastrointestinal irritant Myocardial dysfunction
Aromatic	Benzene, toluene, xylene, naphthalene, aniline Nail polish removers Degreasing cleaners Lacquers	Chemical pneumonitis Cardiac arrhythmias Excitement, delirium, seizure, hypertonicity, hyperreflexia secondary to systemic absorption via lung, skin or gut
Halogenated	Carbon tetrachloride Tetrachloroethane Trichloromethane Polychlorinated biphenyls This group is most commonly used as solvents, antiseptics, propellants, refrigerants, and fumigants	Pulmonary and CNS toxicity less likely Hepatic and renal damage
Hydrocarbons combined with toxic additives		Toxicity dependent on additives
Hydrocarbons (high viscosity)	Lubricating oil Mineral oil Petroleum jelly Grease, tar	Much less likely to cause chemical pneumonitis; minimal absorption secondary to very high viscosity

CNS, Central nervous system.

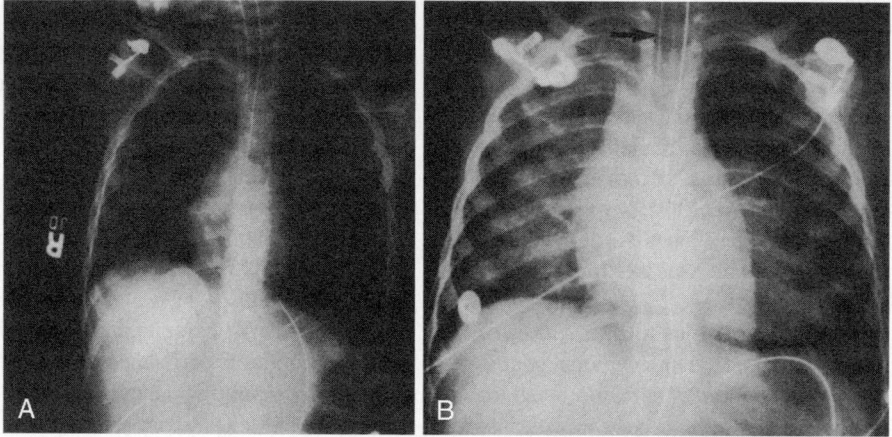

FIG. 9-17 Aspiration pneumonia. **A,** This child aspirated during intubation and so was supine during the aspiration episode. Bilateral infiltrates are present, particularly to the right lung and to the left upper lobe. **B,** This child ingested kerosene and then vomited and aspirated the hydrocarbon. Diffuse bilateral infiltrates are present, consistent with permeability pulmonary edema and early acute respiratory distress syndrome. The endotracheal tube is readily identifiable *(arrow).* (Chest radiographs courtesy Sharon Stein and Dennis Stokes, Vanderbilt University Medical Center, Nashville, TN.)

Initiation of empiric antimicrobial agents in noninfectious aspiration pneumonitis can increase antimicrobial resistance and treatment costs (see section, Other Complications of Mechanical Ventilation for more information on VAP earlier in chapter).[116] The successful use of exogenous surfactant in the treatment of neonates with respiratory distress syndrome and surfactant deficiency has led some clinicians to use exogenous surfactants in the treatment of aspiration pneumonia and other forms of ARDS associated with surfactant deficiency.

Foreign Body Aspiration
Etiology and Pathophysiology
Aspiration of a foreign body (i.e., foreign body aspiration [FBA]) can produce serious complications and may be fatal. The severity of the FBA is determined by the object aspirated and the location and the extent of the airway obstruction produced. Prompt recognition of the problem and effective removal may prevent death and potential complications. The greatest risk of FBA occurs in older infants and toddlers, because children in this age group often put objects in their

mouths. Items aspirated include inorganic objects such as plastic toys and earrings, as well as vegetable matter such as hot dogs, peanuts, seeds, and solid vegetables. Risk of death from FBA is highest in children between 2 months and 4 years of age,[248] likely because children in this age range have narrow airways and immature immunologic protective mechanisms.

Clinical Signs and Symptoms

The most reliable indication of FBA is witnessed aspiration (i.e., known event) with an associated choking episode.[248] Children are more likely to aspirate objects into the right main bronchus compared with the left main bronchus, because the right main bronchus branches less acutely from the trachea (i.e., the left main bronchus branches at a more acute angle from the trachea),[177] so aspirated fluid or an aspirated object will take the more direct path into the right main bronchus.

Laryngotracheal foreign bodies cause dyspnea, cough, and stridor. Tracheobronchial foreign bodies produce cough, decreased air entry, wheezing, and dyspnea. Cyanosis may develop in either group. Other less common findings are hoarseness, chest pain, and recurrent respiratory infection. Foreign body aspiration distally in the lung can cause asymmetric physical findings such as decreased breath sounds and wheezing. This will correlate with asymmetric abnormalities on a radiograph.

Late diagnosis can result in respiratory difficulties ranging from life-threatening airway obstruction to chronic wheezing and cough. The diagnosis of recurrent pneumonia may actually represent inflammation around the foreign body.[215] Misdiagnosis and mismanagement of FBA increases the duration of symptoms, rate of complications, and cost prior to correct diagnosis.[143] Complications from delayed diagnosis include granulation tissue formation surrounding the foreign body, persistent fever, reactive airways disease, or recurrent pneumonia. Diagnosis and removal become more challenging in these patients.[248] Initial diagnostic testing includes anteroposterior and lateral chest radiographs. Radiographic evaluation can confirm FBA but cannot rule it out.[117] Metallic objects will be visible on the chest radiograph; however, objects such as peanuts or plastics usually are not seen. Radiopaque FBA findings have been reported in approximately 20% of patients.[248]

When a single foreign body is lodged in a single bronchus, unilateral obstructive emphysema can be present on a chest radiograph and may be identified more readily if films are taken at both inspiration and expiration (Fig. 9-18), including

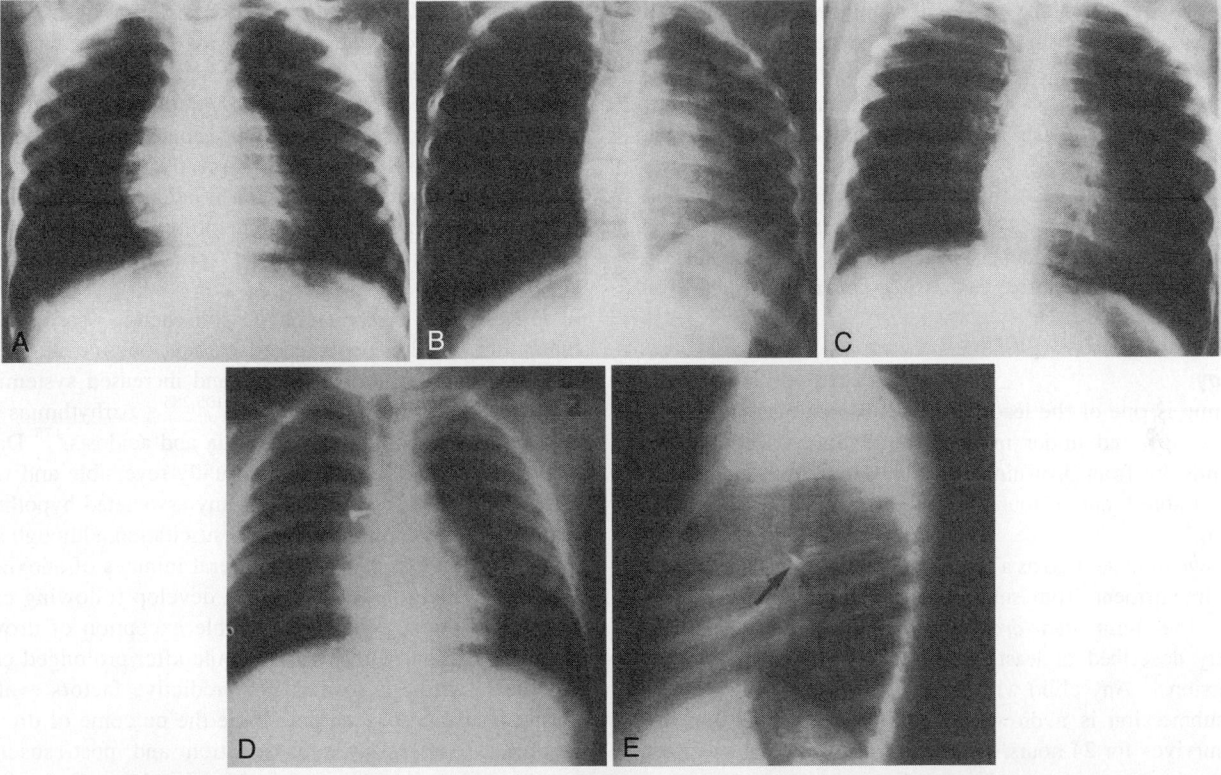

FIG. 9-18 Foreign body aspiration. The child in shown A, B, and C aspirated a peanut. The child shown D and E aspirated a small tack. **A,** Because the aspirated substance is not radiopaque, the diagnosis must be made on the basis of clinical examination and evidence of air trapping on radiographic examination. This posterior-anterior view is relatively normal in appearance. Hyperinflation is not obvious, so decubitus films were obtained. **B,** This left lateral decubitus film (obtained with the patient's left side down) demonstrates normal compression of the left lung in this position. The left diaphragm is elevated, and the mediastinum moves into the left chest. The left lung appears to be more vascular because it is compressed. **C,** This right lateral decubitus film is diagnostic of the right mainstem bronchus obstruction. Despite the fact that the right lung is in a dependent position, there is no evidence of right lung compression, and no mediastinal shift into the right chest. The right lung is hyperinflated, which is suggestive of bronchial obstruction. **D,** The tack was aspirated as this young boy attempted to use a homemade blow-gun. The radiopaque tack is visible in the right chest and appears to be in the right mainstem bronchus. **E,** The lateral view of the same patient as in D confirms the presence of the tack in the right bronchus. (Chest radiographs courtesy Sharon Stein and John Pietsch, Vanderbilt University Medical Center, Nashville, TN.)

anteroposterior and decubitus films. Paired inspiratory and expiratory films are often difficult to obtain in children who are unable to cooperate.[248] Chest fluoroscopy may be considered in patients with normal radiographs but a strong history consistent with FBA. Fluoroscopy often reveals air trapping and an inspiratory shift of the mediastinum to the side contralateral to the foreign body.[248]

Management

Children with FBA are at risk for developing acute airway obstruction. Goals of care include vigilant respiratory assessment, relief of respiratory distress, and general minimization of stimulation. Signs of clinical deterioration include changes in heart and respiratory rates; increased severity of retractions, pallor, or cyanosis; loss of ability to speak; and drooling. Emergency equipment for intubation must be readily accessible.

The most effective intervention for acute aspiration of a foreign body is immediate removal of the object. If FBA is strongly suspected, rigid bronchoscopy is preferable to enable removal of the foreign body. Aspirated vegetable material can break apart during removal and lodge distally. Repeat bronchoscopy may be necessary if symptoms persist. After the foreign body is removed, the child will continue to need frequent assessment. Chest physiotherapy may be helpful for several days, particularly if the object was lodged beyond the mainstem bronchus and signs of infection are present (see Chest Physiotherapy in the Chapter 9 Supplement on the Evolve Website).

Efforts to prevent FBA can target the parents of infants and toddlers. Parents need to be taught the dangers of FBA if young children eat uncooked beans, seeds, or nuts and are allowed to play with beads, buttons, or small toys.

Drowning and Submersion

Etiology

Drowning is one of the leading causes of death in children 4 years of age and under in the United States. Every year, thousands die from drowning and many more are left permanently disabled; one in four of drowning victims are typically children.[42]

Drowning is defined as a process resulting in primary respiratory impairment from submersion or immersion in a liquid.[107] The term *near-drowning* is no longer used, but formerly described at least temporary initial recovery from submersion.[33] Any child who arrives in the critical care unit after submersion is a drowning victim, whether or not the child survives for 24 hours.

Drownings are preventable tragedies, with many occurring in home swimming pools or bathtubs. Most children are under adult supervision at the time of the incident. Parents simply do not realize how quickly or silently children can drown in a bathtub or a pool; often the dangers posed by a home swimming pool are not appreciated.

The single most effective deterrent to unsupervised entrance into a pool area is the presence of a circumferential fence with a self-closing, self-latching gate. The fence must be sufficiently high, and the home cannot form one of the barriers to the pool, because it is easy for a small child to open a house door or window and gain entrance to the pool area. Nonrigid pool covers and warmers merely make the child more difficult to see after a submersion, and they are not effective barriers to the pool. Pool alarms provide a false sense of security and are often found floating next to the child in the pool, with the battery dead or the alarm dismantled.[131]

Pathophysiology

Submersion can occur in either fresh water or salt water, but the tonicity of the fluid aspirated is not usually clinically significant. The rate of survival after drowning is roughly 50%.[128]

Once the child's nose and mouth are below the level of the water, breath holding typically ensues; involuntary aspiration of fluid into the hypopharynx or laryngospasm can then result in hypoxemia, hypercarbia, and acidosis.[107,175] In some victims, laryngospasm (part of the diving reflex) occurs and there is no aspiration of fluid, but asphyxia still develops.[108] In most, however, laryngospasm eventually stops and fluid is aspirated. Vomiting and aspiration often occur, because children often swallow large amounts of water; aspiration of gastric contents causes additional pulmonary injury.

Aspiration of fluid can also occur during active gasping. With loss of consciousness, airway reflexes are abolished and fluid can be aspirated into the airways, leading to airway obstruction, alveolar collapse, and intrapulmonary shunting.[108] Hypercarbia and hypoxemia with combined metabolic and respiratory acidosis may develop quickly. Alveolar permeability, surfactant washout, and inactivation will contribute to atelectasis and intrapulmonary shunting. Other complications of drowning include secondary pneumonia, ARDS, and coagulopathies.

Hypoxemia produces hypoxic-ischemic cardiovascular injury that results in decreased cardiac output, elevated left and right heart filling pressures, and increased systemic and pulmonary vascular resistances[108,285] Arrhythmias may develop in response to hypothermia and acidosis.[175] Damage to the cardiovascular system is usually reversible and will be affected by the period of anoxia, any associated hypothermia, duration of arrest, and quality of resuscitation, although severe hypoxic insult can occur with several minutes of anoxia.

Hypoxic neurologic injury can develop following cardiopulmonary arrest. With the possible exception of drowning in icy water, the neurologic outcome after prolonged cardiopulmonary arrest is dismal. No predictive factors evaluated during resuscitation can determine the outcome of drowning victims, so aggressive resuscitation and postresuscitation care are generally indicated for the first hours following the submersion.[156] If skilled resuscitation is performed at the scene and during transport, and the normothermic child remains asystolic on arrival in the emergency department, neurologic recovery is extremely unlikely.[22,33] Additional poor prognostic indicators include absence of purposeful movement at 24 hours after admission.[156] The time of submersion as reported by bystanders is typically unreliable, and it is often impossible to determine the duration of cardiopulmonary arrest.

Hypothermia generally develops even after submersion in warm water, because the water temperature is usually lower than the child's body temperature and conductive heat loss is rapid and efficient in water. Different degrees of hypothermia produce different clinical consequences. With severe hypothermia (28 to 32° C body temperature), heart rate and blood pressure decrease and oxygen consumption diminishes.[108] Moderate hypothermia (32 to 35° C) results in shivering, increased oxygen consumption, and increased sympathetic tone. When children are profoundly hypothermic (<28° C), there is risk for severe bradycardia, ventricular fibrillation, or asystole.[108]

Although small children may tolerate submersion in extremely cold (icy) water, because rapid development of hypothermia quickly reduces O_2 consumption, submersion beyond a few minutes usually is associated with severe neurologic insult (see section, Clinical Signs and Symptoms). As noted previously, if a perfusing rhythm has not been restored in the normothermic child by the time of arrival in the emergency department, it is extremely unlikely that neurologic recovery will occur.[22,33]

When the child is admitted following drowning, although it may be difficult to do, it is important to try to obtain a good history of the event, including the estimated duration of submersion, the water temperature, the condition of the patient on recovery from the water, the presence of spontaneous respirations at the scene, and the duration and quality of any cardiopulmonary resuscitation attempted.

Clinical Signs and Symptoms

Within 3 minutes of submersion in warm water, most victims will develop sufficient hypoxia and cerebral ischemia to produce loss of consciousness. Most children submerged for several minutes are flaccid with no spontaneous breathing when they are pulled from the water. If the submersion episode is brief, and if skilled CPR is instituted promptly, the child may recover spontaneous respiration and demonstrate a perfusing heart rate and responsiveness at the scene.

If skilled resuscitation is performed at the scene of the submersion and during transport, a child who has suffered a mild anoxic insult will usually demonstrate spontaneous respiration and a perfusing heart rate on arrival at the hospital. Unfortunately there are no absolute predictors of outcome from submersion.[254] Although a variety of articles address this subject, none provide predictors with 100% accuracy. Variables such as Glasgow Coma Scale, fixed and dilated pupils, coma, and even a submersion score at presentation have been studied.[156] In a recent retrospective study, worse outcomes were noted in children who drowned in pools rather than other bodies of water, and better outcomes were noted in younger children.[128] Because outcome predictors have not been established, aggressive resuscitation is generally performed, particularly when the child is hypothermic.

The parents need an honest assessment of the child's clinical condition and possible outcomes so that they can participate in decisions for ongoing medical care for their child. It is extremely difficult to conduct such conversations in the emergency department. Prognostication for children who are submerged in icy water will need to be approached carefully, because outcomes in these children can vary widely.

If the child is breathing spontaneously, pulmonary congestion and airway obstruction can produce signs and symptoms of respiratory distress. The child may exhibit tachycardia, tachypnea, stridor, retractions, nasal flaring, use of accessory muscles of respiration, and excessive respiratory secretions. Auscultation may reveal pulmonary congestion and decreased lung aeration bilaterally. If the child's respiratory distress increases, crackles may be heard on auscultation.

In symptomatic patients, blood gas values are obtained immediately. Most commonly the child demonstrates moderate hypoxemia accompanied initially by hypocarbia. Hypercarbia with respiratory acidosis may be present if ventilation or perfusion abnormalities are severe, and metabolic acidosis will be present if hypoxemia is severe. Pulmonary edema, atelectasis, and chemical pneumonitis also may be present.

The child's level of consciousness may be altered, and there may be changes in pupil response to light. Pupil dilation may be noted, with a decrease or inequality in response to light. Decerebrate and decorticate posturing, seizure activity, and loss of reflexes including cough, gag, and corneal reflex (blink) may be present.

With severe central nervous system injury and cerebral edema, the syndrome of inappropriate antidiuretic hormone (SIADH) secretion or diabetes insipidus (DI) may develop later in the course. With SIADH secretion, free water is retained in excess of sodium, and sodium is lost in the urine; hyponatremia develops, and urine specific gravity increases. With DI, the child loses large amounts of highly diluted urine, hypernatremia develops, and urine specific gravity decreases (see the discussion of SIADH and DI in Chapter 12). If the fluid volume lost in the urine is not replaced in the child with DI, dehydration and hypovolemia can develop rapidly. Central DI is usually a signal of severe brain injury and brain death in these patients.[229]

The chest radiograph of a child after drowning may reveal infiltrates and diffuse pulmonary edema (Fig. 9-19). Fractured ribs or air leaks also may be seen as the result of resuscitative efforts.

Management

By the time the child arrives in the critical care unit, the child usually has received resuscitative efforts consistent with American Heart Association Pediatric Advanced Life Support Guidelines.[15,194] This effort includes treatment for cardiac arrest and respiratory failure, establishing vascular access, and initiating rewarming, if needed.[15,285?]

If the child demonstrates a perfusing cardiac rhythm on arrival in the pediatric critical care unit, the goal of therapy is to maintain O_2 delivery through the support of cardiovascular and pulmonary function. Typically the child in full cardiac arrest will be intubated at the scene or in the emergency department. If the child did not warrant intubation at the scene or in the emergency department, then airway and oxygenation must be assessed and intubation performed if significant

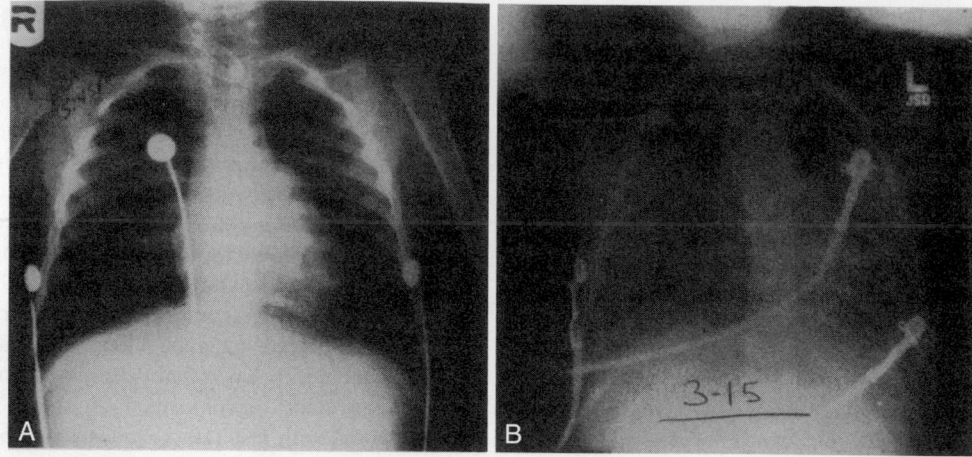

FIG. 9-19 Near-drowning in a toddler. **A,** This first radiograph was taken within hours of the submersion episode. Only some mild perihilar pulmonary edema is apparent, particularly in the right lung. **B,** Within several days, acute respiratory distress syndrome had evolved. The child developed permeability pulmonary edema, intrapulmonary shunting, and decreased lung compliance. Diffuse infiltrates are present bilaterally. (Chest radiographs courtesy of Gordon Bernard, Vanderbilt University Medical Center, Nashville, TN.)

respiratory distress, diminished level of consciousness, hypoxemia, or increased volume of secretions is present.

The most common pulmonary finding in near-drowning victims is bilateral pulmonary edema, likely caused by (1) acute myocardial depression secondary to increased left ventricular afterload, (2) hypoxia and ARDS, (3) interstitial fluid flux secondary to extreme negative pleural pressure generated by respiratory attempts with a closed glottis, and (4) so-called neurogenic pulmonary edema.

Sedation and neuromuscular blockade can be used to control mechanical ventilation, but these drugs preclude effective neurologic assessment and so are typically avoided if at all possible. As long as the child receives mechanical ventilation, the ventilator variables are checked at least every hour when vital signs are assessed (see section, Nursing Care of the Child During Mechanical Ventilation earlier in this chapter).

Analysis of arterial blood gases will help the healthcare team to assess the child's ventilation status and to evaluate response to therapy. In addition, it is important to monitor the patient's A-a O_2 difference or gradient, because this difference will quantitate the amount of intrapulmonary shunting present (see Respiratory Failure, Clinical Signs and Symptoms, earlier in this chapter).

Children with drowning may be hemodynamically unstable and need careful monitoring of systemic perfusion. Signs of poor cardiac output include tachycardia, decreased intensity of peripheral pulses, cool extremities, and decreased urine output, with the excretion of highly concentrated urine. In addition, capillary refill time will be prolonged (greater than 2 seconds). After drowning, a child may demonstrate cardiac arrhythmias, particularly if electrolyte imbalance is present.

Rewarming the patient with severe hypothermia is accomplished gradually and is considered for the child with moderate hypothermia. The primary goal is to rewarm the child by 0.5 to 2° C per h until the child's body temperature reaches 33-36° C, while avoiding hyperthermia.[156,285] Passive rewarming techniques include blankets, preventing further exposure to cold, and removing cold and wet clothing. Active

rewarming includes the use of warmed intravenous fluids and warm gastric lavage. Hot packs, heat lamps, and warming blankets must be used carefully, because their use can result in surface vasodilation leading to further cardiac compromise.[156] The most efficient way of rewarming a child with hypothermia and ongoing cardiac arrest or cardiovascular instability is cardiopulmonary bypass or extracorporeal life support.[156]

Fever contributes to adverse outcomes following cerebral ischemia, because it will increase the cerebral consumption of O_2. As a result, it is important to avoid excessive warming and to treat fever aggressively.

Studies of resuscitation in adults who remain comatose after primary cardiac arrest support induction of mild hypothermia to improve neurologic outcome.[19,106] It is unclear whether hypothermia has a protective effect on neurologic outcome in children after drowning, but it may be considered if the child is hemodynamically stable. Induced (therapeutic) hypothermia after cardiac arrest is the subject of a major study by the National Heart, Lung and Blood Institute (NHLBI).[16] For further information, refer to the NHLBI website (http://clinicaltrials.gov/ct2/show/NCT00880087?term=hypothermia+AND+children&rank=5) and Chapter 6.

For children with mild hypothermia and who are hemodynamically stable, no intervention regarding warming is necessary. Closely monitor these children for the negative effects of hypothermia, including cardiac instability, shivering, coagulopathies, infections, and acid-base imbalances.[19] Increased intracranial pressure following a submersion episode indicates the presence of severe neurologic insult. There is no evidence that treatment to control the increased intracranial pressure using standard therapies (hyperventilation, osmotic diuretics) will improve neurologic outcome.[156]

Excessive fluid administration in children after submersion may accentuate pulmonary edema. The child's fluid intake usually is limited to two thirds of calculated maintenance fluid requirements. A target goal for urine output averages 0.5-1 mL/kg per hour if fluid intake is adequate. An increase in urine specific gravity and a decrease in urine volume may indicate hypovolemia, poor systemic perfusion, or ischemia. The type and volume of intravenous solutions are adjusted based on the child's serum electrolyte concentration, hematocrit, and fluid balance.

The child is at risk for nutritional compromise as the result of prolonged intubation, stress, and bed rest. The healthcare team is responsible for ensuring adequate caloric intake, because it is necessary for lung and wound healing and prevention of infection.

If the child remains comatose, plans are needed to prevent skin breakdown. A specialty bed or, at a minimum, a pressure reduction mattress can be used to decrease the risk of skin breakdown over bony prominences. If the child is comatose or sedated, a physical therapy consultation may be indicated to devise splints and provide motion exercises to prevent contractures.

Finally, the child and family need psychological support. Because drowning is often preventable, the family may feel a great deal of guilt for the child's condition. Throughout the child's illness and recovery it is imperative that the healthcare team use consistent terms so that the family receives consistent information and a consistent prognosis.

Pulmonary Embolus

Pulmonary embolism (PE) occurs when there is mechanical obstruction of pulmonary arterial blood flow from either endogenous or exogenous emboli or local thrombus formation. When the obstruction is severe, PE is a life-threatening disorder.[193] Incidence of PE in the pediatric population has not been well established and depends on underlying conditions and methods of diagnosis. Incidence appears to have a bimodal distribution, with most occurrences taking place in neonates and adolescents. The incidence in African American children may be double that reported in Caucasian children.[193]

Etiology

A PE can arise from many conditions. Most commonly the child has an underlying deep vein thrombus that enters the blood stream and travels to the pulmonary vessels, occluding blood flow distal to the thrombus. PEs can also be caused by small emboli associated with right heart bacterial endocarditis, septic thrombophlebitis, pyomyositis, and osteomyelitis.[41,283] Risk factors for PE in children include obesity, deep vein thrombosis, central venous catheter-related thrombosis, endocarditis, sepsis, and underlying oncologic pathology.[180,193]

Pathophysiology

The obstruction to pulmonary blood flow causes ventilation and perfusion ($\dot{V}/\dot{Q}$) abnormalities. The duration and extent of the obstruction will determine the severity of signs and symptoms. In the acute phase, or the first 48 hours of this process, cardiac output is the main determinate in distribution of $\dot{V}/\dot{Q}$ abnormalities, rather than redistribution of pulmonary blood flow to nonoccluded areas or increasing or redistributing ventilation to areas maintaining perfusion.[257] When cardiac output is maintained or increased, there is increased perfusion to the nonoccluded regions of the lung, which improves blood flow in relation to ventilation. The resulting increase in blood flow to nonoccluded lung segments and reduced or absent blood flow to areas where vessels are occluded will result in less $\dot{V}/\dot{Q}$ mismatch and acute changes in pulmonary function.

If there is a decline in cardiac output, blood flow will decrease through the areas of low ventilation and the $\dot{V}/\dot{Q}$ ratio increases.[257] In addition, acute right ventricular failure and cardiovascular collapse may ensue.

Clinical Signs and Symptoms

The diagnosis of PE can be challenging because signs of PE can mimic other common childhood respiratory illnesses, such as pneumonia. There is a wide spectrum of severity and resulting clinical signs and symptoms, ranging from small segmental PE with no clinical symptoms to large central and/or bilateral clots associated with cardiovascular collapse. A high index of suspicion for PE needs to be entertained when children demonstrate chest pain or dyspnea on exertion.[193]

Optimal strategies for screening of children with PE have not been well established and are extrapolated from data in adults. The D-dimer test has been shown to be highly sensitive in adult patients with PE, but this test has not been shown to be as useful in pediatric patients. This may be explained by clearance of the D-dimer fragments by the liver when diagnosis is delayed. Alternatively, peripheral small pulmonary artery thrombi may not increase the D-dimer level.

Chest radiograph abnormalities may be noted in children with a PE, but these findings are not specific. Although pulmonary angiography has been described as the "gold standard" technique for diagnosing PE, it is infrequently performed. Lack of adequate venous access in children makes this test impractical in many pediatric cases. Spiral CT scan has emerged as an effective diagnostic tool.[159,193,280] This study is rapid, noninvasive, and can detect alternate diagnoses. The main limitation is in the accurate detection of small peripheral artery emboli. Other diagnostic methods include ventilation perfusion scintigraphy, spiral CT angiography, magnetic resonance imaging, and pulmonary angiography.[193]

Management

Thrombolytic therapy and anticoagulation are the major pharmacologic strategies in the treatment of PE.[34,233] Occasionally, anticoagulation is contraindicated because of hemorrhage or recent trauma, or because anticoagulation therapy may be ineffective. In these cases, inferior vena cava (IVC) filters may be considered.[34] IVC filters have been used in adult patients for many years to prevent PE, and their use has increased with percutaneously introduced retrievable filters.[192]

Potential indications for IVC filter placement include presence of a venous thromboembolism (VTE) and contraindication to anticoagulation, proven VTE and complication from anticoagulation, or recurrent VTE despite anticoagulation. Complications from long-term filter use include filter fracture, filter migration, IVC thrombosis, and IVC wall disruption.[192] Use of these devices in children has been limited, but may be increasing with increased identification of VTE in children. Placement and removal of percutaneously placed IVC filters is feasible in pediatric patients and can be performed by clinicians skilled in endovascular procedures.[192]

Thrombectomy, using either a surgical or catheter-based approach, can also be performed in some patients with PE to restore patency of the pulmonary vessel.[233] Long-term complications of pediatric PE are not known, although some patients demonstrate a risk of recurrence.

Congenital Diaphragmatic Hernia
Etiology
Diaphragmatic hernia is a congenital defect in the diaphragm that results in the posterolateral, anterior-midline, or crural diaphragm fusing with the chest wall, with communication between the chest and the abdominal cavity. Acquired diaphragmatic hernia can result from traumatic (typically blunt chest trauma) tearing of the diaphragm (see Chapter 19 for information about acquired or traumatic diaphragmatic hernia).

With congenital diaphragmatic hernia (CDH), there may be complete absence of the diaphragm muscle (agenesis). When this occurs, the abdominal organs are displaced into the chest cavity and interfere with parenchymal and pulmonary vascular development, producing hypoplasia of the lungs and pulmonary vasculature. This condition affects approximately 1 in every 2500 births and may be associated with other major or minor anomalies.[51] It can be diagnosed in utero, and severity can be assessed with ultrasonography or magnetic resonance imaging.[57] Intrauterine diagnosis allows time for both education of the family and staff preparation of the delivery. If untreated the defect is often fatal. Most neonates with diaphragmatic hernia develop severe respiratory insufficiency necessitating critical care support and surgical intervention during the first days of life.

Pathophysiology
The diaphragm is the most important muscle of inspiration. It is composed of a thin, dome-shaped muscle that is inserted in the lower ribs. During contraction of the diaphragm, the abdominal contents are displaced downward and forward, and as a consequence the vertical dimension of the chest cavity is increased.[272]

The diaphragm hernia is on the left side in approximately 80% of all cases.[129] The ipsilateral lung is small and hypoplastic, with decreased pulmonary vascularity and increased pulmonary vascular resistance. The mediastinal structures are shifted to the contralateral side of the chest in utero, and the heart most commonly is shifted into the right chest. The resulting increase in pulmonary vascular resistance produces right-to-left shunting of blood through the patent ductus arteriosus (see the discussion of Patent Ductus Arteriosus and Pulmonary Hypertension in Chapter 8). The contralateral lung is often partially compressed and is usually hypoplastic. Once the child is born, progression of respiratory dysfunction occurs because of both pulmonary hypoplasia and distension of the stomach and intestines with swallowed air.

When the diagnosis of diaphragmatic hernia is made, most patients develop severe hypoxemia and are placed on ECMO. After the patient stabilizes, and ideally when pulmonary hypertension improves, surgical intervention is scheduled (see section, Types of Mechanical Ventilation earlier in this chapter, and Chapter 7).

Clinical Signs and Symptoms
The child with diaphragmatic hernia has a large barrel chest and a suspiciously flat abdomen. Tachypnea, with a respiratory rate exceeding 120/minute, is seen commonly. Respiratory distress is usually noted immediately after birth, or there

may be a period of up to 48 hours before respiratory distress develops. Rarely, signs are delayed for days, weeks, or months. Signs of respiratory distress in addition to tachypnea are nasal flaring, severe chest retractions, cyanosis, absent breath sounds, and severe respiratory acidosis. Bowel sounds may be heard in the chest. The newborn may exhibit extreme respiratory distress when fed. Once the infant is intubated and the lungs are mechanically ventilated, resistance to hand ventilation is noted, and the neonate will need high inspiratory pressures because the lungs are small and stiff. Pulmonary hypertension is often severe.

The diagnosis of diaphragmatic hernia is made clinically and is confirmed with a chest radiograph, which shows air-filled loops of bowel located in the chest (Fig. 10-6). Rarely, further evaluation will be needed with a contrast radiographic study of the upper gastrointestinal tract to confirm the diagnosis. Blood gas analysis will demonstrate the presence of respiratory acidosis and hypoxemia.

An echocardiogram can be obtained to look for pulmonary hypertension, ventricular septal flattening, and right-to-left shunting via the ductus arteriosus. Doppler echocardiography can also be used to evaluate pulmonary vascular resistance.

Management
The optimal medical and surgical management for diaphragmatic hernia continues to evolve. Initial postnatal management includes support of O_2 and ventilation, placement of a nasogastric tube for gastric and bowel decompression, and maintenance of reliable vascular access.

Placing the infant in semi-Fowler's position uses gravity to alleviate pressure of the abdominal contents in the thorax. The involved side of the chest can be placed in a dependent position to increase aeration of the uninvolved lung, although oxygenation may actually improve if the uninvolved lung is placed in a dependent position. NIV is avoided in these patients because these methods may cause gaseous distension in the herniated viscera and worsening of cardiopulmonary status. Endotracheal intubation is typically performed as soon as the neonate becomes symptomatic.

Other medical management strategies include HFOV, inhaled nitric oxide, gentle permissive hypercapnia, and ECMO (see Chapter 7).[51] Ideally the infant is stabilized before surgical intervention. The ideal timing for surgical intervention is still in question. Most centers will wait at least 48 h after initial stabilization. Surgical strategies include primary repair using native tissue or in cases of large defects, repair with a Gore-Tex patch (DuPont). A higher recurrence rate exists with the use of a Gore-Tex patch compared with native tissue patches, because the Gore-Tex patch does not grow with the child. Surgical intervention may be accomplished in the neonatal critical care unit to avoid transport to the operating suite if the neonate is extremely unstable.[70]

Postoperatively, the infant is monitored closely for evidence of respiratory insufficiency, shock, pulmonary hypertension, and bleeding. Neonates with CDH have highly reactive pulmonary vascular beds, and pulmonary hypertension can produce hypoxemia, right ventricular failure, and low cardiac output. Inhaled nitric oxide can be administered during the pre-operative and postoperative periods to promote pulmonary vasodilation. Neonates with diaphragmatic hernia have small, noncompliant lungs that are especially at risk for pneumothorax and tension pneumothorax during the postoperative period.

The availability of ECMO and the utility of preoperative stabilization have improved survival in CDH. ECMO is most commonly used preoperatively (see Chapter 7). The duration of ECMO for neonates with CDH is significantly longer than for those with meconium aspiration or persistent pulmonary hypertension of the newborn.[132] Recurrence of pulmonary hypertension is associated with high mortality, and weaning from ECMO is performed cautiously. If the infant cannot be weaned from ECMO after repair of diaphragmatic hernia, options include discontinuing support or lung transplant in rare cases.[70]

Overall long-term survival for CDH is relatively high. Children with diaphragmatic hernia often have a long-term hospitalization after the initial surgery. The child must receive adequate nutrition (see section, Total Parenteral Alimentation in Chapter 14). Occasionally the child will need subsequent surgical intervention for the release of abdominal adhesions. Sequelae for these neonates include long-term pulmonary function changes, neurodevelopmental delays, and growth retardation. Other common problems are gastroesophageal reflux, pectus excavatum, and scoliosis.[70]

COMMON DIAGNOSTIC TESTS

There are many pulmonary function tests that are clinically useful. Most, however, are impractical for use in the critical care setting because they require maximum effort from cooperative patients. This section focuses only on those tests performed on critically ill children.

Physical Examination

The most important diagnostic tool for assessing respiratory function is the physical examination. A great deal of information can be gained by watching the child's behavior and breathing and noting the child's position of comfort. Carefully observe respiratory rate, effort, work of breathing, and use of accessory muscles of respiration. One must know the normal physical findings for the child's age and typical physical signs of the patient's disease.

Chest Radiograph

The chest radiograph is used frequently to evaluate pulmonary status in critically ill children. See Chapter 10 for a detailed discussion of the radiologic examination.

Bronchoscopy

Bronchoscopy allows direct visualization of the larynx and larger airways using either rigid or flexible instruments. Rigid bronchoscopy is usually performed in the operating room under general anesthesia, whereas flexible bronchoscopy can be performed at the bedside, introduced through the nose, mouth, or artificial airway. These bronchoscopes are small in size (ultrathin flexible scopes are available in diameters as small as 2.5 mm) and do not occlude a small child's airway.

Bronchoscopes have some or all of the following capabilities: fiberoptics for airway visualization and inspection, ventilation ports, suction, and the ability to retrieve objects and collect specimens. Rigid bronchoscopy offers a larger channel and is the preferred method of retrieving foreign bodies. Either a rigid or flexible bronchoscope may be used to evaluate chronically intubated patients for the presence of subglottic stenosis. The bronchoscope can be introduced through a special T adaptor at the end of the tracheostomy or ETT for children with an advanced airway; this allows ongoing mechanical ventilation throughout the procedure.

Complications of bronchoscopy are rare, but they include laryngospasm, hypoxemia, cardiac arrhythmias, laryngeal edema, bronchial tears, pneumothorax, epistaxis, and pulmonary hemorrhage. Monitor the patient to ensure a return to baseline after the procedure. In children with severe pulmonary disease, it may take several hours for the child to return to baseline. (i.e., they may need more mechanical ventilator support and may have higher O_2 requirements).

Noninvasive Monitoring

Pulse Oximetry

The saturation of hemoglobin in arterial blood can be monitored continuously using a pulse oximeter. The pulse oximeter has rapidly become the monitor of choice for the noninvasive monitoring of oxygenation. It continuously monitors and displays the arterial oxyhemoglobin saturation and can quickly indicate hypoxemic events. It is a good indicator of systemic perfusion. For more information on pulse oximetry, please see Respiratory Failure, Management, earlier in this chapter.

Transcutaneous Blood Gas Monitors

The most reliable method for assessing partial pressure of O_2 and CO_2 in the body is analysis of an arterial blood sample. The skin surface Po_2 and PCO_2 monitor is a noninvasive tool that can be used to quantify estimated O_2 and CO_2 tensions either intermittently or continuously.

The use of pulse oximetry has largely replaced skin surface O_2 monitoring, but the skin surface CO_2 monitor is still the most reliable method of noninvasive estimation of $PaCO_2$, (measurement of $P_{ET}CO_2$ reflects alveolar CO_2 tension and can trend with the $PaCO_2$). Transcutaneous devices are modifications of conventional blood gas electrodes, and they have been shown to provide a more accurate estimate of $PaCO_2$ than the $P_{ET}CO_2$ in some patient populations, including children with both cyanotic and acyanotic congenital heart disease.[39,246,277]

Skin surface PCO_2 measurement has also been shown to be an accurate and clinically acceptable estimate of $PaCO_2$ over a wide range of $PaCO_2$ values in pediatric patients during high-frequency oscillatory ventilation and for children undergoing polysomnography.[17,121] This technique is effective because small amounts of O_2 and CO_2 diffuse through the skin. The device warms the skin beneath the electrode membrane to a temperature of 44 to 45° C. Lower temperatures occasionally are used in premature infants to decrease skin injury. Warming the capillaries located beneath the electrode dilates them, and arteriovenous connections within the capillary bed open so that the O_2 and CO_2 tensions of the heated blood beneath the membrane reach arterial levels. In general, the skin surface PO_2 is less than the PaO_2, particularly in older patients.

The minimal requirements for a reliable skin surface O_2 and CO_2 sensor system are the following: (1) measurement of specific gases, with no interference from other gases; (2) uniform heat transfer across the sensing area; (3) drift of less than ±5 mm Hg for 24 h; (4) a machine with mechanical and electrical integrity; and (5) the ability to eliminate discrepancies between the transcutaneous and arterial PO_2 and PCO_2 resulting from hypoperfusion or other factors. The skin electrodes must be applied to skin that is clean, dry, and hairless. Because the electrode causes the surface of the skin to warm, there is a risk for skin irritation or burning. The location of the transcutaneous probe must be rotated intermittently to prevent these effects. These units must be calibrated at intervals specified by the manufacturer.

End-Tidal Carbon Dioxide Monitoring

Measurement of exhaled CO_2 provides real-time evidence of ventilation. The PCO_2 at the end of expiration is approximately equal to the alveolar PCO_2. In patients with normal lungs and pulmonary blood flow, the alveolar PCO_2 is the same as the pulmonary venous and $PaCO_2$. As a result, measurement of $P_{ET}CO_2$ can be used in place of repeated $PaCO_2$ measurements when the child's condition is stable.

Devices are available for end-tidal CO_2 monitoring with the natural airway or with an advanced airway. The amount of CO_2 in the exhaled air is measured using mass spectrometry or infrared absorption. For patients with an advanced airway and on mechanical ventilation, this small device is placed in the ventilator circuit at the proximal airway. If the child does not have an advanced airway or is not on mechanical ventilation, the

sampling catheter can be placed just inside the nostril or at the tracheostomy stoma. As exhaled gas passes through the device, a detector measures the light absorption in the sample. The partial pressure of CO_2 is inversely proportional to the amount of light that is absorbed. Using this information, the device is able to quantify the amount of CO_2 present in exhaled gas.

While it is relatively simple to measure PCO_2, it is extremely difficult to obtain a true alveolar gas sample that is not contaminated by dead space gas or ambient air. If measurement of $P_{ET}CO_2$ is to be used to reflect the $PaCO_2$, simultaneous samples are obtained for measurement of the $PaCO_2$ and the $P_{ET}CO_2$ to assess the relationship between these two measurements. Although many devices can measure the peak PCO_2 in exhaled air (Fig. 9-20) or the end-tidal CO_2, the result may or may not be representative of the alveolar (and arterial) PCO_2. If the patient has severe lung disease, the $P_{ET}CO_2$ does not plateau but varies widely during expiration. As a result, it is difficult to determine which measurement to use.

In general, changes in the $P_{ET}CO_2$ accurately reflect trends in the child's $PaCO_2$, even if a significant lung disease is present. A sudden decrease in the $P_{ET}CO_2$ to zero could indicate extubation, ETT obstruction, esophageal malposition, or a disruption or leak in the system (Fig. 9-21).[21] If cardiac output or lung perfusion falls drastically, the $P_{ET}CO_2$ will fall. A rise in $P_{ET}CO_2$ may be observed with hypoventilation, sepsis, or malignant hyperthermia.[21] Airway obstruction can alter the shape of the expired CO_2 curve and produce a rise in the $P_{ET}CO_2$. This shape is usually demonstrated with an upsloped capnography tracing.[244]

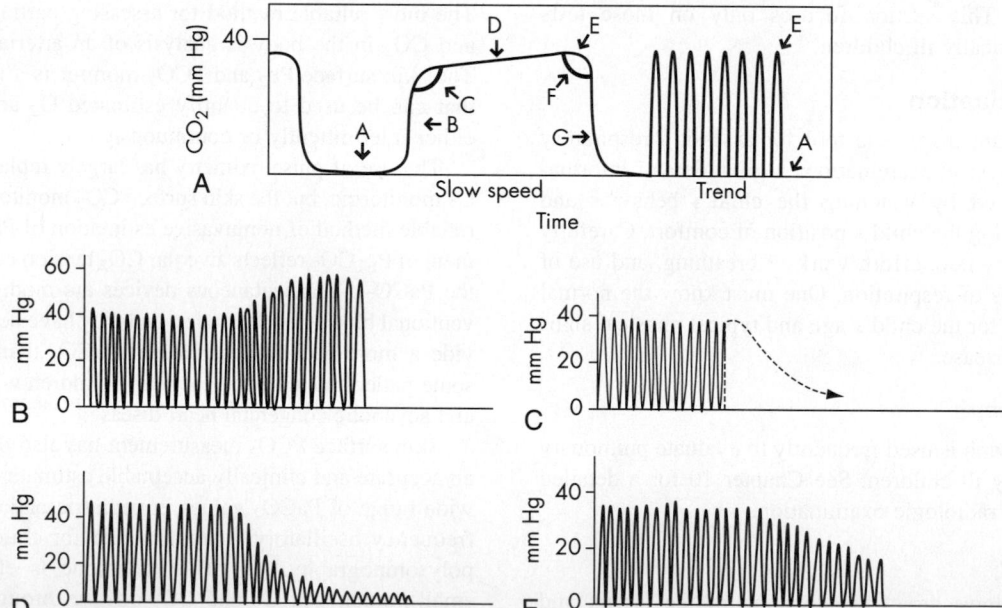

FIG. 9-20 A, Normal features of a capnogram. *A,* Baseline, represents the beginning of expiration and should start at zero. *B,* The transitional part of the curve represents mixing of dead space and alveolar gas. *C,* The alpha angle represents the change to alveolar gas. *D,* The alveolar part of the curve represents the plateau average alveolar gas concentration. *E,* The end-tidal CO_2 value. *F,* The beta angle represents the change to the inspiratory part of the cycle. *G,* The inspiration part of the curve shows a rapid decrease in CO_2 concentration. **B,** Increase in $P_{ET}CO_2$ is consistent with hypoventilation. Diagnosis is confirmed by demonstrating increased $PaCO_2$. **C,** Reduction in $P_{ET}CO_2$ from 40 to 0 mm Hg is consistent with situations in which no alveolar ventilation is occurring (apnea), or the endotracheal tube is malfunctioning of improperly placed. **D,** $P_{ET}CO_2$ tracing demonstrates progressive reduction as cardiac arrest occurs, resulting in decreased pulmonary perfusion. **E,** $P_{ET}CO_2$ tracing is consistent with compromised pulmonary perfusion by hypovolemia, increased pulmonary vascular resistance, or administration of excessive positive end-expiratory pressure. (Adapted from Thompson J and Jaffe M: Capnographic waveforms in the mechanically ventilated patient. *Respir Care* 50:100-109, 2005.)

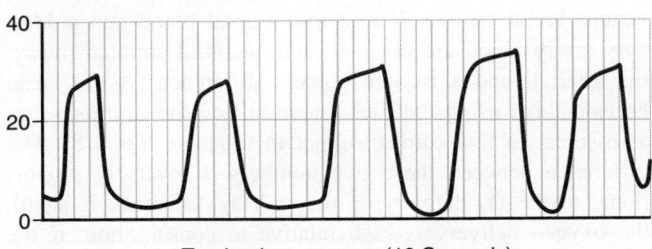

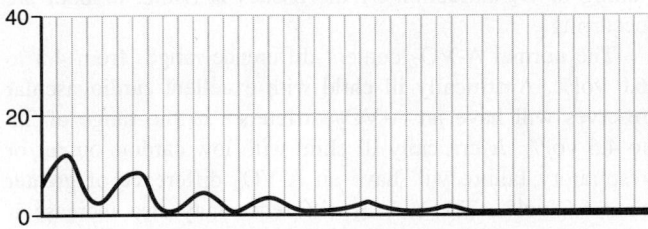

FIG. 9-21 End-tidal CO_2 graphic tracing (capnogram) with tracheal versus esophageal intubation. (From Roberts WA, Maniscalco WM, Cohen AR, Litman RS, and Chhibber A: The use of capnography for recognition of esophageal intubation in the neonatal intensive care unit. *Pediatr Pulmonol* 19:262-268, 1995.)

An increase in the $PaCO_2$-to-$P_{ET}CO_2$ gradient indicates an increase in dead space ventilation ($V_D/V_T = PaCO_2 - P_{ET}CO_2/PaCO_2$). That is, changes in $P_{ET}CO_2$ must be compared with $PaCO_2$. Any time the $PaCO_2$-to-$P_{ET}CO_2$ gradient increases, dead space ventilation has increased. Increased V_D/V_T (dead space ventilation) occurs any time pulmonary perfusion decreases relative to alveolar ventilation. Conditions causing increased dead space ventilation include: (1) pulmonary vascular disease or increased pulmonary vascular resistance, (2) PE, (3) decreased right ventricular output (hypovolemia or arrest), and (4) excessive PEEP.

A more novel use of noninvasive $P_{ET}CO_2$ monitoring is in the child with diabetic ketoacidosis. This monitoring has been shown to reliably reflect acidosis, offering an early warning sign for unexpected changes in acidosis.[5]

Assessment of Arterial Blood Gases
Blood Sampling for Blood Gas Analysis

The adequacy of gas exchange is best evaluated by measuring the pH, PO_2, and PCO_2 of arterial blood. It is also possible to assess arterialized capillary samples, but the analysis of PaO_2 by this method may be unreliable, because it is influenced greatly by the perfusion of the sampled capillary bed.

Arterial Blood Gas Analysis. The vessels most frequently used for blood gas analysis are the umbilical artery in neonates and the radial, femoral, and dorsalis pedis arteries in infants and children. The radial artery is the preferred site for arterial blood sampling, because it is easily accessible and has good collateral circulation.[123] Because an arterial puncture can produce pain and cause anxiety, the blood gas measurements obtained by intermittent sampling in this manner can be unreliable. As a result, arterial catheters usually are placed in children with severe cardiorespiratory disease who need close observation, frequent arterial sampling, or continuous evaluation of blood pressure (see Chapter 21).

An arterial blood sample can be collected in a heparinized syringe. If the blood gas specimen is obtained by arterial puncture, a small-gauge needle or a butterfly needle can be used for the puncture. As little as 0.2 mL of blood can be used to obtain an accurate blood gas analysis. A local anesthetic, intradermal or topical, can be administered immediately over the artery to minimize the child's discomfort during the arterial puncture, although only small volumes of intradermal lidocaine are administered because large volumes can produce arterial spasm. The puncture site is scrubbed with a chlorhexidine, povidone-iodine, or alcohol solution. Before a radial artery puncture is made, an Allen test is performed to assess the adequacy of collateral (nonradial artery) flow to the hand (Box 9-27).

Capillary Sampling for Blood Gas Analysis. Because arterial punctures are sometimes difficult to obtain in infants, capillary samples often are taken. Although an accurate PCO_2 and pH can be obtained with a capillary sample, the PO_2 usually will be lower than the child's PaO_2. If shock or other causes of poor systemic perfusion are present (e.g., hypothermia), the capillary PO_2 probably will not accurately reflect the PaO_2.

The best area for the capillary stick is one that is highly vascularized. The infant's heel, earlobe, or a large finger or toe is typically used. The area must be prewarmed with a warm towel, a heat lamp, or a warm, moist pack for 5 to 10 minutes before the sample is obtained; this will encourage blood flow to the area, thus arterializing the capillary blood. Be careful to avoid applying too much heat that can burn delicate skin. Cleanse the foot with alcohol. A puncture wound is made with a lancet so that blood flows freely from the puncture site. Avoid squeezing the sample area, because squeezing will encourage venous blood to mix with the capillary blood. Figure 9-22 illustrates the circulation of the infant's heel. The best blood gas specimens are obtained from the medial

---

Box 9-27 **Modified Allen Test to Document Adequate Ulnar Arterial Flow to Hand**

1. Elevate the patient's arm and hand well above level of the heart.
2. Clench the patient's fist or open and close the hand (this may be performed actively by the patient or passively by an examiner).
3. Place the thumb of one hand over the ulnar artery and the thumb of the other hand over the radial artery and compress both arteries to occlude flow until the hand becomes pale.
4. Release pressure only on the ulnar side of the wrist.

   The entire hand should regain color in less than 5 s if flow through ulnar artery is sufficient to perfuse the hand; this is a negative result. If reperfusion requires more than 5-10 s, flow through the ulnar artery is sluggish, and hand perfusion probably depends on some flow through the radial artery; this is a positive result. Placing an arterial catheter in the radial artery of a patient with radial artery-dependent hand perfusion can seriously compromise arterial blood flow to the hand.

From Briening E: Arterial catheter insertion: perform. In Verger JT and Lebet RM, editors: *AACN procedure manual for pediatric acute and critical care,* St Louis, 2008, Saunders-Elsevier.

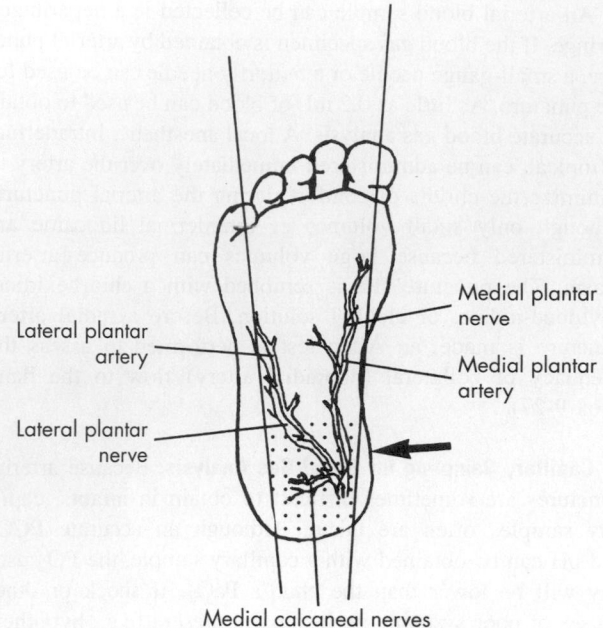

Lateral plantar artery

Medial plantar nerve

Medial plantar artery

Lateral plantar nerve

Medial calcaneal nerves

FIG. 9-22 Vascular anatomy of the infant foot. Heel-stick blood samples for blood gas analysis are best obtained from the medial aspect of the heel *(arrow)*, because this area is highly vascular. To avoid direct injury to the calcaneus or the medial calcaneal nerves, the bottom of the heel should be avoided *(dotted area)*. This area can be identified by drawing imaginary vertical lines along the length of the infant's foot, from the middle of the first and fifth toes. The area of the heel between these two lines must be avoided.

or lateral portion of the heel, because this area is more highly vascular and avoids the calcaneus. Do not obtain heel-stick capillary blood specimens after the infant has begun walking, because calluses have formed on the heel, making the puncture more difficult. In addition, the child may develop an infection once the foot is again used for walking.

Use a heparinized 0.2-mL capillary tube to obtain the specimen. Remove the first drop of blood with gauze and collect the following drop. Try to insert the tip of the tube into the droplet of blood to avoid surface blood, which will begin to equilibrate with air. Once the free-flowing blood has been collected in the tube, seal the tube and placed it on ice. Last, clean the site and apply a dry dressing. Although complications from repeated capillary sticks are rare, infection can occur if the area is not cleaned properly before the puncture. Osteomyelitis has been reported in neonates after only one or two heel punctures.

Venous Samples. Venous blood can be used for blood gas analysis, but interpretation of the PO_2 and PCO_2 is difficult. Venous CO_2 tension (P_VCO_2) is 4 to 6 mm Hg higher than systemic $PaCO_2$, and venous pH is 0.05 lower than arterial pH. Mixed venous saturation ($S\bar{v}O_2$) is a reflection of O_2 delivery. This mixed venous O_2 saturation reflects the balance between O_2 delivery and O_2 utilization. The superior vena caval O_2 saturation ($S_{cv}O_2$) is often used as a surrogate for the mixed venous O_2 saturation (see Chapter 6).

Pulmonary Artery Samples. Pulmonary artery blood obtained through a pulmonary artery catheter provides a true mixed

venous blood sample. If systemic arterial blood and pulmonary artery blood are obtained and analyzed simultaneously, the arterial-venous oxygen content difference (A-VO_2) can be calculated using the Fick equation (see the discussion on assessment of low cardiac output in Chapters 6 and 8). The difference between these two numbers is inversely proportional to the O_2 delivery: if the A-VO_2 difference is small, the oxygen delivery is high relative to consumption; if the A-VO_2 difference is large or increasing, either O_2 delivery is falling or O_2 extraction by the tissues is rising, or both are occurring.

The normal A-VO_2 content difference ranges from 4.5 to 6.0 vol%. A critically ill child with excellent cardiovascular reserves will have an A-VO_2 difference in the range of 2.5 to 4.5 vol%. A critically ill child with low cardiac output or respiratory failure will have an A-VO_2 difference of greater than 6.0 vol%. The A-VO_2 difference may also increase if O_2 consumption is increased in the face of fixed O_2 delivery.

Continuous monitoring of $S\bar{v}O_2$ is possible using a pulmonary artery catheter with fiberoptic light and sensor, but pulmonary artery catheters are rarely used in children. Generally venous O_2 saturation samples are obtained from a central venous catheter, typically from the SVC. Pediatric fiberoptic catheters allow for continuous monitoring of central venous saturation and can facilitate rapid detection of a fall in $S_{cv}O_2$, which can be associated with a compromise in O_2 delivery (i.e., either pulmonary function or cardiac output) or an increase in oxygen consumption.

Lung Volumes and Capacities

Simple measurements of lung volumes and capacities can be performed at the bedside to provide an objective estimate of the child's respiratory status (see section, Essential Anatomy and Physiology at the beginning of this chapter).

Tidal Volume

The measurement of tidal volume is an easy procedure and can be performed at the bedside. This measurement, together with assessment of respiratory rate on a serial basis, can provide an indication of inspiratory effort and tidal volume. To measure tidal volume at the bedside, a handheld spirometer may be used. A mouthpiece is applied to the spirometer, and the child is asked to breathe normally through the mouthpiece. A needle indicator then instantly records the inspiratory tidal volume. The child must breathe for 1 min. To obtain the average inspiratory tidal volume, the total volume recorded is divided by the respiratory rate.

If the child is intubated, the spirometer can be attached easily to the ETT or to the ventilator tubing. A normal predicted tidal volume is 6 to 7 cc/kg. A tidal volume of less than 4 to 5 cc/kg may indicate an inadequate inspiratory effort to sustain spontaneous ventilation, or it may indicate the presence of upper airway obstruction or decreased lung compliance. Measuring a normal tidal volume does not exclude the presence of severe restrictive lung disease. As a result, this test is not clinically useful as a predictor of severity of pulmonary symptoms.

Several devices are available for spirometry measurement; one of the most widely used is the Wright respirometer. Many mechanical ventilators automatically calculate and display delivered and expired (exhaled) tidal volume; however, such calculations will be inaccurate if a significant leak occurs around the ETT.

If the child refuses to cooperate, assessing the tidal volume may be difficult or impossible. Because these bedside tests require a great deal of patient effort, even when they are performed accurately, the results can be highly misleading.

Vital Capacity

VC testing can be used to evaluate readiness for extubation. The VC is the maximal amount of air that can be exhaled after a maximal inspiratory effort. A spirometer is attached to the ETT to quantify the volume, and the child is instructed to take the deepest inspiration possible and then to exhale the air as quickly, forcefully, and completely as possible. This forced expiratory volume measurement is best evaluated in a cooperative patient who is either not sedated or lightly sedated. Normal VC is approximately 65 to 75 cc/kg for infants and young children. Children with significant respiratory disease usually have a VC of approximately 15 to 30 cc/kg, and children with a VC of less than 15 cc/kg often need assisted ventilation. Older children are generally ready for extubation with a VC greater than about 15 cc/kg.[172]

A true decrease in VC is caused by restrictive lung disease processes such as pneumonia, atelectasis, or pulmonary fibrosis. A decrease in VC may also be noted in the absence of lung disease with conditions such as muscle weakness, abdominal distension, or surgical pain.[83] Lower than expected measured VC can result from inadequate effort or from loss of exhaled air as a result of a loose seal around the airway or the patient's mask, so the child's VC is underestimated.

Negative Inspiratory Force

Respiratory muscle strength is evaluated by measuring the maximal positive pressure created by forcefully exhaling after a full inspiration and the maximal negative pressure that can be generated by inhaling after maximal expiration. Clinically this is performed by preventing inspiration by either occluding the inspiratory port of a mask or occluding the inspiratory tubing of the ventilator. The maximal negative pressure generated is measured with a manometer. This information is useful in patients with neuromuscular disease or in patients who are being evaluated for extubation.

Normal inspiratory force is a negative pressure of approximately -60 cm H_2O. Values less forceful than -40 cm H_2O are considered abnormal.[99] The child usually needs assisted ventilation if the negative inspiratory force is less forceful than -20 cm H_2O. Because this measurement also requires patient cooperation, it is subject to error.

Static and Dynamic Lung Compliance

Compliance is how much a compartment will expand if the pressure in the compartment is altered. For example, a partially inflated balloon has high compliance because small pressure increases in the balloon result in the balloon expanding greatly. A rigid cylinder has low compliance because a pressure increase in the cylinder will not result in a significant increase in volume in the cylinder. In humans, tissue elastic forces and surface tension forces contribute to lung compliance.

$$C_L = \Delta V / \Delta P$$

Elastance is the reciprocal of compliance; high elastance is seen in stiff lungs.

$$E_L = \Delta P / \Delta V$$

Static lung compliance is the slope of the pressure-volume curve of the lung that is obtained during deflation from total lung capacity. To obtain a static lung compliance estimate in an intubated child, an inspiratory hold maneuver is performed. At peak inspiration, an inspiratory hold is performed for 1 to 2 seconds. Once the flow is held, a plateau pressure will occur as long as the lungs fall back to resting position at peak inspiration. The plateau pressure reading is used to obtain the patient's static lung compliance. The pressure measured at that volume is recorded and then the tidal volume is divided by the measured pressure. The result reflects the static lung compliance.

Dynamic lung compliance is the ratio of change in the volume compared with the change in pressure over a tidal breath; it represents the ratio of change in volume to a change in pressure between the points of zero flow at the end of inspiration and expiration. In healthy children, the values for static and dynamic compliance are similar. Measurement of dynamic lung compliance can be useful in detecting pneumothorax when the patient's lungs are ventilated with a volume-cycled ventilator. In these patients, higher-than-normal pressures are needed to deliver the desired tidal volume, because the lung compliance is decreased.[89]

Conclusion

All of these diagnostic tests may be clinically useful, but physical examination and arterial blood gas analysis provide the most rapid, complete, and objective estimate of pulmonary function.

References

1. Abd-Allah SA, et al: Helium-oxygen therapy for pediatric acute severe asthma requiring mechanical ventilation. *Pediatr Crit Care Med* 4:353–357, 2003.
2. Aboab J, et al: Effect of inspired oxygen on alveolar decruitment in acute respiratory distress syndrome. *Intensive Care Med* 32:1979–1986, 2006.
3. Acosta B, et al: Hemodynamic effects of noninvasive bilevel positive airway pressure on patients with chronic congestive heart failure with systolic dysfunction. *Chest* 118:1004, 2000.
4. Acute Respiratory Distress Network: Ventilation with lower tidal volumes as compared with conventional tidal volumes for acute lung injury and the acute respiratory distress syndrome. *N Engl J Med* 342:1301–1308, 2000.
5. Agus MS, Alexander JL, Mantell PA: Continuous noninvasive end-tidal CO_2 monitoring in pediatric in patients with diabetes ketoacidosis. *Pediatr Diabetes* 7:196–200, 2006.
6. Al-Sundi S: Acute upper airway obstruction: croup, epiglottitis, bacterial tracheitis, and retropharyngeal abrasions. In Levin DL, Morriss FC, editors: *Essentials of pediatric intensive care*, New York, 1997, Churchill Livingstone.
7. Amato MB, et al: Effect of a protective-ventilation strategy on mortality in the acute respiratory distress syndrome. *N Engl J Med* 338:347, 1998.
8. American Academy of Pediatrics Committee on Fetus and Newborn: Postnatal steroids to treat or prevent chronic lung disease in preterm infant. *Pediatrics* 109:330, 2002.

9. Anas N: Respiratory failure. In Levin DL, Morriss FC, editors: *Essentials of pediatric intensive care*, New York, 1997, Churchill Livingstone.

10. Arnold JH, et al: Prospective, randomized comparison of high-frequency oscillatory ventilation and conventional mechanical ventilation in pediatric respiratory failure. *Crit Care Med* 22:1530–1539, 1994.

11. Ashbaugh DG, et al: Acute respiratory distress in adults. *Lancet* 12:7511, 1967.

12. Bancalari E: Mechanical ventilation. In Rudolph CD, Rudolph AM, editors: *Rudolph's pediatrics*, New York, 2003, McGraw Hill.

13. Baraldi E, Filippone M: Chronic lung disease after premature birth. *N Engl J Med* 357:1946–1955, 2007.

14. Bartlett JG: Aspiration pneumonia. *Clin Notes Respir Disease* 18:3, 1980.

15. Berg MD, Schexnayder SM, Chameides L, et al: Pediatric basic life support. 2010 American heart association guidelines for cardiopulmonary resuscitation and emergency cardiovascular care. *Circulation* 122(18 Suppl. 3):S862-875, 2010.

16. Berg MD: Pediatric in-hospital cardiac arrest and therapeutic hypothermia: where we are and where we are going. *Pediatr Crit Care Med* 10:601–602, 2009.

17. Berkenbosch JW, Tobias J: Transcutaneous carbon dioxide monitoring during high frequency oscillatory ventilation in infants and children. *Crit Care Med* 30:1024–1027, 2002.

18. Bernard GR, et al: The American-European consensus conference on ARDS definitions, mechanisms, relevant outcomes and clinical trial coordination. *Am J Respir Crit Care Med* 149:818, 1994.

19. Bernard SA, et al: Treatment of comatose survivors of out-of-hospital cardiac arrest with induced hypothermia. *N Engl J Med* 346:557, 2002.

20. Bernet VB, et al: Predictive factors for the success of noninvasive mask ventilation in infants and children with acute respiratory failure. *Pediatr Crit Care Med* 6:660, 2005.

21. Bhende MS: End-tidal carbon dioxide monitoring in pediatrics—clinical applications. *J Postgraduate Med* 47:215–218, 2001.

22. Biagas K: Drowning and near drowning: submersion injuries. In Nichols DG, editor: *Rogers' textbook of pediatric intensive care*, ed 4, Philadelphia, 2008, Lippincott Williams and Wilkins.

23. Bindslev L, Hedenstierna G, Santesson J, et al: Ventilation-perfusion distribution during inhalation anaesthesia. Effects of spontaneous breathing, mechanical ventilation and positive end-expiratory pressure. *Acta Anaesthesiol Scand* 25(4):360–371, 1981.

24. Bjornson CL, Johnson DW: Croup. *Lancet* 371:329, 2008.

25. Bledsoe GH, Schexnayder SM: Pediatric rapid sequence intubation. *Pediatr Emerg Care* 20:339, 2004.

26. Boogaard R, et al: Recombinant human deoxyribonuclease for the treatment of acute asthma in children. *Thorax* 63:141–146, 2008.

27. Boyce JAK: Auto positive end-expiratory pressure calculation. In Verger JT, Lebet RM, editors: *AACN procedure manual for pediatric acute and critical care*, St Louis, 2008, Saunders.

28. Branson RD: Secretion management in the mechanically ventilated patient. *Respir Care* 52:1328–1342, 2007.

29. Briassoulis GC, et al: Air leaks from the respiratory tract in mechanically ventilated children with severe respiratory disease. *Pediatr Pulmonol* 29:127–134, 2000.

30. Brochard L, Pluskwa R, Lemaire F: Improved efficacy of spontaneous breathing with inspiratory pressure support. *Am Rev Respir Dis* 136:411, 1987.

31. Bronicki R, Anas N: Cardiopulmonary interaction. *Pediatr Crit Care Med* 10:313–322, 2009.

32. Bryan M, et al: Pulmonary function studies during the first year of life in infants recovering from the respiratory distress syndrome. *Pediatrics* 52:169, 1973.

33. Buford AE, et al: Drowning and near-drowning in children and adolescents. *Pediatr Emerg Care* 21:610, 2005.

34. Cahn MD, et al: Long-term follow up of Greenfield inferior cava filter placement in children. *J Vascular Surg* 34:820–825, 2001.

35. Carlson J, et al: Extubation force: tape versus endotracheal tube holders. *Ann Emerg Med* 50:686–691, 2007.

36. Carroll CL, Schramm CM: Noninvasive positive pressure ventilation for the treatment of status asthmaticus in children. *Ann Allergy Asthma Immunol* 96:454–459, 2006.

37. Carroll CL, Zucker AR: The increased cost of complications in children with status asthmaticus. *Pediatr Pulmonol* 42:914–919, 2007.

38. Carter ER, Webb CR, Moffitt DR: Evaluation of heliox in children hospitalized with acute severe asthma. *A randomized crossover trial.* *Chest* 109:1256–1261, 1996.

39. Casati A, et al: Transcutaneous monitoring of partial pressure of carbon dioxide in the elderly patient: a prospective, clinical comparison with end-tidal monitoring. *J Clin Anesth* 18:436–440, 2006.

40. Caviedes I, et al: Effect of intrinsic positive end-expiratory pressure on respiratory compliance. *Crit Care Med* 14:947, 1986.

41. Celebi S, Hacimustafaoglu S, Demirkaya M: Septic pulmonary emboli in a child. *Indian Pediatr* 45:415–417, 2008.

42. Centers for Disease Control and Prevention, National Center for Injury Prevention and Control. Web-based Injury Statistics Query and Reporting System (WISQARS) [online], 2008, Available at: http://www.cdc.gov/ncipc/wisqars. Accessed July 28, 2008.

43. Chameides LC, Samson RA, Schexnayder SM, Hazinski MF, editors: *Pediatric advanced life support manual*, Dallas, 2011, American Heart Association.

44. Chatte G, et al: Prone position in mechanically ventilated patients with severe acute respiratory failure. *Am J Respir Crit Care Med* 155:473, 1997.

45. Cherry JD: Croup. *N England Med* 358:384, 2008.

46. Choi SJ: Comparison of desaturation and resaturation response times between transmission and reflectance pulse oximeters. *Acta Anaesthesiol Scand* 54:212–217, 2010.

47. Ciarallo L, Brousseau D, Reinert S: Higher-dose intravenous magnesium therapy for children with moderate to severe acute asthma. *Arch Pediatr Adolesc Med* 154:979–983, 2000.

48. Ciarallo L, Sauer AH, Shannon MW: Intravenous magnesium therapy for moderate to severe pediatric asthma: results of a randomized, placebo-controlled trial. *J Pediatr* 129:809–814, 1996.

49. Coalson JJ: Stucture of the respiratory system. In Fuhrman BP, Zimmerman J, editors: *Pediatric critical care*, ed 3, Philadelphia, 2006, Mosby-Elsevier.

50. Collaborative European Multicenter Study Group: Surfactant replacement therapy for severe neonatal respiratory distress syndrome: an international randomized clinical trial. *Pediatrics* 82:683–691, 1988.

51. Colvin J, et al: Outcomes of congenital diaphragmatic hernia: a population-based study in Western Australia. *Pediatrics* 116:e356–e363, 2005.

52. Craven D, et al: Iprtropium bromide plus nebulized albuterol for the treatment of hospitalized children with acute asthma. *J Pediatr* 138:51–58, 2001.

53. Curley MAQ, et al: Effect of prone positioning on clinical outcomes in children with acute lung injury. *J Am Med Assoc* 294:229, 2005.

54. Curley MAQ, Thompson JE, Arnold JH: The effects of early and repeated prone positioning in pediatric patients with acute lung injury. *Chest* 118:156, 2000.

55. D'Ávila RS, et al: Early administration of two intravenous bolus of aminophylline added to the standard treatment of children with acute asthma. *Respir Med* 102:156–161, 2008.

56. Davison C, et al: Efficacy of interventions for bronchiolitis in critically ill infants: a systematic review and meta analysis. *Pediatr Crit Care Med* 5:482, 2004.

57. Datin-Dorriere V: Prenatal prognosis in isolated congenital diaphragmatic hernia. *Am J Obstet Gynecol* 198(1):80–81, 2008.

58. Daya H, et al: Pediatric vocal fold paralysis: a long-term retrospective study. *Arch Otolaryngol Head Neck Surg* 126:21–25, 2000.

59. deCaen A, Duff J, Coovadia AH, et al: Airway Management. In Nichols DG, editor-in-chief: *Roger's textbook of pediatric critical care*, Philadelphia, ed 4, Lippincott, 2008, Williams and Wilkins.

60. Deep A, De Munter C, Desai A: Negative pressure ventilation in pediatric critical care setting. *Indian J Pediatr* 74:483, 2007.

61. DeJonge MH, White M: A comparison of two methods or oral endotracheal tube stabilization in neonatal patients. *J Perinatol* 18:463–465, 1998.

62. deKlerk A: Humidified high-flow nasal cannula: is it the new and improved CPAP? *Adv Neonatal Care* 8:98, 2008.

63. Denne SC: Energy Expenditure in infants with pulmonary insufficiency: is there evidence for increased energy needs? *J Nutr* 131:935S, 2001.

64. Dobyns EL: Assessment and monitoring of respiratory function. In Fuhrman BP, Zimmerman J, editors: *Pediatric critical care*, Philadelphia, 2006, Mosby.

65. Doshi J, Krawiec ME: Clinical manifestations of airway malacia in young children. *J Allergy Clin Immunol* 120:1276, 2007.

66. Drover DW: Gastric versus postpyloric feeding. *Gastrointest Endosc Clin N Am* 17:765–775, 2007.
67. Duffett M, et al: Surfactant therapy for acute respiratory failure in children: a systematic review and meta-analysis. *Critical Care* 11:R66, 2007. Available at: http://pedsccm.org/view.php?id=498. Accessed June 26, 2011.
68. Dullenkopf A, et al: Performance of a novel pressure release valve for cuff pressure control in pediatric tracheal tubes. *Pediatr Anesth* 16:19–24, 2006.
69. Duruisseau O, et al: Endoscopic rehabilitation of vocal cord paralysis with a silicone elastomer suspension implant. *Otolaryngol Head Neck Surg* 131:241–247, 2004.
70. Ehrlich PF: Coran Eventration of the Diaphragm. In Kleigman RM, editor: *Nelson textbook of pediatrics*, ed 18, Philadelphia, 2007, Elsevier/Saunders.
71. Essouri S, et al: Noninvasive positive pressure ventilation: five years of experience in a pediatric intensive care unit. *Pediatr Crit Care Med* 7:329, 2006.
72. Farias JA, et al: An evaluation of extubation failure predictors in mechanically ventilated infants and children. *Intensive Care Med* 28:752, 2002.
73. Farias JA, et al: A comparison of two methods to perform a breathing trial before extubation in pediatric intensive care patients. *Intensive Care Med* 27:1649, 2001.
74. Ferrara TB, et al: Routine use of Dexamethasone for the prevention of postextubation respiratory distress. *J Perinatol* 9:287, 1989.
75. Fewell JE, Abendschein DR, Carlson J, et al: Mechanism of decreased right and left ventricular end-diastolic volumes during continuous positive-pressure ventilation in dogs. *Circ Res* 47:467–472, 1980.
76. Fiastro JF, Habib MP, Quan SE: Pressure support compensation for inspiratory work due to endotracheal tubes and demand continuous positive airway pressure. *Chest* 93:499, 1988.
77. Flori HR, et al: Pediatric acute lung injury: prospective evaluation of risk factors associated with mortality. *Am J Respir Crit Care Med* 171:995–1001, 2005.
78. Foglia E, Meier MD, Elward A: Ventilator-associated pneumonia in neonatal and pediatric intensive care unit patients. *Clin Microbiol Rev* 20:409–425, 2007.
79. Fontán JP, Haddad GG: Respiratory Pathophysiology. In Behrman RE, Kliegman RM, Jenson HB, editors: *Nelson textbook of pediatrics*, Philadelphia, 2004, Saunders.
80. Fontán JP, Lister G: The acutely ill infant and child. In Rudolph CD et al., editors: *Rudolph's pediatrics*, New York, 2003, McGraw-Hill.
81. Frank BS, Lewis RJ: Experience with intubated patients does not effect the accidental extubation rate in pediatric intensive care units and intensive care nurseries. *Pediatr Pulmonol*. 23:424–428, 1997.
82. Frankel L: Respiratory distress and failure. In Berhman RE, Kliegman RM, Jenson HB, editors: *Nelson textbook of pediatrics*, Philadelphia, 2004, Saunders.
83. Gal TG: Pulmonary function testing. In Miller RD, editor: *Miller's Anesthesia*, Philadelphia, 2005, Elsevier.
84. Gardner A, et al: Best practice in stabilization of oral endotracheal tubes: a systemic review. *Aust Crit Care* 18:160–165, 2005.
85. Gawchik SM, et al: The safety and efficacy of nebulized levalbuterol compared with racemic albuterol and placebo, in treatment of asthma in pediatric patients. *J Allergy Clin Immunol* 103:615–621, 1999.
86. Geelhoed GC: Sixteen years of croup in a western Australian teaching hospital: effects of routine steroid treatment. *Ann Emerg Med* 28:621, 1996.
87. Glover ML, Machado C, Totapally BR: Magnesium sulfate administered via continuous infusion in pediatric patients with refractory wheezing. *J Crit Care* 17:255–258, 2002.
88. Goggi N, Macarthur C, Parkin PC: Randomized trial of the addition of ipratropium bromide to albuterol and corticosteroid therapy in children hospitalized because of an acute asthma exacerbation. *Arch Pediatr Adolesc Med* 155:1329–1334, 2001.
89. Gold WM: Pulmonary Function Testing. In Mason RJ, editor: *Murray & Nadel's texbook of respiratory medicine*, Philadelphia, 2005, Elsevier.
90. Gorelick MH, Baker MD: Epiglottitis in children, 1979 through 1992. Effects of haemophilus influenzae type b immunization. *Arch Pediatr Adolesc Med* 148:47, 1994.
91. Grant MJC, Curley MAQ: Pulmonary critical care problems. In Curley MAQ, Maloney-Harmon PA, editors: *Critical care nursing of infants and children*, Philadelphia, 2001, WB Saunders.
92. Grant MJC, Webster HF: Pulmonary system. In Slota MC, editor: *Core curriculum for pediatric critical care nursing*, ed 2, St Louis, 2006, Saunders.
93. Grillo HC, et al: Management of congenital tracheal stenosis by means of slide tracheoplasty or resection and reconstruction, with long term follow-up of growth after slide tracheoplasty. *J Thorac Cardiovasc Surg* 112:145, 2002.
94. Gupta VK, Cheifetz I: Heliox administration in the pediatric intensive care unit: an evidence-based review. *Pediatr Crit Care Med* 6:204–211, 2005.
95. Guyton AC, Jones CE, Coleman TG: Mean circulatory pressure, mean systemic pressure, and mean pulmonary pressure and their effects on venous return. In Guyton AC, Jones CE, Coleman TG, editors: *Circulatory physiology: cardiac output and its regulation*, ed 2, Philadelphia, 1973, WB Saunders, pp. 205–221.
96. Guyton DC, Barlow MR, Besselievre TR: Influence of airway pressure on minimum occlusive endotracheal tube cuff pressure. *Crit Care Med* 25:91–94, 1997.
97. Hales RL: High frequency oscillatory ventilation. In Verger JT, Lebet RM, editors: *AACN procedure manual for pediatric acute and critical care*, Philadelphia, 2008, WB Saunders.
98. Happ MB, et al: Use of the quasi-experimental sequential cohort design in the study of patient-nurse effectiveness with assisted communication. *Contemp Clin Trials* 29:801–808, 2008.
99. Hazinski TA: Tools for Diagnosis and Management of Respiratory Disorders. In Rudolph CD et al., editors: *Rudolph's pediatrics*, ed 21, New York, 2003, McGraw-Hill.
100. Henderson-Smart DJ, et al: Elective high frequency oscillatory ventilation versus conventional ventilation for acute pulmonary dysfunction in preterm infants. *Cochrane Database Syst Rev* Jul 18;3:CD000104, 2007.
101. Henrickson KJ: Cost-effective use of rapid diagnostic techniques in the treatment and prevention of viral respiratory infections. *Pediatr Ann* 34:24, 2005.
102. Herting E, et al: Surfactant improves oxygenation in infants and children with pneumonia and acute respiratory distress syndrome. *ACTA Paediatr* 91:1174, 2002.
103. Heulitt MJ: Physiology of the respiratory system. In Fuhrman BP, Zimmerman J, editors: *Pediatric critical care*, ed 3, Philadelphia, 2006, Mosby-Elsevier.
104. Heyland DK, et al: Optimizing the benefits and minimizing the risks of enteral nutrition in the critically ill: role of small bowel feeding. *J Parenter Enteral Nutr* 28:60, 2002.
105. Hickling KG, Henderson SJ, Jackson R: Low mortality associated with low volume pressure limited ventilation with permissive hypercapnia in severe adult respiratory distress syndrome. *Intensive Care Med* 16:372, 1990.
106. Hypothermia after Cardiac Arrest Study Group: Mild therapeutic hypothermia to improve the neurological outcome after cardiac arrest. *N Engl J Med* 246:549, 2002.
107. Idris AH, et al: Recommended guidelines for uniform reporting of data from drowning the "Utstein Style"*Circulation* 108:2565, 2003.
108. Isben LM, Koch T: Submersion and asphyxia injury. *Crit Care Med* 30:(11 Suppl.):S402–S408, 2002.
109. Jaber S, et al: Volume-guaranteed pressure-support ventilation facing acute changes in ventilatory demand. *Intensive Care Med* 31:1181, 2005.
110. Jardine DS, Crone RK: Specific diseases of the respiratory system: upper airway. In Fuhrman BP, Zimmerman J, editors: *Pediatric critical care*, Philadelphia, 2006, Mosby.
111. Jarog DL: Endotracheal tube: taping. In Verger JT, Lebet RM, editors: *AACN procedure manual for pediatric acute and critical care*, St Louis, 2008, Saunders Elsevier.
112. Jin-Hee K, et al: Elongation of the trachea during neck extension in children: implications of the safety of endotracheal tubes. *Anesth Analg* 101:974–977, 2005.
113. Jobe AH, Bancalari E: Bronchopulmonary Dysplasia (electronic version). *Am J Respir Crit Care Med* 163:1723, 2001. Available at: http://ajrccm.atsjournals.org/cgi/content/full/163/7/1723?ijkey=9885160ff371fb7a8a8b47bf80f44a06e051598c&keytype2=tf_ipsecsha. Accessed June 26, 2011.
114. Johansson F, et al: Effects of albuterol enantiomers on in vitro bronchial reactivity. *Clin Rev Allergy Immunol* 14:57–64, 1999.
115. Joshi VH, Bhuta T: Rescue high frequency jet ventilation versus conventional ventilation for severe pulmonary dysfunction in

preterm infants. *Cochrane Database of Systematic Reviews* 1. Art. No.: CD000437:2006. doi: 10.1002/14651858.CD000437.pub2.

116. Kane-Gill SL, et al: Multicenter treatment and outcome evaluation of aspiration syndromes in critically ill patients. *Ann Pharmacother* 41:549–555, 2007.

117. Karakoc F, et al: Late diagnosis of foreign body aspiration in children with chronic respiratory symptoms. *Int J Pediatr Otorhinolaryngol* 71:241–246, Epub 2006 Nov 27, 2007.

118. Kelley PJ, Arney TD: Use of magnesium sulfate for pediatric patients with acute asthma exacerbations. *J Infus Nurs* 28:329–336, 2005.

119. Kellner JD, Ohlsson A, Gadomski AM, Wang EEL: Bronchodilators for bronchiolitis. *Cochrane Database Syst Rev* 2:CD001266, 2000.

120. Kim IK, et al: Helium/oxygen-driven albuterol nebulization in the treatment of children with moderate to severe asthma exacerbations: a randomized, controlled trial. *Pediatrics* 116:1127–1133, 2005.

121. Kirk VG, Batuyong ED, Bohn SG: Transcutaneous carbon dioxide monitoring and capnography during pediatric polysomnography. *Sleep* 29:1601–1608, 2006.

122. Kissoon N, Rimensberger PC, Bohn D: Ventilation strategies and adjunctive therapy in severe lung disease. *Pediatr Clin N Am* 55:709, 2008.

122a. Kleinman ME, Chameides L, Schexnayder SM, et al: Part 14: pediatric advanced life support: 2010 American Heart Association Guidelines for Cardiopulmonary Resuscitation and Emergency Cardiovascular Care. *Circulation* 122(18 Suppl 3):S876–908, 2010.

123. Kline AM: Arterial Puncture: perform. In Verger JT, Lebet RM, editors: *AACN procedure manual for pediatric acute and critical care*, St Louis, 2008, Saunders-Elsevier.

124. Kregenow DA, et al: Hypercapnic acidosis and mortality in acute lung injury. *Crit Care Med* 34:1, 2006.

125. Krishnan JA, Brower RG: High-frequency ventilation for acute lung injury and ARDS. *Chest* 118:795, 2000.

126. Lacroix J, et al: Transfusion strategies for patients in pediatric intensive care units. *New Engl J Med* 356:1609–1619, 2007.

127. Lee CC, et al: Outcome of vocal cord paralysis in infants. *Acta Paediatr Taiwan* 45:278–281, 2004.

128. Lee LK, Mao C, Thompson KM: Demographic factors and their association with outcomes in pediatric submersion injury. *Acadc Emerg Med* 13:308, 2006.

129. Levin D: Morphological analysis of the pulmonary vascular bed in congenital left-sided diaphragmatic hernia. *J Pediatr* 92:805–809, 1978.

130. Levin DL, et al: A prospective, randomized controlled blinded study of three bronchodilators in infants with respiratory syncytial virus bronchiolitis on mechanical ventilation. *Pediatr Crit Care Med* 9:598–604, 2008.

131. Levin DL: Near-drowning. *Crit Care Med* 8:590–595, 1980.

132. Levin DL, et al: Persistent pulmonary hypertension of the newborn. *J Pediatr* 89:626–630, 1976.

133. Levin DL, Tribuzio W, Green-Wrzesinkit T: Empiric antibiotics are justified for infants with respiratory syncytial virus lower respiratory tract infection presenting with respiratory failure. A prospective slides and evidence review. *Pediatr Crit Care Med* 11:289–294, 2010.

134. Little LA, Koenig JC, Newth CJL: Factors affecting accidental extubations in neonatal and pediatric intensive care patients. *Crit Care Med* 18:163, 1990.

135. Lloyd TC: Effect of inspiration on inferior vena caval blood flow in dogs. *J Appl Phyisol* 55:1701–1708, 1983.

136. Lodato RF: Oxygen toxicity. *Crit Care Clin* 6:749, 1990.

137. Loh LE, Chan YH, Chan I: Noninvasive ventilation in children: a review. *J Pediatr (Rio J)* 83:S91, 2007.

138. Loughead JL, et al: Reducing accidental extubation in neonates. *Jt Comm J Qual Patient Saf* 34:164–170, 2008.

139. Luten RC, et al: Length-based endotracheal tube and emergency equipment in pediatrics. *Ann Emerg Med* 21:900, 1992.

140. Macintyre NR: Principles of mechanical ventilation. In Mason RJ, editor: *Murray and Nadel's texbook of respiratory medicine*, Philadelphia, 2005, Elsevier.

141. MacIntyre NR: Pressure support ventilation: effects on ventilatory reflexes and ventilatory-muscle workloads. *Respir Care* 32:447, 1987.

142. Magnus VS, Turkington L: Communication interaction in ICU—patient and staff experiences and perceptions. *Intensive Crit Care Nursing* 22:167–180, 2006.

143. Mallick MS, et al: Late presentation of tracheobronchial foreign body aspiration in children. *Pediatrics* 51:145–148, 2005.

144. Mancebo J, et al: A multicenter trial of prolonged prone ventilation in severe acute respiratory distress syndrome. *Am J Respir Crit Care Med* 173:1233, 2006.

145. Mannix R, Bachur R: Status asthmaticus in children. *Curr Opin Pediatr* 19:281–287, 2007.

146. Marcin JP, et al: Nurse staffing and unplanned extubation in the pediatric intensive care unit. *Pediatr Crit Care Med* 6:254–257, 2005.

147. Marini JJ: Mechanical ventilation. *Curr Pulmonol* 9:164, 1988.

148. Markovitz BP, Randolph AG, Khemani RG: Corticosteroids for the prevention and treatment of post-extubation stridor in neonates, children and adults. *Cochrane Database Sys Rev* 2:CD001000, 2008.

149. Marraro GA: Innovative practices of ventilatory support with pediatric patients. *Pediatr Crit Care Med* 4:8, 2003.

150. Martins RHG, et al: Endoscopic findings in children with stridor. *Braz J Otorhinolaryngol* 72:649, 2006.

151. McClave SA, et al: Poor validity of residual volumes as a marker for risk of aspiration in critically ill patients. *Crit Care Med* 33:324, 2005.

152. McNamara VM, Crabbe DCG: Traceomalacia. *Paediatr Respir Rev* 5:147, 2004.

153. Meert KL, Daphtary KM, Metheny NA: Gastric vs small bowel feeding in critically ill children receiving mechanical ventilation. *Chest* 126:872–878, 2004.

154. Meissner HC: Selected populations at increased risk from respiratory syncytial virus infection. *Pediatr Infect Dis J* 22:S40, 2003.

155. Mercier J, Dauger S, Durand Javouey E: Acute respiratory distress syndrome. In Fuhrman BP, Zimmerman J, editors: *Pediatric critical care*, Philadelphia, 2006, Mosby-Elsevier.

156. Meyer RJ, Theodorou AA, Berg RA: Childhood drowning. *Pediatr Rev* 27:163, 2006.

157. Mhanna MJ, et al: The "air leak" test around the endotracheal tube, as predictor of postextubation stridor, is age dependent in children. *Crit Care Med* 30:2639–2643, 2002.

158. Michelow IC, et al: Epidemiology and clinical characteristics of community-acquired pneumonia in hospitalized children. *Pediatrics* 113:701, 2004.

159. Michiels JJ, et al: Noninvasive exclusion and diagnosis of pulmonary embolism by sequential use of the rapid ELISA d-dimer assay, clinical score and spiral CT. *Int Angiol* 22:1–14, 2003.

160. Mitchell RB, Kelly J: Adenotonsillectomy for obstructive sleep apnea in obese children. *Otolaryngol Head Neck Surg* 131:104–108, 2004.

161. Mitra A, Bassler D, Ducharme FM: Intravenous aminophylline for acute severe asthma in children over 2 years of age using inhaled bronchodilators. *Cochrane Database Syst Rev* 4:CD001276, 2001.

162. Miyamoto RC, et al: Bilateral congenital vocal cord paralysis: a 16 year institutional review. *Otolaryngol Head Neck Surg* 133:241–245, 2005.

163. Möller JC, et al: Treatment with bovine surfactant in severe acute respiratory distress syndrome in children: a randomized multicenter study. *Intensive Care Med* 29:437, 2003.

164. Moore M, Little P: Humidified air inhalation for treating croup. *Cochrane Database Syst Rev* 3:CD002870, 2006.

165. Morris LG, Zoumalan RA, Roccaforte JD, et al: Monitoring tracheal tube cuff pressures in the intensive care unit: a comparison of digital palpation and manometry. *An Otol Rhinol Laryngol* 116:639–642, 2007.

166. Morrow B, Futter M, Argent A: Effect of endotracheal suction on lung dynamics in mechanically-ventilated paediatric patients. *Aust J Physiother* 52:121–126, 2006.

167. Myers TR: Use of heliox in children. *Respir Care* 51:6, 2006.

168. National Heart, Lung, and Blood Institute Acute Respiratory Distress Syndrome (ARDS) Clinical Trials Network, et al: Comparison of two fluid-management strategies in acute lung injury. *N Engl J Med* 354:2564–2575, 2006.

169. Nawab US, et al: Heliox attenuates lung inflammation and structural alterations in acute lung injury. *Pediatr Pulmonol* 40:524–532, 2005.

170. Nelson HS, et al: Improved bronchodilation with levalbuterol compared with racemic albuterol in patients with asthma. *J Allergy Clin Immunol* 102:943–952, 1998.

171. Newth CJ, et al: The use of cuffed versus uncuffed endotracheal tubes in pediatric intensive care. *J Pediatr* 144:333, 2004.

172. New CJ, et al: Eunice Shriver Kennedy National Institute of Child Health and Human Development Collaborative Pediatric Critical Care Research Network. Weaning and extubation readiness in pediatric patients. *Pediatr Crit Care Med* 10:1–11, 2009.

173. Noda AK, et al: Beneficial effect of bilevel positive airway pressure on left ventricular function in ambulatory patients with idiopathic dilated cardiomyopathy and central sleep apnea-hypopnea: a preliminary study. *Chest* 131:1694, 2007.

174. Northway W, Rosan R, Porter D: Pulmonary disease following respiratory therapy of hyaline membrane disease. *N Engl J Med* 276:357, 1967.

175. Olshaker JS: Submersion. *Emerg Med Clin North Am* 22:357–367, 2004.

176. Openshaw PJM: Potential therapeutic implications of new insights into respiratory syncytial virus disease. *Respir Res* 3:S15, 2002.

177. Paintal HS, Kuschner WG: Aspiration syndromes: 10 clinical pearls every physician should know. *Int J Clin Pract* 61:846–852, 2007.

178. Panitch HB: Viral respiratory infection in children with technology dependence and neuromuscular disorders. *Pediatr Infect Dis J* 23: S222, 2004.

179. Parakininkas D, Rice TB: Pneumonitis and Interstitial Lung Disease. In Fuhrman BP, Zimmerman JJ, editors: *Pediatric critical care*, Philadelphia, 2006, Mosby.

180. Paz-Priel I, et al: Thromboembolic events in children and young adults with pediatric sarcoma. *J Clin Oncol* 25:1519–1524, 2007.

181. Pelosi P, et al: Effects of the prone position on respiratory mechanics and gas exchange during acute lung injury. *Am J Respir Crit Care Med* 157:387, 1998.

182. Perket EA: Lung Growth in Infancy and Childhood. In Rudolph CD, et al., editors: *Rudolph's pediatrics*, ed 21, New York, 2003, McGraw-Hill.

183. Peter JV, Chacko B, Moran JL: Comparison of closed endotracheal suction versus open endotracheal suction in the development of ventilator-associated pneumonia in intensive care units: an evaluation using meta-analytic techniques. *Indian J Sci* 61:201–211, 2007.

184. Peters J, Kindred MK, Robotham JL: Transient analysis of cardiopulmonary interactions. I. Diastolic events. *J Appl Physiol* 64:1506–1517, 1988.

185. Peters J, Kindred MK, Robotham JL: Transient analysis of cardiopulmonary interaction. II. Systolic events. *J Appl Physiol* 64:1518–1526, 1988.

186. Petty TL: A historical perspective of mechanical ventilation. *Crit Care Clin* 6:489, 1990.

187. Phipps LM, et al: Prospective assessment of guidelines for determining appropriate depth of endotracheal tube placement in children. *Pediatr Crit Care Med* 6:519, 2005.

188. Popernack ML, Thomas NJ, Lucking SE: Decreasing unplanned extubations: utilization of the Penn State Children's Hospital sedation algorithm. *Pediatr Crit Care Med* 5:58–62, 2004.

189. Prakash O, Meij S: Cardiopulmonary response to inspiratory pressure support during spontaneous ventilation vs conventional ventilation. *Chest* 88:403, 1985.

190. Priestly MA, Helfaer MA: Approaches in the management of acute respiratory failure in children. *Curr Opin Pediatr* 16:293, 2004.

191. Putensen C, et al: The impact of spontaneous breathing during mechanical ventilation. *Curr Opin Crit Care* 12:13, 2006.

192. Raffini L, et al: A prospective observational study of IVC filters in pediatric patients. *Pediatr Blood Cancer* 51:517–520, 2008.

193. Rajpurkar M, et al: Pulmonary embolism—experience at a single children's hospital. *Thromb Res* 119:699–703, 2007.

194. Ralston M, et al: *PALS provider manual and student CD*, Dallas, 2006, American Heart Association.

195. Randolph AG, et al: Cumulative fluid intake minus output is not associated with ventilator weaning duration or extubation outcomes in children. *Pediatr Crit Care Med* 6:642, 2005.

196. Randolph AG, et al: Effect of mechanical ventilator weaning protocols on respiratory outcomes in infants and children: a randomized controlled trial. *J Am Med Assoc* 288:2561, 2002.

197. Ream RS, et al: Association of nursing workload and unplanned extubations in a pediatric intensive care unit. *Pediatr Crit Care Med* 8:366–371, 2007.

198. Reid C, Chan L, Tweeddale M: The who, where, and what of rapid sequence intubation: prospective observational study of emergency RSI outside the operating theatre. *Emer Med J* 21:296, 2004.

199. Rich JM, et al: The critical airway, rescue ventilation and the combitube: part 1. *AANA J* 72:17, 2004.

200. Roosevelt G: Infectious upper airway obstruction. In Berhman RE, Kliegman RM, Jenson HB, editors: *Nelson textbook of pediatrics*, Philadelphia, 2004, Saunders.

201. Roosevelt GE: Acute Inflammatory upper airway obstruction (croup, epiglottitis, laryngitis, and bacterial tracheitis). In Kleigman RM et al., editors: *Nelson textbook of pediatrics*, Philadelphia, 2007, Saunders.

202. Rosenberg AA: The Neonate. In Gabbe SG et al., editors: *Obstetrics: normal and problem pregnancies*, Philadelphia, 2007, Churchill Livingston.

203. Rothe CF: Mean circulatory filling pressure: its meaning and measurement. *J Appl Physiol* 74:499, 1993.

204. Rotta AT, Steinhorn DM: Conventional mechanical ventilation in pediatrics. *J Pediatr* 83:S100–S108, 2007.

205. Royall JA, Levin DL: Adult respiratory distress syndrome in pediatric patients, I: clinical aspects, pathophysiology, and mechanisms of lung injury. *J Pediatr* 112:169, 1988.

206. Rubens D, Schenkman KA, Martin LD: Noninvasive monitoring in children. In Fuhrman BP, Zimmerman J, editors: *Pediatric critical care,,* ed 3, Philadelphia, 2006, Mosby-Elsevier.

207. Russell K, et al: Glucocorticoids for croup. *Cochrane Database of Syst Rev* 1:CD001955, 2004.

208. Santamore WP, Gray L: Significant left ventricular contributions to right ventricular systolic function. *Chest* 107:1134–1145, 1995.

209. Saragin MJ, et al: Rapid sequence intubation for pediatric emergency airway management. *Pediatr Emerg Care* 18:417, 2002.

210. Sarnaik AP, et al: Pressure-controlled ventilation in children with status asthmaticus. *Pediatr Crit Care Med* 5:133–138, 2004.

211. Sarrell EM, et al: Nebulized 3% hypertonic saline solution treatment in ambulatory children with viral bronchiolitis decreases symptoms. *Chest* 223:2015, 2002.

212. Scharf SM, Ingram RH Jr.: Influence of abdominal pressure and sympathetic vasoconstriction of the cardiovascular response to positive end-expiratory pressure. *Am Rev Respir Dis* 116:661–670, 1977.

213. Schuerer DJE, et al: Extracorporeal membrane oxygenation current clinical practice, coding and reimbursement. *Chest* 134:179, 2008.

214. Sectish TC, Prober CG: Pneumonia, 2008: In Kliegman RM, Behrman RI, Stanton BF, editors: *Nelson textbook of pediatrics*, Philadelphia, 2008, Elsevier, Available at: http:www.mdconsult.com/das/book/body/100677694-7/730226910/1608/939.html. Accessed July 29.

215. Sersar SI, et al: Inhaled foreign bodies: presentation, management and value of history and plain chest radiography in delayed presentation. *Head Neck Surg* 134:92–99, 2006.

216. Severinghaus JW: History of measuring O_2 and CO_2 responses. *Adv Exp Med Biol* 605:3–8, 2008.

217. Shah PS, Ohlsson A, Shah JP: Continuous negative extrathoracic pressure or continuous positive airway pressure for acute hypoxemic respiratory failure in children. *Cochrane Database Syst Rev* 1: DC003699, 2008.

218. Shah RK, Roberson DW, Jones DT: Epiglottitis in the *Hemophilus influenzae* type B vaccine era: changing trends. *Laryngoscope* 114:557, 2004.

219. Shah S, Sharieff GQ: Pediatric respiratory infections. *Emerg Med Clin North Am* 25:961–979, 2007.

220. Shapiro BA, Cane RD, Harrison RA: Positive end-expiratory pressure therapy in adults with special reference to acute lung injury: a review of the literature and suggested clinical correlations. *Crit Care Med* 12:127, 1984.

221. Shekerdemian LS, et al: Cardiorespiratory responses to negative pressure ventilation after tetralogy of Fallot repair: a hemodynamic tool for patients with a low-output state. *J Am Coll Cardiol* 33:549–555, 1999.

222. Siempos II, Vardakas KZ, Falagas ME: Closed tracheal suction systems for prevention of ventilator associated pneumonia. *Br J Anaesth* 299–306, 2008.

223. Siempos II, et al: Impact of passive humidification on clinical outcomes of mechanically ventilated patients: a meta-analysis of randomized controlled trials. *Crit Care Med* 35:2843–2851, 2007.

224. Silvestri JM, Weese-Mayer DE: Apnea and SIDS. In Rudolph CD et al., editors: *Rudolph's pediatrics*, ed 21, New York, 2003, McGraw-Hill, pp. 1934–1937.

225. Simoes EA: Environmental and demographic risk factors for respiratory syncytial virus lower respiratory tract disease. *J Pediatr* 143: (5 Suppl.):S118, 2003.

226. Singer M, et al: Oxygen toxicity in man: a prospective study in patients after open heart surgery. *N Engl J Med* 283:1473, 1970.

227. Smith MM, et al: Flexible fiber-optic laryngoscopy in the first hours after extubation for the evaluation of laryngeal lesions due to intubation in the pediatric intensive care unit. *J Pediatr Otorhinolaryngol* 71:1423–1428, 2007.

228. Stahlman MT: Clinical description of bronchopulmonary dysplasia. *J Pediatr* 8:829, 1979.

229. Staworn D, et al: Brain death in pediatric intensive care unit patients: incidence, primary diagnosis, and the clinical occurrence of Turner's triad. *Crit Care Med* 22:1301–1305, 1994.

230. Steinhorn RH, Green TP: Use of extracorporeal membrane oxygenation in the treatment of respiratory syncytial virus bronchiolitis: the national experience, 1983 to 1988. *J Pediatr* 116:338–342, 1990.

231. Stensballe LG, et al: Atopic disposition, wheezing and subsequent respiratory syncytial virus hospitalization in Danish children younger than 18 months: a nested case-control study [electronic version]. *Pediatrics* 118:1360, 2006.

232. Subirana M, Solà I, Benito S: Closed tracheal suction systems versus open tracheal suction systems for mechanically ventilated adult patients. *Cochrane Database Syst Rev* 4. Art. No.: CD004581. Doi: 10.1002/14651858.CD004581.pub2, 2007.

233. Sur JP, Garg RK, Jolly NJ: Rheolytic percutaneous thrombectomy for acute pulmonary embolism in a pediatric patient. *Catheter Cardiovasc Interv* 70:450–453, 2007.

234. Suter PM, Fairley B, Isenberg MD: Optimum end-expiratory airway pressure in patients with acute pulmonary failure. *N Engl J Med* 292:284, 1975.

235. Swaniker F, et al: Extracorporeal life support outcome for 128 pediatric patients with respiratory failure. *J Pediatric Surgery* 35:197, 2000.

236. Takata M, Robotham JL: Ventricular external constraint by the lung and pericardium during positive end-expiratory pressure. *Am Rev Respir Dis* 143:872–875, 1991.

237. Teague WG: Noninvasive positive pressure ventilation: current status in paediatric patients. *Paediatr Respir Rev* 6:52–60, 2005.

238. Teboul JL, et al: Estimating cardiac filling pressure in mechanically ventilated patients with hyperinflation. *Crit Care Med* 28:3631–3636, 2000.

239. Telford K, et al: Outcome after neonatal continuous negative-pressure ventilation: follow-up assessment. *Lancet* 367:1080, 2006.

240. The Red Book Online: Summaries of Infectious Diseases, Staphylococcal Infections, 2011: http://aapredbook.aappublications.org/cgi/content/full/2006/1/3.121; Accessed on June 30, 2011.

241. Thierbach AR, Pieipho T, Maybauer M: The easytube for airway management in emergencies. *Prehosp Emerg Care* 9:445, 2005.

242. Thill PJ, et al: Noninvasive positive-pressure ventilation in children with lower airway obstruction. *Pediatr Crit Care Med* 5:337–342, 2004.

243. Thompson AE: Pediatric airway management. In Fuhrmans BP, Zimmerman J, editors: *Pediatric critical care*, Philadelphia, 2006, Mosby.

244. Thompson J, Jaffe M: Capnographic waveforms in the mechanically ventilated patient. *Respir Care* 50:100–109, 2005.

245. Tingay DG, et al: Effects of open endotracheal suction on lung volume in infants receiving HFOV. *Intensive Care Med* 33:689–693, 2007.

246. Tobias JD, Meyer DJ: Noninvasive monitoring of carbon dioxide during respiratory failure in toddlers and infants: end-tidal versus transcutaneous carbon dioxide. *Anesth Analg* 85:55–58, 1997.

247. Todisco T, et al: Treatment of acute exacerbations of chronic respiratory failure: integrated use of negative pressure ventilation and noninvasive positive pressure ventilation. *Chest* 125:2217, 2004.

248. Tokar B, Ozkan R, Ilhan H: Tracheobronchial foreign bodies in children: importance of accurate history and plain chest radiography in delayed presentation. *Clin Radiol* 59:609–615, 2004.

249. Tooley WH: Epidemiology of bronchopulmonary dysplasia. *J Pediatr* 85:851, 1979.

250. Truong MT, et al: Pediatric vocal fold paralysis after cardiac surgery: rate of recovery and sequelae. *Otolaryngol Head Neck Surg* 137:780–784, 2007.

251. Truwit JD, Marini JD: Evaluation of thoracic mechanics in the ventilated patient, I: primary measurements. *J Crit Care* 3:133, 1988.

252. Tsugawa J, et al: Development of acquired tracheal stenosis in premature infants due to prolonged endotracheal intubation: etiologic considerations and surgical management. *Pediatr Surg Int* 22:887–890, 2006.

253. Turner DA, Arnold JH: Insights in pediatric ventilation: timing of intubation, ventilatory strategies, and weaning. *Curr Opin Crit Care* 13:57, 2007.

254. Turner GR, Levin DL: Improvement of neurological status after pediatric near-drowning accidents. *Crit Care Med* 13:1080, 1985.

255. Tyler DC: Positive end-expiratory pressure: a review. *Crit Care Clin* 11:300, 1983.

256. Ukleja A, Sanchex-Fermin M: Gastric versus post-pyloric feeding: relationship to tolerance, pneumonia risk, and successful delivery of nutrition. *Curr Gastroenterol Rep* 9:309–316, 2007.

257. Vaughan DJ, Brogan TV: Ventilation/perfusion mismatch. In Fuhrman BP, Zimmerman J, editors: *Pediatric critical care*, ed 3, Philadelphia, 2006, Mosby-Elsevier.

258. Venkataraman ST, Khan N, Brown A: Validation of predictors of extubation success and failure in mechanically ventilated infants and children. *Crit Care Med* 28:2991, 2000.

259. Venkataraman ST: Mechanical ventilation and respiratory care. In Fuhrman BP, Zimmerman JJ, editors: *Pediatric critical care*, ed 4, Philadelphia, 2011, Mosby Elsevier, 657–688.

260. Venkataraman ST: Mechanical ventilation and respiratory care. In Fuhrman BP, Zimmerman JJ, editors: *Pediatric critical care*, ed 4, Philadelphia, 2011, Mosby Elsevier, 657–688.

261. Villar J, et al: A high positive end expiratory pressure, low tidal volume ventilatory strategy improves outcome in persistent acute respiratory distress syndrome: a randomized, controlled trial. *Crit Care Med* 34:1311, 2006.

262. Villeneuve EJ, Zed PJ: Nebulized magnesium sulfate in the management of acute exacerbations of asthma. *Ann Pharmacother* 40:1118–1124, 2006.

263. Ware LB, et al: Pathogenetic and prognostic significance of altered coagulation and fibrinolysis in acute lung injury/acute respiratory distress syndrome. *Crit Care Med* 35:1821, 2007.

264. Ware LB, Matthay MA: The acute respiratory distress syndrome. *N Engl J Med* 342:1334, 2000.

265. Ware LB, Matthay MA: Clinical practice. Acute pulmonary edema. *N Engl J Med* 353(26):2788–2796, 2005.

266. Weber JE, et al: A randomized comparison of helium-oxygen mixture (heliox) and racemic epinephrine for the treatment of moderate to severe croup. *Pediatrics* 107:E96, 2001. Available at: http://www.pediatrics.org/cgi/content/full/107/6/e96. Accessed April 8, 2008.

267. Weber TR, Keller MS, Fiore A: Aortic suspsension (aortopexy) for severe tracheomalacia in infants and children. *Amer J Surg* 184:573, 2002.

268. Webster HF: Weaning from mechanical ventilation. In Verger JT, Lebet RM, editors: *AACN procedure manual for pediatric acute and critical care*, St Louis, 2008, Saunders-Elsevier.

269. Weiss M, et al: Tracheal tube displacement in children during head-neck movement—a radiological assessment. *Br J Anaesth* 96:486–491, 2006.

270. Welliver RC: Review of epidemiology and clinical risk factors for severe respiratory syncytial virus (RSV) infection. *J Pediatr* 143: (5 Suppl.):S112, 2003.

271. West JB: Gas transport by the blood. *Pulmonary pathophysiology: the essentials*, ed 7, Baltimore, 2008, Lippincott Williams & Wilkins.

272. West JB: Challenges in teaching the mechanics of breathing to medical and graduate students. *Adv Physiol Educ* 32:177–184, 2008.

273. Westley CR, Cotton EK, Brooks JG: Nebulized racemic epinephrine by IPPB for the treatment of croup. *Am J Dis Child* 132:484, 1978.

274. Wheeler DS, Dauplaise DJ, Giuliano JS: An infant with fever and stridor. *Pediatr Emerg Care* 24:46, 2008.

275. Wheeler DS, et al: Theophylline versus terbutaline in treating critically ill children with status asthmaticus: a prospective, randomized, controlled trial. *Pediatr Crit Care Med* 6:204–211, 2005.

276. Willson DF, et al: Effect of exogenous surfactant (calfactant) in pediatric acute lung injury: a randomized controlled trial. *J Am Med Assoc* 293:470, 2005.

277. Wilson J, et al: Noninvasive monitoring of carbon dioxide in infants and children with congenital heart disease: end-tidal versus transcutaneous techniques. *J Intensive Care Med* 20:291–295, 2005.

278. Wratney AT, et al: The endotracheal tube air leak test does not predict extubation outcome in critically ill pediatric patients. *Pediatr Crit Care Med* 9:490–496, 2008.

279. Wright ML, Romano MJ: Ventilator-associated pneumonia in children. *Sem Pediatr Infectious Dis* 17:58–64, 2006.

280. Writing Group for the Christopher Study Investigators: Effectiveness of managing suspected pulmonary embolism using and algorithm combining clinical probability, d-dimer testing and computed tomography. *J Am Med Assoc* 295:172–197, 2006.

281. Wunsch J, Mapstone J: High-frequency ventilation versus conventional ventilation for treatment of acute lung injury and acute respiratory distress syndrome. *Cochrane Database Syst Rev* 1: CD004085, 2004.

282. Youngquist S, Gausche-Hill M, Burbulys D: Alternative airway devices for use in children requiring prehospital airway management. *Pediatr Emerg Care* 23:250, 2007.

283. Yuksel H, et al: A pediatric case of pyomyositis presenting with septic pulmonary emboli. *Joint Bone Spine* 74:491–494, 2007.

284. Zelicof-Paul A, et al: Controversies in rapid sequence intubation in children. *Curr Opin Pediatr* 17:355, 2005.

285. Zuckerbraun NS, Saladino RA: Pediatric drowning: current management strategies for immediate care. *Clin Pediatr Emerg Med* 6:2005. Available at: http://www.mdconsult.com/das/article/body/101018360-3/jorg=journal&source=&sp=15573844&sid=731277684/N/473050/1.html?issn=1522-8401. Accessed July 28, 2008.

Chest X-Ray Interpretation

10

Maureen A. Madden • Mary Fran Hazinski

PEARLS

- The chest radiograph must be used in conjunction with careful, clinical examination of the patient.
- Nurses should develop a systematic method of reviewing chest radiographs and use that format for examining every film.
- Loss of the cardiac silhouette indicates lung opacification (e.g., pneumonia, atelectasis).
- Remember that free air shifts or rises to superior portions of the chest, whereas free fluid tends to shift or fall to dependent (inferior) portions of the chest.
- Atelectasis represents a volume loss; therefore, structures are often shifted toward the area of atelectasis.
- Pneumothorax and hemothorax are conditions that represent a volume gain; therefore, structures are often shifted away from the area of pneumothorax or hemothorax.
- Because x-rays, CT scans, and fluoroscopy all use ionizing radiation, they should be used judiciously and with a specific indication or clinical question to be answered. (For more information, refer to the Image Gently campaign, available at: http://www.pedrad.org/associations/5364/ig/.)

INTRODUCTION

The discovery of the technique of radiography in 1895 by Wilhelm Conrad Roentgen provided clinicians with a noninvasive diagnostic method to evaluate internal anatomic structures and changes within the body. Many of the key elements of Roentgen's original technique for the acquisition and development of a chest radiograph are still used today: film is exposed, developed, coded, and stored for review. However, digital radiography and the picture archiving and communication system (PACS) have significantly improved access to images. This system allows images to be viewed remotely almost immediately and manipulated at a workstation by clinicians in different locations. Images can also be viewed at the bedside soon after they are obtained. Often, the nurse is one of the first healthcare providers to see a patient's chest radiograph.

A basic understanding of the chest radiograph can aid in the assessment and care of critically ill children. This understanding can help the nurse to interpret changes in the radiograph; evaluate placement and location of tubes, catheters, and wires; and correlate changes with the patient's response to therapy. This information can assist in prevention or early detection of pulmonary disorders and complications of treatment, and it can help to identify the need for changes in treatment.

The purpose of this chapter is to present the basic concepts used in the interpretation of chest radiographs and the application of these concepts to the care of the critically ill child.

The chest radiograph remains the most important method of chest imaging, providing an easily accessible, inexpensive, quick, and effective diagnostic tool. However, it is important to appreciate the limitations and pitfalls of this technique. It is extremely important that the chest radiograph be used only in conjunction with careful physical assessment. Often the radiograph simply confirms findings of the physical examination, and the child's clinical condition will usually dictate the treatment required. In addition, a radiologist will be responsible for the final interpretation of any radiograph.

This chapter presents a systematic approach to interpretation of the radiograph and highlights the important factors that the nurse evaluates with this approach. This chapter will not discuss treatment of the problems identified on the radiograph. Evaluation of a chest radiograph may appear to be simple, but is in fact a complex task requiring careful observation, sound understanding of chest anatomy, and knowledge of the principles of physiology and pathology. The value of chest radiographs for critically ill pediatric patients is based on the diagnostic efficacy (the influence of a test result on diagnosis) and therapeutic efficacy (the effect of a test result on clinical management).[2] A systematic approach to the review of a chest radiograph will help prevent errors in interpretation and diagnosis.

Radiographs are a common diagnostic study in critical care units, and they can produce scattered radiation during exposure. Healthcare providers often become lax in shielding themselves and their patients from the radiant energy. The clinician should always wear a lead shield if it is necessary to remain at the bedside during x-ray examinations and should always be certain the child has a gonadal shield in place. Pregnant nurses should check hospital policy regarding protection during patient x-ray procedures. It may be necessary for another nurse to assist in obtaining needed radiographs so that the pregnant nurse avoids any risk of radiation. If it is necessary to hold the child during x-ray examinations, clinicians should wear lead gloves.

DEFINITIONS

X-rays are a form of short wavelength radiant energy. Images are produced when an x-ray beam is directed through an object to a film cassette. The image produced on the film is determined by the composition, or density, of the object through which the beam passes. The thickness of components of the body and structures in the body vary in their radiodensity, or ability to block or absorb the x-ray beam. To begin the interpretation of a radiograph, the nurse must be able to recognize the different densities that are produced on a chest radiograph and be aware of terms used to describe these differing densities and their radiographic appearances (Box 10-1). This will help differentiate between normal and abnormal findings on the radiograph.

If the object is extremely dense, it will block or absorb a significant portion of the beam and prevent it from reaching and reacting with the film; this creates a gray or white shadow on the film. The more x-ray beam an object blocks or absorbs the more *radiopaque* or *radiodense* that object is. An object that is not very dense does not block or absorb much of the x-ray beam; it is radiolucent.[19] When the beam passes through such an object, most of the beam reacts with the film, and the resultant image on the film will have a dark gray or black appearance.

Most complex objects are not of uniform density; they contain a variety of substances of varying densities, which produce shadows on a radiograph. There are four major categories of radiographic densities that appear on a radiograph; in order of decreasing density these are metal or bone, water, fat, and gas (or air).[3] Metal is extremely dense, and it is the most radiopaque of materials. Pure metals block or absorb the entire x-ray beam and produce a bright white shadow on the radiograph. Because bones contain a large amount of calcium, they are nearly as dense and radiopaque as metal and also produce white images on the radiograph. Water and other fluids are fairly radiodense; they block a significant amount of the x-ray beam and have a gray appearance. Body tissues or cavities containing water or fluid (such as the heart) will produce a very light or white image on the radiograph. However, because water and fluids are not as dense as bones, bones and metals will still create whiter (more opaque) images than water. Because fat (including muscle) is not as dense as water, it does not block as much of the x-ray beam and consequently is less radiopaque or more radiolucent than bone or fluid. As a result, the radiograph shadow that fat produces is less dense than that produced by bone or water. Fat is contained in subcutaneous tissue and in some muscle; the x-ray image produced by these fat-containing tissues will have a dark gray or charcoal appearance. Gas or air is the least dense of substances visible on the chest radiograph. Because gas does not absorb much of the x-ray beam, it is radiolucent and produces a black image. Gas or air density is normally seen in the lung fields and in the air-filled stomach. The ability to discern muscle, blood, internal organs, fat, and tissues requires the understanding of normal anatomy.[5,7,16,17]

All parts of the body contain one or more of the four densities—metal or bone, fluid, fat, or gas. The juxtaposition of body parts or chambers of differing densities will create contrasts on the radiograph. When objects of varying densities are in contact, their borders will be apparent because of the contrasts in their radiographic images, and the difference in their images creates an edge or silhouette.[3] When structures are visible on a radiograph, it is easy to evaluate their size, shape, and position. When two objects with similar densities are in contact or in the same plane as the x-ray beam, no spectrum of density is seen; therefore, there is no visible border between the objects on the radiograph.[17] This finding may be normal based on normal anatomy. The silhouette sign describes the loss of a normal interface or silhouette, which is suggestive of abnormal tissues densities, often indicating a pathologic condition.[6,16] This observation of abnormal density or silhouette sign can often confirm a diagnosis of inappropriate tissue, fluid, or air accumulation. The silhouette sign is commonly applied to the heart, mediastinum, chest wall, and diaphragm.

An x-ray film creates a two-dimensional image of three-dimensional objects as it compresses the image into one plane. As a result, the depth of structures often cannot be appreciated by evaluation of only one radiograph view. Many times, studies must be taken from two or more views so that the images can be compared to better evaluate the relative position of objects.[14] Healthcare providers are aware that it is impossible to confirm correct placement of a tracheal tube from an anteroposterior (AP) or a posteroanterior (PA) x-ray alone, because such a film compresses the anterior-posterior dimension. The AP film can be used to evaluate depth of insertion and placement in or displacement from the midline. Only on the lateral view of the chest will it be possible to correctly evaluate the position of the tracheal tube relative to the trachea and esophagus.

The radiograph views are typically labeled by patient position (e.g., upright, lateral) and by the body part nearest to the x-ray projection tube. The optimal position for chest radiography is the upright or erect position. The standard chest film is an upright PA film. This film is typically obtained in the radiology department. The patient stands facing the radiographic film cassette, and the x-ray beam is directed from the back of the patient, through the patient, to the film. Thus, the patient's back (posterior aspect) is closest to the x-ray tube.

An AP chest film is the view most frequently obtained in the critical care unit because it can be taken with a portable x-ray machine. When an AP view is obtained, the film cassette is placed under or behind the child and the child faces the x-ray tube. The child optimally should be in a sitting position; however, if there is difficulty in positioning the child because of acute illness or general immobility, the child is positioned supine. The x-ray beam is then directed from in front of the child through the child and to the film. As a result, the front of the child (anterior aspect) is nearest the x-ray tube when the film is taken. The AP film tends to magnify anterior chest structures, including the heart, because of the divergence

---

Box 10-1 Glossary of Terms

- Density: Whiteness or any area of whiteness on an image
- Lucency: Blackness or any area of blackness on an image
- Shadow: Anything visible on an image; any specific density or lucency
- Edge: Any visible demarcation between structures of differing density; sharpest edges are created when there is density on one side and a lucency on the other
- Silhouette: Synonym for edge; the loss of an edge constitutes the silhouette sign
- Line: Thin density with lucency on both sides or a thin lucency with density on both sides

of the x-ray beam; this makes it difficult to compare heart size in an AP versus a PA film. Heart size is most magnified in an AP supine film because of horizontal elongation of the ribs, higher placement of the diaphragm, and the impression of decreased lung volume.[17]

Whenever heart size is evaluated on chest radiographs, it is important to know whether the film was taken with a PA or an AP approach, although the difference is not as significant in infants and small children as it is in older children and adults.[19] Changes in heart size, or in the size of any organ, can best be appreciated by comparing two images obtained using the same approach. Characteristically, chest films obtained in the radiology department under controlled conditions are clearer and of better quality than those obtained with a portable machine. Therefore, the films should be obtained in the radiology department whenever practical.

When PA or AP chest films are obtained, evaluation of lateral relationships of structures is possible, but assessment of AP relationships is not possible because of the compression of the image onto a single plane. If a determination of depth is necessary or if localization of a density is required, a lateral film is taken. Lateral chest films are usually obtained as part of a complete radiographic study of the heart and lungs. To obtain a lateral film, the patient is upright, the film cassette is placed on one side of the patient—typically the patient's left side—and the beam is directed from the other side of the patient. The lateral film is labeled according to the side of the patient that is nearest the x-ray tube. If the patient's left side is against the film cassette and the right side is nearest the x-ray tube, the resultant film is a right lateral film. Conversely, if the patient's right side is nearest the film cassette and left side is nearest the x-ray tube, the film is a left lateral film.[22]

Lateral views allow evaluation of the AP relationships of body structures, but they do not allow determination of their lateral relationships. Therefore, the comparison and evaluation of both a PA and a lateral film provide much more information than either film does separately. An additional advantage of obtaining radiographs in two views is that thin structures (such as fissures) may be visible on only one film if the x-ray beam strikes the structure parallel to its long axis.[9,24] When films of the same object are obtained using two different views, there is a greater chance that small structures will be apparent on one of the views.

A lateral decubitus view is obtained with the patient lying on one side or the other. The film cassette is placed at the patient's back, and the x-ray beam is then aimed horizontally or parallel to the floor.[9] A lateral decubitus view can be obtained in the critical care unit, and it is often helpful in determining the presence of air-fluid levels in the chest, such as those seen when a lung abscess or pleural effusion is present. Positioning has a significant influence on the appearance of air, fluid, and blood vessels within the chest.

INTERPRETATION OF FILM TECHNIQUE

Patient Position and View

The evaluation of a chest radiograph requires knowledge of the exposure conditions of the film, the angle of the x-ray beam, and the alignment and position of the patient. If the

x-ray tube is positioned close to the film and the patient, the x-ray image of the patient will be magnified. Conversely, if the x-ray tube is farther away from the film and the patient, the image of the patient will be smaller but sharper. The x-ray tube should be positioned so that the x-ray beam is exactly perpendicular to the plane of the film. If the patient is positioned properly, the x-ray beam will be perpendicular to the horizontal or vertical axis of the patient. If the x-ray beam or patient is slanted, and not perpendicular, a lordotic (oblique) view will be obtained and will show the body or chest at an angle. An oblique view is undesirable if it is obtained unintentionally, because structures farthest from the beam will be shortened while those closest to the beam will be enlarged.[22] The child's nurse should assist the radiology technologist in ensuring that the child is not rotated during exposure of the image. This can reduce the need for additional radiographs, with the associated increase in radiation to the child.

In a lordotic film, the clavicles are projected higher than normal and may be seen to lie above the lung apices, and the ribs appear more horizontal. In addition, it may cause hazy opacification at the lung bases as a result of overlapping soft tissues with magnification of the heart and mediastinum. If the apices of the lungs are not visible above the clavicles on an AP or a PA chest film, a lordotic view has been obtained, and this must be considered when evaluation of lung size and chest expansion is made.[17]

The alignment and the position of the patient at the time the film is taken also must be considered (Fig. 10-1). To determine whether a patient was positioned appropriately during the radiograph exposure, several structures should be evaluated. This evaluation includes the position of the trachea,

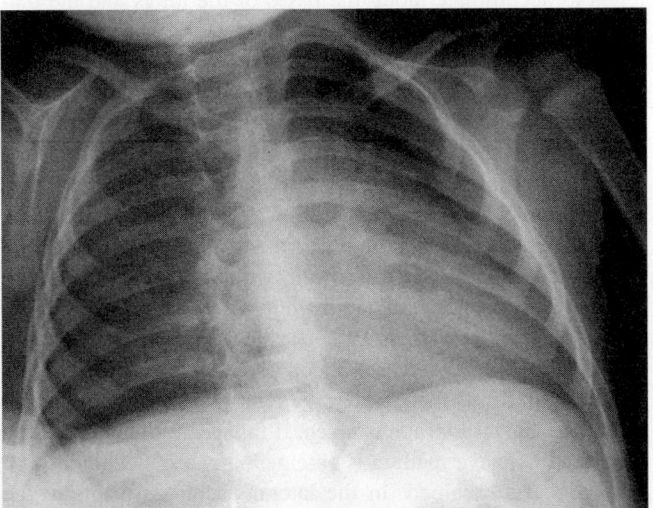

FIG. 10-1 In this chest radiograph the child is rotated to the left. Compared with Fig. 10-2, A, which demonstrates evidence of proper positioning, in this film the proximal ends of the clavicles are not symmetrical in appearance. The patient's left clavicle appears larger. The ribs on the patient's right side are more curved posteriorly, and ribs in the patient's left chest are more elongated with greater visualization of the anterior ribs. The cardiac silhouette is more prominent in the left chest with a normal cardiothoracic ratio, but the heart shape is altered by the rotated view.

curvature of the spine, position of the clavicles, length and symmetry of the ribs, and cardiac landmarks. If the patient is positioned straight and not rotated on the image, the trachea should project in the midline within the upper third of the chest. The spine should be straight with the intervertebral bodies outlined as separate from the disc spaces. With good alignment, the clavicles are of equal size and length. The medial ends of the clavicles should be equidistant from the thoracic spinous processes; they are normally projected over the lung apices and overlap the anterior first ribs. If the clavicles both appear horizontal and of equal size and length, a true AP or PA view was obtained.[14] If, on the other hand, one clavicle appears to be smaller than the other (because it was farther away from the x-ray tube at the time the film was taken), or if one clavicle is at a different angle than the other, the patient was probably rotated, and an oblique view of chest structures appears on the radiograph, creating the appearance that one side of the chest image (and one clavicle) is larger than the other. As noted previously, if the apices of the lungs are not visible above the clavicles on an AP or a PA chest film, a lordotic view has been obtained.[17]

It is important to consider patient alignment when making any observations about heart size. If the patient is rotated, the oblique image changes the heart shape and distorts the image, causing a spurious increase in cardiac size.

When the chest film is obtained, the radiology technologist and the nurse must be sure to note the position of the patient, whether upright (sitting or standing) or supine. The patient's position is important because gravity will influence the appearance, position, and location of any free air or fluid in the chest. Free pleural fluid (such as that accumulating as a result of a hemothorax, chylothorax, or pleural effusion) will assume a dependent position. If the child is upright, free fluid tends to accumulate along the bases of the lungs and the diaphragm, and it will appear as a dense opacification obscuring adjacent structures. The fluid usually reaches a higher point along the lateral chest wall than along the mediastinum, which is referred to as the *meniscus sign*. If the film is taken with the child supine, free pleural fluid will accumulate in the back of the child's pleural cavity, posterior to the lungs, and produce a more diffuse opacification throughout the affected hemithorax. Vascular markings are usually visible within the lung situated anterior to the fluid, which on an AP film can make this fluid difficult to distinguish from intrapulmonary congestion.

To determine the presence, quantity, and location of free intrapleural fluid, the child should be placed upright before and while the radiograph is taken. If this position is impossible or an inconclusive reading is obtained, a lateral decubitus film often will be obtained. In the lateral decubitus position, the patient is positioned with the affected side down, and any free fluid will accumulate in the dependent portion of the lateral pleural space.

Air tends to rise to the highest point within the chest cavity. As a result, in an upright view, free pleural air (such as a pneumothorax) will rise toward the apex of the lung. On a supine film, the highest point in the chest lies adjacent to the heart and mediastinum. When the child is supine for an AP film, free pleural air usually is seen along the diaphragm or the

sides of the lung fields. Free air will typically cause increased lucency at these points, often with no lung edges or lung vascular markings visible.[9,14] If free air is suggested on a supine view, it can be confirmed by a decubitus view. When the child is positioned on the dependent side opposite to the free air, any air in the pleural cavity will rise to lie along the lateral chest wall.[17]

Ideally, chest radiographs should be obtained with the child in the upright position. In this position, air and fluid levels are more readily identified. In addition, when the child is upright, diaphragm excursion is usually better, enabling the child to inspire more deeply so that a better inspiratory film is obtained.

Film Technique

The exposure of the chest film will affect the intensity of the images on the chest radiograph. With the correct exposure, the spinous process of the lower thoracic vertebral bodies should be just visible through the cardiac shadow. If the radiograph is penetrated appropriately, the vertebral bodies will be clear and well delineated behind the heart, and disc spaces will be visible between the vertebral bodies. In addition, some pulmonary vascular markings will be projected over the heart shadow, because they are present behind the heart.

When the exposure of the film is not correct, the change in exposure will affect the entire film appearance. If the chest radiograph is underpenetrated (underexposed), all the structures on the radiograph will appear lighter in appearance or diffusely opaque (i.e., too white). The resulting images are difficult to interpret, preventing a detailed view of the mediastinal, retrocardiac, and spinal anatomy. Pathologic findings in the left lower lobe can be missed easily.[27] In addition, pulmonary vascular markings will appear to be more prominent, with less distinct borders; thus, they may be mistakenly interpreted to be increased or hazy resulting from interstitial edema. If a film is overpenetrated (overexposed), all the images on the radiograph will be darker or diffusely lucent. The lungs will appear blacker than usual. Overpenetration can obliterate shadows and can make pulmonary vascular markings appear to be reduced.[16]

Unless other orders are specifically given, chest radiographs should be obtained during inspiration. This practice maximizes the size of the lung fields, allows detection of intrapulmonary abnormalities, and makes the cardiac image sharp. To determine whether the radiograph was obtained during inspiration or exhalation, the nurse should count ribs visible above the diaphragm and evaluate rib interspaces. With good inspiration and chest expansion, the domes of the hemidiaphragm are forced down to the ninth or tenth ribs posteriorly. In addition, the normal trachea should appear to be straight. If fewer than nine ribs are visible above the diaphragm, the child probably was exhaling while the film was taken.

If the film is obtained during expiration, the heart will appear larger and less well defined. The lung fields will appear to be hazier and the pulmonary vascular markings more prominent. Hypoinflation of the lung fields can lead to misinterpretation of the images and misdiagnosis of a basilar pneumonia or cardiomegaly. Furthermore, if maximal inspiration is not present, the lungs can appear more congested and the trachea

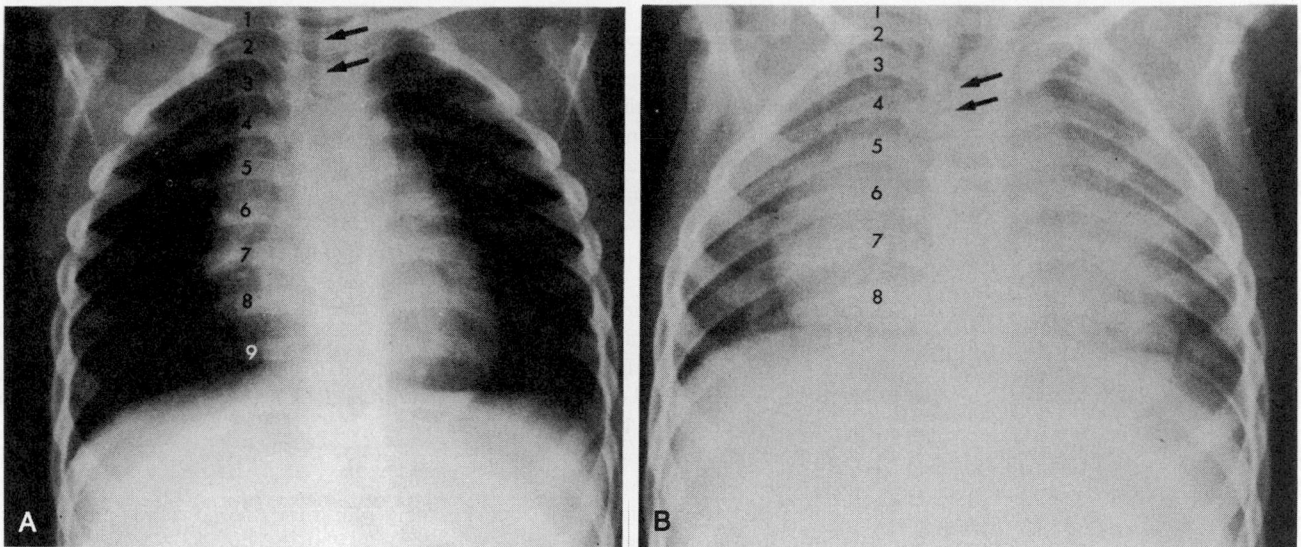

FIG. 10-2 Inspiratory and expiratory chest radiograph. Normal chest films obtained from the same child during inspiration and expiration. **A,** Inspiratory phase. Nine ribs can be counted above the diaphragm, indicating good inspiration. Alignment is good (note similarity of clavicles). Penetration of film is good (all vertebral bodies are visible; some pulmonary vascular markings can be seen). Intercostal spaces are equal; both sides of the diaphragm are visible. The mediastinum and trachea are straight *(arrows)*. Heart borders are sharply defined, and heart size is normal. Pulmonary vascular markings are visible in the proximal two thirds of lung fields (normal). **B,** Expiratory phase. Only eight ribs are visible above the diaphragm (see numbers on ribs), indicating inadequate lung expansion. Alignment is good. Penetration of film is good. Intercostal spaces are narrow because expiration is occurring. Both sides of the diaphragm are hazy, and the left hemidiaphragm is not readily identifiable. The mediastinum appears widened, and the trachea seems to buckle to the right (arrows). Heart appears much larger than in A, and the heart borders are obliterated, but this is caused by expiration and reduction in apparent lung volume. Silhouette sign appears to be present, cardiothoracic size calculated from this view would be large, and pulmonary vascular markings appear prominent, but these are all artifacts caused by expiration. (Courtesy H. Rex Gardner, Rush Presbyterian Saint Luke's Hospital, Chicago, IL.)

will appear to buckle to the right.[21,24] Figure 10-2 illustrates these differences with two views obtained from a normal child during inspiration and expiration.

The child must not move while the film is taken because motion can blur cardiothoracic structures. Blurring of the diaphragm can mimic the appearance of pulmonary infiltrates.[19] If the nurse or radiology technologist suspects that the child moved when the film was taken, this should be noted for consideration when the film is interpreted. If excessive motion artifact is present, another film should be obtained.

Not all opacities on chest films originate in the lungs. Common artifacts that appear on chest radiographs include electrocardiogram leads, jewelry, snaps, ventilator or oxygen tubing, intravenous catheter lines, and wire sutures. When possible, before the chest film is taken, remove any external metal objects or extraneous items that can cause artifacts on the radiograph. Occasionally, long hair, wrinkles in clothing, or skin folds produce artifacts that resemble pulmonary infiltrates, air-fluid interface, or pneumothorax.

INTERPRETATION OF CHEST RADIOGRAPH

It is good practice to develop a routine for reviewing chest radiographs. The first step is to verify that the chest radiograph is the correct film from the correct patient. Verify the patient's name, date of birth, hospital number, and sex. Next, ensure

that the correct film is being reviewed by verifying the date and time that it was taken. Last, confirm that the image is actually the type and view of image to be reviewed: AP, lateral decubitus, or other image type. Examine the film for technical qualities, as described previously. Include verification of the side marker, indicating left or right side of the patient, in addition to supine or lateral view.

Systematic Approach

When an organized systematic approach is used to examine the radiographic image, the nurse will be less likely to overlook significant abnormalities. It is often advisable to initially ignore the most striking or obvious features of a radiograph to avoid overlooking other equally important features. Table 10-1 provides one method of organizing the review of a chest film. Because there are many correct sequences that can be used to interpret the film, the nurse must develop an individual, comfortable style. The most important thing about any approach is that it must include all aspects of the film review. Once a healthcare provider develops a systematic and comprehensive approach to reviewing a film, the provider should use this method every time to ensure that nothing is missed during the review.

Current films should not be reviewed in isolation. They are most valuable when compared with the patient's previous films to better appreciate changes. With the advent of the

Table 10-1 An Organized Approach to Chest Radiograph Examination

Focus of Examination	Aspects of Examination
Technique	1. Check alignment and position (check clavicles) 2. Check degree of inspiration (9 to10 ribs should be visible with full inspiration) 3. Check penetration (vertebral bodies should be easily visualized)
Soft tissues of chest and neck	1. Check for subcutaneous emphysema 2. Examine extrathoracic structures
Bony thorax and intercostal spaces	1. Examine clavicles, scapula, ribs, humeri, and cervical and thoracic vertebrae 2. Check for fractures 3. Evaluate width of intercostal spaces (should be equal)
Diaphragm and area below diaphragm	1. Note clarity of diaphragm and location (check for elevation) 2. Check for location of gastric bubble (normal: patient's left)
Pleura and Costophrenic angles	1. Check for presence of fluid or air between pleural layers (look between bony thorax and lung) 2. Costophrenic angle should be sharp
Mediastinum	1. Borders should be sharp 2. Check for lateral shift
Trachea	1. Should be straight (may buckle to left on expiratory film if right aortic arch is present) 2. Check for narrowing or deviation
Heart and great vessels	1. Borders of heart and aorta should be distinct 2. Obliteration of heart borders is called silhouette sign (see Table 10-2) 3. Measure cardiothoracic ratio—normally approximately 0.5 for children and adults (half the width of the chest)
Lung fields	1. Compare right with left 2. Note presence and location of any opacification; describe it 3. Look for air-fluid levels
Hili and pulmonary vascularity	1. Pulmonary vascularity is most prominent at hili 2. Peripheral pulmonary vascular markings usually are visible in proximal two thirds of lung fields (note if markings are increased or decreased) 3. Prominent but hazy pulmonary vascular markings may result from pulmonary edema or pulmonary venous congestion
Check location and continuity of all tubes, catheters and wires	1. Note position of head when evaluating endotracheal tube position 2. Tip of endotracheal tube should be at level of third rib (1-2 cm above carina)
Compare with previous films	

PACS, previous images are readily available for review and comparison with recent images. PACS allows for the sequential review of older images and can also allow for side-by-side comparison with the most recent image.

After review of the technical aspects of the chest film, the nurse can begin examination of the structures outlined by the radiograph. In this chapter, emphasis is placed on examination of the AP chest film because this is the projection most frequently obtained in the critical care setting.

Soft Tissues and Bony Thorax

Examine the soft tissues of the chest wall for evidence of subcutaneous emphysema (air density between the skin and bony thorax), which can result from an air leak around the chest tube or from a penetrating chest wound. In addition, tissue swelling can indicate the presence of an injury. Check the soft tissues of the neck for subcutaneous emphysema. In addition, if the child is intubated, note the position of the child's head, because flexion or extension of the head can change the position of the tip of the endotracheal (ET) tube.[15]

Examine the bony thorax and the shape of the chest. Infants and young children normally have round chests with a horizontal orientation of their ribs (see Fig. 10-2). However, older children and adults have chests that are wider than they are

deep, and their ribs angle downward from back to front. A round chest in an older child or adult is abnormal and may be the result of chronic respiratory disease with air trapping. As discussed, nine or ten ribs should appear above the dome of the diaphragm if a good inspiratory film has been obtained.

Check the continuity of vertebrae, ribs, scapulas, and clavicles for fractures and bony destruction. The ribs and intercostal spaces should be symmetrical. A fracture often will create a dark line in the bone because of separation of the bone fragments (Fig. 10-3). The vertebral bodies, particularly the cervical vertebrae, should be checked closely for fractures if the child has been admitted following trauma. The presence of multiple rib fractures, especially both posterior and anterior, and in various stages of healing is pathognomonic (positive predictive value of 95% or higher in children 3 years of age and younger) for child abuse.[4] Healing fractures often have an enlarged area consisting of cartilage and woven bone creating a callus. Rib notching, or erosion of the underside of ribs caused by enlargement of the intercostal arteries, can be seen in older children with coarctation of the aorta, because the intercostal arteries become enlarged to carry collateral circulation around the area of coarctation into the descending aorta. Abnormalities of the ribs may be noted if the child has had surgery to alter the size or shape of the rib cage. Splinting

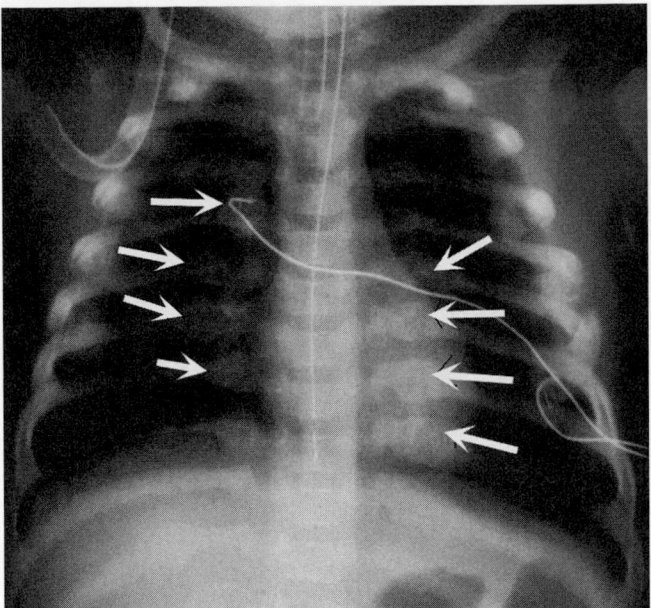

FIG. 10-3 Rib fractures. This chest radiograph of an 18-month-old girl was obtained as part of a series of films to evaluate for evidence of injuries caused by inflicted trauma. The child was admitted to the pediatric critical care unit with altered mental status, subdural hemorrhages, bilateral retinal hemorrhages, and areas of ecchymosis in various stages of healing. There are multiple healing rib fractures of different ages bilaterally, both medially and laterally (some indicated by the *arrows*) with no previous physician visits for trauma and no explanation for the injuries. Note the position of the tip of the nasogastric tube in the distal esophagus.

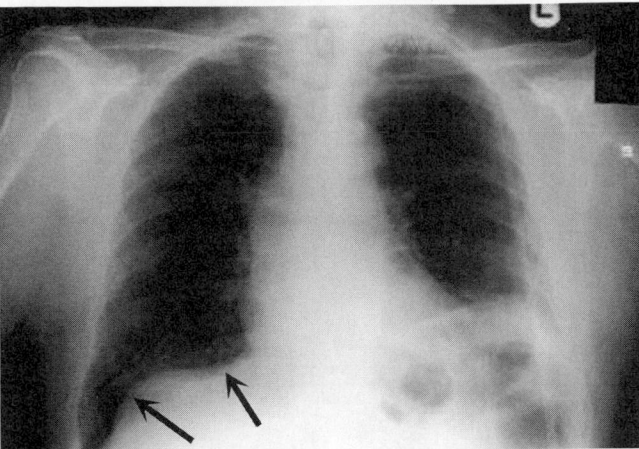

FIG. 10-4 Paralyzed left diaphragm. This patient has congenital paralysis of the left hemidiaphragm. This chest radiograph reveals significant elevation of the left hemidiaphragm. Note the presence of air filled bowel loops under the left hemidiaphragm. The right hemidiaphragm (*arrows*) is flattened with some hyperexpansion of the lung. The number of the ribs visible in the right and left lung fields may be counted to compare the relative lung expansion bilaterally. Note that diaphragm asymmetry may be masked during positive pressure ventilation.

can produce narrowing of the intercostal spaces on one side of the chest.

If the child has undergone previous cardiothoracic surgery, sternal wires or clips may be noted or the appearance of the ribs may be altered. Significant deformities of the chest wall (e.g., pectus excavatum) can alter the location and appearance of the cardiac silhouette.

Evaluate the width of the intercostal spaces. Following a thoracotomy, muscle spasm or sutures can reduce the width of the intercostal space at and near the site of surgery. In addition, significant atelectasis can cause narrowing of the intercostal spaces on the involved side and widening of the spaces on the noninvolved side.[9,14] Hyperinflation, associated with air trapping, will cause widening of the intercostal spaces bilaterally.

Diaphragm and Abdomen

Examine the position and appearance of the diaphragms, including the shape, height, and angles. The patient's right hemidiaphragm is usually approximately 1 to 3 cm higher than the left hemidiaphragm because the liver lies under the right diaphragm. The diaphragms should appear smooth and domed, with sharply defined costophrenic angles (the angle produced by the lateral downward curve of each hemidiaphragm at its periphery). Unilateral elevation of the diaphragm may be caused by diaphragm paralysis; this may be congenital in origin or result from chest trauma or injury to the phrenic nerve during thoracic surgery (Fig. 10-4). The elevation occurs during spontaneous inspiration, but will not occur during positive

pressure inspiration. Atelectasis and abdominal organ distension are additional potential causes of unilateral elevation of the diaphragm. Bilateral elevation of the diaphragm may be observed in the child with hypoventilation, abdominal distension, ascites, intraabdominal mass, or obesity.

If the clear silhouette between the air density of the lungs and the tissue density of the diaphragm is obscured, it is usually caused by basilar atelectasis or accumulation of free pleural fluid along the diaphragm (Fig. 10-5). The accumulation of subpulmonic fluid can create an appearance similar to that produced by an elevated diaphragm if an AP film is taken with the patient upright. The free fluid will be readily apparent, however, when a lateral decubitus film is taken.

The diaphragm can appear to be unusually flat and depressed in any condition that increases the volume of the lung or the contents of the hemithorax. The patient's diaphragm will be unilaterally flattened and displaced downward if the child has a significant unilateral (tension) pneumothorax or if the child has unilateral lung disease and hyperexpansion of one lung (see Fig. 10-4, noting the appearance of the child's right hemidiaphragm).[22]

After evaluation of the diaphragm, examine the structures below the diaphragm. There is usually some air in the child's stomach—in fact, the absence of gastric air in the neonate is one of the pathognomonic radiographic signs of esophageal atresia.[20] The gastric bubble should appear under the patient's left hemidiaphragm. If the gastric bubble is present under the patient's right hemidiaphragm, situs inversus is present (i.e., the abdominal organs are transposed). The bedside nurse should be aware if the child has situs inversus, because this will affect subsequent assessments such as location for auscultation as part of the process of checking placement of the nasogastric tube or palpation of the liver for evidence of hepatomegaly. In addition, situs inversus can be associated with cardiac malpositions, congenital heart defects, or asplenia

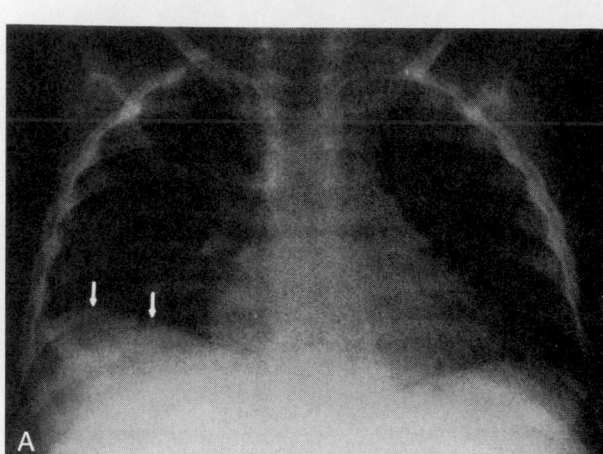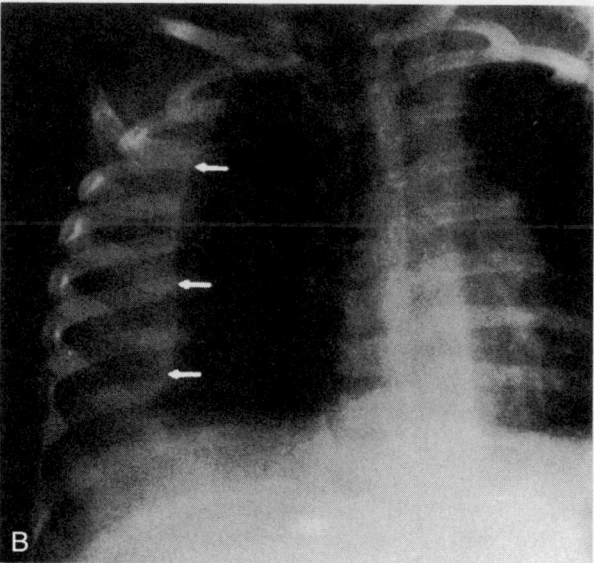

FIG. 10-5 Pleural effusion. These films were obtained when this 3-year-old child developed tachypnea and increased respiratory effort several days after repair of a double-outlet right ventricle. The nurse noted a significant decrease in breath sounds over the right lung fields, particularly the right middle and lower lobes. The right lung fields were dull to percussion. The radiograph was ordered to differentiate between atelectasis and pleural effusion. **A,** The upright anteroposterior film. Despite an apparently good inspiratory film, the right lung field is smaller than the left. This finding could indicate elevation of the diaphragm as a result of atelectasis. It also could represent free pleural fluid accumulation along the diaphragm. The hilar pulmonary vascular markings are somewhat hazy; this is consistent with either atelectasis or compression of the right lung by subpulmonic fluid. The right costophrenic angle is blunted, so the diagnosis of pleural effusion was favored and a decubitus film was ordered to confirm the diagnosis. **B,** The decubitus film. The film was taken with the child lying on his right side so that the free right pleural fluid accumulated along that side. The fluid level is easily discerned *(arrows)*. (Courtesy Andrew K. Poznanski, Children's Memorial Hospital, Chicago, IL.)

(see Chapter 8).[13,23,24] Normally, there should be no free air in the peritoneal cavity although air is usually present in the child's stomach, intestines, and colon.[19]

The newborn with diaphragmatic hernia may demonstrate severe respiratory distress. The chest radiograph reveals multiple abnormal air lucencies within the chest, usually the left hemithorax. This air is caused by the presence of loops of air-filled bowel in the chest (Fig. 10-6). The bowel compresses the lung on the involved side and shifts the mediastinum to the non-involved (usually right) hemithorax, compressing that lung. Until the bowel fills with swallowed air, the newborn with a diaphragmatic hernia may be thought to have a mass in the left chest.

Pleura and Costophrenic Angles

The pleura consist of a double-layered serous membrane; the parietal pleura lines the inside of the thoracic cavity, and the visceral pleura adheres to the outside of the lung. The space between these two layers (the pleural cavity or space) is normally collapsed so that the two layers cast only a thin, white shadow on the radiograph.[22] However, if fluid (hemothorax, effusion) or air (pneumothorax) accumulates in the pleural space, an air-fluid interface or a fluid density may be observed between the bony thorax and the lung. The pleura will cast a thicker white shadow on the radiograph if the pleura thickens as the result of pleural reaction (e.g., following surgery or other irritation). The fluid shadow created by pleural thickening or a loculated pleural effusion will not change when the patient changes position.

When examining the pleura, it is important to follow it and any visible pleural space around the entire margin of each lung. Because free pleural fluid tends to accumulate in dependent portions of the chest, fluid may be noted along the diaphragm in an upright film and behind the lungs in a supine film. On an upright film, small collections of fluid can obscure the costophrenic angle, and more significant collections of fluid tend to obscure the diaphragm and make it appear elevated (see Fig. 10-5, A).[9,14]

On a supine film, free pleural fluid may appear to opacify the lung fields, often making it difficult to distinguish from pulmonary congestion.[9] In this case an upright or lateral decubitus film is usually obtained (see Fig. 10-5, B).

The lungs are divided into lobes by fissures; the right lung has three lobes and the left lung has two lobes. The oblique or major fissures, separating the upper from the lower lobes, are not usually seen on a chest radiograph because they face toward the x-ray beam on AP view. Fluid accumulation in the major fissure is best seen on a lateral film. The minor fissure in the right lung separates the right upper and right middle lobes, and it lies tangential to the beam in an AP view. Fluid can accumulate in the minor fissure; this fluid accumulation often can be observed on both AP and lateral films.[9,21]

A pneumothorax will produce an air-tissue interface in the pleural cavity because the pneumothorax contains only air with no pulmonary vascular markings, whereas the lung contains air, tissues, and vessels. The presence of a significant pneumothorax will cause partial or complete collapse of the

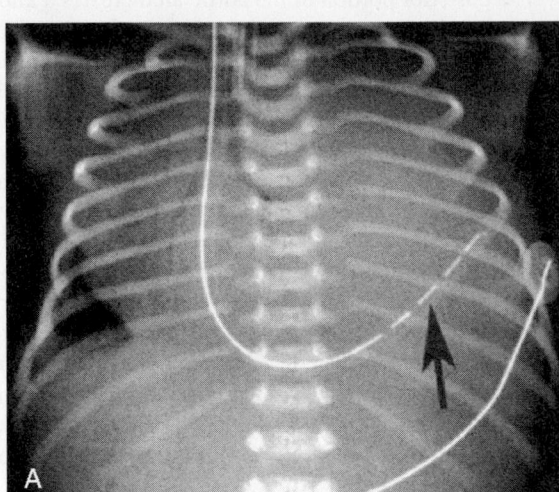
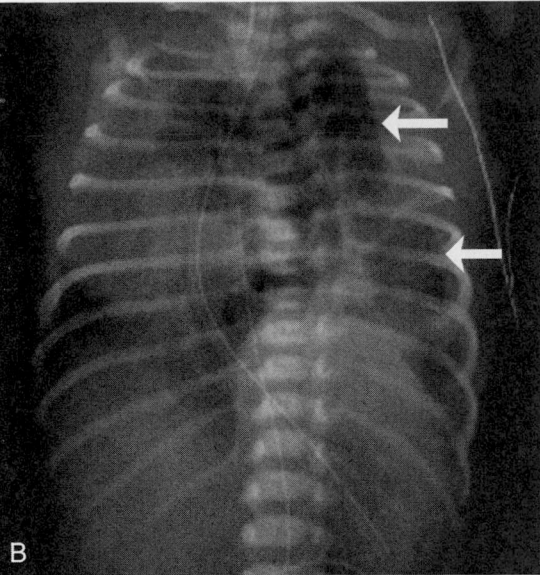

FIG. 10-6 Congenital diaphragmatic hernia. **A,** This chest radiograph was obtained to evaluate a newborn admitted within the first few hours of life to the pediatric critical care unit with respiratory distress and poor feeding. The nasogastric tube can be traced into the left chest *(arrow)*. The mediastinal structures are shifted to the right, and the dense opacity in the left hemithorax is due to the fluid filled stomach and loops of small bowel. There is no air in the stomach or small bowel. The newborn has a left congenital diaphragmatic hernia. **B,** This is a 2-day-old infant with a left congenital diaphragmatic hernia. There are multiple air-filled loops of bowel in the left hemithorax *(arrows),* with a marked shift of the mediastinum to the right. Note that in this case the nasogastric tube ends in the left upper quadrant of the abdomen, indicating that the stomach is in the abdomen and not in the chest. (B, Radiograph courtesy of Sharon Stein, Nashville, TN.)

adjacent (ipsilateral) lung. Note that free pleural air will accumulate in the highest portions of the chest so that the location of the air is influenced by the patient's position when the X-ray is obtained. In an upright film, free pleural air is typically observed above the apex of the lung, whereas in a supine film the air may accumulate along the anterior and lateral aspects of the lung and along the diaphragm (Fig. 10-7).

The costophrenic angle is a sharp angle formed bilaterally from the downward curve of the lateral diaphragm seen on an AP (or a PA) film. The bases of the lower lobe of each lung dip into this recess. Obliteration or blunting of this angle can occur with accumulation of relatively small amounts of free pleural fluid. The angle also can be blunted if pleural reaction or thickening is present.[22]

Mediastinum and Trachea

The mediastinum contains the trachea, the two main bronchi, the esophagus, the ascending aorta, the aortic arch (and major branches), the main pulmonary artery (and the proximal right and left pulmonary arteries), the major veins of the heart, the heart, and the thymus (Fig. 10-8). Because most of these structures contain fluid, the radiographic appearance of the mediastinum is that of a single fluid density between the lungs.

Children older than 6 years have mediastinal structures comparable to those of adults. The thymus shadow, seen in the upper third of the chest at the mediastinum, has bilateral lobes. The thymic silhouette blends almost imperceptibly with the cardiac silhouette, because it occupies contiguous space, giving the appearance of a widened mediastinum. It can

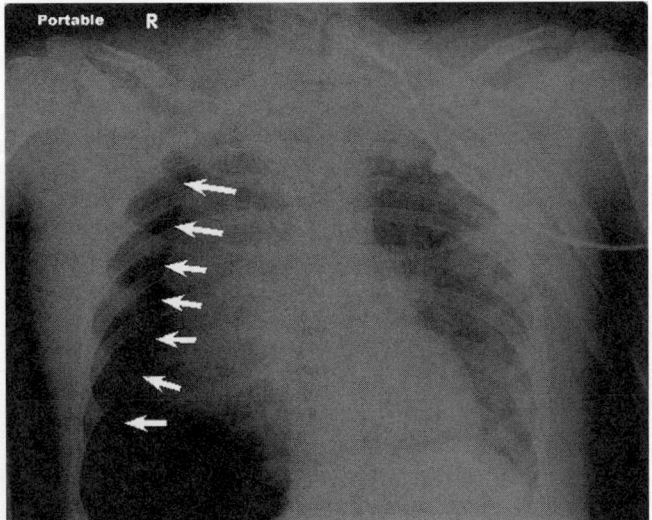

FIG. 10-7 Tension pneumothorax. This film was obtained as part of a routine daily chest radiograph to monitor for endotracheal tube placement in this 18-year-old male with methicillin-resistant *Staphylococcus aureus* necrotizing fascitis. This is a supine AP film that demonstrates near total atelectasis of the right lung. The pneumothorax is visible along the inferior and lateral aspects of the right chest, with a shift of the cardiac silhouette to the left. There is clear visualization of the lung-air interface *(arrows)* seen along the lateral and inferior margins of the right lung. This is a tension pneumothorax because the mediastinum is markedly shifted and the right hemidiaphragm is flattened out of the field of view.

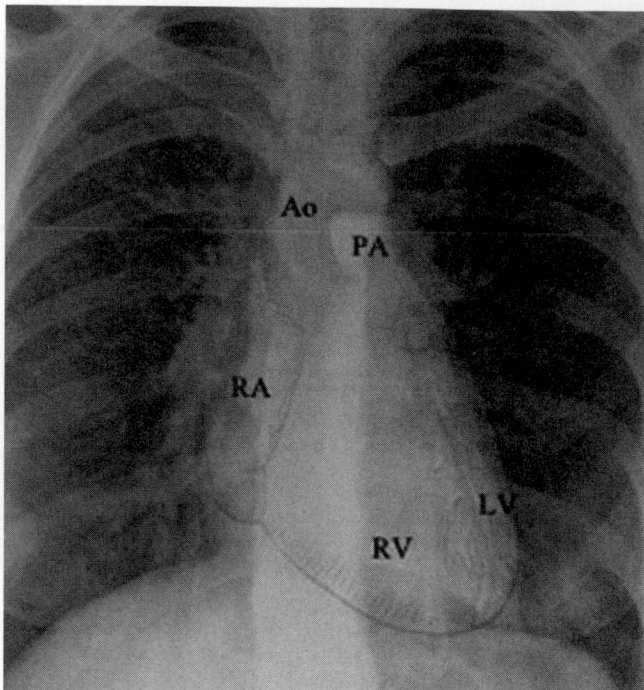

FIG. 10-8 Cardiac anatomy. This chest radiograph has a graphic overlay of the normal location and identification of the pulmonary artery, aorta, aortic knob, right atrium, right ventricle, and left ventricle as they are positioned in the mediastinum.

produce a triangular shadow, resembling the sail of a boat (called the *sail sign*). The thymus is most often visualized on the chest radiograph from birth to 2 years of age, but may persist up to 5 years of age[6,16,17,25] (Fig. 10-9).

The trachea should be straight, and often it is located slightly to the right of the patient's midline. Because the trachea contains air, a dark vertical radiolucent column identifies its position within the mediastinum (see Fig. 10-2). The posterior portion of the aortic arch creates a knob or curve that usually is seen just to the left of the patient's spine. If the aorta arches to the right instead of to the left, the aortic knob can be superimposed on the shadow of the patient's spine on the AP projection, and the trachea is displaced to the patient's left. The incidence of congenital heart disease is higher in patients with a right aortic arch, although a right aortic arch can be seen in otherwise healthy patients.[11,21]

The aortic knob and the trachea will be displaced if a mediastinal shift occurs. When significant atelectasis is present, the trachea and aortic knob usually are displaced toward the area of collapse, because of the volume loss associated with the atelectasis.[22] However, if a large pleural effusion or pneumothorax is present, the trachea and aortic knob typically will be displaced away from the involved lung and toward the unaffected side, because these problems represent volume gain in the chest (Fig. 10-10).

The trachea is identified by a straight vertical air density typically just to the right of the patient's midline. As noted previously, it may appear to buckle to the right on an expiratory film, or it may be displaced toward an area of atelectasis or away from a pneumothorax or pneumomediastinum (see Fig. 10-10). The trachea bifurcates into the right and left mainstem bronchus at approximately the level of the patient's fourth rib. The carina, a portion of the lowest tracheal ridge, is located at the bifurcation of the trachea and is used as a landmark in radiographic assessment of tracheal tube placement. In adults, the angle of branching of the left main bronchus is normally lower than the angle of branching of the right main bronchus. The right main bronchus typically branches off higher with a sharper angle. For this reason, aspirated substances frequently enter the right bronchial tree.[21]

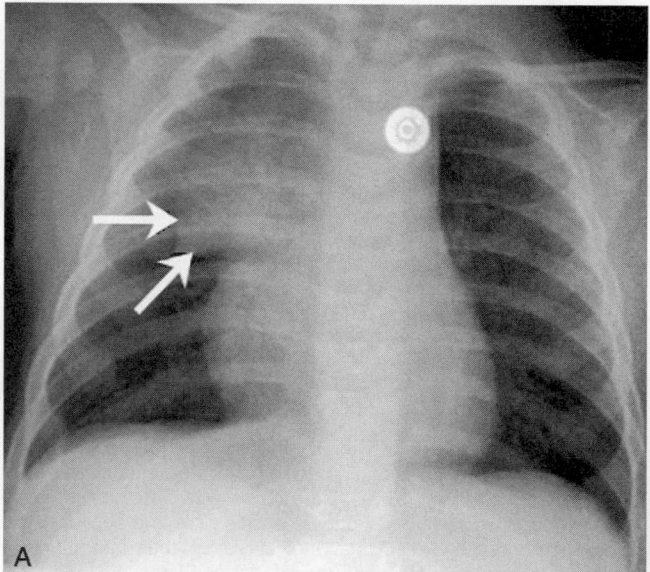

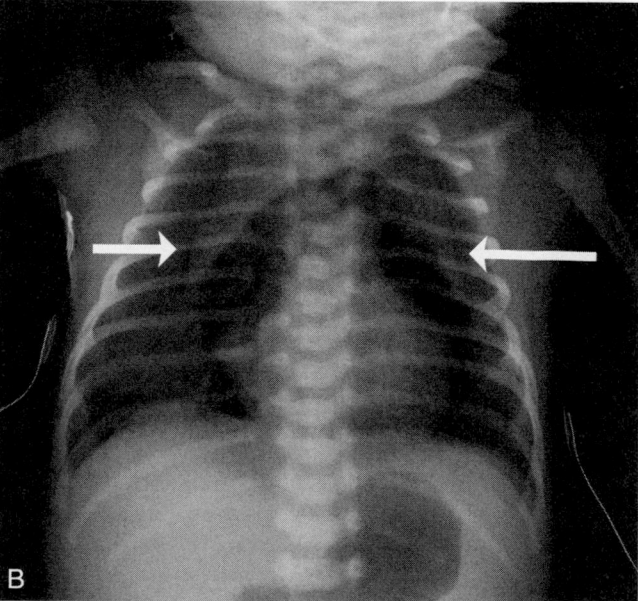

FIG. 10-9 Normal thymus. **A,** This supine anteroposterior film demonstrates the right lobe of the thymus projecting over the right upper lung field, creating the appearance of a widened mediastinum. The triangular shape *(arrows)* is the classic appearance of the sail sign (the right lobe of the thymus forms a triangular shape characteristic of the sail of a boat). **B,** This infant has a pneumomediastinum that has elevated the right and left lobes of the thymus *(arrows)* off the heart. (B, Courtesy Sharon Stein, Nashville, TN.)

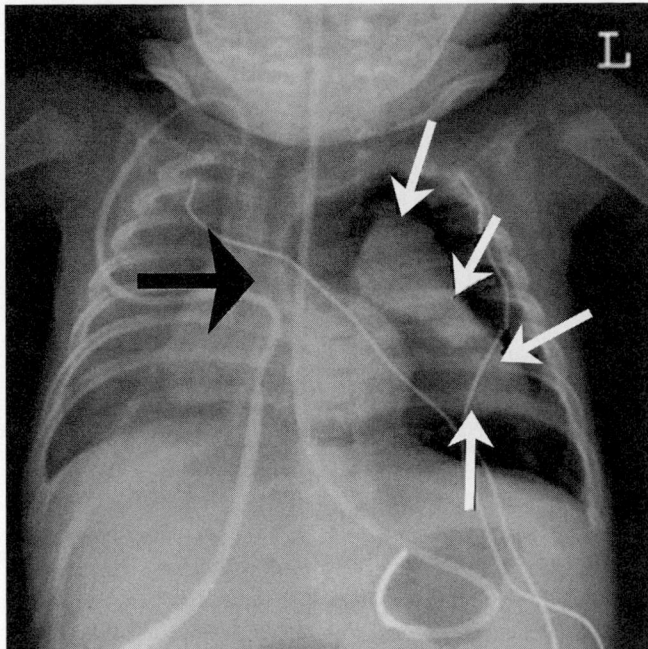

FIG. **10-10** Tension pneumothorax. This 5 month old with complex congenital heart disease was noted by the nurse to have respiratory distress, including tachypnea and nasal flaring. The nurse also noted decreased breath sounds and chest expansion in the left chest and tracheal deviation to the right. This supine anteroposterior film was obtained and demonstrated a left-sided tension pneumothorax *(white arrows)*. The trachea *(black arrow)* and aortic knob are displaced away from the involved left hemithorax and toward the unaffected right side because of the increased volume associated with the pneumothorax.

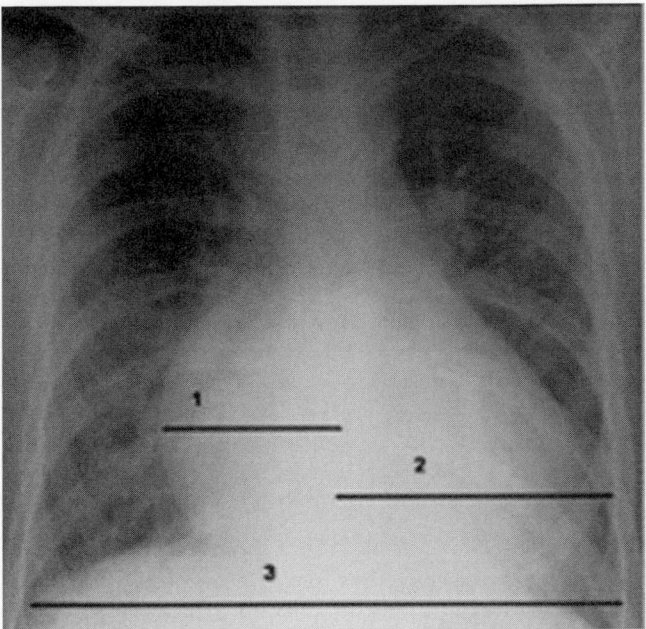

FIG. **10-11** Cardiothoracic ratio measurement. This chest film demonstrates the proper measurement of the cardiac silhouette on the right (from midline to widest point; line 1) and left side (from midline to widest point; line 2) and the inner diameter of the chest (line 3). The added width of the right and left side widest measurement divided by the widest point of the inner diameter of the chest is used to calculate the cardiothoracic ratio.

The left hilum is normally higher than the right because the left side is elevated by the heart. Normal heart position extends approximately two thirds to the left of the midline in the chest. The center of the heart lies under the lower third of the sternum.[10,18] If the child has dextrocardia or dextroversion, the heart will be located in the center of the chest or in the right chest, and additional congenital heart lesions are likely to be present.[21,23] The cardiac shadow on the AP film is created largely by the shadow of the superior vena cava, the right atrium, the aortic knob, the main pulmonary artery, the left pulmonary artery, and the left ventricle.[21] The right ventricle and left atrium normally do not contribute to the margin of the heart shadow in the AP or PA view.

Heart and Great Vessels

The size of the heart is quantified on AP or PA view by calculation of a ratio of the width of the heart to the width of the thorax, called the *cardiothoracic ratio*. To obtain the cardiothoracic ratio, the heart is measured between vertical lines drawn at its widest margins (from the center) on the right and left, and the chest is measured at the costophrenic angles on the inside of the rib cage (Fig. 10-11).

Beyond the newborn period, the heart's width does not normally exceed half the width of the thorax. The cardiothoracic ratio in newborns is normally up to 0.55. In older infants and children up to 6 years of age, a ratio of 0.45 is normal. Between 6 and 12 years of age, a cardiothoracic ratio of up to 0.44 is normal.[21] A convenient rule is that the cardiothoracic ratio in children is normally 0.5, plus or minus 5% to 6%, and it is typically larger in neonates and smaller in older children. An increase in the cardiothoracic ratio suggests the possibility of cardiomegaly. However, a poor inspiratory film and AP (compared with PA) chest radiographs will affect the accuracy of the cardiothoracic ratio.[7,16,17] For practice, calculate the cardiothoracic ratio in Fig. 10-2, A. The ratio is 0.52.

Cardiac enlargement can increase the cardiothoracic ratio. Note that cardiac chamber hypertrophy may not alter heart size appreciably, because the cardiac shadow is determined by the outer border of the heart chambers and is not influenced by the thickness of chamber walls. Cardiomegaly that is apparent on the radiograph is caused by an increase in cardiac chamber volume; thus, it is most often a result of cardiac dilation (Fig. 10-12).[14,21]

Right atrial enlargement will often cause displacement of the right heart border toward the patient's right side. The right atrial portion of the right heart margin also may appear to be more convex. Right ventricular enlargement can be difficult to discern from the AP film alone. When this ventricle enlarges, the rest of the heart is displaced posteriorly and cephalad (upward). Frequently, this enlargement increases the transverse diameter of the heart and pushes the cardiac apex outward and upward, like the upturned toe of a shoe or boot, although this is not an invariable radiologic finding.[14,21] Right ventricular enlargement can be discerned better from a lateral chest film, because the enlarged anterior right ventricle will fill the retrosternal space and rest against the sternum. In small infants, it may be difficult to differentiate between the retrosternal thymus and the retrosternal right ventricle.[14,21]

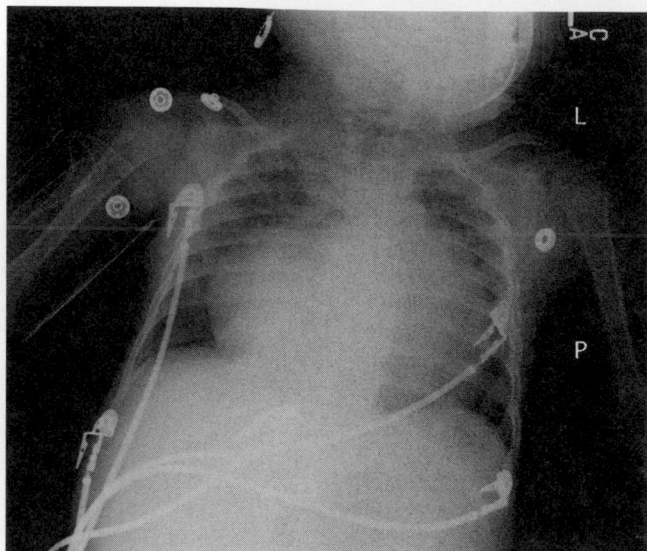

FIG. 10-12 Cardiomegaly. This supine anteroposterior film was obtained preoperatively for this 5-day-old female with a prenatal diagnosis of hypoplastic left heart syndrome. Note the markedly enlarged cardiac silhouette, with the cardiothoracic ratio in excess of 0.5 (it is nearly 0.85).

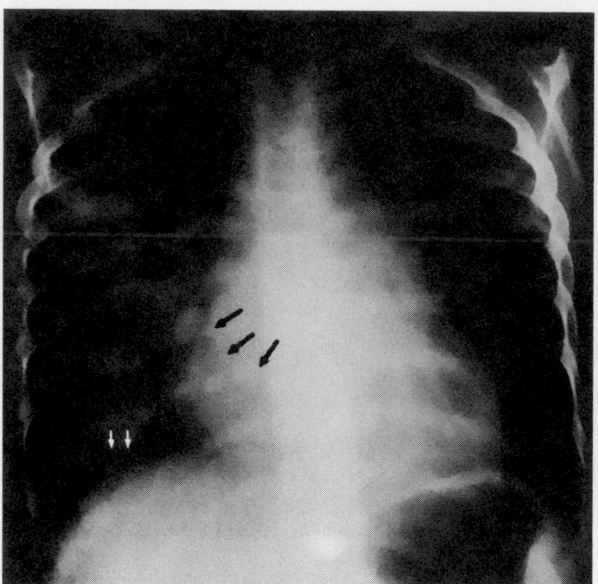

FIG. 10-13 Congestive heart failure with pulmonary edema. This 5-year-old boy with known mitral insufficiency was admitted to the critical care unit with tachypnea and increased respiratory effort. On physical examination, he demonstrated a heart rate of 137/min with a gallop rhythm. The respiratory rate was 54/min with moderate retractions. Breath sounds were adequate and equal bilaterally, and crackles were noted, particularly over the left lung fields. The child's liver was palpable 6 cm below the right costal margin. The child also had cardiomegaly (cardiothoracic ratio of 0.6). The double density seen within the heart (large arrows) is caused by the large left atrium. Pulmonary interstitial markings are prominent and hazy through both lung fields. Kerley B lines are noted in the base of the right lung (*small arrows*). (Courtesy Andrew K. Poznanski, Children's Memorial Hospital, Chicago, IL.)

Left atrial enlargement may be difficult to discern on a chest radiograph, because the left atrium normally does not form a distinct portion of the cardiac margin. With left atrial enlargement, the left heart border below the aortic knob may straighten or become convex instead of concave. In addition, the posterior enlargement of this chamber can elevate the left mainstem bronchus so that the angle of the tracheobronchial bifurcation is widened. A double density also may be observed in the center of the cardiac shadow[14,21] (Fig. 10-13).

Left ventricular enlargement generally increases the transverse diameter of the heart and extends the left heart border toward the left chest wall. Commonly, left ventricular enlargement will displace the cardiac apex downward and outward so that it rests on the diaphragm.[14,21]

After cardiovascular surgery, the mediastinum and cardiac silhouette may be enlarged as the result of bleeding or fluid accumulation around the site of surgery. If the cardiac silhouette widens dramatically in the presence of tachycardia, signs of pulmonary and systemic venous congestion, and decreased systemic perfusion, cardiac tamponade may be present.[22] However, it is important to note that the cardiac silhouette may remain small despite the presence of tamponade if the pericardial sac does not distend.

Cardiac enlargement often is seen when the child has congestive heart failure. Heart failure, often biventricular in children, can produce a global enlargement of all heart chambers.[14] Pulmonary vascular markings also will be indistinct (see Fig. 10-13).

The most reliable way to evaluate radiographic changes in heart size by is by comparison of the most recent film with several previous films made under the same conditions. In addition, the nurse should always correlate clinical assessment with radiographic findings.

The great vessels may be enlarged or reduced in size as the result of congenital heart defects. If the child has a thoracic coarctation of the aorta, a characteristic E configuration of the aortic silhouette may be seen, which is caused by the coarctation. The presence of coarctation of the aorta, patent ductus arteriosus, or aortic valvular stenosis may cause the aortic knob to be more prominent than usual.[11]

The child with an intracardiac left-to-right shunt or a patent ductus arteriosus may demonstrate a large and convex main pulmonary artery shadow on radiograph, because the pulmonary artery is enlarged by the increased pulmonary blood flow. Pulmonary valve stenosis can result in poststenotic dilation of the main pulmonary artery.

Some congenital heart defects, such as severe tetralogy of Fallot or pulmonary atresia, are associated with a small main pulmonary artery. With a small main pulmonary artery, a concavity of the upper portion of the left heart border may be observed, because an extremely small main pulmonary artery will not produce the normal convexity below the aortic knob. This abnormal concavity can make the mediastinum appear to be narrow, because the upper heart shadow is created only by the aorta instead of by the pulmonary artery and aorta. Many children with tetralogy of Fallot or pulmonary atresia have a right aortic arch, so that the aortic knob is located to the right of the patient's trachea. This condition will further decrease the fullness of the left heart border. If significant obstruction to pulmonary blood flow is present, pulmonary vascular markings may be diminished.[11,14,21]

| | Significance of the Silhouette Sign: |
| Table 10-2 | Obliteration of Cardiac Silhouette by Lung Opacification |

Obliterated Heart Border or Structure	Opacified Lung Segment
Upper portion of the right heart border and ascending aorta	Right upper lobe
Most of the right heart border	Right middle lobe
Right diaphragm	Right lower lobe
Aortic knob (and upper left heart border)	Left upper lobe
Most of left heart border	Superior and/or inferior left lingula
Left diaphragm	Left lower lobe

The borders of the heart and great vessels should be sharp. Because the cardiac silhouette is created by the contrast between the fluid density of the heart and the air density of the lung, obliteration of the sharp border between the lung and heart is associated with an abnormality where areas of these organs are normally in contact. This loss of a normal silhouette on a radiograph is referred to as the *silhouette sign*.[9,17] The silhouette sign helps determine the location of the abnormal finding within the chest. Obliteration of the heart border is typically caused by opacification (congestion or atelectasis) of portions of the lung that are in anatomic contact with the heart or great vessels. It also can occur as a result of pleural fluid accumulation, pneumonia, or a lung mass.

To determine the reason for the appearance of the silhouette sign, the nurse must know which areas of the lung are in direct contact with the heart or great vessels. These areas are summarized in Table 10-2. Obliteration of the margins of the upper portion of the right heart border and ascending aorta can occur as a result of opacification of the right upper lobe. Opacification of the right middle lobe can result in loss of most of the right side of the heart border. Because the right lower lobe is posterior and not in direct contact with the heart, opacification of the right lower lobe will overlap the heart border but will not obliterate it.

If the margin of the aortic knob is indistinct, it generally results from opacification of the left upper lobe. Atelectasis or pneumonia of the left lingula will obliterate most of the left side of the heart border. Because most of the left lower lobe is posterior and not in direct contact with the heart, left lower lobe opacification will overlap the heart but will not obliterate its silhouette.[9]

Lungs, Hili, and Pulmonary Vascularity

The lung fields on the chest radiograph are predominantly radiolucent. The soft tissues of the lung normally do not produce radiographic shadows, although some of the blood-filled arteries and veins will produce linear branching fluid density shadows. The right lung is larger than the left and normally is divided into the upper, middle, and lower lobes. Although the thin fissures between the lobes are not usually visible, the minor fissure occasionally is seen as a thin white line on

the chest film. The left lung is smaller because the left chest also contains the heart. The left lung normally contains two lobes, the left upper and left lower lobes. The left lung homologue of the right middle lobe is called the lingula.

The radiolucent lung fields should contain no significant opacifications, other than those created by pulmonary vasculature, or fluid levels. If the nurse notes an opacification, the nurse should describe and localize it.

The air-filled peripheral bronchi normally are not visible on the chest radiograph. Visualization of a bronchus is called an *air bronchogram*. A bronchus is visible only if it is surrounded by an intrapulmonary structure of water or of fluid density. It can be seen as the result of pneumonia, atelectasis, pulmonary edema, consolidation, infarction, or certain chronic pulmonary lesions.[9] In addition, an air bronchogram can be seen within the mediastinum in the radiographs of normal infants and young children, because portions of their lobar bronchi lie within the tissues of the mediastinum (Fig. 10-14). Although an air bronchogram is almost invariably associated with intrapulmonary disease in adults, it may be a normal finding in the mediastinum of infants and young children.[9,21]

The hili of the lungs contain the pulmonary artery and vein for each lung and the right and left main bronchi. Because the bronchi normally do not produce a radiographic shadow, the shadows of the right and left hili are produced by the right and left pulmonary arteries and veins and their major branches. In the majority of patients, the left hilum is slightly higher than the right hilum.[8,9,16,22,24,26] The hili may be

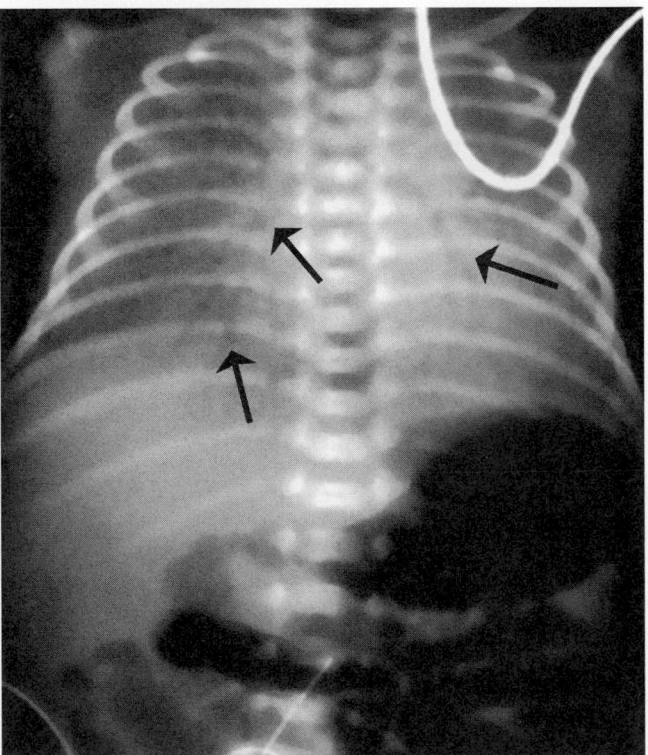

FIG. 10-14 Air bronchograms. This anteroposterior film of a neonate with respiratory distress syndrome demonstrates air bronchograms throughout both lung fields *(arrows)*. There are diffuse reticular granular pulmonary opacities. There is a large gastric bubble under the left diaphragm.

enlarged by congenital heart defects that produce increased pulmonary blood flow and pulmonary artery dilation, such as ventricular septal defect or patent ductus arteriosus. The hili also may be enlarged in the presence of pulmonary venous dilation associated with congestive heart failure or pulmonary venous obstruction. Often, both pulmonary arteries and veins are enlarged (e.g., when the child with a large ventricular septal defect develops congestive heart failure). Enlargement of the hili also may be caused by lymph node enlargement.

The hilum of a lung can be displaced toward an area of lung collapse or away from a significant pneumothorax or pleural effusion.[9] This shift is best appreciated by comparing the film showing suspected displacement with a previous film.

Pulmonary edema, pulmonary hemorrhage, overwhelming infection, aspiration pneumonitis, and pulmonary venous obstruction can cause perihilar opacities,[14] making the lung hili more radiopaque and hazy in appearance (Fig. 10-15). The surrounding lung tissue may be more radiopaque with a reticular appearance caused by interstitial edema. Occasionally, the lung fields are radiolucent, creating a dark halo around the hazy opacity of the hili.

Pulmonary edema, infectious pneumonitis, and pulmonary venous obstruction often produce diffuse changes that are bilaterally symmetrical. Aspiration pneumonitis and partial pulmonary venous obstruction can produce unilateral or localized opacifications. Rarely, pulmonary edema can be segmental.[14,21] Further evaluation of the pulmonary vascularity is made by examination of the peripheral pulmonary vascular markings.

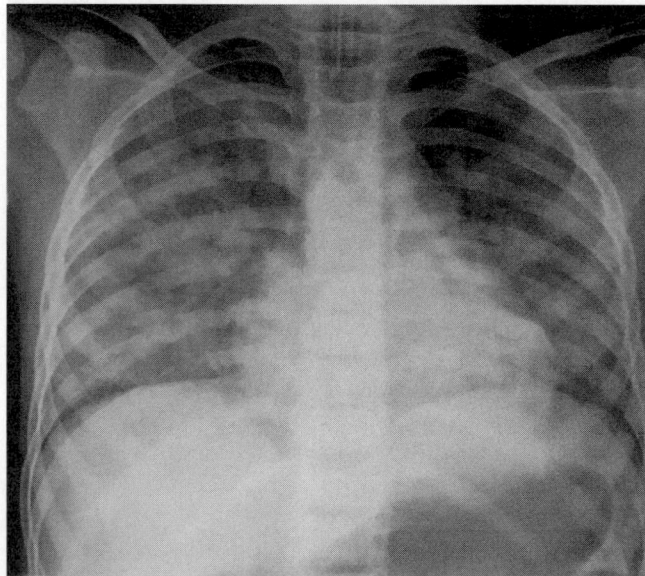

FIG. 10-15 Pulmonary edema. This child was admitted to the pediatric critical care unit after a drowning episode. The child had a respiratory arrest and required cardiopulmonary resuscitation at the scene and subsequent intubation in the field. The child had a return of spontaneous respiratory effort but required mechanical ventilatory support because of progressive respiratory distress, including tachypnea, increased respiratory effort, and hypoxia. The chest radiograph reveals a normal heart size. The pulmonary interstitial markings are all increased and hazy. The interstitial markings are particularly prominent surrounding the hila of the lungs. There was resolution of the edema over the next 48 hours, and the child was extubated without complications.

Normally, the peripheral pulmonary vascular markings are not prominent and generally can be seen only in the proximal two thirds of the lung fields. Prominent pulmonary vascularity can result from the presence of an intracardiac shunt (causing increased pulmonary arterial blood flow), pulmonary venous obstruction, pulmonary hypertension, and increased collateral blood flow to the lungs. Although each of these problems theoretically can produce distinct radiographic changes, it is often difficult to differentiate among them by review of an AP film alone. Although a radiologist may be able to differentiate between the radiographic appearance of pulmonary arterial and pulmonary venous enlargement, this is not a realistic expectation in the critical care setting.

Intracardiac shunt lesions, such as a large ventricular septal defect or a patent ductus arteriosus, initially will produce a dilation of apical vessels on an upright film. (These vessels are normally not prominent in an upright film.) With a significant increase in pulmonary blood flow and possible pulmonary hypertension, the lung hili and the pulmonary arteries and veins become uniformly prominent. Occasionally, the child with anemia or an arteriovenous fistula will develop pulmonary hypervascularity that mimics the appearance of a shunt lesion.

When the newborn has pulmonary venous obstruction associated with left-sided heart failure or obstruction, or total anomalous pulmonary venous connection (TAPVC) below the diaphragm (or other forms of TAPVC with obstruction), and pulmonary venous pressure increases, redistribution of pulmonary blood flow often does not occur. Instead, lung fields become more radiopaque as a result of venous congestion, and the lung fields have a uniform "ground-glass" appearance caused by interstitial edema and pulmonary venous dilation.[27]

When pulmonary venous obstruction is present in the older infant or child and pulmonary venous pressure increases (e.g., caused by left heart failure or obstruction), blood flow in the lungs is redistributed. Normally, when the patient is upright, blood flow in the bases of the lungs is greater than flow to the apices. With an increase in pulmonary venous pressure, blood flow is redistributed and shifted to the upper portions of the lungs, causing a prominence of apical pulmonary venous markings.[21] With progressive pulmonary venous congestion, interstitial edema develops, and the lung hili and all vascular markings begin to become hazy and indistinct. The hili may be particularly opaque.

Kerley-B lines may be seen with severe pulmonary venous congestion. These lines appear as thin, radiopaque, horizontal streaks in the lung bases that are thought to represent lymphatic channels in the interlobular septa of the lungs (see Fig. 10-13).[21,24] If pulmonary venous pressure increases further, transudation of fluid into the tissue can occur. This transudation produces diffuse opacification of both lung fields. Air bronchograms may be visible (see Fig. 10-14).

When the child develops pulmonary hypertension with increased pulmonary vascular resistance, the hilar and proximal pulmonary vessels often appear to be prominent, but peripheral pulmonary vascular markings can be absent. This radiographic appearance of the pulmonary vessels is referred to as the *pruned tree configuration*.[14,21] Because chest radiographs are not the chief method used to confirm or rule out the diagnosis of pulmonary hypertension, the observation of findings consistent with pulmonary hypertension should be used only to provide an index of suspicion. Many children with significant pulmonary hypertension have normal chest radiographs.

Occasionally, children with severe long-standing obstruction of pulmonary arterial blood flow (e.g., caused by uncorrected or palliated pulmonary atresia) develop prominent bronchial collateral vessels that proliferate, thus increasing the absolute amount of pulmonary blood flow. These vessels can be highly dense, but they often do not follow the normal branching pattern. These children are likely to have a normal or diminutive main pulmonary artery shadow and small right and left hili.[14,21] When pulmonary artery blood flow is reduced, the lung fields appear to be abnormally radiolucent (or "empty"), because they do not contain the normal opacities produced by pulmonary vessels.

COMMON RADIOGRAPHIC ABNORMALITIES

The preceding discussion has focused on the systematic review of a chest radiograph, including a brief discussion of abnormalities. The critically ill child can develop pneumonia, atelectasis, or accumulation of free pleural fluid or air. Because these problems require specific changes in nursing care, they are discussed in further detail here.

The term *air space disease* applies to the presence of abnormal (i.e., nonair) densities in the lung fields. These densities can be localized or diffuse and generally indicate the development of lung disease, atelectasis, or tumor or the accumulation of exudate, transudate, or blood in the lung.[14] Often it may be difficult to differentiate between opacification produced by intrapulmonary (air space) disease and that produced by fluid accumulation in the pleural space. The following discussion includes identifying characteristics of each problem and clues to differentiating among them.

Atelectasis produces intrapulmonary opacification as the result of collapse of a portion of the lung tissue (Fig. 10-16). Atelectasis is usually seen as a diffuse increase in density with either a linear, angular, or streaked appearance in the affected area. Atelectasis is typically produced by intrinsic obstruction of an airway (caused by a mucous plug, exudate, or foreign body), extrinsic compression of the airway by another thoracic structure (e.g., enlarged lymph nodes, large heart, tumor), or significant hypoventilation. Because atelectasis represents loss of lung volume (i.e., lung collapse), other intrathoracic structures shift toward the area of atelectasis. The trachea, mediastinum, hilum, and any visible intrapulmonary septa can all shift toward the atelectatic area. If the upper lobe is involved, the loss of volume also elevates the hilum on the affected side. In addition, the hemidiaphragm on the involved side is elevated, and the intercostal spaces on that side become narrow. Air bronchograms may be present within the opacified area, and the visualized bronchi often are crowded together because of lung collapse. The uninvolved lung can become hyperinflated, producing a widening of the intercostal spaces on the nonatelectatic side and subsequent flattening of the hemidiaphragm.

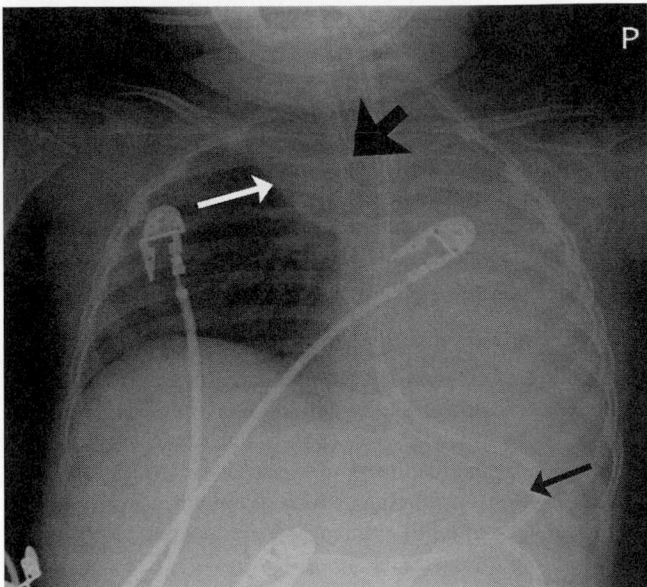

FIG. **10-16** Atelectasis. Note opacification of the right upper lobe *(small white arrow)* and complete opacification of the left lung. Because atelectasis represents pulmonary collapse with associated volume loss, other structures have shifted toward the involved areas. The right hemidiaphragm is elevated, the hilum of the right lung is shifted upward, and the mediastinum is shifted to the left. Note the tracheal tube tip at the level of the third rib *(large black arrow)*. The nasogastric tube ends in the stomach *(small black arrow)*, with decompression of the gastric air bubble.

Pleural fluid accumulation can result from pleural effusion, chylothorax, hemothorax, hydrothorax, empyema (a purulent pleural space infection), or a pleural reaction. The fluid will infiltrate the lung space and appear as a density on the radiograph. The infiltrative process typically is seen at the periphery of the lung and moves inward with a hazy, white appearance without air volume loss. Free pleural fluid characteristically assumes a dependent position so that in the upright chest film it generally accumulates along the diaphragm. With small amounts of fluid accumulation, the costophrenic angles are blunted; with increasing amounts of fluid accumulation, the diaphragm will appear to be elevated and fluid will accumulate laterally as well (see Fig. 10-5, A). On average, more than 150 m of fluid must be present for a pleural effusion to be detected on an upright film. Smaller amounts, greater than 75 mL, can be detected on a lateral decubitus view when the patient is positioned so the affected side is dependent (i.e., the affected side is down).[25,26] Fluid also can accumulate in the fissures between lobes of the lung.

If the free pleural fluid continues to accumulate, the entire hemithorax can be filled; this produces complete opacification of that hemithorax, with compression of the underlying lung and flattening of the involved hemidiaphragm.[14] The trachea, mediastinum, and hilum usually are shifted away from significant fluid accumulation, because it represents an increase in intrathoracic volume (unless concurrent atelectasis is present on the involved side). A lateral decubitus view is not indicated in this case, because there is no air interface to assist in further characterization of the fluid. Ultrasound examination, however, can be extremely helpful.

If the child is supine when the chest radiograph is taken, free pleural fluid will accumulate along the posterior surface of the chest, because it is dependent when the child is supine. This condition will produce a diffuse opacification within the involved thorax that may be difficult to differentiate from interstitial lung disease. An upright film or a lateral decubitus film will help differentiate free pleural fluid from intrapulmonary disease. The lateral decubitus view is often specifically requested to confirm the presence of free pleural fluid, because this view will allow visualization of small amounts of fluid (see Fig. 10-5, B).

Pneumonia can initially produce a patchy infiltration with fluffy margins. The presence of air bronchograms within the infiltrate can confirm the impression that the opacification is caused by intrapulmonary disease.[14] If the pneumonia causes obliteration of the cardiac border, the pneumonia must be in contact with the heart (Fig. 10-17). The portion of the heart that is obliterated will help describe the location of the pneumonia within the lung (see Table 10-2).[14]

Frequently, pneumonia will later cause more segmental or lobar disease, with a more homogenous opacification of the involved area of the lung.[14] The child may develop air trapping with resultant depression of the diaphragm and increased radiolucency of the lung fields.

Some pneumonias cause a characteristic radiographic appearance that correlates with the child's clinical history. Most infectious pneumonia in children, regardless of origin, begins with local or alveolar involvement, which is difficult to differentiate from interstitial disease; it can later progress to lobar disease. Lobar consolidation frequently occurs as the result of *Streptococcus pneumoniae* infection. *Staphylococcus aureus* infection occurs more commonly in infants younger than 1 year; it typically involves the right lung and can cause

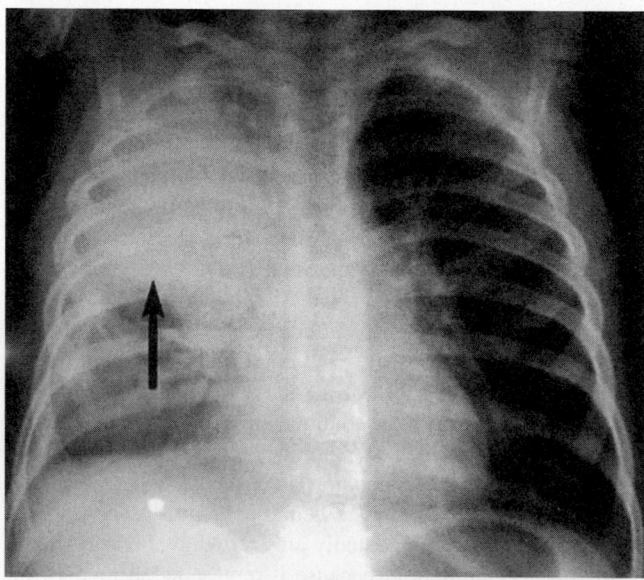

FIG. 10-17 Right upper and middle lobe pneumonia. There is a dense opacity of the right upper lobe consistent with pneumonia. There is also hazy opacification along the right heart border. This opacification is caused by the fluid density of right middle lobe pneumonia obliterating the silhouette of the heart. This silhouette sign enables localization of the pneumonia to the right middle lobe.

development of pneumatoceles (localized collections of intrapulmonary air) or abscesses. *Haemophilus pneumoniae* is nearly always associated with a pleural effusion. Epiglottitis also can accompany this disease, but is uncommon since the advent of the Haemophilus influenzae type B vaccine (Hib) vaccine. *Streptococcus*, *Klebsiella*, and *H. pneumoniae* also may be associated with empyema or pneumatocele formation.[14]

Aspiration pneumonia usually develops in the portion of the lung that is dependent at the time of aspiration. The radiographic changes following the aspiration are related to irritation and inflammation caused by the aspirated material and to the development of pneumonia. A diffuse aspiration process characteristically produces patchy opacification in the lung bases and perihilar infiltrations.[14]

Bronchopneumonia produces perihilar congestion. Pneumonia produced by *Pneumocystis carinii* (most frequently seen in immune compromised patients) can initially produce perihilar congestion and then peripheral intrapulmonary involvement. The disease soon assumes an alveolar and interstitial distribution. In patients with acquired immunodeficiency syndrome (AIDS), *P. carinii* can have virtually any radiographic appearance.

Abnormal areas of radiolucency may also be observed on the chest radiograph as collections of air within soft tissues or surrounded by tissues. They are most frequently caused by a pneumothorax, pneumomediastinum, lung abscess, pneumatocele, or emphysema.

The presence of a unilateral hyperlucency is most often a result of a pneumothorax. A small pneumothorax is more readily observed on an expiratory chest film, because the child's lung volumes are smaller and the normal pulmonary vascular markings are crowded together (see Fig. 10-2, B). Thus, the difference between the vascularized lung fields and the avascular, radiolucent pneumothorax is intensified on an expiratory film. A pneumothorax may also be more readily discerned in an upright film, because free pleural air will rise toward the apex of the lung.

If the child is supine when the radiograph is taken, free pleural air will tend to collect along the diaphragm and the anterior aspects of the thorax (compare Figs. 10-7 and 10-10). In addition, the interface between the pneumothorax and the lung will be in the same plane as the chest radiograph, so a distinct border (or density contrast) between the two may not be apparent. However, a pneumothorax should be considered if an extremely radiolucent area lacking in vascular markings is noted along the diaphragm, along the pleural edge or tracking along the cardiac silhouette.

If the pneumothorax is significant, the underlying lung will collapse, and the trachea and mediastinum will be compressed and shifted away from the side of the pneumothorax. Because the pneumothorax occupies volume, the hemidiaphragm on the involved side of the chest often will be flattened or displaced downward (see Fig. 10-10).

Lung abscesses and pneumatoceles can develop as a result of pneumonia. They both produce circumscribed collections of air within the lungs. The increased radiolucency from an abscess occurs as the result of necrosis. The pneumatocele can also result from necrosis or air trapping.[14]

Emphysematous changes in the lungs may cause localized, circumscribed areas of increased radiolucency within the lungs. The emphysematous lung is distended, and air trapping occurs. The diaphragm on the involved side is flattened, and the trachea and mediastinum are shifted away from the involved side.

A pneumopericardium is a collection of air within the pericardial sac surrounding the heart. It is usually identified easily because it appears as a radiolucent border between the radiopaque pericardial sac and the radiopaque heart, with the radiolucent border tracking underneath the cardiac silhouette outlining the diaphragm (Fig. 10-18, A).[12] In comparison, a pneumomediastinum is a collection of air within the mediastinal space, characterized by streaked radiolucencies over the border of the mediastinum that outline the cardiac silhouette and great vessels. These radiolucencies then extend into the neck and elevate the parietal pleura along the mediastinal borders (Fig. 10-18, B). A pneumomediastinum should be distinguished from a pneumopericardium and a pneumothorax. In pneumopericardium, air can be present underneath the heart, but does not enter the neck.

Children with a diaphragmatic hernia may demonstrate abnormal densities and lucencies within the thorax. Generally, these children have hypoplasia of both lungs. The lung on the side of the diaphragmatic defect is compressed by abdominal contents during fetal life. The heart and other intrathoracic contents shift to the opposite side, thus compressing that lung during fetal life. Even after correction of the diaphragm hernia, the hypoplastic lungs may not completely fill the thorax, so radiolucent areas will surround the lung tissue.[27]

IDENTIFICATION OF TUBES, CATHETERS, AND WIRES

If the child is intubated, the position of the tracheal tube should probably be checked first. The radiopaque tip of the tube should be located approximately 1 to 2 cm above the carina or approximately at the level of the third rib. Because the position of the tracheal tube relative to the carina will change with a change in head position, it is important to note the position of the head when the radiograph is taken. The optimal head position is a neutral and midline position, with no neck flexion or extension. The tip of a tracheal tube will be displaced downward or further into the trachea when the neck is flexed, and it will move upward if the neck is extended or if the head is turned to one side (Fig. 10-19).[15]

If the tip of the tracheal tube is positioned too near the carina, especially if it is near the carina despite extension of the neck, it can easily slip into the right or left mainstem bronchus. Unintentional intubation of the right mainstem bronchus soon results in hyperinflation of the right lung with hypoventilation and possible atelectasis of the left lung (Fig. 10-20). If the tip of the ET tube is positioned too far above the carina, the tube may inadvertently slip out of the trachea with little patient movement.

Check the position and integrity of all central venous, pulmonary artery, or intracardiac catheters. Trace these lines along their entire length, because they can migrate distally or be dislodged to undesirable areas (Fig. 10-21). For example, during percutaneous insertion of a subclavian venous catheter,

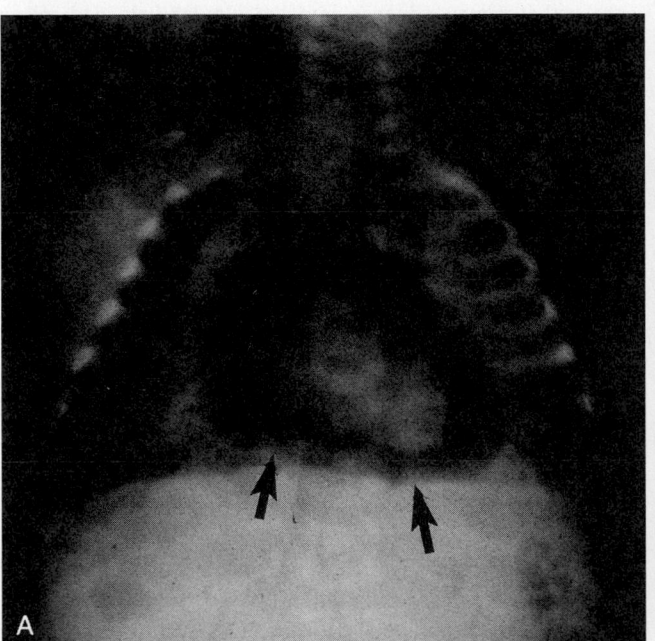
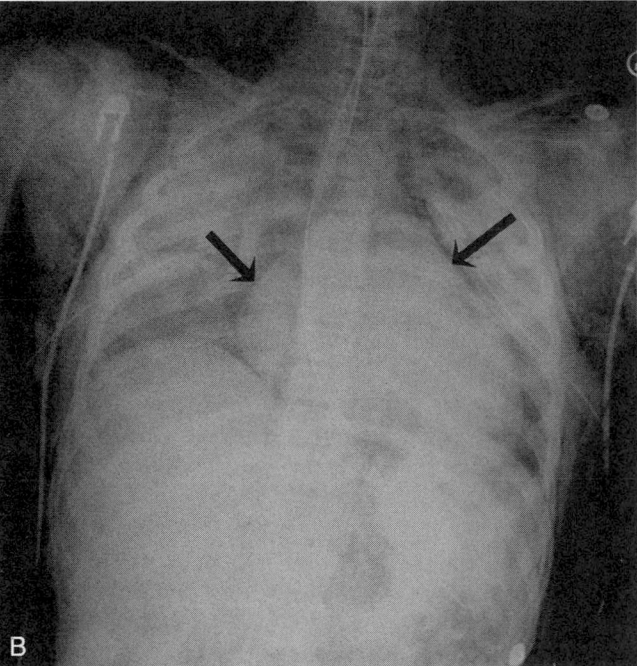

FIG. 10-18 Pneumopericardium and pneumomediastinum. **A,** A pneumopericardium, pneumomediastinum and pneumothorax are present in this supine anteroposterior film. The pneumopericardium creates a dark (air) density surrounding the heart *(arrows).* Note that there is significant compression of the cardiac silhouette. In addition, there are linear air lucencies tracking up into the neck and the left axilla, indicating the presence of pneumomediastinum. There is also a large right pneumothorax. **B,** This supine AP film was obtained from a 10-year-old boy who sustained a traumatic tear to his trachea after colliding with a dumpster. The child had cardiopulmonary arrest in the field and was resuscitated, intubated, and transported to the pediatric critical care unit. He was noted to have pneumomediastinum, creating the bilateral linear areas of radiolucency *(arrows)* tracking along the mediastinum and extending superiorly into the neck.

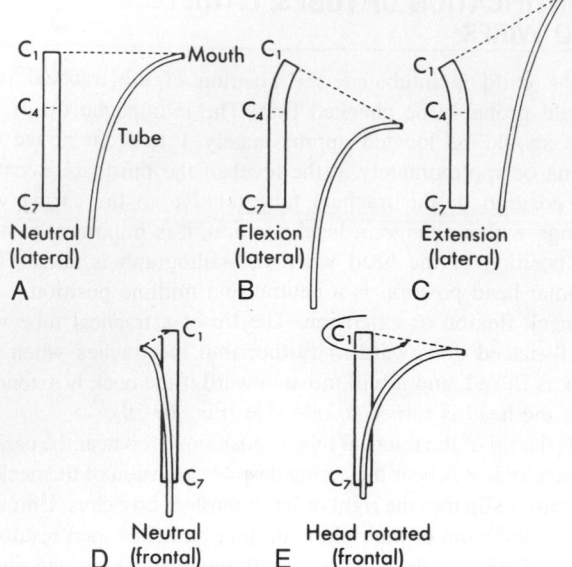

FIG. 10-19 Proposed mechanism of orotracheal tube movement with changes in head position in the infant and young child. This movement must be considered when evaluating tracheal tube position on the chest radiograph. The upper cervical vertebrae (C1 to C4) primarily provide neck flexion and extension and head rotation. The lower cervical spine (C4 to C7) is fairly fixed. A functional lever arm is created between the anterior maxilla and the upper cervical spine; this lever arm moves the tracheal tube when the head moves. **A,** Neutral position, lateral view. **B,** Flexion of the neck, lateral view (pushes endotracheal tube further into trachea). **C,** Extension of the neck, lateral view (pulls endotracheal tube upward by a lever arm effect). **D,** Neutral position, frontal view. **E,** Lateral rotation, frontal view (displaces endotracheal tube upward and further out of trachea). (From Donn SM, Kuhns LR: Mechanisms of endotracheal tube movement with change of head position in the neonate, *Pediatr Radiol* 9:39, 1980.)

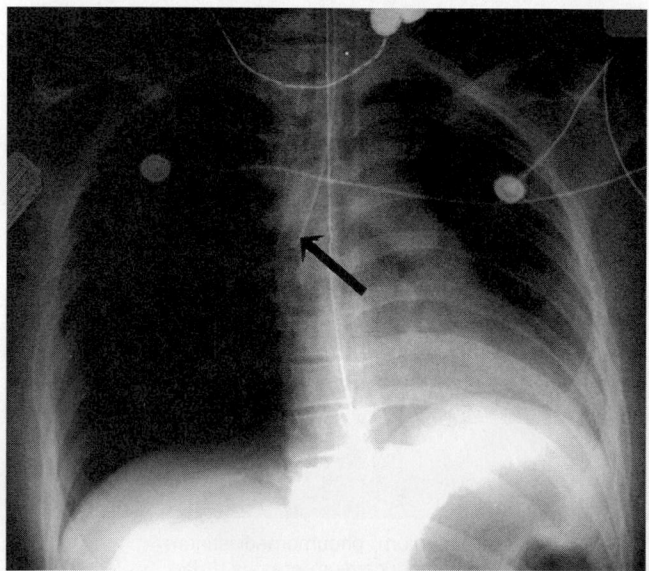

FIG. 10-20 Right mainstem bronchus intubation resulting in left lung atelectasis. The tip of the endotracheal tube is well beyond the level of the carina into the right bronchus *(arrow)*, and the left lung base is opacified with elevation of the left hemidiaphragm resulting from atelectasis. The right lung is hyperinflated with flattening of the hemidiaphragm. The bedside nurse noted decreased breath sounds and chest expansion on the left and loud breath sounds on the right.

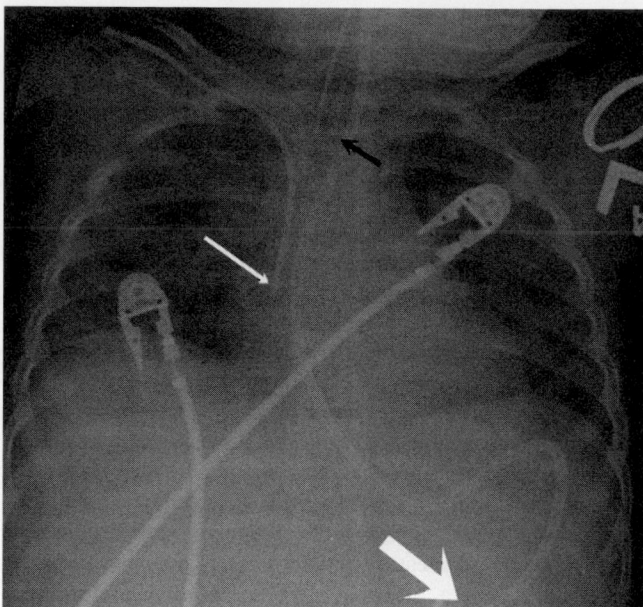

FIG. 10-21 Evaluation of tracheostomy tube, central venous catheter, and nasogastric tube placement. The lungs are difficult to evaluate because inspiration is suboptimal; the right hemidiaphragm is at the level of the right seventh rib posteriorly. Heart size is normal, and pulmonary vascular markings are normal. The tip of the tracheostomy tube is between the clavicular heads *(black arrow)*. A central venous catheter is in place with the tip in the right atrium *(thin white arrow)*. A feeding tube is in place *(thick white arrow)*.

the catheter may advance into the jugular vein and migrate superiorly toward the head instead of inferiorly into the superior vena cava. The right atrial catheter may advance into the right ventricle, which will be obvious from pressure measurements and waveform tracings, or it may rest against the tricuspid valve. The pulmonary artery catheter can migrate distally and become wedged in a small pulmonary artery. Therefore, it is important that the nurse check the location of all catheters and discuss apparent abnormal appearances or the location of these catheters with a member of the medical management team. It is also important to check for pneumothorax following placement, or attempted placement, of a subclavian catheter.

Establish the location of nasogastric or any feeding tubes. In the past, nurses verified the location of the feeding tube with clinical assessment; however, it is now clear that clinical methods alone are inadequate to detect feeding tube misplacement.[1] Therefore, the standard of care is to obtain radiographic confirmation of nasogastric tube placement. The nasogastric tube can migrate, especially if it is taped inadequately or if there is excessive patient movement. If, at any point, there is any concern regarding proper placement of the tube, tube position should be verified with a radiograph. The tip of the nasogastric tube and all ports (identified by breaks in the radiopaque marker line) should reside in the stomach. If the tube extends through the stomach and beyond the midline, it is likely in the duodenum or jejunum, and aspiration of the tube yields fluids with a pH >6 (approximately the same pH as fluids aspirated from the lungs). Nasogastric tubes should be evaluated along their entire length, because occasionally they can become looped in the nasopharynx or cervical region.

Verify the location of any wires. There is a growing population of children with chronic illnesses who have implantable devices such as vagus nerve stimulators, pacemakers, and cardiac pacemaker or defibrillators. In addition, after cardiothoracic surgery the patient will frequently have cardiac pacing wires in place. Occasionally, a wire or lead is dislodged or fractured.

Lateral chest radiographs are often used to evaluate tube placement. As noted earlier in the chapter, AP or PA films are most useful for evaluation of the lateral relationships of structures (Fig. 10-22, A). However, this view occasionally can be misleading because it does not enable evaluation of the AP relationships of structures. The lateral view provides extremely valuable information when evaluating tube placement, because it allows evaluation of the AP relationships of structures (Fig. 10-22, B).

An umbilical venous catheter will curve from the umbilical vein and then into the inferior vena cava (IVC). If the umbilical venous catheter enters the IVC, it should be visible in the right side of the patient's abdomen, moving toward the border between the liver and the heart. Look for the tip along the right side of the patient's vertebral column (Fig. 10-23, A, B). The catheter is typically inserted until a good blood return is obtained (approximately 1-4 cm), or it is advanced to the junction of the IVC and the right atrium. The provider should not allow the tip to remain within the shadow of the liver,

because it will likely reside in the portal vein or hepatic circulation. That tip location is not recommended, because it would allow infusion of hypertonic or alkaline solutions into the portal vein.[27]

An umbilical artery catheter will enter the umbilical artery and the aorta. If the umbilical artery catheter is in the aorta, it will appear on the patient's left side of the vertebral column. The catheter tip is advanced until it enters the descending aorta, to prevent obstruction of the femoral or iliac arteries (Fig. 10-23, C). The tip should reside between the levels of the sixth and tenth thoracic vertebrae; lower placement (at the level of the third or fourth lumbar vertebra) is associated with more complications and is not recommended.[3]

COMMON IMAGING STUDIES OBTAINED IN CRITICALLY ILL CHILDREN

Computed Tomography (CT) Scan

CT is a highly advanced diagnostic procedure that uses x-rays enhanced by a computer to create cross-sectional pictures of the body. Unlike traditional radiographs, the CT rapidly generates a three-dimensional image of the inside of an object from a large series of two-dimensional x-ray images taken around a single axis of rotation. This process creates detailed images of areas surrounded by bone and can show less dense tissues, such as organs and blood vessels (Fig. 10-24). CT completely eliminates the superimposition of structures

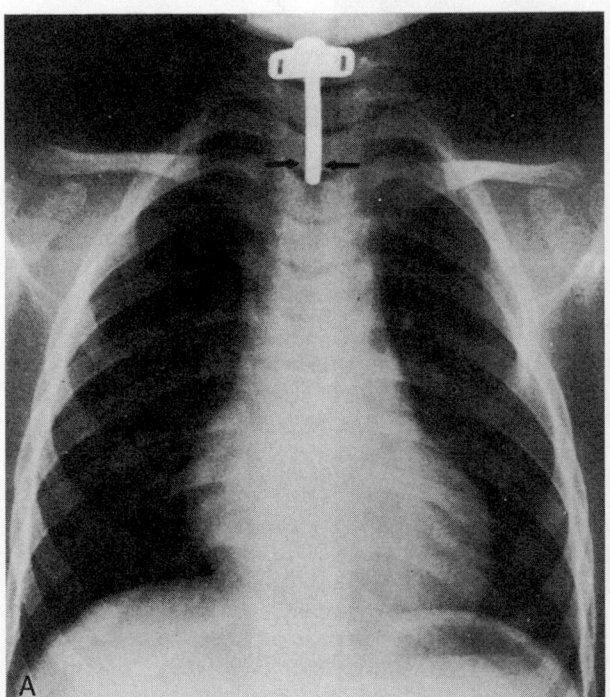
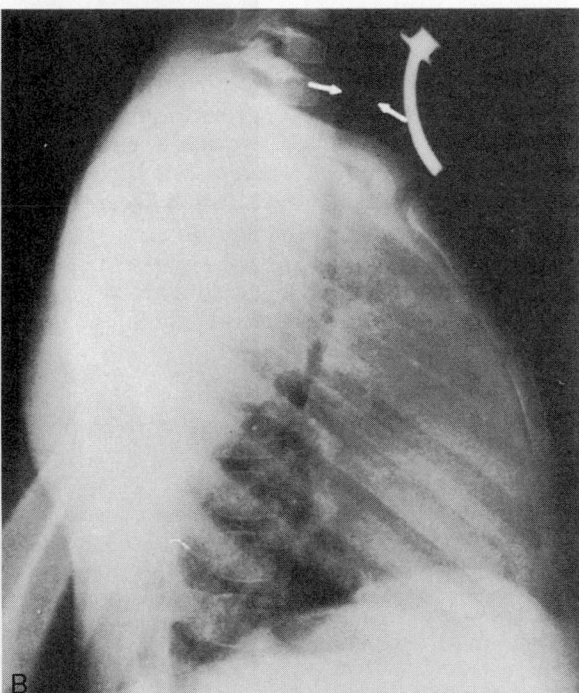

FIG. 10-22 Appearance of tracheostomy tube on anteroposterior and lateral chest radiographs. These films were obtained when the nurse noted difficulty in inserting the tracheostomy tube and noted inadequate breath sounds when hand ventilation was provided via the tube. Breath sounds were adequate during spontaneous ventilation. **A,** Anteroposterior view. Lung expansion appears adequate, and the tracheostomy tube appears to be in the midline of the trachea *(arrows)*. **B,** Lateral view. The air density of the trachea is visible *(arrows)*, and it is apparent that the tracheostomy tube has been inserted subcutaneously (it is not in the trachea at all). (Courtesy Andrew K. Poznanski, Children's Memorial Hospital, Chicago, IL.)

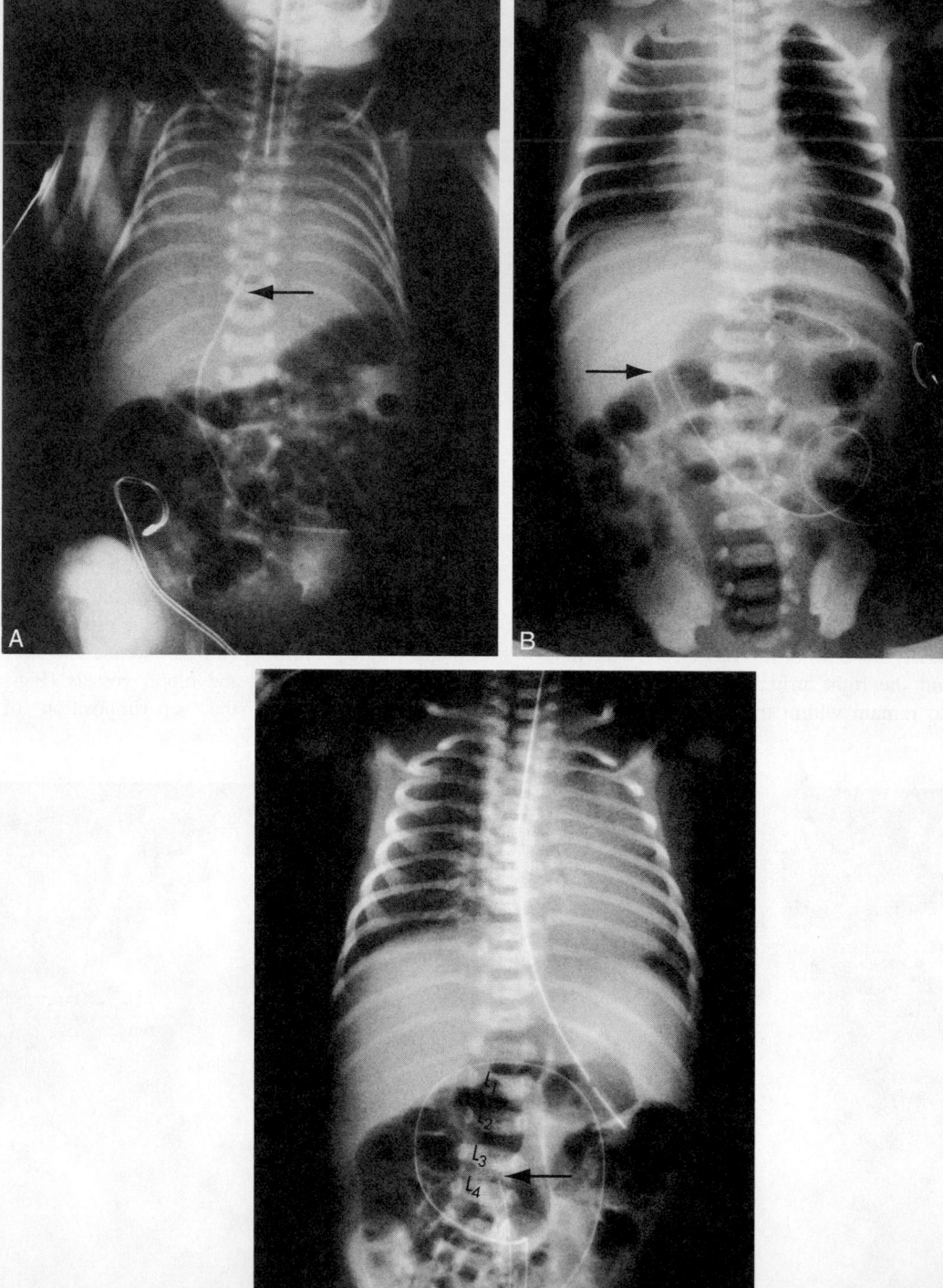

FIG. 10-23 Evaluation of umbilical venous and arterial catheter placement. **A,** Umbilical venous catheter in "high" position at junction of inferior vena cava and right atrium *(arrow)*. This is very high placement, which is acceptable, but not optimal; if the catheter is advanced further, there is a risk of right atrial perforation. If the catheter is withdrawn 1-2 cm, it will reside within the hepatic circulation. **B,** Umbilical venous catheter in hepatic circulation *(arrow)*. This catheter should be withdrawn, because infusion of a high osmolality solution may injure the liver. **C,** Umbilical artery catheter in incorrect position. The tip of this catheter *(arrow)* is at approximately the level of the third or fourth lumbar vertebra; it should be advanced to the level of the sixth through tenth thoracic vertebrae.

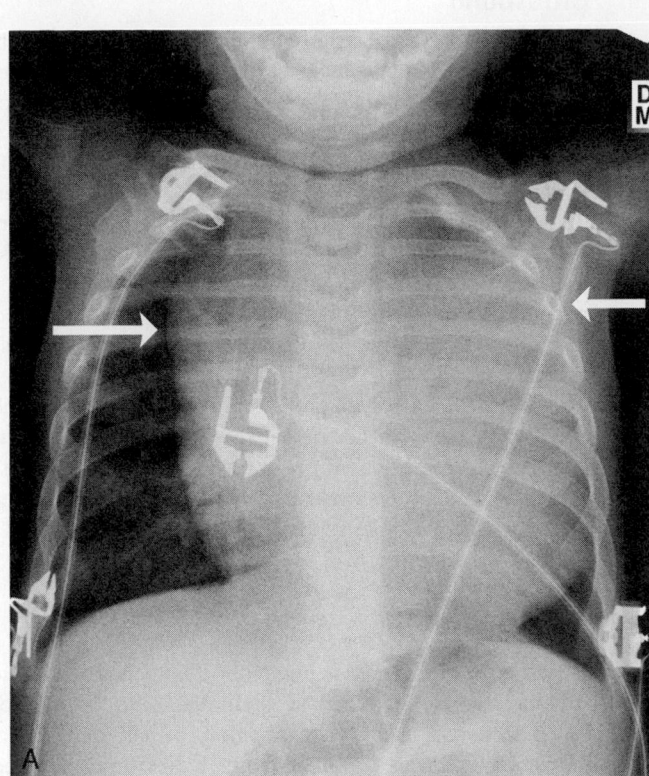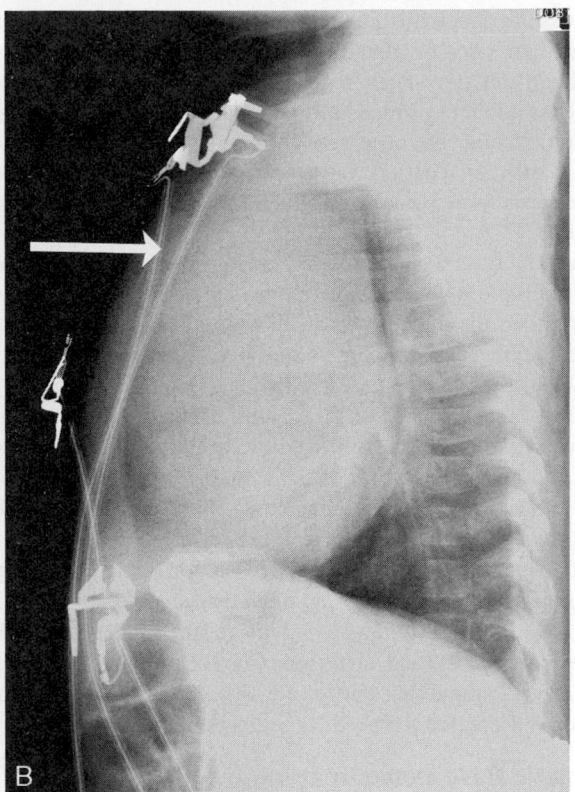
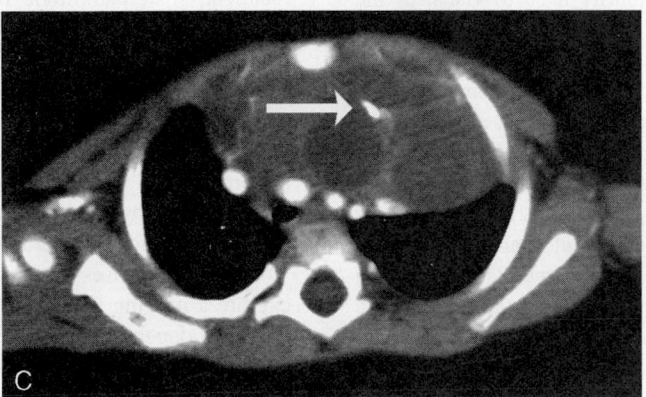

FIG. 10-24 Mediastinal mass: radiographic and computed tomography images. **A,** Anteroposterior radiograph of a 2-year-old child with severe respiratory distress shows marked widening of the mediastinum consistent with a large mediastinal mass *(arrows)*. **B,** Lateral view shows opacity in the retrosternal space *(arrow)* confirming that this mass is in the anterior mediastinum. The trachea is displaced posteriorly and narrowed by the mass. **C,** Computed tomography scan with intravenous contrast shows the large mass with cystic and solid areas, as well as an area of calcification *(arrow)* that was not visible on the plain film. This finding made teratoma the most likely diagnosis, which was confirmed by surgical and pathologic analysis. (Courtesy Sharon Stein, Nashville, Tenn.)

outside the area of interest into the area of focus. Because of the inherent high-contrast resolution of CT, it allows differentiation of structures that differ in physical density by less than 1%. CT can be enhanced by use of intravenous iodinated contrast material, which allows accurate evaluation of the vascular structures and can give information about enhancement of lesions.

Preparation of the patient includes ensuring patent intravenous access if the use of intravenous iodinated contrast material is desired. Before administering the contrast medium, contraindications to the medium must be considered; these include pregnancy, allergic reaction to shellfish or iodinated dye, unstable vital signs, and claustrophobia. The patient must remain motionless, because movement can cause artifact that will affect the clarity of the images. If the patient is likely to move, be agitated, or be uncooperative, then sedation or possible anesthesia may be required. All patients should be ordered "nothing by mouth" status (NPO), based on the American Society of Anesthesiology (ASA) pediatric guidelines, in anticipation of the need for sedation or anesthesia. Before administering contrast medium, check the blood urea nitrogen and creatinine levels for adequate kidney function. Some patients experience flushing or a feeling of warmth, a transient headache, a salty or metallic taste in the mouth, nausea, or vomiting, and they need to be prepared for these possible reactions. After the procedure, patients who receive contrast medium should be observed for signs and symptoms of delayed allergic reaction. Intravenous hydration or oral fluid intake needs to be continued to facilitate clearance of contrast medium.

The data from a single CT imaging procedure consisting of either multiple contiguous or one helical scan can be viewed as images in the axial, coronal, or sagittal planes, depending on the findings and the clinical question. When a typical sagittal view is obtained, the nurse should imagine looking up into the chest from below. The anterior surface of the chest will be at the top of the film, and the posterior surface of the chest will be at the bottom of the film. The patient's left will be on the right side of the image, and the patient's right will be on the left side of the image.

CT scans provide greater resolution than ordinary radiographs and, as a result, can often detect some problems at an earlier stage. CT is often used to image areas of the body such as the brain, chest, and abdomen. Current state-of-the-art CT scanning is so rapid that images are obtained in a few seconds, which has decreased the need for sedation in many cases.

Magnetic Resonance Imaging (MRI)

MRI is an imaging technique primarily used to visualize the structure and function of the body. It provides detailed images of the body in any plane. MRI provides much greater contrast between the different soft tissues of the body than does CT, making it especially useful in neurologic (brain), musculoskeletal, cardiovascular, and oncologic imaging. Unlike CT, it uses no ionizing radiation, but uses a powerful magnetic field to align the nuclear magnetization of (usually) hydrogen atoms in water in the body. Radiofrequency fields are used to systematically alter the alignment of this magnetization, causing the hydrogen-containing nuclei to produce a rotating magnetic field detectable by the scanner. This signal can be manipulated by additional magnetic fields to gather enough information to reconstruct an image of the body. Contrast agents for MRI are those with paramagnetic properties, such as gadolinium and manganese. Some patients who have implanted devices or metallic objects in the body will not be able to have MRI. Nurses or technologists should provide ear protection for the patient during the MRI study, because the magnet and machine create loud noises.

Unlike CT scanning, which is very rapid, MRI is time consuming with most studies taking up to 45 min. Most children require sedation and occasionally general anesthesia. Preparation of the patient includes ensuring patent intravenous access. All patients should be made NPO, based on the ASA pediatric guidelines, in anticipation of the need for sedation or anesthesia. Before administering contrast medium, check the blood urea nitrogen and creatinine levels for adequate kidney function. There have been concerns raised recently regarding the toxicity of gadolinium-based contrast agents and their effects on individuals with impaired kidney function. Adequate hydration is necessary when contrast medium is used, with careful monitoring of urine output and renal function.

Ultrasound

Medical sonography (ultrasonography) is an ultrasound-based diagnostic imaging technique used to visualize the size and shape of internal organs, soft tissues, and other structures and to evaluate possible pathologies or lesions in real time. Ultrasound is particularly useful in the evaluation of pleural effusions and allows the provider to discern whether the fluid is loculated or not. Ultrasound can be used in infants to evaluate diaphragmatic motion if the patient is too unstable to be transported to the radiology suite for fluoroscopy. It is possible to perform diagnostic or therapeutic procedures (e.g., biopsies or drainage of fluid collections) with ultrasound guidance.

Typically a hand-held probe (called a *transducer*) is placed directly on the skin and is moved over the structure to be visualized. A water-based gel is used to couple the ultrasound between the transducer and patient. The equipment is readily available and portable and can be used in the critical care setting or the radiology or emergency department.

Fluoroscopy

Fluoroscopy provides dynamic real-time images of the internal structures being examined; it is similar to an "x-ray movie." Fluoroscopy is used for evaluation of structure or organ movement, such as the diaphragm. It also may be used for localization of pathologic findings. Fluoroscopy generally is performed in the radiology department, although it can be performed at the bedside of the critically ill patient. Modern fluoroscopes couple the screen to an x-ray image intensifier and video camera, allowing the images to be played and recorded on a monitor. Videotapes of the fluoroscopic examination usually are made to allow later viewing and analysis. Gonadal and thyroid shielding, when possible, is required for the child and for the attendant personnel.

Fluoroscopy uses x-rays with the aid of a contrast agent to capture a moving image. Preparation for a fluoroscopy procedure will depend on the type of examination being performed. Barium may be used for gastrointestinal procedures or as intravenous contrast material for cardiac catheterization and insertion of intravenous catheters. The preparation of the patient includes ensuring patent intravenous access. All patients should be made NPO, based on the ASA pediatric guidelines, in anticipation of the need for sedation or anesthesia. Care after the procedure may include restrictions on movement for a specified period of time (such as after cardiac catheterization). Most patients are able to resume their previous diet without restriction and will be encouraged to drink plenty of oral fluids. Otherwise, intravenous fluid hydration will be continued to help rehydrate the patient and facilitate clearance of any remaining contrast or barium material.

CONCLUSIONS

Chest radiographs are valuable adjuncts to assessment of the critically ill patient when they are used in conjunction with a thorough clinical examination and knowledge of the child's condition. If the nurse uses a systematic method of reviewing the radiograph, and if abnormal densities in the chest are identified, the nurse will be able to confirm clinical impressions and better evaluate progress and complications of therapy. Because the nurse is often one of the first healthcare providers to see the chest radiograph, it is important that every nurse is able to recognize significant changes in the radiograph or indications of serious problems.

ACKNOWLEDGMENTS

The authors thank Sharon M. Stein, MD, from the Monroe Carell, Jr., Children's Hospital at Vanderbilt University, Nashville, Tennessee, for her thoughtful review and insights.

References

1. American Association of Critical Care Nurses: *American Association of Critical Care Nurses Practice Alert: verification of feeding tube placement.* Alisa Viejo, CA, 2005, American Association of Critical Care Nurses. Accessed on July 11, 2011 at: http://classic.aacn.org/AACN/practiceAlert.nsf/Files/FT%20Placement/$file/Verification%20of%20Feeding%20Tube%20Placement%2005-2005.pdf.
2. American College of Radiology Panel: *American College of Radiology Thoracic Imaging Expert Panel Report,* Reston, VA, 2002, American College of Radiology.
3. Barrington KJ: Umbilical artery catheters in the newborn: effects of position of the catheter tip. *Cochrane Database Syst Rev* CD000505, 2000.
4. Barsness KA, et al: The positive predictive value of rib fractures as an indicator of non-accidental trauma in children. *J Trauma* 54:1107–1110, 2003.
5. Beckstrand RL: Understanding chest radiographs of infants and children: the AIR systematic approach. *Crit Care Nurse* 21:54–65, 2001.
6. Collins J, Stern E: *Chest radiology: the essentials,* Philadelphia, 2007, Lippincott Williams and Wilkins.
7. Daffner R: *Clinical radiology: the essentials,* Baltimore, 1993, Lippincott Williams and Wilkins.
8. Des Jardin TR: *Cardiopulmonary anatomy and physiology: essentials for respiratory care,* ed 4, New York, 2002, Delmar.
9. Felson B, Weinstein AS, Spitz HB: *Principles of chest roentgenology: a programmed text,* ed 2, Philadelphia, 1970, WB Saunders.
10. Finholt DA, et al: The heart is under the lower third of the sternum: implications for external cardiac massage. *Am J Dis Child* 140:646, 1986.
11. Fink BW: *Congenital heart disease: a deductive approach to its diagnosis,* ed 3, Chicago, 1991, Mosby-Year Book.
12. Fleisher G, Ludwig S, Henretig F, et al: *Textbook of pediatric emergency medicine,* ed 5, Baltimore, 2006, Lippincott, Williams & and Wilkins.
13. Heller RM, et al: *Exercises in diagnostic radiology,* ed 2, Philadelphia, 1987, WB Saunders.
14. Kirks DR: *Practical pediatric imaging,* ed 3, Philadelphia, 1998, Lippincott-Raven.
15. Kuhns LR, Poznanski AK: Endotracheal tube position in the infant. *J Pediatr* 78:991, 1971.
16. Mettler F, et al: *Primary care radiology,* Philadelphia, 2000, Saunders.
17. Novelline R: *Squires's fundamentals of radiology,* ed 6, Cambridge, MA, 2004, Harvard University Press.
18. Orlowski JP: Optimum position for external cardiac compression in infants and young children. *Ann Emerg Med* 15:667, 1986.
19. Poznanski AK: The chest. In Poznanski AK, editor: *Practical approaches to pediatric radiology,* ed 2, Chicago, 1976, Year Book.
20. Raffensperger JG: Esophageal atresia and tracheoesophageal fistula. *Swenson's pediatric surgery,* ed 5, New York, 1992, Appleton-Century-Crofts.
21. Silverman FN, Kuhn JP: *Essentials of Caffey's pediatric X-ray diagnosis,* Chicago, 1996, Chicago Year Book.
22. Squire LF: *Fundamentals of radiology,* ed 6, Cambridge, MA, 2004, Harvard University Press.
23. Stanger P: Cardiac malpositions. In Rudolph AM, editor: *Pediatrics,* ed 18, Norwalk, CT, 1987, Appleton-Century-Crofts.
24. Sutton D: *A textbook of radiology and imaging,* ed 6, New York, 1998, Churchill-Livingstone.
25. Swischuk LR: *Imaging of the newborn, infant, and young child,* ed 5, Philadelphia, 2005, Lippincott Williams and Wilkins.
26. Swischuk LR: *Emergency imaging of the acutely ill or injured child,* ed 4, Baltimore, MD, 2000, Lippincott Williams and Wilkins.
27. Trotter C, Carey B: Radiology basics: overview and concepts. *Neonatal Netw* 19(2):35–47, 2000.

11

Neurologic Disorders

Lisa M. Milonovich •
Valarie Furgeison Eichler

PEARLS

- The major goals of therapy in the treatment of traumatic brain injury (TBI) are preservation of cardiopulmonary and cerebral function and the prevention of secondary brain injury.
- The 5 H's responsible for secondary brain injury in the pediatric patient are: hypotension, hypoxia, hyperthermia, hypo-/hyperglycemia, and hyponatremia.
- Seizures result from abnormal discharges or firing of cerebral neurons that produce alterations in motor function, behavior and consciousness.
- It is important to recognize the difference between posturing and seizure activity. Decorticate and decerebrate posturing typically occur in response to a stimulus, such as a painful stimulus, while seizures can occur at any time and may produce a variety of movements or other evidence of neurologic discharges (e.g., changes in heart rate).
- Decorticate posturing indicates damage along the corticospinal tract, the pathway between the cortex and spinal cord. Decerebrate posturing indicates deterioration of the structures of the nervous system, particularly the upper brain stem; decerebrate posturing has a less favorable prognosis than decorticate posturing.
- Stroke and cerebral vascular disease are among the top 10 causes of childhood death.
- Therapeutic hypothermia has been shown to improve morbidity and mortality following adult cardiac arrest and neonatal hypoxic-ischemic insult. In the pediatric population with TBI, hypothermia remains a controversial therapy. Clinical trials are underway to evaluate the effects of hypothermia in pediatric TBI and hypoxic-ischemic injury.
- When using an extraventricular drainage (EVD) device for CSF diversion, the nurse must maintain the drain at the precise level ordered. If the drain is placed too high, increased ICP may develop before drainage occurs. If the drain is placed too low, excessive drainage of CSF can lead to upward herniation and/or ventricular collapse and intraventricular hemorrhage.

INTRODUCTION

Care of the critically ill child with neurologic disorders is both challenging and rewarding. It requires knowledge of neuroanatomy, neurophysiology, and normal growth and development. In addition, the nurse must be able to recognize subtle changes in the patient's condition and respond, if needed, with appropriate support or therapy. Because the critically ill child with neurologic disease often is admitted under emergent conditions, the medical team usually does not have the benefit of adequate patient history. As a result the accuracy of the nurse's observations and rapidity of detection of changes and response to deterioration are crucial to the child's successful treatment.

This chapter provides an overview of relevant neurologic anatomy, physiology, and pathophysiology. In addition, it provides the information required to perform precise assessment and appropriate interventions for the critically ill child with critical neurologic disease or injury.

ESSENTIAL ANATOMY AND PHYSIOLOGY

The Axial Skeleton

The axial skeleton consists of the bones of the skull and vertebral column. These bones protect the underlying structures of the central nervous system (CNS). The bones of the skull are divided into regions that form the wall of the cranial cavity and that cover the uppermost aspects of the brain and face. The frontal, occipital, temporal, and paired parietal bones form the cranial vault. The floor of this vault defines three bony compartments—the anterior, middle, and posterior fossae.

The anterior fossa contains the frontal lobes of the brain, the middle fossa contains the upper brainstem and the pituitary gland, and the posterior fossa contains the lower brainstem. These fossae and the parts of the brain they contain often are used to designate areas of injury or disease; such a designation allows location of the problem as well as delineation of the brain functions that are affected. Because injury to the area of the posterior fossa potentially disrupts critical brainstem functions, damage in this area is usually more life threatening than damage to the anterior fossa.

Blood vessels and cranial nerves enter and leave the skull through small openings, or foramina. It is useful to know the course of the cranial nerves so that clinical signs and symptoms can be correlated with areas of cranial injury (Fig. 11-1). The posterior fossa contains a large foramen, the foramen magnum, through which the brainstem and spinal cord join. Lesions in this area, such as those produced by cervical neck trauma, can interrupt vital brain functions and nerve pathways to and from the brain. Cerebrospinal fluid (CSF) flows through the foramen magnum as it passes from the brain

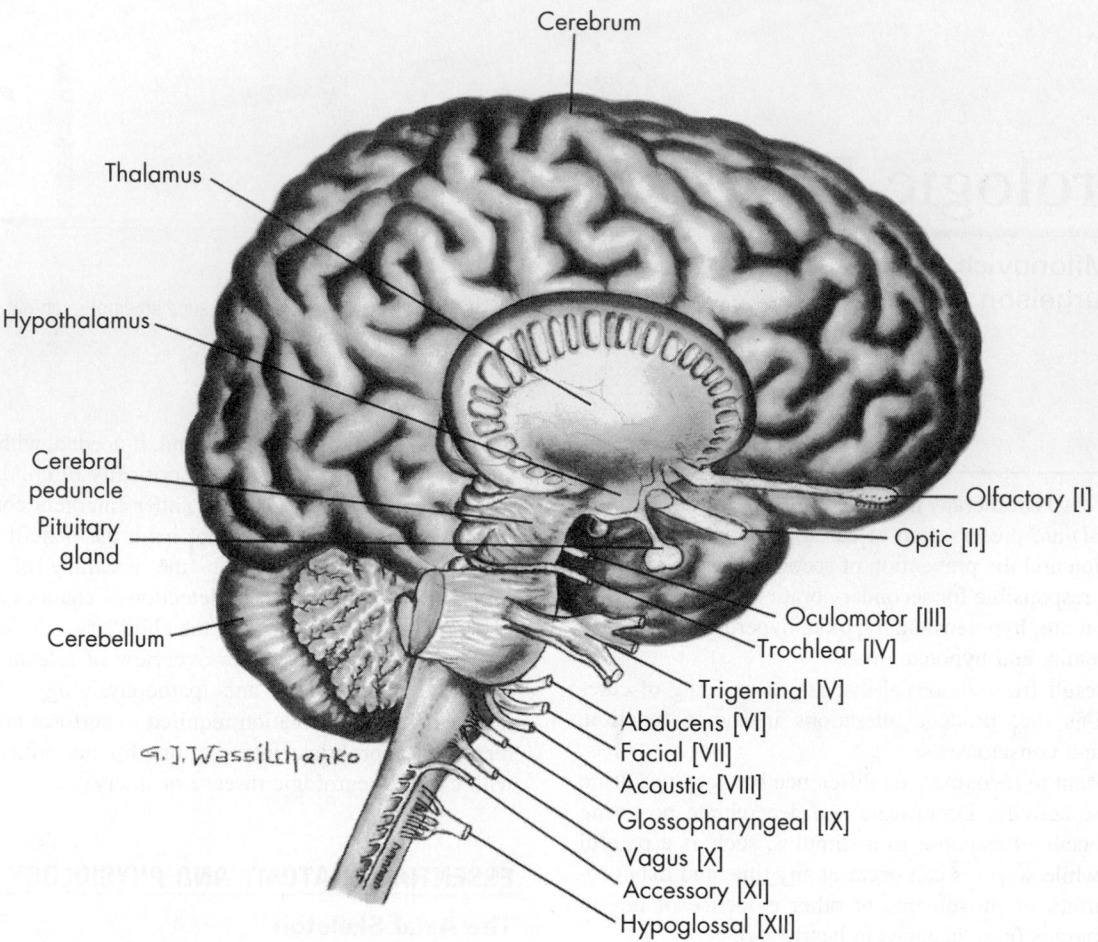

FIG. 11-1 Lateral view of the brain depicting origin of cranial nerves. (From Rudy EB: *Advanced neurological and neurosurgical nursing*, St Louis, 1984, Mosby.)

to the spinal cord and back again, and the vertebral arteries enter the skull through the foramen magnum.

At birth, the skull plates are not fused; they are separated by nonossified spaces called *fontanelles*. The anterior fontanelle is the junction of the coronal, sagittal, and frontal bones. The posterior fontanelle represents the junction of the parietal and occipital bones (see Evolve Fig. 11-1 in the Chapter 11 Supplement on the Evolve Website). Normally, the posterior fontanelle closes at approximately 2 months of age, and the anterior fontanelle closes at approximately 16 to 18 months of age. If the brain does not grow, such as in patients with microcephaly, the cranial bones can fuse early. Conversely, premature fusion of cranial bones, known as *craniosynostosis,* can result in microcephaly unless surgery is performed, because brain growth is inhibited by the restricted intracranial space.

If the infant develops a space-occupying lesion or an increase in intracranial pressure (ICP), the fontanelles will bulge. If intracranial volume or pressure is persistently high or if it increases gradually over a period of time (rather than acutely), the bones of the skull can separate even after fusion; such separation can occur in a child up to 12 years of age.

At birth, the brain is approximately 25% of the adult volume.[76] By 2 years of age, approximately 75% of adult brain volume has been achieved. The cranium itself continues to expand until approximately 7 years of age, when most brain

differentiation is complete. This growth of the brain can be assessed indirectly through measurements of the head circumference. These measurements should always be plotted on a growth chart, because they can aid in the detection of excessive or inadequate head and brain growth that may reflect neurologic disease.

The Meninges

Three highly vascular membranes surround the brain and spinal column; the three membranes collectively are called the *meninges.* The outermost membrane, the dura mater, consists of tough connective tissue that lines the endocranial vault (Fig. 11-2). The dura mater is folded into tents of tissue immediately underneath the skull cap (the periosteum). The most familiar of the many dural folds is the fold that roofs the posterior fossa; this is called the *tentorium cerebelli.* This fold serves as an anatomic landmark; intracranial lesions are divided into those that occur above the tentorium cerebelli (supratentorial lesions) and those that occur below the tentorium cerebelli (infratentorial lesions). The dura not only lines the endocranium, but it also lines the vertebral column. It descends through the foramen magnum to the level of the second sacral vertebra and ends as a blind sac.

The middle membrane, the arachnoid, consists of spiderlike tissue from which it gains its descriptive name. The arachnoid

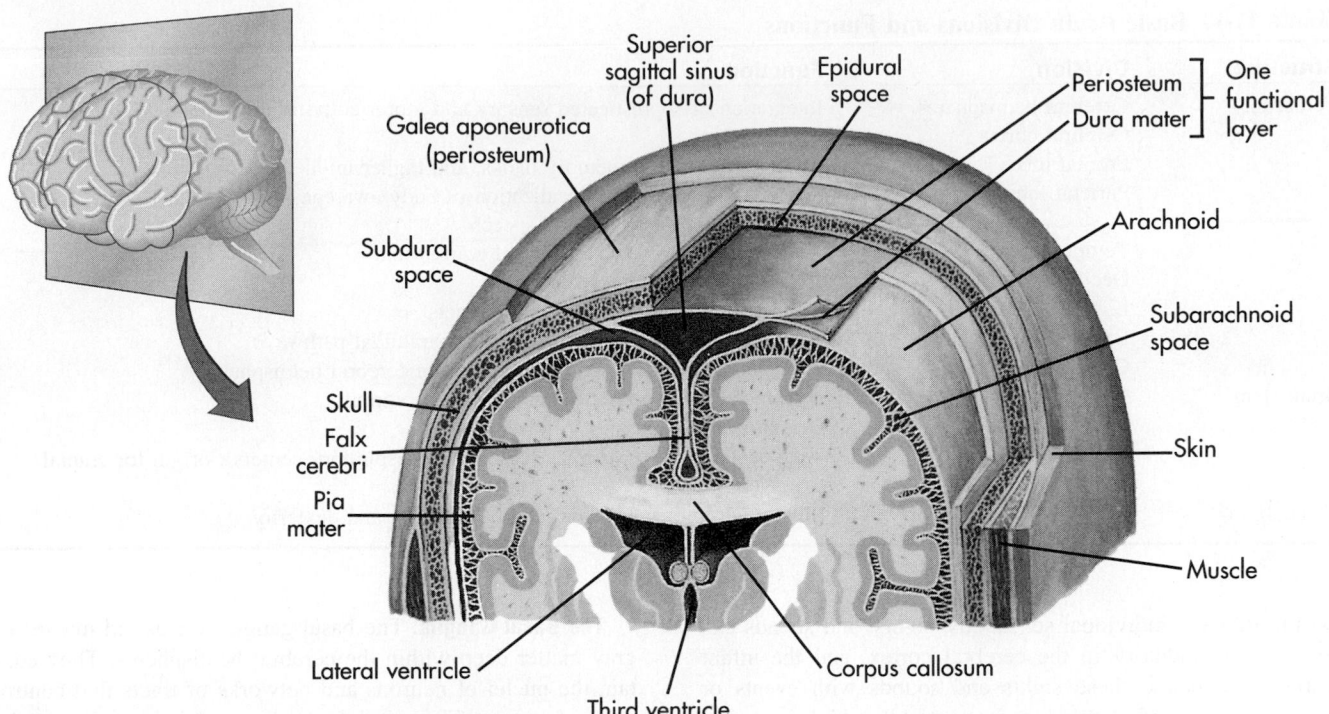

FIG. 11-2 Coverings of the brain. Frontal section of the superior portion of the head, as viewed from the front. The bony and the membranous coverings of the brain can be seen. (From Patton KT, Thibodeau GA: *Anatomy and physiology*, ed 7, St Louis, 2010, Mosby.)

membrane is separated from the dural membrane by the subdural space, which contains cerebral vessels. Because these vessels traverse the subdural space with relatively little support, serious head trauma can cause a rupture of these vessels and the development of a subdural hematoma. This space allows for some cerebral expansion or small hematoma without cerebral compression, but the critical capacity is low. Beneath the subdural space the arachnoid membrane follows the contour of the brain and spinal cord to the end of the spinal cord root.

The pia mater is the third and the innermost membrane. It consists of highly vascular tissue that is separated from the arachnoid membrane by a space called the *subarachnoid space*. This space contains CSF and provides for two major CSF-collecting chambers. The largest chamber, the cisterna magna (also called the *cisterna cerebello-medullaris*), is located between the cerebellum and the medulla. The smallest, the lumbar cistern, is located at the level of the sacrum. Because this space contains CSF, obstruction in this subarachnoid space can obstruct the flow of CSF. Head injury can result in the accumulation of blood in the subarachnoid space; this lesion is called a *subarachnoid hemorrhage*.

The Brain

The brain is contained within the cranial vault and extends through the foramen magnum. It is composed of distinct structures, each having a specific function. The brain can be considered in three major functional areas: the cerebrum, the brainstem, and the cerebellum (see Fig. 11-1). The cerebrum (from the embryologic forebrain) consists of the cerebral hemispheres, the thalamus, hypothalamus, basal ganglia, and the olfactory and optic nerves. The brainstem consists of the midbrain, pons, and medulla. The cerebellum is the final major division of the brain. The brainstem and cerebellum develop from the embryologic hindbrain. Table 11-1 lists the divisions of the brain and their major functions. Each of these brain divisions is presented separately in the following pages.

The Cerebrum

The Cerebral Cortex. The cerebral cortex is the convoluted gray matter that forms the outermost layer of the brain. It consists largely of specialized neurons that process and respond to specific sensory stimuli. The cortex receives electrical discharges from other neurons and converts them into ideas or actions. The cortex is divided into five anatomic divisions: the frontal, parietal, temporal, occipital, and limbic divisions.

The cortical neurons are specialized so that within each major division of the brain, specific areas are devoted to specific functions. Fifty-two specialized areas were identified in the late 1800s by Korbinian Brodmann; these areas are numbered according to histologic appearances and functions. If brain injury is identified in one of these areas, it is possible to predict the resulting sensory or functional impairment. Conversely, a lesion often can be localized according to the motor functions or sensations that are impaired. It is important to note, however, that most functions can be performed through impulses from several areas of the brain.

The cerebral cortex performs the highest functions of the human brain. As a result, it continues to develop beyond infancy and childhood. The newborn responds to the environment with simple awareness and reflex behavior.

Table 11-1   Basic Brain Divisions and Functions

Structure	Division	Function
Cerebrum	Cerebral hemispheres Cerebral cortex	Integration of sophisticated sensory and motor activities and thoughts
	Frontal lobes	Reception of smell, memory banks, and higher intellectual processes
	Parietal lobes	Sensory discrimination, localization of body awareness (spatial relationships), and speech
	Temporal lobes	Auditory functions and emotional equilibrium
	Occipital lobes	Vision and memory of events
	Limbic lobes	Primitive behavior, moods, and instincts
	Basal ganglia	Transmission of motor tracts, linking pyramidal pathways
	Corpus callosum	Provision of intricate connection between cerebral hemispheres
Brain stem	Midbrain	Hypothalamic response to neuroendocrine stimuli
	Pons	Origin of cranial nerves V, VI, VII, VIII
	Medulla	Vital center activity (cardiac, vasomotor, respiratory centers); origin for cranial nerves IX, X, XI
Cerebellum	White and gray matter	Muscle and proprioceptive activity, balance, and dexterity

During infancy, individual sensations, sights, and sounds can be stored in memory in the cerebral cortex, and the infant learns to associate these sights and sounds with events or feelings. As the infant develops into a toddler, higher cortical functions such as imagination and language become apparent.

There is tremendous growth of cortical function during the early years of life. Most developmental and neurologic assessment tools evaluate only basic reflexes and motor skills of the young infant and toddler, and it is not until the preschool and the early childhood years that cognitive functions and learning can be evaluated.

The cerebral hemispheres are two mirror image portions of the brain that consist largely of the cerebral cortex and fiber tracts. In general, each cerebral hemisphere governs the functions of and receives sensations from the contralateral side of the body. Therefore, the right cerebral hemisphere governs movement of and receives sensory input from the left side of the body. The left cerebral hemisphere governs movement of and receives sensory input from the right side of the body.

In most humans, one side of the brain is considered dominant; right-handed people are thought to have a dominant left side of the brain, and left-handed people are thought to have a dominant right side of the brain. Each hemisphere also has primary responsibility for some functions. In most people, the left hemisphere controls language and speech, and the right hemisphere helps interpret three-dimensional images and spaces. Other distinctions have been postulated. For example music understanding is thought to be predominantly controlled by the left hemisphere and arithmetic and design are thought to be controlled by the right hemisphere. To a certain extent, if one side of the brain is injured, the other side of the brain can be taught to assume the dominant functions (this compensation is called *plasticity*). This compensation is more likely when the injury occurs during infancy or early childhood, because cerebral dominance is not established fully until approximately 3 years of age.

The cerebral hemispheres are connected by nerve fibers called the *corpus callosum*. These nerve fibers allow the brain to function as a single unit despite its division into two hemispheres.

The Basal Ganglia. The basal ganglia are paired masses of gray matter deep within the cerebral hemispheres. They contain the nuclei of neurons and networks of tracts that control motor function. These basal ganglia send information to the motor cortex through the thalamus to inhibit unintentional movement. Thus, the basal ganglia regulate the extrapyramidal motor system. This system selects motor messages from lower pathways for interpretation up to the cerebral cortex; thus it influences motor activities, musculoskeletal control, rhythmic movement, and maintenance of an erect posture.

Interference with neurotransmission to the basal ganglia produces disturbances of intentional movement. The uptake of bilirubin by the brain during infancy, known as *kernicterus,* affects this area and can result in the development of neurologic dysfunction.

The Thalamus and Hypothalamus. The thalamus surrounds the third ventricle and is composed of tracts of gray matter. The thalamus is a major integrating center for afferent impulses from the body to the cerebral cortex.[85] The thalamus integrates and modifies messages that come from the basal ganglia and cerebellum and then transmits information up to the cerebral cortex. All sensory impulses, with the exception of those from the olfactory nerve, are received by the thalamus. These impulses are then associated, synthesized, and relayed through thalamocortical tracts to specific cortical areas. The thalamus is the center for the primitive appreciation of pain, temperature, and tactile sensations.

Lying beneath the thalamus and near the optic chiasm is the hypothalamus. It is the chief region for subcortical integration of sympathetic and parasympathetic activities. The hypothalamus secretes hormones that are important in the control of visceral activities, maintenance of water balance and sugar and fat metabolism, regulation of body temperature, and secretion of endocrine glands. The hypothalamus is the source of two hormones: vasopressin (antidiuretic hormone [ADH], also called arginine vasopressin) and oxytocin. These hormones are synthesized by the hypothalamus and are transmitted in nerve tracts to a small mass of tissue suspended below the hypothalamus, called the *posterior pituitary gland or neurohypophysis.* Vasopressin and oxytocin are then released by the posterior pituitary gland as needed.

The anterior pituitary gland, called the *adenohypophysis,* secretes hormones that control glands throughout the body; these hormones include growth hormone (somatotrophin), adrenocorticotropic hormone, thyroid-stimulating hormone, melanocyte-stimulating hormone, follicle-stimulating hormone, luteinizing hormone releasing factor, and prolactin.

Injury to or disease of the hypothalamus or the pituitary can produce a wide variety of neuroendocrine problems and can result in fluid and electrolyte imbalance and growth disturbances (see Chapter 12).

The Brainstem

The brainstem, located at the base of the skull, is the major nerve pathway between the cerebral cortex and the spinal cord. The three major divisions of the brainstem are the midbrain, the pons, and the medulla. Together they control many of the involuntary functions of the body.

The midbrain is a short segment between the hypothalamus and the pons. It contains the cerebral peduncles and the corpus quadrigemina. The midbrain consists of fibers that join the upper and lower brainstem; it is the origin of the oculomotor and trochlear cranial nerves. The midbrain is the center for reticular activity and assimilates all sensory input from the lower neurons before it is relayed to the cortex (see Evolve Fig. 11-2 in the Chapter 11 Supplement on the Evolve Website). It is because of this relay that the cortex can maintain consciousness, arousal, and sleep.

The pons is a round structure located in the anterior portion of the brainstem. It contains fiber tracts that connect the medulla oblongata and cerebellum with upper portions of the brain. It is the origin of the abducens, facial, trigeminal, and acoustic cranial nerves. Disturbances within this area often produce signs of abducens malfunction, including strabismus and visual hemiplegias.

The medulla oblongata lies between the pons and the spinal cord at the level of the foramen magnum. It is the site of decussation (crossing) of many corticospinal motor neurons. In addition, it transmits messages to and from the spinal pathways for interpretation and reaction by the cortex. The medulla is the origin for the glossopharyngeal, vagus, spinal accessory, and hypoglossal cranial nerves. Critical regulatory centers for cardiovascular and respiratory functions are found within this portion of the brain. Severe intracranial injury can result in the loss of medullary control of respirations and cardiac output. A blow to the back of the head can result in respiratory arrest, labile blood pressure, and decreased cardiac output.

Although posture is controlled by the cortex, it is integrated in the medulla, so medullary injury can produce decorticate and decerebrate posturing. Loss of medullary function can lead to decreased gag reflex or swallowing difficulties, because the glossopharyngeal and vagus nerves originate in the medulla. Any disease or injury to the medulla can be life threatening.

The Cerebellum

The cerebellum is located in the posterior fossa, directly below the occipital lobe. It consists of two hemispheres that contain gray matter, and it joins with the basal ganglia and reticular system. This area of the brain integrates voluntary movement. Spatial orientation, fine motor movements, muscle tone, balance, and dexterity are controlled by visual, auditory, and proprioceptive stimuli that are processed by the cerebellum. The cerebral cortex can exert voluntary control over the cerebellum by virtue of cognitive nerve pathways that adjust movement.

The Ventricles

The four ventricles of the brain are cavities that contain CSF. The ventricles are joined to one another by foramina, and the ventricular system ultimately communicates with the subarachnoid spaces of the brain and the spinal column. The ventricles are designed specifically for the production and circulation of CSF.

The first two ventricles are called the *lateral ventricles,* and each is located in a cerebral hemisphere. These ventricles communicate with the third ventricle through the foramen of Monro at the level of the thalamus. The third ventricle joins the fourth ventricle through a channel known as the *Sylvian aqueduct.* This fourth ventricle is located at the level of the pons and medulla. From this last chamber rise three foramina that open into the subarachnoid space to allow distribution of the CSF into the subarachnoid spaces of the brain and spinal cord. Insult or injury to structures surrounding the CSF pathway can cause acute or chronic CSF flow obstruction and can result in the development of hydrocephalus. In addition, the presence of blood or inflammation within this system can obstruct the CSF pathway.

The Cranial Nerves

The cranial nerves are 12 pairs of peripheral nerves that arise from the brain; each has a specific motor or sensory function, and four cranial nerves have parasympathetic functions.[111] Cranial nerve function can be lost as a result of lesions near the origin of the cranial nerve or following direct injury to the cranial nerve itself.

Identification of lost cranial nerve functions can help determine the location and severity of CNS disease or injury. For example, pupil inequality and a unilateral sluggish pupil response to light can develop with uncal herniation of the brain (lateral herniation of the temporal lobe through the tentorial notch) and with compression and stretching of the oculomotor nerve. Assessment of cranial nerve function becomes extremely important when the patient is comatose or unresponsive. (Table 11-2 lists cranial nerve origins and functions; see Fig. 11-1).

The Spinal Cord

The spinal cord is a cylindrical structure composed of neurons and nerve fibers. It joins the medulla at the foramen magnum and extends to the level of the second lumbar vertebra. There are 31 pairs of spinal nerves, which are distributed along the entire spinal cord (Fig. 11-3). These spinal nerves are all multifibered and transmit impulses between the CNS and the rest of the body. When a portion of the spinal cord is viewed in cross section, the cord fills only part of the vertebral column; it is surrounded by the pia mater, the CSF, the arachnoid, and the dura mater.

Table 11-2 **Cranial Nerves: Function, Potential Mechanism of Injury, and Assessment**

Cranial Nerve	Function	Mechanism of Injury	Assessment
I. Olfactory	Smell	Fracture of cribriform plate or ethmoid area (rare)	Provide simple odors (difficult to test reliably in young children).
II. Optic*	Vision	Direct trauma to orbit or globe; fracture involving optic foramen (relatively common); increased ICP	Ask child to describe objects near and far and also ask for identification of colors. Test each eye separately, and assess ability of child to see object moving into visual field from periphery.
III. Oculomotor*	Pupil constriction, movement of eye and eyelid	Pressure of herniating uncus on nerve or fracture involving cavernous sinus	Both pupils should constrict in response to light as light is applied to each. Consensual constriction (constriction in response to light directed to contralateral eye) should also be observed. Eyes should be able to move to follow moving object throughout visual field, and eyelids should raise equally when eyes are open. Damage to sympathetic nervous system fibers (Homer's syndrome) results in parasympathetic dominance and pupil constriction associated with ipsilateral ptosis (drooping eyelid). Ptosis and lateral downward deviation of eye with pupil response to light are typical signs of oculomotor injury. Always record pupil size in millimeters.
IV. Trochlear*	Movement of eye (superior oblique muscle)	Injury near course of nerve in area of brainstem or fracture of orbit (uncommon)	Assess ability of eyes to track object throughout visual field. Damage to this nerve prevents the eyes from moving downward and medially. Diplopia may also be present.
V. Trigeminal	Sensation to most of face and movement of jaw (mastication)	Direct injury to terminal branches, particularly to fibers of second division in roof of maxillary	Apply soft and sharp objects to skin of face (as patient's eyes are covered) and assess sensation (test above eye, upper lip, lower lip, and chin to test all three branches). Motor functions are intact if child can clench and move jaw and chew food.
VI. Abducens*	Lateral movement of eye	Injury near brainstem and course of nerve (uncommon)	Assess eye movement within socket, tracking an object throughout visual field. Assess conjugate eye movement by moving object close to patient. Both eyes should track object and move together as object is tracked throughout visual field. Patient may instinctively turn head toward weakened muscle to prevent diplopia.
VII. Facial	Motor innervation of face (forehead, eyes, and mouth) and sensation to anterior two thirds of tongue (sweet/bitter discrimination). Tearing	Fracture of temporal bone, laceration in area of parotid gland	Ask child to "make faces" (demonstrate) and assess symmetry of face. For a detailed assessment, the provider can use sugar, salt, and vinegar to test taste on front of tongue, but such detailed assessments are not typically performed in the critical care unit. Tearing with cry should be present.
VIII. Vestibulocochlear (Acoustic)	Hearing and equilibrium	Fracture of petrous portion of temporal bone (often injured with cranial nerve VII)	Check gross hearing by clapping hands (startle reflex should be observed in infants, blink reflex should occur with sudden sound). Test fine hearing through use of ticking watch or tuning fork. Vestibular division of this nerve is tested for response to cold water calorics and doll's eyes response. Both of these reflexes require that cranial nerve innervation controlling lateral gaze (cranial nerves III and VI) be intact for normal response. Cold water calorics (oculovestibular reflex)—instillation of cold water in the ear should stimulate cranial

Table 11-2 **Cranial Nerves: Function, Potential Mechanism of Injury, and Assessment—cont'd**

Cranial Nerve	Function	Mechanism of Injury	Assessment
			nerves VIII, III, and VI, producing lateral nystagmus (do not perform this test if patient is conscious; this is typically performed to document absence of any cranial nerve function). The doll's eyes maneuver (oculocephalic reflex) also tests the vestibular portion of cranial nerve VIII as well as cranial nerves III and VI (lateral gaze). As the patient's head is turned, eyes should shift in sockets in direction opposite head rotation.
IX. Glossopharyngeal	Motor fibers to throat and voluntary muscles of swallowing, speech Taste to posterior one third of tongue	Brainstem injury or deep laceration of neck	Evaluate swallow, cough, and gag (tests cranial nerves IX and X simultaneously). Child's clarity of speech should be evaluated.
X. Vagus	Sensory and motor impulses for pharynx, as well as parasympathetic fibers to abdomen	Brainstem injury, deep laceration of neck (rare)	Test as above, particularly cough and gag reflex.
XI. Spinal accessory	Motor innervation of sternocleidomastoid, upper trapezius	Laceration of neck (rare), brain death	Ask child to turn head as you palpate sternocleidomastoid, and to shrug shoulders as you feel trapezius muscles contract.
XII. Hypoglossal	Innervation of tongue	Neck laceration associated with injury of major vessels	Ask child to stick out tongue. Pinch nose of infant; mouth should open and tip of tongue should rise in midline.

Data from McCance K, Huether SE, editors: *Pathophysiology: the biologic basis for disease in adults and children,* ed 6, St Louis, 2009, Mosby; Seidel HM, et al, editors: *Mosby's guide to physical examination,* ed 6, St Louis, 2006, Mosby; Thompson JM, et al, editors: *Mosby's manual of clinical nursing,* ed 5, St Louis, 2002, Mosby; Slota MC: Pediatric neurological assessment. *Crit Care Nurse* 3:106, 1983.
*Innervation to eye muscles is generally tested simultaneously, and cranial nerves controlling lateral gaze (III and VI) must be intact to obtain a normal or positive "Doll's eyes" response (oculocephalic reflex) and "cold water calorics" response (oculovestibular reflex).

The spinal cord contains gray and white material, or matter. The gray matter consists of cell bodies and cell nuclei, and the white matter consists of nerve fibers that are grouped into tracts. The gray matter in the spinal cord is shaped like a butterfly, with anterior and posterior projections called the *anterior* and *posterior* horns or, respectively, the *ventral* or *dorsal* roots.

Peripheral sensory nerves carry impulses to the posterior horn (the dorsal root) of the spinal column where they synapse (i.e., connect or communicate) with other neurons that will carry information up the spinal column or to other neurons at the same level of the spinal column. Lower motor neurons are located in the anterior horn (the ventral root) of the spinal column. The lower motor neurons receive input from the brain and from other neurons within the spinal cord; they affect motor activity.

Spinal cord reflexes do not require any input from higher levels of the CNS. For example, when the lower leg hangs free and the patellar tendon is tapped with a reflex hammer, the rapid stretch of the muscle will produce a reflex contraction of the rectus femoris without the participation of higher CNS structures. As a result of the reflex, the lower leg swings upward. Occasionally, stimulus of a sensory neuron on one side of the body will result in movement on the opposite side of the body. For example, if the right hand is placed on something hot, that hand automatically will be withdrawn, and the left hand and left leg will extend to allow the body to move away from the painful stimulus. These behaviors can all occur at the spinal cord level, and they can continue despite injury to the cerebral cortex or even brain death. If damage to the brain or higher levels of the spinal cord occurs, however, it also can result in loss of inhibition to the lower motor neurons and cause flaccid or spastic paralysis.

Central Nervous System Circulation and Perfusion
The Cerebral Circulation
The brain requires a constant supply of oxygen and substrates (perfusion) to metabolize carbohydrates as an energy source. Adequate perfusion is also necessary to remove carbon dioxide and other metabolites from the brain. The brain requires approximately 20% of the child's cardiac output. A healthy child's brain consumes 5.5 mL of oxygen per 100 g of brain tissue per minute.[37] As a result, if the brain is deprived of oxygen for even a few minutes, brain ischemia can develop and result in permanent neurologic dysfunction or brain death.[32]

The cerebral arterial blood flow is provided by the two vertebral arteries and the right and left internal carotid arteries. The internal carotid arteries enter the skull anteriorly and end in the anterior cerebral and the middle cerebral arteries;

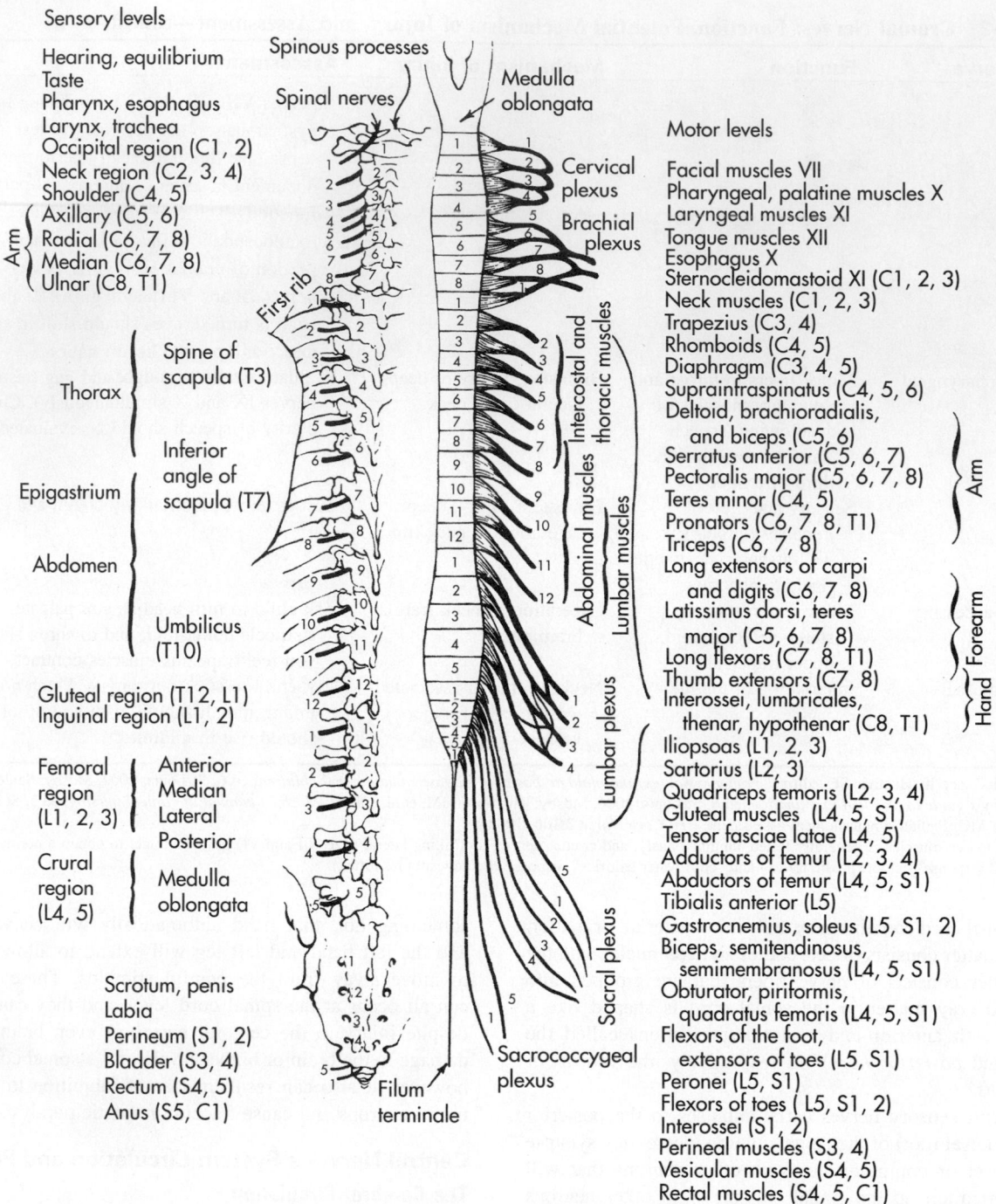

Sensory levels

Hearing, equilibrium
Taste
Pharynx, esophagus
Larynx, trachea
Occipital region (C1, 2)
Neck region (C2, 3, 4)
Shoulder (C4, 5)
Axillary (C5, 6)
Radial (C6, 7, 8) } Arm
Median (C6, 7, 8)
Ulnar (C8, T1)

Spinous processes
Spinal nerves

Medulla
oblongata

First rib

Thorax { Spine of scapula (T3)

Epigastrium { Inferior angle of scapula (T7)

Abdomen {

Umbilicus (T10)

Gluteal region (T12, L1)
Inguinal region (L1, 2)

Femoral region (L1, 2, 3) { Anterior Median Lateral Posterior

Crural region (L4, 5) { Medulla oblongata

Scrotum, penis
Labia
Perineum (S1, 2)
Bladder (S3, 4)
Rectum (S4, 5)
Anus (S5, C1)

Filum terminale

Cervical plexus
Brachial plexus

Intercostal and thoracic muscles

Abdominal muscles
Lumbar muscles

Lumbar plexus

Sacral plexus

Sacrococcygeal plexus

Motor levels

Facial muscles VII
Pharyngeal, palatine muscles X
Laryngeal muscles XI
Tongue muscles XII
Esophagus X
Sternocleidomastoid XI (C1, 2, 3)
Neck muscles (C1, 2, 3)
Trapezius (C3, 4)
Rhomboids (C4, 5)
Diaphragm (C3, 4, 5)
Suprainfraspinatus (C4, 5, 6)
Deltoid, brachioradialis, and biceps (C5, 6)
Serratus anterior (C5, 6, 7)   } Arm
Pectoralis major (C5, 6, 7, 8)
Teres minor (C4, 5)
Pronators (C6, 7, 8, T1)
Triceps (C6, 7, 8)
Long extensors of carpi and digits (C6, 7, 8)
Latissimus dorsi, teres major (C5, 6, 7, 8)   } Forearm
Long flexors (C7, 8, T1)
Thumb extensors (C7, 8)
Interossei, lumbricales, thenar, hypothenar (C8, T1) } Hand
Iliopsoas (L1, 2, 3)
Sartorius (L2, 3)
Quadriceps femoris (L2, 3, 4)
Gluteal muscles (L4, 5, S1)
Tensor fasciae latae (L4, 5)
Adductors of femur (L2, 3, 4)
Abductors of femur (L4, 5, S1)
Tibialis anterior (L5)
Gastrocnemius, soleus (L5, S1, 2)
Biceps, semitendinosus, semimembranosus (L4, 5, S1)
Obturator, piriformis, quadratus femoris (L4, 5, S1)
Flexors of the foot, extensors of toes (L5, S1)
Peronei (L5, S1)
Flexors of toes (L5, S1, 2)
Interossei (S1, 2)
Perineal muscles (S3, 4)
Vesicular muscles (S4, 5)
Rectal muscles (S4, 5, C1)

FIG. 11-3 Motor and sensory innervation from the spinal cord. (From Chusid JG: The spinal nerves. In Feringa ER, editor, *Correlative neuroanatomy and functional neurology*, ed 18, Los Altos, CA, 1981, Lange Medical Publications.)

they supply approximately 85% of cerebral blood flow. The vertebral arteries enter the skull posteriorly and join to form the basilar artery. The basilar artery bifurcates to form two posterior communicating arteries (Fig. 11-4).

The circle of Willis at the base of the brain is formed by a junction of the two internal carotid arteries, the two anterior and two posterior cerebral arteries, and the posterior and anterior communicating arteries (see Fig. 11-4, B). This arterial configuration, present in approximately half of all adults,[85] maintains effective cerebral perfusion despite a reduction in flow from

any single contributory artery. Patients with an alternative form of arterial circulation are considered to have anomalous cerebral circulation, although their arterial circulation typically is not significantly different from that which is considered normal. Congenital anomalies of one or both carotid arteries or of the internal carotid system have been documented. In many of these patients, the development of collateral circulation early in life prevents any compromise in cerebral perfusion.[29]

The cerebral venous circulation is unique in that the cerebral veins have no valves, and they do not follow the course

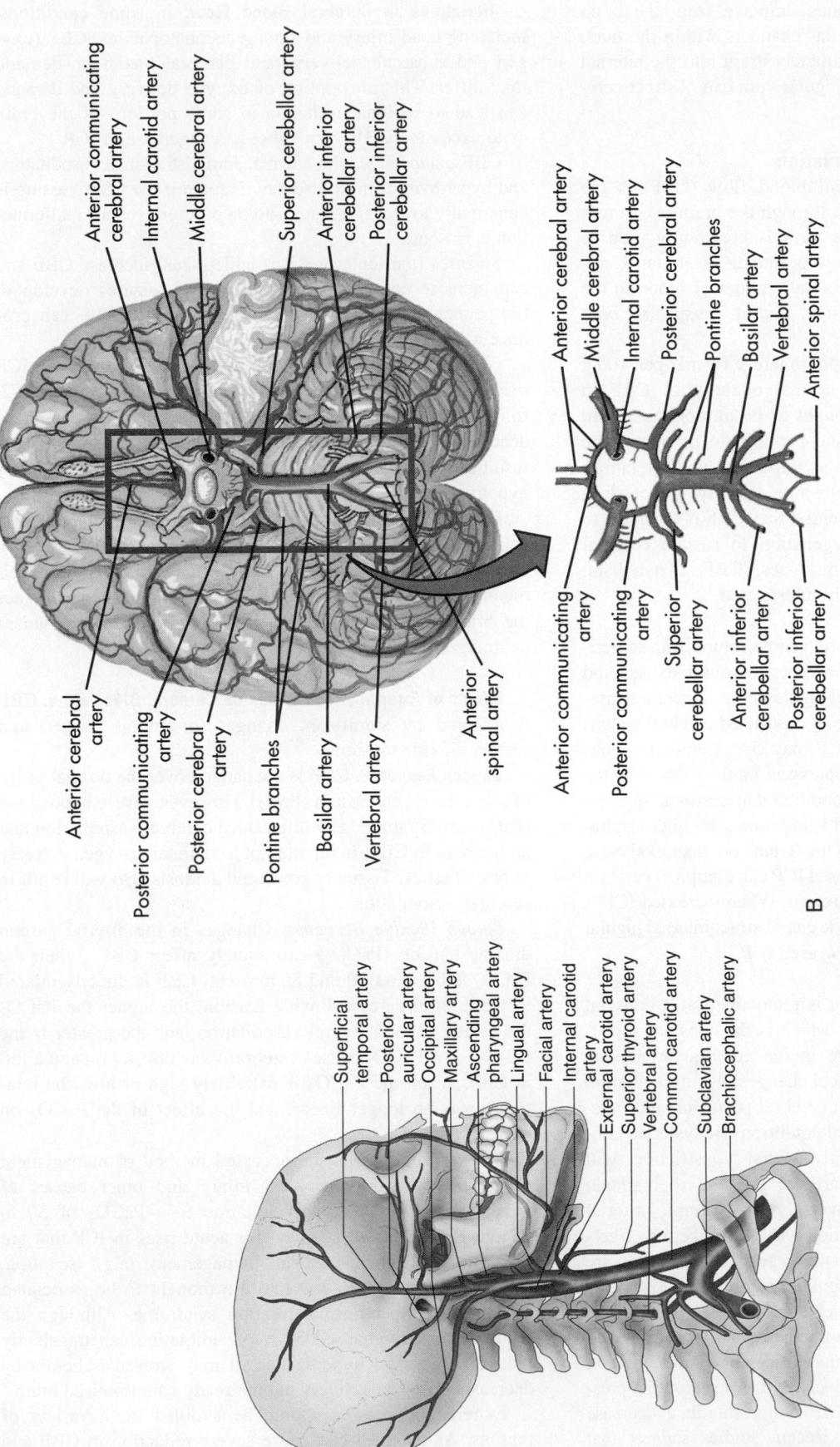

FIG. 11-4 The cerebral circulation. **A,** Major arteries of the head and neck. **B,** Arteries at the base of the brain. The arteries that compose the circle of Willis are the two anterior cerebral arteries, joined to each other by the anterior communicating artery and to the two posterior cerebral arteries, from which the posterior communicating arteries connect to the posterior cerebral arteries. (**A,** From Patton KT, Thibodeau GA: *Anatomy and physiology,* ed 7, St Louis, 2010, Mosby. **B,** Modified from Patton KT, Thibodeau GA: *Anatomy and physiology,* ed 7, St Louis, 2010, Mosby.)

of the cerebral arteries.[85] Venous drainage from the brain flows primarily into large vascular channels within the dura, known as *dural sinuses,* that ultimately drain into the internal jugular veins. Occlusion of the jugular vein can obstruct cerebral venous return.

Cerebral Blood Flow and Regulation

Cerebral Blood Flow. Cerebral blood flow (CBF) is the volume of blood that is in transit through the brain over a unit of time (e.g., per minute); this term is commonly used to describe the cerebral arterial flow perfusing the brain. Cerebral blood volume (CBV) is the total amount of blood in the intracranial vault at any one time, and it consists of both arterial and venous blood.

Normal CBF in adults is approximately 60 mL per 100 g brain tissue per minute. The normal quantity of CBF in children is unknown, but is thought to be approximately 50 to 100 mL per 100 g brain tissue per minute or more. The absolute quantity of CBF is not as important as the relationship between cerebral oxygen, substrate delivery, and cerebral metabolic requirements. It is essential that CBF is adequate to maintain effective cerebral oxygenation to sustain cerebral functions. Under normal circumstances, CBF, metabolism, and oxygen extraction are closely interrelated.[133]

Cerebral Venous Return. Cerebral venous return from superficial and deep cerebral veins flows into venous plexuses and dural sinuses, then into the internal jugular veins. If cerebral arterial flow is maintained in the face of obstructed cerebral venous return, CBV will increase and ICP may rise. Cerebral venous return can be obstructed by compression or thrombosis of the internal jugular vein, or by any condition that obstructs superior vena caval flow (e.g., mechanical ventilation with high inspiratory pressures, the development of a tension pneumothorax, or the Valsalva maneuver). Increased ICP can compress cerebral veins, impeding cerebral venous return. When increased ICP is present, turning the head to one side can obstruct internal jugular venous flow, increase CBV, and worsen ICP.

Autoregulation. CBF normally is maintained at a constant level by cerebral autoregulation, which is the constant adjustment of the tone and resistance in the cerebral arteries in response to local tissue biochemical changes.[72] Autoregulation is essential to the maintenance of cerebral perfusion and function over a wide variety of clinical conditions. If systemic arterial pressure increases, cerebral arterial constriction will prevent a rise in the cerebral arterial pressure to maintain CBF at a constant level. Conversely, if systemic arterial pressures falls, cerebral vasodilation will minimize the effects on CBF. Severe alterations in systemic arterial blood pressure will exceed the limits of autoregulatory compensation, however, and will be associated with changes in CBF.

Autoregulation may be compromised or destroyed with severe traumatic or anoxic brain injury. If cerebral autoregulation is lost, CBF becomes related passively to the mean arterial pressure (MAP) so that a fall in MAP will result in a decrease in cerebral flow and perfusion. Recent studies suggest that impaired autoregulation in traumatic brain injury may correlate with severity of injury and young age.[126]

Alterations in Cerebral Blood Flow. In some conditions, including head injury and some encephalopathies, CBF (oxygen and substrate delivery) and cerebral metabolic demand may differ. This uncoupling of oxygen delivery and demand can lead to regional ischemia in some portions of the brain or to excessive CBV with subsequent increase in ICP.

CBF can increase with anemia, administration of vasodilators, and hyperthyroidism. It also can increase if the CSF pressure is abnormally low or if a hemangioma or arteriovenous malformation is present.

Seizures (particularly status epilepticus) increase CBF and can increase cerebral metabolic rate. If seizures develop in the patient with increased ICP, the additional CBF can produce a further rise in ICP.

CBF will likely be compromised if CSF pressure or ICP rise. The ultimate complication of an accelerating rise in ICP following head injury is the cessation of CBF, producing brain death. CBF also can decrease in the presence of coma or as a result of a rise in cerebral venous pressure, polycythemia, or hypothyroidism.

If CBF is reduced severely, local cerebral metabolism is compromised, and brain cell metabolic functions will be compromised and may cease. If ischemia continues, brain cell membranes will become more permeable, and water will enter the brain cells. Profound ischemia can result in permanent neurologic dysfunction or brain death.

Effects of Arterial Blood Gases on Cerebral Blood Flow. CBF is affected by significant changes in arterial oxygen and carbon dioxide tensions.

Oxygen Response. CBF is unchanged over the normal range of arterial oxygen tension (PaO_2). However, severe hypoxemia (PaO_2 <50-55 mm Hg) will produce cerebral vasodilation and an increase in CBF, in an attempt to maintain oxygen delivery to brain tissues. Tissue hypoxia and acidosis also will result in cerebral vasodilation.

Carbon Dioxide Response. Changes in the arterial carbon dioxide tension ($PaCO_2$) can acutely affect CBF. When the $PaCO_2$ is between 20 and 80 mm Hg, CBF is directly related to the arterial carbon dioxide tension; the higher the $PaCO_2$ the greater is the cerebral vasodilation, and the greater is the CBF. A low $PaCO_2$ causes cerebral vasoconstriction and a fall in CBF. When the $PaCO_2$ is extremely high or low, the relationship is no longer linear, and the effect of the $PaCO_2$ on CBF is blunted.

Normoventilation is the accepted method of management of patients with severe head injury and other causes of increased ICP. Mild hyperventilation to a $PaCO_2$ of 30 to 35 mm Hg should be reserved for acute rises in ICP that are refractory to other medical management (e.g., sedation, hyperosmolar therapy) and that are thought to be associated with acute (impending) herniation syndrome. Although the reduction in CBF caused by hyperventilation can transiently reduce intracranial hypertension, it may worsen ischemia by decreasing oxygen delivery to an already compromised brain.[9]

Extreme hypocarbia should be avoided for a variety of reasons. As noted, it can cause severe reduction in CBF and create cerebral ischemia. It will shift the oxyhemoglobin dissociation curve to the left; although such a shift means that the hemoglobin will be better saturated at lower arterial oxygen tensions, hemoglobin release of oxygen to the tissues is compromised. Decreased oxygen delivery or release to tissues can cause or worsen ischemia. In addition, the effect of changes in the $PaCO_2$ on CBF is transient. Chronic hyperventilation can alter the brain bicarbonate buffering system, with the result that the cerebral circulation becomes hyperresponsive even to small changes in $PaCO_2$.

When increased ICP is present, routine care such as suctioning must be performed skillfully to prevent the development of hypercarbia and cerebral vasodilation and an increase in ICP.[9] The vasoconstrictive response to hypocarbia is unpredictable in patients after traumatic brain injury and the requires careful monitoring of clinical effects of any changes in $PaCO_2$.[9]

Cerebral Perfusion Pressure. Cerebral perfusion pressure (CPP) is calculated as the difference between the systemic mean arterial pressure (MAP) and the ICP:

$$CPP = MAP - ICP$$

The normal range of CPP is thought to be approximately 50 to 150 mm Hg in healthy adults, with a goal of 70 mm Hg following traumatic brain injury. There is a paucity of information to identify the normal range of CPP in children; it is thought to be approximately 40 to 60 mm Hg, but normal ranges vary with age.[9,48] A CPP of at least 40 mm Hg is thought to be necessary for effective cerebral perfusion; however, this number is not absolute because perfusion is determined by blood flow, not blood pressure. It is likely that a CPP of 40 mm Hg is acceptable in an infant, but a CPP of 50 to 65 mm Hg is likely to be necessary in older children and adolescents.

The calculated CPP will fall if the mean systemic arterial pressure falls, if the mean ICP rises, or if both occur simultaneously. The calculated CPP can be maintained despite a rise in ICP if the MAP rises commensurately with a rise in ICP. It is important to note that such compensation may or may not be associated with effective CBF and actual cerebral perfusion (for a Case Study of calculation of CPP, see the Chapter 11 Supplement on the Evolve Website); a normal CPP (40-50 mm Hg or more) has been recorded after brain death was pronounced.[16]

A clinical correlate of CPP in patients with increased ICP might be the MAP in patients with cardiovascular dysfunction. Patients with normal CPP may or may not demonstrate effective cerebral perfusion, just as patients with cardiovascular dysfunction and a normal blood pressure may or may not demonstrate effective systemic perfusion. Shock may be present with a normal blood pressure, and cerebral ischemia may be present with a normal calculated CPP. Therefore, the CPP should be calculated and evaluated in light of the patient's clinical appearance and neurologic function; a low CPP is worrisome, and a high or normal CPP is not reassuring in the presence of intracranial hypertension and clinical, especially neurologic, deterioration.

Evaluation of Cerebral Blood Flow. Qualitative radioisotope scans have been performed for a number of years to determine the presence or absence of CBF. However, quantitative CBF measurements cannot be readily performed at the bedside of the critically ill patient using standard pressure measuring devices. A variety of techniques can detect and monitor trends in CBF.

Jugular Venous Oxygen Saturation. The oxygen (actually oxyhemoglobin) saturation in the jugular venous bulb (SjO_2) is normally 55% to 70%; this measurement reflects the saturation of the hemoglobin leaving the cranial vault, so it reflects trends in the amount of oxygen leaving the brain. Trends in the SjO_2 can reflect changes in global cerebral perfusion in some clinical settings (discussed under Common Diagnostic Tests).

A fiberoptic catheter placed in the jugular bulb can be used to continuously monitor the SjO_2. The jugular bulb fiberoptic catheter must be correctly positioned, calibrated, and functional and correct use requires the ability to troubleshoot its function and potential causes of misleading information. Use of continuous SjO_2 monitoring has been reported for patients with head trauma, encephalopathy, status epilepticus, intracranial hemorrhage, and other conditions that may compromise cerebral perfusion and oxygen delivery.

Because the SjO_2 reflects oxygen (specifically oxyhemoglobin) saturation of blood leaving the cranial vault, it can be affected by any factor influencing oxygen delivery to the brain or oxygen consumption by the brain. As a result, if the SjO_2 changes, providers must attempt to evaluate each component affecting cerebral oxygen delivery and consumption to try to identify and treat the cause of the change. If the fiberoptic is not correctly positioned, calibrated and functional, trends in the SjO_2 may not accurately reflect trends in CBF.

Oxygen delivery to the brain can be altered by cardiac output, arterial oxygen content (which is, in turn, affected chiefly by hemoglobin concentration and its saturation), and factors that affect regional or global CBF (e.g., ICP, arterial pressure, arterial oxygen tension and tissue oxygenation, hemoglobin concentration, arterial and tissue pH, arterial CO_2, cerebral vasoconstriction, vasodilation, and tissue cytokines). Oxygen consumption by the brain can be increased by conditions such as fever and seizures and decreased by therapeutic hypothermia and by drugs such as barbiturates.

The SjO_2 will likely fall if oxygen delivery to the brain falls; in this case, oxygen extraction in the brain will increase so that less oxygen is left in the venous system when it leaves the cranial vault. The SjO_2 will fall if cerebral oxygen consumption increases (e.g., with fever or seizures) and oxygen delivery to the brain remains the same (i.e., it does not increase commensurately with increased consumption). Thus, a fall in the SjO_2 can indicate a fall in oxygen delivery to the brain (caused by a fall in cardiac output or CBF or an uncompensated fall in arterial oxygen content), or a rise in oxygen consumption.

The SjO_2 will rise, typically above 75%,[127] if oxygen delivery to the brain rises in excess of cerebral oxygen consumption. This rise is unlikely to be caused by decreased cerebral oxygen consumption unless a drug such as a barbiturate is administered. The SjO_2 will rise with the development of hypercarbia and associated cerebral vasodilation. An unexpected rise in SjO_2 can indicate hyperemia (excessive CBF) that may signal a loss of cerebral autoregulation.

Calculations Using Jugular Venous Bulb Oxyhemoglobin Saturation

Cerebral extraction of oxygen (normally 20%-42%):

$$\% \ CEO_2 = \frac{SaO_2 - SjO_2}{SaO_2} \times 100 = 20\% \ to \ 42\%$$

Cerebral arteriovenous oxygen content difference (cerebral $AVjDO_2$)*:

$$AVjDO_2 = Arterial \ O_2 \ content - Jugular \ venous \ O_2 \ content$$
$$= (SaO_2 - SjO_2) \times ([Hgb \ in \ g/dL] \times 1.34 \ mL/g)$$
$$= 3.5 \ to \ 8.1 \ mL/dL \ of \ blood$$
$$(average \ approximately \ 6 \ mL \ O_2/dL \ blood)$$

*For simplicity, this equation does not include the calculated dissolved oxygen, typically 0.10-0.3 mL oxygen/dL blood.
CEO_2, Cerebral extraction of oxygen; *SaO_2*, arterial oxygen saturation; *SjO_2*, jugular venous oxygen saturation.

Several calculations can be made using the SjO_2 (Box 11-1). Providers can calculate the cerebral extraction of oxygen (normally 20%-42%) and the cerebral arteriovenous oxygen content difference (normally 3.5-8.1 mL/dL of blood).[127] A rise in these variables indicates a decrease in oxygen delivery versus demand, with increased oxygen extraction or uptake that may signal decreased CBF. A rise in the arterial-jugular lactate difference can indicate a compromise in CBF.

Note that calculations derived from SjO_2 monitoring reflect only global brain oxygenation and cannot identify areas of regional ischemia. In addition, these calculations do not provide absolute values for cerebral metabolic rate and CBF. Sources of inaccurate values include a shift in the oxyhemoglobin dissociation curve—which will change the relationship between oxyhemoglobin saturation and partial pressure of oxygen, thus altering oxygen content at a given saturation—and technical errors related to positioning and calibration, especially in the pediatric population.[96]

Doppler Flow Velocity. Doppler flow velocity can be measured at the carotid artery or through an open fontanelle. In addition, transcranial Doppler flow velocity studies can be performed in older children and adolescents to evaluate cerebral flow velocity within the middle cerebral artery, anterior cerebral artery, and basal artery. Technical limitations of transcranial Doppler include inadequate visualization through available bone windows, the ability to view only medium to large vessels, variations in measurements between studies, and poor correlation with other indices of CBF.[53] There are also limited data regarding pediatric norms. For further information regarding the interpretation of changes in mixed venous oxygen saturations and Doppler flow studies, see the final section of this chapter and Chapters 6 and 8.[96]

Partial Pressure of Oxygen in Brain Tissue. The cerebral tissue oxygen tension ($P_{bt}O_2$) can be monitored using a probe placed through the skull into brain tissue. The probe can be placed in healthy tissue or in an area of the brain in or near a lesion, to monitor trends in oxygenation. Normal $P_{bt}O_2$ is approximately 20 to 35 mm Hg, and critical values are those less than 15 mm Hg. The $P_{bt}O_2$ can be altered by factors that alter CBF and by those that shift the oxyhemoglobin dissociation curve and alter release of oxygen to the tissues.[40]

Noninvasive Near-Infrared Spectroscopy. Noninvasive techniques for detection of trends in CBF, including the near-infrared spectroscopy, have been used more frequently in recent years. These techniques require placement of a light source on the scalp to transmit light through the skin and skull into the brain, and then quantify light reflection from the brain. Light reflection will be affected by tissue or hemoglobin oxygenation. These devices can help to identify trends in cerebral perfusion (see Chapter 21).

The Blood-Brain Barrier

The blood-brain barrier is the name given to the cellular structures that filter (i.e., selectively inhibit) some circulating toxins or potentially harmful substances to prevent their entry into brain tissue and CSF. The cellular structures that are involved include the cerebral capillary wall and the brain cells, especially the glial astrocytes. The astrocytes occupy the space between the relatively impermeable cerebral capillaries and the tissues of the CNS. The low permeability of the capillaries and the surrounding brain cells can protect the cerebral tissue from exposure to wide fluctuations in blood acids or bases (e.g., hydrogen ion or bicarbonate) or ionic composition. Permeability can be altered by widening or narrowing of spaces between endothelial cells and by widening or narrowing of the junctions between the endothelial cells and surrounding brain cells.

Oxygen, carbon dioxide, and lipid-soluble drugs readily cross the blood-brain barrier. The blood-brain barrier is also freely permeable to water, so rapid changes in intravascular osmolality can affect cerebral function (see Chapter 12). The major factor affecting transport across the blood-brain barrier is lipid solubility; the more lipid-soluble the drug is, the more easily it will cross the blood-brain barrier. Many drugs, including some water-soluble contrast agents and some antibiotics, do not cross the blood-brain barrier.

The immature brain does not have adequate development of glial cells; therefore, the blood-brain barrier is incomplete in the preterm infant.[64] This incomplete barrier is thought to contribute to increased risk of intracranial hemorrhage in preterm infants. It also makes the neonatal brain more vulnerable to some circulating drugs and toxins.

The Spinal Cord Circulation

The arterial supply of the spinal cord begins from paired spinal arteries that rise from the vertebral arteries at the level of the foramen magnum. In addition, the spinal cord is perfused from branches of the intercostal arteries that, in turn, branch from the thoracic aorta. This spinal cord circulation can be injured during thoracic surgery (e.g., during repair of coarctation of the aorta), resulting in spinal cord damage and paralysis.

Cerebrospinal Fluid and Its Circulation

CSF is a clear, colorless liquid that is produced in the ventricles and in specialized capillaries within the CNS. CSF circulates in the ventricles, the subarachnoid space, and the central canal of the spinal cord; it provides buoyancy to reduce the effective weight of the brain, and it cushions the CNS from injury.

Table 11-3	Normal Cerebrospinal Fluid Analysis in Children		

	NEONATES		Patients >6 months of Age
	Preterm	Term	
White blood cells per mm³			
Range	0-25	0-22	0-7
Polymorphonuclear leukocytes (%)	57	61-84	5
Protein (mg per 100 mL)			
Range	65-150	20-170	20-45
Glucose (mg per 100 mL)			
Range	24-63	34-119	50-80
Cerebrospinal fluid/blood glucose (%)			
Range	55-105	44-128	60-75

Data from McMillian JA, editor: *Oski's pediatrics principles and practice*, Philadelphia, 2006, Lippincott Williams and Wilkins; Custer JW, Rau RE, editors: *Harriett Lane handbook*, ed 18, Philadelphia, 2008, Mosby.

CSF is not merely a filtrate of plasma. It contains water, oxygen, carbon dioxide, sodium, potassium, chloride, glucose, a small amount of protein, and an occasional lymphocyte (Table 11-3). The CSF glucose is normally approximately 75% of the serum glucose concentration, which is approximately 50 to 80 mg/dL. The normal protein concentration is in the range of 20 to 45 mg/dL (higher normal values, up to 125 mg/dL, are present in neonates), and there are usually less than five white blood cells per cubic millimeter present in children. Again, slightly higher numbers may be normal in the neonate.[58]

Red blood cells are present in a CSF sample only if a traumatic spinal tap was performed or if the patient has suffered a cerebral hemorrhage. Generally, CSF is hypertonic to blood, but changes in CSF osmolality will parallel those of blood (i.e., an increase in serum osmolality will soon be followed by an increase in CSF osmolality). Abnormalities of CSF composition can aid in the diagnosis of some CNS diseases (Table 11-4).

CSF is formed primarily by the choroid plexuses; these plexuses are collections of capillaries located on the floor of each lateral ventricle and in the third and fourth ventricles. Additional CSF is formed by ependymal cells lining the ventricles and meninges and by blood vessels of the brain and spinal cord. CSF formation requires both active transport and simple diffusion between the existing CSF and the secreting surfaces.

In healthy children, the rate of CSF production is approximately 20 mL per hour.[58] The amount of CSF formed is affected by cerebral metabolism, CPP, blood pressure, and changes in the serum osmolality. An increase in the CPP or systemic arterial pressure usually results in an increase in CSF formation.

Once formed, the CSF flows from both lateral ventricles through the foramen of Monro into the third ventricle. From there the fluid passes through the cerebral aqueduct, known as the *Sylvian aqueduct* (or aqueduct of Sylvius), into the fourth ventricle. Some CSF then passes through the two lateral Luschka's foramina into the subarachnoid space to bathe the brain. The remaining CSF passes through Magendie's foramen and enters the subarachnoid space to circulate around the spinal cord. Most CSF ultimately is reabsorbed by venous sinuses that project into the subarachnoid space; these are known as the *arachnoid villi* (Fig. 11-5). Inflammation (e.g., meningitis) or blood in the ventricular system may obstruct CSF flow, often in the narrow aqueduct of Sylvius between the third and fourth ventricle. Subarachnoid hemorrhage can prevent normal reabsorption of CSF.

An obstruction in the flow of CSF, an increase in its production, or a decrease in its reabsorption will result in a condition known as *hydrocephalus*. When hydrocephalus is caused by an obstruction to flow (e.g., with obstruction in the aqueduct of Sylvius or with intraventricular hemorrhage), it is referred to as *obstructive* or *noncommunicating hydrocephalus*. When hydrocephalus is caused by increased CSF production or decreased CSF reabsorption (e.g., with subarachnoid hemorrhage), it is known as *communicating* hydrocephalus. Hydrocephalus causes an increased head circumference in the infant and can produce increased ICP in a patient of any age.

The normal CSF pressure is 7 to 20 cm H_2O or 5 to 15 mm Hg in the quiet, resting child; however, this pressure is not static. The CSF pressure normally varies during the cardiac and respiratory cycles and increases transiently during crying, sneezing, or a Valsalva maneuver (grunting or straining against a closed glottis), but it is normally <27 cm H_2O or <20 mm Hg.

CSF pressure can be measured from the central canal of the spinal cord (during a lumbar puncture), through catheterization of a lateral ventricle, or by insertion of a catheter into the subarachnoid space. All of these techniques measure CSF pressure and are thought to represent the ICP. If the CSF pressure remains above 27 cm H_2O (20 mm Hg), increased ICP is present.

Intracranial Pressure and Volume Relationships
Monroe-Kellie Hypothesis

Monroe (in the eighteenth century) and Kellie (in the nineteenth century) made the observation that the total intracranial volume is relatively constant. In general, the skull is a rigid structure that contains a finite total intracranial volume. The ICP is determined by the total intracranial volume and the intracranial compliance (the change in pressure resulting from a change in volume).

The skull sutures are not fused during infancy, and the skull can expand to accommodate gradual increases in intracranial volume (e.g., hydrocephalus or a slow-growing brain tumor). However, the skull cannot expand rapidly to accommodate acute increases in intracranial volume; therefore, even during infancy the intracranial volume is relatively constant.

The intracranial contents include the brain, the blood, and CSF. Therefore, the intracranial volume is equal to the sum of the volumes of these substances:

$$\text{Intracranial volume} = \text{Brain}_{vol} + \text{Blood}_{vol} + \text{CSF}_{vol}$$

If the volume of any of the intracranial contents increases without a commensurate and compensatory decrease in the volume of other intracranial content, the ICP will rise.

Table 11-4 Cerebrospinal Fluid Findings in Central Nervous System Disorders

Condition	Pressure (cm H$_2$O/mm Hg)	Leukocytes (mm^3)	Protein (mg/dL)	Glucose (mg/dL)	Comments
Healthy	7-20 cm H$_2$O 5-15 mm Hg	<5 (75% or more lymphocytes)	20-45	>50 (or 60-75% serum glucose)	
Common forms of meningitis					
Acute bacterial meningitis	Usually elevated (>27 cm H$_2$O >20 mm Hg)	100-10,000 or more; usually 300-2000; PMNs predominate	Usually 100-500	Decreased, usually <40 (or <50% serum glucose)	Organisms usually seen on Gram stain and recovered by culture
Partially treated bacterial meningitis	Normal or elevated	5-10,000; PMNs usual but mononuclear cells may predominate if pretreated for extended period of time	Usually 100-500	Normal or decreased	Organisms may be seen on Gram stain; pretreatment may render CSF sterile; antigen may be detected by agglutination test
Viral meningitis or meningoencephalitis	Normal or slightly elevated (20-34 cm H$_2$O 15-25 mm Hg)	Rarely >1000 cells; eastern equine encephalitis and lymphocytic choriomeningitis may have cell counts of several thousand; PMNs early but mononuclear cells predominate through most of the course	Usually 50-200	Generally normal; may be decreased to <40 in some viral diseases, particularly mumps (15%-20% of cases)	HSV encephalitis is suggested by focal seizures or by focal findings on CT or MRI scans or EEG; enteroviruses and HSV infrequently recovered from CSF; HSV and enteroviruses may be detected by PCR of CSF
Uncommon forms of meningitis					
Tuberculous meningitis	Usually elevated	10-500; PMNs early, but lymphocytes predominate through most of the course	100-3000; may be higher in presence of block	<50 in most cases; decreases with time if treatment is not provided	Acid-fast organisms almost never seen on smear; organisms may be recovered in culture of large volumes of CSF; *Mycobacterium tuberculosis* may be detected by PCR of CSF
Fungal meningitis	Usually elevated	5-500; PMNs early but mononuclear cells predominate through most of the course; cryptococcal meningitis may have no cellular inflammatory response	25-500	<50; decreases with time if treatment is not provided	Budding yeast may be seen; organisms may be recovered in culture; cryptococcal antigen (CSF and serum) may be positive in cryptococcal infection
Syphilis (acute) and leptospirosis	Usually elevated	50-500; lymphocytes predominate	50-200	Usually normal	Positive CSF serology; spirochetes not demonstrable by usual techniques of smear or culture; dark-field examination may be positive

Condition	Pressure	Leukocytes (differential)	Cell count	Glucose	Comments
Amebic (*Naegleria*) meningoencephalitis	Elevated	1000-10,000 or more; PMNs predominate	50-500	Normal or slightly decreased	Mobile amebae may be seen by hanging-drop examination of CSF at room temperature
Brain and parameningeal focus					
Brain abscess	Usually elevated (>27 cm H_2O >25 mm Hg)	5-200; CSF rarely acellular; lymphocytes predominate; if abscess ruptures into ventricle, PMNs predominate and cell count may reach >100,000	75-500	Normal unless abscess ruptures into ventricular system	No organisms on smear or culture unless abscess ruptures into ventricular system
Subdural empyema	Usually elevated	100-5000; PMNs predominate	100-500	Normal	No organisms on smear or culture of CSF unless meningitis also present; organisms found on tap of subdural fluid
Cerebral epidural abscess	Normal to slightly elevated	10-500; lymphocytes predominate	50-200	Normal	No organisms on smear or culture of CSF
Spinal epidural abscess	Usually low, with spinal block	10-100; lymphocytes predominate	50-400	Normal	No organisms on smear or culture of CSF
Chemical (drugs, dermoid cysts, myelography dye)	Usually elevated	100-1000 or more; PMNs predominate	50-100	Normal or slightly decreased	Epithelial cells may be seen within CSF by use of polarized light in some children with dermoids
Noninfectious causes					
Sarcoidosis	Normal or elevated slightly	0-100; mononuclear	40-100	Normal	No specific findings
Systemic lupus erythematosus with CNS involvement	Slightly elevated	0-500; PMNs usually predominate; lymphocytes may be present	100	Normal or slightly decreased	No organisms on smear or culture; positive neuronal and ribosomal P protein antibodies in CSF
Tumor, leukemia	Slightly elevated to very high	0-100 or more; mononuclear or blast cells	50-1000	Normal to decreased (20-40)	Results of cytologic analysis may be positive

Modified from Prober CG, Dyner L.L.: Central nervous system infections. In: Kliegman RM, et al, editors: *Nelson textbook of pediatrics*, ed 19, Philadelphia, 2011, Saunders, table 595-1. *CFS*, Cerebrospinal fluid; *CT*, computed tomography; *EEG*, electroencephalogram; *HSV*, herpes simplex virus; *MRI*, magnetic resonance imaging; *PCR*, polymerase chain reaction; *PMN*, polymorphonuclear neutrophil.

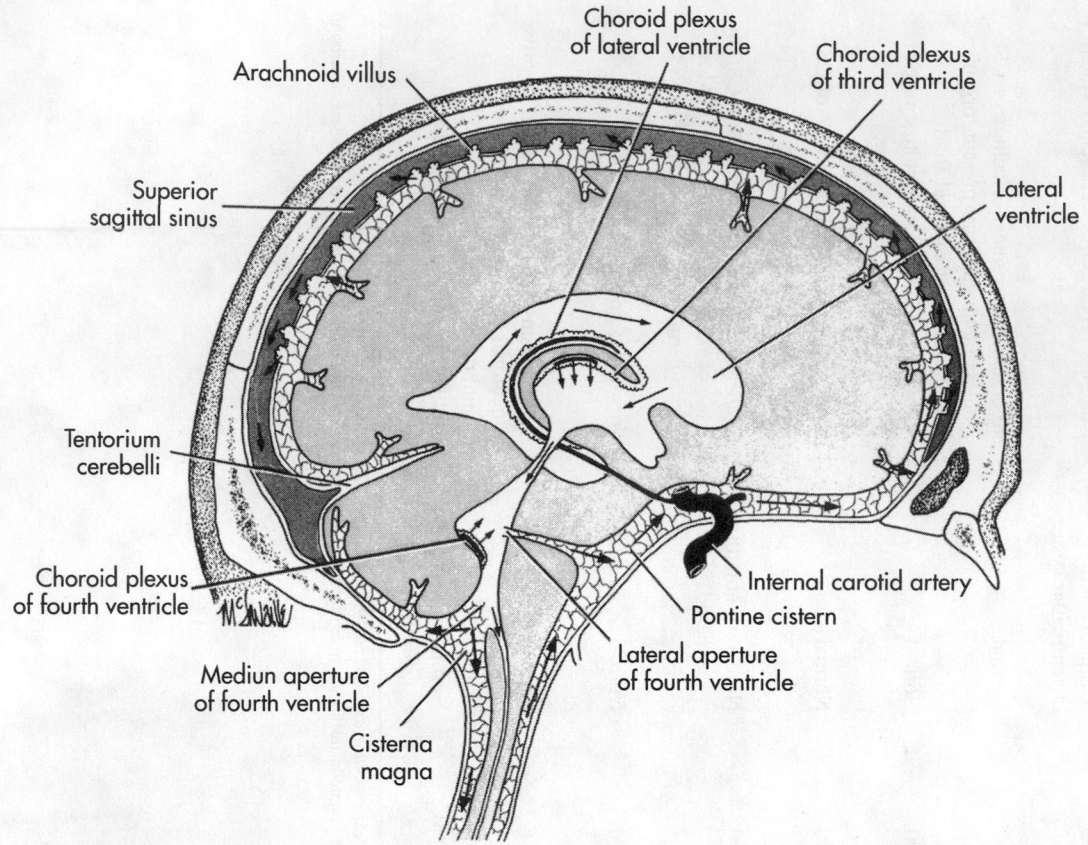

FIG. 11-5 Normal cerebrospinal fluid circulation. CSF is secreted from the floor of the lateral ventricles. After circulation though the ventricles and cisterns and around the spinal cord, the fluid is reabsorbed by the arachnoid villi in the subarachnoid space. (From Nolte J: *The human brain*, St Louis, 1981, Mosby.)

The Brain

The brain occupies the largest portion (80%) of the intracranial space; it is essentially not compressible, but it is somewhat movable within the cranium. If significant pressure gradients develop within the cranium or between the intracranial space and the spinal column, cerebral herniation can occur. A severe increase in ICP can cause herniation of the brainstem through the foramen magnum and brain death (cerebral circulation ceases).

Cerebral edema can increase brain volume. Cerebral edema is an increase in brain water content related to increased cellular membrane permeability or massive extravascular (intracellular) fluid shift. Cerebral edema can develop during some infections, metabolic derangements (e.g., treatment of diabetic ketoacidosis), and asphyxia. This edema may be further categorized as vasogenic, cytotoxic, osmotic, or interstitial edema.

Vasogenic cerebral edema may result from disruption of the blood-brain barrier that allows plasma proteins and fluid to enter the brain parenchyma. Cytotoxic edema results from metabolic derangements that alter sodium-potassium pump function and result in retention of sodium and water by the astrocytes. The blood-brain barrier remains intact in cytotoxic edema. Cytotoxic edema can develop following drug or alcohol intoxication, trauma, hypoxic-ischemic events such as cardiac arrest and in early stroke.

Osmotic cerebral edema occurs when the serum osmolality falls acutely, creating an acute difference between intravascular/extracellular osmolality and intracellular (brain) osmolality. This abnormal pressure gradient leads to movement of water into the brain cells (i.e., from the extracellular—including intravascular—space to the intracellular space) with resultant development of cerebral edema. Causes of osmotic edema include an acute fall in the serum sodium concentration, rapid lowering of blood glucose (such as in treatment of diabetic ketoacidosis) or rapid fall in blood urea nitrogen (BUN) during hemodialysis.

Interstitial edema is a consequence of hydrocephalus. The CSF-brain barrier is disrupted resulting in trans-ependymal flow of CSF into the extracellular space of the brain parenchyma.

Brain volume also can be increased as the result of an increase in CBF, such as occurs in some areas of the brain after head injury. Excessive blood flow is referred to as *hyperemia*.

Cerebral Blood Volume

CBV comprises approximately 7% to 10% of the total intracranial volume. CBF is influenced by the biochemical environment in brain tissue, and changes in CBF normally match changes in cerebral metabolic requirements. As noted previously, CBV can increase or decrease in some areas of the brain after head injury, and cerebral arterial flow may no longer match cerebral metabolic requirements in those areas.

Some cerebral blood is contained in venous capacitance vessels. This blood is dispensable and is shifted from the intracranial vault to reduce total CBV as a compensatory mechanism during periods of increased intracranial volume. Hyperventilation can produce cerebral vasoconstriction; it will decrease cerebral arterial flow and may contribute to displacement of this venous capacitance blood. However, hyperventilation and cerebral vasoconstriction can also produce cerebral ischemia.

If the volume of other intracranial contents increases significantly and ICP rises, CBF and oxygen delivery can be compromised. Cessation of CBF results in brain death.

Cerebrospinal Fluid

CSF normally comprises 7% to 10% of the total intracranial volume and this percentage remains constant if production is matched by absorption. CSF volume will increase if CSF flow pathways are obstructed (e.g., obstructive or noncommunicating hydrocephalus can develop with a brain tumor, after meningitis, or after head trauma associated with intraventricular bleeding), or if CSF reabsorption is diminished (e.g., following head injury with subarachnoid hemorrhage).

CSF is the material most easily displaced from the intracranial vault as compensation for an increase in brain volume or CBV. CSF can be removed from the intracranial vault by a shunt or the placement of a ventricular drain.

Normal Intracranial Pressure

The ICP is the pressure exerted by the intracranial contents. The normal ICP is approximately 5 to 15 mm Hg, but this pressure is not static. It can be increased transiently by anything that acutely increases cerebral venous pressure or by movement from an upright to a reclining position. Typically, the ICP varies by 0.5 to 1.3 mm Hg during respiration.

If the brain, cerebral blood, or CSF volume increases without a compensatory decrease in other intracranial components, the intracranial volume increases. Initially, however, the ICP does not rise (Fig. 11-6). This ability to tolerate an increase

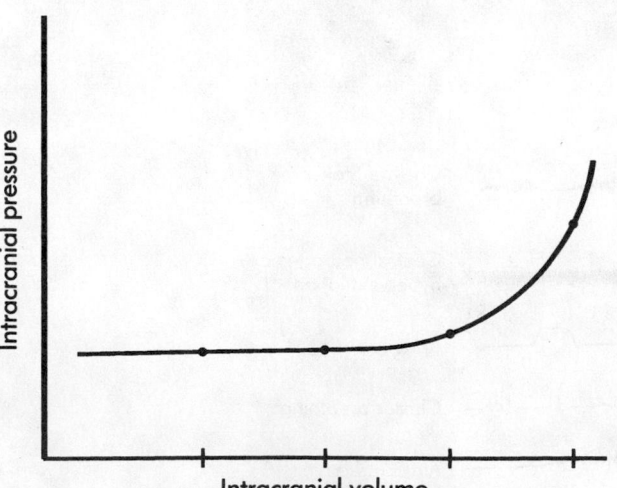

FIG. 11-6 Intracranial pressure (ICP)-volume curve. The change in ICP resulting from an increase in intracranial volume is not linear. Initially, an increase in volume can develop without any increase in pressure. However, once the limits of compliance have been reached, ICP will rise. Note that once the ICP begins to rise, small increases in intracranial volume will produce significant elevations in ICP.

in the volume of one intracranial component results from the compensatory displacement of venous capacitance blood or CSF from the intracranial vault. In addition, intracranial compliance (including a small amount of brain compression) allows for some increase in intracranial volume without an increase in ICP. However, there is a limit to this compliance. If the brain, blood, or CSF volume continues to increase, ICP ultimately will rise. Once the limits of compliance have been reached, progressively smaller incremental increases in intracranial volume will be associated with progressively more significant increases in ICP (see Common Clinical Conditions, Increased Intracranial Pressure).

COMMON CLINICAL CONDITIONS

Nursing care of any child with an actual or potential neurologic problem requires careful and repeated assessments over time. For this reason, before presentation of common clinical conditions themselves, this section begins with a summary of critical bedside neurologic assessment (Box 11-2).

Neurologic assessment and support includes assessment and support of airway, oxygenation, ventilation, and circulation, as well as evaluation of level of consciousness, pupil size and response to light, cranial nerve function, Glasgow Coma Scale score and additional evaluation of motor activity, reflexes, and movement. General neurologic assessment is summarized in Box 11-2. To ensure clear and consistent communication and to facilitate rapid identification of clinical changes, all members of the healthcare team must use consistent terminology and assessment tools and must apply them in a consistent fashion.

Evaluation of Respiratory Pattern

Patients with neurologic disease or dysfunction may demonstrate a wide variety of respiratory patterns. Regardless of the respiratory rate or pattern demonstrated by the patient, the nurse must ensure that the patient's airway and arterial oxygen saturation and carbon dioxide removal are adequate, because hypercapnia, hypoxemia and hypoxia can contribute to cerebral vasodilation, increased CBF, increased ICP, and inadequate cerebral perfusion. If respiratory insufficiency develops, immediately notify the on-call provider and support airway, oxygenation and ventilation.

When intracranial injury or insult occurs, some characteristic breathing patterns may be noted that help identify the level of intracranial problem. Such breathing patterns include Cheyne-Stokes breathing, central neurogenic hyperventilation, apneusis, cluster breathing and ataxic breathing (Fig. 11-7). If the ICP rises to a point that brainstem compression occurs and cerebral herniation is imminent, the Cushing reflex is initiated, producing an abnormal breathing pattern that often includes apnea.

Cheyne-Stokes respirations are defined as alternating hyperpnea and bradypnea, which means that the patient initially breathes faster and deeper, then more shallowly, and then demonstrates a long pause before beginning the cycle again. Cheyne-Stokes respirations can be observed in patients with encephalopathies or cerebrovascular disease and in patients with diabetic ketoacidosis.

Central neurogenic hyperventilation is present when the patient breathes deeply at a constant, rapid rate (hyperpnea)

Box 11-2   Summary of Bedside Nursing Assessment of Neurologic Function

- Airway, Ventilation and Respiratory Pattern, Oxygenation
  - Maintain patent airway (particularly if level of consciousness is decreased).
  - Assess and support adequate ventilation.
  - Monitor for abnormal respiratory patterns (see Fig. 11-7). An irregular respiratory rate or apnea may develop with increased intracranial pressure.
  - Ensure adequate oxygenation.
- Systemic Perfusion
  - If perfusion is poor, cerebral perfusion may be compromised.
  - Evaluate vital signs in light of age and clinical condition. Tachycardia is nonspecific sign of distress, so further assessment is required.
  - Cushing triad (resulting from increased intracranial pressure and impending brainstem herniation) includes: bradycardia, increased systolic blood pressure (with widened pulse pressure), and irregular respiratory pattern (including possible apnea).
- Level of Consciousness
  - Monitor responsiveness in context; watch for unusual irritability or lethargy.
  - If coma is present (no verbal response to stimuli), use consistent terminology (see Table 11-5).
- Pupil Size and Response to Light: notify on-call provider immediately if pupils dilate or have decreased constriction to light
- Cranial Nerve Function
  - Optic Nerve (II): vision
  - Oculomotor (III): pupil constriction in response to light (note size); injury can cause ptosis and lateral downward deviation of eye
  - Trochlear (IV): eye movement downward and medially; injury can also cause diplopia
  - Trigeminal (V): sensation to face, jaw movement, chewing
  - Abducens (VI): lateral eye movement within socket and conjugate eye movement to track object across visual field
  - Facial (VII): movement of facial muscles (especially forehead and around eyes and mouth), sensation on anterior tongue, tearing with cry
  - Vestibularcochlear/Acoustic (VIII): hearing and equilibrium
  - Glossopharyngeal (IX): swallowing, cough, gag and speech
  - Vagus (X): cough and gag reflex
  - Spinal Accessory (XI): shoulder shrug
  - Hypoglossal (XII): tongue movement (sticking tongue out of mouth)
- Glasgow Coma Scale Score (see Table 11-6)
  - Eye opening
  - Verbal response
  - Motor response:
    - *To evaluate ability to obey commands:* Ask the child to hold up two fingers, stick out his or her tongue or (unless spinal cord injury present) wiggle toes.
    - *To evaluate ability to localize painful stimulus:* Rub the child's sternum or pinch trapezius (child's hand should reach toward the site of stimulus).
    - *To evaluate withdrawal in response to pain in each extremity:* Pinch the medial aspect of each extremity (child should abduct each extremity, pulling outward from medial stimulus).
    - *To assess for decorticate or decerebrate posturing (see Fig. 11-9) or no response:* Rub the sternum or pinch the trapezius (observe response).
- Additional Motor Activity and Reflexes
  - Look for abnormal reflexes (e.g., Babinski, see Fig. 11-10).
  - Be aware of developmental milestones achieved or lost (see Table 11-7).
  - Development of incontinence in child with previous bowel or bladder control may indicate neurologic deterioration.
  - Monitor for seizures.

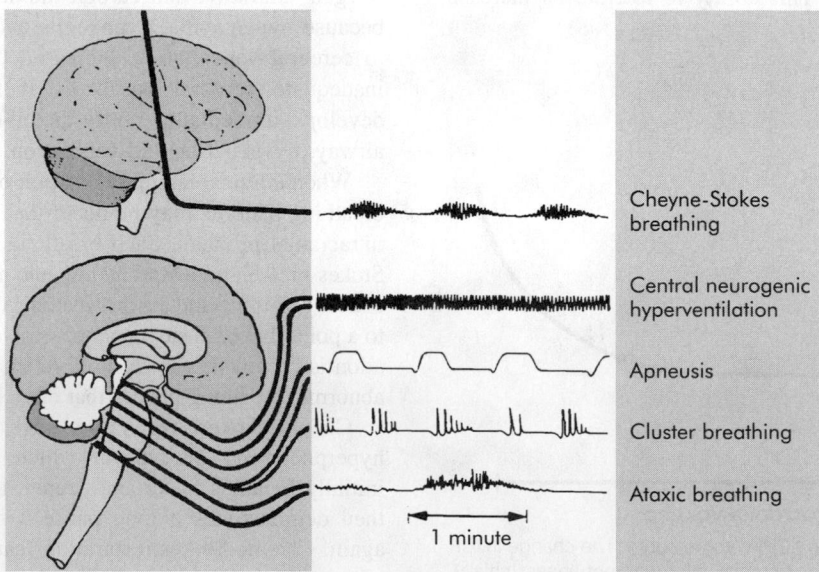

Cheyne-Stokes breathing

Central neurogenic hyperventilation

Apneusis

Cluster breathing

Ataxic breathing

1 minute

FIG. 11-7 Abnormal respiratory patterns with corresponding level of central nervous system activity. (From Boss BJ: Alterations in cognitive systems, cerebral hemodynamics, and motor function. In McCance KE, Huether SE, editors: *Pathophysiology: the biologic basis for disease in adults and children*, ed 6, Philadelphia, 2010, Mosby, p. 531, fig. 16-1.)

despite the presence of adequate arterial oxygenation and hypocapnia. This hyperventilation usually indicates the presence of cerebral hypoxia or ischemia or a midbrain or pontine lesion. Other abnormal breathing patterns include apneustic breathing (pauses after inspiration and possibly after expiration), cluster breathing (irregular breathing associated with irregular pauses), and ataxic breathing (very irregular rate, rhythm, and depth of breaths).

Evaluation of Systemic Perfusion

Careful monitoring of systemic perfusion is required for all critically ill or injured patients. If systemic perfusion is poor, cerebral perfusion may be compromised. This concept is especially true for trauma patients with head injury. Shock resuscitation is essential to optimizing cerebral perfusion.

Vital signs are evaluated in light of the patient's clinical condition (see pages inside front cover for tables of normal heart rates, respiratory rates, and blood pressures in children). Tachycardia and tachypnea are usually more appropriate in critically ill children than are normal heart and respiratory rates. In children who are 1 to 10 years old and of average height, hypotension is present if the child's systolic blood pressure is less than 70 mm Hg plus twice the patient's age in years.[31,56] Hypotension is also present if the MAP is less than 40 mm Hg plus one and one-half times the child's age in years.[56]

Hypertension can develop as a compensatory mechanism to maintain cerebral perfusion in patients with an increase in ICP (see The Cushing Reflex), but hypertension also can be a sign of pain or fear. If hypertension develops, immediately assess and support the child's airway, oxygenation, ventilation, and perfusion. Assess the child's heart rate, level of consciousness, pupil size and response to light, and Glasgow Coma Scale score (see Glasgow Coma Scale Scoring of Neurologic Function, later). Significant hypertension, particularly if associated with any other signs of deterioration, should be reported immediately to the on-call provider; it may signal increased ICP and even impending brain herniation.

The Cushing Reflex

The Cushing reflex is a late and ominous result of increased ICP and ischemia of the vasomotor center.[83] The Cushing reflex indicates profound compromise in brainstem perfusion and may develop only when cerebral brainstem herniation is imminent. This reflex produces the clinical triad of bradycardia, an increase in systolic arterial blood pressure with widened pulse pressure, and abnormal breathing pattern. This clinical triad is referred to as the Cushing triad, a term often used interchangeably with the Cushing reflex. The abnormal breathing pattern that is part of the Cushing triad may consist of an abnormal or irregular respiratory effort or apnea.[83]

The Cushing reflex does not develop until the ICP is elevated significantly. Earlier signs of increased ICP may include tachycardia and fluctuations in arterial blood pressure. A late sign of increased ICP is hypotension.

Evaluation of Level of Consciousness

Detection of neurologic deterioration requires careful monitoring of the patient's level of consciousness, including assessment of behavior and responsiveness that is tailored to each patient. Excessive irritability is a common and nonspecific sign of pain, sleep deprivation, and cardiopulmonary or neurologic dysfunction in the critically ill child. Lethargy is almost always abnormal and is typically a more specific and crucial indicator of deterioration of neurologic function than irritability. However, evaluation of the child's behavior and responsiveness is facilitated by knowledge of the patient's normal behavior and condition.

An infant is expected to be irritable when hungry, tired, or overstimulated, so it is important to be aware of normal feeding times and sleep patterns and to attempt to reduce stimulation of the seriously ill or injured infant. It is normal for the infant to be comforted when swaddled or patted and to be quiet and sleepy after feeding. A healthy infant will not cry or sleep constantly, but a seriously ill infant will likely sleep much of the time. A high pitched cry is usually abnormal.

It is important to evaluate the activity of the infant or child in the context of surrounding events and environmental stimulation. The child is expected to be sleepy if the child was awake throughout the preceding night in the hospital. However, it would be extremely abnormal for the same child to sleep while a venipuncture is performed. A decreased response to frightening or painful procedures is abnormal and probably indicates cardiorespiratory or neurologic compromise.

Assessment of level of consciousness in the verbal child is facilitated if the nursing care plan includes information about the child's normal activities and names of the child's family members, pets, or favorite stuffed animals. This information will assist in assessment of the child's short- and long-term memory and orientation to time and place. For example, a child stating that "Oscar was flying around my room at home" could be demonstrating confusion if Oscar is the child's brother, but can be demonstrating accurate recall if Oscar is the child's pet parakeet that frequently escapes from the cage. It is helpful to document the names of any imaginary friends that the child has if the child normally refers to them.

If acute coma is present, members of the healthcare team should use consistent terminology (Table 11-5) to describe the child's level of response. Coma is present when the patient demonstrates no eye opening or verbal response to any stimuli, demonstrating only motor response to painful or noxious stimuli. Stupor is present when only vigorous and repeated stimulation produces arousal.

When coma is present, careful assessment of the child's motor function is extremely important. Such assessment includes the routine use of a scoring system of neurologic response (see Glasgow Coma Scale Scoring of Neurologic Function).

Evaluation of Pupil Response and Cranial Nerve Function

The pupils are normally of equal size, and they both should constrict briskly in response to light. This constriction reflects function of the third cranial (oculomotor) nerve. *Hippus* is a spasmodic, rhythmic papillary movement, that is often a normal variant.[50] When increased ICP develops, the oculomotor nerve is compressed by general expansion of the brain, by the intracranial lesion, or by uncal herniation; such compression can produce pupil dilation and decreased or absent pupil

Table 11-5   Levels of Acute Coma

State	Definition
Confusion	Loss of ability to think rapidly and clearly; impaired judgment and decision making
Disorientation	Beginning loss of consciousness; disorientation to time followed by disorientation to place and impaired memory; self-recognition is last to be lost
Lethargy	Limited spontaneous movement or speech; easy arousal with normal speech or touch; may not be oriented to time, place, or person
Obtundation	Mild to moderate reduction in arousal (consciousness) with limited response to the environment; falls asleep unless stimulated verbally or tactilely; answers questions with minimal response
Stupor	A condition of deep sleep or unresponsiveness from which the person may be aroused or caused to open eyes only by vigorous and repeated stimulation; response is often withdrawal or grabbing at stimulus
Coma	No verbal response to the external environment or to any stimuli; noxious stimuli such as deep pain or suctioning yields motor movement
Light coma	Associated with purposeful movement on stimulation
Deep coma	Associated with unresponsiveness or no response to any stimulus

From Boss BJ: Alterations in cognitive systems, cerebral hemodynamics, and motor function. In McCance KE, Huether SE, editors: *Pathophysiology: the biologic basis for disease in adults and children*, ed 6, Philadelphia, 2010, Mosby-Elsevier, p. 530, table 16-4.

constriction in response to light. When the intracranial herniation or lesion is unilateral, the pupil dilation will typically occur on the same side as the lesion. The child also may complain of blurred vision or diplopia.

Increased ICP can cause compression of the oculomotor nerve, producing unilateral ptosis with ipsilateral (same side) pupil dilation. However, if unilateral ptosis is noted with ipsilateral pupil constriction, *Horner's syndrome* may be present. This syndrome consists of unilateral ptosis (abnormally low position [drooping] of the upper eyelid), miosis (small pupil), and anhidrosis (lack of sweat on that side of the face). Horner's syndrome is caused by unilateral interruption of sympathetic nervous system fibers, and it can be observed after cardiovascular surgery near the aortic arch.

It is important to differentiate between ptosis caused by third nerve compression and that caused by Horner's syndrome, because the former can indicate the presence of increased ICP (requiring immediate treatment) and the latter requires no treatment. When the third cranial nerve is compressed, the pupil will not constrict normally in response to light and that pupil is typically dilated. When Horner's syndrome is present the involved pupil is small, and both pupils should still react (constrict) in response to light.

Some clinical conditions or medications can modify pupil size or response to light. When the patient has unilateral blindness, the involved pupil will not constrict in response to light. Pupil constriction (miosis) can result from hemorrhage in the pons, poisoning, or administration of large doses of opioids. Pupil dilation can be present with significant pain or hypothermia and can result from administration of atropine or of extremely large doses of sympathomimetic drugs such as dopamine or epinephrine. Pupil dilation will also be present following administration of mydriatic drops to dilate the pupils for examination, so administration of such drugs should be well-documented. Changes in the pupil size and response to light with altered levels of consciousness are summarized in Fig. 11-8.

Evaluation of the function of most cranial nerves can be performed during routine nursing care (see Box 11-2). If the child is verbal and able to count, you can ask the child to tell you the number of fingers you hold in front of the child's face;

if the child can correctly identify the number of fingers, the optic nerve (cranial nerve II) is probably intact. Consensual pupil constriction in response to light requires the oculomotor nerve (cranial nerve III). If the child can track objects across a visual field, the oculomotor, trochlear, and abducens nerves (cranial nerves III, IV, and VI, respectively) are functioning. If wrinkling of the forehead is noted during cough, the facial nerve (VII) is probably intact. If noise startles the child, the acoustic nerve (cranial nerve VIII) is functioning. A gag reflex (cranial nerve X) should be observed during suctioning or insertion of a nasogastric tube, even if the child is comatose. Movement of the shoulders and upper extremities indicates function of the spinal accessory nerve (cranial nerve XI). The hypoglossal nerve (cranial nerve XII) provides tongue movement (e.g., the child can stick out his or her tongue).

If the child demonstrates a loss of previously demonstrated cranial nerve function, notify the on-call provider immediately. When cerebral perfusion is compromised and cessation of brain function occurs, cranial nerve function will disappear (e.g., the child who had a gag reflex will no longer cough or gag during suctioning).

Glasgow Coma Scale Scoring of Neurologic Function

The most widely used neurologic scoring system is the Glasgow Coma Scale (GCS). This scale evaluates motor activity, verbal responses, and motor responses, with a total scale range of 3 to 15. This scale is useful in identifying patients with mild or moderate neurologic dysfunction; it will not reliably differentiate children with profound neurologic dysfunction from those with moderate neurologic dysfunction. The lowest score possible in the scale is a 3—the flaccid unresponsive patient in full cardiopulmonary arrest and the flaccid unresponsive hypothermic but well-perfused patient will both receive a score of 3.

The GCS was validated in adults, and the original GCS verbal section cannot be used in the care of the preverbal or intubated patient. For these reasons, modifications of the GCS have been developed and found to be useful for pediatric patients with neurologic injury or disease (Table 11-6).[34a,83,90,106]

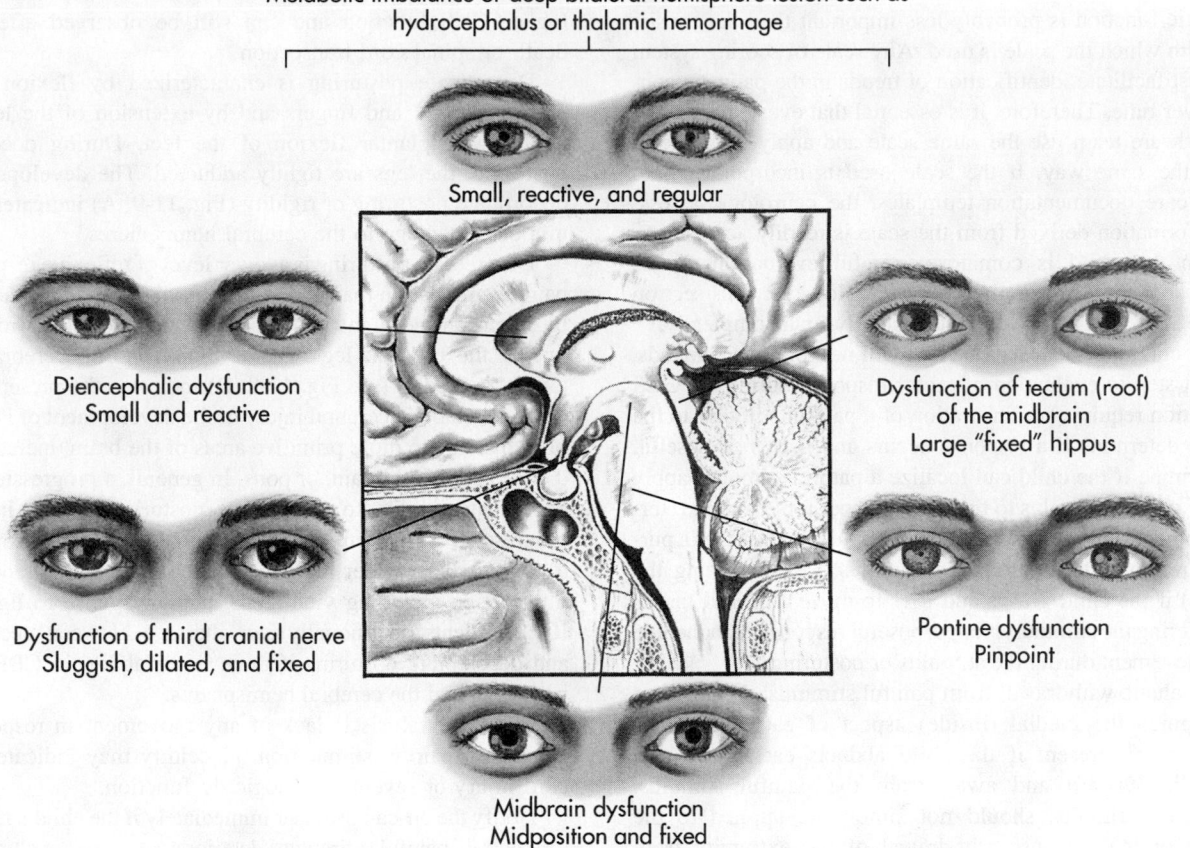

Metabolic imbalance or deep bilateral hemisphere lesion such as hydrocephalus or thalamic hemorrhage

Small, reactive, and regular

Diencephalic dysfunction
Small and reactive

Dysfunction of tectum (roof) of the midbrain
Large "fixed" hippus

Dysfunction of third cranial nerve
Sluggish, dilated, and fixed

Pontine dysfunction
Pinpoint

Midbrain dysfunction
Midposition and fixed

FIG. 11-8 Appearance of pupils associated with common causes of neurologic dysfunction. (From Boss BJ: Alterations in cognitive systems, cerebral hemodynamics, and motor function. In McCance KE, Huether SE, editors: *Pathophysiology: the biologic basis for disease in adults and children*, ed 6, Philadelphia, 2010, Mosby-Elsevier, p. 532, fig. 16-2.)

Table 11-6 Modified Glasgow Coma Scale for Infants and Children

	Child	Infant	Score
Eye opening	Spontaneous	Spontaneous	4
	To verbal stimuli	To verbal stimuli	3
	To pain only	To pain only	2
	No response	No response	1
Verbal response	Oriented, appropriate	Coos and babbles	5
	Confused	Irritable cries	4
	Inappropriate words	Cries to pain	3
	Incomprehensible words or nonspecific sounds	Moans to pain	2
	No response	No response	1
Motor response	Obeys commands (e.g., child holds up two fingers, wiggles toes or sticks out tongue)*	Moves spontaneously and purposefully	6
	Localizes painful stimulus (e.g., child reaches for hand that is rubbing sternum or pinching trapezius)*	Withdraws to touch	5
	Withdraws in response to pain (e.g., child adducts each extremity when medial aspect is pinched)*	Withdraws in response to pain	4
	Flexion in response to pain (i.e., decorticate posturing when sternum rubbed or trapezius muscle pinched)*	Decorticate posturing (abnormal flexion) in response to pain	3
	Extension in response to pain (i.e., decerebrate posturing when sternum rubbed or trapezius muscle pinched)*	Decerebrate posturing (abnormal extension) in response to pain	2
	No response (flaccid)	No response (flaccid)	1
TOTAL			**3-15**

Modified from Tasker RC: Head and spinal cord trauma. In Nichols DG, editor: *Rodgers' textbook of pediatric intensive care*, 4th ed, Philadelphia, 2008, Lippincott Williams & Wilkins; Originally proposed in Morray JP, et al: Coma scale for use in brain-injured children. *Crit Care Med* 12:1018, 1984.
*Additions in parentheses were added to the scale by the chapter authors (LM Milonovich, V Eichler), and editor (MF Hazinski).

The specific scale or modified scale used to score the child's neurologic function is probably less important than the consistency with which the scale is used. Any scale or scoring system used must facilitate identification of trends in the patient's condition over time. Therefore, it is essential that every member of the healthcare team use the same scale and apply the scale in exactly the same way. If the scale used is incorporated into nursing care documentation templates, the neurologic assessment information derived from the scale is readily accessible.

When the child is comatose, careful evaluation of the motor response is extremely important. However, this section of the GCS is often applied inconsistently or incompletely.

If the child is comatose, the child will not follow commands. The next step in evaluation of motor response during the GCS examination requires administration of a painful stimulus to the trunk, to determine if a response occurs and if it is purposeful. To determine if the child can localize a painful stimulus, apply a central painful stimulus to the child's upper torso: rub the sternum or pinch the trapezius muscle. The child demonstrates a purposeful response to central pain stimulus (i.e., localizing the stimulus) if the child grasps and tries to move the hand that is administering the stimulus. Nonpurposeful responses can include vague movement during the stimulus or posturing.

To evaluate withdrawal from painful stimulus, the provider should pinch the medial (inside) aspect of each extremity. Withdrawal is present if the child abducts each extremity, moving it outward and away from the painful stimulus. The painful stimulus should not simply be applied to the fingertip or toe, because withdrawal of the extremity from such a stimulus can be reflexive, accomplished at the spinal cord level. Such spinal reflex withdrawal does not require higher CNS function and can still be observed after brain death or spinal cord transection.

Decorticate posturing is characterized by flexion of the elbows, wrists, and fingers and by extension of the legs and ankles with plantar flexion of the feet. During decorticate posturing, the legs are tightly adducted. The development of decorticate posturing or rigidity (Fig. 11-9, A) indicates ischemia of or damage to the cerebral hemispheres.

Decerebrate posturing is a lower level of reflexive response to painful stimulation than decorticate posturing. It is characterized by extension and slight abduction (movement outward from midline) of the arms and legs. The development of decerebrate posturing or rigidity (see Fig. 11-9, B) indicates the presence of a diffuse metabolic cerebral injury or the development of ischemia of or damage to more primitive areas of the brain, including the diencephalon, midbrain, or pons. In general, a progression from decorticate rigidity to decerebrate posturing usually indicates progression of the neurologic dysfunction and should be reported to an on-call provider immediately (while obtaining additional information including vital signs, pupil response to light, and ICP). Patients occasionally can alternate between decorticate and decerebrate posturing if there is variability in CBF to the brainstem and the cerebral hemispheres.

Flaccid paralysis is lack of any movement in response to even deep painful stimulation. Flaccidity may indicate spinal cord injury or severe neurologic dysfunction.

Notify the on-call provider immediately if the child's response to central painful stimulus deteriorates. Also evaluate any changes in motor response in context with all other assessments.

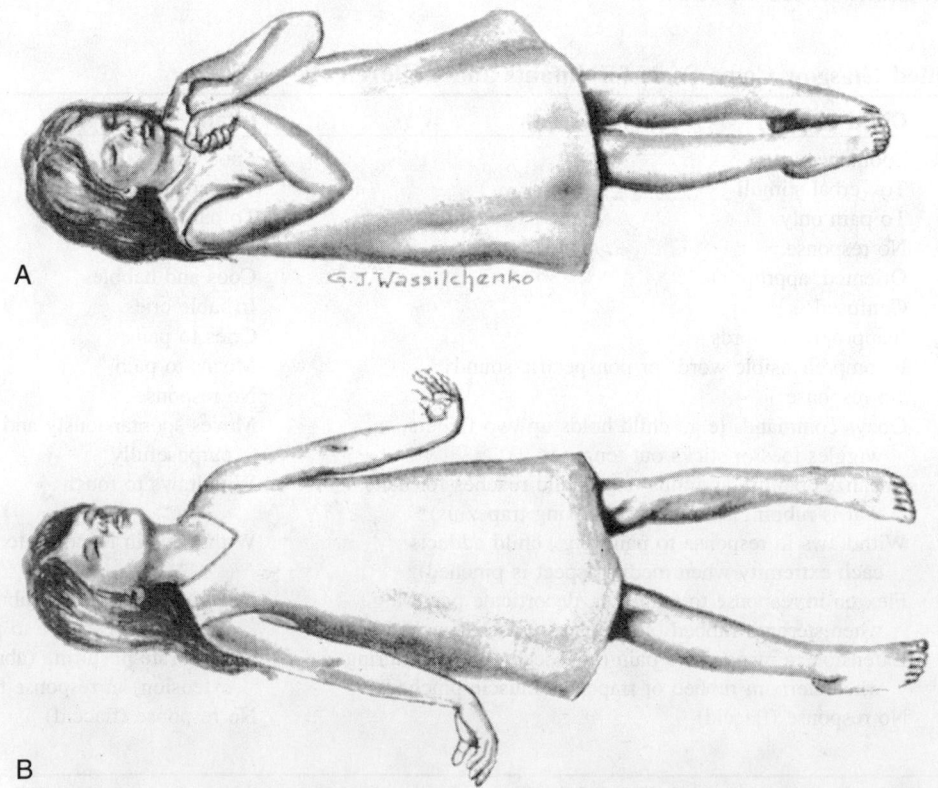

FIG. 11-9 Abnormal posturing. **A,** Decorticate posturing and rigidity. **B,** Decerebrate posturing and rigidity. (From Whaley LF, Wong DL: *Nursing care of infants and children,* ed 2, St. Louis, 1983, Mosby.)

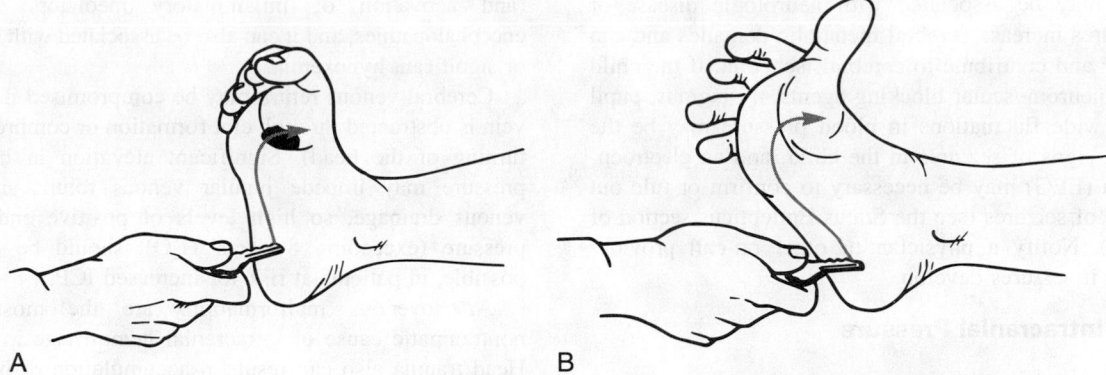

FIG. 11-10 Babinski sign. Test maneuver involves scraping from the heel along the plantar aspect of the foot. A, Normal response (beyond toddler years) or absent Babinski sign. B, Abnormal response or present Babinski sign. (From Mercier LR: *Practical orthopedics*, ed 6, St Louis, 2008, Mosby.)

For example, if a child demonstrates decorticate posturing in response to pain with brisk pupil response to light, an ICP of 18 mm Hg, and appropriate heart rate and respiratory rate for age on admission, and then begins to demonstrate decerebrate posturing, tachycardia, hypertension, pupil dilation, and an ICP of 32 mm Hg, these findings are consistent with significant neurologic deterioration (see Increased Intracranial Pressure).

Additional Assessment of Motor Function and Reflexes

The infant or child with increased ICP will demonstrate decreased motor function and may demonstrate abnormal posturing or reflexes. With progressive neurologic deterioration, flaccid paralysis will result.

When a brain injury or lesion is unilateral, pupil dilation and decreased response to light is likely to occur first on the side of the injury or lesion. However, abnormal decrease in movement or sensation (e.g., hemiplegia or hemiparesis) will typically be present on the side contralateral (opposite) to that of the brain injury.

Neurologic disease or insult can result in abnormal appearance of some other reflexes.

Babinski's reflex is present if the toes fan out and if the great toe extends when the sole of the foot is stroked from the heel to the toes and around to the ball of the foot (Fig. 11-10). Although Babinski's reflex is normally present before the infant or toddler learns to walk, the reflex is abnormal after a child has begun walking, and it may indicate the presence of increased ICP or neurologic dysfunction.

The infant or child with a neurologic problem may demonstrate few spontaneous movements and may be unable to perform motor skills previously demonstrated. For example, the 9-month-old infant may be unwilling or unable to sit without assistance, although such activity was performed previously. The child may demonstrate an abnormal gait or be unwilling to walk without assistance.

Development of incontinence in a child who previously demonstrated bowel and bladder control is a worrisome sign and can indicate significant neurologic deterioration. Deterioration can affect the child's ability to coordinate movement or to follow simple commands. Changes in the child's motor skills will be more readily identified if the nurse is familiar with the normal sequence of achievements of developmental milestones (Table 11-7) and motor skills.

Table 11-7 Typical Age for Attainment of Major Developmental Milestones

Age (Months)	Motor Skill	Language	Social Play
2	Head up in prone		Smiles, fixes and follows
3	Head/chest up in prone, grasps placed object	Coos	
4	Rolls, reaches		
6	Sits with support, transfers	Babbles, turns to sound	Mouthing objects
8	Sits without support, weight bears	Turns to name	
10	Pincer grasp, starting to cruise, crawling	"Bye-bye" wave	Drinks from cup
12	Walks but falls easily	First words	Finger feeds, objects in and out of containers
15	Walks steadily, scribbling	Pointing, multiple single words	Spoon use, assists in dressing
18	Up/down stairs with assistance, climbing, throws ball	Two-word phrases, pointing to body parts	Builds towers, plays with others
24	Up/down stairs one step at a time, kicks ball	Three-word phrases, pronouns	

Adapted from Shevell, M: Office evaluation of the child with developmental delay. *Semin Pediat Neurol* 13:256-261, 2006; Mazumdar M. Clinical approach to neurologic disease. In: Rudolph CD, Rudolph AM, Lister GE, Forst LR, Gershon AA, editors, *Rudolph's Pediatrics*, ed 22, New York, Mc Graw Hill, 2011, p 2141 (table 547-2).

Seizures may be associated with neurologic disease or injury. Seizures increase cerebral metabolic demands and can increase ICP and contribute to cerebral ischemia. If the child is receiving neuromuscular blocking agents, nystagmus, pupil changes, or wide fluctuations in blood pressure may be the only clinical signs of seizures in the child, and an electroencephalogram (EEG) may be necessary to confirm or rule out the presence of seizures (see the Status Epilepticus section of this chapter). Notify a physician or other on-call provider immediately if seizures develop.

Increased Intracranial Pressure

Etiology

Increased ICP results from an uncompensated increase in intracranial volume. Increased ICP can compromise cerebral perfusion, and unchecked severe increases in ICP can result in cerebral herniation and the cessation of cerebral perfusion (brain death).

Normal ICP is approximately 5 to 15 mm Hg, and a pressure exceeding 20 mm Hg is consistent with increased ICP. Transient elevation in ICP is expected with pain, coughing, or other noxious stimuli even under normal circumstances. However sustained elevation in ICP is always abnormal. The ICP can be measured with a variety of devices, including fluid-filled transducer monitoring systems and fiberoptic catheters.

Increased Brain Volume. An increase in brain volume can result from cerebral edema or cerebral swelling. Cerebral edema is categorized as vasogenic, cytotoxic, osmotic and interstitial; the etiology and treatment of each category of edema may vary.

Vasogenic cerebral edema is characterized by increased cerebral capillary permeability and disruption of the blood brain barrier in the absence of neuronal injury.[71] The increased permeability often is caused by inflammatory conditions such as encephalitis and meningitis. When capillary permeability is increased, proteins leak from the vascular space. Because proteins exert osmotic force, when they move from the intravascular to the extravascular space they pull water from the intravascular to the extravascular space, worsening edema and creating further ischemia and further edema.

Cytotoxic cerebral edema or cellular swelling usually is associated with severe neural cell damage. It occurs across the spectrum of brain injuries, but particularly in traumatic brain injury and ischemic injury. The edema occurs secondary to dysfunction of intracellular mechanisms, which promote sodium and water accumulation in the cells, with resultant cell swelling.[71,108]

Osmotic cerebral edema results from an acute fall in serum (and therefore extracellular) osmolality that results in an acute free water shift from the intravascular/extracellular space to the intracellular space. Interstitial cerebral edema results from impaired absorption of CSF.[108] Most commonly, this form of cerebral edema is observed in patients with obstructive hydrocephalus.

Increased Cerebral Blood Volume. Increased CBV can result from increased CBF or obstruction to cerebral venous return. Regional increases in CBF can result from head injury

(and activation of inflammatory mediators) and some encephalopathies, and it can also be associated with hypercarbia or significant hypoxemia.

Cerebral venous return may be compromised if the jugular vein is obstructed through clot formation or compression (e.g., turning of the head). Significant elevation in intrathoracic pressure may impede jugular venous return and cerebral venous drainage, so high levels of positive end-expiratory pressure (exceeding 8-10 cm H$_2$O), should be avoided, if possible, in patients at risk for increased ICP.

Arteriovenous malformations are the most common nontraumatic cause of intracranial hemorrhage in children.[55] Head trauma also can result in accumulation of blood in the subdural or epidural space, or in an intracerebral hematoma. Intraventricular hemorrhage can occur after a traumatic injury or in premature infants.

Cerebral Spinal Fluid Accumulation. CSF will accumulate if there is an obstruction to CSF flow or a compromise in CSF reabsorption. Obstruction to CSF flow may complicate recovery from meningitis if inflammatory cells occlude the aqueduct of Sylvius. If head injury is complicated by intraventricular bleeding, fragments of red blood cells may obstruct the aqueduct of Sylvius. This can produce an acute obstructive hydrocephalus with an acute rise in ICP following a head injury; unlike other causes of posttraumatic hydrocephalus, acute obstructive hydrocephalus may develop during the first hours after injury. It may also be associated with more gradual development of hydrocephalus and increased ICP.

Other causes of obstructive hydrocephalus include tumors and increased ICP that can compress the third and fourth ventricles, obstructing CSF flow. This form of obstructive hydrocephalus will compromise the patient's ability to compensate for additional increases in intracranial volume. Obstructive hydrocephalus may be surgically treated through insertion of a drain or shunt.

Decreased CSF reabsorption causes communicating hydrocephalus. This complication may develop if head trauma is associated with a significant subarachnoid hemorrhage. Because CSF is reabsorbed by the arachnoid villi in the subarachnoid space, the presence of a significant amount of blood can compromise CSF reabsorption. A choroid plexus tumor is a rare cause of communicating hydrocephalus. All of these conditions result in CSF accumulation and can produce increased ICP.

Mass Lesions. Brain tumors are the most common solid tumor of childhood.[55] The tumors are typically infratentorial, located near or in the brainstem, and most contain glial cells (see Intracranial Tumors in the Specific Diseases section of this chapter). Intracranial hypertension can result from the tumor mass itself, from edema generated by the tumor presence, or from obstruction of CSF flow.

Pathophysiology

Intracranial Pressure and Volume. As noted previously in this chapter (see Essential Anatomy and Physiology, Intracranial Pressure and Volume Relationships), the intracranial vault is a relatively fixed space that contains the brain, blood, and

CSF. When the volume of any of these components increases, venous capacitance blood is displaced from the intracranial vault, and, unless hydrocephalus is present, CSF is displaced into the subarachnoid space along the spinal column. Initially, these compensatory mechanisms may prevent a rise in ICP.

Once the limits of compensation and compliance have been reached, however, further increase in intracranial volume will produce a rise in ICP. The increase in ICP then becomes nearly exponential; progressively smaller increases in intracranial volume will produce progressively greater rises in ICP.

Intracranial Compliance. The shape of the intracranial pressure–volume curve reflects intracranial compliance. Intracranial compliance is the change in ICP that occurs with a given increase in intracranial volume (ΔVolume/ΔPressure). Initially, as intracranial volume increases, intracranial compliance is high and the curve is virtually horizontal; an increase in intracranial volume initially will be tolerated without a significant change in ICP. Once the limit of intracranial compliance is reached, intracranial compliance is then very low and the curve becomes virtually vertical; at this point even a small increase in intracranial volume will produce a significant rise in ICP.

Intracranial compliance is affected by time. If the intracranial volume increases gradually, as occurs with a slow-growing brain tumor, a significant volume may be accommodated without a rise in ICP because physiologic compensatory mechanisms have time to develop. In contrast, if the intracranial volume increases rapidly, as occurs following an intracranial hemorrhage, there is little time for compensation, and the ICP is likely to rise rapidly.[103]

Intracranial compliance also is affected by previous rises in intracranial volume and pressure. Frequent spikes in the ICP will decrease intracranial compliance, resulting in a rise in ICP with subsequently smaller and smaller increases in intracranial volume. For example, consider the child with a head injury who develops an increase in CBF and CBV associated with hypercarbia, hypoxemia or seizures. During the initial episode of hypercarbia or hypoxemia or an initial seizure, the increase in CBF and CBV may be tolerated with only a mild rise in ICP. Subsequent similar episodes of hypercarbia or hypoxemia or additional seizures are likely to cause more substantial increase in ICP. A change in compliance alters the relationship between intracranial volume and pressure (Fig. 11-11).

Two terms that are used to quantify the intracranial compliance are the *volume pressure resistance index* and the *pressure-volume index*. These terms can roughly indicate the patient's intracranial compliance (i.e., location on the pressure volume curve) and whether the limits of intracranial compensation have been reached.

The volume pressure resistance index or response was described by Guertin et al. in 1982.[54] Under a research protocol involving children with ICP monitoring in place, physicians gently instilled a known quantity of normal saline (typically 1 mL) into the child's lateral ventricle. The greater the rise in ICP produced by the 1-mL instillation, the lower the intracranial compliance. For example, if instillation of 1 mL of saline produced an approximately 1 mm Hg rise in

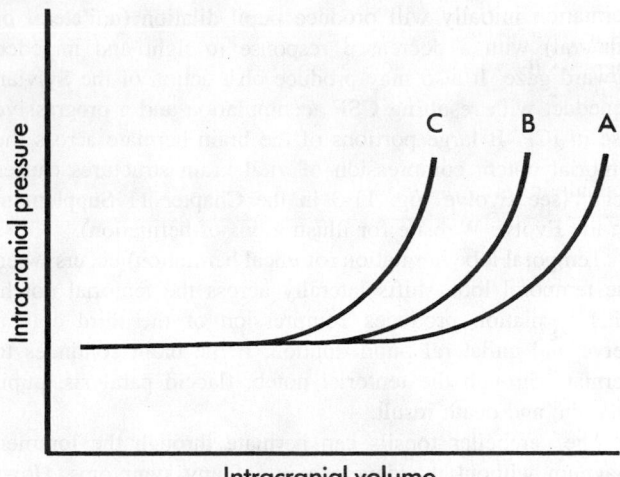

FIG. 11-11 Changes in intracranial pressure (ICP) with changes in intracranial compliance. The relationship between intracranial volume and pressure is not static and is affected by intracranial compliance. Curves A, B, and C depict progressively lower intracranial compliance. When the increase in volume is gradual (curve A), more volume is tolerated before ICP begins to rise because intracranial compliance is initially high. When the intracranial volume increases rapidly, ICP will begin to rise with a smaller volume change (curve B), reflecting lower intracranial compliance. Once the ICP begins to spike, intracranial compliance is low, and progressively smaller increases in volume will produce significant ICP spikes (curve C).

ICP, the patient's intracranial compliance was characterized as high, as depicted on the relatively horizontal part of an intracranial pressure-volume curve. If, however, instillation of 1 mL of normal saline produced a rise in ICP of 7 to 10 mm Hg, the patient's intracranial compliance was characterized as very low, as depicted by the relatively vertical part of an intracranial pressure-volume curve. In patients with low intracranial compliance, instillation of progressively smaller quantities of normal saline resulted in progressively greater rises in ICP (such as shown in Fig. 11-11, curves B and C).

Normal saline is rarely instilled into a lateral ventricle of a critically ill patient with increased ICP. However, it is easy to imagine the addition of 1 mL of CBF and CBV to the intracranial vault (e.g., with vasodilation that results from mild hypoxemia or hypercarbia during suctioning) and its effect on ICP. The change in intracranial compliance that occurs with repeated episodes of increased intracranial volume explains why a patient may tolerate suctioning once with only mild increases in ICP, but the same patient will demonstrate a dramatic elevation in ICP if a second episode of suctioning creates hypercarbia, hypoxia, or increased venous pressure.

Complications of Increased Intracranial Pressure. Unchecked increases in ICP may compromise cerebral perfusion or produce shifting of brain tissue (cerebral herniation). Complete brainstem herniation will produce interruption of cerebral perfusion and brain death.

Transtentorial herniation occurs when part of the brain herniates downward around the tentorium cerebelli. This herniation can occur in the anterior or posterior portions of the brain, and it may be unilateral or bilateral. Transtentorial herniation initially will produce pupil dilation (unilateral or bilateral) with a decreased response to light and impeded upward gaze. It also may produce obstruction of the Sylvian aqueduct with resulting CSF accumulation and a progressive rise in ICP. If large portions of the brain herniate across the tentorial notch, compression of vital brain structures causes death (see Evolve Fig. 11-3 in the Chapter 11 Supplement on the Evolve Website for illustrations of herniation).

Temporal lobe herniation (or uncal herniation) occurs when the temporal lobe shifts laterally across the tentorial notch. This herniation produces compression of the third cranial nerve and unilateral pupil dilation. If the brain continues to herniate through the tentorial notch, flaccid paralysis, pupil dilation, and death result.

The cerebellar tonsils can herniate through the foramen magnum without the development of any symptoms. However, some patients may develop a stiff neck, upper arm and shoulder paresthesia, a change in the respiratory pattern, or a wide fluctuation in heart rate.

Brainstem herniation through the foramen magnum results in compression of the vital cardiorespiratory centers and brain death.

Clinical Signs and Symptoms

The child with increased ICP characteristically demonstrates altered level of consciousness; pupil dilation with decreased reactivity to light; alterations in heart rate, blood pressure, and respiratory rate or pattern; and abnormal motor activity and reflexes. The child may complain of headache or nausea and may vomit, particularly in the morning or after moving from a reclining to an upright position. Because the infant or very young child and the child with decreased level of consciousness will be unable to articulate symptoms, the nurse must be able to recognize signs and symptoms of increased ICP (Box 11-3).

Box 11-3	**Signs of Increased Intracranial Pressure in Children**

Change in Level of Consciousness
Irritability, then lethargy
Confusion, disorientation
Decreased responsiveness (decreased eye contact, decreased response to parents, to pain)
Reduced ability to follow commands (hold up two fingers, wiggle toes, stick out tongue)

Pupil dilation with decreased response to light

Reduced spontaneous movement or deterioration in motor function or reflexive posturing (list below indicates declining level of function):
Purposeful movement deteriorates
Decorticate posturing
Decerebrate posturing
Flaccid response to pain

Cushing's triad (bradycardia, systolic hypertension with widening pulse pressure, altered respiratory pattern, such as apnea) may occur only as late sign.

If an ICP monitoring device is in place, this measurement is used in conjunction with the clinical assessment to determine the severity of the intracranial hypertension. Assessment and support of cardiopulmonary function always precedes assessment of neurologic function.

Evaluation of Airway and Oxygenation. The first step in the evaluation of the patient with increased ICP is the evaluation and support of the airway, oxygenation, and ventilation. Increased ICP may be associated with decreased level of consciousness and an inability to protect the airway. In addition, loss of consciousness can result in airway obstruction by the tongue. Finally, apnea or hypoventilation may produce a rise in $PaCO_2$ and hypoxemia, resulting in an increase in CBF and a possible increase in ICP.

Evaluation of Systemic Perfusion. Monitoring of systemic perfusion is essential for all critically ill or injured patients. If systemic perfusion is poor, cerebral perfusion is likely to be compromised. This concept is especially true for the trauma patient with head injury. Thus, shock resuscitation and support of circulation are essential to optimizing cerebral perfusion.

Children with increased ICP may demonstrate a compromise in systemic perfusion. Tachycardia or bradycardia may be present and the skin may be mottled in appearance.

Hypertension may develop as a compensatory mechanism to maintain cerebral perfusion in patients with an increase in ICP, but hypertension also may be a sign of pain or fear. If hypertension develops, the nurse should immediately assess and support the airway, ventilation, and oxygenation and should evaluate the child's heart rate, level of consciousness, and motor function, and pupil size and response to light. Significant hypertension, particularly if associated with any other signs of deterioration, should be reported to the on-call provider; it may signal increased ICP and even impending herniation.

Level of Consciousness. Evaluation of the child's level of consciousness is probably the single most important aspect of neurologic assessment of the child with increased ICP. The level of consciousness must be evaluated on a regular basis and whenever changes are observed in the child's clinical appearance, or cardiopulmonary function or in the monitored ICP or CPP (see Box 11-2).

Signs of a decreased level of consciousness in infants include lethargy, decreased eye contact, poor visual tracking, and a change in feeding behavior, including vomiting. Children with a decreased level of consciousness may be very irritable or lethargic, may be confused about where they are, may forget the names of family members or pets, or may appear drowsy. Decreased response to painful stimuli is abnormal in infants or children of any age and should be reported to the on-call provider immediately.

Pupil Response and Cranial Nerve Function. The pupils are normally the same size, and brisk pupil constriction in response to light is produced by innervation of the third cranial (oculomotor) nerve. When increased ICP develops, the oculomotor nerve is compressed by either general expansion of the brain, an intracranial lesion, or uncal herniation. Such compression can produce pupil dilation and decreased or absent pupil constriction in response to light. When the intracranial lesion or herniation is unilateral, the pupil dilation will occur on the same side as (ipsilateral to) the lesion. Compression of the third cranial nerve may cause unilateral ptosis in conjunction with pupil dilation. The child also may complain of blurred vision or diplopia.

Evaluation of the function of most cranial nerves can be performed during routine nursing care (see Table 11-2 and Box 11-2). If the child demonstrates a loss of previously demonstrated cranial nerve function, notify the on-call provider immediately. When cerebral perfusion is compromised and cessation of brain function occurs, cranial nerve function will disappear (e.g., the child who had a gag reflex will no longer cough or have a gag during suctioning).

Changes in Motor Function and Reflexes. The infant or child who develops increased ICP may demonstrate few spontaneous movements and may be unable to perform motor skills previously demonstrated. Development of incontinence in a child who previously had bowel and bladder control is a worrisome sign and may indicate significant deterioration.

Increased ICP will produce decreased motor function and possible abnormal posturing or reflexes, such as decorticate or decerebrate posturing (see Fig. 11-9). With progressive neurologic deterioration, flaccid paralysis will result.

If the child is obtunded or comatose, assessment requires evaluation of the child's response to a central painful stimulus to determine whether a response occurs and if it is purposeful. A central painful stimulus is administered over the torso and can include rubbing of the sternum or pinching of the trapezius muscle. A peripheral painful stimulus, such as pinching of the fingernail, should not be used to evaluate purposeful response, because withdrawal of the extremity can occur as a result of only a spinal cord level reflex that requires no higher CNS function. Such withdrawal may still be observed after brain death or spinal cord transection.

The child demonstrates a purposeful response to the central pain stimulus if the child grasps and tries to move the hand that is administering the stimulus. Non-purposeful responses may include vague movement during the stimulus or groaning. To evaluate withdrawal from a painful stimulus, pinch the medial aspect of each extremity; withdrawal will cause abduction (movement outward from midline) of each extremity.

Decorticate posturing is the highest reflexive level of response to stimulus. Decerebrate posturing is a lower level of reflexive response to painful stimulation. Flaccid paralysis is the lack of any movement in response to deep painful stimulation. A provider should be notified immediately if the child's response to central painful stimulus deteriorates.

It is important to evaluate changes in motor response in context with all other assessments of neurologic function. For example, if a child demonstrates decorticate posturing in response to pain with brisk pupil response to light, an ICP of 18 mm Hg, and appropriate heart rate and respiratory rate for age on admission, and then begins to demonstrate decerebrate posturing, tachycardia, hypertension, pupil dilation, and an ICP of 32 mm Hg, these findings are consistent with neurologic deterioration. Immediately notify an on-call provider of

deterioration in motor activity and response. Flaccidity in response to painful stimulus can indicate spinal cord injury or severe neurologic dysfunction.

Alterations in Respiratory Pattern. The patient with increased ICP may demonstrate a wide variety of respiratory patterns (see Fig. 11-7). When ICP rises and the Cushing reflex is initiated, respirations become irregular, and apnea then respiratory arrest can develop. However, other breathing patterns also may be noted before the Cushing reflex develops.

The Cushing Reflex. The Cushing reflex produces the Cushing triad, three late and ominous signs of increased ICP that result from ischemia of the vasomotor center.[83] The Cushing triad may appear only when cerebral brainstem herniation is imminent. This triad consists of bradycardia, an increase in systolic arterial blood pressure (as an attempt to maintain CPP) with widened pulse pressure, and abnormal breathing pattern, typically apnea.[83]

This reflex does not develop completely until ICP is elevated significantly. Earlier signs of increased ICP may include tachycardia and fluctuations in arterial blood pressure. Hypotension can develop late with increased ICP.

Papilledema. Papilledema is edema around the optic nerve and disc that results from increased ICP and compression of these structures. When an ophthalmoscope is used to examine the retina, the optic disc appears indistinct and the retinal veins are engorged and pulseless. Papilledema develops when ICP has been elevated for 48 hours or more (e.g., caused by a brain tumor). Therefore, papilledema indicates that the increased ICP is not a recent development, but has been present for a considerable period of time; this may aid in the identification of inflicted trauma.

When mild papilledema is present, the child's vision should be normal. With progressive compression of the optic disc, however, hemorrhages can develop in the optic disc and the child may complain of headaches, blurred vision, or diplopia.

Scoring Neurologic Function. The most widely used neurologic scoring system is the GCS. This scale evaluates motor activity, verbal responses and motor responses, with a total scale range of 3 to 15 (see Table 11-6)

The GCS was validated in adults, so the verbal section cannot be used as written in the care of the preverbal patients. As a result, modifications of the GCS have been developed and found to be useful for pediatric patients with neurologic injury or disease (see Table 11-6).[34a,83,93,106] The verbal section can't be used as written for intubated patients. When the patient is intubated, it is very important for healthcare providers to identify a consistent approach to either modified application or omission of the verbal portion of the GCS.

The specific scale or modified scale used to score the child's neurologic function is probably less important than the consistency with which the scale is used. Any scale or scoring system is most useful if it enables identification of trends in the patient's condition over time. Therefore, it is essential that every member of the healthcare team use the same scale and apply the scale in exactly the same way.

If the scale used is incorporated into the medical and nursing care documentation templates, the assessment information derived from the tool is readily accessible.

When the child is comatose, careful evaluation of the motor response is extremely important. However, this section of the GCS is often applied inconsistently or incompletely. For this reason, details about assessment of motor function are listed under the GCS Score in Table 11-6 and Box 11-2.

Other Signs of Increased Intracranial Pressure. The infant with increased ICP is often extremely lethargic, with a high pitched cry. The infant's anterior fontanelle is usually full and tense. With chronic increased ICP, the scalp veins may appear distended. The infant's eyes may deviate downward, with sclera visible above the irises; this is often referred to as *sunset eyes*. The infant may become extremely irritable when the head is moved or the neck is flexed, and the infant may be uninterested in feeding, or may vomit frequently. If the increased ICP is of longer duration, the nurse may be able to palpate spaces between the cranial bones as the cranial sutures widen.

The verbal child with intracranial hypertension may complain of headache, nausea, vomiting, blurred vision, or diplopia. The child may demonstrate mood swings and also may be more lethargic, with periods of confusion. Slurred speech is common. Clinical signs of increased ICP are summarized in Box 11-3.

Neurogenic pulmonary edema occasionally complicates increased ICP. This pulmonary edema can develop suddenly and without warning. The mechanism of the pulmonary edema is unclear, but it appears to be related to development of increased systemic and pulmonary artery pressure in response to the intracranial hypertension. The pulmonary edema usually produces respiratory failure (i.e., hypoxemia with decreased lung compliance and increased respiratory effort). For further information about pulmonary edema, refer to Chapter 9.

Helpful Diagnostic Tests. Careful clinical assessment, ICP monitoring, and evaluation of cerebral venous or tissue oxygen saturation provide the most useful bedside information about the child's neurologic status. In addition, the EEG may be used during barbiturate therapy to assess cerebral activity or to evaluate for subclinical seizure activity.

Computed tomography (CT) is extremely helpful in localizing mass lesions or intracranial bleeding or in determining the presence of diffuse cerebral edema or infarction. (See the Common Diagnostic Tests section, later in this chapter, for further discussion of EEG and CT). The CT scan may be used in the acute management of the patient with increased ICP to evaluate potential causes of deterioration and to assess for the presence and severity of cerebral edema. If the third and fourth ventricles are widely patent and visible on a CT scan, the patient's intracranial volume has not yet reached the limits of intracranial compensation (Fig. 11-12, A). If the third and fourth ventricles are collapsed and the basilar cisterns are obliterated, CSF has been displaced from the intracranial vault and the patient probably is reaching the limits of intracranial compensation, so intracranial compliance is low. Further increase in intracranial volume is likely to produce a significant increase in ICP, and cerebral herniation is possible. Collapse of the lateral ventricles (in the absence of an external CSF drain) also indicates that intracranial compliance is low (see Fig. 11-12, B and C).

Magnetic resonance imaging (MRI) or magnetic resonance angiography may be helpful in the evaluation of stroke and other intracranial lesions. MRI also enables more definitive evaluation of intracranial masses and potential metastatic disease. It can provide useful information in confirmation of infectious disease of the brain and spinal cord.

If cerebral ischemia is suspected or brain death is thought to be present, a quantitative or qualitative radioactive cerebral perfusion scan may be performed. This study requires the injection of radioactive ^{99m}Tc pertechnetate into the venous system and documentation of the absence of this substance in the cerebral vessels. For further information, see Cerebral Angiography in the Common Diagnostic Tests section of this chapter.

Management

The goals of management of increased ICP are as follows: (1) maintain effective cerebral perfusion by supporting effective oxygenation, ventilation, and systemic perfusion and by controlling ICP; (2) preserve cerebral function; and (3) prevent secondary insults to the brain. Adequate cerebral perfusion requires maintenance of a patent airway, effective oxygenation and ventilation, and support of adequate systemic perfusion—too often the child with increased ICP deteriorates as the result of inadequate support of cardiopulmonary function.

Optimal management of increased ICP ultimately requires the identification and treatment of the specific cause of the increased ICP. The treatment of traumatic head injury will not be identical to the treatment of anoxic cerebral injury, and the reader is referred to specific management of causes of increased ICP (e.g., brain tumors) in the Specific Diseases section of this chapter.

Anoxic cerebral injury produces cytotoxic cerebral edema. Signs of increased ICP often do not develop for approximately 48 to 72 hours or longer after the anoxic insult—too late to reverse the damage. In fact, longitudinal studies of drowning victims have demonstrated that a rise in ICP following an anoxic insult is generally an indication of overwhelming neurologic insult, and patients who develop such an increase in ICP may deteriorate despite efforts to control the ICP.[26,27,43]

The pathophysiology, management, and outcome of anoxic injury differ from increased ICP of traumatic or inflammatory origin. In traumatic or inflammatory increased ICP, the initial insult may not be devastating, and the patient may recover completely if complications of increased ICP are avoided. Untreated rises in ICP or other secondary insults, however, can be fatal.

Assessment and Support of Airway and Ventilation. Whenever the child is at risk for increased ICP, the healthcare team must continually monitor the child's airway and ventilation. If the child is obtunded or demonstrates a decreased response to painful stimulation, intubation with mechanical ventilation are indicated to prevent possible airway obstruction or respiratory

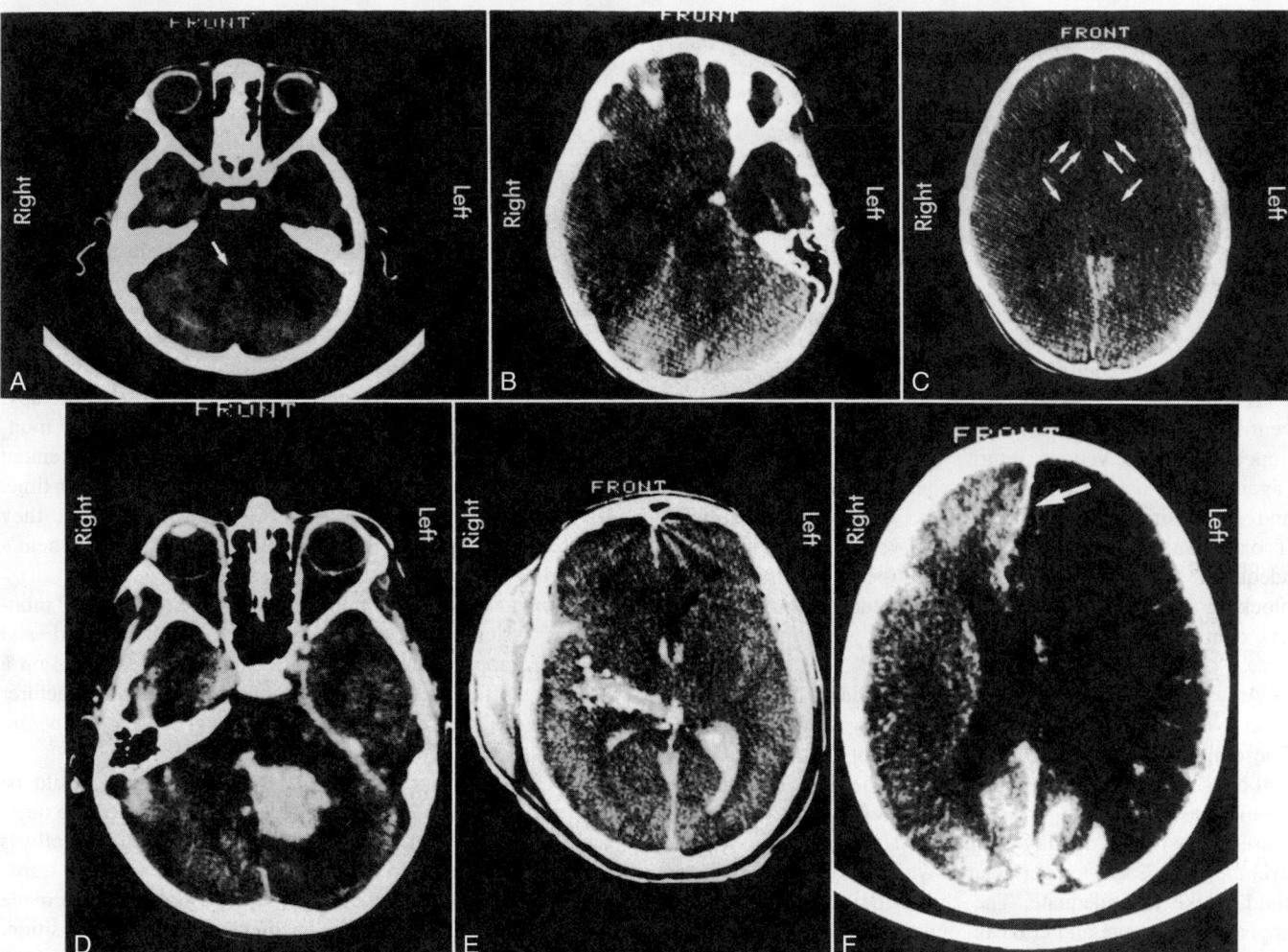

FIG. 11-12 Computed tomography (CT) scans. The front of the patient's head is at the top of each image (indicated), and the patient's right and left sides are labeled. The viewer should imagine looking up into the intracranial vault (patient's left is on the viewer's right). **A,** The fourth ventricle is widely patent in this 11-year-old girl. It is visible as a horseshoe-shaped fluid-filled density *(arrow)*. **B,** In contrast, a similar view from a 5-year-old boy shows no fourth ventricle. This child sustained a massive head injury and arrived at the hospital with signs of increased intracranial pressure and dilated and fixed pupils. The fourth ventricle is completely collapsed. White patches in occipital area are areas of subarachnoid hemorrhage (also present in C). **C,** This CT scan is from the patient in B. The lateral ventricles are visible but collapsed *(small arrows)*, indicating displacement of cerebrospinal fluid from the intracranial vault with severe increase in intracranial pressure. **D,** In this CT scan of a 5-year-old boy who suffered a sudden intracranial hemorrhage, blood is visible in the fourth ventricle as a white or radiopaque density. **E,** In this CT scan of a young man with a self-inflicted gunshot wound to the right temple, the soft-tissue swelling is apparent over the right temple, and the track of the bullet fragments (the metal of the bullet is radiopaque) can be seen easily. The bullet crossed the midline, and blood (white or radiopaque) is visible in the lateral ventricles and between the cerebral hemispheres. **F,** The CT scan also will demonstrate significant alteration in cerebral circulation or tissue viability. This CT scan of a 6-year-old girl with acute nonlymphocytic leukemia and hyperleukocytosis was performed because the nurse noted the sudden onset of the right-sided weakness during examination. Soon afterward, the child's left pupil dilated. A left cerebral infarction is apparent, producing a midline shift (arrow). Whitened areas of calcification indicate old embolic events. This child suffered a left hemisphere cerebral infarction secondary to embolism of adherent white blood cells. The right lateral ventricle is visible and dilated.

arrest (Box 11-4). Intubation is also indicated if the child demonstrates hypoventilation or if signs of increased ICP are present.

Intubation of the child with increased ICP requires coordination of team activities to provide adequate preoxygenation, prevent development of hypoxia or hypercarbia during the attempt, and verify correct tube placement. Medications chosen for intubation should suppress awareness of and reflexes during direct laryngoscopy, to prevent a cough or gag that will further increase ICP. Succinylcholine is generally not the neuromuscular blocking agent of choice, because it can increase CBF and ICP. Other rapid onset neuromuscular blocking agents such as rocuronium are preferred (see Chapter 9 for additional information about Rapid Sequence Intubation).

Support of effective oxygenation and ventilation are critical throughout the treatment of increased ICP. Suctioning of the

Box 11-4 **Indications for Intubation in the Child with Increased Intracranial Pressure**

Impaired airway clearance or compromise in airway protective reflexes (e.g., weak or absent cough, gag)
Glasgow Coma Scale score ≤8
Hypoventilation
Evidence of increased intracranial pressure
Associated shock, cardiopulmonary failure

endotracheal tube may require two providers in order to prevent the development of hypercarbia and hypoxemia.

If the child coughs frequently or struggles against the ventilator, peak and mean airway pressures will rise and will impede cerebral venous return. If the child is struggling "against" the ventilator, verify oxygenation and tube patency and the position and appropriateness of ventilator settings. If oxygenation, airway patency and ventilator settings are adequate, sedation, analgesia, and possibly neuromuscular blocking agents with sedation may be needed to ensure effective control of ventilation (see Chapter 5).

Assessment and Support of Systemic Perfusion. The healthcare team will constantly assess the child's systemic perfusion. The child's color should be consistent, not mottled, and the nail beds and mucous membranes should be pink. Extremities should be warm with brisk capillary refill, and peripheral pulses should be readily palpable. Urine volume should average 1 to 2 mL/kg per hour if volume resuscitation and fluid intake are adequate. The child's heart rate should be appropriate for age and clinical condition, and the blood pressure should be appropriate for age. Continuous monitoring of heart rate is required. Intraarterial pressure monitoring is indicated if intracranial hypertension is present or likely to develop.

Signs of poor systemic perfusion include a mottled color or pallor. The extremities will cool in a peripheral-to-proximal direction, and capillary refill will become sluggish. Oliguria will be observed, and the heart rate may be excessive or inadequate for clinical condition. The blood pressure may be normal or low in the presence of inadequate cardiac output and systemic perfusion. Alternatively, the blood pressure may be high if the child is agitated or in pain. A high systolic blood pressure with widened pulse pressure may indicate that ICP is high and cerebral herniation is imminent.

Treatment of inadequate systemic perfusion requires support of the heart rate, maintenance of an adequate intravascular volume relative to the vascular space, support of myocardial function, and manipulation of vascular resistance. Volume therapy is administered as needed to ensure adequate preload and intravascular volume. Inotropic support may be necessary if myocardial dysfunction is present.

If the patient remains hypotensive despite the presence of an adequate intravascular volume, vasopressors are indicated, and neurogenic shock may be present. If ICP increases every time the systemic arterial pressure rises, cerebral autoregulation has likely been lost; loss of autoregulation is a poor prognostic sign.

Intracranial Pressure Monitoring. ICP monitoring is a useful adjunct to clinical assessment of the child with neurologic insult or disease. Accurate ICP monitoring requires knowledge of the system and ability to troubleshoot the devices.

Purposes. If the child is responsive, signs of increased ICP may be detected from clinical examination. However, if the child is comatose, early signs of increased ICP will not be apparent. If the comatose patient is at risk for the development of increased ICP (e.g., following traumatic brain injury), ICP monitoring is indicated. ICP monitoring through a ventricular catheter will facilitate CSF drainage if necessary.

ICP monitoring is most useful as an adjunct to the clinical assessment. It is extremely helpful in the evaluation of trends in the patient's condition, particularly in response to therapy. Therefore, it is imperative that every nurse perform ICP monitoring in exactly the same way so that the ICP measurement will contribute to the evaluation of patient progress over time. ICP measurements cannot be evaluated in isolation; they should always be interpreted in conjunction with the patient's clinical appearance.

Zeroing and Calibration. Regardless of the type of ICP monitoring system used, every system must be zeroed and calibrated appropriately. Fluid-filled systems are zeroed on a daily or shift basis (per unit protocol or device manufacturer recommendation), and fiberoptic catheters are zeroed before insertion.

If a fluid-filled system is used, the transducer should be leveled at about the level of the foramen of Monroe. The outer canthus of the eye or the external auditory canal typically is used as a landmark for this zero reference point. The transducer level should be verified when measurements are made and should be re-leveled with each change in patient position.

The CPP is the difference between the MAP and the ICP. However, this calculated difference will be affected by the position of the arterial and ICP transducers, which should be leveled based on unit protocol. Typically, the transducers are each placed at their typical reference points (ICP catheter at the level of the outer canthus of the eye or the external auditory canal, and the arterial catheter at the level of the right atrium). Some institutions prefer to have both transducers, (ICP/ventricular and arterial), at the same level, usually the level of the right atrium, so that the pressures used to calculate the CPP have the same zero reference point. Either practice is acceptable provided there is consistency in the positioning of the transducers from nurse to nurse and patient to patient.

Methods. The ICP can be monitored in a variety of ways (for additional information, see Chapter 21). The most accurate method of ICP monitoring is through an intraventricular catheter (Fig. 11-13) using a fiberoptic or standard intraventricular catheter inserted into a lateral ventricle. Intraventricular monitoring is typically performed in combination with drainage of CSF.

Complications of intraventricular monitoring include infection, excessive drainage, difficulty in placement, and technical complications of a fluid filled system. Drains that are in place longer than 5 days increase the risk of infectious complications (this risk is about 5%).[123] Ventricular bleeding may develop during catheterization. Aspiration of the ventricular catheter is not recommended, because application of

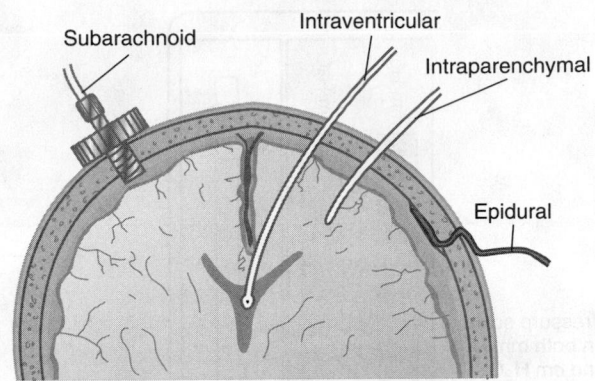

Subarachnoid   Intraventricular   Intraparenchymal   Epidural

FIG. 11-13 Locations for intracranial pressure monitoring. (From Kee KR, Hoff JT: *Youman's neurological surgery*, ed 4, Philadelphia, 1996, Saunders.)

suction can tear or injure the choroid plexus, producing intracranial hemorrhage.

The intraparenchymal fiberoptic catheter is easier to place than the intraventricular catheter and offers accuracy that rivals intraventricular pressure monitoring, with a similar risk of infection. One disadvantage of this catheter is that it cannot be readjusted to a zero reference point after insertion, and its zero reference has a tendency to drift over time.[123]

The subarachnoid bolt or screw can be placed through a burr hole in the skull into the subarachnoid space. Although this form of ICP measurement cannot be used in infants, it can provide a relatively reliable form of ICP monitoring with a low complication rate for children. Epidural catheters are occasionally used.

Nursing Responsibilities. When an ICP monitor is in place, the nurse is responsible for monitoring trends in the ICP, identifying worrisome changes in ICP, evaluating accuracy of the ICP measurements, and ensuring safety of the system (see Chapter 21 for information regarding the insertion and maintenance of ICP monitors). Throughout ICP monitoring, the nurse should immediately notify the appropriate physician or on-call provider of any deterioration in the child's clinical status, an increase in the child's ICP above the threshold reporting request, dampening of the ICP waveform, or malfunction of the ICP system.

If an extraventricular drainage (EVD) system is in place, the nurse should obtain orders regarding the height for placement of the drainage chamber (above the level of the child's lateral ventricles), whether CSF drainage is to be continuous or intermittent, and actions to take if the ICP rises. Typically, the drainage port is placed at a specified height (typically ordered in centimeters) above the patient's lateral ventricles, and the drainage stopcock is open to allow drainage (Fig. 11-14). If the system is functioning and the stopcock is turned "open" to drainage, CSF will drain from the child's ventricle into the collection chamber and ultimately into the drainage bag once the patient's ICP is sufficiently high to equal or exceed the equivalent of centimeters of water (cm H_2O) pressure.

If the EVD system is functioning correctly and the ventricles are not collapsed, the patient's ICP during continuous drainage should never exceed the equivalent of the cm

H_2O elevation of the drainage port above the child's ventricles, because CSF will drain at that pressure. Note that the child's ICP is typically monitored in millimeters of mercury, and the fluid-filled EVD system is operating with centimeters of water pressure. The following conversion factor is used:

$$1.36 \text{ cm } H_2O \text{ pressure} = 1.0 \text{ mm Hg}$$

Therefore, if the drainage chamber is placed 13.6 cm above the child's ventricles and the stopcock is open to drainage, CSF should drain whenever the child's ICP begins to exceed 10 mm Hg, and the ICP should not exceed 10 mm Hg unless the drain stopcock is closed. If the drainage chamber is placed 27.2 cm above the child's ventricles, CSF will drain whenever the child's ICP begins to exceed 20 mm Hg; therefore, the ICP should not exceed 20 mm Hg unless the drain stopcock is closed. If the ICP exceeds the drainage pressure with the stopcock open to drain, the nurse should search for obstruction in the tubing system and notify the appropriate on-call provider.

When intermittent drainage is ordered, the drainage stopcock is maintained in the closed position, and the nurse opens it to allow drainage of CSF if the ICP exceeds a specified pressure, typically 20 mm Hg. Such intermittent CSF drainage enables better evaluation of the patient's intrinsic ICP and the severity (magnitude) of any ICP spikes.

If drainage is intermittent, specific orders are needed regarding actions to be taken when the ICP rises (e.g., exceeds 20 to 25 mm Hg). For example, the provider may request that the child's ventricular drain be opened for 5 minutes to drain CSF if the ICP rises above 20 mm Hg for more than 10 minutes, or that drainage continue until the child's ICP is below a threshold. Any such orders must be clear (unambiguous) to protect the patient, the nurse, and the provider.

Transducers used for ICP monitoring must not be connected to standard infusion devices, because solution is not routinely infused into the subarachnoid space or ventricles. Occasionally, a provider may order instillation of a small amount of solution into the ICP catheter, but such instillation is performed only in the presence of the on-call provider with a specific order. A physician typically instills the solution. The ventricular catheter should not be aspirated, because application of suction can cause injury to the choroid plexus and intracranial hemorrhage.

The scalp entrance site of the intraventricular catheter should be covered with a clear biocclusive dressing; this allows the nurse to examine the entrance site for evidence of inflammation while maintaining an airtight dressing. The dressings covering intradural, subdural, and epidural monitors should be as occlusive as possible.

Tubing and drainage systems used for ICP monitoring should be changed per institutional policy and manufacturer's recommendations, using sterile technique. This procedure usually requires two people, with one person maintaining sterility during the process (the other person assisting). Care must be taken to avoid any break in sterile technique that could contaminate the system; contamination can lead to ventriculitis or meningitis and worsening of the patient's condition.

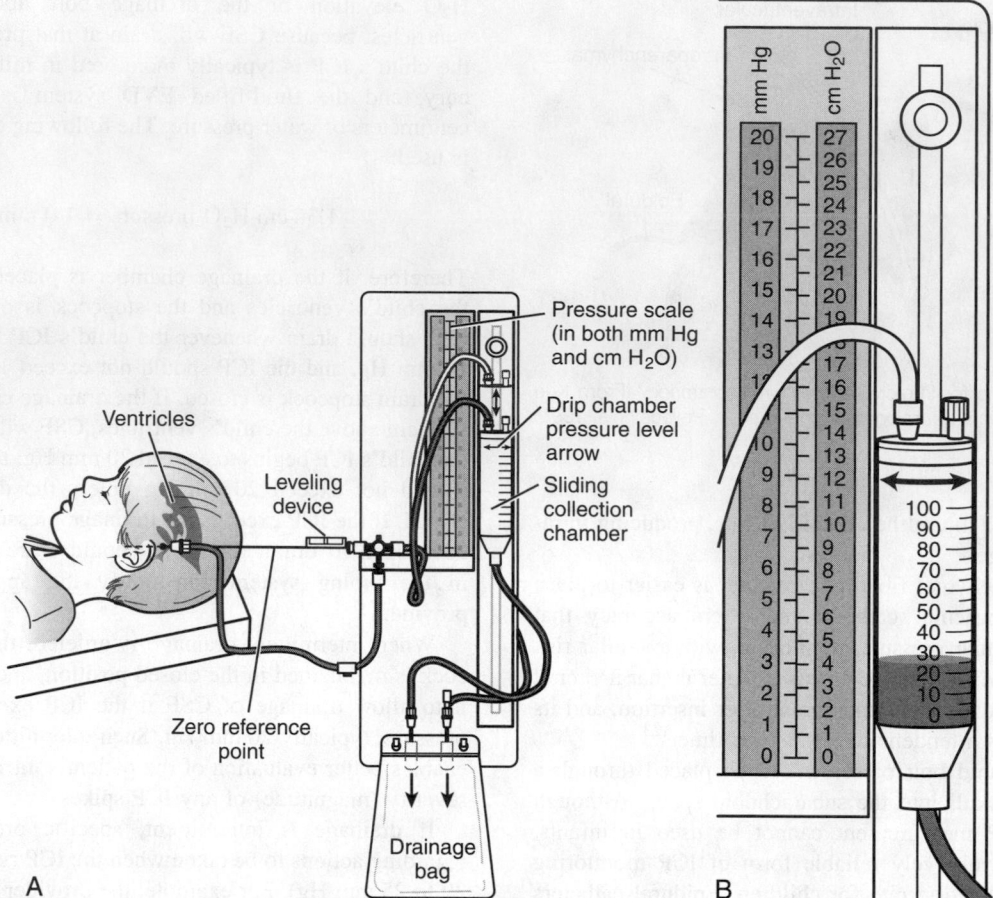

FIG. 11-14 Intraventricular intracranial pressure (ICP) monitoring system with an external ventricular drainage system for controlled drainage of cerebrospinal fluid. **A,** The system consists of an intraventricular catheter joined by tubing to a drainage system with adjustable height and a drainage bag. The system also typically has a stopcock, an injection sampling port, and a clamp. The zero reference point for the system is typically between the outer canthus of the eye and the external auditory canal (see leveling device placed at that level). **B,** The drip chamber pressure level (horizontal arrow) is placed a prescribed height (in cm) above this zero reference point. The drainage stopcock can allow continuous drainage or be turned to allow only intermittent drainage when the child's ICP exceeds a prescribed threshold. If the system is functioning and the stopcock is turned to drainage, CSF will drain from the child's ventricle into the collection chamber and ultimately into the drainage bag once the patient's ICP is sufficiently high. If the drip chamber is placed 27.2 cm (rounded to 27 cm) above the child's ventricles, drainage should occur if the child's ICP equals 27.2 cm H_2O or 20 mm Hg (1.36 cm H_2O pressure = 1 mm Hg pressure; 27.2 cm H_2O pressure = 20 mm Hg pressure). (Redrawn and modified from Owen A: *Clinical guideline: external ventricular drainage.* Great Ormond Street Hospital for Sick Children, Institute of Children's Health and University College of London, Revised, September, 2009.)

Dangerous Trends in the ICP. A rise in ICP alone is not problematic. Intracranial hypertension can be harmful because it can result in a compromise in cerebral perfusion or shifting (herniation) of the brain. There is no single ICP that is universally considered to be deleterious; the level at which the ICP becomes harmful is determined by intracranial compliance, the patency of the CSF spaces, the function of cerebral autoregulation and carbon dioxide responsiveness, the cerebral metabolic rate, and the rapidity and duration of the rise in ICP. For further information, see the Intracranial Pressure section earlier this chapter (see Figs. 11-6 and 11-11).

Trends in the ICP may indicate the need for further assessment and probable intervention. These trends include any rise in ICP associated with clinical deterioration (e.g., pupil

dilation, decreased level of consciousness, reduced response to painful stimulus), any spontaneous spikes above 20 to 25 mm Hg, any spikes associated with an inadequate CPP for age, or any severe or persistent elevation in ICP.

Documenting the ICP. The ICP documented on the nursing flow sheet or in the electronic record should reflect the peak ICP as well as the typical ICP that hour and the CPP during a monitoring interval (see Box 11-5 for one nurse entry method and Fig. 11-15 for sample screen from an electronic record). Such documentation provides more information than simple documentation of the ICP at one point in time, particularly if the ICP varies throughout the monitoring interval. If the nurse either documents or downloads the ICP measurement at a convenient time without ensuring that the pressure is

Box 11-5 Hourly Documentation of Intracranial Pressure

↑ 42 * /$\overline{18}$

↑42 = highest ICP observed that hour

* = ICP peak occurred only with stimulation (if no asterisk indicated, the ICP peak occurred without stimulation)

$\overline{18}$ = typical (average) ICP during that hour (this number used to calculate CPP)

CPP, Cerebral perfusion pressure; *ICP*, intracranial pressure.

representative, it will be more challenging to identify trends in the patient's condition. The healthcare team can also examine graphic images or trends in the ICP over hourly, daily, or longer intervals; such evaluation is better than review of isolated pressure measurements.

If the child's ICP is elevated, it is helpful to note whether the ICP spikes are spontaneous or occur only with stimulation. If a spike in ICP with stimulation (e.g., suctioning, painful stimulus) is recorded, the source of stimulation should be noted in the record. The healthcare team should be aware of trends in the patient's ICP, including spikes and typical ICP.

If the patient's intracranial compliance is low, the ICP will peak at higher levels, even without stimulation, and the average ICP will be higher than if the intracranial compliance is high. As the patient recovers, the ICP peaks will be lower and may occur only with stimulation. In addition, the average ICP will fall as intracranial compliance improves.

One or more of three distinct pressure waveforms, designated *A*, *B*, and *C*, may be visible when the ICP waveform is displayed on an oscilloscope. *A waves* are commonly called *plateau waves,* and they usually range in amplitude from 50 to 100 mm Hg. These plateau waves usually appear in patients who already have elevated ICP; they represent a further critical rise in the ICP associated with factors such as hypercapnia, hypoxia, or cerebral edema. Because the appearance of A waves is extremely worrisome and usually is associated with other signs of neurologic deterioration, their appearance warrants immediate notification of an on-call provider.

B waves are sharp, rhythmic, low-amplitude waves that fluctuate during the respiratory cycle. These waves usually range in amplitude from 20 to 50 mm Hg and indicate decreased cerebral compliance. They may precede the development of A waves.

C waves are also rhythmic, low amplitude waves. They are related to normal changes of the systemic arterial blood pressure and ventilation, and their clinical significance is not clear.[62]

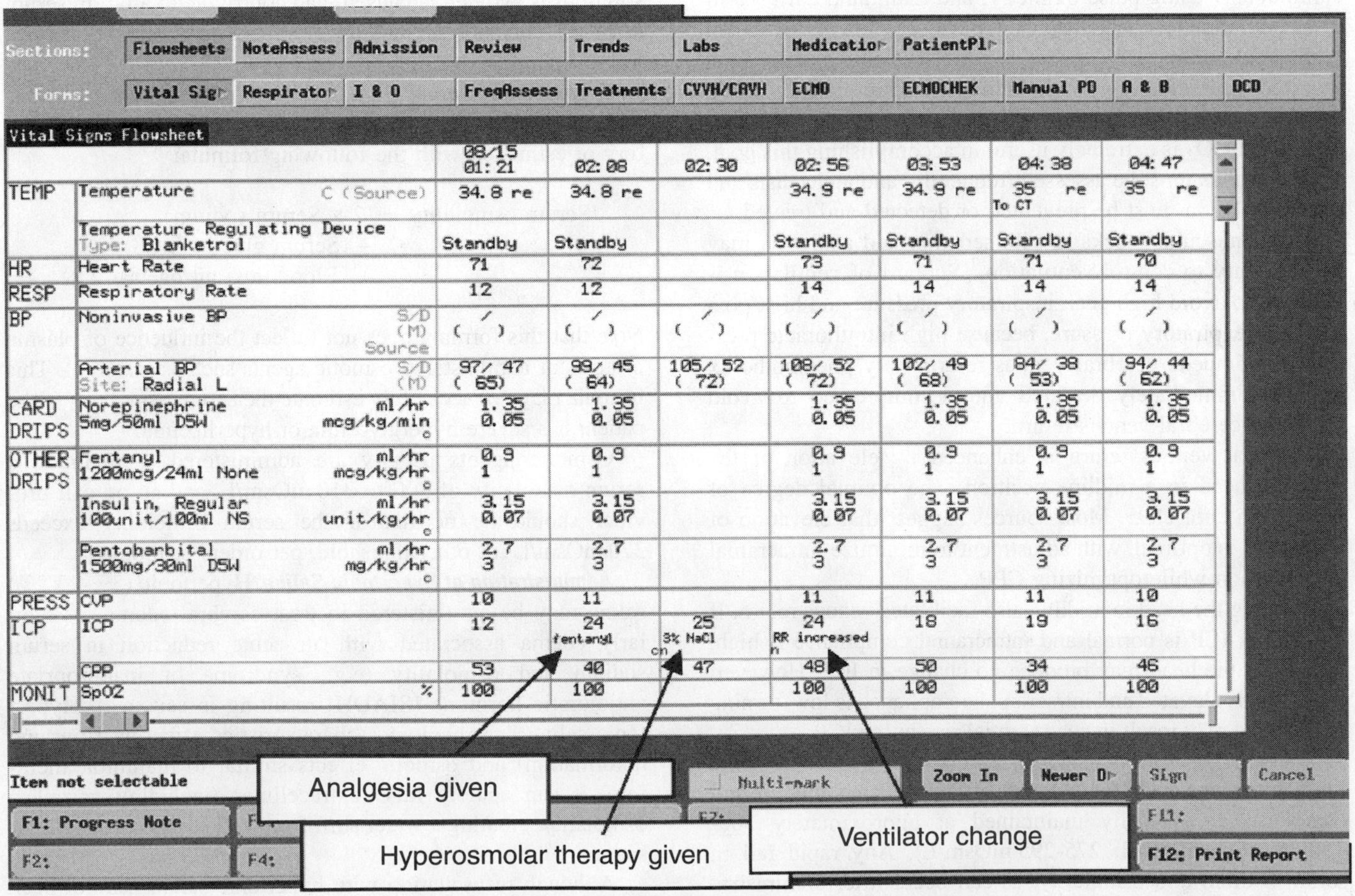
Vital Signs Flowsheet

			08/15 01:21	02:08	02:30	02:56	03:53	04:38	04:47
TEMP	Temperature	C (Source)	34.8 re	34.8 re		34.9 re	34.9 re	35 re To CT	35 re
	Temperature Regulating Device Type: Blanketrol		Standby	Standby		Standby	Standby	Standby	Standby
HR	Heart Rate		71	72		73	71	71	70
RESP	Respiratory Rate		12	12		14	14	14	14
BP	Noninvasive BP	S/D (M) Source	/ ( )	/ ( )	/ ( )	/ ( )	/ ( )	/ ( )	/ ( )
	Arterial BP Site: Radial L	S/D (M)	97/ 47 (65)	99/ 45 (64)	105/ 52 (72)	108/ 52 (72)	102/ 49 (68)	84/ 38 (53)	94/ 44 (62)
CARD DRIPS	Norepinephrine 5mg/50ml D5W	ml/hr mcg/kg/min	1.35 0.05	1.35 0.05		1.35 0.05	1.35 0.05	1.35 0.05	1.35 0.05
OTHER DRIPS	Fentanyl 1200mcg/24ml None	ml/hr mcg/kg/hr	0.9 1	0.9 1		0.9 1	0.9 1	0.9 1	0.9 1
	Insulin, Regular 100unit/100ml NS	ml/hr unit/kg/hr	3.15 0.07	3.15 0.07		3.15 0.07	3.15 0.07	3.15 0.07	3.15 0.07
	Pentobarbital 1500mg/30ml D5W	ml/hr mg/kg/hr	2.7 3	2.7 3		2.7 3	2.7 3	2.7 3	2.7 3
PRESS	CVP		10	11		11	11	11	10
ICP	ICP		12	24 fentanyl	25 3% NaCl	24 RR increased	18	19	16
	CPP		53	40	47	48	50	34	46
MONIT	SpO2	%	100	100		100	100	100	100

FIG. 11-15 Documentation of intracranial pressure in electronic record.

Reduction in Cerebral Blood Volume. Support of mechanical ventilation is generally provided to maintain the arterial carbon dioxide tension at approximately 35 to 40 mm Hg, the arterial oxygen tension at 80 to 100 mm Hg, and the oxyhemoglobin saturation at 95% to 97%. Hypercarbia and hypoxemia must be prevented, because they cause cerebral vasodilation that will increase CBF and will likely contribute to a further rise in the ICP.

An acute reduction in CBV can be achieved through hyperventilation and the creation of hypocarbia. Hyperventilation is not recommended for long-term management of increased ICP. Mild hyperventilation (to a $PaCO_2$ of 30-35 mm Hg) can be used in the presence of an acute neurologic deterioration and fear of impending herniation.[9] If the child is not intubated, the CBV may be acutely reduced using bag-mask ventilation, but intubation and mechanical ventilation are ultimately required.

If the child develops alkalosis (respiratory or metabolic), the child's oxyhemoglobin dissociation curve will be shifted to the left; this increases the risk of cerebral hypoxia and reflex cerebral vasodilation for two reasons. A shift in the curve to the left increases hemoglobin saturation at any arterial oxygen tension (PaO_2), so that even mild-to-moderate hemoglobin desaturation (e.g., 90%) may be associated with significant hypoxemia (e.g., PaO_2 of 50-60 mm Hg). In addition, a left shift of the oxyhemoglobin dissociation curve results in compromise of oxygen release at the tissue level. Therefore, the hemoglobin saturation should be monitored continuously using pulse oximetry, and maintained at 95% to 97% saturation, and alkalosis is avoided.

Skillful pulmonary support and suction technique is required to prevent hypoxemia and any rise in arterial carbon dioxide tension. Monitoring of pulse oximetry and end-tidal or exhaled CO_2 is extremely useful in accomplishing this goal. Breath sounds must be assessed frequently, and atelectasis and hypoventilation must be prevented or detected and treated.

Neuromuscular blockade with sedation and analgesia may be necessary to control ventilation.[7] Support of ventilation is adjusted to avoid high peak inspiratory pressure and high positive end-expiratory pressure, because high intrathoracic pressure will impede cerebral venous return. Any pneumothorax must be immediately detected and decompressed to avoid impeding cerebral venous return.

Cerebral venous return is enhanced by elevation of the patient's head in a midline position. The optimal degree of elevation is not clear. Most sources suggest that elevation of 15° to 30° is optimal, with adjustment to minimize intracranial hypertension while optimizing CPP.

Keeping the head in midline also facilitates venous return. If the child's ICP is normal and intracranial compliance is high, turning of the head may produce no change in ICP. However, if the ICP is elevated and intracranial compliance is low, turning of the head may result in a substantial rise in the ICP.

Maintenance and Manipulation of Serum Osmolality. Serum osmolality is typically maintained at approximately 300-310 mOsm/L (normal: 275-295 mOsm/L). Any rapid fall in serum sodium and osmolality, as can occur after administration of a large volume of hypotonic fluid, must be avoided because such a fall will produce a sudden shift of free water into the cells, contributing to cerebral edema.

Serum osmolality exceeding 320 to 340 mOsm/L has been associated with renal dysfunction and increased mortality in patients with head injury when using mannitol as the osmotic agent.[8,70] However, recent studies suggest that when using hypertonic saline solution, serum osmolality as high as 360 mOsm/L may be acceptable without adverse effects.

The healthcare team must closely monitor the child's serum electrolytes during therapy. The osmotic diuretic effect of mannitol can produce the loss of free water and electrolytes, leading to fluid and electrolyte imbalance and possible hypotension. This hypotension can compromise cerebral perfusion, producing secondary injury in an already compromised brain. Hypertonic saline does not cause the same diuresis and may improve hemodynamics.[8,70]

Fluid administration. The key goals of fluid administration are to support adequate intravascular volume and systemic perfusion. If intravascular volume and systemic perfusion are adequate (i.e., euvolemia) in the child with increased ICP, fluid administration is typically calculated to provide approximately 75% of estimated maintenance fluids requirements (Table 11-8), typically administered as normal saline. This approach maintains the serum sodium and osmolality even if the child develops the syndrome of inappropriate antidiuretic hormone (see Syndrome of Inappropriate Antidiuretic Hormone in Chapter 12), a common complication of head injury and other neurologic disorders. Administration of hypotonic solutions is avoided because it can contribute to a fall in serum sodium and osmolality and development or worsening of cerebral edema.

Estimation of Serum Osmolality. The patient's serum osmolality is monitored closely; it may be measured in the laboratory or estimated with the following formula:

$$Serum\ osmolality = (2 \times Serum\ sodium) \\ + (Serum\ glucose \div 18) \\ + (Blood\ urea\ nitrogen \div 2.8)$$

Note that this formula does not reflect the influence of plasma proteins or administered osmotic agents such as mannitol. This formula may not accurately estimate the serum osmolality if the patient has severe hyperglycemia or hyperlipemia.

Osmotic agents usually are administered to maintain a serum osmolality of 300 to 310 mOsm/L, and an on-call provider should be notified if the serum osmolality exceeds 320 mOsm/L (or other threshold, per orders or protocol).

Administration of Hypertonic Saline. Hypertonic (3%-23.5%) saline may be administered to treat cerebral edema, particularly edema associated with an acute reduction in serum sodium and osmolality (e.g., syndrome of inappropriate antidiuretic hormone [SIADH] resulting in seizures). Hypertonic saline has rheologic (characteristics affecting flow and deformation) and osmotic effects similar to mannitol; therefore, it can acutely raise extracellular (including vascular) osmolality, creating a water shift from cells to the extracellular space.

Although resuscitation with hypertonic saline has not been shown to improve survival when compared with use of

Table 11-8 **Formulas for Estimating Daily Maintenance Fluid Requirements for Children**

	Daily Requirements	Hourly Requirements
Fluid Requirements Estimated from Weight*		
Newborn (up to 72 h after birth)	60-100 mL/kg (newborns are born with excess body water)	–
Up to 10 kg	100 mL/kg (may increase up to 150 mL/kg to provide caloric requirements if renal and cardiac function adequate)	4 mL/kg
11-20 kg	1000 mL for the first 10 kg + 50 mL/kg for each kg over 10 kg	40 mL for first 10 kg + 2 mL/kg for each kg over 10 kg
21-30 kg	1500 mL for the first 20 kg + 25 mL/kg for each kg over 20 kg	60 mL for first 20 kg + 1 mL/kg for each kg over 20 kg
Fluid Requirements Estimated from Body Surface Area (BSA)		
Maintenance	1500 mL/m^2 body surface area	–
Insensible losses	300-400 mL/m^2 body surface area	–

*The "maintenance" fluids calculated by these formulas must only be used as a starting point to determine the fluid requirements of an individual patient. If intravascular volume is adequate, children with cardiac, pulmonary, or renal failure or increased intracranial pressure should generally receive less than these calculated "maintenance" fluids. The formula utilizing body weight generally results in a generous "maintenance" fluid total.

conventional fluids in studies of adults with head trauma, in these studies the patients who received hypertonic saline required fewer interventions to treat ICP. For this reason, hypertonic saline may be used instead of mannitol for treatment of increased ICP; it can be administered intermittently or as a continuous infusion to produce an extracellular fluid shift, reduce cerebral edema, and control ICP. Use of hypertonic saline may improve CPP and brain tissue oxygenation (P$_{bt}$O$_2$). Hypertonic saline can also have additional benefits, including restoration of normal cell volume and resting membrane potential, stimulation of atrial natriuretic peptide release, inhibition of inflammation, and enhancement of circulating blood volume and cardiac output.[70]

Potential complications of hypertonic saline administration include a rebound intracranial hypertension and higher incidence of subarachnoid hemorrhage and pontine myelinolysis.[8] Hypertonic saline is a vesicant and for that reason should be administered via a large vein or central venous catheter.

Mannitol. Mannitol is widely accepted and has long been used as an osmotic agent for treatment of intracranial hypertension. Although precise mechanisms of beneficial effects have not been completely established, mannitol produces both osmotic and vasoactive effects that aide in decreasing ICP. Its initial effect on intracranial hypertension is likely related to its rheologic properties, including characteristics of flow and deformity. The osmotic effects of mannitol create a shift of water from the cellular to the extracellular (including intravascular) space that rapidly decreases blood viscosity, leading to an increase in CBF and tissue oxygen delivery. This acute fluid shift likely explains the immediate effect in reduction of ICP.[8]

The diuretic effect of Mannitol occurs approximately 15 to 30 minutes after administration when it is filtered out of the blood by the kidneys, causing an osmotic diuresis (i.e., it draws water with it and is excreted in urine).[8] Mannitol is excreted essentially unchanged by the kidneys. Care must be taken to prevent hypovolemia and associated hypotension caused by the diuretic effects of mannitol, because these complications can lead to further cerebral ischemia.

Mannitol should be filtered before use to prevent the infusion of crystals. It is generally administered over 5 to 20 minutes, in a dose of 0.25 to 0.5 g/kg per dose. Higher doses of mannitol (0.5-1 g/kg) are generally reserved for the emergency control of intracranial hypertension.

Other Osmotic Agents. Glycerol, urea, and hypertonic glucose are no longer part of standard hyperosmolar therapy.

Diuretic Therapy. The role of diuretic therapy in the management of cerebral edema is somewhat controversial. Loop diuretics, primarily furosemide, can be used alone or in combination with mannitol. The patient's intravascular volume and systemic perfusion must be monitored closely, because hypovolemia and hypotension may compromise CBF, further impairing the already compromised brain.

Drainage of Cerebrospinal Fluid. A reduction in CSF volume is necessary if hydrocephalus is present. This reduction is achieved by surgical insertion of a ventriculoperitoneal shunt or other form of ventricular drain. If the child has such a shunt in place, the healthcare team must determine and document whether the shunt must be pumped regularly to maintain function. Shunts should be pumped only with an order from the physician or other on-call provider or per institutional policy. Shunts can malfunction, become obstructed, or become disconnected during the immediate postoperative period or anytime after insertion, resulting in a gradual or acute increase in ICP.

Even if CSF volume is not increased or excessive, reduction in CSF volume can be used to reduce intracranial volume and pressure. This can be accomplished using an intraventricular catheter to drain CSF. This extraventricular drain (EVD) can be intermittent or continuous (see Fig. 11-14). The collection chamber is positioned at a constant prescribed level above the patient's lateral ventricles (leveled at the anatomic landmark of the outer canthus of the eye, the external auditory canal, or a space between these points); the higher the collection chamber above the lateral ventricles, the higher the ICP required to produce CSF drainage. Rapid drainage of a large volume of CSF is not recommended, because upward herniation of the brain can occur. If an EVD is in place, strict sterile technique is used whenever the drainage system is entered (per provider order or unit policy), for example, to change drainage bags.

A malfunctioning or infected shunt may be externalized distal to the valve and attached to an EVD system. While the set-up and general care are similar to those described for use of an intraventricular catheter, the nurse must understand that CSF drainage is also influenced by the valve function.

CSF drainage should be performed with some caution. The most common complication of external CSF drainage is infection, although the incidence is low. The other common complication is loss of waveform transmission, typically secondary to obstruction of the catheter or drainage system. This complication can result from the presence of tissue or a clot within the system or from complete collapse or compression of the ventricular system in the setting of extremely elevated ICP. There are no pediatric data documenting the incidence of complications such as brain injury, hemorrhage, or seizure related to the placement of these drains, although the incidence of these noninfectious complications is thought to be low.[6]

A less commonly used device for removal of CSF is the lumbar drain. The lumbar drain is a sterile, continuous drainage device that diverts CSF from the subarachnoid space. While the lumbar drain is used primarily for the management of postoperative CSF leak, management of shunt infections, and for the diagnosis of idiopathic normal pressure hydrocephalus, it has been used in the operating room during a craniotomy to reduce ICP and as adjuvant therapy in patients with increased ICP secondary to traumatic brain injury. Experimentally lumbar drains have been used in the management of subarachnoid hemorrhage (SAH).

As with the EVD, the lumbar drain collection device is leveled at a predetermined position. The level of the transducer is dependent on the goal of therapy: draining at a precise level, draining at a specified volume, or draining at an established pressure. If the lumbar drain is being utilized in conjunction with an EVD for treatment of increased ICP then the collection chamber should be raised to the same level as the drain of the EVD. The tragus is typically used as the zero reference point.[125a]

General Supportive Care and Control of Oxygen Requirements and Nutrients. As noted previously, the patient with increased ICP should be intubated and mechanically ventilated. If the patient is agitated, sedation is indicated. Adequate analgesia must always be provided, because pain can contribute to a rise in ICP. If work of breathing is increased or agitation continues, sedation and analgesia with neuromuscular blockade may be required during mechanical ventilation. Of course, providers should closely monitor oxygenation and ventilation to ensure that both are adequate. Auditory stimulation should be minimized, because it can also contribute to a rise in ICP.

The child's temperature should be controlled to maintain normothermia and prevent elevation in temperature. Fever is detrimental to the injured brain because it increases the metabolic and oxygen requirements, so it is important to prevent and immediately treat any elevation in temperature above normal. Fever is typically treated with antipyretics and possibly a cooling device. If a cooling device is used, monitor for shivering. Shivering will increase metabolic demand and increase ICP; if shivering develops, it may be necessary to adjust cooling or (assuming mechanical ventilation is provided) administer a neuromuscular blocking agent with sedation.

The role of therapeutic hypothermia remains controversial in pediatric traumatic brain injury (see Additional Controversial Therapies). If therapeutic hypothermia is utilized, the child is cooled to approximately 32° to 34° C; sedation or sedation with neuromuscular blockade is generally required to prevent shivering.

Seizures can complicate the management of the child with increased ICP. Because seizures increase CBF and metabolic rate, they require treatment. Status epilepticus can create an acute and severe rise in ICP and should be suspected in any child with head injury who demonstrates sudden neurologic deterioration, pupil dilation, and fluctuation in vital signs.

The use of prophylactic anticonvulsants in pediatric patients with head injury is controversial. Current guidelines recommend the use of anticonvulsant therapy to prevent seizures in high-risk pediatric patients during the first week following a traumatic brain injury, noting that infants and small children are at greater risk for early posttraumatic seizure activity than are older children and adults.[14] Late prophylaxis (after the first week) should not be used.

Anesthetic, sedative, analgesic, and neuromuscular blocking agents (lidocaine, fentanyl, midazolam, vecuronium) are often administered to reduce the cerebral metabolic rate and improve the cerebral oxygen delivery and supply relationship (see Chapter 5 for information about the drugs). The use of barbiturates is reviewed in "Barbiturate therapy," below.

If the child appears agitated but does not respond in a purposeful manner to questions, it may be difficult to determine whether the child is in pain or is simply agitated as the result of a decreased level of consciousness. Treatment of pain is always important, and treatment of episodes of agitation will be necessary if they contribute to increased ICP or interfere with care. The healthcare team should have an organized and consistent approach to this challenge (e.g., sedative administration, reassessment, and administration of an analgesic if agitation continues).

Once the child is stable, nutritional support is needed. Gastric feedings may be initiated if the child demonstrates an effective cough and gag reflex. Transpyloric feeding may be undertaken if the child is intubated and sedated or the patient is thought to be at risk of aspiration. Parenteral alimentation should be reserved for patients who cannot tolerate enteral feeding or who have other injuries for which enteral feeding is contraindicated. Some nutritional support should be initiated by 48 to 72 hours after admission and full support should be provided by the end of the first week.

Gastrointestinal function should be monitored closely, and stress ulcer prophylaxis provided until feedings are initiated. Stool softeners should be administered as needed. Unless contraindicated, the head of the bed should be elevated to 30 degrees, to decrease risk of aspiration and ventilator-associated pneumonia. Regular oral care and frequent assessment of endotracheal secretions should be instituted (per protocol to prevent ventilator-associated pneumonia) to detect, prevent, or minimize the risk of pneumonia associated with aspiration (see Chapter 9).

Uncontrolled endogenous or exogenous hyperglycemia can be harmful to critically ill patients and can increase complications and decrease survival. Hyperglycemia is associated with a worse outcome in children with head injury and following cardiac arrest, but it is unclear whether the hyperglycemia is the cause or a symptom of the problem. Insulin infusion to prevent hyperglycemia has been associated with reduced ICU mortality in adult studies and in one multicenter pediatric study,[128] but it will increase hypoglycemic episodes. The relative risk of hyperglycemia and potential harm from hypoglycemia must be considered when contemplating insulin infusion for glucose control. If an insulin infusion is provided to control hyperglycemia, it is typically used during the first 12 to 18 hours of critical care, with careful monitoring of serum glucose concentration (using point of care testing, if possible). A glucose infusion may be added and titrated to prevent significant hypoglycemia during the insulin infusion.

Barbiturate Therapy. Barbiturate therapy may be prescribed for children with severe intracranial hypertension that is refractory to hyperosmolar therapy, sedation, analgesia, neuromuscular blockade, and CSF drainage. There are currently no data to support the use of barbiturates for prophylactic neuroprotection or prevention of intracranial hypertension.

Barbiturates lower ICP by suppression of metabolism and alteration in vascular tone, thereby improving the oxygen delivery-to-consumption ratio in patients with compromised cerebral perfusion. The anesthetic effect of the barbiturate will lower ICP. However, if the vasodilatory effect of the barbiturate reduces the MAP, cerebral perfusion will likely be compromised. Therefore, when barbiturates are administered, cardiovascular function must be closely monitored and supported.

If a barbiturate-induced coma is planned, an arterial and a central venous pressure monitoring catheter should be in place. Intravascular volume must be adequate before the infusion of the barbiturate is initiated, or hypotension will likely ensue. A continuous infusion of dopamine or epinephrine should be prepared and available at the bedside, to be administered as needed (with provider order) to maintain the MAP (and CPP).

As noted previously, barbiturates can produce hypotension and myocardial depression with a resultant fall in cardiac output and compromise in systemic and cerebral perfusion. Cardiac output can be maintained during barbiturate therapy with volume infusion and inotropic drug support. The goal of barbiturate therapy is to improve cerebral perfusion. As a result, the ICP should fall while the MAP is maintained. The child's systemic perfusion should be monitored constantly during barbiturate therapy.

Thiopental, phenobarbital, or pentobarbital may be administered to induce coma. Thiopental is used most often for short-term anesthesia. Pentobarbital usually is preferred for continuous infusion because it has a shorter half-life than phenobarbital, so a shorter time is needed between cessation

of therapy and drug elimination (i.e., drug concentration becomes subtherapeutic—and the patient should awaken—more rapidly after infusion is discontinued). An initial pentobarbital loading dose of 10 to 15 mg/kg is administered, followed by a continuous infusion of 1 mg/kg per hour.[10,120] The dose is increased until coma is achieved.

A rare complication of pentobarbital infusion is propylene glycol toxicity. Propylene glycol is the vehicle in which pentobarbital intravenous (IV) formulation is prepared. If large amounts of pentobarbital are administered in a short period of time, propylene glycol toxicity may result. Initial signs of toxicity include hyperosmolarity and lactic acidosis, which can cause renal dysfunction and multisystem organ failure.[24,88] During barbiturate therapy, the healthcare team should monitor for signs of toxicity.

Once coma is induced, the presence of coma is verified by observation of a "burst suppression" pattern on a bedside EEG monitor or the obliteration of any response to painful stimulation. In general, cranial nerve function is abolished, although some pupil constriction in response to light may be observed during barbiturate coma. Brain stem-evoked potentials can be evaluated during this therapy.

If ICP is controlled effectively, the barbiturate therapy can be reduced approximately 24 to 36 hours later. During reduction in the barbiturate dose, the patient's ICP, MAP, CPP, and neurologic function must be monitored closely.

Because barbiturates obliterate most neurologic function, the diagnosis of brain death will require the withdrawal of the barbiturate and/or the performance of confirmatory tests (e.g., cerebral perfusion scan) as dictated by institutional policy. If an EEG or clinical examination is used for confirmation of brain death, the serum barbiturate concentration must be subtherapeutic before the confirming EEG or examination is performed. Typically several days are needed between discontinuation of the barbiturate infusion and the fall in the barbiturate concentration to subtherapeutic levels.

Once medical therapy is maximized the only additional alternative to control increased ICP is decompressive craniectomy. This procedure is controversial and not employed in all centers. However, for patients with severe traumatic brain injury and refractory intracranial hypertension the procedure lowers ICP and may improve outcome. Removal of a portion of the skull, especially over the injured area allows additional room for the brain to swell without further restricting blood flow to the parenchyma. A decompressive craniectomy may be most beneficial in young patients with severe TBI and refractory intracranial hypertension from inflicted head trauma or those with some or all of the following: diffuse edema on CT scan, <48 hours post injury, no episodes of ICP >40 mm Hg prior to surgery and a GCS of >3 at some point after injury.[11a]

Additional Controversial Therapies. Steroid administration does not improve survival or recovery from increased ICP caused by trauma or ischemia. It can, however, reduce cerebral edema in patients with mass lesions, specifically brain tumors or discrete hematoma[12]; these problems remain the only indications for the use of steroids in the treatment of increased ICP. Complications of steroid administration include gastrointestinal bleeding, hyperglycemia, and increased susceptibility to infection. When discontinuing steroid therapy that has been used for more than a few days, taper the dose gradually.

The use of therapeutic hypothermia is controversial for pediatric patients with increased ICP following traumatic brain injury. There are currently no data to support the use of therapeutic hypothermia except as treatment to be considered in cases of refractory intracranial hypertension.[11] There is some support for the use of therapeutic hypothermia in the adult and neonatal patients with presumed hypoxic-ischemic injury following cardiopulmonary resuscitation; its role in the pediatric population remains unclear and is currently under investigation.[63]

Weaning from Support. As the child's condition improves, neuromuscular blockade, sedatives, and analgesics are weaned and the child is allowed to wake, move, and begin gradual weaning from mechanical ventilation. To wean treatment, one change in treatment is made at a time to allow for thorough evaluation of the child's response before a second change is made. If the child's ICP begins to rise again, an on-call provider should be notified immediately and resumption of recently discontinued therapy should be considered. The development of hypercapnia, hypoxia, and hypoventilation must still be avoided, because these factors may still result in a rise in ICP.

Psychosocial Support. The child and family will require sensitive support. While the child is unstable, it is often necessary to focus on the technical aspects of the child's care; however, the psychosocial aspects obviously cannot be neglected. If the nurse is unable to allow time or attention for supportive interaction with the family, an additional nurse, chaplain, or social worker should be called to provide the parents with the support they will need.

Throughout care, the child should receive explanations of all procedures performed and of all the things that will be seen, felt, or heard. Comatose children and those receiving neuromuscular blockade, sedation, and analgesia are still able to hear bedside conversation; therefore, the staff members should minimize technical discussions near the bedside and avoid discussion of a poor prognosis in the child's presence. Too often severely ill children are treated as though they are unconscious when they are merely immobile. As the child becomes able to move, simple signals should be devised to allow the child to communicate, and all signals should be recorded carefully in the plan of care.

As children with intracranial hypertension recover, they should receive repeated explanations of where they are and how they are progressing, because they may be disoriented from the effects of medications or when waking from a sound sleep. It is natural for children to be frightened during this time.

If the child will require rehabilitative therapy, such therapy should be initiated as soon as possible so that the child's progress or discharge from the unit is not delayed unnecessarily. Physical and occupational therapists should be consulted on admission to assist with prevention of contractures, foot drop, and other

complications of long-term immobility. Prior to initiating oral intake, speech therapists should be consulted for evaluation of swallow. If the child is not expected to recover, each member of the healthcare team should be aware of the prognosis, the information provided to the family, and the family's response to this information, so that consistent and constructive intervention can be planned (see the Brain Death and Organ Donation section in this chapter and see Chapter 3).

Coma
Etiology
Normal responsiveness to environmental stimuli requires normal functioning of the cerebral hemispheres and the reticular system. A normal state of consciousness is present when the patient is aware of the environment, can be aroused from sleep, and is oriented (as age appropriate) to time, place, and person. A decreased level of consciousness is present if the child is abnormally lethargic or confused or if the child (as age-appropriate) is not oriented to time and place. Stupor is a state of decreased consciousness from which the child can be aroused only through the application of vigorous and repeated external stimuli. Coma is a state of decreased consciousness in which the child demonstrates no verbal response despite the provision of strong external stimuli (see Table 11-5). Children in coma may, however, demonstrate motor response to noxious stimuli (e.g., deep pain or suctioning).

Coma in children can occur as the result of any of the following disorders: CNS inflammation, cerebral edema, head injury, intracranial bleeding, intracranial tumors or other mass lesions, hypoxia, hypercapnia, acid-base imbalance, electrolyte imbalance (e.g., hyponatremia or hyperglycemia), disturbances of water balance, or Reye's syndrome. Coma in children also can result from intentional or inadvertent overdose of therapeutic drugs (e.g., aspirin, barbiturates, antihistamines, ferrous sulfate) and from the ingestion of street drugs (e.g., phencyclidine [PCP], methaqualone [Quaaludes], marijuana, heroin).

It is probably helpful to divide the causes of coma into structural and toxic or metabolic problems. Structural coma results from actual physical injury to the brain. Treatment is aimed at preventing or limiting cerebral swelling or edema and preventing or treating increased ICP. Structural coma may also be caused by a space occupying lesion or an intracranial hemorrhage. Toxic or metabolic coma results from electrolyte or acid-base imbalances, liver or renal failure, or the ingestion of toxic substances. Treatment of this type of coma is aimed at removing or neutralizing the toxin.[102]

Pathophysiology
Coma is a lack of consciousness. Consciousness is a set of neural processes that allow perception and comprehension of and action on the internal and external environment.[23,100,102] Comatose patients lack two neurophysiologic processes that occur in consciousness: arousal and awareness.

Clinical Signs and Symptoms
As noted, comatose children demonstrate no verbal response to external stimuli, but may demonstrate motor response to noxious stimuli (e.g., deep pain or suctioning). In addition,

painful stimulus can trigger abnormal posturing. The child may demonstrate impaired cranial nerve function, loss of oculocephalic and oculovestibular reflexes, and progressive brainstem dysfunction. Ultimately, cardiorespiratory compromise may develop.

Assessment of comatose children should include all aspects presented in the section on the clinical signs and symptoms of increased ICP. This includes frequent evaluation of the child's level of consciousness and neurologic function. The child's pupil size and reaction to light should be assessed hourly and whenever the clinical condition changes. Although there are no characteristic changes in pupil response associated with coma, characteristic changes may occur as a result of the underlying cerebral insult or the development of increased ICP (see Fig. 11-8 and Table 11-9). The use of a standardized tool such as the GCS (see Table 11-6) will facilitate consistent, objective scoring by different providers and identification of changes over time.

The assessment of cranial nerve function is important, because the evaluation of higher brain function is impossible in unresponsive children. Thorough cranial nerve evaluation is typically performed by the physician or advanced practice nurse. The bedside nurse will also evaluate cranial nerve function. The nurse assesses function of the oculomotor nerve (third cranial nerve) when evaluating pupil constriction to light, the acoustic nerve (eighth cranial nerve) when monitoring the child's response to voice or noise, and the glossopharyngeal and vagus nerves (ninth and tenth cranial nerves that produce a gag reflex) when suctioning the child's airway. (See Table 11-2 for a list of cranial nerve functions.)

Two reflexes that may be absent in the comatose child are the oculocephalic reflex and the oculovestibular reflex. Evaluation of the oculocephalic reflex is often called *testing of doll's eyes*. This test must not be performed on any patient suspected of having a cervical spine injury. The reflex is evaluated when the child's eyes are held open and the head is turned sharply from the midline to one side and then turned to the other side. If the child's brainstem is intact, the normal doll's eyes reflex is present: the eyes will seem to turn (rotate) toward midline when the head is turned to the side. The eyes will move in the direction opposite that of the head movement; if the patient's head is turned sharply to the left, the patient's eyes will deviate toward the right.

When the doll's eyes reflex is absent, the eyes remain fixed in the middle of their sockets so they face wherever the head is pointed (as though the eyes are painted on the face). Loss of the doll's eyes reflex can result from severe drug intoxication, increased ICP, metabolic dysfunction, or the presence of a severe lesion in the area of the midbrain or brainstem.

The elicitation of the oculovestibular reflex is commonly referred to as the *cold water calorics* test. Testing of this reflex usually is performed by a physician or advanced practice nurse, and it is contraindicated in the patient with a ruptured tympanic membrane. The test is reserved for evaluation of unconscious patients. The head is elevated at a 45- to 60-degree angle and positioned in midline with the eyes held open. Approximately 10 to 20 mL of ice water is instilled into the external auditory (ear) canal. If the brainstem is intact, both eyes should deviate toward the side of the irrigation.

The eye deviation in response to the cold water instillation often is associated with slow and then rapid nystagmus. If the child's eyes do not deviate together toward and then away from the side of the irrigation, brainstem injury or metabolic dysfunction is present. (Testing for these reflexes is summarized and illustrated in the Brain Death and Organ Donation section in this chapter.)

The corneal reflex can be tested in the comatose child. Normally, gentle stroking of the eyelashes or of the peripheral portion of the cornea with a wisp of cotton will produce a brisk blink response. If no blink is seen, brainstem injury is probably present.

The tonic neck reflex is normally present in infants between 2 and 6 months of age. This reflex can be elicited by rapidly turning the infant's head to the side while the infant is supine. When the tonic neck reflex is present, the ipsilateral arm and leg will extend, and the contralateral arm and leg will flex. Persistence of this reflex beyond 9 months of age usually indicates neurologic disease or injury.

Table 11-9 **Reflex Responses in Altered States of Consciousness**

Level of CNS Lesion	Level of Consciousness	Pupil Size and Reactivity	Oculocephalic and Oculovestibular Reflexes	Respiratory Pattern	Motor Responses
Thalamus	Lethargy, stupor	Small, reactive	Increased or decreased	Cheyne-Stokes*	Normal posture, tone slightly increased
Midbrain	Coma	Midposition, fixed	Absent	Central neurogenic, hyperventilation[†]	Decorticate,[‡] tone markedly increased
Pons	Coma	Pinpoint	Absent	Eupnea[§] or apneustic[ǁ] breathing	Decerebrate,[¶] flaccid
Medulla	Coma	Small, reactive	Present	Ataxic breathing	No posturing, flaccid

From Morriss FC: Altered states of consciousness. In: Levin DL, Morriss FC, Moore GC: *A practical guide to pediatric intensive care*, ed 2, St Louis, 1984, Mosby.
*Cheyne-Stokes respiration: type of regular periodic breathing characterized by crescendo-decrescendo breaths interspersed with periods of apnea.
[†]Central neurogenic hyperventilation: hyperventilation with forced inspiration and expiration.
[‡]Decorticate posturing: upper extremities flexed against chest, lower extremities extended.
[§]Eupnea: normal breathing.
[ǁ]Apneustic breathing: pattern of breathing in which there is cessation of respiration in inspiratory position, usually rhythmical.
[¶]Decerebrate posturing: arms and legs extended with arms internally rotated, neck extended.

Deep tendon reflexes, such as the patellar reflex, can be thoroughly checked by the physician or advanced practice nurse. The bedside nurse or provider can attempt to elicit clonus by briskly flexing the wrists and ankles. Clonus is present if the extremities then rhythmically flex and contract. Exaggerated deep tendon reflexes, sustained clonus, or spasticity may be present if the child is fatigued, but they also may indicate the presence of upper motor neuron lesions (cerebral cortex injury).[111]

The nurse will also evaluate and document the child's posture and limb movements. The development of decorticate rigidity or decerebrate posturing should be reported to an on-call provider. Decerebrate posturing usually indicates damage to lower (more basic) brain centers; however, some comatose patients demonstrate alternating decorticate rigidity and decerebrate posturing (see Fig. 11-9).

Limb movements should be described as purposeful, nonpurposeful, or consistent with seizure activity. Purposeful movements are present if the child responds to a central applied painful stimulus or withdraws an extremity from painful stimulation. A sternal rub is an example of a central pain stimulus; the child responds purposefully if the child attempts to grab the hand that is applying the stimulus. To elicit withdrawal of an extremity, pinch the medial aspect of the extremity; purposeful movement is present if the limb is abducted or drawn outward from the midline (i.e., the extremity is withdrawing from the painful stimulus).

Flexion and adduction of extremities in response to painful stimuli are not necessarily purposeful and may represent decorticate posturing. Furthermore, arm or leg withdrawal from a peripheral painful stimulus can result from a spinal cord reflex only; such withdrawal may be observed despite the presence of brain death or spinal cord transection.

Rhythmic or bizarre movements of the limbs or eyes should be investigated thoroughly, because they may represent seizure activity. If the child has received neuromuscular blocking agents, seizures may be impossible to confirm or rule out unless an EEG is performed. It is important to identify seizures and to document their frequency, duration, and severity because status epilepticus can compromise cerebral perfusion and result in cerebral ischemia (see Status Epilepticus later in this chapter).

The nurse caring for the child in coma must carefully assess the child's respiratory rate and pattern and the effectiveness of the child's airway, oxygenation and ventilation. Potential abnormalities in respiratory pattern have been summarized previously (see Alterations in Respiratory Pattern in the Clinical Signs and Symptoms section of Increased Intracranial Pressure). The most common respiratory patterns observed in the comatose patient include Cheyne-Stokes respirations (alternating bradypnea and hyperpnea), central neurogenic hyper-ventilation (constant rapid respiratory rate in the absence of hypercapnia or hypoxemia), apneustic breathing (pauses after inspiration and possibly after expiration), cluster breathing (irregular breathing associated with irregular pauses), and ataxic breathing (extremely irregular rate, rhythm and depth of breaths). Table 11-9 correlates abnormal breathing patterns with levels of cerebral injury (see, also, Fig. 11-7 for an illustration of abnormal breathing patterns).

Regardless of the respiratory pattern observed, the nurse must ensure that the child's airway, oxygenation, and ventilation are adequate; this requires clinical assessment of the child's chest expansion and breath sounds, as well as assessment of the child's color and systemic perfusion, and monitoring of arterial oxyhemoglobin saturation. Clinical signs of hypoxemia include tachycardia and peripheral vasoconstriction, and late signs of hypoxemia include cyanosis and bradycardia. Hypercapnia and hypoxia can contribute to the development of increased CBF and ICP; therefore, respiratory dysfunction must be avoided.

Thorough evaluation of the child's respiratory status includes the assessment of cough and gag reflexes. These reflexes require function of the glossopharyngeal (ninth cranial) and vagus (tenth cranial) nerves, for maintenance of a patent airway and prevention of aspiration. The child who does not possess adequate cough and gag reflexes is at risk for aspiration or airway obstruction and will require intubation and frequent pharyngeal or tracheal suctioning. A tracheostomy ultimately may be performed.

When any child is admitted with coma of unknown origin, the first urine specimen obtained should be sent for toxicologic screening. In addition, blood samples are taken for analysis of arterial blood gases, serum electrolyte and glucose concentrations, and blood cultures. A thorough neurologic examination is performed, and a lumbar puncture may be obtained. Additional useful diagnostic tests for evaluation of the comatose child include an EEG, a CT scan and/or MRI. These studies may help confirm the presence of local or diffuse cerebral injury, and they may be helpful in identifying treatable conditions and predicting the child's recovery (see Common Diagnostic Tests at the end of this chapter for further information).

Management

The management of the comatose child is largely supportive. This care includes: assessment of neurologic and cardiorespiratory function, prevention or early detection of any deterioration in neurologic function, support of vital functions, maintenance of adequate nutrition, and prevention of the complications of immobility.

The assessment of neurologic function has been discussed in the preceding section. It is important to report any deterioration in the patient's clinical status to an on-call provider. The child at risk for the development of increased ICP requires continuous monitoring of systemic perfusion, including urine output, warmth of extremities, strength of peripheral pulses, and briskness of capillary refill. The child's level of consciousness, pupil response to light, blood pressure, heart rate, respiratory rate and pattern, and motor function or posturing are also closely monitored.

If the patient develops signs of poor systemic perfusion or signs of increased ICP (including lethargy, increase in systolic blood pressure, widening of pulse pressure, and bradycardia), immediately notify the on-call provider and begin assessment and support of airway, breathing, and circulation. Endotracheal intubation for airway protection may be necessary if it has not already been performed. If the patient is already intubated, the management protocol for intracranial hypertension should be initiated as appropriate.

Support of Vital Functions. The patient's airway must be kept patent and free of secretions. The comatose patient may be unable to cough effectively to keep the oropharynx and trachea free from obstruction by secretions. In addition, ineffective gag and uncoordinated swallow reflexes will increase the risk of aspiration of vomitus, oral secretions, or mucus.

The nurse should suction the pharynx as needed and position the patient so that oral secretions pool in the side of the mouth instead of in the pharynx. The tongue of the unconscious patient can obstruct the pharynx when the patient is supine; therefore, the patient is typically positioned with the head of the bed elevated and the patient's head turned to the side (unless increased ICP is present). If secretion control or maintenance of a patent airway becomes difficult, intubation may be required.

If the child is breathing spontaneously, the nurse must constantly assess the effectiveness of the child's ventilation and oxygenation. Air movement should be adequate and equal bilaterally, and signs of increased respiratory effort (retractions, nasal flaring, or grunting) should be absent. Elevation of the head of the child's bed will allow maximal inspiratory effort by allowing abdominal contents to drop away from the diaphragm. Placement of a small linen roll under the child's shoulders will support a patent airway.

If the comatose child is apneic, bag-mask ventilation and then intubation with mechanical ventilation are required. This assistance also is needed if the child develops hypercapnia, hypoxia, or inadequate inspiratory effort.

After the institution of mechanical ventilation, the child will require excellent pulmonary toilet using aseptic technique. Supplementary ventilation and preoxygenation must be provided before and immediately after suctioning to prevent carbon dioxide retention and hypoxemia during the suctioning attempt; this is especially important if the child is at risk for the development of increased ICP.

If the child has severe pulmonary dysfunction and alveolar hypoxia, attempts should be made to determine the position associated with the best arterial oxygen saturation and most efficient carbon dioxide removal. Dependent portions of the lung will receive the greatest blood flow, whereas the best aerated portions of the lung are often the nondependent lung segments. As a result, the nurse should document the child's position when blood gases are drawn in an attempt to determine what effect, if any, the child's position has on oxygenation and carbon dioxide elimination.

The comatose patient may not become agitated or restless when hypoxic and will be unable to articulate complaints. It is therefore extremely important that the nurse recognize signs of poor systemic perfusion or inadequate respiratory function.

When the child is comatose or when pharmacologic coma is induced, venous pooling of blood occurs[41] and can produce a relative hypovolemia. The administration of additional IV fluids may be required to maintain an adequate central venous pressure and systemic perfusion.

If the comatose child is always kept in the recumbent position, orthostatic hypotension can result when the child initially resumes the upright position.[41] In addition, the recovering child may be extremely frightened when immobilized in the supine position, with caretakers looming overhead. If possible

the child should be placed in the semi-Fowler's position several times each day. This position provides the recovering child with a different view of the unit, helps to prevent the development of orthostatic hypotension, and allows maximal diaphragm excursion and chest expansion. This positioning can be provided for the small infant through the elevation of the head of the crib mattress or the use of an upright infant's seat.

The child's hourly fluid intake and daily weight should be assessed carefully. Urine output should average 1 mL/kg per hour if fluid intake is adequate. If the child's fluid intake or output is inadequate, it should be discussed with a provider.

Maintenance of Adequate Nutrition. As soon as the comatose child is admitted to the critical care unit, the healthcare team should plan to provide adequate nutrition. Fluid requirements can be delivered easily in the form of IV solutions, but maintenance calories may be more difficult to provide. If inadequate caloric intake is provided, the child will develop a negative nitrogen balance and a protein deficiency, wound healing will be delayed, the young infant will not be able to make the brown fat needed to generate heat, and general recovery will be slowed. Therefore, the team should plan to provide some form of enteral or parenteral alimentation.

If enteral feedings are attempted, small amounts of formula are initially provided, and the amount and concentration is then advanced slowly as tolerated. When continuous nasogastric feeding is tolerated, the child can be advanced to small bolus feedings. During this time, the nurse should measure and record the residual formula remaining in the stomach before feeding and should assess the child's abdominal girth and firmness throughout the feeding. The comatose child might not tolerate enteral feedings, because immobilization may produce a paralytic ileus. If gastric distension, diarrhea, vomiting, or gastric reflux develops, enteral feedings should be discontinued, and parenteral alimentation should be instituted (see Parenteral Nutrition in Chapter 14).

Care should be taken to monitor the child's acid-base and electrolyte status, supporting electrolyte and acid-base balance. This support includes the provision of daily electrolyte requirements and checking electrolyte concentrations at regular intervals or with changes in the patient's condition.

A bowel regimen should be instituted to prevent constipation or bowel impaction. Stool output must be charted consistently so that the healthcare team does not overlook the absence of a bowel movement for several days. Use of glycerin suppositories or enemas may be required occasionally to promote the evacuation of stools.

Prevention of the Complications of Immobility. As soon as the status of the comatose child is stable, a referral should be made to occupational and physical therapists. Passive range-of-motion exercises are needed on a regular basis, and splints or ankle pads should be used to prevent ankle and wrist contractures, foot drop, and pressure sores.

Comatose children require excellent skin care. Foam or alternating-pressure mattresses or other pressure-relieving devices will help prevent the development of pressure sores over bony prominences. Careful assessment includes complete inspection of the child's skin at least once every shift, unless the child is extremely unstable. Gentle massage over any reddened areas will promote circulation and reduce ischemia. The skin should be kept as dry as possible, and the sheets should be free of wrinkles. The development of skin breakdown signals inadequate attention to skin care.

The insertion of multiple invasive monitoring lines and drains and other tubes increases the patient's risk of hospital-acquired infection. Good hand washing technique is one of the best ways to avoid the transmission of infection. Strict hand washing technique must be used when handling the patient catheters and tubes. Aseptic technique must be used when suctioning the ET tube. For additional measures to prevent ventilator associated pneumonias, see Chapter 9.

All skin puncture sites require inspection at least once each shift, with wound drainage, wound fluctuance, erythema, or odor reported to an on-call provider. Other signs of infection include an elevation in white blood cell count and fever. In small children, a decrease in platelet count can indicate the presence of sepsis and the development of disseminated intravascular coagulation (see Chapters 6 and 16). If infection is suspected, obtain appropriate wound, serum, or catheter cultures per order or protocol, and administer antibiotics as needed.

Comatose children typically have both bowel and bladder incontinence. However, a urinary catheter should not be inserted merely to simplify urine collection. Diapers, condom catheters, or padded rubberized sheets can enable measurement of urine output and minimize need for linen changes. If the use of a urinary catheter is required for ongoing evaluation of renal function and urine output, meticulous catheter and meatus care is required. If cloudy or foul smelling urine develops, notify an on-call provider and obtain urinalysis and urine culture (and Gram's stain, if indicated) per order or protocol.

If the child's blink reflex is not intact, apply ophthalmic ointment to lubricate the cornea and prevent corneal abrasions. It may be necessary to patch the eyes to protect the corneas. Before patch placement, both the child and the family should be told about the purpose of the patches.

The child's mouth requires lubrication and cleaning several times each shift to prevent the development of gingivitis or dental caries. The child's mouth and lips should be kept clean, even if they are covered with the tape holding the ET or nasogastric tube in place.

Immobilized adolescents and preadolescents are at risk for development of deep venous thrombosis. This subpopulation of pediatric patients requires deep venous thrombosis prophylaxis using thromboembolic deterrent (TED) hose, sequential compression devices and/or low-molecular weight heparin (per order or institutional preference or protocol). This prophylaxis is also indicated for younger patients with a patient or family history of hypercoagulable states.

Psychosocial Support. The comatose child may hear any or all of the conversations held near the bedside. Therefore, all members of the healthcare team must avoid conversation and complex terminology that could be heard or misunderstood by the child, particularly discussions of a pessimistic prognosis.

At all times, the nurse should assume that the comatose child is able to hear and is frightened. Begin and end each shift by speaking gently to the child and orienting the child (if age-appropriate) to time and place. Throughout the day, talk to the child about the time of day and prepare the child before treatments or procedures are performed and before the child is moved. As the child is recovering, he or she may be awake yet unresponsive to surroundings and unable to ask questions; for such patients, a nurse's daily support and review of the child's progress (as appropriate) can be extremely helpful.

The family will require consistent information and support from the healthcare team to help them have a realistic understanding of the child's prognosis. If the child's recovery is doubtful, it will be necessary to prepare the family for the news, yet convey continued concern about the child's care. The medical team must strike a fine balance to be realistic but avoid suggesting they have given up hope for recovery unless or until the child meets the legal definition of brain death. If withdrawal of support is considered, the family will be included in the decisions reached, but the pronouncement of brain death or futility and the recommendation of discontinuation of medical care will appropriately come from the medical providers (see Psychosocial Support of the Family in the Brain Death and Organ Donation section in this chapter).

Significant work has been completed in recent years to develop helpful tools to predict functional outcome after severe brain injury. These tools may be helpful in discussing long term outcomes with families.[1]

As a rule, children demonstrate faster and more complete recovery from coma than do adults. However, it is important to note that the child's brain is growing rapidly (particularly through the age of seven), making it extremely difficult to predict the degree of permanent neurologic damage that will result from a neurologic injury. Neurologic sequelae often are not manifest for months or years after the insult has occurred.[1] Recovery, too, can occur over years.

Status Epilepticus

Etiology

Status epilepticus is defined as a continuous seizure lasting longer than 30 minutes or more than two seizures without return to a baseline level of consciousness between events.[119] The most common causes of status epilepticus in children include high fever secondary to a non-CNS infection and sudden discontinuation of an anticonvulsant drug.[46] Approximately 20% of children with status epilepticus have a chronic encephalopathy or seizure disorder. In approximately half of children who develop status epilepticus, no specific cause can be identified. The remaining causes of status epilepticus in children include acute encephalopathy (such as that resulting from meningitis or encephalitis), metabolic disorders (including hypoxia, acidosis, sepsis, dehydration, hypocalcemia, hypoglycemia, hyponatremia, and hypernatremia), ingestion of toxic substances, and head injury.[119]

Causes of status epilepticus vary somewhat depending on the age of the child. The most common cause of seizures in the neonatal period is intrauterine or perinatal hypoxia. Metabolic disorders, intraventricular hemorrhage, and infection can also cause neonatal seizures. High fever, toxic ingestion, and preexisting seizure disorders are more common causes of status epilepticus during later infancy and early childhood. Status epilepticus during adolescence often is caused by metabolic disorders, toxic ingestions, and head injury.[78] Status epilepticus is most common in children younger than 3 years; the incidence then decreases with advancing age.[25]

Pathophysiology

Seizures are characterized by a spontaneous, repetitive, electrical discharge from abnormal neurons. If the abnormal electrical activity remains localized within a small area of the cerebral cortex, a focal or partial seizure will occur, producing unilateral tonic-clonic activity. If this activity spreads throughout the subcortical area, a generalized seizure and bilateral tonic-clonic activity will occur; this can be associated with loss of consciousness or coma. Localized seizure activity can affect adjacent neurologic tissue so that the focal seizure becomes a generalized seizure.

Sustained seizure activity increases the adenosine triphosphate requirements of neurons, because the constant electrical activity requires an extremely active sodium-potassium pump. In addition, the constant muscle contraction and relaxation produced by tonic-clonic seizures will increase tissue oxygen requirements. Thus, cerebral and tissue metabolic requirements are maximal at this time. If CBF cannot increase sufficiently to meet cerebral cell substrate requirements, cerebral ischemia and death can result. If tissue oxygenation is not maintained adequately, hypoxemia, lactic acidosis, and hypoglycemia can develop.

Seizures may cause a Valsalva maneuver and increased intrathoracic pressure that impedes cerebral venous return. This will increase ICP in patients with cerebral edema or increased intracranial volume.

Some clinical conditions may predispose the child to the development of seizures. These conditions include fatigue, pain, specific photic stimuli (usually rapidly and regularly flickering lights or images), or abrupt changes (particularly a fall) in serum sodium concentration (see Hyponatremia in Chapter 12).

Clinical Signs and Symptoms

Whenever seizure activity is suspected, the nurse should note the time of the onset of seizure activity, any precipitating factors, the location and type of the seizure activity, any progression of the seizure, and its duration. Although it is best for the nurse to describe rather than label the seizure activity, a few descriptive terms are used widely.

Generalized myoclonic, or tonic-clonic, status epilepticus is characterized by bilateral extensor or flexor (or both) muscular contractions that occur continuously or in a series lasting for hours or days. This form of status epilepticus is typically related to degenerative brain disease, toxic encephalopathy, or anoxic brain damage. The EEG usually reveals the presence of many spikes with slow background activity.[112,119]

Generalized absence status epilepticus is associated with periods of confusion and with a decreased level of consciousness or stupor that is not associated with any abnormal muscle activity. This form of status epilepticus most commonly develops in children with persistent petit mal seizures.

It is rarely associated with acute CNS pathology. The EEG shows bilateral, regular, generalized, symmetrical spikes.[112,119]

Focal motor status epilepticus is produced by a localized area of cortical injury or by metabolic disease. It produces rapid, focal, clonic movements of one part or one side of the body without loss of consciousness. The EEG reveals focal spikes.[112,119]

The presence of seizure activity or of status epilepticus may be impossible to detect clinically in the patient receiving a neuromuscular blocking agent, and an EEG is needed to confirm the seizure activity. The critically ill child typically has severe neurologic, cardiac, respiratory, or multisystem disease, so is at risk for the development of cerebral injury, anoxia, or metabolic imbalances that can produce seizures. However, when a child receives neuromuscular blocking agents, myoclonic or tonic-clonic muscle activity will be suppressed and seizure activity will not be apparent. In these patients, the only evidence of seizure activity may be tachycardia or alternating tachycardia and bradycardia, wide fluctuations in blood pressure, poor systemic perfusion, nystagmus, or pupil dilation. Therefore, it is extremely important that an EEG be obtained whenever seizures are suspected in the child receiving neuromuscular blockade so that status epilepticus does not develop or progress undetected.

Management

Treatment of the child with status epilepticus requires support of vital functions, abolition of the seizures, and elimination of any precipitating factors. A protocol is needed for the treatment of status epilepticus, so that care is organized and orderly and therapy does not produce more complications than the seizures themselves.

Support of Vital Functions. During status epilepticus, priorities of care include maintenance of systemic perfusion and cerebral oxygenation. During the seizure activity, place the child on a flat soft surface with no hard or sharp objects nearby. The patient's bed is an appropriate surface, although the side rails should be padded. If the child is breathing spontaneously, position the child to prevent upper airway obstruction and to maximize diaphragm excursion. Place a roll under the child's shoulders to extend the neck, and elevate the head of the bed approximately 30°.

In general, there is no need to stick anything in the patient's mouth during seizures, particularly if the child's aeration is adequate and if there is no obvious oral bleeding from lacerations of the mouth or tongue. In fact, forced insertion of a tongue blade or airway can cause broken teeth or oral lacerations. Placement of an oral airway is only recommended if tongue-biting or cheek-biting results in significant bleeding in the unconscious child.

If the child becomes apneic or demonstrates respiratory distress or inadequate aeration, provide bag-mask ventilation until intubation can be accomplished. Before endotracheal intubation is attempted, a nasogastric tube is inserted and suction is applied, and then the nasogastric tube is withdrawn. This procedure will allow emptying and decompression of the stomach to reduce the risk of vomiting during the intubation. It is extremely important that all members of the healthcare team be notified if neuromuscular blocking agents or sedatives are administered during the intubation, because these agents will affect or eliminate motor activity and neurologic responses after the intubation.

Throughout the episode of status epilepticus, carefully assess and support systemic perfusion. Treat hypotension or bradycardia promptly because they can result in inadequate systemic and cerebral perfusion (see Treatment of Shock in Chapter 6). If vascular access is not present, insert a large-bore venous catheter as quickly as possible to allow the infusion of IV fluids and medications. Obtain blood samples for analysis of arterial blood gases, electrolytes, glucose, calcium, and BUN, and to evaluate serum concentration of anticonvulsants, as indicated. If the child has just been admitted to the critical care unit, obtain a urine specimen for toxicology screening.

Perform a rapid neurologic examination to determine whether there is a reversible or accelerating neurologic problem responsible for the status epilepticus. Increased ICP, brain herniation, and intracranial hemorrhage can all produce seizures. If signs of intracranial hypertension are present, treat this problem at the same time that the status epilepticus is treated.

Rapid correction of any existing metabolic derangement is needed and may abolish the seizure activity. Because hypoglycemia is a relatively common and rapidly treatable cause of seizures in critically ill children, evaluate the serum glucose concentration, using point-of-care testing if available. Administration of hypertonic glucose (D_{25}:1.0-2.0 mL/kg or D_{50}:0.5-1.0 mL/kg), may be ordered empirically after blood samples are drawn, but before the results of serum electrolyte and glucose analyses are available. Hyponatremia, hypernatremia, hypocalcemia, or hypomagnesemia should be treated if present (see Chapter 12).[119]

Evaluate the infant's rectal temperature, because febrile seizures are relatively common during infancy. If a high fever (body temperature >40° C) is present, administer an antipyretic suppository such as acetaminophen, and use a cooling blanket to slowly reduce the child's temperature.

Anticonvulsant Therapy. The most popular drugs for the treatment of status epilepticus include lorazepam, diazepam, phenobarbital, and phenytoin or fosphenytoin. Each of these drugs is addressed separately in this section. The choice of drug will depend on provider preference and on the previous effectiveness of the drug for the patient. Intravenous, rather than intramuscular, drug administration is needed during status epilepticus to ensure maximal absorption and rapid CNS penetration.

If the child with a known seizure disorder presents with status epilepticus, it is important to ask the child's parents or care providers about the child's daily drug regimen and the last doses of anticonvulsants taken. In such patients determination of the serum concentration of anticonvulsants will assist in evaluation of the potential cause of and in treating the status epilepticus,

Any anticonvulsant agent can depress respiratory or cardiovascular function, so the bedside nurse plays a crucial role in assessing and supporting airway, oxygenation, ventilation, and perfusion as well as monitoring drug effect on seizures

and neurologic function. In general, the patient requires intubation, mechanical ventilation, and establishment of hemodynamic monitoring. Volume expanders and vasoactive medications should be available at the bedside.

Lorazepam (Ativan) is the first-line treatment for all types of status epilepticus beyond the neonatal period.[119] It has a rapid onset of action and stops seizure activity in most patients within 2 to 5 minutes.[112] Its effects last longer than those of diazepam; therefore, it may be preferable to diazepam. It is administered intravenously in a dose of 0.05 to 0.1 mg/kg (maximum single dose: 4 mg) over 2 to 5 minutes; the dose may be repeated in 10 to 15 minutes if needed. This drug may produce respiratory depression, although the incidence of this complication is lower than with diazepam. The nurse must be prepared to institute respiratory support if needed.

Diazepam (Valium) is used commonly in the initial treatment of seizures. The initial dose of 0.05 to 0.5 mg/kg (maximum: 5 mg for children under 5 years if age, and 10 mg for children over 5 years of age) is typically administered by slow IV push over several (3-5) minutes. The drug should be effective within minutes; peak diazepam concentrations are reached in the brain within 1 to 5 minutes. Because the serum half-life of the drug is relatively short, seizures often return and may require repeat dosing at 15-minute intervals. It is often necessary to add a second, longer acting anticonvulsant at this point.[112]

Side effects of diazepam include hypotension, cardiac arrest, laryngospasm, respiratory depression, respiratory arrest, sedation, and local vascular irritation at the site of infusion. Disadvantages of this drug are its relatively short effective period and the potentially significant respiratory depressant effects. One potential advantage of diazepam is that it is available in a formulation for rectal administration (Diastat) which may be used if the patient does not have intravenous access. This formulation is available in a pre-filled syringe (5 mg/mL). The dose for treatment of status epilepticus in infants and children 2 to 5 years of age is 0.5 mg/kg, for children 5 to 11 years of age the dose is 0.3 mg/kg, and for children over 12 years of age is 0.2 mg/kg.

Fosphenytoin (Cerebyx), the water soluble prodrug of phenytoin, is often used in the management of status epilepticus and is preferred to phenytoin because it is less caustic to the veins and is compatible with most IV fluids.[126] It is given as a loading dose of 10 to 20 mg phenytoin equivalents (PE) followed by a maintenance dose of 5 to 7 mg PE/kg per day in two to three divided doses. The therapeutic serum level is 10 to 20 mcg/mL. Side effects are similar to those of phenytoin and include hypotension, if the drug is administered too rapidly, bradycardia, tachycardia, and vasodilation.[120]

Phenobarbital is used widely in the treatment of seizures in children, particularly infants, because it has a relatively long serum half-life and a wide therapeutic range. If phenobarbital is administered without diazepam, a loading dose of 10 to 20 mg/kg (given as a single dose or in divided doses; maximum total loading dose, 20 mg/kg) is administered intravenously at a rate no faster than 1 mg/kg per minute (or maximum rate, 50 mg/minute).[112,120]

Phenobarbital is often administered with diazepam during the treatment of status epilepticus, because they seem to act synergistically. If phenobarbital is administered with diazepam, a lower phenobarbital dose (5.0 mg/kg; maximum dose, 390 mg) may be given initially by slow IV push. This dose usually is repeated twice (at 20-minute intervals), even if the seizures are controlled, to provide a total initial dose of 15.0 mg/kg and establish a therapeutic serum level (15-30 mcg/mL).

Peak concentrations of phenobarbital can develop in the brain within approximately 5 minutes, although the drug usually is not maximally effective for approximately 30 minutes. Side effects of phenobarbital include respiratory depression, bronchospasm, apnea, bradycardia, hypotension, and sedation. Occasionally, phenobarbital produces CNS irritability in children.[120] The major disadvantage of this drug is the long-term sedation it produces, making further neurologic evaluation difficult.

Valproic acid (valproate, Depakene) has long been used in the treatment of seizures refractory to first line agents. However, new information suggests that IV valproate may have a role in initial treatment of status epilepticus and may be as effective as phenytoin or fosphenytoin.[124,130] It is available in oral and IV formulations. A rectal formulation can be prepared by diluting valproate syrup (250 mg per 5 mL) with tap water in a 1:1 ratio.

An initial IV loading dose is 10-15 mg/kg per day divided into four doses (given every 6 hours for the IV formulation). The dose is then increased by 10 to 15 mg/kg per day on a weekly basis until a therapeutic level is obtained (50-100 mcg/mL). Generally a maintenance dose of 30 to 60 mg/kg per day is necessary to achieve therapeutic levels. Potential complications of this drug include the development of liver dysfunction (closely monitor liver enzyme concentrations), pancreatitis, and a possible increase in the plasma concentrations of other anticonvulsants.

Levetiracetam (Keppra) is used primarily for the treatment of partial onset seizures, but more recently it has been used in the treatment of status epilepticus refractory to first line agents.[130] The usual dose is 5 to 20 mg/kg per day divided into two doses per day, with weekly increases of 10 mg/kg per day to a maximum dose of 60 mg/kg per day. Dose recommendations for status epilepticus vary and firm recommendations do not currently exist; therefore, providers will need to titrate doses and closely monitor patient response.[124,130]

Barbiturate Coma. If status epilepticus is unresponsive to the drugs listed previously, it may be necessary to transfer the patient to a facility where intensive and continuous hemodynamic and electroencephalographic monitoring can be performed. Control of status epilepticus may then be attempted by administration of barbiturates to induce coma.

Before coma is induced, providers must initiate adequate monitoring. The child is intubated and ventilated mechanically, an arterial line is inserted, and a central venous catheter is placed. Because high doses of barbiturates frequently produce hypotension, the child's intravascular volume must be adequate and volume expanders must be available at the bedside. An infusion of an inotropic agent such as dopamine or epinephrine must also be available at the bedside for immediate use if hypotension develops.

Once adequate monitoring and support are established, phenobarbital or pentobarbital is administered in doses sufficient to induce coma. Thiopental sodium often is preferred because it has a shorter half-life, so that the effects will disappear in a shorter period of time following discontinuation of the drug. A loading dose is required, followed by a continuous infusion or hourly dose titrated to maintain burst suppression (associated with a reduced cerebral metabolic rate) on the EEG.[120] The child's blood pressure and systemic perfusion must be monitored closely as the barbiturate dose is increased, and appropriate therapy must be provided to maintain systemic perfusion.

Table 11-10 includes a list of common anticonvulsant therapies for status epilepticus. Once the child's seizures are controlled, long-term anticonvulsant prophylaxis and patient and family education is planned.[112]

Non-pharmacologic Management of Seizures. Several forms of ketogenic diets have been used for centuries to reduce seizures. These diets have gained in popularity in recent years, particularly for patients who are refractory to antiepileptic agents. The precise mechanism by which the diet inhibits seizures is unclear.[132] The diet induces ketosis by providing most daily calories from fat sources, so the classic diet strictly limits carbohydrate and protein intake to minimum daily quantities. Recently, more liberal forms of the diet have emerged, allowing for slightly more protein and carbohydrate intake.

The goal of all forms of ketogenic diet is to control seizure activity through strict dietary control; such control may be challenging, particularly for toddler and adolescent patients. Seizure control is generally observed 1 to 3 months after initiation of the diet. The diet is continued for approximately 3 years if tolerated, and then it is gradually weaned. Side effects of the diet are primarily gastrointestinal in nature; the high fat intake can contribute to constipation and reflux. Patient growth is monitored closely, with assessment for micronutrient deficiencies and elevated serum lipids. During initiation of the diet, serum glucose concentrations are monitored on a frequent basis.

When a patient receiving the ketogenic diet is admitted to the critical care unit, care should be taken to preserve the ketotic state. This state requires either continuing the patient's home dietary regimen or providing IV fluids and nutrition containing little protein and dextrose but high fat content. Medications must be evaluated because many oral solutions are provided in a high-glucose vehicle; these solutions are avoided if at all possible.

Vagal Nerve Stimulators. The vagal nerve stimulator may be implanted to control seizures in pediatric patients with medically and/or surgically refractory epilepsy. The precise mechanism by which vagal stimulation controls seizure activity is unknown. Stimulation of the afferent tract of the vagus nerve may desynchronize electroencephalographic activity and alter epileptic activity. Common side effects of vagal nerve stimulator insertion include hoarseness, shortness of breath, paresthesia, and cough. Infection of the generator pocket is also a concern in the immediate post operative period.

Wound care is similar to that needed following cardiac pacemaker implantation. In addition, electromagnetic and

Table 11-10   Anticonvulsant Therapy in Treatment of Pediatric Status Epilepticus

Drug (Trade Name)	Dose	Onset and/or Peak Effect	Therapeutic Serum Level
Diazepam (Valium)	IV: 0.05-0.5 mg/kg Maximum: 5 mg for < 5 years, 10 mg for > 5 years	1-3 min	0.2-1.5 mcg/mL
Lorazepam (Ativan)	IV: 0.05-0.1 mg/kg slow IV (maximum: 4 mg)	Onset: 2-5 min Peak: 60-90 min	20-40 nanog/mL
Phenobarbital (Luminal)	IV: 10-20 mg/kg in a single or divided doses Maximum: 20 mg/kg (less if given with diazepam)	Onset: 5 min Peak: 30 min	15-30 mcg/mL
Phenytoin (Dilantin)	IV: 15-20 mg/kg		10-20 mcg/mL
Fosphenytoin (Cerebyx)	IV: 10-20 mg (PE)/kg in single or divided doses	10 min (range: 24 hours)	phenytoin: 10-20 (mcg/mL)
Valproic acid (Depakene)	IV: 10-15 mg/kg per day given in 1-3 doses; dose increased weekly as needed	1-4 hours	50-100 mcg/mL or 5-10 mg/L
Levetriacm (Keppra)	IV: 5-20 mg/kg per day in divided doses; dose increased weekly as needed	1 hour	6-20 mg/L (from adult studies)
General anesthesia*			
Thiopental sodium (Pentothal) or sodium pentobarbital (Nembutol)	IV: 3-10 mg/kg loading plus continuous infusion to maintain EEG burst suppression (typically 0.5-3.0 mg/kg per hour)	Onset: 30-60 seconds	Thiopental coma: 30-100 mcg/mL; pentobarbital coma: 20-40 mcg/mL

Data from Blumstein MD, Friedman MJ: Childhood seizures. *Emerg Med Clin North Am* 25:1061-1086, 2007; Taketomo CK, Hodding JH, Kraus DM, editors: *Pediatric dosage handbook*, ed 15, Hudson, OH, 2008, Lexicomp.
*Not to be instituted without proper monitoring of hemodynamic status. Monitor closely for hypotension, compromise of cardiovascular function.
IV, Intravenous; *PE*, phenytoin equivalents.

electrostimulation devices, including magnetic resonance imaging are avoided.[73,115]

Surgical Interventions. Surgical intervention may be provided for intractable seizures. This seemingly radical approach has rendered many children free of seizures or has vastly improved their seizure control and quality of life. Preoperative testing including MRI, video electroencephalogram, and often subdural electrode placement (grids and strips) is necessary to define the seizure focus before surgical resection.

The surgical procedure is tailored to the location of the seizure focus, surrounding tissue, and goal of the surgery. For example, if the patient has a localized lesion that is amenable to resection, a targeted resection may render the patient completely seizure free. If the seizure focus is not resectable or diffuse in nature, a palliative procedure such as complete or partial hemispherectomy, corpus callosotomy, or multiple subpial transection may be performed. In these cases, seizure activity should be better controlled but will likely not be eliminated completely.

Care for these patients is similar to general postoperative neurosurgical critical care (see the Postoperative Care of the Pediatric Neurosurgical Patient, later in this chapter). Anticonvulsants are generally continued in the initial postoperative period and then gradually weaned as tolerated. The nursing care plan must include a description of the patient's baseline seizure activity, the procedure performed, and any anticipated postoperative deficits.[94,95]

Endocrinopathies Associated with Neurologic Insults. Diabetes insipidus (DI), the syndrome of inappropriate antidiuretic hormone (SIADH), and cerebral salt wasting (CSW) are common endocrine complications of neurologic injury or surgical procedures. CSW associated with head injury or neurosurgical procedures usually develops later (2-7 days) after injury. Please see Chapter 12 for a complete discussion of the pathophysiology, clinical presentation and management of these disorders. Table 12-7 compares and contrasts the presentation and effects of DI, SIADH, and CSW.

Brain Death and Organ Donation

Etiology

Brain death is the total cessation of brainstem and cortical brain function that can result from irreversible traumatic, anoxic, or metabolic conditions. Brain death represents the end result of a compromise in cerebral perfusion or cerebral herniation. If the child is intubated and receiving mechanical ventilation and possible vasopressor support at the time of brain death, then heart rate, systemic oxygenation, and systemic perfusion may initially be adequate. It is important to note that mechanical ventilation is not considered "life support" for such children, because the child is dead.

Traditionally, the pronouncement of brain death was required before transplantation of solid organs from the donor. However, donation after cardiac death protocols do not require brain death pronouncement. The Joint Commission (formerly the Joint Commission on Accreditation of Healthcare Organizations [JCAHO]) now requires that hospitals have policies regarding donation after cardiac death. This requirement is expected to increase the number of potential organ donors by as much as 20%.[84] Care of the donor presents a number of unique challenges for the healthcare team; these are discussed in Chapters 3 and 24.

The declaration of brain death requires appropriate clinical examination and testing per institutional policy. Documentation

<table>
<tr><td>**Box 11-6**</td><td>**Public Law 99-509: "Required Request" Law**</td></tr>
</table>

I. Hospitals receiving federal funding must establish written protocols for identification of potential donors that:
  1. Ensures that families of potential organ donors are made aware of the option of organ or tissue donation and their option to decline
  2. Encourages discretion and sensitivity with respect to circumstances, views, and beliefs of family
  3. Requires that a federally funded and approved organ procurement agency be notified of potential donors
II. Local organ procurement agencies must abide by rules and requirements of Organ Procurement and Transplantation Network

<table>
<tr><td>**Box 11-7**</td><td>**Criteria for Pediatric Brain Death Determination**</td></tr>
</table>

Irreversible Condition
Requires observation over time (proposed length of observation time increases during infancy)
Absence of complicating factors
Adequate resuscitation provided

Absence of Brain Function
Flaccid paralysis (no posturing, no response to central pain stimulus)
Absence of brain stem and cranial nerve function:
  No pupil response to light
  No corneal (blink) reflex
  No oculocephalic reflex (doll's eyes)
  Absence of eye movements
  No oculovestibular reflex (cold water calorics)
  No cough or gag reflex
  Apnea despite documented $PaCO_2$ >55-60 mm Hg or despite rise in $PaCO_2$ of >20 mm Hg

Possible Confirmatory Tests
Electroencephalogram (requires special electrode placement and amplitude, absence of sedative drug levels, normothermia)
Radionuclide angiogram
Carotid arteriogram
Magnetic resonance angiography
Reliability of additional tests in children, including cold xenon blood flow study, brain stem-evoked potentials, and Doppler cerebral blood flow studies are under investigation

of the pronouncement of brain death must be provided in the patient's chart. Federal legislation (Box 11-6) requires that the local federally funded organ procurement agency be informed about the presence of a potential organ donor, and that the family of a potential organ donor be informed about the option of organ and tissue donation.[42] This notification must also be documented in the patient chart.

Every state has a law or a precedent set by the appellate court that recognizes the cessation of brain function as a legal definition of death. In addition, every hospital receiving Medicaid reimbursement is required to have protocols in place for the identification of potential organ donors to the local organ procurement agency. Each nurse must be familiar with state law and hospital policy regarding the pronouncement of brain death and responsibilities in discussing potential organ and tissue donation with the family.[59]

Criteria for Pronouncement of Brain Death
The pronouncement of brain death has two requirements: (1) an irreversible condition and (2) complete cessation of clinical evidence of brain function. The cause of brain death should be known. A variety of criteria for brain death pronouncement in children have been proposed, but most are consistent in the clinical indications of brain death. These criteria differ in their requirements of adjunctive tests.[2,3,16,17,121] The healthcare team must apply these criteria consistently.

Irreversible Condition. The cause of the cessation of brain function must be irreversible. For example, devastating closed head injury or anoxic insult can be irreversible causes of brain death. Metabolic conditions such as hypotension, hypoglycemia, or hypothermia are reversible conditions and must be corrected if they are thought to be contributing to the depression of CNS function. In the past, sedative levels of barbiturates or narcotics could not be present because they could cause a reversible depression of brain function; in some institutions, if cerebral perfusion studies are used as an adjunctive test, barbiturates or narcotics may be detectable in serum samples, because they are not known to affect the results of cerebral perfusion studies.

Physical Examination to Document the Absence of Brainstem Function. The child must have no voluntary movement or response to stimuli in the absence of neuromuscular blockade. All brain stem function must be absent. The cranial nerve functions will be evaluated as possible through the testing of the following reflexes: oculocephalic, oculovestibular, cough and gag, corneal and pupil response to light. The pupils must be dilated or fixed in midposition, and apnea must be present. Flaccid paralysis must be present (Box 11-7).

The oculocephalic reflex is tested (testing of "doll's eyes" reflex) by briskly rotating the head from midline to the side while holding the eyelids open to observe eye movement. If the oculocephalic reflex is intact, head rotation is detected by the semicircular canals (innervated by the vestibular branch of the acoustic nerve) and neck proprioceptors, and they will stimulate the third (oculomotor) and sixth (abducens) cranial nerves to rotate the eyes in the sockets in the direction opposite head rotation (i.e., if the head is turned from midline to the right, the eyes will rotate to the left). This normal eye rotation is designed to help focus on objects despite head rotation. When the oculocephalic reflex is absent, the eyes will remain fixed in their sockets, despite rotation of the head (Fig. 11-16). The nurse can imagine the eyes painted on the face of a doll—that is, they will not move in the sockets. The reflex will not be present when brain function ceases.

Testing of the oculovestibular reflex (the cold water calorics test) tests brainstem function by stimulating the vestibular branch of the eighth (acoustic) cranial nerve as well as the function the third (oculomotor) and sixth (abducens)

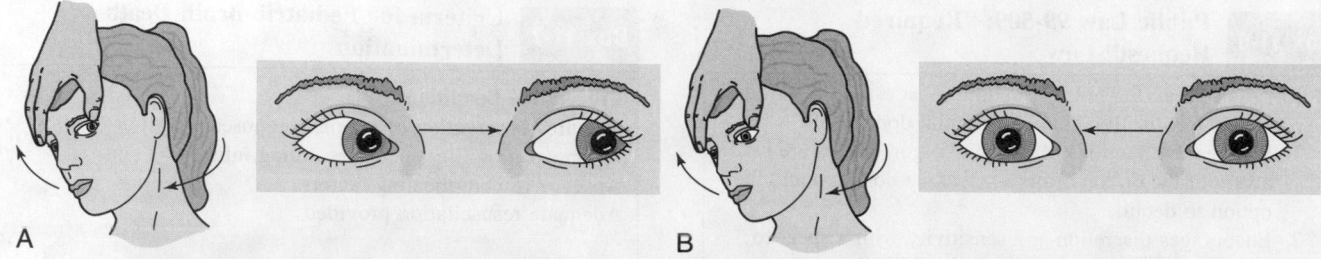

FIG. 11-16 Oculocephalic reflex ("doll's eyes"). **A,** Normal response: eyes move to the left as the head is briskly rotated to the right. **B,** Abnormal response: eyes do not rotate in the sockets as the head is turned, but passively follow the head (i.e., as eyes would appear if painted on a doll's face). (From Monahan, Frances Donovan. *Phipps' medical-surgical nursing: health and illness perspectives*, ed 8, Saint Louis, Mosby, 2006, fig. 48-3.)

cranial nerves. If the brain stem is intact, the cold water will have the same effect on the semicircular canals as head rotation, resulting in stimulation of eye movement. This test should be performed only if the tympanic membrane is intact and the patient is unconscious. If the reflex is tested/elicited in conscious patients, it will produce eye movement, but typically produces severe vertigo and nausea.

To perform the test, the head of the bed is elevated 30 degrees and ice water is quickly instilled by syringe (without a needle) deep into the ear canal. If the oculovestibular reflex is intact, bilateral conjugate eye movement will occur with slow horizontal nystagmus initially toward the stimulus, and then rapid nystagmus away from the stimulus. If the reflex is abnormal, disconjugate or asymmetrical eye movements will occur. If the reflex is absent, the eyes will remain fixed in midposition (Fig. 11-17).

Testing of the cough, gag, cornea, and pupil reflexes is relatively simple. A suction catheter inserted into the back of the pharynx normally will stimulate a cough or gag reflex; if brain stem function is absent, neither response is observed. When the brain stem is intact, an automatic blink will occur when any object approaches the eye; when brain stem function is absent, the cornea can be stroked lightly with a cotton-tipped applicator, and a blink will not be observed. When the brain stem is intact, the pupils will constrict in response to light; when brain stem function is absent, the pupils will be fixed and unresponsive to light. The pupils typically are

fully dilated when brainstem function ceases, although they may be midsize.

The presence of apnea must be carefully assessed and documented (Box 11-8). Apnea can be documented if the patient fails to demonstrate spontaneous ventilation despite an arterial carbon dioxide tension exceeding 55 to 60 mm Hg. The arterial carbon dioxide tension must be documented to be sufficiently high to stimulate ventilation. Before initiating the test, support of ventilation is adjusted to ensure normocarbia, and preoxygenation (using 100% oxygen) is provided to ensure adequate oxygenation. The apnea test should begin, if possible, with an arterial carbon dioxide tension of 35 to 40 mm Hg.

Oxygen must be provided during the apnea test to avoid hypoxemia; pulse oximetry should be used to monitor systemic oxygenation during the study. Supplementary oxygen can be delivered with a T-connector joined to the endotracheal tube. However, many providers prefer to administer the oxygen directly into the endotracheal tube. To accomplish this, a suction catheter is joined to standard green oxygen tubing, and the suction catheter is inserted into the endotracheal tube. Oxygen then flows through the suction catheter into the endotracheal tube. If the child becomes hypoxemic during the test, it may be necessary to interrupt the test and resume support of mechanical ventilation.

An arterial blood gas sample usually is obtained at the beginning of the study to document normocarbia. Correlation

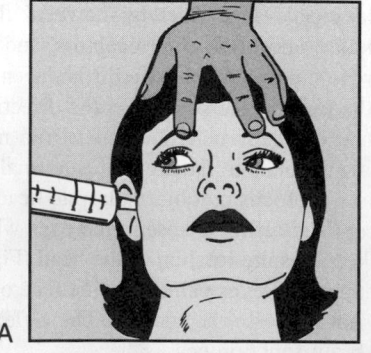 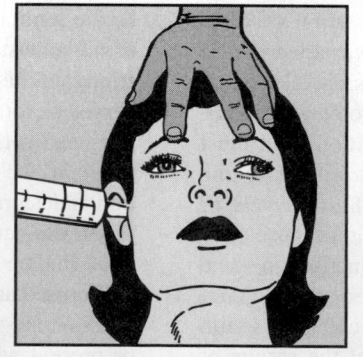 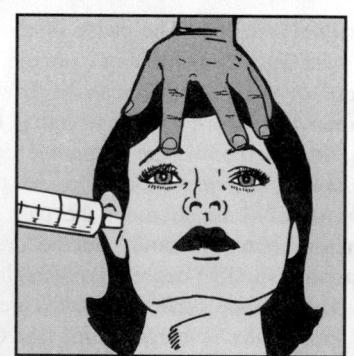

FIG. 11-17 Oculovestibular reflex (cold water calorics) test. **A,** Normal response—conjugated eye movements. **B,** Abnormal response—disconjugate or asymmetrical eye movements. **C,** Absent response—no eye movements. (From Boss BJ: Alterations in cognitive systems, cerebral hemodynamics, and motor function. In McCance KE, Huether SE, editors: *Pathophysiology: the biologic basis for disease in adults and children*, ed 6, Philadelphia, 2010, Mosby-Elsevier, p. 534, fig. 16-4.)

| Box 11-8 | Apnea Test to Document Absence of Spontaneous Respirations |

1. Before study, adjust mechanical ventilation support (if needed) to ensure normal oxygenation and normocarbia ($PaCO_2 = 35$-45 mm Hg). Obtain arterial blood gases before and at conclusion of study. Monitor pulse oximetry throughout study to ensure effective oxygenation. Monitor exhaled CO_2 monitoring, if possible, to estimate $PaCO_2$ during study.
2. Before study, preoxygenate patient for 5-10 min using 100% oxygen.
3. Remove patient from ventilator and provide passive oxygenation with 100% oxygen (6 L/min or twice the minute ventilation appropriate for child's weight) delivered to endotracheal tube (using blow-by tubing or T-piece) or via suction catheter (joined to green oxygen tubing) inserted into endotracheal tube.
4. Closely observe patient during 5-10 min duration of study. No chest movements or respiratory effort will be present if brain function has ceased. Abort study if cardiovascular deterioration occurs.
5. During the study, titrate oxygen support as needed to ensure effective oxygenation (per pulse oximetry). When exhaled CO exceeds 60 mm Hg or the 5-10-min observation period has elapsed, draw arterial blood gas sample. The $PaCO_2$ will rise approximately 4 to 5 mm Hg/min during apnea.
6. To confirm apnea, no respiratory effort can be noted, and the $PaCO_2$ at end of study should exceed 55-60 mm Hg.

between the exhaled carbon dioxide ($P_{ET}CO_2$) and the $PaCO_2$ can be established with the initial blood gas, and then the $P_{ET}CO_2$ can be monitored during the study. Based on the initial $PaCO_2$, providers can predict the length of time needed to raise the $PaCO_2$ to 60 to 65 mm Hg. During apnea, the $PaCO_2$ will rise approximately 4 to 5 mm Hg for each minute of apnea[97]; therefore, it will require approximately 4 minutes of apnea to raise the $PaCO_2$ from 40 mm Hg to 56 to 60 mm Hg. Remember that this is an estimate however, and formal documentation is necessary for the apnea test to be valid.

During the apnea test, the nurse must remain at the bedside, watching the child closely for any evidence of respiratory effort. In addition, the nurse must monitor the child's heart rate and systemic perfusion. At the end of a 5- or 10-minute observation period, an arterial blood gas sample is taken and mechanical ventilation is resumed.

Confirmatory and Adjunct Tests. Confirmatory tests are unnecessary in children older than 1 year when the cause of brain function cessation has been established and is irreversible, and there is no evidence of brain function on clinical examination. These patients may be examined twice (with the examinations separated by 12-24 hours) and pronounced brain dead at the time of the second examination.

The Task Force on Brain Death Determination in Children (TFBDDC) recommends electroencephalography as the confirmation test of choice for children younger than 1 year and for those with hypoxic ischemic cerebral insult.[121] The EEG

was favored at the time of the recommendations because clinical experience with the EEG during childhood was more extensive than the clinical experience with xenon perfusion scans or brainstem evoked potentials. However, a "technically satisfactory radionuclide angiogram" also was noted as being acceptable by the Task Force.

If the EEG is performed to confirm brain death, the technician must be informed that the study has been ordered to confirm brain death. For such studies, the electrodes are placed farther apart than for a normal EEG, and the voltage is increased. A long, uninterrupted recording is made at the end of the EEG brain death study to document 30 minutes of electrocerebral silence.

Slow EEG activity can persist despite brain death. EEG activity persisted in as many as 25% of adult donors following the pronouncement of brain death.[51] EEG activity has also been shown to persist in children, despite the absence of CBF on angiography.[15-17] A case study documented the return of cerebral activity following a flat EEG during the neonatal period.[15] These reports of false positive and false negative EEGs raise doubts about the reliability of the EEG as a confirmatory test of brain death.

An added disadvantage to the use of the EEG as a confirmatory test is that serum concentrations of any sedative drugs and barbiturates present must be subtherapeutic, and electrolytes must be normal. The body temperature must be higher than 32° C. If a barbiturate coma has been induced, several (3-5) days may elapse before the serum barbiturate concentration is sufficiently low to allow the first EEG.

Many centers use cerebral angiography or radionuclide brain flow scans to determine the presence or absence of cerebral perfusion[131] (Fig. 11-18) as an adjunct to the clinical determination of brain death. Although the reliability of these studies has not been reported with a large series of children, no significant issues of reliability have been raised for older infants and children. These blood flow studies are not influenced by the presence of electrolyte imbalance or barbiturates. Additional data suggest that brain stem-evoked potential, transcranial Doppler, and magnetic resonance angiography may be useful adjunctive tests.[19]

Observation Period. The Task Force on Brain Death Determination in Children recommended repeated clinical examinations, separated by an observation period, to ensure that irreversible cessation of brain function has occurred. The younger the child, the longer the suggested interval between examinations.[125] Some institutions adhere strictly to these criteria, and others use cerebral perfusion studies to shorten the observation time or replace the EEG. It is important for the nurse to be familiar with the hospital protocol and ensure strict adherence to and documentation of the protocol.

Infants 7 Days to 2 Months of Age. The Task Force recommends two examinations separated by at least 48 hours. Additional confirmation is recommended using two EEGs separated by at least 48 hours.[121]

Infants 2 Months to 1 Year of Age. The Task Force recommends two examinations separated by 24 hours. One EEG consistent with brain death is recommended, and a

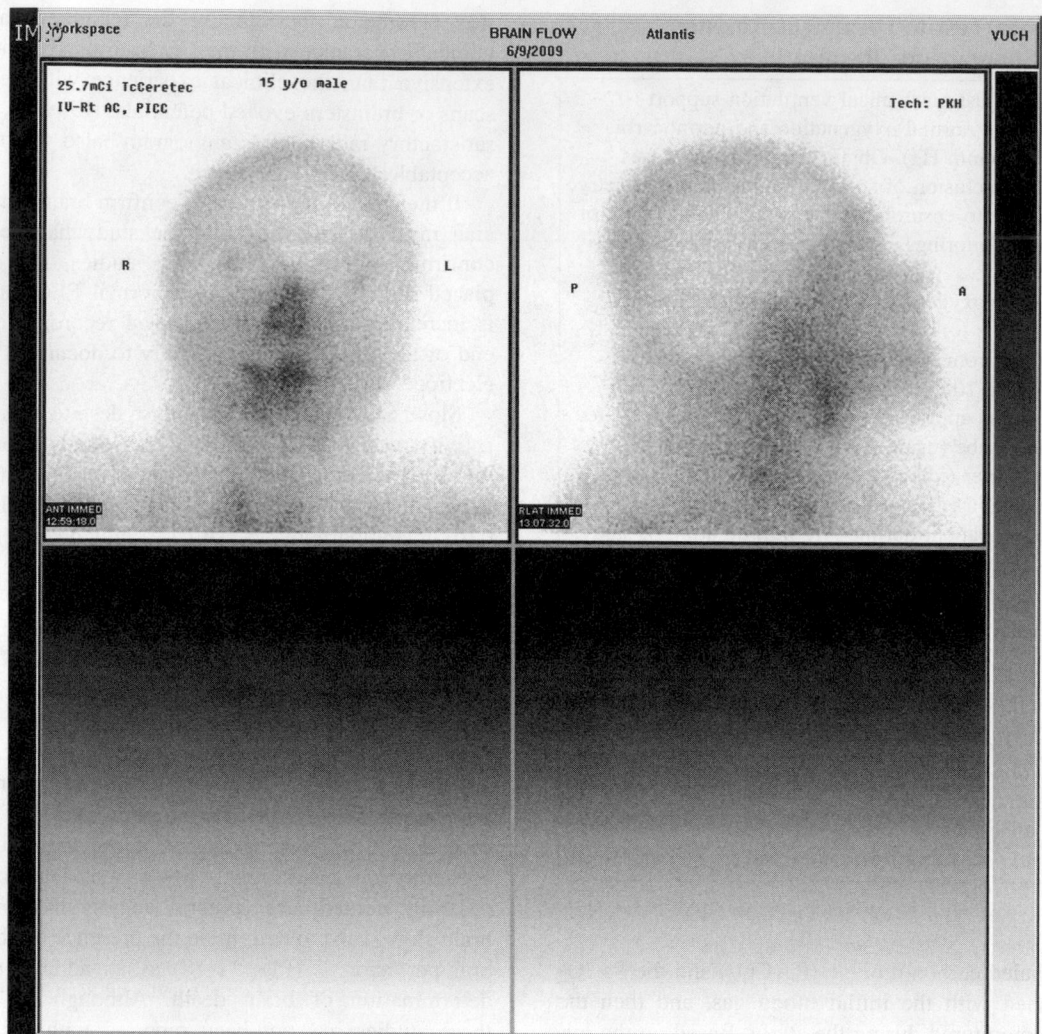

FIG. 11-18 Abnormal cerebral perfusion scan, consistent with brain death (15-year-old male). A radiotracer has been injected intravenously. Anterior (left) and lateral (right) delayed static images of the head and neck depict blood pooled in soft tissues of the scalp and face, supplied by the external carotid arteries. There is no perfusion of the brain by the internal carotid arteries. Pooling of the tracer is visible in the nose ("hot nose" sign) and reflects perfusion of the face from the external carotid arteries. The initial dynamic images from this study are included in Evolve Fig. 11-4 in the Chapter 11 Supplement on the Evolve Website. (Courtesy Stephanie E. Spottswood, Vanderbilt Children's Hospital, Nashville, Tenn.)

cerebral radionuclide angiographic study can be substituted for the second EEG.[121]

Beyond 1 Year of Age. The Task Force recommends two examinations separated by at least 12 hours. A 24-hour observation period is suggested if the cause of death is a hypoxic-ischemic insult. Confirmatory tests or adjunct studies are not suggested.[121]

Brain Death in the Neonate. Standards are still evolving for the pronouncement of brain death in the neonate.[18,19,121] After the Task Force on Brain Death Pronouncement in Children guidelines became available, additional studies suggested that brain death can be pronounced in the neonate and preterm infant older than 34 weeks' gestation.[18] Diagnosis of brain death in this group can use the standard clinical examination and confirmatory testing, but the clinician should be knowledgeable about the challenges of declaring brain death in the neonate. A 48-hour observation period is recommended between examinations. The cause of brain death should be

determined and the timing of cessation of brain function established, if possible. Repeated examinations are performed, and confirmatory or adjunct studies are almost always performed, although EEG activity may be present despite the absence of CBF.[18]

Contact with the Local Organ Procurement Organization

Federal law requires that the hospital notify the local organ procurement organization (OPO) about a potential organ donor. A coordinator from the OPO will determine whether there are any absolute or relative contraindications to organ donation. Such contraindications are few, but they should be ruled out so that the family does not become hopeful about organ donation that is not feasible (Box 11-9).

The OPO coordinator will explain the donation process to the parents and answer their questions. The coordinator is skilled in dealing with parents during an extremely stressful

Box 11-9	Donor Contraindications to Solid Organ Donation

Untreated sepsis

Organ ischemia, inadequate resuscitation

Some systemic diseases (always consult with local federally funded organ procurement agency)

Significant organ dysfunction

time and can provide the parents with current, accurate information. The coordinator will write to the family months after the donation (if the family desires), to inform them in general terms about the recipient of their child's organs. Parents often find this information extremely comforting. Parents should be aware that there is no cost to them for the organ donation, and that the process will not delay or alter standard funeral arrangements.

If the child's parents consent to organ donation, a written consent is required and the OPO assumes all financial responsibility for donor care once the child is pronounced brain dead. If any diagnostic studies are obtained before the pronouncement of death that will contribute to the donation process, those costs also are assumed by the OPO. Once pronouncement of death has occurred, the donor coordinator participates in the management of systemic and organ perfusion until actual donation takes place. Some OPOs will reimburse the hospital for the cost of nursing care of the donor between brain death pronouncement and recovery of the organs.

Once the parents sign the consent for organ donation, the child's age, weight, blood type, and available organs are listed on a national website via the United Network for Organ Sharing. If the organs are compatible with several potential recipients, priority is given to the most severely ill local recipient. Organs are distributed at a regional level before they are available at a national level. It is extremely important that both donor and recipient families realize that these organs are distributed fairly according to strict criteria developed by the United Network for Organ Sharing.

Psychosocial Support of the Family

The death of a child is always tragic. Because brain death often is the end result of a tragic injury or illness, the parents are often physically and emotionally exhausted when death is pronounced. When brain function ceases, it can be extremely difficult for the parents to wait for confirmation that their child has, in fact, died. Often, brain death pronouncement is attempted to remove the burden of the decision to withdraw support and to enable donation of the child's organs. Therefore, it is important that the parents be approached in a sensitive and compassionate manner about this issue (see Chapters 3 and 24).

Organ donation can be life saving for the recipients who are dying of organ failure. Since the inception of the Health Resources Services Administration's Organ Donation and Transplantation Breakthrough Collaboratives in 2003, the number of organ donors has increased. Yet, hundreds of children awaiting organ transplantation will die each year before a donor is located.[129] Organ donation does not benefit only the recipient, however. Parents have expressed gratitude that something positive could come out of the tragic death of their child. Parents have stated that they feel a part of their child is able to survive

through the gift of organ donation. In a national survey of pediatric organ donation, approximately two-thirds of families (range, 63%-75%) of eligible pediatric donors consented to donation, with highest consent rates occurring when the potential donor was 12 years of age or older.[129]

The family's decision about organ donation can be influenced by religious or cultural beliefs.[45] However, the family's interaction with healthcare providers and the manner in which the subject of organ donation is introduced can have a profound effect on the family's decision and memories of the child's death (see Chapter 3).

The nurse is typically the member of the healthcare team who is closest to the family of the dying child. Although it is necessary to offer hope to parents of dying children, the nurse is often the best member of the healthcare team to help the family prepare for their child's death. If open visitation is in place and parents are allowed to participate in their child's care, they can see that everything possible was done for their child. However, if parents are separated from the child for most of the child's final hours, it will be more difficult for the parents to be aware of the efforts to save the child's life.

Each healthcare team and OPO will determine the best person to approach the family about organ donation. Often, family members will introduce the subject of organ donation; if not, the nurse will be aware of the best time to begin to discuss potential organ donation with the family. This discussion must be compassionate and accurate. Parents should not be approached about organ donation if there is still hope that the child will survive. The bedside nurse should be aware of the hospital and unit protocol and be available to support the family through this difficult period.

Understandably, the family will be easily confused by inconsistent statements and terminology from members of the healthcare team. When a child is brain dead, it is possible to maintain oxygenation, ventilation, and perfusion, but the ventilator does not keep the child alive. The ventilator is merely moving air into and out of the child's lungs. Parents must be aware that the diagnosis of brain death is made according to established protocols, and there is no possibility of error when these protocols are followed strictly.

Parents should be allowed to remain with the child as much as possible during the time preceding the child's death, and they should be asked whether they would like to stay with the child while the brain death examinations are performed. Many parents express the wish to be alone with the child before the final examinations and studies are performed, to say goodbye before they are informed that the child has died.

Support of the Cadaveric Donor

Maintenance of the cadaveric donor requires expert critical care to support excellent perfusion to solid organs. This care requires close coordination among members of the healthcare team and with the organ donation coordinator. If medications are administered to the donor, the recipient transplant surgeons may be consulted regarding potential effects of the drugs on the organs to be donated.

Because several transplant teams may be coming to obtain organs from the same donor, the organ procurement coordinator and the bedside nurse are often responsible for integrating the orders of teams from several hospitals. This responsibility requires skill and flexibility. The nurse should be aware that the goals of management change after brain death is pronounced. The goal then becomes provision of adequate substrate and oxygen delivery to the organs to be donated, rather than maintenance of brain perfusion and function.

At the time of brain death pronouncement, most organ donors are relatively hypovolemic for several reasons. They usually have been treated for increased ICP with fluid limitation and osmotic diuretics, and the loss of brain stem regulation of vascular tone and blood pressure results in the vasodilation and expansion of the vascular space. Finally, diabetes insipidus (DI) can develop in as many as 90% of donors,[75] and unreplaced fluid lost in the urine can result in the rapid development of hypovolemia and inadequate organ perfusion.[75] Fluid administration with frequent bolus therapy of isotonic crystalloid (20 mL/kg) is generally required.[68]

Cardiovascular dysfunction is common in the pediatric donor. Arrhythmias and hypotension are encountered in more than half of donors. The most common arrhythmias include bradycardia and ventricular arrhythmias.[68]

Electrolyte imbalances also are encountered frequently, particularly hypokalemia, hypernatremia, and hyperglycemia. If DI is present, urine losses should be replaced with an equal volume of 0.2% or 0.45% sodium chloride in order to minimize hypernatremia and maintain euvolemia. If urine losses are excessive, exogenous antidiuretic hormone (ADH or vasopressin) often is administered. Although the administration of this hormone can result in reduced liver and renal perfusion, this condition is usually preferable to the fluid and electrolyte imbalances that can accompany urine volume loss and attempted replacement.

If possible, blood pressure and systemic perfusion are maintained through volume administration alone. If it is necessary to administer an inotropic or vasopressor medication, a low dose of dopamine (<10 mcg/kg per minute) has traditionally been used; however, more recent data support the use of vasopressin as the therapy of choice for both hemodynamic instability and DI.[75] If large doses of vasoactive medications are required to maintain systemic perfusion, myocardial injury or dysfunction may be present. Thyroid hormone may be administered to help stabilize hemodynamic status and allow for weaning of inotropic and vasopressor medications.[109,110]

The temperature of the donor must be maintained. An overbed warmer or warming blanket usually is required because the hypothalamus is no longer functional. Hypothermia should be prevented because it may further depress myocardial function.[68]

Care of the Donor after Cardiac Death

The protocol for care of patients who become candidates for donation after cardiac death varies by institution. This donation often follows a devastating neurologic injury that does not result in brain death. In this population, the family is approached about potential organ donation only after a decision has been made by the family and healthcare team to withdraw support.

The subject of donation is usually introduced by a member of the OPO staff or others trained in this discussion. If the family agrees, arrangements are made to withdraw support as would normally occur. Once cardiac death is pronounced, the patient is then taken to the operating room for removal of organs, usually the kidneys and liver. The amount of time between pronouncement of death and retrieval of organs is usually approximately 5 minutes, making team coordination crucial.

Withdrawal of care can take place in the critical care unit, operating suite, or another location. The role of the nurse is to provide the same care normally provided for the patient, including support the grieving family and assistance in transporting the donor to the operating room, if necessary, after cardiac death occurs (see Chapter 3 for more information).

The concept of and procedures for donation after cardiac death are evolving. This issue remains one of ethical concern for many, and widespread acceptance and implementation remains a challenge for the future (see Chapter 24).

The Emotional Toll on the Nurse

It is extremely difficult to care for a dying child and to support the family. At the very time that the child requires the most attentive physical care, the family requires the most sensitive emotional support. The bedside nurse should ask for help at the bedside to be able to spend time with the family. Additional support from chaplain services or social work specialists can be utilized.

When a nurse is closely involved with the child and family, the nurse must have the opportunity to grieve about the child. If at all possible, before the nurse begins to care for the organ donor, the nurse should take a few minutes to think about the child and family and derive some comfort from the fact that they were given the best support possible.[60]

Care of the organ donor is extremely hectic, but it can also be rewarding. Many nurses have voiced satisfaction about participation in the donor process because they could see something wonderful come from a tragedy. For further information about the care of the dying child and family see Chapter 3.

POSTOPERATIVE CARE OF THE PEDIATRIC NEUROSURGICAL PATIENT

Care of the child after neurosurgery requires maintenance of vital functions, assessment of neurologic function, recognition and treatment of potential complications of neurosurgery, regulation of fluid and electrolyte balance, and emotional support of the child and family.

Postoperative assessment is facilitated if the nurse is able to perform a thorough preoperative examination of the child. This examination enables the nurse to quickly recognize changes in the child's condition or level of response. When a detailed preoperative assessment is not available, it is important to determine what the child's baseline status was before surgery in order to determine recovery goals. Thus, the following discussion includes the preoperative assessment.

Preoperative Assessment

The nurse must obtain as much information as possible about the child's preoperative neurologic function from the parents or primary caretaker. If the child is transported to the hospital by medical personnel, the nurse should receive a report from the medical team that cared for the child before transport and from the transport providers. The nurse will also obtain information from medical records from the transferring hospital, emergency medical services providers or transport team and from the parents or primary caretaker in person or by telephone.

It is important to know the child's normal motor activity, self-comforting measures, communication, cognitive and motor skills, sleep patterns, feeding preferences, and behavior when frightened or angry; all of this information will be helpful during the postoperative period. The names of family members, special friends, pets, and favorite activities should be noted in the nursing plan of care to enable the evaluation of level of consciousness through questions about familiar people or things.

The nurse also should note the presence and severity of any preoperative neurologic symptoms or deficits such as seizures, coma, blindness, cranial nerve palsies, delayed developmental milestones, abnormal posturing or motor activity, or abnormal or absent reflexes, to establish a baseline for evaluating postoperative progress or deterioration. The preoperative head circumference should be recorded in the care plan of every infant and young child.

The nurse will carefully evaluate and document the child's preoperative level of consciousness. Whenever possible, use descriptions rather than general classifications to avoid confusion. When the child is older and responsive, the nurse should ask the child specific questions about name, age, birthday, and normal activities. Alert, accurate answers are normal; confused answers and lack of response to painful stimuli are clearly abnormal. During infancy, evaluation of the level of consciousness will be made through observation of the infant's cry, response to auditory and tactile stimuli, feeding and sleeping behavior, and through evaluation of the infant's achievement of developmental milestones. A high-pitched, breathless cry is considered abnormal in an infant; extreme lethargy, poor feeding, and delay in achieving developmental milestones are all abnormal.

The nurse will evaluate and document the child's motor ability, including head control, grasp, strength and movement of extremities, and symmetrical withdrawal of all extremities following painful stimulus. The older child should be able to move all extremities, follow commands, and squeeze the observer's fingers upon request. In addition, hand use and strength should be symmetrical and equal bilaterally. Evaluation of antigravity muscles is important, because discrepancies can be appreciated most readily in these muscles. If the child is walking, abnormalities of gait and balance are important to note.

The child's reflexes will be evaluated preoperatively, including the child's pupil size and response to light. The presence of papilledema should also be noted (see the Increased Intracranial Pressure section of this chapter). The complexity and extent of the assessment will be determined by the child's general condition. If time permits, the nurse should observe or perform an assessment of the child's cranial nerve function (see Table 11-2). In general, it is too difficult to test the olfactory nerve in infants and young children. If tested, strongly pungent substances should be avoided, and familiar odors such as lemon, orange, or peppermint should be used.[58]

The evaluation of some reflexes, such as the oculomotor or oculovestibular reflexes, should not be performed in an alert, mobile, responsive child, but may be required if the child is comatose.

It is important to assess and document the child's preoperative cardiovascular function and systemic perfusion. Signs of adequate perfusion include warm skin with brisk capillary refill, consistent color tones, pink nail beds and mucous membranes, and strong peripheral pulses, with heart rate and blood pressure appropriate for age and clinical condition. If systemic perfusion is poor, cerebral perfusion can be compromised and the child's level of consciousness can deteriorate. The child's typical heart rate and blood pressure should be noted carefully for comparison with postoperative values (see pages inside front cover for normal pediatric heart and respiratory rate ranges and blood pressure ranges for age). The median systolic blood pressure for a child 1 to 10 years old is estimated by adding 90 mm Hg to twice the child's age in years; a systolic blood pressure lower than the sum of 70 mm Hg plus twice the child's age in years (for children 1-10 years of age) is definitely hypotensive.[104] Signs of increased ICP are discussed in the Increased Intracranial Pressure section earlier in this chapter.

The child's respiratory status is assessed carefully preoperatively, because neurologic disease can produce characteristic respiratory patterns (such as Cheyne-Stokes respirations), apnea, or respiratory arrest (see Fig. 11-7). It is important to note the presence and strength of the child's gag and cough reflexes, because they will affect the child's ability to maintain a patent airway and handle respiratory secretions and oral or enteral feedings postoperatively. Increased ICP may produce central hypoventilation or apnea. Serious hypercapnia or hypoxemia must be corrected preoperatively, and the reports of the child's preoperative arterial blood gases must be readily available to serve as a basis for comparison during the postoperative period.

Evaluation of the child's preoperative fluid balance and general nutrition is important. The child who is admitted with SIADH will demonstrate hyponatremia and water intoxication (with potential cerebral edema). The child with diabetes insipidus (DI) may demonstrate massive intravascular volume depletion and hypernatremia. Careful evaluation of the child's preoperative fluid balance will aid in both perioperative and postoperative fluid administration. It is extremely helpful if the child's normal feeding behavior, food preferences, and sleep patterns are documented in the nursing plan of care so that attempts can be made to provide these postoperatively.

If neurosurgery is planned on an elective basis, the child (as age appropriate) can be prepared for the sights, sounds, and sensations encountered during postoperative care through a visit to the postoperative unit. A child life specialist, if available, can assist in the preoperative teaching process and address specific questions and concerns that the child or siblings may have. During these sessions the parents can clarify some of the child's concerns and reassure the child that they will be present throughout the child's postoperative care (see Chapter 2).

If the child is admitted to the critical care unit following trauma, intracranial hemorrhage, or acute illness, the nurse may want to spend a few moments with the parents and family before they enter the critical care unit for the first time. These moments may help prepare the parents for the sights and sounds of the critical care unit. At a later time it will be important to verify that the critical care unit policies and procedures have been discussed with the parents; however, such discussion should take place later, after the parents and family have visited the child. If the child has suffered major multisystem trauma, the family should be warned about the child's altered appearance. Too often the medical team welcomes the parents to the bedside of a recently stabilized child with the comment, "He looks good," when the parents are confronted with the sight of a bruised or bloodied, puffy, unconscious child covered with tubes and bandages. The parents should be reassured that the child is not aware of his or her appearance, and that the phrase *looks good* refers to the child's neurologic status and vital functions. If at all possible, the nurses should clean the child as much as possible and partially cover the child with a colorful blanket so that tubes and incisions are not all immediately visible.

Preparation for Admission or Transfer to the Critical Care Unit

The nurse and respiratory therapists will assemble all equipment necessary for postoperative care at the bedside so it is ready for use before the child returns from neurosurgery. All IV administration equipment is ready for use at the bedside. Arterial and central venous pressure transducers, flush systems, and an ICP monitoring system should be prepared per unit policy if they will not arrive with the child.

Equipment to support airway and ventilation must be set up and ready for use at the bedside, including a pediatric mechanical ventilator, face mask or oxygen administration device, a functional bag and mask connected to an oxygen source, and pediatric intubation equipment. Resuscitation drugs and drugs used in the prevention or treatment of increased ICP (e.g., lidocaine, 3% saline and mannitol), those used to control status epilepticus (e.g., lorazepam, phenobarbital, and phosphenytoin), analgesics, sedatives and neuromuscular blockers (see Chapter 5) and steroids (i.e., dexamethasone) for control of local edema associated with brain tumors must be readily available.[50,96,120] Most nurses prepare or obtain a computerized, precalculated emergency drug sheet based on the child's age and body weight. The pharmacy may provide such a sheet. The Broselow Resuscitation Tape is a quick reference that assists in determining proper equipment sizes and emergency drug doses (see Fig. 1-1).[79]

The neurosurgeon discusses the planned surgery and potential postoperative complications with the family to obtain informed consent before the procedure. It is extremely useful if the nurse who will care for the patient postoperatively is present for these discussions.

Postoperative Care

Initial Assessment

When the child returns from neurosurgery, the nurse receives a report from the surgical team while assessing the child's airway, oxygenation, and respiratory function or ventilation support, systemic perfusion, and evidence of neurologic function. First priority must be given to establishing airway, oxygenation, ventilation, and perfusion.

If the child is breathing spontaneously, the child is generally positioned to extend the neck, avoiding flexion or hyperextension. If the blood pressure is adequate and no spine injury is present, the head of the child's bed can be elevated approximately 30 degrees to maximize chest expansion and diaphragm excursion. Although this position will enhance cerebral venous return, its effect on actual cerebral perfusion varies so the position must be reevaluated based on the child's progress.

If ventilation is effective, the child's aeration will be equal and adequate bilaterally, and the respiratory rate will be appropriate for the child's age and clinical condition (see Chapter 9). A respiratory rate of 50/minute can be appropriate in a crying, vigorous infant, but this rate is fairly rapid for an adolescent. Conversely, a respiratory rate of 12/minute in a sleeping but arousable adolescent may be appropriate, but it is too slow for an infant.

Evidence of respiratory distress such as retractions, nasal flaring, grunting, stridor, apnea, gasping, or cyanosis should be reported immediately to an on-call provider. Inadequate ventilation can produce hypercapnia, hypoxemia, cerebral vasodilation, and increased cerebral blood flow (CBF) and increased cerebral blood volume (CBV), leading to increased ICP. If ventilation is inadequate, hand ventilation is provided with a bag and mask until intubation can be accomplished and mechanical ventilation can be provided. If the intubated child deteriorates suddenly, the nurse must check for tube displacement, tube obstruction, pneumothorax and equipment failure (recalled with the mnemonic "DOPE").[104]

As soon as possible after admission of the unstable child, a blood sample is taken for blood gas analysis to confirm or rule out the presence of hypercapnia, hypoxemia, or acidosis. Based on the blood gas analysis results, oxygen administration and support of ventilation are initiated or adjusted.

The nurse should quickly assess the child's systemic perfusion. Signs of adequate perfusion include warm skin with brisk capillary refill, consistent color tones, pink nail beds and mucous membranes, and strong peripheral pulses, with heart rate and blood pressure appropriate for age and clinical condition. Hypotension may be the result of bleeding or hypovolemia and can compromise the child's CPP (CPP = MAP − ICP). Hypertension may be an early sign of increased ICP; if present, it should not be corrected unless an extremely high blood pressure raises concern about the development of hypertensive encephalopathy, because hypertension may be necessary to maintain the CPP.

If an ICP monitoring device is in place, the ICP should be monitored closely and the nurse should be alert for the development of clinical signs of increased ICP (see earlier sections of this chapter). If intraarterial pressure monitoring was not established during surgery and the child's condition is unstable, the nurse should request the insertion of an arterial catheter to enable continuous monitoring of the arterial blood pressure, calculation of CPP, and sampling of blood for laboratory analysis. If the child requires frequent venipunctures for blood sampling, vigorous crying can result in a rise in ICP every time blood samples are drawn.

The child's heart rate may vary if increased ICP develops, so close continuous observation of heart rate is required. Although bradycardia is one of the signs of a severe increase in ICP with imminent brainstem herniation, tachycardia may be an early sign of increased ICP. The heart rate should be appropriate for age and clinical condition; tachycardia is appropriate if the child is apprehensive, crying, febrile, or in pain.

A quick but thorough assessment of the child's neurologic status is needed as soon as possible after the child returns from surgery. Pupils should be equal and reactive to light; pupil inequality or sluggish response to light should be reported immediately to an on-call provider, because these signs can indicate the development of increased ICP. When pupil size and responsiveness are checked, the nurse should assess the corneal reflex and notify a physician immediately if it is absent.

The nurse should notify an on-call provider immediately of decorticate rigidity, decerebrate posturing, or absence of normal reflexes such as gag and cough reflexes assessed during suctioning of the child's airway. Normal withdrawal of an extremity is demonstrated by abduction (movement outward or away from the midline) when a painful stimulus is applied to the medial aspect of the extremity; lack of this withdrawal is abnormal and worrisome. The patient normally moves purposefully (grabs toward the nurse's hand) in response to a central painful stimulus (i.e., one applied to the trunk or by pinching the trapezius muscle).

The child is monitored at all times for seizure activity because seizures can develop following intracranial surgery or traumatic brain injury.[83,96] If neuromuscular blocking agents are administered postoperatively, seizures may progress unrecognized because the neuromuscular blocking agents will prevent tonic-clonic movements. Whenever seizures are suspected in the paralyzed child or whenever unexplained fluctuations in heart rate or blood pressure, poor systemic perfusion, nystagmus, alternating dilation and constriction of pupils, or a disconjugate gaze develops, notify an on-call provider immediately; it may be necessary to obtain an EEG to confirm that seizures are present. Continuous EEG monitoring may be indicated to detect seizure activity or status epilepticus.

If an ICP monitoring system is in place, both the ICP and the calculated CPP are recorded. The nurse will need specific orders for actions to take if the ICP exceeds 20 mm Hg for more than 10 minutes or if the CPP falls significantly; a fall near or below 40 mm Hg is extremely worrisome and requires immediate treatment. (Additional management is discussed in the Increased Intracranial Pressure section earlier in this chapter.)[5,13]

Maintenance of Cardiorespiratory Function

As noted earlier, optimal cerebral perfusion requires adequate systemic oxygenation and ventilation (including normocarbia). If the child demonstrates increased ICP postoperatively, the child will remain intubated with mechanical ventilation. The child's $PaCO_2$ is maintained between 35 and 40 mm Hg and the PaO_2 at 100 mm Hg. Appropriate analgesia will be needed

and sedation with or without neuromuscular blockade may be required (see Chapter 5).

Preoxygenation is needed before endotracheal suctioning, and the child may require premedication with lidocaine (1 mg/kg IV bolus) before suctioning or other noxious stimuli to prevent or limit increases in ICP. Suctioning should be brief with careful assessment of the child's color, arterial blood pressure, and ICP (if monitored). Generally, two nurses are needed to suction efficiently yet provide appropriate monitoring and minimize hypoxia and hypercarbia. If an inline suction system is used, careful airway suctioning may be accomplished with only one care provider. Suctioning of the airway should be interrupted if the child develops bradycardia, hypotension, hypertension, deterioration in systemic perfusion, or increased ICP.

If the child's condition is relatively stable and the child is breathing spontaneously upon arrival in the critical care unit, the goals of respiratory care are maintenance of adequate respiratory function and detection of early signs of respiratory insufficiency. Oxygenation is monitored by pulse oximetry and blood gas analysis. The child's airway is assessed and supported as needed, and ventilation is evaluated through clinical examination, monitoring of exhaled CO_2 ($P_{ET}CO_2$), and arterial blood gas analysis.

A nasogastric tube is inserted to decompress the stomach and prevent vomiting that may result in aspiration. Gastric decompression and drainage is especially important if the patient demonstrates inadequate cough and gag reflex.

Assessment of systemic perfusion, heart rate, and blood pressure will continue throughout the postoperative period. Extreme tachycardia, bradycardia, and systolic hypertension with a widened pulse pressure should be reported to an on-call provider immediately, because these signs can indicate the development of increased ICP.

After neurosurgery, most children will receive 80%-100% of maintenance fluid requirements consisting of 0.9% sodium chloride with appropriate dextrose added to maintain normoglycemia (Table 11-8). The child can develop hypovolemia if this fluid volume is inadequate to provide for maintenance requirements plus replace fluid lost via insensible losses, bleeding, urine output, and gastric suction. Hypotension and hypovolemia require prompt treatment, because poor systemic perfusion can significantly compromise cerebral perfusion. Occasionally, vasopressors may be required to increase the MAP and maintain the CPP.

Aggressive fluid administration is avoided unless it is needed to maintain systemic perfusion during treatment of shock. If shock resuscitation is required, bolus therapy with isotonic crystalloid or 3% saline is provided until systemic perfusion is adequate. Hypotonic fluids are not used because they are likely to produce a fall in the child's serum sodium concentration (see Chapter 12). Neurosurgery patients are likely to retain free water as the result of ADH secretion or SIADH; therefore, the child's fluid balance, urine output, and serum sodium concentration require close monitoring. If a central venous catheter is in place, the child's central venous pressure can provide helpful information about the child's intravascular volume status.

Neurologic Assessment

The nurse must be able to perform a rapid but thorough neurologic assessment to detect potential complications of neurosurgery, including acute neurologic deterioration. These potential complications include increased ICP, status epilepticus, SIADH, diabetes insipidus (DI), CSF otorrhea or rhinorrhea, and CNS infection. In most cases a thorough neurologic examination, ongoing assessment of vital signs and fluid intake and output, and evaluation of the child's complete blood count, serum electrolytes, and acid-base balance should alert the nurse to the development of any of these complications.

Because assessment, pathophysiology, and treatment of each of the major postoperative complications have been summarized in the Common Clinical Conditions section of this chapter, the following discussion is designed to highlight important aspects of the neurologic examination of the critically ill child and to provide a brief discussion of the major complications of neurosurgery. For more detailed information about these complications, please refer to the Common Clinical Conditions section earlier in this chapter.

Highlights of the Neurologic Examination. Evaluation of the level of consciousness is one of the most important aspects of the neurologic examination of a nonsedated infant or child. Because the infant is unable to communicate verbally, the nurse must evaluate the infant's alertness and response to the environment. The alert infant will awaken to auditory or tactile stimuli, visually track bright objects or lights, cry in response to painful stimuli, be comforted when held or fed, suck vigorously, and sleep when not disturbed, stimulated, or in pain.

The critically ill infant may be extremely irritable, reacting strongly to even mild stimulation. The irritable infant may cry often, will not be comforted when held or fed, will sleep or feed only for short periods, and may hold extremities rigidly. Lethargy is also a potential sign of neurologic dysfunction. When lethargy is present, the infant is difficult to arouse, seems uninterested in surroundings or feeding, will fail to maintain eye contact or respond to parents, and may demonstrate poor muscle tone and a weak suck.

Evaluation of the level of consciousness in the nonsedated child can rely heavily on the child's response to questions and ability to follow commands—ask the child to hold up two fingers, stick out his or her tongue, or wiggle toes. Sluggish or confused responses are usually signs of decreased level of consciousness. However, if the child is suffering from sleep deprivation, then drowsiness, confusion, or irritability can be appropriate. If questions used to evaluate the child's alertness include questions about familiar family members or activities (using information obtained from the parents or primary caretaker) the child may be more likely to respond, because such questions are less likely to be intimidating.

The intubated but ordinarily verbal child will be able to answer questions by nodding or shaking his or her head (or the child may hold up one finger for *yes* and two fingers for *no*). Rating of the child's level of consciousness should be performed using a standard rating scale, such as the GCS score (see Table 11-6).

The child's pupil size and response to light can be extremely sensitive indicators of intracranial events. With the development of increased ICP, one or both pupils dilate and begin to react sluggishly to light. If drugs are administered that can cause pupil dilation (e.g., large doses of atropine or atrovent) or the pupils have been medically dilated, then this should be noted prominently in the patient record and with a sign placed at the bedside. The pupils will dilate with pain, but they will remain reactive to light (see Fig. 11-8 for variations in pupil size that can result from neurologic disorders).

As noted previously, assessment of the child's vital signs is an essential part of the neurologic examination. *Cushing's reflex* causes a triad (often called Cushing's triad) of late clinical signs of increased ICP; these signs develop when brain stem herniation is imminent. The classic clinical triad includes bradycardia, systolic hypertension with widening pulse pressure, and irregular respirations. In children the change in heart rate can include tachycardia or bradycardia, and irregular respirations can include respiratory depression or apnea.

An important component of the neurologic examination and of the GCS score is assessment of motor function and reflexes (see Table 11-6); this assessment is particularly important if the child is unconscious (i.e., with no eye opening or verbal response). Decorticate rigidity and decerebrate posturing are abnormal (see Fig. 11-9). A positive Babinski's reflex is abnormal after the infant has begun walking (see Fig. 11-10).

The child should withdraw extremities in response to pain, and he or she should demonstrate corneal, gag, and cough reflexes (described under Clinical Signs and Symptoms for Increased Intracranial Pressure and for Coma). Any deterioration in responsiveness or motor function should be reported to an on-call provider immediately.

If the child has been awake and alert and is old enough to follow commands, the nurse can assess muscle strength by asking the child to move all extremities and to move each extremity against resistance. Testing strength of antigravity muscles may reveal unilateral muscle weakness (e.g., ask the child to extend both arms and close eyes; if the right arm falls, a left hemisphere lesion is suspected).

The nurse should ensure that the child moves all four extremities equally and appropriately and is able to sense light touch and pain. The nurse can evaluate motor coordination by asking the child to touch the nurse's index finger and then his or her own nose—even toddlers will perform this activity. Seizure activity should be reported to the provider and must be treated promptly.

Many of the cranial nerves can be evaluated while other nursing care is performed (see Table 11-2 and Box 11-2). For example, the glossopharyngeal (ninth cranial) nerve and vagus (tenth cranial) nerve are probably intact if the child coughs and gags during suctioning of the airway and if the child is able to swallow.

The child may complain of headaches, nausea, malaise, vomiting, blurred vision, diplopia, and poor feeding; these can be nonspecific symptoms of increased ICP and should be reported to the on-call provider. Unless a large head dressing is in place, the infant's head circumference is measured when the infant returns from surgery and at daily or other intervals per hospital protocol. An increase in head circumference can be caused by a gradual increase in intracranial volume, such as occurs with hydrocephalus or a subdural empyema.

Postoperative Complications. Increased ICP results from an uncompensated increase in the volume of blood, brain, or CSF within the skull. Hemorrhage, cerebral venous obstruction, or cerebral vasodilation can increase the child's CBV. The brain size can increase with cerebral edema, and the CSF volume can increase with obstruction to CSF flow or decreased CSF reabsorption. Although intracranial volume can initially increase without a rise in ICP, further small increases in intracranial volume will produce significant increases in ICP once a critical volume is reached (see Increased Intracranial Pressure).

Signs and symptoms of increased ICP are summarized in Box 11-3, and they include a decrease in the level of consciousness, pupil dilation and sluggish response to light, decreased motor function, hypertension, tachycardia or bradycardia, altered respiratory pattern, and ultimately apnea and cardiorespiratory arrest. If ICP monitoring is used, an on-call provider should be notified of rises in ICP or a compromise in calculated CPP.

The treatment of increased ICP includes control of CBV through maintenance of adequate oxygenation and normocarbia. If an extraventricular drainage (EVD) system is in place, CSF drainage (if ordered) can reduce CSF and intracranial volume. The use of hypertonic agents such as 3% saline or hyperosmolar agents such as mannitol can reduce cerebral edema. Analgesics, such as fentanyl, and sedatives, such as midazolam, can also help control increased ICP.

Acute hyperventilation is reserved for management of increased ICP when signs of impending herniation (i.e., Cushing triad of bradycardia, systolic hypertension with widening pulse pressure, and irregular respirations) develop.[83] When all other methods of medical treatment fail, the child may be placed in a barbiturate coma to reduce cerebral metabolic requirements and ICP (see Management, Barbiturate Therapy, in the Increased Intracranial Pressure section of this chapter).

Status epilepticus is repetitive or continuous seizure activity for more than 30 minutes without a return to consciousness. Status epilepticus requires immediate treatment because it can produce cerebral vasodilation, an increase in cerebral metabolic requirements, and in an increase in ICP.

When the child receives neuromuscular blocking agents during the postoperative period, clinical evidence of seizure activity is masked. Therefore, the presence of seizures or status epilepticus should be considered if the child receiving neuromuscular blockade demonstrates wide fluctuations in blood pressure, sudden pupil dilation, or other unexplained deterioration in clinical status. Once herniation has been ruled out, an EEG will likely be necessary to identify seizures.

An individual seizure does not require treatment. Status epilepticus, however, must be treated immediately. In children,

lorazepam (0.05-0.1 mg/kg IV), phenobarbital (10-20 mg/kg IV), fosphenytoin (15-20 mg (PE)/kg IV), are used most commonly[120] (see Status Epilepticus, in the second part of this chapter). Monitoring and support of therapeutic serum drug levels is also needed.

SIADH frequently develops after neurosurgery. Clinical signs and symptoms of this syndrome include hyponatremia, persistently high urine sodium concentration, high urine osmolality, and low urine volume. Treatment of SIADH includes water restriction to approximately ½ to ⅔ of maintenance fluid requirements and administration of isotonic fluid, such as 0.9% sodium chloride. If the serum sodium concentration is dangerously low or if neurologic signs of water intoxication (e.g., lethargy, irritability) are present, 3% sodium chloride may be administered to reach a target sodium of 125 mEq/L or to elevate the child's serum sodium concentration approximately 0.5 to 1 mEq/L. The remaining sodium deficit is replaced over the next 12 to 24 hours. The following formula can be used to calculate sodium requirements:

$$(0.6^* \times \text{Body weight [kg]}) \times (\text{Desired-Actual [Na+]}) = \text{mEq Na+ required to correct}$$

*Use 0.5 in females.

Diabetes insipidus most commonly results from decreased production of ADH, also called central or neurogenic DI. The child with DI has massive free water loss in the urine. If DI progresses unrecognized, fluid depletion can rapidly cause shock, hypernatremia, and neurologic deterioration. Clinical signs of DI include excretion of large quantities of dilute urine often in excess of 10 to 15 mL/kg per hour, hypernatremia, low urine sodium concentration, and low urine osmolality. Treatment of DI includes replacement of urinary fluid and electrolyte losses and administration of IV vasopressin (for further discussion of management of Diabetes Insipidus and SIADH, see Chapter 12).

General Supportive Care

Fluids and Nutrition. Serum electrolytes, serum osmolality, urine output, specific gravity, and urine osmolality must be closely monitored to determine ongoing fluid and electrolyte needs. The child's level of hydration should be monitored closely. Signs of adequate hydration include evidence of good systemic perfusion, moist mucous membranes, adequate urine output (1 mL/kg per hour) and tearing with cry. The infant's fontanelle will not be depressed if hydration is adequate.

The dehydrated infant will demonstrate dry mucous membranes, a sunken fontanelle, decreased urine output with increased specific gravity, poor skin turgor, and an elevation in blood urea nitrogen (BUN). With more severe levels of dehydration, hemoconcentration produces a rise in serum electrolyte concentrations and signs of circulatory compromise (see Chapters 6 and 12).

IV fluids containing 5% to 10% glucose will not provide maintenance caloric requirements. Plans should be made to provide parenteral nutrition if the child does not tolerate enteral feedings within 1 to 2 days after surgery.

Analgesia. Relief of pain during the postoperative period is mandatory for all neurosurgery patients; however, the degree of analgesia and sedation must be balanced with the need to evaluate the patient's neurologic status. If the child is tolerating an enteral feeding, codeine (0.5-1 mg/kg per dose, orally) is often the preferred analgesic because it does not produce the respiratory depression associated with morphine sulfate or fentanyl. If the child is intubated, and receiving mechanical ventilatory support, fentanyl (0.5-2 mcg/kg per dose as an IV bolus or a continuous infusion of 0.5-2 mcg/kg per hour), or morphine sulfate (0.05-0.1 mg/kg per dose IV) may be administered (see Chapter 5). These medications are titrated to clinical effect. If the child becomes agitated, it is important to verify that the child's airway, oxygenation, and ventilation are adequate, and identify and treat any increased ICP before assuming that analgesia or sedation are needed for simple agitation.

Sedation. Agitation during the immediate postoperative period can be treated with midazolam, (0.05-0.1 mg/kg per dose IV bolus [maximum dose, 2-5 mg] or by continuous infusion of 0.05-0.1 mg/kg per hour). Sedatives are especially helpful if it is anticipated that the child will be intubated with mechanical ventilation for any length of time. It is important to determine whether agitation is caused by hypoxia or increased ICP before sedation is administered.

Prevention of Infection. Routine postoperative administration of prophylactic antibiotics is no longer recommended for prevention of infection. However, some patients will receive intraoperative antibiotics.

The single most effective tool for prevention of hospital-acquired infection is good handwashing technique. Stellar wound care and judicious use of central and arterial access also minimizes the risk of postoperative infection (see Chapters 16 and 22).

Infection risk increases if the surgery was performed to repair a cerebral contusion or skull penetration by a foreign object or if the child develops a CSF leak from the nose or ears (see the Head Trauma section of this chapter). The child's temperature and white blood cell count are monitored to detect evidence of infection; appropriate blood, wound, and catheter cultures are taken (per order or protocol) if infection is suspected.

Treatment of Fever. Fever increases metabolic rate, so will increase cerebral oxygen consumption. Such an increase in oxygen consumption can be extremely detrimental in the face of limited oxygen delivery to the brain. As a result, it is especially important to prevent or promptly treat fever in the child with head injury. Fever should be treated with antipyretics such as acetaminophen (10-15 mg/kg per dose orally, nasogastric or rectally with a maximum of 650 mg every 6 hours) or ibuprofen (10 mg/kg per dose orally or via nasogastric tube every 4-6 hours) if bleeding is not a risk.

It is important to rule out sources of infection if high or persistent fever develops. If antipyretics are not effective, a hypothermia blanket may be used to reduce fever if it does not cause shivering. Shivering can increase cerebral metabolism and contribute to increased ICP.[83,96]

Prevention of the Complications of Immobility. The comatose or paralyzed child can quickly develop atelectasis, pulmonary infiltrates, contractures, deep vein thrombosis, and other complications of immobility unless the nurse provides good pulmonary toilet, passive range-of-motion exercises, and other preventive care (for further information see Management in the Coma section of this chapter).

Psychosocial Support

Neurosurgery is likely to be extremely frightening for the child and parents. In recent years, the general public has become more aware that a patient can survive a neurologic insult in a chronic vegetative state. Many parents have expressed the willingness to cope with their child's physical handicap as long as a chronic vegetative state does not develop. Thus, the prospect of neurosurgery and its possible complications can be extremely threatening. If the child requires surgery after head trauma, the parents may be overwhelmed by the acuity and severity of the injury and by guilt for not having prevented it.

If possible before the surgery, the nurse should determine the parents' and child's understanding of and response to the child's condition. If the parents have major misconceptions, the nurse can attempt to clarify them. If the child or parents have unanswered questions before surgery, the nurse should notify the neurosurgeon or on-call provider to ensure that these questions are answered. Providing informed consent for surgery requires that the parents be aware of the child's condition, potential postoperative complications, and alternatives to surgery.

During the surgery, it is helpful for the nurse to keep the parents informed about the progress of surgery. It is not necessary for the parents to be made aware of each aspect of the surgical technique or specifics of dissection, suturing, or debridement, but it is helpful for the parents to know of the general progress of the surgery. The nurse also can provide the parents with interim reports of the child's condition during surgery; however, these reports must be carefully worded and require the consent and input of the surgeon. Such interim reports can reduce the parents' anxiety during the waiting period and also provide the opportunity to prepare the family for bad news if the child's condition deteriorates. If the family's first hint of trouble comes when the surgeon arrives to inform them that the child suffered a catastrophic cerebral insult, the parents can be overwhelmed by grief or anger and be too shocked to respond or ask questions.

After surgery, the parents will require support when visiting their child for the first time. They should be given consistent reports of the child's condition and prognosis throughout postoperative care. The child will require gentle care and encouragement. When discussing a child's condition and prognosis with the child and the child's siblings, a child life specialist is often very helpful (see Chapters 2 and 24 for further information). Box 11-10 summarizes the important aspects of nursing care of the postoperative pediatric neurosurgery patient.

Box 11-10 | **Postoperative Care of the Pediatric Neurosurgery Patient and the Patient with Increased Intracranial Pressure**

Postoperative care of the neurosurgery patient includes assessment for deterioration (particularly development or worsening of increased ICP) and prevention or detection and treatment of potential surgical complications of the surgical procedure. This box highlights nursing care priorities.

I. Potential Respiratory Insufficiency, Related to:

Anesthesia
Airway obstruction
Hypoventilation, atelectasis
Increased intracranial pressure
Neurogenic pulmonary edema
Pneumonia

Expected Patient Outcomes

1. Patient will demonstrate appropriate respiratory rate for age and clinical condition.
2. Patient will demonstrate no evidence of airway obstruction.
3. Patient will demonstrate equal and adequate breath sounds and lung expansion bilaterally, with no evidence of increased respiratory effort or distress.
4. Oxygenation and ventilation as evaluated by arterial blood gases and arterial oxygen saturation (pulse oximetry) and exhaled CO_2 will be appropriate for clinical condition. Hypoxemia and hypercarbia will be prevented or promptly treated (both increase cerebral blood flow and can contribute to potential rise in ICP).
5. Systemic oxygen delivery (arterial oxygen content × cardiac output) will be adequate and metabolic acidosis will be absent.

Nursing Interventions

1. Obtain report of patient condition and surgical procedure before the child's arrival. Prepare all equipment and support needed in the postoperative care unit.
2. If child is intubated and receiving mechanical ventilation:
   a. Assess airway and effectiveness of ventilation. If positive pressure ventilation is adequate, chest expansion will be equal and adequate bilaterally. If the chest does not expand during positive pressure ventilation, ventilation is not adequate.
   b. Evaluate oxygenation through pulse oximetry, arterial blood gases, and ventilation (carbon dioxide elimination) through exhaled carbon dioxide.
   c. Monitor child's heart rate, spontaneous respiratory effort, color, and general appearance; notify physician/provider of signs of distress.
   d. Adjust ventilation support as indicated and ordered to maintain oxygenation and normocarbia. Monitor for hypoxemia and hypercarbia and treat immediately.
   e. Once child's condition is stable, wean mechanical ventilation as indicated (and per order or protocol); closely monitor neurologic function.
   f. Keep emergency hand ventilator (bag), oxygen source, mask, and reintubation equipment readily available
3. If child is breathing spontaneously, evaluate and support airway, oxygenation, and ventilation:
   a. Be alert for signs of airway obstruction, hypoventilation, or inadequate gas exchange.

   b. Monitor level of consciousness and responsiveness; if child's response to painful stimulus is compromised, airway protective mechanisms (cough, gag) may also be depressed; consider elective intubation.
4. Monitor vital signs and report excessive tachycardia, bradycardia, systolic hypertension, or irregular breathing to physician; be prepared to treat increased ICP.
5. Auscultate breath sounds bilaterally, and report decreased intensity or change in pitch of breath sounds (may be associated with unilateral pulmonary pathology) to provider. Monitor for clinical evidence of pulmonary edema (see Chapter 9), pulmonary edema on chest radiograph (see Chapter 10), or hypoxemia (and report findings to on-call provider).
6. Evaluate presence of cough and gag; if these reflexes are depressed, withhold oral fluids and discuss potential intubation with on-call provider.
7. Monitor for signs of increased ICP: deterioration in level of consciousness, decreased responsiveness, pupil dilation with decreased response to light. Be prepared to treat increased ICP as needed and ordered.
8. Administer analgesics and sedatives as needed to maintain patient comfort and ensure effective mechanical ventilation (see Chapter 5). If agitation develops, assess for hypoxia, increased ICP and pain.

II. Potential Compromise in Systemic Perfusion Related to:

Hemorrhage
Increased intracranial pressure
Inadequate fluid administration or excessive diuretic therapy
Fluid loss associated with diabetes insipidus
Electrolyte imbalance
Hypoventilation and hypoxemia

Expected Patient Outcomes

1. Patient will demonstrate a heart rate and blood pressure appropriate for age and clinical condition.
2. Systemic perfusion will remain adequate, as demonstrated by urine output approximately 1-2 mL/kg per hour (if fluid intake adequate), warm skin with brisk capillary refill, strong peripheral pulses, normal serum lactate (no lactic acidosis).

Nursing Interventions

1. Monitor systemic perfusion: heart rate, blood pressure, warmth of extremities and trunk, capillary refill, quality of peripheral pulses and urine output. Notify the provider immediately of any deterioration.
   a. Assess intravascular volume status; administer fluid or blood as needed.
   b. Assess neurologic function.
   c. Assess and support fluid and electrolyte balance.
   d. Ensure that oxygenation and ventilation are adequate; be prepared to provide supplementary oxygen and ventilation as needed (and ordered).
2. Administer isotonic (e.g., normal saline) intravenous fluids as ordered:
   a. Avoid hypotonic fluids (they may contribute to a fall in serum sodium with development of cerebral edema).

Continued

Box 11-10	Postoperative Care of the Pediatric Neurosurgery Patient and the Patient with Increased Intracranial Pressure—cont'd

b. If intravascular volume and systemic perfusion are adequate, typical fluid administration volume is less than maintenance fluids (see Table 11-8).

c. Plan to provide adequate nutrition (see Chapter 14).

d. Monitor for evidence of SIADH: fall in serum sodium concentration (with possible associated change in mental status) and serum osmolality, oliguria with high urine sodium concentration. Treatment: restrict water intake to approximately 50%-75% of calculated maintenance requirements (see Chapter 12).

e. Monitor for evidence of diabetes insipidus: extremely high urine volume with low urine specific gravity. Treatment: replace urine losses (milliliter for milliliter), monitor for and treat hypovolemia or electrolyte imbalance, administer ADH (see Chapter 12).

3. Monitor fluid balance closely and be aware of potential sources of increased insensible water loss (including fever); notify provider of positive or negative fluid balance.

4. Monitor electrolyte balance; notify provider of imbalance.

5. Administer hypertonic saline and osmotic agents as ordered; monitor result and notify provider of effect on ICP and neurologic function.

6. Ensure that oxygen delivery (arterial oxygen content × cardiac output) is adequate (inadequate oxygen delivery will result in development of metabolic acidosis), and treat reversible causes of increased oxygen consumption (fever, pain, anxiety).

III. Potential Cerebral Ischemia or Dysfunction Related to:

Increased intracranial volume (caused by increased blood volume, brain volume or CSF volume) and pressure and reduction in cerebral perfusion pressure

Status epilepticus

Cerebral oxygen consumption in excess of oxygen and substrate delivery

Expected Patient Outcomes

1. Patient will demonstrate no deterioration in neurologic function.

2. Complications of increased ICP, such as a compromise in cerebral perfusion or brain death, will not develop.

3. Seizure activity will be detected promptly and treated as needed.

Nursing Interventions

1. Closely monitor neurologic function including (see Box 11-2):
   a. Level of consciousness and responsiveness
   b. Pediatric Glasgow Coma Scale score (see Table 11-6)

Note: Notify the provider immediately of deterioration in child's responsiveness. Responsiveness should be assessed whenever clinical condition changes.
   c. Pupil size and response to light
   d. Evidence of cranial nerve function during nursing care activities

2. Monitor systemic perfusion; report compromise to provider immediately.

3. Monitor patient for signs of increased intracranial pressure, including: deterioration in level of consciousness, decreased responsiveness and ability to follow commands, pupil dilation with decreased response to light. Late signs of increased intracranial pressure (and impending herniation) include: bradycardia (note that tachycardia may be present early), systolic hypertension with widened pulse pressure, and irregular respirations with possible apnea. Notify on-call provider immediately if these signs are observed, and be prepared to provide mild hyperventilation if signs of impending herniation develop.

   a. Maintain normocarbia (arterial carbon dioxide tension approximately 35-40 mm Hg) with mechanical ventilation to control cerebral blood flow

   b. Prevent development of hypoxemia (maintain PaO_2 ≥100 mm Hg).

   c. Maintain serum sodium concentration and serum osmolality.

   d. Administer analgesics and sedatives as ordered (see Chapter 5)

   e. If deterioration in clinical condition is observed, quickly assess neurologic function and report any change to provider immediately.

4. Maintain head in midline position (to enhance cerebral venous return). Avoid any condition that will impede cerebral venous return, such as extremely high levels of positive end-expiratory pressure. If systemic arterial pressure is adequate, elevate head of the bed to enhance cerebral venous return (per order or protocol).

5. Administer hypertonic saline or osmotic diuretics as ordered. Monitor serum sodium concentration and evaluate serum osmolality (via laboratory) and estimate according to the following formula:

$$(2 \times serum\ Na^+) + (serum\ glucose \div 18) + (BUN \div 2.8)$$

Normal serum osmolality is approximately 275-295 mOsm/L. As a rule, diuresis is performed to maintain serum osmolality at approximately 300-310 mOsm/L, with the serum sodium concentration maintained at approximately 145-150 mEq/L. Prevent an abrupt fall in serum sodium concentration or serum osmolality that can contribute to intracellular fluid shift and cerebral edema.

6. If intracranial pressure monitor is in place, verify calibration and accuracy of system.

7. Chart the ICP to reflect the peak (hourly) intracranial pressure, whether this peak occurred with stimulation, and the average ICP (see Fig. 11-15 and Box 11-5)

8. Calculate CPP; notify provider of rise in ICP (>20 mm Hg) or compromise in CPP. For further information regarding ICP monitoring, see below

9. If intracranial pressure monitoring is performed, discuss plan with the provider for response to rises in ICP (e.g., draining of CSF through EVD, administration of osmotic diuretics, administration of anesthetic agents). Report significant or spontaneous rises in intracranial pressure to on-call provider

Box 11-10 **Postoperative Care of the Pediatric Neurosurgery Patient and the Patient with Increased Intracranial Pressure—cont'd**

immediately; be prepared to report any associated changes in neurologic function.

10. Maximize oxygen delivery (arterial oxygen content × cardiac output) and eliminate treatable causes of increased oxygen consumption (e.g., fever, pain, seizures).

11. Monitor for evidence of seizure activity, including lateral eye deviation, a rise in ICP, or a sudden change in vital signs. Posttraumatic seizures are most likely to develop in patients with severe head injury, diffuse cerebral edema, acute subdural hematoma, or an open depressed skull fracture.

12. If ICP continues to rise despite provision of mild hyperventilation, and osmotic therapy, administration of anesthetic agents may be prescribed. This will require transfer to appropriate facility. See Increased Intracranial Pressure, Management)

IV. Maintain ICP Monitoring System and Verify Function
Expected Patient Outcomes

1. Intracranial pressure measurements will be accurate and trends recorded on patient flow chart will reflect trends in patient ICP and cerebral perfusion pressure accurately.

2. Longevity of intracranial pressure monitoring device will be maximized.

3. Infection will be prevented.

Nursing Interventions

1. Assemble, zero, and calibrate ICP monitoring system according to manufacturer's specifications.
   a. Fluid-filled monitoring systems use standard pressure transducers, which must be properly leveled (at the level of the intracranial ventricle), zeroed, and calibrated per the manufacture's instruction and unit policy.
   b. If fiberoptic catheter is used, zero and calibrate per the manufacturer's instruction before insertion. Calibrate waveform after insertion. Damage to the transducer or faulty signal will result in dampening of the waveform signal.
   c. Notify provider of any dysfunction.

2. Support insertion of ICP monitoring catheter under sterile conditions, apply dressing over the skin entrance site. Discuss removal of monitoring catheter as soon as possible, to reduce infection.

3. If a ventricular catheter is placed with EVD system, obtain specific information from the provider regarding the technique of CSF drainage, including:
   a. Continuous versus intermittent drainage (and pressure for intermittent drainage)
   b. Position of drainage drip chamber above lateral ventricles
   c. Placement of the head of the bed

Note: If the ventricular catheter is open to drainage at all times, CSF drainage should automatically occur when the ICP exceeds the pressure above the mm Hg (or cm H$_2$O) corresponding to the height at which drip chamber set. For example, if the drainage drip chamber is set at the 27 cm mark above the lateral

ventricles, the CSF should automatically drain when the ICP exceeds 27 cm H$_2$O (or 20 mm Hg). If the system is patent, the ICP should never exceed that pressure.

4. Monitor volume of CSF drainage; change the drainage bag (using sterile technique) when it is half full (or per unit practice). If obstruction of CSF drainage is suspected, notify provider.

5. If the nurse is uncertain of the accuracy of ICP monitoring results, or if the ICP rises, the nurse should assess patient's neurologic function and report changes to provider.

6. For further information, see Increased Intracranial Pressure in this chapter, and Intracranial Pressure Monitoring in Chapter 21.

V. Potential Infection, Related to:
Breaks in skin barrier
Invasive monitoring catheters
Multiple trauma
Contamination of surgical wound

Expected Patient Outcomes

1. Patient will demonstrate no signs of infection such as fever, localized inflammation, leukocytosis or leukopenia, or positive wound or blood cultures.

2. Existing infection will resolve promptly.

Nursing Interventions

1. Ensure strict handwashing

2. Ensure that sterile and aseptic procedures are used as needed for insertion and maintenance of monitoring catheters and systems.

3. Change dressings, transducer tubing, and catheters according to unit policy. Maintain occlusive dressings over central venous catheter skin entrance sites.

4. Monitor for signs of infection, including localized signs of inflammation, fever, leukocytosis or leukopenia. Notify physician of cloudy urine, CSF drainage, or drainage from wounds or catheter insertion sites. Obtain cultures as ordered or per unit policy.

5. Administer antibiotics as ordered; monitor peak and trough levels as ordered.

6. Be alert for signs of ventriculitis following intraventricular pressure monitoring. Signs can include deterioration in level of consciousness, sluggish pupil response to light, fever, and headache. Notify a provider immediately if these are observed.

VI. Fluid and Electrolyte Imbalance, Related to:
Alterations in ADH secretion, including SIADH
Diabetes insipidus (DI)
Limited fluid intake
Administration of diuretic agents

Expected Patient Outcomes

1. Fluid balance will be appropriate for patient clinical condition.

2. Electrolyte balance will be normal or appropriate for clinical condition (e.g., serum sodium will be maintained at approximately 145-150 mEq/L). Abrupt fall in serum sodium and osmolality will not develop.

Continued

| Box 11-10 | **Postoperative Care of the Pediatric Neurosurgery Patient and the Patient with Increased Intracranial Pressure—cont'd** |

Nursing Interventions

1. Monitor and accurately record all sources of fluid intake and output. Monitor effects of diuretic agents on urine volume and neurologic function. Monitor urine specific gravity and serum osmolality (estimate serum osmolality according to formula in III., 5., above). Notify provider of fall in the serum sodium concentration or osmolality.

2. Administer intravenous fluids as ordered (see Table 11-8). Avoid hypotonic fluids or excessive fluid administration.

3. Monitor for signs of SIADH, including a fall in the serum sodium concentration, oliguria, and high urine sodium concentration. Notify a provider if these signs develop. Treatment requires restriction of water intake. Treat symptomatic hyponatremia with 2-4 mL of 3% saline as ordered.

4. Monitor for signs of diabetes insipidus, including increased urine volume with a low urine specific gravity (<1.005). If urine volume increases and diabetes insipidus is suspected, replace fluid lost in the urine and administer ADH as ordered.

5. If ADH administered, monitor urine output before and after administration.

6. Monitor serum electrolyte concentration and notify provider of imbalance.

7. Assess systemic perfusion and notify physician of signs of dehydration, hypovolemia or hypervolemia.

8. When the patient begins oral fluid intake, restrict fluid intake as ordered and needed.

9. Monitor neurologic function closely and notify the provider of any deterioration.

Additional Nursing Diagnoses or Patient Problems

Patient or family anxiety or anger related to: severity of patient condition, potential sequelae of neurosurgery or underlying disease or injury, unknown aspects of treatment or prognosis

Knowledge deficit regarding: patient's condition, long-term treatment and home care required

Impaired patient mobility related to: neurologic deficit, associated injuries, complications of the underlying disease or initial trauma

Potential pain related to: underlying disease or initial trauma, multiple invasive catheters, surgical incision

ADH, Antidiuretic hormone; *BUN*, blood urea nitrogen; *CPP*, cerebral perfusion pressure; *CSF*, cerebrospinal fluid; *EVD*, extraventricular drainage; *ICP*, intracranial pressure; *SIADH*, syndrome of inappropriate antidiuretic hormone.

SPECIFIC DISEASES

Head Trauma

Etiology

CNS injury is the leading cause of death in children. In children younger than 2 years, serious head injuries (traumatic brain injuries [TBIs]) are commonly intentional (also called *inflicted* or *non-accidental trauma*). Children older than 3 years of age sustain head injuries secondary to falls or to motor vehicle, all terrain vehicle, bicycle, and pedestrian collisions. In high school-aged adolescents, football is the team sport most commonly linked with head injury.

Each year 1.5 million head injuries occur in the United States. Of this number approximately 300,000 children are hospitalized with head trauma. Nearly 90% of injury-related deaths are associated with head trauma. Males are twice as likely as females to sustain head trauma. Severe TBI or associated cardiorespiratory arrest can cause death within a few hours of injury.[20]

Pathophysiology

The rigid cranium and the CSF cushion can protect the child's brain from injury during minor trauma. However, if distortion of the skull, shear injury, actual tissue damage, intracranial hemorrhage, or cerebral edema develop, the injury is likely to be complicated by increased ICP. Therefore, the child with head trauma requires assessment and treatment of the primary (or direct) injury, as well as careful assessment and treatment of secondary complications.

The types of cerebral injuries occurring with head trauma include concussions, contusions, skull fractures, vascular injuries, diffuse axonal injuries, penetrating injuries, and cerebral edema. Each lesion is summarized below.

Concussion. A concussion is associated with mild to moderate cerebral injury. It results from a blow to the head or a shearing rotational injury of the brain within the skull that produces no structural brain damage. The concussion is more likely to occur if the head moves freely after impact; an acceleration-deceleration injury produces shearing stresses on the brainstem and results in injury to the reticular activating system. Many patients with concussion experience loss of consciousness for a few seconds or several hours, although some may never lose consciousness.

After the impact, the CSF pressure rises transiently, and electroencephalographic evidence of slow brain wave activity has been documented.[62] Infants may exhibit less specific signs than those of older children; the infant may develop seizures, nausea, emesis, and lethargy, but usually no loss of consciousness. Older children may complain of headache, dizziness, fatigue, and amnesia. Generally, symptoms of a concussion will resolve in approximately 1 week. However, some symptoms may persist for up to 1 year. The diagnosis of concussion is generally made based on a history of a temporary loss of consciousness with no other findings.[50,78]

Contusion. A cerebral contusion is a localized brain injury that consists of bruising, hemorrhage, and cerebral edema.

The hemorrhage may be epidural, subdural, or subarachnoid (see the section on vascular injuries that follows), and it can produce an increase in ICP or loss of consciousness.

The injury can occur directly beneath the site of impact (the coup injury) or on the side of the brain opposite the impact (the contrecoup injury). The contrecoup injury is thought to occur as the brain strikes the skull on the side of the head opposite the initial impact. The severity of the cerebral contusion is determined by the amount of direct tissue injury, bleeding, and edema that result.[50]

Posttraumatic seizures occur in approximately 10% of children with cerebral contusions. Prophylactic anticonvulsant drugs are of little benefit in preventing seizures. These delayed effects of head injury can be classified as early or late seizures. Early seizures typically occur within the first week after injury, usually seen within the first 24 hours. Factors associated with increased risk include age <5 years, prolonged course of posttraumatic amnesia, intracranial (particularly intraventricular) hemorrhage, and compound depressed skull fractures.

Late seizures develop in approximately 5% of children with TBI, typically developing between the first week and 1 year after injury. Risk factors include early seizures, intracranial hemorrhage, and compound depressed skull fractures.[78]

Skull Fractures. A skull fracture is a break in the continuity of the cranial bones that may or may not be associated with displacement of the bone fragments. Skull fractures are present in approximately one fourth of all patients hospitalized with head injury and can be further classified as simple (closed injury) or compound (open injury). Compound fractures are frequently associated with dural tears; these increase the risk of abscess formation and meningitis.[78] The fracture itself may be benign, but is often associated with injury to the underlying meninges or vasculature.

Approximately three fourths of all skull fractures in children are simple or linear skull fractures. In this form of skull fracture, the bone fragments remain approximated and the dura mater is not penetrated.

A depressed skull fracture is present when one or more bone fragments are indented below the normal contour or table of the cranium. As a result, the skull is indented, and the brain tissue below the fracture is injured. A hematoma may cover the area of injury, and a cerebral contusion may be present below the fracture. The dura usually is not penetrated when a depressed skull fracture is present.

A compound skull fracture exists when a scalp laceration and depressed skull fracture are present, allowing direct communication from the scalp through the skull and into the cranium. The dura often is penetrated when a compound fracture is present, and the skull fragment can be displaced into the brain tissue.

Basilar skull fractures are those that involve a break in the posteroinferior portion of the skull. These fractures do not typically produce cerebral tissue damage, but they frequently produce dural tears. As a result, basilar skull fractures are commonly associated with leak of CSF. When a dural tear and CSF leak are present, contamination of the CSF by ascending upper respiratory tract infection is also possible and can result in the development of meningitis.

Basilar skull fractures can occur over the paranasal sinuses of the frontal bone, over the temporal bone, or over the entrance of the internal carotid artery into the skull. A fracture over the internal carotid artery can result in hemorrhage, aneurysm, or a fistula.[62,78]

Petrous bone fractures can involve injury of cranial nerves V, VII, and VIII and sometimes are associated with injury to the nerve, cochlea, or ossicles. Cranial nerve involvement can be acute or delayed. Treatment may involve the administration of steroids, surgical decompression, or both. Acute presentations are usually associated with poor outcome, whereas children with delayed presentation usually recover. Neuronal deafness is often permanent, but conductive deafness usually improves gradually.[78]

Vascular Injuries and Hemorrhage. Vascular injuries resulting from head trauma can produce epidural hematoma, subdural hematoma, or a subarachnoid hemorrhage. Each of these vascular injuries is discussed separately.

An epidural hematoma (EDH) results from hemorrhage into the extradural space secondary to a tear in the middle meningeal artery or dural veins. Arterial bleeding is the most common source of bleeding and is responsible for 85% of EDHs; the remaining 15% of EDHs arise from the middle meningeal vein or dural sinus. An EDH usually results from direct trauma in the region of the temporal bone and approximately half of patients with EDH have an associated with a skull fracture. Because the hematoma often develops from the artery, blood can rapidly accumulate between the skull and the dura. For this reason EDHs are considered neurosurgical emergencies.

The child with EDH may demonstrate a lucid period that can last minutes to several days after the head injury. As the hematoma expands it compresses the temporal lobe, leading to an acute rise in ICP. The child may abruptly lose consciousness and demonstrate ipsilateral pupil dilation and contralateral hemiparesis. Left untreated, uncal herniation and death will result. Because an EDH is usually detected on an initial CT scan, the classic presentation is somewhat uncommon. Significant mortality and morbidity results if recognition or treatment is delayed.[50,125]

A subdural hematoma (SDH) is a collection of blood between the dura and the arachnoid membranes, resulting from tearing of bridging veins that drain the cortex.[125] An SDH is usually associated with some damage to the underlying brain tissue from the initial injury.

An SDH can be classified as acute, subacute, or chronic. An acute subdural hematoma usually develops after severe head injury or cerebral laceration and results in accumulation of blood within hours of the injury. A subacute subdural hematoma occurs early after a less severe cerebral contusion and usually produces a rise in ICP that prevents the patient from regaining consciousness after the head injury.[62] A chronic subdural hematoma develops weeks or months after a relatively minor head injury. The injury typically produces a venous tear, and blood slowly accumulates in the subdural space. Subdural hematomas are often present bilaterally, and they are frequently present in victims of inflicted trauma under the age of 2 years (see Chapter 19).

Children with subdural hematomas will often exhibit symptoms of increased ICP. These symptoms are secondary to direct injury to the brain tissue, often associated with vasogenic cerebral edema. Many patients who sustain subdural hematomas develop early or late seizures as a result of the injury.[50,83]

A subarachnoid hemorrhage (SAH) results from a severe head injury. Hemorrhage occurs when shear forces producing the massive head injury tear the subarachnoid vessels. Children with an SAH can demonstrate seizures or rapid development of increased ICP. Because subarachnoid hemorrhages frequently are present in children with inflicted trauma, the presence of an SAH warrants careful examination for evidence of other injuries, including healed fractures or retinal hemorrhages (see Inflicted Injuries in Chapter 19).

Diffuse Axonal Injury. Diffuse axonal injury results from an acceleration-deceleration brain injury. This movement creates pressure that begins at the brain surface, and as greater force is transmitted it can extend deep into the brain. This pressure creates a shearing force that tears the axons (long projections of the cell bodies that carry nerve impulses). Traumatic diffuse axonal injury (TDAI) appears to be age independent and may be devastating to the developing brain. It appears to be more widespread in the victim of inflicted trauma.

Traumatic diffuse axonal injury can be further categorized into three subsets: grade 1, microscopic damage to the axons without gross hemorrhage; grade 2, microscopic damage to axons with hemorrhage in the corpus callosum; and grade 3, microscopic damage to axons with hemorrhage in the dorsal aspect of the brainstem. Hemorrhages associated with shearing are often initially microscopic (measuring approximately 1 mm); they can be described as streak or punctuate hemorrhages. However, as the bleeding continues over several days the size can easily reach several centimeters. Hemorrhage is rarely seen in infants or younger children because the cerebral vasculature is relatively elastic. The result of this elasticity is that vessels do not appear to tear as easily as the axons and surrounding tissue. Treatment is largely supportive with intensive long-term rehabilitation.[30,122]

Penetrating Injuries. A small percentage of pediatric TBI is related to penetrating head trauma. Although injuries from motor vehicle crashes and falls are still leading causes of TBI and death in children, there are other common mechanisms of TBI. These mechanisms include but are not limited to bullets, pellets, knives, pencils, sticks, coat hangers, glass, and objects propelled from lawnmowers.

Initial management for penetrating head trauma is the same as for any TBI: assess and support airway, breathing, and circulation. Once initial vital functions are supported, a CT scan may be obtained to document the involved areas and assist the surgeon in making operative decisions. Any object protruding from the skull should not be removed before surgery—support with gauze and tape will keep it in place. Care should be taken to avoid dislodging the object.

Management usually requires a multidisciplinary approach. Depending on the area of involvement, the surgical team may be composed of specialists in neurosurgery, plastic surgery, maxillofacial surgery, otolaryngology, ophthalmology, and vascular surgery. A medical examiner may be helpful to determine patterns of injury.

Postsurgical management is dependent on the area of injury. Penetrating trauma is often associated with skull fractures, pneumocephalus, SDH, intraventricular hemorrhage, and intraparenchymal hemorrhage. These associated injuries can produce traumatic seizures, cerebral edema, increased ICP, meningitis, or intracranial abscess formation.

BB guns are generally thought to fire with low velocity that will likely cause only superficial injury. As a result, children with these injuries may be discharged from the emergency department without evaluation for intracranial injury. Because serious intracranial injuries (including intraparenchymal hemorrhage) have been documented hours after BB gun injury, it is reasonable to admit children with these injuries for short-term observation.[69,74,92,116]

Inflicted (Intentional/Non-accidental) Injuries and Shaken Baby Syndrome. Shaking injury is the most common form of inflicted (intentional/non-accidental) brain injury in infants up to 12 months of age. The infant's head is large in proportion to the body, and the muscles and ligaments in the neck are immature and weak. Shaken baby syndrome results from a violent whiplash acceleration-deceleration of the head that causes significant brain injury. In some instances there is additional impact injury from striking the infant's head on a hard surface. Brain injuries include subdural or subarachnoid hemorrhages or chronic subdural fluid collections (see Vascular Injuries and Hemorrhage).

Infants with inflicted trauma (including shaken baby syndrome) may present with what appears to be new onset seizures, sudden infant death syndrome, or an apparent life-threatening event (ALTE). The provider should be suspicious of inflicted injuries if the history given by the caretaker does not match the presentation or if there are suspicious findings such as retinal hemorrhages, bilateral chronic subdural hematomas, skull fractures, and significant neurologic injury without external signs of trauma. Many victims die from uncontrollable intracranial hypertension, and survivors may be neurologically devastated.[50,122]

Cerebral Edema. Cerebral edema is an immediate consequence of TBI, intracerebral hemorrhage, or other brain insult. This increase in brain volume can develop up to 72 hours after the injury. Cerebral edema can be categorized into four subsets: cytotoxic, vasogenic, osmotic and interstitial.[83,108] Children may develop any or a combination of these types of cerebral edema following direct cerebral or vascular injury or secondary hypoxia. The pathophysiology of cerebral edema is reviewed in detail in the Increased Intracranial Pressure section earlier in this chapter.

Clinical Signs and Symptoms
The child with head injury requires frequent neurologic examinations and monitoring of neurologic function and responsiveness. Recently, evaluation of cerebral biomarkers

has been shown to be helpful in the identification of head injury.

This section describes the use of serum biomarkers and the clinical signs and symptoms of each of the major forms of head injury. A review of the initial assessment of children with head trauma is included in the following section, Management.

Cerebral Biomarkers. Cerebral biomarkers are proteins that are normally present in low concentrations in the serum and cerebral spinal fluid (CSF), but concentrations increase following specific types of brain injury. Evaluation of these biomarkers can be helpful in establishing the diagnosis and prognosis of pediatric traumatic brain injury (TBI), hypoxic-ischemic encephalopathy (HIE), and TBI from inflicted (intentional/non-accidental) trauma.[72b]

Three cerebral biomarkers shown to be useful in the care of pediatric patients with CNS insults are: neuron specific enolase (NSE), S100-Beta (S100B), and myelin basic protein (MBP).[21b,72a,110a] NSE is a marker of neuronal death, S100B is a marker of astrocyte injury or death and MBP marks axonal injury.[72a]

NSE is only released during cell destruction, and shows different patterns in children with inflicted TBI and HIE versus children with non-inflicted TBI.[72a] The NSE serum concentration peaks early (within 12 hours) after TBI but the rise in serum concentration is delayed (3-5 days) in HIE and inflicted trauma. Bell & Kochanek[21b] suggest that this delay in the rise in NSE could be related to additional apoptosis that occurs following HIE and inflicted trauma. Higher concentrations of NSE are associated with worse outcome following TBI in children.[72a]

MBP is elevated in patients with TBI and inflicted trauma. HIE does not appear to produce elevated levels of MBP.[21b] This is likely related to the fact that the white matter is resistant to ischemic injury while there is greater axonal injury seen in TBI.[21b,110a]

S100Beta (S100B) is a calcium-binding protein molecule that is primarily found in the cytoplasm of cells in the CNS, although it may be present in some non-CNS cells. S100B crosses into the systemic circulation when there is a breech in the blood-brain barrier. It is metabolized by the renal system and excreted in the urine.[110a] The sensitivity and specificity of S100B in separating inflicted versus non-inflicted TBI and in differentiating severe from mild TBI has varied in the relatively small pediatric case series published to date.[72a] In a study by Bechtel et al,[21a] S100B levels were higher in pediatric patients with than without closed head injury (CHI) if the child with CHI presented to the emergency department (ED) within 6 hours of the injury. Although there was a relationship between elevated S100B levels and CHI, S100B may not be the most sensitive and specific screening marker in CHI because the half-life of the protein is approximately 6 hours, an elevated S100B may also be associated with long bone fractures (so it is less useful in patients with multiple trauma), and non-Caucasian children normally have higher levels of S100B proteins than Caucasian children.[21a, 72a]

Biomarkers can be helpful in screening patients with TBI. In combination with the clinical examination, these markers may be useful in establishing the prognosis of head injuries. However, further studies in pediatric patients are needed. If these markers are monitored, the provider must be familiar with the laboratory normal ranges for the biomarker concentrations, and potential causes of elevations in these biomarkers.[110a] Assays for cerebral biomarkers may not be available in all institutions.

Concussion. The patient who sustains a concussion loses consciousness for a variable period of time. This loss of consciousness typically is associated with a brief slowing of respirations (possibly accompanied by apnea), bradycardia, and hypotension. All reflexes should be present after the injury, but some (e.g., corneal or gag reflex) may initially be depressed. The patient may demonstrate reduced response to painful stimuli.[83]

Upon waking, the patient slowly becomes oriented to surroundings (over a period of hours or days) and is gradually able to respond to questions and follow commands. Patients often experience delayed effects of head injury and may suffer temporary memory loss, called posttraumatic amnesia. After a concussion, there is no evidence of further neurologic injury unless a second impact occurs within a few days or weeks (see Contusion). Patients occasionally complain of headache, malaise, vertigo, anxiety, or fatigue for several days or weeks following a concussion. These symptoms, known as *postconcussion syndrome,* may require several weeks to resolve. Injury to the vestibular region may be responsible for symptoms of dizziness and vertigo.[78,125]

Contusion. The clinical signs and symptoms that result from a cerebral contusion are dependent on the extent of the cranial injury, the volume of bleeding present, and the amount of cerebral edema that develops. The associated hemorrhage may be epidural, subdural, or subarachnoid (see Vascular Injuries and Hemorrhage). The resultant cerebral edema can produce increased ICP (see Increased Intracranial Pressure).

Patients who suffer a cerebral contusion may or may not lose consciousness, and they may demonstrate mild motor and sensory weakness or coma. Children may demonstrate a vacant stare or puzzled expression, slurred or incoherent speech, memory deficits, or difficulty focusing, and they may be slow to answer questions or follow commands. Because at least 10% of children with cerebral contusion develop posttraumatic seizures, most are hospitalized for observation after the injury.[50,78]

Second impact syndrome is a rare condition described primarily in athletes who sustain a second head injury after a recent (generally within 7-10 days) concussion. During the days after the concussion, the brain is particularly vulnerable, and repeated injury can cause malignant cerebral edema, hyperemia, intracranial hypertension, and herniation[50] that often occur within minutes and are refractory to most therapy. The mortality of second impact is extremely high. The classic presentation of second impact injury is the athlete who walks off the field without assistance and then abruptly deteriorates into a coma within a few minutes. Attempts to prevent these second impact injuries have led to playing restrictions for athletes who sustain concussions.

Skull Fractures. The clinical signs and symptoms associated with any skull fracture will depend on the location of the fracture and on the extent of the underlying cranial injury. Most skull fractures are diagnosed by radiographic examination rather than by clinical examination, because the vast majority of skull fractures are linear (i.e., the bone fragments remain approximated).

A basilar skull fracture is often not detectable on a radiograph, unless a blood-air level develops in the sphenoid sinus. A CT scan may be required to identify a basilar skull fracture. Approximately 40% of patients with EDH have no identified fractures.[50]

Depressed or compound skull fractures should be suspected whenever the contour of the patient's head is altered or whenever an obvious indentation in the skull is observed or palpated. If a depressed skull fracture is located over the sagittal or lateral sinus, profuse bleeding can develop from injury to these venous channels, and hypovolemic shock can result.

If a basilar skull fracture is present, the patient can develop a CSF leak from the floor of the brain into the nose or ears. Although the CSF leak itself is not harmful, it indicates that communication is present between the upper respiratory tract and the subarachnoid space; this communication increases risk of CNS infection either in the form of meningitis or an intracranial abscess.

Detection of a CSF leak is extremely difficult; various bedside techniques have been described, but none are reliable and all can provide false-positive results. For example, if a yellow halo forms around serosanguineous drainage that has been collected from the nose or ear, the halo is thought to be produced by CSF; however, plasma frequently can produce a similar halo. Nasal or ear drainage can be tested for glucose, because theoretically the presence of glucose in the drainage indicates that CSF is present; however, nasal drainage also can contain glucose. If confirmation of CSF drainage is desired, a sample of the fluid can be sent to the laboratory for a beta-2 transferrin (a protein found only in CSF and perilymph fluid) level. This beta-2 transferrin has >94% sensitivity and 98% specificity, and it has become the gold standard test for detection of CSF leak.[57]

In general, a CSF leak may be present in any child with a basilar skull fracture, so the child with such a skull fracture usually is admitted to the hospital for observation. Signs of deterioration in clinical status or signs of CNS infection (e.g., fever, irritability, nuchal rigidity, leukocytosis) must be reported to an on-call provider immediately. Other signs associated with basilar skull fracture include the presence of ecchymotic lesions over the mastoid (Battle's sign) or around the eyes (raccoon sign), bleeding at the tympanic membrane, and palsies of the first, seventh, and eighth cranial nerves (see Table 11-2).[50,78]

Vascular Injuries and Hemorrhage. The classic presentation of an EDH includes brief loss of consciousness after an injury, regaining consciousness with a lucid interval lasting minutes to several hours, and then abruptly developing a headache, obtundation, ipsilateral pupil dilation, and contralateral hemiparesis. If EDH goes unrecognized and untreated, the child will experience decerebrate posturing, signs of increased ICP, and death. (see the Increased Intracranial Pressure section of this chapter).[35,50] However, fewer than one third of the children sustaining an epidural hematoma lose consciousness and do not awaken spontaneously, and 60% of children with EDH never lose consciousness. Thus, the classic presentation of an EDH occurs infrequently.[50]

The healthcare team should suspect an EDH in any child who develops headache, a rapid deterioration in level of consciousness, a decrease in the hematocrit by 10%, and unilateral pupil dilation. The pupil usually dilates on the same side (ipsilateral) as the injury. However, because an EDH can result from a contrecoup injury, the pupil contralateral to the initial side of impact may dilate. A fever also may be present.[74] As the child's symptoms progress, decerebrate posturing may be observed, and approximately half of involved children develop hemiparesis (usually on the side contralateral to that of pupil dilation). If immediate surgical decompression of the hematoma is not provided, the child will develop bilateral pupil dilation, respiratory depression, bradycardia, apnea, and death from increased ICP.[50,125]

The best diagnostic test to confirm the presence of an EDH is a CT scan. Because the hematoma often is located directly under the skull fracture, plain skull radiographs may be adequate to localize the hematoma in a severely ill child. Most EDHs have the classic biconvex appearance on CT. A small percentage of EDHs have a crescent shape, and resemble an SDH. However, the edges of an EDH are usually sharp and the EDH has uniform density. Because the hematoma develops rapidly, there is almost always mass effect apparent on the CT scan. In rare cases the EDH may be isodense with the brain tissue and IV contrast must be used to identify the hemorrhage.[50]

The patient with an acute SDH may demonstrate bilateral hematomas and evidence of diffuse neurologic injury. Because acute subdural hematomas are associated with underlying parenchymal injury, they are generally considered more lethal than EDHs. Approximately two thirds of all children with SDHs lose consciousness immediately after the cranial trauma. Frequently, the child demonstrates focal signs of injury, such as unilateral pupil dilation, focal seizures, or hemiparesis. Because most of these patients sustain additional cerebral injuries, including cerebral lacerations, contusions, and intracerebral hematomas, intracranial hypertension can develop rapidly and progress to severe levels.

Diagnosis of an acute or chronic SDH can be confirmed with a CT scan or angiography. The acute SDH is a crescent-shaped mass, and edema is usually present. The SDH is usually more diffuse than an EDH, the borders are less sharp, and the EDH may be less isodense because the blood mixes with CSF. Radiographic studies are extremely important because they can help determine the need for surgery.[50]

The patient with a chronic SDH may develop a minor headache, confusion, and a progressive decrease in level of consciousness weeks or months after a relatively minor head injury. Because the hematoma is present for a long period of time, papilledema may be present. The ipsilateral pupil will be large with a sluggish response to light. Hemiparesis and focal seizures can develop.[62] Treatment of chronic subdural hematomas includes seizure control (anticonvulsants), correction of coagulopathies, and surgical evacuation.[50]

The patient with an SAH may experience a sudden onset of a severe headache (the most common symptom and present in nearly all cases), emesis, syncope, meningismus, and photophobia. These symptoms are associated with a rapid rise in ICP. Left untreated, the child will progress to coma and possibly death. Although spontaneous SAHs can arise from a variety of sources, including aneurysms, coagulation disorders, and small artery ruptures, trauma remains the leading cause of an SAH in children. CT scans performed within 48 hours of a hemorrhage will detect the vast majority of subarachnoid hemorrhages. The blood will appear as a white, hyperdense area in the subarachnoid spaces (see Fig. 11–12, B and C).

Complications of SAHs include rebleeding, hydrocephalus, hyponatremia, hypovolemia, arrhythmias, embolism, and seizures. Approximately half of patients with acute hydrocephalus have spontaneous resolution, whereas the remainder if symptomatic may require a ventriculostomy or ventricular shunt. If a ventriculostomy is placed, the recommended range of ICP for drainage is 15 to 25 mm Hg (20-34 cm H$_2$O). Drainage should be gradual to avoid rapid decreases in the ICP that may increase the risk of rebleeding.[50]

Cerebral Edema. Signs of cerebral edema are those associated with increased ICP (see the Increased Intracranial Pressure section earlier in this chapter).

The "Talk and Die" Phenomenon. A small number of children who sustain closed head injury initially are awake and lucid, but then suddenly deteriorate and may develop cerebral herniation and death. This clinical picture may develop in the absence of any mass lesion (such as an EDH) or any initial symptoms of severe injury. This phenomenon has been referred to as the *talk and die injury* or the *pediatric concussion syndrome*.

Most children who "talk and die" sustain a potentially significant head injury; they usually are involved in a motor vehicle crash or a serious fall. Initially the child is alert, with a high GCS score (9 or more). Within 48 hours of the injury there is a sudden deterioration in the child's neurologic status. The child is restless, irritable, or difficult to arouse, with pupil dilation with decreased response to light. Seizures also may be associated with the deterioration.[52]

Postmortem examination reveals the presence of cerebral hyperemia, often associated with multiple cerebral contusions. The ultimate causes of death are cerebral herniation and ischemia. This phenomenon is thought to be related to the rapid development of cerebral swelling following significant head injury. It is important to note that the severity of the head injury may not be discernable from clinical examination, but usually will be apparent on CT scan.

Management

All children with moderate or severe head injury require critical care. Children with mild head injury usually are admitted to the critical or intermediate care unit for skilled continuous nursing observation. Because a small number of patients with apparently minor head injuries may deteriorate acutely as the result of rapid brain swelling and increased ICP, a CT scan is indicated when the child has a history or mechanism of injury consistent with a serious head trauma (e.g., a fall from a significant height, unrestrained occupant in a severe motor vehicle crash). This scan should be performed even if the child initially appears alert and oriented.[50]

All children with serious head trauma are presumed to have a spinal cord injury until it has been ruled out. The cervical spine should be immobilized, and the child should be log rolled whenever turning is necessary. Until definitive radiographic studies and clinical examination can be performed, the nurse must frequently and carefully evaluate the patient's movement and sensation in all four extremities. The development of a progressive neurologic deficit in the patient with a spinal cord injury is a neurosurgical emergency that will require urgent intervention (see Spinal Cord Injury). When assessing movement and sensation, it is important to verify that movement is voluntary and intentional; the reflex withdrawal of an extremity may occur in response to stimulation of a spinal reflex arc despite complete spinal cord transection.

Support of Cardiopulmonary Function. When the child with head trauma is admitted to the critical care unit, the first priority is establishing and maintaining adequate airway, oxygenation, ventilation, and systemic perfusion. Because increased ICP can cause decreased airway protective mechanisms, and because apnea and hypoventilation can cause hypoxia and hypercapnia that will contribute to increased CBF and increased ICP, establishing an effective airway, oxygenation, and ventilation are essential. If there is any doubt about the child's ability to maintain a patent airway or breathe spontaneously, intubation is performed and mechanical ventilation is provided.

If a cervical spine injury has been ruled out, the child's should be placed in a "sniffing" position to prevent upper airway obstruction. If the child is severely injured, intubation is performed and mechanical ventilation provided. Rapid sequence intubation is typically performed to prevent cough and gag and to reduce the risk of vomiting during the intubation (see Chapter 9). A nasogastric tube is inserted to decompress the stomach and prevent vomiting; if a basilar skull fracture or facial fractures are suspected the gastric tube is placed orally.

The entire healthcare team will carefully assess the child's systemic perfusion. Extremities should be warm with pink nail beds and brisk capillary refill. Peripheral pulses should be strong, urine output should average 1-2 mL/kg per hour, and the child's blood pressure should be appropriate for age. (The systolic blood pressure should average 90 mm Hg + twice the child's age for children 1-10 years old.) Hypotension (a systolic blood pressure less than 70 mm Hg + twice the child's age in years) is rarely caused by head injury; if it is present, hypovolemic shock is the likely cause. Tachycardia may indicate the presence of hemorrhage or the development of increased ICP; it also may indicate that the child is frightened, agitated, or in pain.

Hypovolemic shock is treated immediately (see Chapter 6). As soon as possible, at least one large-bore central venous catheter is inserted to allow measurement of the central venous pressure and administration of blood products, colloids, medications, or IV fluids.

Because head trauma frequently is associated with the injury of other major organs, the team will assess for signs of abdominal trauma, hemothorax, flail chest, and pneumothorax (see Chapter 19). Cerebrovascular injury alone usually will not account for a significant blood loss unless a massive intracranial hemorrhage and increased ICP develop. Severe cerebral injury will result in the release of tissue thromboplastin that may produce disseminated intravascular coagulation,[61] which is treated with blood products (see Chapter 15).

The healthcare team will estimate the child's circulating blood volume (approximately 75 mL/kg in infants and children and 70 mL/kg in adolescents), and evaluate blood losses in light of that total estimate. Acute symptomatic traumatic blood loss is replaced immediately. Nurses will total all blood lost or obtained for laboratory analysis, and replacement is considered when blood loss totals 5% to 7% of the child's total circulating blood volume.

Assessment of Neurologic Function. Once adequate cardiopulmonary function has been established, the nurse should perform a careful neurologic assessment. This assessment includes an evaluation of the systemic perfusion and vital signs, including blood pressure, respiratory function, and level of consciousness (including the ability to follow commands, pupil size and response to light) and a careful assessment of motor activity and reflexes (see Box 11-2).

The healthy child will be awake, alert, and frightened in the hospital. The comatose child demonstrates no verbal response to external stimuli. To evaluate neurologic function and responsiveness, a standard rating scale, such as the GCS, should be applied in a consistent fashion by everyone who examines the child with head injury (see Table 11-6).

The child's pupil size and constrictive response to light should be evaluated frequently. The pupils normally are equal in size and constrict briskly and equally to light. Consensual pupil constriction also should be present (i.e., the right pupil constricts when light is shined into the left eye). High doses of morphine sulfate can cause pupil constriction, and high doses of atropine and atrovent can produce pupil dilation. The presence of fixed and dilated pupils during the initial evaluation of the child with a head injury often is regarded as a poor prognostic sign; however, children who have fixed pupils after a head injury have a better rate of recovery than do adults.[26]

Although the classic Cushing's triad (bradycardia, elevation in systolic blood pressure with widening of pulse pressure, and irregular respirations, including apnea) indicates the development of a severe increase in ICP, children rarely demonstrate such classic findings unless cerebral herniation is occurring. Often, the child exhibits tachycardia and hypertension. The widening of the pulse pressure and irregular respirations are typically late signs of deterioration in neurologic status.

Report the presence of any seizures to an on-call provider, and protect the child from injury during any seizure activity. A significant risk (30%-40%) of posttraumatic seizures is associated with the following conditions: severe head injury,

diffuse cerebral edema, acute subdural hematoma, or an open depressed skull fracture with parenchymal damage.[50] The routine use of prophylactic anticonvulsants has not been shown to prevent the development of seizures.

Status epilepticus should be reported and treated immediately, because it compromises CBF.[58] Any abnormal posturing, such as decorticate posturing or decerebrate rigidity (see Fig. 11-9), should also be reported to an on-call provider.

As soon as the patient's condition is stable, the nurse should attempt to evaluate the child's cranial nerve function (see Table 11-2 and Box 11-2), and notify the on-call provider if any cranial nerve function is absent.

Key reflexes evaluated during critical care are the cough and gag reflex and the corneal reflex. The child should demonstrate a cough during suctioning of the airway, and a gag is typically observed during insertion of an orogastric or nasogastric tube. If the corneal reflex is intact, stroking of the eyelashes or the outer edge of the child's eye with a sterile cotton applicator will cause a blink. If this blink is absent, the brain stem is probably injured, and the child will require the regular application of ophthalmic ointment and eye patching to prevent corneal drying and lacerations.

When the child's condition is stable, CT scan, MRI and skull radiography may be performed to aid in the evaluation of the extent of the head injury (see Diagnostic Tests, later in this chapter). A nurse should always accompany the child to the CT scan to monitor the child's level of consciousness and to monitor and support cardiorespiratory function. Appropriate resuscitation equipment and medications should accompany the patient. If the child is extremely unstable with an elevated ICP, a provider who can perform intubation and direct management of increased ICP should accompany the nurse and the patient.

Increased ICP following head injury is treated with support of oxygenation and normocarbia, sedatives, analgesics, paralytics, and hyperosmolar therapy (e.g., hypertonic saline, mannitol); if refractory elevation in ICP is present, the child may be placed in a barbiturate coma. Diuretic therapy and therapeutic hypothermia currently are controversial, because clear benefit has not yet been documented from these therapies in children with TBI. (See Management in the Increased Intracranial Pressure section of this chapter.)

Throughout the child's care, the nurse must be alert for signs of increased ICP (see Increased Intracranial Pressure). The sudden appearance of irritability, confusion, lethargy, and pupil dilation must be reported to a physician or other on-call provider immediately. Emergency acute management of sudden increases in ICP requires immediate intervention with support of the airway, oxygenation, and ventilation and administration of mannitol (0.5-1 gm/kg IV) or 3% saline (3-5 mL/kg IV bolus), or both. A CT scan is typically performed to detect any mass lesion requiring surgical intervention; the CT scan also will enable the evaluation of cerebral edema (see Fig. 11-12).[20]

Poor prognostic findings following pediatric head injury include the following (assuming normothermia is present): cardiovascular instability despite adequate shock resuscitation, absence of spontaneous respirations, fixed pupils, flaccid extremities with no response to painful stimuli, the presence of diabetes insipidus on admission, severe disseminated intravascular coagulation and elevation of fibrinogen on admission, a GCS score of 4 or less, and persistent elevation in ICP (>20 mm Hg).[61]

Children who have an initial GCS score >8 usually have good long term outcomes, and those children with initial GCS score of 3-4 have significantly higher morbidity and mortality. Overall, children with head injuries have better outcomes than the adults with similar injuries, and a child's neurocognitive function may continue to improve for years after the initial injury.[61]

Temperature Control. In recent years, there has been increasing interest in the use of therapeutic hypothermia for children with TBI. In a large multicenter trial conducted by Hutchison and others, hypothermia initiated within 8 hours of injury and continued for 24 hours did not improve either survival or neurologic outcome in the pediatric patient.[63] There were significantly more hypotensive episodes and lower average CPP in the hypothermic group, necessitating the use of inotropic drugs and fluid boluses. An earlier study of hypothermia in adult patients with TBI also failed to show improvement in survival or neurologic outcomes,[33] although results of another study are anticipated.[34] Additional pediatric hypothermia trials are in progress. Current recommendations for children are to maintain normothermia, avoid or rapidly treat hyperthermia, and consider therapeutic hypothermia for refractory intracranial hypertension.[11,96]

Supportive Care. The healthcare team will assess all major organ systems in the child with TBI (see Chapter 19) and assess the child's airway, oxygenation, ventilation, and perfusion at regular intervals and whenever the child's neurologic condition changes. Once the child's condition is stable, more complete examinations are performed to look for fractures or major lacerations that may require sutures. The examinations include inspection of the skin and body for signs of edema, contusions, petechiae, or hematomas and palpation of the scalp for evidence of depressed or compound skull fractures.

The child's skin and rectal temperature must be monitored closely; a high rectal temperature and low skin temperature can indicate poor systemic perfusion, and fever can indicate EDH or infection. Fever is treated with antipyretics and a cooling blanket if needed. Hypothermia may develop in children with severe head injury; however, hyperthermia blankets or warming lights should be used only to restore normothermia (or a temperature slightly below normal) while avoiding hyperthermia.

A urinary catheter is inserted whenever multisystem trauma or shock is present, unless blood is present at the urinary meatus, which suggests a urethral tear (see Chapter 19). Report any difficulty inserting the catheter or the presence of bloody urine to an on-call provider immediately, because these findings can indicate the presence of genitourinary trauma. The child's urine output normally averages 1 mL/kg per hour if fluid intake is adequate. Inadequate urine output can be caused by prerenal failure (e.g., inadequate systemic perfusion), renal failure (e.g., renal ischemic tubular injury or renal contusion), or postrenal failure (e.g., urethral obstruction).

Oliguria requires immediate investigation and prompt treatment of the cause (see Chapter 13). As noted previously, hypertonic saline or hyperosmotic agents may be administered if increased ICP develops.

During the initial assessment and treatment of the child with head trauma, a nurse, social services member, chaplain or other resource typically remains with the parents to answer questions at the bedside. Although it can be difficult for the nurse to arrange the time to speak with the parents, brief updates are extremely helpful. Most parents understand the need for the nurse to focus attention on the physical care of the child. The parents often are reassured to see the careful treatment their child receives, seeing that every effort is being undertaken to stabilize and care for their child.

Injury-Specific Management. Once the child is stable, treatment of the child's specific injury is undertaken. The following information includes the specific management of the most common forms of pediatric TBI.

Concussion. Concussions are not associated with abnormalities on a CT scan, and they usually require no treatment. However, because the history of loss of consciousness followed by recovery and responsiveness also can be consistent with that of the development of an EDH, the child with concussion is often admitted to the hospital for observation. As noted earlier, children occasionally complain of headache, dizziness, malaise, and fatigue for days or weeks following a concussion. It is important that the parents be aware of this postconcussion syndrome so that the child will not be suspected of malingering. However, the healthcare team should not suggest to the child that symptoms are an expected part of the child's behavior.

Contusion. The appropriate treatment of a cerebral contusion is determined by the extent of the primary cerebral injury and the severity of secondary injuries, such as hemorrhage or cerebral edema. Treatment of skull fractures, EDHs, SDHs, and SAHs is reviewed in the sections immediately following. Approximately 10% of children with a cerebral contusion will develop posttraumatic seizures beginning hours, months, or years after the head injury.[78]

Skull Fractures. Most children with simple or linear skull fractures require no treatment. However, children should be observed carefully for signs of the development of an EDH or SDH.[50]

Depressed skull fractures are elevated surgically if the skull fragment is 5 mm or more (or a distance greater than the thickness of the skull) below the contour of the skull or if serious underlying cerebral injury or hemorrhage is present. Depressed skull fractures also can be elevated surgically for cosmetic reasons. Before any surgery is performed, the child's cardiorespiratory status is assessed thoroughly and shock resuscitation is provided, if needed. If the depressed skull fracture is located near the sagittal or lateral sinus, this venous channel might tear, causing profuse external or intracranial bleeding. In such a case, treatment of hypovolemic shock will be required (see Shock in Chapter 6). Immediate surgical control of the bleeding site is also necessary. The surgeon will elevate the depressed bone fragment and debride the wound in the operating suite.

When a compound (open, depressed) skull fracture is present, surgical elevation and repair is necessary. Because portions of the scalp or other foreign material can enter the wound and the intracranial space, the wound is carefully debrided. In addition, the surgeon will repair any dural tears.

Children with basilar skull fractures are hospitalized for observation. Because CSF drainage from the nose or ear indicates communication between the subarachnoid space and the nasal passages or external ear, such children are at risk for developing meningitis or intracranial abscess formation. Antibiotic therapy in CSF leaks is reserved for patients who show symptoms of CNS infection. The head of the patient's bed is typically kept level, unless the ICP is elevated, in an effort to decrease pressure and allow the CSF leak to spontaneously seal. In some cases, a lumbar drain can be placed in an effort to decrease pressure and allow the CSF leak to seal. Most CSF leaks will seal spontaneously within a few weeks, but occasionally children develop a chronic CSF leak as the result of entrapment of the dura between skull fragments during healing. This leak increases risk of meningitis and eventually will require surgical repair.

If a basilar skull fracture or head injury with facial bone fractures is present, the nurse should not attempt to insert a nasogastric tube, because as the tube may be directed intracerebrally. An orally inserted gastric tube is appropriate in this situation (see Chapter 19). Prophylactic antibiotics are frequently given if pneumocephalus is detected on the CT scan. Facial fractures involving the sinus cavities or producing pneumocephalus indicate a dural breach and are associated with increased risk of meningitis or abscess formation. Vaccines are given for pneumococcal and meningococcal meningitis prophylaxis.[74]

Intracranial hematoma and other forms of significant cerebral injury frequently are associated with a skull fracture.[50,78] Any child admitted with a skull fracture must be closely monitored for seizures, evidence of hemorrhage, or increased ICP.

Vascular Injuries. When the child with an EDH demonstrates a sudden decreased level of consciousness, immediate surgical decompression of the hematoma is required. A CT scan will assist in the diagnosis of an epidural hematoma before deterioration in the child's clinical status.[50,78] Before surgery the child requires treatment of increased ICP. After surgery many patients will demonstrate elevation in ICP, requiring aggressive medical management.[50] The perioperative mortality is proportional to the degree of neurologic deterioration that develops preoperatively; if surgical decompression is performed before significant herniation or pupil dilation occurs, perioperative mortality is typically less than 10%.[50] If, however, significant elevation in ICP, brain herniation, and ischemia develop before surgical relief is provided, perioperative morbidity and mortality will be high.[50]

The patient with an acute SDH requires careful assessment for and prevention of increased ICP. Generally, small subdural hematomas do not require surgical intervention; however, surgery may be considered if a large, acute SDH is producing significant signs of increased ICP (i.e., the hematoma is creating a significant mass effect exceeding that produced by cerebral edema or if a midline shift is present). Immediate surgical evacuation of a symptomatic hematoma is warranted if it is >5 mm at the thickest point. A delay in surgical intervention increases mortality to approximately 90%.[50]

Often, children with an SDH also have diffuse hyperemia and vasogenic cerebral edema that can be aggravated by surgery and will continue to progress even after removal of the hematoma. These children will require aggressive management of increased ICP. Because extremely high ICP has been recorded in both surgically treated and untreated patients, initiation of a barbiturate coma may be indicated.[83,108]

Mortality following an SDH is significant, and both morbidity and mortality seem to be closely related to the patient's level of consciousness at the time of surgery (if operated) and the degree and duration of intracranial hypertension.

The child with an SAH can develop a rapid increase in ICP requiring aggressive medical management. The presence of blood in the subarachnoid space can interfere with CSF reabsorption. As a result, children with an SAH are at risk for developing communicating hydrocephalus days or weeks after the injury.

Intracerebral hemorrhage can be the most damaging form of cerebral vascular injury, because it results in a rapid increase in ICP and in direct damage to surrounding brain tissue. When the diagnosis of an intracerebral hematoma (clot) with a mass effect is confirmed by CT scan or arteriography, surgery is performed immediately. The bleeding site is controlled, the clot is evacuated, and the area is debrided. Cerebral contusions are rarely removed, but they can contribute to the development of increased ICP. Postoperative management often is complicated by increased ICP, seizures, and motor or sensory deficits.[62,96,110]

Cerebral Edema. Children with head injury usually develop hyperemic cerebral edema for 24 to 48 hours after the injury. In addition, direct cerebral injury may produce vasogenic cerebral edema, and cytotoxic cerebral edema can result from hypoxia secondary to hypovolemic shock.[83] Therefore, children with TBI are at risk for increased ICP and should be transferred to or cared for at a trauma center with experience in pediatric ICP monitoring and the management of intracranial hypertension. Medical and nursing management of this complication has been discussed previously.

Psychosocial Support. Children with head injury can be extremely agitated as the result of fear, pain, or increased ICP. It is important that the nurse be able to provide calm, efficient care, including assessment and physical and emotional support. The nurse is also the best person to recognize changes in the child's level of consciousness and separate these signs from those produced by fear, pain, or sleep deprivation.

The parents may feel extremely guilty if the child's injury occurred during a motor vehicle crash while they were driving the car, or if the child was injured from a preventable fall or sports activity. Parents often are inclined to think that they could or should have prevented the injury. If the child's injury is inflicted, the parents may feel distraught and guilty. If inflicted injury is suspected, the hospital child abuse team must be notified immediately so that the child is protected throughout recovery, documentation is accurate and complete, family support is provided and appropriate legal action is taken.

Children with TBI require close follow up care and appropriate referrals for supportive care after discharge. Many children demonstrate functional morbidity following TBI and may have difficulty returning to school, behavioral problems, sleep disturbances, and discipline problems.

Poor outcomes are thought to be closely related to periods of uncontrolled intracranial hypertension and inadequate cerebral perfusion. As a result, it is imperative that the nurse notify an on-call provider of sharp or prolonged increases in ICP or hypotensive episodes that lead to a prolonged decrease in calculated CPP.[123]

If the child's neurologic status deteriorates and the child dies, the parents require compassionate and consistent preparation and support (see Brain Death and Organ Donation in this chapter and in Chapter 3, and Withholding and Withdrawing Therapy in Chapter 24).

Spinal Cord Injury

Etiology

Any trauma victim can sustain spinal cord injury (SCI). Traumatic SCI can be primary or can result from a secondary insult. The mechanisms most commonly associated with pediatric SCI include falls and pedestrian-related motor vehicle crashes. In adolescents, motor vehicle crashes, sports and diving injuries and gunshot wounds are common causes of SCI. Intentional injury may also cause SCI.

Pathophysiology

The young child's head is large and heavy in proportion to the rest of the body. The child ejected from or struck by a car often is propelled head-first into the ground or another object, and resulting hyperextension or flexion of the neck is likely to produce cervical spine injury. Flexion-rotation or hyperflexion injuries can cause dislocation or locking of the facets (articulation surfaces) of two contiguous vertebrae with resulting spinal cord compression.

The cervical spine is relatively unstable and is still developing in young children. As a result, SCI patterns in children differ from those in adults. The ligaments along the child's cervical vertebrae are relatively lax, and the paraspinous muscles are incompletely developed. The child's vertebral bodies are wedge-shaped and not completely ossified. In addition, the facet joints of the cervical vertebrae are relatively flat. For these reasons, the vertebrae can shift several centimeters during injury or the application of force to the spine, resulting in spinal cord injury without evidence of injury to the vertebrae. Although the pediatric spine is relatively more elastic than the adult spine, it will be injured if significant cervical subluxation occurs (Fig. 11-19).

The most common areas of SCI in children younger than 9 years include the atlas, axis, and upper cervical spine. Generally, ligamentous injuries are more common than bone injuries. In patients older than 9 years, injury patterns resemble those of the adult, with less cervical involvement.[123]

Pediatric spinal cord injuries occur when vertebral bodies are fractured, or when vertebral subluxation (partial dislocation) occurs. Subluxation results in anteroposterior misalignment of contiguous vertebrae, with narrowing of the spinal canal and spinal cord compression. Young children are likely to sustain subluxation injuries without associated fractures. The severity of the neurologic deficit is related to the location and severity of the subluxation.[123]

The neurologic dysfunction associated with SCI can result from the injury itself or from secondary compromise of spinal cord perfusion (ischemia or infarction), edema and necrosis. In laboratory experiments, SCI produces altered permeability of neuron membranes, electrolyte flux across the membranes, and the release of catecholamines and endorphins. Vasospasm and thrombosis in spinal cord vessels can contribute to ischemia, infarction, and dysfunction.[91]

Severe traumatic cervical spine injury (especially to the upper cervical spine) usually produces respiratory arrest at the scene of the injury, and the patient dies unless immediate resuscitation is provided. Occasionally, children with a cervical spinal injury sustain injury to the cervical vertebrae, rendering them unstable. These children can move all four extremities and breathe at the scene of the accident; however, if the cervical spine is not immobilized (particularly during intubation), spinal cord injury, respiratory arrest, and tetraplegia can result.

If a spinal cord injury is mild or moderate, complete recovery of neurologic function is possible despite the presence of complete neurologic deficit on admission.[123] However, if the initial insult is severe (particularly if severe subluxation occurred) or is associated with the development of edema, permanent loss of function and sensation below the level of injury can occur.

Traumatic atlantooccipital dislocation is the disruption of the supporting ligaments between the skull and the vertebral column, occurring in a transverse or vertical direction and resulting in complete transection of the spinal cord. Although this type of SCI is rare in children and adolescents, traumatic atlantooccipital dislocation is seen in infants and toddlers. Most children do not survive this initial insult, but as prehospital care has improved over recent years there are reports of survival when immediate CPR is provided at the scene or emergency responders arrive within a few minutes of the injury.[123]

Clinical Signs and Symptoms

Physical Examination. Approximately half of all children with SCIs demonstrate signs of neurologic deficit on initial examination.[123] The most consistent sign of SCI is the loss of some or all movement and sensation below the level of injury. The degree of deficit is used to assess the severity of injury. Complete injury is present if the child demonstrates complete absence of all movement and sensation below the level of injury. Rectal sphincter tone is also lost. Partial injury is present if the child demonstrates transient weakness or paresthesias.[123] Careful repeated clinical evaluation of movement and sensation in all extremities must be performed until definitive studies are completed, because many children demonstrate a delayed onset of symptoms.[123]

The clinical signs of cervical SCI include the development of respiratory depression or apnea and weakness in the upper arms. Complete cervical spine injury is associated with flaccid paralysis (usually tetraplegia) and anesthesia below the level of the injury. Paradoxic respirations may be observed if an

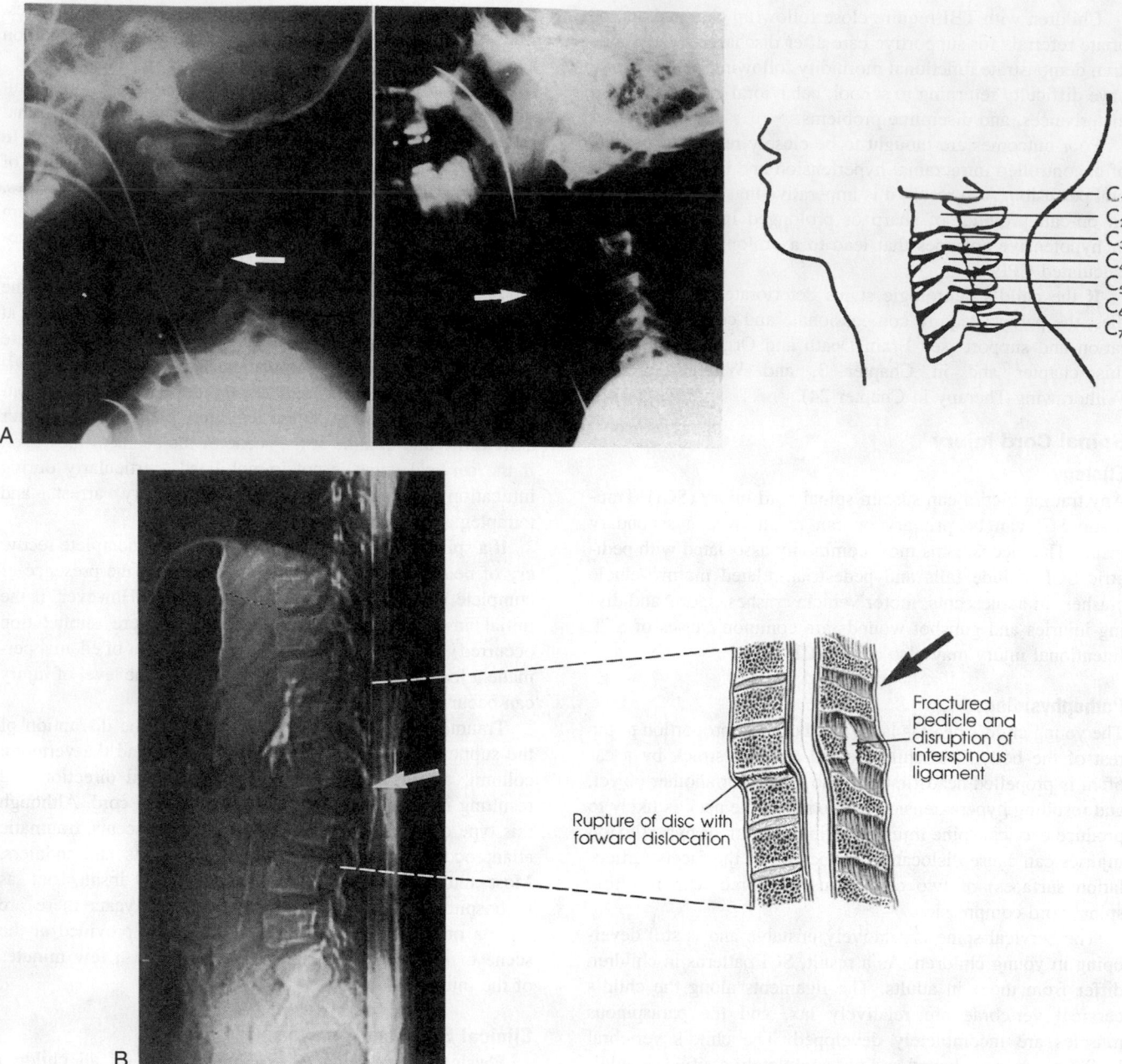

FIG. 11-19 Spinal cord injury. Many injuries resulting in spinal cord damage produce visible radiographic changes, although a significant number (20%-60%) are not associated with any skeletal fracture or dislocation. **A,** Lateral cervical spine radiographs demonstrating skeletal abnormalities associated with cervical spine injury. The first radiograph is from a 4 year old who was restrained in a car seat that was not anchored in the car. The separation between the fifth and sixth cervical vertebrae is subtle but detectable (arrow), especially when compared with the line drawing of normal anatomy (far right). Radiopaque orogastric and nasogastric tubes are visible; they are slightly displaced anteriorly, indicating a small amount of edema surrounding the spinal cord injury. The location of the injury is unusual for this age. The second radiograph shows a 5-year-old pedestrian struck by an automobile and demonstrates significant separation between the first and second cervical vertebrae. This is a more common site of cervical spine injury in young children. Note the anterior displacement of the nasogastric tube (*arrow*) produced by edema surrounding the injury. An endotracheal tube is present but not visible. The line drawing depicts normal cervical spinal anatomy in a 3- to 4-year-old child. **B,** This scan film performed before a computed tomography scan demonstrates lumbar vertebral and spinal cord trauma associated with a lap belt injury. Separation of the lumbar vertebrae can be seen (arrow) and resulted in paraplegia. This injury resulted from flexion of the lumbar spine (see drawing).

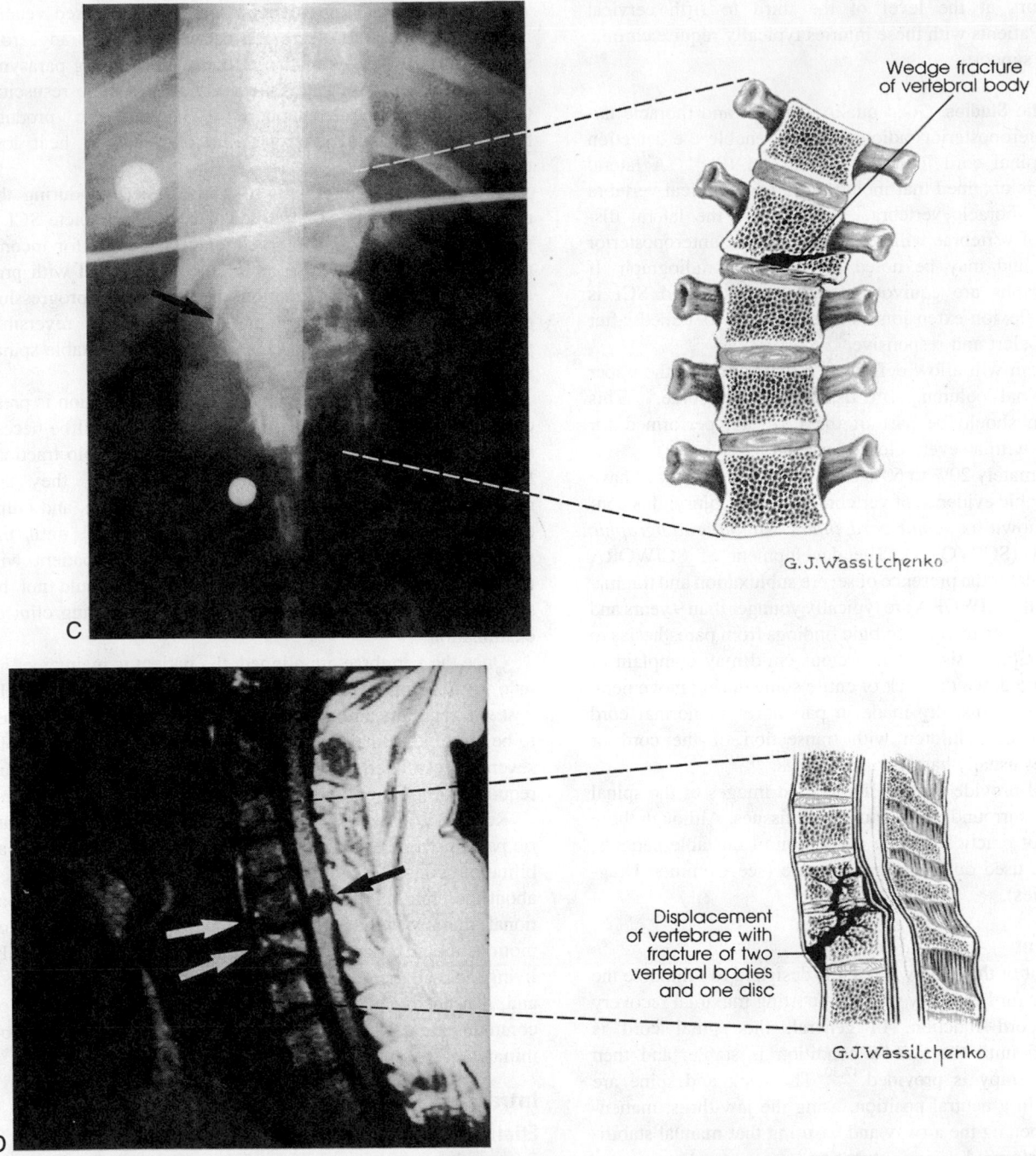

Wedge fracture
of vertebral body

G.J.Wassilchenko

Displacement
of vertebrae with
fracture of two
vertebral bodies
and one disc

G.J.Wassilchenko

FIG 11.19, cont'd C, Flexion injury of the lower thoracic vertebrae and spine is visible on this anteroposterior chest radiograph. This radiograph shows an unrestrained 16-year-old driver who was thrown from the car. The lateral flexion resulted in compression of the spinal cord and fracture of the thoracic vertebrae (see *arrow* and corresponding illustration). The rod placed during surgery is visible. **D,** This magnetic resonance imagery scan shows in detail the skeletal and spinal damage resulting from a flexion-rotation injury. This 16-year-old motorcycle driver sustained displacement of two vertebrae (white arrows) and fracture of two vertebrae and one disc. Resulting compression of the cervical spine produced a complete spinal cord injury. A contusion is visible in the spinal cord *(black arrow)*. The line drawing depicts the injury. (A, courtesy Carol Gilbert and John Feldenzer, Roanoke, Va. Drawing reproduced from Riviello JJ, et al: Delayed cervical central cord syndrome after trivial trauma, *Pediatr Emerg Care* 6:116, 1990. B, courtesy Bennett Blumenkopf, Vanderbilt University Medical Center, Nashville, Tenn. Line drawing reproduced from Rudy EB: *Advanced neurological and neurosurgical nursing,* St Louis, 1984, Mosby. C, courtesy Noel Tulipan, Vanderbilt University Medical Center, Nashville, Tenn. Illustration reproduced from Rudy EB: *Advanced neurological and neurosurgical nursing,* St Louis, 1984, Mosby. D, courtesy Bennett Blumenkopf, Vanderbilt University, Nashville, Tenn. Line drawing reproduced from Rudy EB: *Advanced neurological and neurosurgical nursing,* St Louis, 1984, Mosby.)

injury occurs at the level of the third to fifth cervical vertebrae. Patients with these injuries typically require chronic ventilatory support.

Diagnostic Studies. Good quality cervical and thoracic lateral and anteroposterior radiographs will enable the detection of many spinal cord injuries (see Fig. 11-19).[123] A lateral radiograph is obtained that includes the first cervical vertebra to the first thoracic vertebra.[6] Occasionally the lateral displacement of vertebrae will be apparent on the anteroposterior radiograph and may be noted on the chest radiograph. If the radiographs are equivocal, or if nonvisualized SCI is suspected, flexion-extension radiographs are obtained after the child is alert and responsive.[50]

A CT scan will allow definitive visualization of the upper cervical spinal column, soft tissue, and vertebrae.[50] This examination should be part of the CT scan performed for every child with a severe closed head injury.

Approximately 20% to 60% of children with SCIs will have no radiographic evidence of vertebral or spinal injury; this condition is known as *spinal cord injury without radiographic abnormality* (SCIWORA). The development of SCIWORA usually indicates the presence of severe subluxation and trauma. Children with SCIWORA are typically younger than 9 years and exhibit a wide range of neurologic findings from paresthesias to weakness or paralysis. The conscious child may complain of pain radiating down the neck or entire spine during movement. Full recovery is usually made in patients with normal cord signals, whereas children with transection of the cord or hemorrhages usually have poor outcomes.[123]

MRI will provide beautifully detailed images of the spinal cord and all surrounding structures and tissues. Although these scans are not practical for the evaluation of unstable patients, they can be used during follow-up care (see Common Diagnostic Studies).

Management

Management of the child with SCI is designed to minimize the potential for further injury while supporting maximal recovery of spinal cord function. In general, the spinal cord is immobilized until the child's condition is stable, and then definitive therapy is provided.[47,50] The neck and spine are maintained in a neutral position, using the jaw-thrust maneuver when opening the airway and ensuring that manual stabilization is performed during intubation.

Steroid administration is advocated within the first 8 hours after injury to prevent secondary spinal cord edema and inflammation. A Cochrane meta-analysis of three studies documented that large dose methylprednisolone administration (a bolus dose of 30 mg/kg, followed by continuous infusion of 5.4 mg/kg per hour for 23 hours) significantly increased functional recovery of adult patients with SCI.[28] Although this steroid administration has now become standard,[50] controlled trials of this therapy have not been performed in children. There are no class I data to support the use of steroids in children younger than 18 years with SCI, and it should be avoided in children with brain injury.[13,123]

Children with SCI require close observation for signs of neurogenic shock. These children experience a loss of

vasomotor tone leading to venous pooling, decreased venous return, and ultimately decreased cardiac output. Bradycardia results from loss of sympathetic tone with resulting parasympathetic dominance. Management includes volume resuscitation and vasopressor support. SCI will also produce hypothermia, because the vasodilation leads to heat loss through the skin.

Urgent surgical intervention is rarely needed during the acute management of SCI, particularly when complete SCI is present. Urgent surgical intervention is indicated for incomplete SCI with compromise or for incomplete SCI with progressive neurologic dysfunction, because such progression often indicates the presence of an emerging but reversible problem, such as an epidural hematoma, or an unstable spinal injury.[50]

If a cervical spine injury is unstable or subluxation is present, immobilization and alignment of the spine will be necessary through the use of Gardner-Wells tongs or halo traction. If the vertebral bodies are not reduced (i.e., they are misaligned), weight is added to the traction device, and clinical and radiographic examinations are repeated until the vertebrae are realigned or reduced. The alert patient will require analgesia during this procedure, but should not be sedated because the child must be responsive during clinical examination.[50,123]

Once the vertebrae are aligned, the patient is maintained in halo traction for several weeks. In children, the use of a halo vest will facilitate ambulation.[50] If the area of injury continues to be unstable, spinal fusion occasionally is required, possibly several weeks later. Surgical stabilization is most likely to be required for children with SCI who are younger than 3 years.

Rehabilitation services should begin as soon as the pediatric patient with a SCI is stable. A physical medicine and rehabilitation consult should be obtained to provide guidance about the child's long term care needs. Physical and occupational therapy will be beneficial in maintaining range of motion, mobilization and integration into activities of daily living. Speech therapists will evaluate tolerance of oral intake and, if needed, can assist in providing alternative methods of communication. A bowel and bladder regimen should be initiated early and re-evaluated on a routine basis.

Intracranial Tumors
Etiology
Primary brain tumors are one of the most common forms of cancer in children, and medulloblastoma is the most common malignant brain tumor. Survival from brain tumors has now risen from approximately 60% in the 1980s to 80% to 85% in recent years.[98] This improved survival can be attributed to earlier and more complete tumor resection (particularly for medulloblastomas) as well as more aggressive and targeted chemotherapy and radiation therapy. The involvement of the disease at presentation, the amount of tumor resection possible, and tumor grades are part of the prognostic factors involved in the outcomes of most brain tumors (e.g., ependymoma).[21]

Tumors are abnormal masses that can arise from any tissue in the body. Their cause is unknown, although the role of hereditary factors and environmental carcinogens continues to be explored. Although few tumors are present from birth, many tumors of childhood arise from the inappropriate development of primitive neuroepithelial cells. Astrocytomas are the most common primary intraaxial brain tumor, and pilocytic astrocytomas typically manifest in the second decade of life.[50]

Pathophysiology

Intracranial tumors in children produce an increase in intracranial volume; unless the skull can expand commensurately, the child will develop increased ICP. In addition, the tumor causes compression of the surrounding brain tissue, compromising important cerebral functions.

Tumors are classified according to their location, degree of malignancy, and histologic features. Classification by location is used here because it enables more straightforward prediction of the clinical consequences of tumor expansion and the possibility and risks of surgical tumor excision (Box 11-11).

Supratentorial tumors involve the cerebral hemispheres and all structures located above the tentorium cerebelli. Infratentorial tumors are those that involve the brain stem and cerebral structures located below the tentorium cerebelli.

Classification of tumors by cell type allows some predictions about the speed of tumor growth and spread and about recurrence risks. It is important to note that intracranial tumors in children may be malignant by position as well as by cell type. This means that the tissue itself is not malignant, but tumor growth can compress or erode vital brain tissue, resulting in serious neurologic compromise or death.

In the following section, the most common intracranial tumors in children are described. This description includes the clinical consequences of tumor growth.

Supratentorial Tumors. The two most common supratentorial tumors in children are the astrocytoma and the craniopharyngioma. The astrocytoma is the most common of all supratentorial tumors accounting for approximately 12,000 new cases per year.[50] This tumor arises from abnormal proliferation of the cerebral astrocytes. Astrocytomas can develop in

---

Box 11-11	**Pediatric Central Nervous System Tumors Classified By Location**

1. Supratentorial
   a. Hemispheres: astrocytoma, sarcoma, meningioma
   b. Midline tumors: craniopharyngioma, optic glioma, pinealoma, ependymoma
2. Infratentorial
   a. Cerebellar and fourth ventricle: astrocytoma, medulloblastoma, ependymoma
   b. Brainstem: brainstem glioma
3. Spinal cord tumors: ependymoma, astrocytoma
4. Generalized disease with brain tumor components: von Recklinghausen disease, tuberous sclerosis, Sturge-Weber disease, von Hippel-Lindau disease, ataxia telangiectasia, nevoid basal cell carcinoma syndrome
5. Metastatic tumors

From Van Eys J: Malignant tumors of the central nervous system. In Sutow WW, Fernbach DJ, and Vietti TJ, editors: *Clinical pediatric oncology*, ed 3, St Louis, 1984, Mosby.

---

the frontal, temporal, and central parietal areas of the cerebral hemispheres, and tumor growth can extend across the corpus callosum from one parietal lobe to the other. These tumors also can invade the brainstem or third ventricle and may cause hydrocephalus.[50]

Astrocytomas can grow slowly or rapidly. Tumor specimens are typically graded on a scale of one to four according to the degree of cell differentiation present in the tumor.[50] When an astrocytoma is located above the tentorium, it is usually diffuse and expands into surrounding tissue or along long nerve fiber tracts. Expansion through metastases (transfer to other organs) is rare.

The craniopharyngioma is responsible for approximately 4% of all intracranial tumors in children and generally occurs between the ages of 5 and 10 years.[50] It results from the growth of displaced neuroepithelial cells. The tumor consists of a solid mass or cyst that contains fluid, cellular debris, and calcified material. It develops within or just above the sella turcica (the skull pouch containing the pituitary) or within the third ventricle. As the craniopharyngioma grows, it can obstruct the foramen of Monro, producing hydrocephalus, or it can compress the optic chiasm, the pituitary, or the hypothalamus, producing visual disturbances, fever, hypoglycemia, diabetes insipidus (DI), or occasional hypotension.[50]

Infratentorial Tumors. Infratentorial tumors account for nearly two thirds of all pediatric brain tumors and for nearly half of all tumors in children.[50] These tumors are typically detected early in their development because they can rapidly produce changes in vital body functions. The most common forms of infratentorial tumors in children are medulloblastomas, astrocytomas, ependymomas, and brain stem gliomas.

The medulloblastoma accounts for 15% to 20% of all intracranial tumors and one fourth of primary intracranial tumors in children.[50] It is the most malignant of the posterior fossa tumors because it grows rapidly and tends to recur after surgical excision. The tumor rises from neuroepithelial cells located in the roof of the fourth ventricle, so it may cause early development of hydrocephalus.[50] The tumor is usually a soft, gray mass that extends from the medulla along CSF pathways into the fourth ventricle, subarachnoid space, third ventricle, or spinal column. Symptoms include stiff neck or neck pain, increased ICP, obstructive hydrocephalus, ataxia, and fatigue. Hypotension or hypertension can result from compression of the medulla, and backache, limb weakness, or loss of bladder control will indicate spinal cord involvement. Medulloblastomas occur most commonly in children in the first decade of life. Five-year survival rates vary widely in published reports (21%-70%), but late relapses do occur.[50]

Astrocytomas also can grow in the brain stem, although they usually are confined to the pons. They produce sequential and multiple cranial nerve palsies, ataxia, and pyramidal (voluntary movement) dysfunction; headache and diplopia also occur frequently. The mean age at diagnosis of brainstem astrocytoma is 7 years. Five-year survival is approximately 40% despite aggressive chemotherapy and radiation therapy.[50]

Ependymomas account for approximately 5% to 6% of all intracranial tumors in children.[50] This tumor rises from neuroepithelial cells, and it forms a fleshy gray mass that most frequently obstructs the fourth ventricle, producing hydrocephalus and cranial nerve palsies. These tumors can occur anywhere along the neuraxis.[50]

Brain stem gliomas are cysts that compress the cranial nerves, the pons, and medulla. If the glioma expands into the cerebellum, relatively large tumor growth can be accommodated without symptoms of cerebellar compression. The first symptoms of the brain stem glioma are usually those of cranial nerve dysfunction. Initially, compression of the abducens nerve (sixth cranial nerve) will cause nystagmus, facial nerve (seventh cranial nerve) compression will cause a facial palsy, and oculovestibular nerve (eighth cranial nerve) compression will result in hearing loss. As the glossopharyngeal and vagus nerves (ninth and tenth cranial nerves) become involved, the child will develop hoarseness and experience difficulty in swallowing. Increased ICP develops during the terminal stages of tumor expansion, producing headache, vomiting, and other signs of intracranial hypertension. The prognosis of this tumor is extremely poor, and most children with malignant brainstem gliomas die within 6 to 12 months of diagnosis. Treatment is usually not surgical, and a biopsy should not be performed if there is diffuse infiltrating brainstem lesion.[50]

Spinal cord tumors account for approximately 15% of all primary CNS tumors. They may be primary or secondary. Spinal tumors can be classified into three categories: extradural, intradural/extramedullary, and intramedullary. Extradural tumors typically arise within the vertebral bodies and are often metastatic. Intradural/extramedullary tumors arise inside the dura but outside of the spinal cord itself. Meningiomas and spinal cord sheath tumors are examples of intradural/extramedullary tumors. Intramedullary tumors arise within the spinal cord tissue. Typical tumor types are ependymomas and astrocytomas. These tumors may be metastatic.

Spinal cord tumors typically compress rather than invade the cord. Pain is the most common presenting symptom, and motor disturbances (typically weakness) are the second most common complaint. High-grade astrocytomas are typically treated with surgical excision and postoperative chemotherapy. Surgical removal is the only recommended treatment for ependymomas.

Prognosis is determined by the aggressiveness and resectability of the initial tumor. Astrocytomas have poorer outcomes than ependymomas and have a 50% recurrence rate within 4 to 5 years.[50]

Clinical Signs and Symptoms
Intracranial tumors in children can grow to a large size without producing significant symptoms until they invade vital brain tissue or cause increased ICP. In children up to 12 years of age, the skull can expand to accommodate a gradual increase in intracranial volume. Tumors may not be diagnosed in the young child with nonspecific signs of neurologic compromise, because testing of cognitive functions, fine motor skills, and sensation is very difficult in very young patients.

Signs and symptoms of any neoplasm in the child include a change in the child's appearance or growth patterns, swelling, lumps, masses, vague pains, or persistent irritability. The child may also change feeding patterns or bowel or bladder function or may develop unexplained clumsiness or stumbling or unexplained or persistent bleeding. General signs of an intracranial tumor during childhood include signs of increased ICP, headache, emesis, anorexia, ataxia, cranial nerve palsies, nystagmus, paresis, seizure activity, and hydrocephalus.

Specific signs of increased ICP caused by an intracranial tumor include papilledema, altered level of consciousness, visual disturbances (diplopia and blurring of vision), headache, and emesis. The headache is characteristically intermittent but progressive. It tends to be present after awakening, and it often is associated with vomiting. The child usually does not feel nauseated before vomiting. If vomiting or headaches are persistent, anorexia may develop.

As the tumor grows, an infant will develop a bulging fontanelle, and torticollis may result from the asymmetric compression of neck muscles by the tumor. Nuchal rigidity may be noted.[35]

If the tumor compresses the sixth cranial nerve or if uncal (temporal-lateral) herniation develops from increased ICP, the child may develop strabismus, diplopia, or blurring of vision. Ataxia or nystagmus will develop if the tumor compresses or erodes the cerebellum.[50] Paresis will develop if the tumor compresses the brainstem or pyramidal tract. Seizures are rarely an early sign of an intracranial tumor, although they can develop late in the clinical course. If hydrocephalus is present, the tumor is obstructing CSF pathways.

The best means of diagnosing an intracranial tumor is with a thorough neurologic examination and a CT scan with and without contrast. MRI is also an essential tool in the diagnosis of brain tumors and is the preferred method of scanning for some brain stem tumors. (See Common Diagnostic Tests later in this chapter.) A plain skull radiograph may demonstrate characteristic changes associated with some tumors (e.g., calcification near the sella turcica that occurs with craniopharyngioma), but often the radiographs are not helpful. Arteriography can be performed to better locate and define the tumor.

Management
Care of the child with an intracranial tumor requires treatment of intracranial hypertension (see Increased Intracranial Pressure in the Common Clinical Conditions section of this chapter), surgical resection if possible, and initiation of chemotherapy or radiation therapy. Laser, stealth, and gamma knife surgeries are surgical techniques that have improved the efficacy of surgical intervention for intracranial tumors. Stealth or stereotactic guidance is especially useful in transsphenoidal tumor resection. Over the past decade, the development of frameless stereotaxy in combination with fluoroscopy assists the neurosurgeon in staying midline. It is considered safe and accurate and adds little cost and time to conventional surgical approaches.[44]

Radiation therapy is typically prescribed for intracranial tumors, and chemotherapy recently has been found to be helpful in the treatment of some intracranial tumors in children.[50] Steroid therapy such as dexamethasone may be used for treatment of localized edema surrounding the tumor. Although the mechanism of action is unclear, the working theory is that the drug decreases the blood-tumor barrier permeability or it may increase parenchymal resistance to fluid transport.[50]

The child with a brain tumor is typically admitted to the critical care unit following neurosurgery. The child may also require critical care for management of sepsis or infections secondary to chemotherapy-induced immunosuppression (see Chapters 6 and 16).

The child and family will require long-term physical and emotional support. If the tumor initially produced vague clinical signs and symptoms, and the parents ignored the child's initial complaints, they may feel guilty and frustrated. Unless deterioration is rapid, the child will require surgery, radiation, and possible chemotherapy with frequent hospitalizations. The child may, in fact, have a chronic neurologic disease and require prolonged treatment. The child and family will require long-term follow-up and ongoing support.

Meningitis
Etiology
Meningitis is an acute inflammation of the meninges and CSF. It occurs far more commonly in children than in adults, and it is seen most frequently in children between 1 month and 5 years of age. Meningitis most commonly is produced by bacteria (called *purulent meningitis*) or viruses (usually called *aseptic meningitis*), although it can also result from fungi, parasites, or mycobacteria.

Over the past decade there have been advances in testing technology. The addition of pneumococcal and meningococcal vaccines into the routine immunization schedule and the adjunctive use of steroids have changed the management of meningitis. However, meningitis remains a leading cause of infection in children, with significant morbidity and mortality.

The three major organisms responsible for meningitis worldwide are *Haemophilus influenzae, Neisseria meningitidis,* and *Streptococcus pneumoniae,* but the causative organisms vary depending on the geographic location and age of the child. In the United States, meningococcus and pneumococcus account for approximately 95% of acute bacterial meningitis in children. Group B streptococcus remains a leading cause of meningitis in the neonatal population. These forms of meningitis usually result from the extension of a localized infection, with transient bacteremia and CNS spread of the organism. Staphylococcal meningitis occurs most commonly after neurosurgery or after a skull fracture with a dural tear.[81,114]

Pathophysiology
Most pathogens responsible for bacterial meningitis are introduced via the respiratory system. Colonization of the organism in the mucous membranes of the nasal passages causes injury to the epithelial cells, allowing access into bloodstream. After this hematogenous spread of bacteria (i.e., it is spread by blood), the bacteria then penetrate the blood-brain barrier, infecting the meninges. Once the CNS has been breached, the bacteria will multiply freely and rapidly spread throughout the entire surface of the spinal cord and brain. Inflammatory mediators and cytokines are then released causing an inflammatory response. Cerebral edema, inflammation, and ensuing increased ICP are frequently seen after bacterial invasion of the brain parenchyma. Cerebral vasculitis, thrombosis, and infarction are the consequence of endothelial damage at the vascular level. Edema or scarring of the outlet of the third ventricle produces stenosis of the Sylvian aqueduct and results in obstruction to CSF flow and hydrocephalus.[50]

Clinical Signs and Symptoms
Clinical presentation depends on the age of the child, the time lapse between initial symptoms and medical treatment, the immunity of the child, and the infecting organism. Onset can be acute or slow. In the neonate or infant of younger than 6 months, the signs of meningitis are often nonspecific. The infant may be extremely irritable or lethargic with a history of poor feeding, vomiting, and fever. Seizures may develop. A high-pitched cry may be observed in infants with increased ICP.

Extremely malnourished or very small infants with meningitis may be afebrile.[114] If the ICP is high, the anterior fontanelle will be full and may be tense. Although the presence of nuchal rigidity (stiff neck) provides an index of suspicion, it is often not present in the young infant. The diagnosis is only confirmed by the results of the spinal tap.

Older children with meningitis usually complain of headache and exhibit nausea, vomiting, anorexia, photophobia, acute onset of fever, decreased level of consciousness or seizures.[114] Nuchal rigidity, neck pain, and sensitivity to touch are also present. Kernig's sign (pain with extension of the legs) and Brudzinski's sign (flexion of the neck stimulates flexion at the knees and hips) also may be present. Often there is a history of an antecedent upper respiratory or gastrointestinal infection.[114]

When meningitis is suspected, blood samples are obtained for a complete blood cell count with white blood cell differential, glucose, electrolytes, and blood cultures. The results will help detect evidence of a localized infection or sepsis. Additional urine, serum, or wound cultures are obtained as indicated.

A lumbar puncture is the definitive diagnostic test for meningitis. During the lumbar puncture, CSF samples are taken. From these samples, a culture, Gram staining, and cell count will be performed, and protein and sugar levels will be measured. The general appearance of the fluid and the opening and closing CSF pressures should be noted in the nursing record.

When bacterial meningitis is present, the glucose concentration of the CSF is low, but the protein content is high. In addition, there will be a large number of cells present in the fluid, predominantly neutrophils (Table 11-11). The culture and Gram stain will be positive.[114]

When aseptic (viral or fungal) meningitis is present, the CSF glucose concentration is usually normal, and the protein content is only slightly elevated. In aseptic meningitis, there may be a moderate or large number of cells, predominantly polymorphonuclear leukocytes early in the course, and lymphocytes later in the course. The Gram stain is usually

Table 11-11 Cerebrospinal Fluid Analysis in Bacterial and Viral Meningitis

	NORMAL			MENINGITIS	
	Preterm	**Term**	**>6 months**	**Bacterial**	**Viral**
Cell count (WBCs/mm³)*					
Mean	9	8	0	>500	<500
Range	0-25	0-22	0-4		
Predominant cell type	Lymph	Lymph	Lymph	80% PMN leukocyte	PMN leukocyte initially; lymphocyte later
Glucose (mg/dL)					
Mean	50	52	>40	<40	>40
Range	24-63	34-119			
Protein (mg/dL)					
Mean	115	90	<40	>100	<100
Range	65-150	20-170			
CSF/blood glucose (%)					
Mean	74	81	50	<40	>40
Range	55-150	44-248	40-60		
Tests					
Gram's stain	Negative	Negative	Negative	Positive[†]	Negative
Bacterial culture	Negative	Negative	Negative	Positive[‡]	Negative

From Barkin RM and Rosen P: *Emergency pediatrics: a guide to ambulatory care*, ed 3, St Louis, 1990, Mosby-Year Book.

*Total WBC/mm³ by age in the healthy child can be further delineated as follows (mean ± 2 SD): <6 weeks, 3.7 ± 6.8; 6 weeks-3 months, 2.9 ± 5.7; 3-6 months, 1.9 ± 4.0; 6-12 months, 2.6 ± 4.9; >12 months, 1.9 ± 5.4.

[†]If Gram's stain is negative, a methylene blue stain may distinguish intracellular bacteria from nuclear material.

[‡]Eighty-five percent of partially treated patients will have a positive Gram's stain and >95% have positive cultures. Counterimmunoelectrophoresis may be helpful if the culture is negative.

CSF, Cerebrospinal fluid; *PMN,* polymorphonuclear; *WBC,* white blood cell.

negative, and, with viral meningitis, the serologic culture is usually positive for virus.[114]

Untreated meningitis can cause rapid deterioration. The child may demonstrate mild irritability and fever and quickly progress to high fever, seizures, a decreased level of consciousness, and coma. Thus, the effectiveness of treatment can be related directly to the speed of diagnosis and the early initiation of appropriate treatment.

Management

Bacterial Meningitis. If the child is critically ill, support of airway, ventilation, and perfusion will be needed. However, the treatment of bacterial meningitis requires the prompt initiation (in less than 1 hour of first medical contact) and uninterrupted administration of appropriate IV antimicrobial agents. Vascular access must be established immediately and carefully maintained throughout therapy. Broad spectrum antibiotics are administered even before the results of the CSF cultures and sensitivities have been obtained. The infant or child is given nothing by mouth until systemic perfusion and neurologic function are acceptable.

Accurate recording of fluid intake and output and serum electrolyte concentrations is important, because many children will develop SIADH during or after the meningitis (see Chapter 12). The infant or child is typically given nothing by mouth, and IV maintenance fluids are administered. Fluid boluses may be required because these children usually are somewhat dehydrated related to fever and poor oral intake.

The infant's head circumference should be measured on admission and at least every 8 hours, because subdural effusions and obstructive hydrocephalus can develop after meningitis and can be detected by an increase in head circumference. The infant or child with *H. influenzae* or *N. meningitidis* meningitis is placed in respiratory isolation until antibiotic therapy has been administered for 24 hours.[101]

Treatment of bacterial meningitis should begin as soon as there is suspicion of infection. It is ideal to collect all cultures before beginning antibiotic therapy, but antibiotic administration should not be delayed if samples are difficult to obtain. Antibiotics should be given immediately, and the cultures can be obtained at a later time. Initially, broad spectrum antibiotics should be administered that will cover likely causative organisms for age (Table 11-12). The Gram stain is a guide for initial therapy, but coverage should not be narrowed based on this single test result. The CSF culture remains the gold standard for diagnosis of bacterial meningitis. The antimicrobial therapy can be modified once culture results (including organism and sensitivities) have been completed.

The duration of antibiotic therapy is determined by the specific pathogen, but typically CNS infections are treated for 10 to 14 days. Infants infected with herpesvirus are generally treated for 28 days. In the neonate younger than 6 weeks, acyclovir is added because herpesvirus is a concern for CNS infection in the population. Vancomycin is added if the Gram stain is suggestive of pneumococcus. In the infant older than 2 months, vancomycin is added for empiric coverage because

Table 11-12 Recommendations for Antimicrobial Therapy in Bacterial Meningitis Based on Predisposing Conditions or on Isolated Pathogen and Susceptibility Testing

Predisposing Factor	Common Bacterial Pathogens	Antimicrobial Therapy
Age		
<1 month	*Streptococcus agalactiae, Escherichia coli, Listeria monocytogenes, Klebsiella* species	Ampicillin plus cefotaxime or ampicillin plus an aminoglycoside
1-23 months	*Streptococcus pneumoniae, Neisseria meningitidis, S. agalactiae, Haemophilus influenzae, E. coli*	Vancomycin plus a third-generation cephalosporin*,†
2-50 years	*N. meningitidis, S. pneumoniae*	Vancomycin plus a third-generation cephalosporin*,†
>50 years	*S. pneumoniae, N. meningitidis, L. monocytogenes,* aerobic gram-negative bacilli	Vancomycin plus ampicillin plus a third-generation cephalosporin*,†
Head trauma		
Basilar skull fracture	*S. pneumoniae, H. influenzae,* group A β-hemolytic streptococci	Vancomycin plus a third-generation cephalosporin*
Penetrating trauma	*Staphylococcus aureus,* coagulase-negative staphylococci (especially *Staphylococcus epidermidis*), aerobic gram-negative bacilli (including *Pseudomonas aeruginosa*)	Vancomycin plus cefepime, vancomycin plus ceftazidime, or vancomycin plus meropenem
Postneurosurgery	Aerobic gram-negative bacilli (including *P. aeruginosa*), *S. aureus,* coagulase-negative staphylococci (especially *S. epidermidis*)	Vancomycin plus cefepime, vancomycin plus ceftazidime, or vancomycin plus meropenem
CSF shunt	Coagulase-negative staphylococci (especially *S. epidermidis*), *S. aureus,* aerobic gram-negative bacilli (including *P. aeruginosa*), *Propionibacterium acnes*	Vancomycin plus cefepime,‡ vancomycin plus ceftazidime,‡ or vancomycin plus meropenem‡

Microorganism, Susceptibility	Standard Therapy	Alternative Therapies
Streptococcus pneumoniae		
Penicillin MIC		
<0.1 mcg/mL	Penicillin G or ampicillin	Third-generation cephalosporin,* chloramphenicol
0.1-1.0 mcg/mL§	Third-generation cephalosporin*	Cefepime (B-II), meropenem (B-II)
≥2.0 mcg/mL	Vancomycin plus a third-generation cephalosporin*,‖	Fluoroquinolone¶ (B-II)
Cefotaxime or ceftriaxone MIC ≥1.0 mcg/mL	Vancomycin plus a third-generation cephalosporin*,‖	Fluoroquinolone¶ (B-II)
Neisseria meningitidis		
Penicillin MIC		
<0.1 mcg/mL	Penicillin G or ampicillin	Third-generation cephalosporin,* chloramphenicol
0.1-1.0 mcg/mL	Third-generation cephalosporin*	Chloramphenicol, fluoroquinolone, meropenem
Listeria monocytogenes	Ampicillin or penicillin G#	Trimethoprim-sulfamethoxazole, meropenem (B-III)
Streptococcus agalactiae	Ampicillin or penicillin G#	Third-generation cephalosporin* (B-III)
Escherichia coli and other Enterobacteriaceae ††	Third-generation cephalosporin (A-II)	Aztreonam, fluoroquinolone, meropenem, trimethoprim-sulfamethoxazole, ampicillin
Pseudomonas aeruginosa††	Cefepime# or ceftazidime# (A-II)	Aztreonam,# ciprofloxacin,# meropenem#
Haemophilus influenzae		
β-Lactamase negative	Ampicillin	Third-generation cephalosporin,* cefepime, chloramphenicol, fluoroquinolone
β-Lactamase positive	Third-generation cephalosporin (A-I)	Cefepime (A-I), chloramphenicol, fluoroquinolone
Staphylococcus aureus		
Methicillin susceptible	Nafcillin or oxacillin	Vancomycin, meropenem (B-III)
Methicillin resistant	Vancomycin**	Trimethoprim-sulfamethoxazole, linezolid (B-III)
Staphylococcus epidermidis	Vancomycin**	Linezolid (B-III)
Enterococcus species		
Ampicillin susceptible	Ampicillin plus gentamicin	
Ampicillin resistant	Vancomycin plus gentamicin	
Ampicillin and vancomycin resistant	Linezolid (B-III)	

Note: All recommendations are A-III, unless otherwise indicated.
Adapted from Tunkel, AR, Hartman BJ, Kaplan SJ, et al: Practice guidelines for the management of bacterial meningitis. *Clin Infect Dis*39:1267-1284, 2004.
*Ceftriaxone or cefotaxime.
†Some experts would add rifampin if dexamethasone is also given.
‡In infants and children, vancomycin alone is reasonable unless Gram stains reveal the presence of gram-negative bacilli.
§Ceftriaxone/cefotaxime-susceptible isolates.
‖Consider addition of rifampin if the MIC of ceftriaxone is 12 mg/mL.
¶Gatifloxacin or moxifloxacin.
#Addition of an aminoglycoside should be considered.
**Consider addition of rifampin.
††Choice of a specific antimicrobial agent must be guided by in vitro susceptibility test results.

pneumococcal resistance to third-generation cephalosporins has emerged.[81,114]

Additional days of therapy are indicated if the patient fails to demonstrate clinical improvement or if additional CSF findings indicate partially treated meningitis. Throughout therapy the nurse must monitor for side effects of the antibiotics.

The use of steroids (dexamethasone is 0.6 mg/kg per day divided into four doses for 4 days) in bacterial meningitis has been shown to reduce the incidence of hearing loss and decrease CNS inflammation. However, the first dose must be administered before or in conjunction with the first dose of antibiotics. The targeted bacteria include *H. influenzae* and pneumococcus. The use of steroids in the neonatal population is yet to be established. Although recommended by the American Academy of Pediatrics, widespread use has not been adopted. Often the infant has already received the first dose of antibiotics before the diagnosis of meningitis is made, so this may partially account for the lack of steroid use in this population. Steroids are not recommended in cases of viral meningitis.

Gastrointestinal prophylaxis with ranitidine or a proton pump inhibitor should be administered when steroids are used.[81,114] The nurse should be alert for signs of gastrointestinal hemorrhage or secondary infection that could complicate steroid administration.

A repeat lumbar puncture is not typically recommended at the end of therapy if the child's condition has improved and the child is afebrile. However, if the child is receiving appropriate therapy and does not show clinical improvement within 3 to 4 days of treatment, is experiencing new symptoms, culture results are positive for an unusual or resistant pathogen, or there is no improvement (i.e., in neurologic signs) or child remains febrile on specific therapy after 24 to 48 hours, then the lumbar tap should be repeated. In the neonate, Gram-negative meningitis is an indication for repeat lumbar puncture.[81,114]

Prophylactic antibiotic administration is recommended for household, daycare, and nursery-school contacts of the patient with *Neisseria* spp. meningitis. These contacts should begin taking antibiotics within 24 hours of the patient's diagnosis. Prophylaxis also is recommended for anyone having intimate contact with the patient, including babysitters who may have kissed the child. Ceftriaxone, ciprofloxacin, and rifampin are used for prophylaxis in adults, and rifampin is the drug of choice for prophylaxis in most children.[101]

Viral Meningitis. Supportive care is provided for the child with viral meningitis. Antibiotic administration is not indicated unless a concurrent bacterial infection is present.

Fungal Meningitis. Although rare in the pediatric population, fungal meningitis does occur. It most often occurs in immunosuppressed patients in the setting of HIV, lupus, diabetes, transplant, or cancer. It may also be seen in the premature neonatal population, typically caused by *Candida albicans*. Fungal meningitis can also complicate invasive neurosurgical procedures.[81]

Supportive Care. Throughout the first days of therapy, the infant or child should be monitored closely for signs of increased ICP, continued fever, or neurologic deterioration. These findings should be reported to a provider immediately. If the child does develop signs of increased ICP, then ICP monitoring and mechanical ventilation may be required (see Increased Intracranial Pressure in the Common Clinical Conditions section of this chapter).

Because SIADH is a known risk factor in meningitis, the child's serum sodium concentration and osmolality are closely monitored throughout therapy (see Chapter 12). Antipyretics are administered to reduce fever and decrease the risk of febrile seizures. If seizures develop and progress to status epilepticus, prompt anticonvulsant therapy is essential (see Status Epilepticus earlier in chapter). If bacteremia is present, septic shock and disseminated intravascular coagulation may develop (see Septic Shock, Chapter 6 and Immunology and Infectious Diseases, Chapter 16).

Prognosis varies in every patient. Mortality rates are as high as 20% and survivors, especially those with pneumococcal meningitis, often have neurologic deficits. These deficits can include decreased cognitive and motor skills, hydrocephalus, spasticity, hearing loss, and blindness. Hearing screens should be obtained on all children treated for bacterial meningitis, because risk of hearing loss is significant.[81,114]

Brain Abscess

Etiology

A brain abscess is an isolated intracranial collection of purulent fluid, typically located in the cerebral hemispheres or the cerebellum. The abscess usually develops after bacteremia, but it also can result from chronic sinusitis or following a head injury with a skull fracture. Children with cyanotic congenital heart disease (especially if untreated and older than 2 years) or those with bacterial endocarditis are at increased risk for developing brain abscesses.

Pathophysiology

The pathogen enters the cerebral circulation at the site of intracranial surgery or compound skull fracture or as the result of a systemic or blood-borne infection. Abscesses also can spread into adjacent cerebral tissue from middle ear or mastoid infections.

The infected tissue initially is localized and is invaded quickly by white blood cells. Over a period of several weeks, necrotic tissue within the abscess liquefies, and the abscess becomes encapsulated by fibroblasts.[62] As the abscess grows, it can produce signs of increased ICP. If it ruptures, it can produce diffuse meningoencephalitis.

Clinical Signs and Symptoms

The child with a brain abscess may be asymptomatic during the initial period or may demonstrate nonspecific signs and symptoms including headache, fever, malaise, vomiting, confusion, seizures, motor deficits, sensory deficits, speech deficits, and leukocytosis. As the brain abscess enlarges, it produces signs of increased ICP, including a progressive headache, decreased level of consciousness, pupil dilation with sluggish or absent response to light (especially if uncal herniation develops), papilledema, cranial nerve deficits, and seizures. With enlargement of the abscess, progressive signs of increased ICP develop (see Increased Intracranial Pressure section in this chapter).

A brain abscess also can produce localizing symptoms. The child with a frontal lobe abscess may have contralateral hemiparesis, frontal headache, aphasia, or seizures. Temporal lobe abscesses can produce a temporal lobe headache and contralateral facial weakness. A cerebellar abscess often produces a postoccipital headache, nystagmus, ipsilateral ataxia, and limb weakness.[62,114]

A lumbar puncture will reveal an extremely high CSF pressure, a normal or increased cell count (with polymorphonuclear lymphocytes), an increased protein concentration, and a normal glucose concentration (see Table 11-4). The brain abscess can be localized with a CT scan or MRI.

Management

Prompt initiation and continued administration of IV antibiotics is the key treatment for a brain abscess. Treatment of increased ICP also may be required (see Management in the Increased Intracranial Pressure section of this chapter).[114]

The most common pathogens causing brain abscesses include anaerobic bacteria, Gram-negative organisms, streptococci, and staphylococci. The underlying cause of the abscess usually determines the causative organism. In children with heart disease, α-hemolytic streptococcus is the most common organism, whereas streptococcus and *Staphylococcus aureus* are common organisms associated with subacute bacterial endocarditis. *S. aureus* is commonly seen in abscesses associated with trauma, whereas streptococci, pseudomonas, or *H. influenzae* are the typical pathogens isolated in patients with otitis or sinusitis (see the Table 11-12 for specific antibiotic choices).

If the abscess appears to be well encapsulated, surgical excision may be attempted. If complete excision is not possible, serial aspiration and irrigation of the abscess may be required.

Throughout the child's care, it is important for the nurse to monitor for signs of neurologic deterioration, because increased ICP can develop and progress rapidly. Even with aggressive medical and surgical treatment of brain abscess, mortality is significant, and survivors may have neurologic deficits and seizures.[62,114]

Encephalitis
Etiology

Encephalitis is defined as an inflammation of the brain parenchyma. It can be associated with other CNS infections such as meningitis, or it can be related to viral illness such as rabies or herpes simplex. In the neonatal population, enterovirus and adenovirus are responsible pathogens. In children, arboviruses and enteroviruses are common causes of encephalitis. Adenovirus, Epstein-Barr virus, West Nile virus, measles, mumps and varicella are responsible for a small portion of pediatric encephalitis cases.

Encephalitis may appear during the course of an acute viral illness, or it may follow an infection. The term *encephalitis* is used to indicate an infective or inflammatory cerebral disorder. The term *encephalopathy* is used to refer to any neurologic disorder of unknown or noninfectious cause associated with a change in level of consciousness, irritability, seizures, and motor or sensory deficit.[114]

Pathophysiology

Encephalitis probably results from a toxic or infectious agent that enters the brain. The inflammatory mediators released or triggered by the agent produce an inflammatory response that results in cerebral edema, cellular damage, neuronal destruction, and transient neurologic dysfunction.

In the temporal region an acute inflammatory demyelination may be seen in association with viral infections or post immunization. In this circumstance if there is no direct viral involvement of the CNS it is called postinfectious encephalitis. In cases where the spinal cord is involved, it is referred to as acute disseminated encephalomyelitis (ADEM).[114]

Clinical Signs and Symptoms

Children with encephalitis demonstrate symptoms during or immediately after an acute viral illness or following exposure to a toxic or inflammatory agent. Affected children usually complain of a headache and may demonstrate irritability, lethargy, a change in level of consciousness, nuchal rigidity, visual, auditory and speech disturbances, seizures, or loss of consciousness. High fever is usually not present.

Herpes simplex virus encephalitis generally presents in children 6 months to 18 years of age and is equally distributed between males and females. Herpes simplex virus usually produces an acute, hemorrhagic, necrotizing encephalitis with associated cerebral edema.[50,62]

A lumbar puncture usually is performed to rule out a bacterial cause of the neurologic symptoms. It reveals normal CSF pressure, normal or increased cell count (lymphocytes may be elevated), normal or slightly increased protein concentration, and normal glucose concentration. The CSF culture and Gram stain will yield no bacterial growth, but serologic tests can aid in the diagnosis of a viral agent (see Table 11-4).

An EEG will reveal diffuse cortical inflammation with high-voltage discharges, usually from the temporal lobes. CT scans typically fail to demonstrate localized areas of infection, but they will show defined areas of edema, predominantly in the temporal lobes. Hemorrhagic lesions are seen on approximately 12% of scans.[50,62] MRIs are more sensitive than CT scans, revealing edema as high signals on T2 weighted images, primarily in the temporal lobes.[50]

Management

Treatment of encephalitis is largely supportive, but acute encephalitis is considered an emergency. The child should be admitted to the pediatric critical care unit for close neurologic monitoring. These children can develop rapid neurologic deterioration, including coma. As always, support of airway, oxygenation, ventilation, and perfusion are priorities. Antibiotic administration is not indicated if the disease is viral or toxic in origin. If the toxic agent can be identified (e.g., a drug) and an antidote is available, it should be administered. Antiviral agents such as amantadine and rimantadine can be used in cases influenza infection.

Steroid use has not been shown to change outcomes in cases of acute viral encephalitis; however, they may be used in an effort to decrease cerebral and neuronal inflammation.[114] In cases of acute disseminated encephalomyelitis, steroid administration is the initial treatment of choice.[67]

If seizures are present, they may be refractory to typical anticonvulsant therapy. Refractory status epilepticus in the child with encephalitis may require a induction of a barbiturate coma using either pentobarbital or thiopental (see Barbiturate Coma in the Management section under Status Epilepticus).

Plasmapheresis to remove circulating cytokines and other inflammatory mediators is an accepted mode of therapy in children with acute disseminated encephalomyelitis who are refractory to steroid therapy.[67,89,105] Before initiating this mode of therapy, a large-bore double-lumen central venous catheter (e.g., a hemodialysis catheter) is placed. Intravenous immune globulin (IVIG) may also be used in children with encephalitis who are unable to produce an effective immune response.[32,114]

Children with encephalitis should be monitored closely for signs of neurologic deterioration that may indicate greater inflammation or the development of increased ICP. Analgesics that do not produce respiratory depression (e.g., codeine) can be prescribed to relieve a persistent or severe headache. If the child complains of sensitivity to light or noise, a private room or isolated bed space is usually necessary to enable reduction of room light and noise and to minimize stimulation.

Children with encephalitis may demonstrate mild symptoms and a rapid recovery or may develop progressive and fatal neurologic deterioration. The prognosis is determined by the causative agent and the general health of the patient.

Metabolic Encephalopathies

Etiology

Metabolic encephalopathies can be divided into three subgroups: endogenous intoxication related to accumulation of neurotoxic metabolites, energy failure related to a lack of metabolites needed for brain function, and acute water-electrolyte-endocrine disturbances.

Pathophysiology

In several disease processes, including liver failure and inborn errors of metabolism, the products of amino acid catabolism are not cleared or detoxified by either the liver or kidneys. These waste products (e.g., ammonia and urea) accumulate and affect organ function, often causing neurologic problems such as cerebral edema. Examples of these disorders include maple syrup urine disease, methylmalonic aciduria, and propionic aciduria.

Energy failure encephalopathies include hypoglycemia, thiamine deficiency, and mitochondrial energy metabolism defects. Water and electrolyte encephalopathies include diabetic ketoacidosis, nonketotic hyperosmolar coma, hyponatremia, and hypernatremia (see Chapter 12). Cerebral edema again is the cause.[66,117]

Clinical Signs and Symptoms

Children with metabolic encephalopathy can exhibit progressive confusion, motor and sensory deficits, hallucinations, and seizures. Respiratory failure develops as the level of consciousness deteriorates. Signs and symptoms of cerebral edema and increased ICP may also be present. (See Increased Intracranial Pressure in the Common Clinical Conditions section of this chapter.)

Management

Treatment is determined by the etiology of the encephalopathy. Patients usually are admitted to the critical or intermediate care unit for skilled continuous nursing observation. Initial priorities of care include establishing and maintaining an adequate airway, ventilation, oxygenation, and systemic perfusion. Careful monitoring for signs of increased ICP is imperative. Hypoventilation and hypercapnia will further exacerbate the already increased ICP. If the child is unable to maintain a patent airway or breathe spontaneously, elective intubation and mechanical ventilation are indicated before the development of airway obstruction, hypoxia, and hypercarbia (see Chapter 9).

Ischemic and Hemorrhagic Stroke

Etiology

Stroke is an acute loss of blood flow to a region of the brain that results in a loss of neurologic function. More than 3200 new strokes are diagnosed annually in children younger than 18 years.[38,107] Approximately 30 neonates per 100,000 births are affected; in the pediatric population stroke incidence is approximately 2 to 13 per 100,000 children per year.[38] The remainder of this section addresses stroke in infants beyond the neonatal period and in children.

Ischemic strokes usually occur within the first year of life, and subarachnoid hemorrhages are more common in the teenage population.[39] Those at high risk are males and African-Americans.[38,39] Prognosis in children is much better than in adults.

Cerebral vascular accidents and strokes are rare occurrences in children, but carry significant morbidity and mortality. Stroke is among the top 10 causes of childhood deaths, and more than 50% of survivors have cognitive and motor dysfunction. Increasing prevalence is likely related to improved imaging and recognition in addition to advances that allow children with predisposing conditions such as cancer, sickle cell disease, heart disease and neurologic disease to survive longer.[38,39,65,99]

Pathophysiology

Many factors and disease processes predispose children to strokes. A preexisting condition that increases the child's risk of stroke is identified in only about half of pediatric stroke victims. Common preexisting conditions include congenital heart disease and sickle cell anemia. Other known causes are leukemia, brain tumors, Down syndrome, trauma, recent infection, vasculitis, and bleeding disorders. Strokes can be classified as either ischemic or hemorrhagic.

Ischemic strokes are the result of either a thrombus or embolism and are responsible for approximately 85% of all strokes. Emboli generally originate in the heart, but extracranial arteries are another source. Thrombi are occlusive, and the most common sites are in the cerebral artery branches. Turbulent blood flow can also increase the risk for thrombus formation. Other causes include sickle cell disease, protein C disorders, polycythemia, hypoperfusion, anemia, and prolonged vasoconstriction.

Hemorrhagic strokes are intracerebral hemorrhages affecting the brain parenchyma. These hemorrhages can occur in small arteries damaged from hypertension, or they result from rupture of aneurysms, arteriovenous malformations, bleeding disorders, or cocaine abuse.[99]

Clinical Signs and Symptoms

Acute stroke in children can produce signs and symptoms such as nausea, emesis, headache, altered mental status, abrupt onset of hemiparesis, visual disturbances, ataxia, and aphasia. Symptoms may be single or occur in combination. It is imperative to establish the precise time of the onset of symptoms, because it can affect the potential use of thrombolytics for ischemic stroke.

Management

All children suspected of having an acute stroke require blood sampling on admission for initial serum chemistries (electrolytes, glucose, calcium, and BUN), complete blood count, and coagulation studies, including activated partial thromboplastin time (aPTT). A comprehensive urine toxicology screen is performed to rule out any toxins or drugs that can produce signs similar to a stroke. Additional testing may include lupus anticoagulant; antiphospholipid antibody; dilute Russell viper venom time; anticardiolipin immunoglobulin (Ig) G, IgM, IgA; antiphosphotidyl serine IgG, IgM, IgA; anti-β2 glycoprotein IgG, IgM, IgA; fasting lipid profile; cholesterol; lipoprotein A; plasma homocysteine; varicella titers; organic and amino acids; factor V Leiden; antinuclear antibody, erythrocyte sedimentation rate; and C-reactive protein. The child is evaluated for mitochondrial myopathy, encephalomyopathy, lactic acidosis, and stroke—a family of inherited mitochondrial cyopathies.

Noncontrast CT, CT angiography, and MRI are the mainstays of imaging for stroke diagnosis. The noncontrast CT is completed and read soon after the child's arrival to quickly differentiate ischemic from hemorrhagic insults. In adult acute stroke guidelines, the recommended goal for completion of the CT image is 25 minutes or less from the time of hospital arrival, with CT image interpretation within 45 minutes of hospital arrival.[4] Although the sensitivity and specificity of CT has not been shown in children, expert consensus supports its use.[107] However, it is often necessary to stabilize the child's condition before the CT scan.

CT angiography can identify filling defects and localize specific portions of the vessel that may be the cause of the stroke. MRI is sensitive in detecting both acute ischemic and hemorrhagic strokes. A cardiac echocardiogram should be obtained to rule out cardiac embolism as a cause of the stroke. Children with suspected strokes are admitted to the critical care unit for skilled continuous nursing observation. Obviously, establishing and maintaining an adequate airway, ventilation, and systemic perfusion are priorities.

Thrombolysis. A neurologist should be consulted to assist with both acute and long-term management of the pediatric stroke patient. Treatment with tissue plasminogen activator (tPA) has become a standard of care for adult ischemic stroke treated within hours of the event. No randomized studies have evaluated the use of tPA for stroke in children <18 years of age, so the FDA has not yet approved tPA for this use. Although small case series have documented tPA clot dissolution in children with systemic thromboses, the complication rate was high.[107]

If given within 3 hours of stroke symptom onset, tPA may be considered for some patients with occlusive ischemic stroke. In carefully selected adult patients, IV tPA may be given up to 4.5 hours after symptom onset, and intraarterial tPA may be administered up to 6 hours after symptom onset in carefully selected adult patients with anterior circulation strokes.[107]

Heparin therapy is the mainstay for anticoagulation in the pediatric stroke patient. The use of heparin can prevent repeat cardiac embolic events and inhibit further development of cerebrovascular thrombi. After imaging has ruled out hemorrhage, the child will be given a bolus dose of heparin (75 units/kg; maximum, 10,000 units) and given a heparin infusion of 15 units/kg per hour. Blood should be obtained for an aPTT 1 hour after the heparin infusion. The infusion will be adjusted with the goal maintaining the aPTT in the range of 60 to 85 seconds. Hematologists should be consulted to assist with transition to low molecular weight heparin or warfarin.

Children with hemorrhagic stroke require immediate transfer to the pediatric critical care unit for close neurologic and hemodynamic monitoring. An emergency craniectomy may be required if the lesion has a mass effect on the brain. Failure to intervene quickly can lead to increased ICP and subsequent brain death (see Increased Intracranial Pressure earlier in this chapter).[99]

Drowning

Etiology

The term *drowning* is used to describe a submersion event producing primary respiratory impairment.[87] The victim typically requires some form of resuscitation (stimulation, rescue breathing, or compressions and ventilations). After a drowning event, the child may survive with or without significant neurologic impairment.

There are three categories of children at risk for drowning injuries: infants, children 1 to 4 years of age (toddlers and preschoolers), and adolescents. Infants usually drown in bathtubs and children 1 to 4 years of age are typically found submerged in shallow wading pools, home swimming pools, or spas.[22,33] Adolescents often drown in natural bodies of water, and alcohol or diving injuries are often involved.

Pathophysiology

The pulmonary complications of submersion are summarized in Chapter 9. The following paragraphs address only the potential neurologic complications of submersion. Within 3 minutes of submersion, most patients will develop sufficient hypoxia and cerebral ischemia to produce loss of consciousness. If submersion continues, CNS dysfunction develops; further ischemia and hypoxia can produce brain death.

The hypoxic-ischemic insult during the submersion may not be immediately fatal. Cardiopulmonary resuscitation can produce the return of spontaneous circulation. However, profound cerebral cellular damage, cerebral edema, and reperfusion injury may develop. This edema may produce signs of increased ICP as late as 48 to 72 hours or longer after the submersion episode.

The severity of neurologic sequelae following submersion is related to the severity of the primary hypoxic insult and any secondary insults that occur. The severity of the primary insult is affected by the duration of immersion, the temperature of the submersion water, and the time that elapsed before effective cardiopulmonary resuscitation was provided. Secondary neurologic insults (e.g., hypotension, further hypoxic episodes, hyperthermia, decreased CBF) may occur after initial return of spontaneous circulation.[87] The time of submersion as reported by bystanders is notoriously unreliable, so it is often impossible to determine the duration of cardiopulmonary arrest.

Submersion can stimulate the diving reflex. This reflex results in initial apnea, loss of consciousness, bradycardia, hypertension, and shunting of blood to vital organs and away from the skin and splanchnic vascular beds. When very small children are submerged in very cold water ($<5°$ C), the diving reflex can slow metabolic rate and redistribute blood flow sufficiently to prevent profound neurologic injury. However, such protection cannot be assured, and intact survival following prolonged submersion is rare.[22]

Clinical Signs and Symptoms

Unless the submersion is extremely brief, most children are apneic and flaccid when pulled from the water. If high-quality cardiopulmonary resuscitation is immediately initiated, many of these children will demonstrate a perfusing cardiac rhythm and spontaneous respirations on arrival in the emergency department; these children are likely to recover completely from the episode. The presence of any spontaneous movement or posturing on arrival in the emergency department and even within the first 24 hours after submersion is consistent with neurologic recovery.[87]

No predictive factors evaluated during resuscitation can determine the outcome of drowning victims, so aggressive resuscitation and post-resuscitation care are generally indicated for the first hours following the submersion.[87]

If skilled resuscitation was performed at the scene and during transport, and the normothermic child is asystolic on arrival in the emergency department, reported outcome is poor.[22] Additional poor prognostic indicators include absence of purposeful movement at 24 hours after admission.[87]

Serial neurologic examinations are required for children who remain comatose or severely impaired after return of spontaneous circulation and admission to the critical care unit.[87] If these children receive aggressive hemodynamic support, it may be possible to restore effective systemic perfusion, but the child with severe hypoxic brain injury may never recover significant neurologic function. Therefore, the indication for aggressive or prolonged resuscitation beyond the first 24 hours should be considered carefully, and the parents should be included in these discussions.

Management

If the drowning victim is responsive after resuscitation, further neurologic support is typically not required. The child should be monitored closely, and aggressive respiratory support may be needed to treat pulmonary complications (see Chapter 9).

If the child with severe neurologic injury is supported vigorously during the first hours after the drowning episode, the child may demonstrate some gasps within 12 to 24 hours. However agonal gasps indicate brain stem function and do not indicate neurologic recovery.

Signs of increased ICP can develop 48 to 72 hours after submersion. There is currently no evidence that aggressive therapy to treat increased ICP and limit secondary neurologic injury is beneficial for drowning victims with increased ICP.[22,87] At this time, immediate resuscitation and therapeutic hypothermia are the only therapies that have been shown to improve neurologic outcome following hypoxic-ischemic brain injury, and evidence comes largely from the neonatal population. More data are needed regarding effectiveness of therapeutic hypothermia in children following resuscitation.

The parents of the drowning victim will need a great deal of compassionate support. They should be included in discussions and decisions to limit care or to pursue aggressive resuscitation and postresuscitation support (see Withholding and Withdrawing Care in Chapter 24).

If the child develops brain death, the parents should be offered the option of organ donation (see the Brain Death and Organ Donation section of this chapter). Support of the parents is reviewed in Chapter 3.

COMMON DIAGNOSTIC TESTS

One of the best methods for evaluating neurologic function in the child is a thorough neurologic examination (Box 11-2). However, when the child is critically ill and unresponsive, it is often difficult to determine the severity of a neurologic injury or deficit, and it may be difficult to separate the signs of neurologic disease from neurologic depression associated with failure of other body systems. As a result, a few diagnostic studies can provide additional important information about the child's diagnosis, clinical status, or prognosis.

Lumbar Puncture
Definition and Purpose

A lumbar puncture, or spinal tap, is performed by introducing a needle into the subarachnoid space of the lumbar spinal canal. The needle is inserted with a stylette into the interspace between the third and fourth lumbar vertebrae; puncture at this level avoids damage to the spinal cord.[36,118]

The lumbar puncture can be performed to examine the CSF, to measure CSF pressure, or to introduce medication, air, or radiopaque contrast material into the subarachnoid space. The lumbar puncture will aid in the diagnosis of intracranial or intraventricular hemorrhage if blood is present in the CSF.

The CSF can be sent for culture, Gram staining, cell count, and glucose and protein content to aid in the diagnosis of CNS infection or inflammation. In addition, anesthesia or antibiotics can be introduced into the subarachnoid space to reduce pain or treat infection, respectively. Finally, injected air or radiopaque contrast material can be used to outline subarachnoid structures or identify CSF obstructions or leaks. In the pediatric critical care unit, the lumbar puncture is used most often to confirm the diagnosis of CNS infection.[118]

Procedure

The lumbar puncture is safe when it is performed correctly by an experienced provider. Before the procedure, the child should be examined carefully for signs of increased ICP. If these signs are present in the infant, the lumbar puncture may proceed with caution if a CSF sample is absolutely necessary to identify and treat CNS disease. If, however, signs or suspicion of increased ICP are present in an older child with fused cranial sutures, the lumbar puncture should be postponed because the sudden release of CSF and pressure by the lumbar puncture can result in herniation of the medulla through the foramen magnum.

The procedure should be explained to the child carefully and in an age-appropriate manner. The child is placed in the knee-chest position, either sitting or lying on the side with the neck flexed toward the knees; this position maximizes separation of the vertebral bodies. The position must be modified if the child is intubated or has major trauma and fractures. The child should be held firmly to prevent excessive movement during the lumbar puncture.[36,118]

Once the child is positioned, the back is draped and the puncture area is identified and scrubbed with a surgical preparation, such as chlorhexidine. The remainder of the procedure is then performed using strict sterile technique. Local anesthesia may be obtained by infiltrating lidocaine intradermally around the puncture site. If time is not a factor in obtaining samples, alternative anesthesia can be provided by using topical analgesic ointments (see Chapter 5). Such agents typically provide local numbness in 15 to 30 minutes.

The needle and stylette are inserted firmly into the subarachnoid space. Frequently a sharp sound is heard when the dura is pierced. The stylette should always remain in place when advancing the needle into the skin and past the subcutaneous tissue. This technique avoids introducing epidermal cells into the spinal canal that can lead to an iatrogenic epidermoid tumor. Once the needed is inserted into the subarachnoid space, the stylette is withdrawn.[50]

As soon as the subarachnoid space is entered, the opening CSF pressure is obtained with a manometer. A few drops of CSF are then allowed to drain from the needle. Additional CSF is collected in three or more sterile sampling tubes as follows:

1. Culture and Gram stain analysis
2. Protein and sugar analysis
3. Cell count

Additional tubes are used as needed for viral cultures or other special studies.

The nurse and provider performing the lumbar puncture will observe and later record the appearance of the CSF in the sampling tubes. If red blood cells result from a traumatic tap, the fluid should be clear by the time the final tube is filled. If intracranial hemorrhage is present, the final CSF sampling tube will still contain red blood cells. CSF cloudiness is usually abnormal and often indicates the presence of infection. Xanthochromia (yellow discoloration of the CSF) may be caused by hyperbilirubinemia or the presence of hemolyzed red blood cells. Changes in the CSF content with common CNS diseases are listed in Table 11-4.[62]

After samples are obtained, the CSF closing pressure is measured, the needle is withdrawn, and a small dressing is placed over the area of the puncture site. If iodine was used as a preparation, it is removed before placing a dressing or adhesive bandage.

Nursing Responsibilities and Complications

It is the nurse's responsibility to prepare the child (as age appropriate) and family for the procedure. The nurse is also responsible for positioning, monitoring, and comforting the child throughout the procedure. The nurse will administer analgesics as ordered and monitor the child closely for effects and side effects of these drugs (see Chapter 5). In addition, the nurse is responsible for verifying the accurate labeling of all CSF samples and ensuring that samples are sent for analysis.

An uncommon but devastating potential complication of a lumbar puncture is brain stem herniation. Therefore, during and after the lumbar puncture, the nurse must monitor for signs of deterioration of neurologic status that could indicate brain stem herniation. These signs include decreased responsiveness, tachycardia or bradycardia, unilateral or bilateral pupil dilation with sluggish constrictive response to light, hypertension with widening pulse pressure, irregular breathing (including apnea), and abnormal posturing. These signs should be reported immediately to an on-call provider, and efforts should be made to reduce ICP.

Additional complications of the lumbar puncture include severe headache and bleeding from the puncture site.[50,62] The child should lie flat (unless signs of increased ICP are present) for 4 to 6 hours after the procedure to reduce the possibility and severity of headaches. Analgesics and intravenous fluids (unless contraindicated) will be given as needed to treat the headache, per provider order.

Electroencephalography

Definition and Purpose

The EEG is a recording of the electrical potentials that arise from the brain. These potentials can be quantified, localized, and compared with established, normal EEGs for the patient's age to aid in the diagnosis of seizure activity or CNS injury or dysfunction.[62] An isoelectric (flat) EEG in the nonhypothermic, nonsedated patient is one of the criteria used to confirm cerebral death in patients with no clinical evidence of brain function.

Procedure

The EEG is recorded by placing approximately 17 to 21 electrodes on the surface of the frontal, parietal, occipital, and temporal areas of the scalp and over the ear. A unique electrode placement is required if the EEG is performed to confirm brain death (see Confirmatory Tests in the Criteria for Pronouncement of Brain Death section of this chapter). The EEG electrodes are fixed with an acetone-soluble paste to prevent electrode movement during the study. The EEG is performed when the patient is reclining and still. When this study is required in critically ill patients, it is usually performed in the critical care unit.

The EEG is typically recorded continuously for 20 minutes; longer recordings will be necessary if additional studies, such as the measurement of brain-stem evoked auditory potentials or the confirmation of brain death, are requested. Because the cerebral electrical activity must be magnified to provide a visible recorded signal, patient movement and electrical (equipment) artifact must be reduced to a minimum. Because extraneous or sudden noise or lights can stimulate cranial nerve electrical activity, they should also be minimized during the recording. If the child is alert and mobile, sedation may be required (see Chapter 5).

The EEG usually is recorded during sleep (or coma), and the recording often is continued during hyperventilation and with photic (rhythmic light flash) stimulation. The sleep EEG allows analysis of baseline activity, and hyperventilation is used to accentuate abnormal EEG findings. A 2-minute, rhythmic light flash (photic stimulation) may be used to attempt to induce seizure activity during the recording.

Brain stem-evoked responses can be tested to evaluate cranial nerve responses and to detect early evidence of cranial nerve damage. This testing is particularly useful in the newborn or comatose patient when response to painful stimuli is difficult or impossible to detect.

The brain stem-evoked auditory response is obtained by recording electrical activity over the auditory pathway after provision of a standard auditory stimulus. If the acoustic nerve itself is damaged, early conduction of the impulse through the nerve will be prolonged or diminished; this can occur, for example, as a complication of drug therapy and resultant ototoxicity. If brainstem disease or dysfunction is present, conduction of the auditory impulse through the nerve will be normal, but the time required for the impulse to travel between the auditory nerve and the brainstem will be prolonged.

Nursing Responsibilities and Complications

Before the EEG is obtained, the nurse will describe the procedure to the child (as age appropriate) and the parents. Important points to emphasize include the fact that the procedure is painless, and (if applicable) that the child will be given medication to make him or her drowsy during the procedure. In addition, the child should be told that some special soap (acetone) is used to clean the hair after the procedure, because the acetone has a distinctive and noxious odor. If the child is awake and alert, the nurse may administer a sedative if ordered. Care should also be taken to fully remove all traces of the electrode gel from the child's head after the EEG, because the paste can cause superficial burns if it remains in place during an MRI.

During the EEG, it is important that the nurse avoid touching or stimulating the patient more than is absolutely necessary. Lights should be dimmed and noises should be reduced to a minimum. The nurse should remain near the child's bedside throughout the EEG to monitor the child, answer questions, and provide hyperventilation or additional sedation as ordered and indicated. There are no complications resulting from a standard EEG.

Computed Tomography
Definition and Purpose

The CT scans the head in successive layers, using x-ray beams passing throughout the head in multiple directions. For a traditional CT, the information obtained is then constructed into images in a cross-sectional format. Each picture is referred to as a *slice* or *cut*. Multi-view imaging is now used to create 3-dimensional CT volume rendering images to evaluate structures of the head and brain (Fig. 11-20) and to create images in many views.

The CT scan is a reliable, painless, safe, and noninvasive method of visualizing a variety of neurologic disorders, including space occupying lesions, hematomas, hemorrhage, hydrocephalus, brain abscess, and cortical atrophy. The images produced by the scan allow differentiation of intracranial spaces and normal gray and white matter.[62,86] This scan has eliminated or reduced the need for many other more invasive diagnostic neurologic tests; it is the most useful test available in the evaluation of children with head trauma (see Fig. 11-12).[80]

Procedure

This procedure must be performed in the neuroradiology department. The child is positioned supine on a mobile platform that is slid toward and into the scanner so the child's head is positioned within the scanner. A portion of the scanner will move around the child's head to direct the x-ray beam at many different angles; hundreds of radiographs are obtained and reconstructed during the scan.

The CT scan takes approximately 15 minutes. Occasionally, contrast agents are administered intravenously immediately before the scan to enable better visualization of intracranial structures.[80]

Nursing Responsibilities and Complications

The nurse will prepare the child and family for the procedure, including a discussion of the noises that the child will hear during the scan. The nurse accompanies the child to the scanner, ensures that all tubes and catheters are secure during any movement into and out of the scanner and during the scan itself, and monitors the child during the procedure itself. Because the child must remain absolutely still throughout the procedure, sedatives and/or analgesics are administered before the procedure is performed on a conscious and alert child (see Chapter 5).

During the procedure, healthcare personnel and radiology technicians are positioned behind a lead screen to minimize stray radiation exposure. The nurse must be able to see the child throughout the procedure and ensure proper functioning of the child's IV equipment and mechanical ventilation support. Children in unstable condition must be monitored closely throughout the procedure.

The risk of complications associated with CT scans is relatively low. The typical dose of radiation emitted during a scan is essentially equivalent to natural sources of radiation.[62,86]

If a contrast agent is injected before the scan, the nurse must monitor for signs of a reaction to the contrast material

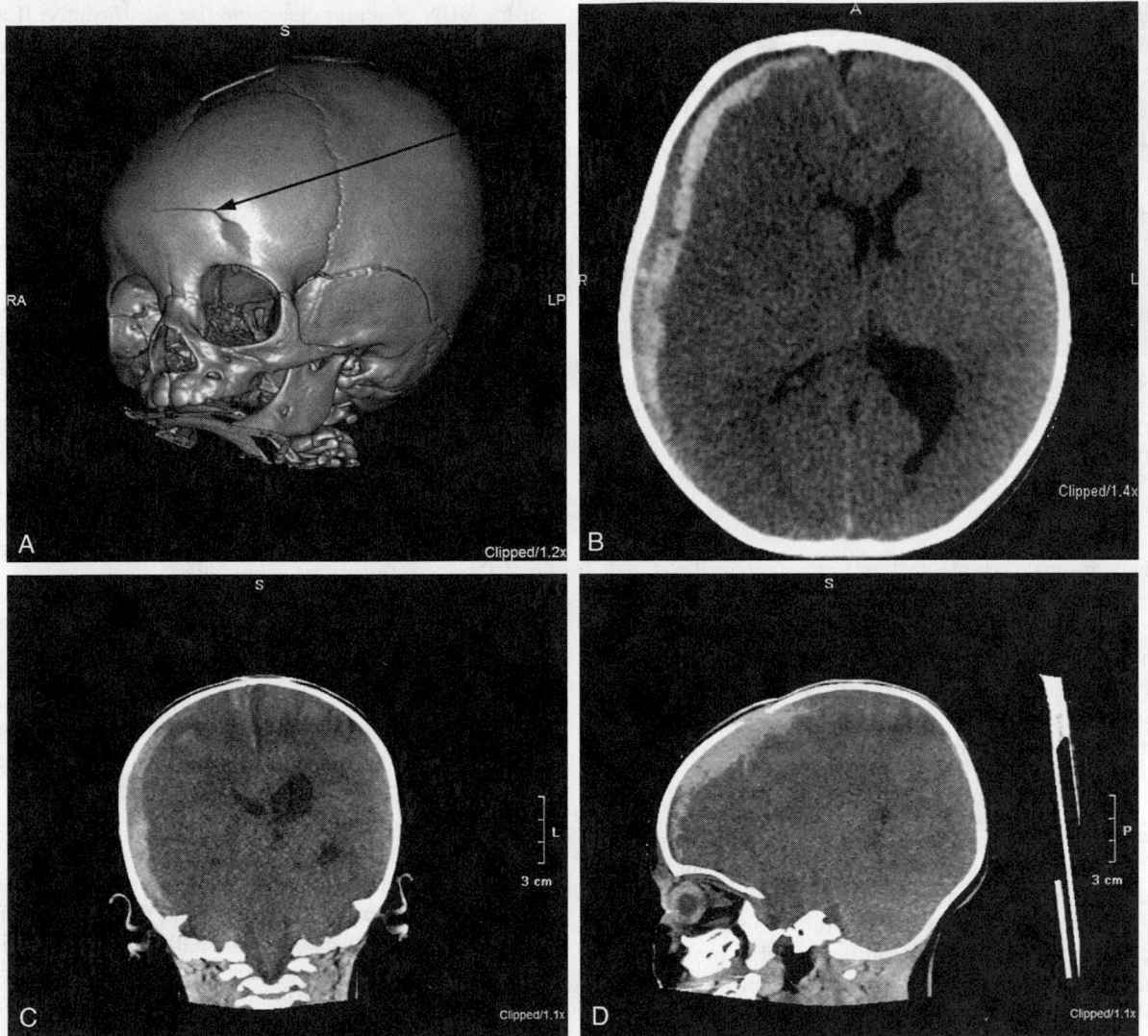

FIG. 11-20 Multi-view imaging of 10 month-old girl with head injury from a motor vehicle collision. **A,** Three-dimensional (3D) computed tomography (CT) volume rendering image shows a fracture of the frontal bone (see arrow). **B,** This traditional axial CT image provides a view looking up to the patient's head (so the patient's left side appears on the right of this image and the patient's right side appears on the left side of this image; the front of the patient is at the top of the image and the back of the patient's head is at the bottom of the image). Severe compression of the right lateral ventricle (CSF appears as a black density) is apparent, and a midline shift (toward the patient's left side) is present. A large subdural hemorrhage is visible as a white density along the outer edge of the patient's right cerebral hemisphere. **C,** Coronal CT image is interpreted as if the viewer is facing the patient. It shows the large subdural hemorrhage on the patient's right side (the white density), the compression of the patient's right lateral ventricle, and the midline shift toward the patient's left. **D,** Sagittal CT image (from the side), shows the large subdural hemorrhage (it appears as white against the grey-white matter of the brain). In B, C, and D, there is diffuse loss of normal grey-white differentiation due to cerebral infarction. (Images courtesy of Dr. Chetan Shah, Department of Pediatric Radiology, Arkansas Children's Hospital.)

and for evidence of complications similar to those occurring after cerebral angiography. Before contrast agents are administered, it is important to identify any previous reaction to contrast agents. In addition the healthcare team must be aware of the patient's baseline renal function, including BUN and creatinine concentrations, because these may rise after the use of contrast media. After the procedure, the nurse must monitor the child's urine output and serum BUN and creatinine and notify an on-call provider if urine output

is inadequate or if the BUN or serum creatinine rise significantly.

Magnetic Resonance Imaging
Definition and Purpose
MRI is the application of a strong external magnetic field around the patient to generate images of the body. This magnetic field causes rotation of the cell nuclei in a predictable direction at a predictable speed. The result of this rotation of

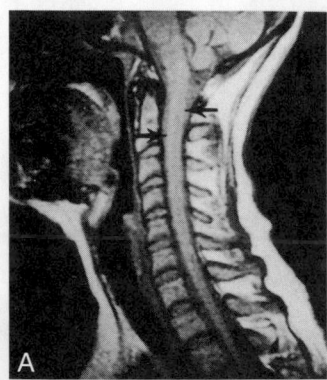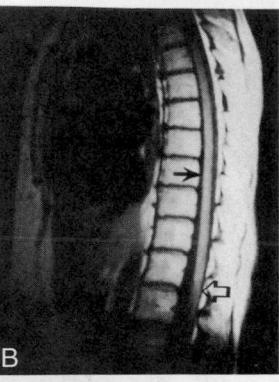

FIG. 11-21 Magnetic resonance imaging. Normal midline sagittal magnetic resonance imaging scan of the entire spine. **A,** Cervical spine. **B,** Thoracic spine. Note in detail the cord (*closed arrows*), the conus medullaris (*open arrow*), and the bones and intervertebral discs. (From Mercier LR: *Practical orthopedics,* ed 6, St Louis, 2008, Mosby, fig. 16-84, A-C.)

nuclei is a resonant image that is extremely well defined, enabling visualization of soft tissues better than any other non-invasive device. Visualization of tumors, shunts, and organ or tissue thickness is excellent using MRI. The MRI scan enables detailed visualization of areas of spinal cord compression after trauma. Because this device does not use any radiation, there are no complications related to radiation exposure (Fig. 11-21).

Procedure

The MRI scanner typically is located well away from critical care units. At present, scanning can be performed only on patients in relatively stable condition, because no metal-constructed mechanical devices can be placed in proximity to the magnetic field. Although all-plastic mechanical ventilators are available for use in the MRI scanner, monitoring systems cannot be used. Thus, MRI is most likely to be used in pediatric patients recovering from critical illness or injury.

Nursing Responsibilities

There are no known complications of MRI scanning. The nurse must be able to monitor the patient closely during the procedure, and this may be difficult with some units. MRI scanning is time consuming and requires the nurse and patient to be away from the unit for long periods of time. Prior to placing the patient in the MRI scanner, the nurse should insure that all metal objects have been removed from the patient and that appropriate MRI monitoring equipment is available.

Depending in the size of the child and the study ordered, a scan of the brain and entire spine with and without contrast can take up to hours to complete. The nurse should anticipate the need for additional doses of sedation and analgesia and possibly neuromuscular blockers if the patient is not receiving continuous infusions of these drugs (see Chapter 5).

When contrast media are used, it is important for the nurse to identify any history of previous reactions to contrast agents, and the child's current renal function, including BUN and serum creatinine. After the procedure, the nurse must monitor the child's urine output and serum BUN and creatinine and then notify an on-call provider if urine output is inadequate

or the BUN or serum creatinine rise significantly. If a patient has a programmable ventriculoperitoneal shunt, the shunt programming is checked by a member of the neurosurgery team after the procedure to verify correct settings and function.

Skull Roentgenography (Skull Films)

Definition and Purpose

Skull roentgenography (or a skull radiographs or films) enable evaluation of cranial bone relationships and densities and the size and shape of the skull. Skull radiographs are helpful in the diagnosis of skull deformities or fractures, head injuries, and bone erosion or calcification secondary to space occupying lesions. Skull radiographs, however, are often not helpful in the identification of intracranial abnormalities, such as brain tumors or head injury unless they also affect the bony structures.

A complete radiographic study of the skull includes anteroposterior and lateral views of the skull and an oblique anteroposterior view or other special angles as indicated by the child's presumed diagnosis.[62,78]

Procedure

Preferably, skull radiographs are obtained in the radiology department so that the patient's head can be immobilized and good quality radiographs can be obtained. If this is impossible, portable radiographs are obtained in the critical care unit. The radiology technician will assist in positioning the child appropriately for each film.

Nursing Responsibilities and Complications

The child (as appropriate for age and clinical condition) and family require explanations about the need for radiographs and about any special positioning required. The nurse must monitor the child closely throughout the procedure. If an ICP monitoring system is in place, it is especially important to monitor the effects of changes in head position on the ICP and request modifications in these positions as needed to maintain the ICP under appropriate thresholds. The procedure is painless.

Cerebral Angiography

Definition and Purpose

In cerebral angiography, a radiopaque contrast agent is injected into the cerebral arterial system to enable radiographic visualization of the cerebral circulation. The progress of the contrast material through the cerebral circulation is recorded with radiographs for further study. Angiography is helpful in the diagnosis of intracranial tumor, hematoma, arterial aneurysm, and arteriovenous fistula and is the definitive diagnostic procedure for arteriovenous malformation (AVM).[62]

Procedure

Contrast material, usually an iodine-containing material is injected into a selected cerebral vessel—typically the internal carotid artery. Sequential radiographs of the head are then made. This procedure usually is performed in the radiology department.

Nursing Responsibilities and Complications

The child (as appropriate for age and clinical condition) and parents require a brief explanation of the procedure. It is usually best to limit the explanation to the child to only those things that will be seen, heard, or felt; the alert child may be frightened or intrigued by the x-ray equipment.

Because the child will be transported to the radiology department for the angiography, the nurse is responsible for monitoring the child's condition during transport to and from the radiology department and throughout the procedure itself. If the child is intubated or in unstable condition, a provider able to re-intubate and prescribe drugs will accompany the bedside nurse and the child.

If contrast media are used, it is important for the nurse to be aware of the child's baseline renal function and current BUN and creatinine levels. A reaction to the contrast agent can occur after angiography. Mild symptoms may include urticaria, rhinorrhea, nausea, retching and/or vomiting, diaphoresis, coughing, and dizziness. Moderate symptoms may include vomiting, diffuse urticaria, headache, facial edema, laryngeal edema, mild bronchospasm, or dyspnea, tachycardia, bradycardia, hypertension, and abdominal cramps. Severe symptoms include life-threatening arrhythmias, hypotension, bronchospasm, pulmonary edema, seizures, syncope, and even death.[82,113] Treatment of anaphylactic shock requires volume administration and administration of vasopressors and antihistamines (see Chapter 6).

After the procedure, the nurse must monitor the child's urine output and serum BUN and creatinine levels. An on-call provider should be notified if urine output is inadequate or the BUN or serum creatinine levels rise significantly

Radionuclide Brain Scanning

A radionuclide brain scan is used as an adjunct to clinical examination to pronounce brain death; it reveals absence of CBF (brain death). To eliminate scalp circulation, a tourniquet can be placed around the patient's forehead, but this is often impractical when the patient has head injury.

A radiotracer (also called a *radiopharmaceutical*), ^{99m}Tc pertechnetate (an isomer of technecium-99), is injected intravenously and ultimately enters the circulation of the cranial vault. At this point, pictures are obtained using a gamma camera. Multiple, postinjection dynamic images are obtained over 1 minute, immediately after injection to provide dynamic perfusion images (see Evolve Fig. 11-4 in the Chapter 11 Supplement on the Evolve Website). Delayed anterior and lateral projection static images are obtained a few minutes later. These static pool images refer to radiolabeled blood now pooling in the soft tissues, rather than located only in blood vessels (see Fig. 11-18).

Absence of cerebral flow within the cranium is an adjunctive test used with the clinical exam to confirm the diagnosis of brain death. Although this technique is simple, its reliability in preterm and young infants (<2 months of age) has not been established, and there are several problems inherent in interpreting these scans in young infants. For example, decreased perfusion in the frontal or parietal cortex may be present as a nonpathologic normal variant in young infants, and infants may maintain some brain perfusion despite extensive brain injury. However, in the older infant to adolescent age group there was 100% correlation between four-vessel cerebral angiography and radionuclide cerebral scanning.[77]

References

1. Abend SN, et al: Evaluation of the comatose child. In: Nichols DG, editor: *Rogers' textbook of pediatric intensive care*, ed 4, Philadelphia, 2008, Lippincott, Williams and Wilkin.
2. Ad Hoc Committee on Brain Death—The Children's Hospital: Determination of brain death. *J Pediatr* 110:15, 1987.
3. Ad Hoc Committee of Harvard Medical School to Examine the Definition of Brain Death: A definition of irreversible coma. *J Am Med Assoc* 205:85, 1968.
4. Adams HP Jr, et al: Guidelines for the early management of adults with ischemic stroke: a guideline from the American Heart Association/American Stroke Association Stroke Council, Clinical Cardiology Council, Cardiovascular Radiology and Intervention Council, and the Atherosclerotic Peripheral Vascular Disease and Quality of Care Outcomes in Research Interdisciplinary Working Groups: the American Academy of Neurology affirms the value of this guideline as an educational tool for neurologists. *Stroke* 38(5):1655–1711, 2007.
5. Adelson PD, et al: Guidelines for the acute medical management of severe traumatic brain injury in infants, children, and adolescents. Chapter 6. Threshold for treatment of intracranial hypertension. *Pediatr Crit Care Med* 4(3 Suppl):S25–S27, 2003.
6. Adelson PD, et al: Guidelines for the acute medical management of severe traumatic brain injury in infants, children, and adolescents. Chapter 7. Intracranial pressure monitoring technology. *Pediatr Crit Care Med* 4(3 Suppl):S28–S30, 2003.
7. Adelson PD, et al: Guidelines for the acute medical management of severe traumatic brain injury in infants, children, and adolescents. Chapter 9. Use of sedation and neuromuscular blockade in the treatment of pediatric traumatic brain injury. *Pediatr Crit Care Med* 4(3 Suppl):S34–S37, 2003.
8. Adelson PD, et al: Guidelines for the acute medical management of severe traumatic brain injury in infants, children, and adolescents. Chapter 11. Use of hyperosmolar therapy in the management of severe pediatric traumatic brain injury. *Pediatr Crit Care Med* 4(3 Suppl):S40–S44, 2003.
9. Adelson PD, et al: Guidelines for the acute medical management of severe traumatic brain injury in infants, children, and adolescents. Chapter 12. Use of hyperventilation in the acute management of severe pediatric traumatic brain injury. *Pediatr Crit Care Med* 4(3, Suppl):S45–S48, 2003.
10. Adelson PD, et al: Guidelines for the acute medical management of severe traumatic brain injury in infants, children, and adolescents. Chapter 13. The use of barbiturates in the control of intracranial hypertension in severe pediatric traumatic brain injury. *Pediatric Crit Care Med* 4(3Suppl):S49–S52, 2003.
11. Adelson PD, et al: Guidelines for the acute medical management of severe traumatic brain injury in infants, children, and adolescents. Chapter 14. The role of temperature control following severe pediatric traumatic brain injury. *Pediatr Crit Care Med* 4(3 Suppl):S53–S55, 2003.
11a. Adelson PD, et al: Guidelines for the acute medical management of severe traumatic brain injury in infants, children, and adolescents. Chapter 15. Surgical treatment of pediatric intracranial hypertension. *Pediatr Crit Care Med* 4(3 Suppl):S56–S59, 2003.
12. Adelson P, et al: Guidelines for the acute medical management of severe traumatic brain injury in infants, children, and adolescents. Chapter 16. The use of corticosteroids in the treatment of severe pediatric traumatic brain injury. *Pediatr Crit Care Med* 4(3 Suppl):S60–S64, 2003.
13. Adelson PD, et al: Guidelines for the acute medical management of severe traumatic brain injury in infants, children, and adolescents. Chapter 17. Critical pathway for the treatment of established intracranial hypertension in pediatric traumatic brain injury. *Pediatr Crit Care Med* 4(3 Suppl):S65–S67, 2003.
14. Adelson PD, et al: Guidelines for the acute medical management of severe traumatic brain injury in infants, children, and adolescents. Chapter 19. The role of anti-seizure prophylaxis following severe pediatric traumatic brain injury. *Pediatr Crit Care Med* 4(3 Suppl):S72–S75, 2003.

15. Ashwal S: Clinical diagnosis and confirmatory tests of brain death in children. In: Wijdicks EFM, editor: *Brain death*, New York, 2001, Lippincott Williams and Wilkins.

16. Ashwal S, Schneider S: Brain death in children: Part I. *Pediatr Neurol* 3:5, 1987.

17. Ashwal S, Schneider S: Brain death in children: Part II. *Pediatr Neurol* 3:69, 1987.

18. Ashwal S, Schneider S: Brain death in the newborn. *Pediatrics* 84:429, 1989.

19. Ashwal S, Serna-Fonseca T: Brain death in infants and children. *Crit Care Nurse* 26(2):117–128, 2006.

20. Atabaki SM: Pediatric head injury. *Pediatr Rev* 28:215–224, 2007.

21. Babcock MA, et al: Tumors of the central nervous systems: clinical aspects, molecular mechanisms, unanswered questions, and future research directions. *J Child Neurol* 23(10):1103–1121, 2008.

21a. Bechtel K, Frasure S, Marshall C, et al. Relationship of serum S100B levels and intracranial injury in children with closed head trauma. *Pediatrics* 124(4):697–704, 2009.

21b. Bell MJ, Kochanek PM: Traumatic brain injury in children: recent advances in management. *Indian J Pediatr* 75(11):1159–1165, 2008.

22. Biagas K: Drowning and near drowning: submersion injuries. In: Nichols DG, editor: *Rogers' textbook of pediatric intensive care*, ed 4, Philadelphia, 2008, Lippincott Williams and Wilkins.

23. Bleck TP: Level of consciousness and attention. In: Goetz CG, editor: *Textbook of clinical neurology*, Philadelphia, 1999, Saunders.

24. Bledsoe KA, Kramer AH: Propylene glycol toxicity complicating use of barbiturate coma. *Neurocrit Care* 9:122–124, 2008.

25. Blumstein MD, Friedman MJ: Childhood seizures. *Emerg Med Cin N Am* 25:1061–1086, 2007.

26. Bohn DF: Near-drowning: when to resuscitate. *Pediatr Trauma Acute Care* 2:49 (Commentary), 1989.

27. Bohn DF: Near drowning: saving the brain. *Pediatr Trauma Acute Care* 1:5 (Commentary), 1988.

28. Bracken MB: Steroids for acute spinal cord injury. *Cochrane Database Syst Rev* (3):CD001046, 2002.

29. Capildeo R: Cerebrovascular disease. In: Rose FC, editor: *Paediatric neurology*, Oxford, 1979, Blackwell Scientific.

30. Case ME: Traumatic diffuse axonal injury. *Brain Path* 18(4):571–582, 2008.

31. Callas HJ: Drowning and near drowning. In: Behrman RE et al., editors: *Nelson textbook of pediatrics*, ed 18, Philadelphia, 2007, Saunders.

32. Cheng M-F, et al: Clinical application of reverse-transcription polymerase chain reaction and intravenous immunoglobulin for enterovirus encephalitis. *Jpn J Infect Dis* 61:18–24, 2008.

33. Clifton GL, et al: Lack of effect of induction of hypothermia after acute brain injury. *N Engl J Med* 344:556–563, 2001.

34. Clifton GL, et al: Multicenter trial of early hypothermia in severe brain injury. *J Neurotrauma* 26(3):393–397, 2009.

34a. Cohen J, Cohen J: Interrater reliability and predictive validity of the FOUR score coma scale in a pediatric population. *J Neurosci Nurs* 41(5):261–267, 2009.

35. Cross JH, Neal EG: The ketogenic diet-update on recent clinical trials. *Epilepsia* 49(Suppl 8):6–10, 2008.

36. Custer JW, Rau RE, editors: *The Harriett lane handbook*, ed 18, Philadelphia, 2008, Mosby.

37. Davis A, Ravussin P, Bissonnette B: Central nervous system anatomy and physiology. In: Bissonett B, Dalens B, editors: *Pediatric anesthesia: principles and practice*, New York, 2002, McGraw-Hill.

38. deVeber G: Stroke and the child's brain: an overview of epidemiology, syndromes and risk factors. *Curr Opin Neurol* 15:133–138, 2002.

39. deVeber G: Risk factors for childhood stroke: little folks have different strokes. *Ann Neurol* 53(2):149–150, 2003.

40. Enix A, et al: Traumatic brain injury. In: Cartwright CC, Wallace DC, editors: *Nursing care of the pediatric neurosurgery patient*, New York, 2007, Springer.

41. Faria SH: Assessment of immobility hazards. *Home Care Prov* 3 (4):189–191, 1998.

42. Federal Law: Public Law 99-509, Omnibus budget reconciliation act of 1986, Approved October 21, 1986 (100 Stat. 1874).

43. Fink EL, Manole MD, Clark RSB: Hypoxic-ischemic encephalopathy. In: Nichols DG, editor: *Rogers' textbook of pediatric intensive care*, ed 4, Philadelphia, 2008, Lippincott Williams and Wilkins.

44. Fox WC, Wawrzyniak S, Chandler WF: Intraoperative acquisition of three-dimensional imaging for frameless stereotactic guidance during transsphenoidal pituitary surgery using the Arcadis Orbic System. *J Neurosurg* 108:746–750, 2008.

45. Frauman AC, Miles MS: Parental willingness to donate the organs of a child. *ANNA J* 14:1, 1987.

46. Fuchs S: Seizures. In: Barkin R et al., editors: *Pediatric emergency medicine*, ed 2, St Louis, 1997.

47. Furlan JC, et al: Timing of decompressive surgery after traumatic spinal cord injury: an evidence-based examination of pre-clinical and clinical studies. *J Neurotrauma* 8(28):1371–1399, 2011 [epub ahead of print, March 4, 2010].

48. Giza CC, Mink RB, Madikians A: Pediatric traumatic brain injury: not just little adults *VC Curr Opin Crit Care* 13:143–152, 2007.

50. Greenberg MS, editor: *Handbook of neurosurgery*, ed 6, New York, 2006, Thieme.

51. Grigg MM, et al: Electroencephalographic activity after brain death. *Arch Neurol* 44:948, 1987.

52. Goldschlager T, Rosenfeld JV, Winter CD: Talk and die patients presenting to a major trauma centre over a 10 year period: a critical review. *J Clin Neurosci* 14:618–623, 2007.

53. Goldstein B, Aboy M, Graham A: Neurologic monitoring. In: Nichols DG, editor: *Rogers' textbook of pediatric intensive care*, ed 4, Philadelphia, 2008, Lippincott Williams and Wilkins.

54. Guertin SR, et al: Intracranial volume pressure response in infants and children. *Crit Care Med* 10:1, 1982.

55. Guertin SR: Neurosurgical intensive care: selected aspects. In: Fuhrman BP, Zimmerman JJ, editors: *Pediatric critical care*, ed 2, St Louis, 1998, Mosby, Inc.

56. Haque IU, Zaritsky AL: Analysis of the evidence for the lower limit of systolic and mean arterial pressure in children. *Pediatr Crit Care* 8:138–144, 2007.

57. Haft GF, et al: Use of beta-2-transferrin to diagnose CSF leakage following spinal surgery: a case report. *Iowa Orthopaedic J* 24:115–118, 2004.

58. Haslam RHA: Neurologic evaluation. In: Behrman RE et al., editors: *Nelson Textbook of Pediatrics* ed 18, Philadelphia, 2007, Saunders.

59. Hazinski MF: Organ donation: what the new "required request" law means to you. *Pediatr Nurs* 13:415, 1987.

60. Hazinski MF: Pediatric organ donation: responsibilities of the critical care nurse. *Pediatr Nurs* 13:354, 1987.

61. Heegaard WG, Biros MH: Head. In: Marx JA, editor: *Rosen's emergency medicine*, Philadelphia, 2006, Mosby-Elsevier.

62. Hickey JV: *The clinical practice of neurological and neurosurgical nursing*, ed 5, Philadelphia, 2003, Lippincott Williams and Wilkins.

63. Hutchison JS, et al: Hypothermia therapy after traumatic brain injury in children. *N Engl J Med* 358:2447–2456, 2008.

64. Johnston MV: Development, structure and function of the brain and neuromuscular system. In: Fuhrman BP, Zimmerman JJ, editors: *Pediatric intensive care*, ed 3, Philadelphia, 2006, Mosby.

65. Jordan LC, et al: Ischemic stroke in children with critical illness: a poor prognostic sign. *Pediatr Neurol* 36:244–246, 2007.

66. Jouvet P, et al: Metabolic encephalopathies in children. In: Nichols DG, editor: *Rogers' textbook of pediatric intensive care*, ed 4, Philadelphia, 2008, Lippincott Williams and Wilkins.

67. Keegan M, et al: Plasma exchange for severe attacks of CNS demyelination: predictors of response. *Neurology* 58:143–146, 2002.

68. Kissoon N, et al: Pediatric organ donor maintenance: pathophysiologic derangements and nursing requirements. *Pediatrics* 84:688, 1989.

69. Klinker DB, et al: Pediatric vascular injuries: patterns of injury, morbidity, and mortality. *J Ped Surg* 42(1):178–183, 2007.

70. Knapp JM: Hyperosmolar therapy in the treatment of severe head injury in children. *AACN Clin Issues* 18(2):199–211, 2005.

71. Kochanek PM, et al: Molecular biology of brain injury. In: Nichols DG, editor: *Rogers' textbook of pediatric intensive care*, ed 4, Philadelphia, 2008, Lippincott Williams and Wilkins.

72. Kontos HA: Regulation of the cerebral circulation. *Ann Rev Physiol* 43:397, 1981.

72a. Kovesdi E, Luckl J, Bukovics P, Farkas O, et al: Update on protein biomarkers in traumatic brain injury with emphasis on clinical use in adults and pediatrics. Acta Neurochir 152:1–17, 2010.

73. Krapohl BD, Deutinger M, Komurcu F: Vagus nerve stimulation: treatment modality for epilepsy. *Medsurg Nurs* 16(1):39–44, 2007.

74. Kulkarni MS, Baum CR: Traumatic pneumocephalus. *Clin Ped Emerg Med* 1(1):70–73, 1999.

75. Kutsogiannis DJ, et al: Medical management to optimize donor organ potential: review of the literature. *Can J Anesth* 53 (8):820–830, 2006.

76. Larsen WJ, editor: *Human embryology*, Philadelphia, 2001, Churchill-Livingstone.

77. Levin DL: Brain death. Nichols DG, editor: *Rogers' textbook of pediatric intensive care,* ed 4, Philadelphia, 2008, Lippincott Williams and Wilkins.

78. Lindsay KW, Bone I: *Neurology and neurosurgery illustrated,* ed 4, Edinburgh, 2004, Churchill-Livingstone.

79. Lubitz DS, et al: A rapid method for estimating weight and resuscitation drug dosages from length in pediatric age group. *Am Emerg Med* 17:576, 1988.

80. Maguire JL, et al: Should a head-injured child receive a head CT scan? A systematic review of clinical prediction rules. *Pediatrics* 124(1):e145–e154, 2009.

81. Mann K, Jackson MA: Meningitis. *Pediatr Rev* 29:417–430, 2008.

82. Mansfield RT: Severe traumatic brain injuries in children. *Clin Ped Emerg Med* 8:156–164, 2007.

83. Marcoux KK: Management of increased intracranial pressure in the critically ill child with an acute neurological injury. *AACN Clin Issues* 16(2):212–231, 2005.

84. Mathur M, et al: Pediatric critical care nurses' perception, knowledge, and attitudes regarding organ donation after cardiac death. *Pediatr Crit Care Med* 9(3):261–269, 2008.

85. McCance KL, Huether SE: *Pathophysiology: the biologic basis for disease in adults and children,* ed 5, Philadelphia, 2005, Mosby.

86. McCollough CH, et al: Strategies for reducing radiation dose in CT. *Radiol Clin North Am* 47:27–40, 2009.

87. Meyer RJ, Theodorou AA, Berg RA: Childhood drowning. *Pediatr Rev* 27:163–169, 2006.

88. Miller MA, Forni A, Yogaratnam D: Propylene glycol-induced lactic acidosis in patient receiving continuous infusion pentobarbital. *Ann Pharmacother* 42:1502–1506, 2008.

89. Miyazawa R, et al: Plasmapheresis in fulminant acute disseminated encephalomyelitis. *Brain Dev* 23:424–426, 2001.

90. Morray JP, et al: Coma scale for use in brain-injured children. *Crit Care Med* 12:1018, 1984.

91. Nance JR, Golomb MR: Ischemic spinal cord infarction in children without vertebral fracture. *Pediatr Neurol* 36:209–216, 2007.

92. Nilles EJ, Spiro DM: Delayed intracerebral hemorrhage from an extracranial ball bullet pellet. *Ped Emerg Care* 23(6):408–411, 2007.

93. Norwood SH, et al: Early venous thromboembolism prophylaxis with enoxaparin in patients with blunt traumatic brain injury. *J Trauma* 65:1021–1027, 2008.

94. Obeid M, et al: Approach to pediatric epilepsy surgery: state of the art, part I: general principles and presurgical workup. *Eur J Paediatr Neurol* 13:102–114, 2009.

95. Obeid M, et al: Approach to pediatric epilepsy surgery: state of the art, part II: approach to specific epilepsy syndromes and etiologies. *Eur J Paediatr Neurol* 13:115–127, 2009.

96. Orliaguet GA, Meyer PG, Baugnon T: Management of critically ill children with traumatic brain injury. *Pediatr Anesth* 18:455–461, 2008.

97. Outwater KM, Rockoff MA: Apnea testing to confirm brain death in children. *Crit Care Med* 12:357, 1984.

98. Packer RJ: Childhood brain tumors: accomplishments and ongoing challenges. *J Child Neurol* 23(10):1122–1127, 2008.

99. Pappachan J, Kirkham F: Cerebral vascular disease and stroke. In: Nichols DG, editor: *Rogers' textbook of pediatric intensive care,* ed 4, Philadelphia, 2008, Lippincott Williams and Wilkins.

100. Pearson-Shaver AL, Mehta R: Coma and depressed sensorium. In: Fuhrman BP, Zimmerman JJ, editors: *Pediatric intensive care,* ed 3, Philadelphia, 2006, Mosby.

101. Pickering LK et al, editors: *Red book: 2006 report of the committee on infectious diseases,* ed 27, Elk Grove Village, IL, 2006, American Academy of Pediatrics.

102. Plum F, Posner JB: *The diagnosis of stupor and coma,* ed 3, Philadelphia, 1980, FA Davis.

103. Poss WB, Moss SD, Dean MJ: Intracranial hypertension. In: Fuhrman BP, Zimmerman JJ, editors: *Pediatric critical care,* ed 2, St Louis, 1998, Mosby.

104. Ralston M, et al: *Pediatric advance life support,* Dallas, 2006, American Heart Association.

105. RamachandranNair R, Parameswaran M, Girija AS: Acute disseminated encephalomyelitis treated with plasmapheresis. *Singapore Med J* 46(10):561–563, 2005.

106. Reilly PL, et al: Assessing the conscious level in infants and young children: a paediatric version of the Glasgow Coma Scale. *Childs Nerv Syst* 4:30, 1988.

107. Roach ES, et al: Management of stroke in infants and children: a scientific statement from a special writing group of the American Heart Association Stroke Council and the Council of Cardiovascular Disease in the Young. *Circulation* 39(9):2644–2691, 2008.

108. Raslan A, Bhardwaj A: Medical management of cerebral edema. *Neurosurg Focus* 22(5):E12, 2007.

109. Salim A, et al: Using thyroid hormone in brain-dead donors to maximize the number of organs available for transplantation. *Clin Transplant* 21:405–409, 2007.

110. Salim A, et al: Aggressive organ donor management significantly increases the number of organs available for transplantation. *J Trauma* 58:991, 2005.

110a. Sandler SJ, Figaji AA, Adelson PD: Clinical applications of biomarkers in pediatric traumatic brain injury. *Childs Nerv Syst* 26:205–213, 2010.

111. Seidel HM, et al: *Mosby's guide to physical examination,* ed 6, St Louis, 2006, Mosby.

112. Shields WD: Status epilepticus. *Pediatr Clin North Am* 36:383, 1989.

113. Siddiqi NH: Contrast medium reactions, recognition and treatments. Available at http://emedicine.medscape.com/article/422855-overview Updated April 20, 2011. Accessed August 28 2011.

114. Singhi PD, et al: Central nervous system infections. In: Nichols DG, editor: *Rogers' textbook of pediatric intensive care,* ed 4, Philadelphia, 2008, Lippincott Williams and Wilkins.

115. Smyth MD, et al: Complications of chronic vagus nerve stimulation for epilepsy in children. *J Neurosurg* 22:500–503, 2003.

116. Solarine B, Rechentwald K, Burrows-Beckham AM: An unusual case of child head injury by coat hanger. *J Forensic Sci* 53 (5):1188–1190, 2008.

117. Sperling MA: Diabetes mellitus. In: Behrman RE et al., editors: *Nelson textbook of pediatrics,* ed 18, Philadelphia, 2007, Saunders.

118. Sorcher MA: Lumbar puncture: perform. In: Verger JT, Lebet RM, editors: *AACN procedure manual for pediatric acute and critical care,* St Louis, 2008, Saunders.

119. Statler DK, Van Orman CB: Status epilepticus. In: Nichols DG, editor: *Rogers' textbook of pediatric intensive care,* ed 4, Philadelphia, 2008, Lippincott Williams and Wilkins.

120. Taketomo CK, Hodding JH, Kraus DM, editors: *Pediatric dosage handbook,* ed 14, Hudson, Ohio, 2007, Lexicomp.

121. Task Force for Brain Death Determination in Children: Guidelines for the determination of brain death in children. *Pediatrics* 80:298, 1987.

122. Tasker RC: Head and spinal cord trauma. In: Nichols DG, editor: *Rogers' textbook of pediatric intensive care,* ed 4, Philadelphia, 2008, Lippincott Williams and Wilkins.

123. Tasker RC, Czosnyka M: Intracranial hypertension and brain monitoring. In: Fuhrman BP, Zimmerman JJ, editors: *Pediatric intensive care,* ed 3, Philadelphia, 2006, Mosby.

124. Trinka E: The use of valproate and new antiepileptic drugs in status epilepticus. *Eplipesia* 48(Suppl 8):49–51, 2007.

125. Thompson G, Scoles P: Bone and joint disorders. In Behrman RE, et al, editors: *Nelson Textbook of pediatrics* ed 18. Philadelphia, 2007, Saunders.

125a. Thompson H, Avanecean D: Care of the patient with a lumbar drain. *AANN Ref Ser Clin Pract* 2:4–15, 2007.

126. Vavilala MS, et al: Cerebral autoregulation in pediatric traumatic brain injury. *Pediatr Crit Care Med* 5(3):257–263, 2004.

127. Velasco AJ: Jugular venous saturation monitoring: insertion, assist, monitoring and care. In: Verger JT, Lebet RM, editors: *AACN procedure manual for pediatric acute and critical care,* St Louis, 2008, Saunders.

128. Vlasselaers D, et al: Intensive insulin therapy for patients in paediatric intensive care: a prospective, randomised controlled study. *Lancet* 373:547–556, 2009.

129. Webster PA, Markham L: Pediatric organ donation: a national survey examining consent rates and characteristics of donor hospitals. *Pediatr Crit Care Med* 10:1–5, 2009.

130. Wheless JW, Treiman DM: The role of the newer antiepileptic drugs in the treatment of generalized convulsive status epilepticus. *Epilepsia* 49(Suppl 9):74–78, 2008.

131. Zuckier LS, Kolano J: Radionuclide studies in the determination of brain death: criteria, concepts, and controversies. *Semin Nucl Med* 38:262–273, 2008.

132. Zupec-Kania BA, Spellman E: An overview of the ketogenic diet for pediatric epilepsy. *Nutr Clin Pract* 23:589–596, 2008.

133. Zwienenberg M, Muizelaar JP: Cerebral perfusion and blood flow in neurotrauma. *Neurol Res* 23:167–174, 2001.

Fluid, Electrolyte, and Endocrine Problems

12

Kathryn E. Roberts

ⓔvolve Be sure to check out the supplementary content available at http://evolve.elsevier.com/Hazinski.

PEARLS

- The term *osmolality* refers to the concentration of solute (electrolytes and proteins) per liter of fluid. Serum osmolality reflects extracellular fluid osmolality. It can be estimated with the following formula:

$$
\begin{aligned}
\text{Serum osmolality} = \ &(2 \times \text{Serum sodium}) \\
&+ (\text{Serum glucose} \div 18) \\
&+ (\text{Blood urea nitrogen} \div 2.8)
\end{aligned}
$$

Note: This formula does not reflect the influence of plasma proteins or administered osmotic agents such as mannitol. It may be inaccurate in the presence of severe hyperglycemia and hyperlipemia.

- Acute changes in serum sodium and osmolality can cause acute water shifts between the intracellular and extracellular spaces. An acute fall in serum sodium concentration and osmolality and the resulting intracellular water shift can cause cerebral edema. If neurologic symptoms develop, urgent treatment is needed. In general, significant water shifts into and out of the vascular space are poorly tolerated.
- Critical care practitioners use the child's estimated maintenance fluid requirement as a baseline and individualize administered fluid and electrolytes to meet patient needs.
- With the development of acidosis or alkalosis, the serum potassium concentration will change in a direction opposite the change in serum pH, in response to reciprocal potassium and hydrogen ion shifts into and out of the cell.
- If the level of consciousness of the child with diabetic ketoacidosis (DKA) deteriorates during treatment, cerebral edema may be present and urgent intervention is needed. If clinical signs of cerebral edema develop, immediate treatment with intravenous (IV) mannitol or hypertonic saline is needed. If the child's ability to protect the airway or spontaneous ventilation deteriorates, intubation and mechanical ventilation are indicated.

INTRODUCTION

Small disruptions in fluid or electrolyte homeostasis or endocrine function can result in significant clinical changes in critically ill infants and children. These disruptions may be a primary problem, or they may be secondary to critical illness, critical injury, or therapeutic interventions (e.g., medication administration, fluid resuscitation).

ANATOMY AND PHYSIOLOGY

Body fluids contain water and solutes. These solutes are positively or negatively charged electrolytes (e.g., Na^+, K^+, Cl^-) and nonelectrolytes (e.g., glucose, urea). Fluid and electrolyte homeostasis is present when fluid and electrolyte balance is maintained within narrow limits despite significant variations in dietary intake, metabolic rate, and renal function.

Fluid Compartments

Water accounts for 65% to 80% of total body weight. The total body water (TBW) volume and distribution are influenced by factors such as age, gender, adipose content, and skeletal muscle mass (Table 12-1). TBW is divided into two compartments (see Evolve Table 12-1 and Evolve Fig. 12-1 in the Chapter 12 Supplement on the Evolve Website for more information): intracellular fluid (ICF) and extracellular fluid (ECF) compartments (Fig. 12-1).

ICF Compartment

The ICF is within the cell membranes. It is the largest fluid compartment, comprising approximately 33% of body weight by 1 year of age. Potassium and phosphate are the primary intracellular electrolytes.

ECF Compartment

The ECF is composed of intravascular fluid (plasma or serum), interstitial fluid (lymph), and transcellular water. The ECF comprises almost half of the body weight in the full-term infant; this percentage declines as the child grows.

Table 12-1	Developmental Changes in Total Body Water, Extracellular Fluid, and Intracellular Fluid		
Age	Total Body Water (% Body Weight)	Extracellular Fluid (% Body Weight)	Intracellular Fluid (% Body Weight)
Neonate	72-79	32-44	35-40
1-2 years	59	25	33
3-5 years	62	21	41
10-16 years	58	18	39

Adapted from Finberg L, et al, editors: *Water and electrolytes in pediatrics: physiology, pathophysiology and treatment*, Philadelphia, 1993, WB Saunders, pp. 12-15.

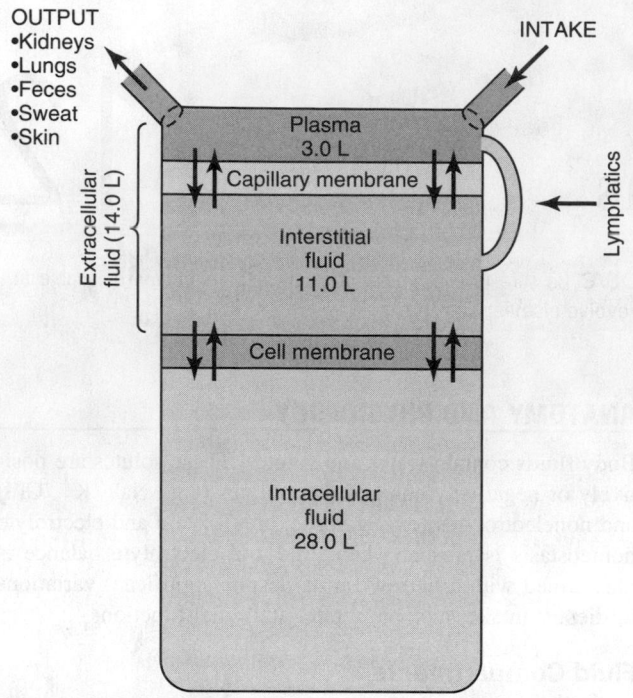

FIG. 12-1 Body fluid compartments showing values for an average 70-kg person. (From Guyton AC, Hall JE, editors: *Textbook of medical physiology*, ed 11. Philadelphia, 2006, WB Saunders, p. 292, Fig. 29-1.)

Sodium and chloride are the primary electrolytes of the ECF. Although the largest volume within the ECF is interstitial fluid (20% of TBW), it is the plasma or intravascular volume that is essential to cardiac output and systemic perfusion. Transcellular water typically accounts for a small percentage of TBW and is found in the pleural, pericardial, peritoneal, and joint spaces. During some disease states, the volume of transcellular fluid increases.

Fluid Shifts

Fluid compartments are separated by selectively permeable membranes. These membranes permit movement of water and some solutes (e.g., electrolytes) from one compartment to another. This movement of fluids and electrolytes occurs through osmosis, diffusion, active transport, and filtration. If osmolality becomes unequal between compartments, water shifts to restore equilibrium (see section, Role of Osmolality).

Developmental Considerations

Renal function, metabolic rate, body surface area (BSA), and fluid requirements change with development. The infant kidney is unable to concentrate urine until approximately 3 months of age, and it is relatively inefficient at concentrating urine until approximately 2 years of age. In the first years of life the kidneys are also inefficient at excreting electrolytes and waste products, and they are unable to effectively conserve or excrete sodium, acidify urine, or handle large quantities of solute-free water. As a result, infants and small children are less able to maintain homeostasis with sudden, acute changes in fluid and electrolyte intake or output.

Energy requirements (per kilogram body weight) and metabolic rate are higher in infancy and childhood (for further information, see Chapter 14). The ratio of BSA to volume is significantly higher in infants and children than in adults. As a result, pediatric evaporative fluid losses and fluid requirements per kilogram body weight are higher than those of adults.

Insensible water loss (IWL) is fluid lost through the skin, via evaporation and sweat, and through the respiratory tract. Normal IWL is approximately 300 to 400 mL/m^2 BSA per day (for more detailed information, see Evolve Table 12-2 in the Chapter 12 Supplement on the Evolve Website). Fever increases IWL by approximately 0.42 mL/kg per hour for each degree Celsius increase above 37° C. Increased IWL can occur

Table 12-2   Formulas for Estimating Daily Maintenance Fluid and Electrolyte Requirements for Children

	Daily Requirements	Hourly Requirements
Fluid Requirements Estimated from Weight*		
Newborn (up to 72 hr after birth)	60-100 mL/kg (newborns are born with excess body water)	–
Up to 10 kg	100 mL/kg (can increase up to 150 mL/kg to provide caloric requirements if renal and cardiac function are adequate)	4 mL/kg
11-20 kg	1000 mL for the first 10 kg + 50 mL/kg for each kg over 10 kg	40 mL for first 10 kg + 2 mL/kg for each kg over 10 kg
21-30 kg	1500 mL for the first 20 kg + 25 mL/kg for each kg over 20 kg	60 mL for first 20 kg + 1 mL/kg for each kg over 20 kg
Fluid Requirements Estimated from Body Surface Area (BSA)		
Maintenance	1500 mL/m^2 BSA	–
Insensible losses	300-400 mL/m^2 BSA	–
Electrolytes		
Sodium (Na)	2-4 mEq/kg	–
Potassium (K)	1-2 mEq/kg	–
Chloride (Cl)	2-3 mEq/kg	–
Calcium (Ca)	0.5-3 mEq/kg	–
Phosphorous (Phos)	0.5-2 mmol/kg	–
Magnesium (Mg)	0.4-0.9 mEq/kg	–

*The "maintenance" fluids calculated by these formulas must only be used as a starting point to determine the fluid requirements of an individual patient. If intravascular volume is adequate, children with cardiac, pulmonary, or renal failure or increased intracranial pressure should generally receive less than these calculated "maintenance" fluids. The formula utilizing body weight generally results in a generous "maintenance" fluid total.

with increased air movement across the skin, and with tachypnea, unless inspired air is humidified. IWL decreases when ambient and inspired air are humidified.

Fluid and electrolyte requirements will vary with age and clinical condition. Normal baseline fluid and electrolyte requirements are listed in Table 12-2. Critical care practitioners use estimated maintenance fluid requirements as a baseline and individualize administered fluid and electrolytes to meet patient needs.

Fluid, Electrolyte, and Glucose Balance

Role of Osmolality

The term *osmolality* refers to the concentration of solute (electrolytes and proteins) per liter of fluid. Serum osmolality reflects ECF osmolality. It can be estimated with the following formula*:

$$\text{Serum osmolality} = (2 \times \text{Serum sodium}) + (\text{Serum glucose} \div 18) + (\text{Blood urea nitrogen} \div 2.8)$$

*This formula does not reflect the influence of plasma proteins or administered osmotic agents such as mannitol. It may be inaccurate in the presence of severe hyperglycemia and hyperlipemia.

Because sodium is the primary electrolyte that determines serum osmolality, a major increase or decrease in serum sodium concentration will increase or decrease the serum osmolality, respectively.

Changes in the osmolality of one body fluid compartment will affect all other compartments. Water shifts between the ICF and the ECF compartments in response to changes in the osmolality of either compartment, moving from the compartment of lower osmolality to the compartment of higher osmolality until osmolality equilibrates. When the osmolality of the extracellular compartment (including the vascular space) decreases, water will shift from the extracellular compartment into cells (Fig. 12-2). Conversely, when the osmolality of the extracellular compartment (including the vascular space) increases, water will shift from the intracellular to the extracellular compartment (including into the vascular space). The volume and acuity of the water shift, as well as likely clinical significance, is determined by the magnitude and acuity of the osmolality gradient between compartments. Significant water shifts can cause neurologic complications.

Renal Influences

The kidneys help maintain fluid balance through filtration and selective reabsorption. Changes in the glomerular filtration rate (GFR) alter the amount of water and sodium excreted or reabsorbed by the kidneys. Expansion of intravascular volume normally increases the GFR, increasing sodium and water excretion. When intravascular volume is depleted, the GFR falls and sodium and water excretion decrease (i.e., more sodium and water are reabsorbed into plasma from the renal filtrate). As noted previously, the kidney is less able to concentrate urine during the first months of life. (See Chapter 13 for more detailed information.)

Endocrine Influences

Several hormones contribute to regulation of fluid and electrolyte balance.

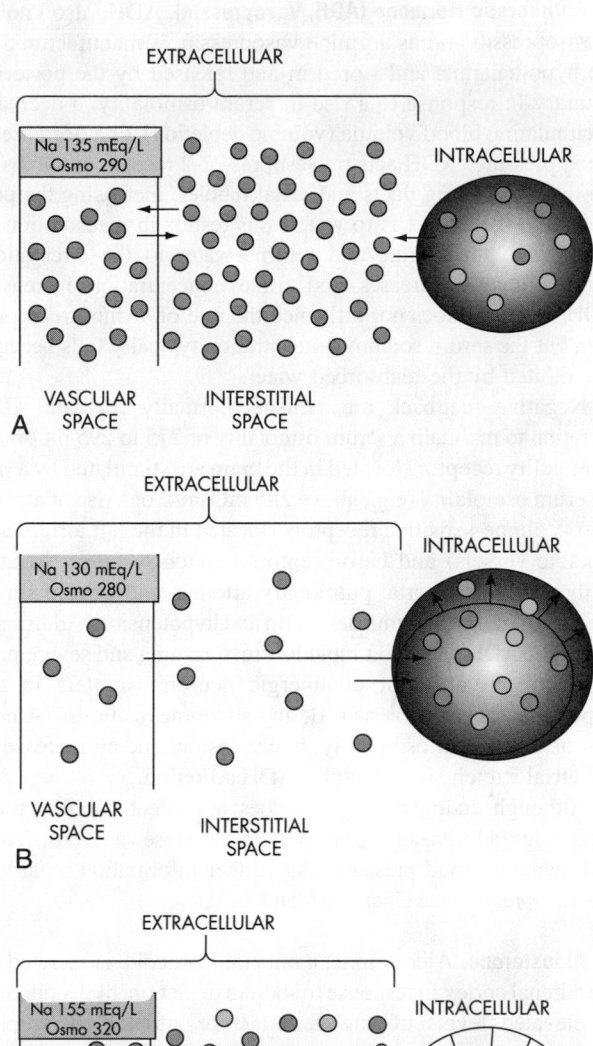

FIG. 12-2 Water shifts with changes in serum sodium and osmolality. **A,** Normal. Free water shifts between extracellular and intracellular compartments and across the semipermeable vascular membrane (between the vascular and interstitial spaces) to maintain osmotic equilibrium. **B,** Effects of acute fall in serum osmolality. An acute fall in serum sodium and osmolality cause water to shift from the extracellular (including the vascular space) to the intracellular compartment. Intracellular water volume increases until osmolality equilibrates. The *smaller inside circle* (under the word "Intracellular") represents original cell size. The black arrows schematically represent the effects of the shift of water into the intracellular compartment. **C,** Effects of acute rise in serum osmolality. An acute rise in serum sodium and osmolality cause water to shift from the intracellular to extracellular (including into vascular space) compartment. Intracellular water volume decreases until osmolality equilibrates. The *larger outside circle* (under the word "Intracellular") represents original cell size. The arrows schematically represent the effects of the shift of free water from the intracellular to the extracellular compartment.

Antidiuretic Hormone (ADH, Vasopressin). ADH, also known as vasopressin and as arginine vasopressin, is manufactured in the hypothalamus and stored in and released by the posterior pituitary in response to a rise in serum osmolality, a decrease in circulating blood volume (volume depletion), or a decrease in blood pressure. ADH acts on vasopressor-2 receptors of cells in the renal collecting ducts and distal tubules, increasing the permeability of these cells to water; this results in reabsorption of water from the filtrate and returns water to the circulation. Urine volume decreases and urine concentration increases. ADH secretion does not influence the rate of sodium reabsorption, but the serum sodium concentration typically falls because it is diluted by the reabsorbed water.

Negative feedback mechanisms normally regulate ADH secretion to maintain a serum osmolality of 275 to 295 mOsm/L. Osmolality receptors located in the brain are stimulated by a rise in serum osmolality (e.g., above 285 mOsm/L or a rise of at least 2%). Volume-sensitive receptors (located in the left atrium and thoracic vessels) and baroreceptors (stretch receptors located in the ascending aorta, pulmonary arteries, and carotid sinus) are stimulated by volume depletion and hypotension. Additional causes of ADH secretion include stress, trauma and severe pain (through activation of cholinergic neurotransmitters in the hypothalamus), angiotensin II, and some medications.[3] A normal or low serum osmolality, hypertension, and an increase in left atrial stretch should inhibit ADH secretion.

Although endogenous ADH does not affect vascular tone, exogenous (administered) vasopressin can cause vasoconstriction and increase blood pressure. For further information regarding use vasopressin, see Chapters 6 and 14.

Aldosterone. Aldosterone, a mineralocorticoid, is secreted by the adrenal cortex in response to sodium depletion, hyperkalemia, or elevated levels of angiotensin II or adrenocorticotrophic hormone. Aldosterone increases sodium reabsorption by the intestine, the renal distal tubules, and collecting ducts; this increases both sodium and water reabsorption. Aldosterone increases renal secretion of potassium and hydrogen ions.

Natriuretic Peptides. The natriuretic peptides are salt-losing hormones that influence blood volume and blood pressure. Atrial natriuretic peptide (ANP) is synthesized, stored, and released by atrial myocytes in response to atrial distension, endothelin, and sympathetic nervous system and angiotensin II stimulation. Increased ANP is present during hypervolemia and congestive heart failure.

Brain natriuretic peptide is synthesized in the brain and in the ventricles of the heart. Brain natriuretic peptide release is triggered by the same conditions that trigger ANP release, and it has similar physiologic actions. Brain natriuretic peptide is a sensitive diagnostic marker for heart failure (see Congestive Heart Failure in Chapter 8).

Natriuretic peptides are involved in the long-term regulation of sodium and water balance, blood volume, and blood pressure. These hormones decrease aldosterone release, increase GFR, produce natriuresis (sodium excretion in urine) and diuresis (potassium sparing), and they decrease renin release, thereby decreasing angiotensin II. These actions reduce blood volume and central venous pressure, cardiac output, and arterial blood pressure. Chronic elevation of natriuretic peptides appears to decrease arterial blood pressure primarily by decreasing systemic vascular resistance.

Serum Glucose in Critically Ill or Injured Children

Although a serum glucose concentration of 60 to 180 mg/dL is normally maintained over a wide range of conditions, critically ill or injured children often develop hypoglycemia or hyperglycemia. Infants have high glucose needs and low glycogen stores, so they can rapidly become hypoglycemic during critical illness or injury.[24] Providers should monitor serum glucose concentration with point-of-care testing, if possible, and treat hypoglycemia as needed. Treatment of hypoglycemia should avoid frequent, intermittent bolus administration of large quantities of glucose; provision of a continuous source of glucose is preferable.

Hyperglycemia can result from steroid administration, stress response, relative hypoinsulinemia, or insulin resistance and has been associated with increased mortality in critically ill children in some studies. A prospective, randomized study of tight control of serum glucose concentration in critically ill children (targeted to age-adjusted normal fasting glucose concentration) reduced critical care unit mortality,[37] but was associated with episodes of hypoglycemia. In general, an insulin infusion (0.5-1 unit regular insulin/kg per hour) is often titrated during the first 18 to 24 hours of critical care therapy to maintain the serum glucose concentration less than 150 mg/dL (range will vary; use your unit protocol). Careful monitoring is required to avoid and treat episodes of hypoglycemia. The ultimate value versus risk of this approach is still under investigation.

ELECTROLYTE HOMEOSTASIS AND COMMON IMBALANCES

Table 12-3 presents a summary of electrolyte imbalances and associated clinical manifestations in critically ill infants and children. In the following sections, approximate ranges for normal and abnormal serum electrolyte concentrations are listed, but providers should use normal ranges referenced by the clinical laboratory in their practice settings.

Sodium Homeostasis

Sodium (Na^+), the primary extracellular cation, plays an important role in the regulation of action potentials in skeletal muscles, nerves, and the myocardium; maintenance of acid-base balance; and maintenance of ECF balance. The normal serum sodium concentration is approximately 135 to 145 mEq/L.

Alterations in sodium and fluid balance often occur concurrently and can alter serum osmolality. An abnormal serum sodium concentration often results from fluid volume deficit or excess. GFR and aldosterone secretion both affect sodium balance.

Sodium Imbalance: Hyponatremia
Etiology
Hyponatremia is a low serum sodium concentration, typically less than 130 to 135 mEq/L. It often develops as a complication of disease or therapy. The critically ill infant or child can develop hyponatremia from excessive water intake relative to sodium, excess water retention, increased sodium loss, or a combination of these factors.[10]

Hyponatremia can occur in conjunction with hypervolemia, euvolemia, or hypovolemia. Hypervolemic hyponatremia is associated with water intoxication, nephrotic syndrome, cardiac failure, renal failure, and the syndrome of inappropriate antidiuretic hormone (SIADH). Hypovolemic hyponatremia can occur with renal losses (e.g., osmotic diuresis, renal tubular acidosis) or extrarenal losses (e.g., diarrhea, vomiting, burns).[10] Other potential causes include adrenal insufficiency, excessive use of diuretics, and cerebral salt-wasting syndrome.

A laboratory report of a low serum sodium concentration can be misleading. These pseudohyponatremic states are associated with hyperlipidemia, hyperproteinemia, or hyperglycemia. In hyperlipidemia or hyperproteinemia, the lipid or protein displaces fluid from serum, decreasing the relative volume of water and electrolytes. As a result, the reported serum sodium concentration will be low. The total body sodium actually may be normal, although its concentration (in milliequivalents per liter of plasma, or mEq/L) is reduced. Hyperlipidemia of this degree usually produces a milky white plasma.

Because the serum osmolality is determined by the combined effects of particles (solutes) in the serum—especially the sodium, glucose, and blood urea nitrogen—the serum osmolality can be normal if a fall in the concentration of one solute is accompanied by a commensurate (in osmotic effect) increase in the concentration of another solute. With significant hyperglycemia, the high glucose concentration increases serum osmolality, drawing fluid into the vascular space; this may artificially reduce the serum sodium concentration. The significance of this dilutional effect is debatable—the serum sodium concentration may still influence osmotic changes to which the cells are exposed. To estimate the potential effect of severe hyperglycemia on the serum sodium concentration, for every 100 mg/dL rise in serum glucose above normal, the serum sodium concentration is likely to be depressed approximately 1.6 mEq/L below 135 mEq/L.

Pathophysiology and Clinical Signs and Symptoms

An isolated decrease in serum sodium concentration (i.e., without a rise in glucose or blood urea nitrogen) reduces serum osmolality; an acute fall in serum osmolality produces a shift of water from the extracellular compartment (including vascular space) to the intracellular compartment. This fluid shift can cause swelling of cells (edema). Because there is limited capacity for volume expansion within the skull, swelling of brain cells (cerebral edema) can have catastrophic consequences, such as brain herniation and death.

The volume of water shift and the severity of clinical manifestations with hyponatremia are directly related to the acuity and the magnitude of the fall in serum sodium and osmolality. Infants and children who develop hyponatremia that gradually worsens over several days or weeks (e.g., with adrenocortical insufficiency) typically have milder clinical manifestations and may be asymptomatic until the serum sodium is very low.[26]

Acute hyponatremia that develops within hours or days (i.e., <48 hours) is more likely to produce cerebral edema.[26] Seizures and coma are associated with a serum sodium concentration less than 120 mEq/L.

Management

If the child is at risk for hyponatremia, providers should closely monitor the child's serum sodium concentration to detect and promptly treat hyponatremia before it becomes severe. Frequent neurologic assessments are indicated. Notify an on-call provider immediately if the child develops altered level of consciousness, seizures, or signs of increased intracranial pressure.

Hyponatremia associated with neurologic symptoms is a neurologic emergency. Urgent treatment includes administration of 2 to 4 mL/kg of 3% saline (513 mEq sodium/L, or 0.513 mEq/mL); this will typically raise the child's serum sodium concentration approximately 1 to 2 mEq/L and raise serum osmolality sufficiently to slow the intracellular water shift. If the SIADH produces seizures or other severe symptoms, hyponatremia and water intoxication can be treated acutely by administration of hypertonic saline (2-4 mL/kg of 3% saline) and furosemide (1-2 mg/kg). These medications will increase the serum sodium concentration and eliminate excess free water (see section, Specific Diseases, Syndrome of Inappropriate Antidiuretic Hormone).

Management of hyponatremia includes restoration of appropriate intravascular volume, replacement of the sodium deficit, and identification and treatment of the underlying cause. Symptomatic hypovolemia is treated with boluses of normal saline or lactated Ringer's solution. Management of hypervolemic hyponatremia may include fluid restriction and administration of loop diuretics.

Once the child's neurologic status is stable and perfusion is adequate, plans are made to replace the sodium deficit. The following formula[36] is used to calculate the sodium deficit:

$$\text{Sodium deficit} = \text{Weight in kg} \times 06^\dagger \\ \times (135 - \text{observed sodium mEq/L})$$

†Use 0.5 as multiplier for females.

During treatment of hyponatremia, providers must closely monitor the serum sodium concentration and the rate of rise in the concentration. If the serum sodium and osmolality are raised too rapidly, the resulting water shifts from the cellular to the extracellular (including intravascular) compartments can produce neurologic complications including intracranial bleeding (Box 12-1). In general, the serum sodium should be raised no faster than approximately 0.5-1.0 mEq/L per hour.[35] Additional important assessments include strict monitoring of intake and output, urine specific gravity, serum electrolytes, serum osmolality, and daily weights.

Sodium Imbalances: Hypernatremia
Etiology

Hypernatremia (serum Na^+ >145-150 mEq/L) occurs less frequently than hyponatremia. One of the body's major defenses against hypernatremia is thirst. Infants, small children, and any children with significant developmental delay, decreased level of consciousness, or critical illness have an increased risk of hypernatremia during episodes of fluid loss, because they may not be able to signal caregivers of thirst or drink additional fluids.

Table 12-3   Electrolyte Imbalances in Critically Ill Infants and Children

Electrolyte Imbalance	Causes	Clinical Manifestations	ECG Findings	Management
Hyponatremia Na^+ <130 to 135 mEq/L (same in mmol/L)	• Vomiting/diarrhea • Nasogastric suction • ↓ Na^+ intake • Fever • Excessive diaphoresis • ↑ Water intake • Burns and wounds • Renal disease • SIADH • DKA • Malnutrition	• Lethargy • Muscle cramps • Nausea and vomiting • Disorientation • Seizures • Coma • Increased intracranial pressure	• N/A	• Treat underlying cause • Fluid replacement or restriction depending on fluid status • ± Hypertonic saline • Monitor Na^+ concentration • Frequent neurologic assessments
Hypernatremia Na^+ >145 to 150 mEq/L (same in mmol/L)	• ↑ Na^+ intake • Renal disease • ↑ Insensible water loss • Diabetes insipidus • Fever • Vomiting/diarrhea • Excessive use of diuretics	• Intense thirst • Flushed skin • "Doughy" skin • Irritability, agitation • Dry, tacky mucous membranes • Lethargy, confusion • Muscle weakness • Muscle twitching • Seizures • Coma • Intracranial bleed	• N/A	• Treat underlying cause • Strict monitoring of intake and output • Slow correction of fluid deficit • Monitor Na^+ concentration • Frequent neurologic assessments
Hypokalemia K^+ <2.5 to 3.0 mEq/L (same in mmol/L)	• ↓ K^+ intake • Starvation • Malabsorption syndromes • Gastrointestinal losses • Diuresis • Nephritis • Alkalosis	• Muscle weakness, cramping, stiffness, paralysis, hyporeflexia • Hypotension • Lethargy • Irritability • Tetany • Nausea, vomiting • Abdominal distension • Paralytic ileus • Irregular, weak pulse	• Increased P wave amplitude • Prolonged PR interval • Flattened, inverted T waves • Presence of U-waves • PVCs	• Determine and treat cause • K^+ replacement • Monitor acid-base status • Monitor ECG; be prepared to support CV function • Monitor respiratory status
Hyperkalemia K^+ >5.0 to 5.5 mEq/L (same in mmol/L)	• ↑ K^+ intake • Renal disease, failure • Adrenal insufficiency • Metabolic acidosis • Severe dehydration • Burns • Crushing injuries • Hemolysis	• Muscle weakness • Ascending paralysis • Hyperreflexia • Confusion • Apnea • Nausea/vomiting • Diarrhea • ↓ Cardiac function	• Tall, peaked T waves • Widened QRS • ST-segment depression • Prolonged PR interval • Ventricular arrhythmias • Asystole • Cardiac arrest	• Determine and treat cause • Administer IV fluids • Discontinue K^+ containing fluids and medications • Give IV calcium • Insulin 0.1 units/kg + glucose 0.5 g/kg • Na^+ bicarbonate • Kayexalate • Furosemide • Albuterol • Dialysis • Monitor serum K^+ concentration • Monitor ECG; support CV function • Evaluate acid-base status

Table 12-3   Electrolyte Imbalances in Critically Ill Infants and Children—cont'd

Electrolyte Imbalance	Causes	Clinical Manifestations	ECG Findings	Management
Hypocalcemia Ca^{2+} <8 to 8.5 mg/dL (<2 mmol/L) Ionized Ca <4.0 mg/dL (<1 mmol/L)	• ↓ Dietary Ca^{2+} • Vitamin D deficiency • Renal insufficiency • Diuretics • Hypoparathyroidism • Alkalosis • ↑ Serum protein	• Neuromuscular irritability • Tingling sensation • Chvostek's sign • Trousseau's sign • Tetany • Muscle cramps • Lethargy • Seizures • Hypotension	• Prolonged QT interval	• Treat, control cause • Monitor ECG • Give IV calcium • Monitor ECG • Monitor Ca^{2+} and Mg^{2+} concentrations
Hypercalcemia Ca^{2+} >11 to 12 mg/dL (>2.75 mmol/L) Ionized Ca >5.3 mg/dL (>1.33 mmol/L)	• Acidosis • Prolonged immobilization • Kidney disease • Hyperparathyroidism • Excessive administration	• Lethargy • Stupor • Coma • Seizures • Anorexia • Nausea/vomiting • Constipation • Hypotonicity	• Shortened QT interval • Bradycardia • Cardiac arrest	• Treat underlying cause • Monitor ECG • Give IV fluids • Consider loop diuretics
Hypomagnesemia Mg^{2+} <1.3 mEq/L (<0.65 mmol/L)	• ↓ Intake (NPO) • Malabsorption syndromes • ↑ Renal excretion	• Cardiac arrest • Neuromuscular excitability • Tetany • Confusion • Dizziness • Headache • Seizures • Coma • Respiratory depression • ↑ HR	• PVCs • Ventricular arrhythmias (including Torsades de pointes, pulseless arrest)	• Treat cause, provide CPR as needed • Give IV Mg^{2+} • Monitor ECG • Neuromuscular assessments • Assess serum sodium, potassium, calcium and phosphate; administer sodium, potassium, and calcium as needed
Hypermagnesemia Mg^{2+} >2.5 mEq/L (>1.25 mmol/L)	• Chronic renal disease • ↓ GFR, ↓ excretion • ↑ Administration of Mg^{2+} containing drugs (e.g., antacids, laxatives)	• Lethargy • Muscle weakness • Seizures • ↓ Swallow • ↓ Gag • ↓ HR • ↓ BP	• Prolonged PR interval • Prolonged QRS • Prolonged QT • Atrioventricular block	• Treat cause • Monitor ECG • Administer Calcium • Give IV fluids • Furosemide • Dialysis
Hypophosphatemia PO_4^{-3} <3 mg/dL (<0.97 mmol/L)	• Limited intake • Shift of PO_4^{-3} from ECF to ICF • ↓ GI tract absorption • ↑ renal excretion	• Irritability • Disorientation • Tremors • Seizures • Hemolytic anemia • ↓ Myocardial function • Potential respiratory failure • Coma	• Premature ectopic beats	• Treat underlying cause • Slow PO_4^{-3} replacement • Monitor for other electrolyte imbalances
Hyperphosphatemia PO_4^{-3} >5.5 mg/dL (>1.78 mmol/L) children 2-12 years	• Chronic renal failure • Rapid cell catabolism • Excessive intake • Neoplastic disease • Hypoparathyroidism	• Tachycardia • Hyperreflexia • Abdominal cramps • Nausea • Diarrhea • Muscle tetany • Hypocalcemia	• N/A	• Treat underlying cause • Monitor PO_4^{-3} and Ca^{2+} • Dietary restrictions • Antacid administration • Hydration • Correction of hypocalcemia • Dialysis

BP, Blood pressure; *CPR,* cardiopulmonary resuscitation; *CV,* cardiovascular; *DKA,* diabetic ketoacidosis; *ECF,* extracellular fluid; *ECG,* electrocardiogram; *GFR,* glomerular filtration rate; *GI,* gastrointestinal; *HR,* heart rate; *ICF,* intracellular fluid; *IV,* intravenous; *N/A,* not applicable; *NPO,* nothing by mouth; *PVCs,* premature ventricular contractions; *SIADH,* syndrome of inappropriate antidiuretic hormone; ±, considered but not used in all cases.

Box 12-1	**Advanced Concepts: Potential Central Nervous System Complications of Rapid Changes in Serum Sodium and Osmolality**

The brain does not tolerate rapid or significant water shifts into and out of the cells. A shift of water into brain cells—such as that occurring with an acute fall in serum sodium concentration and serum osmolality—is likely to produce cerebral edema. A rapid shift of water from cells, including brain cells, can cause the cells to shrink and can result in cerebral dysfunction. Cells in the gray matter and tissue in the white matter in the brain swell and shrink at different rates when water shifts occur. As a result, significant water shifts between intracellular and extracellular compartments in the brain can cause tearing of cerebral bridging veins and intracranial bleeding.

Rapid correction of hyponatremia has been shown to result in cerebral dysfunction, linked with damage to the myelin sheath of neurons. This myelinolysis is called *central pontine myelinolysis* if it occurs in the pons (brainstem) and *osmotic demyelinization syndrome* if it occurs elsewhere in the brain. Signs of brain dysfunction can include decreased level of consciousness, lack of coordination, paralysis, and dysphagia. Because there is no known treatment for such cerebral dysfunction, and it can cause permanent disability, prevention is critical. In general, unless neurologic symptoms indicate the need for more aggressive treatment, providers should aim to correct hyponatremia or hypernatremia no faster than approximately 0.5 mEq/L per hour (or 10-12 mEq/L per day). For more information, consult the National Institutes of Health Web site: http://www.ninds.nih.gov/disorders/central_pontine/central_pontine_myelinolysis.htm.

Box 12-2	**Advanced Concepts: The Role of Idiogenic Osmoles in Brain Cells**

When extracellular (including serum) osmolality rises, water shifts from the intracellular to the extracellular compartment, and cells typically shrink. When the serum osmolality is chronically elevated, brain cells generate idiogenic osmoles (e.g., glycine and taurine) to help brain cells maintain normal cell volume despite a water shift to the extracellular space. These idiogenic osmoles, however, may contribute to cerebral edema if a high serum osmolality is lowered too rapidly.

Patients who are unable to produce and/or respond to ADH (e.g., patients with DI) are at risk for development of significant hypernatremia and hypovolemia. These patients must be closely monitored to detect and treat these complications before they become severe.

Management

If the patient with hypernatremia has signs of inadequate tissue perfusion (i.e., shock), administer isotonic crystalloid by bolus (20 mL/kg) until perfusion is adequate. Avoid excessive bolus fluid administration (i.e., beyond that needed to treat shock), because it can contribute to a rapid fall in serum sodium and osmolality resulting in cerebral edema and other neurologic complications (see Box 12-2).

Once shock is corrected, estimate the fluid deficit and plan to replace the deficit over 48 to 72 hours, while providing for maintenance fluid requirements as well as for replacement of any ongoing additional fluid losses (e.g., persistent diarrhea). The type of IV fluids administered will vary depending on the rate at which the serum sodium is falling during therapy. Generally, the serum sodium should decrease at a rate no faster than 0.5 to 1.0 mEq/L per hour.

Monitor patients for the clinical manifestations of cerebral edema throughout the course of their treatment. Management of the child with hypervolemic hypernatremia will typically involve loop diuretics and decreased sodium administration.

Potassium Homeostasis

Potassium is the primary intracellular cation (i.e., a positively charged ion). The magnitude of the transmembrane (i.e., between intracellular and extracellular) potassium gradient determines the excitability of nerve and muscle cells (including skeletal and heart muscle) and the rate of conduction of nerve impulses. Potassium also plays a significant role in the maintenance of acid-base balance.

The normal serum potassium (K^+) concentration is 3.0 to 5.0 mEq/L. The intracellular potassium concentration is much higher, approximately 150 mEq/L.[28] Small alterations in serum potassium concentration can significantly affect the transmembrane gradient and therefore neuromuscular and cardiac function. The serum K+ concentration is affected by potassium intake and excretion, renal regulation, and serum pH. Because the intravascular (serum) potassium concentration represents only a small proportion of the total body potassium, accurate interpretation of the child's potassium balance requires consideration of the child's clinical status and acid-base balance.

Hypernatremia is most likely to result from a water deficit (e.g., dehydration, diuretic use, diabetes insipidus, DI). Less commonly, hypernatremia can result from excessive sodium intake, such as if powder for infant formula is incorrectly diluted. The child with hypernatremia may be hypovolemic, euvolemic, or hypervolemic; therefore, it is important to assess the child's fluid volume status when determining the cause of the hypernatremia.

Pathophysiology and Clinical Signs and Symptoms

Hypernatremia typically increases the serum osmolality. The rise in osmolality stimulates the posterior pituitary to release ADH, which increases renal water reabsorption until the osmolality returns to normal. The increased osmolality associated with hypernatremia also leads to a shift in water from the intracellular to the extracellular compartment, including into the vascular space. This water movement from the cells can cause cellular dehydration and central nervous system dysfunction. Complications including subdural, subarachnoid, and intracerebral bleeding and sinus vein thrombosis can develop with acute and severe increases in serum sodium concentration and the resulting water shift (see Box 12-1). Permanent central nervous system dysfunction can result when the serum sodium concentration is extremely high (e.g., >165-170 mEq/L).[12] When serum osmolality is chronically elevated, brain cells will generate idiogenic osmoles to maintain cell volume (Box 12-2).

Potassium ions normally shift between the intra- and extracellular compartments with changes in the serum pH (see Evolve Fig. 12-2 in the Chapter 12 Supplement on the Evolve Website). When the serum hydrogen ion concentration increases (i.e., with acidosis or a fall in pH), hydrogen moves from the extracellular to the intracellular compartment, where it is buffered. To maintain a balance of cation movement across cell membranes, the intracellular movement of hydrogen ions is associated with an extracellular shift of potassium. Thus, acidosis or a fall in pH (e.g., with correction of alkalosis) is associated with a rise in serum potassium concentration. In contrast, alkalosis or a rise in serum pH (e.g., with treatment of acidosis) is associated with a fall in serum potassium, because hydrogen ion shifts out of cells and is replaced by potassium.

The change in serum potassium concentration associated with changes in serum pH will always be in the direction opposite the change in pH. That is, if the pH falls (as in acidosis) the serum potassium usually rises; as acidosis is corrected (the pH rises) the serum potassium should fall. Hypokalemia with acidosis is particularly dangerous: as acidosis is treated and the serum pH rises, the serum potassium concentration will fall further. Thus, correction of acidosis in the child with hypokalemia and acidosis may result in a dangerously low serum potassium concentration. The potassium concentration should always be evaluated in light of the patient's present acid-base status, and likely changes in potassium concentration should be anticipated in response to changes in acid-base status that will result from planned therapy.

The kidneys play a critical role in potassium homeostasis. Renal failure limits the kidney's ability to excrete potassium and may result in hyperkalemia (see Chapter 13).

Potassium Imbalances: Hypokalemia

Etiology

Causes of hypokalemia (serum K+ concentration <2.5 to 3.0 mEq/L) can be classified into three general categories: inadequate potassium intake (rare, but may be iatrogenic), shifts of potassium from the extracellular to the intracellular compartment (e.g., with alkalosis or a rise in serum pH), or excessive losses of potassium (see Evolve Fig. 12-3 in the Chapter 12 Supplement on the Evolve Website for more information). Critically ill patients often develop true potassium deficit following the use of diuretics, especially loop and thiazide diuretics. Some antimicrobial agents (e.g., amphotericin B or carbenicillin) can increase renal potassium losses. Hypokalemia also is associated with severe hypochloremia and the potassium-wasting Bartter's syndrome.

Because gastrointestinal fluids all contain significant amounts of potassium in the form of potassium chloride salt, vomiting, diarrhea, intestinal fistulas of the small intestine or colon, ileostomy drainage, or gastric suctioning can all result in potassium losses as well as loss of hydrogen ions and chloride.

Pathophysiology and Clinical Signs and Symptoms

The large quantity of intracellular potassium serves as a reservoir to help maintain intravascular potassium concentration despite potassium loss. When the serum potassium concentration begins to decline, some intracellular potassium, known as the *exchangeable potassium,* moves from the intracellular

space to the extracellular compartment (including the vascular space). Only when this amount of exchangeable potassium is depleted will further extracellular potassium loss produce a fall in serum potassium concentration. Thus, the serum potassium concentration may be normal or even elevated when a total body potassium deficit is present.

Evaluation of the patient's potassium balance is further complicated by potassium shifts between the intracellular and extracellular compartments that result from administration of some medications and with changes in acid-base balance. β-Adrenergic agonists (e.g., inhaled albuterol) can cause a fall in serum potassium, whereas α-adrenergic agents can cause a rise in serum potassium. β-Adrenergic agonists increase intracellular sodium ion movement that stimulates the sodium-potassium pump to move sodium out of the cells. For every three sodium ions pumped out of cells, two potassium ions are allowed to enter cells. Thus, potassium shifts from the extracellular (including vascular) to the intracellular space.

Alpha-adrenergic agents can cause a rise in serum potassium, because potassium shifts from the intracellular to the extracellular (including vascular) space. Insulin administration can produce a fall in the serum potassium concentration, because insulin stimulates cellular uptake of potassium.

Acute alkalosis or a rise in serum pH (e.g., during treatment of acidosis) will cause a fall in serum potassium concentration, because hydrogen ion shifts out of the cell and is replaced by potassium (i.e., potassium moves into the cells). If the serum potassium concentration is within the normal range and the child's serum pH then rises (e.g., as occurs with treatment of acidosis) hypokalemia may result.

Hypokalemia may also result from increased renal potassium excretion. This hypokalemia can be associated with metabolic alkalosis, renal tubular acidosis, and DKA. Hypokalemia can perpetuate metabolic alkalosis, particularly if either condition is chronic. When the serum potassium concentration is low, the kidney vigorously reabsorbs potassium and must excrete hydrogen ions. As a result, it may be necessary to treat the child's hypokalemia to correct significant alkalosis.

Excessive renal potassium losses can also result from increased mineralocorticoid activity and increased delivery of sodium to the distal nephron. Excessive renal potassium losses have been associated with administration of antibiotics such as carbenicillin (and other penicillins), amphotericin B, gentamicin and aminoglycosides. A common cause of hypokalemia in the critically ill patient is the use of diuretics, especially loop and thiazide diuretics.

Chronic hypokalemia can change renal concentrating ability and cause polyuria. The kidney has little ability to conserve potassium when body potassium stores become low; as a result, urinary potassium excretion will remain greater than 20 mEq/L once hypokalemia persists for 10 to 20 days.

Although some potassium is lost with vomiting, diarrhea, and loss of other gastrointestinal fluids, potassium losses are exacerbated by intravascular volume contraction. Hypovolemia stimulates aldosterone secretion, which produces sodium and water retention, but it increases hydrogen ion and potassium excretion.

Hypokalemia can cause hyperpolarization of nerve and muscle cells, leading to muscle weakness, slowed nerve

SERUM K

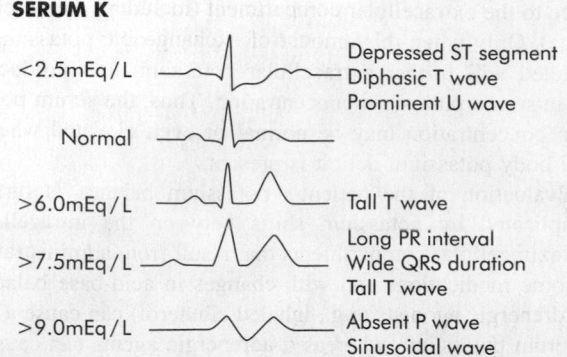

FIG. 12-3 Electrocardiogram changes with hypokalemia and hyperkalemia. (From Park MK, Guntheroth WG: *How to read pediatric ECGs*, ed 3, St. Louis, 1992, Mosby, p. 108.)

impulse conduction, and decreased muscle contraction. Hypokalemia can cause characteristic electrocardiogram (ECG) changes, including development of a U-wave (Fig. 12-3).

Management

Nurses should watch for ECG changes in patients with or at risk for development of hypokalemia. Patients with preexisting cardiac disease may be particularly likely to develop arrhythmias with even mild hypokalemia. Because hypokalemia will potentiate the effects and potential toxic effects of digitalis glycosides (as the result of depressive effects on the sodium-potassium adenosine triphosphatase pump), it is very important to monitor and maintain serum potassium concentration and promptly treat hypokalemia in patients receiving digitalis.

The appropriate speed and method of potassium replacement is based on the severity of the hypokalemia and the child's clinical condition (including acid-base balance, renal function and urine output). Replacement is typically indicated if the serum potassium concentration is below 3 mEq/L or if the child becomes symptomatic. Enteral replacement in a dose of 0.5-1 mEq/kg will usually correct mild, asymptomatic hypokalemia.[17] The dose may be repeated every 4 to 8 hours.

IV potassium administration is indicated when the serum potassium concentration is less than 2.5 mEq/L or when milder levels of hypokalemia are present in patients who cannot receive enteral replacement (Box 12-3). A typical IV supplement dose is 0.5 to 1.0 mEq/kg, infused over approximately 1 to 3 hours.[6,17] Dilute the potassium adequately and administer it over several hours to prevent bolus or rapid delivery that can produce lethal arrhythmias. Closely monitor the child's serum potassium concentration and ECG.

The Institute for Safe Medication Practices lists IV potassium among drugs with heightened risk of causing patient harm when administered in error. Most institutions have developed policies regarding IV potassium supplement infusions that incorporate patient safety checks, frequent laboratory verification of serum potassium concentration, and pharmacy preparation of solutions.

If hypokalemia is induced by an acute respiratory or metabolic alkalosis, the treatment of choice is correction of the alkalosis. Potassium administration is rarely necessary.

Box 12-3   Recommended Intravenous Potassium Dose and Administration Guidelines*

- Daily: 2-5 mEq/kg per day in parenteral nutrition fluid or in divided doses
- Supplement: 0.5-1.0 mEq/kg per dose administered over 1-3 hours via syringe or infusion pump
- Typical maximum concentration
  ○ Peripheral: 0.08 mEq/mL
  ○ Central: 0.4 mEq/mL
- Typical maximum infusion rate: 0.5 to 1 mEq/kg per hour
- Monitor EKG for doses > 0.3 mEq/kg per hour

Information consistent with Lacy CF, et al: *Lexicomp's drug information handbook*, ed 18. Hudson, OH, 2009, Lexicomp; and Custer JW, Rau RE: *The Harriet Lane handbook*, ed 18, Philadelphia, 2009, Mosby-Elsevier. *See also institutional guidelines.

Potassium Imbalances: Hyperkalemia
Etiology

Hyperkalemia (serum potassium >5.0-5.5 mEq/L) can cause life-threatening arrhythmias; it can result from potassium administration, extracellular (including into the intravascular space) shift of potassium ions associated with a fall in serum pH, significant cell destruction (and release of intracellular potassium), or reduced renal excretion of potassium ions.

Pseudohyperkalemia is a high reported serum potassium concentration caused by release of intracellular potassium at the time of phlebotomy or in the specimen after collection.[28] Intracellular potassium is released during fingerstick or other traumatic blood sampling and can be released in a blood specimen after collection in patients with severe leukocytosis or thrombocytosis. Pseudohyperkalemia should be considered when an unexpected high serum potassium concentration is reported by the laboratory in patients who are asymptomatic and have an otherwise normal electrolyte and/or acid-base status. If there is a question about the accuracy of a high reported serum potassium concentration in an asymptomatic patient, the concentration should be rechecked before therapy is initiated to reduce the serum potassium.

Pathophysiology and Clinical Signs and Symptoms

A rise in serum potassium concentration in the healthy patient is usually transient because enhanced renal excretion can quickly return the serum potassium concentration to normal. However, if the rate of potassium accumulation exceeds the rate of renal potassium excretion, the serum potassium concentration will rise.

A rise in serum potassium is associated with a fall in serum pH, because potassium shifts from the intracellular to the extracellular compartment (including into the vascular space). Theoretically, for each 0.1 fall in the arterial pH, the serum potassium concentration can be expected to rise 0.6 to 0.8 mEq/L. When the acidosis is corrected (i.e., the serum pH rises), the serum potassium concentration should fall. In this situation, hypokalemia with acidosis is particularly dangerous, because correction of the acidosis can be associated with development of severe hypokalemia. Conversely, because alkalosis lowers the serum potassium concentration (see Hypokalemia, earlier), a high serum potassium concentration in an alkalotic patient is significant and will likely rise further when the alkalosis is corrected.

Additional causes of extracellular (including intravascular) shifts in potassium are: insulin deficiency, rapid cell breakdown, burns, trauma, hyperosmolality (e.g., hyperglycemia, mannitol administration), rhabdomyolysis, and the administration of succinylcholine.[23] Unless the amount of cellular potassium release is excessive, such as in crushing injuries, tumor necrosis syndrome, or administration of succinylcholine, such an extracellular potassium shift alone rarely causes clinically significant hyperkalemia.[23]

Decreased potassium elimination can result from renal dysfunction or the administration of medications such as potassium-sparing diuretics. Although both acute and chronic renal failure can cause hyperkalemia, patients with acute renal failure are at higher risk for life-threatening hyperkalemia because the potassium concentration often rises quite rapidly, before the body is able to mount a compensatory response.[28] Acidosis or cell injury in these patients will likely worsen the severity of the hyperkalemia.

Hyperkalemia can produce characteristic changes in the ECG such as a tall, peaked T wave, followed by widening of the QRS complex, S-T segment depression, and decreased R-wave amplitude (see Fig. 12-3). If the serum potassium concentration continues to rise, the P-R interval is prolonged, the amplitude of the P wave decreases, and finally the P wave disappears. Ultimately the patient's rhythm deteriorates into a classic sine wave. Ventricular arrhythmias or fibrillation can occur at any point during this progression.

Management

Critical care management of hyperkalemia includes recognition of at-risk patients, and rapid identification and correction of the hyperkalemia. Priorities of management are determined by the child's clinical presentation (for more information regarding treatment of hyperkalemia in the patient with renal failure, see Chapter 13).

If the serum potassium concentration is less than 6.5 mEq/L and no ECG changes are present, it may be sufficient to discontinue potassium in IV fluids and medications and closely monitor the patient and the serum potassium concentration. Administration of polystyrene sulfonate (Kayexalate) may be warranted to increase intestinal potassium removal (it results in the exchange of sodium for potassium in the intestinal lumen). Polystyrene sulfonate may also bind calcium and magnesium; therefore, providers should monitor serum concentration of these electrolytes and assess patients for the clinical manifestations of hypocalcemia and hypomagnesemia.

Immediate intervention is required when the serum potassium concentration is greater than 6.5 to 7.0 mEq/L or is associated with ECG changes (see Fig. 12-3). Although the evidence supporting emergent therapies for hyperkalemia is largely anecdotal, widely accepted goals are to stabilize the myocardial cellular membrane, expand the ECF volume, shift potassium into the cells, and remove potassium from the body (Table 12-4).[16,19,20,24]

Table 12-4 Emergent Management of Hyperkalemia

Management Goal	Intervention	Comments
Stabilize myocardium	Calcium salts • Calcium gluconate • Calcium chloride	Onset of action occurs within minutes and lasts for approximately 30 min*
Expand ECF volume	Intravenous fluids	Decrease serum concentration of potassium
Shift potassium into the ICF	Sodium bicarbonate	Results in an intracellular shift of potassium; it may take up to 60 min for this to occur,* and the effects can last several hours; acid-base status must be monitored closely.† Monitor children with respiratory failure carefully, because buffering of sodium bicarbonate increases CO_2 and may worsen respiratory acidosis if the lungs cannot clear CO_2. Hypernatremia may develop as complication of this therapy.
	Insulin and glucose/dextrose	Administration of insulin (0.1 unit regular insulin/kg) will activate the sodium-potassium pump, resulting in increased cellular uptake of potassium; insulin should be administered in conjunction with glucose/dextrose.† The decrease in serum potassium occurs within 15 min and lasts approximately 60 min.*
	Albuterol	Activates the sodium-potassium pump and stimulates the pancreas to release insulin, thereby causing an intracellular shift of potassium; administer albuterol in conjunction with insulin to produce cumulative effect in lowering serum potassium‡
Remove potassium from the body	Kayexalate	Decreases potassium absorption in the intestine
	IV furosemide (thiazide diuretic)	May not be a viable option in infants or children with hyperkalemia and impaired renal function
	Dialysis	Indicated for hyperkalemia refractory to medical management

*Ahee P, Crowe AV: The management of hyperkalemia in the emergency department. *J Accid Emerg Med* 17:188-191, 2000.
†Jones RE, Brashers VL, Huether SE: Alterations of hormonal regulation. In: McCance KL, Huether SE, editors: *Pathophysiology: the biologic basis for disease in adults and children*, ed 6. Philadelphia, 2009, Mosby-Elsevier.
‡Chmielewski CM: Hyperkalemic emergencies: mechanisms, manifestations and management. *Crit Care Nursing Clin North Am* 10:449-458, 1998.
ECF, Extracellular fluid; *ICF*, intracellular fluid; *IV*, intravenous.

Calcium Homeostasis

Calcium (Ca^{2+}) is the most abundant mineral in the body. Calcium, phosphorous, and magnesium are important in nerve impulse transmission, smooth and cardiac muscle contraction, bone composition, and activation of cellular enzymatic processes.

Most of the body's calcium stores are found in bones and teeth, with the remainder in soft tissue and serum. Approximately 50% of serum calcium is bound to anions or protein and is unavailable for use by the body. The remaining 50% is ionized; it is this ionized serum calcium that influences cardiac function, muscle contraction, nerve impulse transmission, and coagulation.

The serum albumin concentration and acid-base status will affect the serum ionized calcium concentration. An increase in serum albumin will decrease the portion of the total serum calcium that is ionized, because more calcium will bind albumin. The serum ionized calcium concentration will rise with acidosis (a fall in serum pH) and fall with alkalosis (a rise in serum pH). Thus, the serum ionized calcium concentration changes in a direction opposite the pH.

Serum calcium concentration is tightly regulated through the effects of parathyroid hormone (PTH), calcitonin, and vitamin D and their effects on calcium and phosphate deposition and resorption from bone, absorption in the intestine, and reabsorption and excretion in the kidney. A fall in serum ionized calcium concentration stimulates PTH production and secretion, which in turn increases intestinal calcium absorption, increases renal calcium reabsorption, and inhibits renal phosphate reabsorption; therefore, more phosphate is excreted in the urine. PTH also mobilizes calcium from bone, so the serum calcium rises and the serum phosphate falls. These activities increase renal activation of vitamin D, which enhances calcium absorption in the intestines, calcium liberation from bone, and calcium reabsorption in the kidneys.

When the serum ionized calcium concentration rises, PTH is suppressed, vitamin D is not activated, and calcitonin decreases intestinal calcium absorption and renal tubular calcium reabsorption and decreases osteoclastic activity in the bone.

Calcium Imbalances: Hypocalcemia
Etiology

Hypocalcemia (total Ca^{2+} <8.0 to 8.5 mg/dL [<2.0 mmol/L]; ionized Ca^{2+} <4.0 mg/dL [<1.0 mmol/L]) is associated with significant morbidity and mortality in critically ill infants and children. Hypocalcemia can result from inadequate calcium intake, reduced calcium absorption, or excessive calcium excretion (Box 12-4).

The serum ionized calcium concentration will fall if the serum albumin concentration or serum pH rise (e.g., during correction of acidosis or with development of alkalosis). Hypocalcemia can develop after administration of stored whole blood or packed cells preserved with citrate, phosphate, and dextran, because serum ionized calcium can precipitate with the phosphate anticoagulant and can be bound by the citrate. Hyperphosphatemia will also produce hypocalcemia because the phosphate precipitates with calcium.

Pathophysiology and Clinical Signs and Symptoms

When the serum ionized calcium falls, PTH secretion and vitamin D act to increase the serum calcium and lower the serum phosphate. Both PTH and vitamin D increase intestinal

---

Box 12-4 Causes of Hypocalcemia

Hypoparathyroidism
Altered vitamin D production or action
Hyperphosphatemia
Hypomagnesemia
Malabsorption syndromes
Transfusion with citrate-preserved blood products
Medications (e.g., aminoglycosides, glucagons, phenytoin, phenobarbital)
Protein malnutrition
Nephrotic syndrome
Renal failure
Acute pancreatitis
Burns
Chemotherapy

---

calcium absorption and renal calcium reabsorption and decrease renal phosphate reabsorption. Both contribute to the liberation of calcium and phosphate from bone (osteoclastic activity).

Signs and symptoms of hypocalcemia result from increased neuromuscular excitability and can include tingling, muscle cramps, lethargy, carpal-pedal spasm, seizures, and prolonged QT interval on ECG. A classic sign of hypocalcemia is Chvostek's sign, which is elicited by tapping on the facial nerve at the temple. A positive sign is a twitch of the lip or facial muscles near the nose. Trousseau's sign is the development of carpal pedal spasm after an extremity artery is occluded for 3 minutes. Severe hypocalcemia can produce muscle tetany.

Management

Management of hypocalcemia includes correction of the cause, administration of calcium supplements as needed, and monitoring for cardiac, neuromuscular, and neurologic dysfunction. Any concurrent conditions (e.g., hyperphosphatemia, hypomagnesemia, respiratory alkalosis) must be identified and treated as indicated.

The healthcare team should immediately treat any acute episode of hypocalcemia in children at risk for impending cardiovascular or neurologic failure. Calcium chloride is the calcium supplement of choice for infants and children, because it provides greater bioavailability of calcium.[11,16a] An IV dose of 20 mg/kg of 10% calcium chloride provides 5.4 mg/kg of elemental calcium. Calcium gluconate can be used in neonates (IV dose of 60-100 mg/kg of 10% calcium gluconate provides approximately 5.4-9 mg/kg). Administer IV calcium by slow push or infusion and monitor for arrhythmias. Rapid administration of calcium salts (faster than 100 mg/min) is not recommended because it may produce bradycardia and asystole.[24,32]

Calcium Imbalances: Hypercalcemia
Etiology

Hypercalcemia (total serum calcium >11-12 mg/dL [>2.75 mmol/L]) is an excess of calcium in the extracellular (including vascular) compartment. A serum calcium concentration greater than 15 mg/dL can be life threatening. Although hypercalcemia is not common, it may be seen in critically ill infants and children with hyponatremia, hyperkalemia, resolution of chronic renal failure, and prolonged immobility. Children with acute leukemias or a large tumor burden can also develop clinically significant hypercalcemia. Hemoconcentration can cause pseudohypercalcemia in hypovolemic patients. In addition, excessive calcium administration to treat hypocalcemia can cause iatrogenic hypercalcemia.

Pathophysiology and Clinical Signs and Symptoms

Hypercalcemia develops when an excessive amount of calcium moves from the bones and intestines into the ECF, overwhelming the regulatory hormones (vitamin D and PTH) and renal excretory systems, and if the function of either of these systems is compromised. Both serum albumin (protein) and pH can affect the serum ionized calcium concentration. An increase in serum protein concentration will increase total serum calcium concentration, but will reduce the ionized calcium concentration because more calcium is bound to protein. A fall in serum pH (acidosis) will decrease serum binding of calcium, so will increase ionized calcium.

Hypercalcemia produces a reciprocal fall in serum phosphate and can produce complications similar to hyperparathyroidism, including renal stones and osteoporosis. Severe hypercalcemia can produce a polyuria-polydipsia syndrome with dehydration. If the polyuria produces dehydration, renal excretion of calcium is reduced, exacerbating the hypercalcemia.

Hypercalcemia decreases excitability of nerve and muscle cells and can cause neuromuscular pain and tingling. Symptoms are often vague and may not be significant until the serum calcium concentration exceeds 12 mg/dL.

Management

Management of hypercalcemia includes identifying the underlying cause, reducing the concentration of calcium in the ECF, and managing clinical manifestations. In patients with known hypercalcemia or in those at risk for its development, it is essential to closely monitor neuromuscular and cardiac function.

A serum calcium concentration greater than 15 mg/dL can be life threatening and requires immediate treatment. Treatment is typically achieved through administration of IV fluids to expand the ECF and loop diuretics to enhance calcium excretion. Thiazide diuretics are contraindicated because they limit calcium excretion.

With life-threatening hypercalcemia, aggressive therapy is needed to reduce the serum calcium. Drugs are typically administered to reduce the serum calcium concentration over several days: biphosphonate inhibits bone reabsorption, calcitonin inhibits calcium reabsorption from bone, mithracin reduces osteoclast activity, and gallium nitrate interferes with osteoclast function (for more information, see Table 15-2).[4] Administration of a biphosphate such as pamidronate (1 mg/kg) may be indicated in severe hypercalcemia. It can cause mild to moderate hypophosphatemia, hypomagnesemia, and transient hypocalcemia at 2 to 10 days after administration[9]; therefore, it will be important to monitor these electrolytes.

Magnesium Homeostasis

Magnesium (Mg^{2+}) is the second most abundant cation inside cells; less than 1% of total magnesium is located in the extracellular (including intravascular) compartment. The normal serum magnesium concentration ranges from 1.5 to 2.5 mEq/L.

The three primary roles of magnesium are enzyme and biochemical activation, mediation of skeletal muscle tension, and inhibition of electrical activity at the neuromuscular junction. Magnesium plays an essential role in the metabolism of adenosine triphosphate (ATP), the source of cellular energy.

Magnesium is absorbed in the gastrointestinal tract (absorption varies directly with intake) and eliminated or reabsorbed by the kidney as needed. Calcitriol and PTH enhance magnesium intestinal absorption and renal reabsorption. Renal magnesium reabsorption appears to vary directly with the GFR; therefore, renal failure can produce hypomagnesemia. Hypomagnesemia is often associated with hyponatremia, hypokalemia, hypocalcemia, and hyperphosphatemia (see Hypomagnesemia).

Magnesium Imbalances: Hypomagnesemia

Etiology

Hypomagnesemia (serum magnesium <1.3 mg/dL [0.65 mmol/L]) is common in hospitalized patients, especially those with chronic illness. Hypomagnesemia results from decreased intestinal magnesium absorption or renal failure with increased renal magnesium losses. Diuretics and DKA with osmotic diuresis can produce hypomagnesemia.

Pathophysiology and Clinical Signs and Symptoms

Decreased intestinal absorption of magnesium may be intrinsic or induced by medications (e.g., laxatives) or disease.[30] Medical conditions associated with decreased absorption include pancreatitis, severe or chronic diarrhea, prolonged vomiting, malabsorption syndromes, and intestinal and biliary fistulas. Prolonged gastric suctioning can reduce serum magnesium.

Increased renal excretion of magnesium can also be caused by medications such as diuretics (especially loop diuretics), aminoglycosides, amphotericin B, cisplatin, and cyclosporine. Medical conditions that cause rapid diuresis (e.g., DKA; hyperosmolar, hyperglycemic, or nonketotic coma) can also cause an increase in magnesium excretion.

Hypomagnesemia can cause lethal ventricular arrhythmias, including torsades de points and ventricular fibrillation. Because magnesium is essential to ATP metabolism, hypomagnesemia can damage the sodium-potassium pump, which depends on ATP to function properly.

Hypomagnesemia can be associated with additional electrolyte imbalances and with complications of the primary disease (e.g., renal failure). Hypomagnesemia causes an extracellular potassium shift that may transiently increase serum potassium. However, hypomagnesemia also causes increased urinary losses of sodium, potassium, phosphate, and hydrogen; therefore, it typically causes deficiency of these electrolytes. Hypomagnesemia can also produce hypocalcemia and hyperphosphatemia through impairment of PTH synthesis or secretion. Signs of hypomagnesemia are similar to signs of hypocalcemia, including possible tingling, muscle cramps, Chvostek's sign, tetany, and seizures (see under Hypocalcemia).

Management

If hypomagnesemia produces ventricular arrhythmias, cardiopulmonary resuscitation is needed (see Chapter 6) with bolus magnesium administration.[24] Acute hypomagnesemia in children at risk for impending cardiovascular or neurologic failure is treated immediately with IV administration of magnesium sulfate (25-50 mg/kg infusion over 10-20 minutes or longer).[24] Monitor for arrhythmias and hemodynamic instability during administration of magnesium supplements.[30]

Additional critical care management of an acute episode of hypomagnesemia includes correction of the cause and administration of other electrolyte supplements as needed. Treatment of hyponatremia, hypokalemia, and hypocalcemia is often necessary (see sections on Hyponatremia, Hypokalemia, and Hypocalcemia in this chapter for more information).

Monitor cardiac, muscular, and neurologic function throughout therapy. Although altered neuromuscular excitability is the most common feature of hypomagnesemia, patients can develop respiratory muscle depression and hypoventilation, requiring mechanical ventilation.

Magnesium Imbalance: Hypermagnesemia

Etiology

Hypermagnesemia (serum magnesium >2.5 mg/dL [1.25 mmol/L]) is far less common than hypomagnesemia. Hypermagnesemia can result from decreased renal excretion of potassium or, less commonly, an increase in magnesium intake through the intestine.

Pathophysiology, Clinical Signs, and Symptoms

Hypermagnesemia usually results from decreased renal excretion of magnesium, most commonly caused by chronic renal failure. Increased magnesium load and intestinal absorption may complicate the use of magnesium-containing laxatives or antacids.

Clinical signs and symptoms are associated with decreased neuromuscular and cardiovascular function. These signs and symptoms can include weakness, neurologic or respiratory depression, bradycardia, and hypotension.

Management

Patients at risk for hypermagnesemia should be monitored closely, because severe hypermagnesemia can lead to coma or cardiac arrest.[27] Management of the pediatric patient with hypermagnesemia includes identification and correction of the cause and administration of calcium salts and IV fluids. Calcium salts antagonize magnesium and can reverse cardiac complications.

If renal function is normal, administration of IV fluids will facilitate renal excretion of magnesium. Dialysis may be indicated, particularly for children with renal failure.

DEHYDRATION AND HYPOVOLEMIA

Dehydration occurs when the loss of all fluids and electrolytes exceeds intake. Hypovolemia is intravascular volume depletion, and can cause circulatory collapse.

Etiology

Dehydration with resulting hypovolemia is common in critically ill infants and children. Dehydration can result from excessive loss of fluids and electrolytes (e.g., diarrhea or vomiting), shifts of fluids and electrolytes into nonaccessible third spaces (e.g., burns or after abdominal surgery), and decreased intake of fluid and electrolytes (e.g., impaired thirst mechanism, dysphagia, or prolonged NPO status with inadequate IV therapy).

Gastrointestinal fluid loss from diarrhea is the most common cause of dehydration in infants and children. Increased insensible fluid losses can also contribute to dehydration.

In the critically ill child, "third spacing" is a common cause of intravascular volume loss.[31] "Third spacing" is a shift of fluid from the vascular space to a space that is neither intravascular nor intracellular. The third space may be interstitial (e.g., with septic shock), on the surface of a burn, or even into the bowel lumen. With third spacing of fluid, a significant volume of fluid is unavailable to the circulation to support cardiac output and systemic perfusion. Third spacing of fluid can develop in conditions such as ascites, pancreatitis, burns, peritonitis, sepsis, and intestinal obstruction. Such third-spacing results in inadequate intravascular volume that can compromise systemic perfusion.

Pathophysiology

Dehydration is classified by severity and by its effect on serum sodium concentration. Hyponatremic dehydration (serum Na^+ <130 mEq/L) occurs when there is a relatively greater loss of sodium than water, so the serum sodium concentration falls. This effect is often seen when gastrointestinal fluid losses are replaced with water or other hypotonic solution (e.g., 5% dextrose and water).[22] The resulting hyponatremia creates an osmolality gradient between the extracellular (including vascular) and intracellular compartments, so that water shifts from the vascular and interstitial spaces to the intracellular compartment. This water shift increases the severity of the clinical signs of (intravascular) volume depletion at any given volume deficit.

Hypernatremic dehydration (serum Na^+ >150 mEq/L) develops when there is a relatively greater loss of water than sodium (e.g., untreated DI). The resulting hypernatremia increases the extracellular osmolality, so that water shifts from the cellular to the extracellular compartment (i.e., intravascular and interstitial spaces). This free water shift decreases the severity of the clinical signs of volume depletion that will be present at any given volume deficit.

Clinical Signs and Symptoms

The clinical manifestations of dehydration will vary based on the severity of the fluid deficit and the serum sodium concentration. Table 12-5 shows a comparison of the clinical manifestations of mild, moderate and severe dehydration.

Management

The severity of a child's fluid volume deficit is estimated on the basis of weight loss, clinical manifestations and diagnostic studies. If a weight before illness is available, 1 kg of weight loss is equivalent to 1000 mL (1 L) of fluid loss.

If signs of shock are present (i.e., signs of poor peripheral perfusion or hypotension), initial management focuses on restoring intravascular volume to treat shock. Typically, 20 mL/kg IV boluses of isotonic crystalloid are administered until signs of shock are corrected. Infants or children with a severe fluid volume deficit may require resuscitation with 60 mL/kg or more of isotonic crystalloid.[11]

Table 12-5 Clinical Manifestations of Mild, Moderate, and Severe Dehydration

Clinical Manifestations	Mild Dehydration	Moderate Dehydration	Severe Dehydration
Mental status, general appearance*			
• Infants and young children	Thirsty, alert, restless	Thirsty, restless or lethargic but irritable to touch	Lethargic, somnolent
• Older children and adults	Thirsty, alert, restless	Thirsty, alert	Usually conscious, apprehensive
Radial pulse	Normal rate and strength	Rapid and weak	Rapid, feeble, sometimes impalpable
Heart rate	Normal or mild tachycardia	Tachycardia	Severe tachycardia that may progress to bradycardia
Respirations	Normal	Normal to rapid	Deep and rapid
Fontanelle and eyes	Normal	Slightly depressed	Severely sunken
Systolic blood pressure	Normal	Orthostatic hypotension	Severe hypotension
Skin elasticity	Pinch retracts immediately	Pinch retracts slowly	Pinch retracts very slowly (>3 seconds)
Tears*	Present	Present or absent	Absent
Mucous membranes*	Moist	Dry	Very dry
Urine output	Normal	Oliguria	Oliguria or anuria
Body weight loss (%)	3-5	6-9	≥10

Data from Friedman A: Nephrology: fluids and electrolytes. In: Behrman RE, Kliegman RM, editors: *Nelson essentials of pediatrics*, ed 4. Philadelphia, 2002, WB Saunders, p. 680; *AACN Pediatric Critical Care Pocket Reference Card* 1998, AACN, 1998, Aliso Viejo, CA; and Gorelick MH, Shaw KN, Murphy KO: Validity and reliability of clinical signs in the diagnosis of dehydration in children, *Pediatrics* 99:E6, 1997.
*Best indicators of fluid status.

During volume resuscitation, providers should closely monitor signs of systemic perfusion (including mental status, skin perfusion and urine output), heart rate and blood pressure, to evaluate response to therapy. The fluid bolus administration is repeated, as needed. If volume resuscitation is adequate, the blood pressure and signs of systemic perfusion and blood pressure should improve and the heart rate should decrease toward normal; if the child fails to improve, additional boluses are needed or there may be other causes of the child's shock. See Chapter 6 for further details of the management of hypovolemic shock.

Once initial fluid resuscitation is complete, ongoing management includes estimation and replacement of water and electrolyte deficits. In isotonatremic or hyponatremic dehydration, the fluid and electrolyte deficit is typically replaced over a period of 24 to 36 hours to restore intravascular volume within a short period of time while preventing overexpansion of the ECF.[10] In the presence of hyponatremic dehydration, the need for sodium replacement should be carefully evaluated.

In hypernatremic dehydration, replacement of fluid and electrolyte deficit is typically accomplished more slowly, over a period of 48 to 72 hours. The goal is to prevent rapid decreases in the serum sodium and osmolality during rehydration because such decreases can produce an intracellular water shift and neurologic complications. Replacement fluids to treat the fluid deficit are administered in addition to routine maintenance fluids (see Table 12-2) and replacement of any ongoing fluid losses (e.g., emesis or diarrhea).

GUIDELINES FOR PARENTERAL FLUID THERAPY

Parenteral fluid therapy is ubiquitous in pediatric critical care. See Table 12-6 for a comparison of common parenteral fluid solutions.

IV maintenance fluids are administered to provide daily free water and electrolyte requirements in a fasting patient. Fluid administration rate for each patient begins with an estimation of maintenance fluid requirements based on the formula developed by Holliday and Segar in 1957.[13] These estimated requirements are then tailored to meet the needs of the patient.

For many years, hypotonic crystalloids (e.g., 5% dextrose with 0.2% sodium chloride) were routinely used for maintenance and replacement fluids for critically ill infants and children, based on the assumption that critically ill patients were likely to have a tendency to retain sodium and water. However, after reports of fatal hyponatremia in hospitalized children,[1,2,21] a systematic review of the literature by Choong et al.[5] estimated that the odds of developing hyponatremia after administration of hypotonic solutions were 17-fold higher than with administration of isotonic solutions. In addition, the administration of isotonic solutions was not associated with hypernatremia; in fact, some patients receiving isotonic fluids still developed hyponatremia.[5]

Currently, there is insufficient evidence to identify use of a single IV fluid (e.g., hypotonic or isotonic) as the standard of care for pediatric maintenance therapy. Until clinical trials compare the safety and efficacy of different IV fluid regimens, practitioners must continue to individualize IV fluid selection and administration rate for each patient.[3,5] Providers should monitor serum electrolytes and clinical status during parenteral fluid therapy to prevent or rapidly detect and treat any imbalances that develop.

SPECIFIC DISEASES

Syndrome of Inappropriate Antidiuretic Hormone
Etiology

SIADH is characterized by ADH secretion in the absence of a physiologic stimulus. Patients with SIADH demonstrate low serum osmolality, hyponatremia, and hypervolemia. Causes of SIADH include central nervous system injury (e.g., surgery, tumor, traumatic brain injury) or infection, disease or damage to the pituitary stalk or hypothalamus, holoprosencephaly, spinal

Table 12-6   Comparison of Common Parenteral Fluid Solutions

Solution	Solute	Concentration (g/dL)	pH	Na+	K+	Ca2+	Cl	Lactate	Calculated OSM (mOsm/L)
Dextrose in Water									
5%	Glucose	5	4.7	–	–	–	–	–	250
10%	Glucose	10	4.6	–	–	–	–	–	505
Saline									
0.45% NaCl (hypotonic)	NaCl	0.45	5.3	77	–	–	77	–	155
0.9% NaCl (isotonic)	NaCl	0.9	5.3	154	–	–	154	–	310
Dextrose in Saline									
2.5% in 0.45% NaCl	Glucose	2.5							
	NaCl	0.45	4.9	77	–	–	77	–	280
5% in 0.2% NaCl	Glucose	5							
	NaCl	0.20	4.6	34	–	–	34	–	320
5% in 0.45% NaCl	Glucose	5							
	NaCl	0.45	4.6	77	–	–	77	–	405
5% in 0.9% NaCl	Glucose	5							
	NaCl	0.90	4.6	154	–	–	154	–	560
Polyionic									
Ringer's lactate (RL)	Lactate	0.31							
	NaCl	0.60	6.3	130	4	3	109	28	275
	KCl	0.03							
	CaCl2	0.02							
Dextrose in Polyionic									
2.5% in ½ RL	Glucose	2.5							
	Lactate	0.155	5.1	65	2	.015	54	14	265
	NaCl	0.30							
	KCl	0.015							
	CaCl2	0.01							
4% in modified RL	Glucose	4							
	Lactate	0.062	5.0	26	0.8	0.5	22	5.5	280
	NaCl	0.12							
	KCl	0.006							
	CaCl2	0.004							
5% in RL	Glucose	5							
	Lactate	0.31	4.7	130	4	3	109	28	515
	NaCl	0.60							
	KCl	0.03							
	CaCl2	0.02							
5% in albumin (Plasmanate)	Albumin	5	6.9	154	1		154	–	310
	NaCl	0.9							

From Roberts KE: Fluid and electrolyte regulation. In: Curley MAQ and Moloney-Harmon P, editors: *Critical care of nursing of infants and children*, ed 2, Philadelphia, 2001, WB Saunders, p. 377; Based on data from Krau SD: Selecting and managing fluid therapy: colloids versus crystalloids. *Crit Care Nurs Clin North Am* 10:401-410, 1998; and Perkin RM, Levin DL: Common fluid and electrolyte problems in the pediatric intensive care unit. *Pediatr Clin North Am* 27: 567-586, 1980.

cord injury or surgery, chemotherapy, pulmonary disease, and liver disease.[34] The critically ill patient with any of these conditions requires close monitoring for the development of SIADH.

Pathophysiology

ADH secretion results in increased permeability of the renal collecting ducts and distal tubules to water, resulting in increased water reabsorption, increased intravascular volume, and decreased urine volume. As a result, patients with SIADH develop a state of hypervolemia with dilutional hyponatremia (i.e., the dilutional effect of increased intravascular water).

Clinical Signs and Symptoms

Clinical manifestations of SIADH include adequate circulating volume, signs of hyponatremia, and decreased serum osmolality discussed in the second section of this chapter (see Hyponatremia). Urine volume is low (output typically <0.5 mL/kg per hour), with inappropriately high urine osmolality.

Laboratory studies consistent with SIADH include a low serum sodium (typically <130 mEq/L) and osmolality (<275 mOsm/L) with high urine sodium, specific gravity, and osmolality.

Management

Management of SIADH is targeted at the prevention of complications associated with hyponatremia. Early detection of neurologic deterioration is critical; therefore, frequent neurologic assessments are needed. If neurologic complications develop, including a change in mental status or seizure activity, immediate treatment includes administration of hypertonic saline (e.g., 2-4 mL/kg of 3% saline should raise serum sodium approximately 1 to 2 mEq/L) and loop diuretics (e.g., furosemide).[34] These therapies should raise the serum sodium sufficiently to slow the intracellular water shift.

Treatment of SIADH includes restriction of free water intake (to approximately half or two-thirds of estimated maintenance fluid requirements) and close monitoring of neurologic function, fluid intake and output, urine specific gravity, and serum sodium.

Cerebral Salt Wasting

Etiology

Cerebral salt wasting (CSW) is caused by increased circulating levels of ANP with resulting natriuresis and contraction of intravascular volume, including potential hypovolemia. Causes of CSW are the same as those causing SIADH (see sections, Specific Diseases and Syndrome of Inappropriate Antidiuretic Hormone). When CSW is associated with a head injury, it typically develops 2 to 7 days after the injury. CSW can also complicate congestive heart failure, Cushing's syndrome, DKA, and hyperaldosteronism.[33]

Pathophysiology

Intracranial disease or injury and complications of other disease are thought to alter neurologic secretion of ANP and other natriuretic peptides.[25] Increased circulating levels of ANP lead to increased excretion of a large amount of sodium in a high volume of urine. Like SIADH, CSW produces hyponatremia with a low serum osmolality and a high urine sodium and urine osmolality. However, because ANP and other natriuretic peptides produce a high urine volume, the patient also develops mild to moderate dehydration.[34]

Clinical Signs and Symptoms

Clinical manifestations of CSW include the signs and symptoms of hyponatremia (see "Hyponatremia" earlier in chapter) and those of mild to moderate dehydration (see Table 12-5). Laboratory studies confirm hyponatremia (serum Na^+ <130 mEq/L) and increased urinary sodium (urine Na^+ >80 mEq/L). Although not routinely monitored, serum levels of ANP are increased.[33]

Management

Because the priorities of management differ, it is important to distinguish CSW from SIADH (Table 12-7).[14,33] Treatment of CSW includes sodium replacement with oral salts or hypertonic saline, volume replacement with isotonic crystalloids, and vigilant monitoring for and prompt treatment of adverse effects of hyponatremia and hypovolemia.[25] Mineralocorticoid therapy (fludrocortisone) can enhance sodium reabsorption and expand intravascular fluid volume in patients with CSW.[29]

Diabetes Insipidus

Etiology

DI is caused by a deficiency of ADH secretion (neurogenic or central DI) or an insensitivity of renal receptors to ADH (nephrogenic DI). Neurogenic DI is caused most commonly by lesions of the central nervous system (pituitary tumors, Langerhans cell histiocytosis, germinoma, craniopharyngioma, suprasellar tumors) or the resection of these lesions. DI also occurs as a complication of brain death from severe traumatic brain injury. Inherited mutations in the vasopressin gene are uncommon causes of central DI without associated central nervous system pathology.

Nephrogenic DI can be hereditary or acquired. The renal ADH receptor is carried on the X chromosome, resulting in a male predominance of inherited (X-linked) nephrogenic DI. DI can complicate drug administration or damage to the renal tubules. Amphotericin B, loop diuretics, and some anesthetics have been reported to cause reversible DI. Irreversible nephrogenic DI results from a loss of ADH sensitivity secondary to renal disease or an insult that interferes with the kidneys' ability to concentrate water.

Table 12-7 Comparison of DI, SIADH, and CSW

Clinical Manifestation	DI	SIADH	CSW
Serum Na+	Increased	Decreased	Decreased
Serum osmolality	Increased	Decreased	Decreased
Urine output	Increased	Normal or decreased	Normal or increased
Urine osmolality	Decreased	Increased	Increased
Body weight	Stable or decreased	Stable or increased	Stable or decreased
Blood urea nitrogen	Normal or increased	Normal or decreased	Normal or increased
ECF volume	Decreased	Increased	Decreased
Management	Vasopressin, DDAVP, fluid replacement	Fluid restriction; sodium administration only if neurologic complications of hyponatremia develop; possible use of diuretics	Fluid replacement, sodium replacement, fludrocortisone

CSW, Cerebral salt wasting; *DDAVP,* 1-deamino-8-D-arginine vasopressin; *DI,* diabetes insipidus; *ECF,* extracellular fluid; *SIADH,* syndrome of inappropriate antidiuretic hormone.

Pathophysiology

A deficit of ADH or lack of renal response to ADH results in decreased reabsorption of water by the renal distal tubules, so a significant volume of water is lost in the urine. As a result of this free water loss, unless fluid replacement is provided, patients can rapidly develop significant hypovolemia and hypernatremia (concentration effect).

Clinical Signs and Symptoms

The classic clinical manifestations of DI include polyuria, hypernatremia, and intense thirst. If not recognized early, the infant or child with DI can rapidly develop hypovolemic shock. In the chronic state, the excessive water intake associated with DI leads to anorexia, weight loss, and a catabolic state.

Patients at risk should be monitored closely for the clinical manifestations of hypovolemia and hypernatremia. Laboratory studies consistent with DI (see Table 12-7) include elevated serum sodium (Na^+ >150 mEq/L) and osmolality (>295 mOsm/L) and low urine osmolality (<100-200 mOsm/L).[33]

Management

Critical care management of DI includes administration of exogenous vasopressin (aqueous vasopressin [5-10 units subcutaneously] or lysine vasopressin [2-4 units IV]) or the vasopressin analog, 1-Deamino-8-d-Arginine Vasopressin (DDAVP [5-20 mcg intranasally every 12-24 hours]), careful fluid replacement, close monitoring of fluid intake and output, and close monitoring of serum sodium and other electrolytes.[33,34] While urine volume is high, it is also important to monitor for the signs and symptoms of hypovolemic shock and support electrolyte balance.

When urine output is high, urine output is totaled typically every 10 or 15 minutes. In the next equal time interval (i.e., the next 10 or 15 minutes), the volume lost in the urine is replaced milliliter for milliliter (typically alternating 5% dextrose and water with 5% dextrose and 0.2% sodium chloride). Replacement fluid is added to maintenance fluid requirements and must also include replacement of any additional sources of fluid loss (e.g., gastric drainage).

Diabetic Ketoacidosis

Etiology

DKA is a life-threatening complication of diabetes mellitus that includes the combination of severe hyperglycemia and ketoacidosis. Approximately 40% of children with diabetes mellitus present with DKA as their first clinical manifestation of diabetes mellitus.[25]

Type I diabetes mellitus in children results from a loss of insulin-secreting pancreatic beta cells. The most common form of type I diabetes is triggered by a combination of genetic susceptibility and environmental factors, including some viruses, that produce autoimmune destruction of beta cells.[15]

Pathophysiology

DKA results from a severe deficiency of insulin that impairs glucose uptake into the cell. To correct the ensuing energy deficit, there is an increase in counter-regulatory hormones such as glucagon, catecholamines, cortisol, and growth hormone in an attempt to produce more glucose. As

a result, the serum glucose concentration is extremely high, but glucose uptake by the cells continues to be impaired. A state of intracellular energy debt ensues, resulting in derangements in the metabolism of fat, protein, and carbohydrates. Gluconeogenesis occurs, with the breakdown of proteins and lipids to make amino acids and fatty acids available as energy substrates.

Ketoacids—acetoacetic acid and beta-hydroxybutyric acid—are released from adipocytes in instances of prolonged insulin deficiency. The presence of high levels of these circulating ketoacids results in ketoacidosis.[34] Children with DKA always experience acidosis and hyperosmolar dehydration with glucosuria and osmotic diuresis.

Deficits of sodium, potassium, and phosphate are always present. Although there are urinary losses of these electrolytes, the presence of severe dehydration and hemoconcentration with acidosis (producing an extracellular potassium shift) may initially mask these deficiencies. As a result, the child may have normal or even elevated serum sodium, potassium, and phosphate concentrations despite total body deficits of these electrolytes. After treatment and rehydration, the serum electrolyte concentrations fall, and hyponatremia and hypokalemia develop. Hypokalemia can contribute to cardiac arrhythmias and death on rare occasions if it is not corrected quickly (see section, Clinical Signs and Symptoms).

Finally, dehydration, acidosis, and osmotic water shifts into brain cells (see Box 12-1) can contribute to life-threatening cerebral edema or intracranial thrombotic events.[18] A major difference between children and adults with DKA is the susceptibility of the young to potentially fatal episodes of cerebral edema. Proposed mechanisms of cerebral edema include: accumulation of intracellular idiogenic osmoles (see Box 12-2); vasopressin and atrial natriuretic factor producing water retention, natriuresis, and hyponatremia; disruption in cell membrane ion exchange processes, causing intracellular ion movement and cell swelling; hypoxia and ischemia; ketones and acidosis contributing to the inflammatory cascade; and abnormalities in water (aquaporin) channels in the glial cells of the brain.[18]

Symptomatic cerebral edema in children with DKA can cause death or neurologic devastation.[20] Additional intracranial pathologic conditions—including bleeding, thrombosis, infarction or emboli—can cause altered mental status in children with DKA.[18]

Clinical Signs and Symptoms

Children with DKA have severe hyperglycemia (serum glucose ≥180 mg/dL or >10 mmol/L) and ketoacidosis. Additional signs and symptoms are related to the severity of the resulting hyperosmolality, volume depletion, and acidosis. Children with DKA generally present with a 5% to 10% fluid deficit[7] caused by the massive water losses secondary to glucosuria.

Acidosis results from the extremely large quantity of ketoacids in the blood. Acetoacetic acid may be reduced to beta-hydroxybutyric acid or decarboxylated to acetone. This ketonemia produces the classic "fruity breath" in children with DKA. The resulting urinary excretion of these ketone bodies, ketonuria, causes further osmotic loss of fluids and electrolytes. In the presence of acidosis, the body develops compensatory hyperpnea or Kussmaul breathing, a classic sign of DKA.

As noted previously, the serum sodium, potassium, and phosphate concentrations may be low, normal, or high but deficits of these electrolytes are present. The serum sodium should be interpreted in light of the serum glucose concentration (each 100 mg/dL rise in serum glucose above 180 mg/dL is likely to depress the serum sodium 1.6 mEq/L below 135 mEq/L). The serum potassium should be evaluated in the context of the serum pH: acidosis causes an extracellular shift in potassium, so the serum potassium rises. After treatment and rehydration, serum electrolyte concentrations fall; therefore, hyponatremia and hypokalemia can develop with attendant complications (see the Chapter 12 Supplement on the Evolve Website for a case study that demonstrates typical serum sodium and glucose values in a patient with DKA).

Dehydration, acidosis and osmotic fluid shifts in the brain can contribute to life-threatening cerebral edema or intracranial thrombotic events. These central nervous system complications can produce decreased responsiveness, posturing, abnormal respiratory patterns, and signs of increased intracranial pressure and cerebral herniation.[18] Table 12-8 shows a summary of the clinical manifestations of DKA and their underlying mechanisms.

Management

Priorities of management of DKA in order of importance are: assessment and support of neurologic function (including support of patent airway and effective ventilation), assessment and support of circulation (including volume resuscitation), insulin therapy, and restoration and maintenance of electrolyte, glucose and acid-base balance (Box 12-5). Consideration is also given to confounding factors, such as infection, injury or other patient problems.

Although very few children present with neurologic compromise (primarily cerebral edema) this can be a very poor prognostic indicator. Most who present with this finding perish and those who survive are often severely neurologically compromised with little or no independent function.[20]

If the child's level of consciousness deteriorates, cerebral edema may be present, and urgent intervention is needed (see diagnostic criteria for cerebral edema[21a] in Box 12-6). If clinical signs of cerebral edema develop, immediate treatment with IV mannitol (0.2-1.0 g/kg over 30-60 minutes) is indicated. Hypertonic saline (e.g., 3% sodium chloride, 10 mL/kg, administered IV over 30 minutes) may be used as an alternative to mannitol. If the child's ability to protect the airway or spontaneous ventilation deteriorates, intubation and mechanical ventilation are indicated.

The child's volume deficit is initially treated with the administration of normal saline or lactated Ringer's. The quantity of fluid administered is determined by the patient's clinical severity; if shock is present, bolus administration of isotonic crystalloids is needed. For less significant volume deficit, typically 10 to 20 mL/kg is administered over 1 to 2 hours and repeated as needed.[18] Replacement of the total fluid deficit is planned over approximately 48 hours or longer. Isotonic crystalloids are used for initial fluid replacement; the

Table 12-8	Clinical Manifestations of Diabetic Ketoacidosis
Signs and Symptoms	**Underlying Mechanisms**
Hyperglycemia, dehydration, cardiovascular collapse	Osmotic diuresis secondary to hyperglycemia
Acidosis	Accumulation of ketoacids and lactic acid in serum from lipolysis, resulting in increased H^+ concentration in serum
Electrolyte imbalance: sodium	Total body hyponatremia because of passive loss of electrolytes as a result of osmotic diuresis; however, serum sodium may be high as a result of hemoconcentration
Electrolyte imbalance: potassium	In acidosis, potassium shifts from ICF to ECF; therefore, initially serum potassium may be normal or even high, but will decrease as a result of osmotic diuresis and correction of acidosis
Cardiac arrhythmia	Hypokalemia or hyperkalemia
Ketonuria	Serum ketone levels rise above the renal threshold and are spilled in the urine
Hyperpnea	Compensatory mechanism; effort to blow off excess CO_2 and thereby correct the degree of acidosis
Mental status changes, cerebral edema	Possibly related to rate of correction of hyperglycemia, level of acidosis, fluid shifts

From Trimarchi T: Endocrine critical care problems. In: Curley MAQ, Moloney-Harmon PA, editors: *Critical care nursing of infants and children*, ed 2, Philadelphia, 2001, WB Saunders, p. 817.
ECF, Extracellular fluid; *ICF*, intracellular fluid.

Box 12-5	Priorities of Management of Diabetic Ketoacidosis in Order of Importance*

1. Assess and support neurologic function, including support of patent airway and effective ventilation
2. Assess and stabilize circulation (including fluid resuscitation)
3. Treat with insulin
4. Restore and maintain electrolyte, glucose and acid-base balance
5. Identify confounding factors (infection, drugs, injury, other diagnoses)

*Perform serial assessments throughout care and immediately notify provider of any deterioration.

sodium content may then be reduced to 0.45% sodium chloride with potassium added as the child's condition stabilizes.

Replacement of insulin is generally accomplished by continuous IV infusion. An infusion of regular insulin (0.05 to 0.1 unit/kg per hour) is titrated to gradually reduce the serum

Box 12-6	**Bedside Neurologic Evaluation of Children with Diabetic Ketoacidosis**

Diagnostic Criteria for Possible Cerebral Edema*

- Abnormal motor or verbal response to pain
- Decorticate or decerebrate posturing
- Cranial nerve palsy (especially cranial nerves III, IV, and VI)
- Abnormal neurologic respiratory pattern (e.g., grunting, tachypnea, Cheyne-Stokes respiration, apneusis)

Major Criteria

- Altered mentation, fluctuating level of consciousness
- Sustained heart rate deceleration (decline in HR by more than 20/min) not attributable to improved intravascular volume or sleep state
- Age-inappropriate incontinence

Minor Criteria[†]

- Vomiting
- Headache
- Lethargy or decreased arousability from sleep
- Diastolic blood pressure >90 mm Hg
- Age <5 years

From Muir AB, et al: Cerebral edema in childhood diabetic ketoacidosis. *Diabetes Care* 24:1541-1546, 2004.
*Signs that are present before treatment should not be considered in the diagnosis of cerebral edema.
[†]Minor criteria are frequently present in children who do not develop symptomatic cerebral edema.[20]

glucose at the rate of approximately 50 to 100 mg/dL per hour. Simultaneous infusion of 10% glucose IV can be titrated to control the maximum rate of decline in the serum glucose to no more than 100 mg/dL per hour. Glucose infusion is preferable to slowing the insulin infusion, because reducing the insulin dose can worsen the patient's acidosis.[18]

As noted previously, patients with DKA typically have deficits of water, sodium, potassium, and phosphate. Although serum electrolyte concentrations may be normal at the time of initial clinical presentation, with treatment hyponatremia, hypokalemia, and hypophosphatemia are likely to be present. Replacement fluids are selected to address these deficits. Some landmark studies suggest that phosphate replacement is of no clinical value.[8,38] There is no evidence that the addition of sodium bicarbonate to correct acidosis is of value, and it may contribute to hypokalemia and cerebral edema.[18] To prevent a fall in serum osmolality when the serum glucose is reduced, the serum sodium concentration should rise approximately 1.6 mEq/L for every 100 mg/dL fall in serum glucose concentration.

Providers should look for evidence of confounding factors in a child with DKA. These factors include infection, illicit use of drugs or other medications, injury, or other intracranial pathologic finding. Most of these factors will aggravate acidosis and slow the recovery from DKA.

Box 12-7 contains a typical management plan for children with DKA. As a general rule, patients in DKA recover from acidosis within 24 hours after presentation.

Adrenal Insufficiency

Etiology

Adrenal insufficiency can be either primary or secondary and includes several conditions that result in a deficiency of glucocorticoids (cortisol) and mineralocorticoids (aldosterone). Adrenal insufficiency also results in decreased production and release of catecholamines.

Primary adrenocortical deficiency (Addison's disease) results from disease states that prevent the adrenal glands from producing cortisol or aldosterone. These diseases include: congenital adrenal hypoplasia, tuberculous adrenalitis, autoimmune adrenalitis, adrenoleukodystrophy, and adrenal hemorrhage. In addition, recessively inherited defects in the synthesis of cortisol and aldosterone constitute the congenital adrenal hyperplasia syndromes and are among the most common causes of primary adrenocortical insufficiency in neonates (1 in 16,000 births).

Secondary adrenocortical deficiency occurs as the result of interrupted communication in the hypothalamic-pituitary-adrenal axis. Secondary adrenal insufficiency is due to deficiencies in corticotrophin releasing hormone (CRH) from the hypothalamus or adrenocorticotropic hormone from the anterior pituitary.[15] The most common cause of adrenal insufficiency in children is the abrupt cessation of administration of exogenous corticosteroids.[34] Adrenal insufficiency should be considered in any critically ill child with persistent shock despite fluid resuscitation and vasopressor therapy (e.g., unresponsive or fluid-refractory septic shock).

Pathophysiology

With primary adrenal disease, there is frequently a deficiency of both aldosterone and glucocorticoids, whereas pituitary disease can lead to diminished adrenocorticotropic hormone secretion and an isolated deficiency of glucocorticoids only.

- Aldosterone deficiency leads to decreased renal reabsorption of sodium and water and increased reabsorption of potassium.
- Isolated glucocorticoid deficiency results in hypoglycemia, elevated levels of ADH (as in SIADH, producing hypervolemia and dilutional hyponatremia), and decreased secretion of and responsiveness to catecholamines. This condition in turn results in the development of myocardial depression, hypotension, and diminished arterial tone.

The combination of aldosterone and glucocorticoid deficiencies can cause severe hypotension. Isolated deficit of glucocorticoids in the presence of a significant stressor (e.g., sepsis) can also produce vasodilation and shock.

Clinical Signs and Symptoms

The initial presentation of acute adrenal insufficiency is often that of profound circulatory failure with the clinical manifestations of hypovolemic, distributive, and cardiogenic shock (see Chapter 6.) Children may also exhibit hyponatremia, hyperkalemia, and hypoglycemia and their corresponding clinical manifestations, as presented earlier in this chapter.

Management

Management of children with adrenal insufficiency is directed at preventing the complications associated with shock and hypoglycemia and correcting electrolyte imbalances. Emergent

Text continues on p. 700

| Box 12-7 | **Management Plan for Children with Diabetic Ketoacidosis** |

1. First Priority: Perform repeat assessments of neurologic function, airway and ventilation
   - Notify on-call provider of a deterioration in neurologic function, airway patency, or ventilation
   - If level of consciousness decreases, be prepared to immediately support airway and ventilation
2. Second priority: Assess and stabilize circulation (including acute management of severe hyperkalemia associated with acidosis).
   - Bolus with normal saline.
     - Give 10 to 20 mL/kg for circulatory failure—repeat as needed to regain circulation, but proceed with caution and avoid >40 mL/kg when possible.
     - Without ongoing circulatory collapse, bolus 5 to 20 mL/kg over 1 to 2 hours.
   - Calculate volume deficit (typically 10%-20% dehydration) and replace.
     - Administer 0.9% saline at maintenance plus deficit correction over next 24 to 72 hours.
   - Establish vascular access.
     - Minimum of two peripheral IV catheters (largest bore possible)
     - Consider a separate "blood-drawing IV."
   - Arterial line is indicated when patient has:
     - Profoundly altered mental status
     - Signs of uncompensated shock
     - Severe acidosis (pH<7.0)
3. Third priority: Insulin administration
   - Use regular insulin 0.05-0.1 unit/kg per hour.
     - Start with low dose insulin infusion (do not bolus).
     - Titrate according to drop in serum glucose.
   - Do not allow glucose to drop faster than 50-100 mg/dL per hour.
     - Add 5% dextrose to intravenous fluids when serum glucose reaches 300 mg/dL.
     - Add 10% dextrose to intravenous fluids when serum glucose reaches 200 mg/dL.
   - Convert from regular insulin infusion to subcutaneously administered insulin preparations when ketoacidosis has resolved, as evidenced by the absence of ketones in the urine.

        Use of an infusion of regular insulin without a bolus loading dose is recommended to allow for careful titration of intravenous fluids as serum glucose concentration begins to decrease. The infusion enables control of the rate of decrease and helps prevent iatrogenic hypoglycemia. A rapid decrease in serum glucose level is known to precipitate central pontine myelinolysis and may also be associated with development of global cerebral edema in patients with diabetic ketoacidosis (DKA).

4. Assess and maintain serum sodium concentration.
   - Evaluate child's serum sodium in light of serum glucose concentration: every 100 mg/dL elevation in serum glucose above 180 mg/dL typically produces a fall in serum sodium by 1.6 mEq/L (<135 mEq/L)
   - As you correct hyperglycemia, serum sodium concentration should rise approximately 1.6 mEq/L for every 100 mg/dL fall in serum glucose concentration
5. Treat potassium and phosphate imbalance.
   - Replace potassium and phosphorous as needed by adding to IV fluid bag (avoid single-dose administration to allow for more careful titration of supplementary electrolyte needs. Potassium will move between intracellular and extracellular compartments as insulin dosing is adjusted and acidosis resolves, and thus may result in rapid fluxes in serum levels). Guidelines for adding potassium supplements:
         K^+ <3.5 mEq/L: Add 40 mEq/L to IV fluids.
         K^+ 3.5-5 mEq/L: Add 30 mEq/L to IV fluids.
         K^+ >5.5 mEq/L: Do not add potassium to IV fluids.
     - Use potassium chloride, add potassium phosphate if phosphorous <3 mg/dL.
     - Add potassium supplementation only after a patient is assessed to have sufficient renal function.
   - Patients may present with hyperkalemia. Potassium will return to intracellular space with administration of insulin and correction of acidosis.
     - Treat severe hyperkalemia (>7 mEq/L and ECG changes) with calcium and consider sodium bicarbonate administration (see Table 12-4).
6. Serial assessments
   - Serum glucose every 1 hour
     - Also check serum glucose after the initial fluid administration.
   - Check urine for ketones with every void.
     - The absence of ketones and serum glucose <200 mg/dL indicates readiness for transition to subcutaneous closing.
   - Measure serum electrolytes every 2 hours.
   - Continuous cardiac-respiratory monitoring, strict monitoring of fluid intake and output and neurologic checks (minimum of every 1 hour during acute phase of illness)
7. Assess for infection (most frequent cause of DKA)
   - Obtain complete blood count with differential.
   - Obtain urine and blood cultures (and possibly respiratory samples).
   - Defer lumbar puncture for cerebrospinal fluid culture unless suspicion of meningitis is very strong and head computed tomography demonstrates no cerebral edema.
   - Consider broad-spectrum empiric IV antibiotics.
   - Monitor body temperature closely.
   - Evaluate for signs and symptoms of infection on history and physical examination.
8. Assess for chronic hyperglycemia
   - Obtain glycosylated hemoglobin (Hgb A1c) level.
   - In a patient with known diabetes, high percentage of Hgb A1c (e.g., 7% or higher) suggests chronic hyperglycemia due to poor compliance with insulin administration.
9. Provide patient-family teaching

Modified from Trimarchi T: Endocrine problems in critically ill children: an overview. *AACN Clin Issues* 17:66-78, 2006.

Table 12-9   Diagnostic Studies to Consider when Evaluating Fluid Imbalances

Diagnostic Study	Normal Values	Causes of an Elevated Level	Causes of a Decreased Level	Comments
Serum				
BUN	8-25 mg/dL	Decreased renal blood flow related to hypovolemia; also seen with increased protein intake	Fluid volume excess, malnutrition, hepatic failure	
Creatinine	0.6-1.2 mg/dL	Hypovolemia, impaired renal function, muscle injury	Fluid volume excess	More specific indicator of renal function than BUN
BUN:creatinine ratio	10:1-15:1	Decrease in renal perfusion, increased protein metabolism	Decreased protein intake, hepatic insufficiency, repeated dialysis	
Sodium	135-145 mEq/L	Excess of total body sodium; concentrated effect of hypovolemia	Depletion of total body sodium; dilutional effect of hypervolemia	Must evaluate in light of physical findings as serum sodium can increase or decrease with changes in fluid balance
Osmolality	275-295 mOsm/L	Hypernatremic dehydration, hyperglycemia, elevated BUN	Hyponatremia	Decreased osmolality may be seen in hypovolemia, euvolemia and hypervolemia
Hematocrit	Males, 40%-52%; females, 37%-46%	Hypovolemia	Hypervolemia	Must be evaluated in terms of changes in red cell mass
Total protein	6.3-8.2 g/dL	Hypovolemia	Hypervolemia	Affected by changes in volume status
Urine				
Specific gravity	1.010-1.030	Hypovolemia associated with normal renal function	Hypervolemia	Reflection of the kidney's ability to concentrate and dilute
Osmolality	50-1200 mOsm/L	Hypovolemia associated with normal renal function	Hypervolemia	Reflection of the kidney's ability to concentrate and dilute

Data from Roberts KE: Fluid and electrolyte balance. In: Curley MAQ, Moloney-Harmon PA, editors: *Critical care nursing of infants and children*, ed 2, Philadelphia, 2001, WB Saunders, p. 376.
BUN, Blood urea nitrogen.

resuscitative measures include bolus fluid administration as needed and administration of vasoactive agents to increase heart rate, cardiac contractility, peripheral vascular resistance, and systemic perfusion.

Treatment for aldosterone deficiency and volume depletion includes judicious fluid resuscitation with an isotonic crystalloid (typically normal saline, possibly with 5% or 10% dextrose) to expand intravascular volume. Excessive fluid replacement can be harmful in instances of isolated glucocorticoid deficiency when SIADH is already present. If the child exhibits the clinical manifestations of hyperkalemia, urgent treatment with calcium, glucose plus insulin, and other strategies listed in Table 12-4 are needed.

Emergent replacement of glucocorticoids is accomplished through IV administration of stress doses of hydrocortisone ($25-50$ mg/m^2 body surface area per day by IV continuous infusion or divided into 4-8 doses). Vigilant monitoring of fluid and electrolyte balance is a key component of the nursing care of the child with acute adrenal insufficiency.

DIAGNOSTIC TESTS

Diagnostic studies are a key component in identifying disruptions in fluid or electrolyte balance. Table 12-9 provides an overview of the most common diagnostic tests used to evaluate fluid balance. However, these diagnostic studies are just one piece of the puzzle when evaluating a child with a disruption in fluid or electrolyte balance. The laboratory results should be evaluated in light of the child's history and clinical presentation.

References
1. Arieff AI, Ayus JC, Fraser CL: Hyponatraemia and death or permanent brain damage in healthy children. *BMJ* 304:1218–1222, 1992.
2. Armon K, et al: Hyponatremia and hypokalemia during intravenous fluid administration. *Arch Dis Child* 93:285–287, 2008.
3. Beck CE: Hypotonic versus isotonic maintenance intravenous fluid therapy in hospitalized children: a systematic review. *Clin Pediatr* 46:764–770, 2007.
4. Brashers VL, Jones RE: Mechanisms of hormonal regulation. In McCance KL, Huether SE, editors: *Pathophysiology: the biologic*

basis for disease in adults and children, ed 6, Philadelphia, 2009, Mosby-Elsevier.

5. Choong K, et al: Hypotonic versus isotonic saline in hospitalized children: a systematic review. *Arch Dis Child* 91:828–835, 2006.
6. Custer JW, Rau RE: *The Harriet Lane handbook,* ed 18, Philadelphia, 2009, Mosby-Elsevier.
7. Dunger DB, et al: European Society for Paediatric Endocrinology/ Lawson Wilkins Pediatric Endocrine Society consensus statement on diabetic ketoacidosis in children and adolescents. *Pediatrics* 113: e133–e140, 2004.
8. Fisher JN, Kitabchi AE: A randomized study of phosphate therapy in the treatment of diabetic ketoacidosis. *J Clin Endocrinol Metab* 57: 177–180, 1983.
9. Elisaf M, Kalaitzidis R, Siamopoulos KC: Multiple electrolyte abnormalities after pamidronate administration. *Nephron* 79:337–339, 1998.
10. Friedman AL: Nephrology: fluid and electrolytes. In Behrman RE, Kliegman RM, editors: *Nelson essentials of pediatrics,* ed 4, Philadelphia, 2002, WB Saunders, pp. 671–709.
11. Hazinski MF, et al: Fluid therapy and medications for shock and cardiac arrest. *PALS provider manual,* Dallas, 2002, American Heart Association.
12. Hellerstein S: Fluids and electrolytes: clinical aspects. *Pediatr Rev* 14: 103–115, 1993.
13. Holliday MA, Segar WE: The maintenance need for water in parenteral fluid therapy. *Pediatrics* 19:823–832, 1957.
14. Jimenez R, et al: Cerebral salt wasting syndrome in children with acute central nervous system injury. *Ped Neuro* 35:261–263, 2006.
15. Jones RE, Brashers VL, Huether SE: Alterations of hormonal regulation. In McCance KL, Huether SE, editors: *Pathophysiology: the biologic basis for disease in adults and children,* ed 6, Philadelphia, 2009, Mosby-Elsevier.
16. Kamel KS, Wei C: Controversial issues in the treatment of hyperkalemia. *Nephrol Dial Transplant* 18:2215–2218, 2003.
17. Lacy CF, et al: *Lexicomp's drug information handbook,* ed 18, Hudson, OH, 2009, Lexicomp.
17a. Kleinman ME, Chameides L, Schexnayder SM, et al: Part 14: pediatric advanced life support: 2010 American Heart Association Guidelines for Cardiopulmonary Resuscitation and Emergency Cardiovascular Care. *Circulation* 122(18 Suppl 3):S876–908, 2010.
18. Levin DL: Cerebral edema in diabetic ketoacidosis. *Pediatr Crit Care Med* 9:320–329, 2008.
19. Mahoney BA, et al: Emergency interventions for hyperkalaemia. *Cochrane Database Syst Rev April 18 (2) CD003235,* 2005.
20. Marcin JP, et al: American Academy of Pediatrics: The Pediatric Emergency Medicine Collaborative Research Committee: factors associated with adverse outcomes in children with diabetic ketoacidosis-related cerebral edema. *J Pediatr* 141:793–797, 2002.
21. Moritz ML, Ayus JC: Prevention of hospital-acquired hyponatremia: a case for using isotonic saline. *Pediatrics* 111:227–230, 2003.
21a. Muir AB, et al: Cerebral edema in childhood diabetic ketoacidosis. *Diabetes Care* 24:1541–1546, 2004.
22. Neville KA, et al: Isotonic is better than hypotonic saline for intravenous rehydration of children with gastroenteritis: a prospective randomized study. *Arch Dis Child* 91:226–232, 2006.
23. Nyirenda MJ, et al: Clinical review: hyperkalemia, *Br Med J* 339: 4114.
24. Ralston M, et al: *PALS provider manual,* Dallas, 2006, American Heart Association.
25. Relvas MS: Endocrine emergencies. In Conway EE, editor: *Pediatric multiprofessional critical care review,* Des Plaines, IL, 2006, Society of Critical Care Medicine, pp. 365–376.
26. Reynolds M, Padfield PL, Seckl JR: Disorders of sodium balance. *Br Med J* 332:702–705, 2006.
27. Roberts KE: Fluid and electrolyte regulation. In Curley MAQ, Moloney-Harmon P, editors: *Critical care nursing of infants and children,* ed 2, Philadelphia, 2001, WB Saunders.
28. Schaefer TJ, Wolford RW: Disorders of potassium. *Emerg Med Clin North Am* 23:723–747, 2005.
29. Springate J: Cerebral salt wasting, Available at: http://www.emedicine.com/ped/topic354.htm. Accessed July 4, 2008.
30. Springate JE, Kala GK: Hypomagnesemia, 2010: Available at: http://emedicine.medscape.com/article/922142-overview. Accessed January 4.
31. Stark J: A comprehensive analysis of the fluid and electrolytes system. *Crit Care Nursing Clin North Am* 10:471–475, 1998.
32. Styne DM, Glaser NS: Endocrinology. In Behrman RE, Kliegman RM, editors: *Nelson essentials of pediatrics,* ed 4, Philadelphia, 2002, WB Saunders, pp. 711–766.
33. Trimarchi T: Endocrine critical care problems. In Curley MAQ, Moloney-Harmon PA, editors: *Critical care nursing of infants and children,* ed 2, Philadelphia, 2001, WB Saunders, pp. 805–819.
34. Trimarchi T: Endocrine problems in critically ill children: an overview. *AACN Clin Issues* 17:66–78, 2006.
35. Vellaichamy M: Hypernatremia, 2008: Available at: http://www.emedicine.com/ped/topic1082.htm. Accessed July 4.
36. Vellaichamy M: Hyponatremia, 2008: Available at: http://www.emedicine.com/ped/topic1124.htm. Accessed July 4.
37. Vlasselaers D, et al: Intensive insulin therapy for patients in paediatric intensive care: a prospective, randomised controlled study. *Lancet* 373:547–556, 2009.
38. Wilson HK, et al: Phosphate therapy in diabetic ketoacidosis. *Arch Intern Med* 142:517–520, 1982.

Renal Disorders

Frances Blayney

PEARLS

- Urine output will decrease if cardiac output and renal blood flow are compromised; as a result, urine output is a sensitive indicator of cardiac output.
- The normal hourly volume of urine output in children is small, and a small compromise in urine volume may indicate a significant compromise in renal perfusion or function.
- A child's glomerular filtration rate will approach adult values by about 3 years of age.
- Renal failure may be present in a child with a low, normal, or high volume of urine output.
- Accurate measurement of urine volume and composition provide fundamental data on which clinical decisions are made.
- The modified pRIFLE is a classification system to standardize the definition of acute kidney injury (AKI) in pediatric patients. The acronym, pRIFLE stands for: pediatric risk of renal dysfunction, injury to the kidney, failure of kidney function, loss of kidney function, and end-stage kidney disease. Studies have shown that use of the pRIFLE enhances the classification of AKI epidemiology and the course of AKI in critically ill pediatric patients.
- Renal replacement therapies differ significantly in their effectiveness in treating AKI and its complications. It is therefore helpful for the nurse to be aware of the advantages and disadvantages of each therapy so that the nurse can participate in decisions regarding the best treatment modality for each patient.

INTRODUCTION

The kidney is an amazing organ system. It continuously adjusts extracellular fluid volume, solute concentration, and pH; it secretes organic acids, bases, and most ingested food additives and chemicals; it helps maintain calcium and phosphate balance and production of erythropoietin for red blood cell (RBC) synthesis; and it contributes to a variety of feedback systems. Because the kidney receives a large percentage of the cardiac output to perform all these vital functions, urine output is a sensitive indicator of cardiac function.

ESSENTIAL ANATOMY AND PHYSIOLOGY

Kidney Structure

Gross Anatomy

The kidneys lie anterior and lateral to the twelfth thoracic and first, second, and third lumbar vertebrae and behind the abdominal peritoneum; therefore they are retroperitoneal structures. The kidneys are embedded in a mass of fatty tissue called the *adipose capsule,* and each capsule is enclosed in the renal fascia (Fig. 13-1). The kidneys are not secured to the abdominal wall, but are held in position by the renal fascia and the large renal arteries and veins. The adipose capsule and the pararenal fat help to protect the kidney and keep it in place.

The medial aspect of each kidney is curved away from the midline; at the center of this concavity is the hilus, where the renal artery and nerves enter the kidney and where the renal vein and ureter exit the kidney. Surrounding each kidney is a tough, nearly indistensible fibrous capsule, which becomes the outer lining of the renal calyces, renal pelvis, and ureter.

A longitudinal section of the kidney shows the three general areas of renal structure: the cortex, the medulla, and the pelvis (Fig. 13-2). The renal cortex is the outer portion of the kidney. It has a granular appearance and extends in finger-like projections into the medullary areas. The cortex contains most of the nephrons, the smallest functioning unit of the kidney. The cortex also contains all glomeruli, the proximal and distal convoluted tubules, and the first parts of the loop of Henle and the collecting ducts.

The renal medulla is composed predominately of the long loops of Henle from the juxtamedullary nephrons and the collecting ducts that grow progressively larger as they approach the renal pelvis. These structures give the medulla a striated, pyramidal appearance, with the apex of the pyramid pointing toward the renal pelvis and the base pointing toward the renal cortex.

The renal pelvis contains the outflow tract and a small amount of surrounding fat that acts as a cushion. The renal outflow tract begins with the minor calyces (Greek for *cup*) that receive urine from the collecting ducts. The urine flows from the minor calyces into the major calyces, into the renal pelvis, into the ureters and bladder, out of the bladder, and through the urethra to exit the body through the urethral meatus.

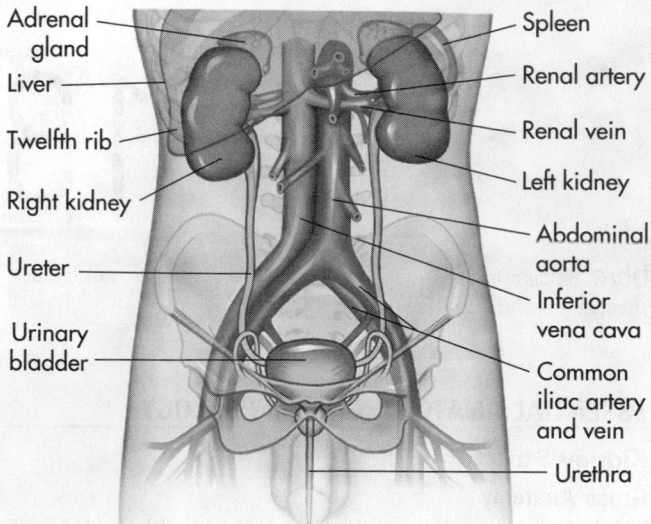

FIG. 13-1 Components of the urinary system. (From Patton KT, Thibodeau GA: *Anatomy and physiology*, ed 7. St Louis, 2010, Mosby.)

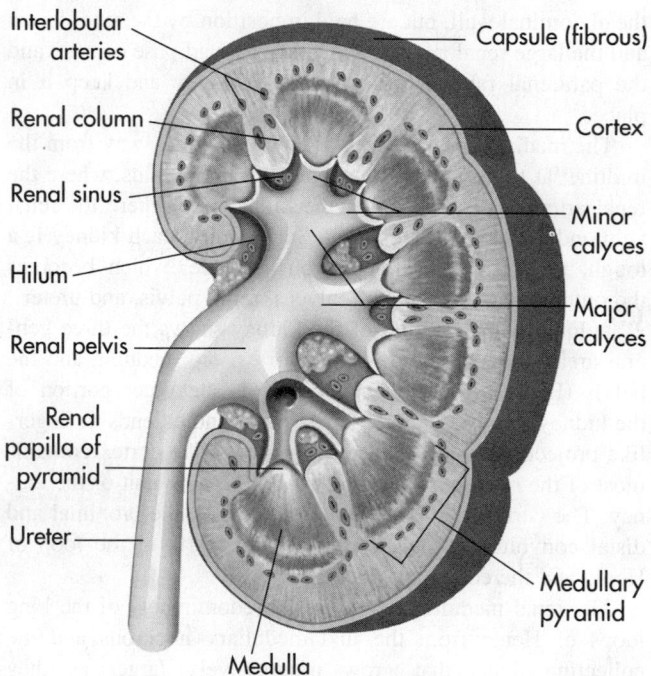

FIG. 13-2 Cross-section of the kidney. (From Patton KT, Thibodeau GA: *Anatomy and physiology*, ed 7. St Louis, 2010, Mosby.)

The functioning unit of the kidney is the nephron, which consists of a vascular component and a tubular component (Fig. 13-3). Each kidney contains approximately 1 million distinct nephrons. Eighty-five percent of all nephrons originate in the outermost area of the cortex. The remaining nephrons are the juxtamedullary nephrons that originate in the inner cortical area. The long loops of Henle from the juxtamedullary nephrons that extend deep into the medulla lie parallel to the medullary collecting ducts and play an important role in the concentration of urine (see Evolve Fig 13-1 in the Chapter 13 Supplement on the Evolve Website).

Renal Vasculature

In most patients, each kidney is supplied with systemic arterial blood from a single artery. The renal arteries branch from the aorta at the level of the second or third lumbar vertebrae; together they receive approximately 20% of the total cardiac output. Each artery divides into an anterior and posterior artery. These arteries continue to branch into small arterioles. Some of these arterioles will supply nutrients to the renal medulla, cortical tissue, and capsule, while other arterioles enter the glomerular capsule.

The *afferent arteriole* enters the glomerular capsule and divides to form the glomerulus, a tuft of capillaries that allows filtration of plasma through the capillary membranes. The glomerular capillaries do not recombine into venous channels, but instead recombine into a second arteriole called the *efferent arteriole* (Fig. 13-4). Because arterioles are present at either end of the glomerular capillary system, constriction or dilation of these arterioles will alter the resistance to flow through the glomerular capillaries and thus will regulate glomerular filtration.

After leaving the glomerulus, the efferent arterioles branch to form a network of capillaries that surround the convoluted tubules and the loop of Henle. These peritubular capillaries then converge into venules that will return renal venous blood to the systemic circulation via the inferior vena cava. Elements that the kidney reabsorbs from the filtrate to return to the circulation are reabsorbed into this peritubular capillary system.

Renal Tubules and Collecting Ducts

The tubular component of the nephron begins as a single layer of flat epithelial cells surrounding the glomerulus. This layer is known as *Bowman's capsule* (Fig. 13-4, B). Filtered plasma from the glomerular capillaries will enter Bowman's capsule and flow into a coiled tubule called the proximal tubule, also known as the *proximal convoluted tubule* (Fig. 13-5).

The structure and appearance of the proximal tubule changes as it descends toward the renal medulla. The tubular lumen narrows and the cells become flattened as the tubule makes a hairpin turn, called the *loop of Henle*. As the loop of Henle ascends from the medulla into the renal cortex, the tubular cells enlarge and again become cuboidal; in addition, the tubule coils, forming the *distal convoluted tubule*. The tubule then straightens and joins the collecting duct.

Collecting ducts are the terminus of many distal tubules; they are formed in the inner and outer renal cortex. These small collecting ducts enter the renal medulla where they form larger ducts, which in turn drain into a minor calyx in the renal pelvis. Approximately 8 to 10 minor calyces join into the major calyces, which combine to form the renal pelvis. The renal pelvis is the largest portion of the outflow tract proximal to the bladder.

Ureters

The two ureters conduct urine from the renal pelvis to the urinary bladder; they are located behind the peritoneum and they descend through the pelvic cavity, crossing over the common iliac arteries. The ureters are attached to the bladder at an oblique angle; they enter the bladder laterally and tunnel

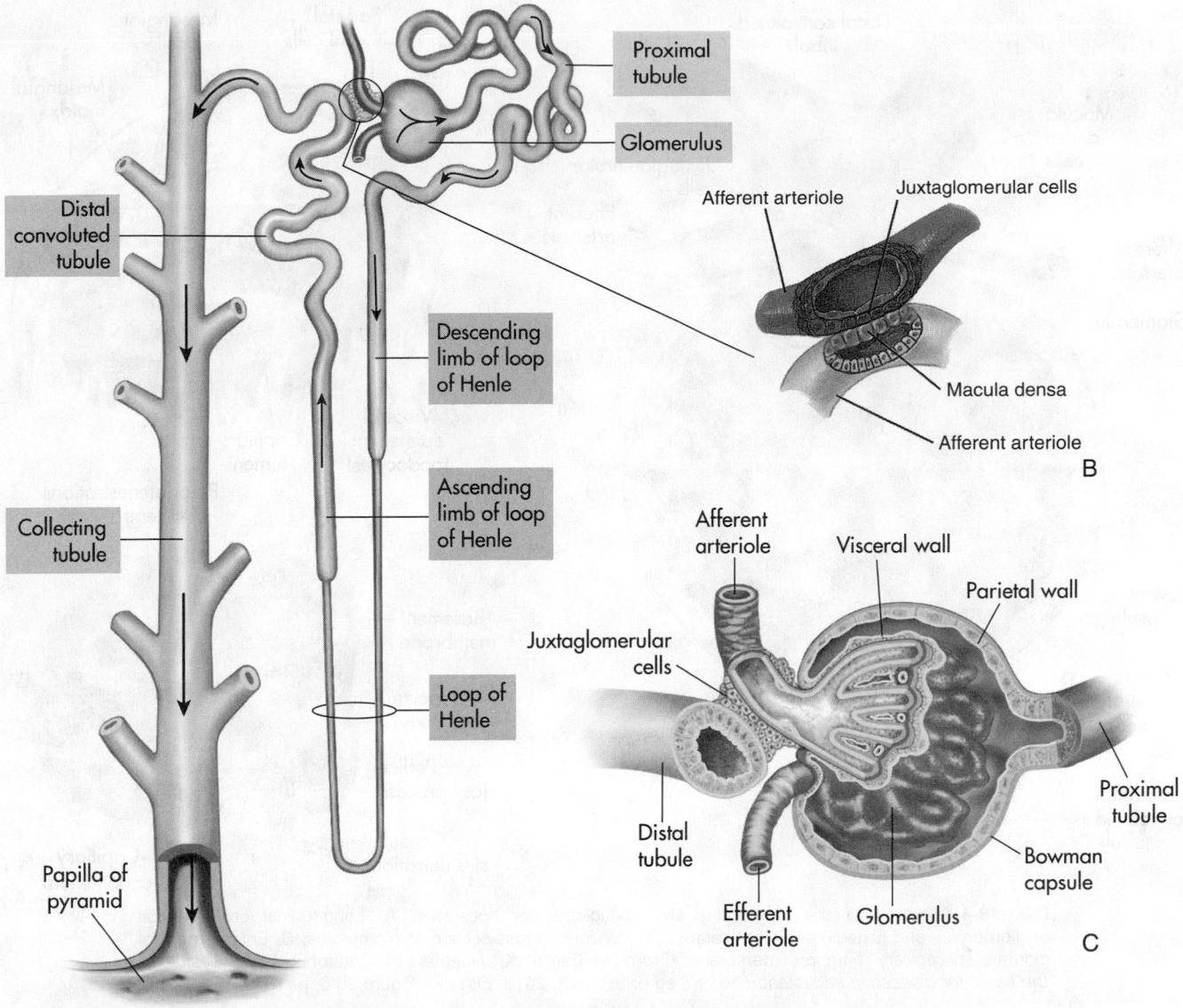

FIG. 13-3 Components of the nephron. A, One nephron. B, Cells of juxtaglomerular apparatus. C, Glomerulous and juxtaglomerular apparatus. (A from Patton KT, Thibodeau GA: *Anatomy and physiology*, ed 7. St Louis, 2010, Mosby; B from Applegate E: *The anatomy and physiology learning system*, St Louis, 2011, Saunders; C from McCance K, Huether SE, editors: *Pathophysiology: the basis for disease in adults and children*, ed 6. St Louis, 2010, Mosby.)

between the bladder mucosa and detrusor muscle, creating a flap-valve design that normally prevents reflux of urine into the ureters during bladder contraction.[30]

Each ureteral wall has three layers: an inner epithelial lining, a middle muscular layer, and the outer fibrous layer that is continuous with the renal capsule. The middle muscular portion of the ureter consists of both a circular and a longitudinal muscle layer. The circular muscles propel the urine toward the bladder by peristaltic contraction, and they generate enough pressure to overcome the resistance caused by the oblique ureteral insertions into the bladder. Contraction of the longitudinal fibers opens the lumen of the ureter. These ureteral muscle fibers are innervated by fibers from the aortic, spermatic or ovarian, and hypogastric plexuses. Peristalsis persists even when the ureter is denervated, allowing ureters to be transplantable.[55]

The Bladder and Urethra

The urinary bladder is a hollow, muscular organ that stores urine. There are three openings in the bladder wall: the entrances of the two ureters and the exit of the urethra. These openings form the corners of a triangle, called the *trigone*. There is a dense area of smooth (involuntary) muscle around the neck of the bladder at the orifice of the urethra; this muscle constitutes the internal sphincter. The urethra extends from the urinary bladder to the body surface. At the point where the urethra passes through the muscles of the pelvic floor, striated (voluntary) circular muscles form an external sphincter.[55]

Micturition is the emptying of the stored urine from the bladder. The process normally involves both voluntary and involuntary nervous system activities in children beyond approximately 2 to 3 years of age. Once an adequate volume of urine has accumulated in the bladder, the bladder wall stretches,

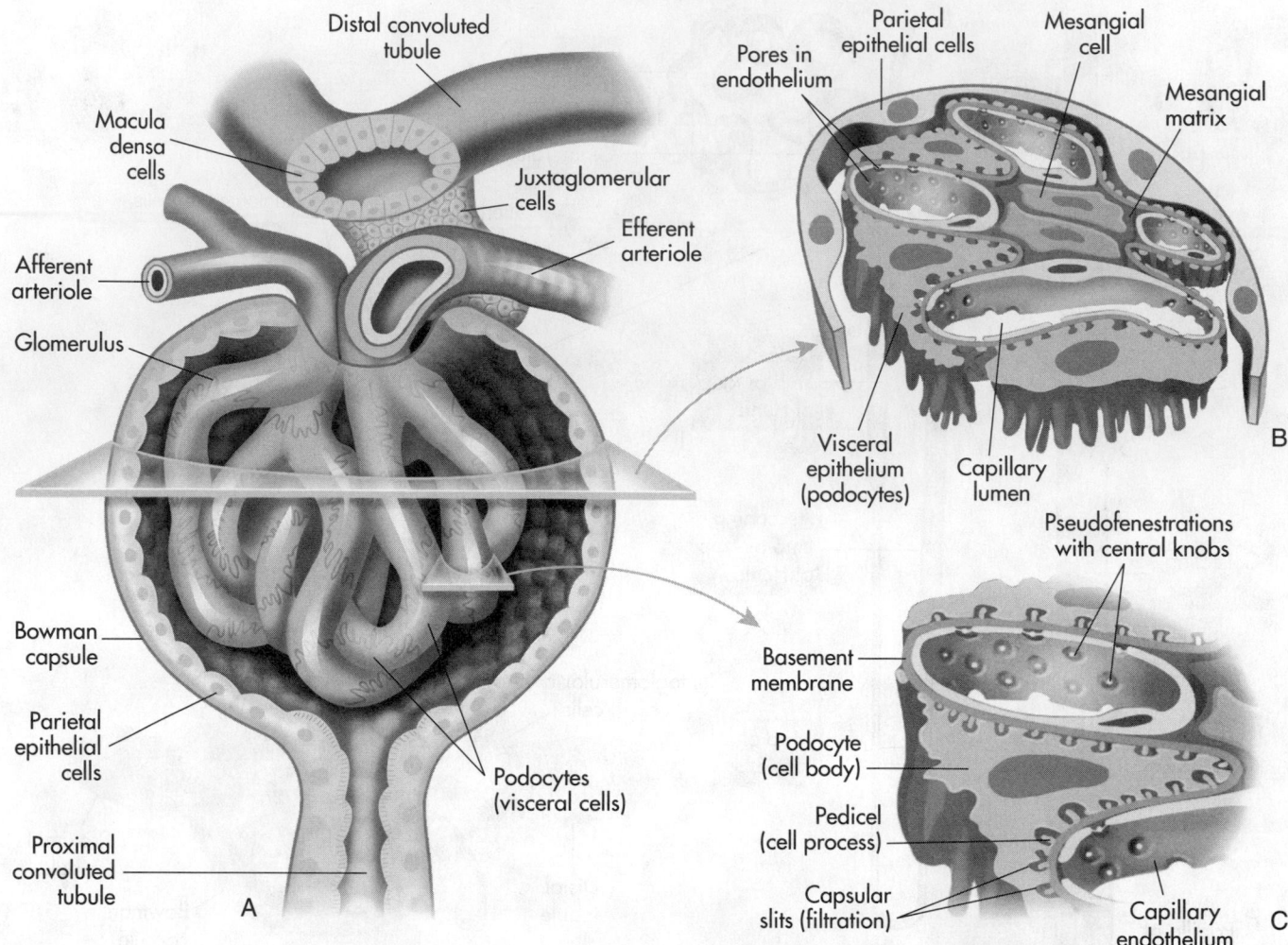

FIG. 13-4 Anatomy of the glomerulus and juxtaglomerular apparatus. **A,** Longitudinal cross-section of glomerulus and juxtaglomerular apparatus. **B,** Horizontal cross-section of glomerulus. **C,** Enlargement of glomerular capillary filtration membrane. (From McCance K, Huether SE, editors: *Pathophysiology: the basis for disease in adults and children*, ed 6. St Louis, 2010, Elsevier, Figure 35-6, p. 1349).

stimulating stretch receptors. Sensory signals are then conducted through afferent pelvic nerves to the spinal cord. Efferent nerves from the spinal cord return impulses through the parasympathetic fibers in the pelvic and hypogastric nerves to the bladder wall muscle and the neck of the bladder. Efferent nerve stimulation causes contraction of the bladder and relaxation of the internal sphincter. In addition, impulses from the central nervous system through the pudendal nerves innervate the voluntarily controlled external sphincter. If the external sphincter also relaxes, the bladder will then empty.

Appropriate contraction and voluntary intermittent emptying of the bladder require both inhibitory and facilitory impulses from the upper pons, the hypothalamus, the midbrain, and the cortex. The inhibitory centers prevent constant voiding, and the facilitory centers allow micturation to occur voluntarily (once bladder control is learned). If the inhibitory centers are injured, the patient can demonstrate an uninhibited neurogenic bladder and nearly constant urination.

Reflex bladder contraction and sphincter relaxation also require the presence of intact afferent nerves from the bladder to the second and third sacral spinal cord level and intact

efferent nerves (including the hypogastric, pelvic, and pudendal nerves) from the first through the third sacral spinal level. If afferent nerves from the bladder to the spinal cord are injured or malformed, the patient can develop an atonic bladder, with loss of voluntary sphincter control. When an atonic bladder is present, the bladder fills to capacity and then overflow voiding begins.

If the spinal cord is damaged above the sacral spinal level, the patient initially loses all micturation reflexes because inhibitory and facilitory reflexes from the brain cannot be transmitted through the injured spinal cord. Later, however, simple spinal reflexes can return and the patient can void when bladder distension is sufficient. In this case, the bladder reflex will be initiated at the volume of urine that is usually present in the bladder during the patient's convalescent period.[45]

Urine Formation

Physiologic Processes

The production of urine by the kidneys is accomplished through three physiologic processes: glomerular filtration, reabsorption, and secretion. The first and most important step

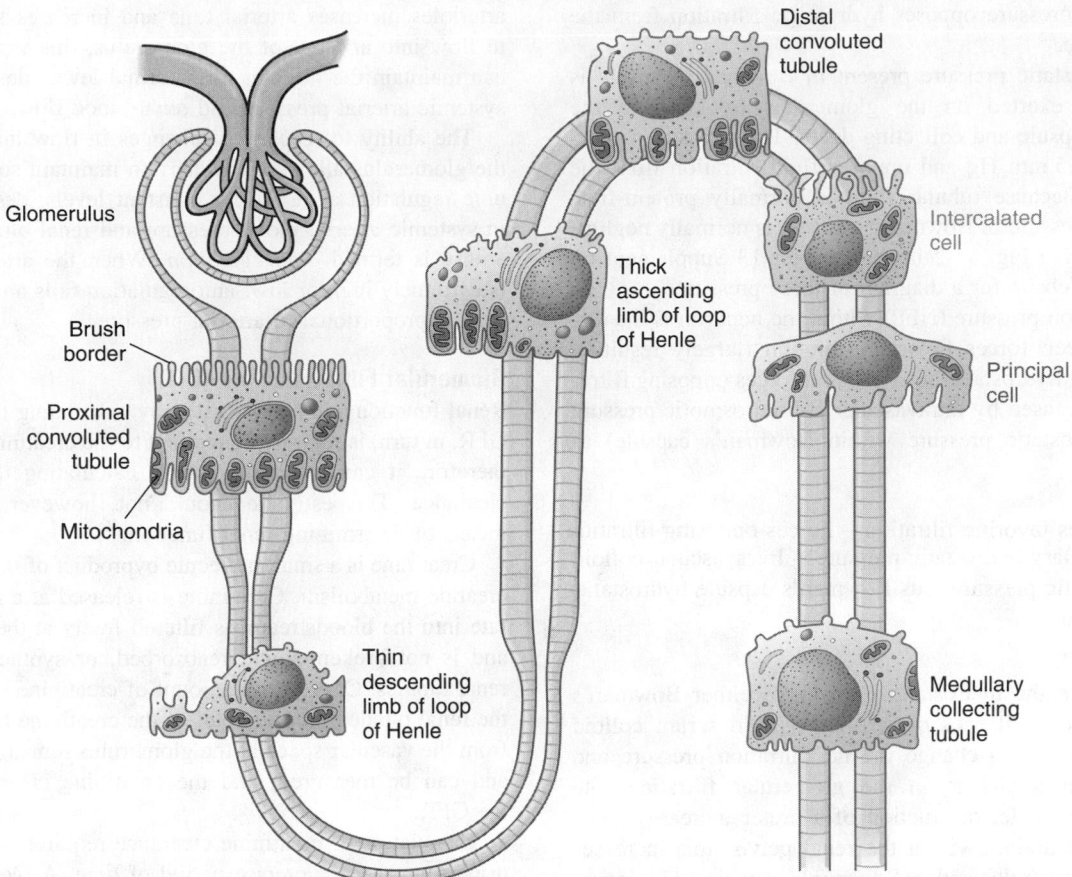

FIG. 13-5 Epithelial cells of the various segments of nephron tubules. The brush border and high number of mitochondria in the cells of the proximal convoluted tubule permit reabsorption of the 60% of the glomerular filtrate. Intercalated cells (rectangles) secrete either H^+ (reabsorb HCO_3^-) or HCO_3^- reabsorb K^+. Principal cells (enlarged figures) reabsorb Na^+ and water and secrete K^+. (From McCance K, Huether, SE, editors: *Pathophysiology: the basis for disease in adults and children*, ed 6. St Louis, 2010, Elsevier).

in urine formation is the filtration of plasma out of the glomerular capillaries into Bowman's capsule. The fluid that is filtered from the plasma, called filtrate, is then "acted on" by the renal tubular cells, through reabsorption or secretion.

Reabsorption is the process by which essential elements from the filtrate pass through the tubular cell back into the peritubular capillary plasma. Secretion is the transfer of substances from the peritubular capillary or the renal tubular cells to the filtrate so that it will be excreted. Secretion may be seen as an adjunct to filtration.

As the filtrate flows into the renal pelvis it becomes urine. The following discussion will detail the mechanisms involved in these three processes, glomerular filtration, reabsorption and secretion.

Glomerular Function

Filtration Physiology

The kidney receives its sympathetic nerve supply from the tenth through twelfth thoracic nerves and its parasympathetic nerve supply from branches of the vagus nerve. The renal blood vessels are innervated, but the renal tubules are not. Adjustment in the diameter of either or both of the afferent and efferent arterioles will affect the amount of fluid filtered in the glomerulus. As with any capillary, filtration of fluid in

the glomerulus is affected by pressure gradients across the capillary bed and the intrinsic properties of the glomerular capillary membrane.

Capillary hydrostatic pressure is the pressure generated by the pumping action of the heart; it is maintained or altered by arterial resistance. Hydrostatic pressure in most capillaries is higher at the arterial end than at the venous end. This difference favors filtration of fluid out of the vascular space at the arterial end and favors reabsorption of fluid into the vascular space at the venous end. Because the glomerulus has an afferent arteriole at the proximal end and an efferent arteriole at the distal end, the glomerular capillary pressure is higher than in other capillary beds and is approximately equal to systemic arterial pressure. This high pressure favors fluid filtration out of the vascular space. The glomerular capillary pressure is altered by constriction or relaxation of the afferent or efferent arteriole.

Intravascular colloid osmotic pressure, or oncotic pressure, is the pressure opposing free water movement out of the vascular space. It is generated by dissolved proteins, ions, and other particles that are normally present in the blood. Larger particles such as proteins cannot move readily across a capillary membrane; therefore they remain in the vascular space, exerting an osmotic pressure of approximately 35 mm Hg.

This oncotic pressure opposes hydrostatic filtration from the vascular space.[55]

The hydrostatic pressure present in Bowman's capsule is the pressure exerted on the glomerulus by fluid in the Bowman's capsule and collecting ducts. This pressure is normally 10 to 15 mm Hg and opposes fluid filtration from the glomerulus. Because tubular fluid is normally protein-free, the oncotic pressure in Bowman's capsule is normally negligible. (See Evolve Fig. 13-2 in the Chapter 13 Supplement on the Evolve Website for a diagram of these pressures.)

Net filtration pressure (NFP) within the nephron is the difference between forces favoring filtration (largely resulting from capillary hydrostatic pressure) and forces opposing filtration (largely caused by intravascular colloid osmotic pressure and the hydrostatic pressure within Bowman's capsule) as follows:

NFP = Forces favoring filtration − Forces opposing filtration

NFP = Capillary hydrostatic pressure − Intravascular colloid osmotic pressure plus Bowman's capsule hydrostatic pressure

Any change in the hydrostatic pressure in either Bowman's capsule or the capillaries or any changes in serum colloid osmotic pressure can change the net filtration pressure and may result in a change in the glomerular filtration rate (GFR). For example, obstruction of a ureter increases resistance to urine drainage from the renal pelvis; this increases pressure in the tubules and in Bowman's capsule and opposes filtration. The loss of a large volume of hypotonic fluid caused by diarrhea or unreplaced insensible losses during high fever will produce dehydration and hemoconcentration; this increases the colloid osmotic pressure and opposes filtration. If the child develops severe hypotension, capillary hydrostatic pressure will fall. All these changes oppose filtration and reduce the amount of glomerular filtrate. As noted previously, capillary hydrostatic pressure is determined by cardiac output (blood flow) and resistance in the arterioles. The relationship of flow, pressure, and resistance is described by the following equation (Poiseuille's Law):

$$P = \text{Flow} \times \text{Resistance}$$

$$\frac{\text{Pressure}}{\text{Resistance}} = \text{Flow}$$

P = mean arterial pressure − venous pressure for that organ

This equation predicts that an increase in mean arterial pressure will increase blood flow if the resistance to flow remains constant. The kidney is designed to maintain glomerular hydrostatic pressure so it can create urine over a wide range of blood pressures. As a result, resistance to flow does not remain constant when the systemic arterial pressure changes. Instead, when mean arterial pressure increases, the afferent arterioles constrict; this constriction restricts renal blood flow and prevents transmission of the entire increase in arterial pressure to the glomerulus. When arterial pressure falls, sympathetic innervation to the afferent and efferent arterioles increases arterial tone and increases the resistance to flow into and out of the glomerulus; this vasoconstriction can maintain the GFR at near-normal levels despite a fall in systemic arterial pressure and renal blood flow.

The ability to respond to changes in flow into and out of the glomerulus allows the kidney to maintain solute and volume regulation at relatively constant levels, despite changes in systemic arterial blood pressure and renal blood flow; this ability is termed *autoregulation*. When the arterial pressure is extremely high or low, autoregulation fails and renal blood flow is proportional to arterial pressure.

Glomerular Filtration Rate (GFR)

Renal function can be evaluated by calculating the GFR. The GFR, in turn, is roughly equivalent to the creatinine clearance; therefore it can be estimated by calculating the creatinine clearance. This estimate should not, however, be the sole means of determining renal function.[56]

Creatinine is a small molecule byproduct of skeletal muscle creatine metabolism. Creatinine is released at a near constant rate into the bloodstream, is filtered freely at the glomerulus, and is not broken down, reabsorbed, or synthesized by the renal tubules. Only a tiny amount of creatinine is secreted by the renal tubules. In effect, all of the creatinine that is filtered from the vascular space at the glomerulus remains in the urine and can be measured, and the creatinine clearance mirrors the GFR.[62]

Calculation of creatinine clearance requires collection of a urine sample for a precise period of time. A blood sample is collected during that same time period. The sampling of blood and urine enables simultaneous determination of the concentration of creatinine in the plasma and in the urine, as well as calculation of creatinine clearance.

The relationship between the plasma and urine concentrations of creatinine (Cr), the urine volume formed per unit of time, and the glomerular filtration rate is expressed as follows:

$$\text{GFR} = \frac{\text{Urine [Cr]} \times \text{Volume of urine per minute}}{\text{Plasma [Cr]}}$$

It is important to note that laboratory determination of serum creatinine concentration may be affected by some cephalosporin antibiotics. For this reason the blood sample for analysis of the serum creatinine level should be obtained when antibiotic drug levels are at their lowest.[7]

The GFR is expressed as milliliters per minute per 1.73 square meter of body surface area, which allows a comparison of renal function among children and adults. The child's GFR is approximately 55 to 65 mL/minute per 1.73 m^2 and will approach adult values (120 mL/minute per 1.73 m^2) by approximately 3 years of age.

When the amount of fluid filtered by the glomerulus is expressed as a fraction (ratio) of the total renal plasma flow (600 mL/minute per 1.73 m^2 in the adult), this provides an estimate of the percentage of total renal plasma flow that is filtered into Bowman's capsule. This ratio is termed the *filtration fraction* and equals approximately 20% of total renal plasma flow. Plasma that is not filtered (i.e., plasma that remains in the vascular space) continues through the glomerulus into the efferent arteriole, through the peritubular capillaries, and into venules and interlobular veins.

The glomerular filtrate in Bowman's capsule is an ultrafiltrate of blood. Its composition, like interstitial fluid from other capillaries, is usually free of proteins and cells. Animal micropuncture studies have established that all of the solutes (such as ions and amino acids) measured in the glomerular filtrate are present in virtually the same concentrations as their free, unbound concentrations in the plasma. If a substance is bound even partially to protein, that restricts its glomerular filtration because proteins normally cannot pass through the glomerular capillary membrane.

The urine that ultimately is formed by the kidneys is not merely the ultrafiltrate of plasma, because excretion of an ultrafiltrate through the urine would soon deplete the body of solutes and water. To modify the volume and content of the urine, the tubules selectively reabsorb and secrete substances.

Tubular Function

Reabsorption

Table 13-1 summarizes the work of the renal tubular cells in the process of reabsorption. An average of 180 L of water (protein-free plasma) is filtered through the glomerulus of an adolescent per day, and yet the average urine output is 1.5 L/day. This means that 178.5 L of water is reabsorbed out of the tubular lumen back into the body's circulation per day.

Passive and Active Reabsorption. Reabsorption of substances from the renal tubular fluid is described as *passive* if no energy-requiring reactions are necessary. Passive reabsorption occurs if a substance is reabsorbed as the result of an electrical or concentration gradient. An electrical gradient causes charged particles to move toward particles of opposite charge and away from particles of similar charge, or it may cause an exchange of similarly charged particles across a membrane to maintain an electrical balance.

A concentration gradient is created by the tendency of substances in solution to be distributed equally throughout that solution. Substances will tend to move across a semipermeable membrane from an area of high concentration to an area of lower concentration.

Active reabsorption or active transport of substances moves substances against a concentration or electrical gradient. Active reabsorption requires energy expenditure by the transporting cells. Both active and passive reabsorption from the renal tubules require diffusion of substances from the lumen through the tubular luminal cell membrane. Once the substances enter the cell, they traverse the cytoplasm of the tubular cell and exit through the cell membrane on the opposite side of the cell into the interstitial fluid. These substances can then pass into the adjacent peritubular capillaries for return to the systemic venous circulation. If energy is required in any of these steps, the process is considered active transport. Sodium, chloride, glucose, and bicarbonate are important substances that are reabsorbed actively, whereas water is reabsorbed passively.

Transport Maximum and Thresholds. Many of the substances that are transported actively out of the tubules can be reabsorbed only in limited quantity over time. These substances exhibit a transport maximum (Tm). This transport maximum is relatively fixed for each substance, although it can be affected by hormones or drugs. The renal threshold of a substance is the plasma and filtrate concentration at which some of the active transport tubular carriers become saturated and are unable to reabsorb all of the substance present in the filtrate. At this point, some of the substance will begin to appear in the urine because it cannot all be reabsorbed from the filtrate.

The tubular transport maximum is reached when all of the tubular carriers for that substance are saturated. Any further increase in the serum and filtered concentration of the substance beyond the transport maximum will produce a proportional increase in the urine concentration of the substance.

Glucose is a familiar substance that can be used to illustrate this concept of renal threshold and tubular transport maximum. Under normal conditions, glucose is not excreted in the urine. All the glucose filtered by the glomerulus is reabsorbed by the tubules and returned to the blood. When the serum glucose concentration exceeds approximately 180 mg/dL, some glucose tubular carriers are saturated and glucose begins to appear in the urine. The appearance of glucose in the urine indicates that the renal threshold for glucose reabsorption has been reached. If the serum glucose concentration exceeds approximately 300 mg/dL, all the tubular carriers are saturated and

Table 13-1 **Filtration, Excretion, and Reabsorption of Water, Electrolytes, and Solutes by the Kidneys**

Substance	Measure	Filtered*	Excreted	Reabsorbed	Filtered Load Reabsorbed (%)
Water	L/day	180	1.5	178.5	99.2
Na^+	mEq/day	25,200	150	25,050	99.4
K^+	mEq/day	720	100	620	86.1
Ca^{++}	mEq/day	540	10	530	98.2
HCO_3^-	mEq/day	4320	2	4318	99.9+
Cl^-	mEq/day	18,000	150	17,850	99.2
Glucose	mmol/day	800	0	800	100.0
Urea	g/day	56	28	28	50.0

From Koeppen BM, Stanton BA. Renal transport mechanisms: NaCl and water reabsorption along the nephron. In *Renal Physiology*, ed 4. Philadelphia, 2007, Elsevier.
*The filtered amount of any substance is calculated by multiplying the concentration of that substance in the ultrafiltrate by the glomerular filtration rate (GFR).
For example, the filtered load of Na^+ is calculated as $[Na^+]_{ultrafiltrate}$(140 mEq/L) × GFR (180 L/day) = 25,200 mEq/day.

the transport maximum for glucose is reached. Further increase in the serum glucose concentration will produce a proportional increase in the urine glucose concentration. The difference between the renal plasma threshold and the transport maximum for glucose is caused by different transport maximums of individual nephrons and tubules.

For many substances, there is a large difference between the normal serum concentration of a substance and the renal threshold and transport maximum of that substance. This difference indicates that the kidney conserves the substance but does not regulate its serum concentrations. Once the serum concentration of the substance far exceeds the homeostatic requirements, that substance will be lost into the urine. Glucose is an example of a substance that is conserved by the kidneys, although the serum glucose concentration is not regulated by the kidneys.

If the renal threshold and transport maximum are approximately equal to the daily filtered load of a substance, then the kidneys participate in regulation of the serum concentration of the substance. In such a case, a slight increase or decrease in plasma and filtered concentration of the substance changes its rate of renal reabsorption and excretion, so the serum concentration returns to normal. The renal threshold and transport maximum for phosphate are close to the normal daily filtered load of phosphate, so the serum phosphate concentration is regulated by kidney tubular function. Phosphate transport and reabsorption also will be affected by the serum calcium concentration, parathyroid hormone (PTH), and adrenal cortical hormones.[63]

Secretion

Although most substances enter the tubules through filtration at the glomerulus, other substances actually can be secreted into the urine by the tubular cells. Like tubular reabsorption, tubular secretion can be either an active or a passive transport process. Substances dissolved in the serum of the peritubular capillaries cross into the tubular cell and then can be transported into the tubular lumen and excreted in the urine.

Substances most commonly secreted by the tubules include organic acids and bases, food additives, and many drugs and chemicals. A transport maximum for secretion is known for only three substances; therefore tubular secretory functions may be less limited than reabsorptive functions.

Reabsorption and Secretion in the Proximal Tubule

The selective reabsorption of solute begins in the proximal tubules. Approximately 67% of the filtered water, Na^+, Cl^-, K^+, and other solutes such as bicarbonate are reabsorbed in the proximal tubule. In addition, the proximal tubules normally reabsorb all filtered amino acids and glucose.[63]

The most important function of the proximal tubule is the reabsorption of the filtered sodium and water. The proximal tubule neither concentrates nor dilutes the urine; its primary responsibility is the reabsorption of sodium, water, and electrolytes.

Sodium. The primary mechanism for regulation of intracellular and extracellular fluid volume involves renal sodium excretion.[63] Sodium is filtered freely at the glomerulus,

so its concentration in the proximal glomerular filtrate is identical to its plasma concentration. Sodium is reabsorbed by an active transport mechanism; the mechanism is carrier-mediated and requires energy so the sodium can move against a gradient. Sodium is not secreted into the tubules.

Once sodium is filtered into the tubules, it moves passively through the extremely sodium-permeable brush border of the proximal tubular cell. Sodium diffuses across this cell in response to a concentration gradient to the opposite cell membrane that is impermeable to sodium. This cell membrane then actively pumps sodium out of the tubular cell into the surrounding interstitial fluid. The movement of sodium out of the tubular lumen into the interstitial fluid creates an osmotic gradient between the tubule and the interstitial fluid. Because the epithelium of the proximal tubule is highly permeable to water, water follows the movement of the sodium ion. As water moves out of the tubule, the relative concentration of the other solutes within the tubular lumen increases, establishing a concentration gradient for the solutes between the tubular lumen and the interstitial fluid. As a result, solutes such as chloride, calcium, and urea will diffuse passively out of tubules and into the tubular cells and interstitial fluid.

Diffusion and transport of the sodium ion from the tubule also creates an electrical gradient between the tubular lumen and the inside of the tubular cell; the tubular cell now contains more positively charged (sodium) ions, and the tubular lumen (which has lost positive ions), becomes more negatively charged. This electrical gradient causes passive reabsorption of negatively charged substances such as chloride.

As the ultrafiltrate reaches the end of the proximal tubule, 65% of the filtered sodium and water has been reabsorbed into the renal interstitial space, predominantly through the active transport of sodium. Because water is being reabsorbed at almost the same rate as sodium is being pumped out of the proximal tubule, the osmolality of the proximal tubular fluid will be virtually the same as the plasma osmolality (normally 275-295 mOsm/L).

Sodium and water reabsorption in the proximal tubule and in the loop of Henle varies proportionately with the glomerular filtration rate. Increases in GFR are accompanied automatically by increases in sodium and water reabsorption. This coupling between the quantity of filtrate and the amount of reabsorption is termed *glomerulotubular balance*. This balance means that if renal blood flow remains constant, sodium and water reabsorption will vary directly with the GFR; if the GFR increases, sodium and water reabsorption will increase. Conversely, if renal blood flow remains constant and the GFR falls, sodium and water reabsorption will decrease. This mechanism maintains sodium balance despite changes in the GFR. If there is a severe reduction in renal arterial pressure and GFR, sodium will be reabsorbed almost completely from the proximal tubule.

Bicarbonate and Hydrogen Ions. Because the kidney is responsible for bicarbonate reabsorption and is also responsible for generating new bicarbonate ions, it plays an important role in the regulation of acid-base balance. Sodium and bicarbonate ions in the glomerular filtrate enter the proximal tubule. There, as noted previously, the sodium passively diffuses by concentration gradient into the proximal tubular cell and then is actively transported out of the tubular cell. To maintain electrical balance, another positively charged ion—hydrogen—is pumped actively from the tubular cells into the tubular lumen.

Once the hydrogen ion enters the tubular lumen, it combines with the bicarbonate in the filtrate to form carbonic acid. The carbonic acid in the tubule quickly disassociates to form carbon dioxide and water. The carbon dioxide easily diffuses back through the tubular cell membrane where it recombines with water, forming carbonic acid. Subsequent disassociation of the carbonic acid within the tubular cell again forms the hydrogen ions and bicarbonate ions; and the process is repeated. The tubular cell will again actively secrete the hydrogen ions into the lumen in exchange for sodium ions, and the bicarbonate ions will then diffuse passively out of the tubule cell into the peritubular interstitial fluid in response to concentration and electrical gradients.

As a result of this process, for every bicarbonate ion that combines with a hydrogen ion in the lumen of the tubule, a bicarbonate ion ultimately will diffuse into the peritubular capillaries (Fig. 13-6). This secretion of hydrogen ions and reabsorption of bicarbonate ions occurs along the length of the renal tubules, but 90% of bicarbonate reabsorption occurs in the proximal tubule. (See section, Regulation of Acid-Base Balance.)

Potassium. Although the extracellular concentration of potassium is low, this concentration is regulated closely by renal and nonrenal mechanisms. Potassium is filtered freely by the glomerulus into the filtrate; therefore the tubular concentration of potassium is equal to the serum potassium concentration in the postglomerular vessels. The tubular reabsorption of potassium is an active transport process that occurs in all segments of the tubule, with the exception of the descending limb of the loop of Henle. The active transport of the potassium ion from the tubular lumen into the tubular cell occurs against a large concentration gradient, because the potassium concentration is high in the tubular cell.

Nearly all filtered potassium is reabsorbed by the proximal tubule, and the remaining potassium is reabsorbed in the ascending limb. The proximal reabsorption of the filtered potassium occurs at a constant rate and does not alter, despite the presence of hyperkalemia or hypokalemia. Potassium is also secreted by the distal convoluted tubule and cortical collecting duct, and the rate of K^+ reabsorption or secretion in these tubular segments depends on a variety of hormones and factors. Overall, the rate of renal K^+ excretion is determined by the distal convoluted tubule and the cortical collecting duct.[63] The net result is normally a continuous loss of potassium in the urine.

Calcium. A low amount of calcium is excreted in the urine. Forty percent of total serum calcium is bound to serum proteins, such as albumin, and is not able to pass through the glomerular capillary membrane; consequently it is not filtered in the glomerulus. The remaining 60% of total serum calcium is not bound to protein; it is filtered and present in the filtrate as either ionized calcium (the biologically active

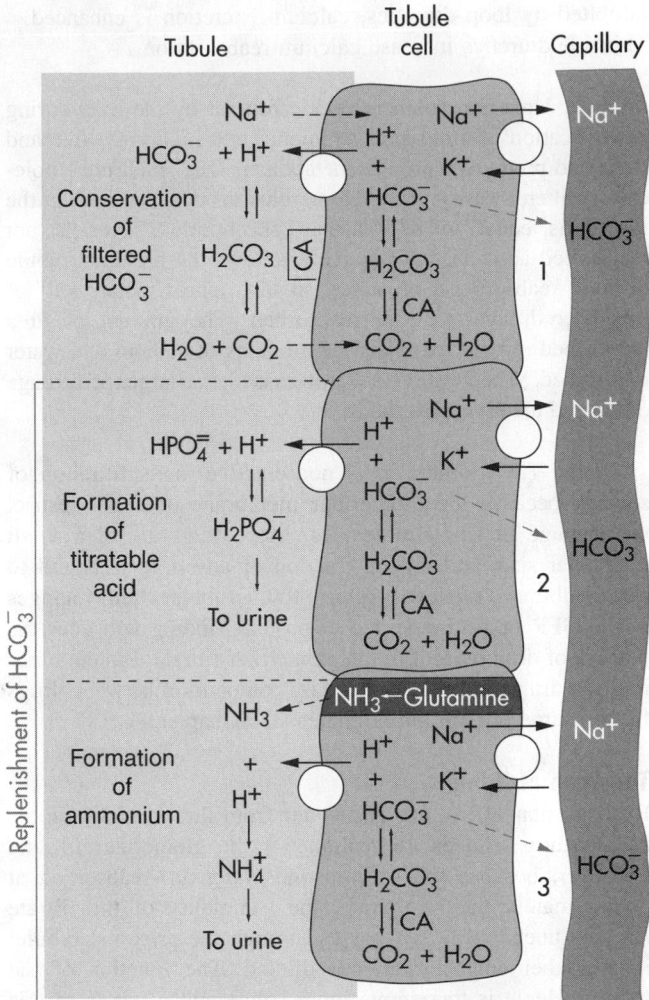

FIG. 13-6 Renal excretion of acid. 1. Conservation of filtered bicarbonate. Filtered bicarbonate combines with secreted hydrogen in the presence of carbon anhydrase (CA) to form carbonic acid (H_2CO_3), which then dissociates to water (H_2O) and carbon dioxide (CO_2); both diffuse into the epithelial cell. The CO_2 and H_2O combine to form H_2CO_3 in the presence of CA, and the resulting bicarbonate (HCO_3^-) is reabsorbed into the capillary. 2. Formation of titratable acid. A hydrogen ion is secreted and combines with dibasic phosphate (HCO_4^-) to form monobasic phosphate ($H_2PO_4^-$). The secreted hydrogen is formed from the dissociation of H_2CO_3, and the remaining HCO_3^- is reabsorbed into the capillary. 3. Formation of ammonium. Ammonia (NH_3) is produced from glutamine in the epithelial cell and diffuses to the tubular lumen, where it combines with H^+ to form ammonium (NH_4^+). Once NH_4^+ has been formed, it cannot return to the epithelial cell (diffusional trapping), and the bicarbonate remaining in the epithelial cell is reabsorbed into the capillary. (From McCance K, Huether SE, editors: *Pathophysiology: the basis for disease in adults and children*, ed 6. St Louis, 2010, Elsevier).

form) or as complex calcium (calcium bound in reactions with other ions).

Calcium reabsorption is controlled by parathyroid hormone. Just as for sodium reabsorption, 80% to 90% of filtered calcium is reabsorbed in the proximal tubule and loop of Henle; only 10% of filtered calcium enters the distal tubule for concentration adjustments. When sodium reabsorption is inhibited by loop diuretics, calcium excretion is enhanced.[79] Thiazide diuretics increase calcium reabsorption.

Urea. Urea is a small molecule formed by the liver during detoxification of ammonia. Ammonia is a highly reactive and toxic end product of protein metabolism. The small urea molecule is filtered easily in the glomerulus; its concentration in the filtrate is equal to its plasma concentration. Urea is not reabsorbed actively, but passively follows the proximal tubule osmotic reabsorption of water, so that approximately half of the filtered urea will be reabsorbed. The amount of urea reabsorbed directly parallels the amounts of sodium and water reabsorbed. When water reabsorption is high, a larger percentage of filtered urea is reabsorbed.

Drugs. The glomerulus is nonselective in its filtration of solutes, because the glomerular membrane does not restrict the passage of small molecules. Most drugs are of a small molecular size, and only a fraction of any drug is bound to serum albumin; most will filter into the tubular fluid. Changes in the GFR or in the degree of protein binding will alter the amount of drug present in the glomerular filtrate. Protein binding of a drug can be influenced by competition between drugs for the same protein binding sites (see Chapter 4).

The Loop of Henle

Reabsorption of sodium and water from the proximal tubule significantly reduces the volume of the glomerular filtrate. However, because the sodium and water are reabsorbed at approximately the same rate, the osmolality of the filtrate remains unchanged as it passes through the proximal tubule; it is neither concentrated nor diluted. The function of the loop of Henle is to remove more solute and water from this filtrate.

The loop of Henle, located within the renal cortex and the medulla, provides a countercurrent mechanism for urine concentration. The descending limb of the loop of Henle does not transport sodium or chloride actively, but it is highly permeable to sodium and water. Thus, as the filtrate passes through the descending limb of the loop, it becomes progressively more concentrated. The osmolality can increase from 300 to 1200 mOsm/L between the beginning of the descending limb and the tip of the loop of Henle (Fig. 13-7).

As the filtrate begins to pass through the ascending limb of the loop of Henle, chloride is actively pumped out of the tubule, and sodium follows passively. Water, however, must remain in the tubule because the ascending limb is impermeable to water. The solute loss from the tubule produces a fall in the osmolality of the filtrate and a rise in the osmolality of the interstitial fluid surrounding the loop. Thus, the osmolality of filtrate arriving in the distal tubule is lower than that of filtrate entering the loop of Henle and lower than that of interstitial fluid in the medulla.

The loop of Henle removes approximately 25% of filtered sodium and 15% of filtered water from the tubule, leaving approximately 10% of the filtered sodium and 20% of the filtered water to enter the distal tubule.

The blood vessels surrounding the loop of Henle form a hairpin loop structure, called the *vasa recta*. The vasa recta consists of capillaries that run parallel to the loop of Henle and the collecting ducts (for an illustration, see Evolve Fig. 13-1 in the Chapter 13 Supplement on the Evolve Website). As these capillaries follow the loop of Henle into the interstitium of the renal medulla, where osmolality is high (as the result of the tubular countercurrent mechanism), water shifts out of capillaries into the interstitial fluid, and sodium and chloride move from the interstitial fluid into the capillaries.

The vasa recta does not contribute to the creation of a concentration gradient; its content is affected by the osmotic gradients surrounding the loop of Henle. This capillary loop mechanism is termed a *countercurrent exchanger;* the term reflects its passive nature. By this mechanism, the solute and

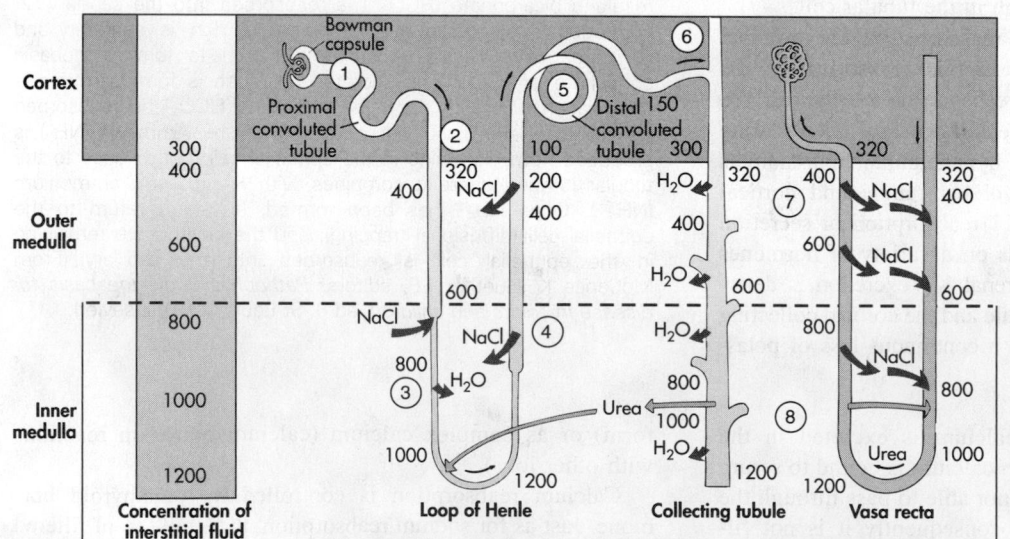

FIG. 13-7 Countercurrent mechanism for concentrating and diluting urine. *ADH,* Antidiuretic hormone (*Note:* Numbers in illustration represent milliosmoles). (From McCance K, Huether, SE, editors: *Pathophysiology: the basis for disease in adults and children,* ed 6, St Louis, 2010, Elsevier).

water in the interstitial fluid surrounding the loop of Henle and the collecting ducts are reabsorbed into the circulation while maintaining the interstitial osmolality.

The Distal Tubule and Collecting Ducts

The distal tubule arises from the ascending limb of the loop of Henle; its thick cellular structure is distinct from the thin cells of the ascending loop. Thick cuboidal cells continue up through the renal cortical area to a point where the distal tubule is in direct contact with the afferent arteriole of its glomerulus. At this junction, the distal tubule cells become more densely packed and more columnar, and the muscle cells of the arteriole enlarge and take on a granular appearance. This point of contact between the distal tubule and the glomerular afferent arteriole is called the *juxtaglomerular apparatus* (see Fig. 13-3).

The juxtaglomerular apparatus consists of the columnar cells of the distal tubule (called the *macula densa* because of their prominent nuclei) and large cells of the afferent arteriole (called *polkissen* or *polar cushion*). The term *juxtaglomerular cells* most commonly refers to the cells of the afferent arteriole; these cells are able to sense pressure and secrete the hormone renin.

Beyond the juxtaglomerular apparatus, the distal tubule joins the collecting duct. The collecting duct will in turn descend from the renal cortex through the medulla and into the renal calyces. The filtrate present in the early distal tubule has a lower osmolality and lower sodium concentration than the plasma and the surrounding interstitial fluid. As the urine filtrate passes through the distal tubule and the collecting ducts, more water will be removed to further concentrate

the urine. The final concentration of urine in the distal tubule and the collecting ducts is adjusted by the active transport of sodium out of the distal tubule and changes in the relative permeability of the collecting ducts to water (e.g., under the influence of antidiuretic hormone).

The distal tubule is the site of final adjustments in the urine sodium and potassium content. The distal tubule actively reabsorbs approximately 10% of the filtered sodium. This active transport process occurs against a high electrical and concentration gradient and is influenced by the volume and character of the fluid arriving from the loop of Henle, as well as by hormones, especially aldosterone.

Renin, Aldosterone, and Antidiuretic Hormone

Renin is secreted from the polkissen cells of the afferent arteriole in the juxtaglomerular apparatus. In turn, renin forms angiotensin I from renin substrate (a circulating peptide from the liver). The amounts of renin released and angiotensin formed are determined by the renal perfusion pressure, sympathetic nervous system stimulation, circulating vasoactive substances, and changes in electrolyte concentration.[55]

Angiotensin I circulates to the lung and is converted enzymatically to angiotensin II. Angiotensin II produces peripheral vasoconstriction and an increase in aldosterone secretion, which increases renal sodium and water reabsorption. These effects should increase intravascular volume (Fig. 13-8). Angiotensin I and II are destroyed by angiotensinase, an enzyme that is present in plasma and secreted by a variety of organs, such as the kidney, intestine, and liver.

The quantity of sodium that is excreted in the urine when aldosterone is absent totals approximately 2% of the total

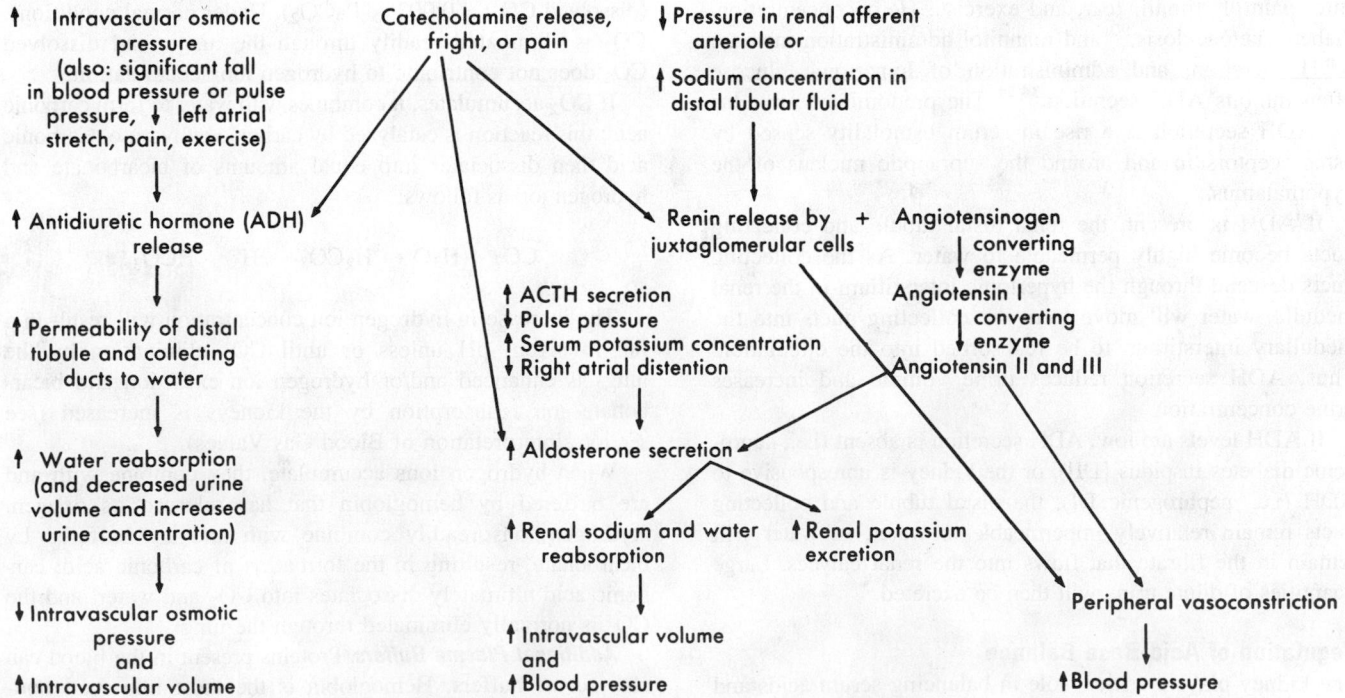

FIG. 13-8 Renal response to changes in extracellular fluid volume and electrolyte concentration or stress.

filtered sodium. If aldosterone is absent (e.g., in patients with untreated adrenal insufficiency), excretion of that sodium will be associated with excretion of a large volume of water that can produce hypovolemic shock. Thus, aldosterone is responsible for the reabsorption of a very small but significant portion of the filtered sodium.

Aldosterone is secreted by the adrenal cortex in response to pituitary adrenal corticotropic hormone (ACTH) secretion and a variety of other stimuli. A fall in the pulse pressure, decreased stretch of the right atrium, and an increased serum potassium concentration all stimulate aldosterone secretion.[63] An important stimulus for aldosterone is formation of angiotensin from renin released by the juxtaglomerular apparatus. Aldosterone stimulates epithelial cell transport of sodium in the renal tubular epithelium, along the intestinal lumen, and in sweat and saliva. Increased aldosterone levels increase the active reabsorption of sodium and decrease potassium reabsorption. The increased sodium reabsorption produces water reabsorption; this increases intravascular volume and reduces the juxtamedullary secretion of renin. The reduction in potassium tubular reabsorption increases potassium excretion in the urine and should result in a fall in the serum potassium concentration. These responses to aldosterone should in turn reduce the stimulus for aldosterone secretion (see Fig. 13-8).

Antidiuretic hormone (ADH), or arginine vasopressin (AVP), secretion also affects the final concentration of urine. ADH is produced by the supraoptic and paraventricular nuclei in the hypothalamus and is transported to the posterior lobe of the pituitary, where it is released in response to an increase in serum osmolality. ADH secretion is stimulated by serum osmolality greater than 280 to 285 mOsm/L (or a rise in serum osmolality of 2% or more). It also is secreted in response to significant (10%-15%) volume depletion, a fall in blood pressure, painful stimuli, fear, and exercise. Hemoconcentration, diabetic ketoacidosis,[90] and mannitol administration increase ADH secretion, and administration of hypertonic glucose often inhibits ADH secretion.[34,54] The predominant stimulus for ADH secretion is a rise in serum osmolality sensed by osmoreceptors in and around the supraoptic nucleus of the hypothalamus.

If ADH is present, the renal distal tubule and collecting ducts become highly permeable to water. As the collecting ducts descend through the hypertonic interstitium in the renal medulla, water will move from the collecting ducts into the medullary interstitium to be reabsorbed into the circulation. Thus, ADH secretion reduces urine volume and increases urine concentration.

If ADH levels are low, ADH secretion is absent (i.e., neurogenic diabetes insipidus [DI]), or the kidney is unresponsive to ADH (i.e., nephrogenic DI), the distal tubule and collecting ducts remain relatively impermeable to water, so water will remain in the filtrate that flows into the renal calyces. Large quantities of dilute urine will then be excreted.

Regulation of Acid-Base Balance

The kidney plays a critical role in balancing serum acids and bases. A substance is labeled as an acid or a base according to its ability to lose or gain a hydrogen ion (a proton). Strong acids dissociate freely in solution, readily yielding a hydrogen ion; therefore they will contribute to the development or progression of acidosis. Weak acids only partially dissociate into a solution that will then contain both acid and base; thus, they do not contribute to changes in acidity. Bases are substances that will accept a free hydrogen ion; they reduce the hydrogen ion concentration, increasing the pH.

The pH is the inverse of the logarithm (log) of the hydrogen ion concentration; as the hydrogen ion concentration rises, the pH falls (the serum becomes more acid). The normal range of pH is 7.35 to 7.45. If the pH is less than 7.35, acidosis is present; if the pH exceeds 7.45, alkalosis is present. Even slight changes in hydrogen ion concentration or serum pH can alter metabolic and cell functions.

Buffering Systems. All body fluids contain buffers. These buffers are compounds that combine with any acid or base so the acid or base does not significantly alter the serum or tissue pH. Effective buffering requires interaction of serum and cell buffers. When the hydrogen ion concentration changes significantly, plasma, respiratory, and renal buffering systems are activated.

The Bicarbonate-Carbonic Acid Buffering System. The bicarbonate-carbonic acid buffering system operates in both the lung and the kidney and is the most important plasma buffering system. It consists of the buffer pair of carbonic acid (H_2CO_3—a weak acid) with sodium, potassium, or magnesium bicarbonate. Because two end products of the system (carbon dioxide and bicarbonate) are closely regulated, this buffering system maintains the serum pH within a narrow range.

Carbon dioxide (CO_2) is produced by tissue metabolism and is dissolved in plasma. The plasma concentration of CO_2 is proportional to the partial pressure of carbon dioxide in the gas phase with which the solution is equilibrated (dissolved $CO_2 = 0.003 \times PaCO_2$). Under normal conditions, CO_2 is eliminated readily through the lungs, and dissolved CO_2 does not contribute to hydrogen ion accumulation.

If CO_2 accumulates, it combines with water to form carbonic acid; this reaction is catalyzed by carbonic anhydrase. Carbonic acid then dissociates into equal amounts of bicarbonate and hydrogen ion as follows:

$$CO_2 + H_2O \leftrightarrow H_2CO_3 \leftrightarrow H^+ + HCO_3^-$$

The increase in hydrogen ion concentration will result in a fall in serum pH unless or until CO_2 elimination by the lungs is enhanced and/or hydrogen ion excretion and bicarbonate ion reabsorption by the kidneys is increased (see section, Interpretation of Blood Gas Values).

When hydrogen ions accumulate, they combine with and are buffered by hemoglobin that has released its oxygen. Hydrogen ions readily combine with and are buffered by bicarbonate, resulting in the formation of carbonic acid; carbonic acid ultimately dissociates into CO_2 and water, and the CO_2 is normally eliminated through the lungs.

Additional Plasma Buffers. Proteins present in the blood can also act as buffers. Hemoglobin is the most important nonbicarbonate buffer. It binds with hydrogen ions and transports CO_2 from the tissues to the lungs for elimination.[34]

Inorganic phosphate contributes in only a minor way to plasma buffering, but it is a significant urinary buffer. Organic phosphates are significant intracellular buffers.

Renal Hydrogen Ion Excretion and Bicarbonate Reabsorption.

The kidneys regulate serum pH and HCO_3^- concentration through hydrogen ion secretion and bicarbonate reabsorption and reclamation. Renal compensation for respiratory acidosis requires several hours to begin and will not be fully effective for several days; it requires reabsorption of all filtered bicarbonate and generation of new bicarbonate through the formation of titratable acids.

The major stimulus for increased bicarbonate reabsorption or reclamation in the proximal tubule is the presence of increased hydrogen ion concentration in the cells of the proximal tubule, as occurs with the development of metabolic acidosis. It is important to note, however, that bicarbonate reabsorption is also affected by changes in serum potassium and chloride concentrations. Both hypokalemia and hypochloremia increase hydrogen ion concentration in the renal tubular cells, so that hydrogen ion secretion into the proximal tubule and bicarbonate reabsorption are enhanced. This process is the mechanism for development of alkalosis with hypokalemia or hypochloremia (i.e., hypokalemic or hypochloremic metabolic alkalosis).

A hydrogen ion is secreted into the proximal renal tubule in exchange for a sodium ion. Once in the tubule, the hydrogen ion combines with filtered bicarbonate to form carbonic acid and then quickly dissociates into CO_2 and water. The CO_2 diffuses back into the renal tubular cell, where it recombines with water to form carbonic acid, and then quickly dissociates into hydrogen ion and bicarbonate. The bicarbonate diffuses out of the tubular cell into the interstitial fluid and ultimately into the plasma while the hydrogen ion is again secreted into the renal tubule. This method of reclaiming bicarbonate ions results in a net reabsorption of filtered bicarbonate ions from the renal tubule, without any net reabsorption of hydrogen ions.

New bicarbonate can be formed when CO_2 combines with water, yielding carbonic acid. The carbonic acid then dissociates into hydrogen ions and bicarbonate; the hydrogen ion is bound to phosphate buffers or ammonia to form hydrogen phosphate or ammonium (NH_4^+). Hydrogen phosphate and ammonium are nonreabsorbable, and they are excreted unchanged in the urine. When hydrogen ions are excreted in this way, a quantity of acid can be measured in the urine; this buffering mechanism results in the formation of titratable acids (see Fig. 13-6). The amount of hydrogen ion excreted in the urine is limited, because the kidney cannot secrete urine with a pH lower than approximately 4.4. In addition, the formation of titratable acid will be limited by the amount of ammonia, phosphate, and other inorganic buffers available.

To determine the quantity of hydrogen ions present in the urine in combination with buffers, sodium hydroxide (NaOH) is titrated into the urine sample. The number of milliequivalents of NaOH needed to restore the pH to 7.4 will equal the number of milliequivalents of hydrogen ions present in the urine in combination with buffers. This quantity of hydrogen ion is referred to as the *titratable acid in the urine*.

Respiratory Buffering.

In the alert patient with normal neurologic function, carbon dioxide accumulation or metabolic acidosis will stimulate ventilation. Increased carbon dioxide elimination by the lungs lowers the amount of plasma carbonic acid; this encourages hydrogen ions to combine with bicarbonate ions. The result is elimination of hydrogen ions and compensation for metabolic acidosis. Hypoventilation can partially compensate for metabolic alkalosis, although this response may be limited if hypoxemia develops. The respiratory buffering system requires minutes or hours to take full effect.

Interpretation of Blood Gas Values.

When evaluating acid-base disturbances, it is important to identify the effects of the primary disorder and the results of respiratory or renal compensation. If an acute problem is present, treatment must focus on the underlying disorder, while supporting whatever compensation is occurring. By definition, compensatory mechanisms will strive to restore the pH to near-normal levels; therefore compensation will never result in overcorrection or a change in the pH in a direction opposite the initial stimulus. For example, renal compensation for chronic respiratory acidosis can restore the pH to near the 7.35 to 7.45 range, but will not create an alkalotic condition (pH above 7.45). If a patient with chronic respiratory acidosis has an alkalotic pH, that patient has an additional condition causing the metabolic alkalosis.

Treatment of acid-base disorders often complicates the interpretation of acid-base imbalance. For example, if the patient with metabolic acidosis arrives in the pediatric critical care unit breathing spontaneously, with appropriate respiratory compensation, the patient's pH may be near normal (e.g., 7.31). If aggressive treatment of the metabolic acidosis is provided, spontaneous hyperventilation can continue for several hours after effective treatment of the acidosis, because it takes several hours for ventilatory response to pH changes to be maximal. Continued hyperventilation can produce a transient alkalosis that results not from respiratory overcorrection of the acidosis, but from combined intrinsic respiratory compensation coupled with extrinsic buffering of the patient's pH (therapy).

Evaluation of the pH and PaCO₂.

Blood gas analysis requires evaluation of the pH, the $PaCO_2$, the calculated base deficit or excess, and the serum bicarbonate. The first step is evaluation of the pH. If the pH is less than 7.35, acidosis is present; if the pH is greater than 7.45, alkalosis is present. The second step is evaluation of the $PaCO_2$ in light of the pH to determine whether any existing change in pH can be explained by the alteration in $PaCO_2$. For every uncompensated torr unit rise in $PaCO_2$ above 45, the pH should fall 0.008 units below 7.35, and for every uncompensated torr unit fall in $PaCO_2$ below 35, the pH should rise 0.008 units above 7.45. Acidosis or alkalosis in excess of that predicted from the $PaCO_2$ must be metabolic in origin (Box 13-1).

The use of the $PaCO_2$ to interpret the pH does not indicate the primary versus the compensatory alteration, but careful evaluation of the child's pH may help distinguish these alterations. When the primary problem is alkalosis, the pH

Box 13-1   **Evaluation of pH and PaCO$_2$ and Calculation of Base Deficit or Excess**

1. Subtract the child's PaCO$_2$ from 45 (result can be a negative or positive number)
2. Multiply difference obtained in Step 1 by 0.008 (result can be a negative or positive number).
3. Add the product obtained in Step 2 and 7.35; this yields the pH predicted from the PaCO$_2$ alone. If child's pH is lower than predicted, metabolic acidosis is present; if the pH is higher than predicted from the PaCO$_2$, metabolic alkalosis is present.
4. To calculate base deficit, subtract the predicted pH (calculated in Step 3) from the child's actual pH and multiply this difference by 0.66. A base deficit more negative than (larger than) −2 indicates the presence of metabolic acidosis, and a base excess greater than 2 indicates the presence of metabolic alkalosis.

PaCO$_2$, Partial pressure of carbon dioxide.

Box 13-2   **Rules for Assessment of Respiratory and Renal Compensatory Responses in Acid-Base Disturbances**

Compensatory mechanisms bring pH toward but not to a normal level.

If *respiratory* compensation is intact in metabolic disturbances:

1. [HCO$_3^-$] + 15 = 2 digits of pH after the decimal point, or
2. PaCO$_2$ = Last 2 digits of pH

If *metabolic* compensation is intact in respiratory disturbances:

In acute respiratory acidosis

$$\Delta[\text{HCO}_3^-] = 0.1 \times \Delta\text{PaCO}_2$$

In chronic respiratory acidosis

$$[\text{HCO}_3^-] = 0.35 \times \Delta\text{PaCO}_2$$

In acute respiratory alkalosis

$$\Delta[\text{HCO}_3^-] = 0.2 \times \Delta\text{PaCO}_2$$

In chronic respiratory alkalosis

$$\Delta[\text{HCO}_3^-] = 0.5 \times \Delta\text{PaCO}_2$$

here Δ indicates the degree of deviation from normal value.

From Ichikawa I, Narins RG, Harris HW Jr: Regulation of acid-base homeostasis. In Ichikawa I, editor: *Pediatric textbook of fluids and electrolytes,* Baltimore, 1990, Williams and Wilkins, p. 84.
PaCO$_2$, Partial pressure of carbon dioxide.

will remain in the alkalotic range despite the presence of compensation. If the primary problem is acidosis, the pH will remain in the slightly acidotic range despite the presence of compensation.

The Base Deficit or Excess. The base deficit or excess is a calculated number that is indicative of acidosis (base deficit) or metabolic alkalosis (base excess). The normal base deficit or excess is −2 to 2. A number more negative than (larger than) −2 indicates a base deficit and the presence of metabolic acidosis. A positive number higher than 2 indicates a base excess and the presence of metabolic alkalosis. The base deficit or excess is calculated by subtracting the pH predicted from the PaCO$_2$ (see Box 13-1) from the actual pH and multiplying the result by 0.66.

The Serum Bicarbonate. The normal serum bicarbonate is approximately 24 to 28 mmol/L. The serum bicarbonate is elevated in the presence of primary metabolic alkalosis or with metabolic compensation for chronic respiratory acidosis. If metabolic alkalosis is present, the pH will be in the alkalotic range. If metabolic compensation for chronic respiratory acidosis is present, the pH will remain in the acidotic range.

If the serum bicarbonate is less than 24 mmol/L, a metabolic acidosis or metabolic compensation for chronic respiratory alkalosis is present. If a metabolic acidosis is present, the pH will remain in the acidotic range. If metabolic compensation for chronic respiratory alkalosis is present (a rare condition), the pH will remain in the alkalotic range.

Rules to Assess Effectiveness of Compensation. A few rules are helpful in the evaluation of compensation for acid-base disorders. These are summarized in Box 13-2.

During any interpretation of blood gases, providers should consider the child's intravascular volume and hydration. Dehydration can exacerbate acidosis, because the hydrogen ion concentration is increased. Rehydration of the acidotic patient will partially correct this acidosis even before buffering agents are administered. Dehydration can exacerbate alkalosis, but this is less common.

Acidosis. Acidosis is a condition produced by a relative increase in hydrogen ion concentration or a deficit of bicarbonate.

Respiratory Acidosis. Respiratory acidosis is present when CO$_2$ accumulation is sufficient to lower the serum pH below 7.35. Uncompensated respiratory acidosis usually will occur with a PaCO$_2$ exceeding 50 torr. Carbon dioxide accumulation may result from central nervous system depression or another cause of inadequate respiratory drive, such as intrinsic airway disease, chest wall instability, compromise in diaphragm or upper airway muscle function, or alveolar disease. Metabolic compensation for chronic respiratory acidosis will result in an elevation of serum bicarbonate and a return of pH to near normal, although it will remain slightly acidotic. The CO$_2$ will remain elevated until the cause of respiratory dysfunction resolves.

Metabolic Acidosis. Metabolic acidosis results from either excess hydrogen ions (acids) or a deficit in bicarbonate. Excess hydrogen ion concentration can result from incomplete oxidation of fatty acids (as occurs in diabetic ketoacidosis or salicylate poisoning), lactic acid production (resulting from inadequate systemic perfusion and tissue oxygen and substrate delivery), or accumulation of inorganic acids (resulting from renal failure).

Loss of bicarbonate can result from inappropriate renal bicarbonate loss (renal acidosis) or the intestinal loss of any fluid distal to the pylorus, especially pancreatic or small intestine secretions. Metabolic acidosis is enhanced by the development of dehydration, because this will increase hydrogen ion concentration.

Serum buffers initially will attempt to compensate for the acidosis, and respiratory compensation should be effective within hours, provided that neurologic function and pulmonary function are adequate. As CO_2 elimination is increased, the serum pH should approach normal. The combination of a decrease in $PaCO_2$ and a decrease in serum bicarbonate indicates the presence of metabolic acidosis with respiratory compensation.

Spontaneous respiratory compensation is the most effective method of treating metabolic acidosis. However, if respiratory effort or function is compromised or if profound acidosis is present, administration of a buffering agent may be required. Before administration of sodium bicarbonate, providers should assess and support the patient's airway and ventilation, because the buffering action of the sodium bicarbonate will result in the formation of CO_2. The sodium bicarbonate dose that should correct acidosis to a total CO_2 of 15 mEq/L is estimated using the following formula[76]:

$$\text{mEq NaHCO}_3 = (15 - \text{Patient's total CO}_2) \times (\text{Weight in kg} \times 0.3)$$

Half of the calculated bicarbonate dose can be administered immediately, with the second half administered over the next 2 to 3 hours, if needed. Providers should assess the patient's pH and effectiveness of ventilation.

An alternative formula for determination of the sodium bicarbonate dose utilizes the base deficit. This formula estimates that the bicarbonate deficit equals the base deficit, distributed chiefly in the extracellular space (one third of the total body weight) as follows[66]:

$$\text{mEq NaHCO}_3 = \text{Base deficit} \times 0.3 \times \text{Body weight in kg}$$

Total correction with exogenous buffering agents should not be necessary if ventilation is supported effectively.

Alkalosis. Alkalosis is a relative excess of bicarbonate or a deficit of hydrogen ions that results from hyperventilation, loss of acid, or accumulation of bicarbonate.

Respiratory Alkalosis. Primary respiratory alkalosis is uncommon in the pediatric critical care unit. It requires an increase in alveolar ventilation with a significant reduction in $PaCO_2$, so the pH rises above 7.45. Respiratory alkalosis usually results from central nervous system disorders, drug toxicity, salicylate poisoning, advanced liver failure, or emotional hyperventilation. Profound hypoxemia can stimulate hyperventilation, but usually it will not be sufficient to produce alkalosis. Chronic respiratory alkalosis will stimulate renal bicarbonate excretion, which occurs in conjunction with sodium or potassium excretion.

Metabolic Alkalosis. Metabolic alkalosis results from a loss of acid or a gain of bicarbonate. A loss of acid typically occurs with prolonged vomiting and is exacerbated by dehydration. A gain in bicarbonate most commonly occurs in the presence of hypochloremia or hypokalemia after diuretic therapy with inadequate electrolyte replacement. Metabolic alkalosis also can result from overzealous administration of sodium bicarbonate.

With both hypochloremia and hypokalemia, the renal tubule cells increase sodium and bicarbonate reabsorption and hydrogen ion excretion. A profound chloride deficit enhances renal tubular bicarbonate reabsorption, occurring at the expense of hydrogen ion excretion. Profound potassium depletion causes tubule cells to excrete a hydrogen ion into the tubule in exchange for potassium. The more hydrogen ions present in the tubule, the more bicarbonate is ultimately reabsorbed, thus worsening the alkalosis. Patients with hypochloremic or hypokalemic alkalosis demonstrate acid urine and an alkalotic pH.

Respiratory compensation for metabolic alkalosis should be apparent within a few hours and will result in hypoventilation and an increase in the $PaCO_2$. Respiratory compensation cannot occur if the patient is receiving mechanical ventilation (particularly if ventilation is totally controlled), and it may not occur if the patient is sedated or has decreased level of consciousness.

Calcium Regulation

The serum (extracellular) ionized calcium concentration normally is maintained within very narrow limits by renal regulatory mechanisms and by adjustments in bone deposition or demineralization and vitamin D reabsorption in the gastrointestinal tract. Serum ionized calcium concentrations also are affected by serum albumin concentration and acid-base balance.

Precise regulation of the serum extracellular calcium is necessary because calcium imbalance can exert a profound effect on neuromuscular excitability and cardiovascular function. In addition, calcium plays an important role in the chemical reactions necessary for thrombin formation and coagulation. Finally, calcium ions react with phosphate ions to form bone salts; these bone salts give the bones rigidity.

Approximately 99% of the total body calcium stores are deposited in the bones, and the remaining 1% resides in the plasma and the interstitial fluid. If the serum pH is normal, approximately half of the total plasma calcium is bound to serum albumin, does not enter into chemical reactions, and does not filter into the glomerular filtrate. The remaining half of the total plasma calcium is present in the ionized form; this constitutes the biologically active form of calcium.

The normal total serum calcium concentration is 9 to 11 mg/dL, and normal ionized calcium concentration is approximately 4.4 to 5.3 mg/dL.[80] The serum calcium concentration is evaluated in light of the serum protein concentration. An increase in the serum albumin and globulin will increase the amount of calcium bound to proteins, so will reduce the amount of the serum calcium that is present in the ionized form. For each 1 g/dL increase in serum albumin, 0.8 mg/dL of calcium is removed from its ionized state and is bound to the albumin. Increases in serum globulin level, however, will lower the ionized calcium concentration by only 0.16 mg/dL. If serum albumin and globulin concentrations are reduced, a relatively greater portion of the patient's total serum calcium will be present in the ionized form. As a result, the patient with a low total serum calcium concentration and a reduction in serum albumin may have a normal serum ionized calcium concentration.

Changes in the serum pH also will affect the amount of calcium bound by proteins. An increase of 0.1 in serum pH will increase protein-bound calcium by 0.12 mg/dL. Conversely, when the serum pH falls, more calcium is removed from the protein binding sites and is ionized, and available to participate in chemical reactions. Thus, when a decreased total serum calcium concentration is present in a patient with alkalosis, the serum ionized calcium concentration is probably extremely low. Alternatively, if the total serum calcium concentration is low in a patient with acidosis, the serum ionized calcium concentration may not be reduced significantly.[103]

Calcium homeostasis requires regulation of the amount of calcium filtered and reabsorbed by the kidneys, the amount of calcium absorbed from and excreted by the gastrointestinal tract, and the mobilization or deposition of calcium phosphate and other minerals in the bone matrix. These three methods of calcium regulation are controlled by parathyroid hormone (PTH), which is secreted by the four parathyroid glands. When serum ionized calcium levels fall, PTH is released, increasing the renal reabsorption of calcium and the gastrointestinal absorption of calcium. PTH enhances the movement of calcium and phosphate from the bone into the extracellular fluid. In addition, PTH decreases renal tubular reabsorption of phosphate, resulting in excretion of the phosphate that was released when calcium was mobilized from the bone.[54]

Renal Regulation of Calcium. Renal calcium reabsorption is an active process that occurs throughout the nephron. Normally, only 1% of filtered calcium is excreted in the urine, although this amount can be altered by changing either the filtered load of calcium or its rate of reabsorption. If calcium intake is increased, the serum calcium concentration increases and will be reflected in an increased amount of calcium filtered into the tubule, resulting in increased calcium excretion in the urine. The renal capacity to excrete calcium is compromised by a reduction in the GFR, by volume depletion, and by chronic expansion of the extracellular fluid associated with mineralocorticoid administration.

The rate of calcium reabsorption from the renal tubules also can be altered through exchange for sodium. When PTH is secreted, renal calcium excretion is reduced and urinary excretion of sodium is enhanced. Calcium retention also is increased by the continued administration of thiazide diuretics; these drugs produce a distal tubular natriuresis so that sodium is excreted and calcium is retained.

Gastrointestinal Absorption of Calcium. The intestinal absorption of calcium occurs through an active transport system controlled by PTH. When the serum calcium concentration falls and PTH is released, intestinal absorption of calcium will increase somewhat. More importantly, PTH will stimulate renal activation of vitamin D_3. The presence of activated vitamin D_3 will greatly accelerate gastrointestinal absorption of ingested calcium (see Chapters 12 and 14).

Mobilization of Calcium from Bone. When PTH levels are increased, bone is reabsorbed, liberating calcium and phosphate and raising the serum concentrations of both. Because PTH enhances renal calcium reabsorption but reduces phosphate absorption, the ultimate effect of PTH release is an increase in serum ionized calcium concentration. The full effect of PTH in bone reabsorption requires the simultaneous presence of vitamin D_3, which must be activated in the kidneys.

Prenatal and Postnatal Development of Renal Function

During fetal life, the placenta performs many of the functions of the kidney, so congenital renal malformations may not cause fetal distress. Urine secretion into the amniotic fluid begins during the ninth through twelfth weeks of gestation. Most kidney growth occurs during the last 20 weeks of gestation, and the GFR increases rapidly between the twenty-eighth and thirty-fifth weeks of gestation. All nephrons of the mature kidney are formed by the twenty-eighth week of gestation.[40]

After birth, kidney size increases in proportion to body length. Kidney weight doubles in the first 10 months of life, more as the result of proximal tubular growth than from an increase in glomerular size. The GFR also increases significantly after birth. The GFR of the full-term neonate (per square meter of body surface area) is approximately one third the GFR of an adult. Renal blood flow and the GFR double during the first 2 weeks of life, and GFR is nearly equal to adult values within the first 3 years of life.[40]

Immediately after birth, the neonate normally has a high urine volume with low osmolality, thought to be the result of immaturity of renal sodium and fluid regulatory mechanisms. Because increases in systemic arterial pressure and systemic vascular resistance also result in an increase in renal blood flow and GFR during this time, these factors also may be responsible for the high urine volume. Beyond the first several hours of life, urine volume normally falls and urine concentration gradually rises.[40]

The newborn kidney is able to excrete amino acids and conserve sodium and glucose as well as the adult kidney. However, the newborn kidney is less able to excrete free water and to concentrate urine than is the adult kidney.[40] As a result, the infant kidney may be less able to excrete a large water load and may be unable to concentrate urine in response to dehydration.

Regulation of the acid-base balance by the newborn kidney is relatively efficient, although it has less ability to secrete hydrogen ions or fixed acid than does the adult kidney; this is exacerbated by limited dietary protein intake. As a result, renal compensation for metabolic acidosis may be limited in the neonate. Dehydration, hypotension, and hypoxemia all produce a marked fall in the infant's GFR; therefore renal function may become compromised quickly during critical illness.

Factors Influencing Body Fluid Composition and Distribution

Serum Osmolality

Osmotic pressure in a fluid is measured in milliosmoles and is the force exerted by particles in solution that will draw water across a semipermeable membrane. The normal serum osmolality is approximately 275 to 295 mOsm/L. Sodium and its chief anions, chloride and bicarbonate, account for 90% of the total osmolality of the plasma. The serum osmolality can be calculated by adding the concentrations of the solutes (including sodium, potassium, calcium, magnesium, sulfate, creatinine, glucose, protein, and urea) per unit of solvent. For simplicity, the total serum osmolality is estimated using the serum concentrations of sodium, glucose, and blood urea nitrogen (BUN) as follows[86]:

$$\text{Serum osmolality} = (\text{Serum sodium} \times 2)$$
$$+ (\text{Serum glucose} \div 18)$$
$$+ (\text{BUN} \div 2.8)$$

*This formula does not reflect the influence of plasma proteins or administered osmotic agents, such as mannitol. It may be inaccurate in the presence of severe hyperglycemia and hyperlipemia.

If the serum glucose and BUN are normal, the serum osmolality will be slightly more than double the serum sodium concentration.

Factors Influencing Water Movement Between Body Compartments

Under normal conditions, free water is distributed within the intracellular and the extracellular (including intravascular and interstitial) compartments, so that osmolality is equal within all spaces.[34] Acute changes in the osmolality of any one body fluid compartment will result in free water movement across the semipermeable vascular and cell membranes until osmotic equilibrium is restored. Acute changes in serum sodium and osmolality can cause acute water shifts between the intracellular and extracellular spaces. Sudden, significant water shifts are tolerated poorly.

An acute fall in serum sodium and the resulting intracellular water shift can cause cerebral edema. If neurologic symptoms develop, urgent treatment is needed. An acute rise in serum sodium and osmolality can cause a water shift from the cells to the extracellular space. A significant extracellular water shift can cause cerebral dysfunction and intracranial bleeding. For further information, see Chapter 12.

Changes in Body Fluid Composition and Distribution During Critical Illness

Critically ill patients have a tendency to retain fluids, because antidiuretic hormone and aldosterone secretion are typically increased. Catecholamine release, hypotension, fright, or pain can stimulate antidiuretic hormone (ADH), renin, and aldosterone release. ADH release also is known to be stimulated by any condition that reduces left atrial pressure (including hemorrhage, positive pressure ventilation, and severe pulmonary hypertension), and the administration of general anesthetics, morphine, or barbiturates.[54]

ADH secretion promotes water reabsorption in the renal tubules and collecting ducts, so that intravascular volume will increase and intravascular osmolality will fall. Aldosterone secretion enhances renal sodium reabsorption; water follows, contributing to an increase in intravascular volume. As a result of the actions of these hormones, postoperative patients often demonstrate decreased urine volume and increased urine concentration in the presence of hemodilution. Because the newborn kidney has a limited ability to concentrate urine, neonates may demonstrate decreased urine volume and only moderate urine concentration.

Postoperative fluid administration must be tailored to prevent fluid overload or sodium imbalance. Typical fluid and electrolyte losses in the urine most closely resemble 0.45% sodium chloride, whereas insensible losses through the skin and respiratory tract are more similar to 0.2% sodium chloride. For this reason, 0.2% or 0.45% sodium chloride with 5% or 10% glucose may be administered during the postoperative period to replace insensible and urine losses only, but not for the provision of maintenance fluids. Recent reports of hyponatremia in critically ill children have led to caution in the use of hypotonic fluids, and greater use of isotonic crystalloids (see Chapter 12).

The stressed patient will tend to retain sodium and water as a result of renin, aldosterone, and ADH secretion; therefore administration of hypotonic solutions (e.g., 5% dextrose and water) should be avoided unless sodium intake is restricted (e.g., in postoperative patients with congenital heart disease). Excessive gastrointestinal fluid and electrolyte losses should be replaced with a solution approximating the electrolyte concentration in the gastrointestinal fluid lost.[43] These recommendations should serve only as guidelines and must, of course, be adjusted to meet the patient's individual requirements.

Urine volume should be monitored closely and should average more than 1 mL/kg per hour if fluid administration is adequate. If severe fluid restriction is imposed, urine volume will likely be lower and can average 0.5-1.0 mL/kg per hour. Urine concentration is evaluated through measurement of urine specific gravity and osmolality. The specific gravity of the urine reflects the combined weight of all the particles in the urine. The specific gravity of water is 1.000, and the specific gravity of normal urine ranges from 1.010 to 1.030. The higher the solute content of urine, the higher the urine specific gravity.

The urine specific gravity usually correlates with the urine osmolality. However, if an excessive number of large particles such as glucose, protein, mannitol, or contrast agent is present in the urine, then the urine specific gravity will increase disproportionate to its true osmolality, rendering the specific gravity measurement useless. Because the urine osmolality best indicates the renal ability to concentrate urine above the serum osmolality, it is a more reliable indicator of renal function than the measurement of urine specific gravity.

Normal urine osmolality is approximately 300 mOsm/L when plasma osmolality is approximately 275 to 295 mOm/L. If renal function is good, the ratio of urine to plasma osmolality should be 1.1:1 or higher (i.e., urine osmolality should always be higher than plasma osmolality). When renal failure is present, urine osmolality often is equal to plasma osmolality.

Potential Effects of Drugs and Solutions on Renal Function

Some drugs and solutions used in the evaluation or treatment of critically ill patients may be nephrotoxic. Antibiotics such as the cephalosporins, the aminoglycosides, and the sulfonamides may be nephrotoxic in infants and children.[23,99] Alpha adrenergic medications that produce renal vasoconstriction can result in decreased renal perfusion and oliguric renal failure. Indomethacin administration to promote constriction of the neonatal ductus arteriosus can produce a fall in GFR or a decrease in urine output.

The use of hypertonic angiographic contrast agents can result in renal vein thrombosis, medullary hypoperfusion, renal ischemia, and renal insufficiency. Because these agents have an osmolality of 1300 to 1940 mOsm/L, they should be administered carefully in low doses and only to well-hydrated infants. If possible, low-osmolality radiocontrast agents should be used, and other nephrotoxic drugs should be avoided.[23] Use of nephrotoxic drugs in children also should be restricted if circulatory compromise or renal insufficiency is present.

Diuretics

Diuretic agents increase urine volume. The primary effect of such drugs is to decrease tubular reabsorption of sodium and chloride; this indirectly decreases water reabsorption so water loss in the urine is increased. Diuretics usually do not exert a primary effect on water reabsorption itself.

Diuretics can be classified according to their renal site of action and their chemical groups.[31] The osmotic agents and carbonic anhydrase inhibitors are proximal tubule diuretics that are less commonly used than the more popular thiazides and sulfonamide derivatives. Potassium-sparing diuretics act in the distal tubule. Furosemide (Lasix) and ethacrynic acid exert their effect on the loop of Henle (Box 13-3).

The classifications, effects, doses, and side effects of the most frequently used pediatric diuretics are included in Table 13-2.

Box 13-3 Classification of Diuretics by Nephron Site of Action

Filtration Diuretics
- Aminophylline
- Glucocorticoids

Proximal Tubular Diuretic
- Mannitol

Carbonic Anhydrase Inhibitors
- Acetazolamide (Diamox)
- Metolazone (Zaroxolyn)

Loop of Henle Diuretics
- Bumetanide (Bumax)
- Ethacrynic acid (Edecrin)
- Furosemide (Lasix)

Distal Tubular Diuretics
Potassium-Losing
- Thiazides
- Chlorthalidone
Potassium-Retaining
- Triamterene
- Spironolactone
- Metolazone (Zaroxolyn)

Proximal Tubule Diuretics

Osmotic Agents. Osmotic agents such as mannitol, urea, and glucose cause diuresis as a result of their high osmolality. Once these agents are filtered through the glomerulus, they pull additional free water into the filtrate. They result in increased glomerular filtrate volume, they retard sodium and water reabsorption in the proximal tubule and result in increased urine volume.

Hypertonic glucose and mannitol are not the drugs of choice for routine diuresis. However, they can be extremely useful in promoting diuresis in children with marginal renal function, because their effect is produced as soon as they are filtered through the glomerulus, and they do not depend on renal tubular excretory or reabsorptive functions. In the setting of rhabdomyolysis, radiocontrast administration, and cardiopulmonary bypass, osmotic diuretics have been used in an attempt to prevent acute kidney injury.[3]

Intravenous administration of any osmotic agent can produce a temporary but significant increase in intravascular volume, because the intravenous osmotic agent produces an intravascular fluid shift. Use of these agents typically is contraindicated in patients with congestive heart failure or hypervolemia, because they can cause further increase intravascular volume. However, these drugs can be extremely useful in the treatment of patients with increased intracranial pressure (see Chapter 11).

Carbonic Anhydrase Inhibitors. Carbonic anhydrase inhibitors (e.g., acetazolamide) limit the rate at which the proximal cells hydrate CO_2 to carbonic acid. As a result, fewer hydrogen ions are available beyond the proximal tubule cell to exchange for sodium, sodium reabsorption is reduced, and diuresis occurs. This reduced hydrogen ion-sodium exchange also limits the amount of urinary bicarbonate returned to the blood as sodium bicarbonate, and a mild metabolic acidosis can result.

Metolazone. Metolazone (Zaroxolyn) is a nonthiazide sulfonamide diuretic that works in the proximal and distal tubule. Metolazone blocks sodium, chloride, and water reabsorption at the cortical diluting segments and may be particularly effective when administered with furosemide.

Distal Tubule Diuretics

Most agents that act on the distal convoluted tubule will be ineffective if the GFR less than 40 mL/min or less than 40% of normal.[31]

Thiazide Diuretics. Thiazide diuretics block the reabsorption of sodium and chloride in the cortical segment of the distal tubule. They do not interfere with the nephron's ability to concentrate the urine, but they do limit the excretion of a maximally dilute urine. All thiazide diuretics produce significant potassium and calcium loss in the urine. Because these diuretics can depress the glomerular filtration rate, administration can result in a reversible rise in BUN.

Oral thiazide diuretics are absorbed promptly from the gastrointestinal tract, usually produce diuresis within 1 h, and are usually effective for 12 to 24 hours before they are excreted in

Table 13-2 Diuretic Therapy for Children

Drug (trade name)	Peak Effect	Action	Dose	Effect on Serum [K$^+$]
Bumetanide (Bumex)	IV: 15-30 min PO: 1-2 hours	Inhibits sodium reabsorption in ascending limb of the loop of Henle; also blocks chloride reabsorption	IV/PO: 0.015 to 0.1 mg/kg per dose	↓↓↓
Chlorothiazide (Diuril)	2-4 hours	Inhibits tubular reabsorption of sodium primarily in the distal tubule but also in the loop of Henle; also inhibits water reabsorption in cortical diluting segment of ascending limb of loop	IV: 4 mg/kg per day PO: 20-40 mg/kg per day	↓↓
Ethacrynic acid (Edecrin)	IV: 5-10 min PO: 0.5-8 hours	Same as furosemide	IV: 1-2 mg/kg PO: 2-3 mg/kg	↓↓↓
Furosemide (Lasix)	IV: 5-20 min PO: 0.5-2 hours	Inhibits sodium chloride transport in ascending limb of loop of Henle and in proximal and distal tubules	IV: 1-2 mg/kg PO: 1-4 mg/kg	↓↓↓
Hydrochlorothiazide (Hydrodiuril)	2-4 hours	Inhibits sodium reabsorption in distal tubule and loop of Henle and inhibits water reabsorption in cortical diluting segment of ascending limb of loop	PO: 2-3 mg/kg per day divided into two doses (every 12 hours)	↓↓
Hydrochlorothiazide + Spironolactone (Aldactazide)	2-4 hours (prolonged effects)	Hydrochlorothiazide functions as noted above; the spironolactone functions as an aldosterone antagonist and inhibits exchange of sodium for potassium in distal tubule	PO: 1.65-3.3 mg/kg per day	K$^+$ remains approximately unchanged
Metolazone (Zaroxolyn)	2 hours (prolonged effects)	Inhibits sodium reabsorption at the cortical diluting site and in the proximal convoluted tubule; results in approximately equal excretion of sodium and chloride ions; may increase potassium excretion as a result of increased delivery of sodium to distal tubule (and Na-K exchange)	PO: 0.2 to 0.4 mg/kg per day given in divided doses (every 12 hours)	↓↓
Spironolactone (Aldactone)	1-4 days (prolonged effects)	Aldosterone antagonist; inhibits exchange of sodium for potassium in distal tubule	PO: 1.3-3.3 mg/kg per day	K$^+$ is saved

IV, Intravenous; *PO,* by mouth.

the urine. Patients who receive thiazide diuretics may require simultaneous potassium supplementation to prevent hypokalemia.

Potassium-Sparing Diuretics. Potassium-sparing diuretics constitute a separate class of diuretics and include spironolactone, triamterene, and amiloride. These drugs inhibit distal tubule sodium reabsorption and potassium secretion. Consequently, sodium and water are excreted, and potassium is spared. This action is the most common reason for the use of these drugs—preserving the serum potassium. These diuretics are often administered in combination with other more potent diuretics such as furosemide.[31]

Loop of Henle Diuretics

The loop diuretics, furosemide (Lasix) and ethacrynic acid (Edecrin) are the most potent and popular diuretics used in the care of critically ill children. Both drugs inhibit sodium chloride transport in the ascending limbs of the loop, so that natriuresis and diuresis result. These drugs are often effective in patients responding maximally to other diuretics, and they

will be effective despite a decrease in glomerular filtration rate.[31] Both drugs can be administered intravenously, and they have a rapid onset.

Loop diuresis results in increased urinary potassium, hydrogen, and calcium ion loss. Potassium supplementation often will be required to prevent hypokalemia. The child's serum electrolytes should be monitored closely.

Large diuresis can decrease plasma volume, causing a contraction alkalosis. The increased hydrogen ion excretion that results from the administration of loop diuretics can further contribute to the alkalotic state (Box 13-4).

In large doses, both furosemide and ethacrynic acid can cause an increase in renal blood flow with an accompanied increase in perfusion to the outer renal cortical areas. These drugs are useful in patients with marginal renal perfusion or in patients with both cardiovascular and renal disease. Both drugs have been associated with ototoxicity, although the reported incidence of this complication seems to be higher with ethacrynic acid. The ototoxicity may not be reversible even after the drug is discontinued.

Box 13-4 **Factors Contributing to Development of Metabolic Alkalosis with Administration of Loop Diuretics**

Losses	Increased
Potassium chloride	Titratable acid
	Ammonium
Hydrogen	New bicarbonate added to plasma
	Contraction of plasma volume

COMMON CLINICAL CONDITIONS

Hyponatremia

Hyponatremia can develop in patients with renal dysfunction after aggressive use of diuretics. A pseudohyponatremia may be reported in patients with significant hyperlipidemia or hypoproteinemia,[96] and severe hyperglycemia may depress the serum sodium concentration (see Hyponatremia in Chapter 12). An acute fall in the serum sodium and osmolality is problematic because it can produce an acute intracellular shift of water, causing cerebral edema.

In any patient with renal failure, serum electrolytes and serum and urine osmolality will be assessed frequently; hyponatremia or other electrolyte imbalances should be promptly detected and treated. Hyponatremia producing neurologic symptoms is treated urgently with hypertonic (3%) saline (2-4 mL/kg). Hyponatremia not associated with neurologic symptoms is treated more slowly, raising the serum sodium at a rate of approximately 0.5 mEq/L per hour (see Chapter 12).[14,103]

Hypokalemia

Hypokalemia can develop in patients with renal tubular acidosis or if a hypokalemic dialysate is used after the child's serum potassium concentration normalizes. Hypokalemia can also develop if a 4.25% glucose dialysate is used for prolonged periods.

Severe hypokalemia can produce ventricular irritability and arrhythmias such as premature ventricular contractions, ventricular tachycardia and ventricular fibrillation. In addition, the electrocardiogram may reveal flattened or inverted T waves, ST-segment depression, and the appearance of a U wave. The child may also develop vomiting and a paralytic ileus.[85]

If hypokalemia develops, small doses of potassium can be added to the dialysate, or small doses of potassium chloride can be administered intravenously (0.5-1.0 mEq/kg, administered over several hours). If the hypokalemia is related to prolonged use of 4.25% glucose dialysate, and the child's condition permits it, the treatment of choice is to change the dialysate solution.[42,50,89] For further information, see Chapter 12.

Hyperkalemia

Etiology

An increase in serum potassium can result from excessive potassium administration, intravascular accumulation of potassium ions caused by changes in the acid-base balance or significant cell destruction (and release of intracellular potassium), or reduced renal excretion of potassium ions.

Pathophysiology

The serum potassium concentration should be evaluated in light of the serum pH. Acidosis (or a fall in serum pH) produces a rise in the intravascular potassium ion concentration, because potassium ions will move from the cells into the vascular space in exchange for hydrogen ions. Thus, a modest elevation in the serum potassium concentration in the acidotic patient may not represent significant hyperkalemia. When acidosis is corrected (i.e., the serum pH rises), the serum potassium concentration will fall.

Alkalosis (or a rise in serum pH) produces a fall in the serum potassium concentration. Therefore if the serum potassium concentration is high despite the presence of alkalosis, significant hyperkalemia is present.

Hyperkalemia can complicate renal failure because renal potassium excretion decreases. When chronic renal failure is present, the serum potassium concentration can remain normal if the child does not have a high potassium load (such as can result from increased potassium intake, acidosis, or potassium release from injured cells). If the child has acute kidney injury and decreased urine volume, the child's serum potassium concentration may rise quickly.

Clinical Signs and Symptoms

The manifestations of hyperkalemia affect neuromuscular function, because the membrane potential in excitable tissue is determined by the ratio of extracellular to intracellular potassium concentration. Therefore hyperkalemia causes muscle weakness and paralysis.

Hyperkalemia can produce characteristic changes in the electrocardiogram. Initially a tall, peaked T wave develops; this is followed by a widening of the QRS complex, ST-segment depression, and decreasing amplitude of the R wave. As the serum potassium concentration continues to rise, the P-R interval is prolonged, the amplitude of the P wave decreases, and finally the P wave disappears. Ventricular arrhythmias or ventricular fibrillation can develop at any point during this progression (Fig. 12-3).

Management

The best way to prevent hyperkalemia is to identify at-risk patients so that potassium administration can be curtailed. In addition, providers should frequently assess the at-risk child's serum potassium concentration and monitor for signs of clinically significant hyperkalemia. Finally, the child's fluid intake and output and acid-base status should be monitored, because these also affect serum potassium concentration.

Once the child's serum potassium concentration exceeds 6.5-7.0 mEq/L, there is a high risk of serious cardiac arrhythmias, and immediate intervention is required. Although the evidence supporting emergent therapies for hyperkalemia is largely anecdotal, widely accepted goals are: stabilize the myocardial cellular membrane, expand the extracellular fluid volume, shift potassium into the cells, and remove potassium from the body (see "Acute Kidney Injury" later in this chapter and Chapter 12, Table 12-4 for more information).

Calcium chloride or calcium gluconate is administered to transiently counteract adverse effects of hyperkalemia on cardiac cells. Calcium chloride (20 mg/kg) is infused intravenously over 1 to 5 minutes (calcium gluconate is used in neonates). During the calcium infusion, the nurse should monitor for bradycardia. In the presence of arrhythmias, an immediate improvement in the patient's electrocardiogram (ECG) may be observed as the calcium is given; these effects last approximately 30 min.[50] During this 30-minute window, additional therapy is provided to reduce the serum potassium concentration.

If hyperkalemia is associated with contraction of intravascular volume or hemoconcentration (e.g., with hypovolemic shock or severe dehydration), reexpansion of the intravascular volume should produce a dilutional reduction in the serum potassium concentration.

Because a rise in serum pH produces a shift of potassium ions into the cells, sodium bicarbonate may be administered (1.0 mEq/kg) over a 30- to 60-minute period to alkalinize the serum and enhance the intracellular potassium shift. Full-strength (8.4%) sodium bicarbonate typically is diluted to half strength before administration to infants and young children, to prevent vascular irritation and the development of increased intravascular osmolality and hypernatremia. Sodium bicarbonate should not be used to treat hyperkalemia in patients with respiratory failure and hypercarbia, because the buffering action of the bicarbonate will result in more carbon dioxide formation.

The administration of sodium bicarbonate does not reduce the total body potassium and may have a minimal effect on the serum potassium concentration of the nonacidotic patient. If the drug is effective, the serum potassium should begin to fall within 5 to 10 minutes, and the effects usually are apparent for several hours.

Cellular uptake of potassium from the extracellular (including intravascular) fluid is enhanced with the infusion of glucose plus insulin, one of the most effective methods of reducing hyperkalemia in critically ill children. A hypertonic glucose solution is administered (1-2 mL/kg of 25% dextrose [1 g/kg]) with a dose of regular insulin (0.1 U/kg).[50] The serum potassium concentration should begin to fall within 15 to 30 minutes, and effects may be apparent for about an hour.

The half-life of regular insulin is longer than the half-life of hypertonic glucose. Therefore late hypoglycemia often is observed after administration of the glucose and insulin. The child's serum glucose concentration should be monitored and point-of-care glucose testing should be used (if available), especially 1 to 2 hours following administration. Supplementary glucose should be administered as needed.[5]

Removal of potassium from the body can be accomplished via the gastrointestinal tract because potassium is present in intestinal fluids. The ion exchange resin, sodium polystyrene sulfonate (Kayexalate) will exchange potassium for sodium ions on an ion-for-ion basis when it is administered orally or as a retention enema.

Sodium polystyrene sulfonate is administered as a 20% suspension in a 5% glucose solution. The dose of 1.0 g/kg can be repeated as often as two or three times in 24 hours.[52] Because the greatest exchange of sodium for potassium occurs in the large intestine, an oral or nasogastric dose of 1.0 g/kg (given in divided doses) can reduce the serum potassium 1 mEq/L over a 24-hour period. The enema dose is somewhat higher and usually totals 2 g/kg, given once or twice per day.

The serum sodium will rise following sodium polystyrene sulfonate administration, and fluid retention may develop.

Inhaled albuterol causes rapid movement of potassium into the cells by stimulating the beta 2 adrenergic receptors, which in turn increase activity of the sodium-potassium-adenosine triphosphatase pump in the cell membrane, increasing cellular uptake of potassium. Albuterol stimulates the release of insulin, which also promotes cellular uptake of potassium.[83] Albuterol may provide rapid but unpredictable lowering of the serum potassium.

If all other measures to reduce serum potassium concentration fail, then hemofiltration, exchange transfusion, or hemodialysis may be required (see section, Care of the Child During Dialysis, Hemoperfusion, and Hemofiltration).

Acute Renal Failure and Acute Kidney Injury

Acute renal failure is a sudden reduction in renal function characterized by progressive accumulation of nitrogenous waste products of protein metabolism, urea, and creatinine in the blood. This condition is called *azotemia*. Oliguria is present in 30% to 70% of patients with acute renal failure (ARF).[47]

ARF is a multifaceted and often severe disorder that results in complicated imbalances in fluid and electrolytes, acid-base status, and the function of other organ systems. Critically ill patients further complicated with ARF continue to have a high mortality rate despite treatment and technological advances. The occurrence of ARF (depending on the definition used) is estimated to range from 1% to 25% of critically ill patients.[2,60]

An extremely important milestone regarding the definition of ARF was published in 2004 as a result of the Second International Consensus Conference of the Acute Dialysis Quality Initiative Group. One of the goals of this conference was to arrive at a consensus definition of ARF, because more than 30 different definitions existed in the literature.[11] The multiple definitions confounded research studies, their comparisons, and any meaningful interpretation of best treatment practices.

The Acute Dialysis Quality Initiative Group defined ARF for clinical research as "an abrupt and sustained decrease in glomerular function, urine output, or both."[2] The group then developed consensus criteria for essential features of ARF. The consensus criteria are known collectively as the *RIFLE criteria,* using the acronym indicating: risk of renal dysfunction, injury to the kidney, failure of kidney function, loss of kidney function, and end-stage kidney disease. These criteria have gained wide acceptance.[53] In this classification, there are separate criteria for creatinine and urine output to enable accurate and reproducible staging of the progression of renal dysfunction.[11] Changes in serum creatinine or changes in urine output, or both, will place a patient in a classification level of acute kidney injury (AKI).

Akcan-Arikan et al. published modified RIFLE criteria (pRIFLE) "for use in critically ill children (Table 13-3), assessing acute kidney injury incidence, and course along with renal and/or nonrenal comorbidities."[4] The pediatric criteria are based on (1) the patient's estimated creatinine clearance using the Schwartz formula, (2) the constant *k* values[4] determined by age (Box 13-5), and (3) urine output (see Evolve

Table 13-3 **Pediatric-Modified Acute Renal Failure (pRIFLE) Criteria**

Criteria	Estimated Creatinine Clearance	Urine Output
Risk	Decreased by 25%	<0.5 L/kg per hour × 8 hours
Injury	Decreased by 50%	<0.5 mL/kg per hour × 16 hours
Failure	Decreased by 75% or <35 mL/min per 1.73 m^2	<0.3 mL/kg per hour × 24 hours or anuric for 12 hours
Loss	Persistent failure >4 weeks	
End-stage	Persistent failure >3 months	

Reproduced from Akcan-Arikan A, et al: Modified RIFLE criteria in critically ill children with acute kidney injury, *Kidney Int* 71:1028-1035, 2007. *pRIFLE*, Pediatric modified RIFLE.

Box 13-5 **Schwartz Formula and *K* Values for Calculating Estimated Creatinine Clearance**

Schwartz Formula

$$eCrCl \text{ (mL/min per 1.73 m}^2) = K \times \text{Height (cm)} \div SCr \text{ (mg/dL)}$$

That is, estimated creatinine clearance (eCrCl) in milliliters per minute per 1.73 meter squared is equal to *K*—a constant value that varies with age*—times the height in centimeters divided by serum creatinine (SCr) in milligrams per deciliter

*K values to be used in conjunction with the Schwartz formula: <2 years, 0.45; 2 to <13 years, 0.55; 13 to <20 years, 0.70 for males, 0.55 for females.

Box 13-1 for an example of the calculation of the pediatric RIFLE score in the Chapter 13 Supplement on the Evolve Website).

The pediatric modified pRIFLE criteria provide a systematic, standard method of defining and classifying acute kidney injury in children. The criteria have been shown to reliably predict increased cost, length of stay, mortality, and need for renal replacement therapy.[8]

In this chapter, the term *AKI* is used "to represent the entire spectrum of acute renal failure" as proposed by the Acute Kidney Injury Network in their report of an initiative to improve outcomes in acute kidney injury.[70] The use of a standard definition of AKI and the pRIFLE classification help focus on early changes and recognition, which may lead to prevention.

Etiology

There are many causes of AKI in critically ill children. Critically ill neonates can develop AKI as a result of asphyxia, hypoxia, shock, and sepsis.[6] AKI also can occur as a complication of umbilical artery or vein catheterization and subsequent thrombosis of the aorta, the renal artery, or the renal vein. Critically ill children most commonly develop AKI as a complication of major surgical procedures, multisystem organ failure, drug toxicity, or toxic ingestions.[9,27]

Causes of AKI are classified according to the location of the primary disorder. The categories to describe these etiologies are prerenal, postrenal and intrarenal (intrinsic). Ostensibly, prerenal and postrenal causes of AKI, if not prolonged, do not involve damage to the renal parenchyma, and correction or reversal of these causes should allow renal function to return to normal. However, severe prerenal or postrenal failure can produce damage to the nephron unit, so that normal renal function might not return after correction of the underlying cause, and intrinsic renal failure occurs. Intrinsic renal failure can also result from primary kidney disease.

Prerenal Failure. Prerenal failure results from compromise in renal perfusion. The most common cause of prerenal failure is poor systemic perfusion secondary to hypovolemia or poor cardiac function. Bilateral embolus or thrombosis in the renal arteries can also produce prerenal failure, and it can be caused by intravascular fluid loss, sepsis, cardiovascular disease, asphyxia, or shock. In each case, renal blood flow and renal perfusion are compromised, the glomerular filtration rate falls, and AKI develops.

A fall in renal blood flow and the GFR frequently is encountered among patients with moderate to severe dehydration. Unless the compromise in renal perfusion is severe or prolonged, damage to the renal parenchyma typically does not occur and renal function returns once perfusion is restored.

Postrenal Failure. Postrenal causes of AKI include disorders that obstruct urine flow and prevent the elimination of urine. The obstruction to flow must involve both ureters, because a single normal kidney can maintain fluid and electrolyte balance adequately, or the obstruction must be severe enough to produce a decrease in renal function. Obstruction of urine flow can result from compression by an extrarenal mass, such as a Wilms' tumor or a neuroblastoma.

Congenital disorders such as posterior urethral valves and bilateral ureteropelvic junction strictures are the most common postrenal causes of AKI in neonates and infants.[98] Blood clots, calculi, inflammation or edema, tumors, and hemorrhagic cystitis are a few of the additional conditions that can prevent urine flow into the bladder or prevent adequate bladder evacuation.

Intrinsic Renal Failure. Intrinsic forms of AKI include all causes of renal dysfunction associated with damage to renal parenchymal cells. The most common causes of intrinsic AKI are associated with acute tubular necrosis (ATN) from ischemia and nephrotoxic substances or drugs. ATN is the most frequent cause of intrinsic renal failure in children.[27]

Intrarenal AKI may be secondary to a prolonged and severe prerenal or postrenal problem, it may involve chemicals that have a toxic effect upon the kidney, or it may be associated with primary renal disease such as glomerulonephritis. Intrarenal failure may develop after profound circulatory disturbances, hypoxia, septicemia, or ingestion of drugs or poisons.

AKI in the neonate can be associated with renal structural anomalies. Because the placenta performs the excretory functions of the kidneys, neonates with significant renal malformations can have normal plasma electrolyte concentrations at birth. Ninety-five percent of all preterm and term infants excrete urine within the first 24 hours of life[85]; therefore failure of micturation in the first 2 days of life is strongly suggestive of severe congenital renal anomalies. A history of oligohydramnios, limb deformities, and characteristic facial features suggest the presence of Potter's syndrome, which includes renal dysplasia or bilateral renal agenesis. Many neonates with oligohydramnios also have associated pulmonary hypoplasia.

Pathophysiology

The most common cause of AKI is an acute reduction in renal perfusion. As noted in the Etiology section above, this reduction can be caused by hypovolemia, hypotension, other forms of shock, or renal artery or aortic thrombosis. When renal perfusion is compromised, renal efferent arteriolar constriction can initially maintain glomerular filtration. However, if the compromise in perfusion is severe or acute, efferent arteriolar constriction cannot maintain glomerular capillary pressure sufficiently, and glomerular filtration falls.

Postrenal failure can develop as the result of obstruction to the ureters or urethra with obstruction to urine flow. Urine obstruction increases the volume and pressure of fluid in the collecting system and ultimately will increase the pressure in Bowman's capsule. This increase in pressure will impede glomerular filtration. Once the obstruction to urine flow is relieved, a natriuresis often is present for several days or weeks (up to 2 weeks is common). Renal function ultimately is restored unless the obstruction has been prolonged.

If both prerenal and postrenal causes have been ruled out in the patient with AKI, the cause is assumed to be injury to the kidney's functional components—the renal parenchymal cells. This damage can occur through direct injury to the glomeruli, tubules, or renal vasculature. Glomerular damage is associated more commonly with the glomerulonephropathies; tubular damage is more commonly a result of ischemia or nephrotoxins.

Obstruction and damage to the renal vasculature can complicate umbilical artery or vein catheterization in the neonate; however, this is an uncommon cause of ARF in children. Renal vasculature pathology in children is most frequently the result of hemolytic uremic syndrome and other pathologies, including sickle cell disease, Kawasaki disease, and Henoch-Schonlein Purpura.[58]

Tubular lesions caused by nephrotoxins temporarily disrupt the tubular structure, because they produce necrosis of the tubular epithelium down to, but not including, the supporting basement membrane. Ischemic lesions may affect any segment of the nephron, and injured areas may be interspersed with normal segments of tubular epithelium. Healing of both ischemic and nephrotoxic injury occurs through re-epithelialization. If the basement membrane is intact, tubular morphology can be reestablished after healing. If the basement membrane has been fragmented, however, the lack of supportive structure prevents regrowth of organized tubules. Connective tissue can extend through the ruptured basement membrane and fibrosis can replace the tubules.

The unpredictability of tubular healing makes it impossible to predict the rate of recovery of nephron function after ischemic or nephrotoxic injury.[27] Renal failure can be complicated by the development of backleak of fluid through the damaged tubular basement membrane. Backleak prevents elimination of the filtrate and results in reabsorption of the creatinine and other nitrogenous wastes back into the circulation.[79]

Although the precise pathophysiology of AKI is not understood, almost all theories include a severe reduction in renal blood flow by 25% to 50%. This reduction in renal blood flow often occurs despite a normal systemic arterial pressure and is thought to result from intense renal vasoconstriction[27] that reduces GFR and renal cortical blood flow. This reduction stimulates renin and aldosterone secretion and produces sodium and water retention and decreased urine volume.

The development of AKI usually indicates the presence of renal tubular damage and reduced renal blood flow. In addition, there may be destruction of the glomerular capillary membrane, increased tubular permeability, or obstruction of the tubules.

Clinical Signs and Symptoms

AKI is characterized by a steady increase in the BUN and serum creatinine levels. Oliguria (urine output <300 mL/m^2 body surface area per day) is a common but not a constant clinical sign of AKI. Anuria is less common, and it often indicates more severe renal damage. Some children who develop AKI have nonoliguric renal failure, which is characterized by a rise in serum BUN and creatinine without a fall in urine volume. Children with AKI may even exhibit polyuria.

Clinical signs produced by uremia include an altered level of consciousness, seizures, anorexia, nausea, vomiting, abnormal platelet function, diminished white blood cell function, and pericarditis.[71] Once AKI develops, the ability of the kidneys to regulate fluid volume and potassium, calcium, and glucose concentrations is severely impaired. In addition, renal regulation of acid-base balance is reduced. Finally, many patients with AKI develop anemia and coagulopathies, and they are at risk for the development of gastrointestinal hemorrhage and infection.[71] As a result, assessment of children with AKI must include assessment of the reversible causes of renal failure as well as the recognition and management of its complications.

Disorders of Fluid Balance. If oliguria develops in patients with AKI and fluid administration is not tapered appropriately, hypervolemia will develop. Hypervolemia will complicate the management of children with cardiovascular problems and may produce hypertension. To evaluate the child's fluid status, the nurse should assess for hypertension and for signs of congestive heart failure, including hepatomegaly, high central venous pressure (CVP), periorbital edema, tachycardia, and increased respiratory effort or oxygen requirements.

If congestive heart failure is present, the cardiac silhouette will be enlarged on the chest radiograph. These findings usually indicate the need for urgent dialysis or hemofiltration. The child's mucous membranes will be moist, and ascites or edema of dependent areas or extremities may also be noted. When the infant is younger than 16 to 18 months of age, the fontanelle should be palpated; it will be full or tense in this setting.

The hypervolemic child will also have a positive fluid balance when fluid intake, output, and insensible water loss are calculated. In addition, the child's weight will increase. If these signs are noted, the child probably has hypervolemia.

Signs of inadequate intravascular volume include dry mucous membranes, poor skin turgor, poor systemic perfusion, and low (less than 5 mm Hg) CVP. Late findings include hypotension and metabolic (lactic) acidosis. A negative fluid balance is often apparent when total fluid intake, output, and insensible losses are calculated. The child with inadequate intravascular volume may require fluid administration. It is important to note that the child's intravascular volume may be inadequate, despite the administration of adequate fluids and the presence of edema; this occurs if the child is losing fluid from the vascular space or to the peritoneal cavity (this is known as *third spacing* of fluid and may be seen in the child with sepsis, burns, or ascites).

Disorders of Electrolyte and Acid-Base Balance. *Hyperkalemia* is one of the most serious complications of acute kidney injury, because it can result in fatal cardiac arrhythmias. Hyperkalemia develops because distal tubular injury impairs potassium secretion, and reduced glomerular filtration limits the formation of urine; therefore potassium secretion in the cortical collecting tubule is reduced.[77]

Acidosis results from the damaged kidney's inability to excrete acid, and the acidosis will worsen existing hyperkalemia. In the presence of acidosis, the serum potassium concentration is further elevated as hydrogen ions are taken up by the RBCs to be buffered by intracellular proteins, and potassium ions shift to the extracellular (including intravascular) space in exchange for the hydrogen ions.

Normally, the serum potassium concentration will not rise to dangerous levels for 2 or 3 days after the development of oliguric renal failure. However, in critically ill children, the rate of serum potassium rise is accelerated by the presence of acidosis, hemolysis, infection, gastrointestinal bleeding, or trauma. Adverse effects of hyperkalemia are enhanced as the result of hypocalcemia, hypomagnesemia, and the use of digitalis.

Signs of hyperkalemia include generalized muscle weakness, peaking of the T wave on the ECG, widening of the QRS complex, ventricular arrhythmias, heart block, and ventricular fibrillation.

Hyperphosphatemia develops as a result of a reduction in the GFR. The tubular maximum for phosphate reabsorption varies inversely with the GFR; as the GFR falls, the tubular maximum rises, and more phosphate is transported actively out of the tubules and returned to the circulation. If chronic kidney disease develops, hyperparathyroidism will partially compensate for this hyperphosphatemia by increasing calcium mobilization from bone so that phosphate is precipitated. Although hyperphosphatemia itself may produce no symptoms until the phosphate level is extremely high (e.g., much higher than 5.5 mg/dL), it will produce hypocalcemia that can result in neuromuscular or cardiovascular complications.[77]

Hypocalcemia develops frequently among patients with AKI, because renal clearance of phosphate is impaired and renal activation of vitamin D is reduced. Hypocalcemia is more likely to develop after administration of stored whole blood or packed red blood cells preserved with citrate, phosphate, and dextran, because serum ionized calcium can precipitate with the phosphate anticoagulant and bind with the citrate. Signs of hypocalcemia include a low serum calcium concentration, decreased cardiovascular function (including arrhythmias and evidence of decreased cardiac contractility), muscle cramps, tetany, and seizures.

Metabolic acidosis often develops in children with AKI because the kidney is less able to secrete hydrogen ions, form titratable acids or ammonia, or reabsorb bicarbonate ions. Metabolic acidosis can be caused or exacerbated by lactic acidosis resulting from poor systemic perfusion, and it can compromise cardiac contractility and rapidly contribute to deterioration in cardiovascular function.

Hypoglycemia is more likely to develop in critically ill infants because they have high glucose needs and low glycogen stores. Signs of hypoglycemia include a low serum glucose concentration, irritability, and late findings such as seizures or poor systemic perfusion.

Hematologic Complications and Infections. Anemia and bleeding can be serious problems in critically ill pediatric patients with AKI. These children often have thrombocytopenia and thrombocytopathia (decreased platelet function). Coagulopathies may be detected by a coagulation screening panel, or they may produce clinical signs such as the development of petechiae or ecchymoses. Gastrointestinal hemorrhage occurs in a significant number of patients with AKI, and stress ulcers also may develop.

Because infection can produce such serious complications in the child with AKI, the child should be monitored closely for evidence of infection. Potential signs of infection include the development of fever (or hypothermia in infants), lethargy, irritability, localized signs of infection (such as erythema or drainage from venous access sites or wounds), an elevation in white blood count, or the presence of white blood cells or glucose in the urine. These signs should be reported to an on-call provider immediately.

Evaluation of Renal Function. During initial assessment of the child with AKI, it is important to attempt to differentiate between reversible prerenal or postrenal AKI and renal injury resulting from renal parenchymal damage. The tests to differentiate between prerenal and intrinsic renal injury basically evaluate the ability of the kidney to conserve sodium and concentrate urine (Table 13-4).

If prerenal failure is present, the healthy kidney attempts to maintain intravascular volume by reabsorbing sodium and water and excreting a small volume of concentrated urine. As a result, the urine sodium concentration will be low (<10 mEq/L) and the urine osmolality will be greater than the serum osmolality. When prerenal oliguria is present, the urine osmolality should exceed 500 mOsm/L, with the serum osmolality less than 300 mOsm/L.

The serum BUN will be increased out of proportion to the serum creatinine in prerenal failure, because urea is a small molecule that is reabsorbed as the kidneys reabsorb sodium and water. At the same time, the renal tubular excretion of creatinine continues in a normal fashion. For these reasons, the ratio of serum BUN to creatinine ratio will be greater than 20:1.

Table 13-4 Laboratory Tests in Differential Diagnosis of Prerenal and Intrinsic Renal Failure

Characteristic	Prerenal	Intrinsic Renal
Urine specific gravity	>1.020	≤1.010
Urine osmolality (mOsm/L)	>500	<400
Urine creatinine (mg/dL)	>100	<70
Creatinine urine:plasma ratio	>30	<20 (<10 in neonates)
Urea urine:plasma ratio	>14	<6
Urine urea (mEq/L)	>2000	<400
Urine sodium (mEq/L)	<10 mEq/L	>30 mEq/L (>25 mEq/L in neonates)
Urine potassium (mEq/L)	30-70	<20-40
Urine Na:K ratio	<1.0	0.8-1.0
Urine appearance (microscopic)	Hyaline casts	Cellular casts
Serum BUN:creatinine ratio	>20:1	<10:1
FE_{Na}	<1% (<2.5% in neonates)	>1% to 3% (>3.5 in neonates)
Fluid status	Dry, hypovolemic or inadequately perfused	Euvolemic

BUN, Blood urea nitrogen; *FE_{Na},* fractional excretion of filtered sodium.

The most accurate test to separate prerenal failure from AKI caused by renal factors is the fractional excretion of filtered sodium (FE_{Na}), which is calculated as follows:

$$FE_{Na} = \frac{\text{urine sodium concentration/serum sodium concentration}}{\text{urine creatinine concentration/serum creatinine concentration}} \times 100$$

When prerenal azotemia is present, the FE_{Na} is less than 1% (<2.5% in neonates)[40]; when AKI is caused by renal damage the FE_{Na} is greater than 1% to 3%.[82] It is important to note that evaluation of renal function using the FE_{Na} is not reliable if the urine sample is collected after diuretic therapy, because diuretics increase the urine sodium concentration.

When AKI results from renal damage, the child's urine usually is not concentrated, and it often contains casts of renal tubular cells. If the test result for blood in the urine is positive with a bedside reagent strip, but the urine contains no RBCs on microscopic examination, providers should suspect the presence of hemoglobinuria or myoglobinuria.[44]

If the newborn has evidence of AKI, it is important to determine if the neonate has voided, because lack of micturation within the first 48 hours of life is associated with congenital renal anomalies. Any fetal ultrasound examination results should be obtained; they can aid in the identification of urinary obstruction. Other clinical signs frequently associated with renal anomalies in the neonate include persistent bladder distension, ascites, ambiguous genitalia, epispadias, single umbilical artery, hypospadias, abnormalities of the abdominal muscles (prune belly), or off-set or low-set ears.

Postrenal failure is unusual in children. However, it should be suspected in any anuric patient. The presence of obstruction to urine flow can be confirmed readily with an ultrasound examination.

Management

Fluid balance and Renal Perfusion. Early recognition of AKI is essential so that fluid, drug, and electrolyte administration can be adjusted to prevent fluid overload and minimize drug and potassium accumulation. Whenever any critically ill child becomes oliguric, providers should suspect AKI, and immediate efforts should be made to determine and eliminate any reversible causes. The nurse should frequently verify the patency of the urinary catheter and drainage system.

Assessment of Fluid Balance. Maintenance of fluid balance is vital in the management of AKI, and the bedside nurse plays an invaluable role in the assessment of fluid balance. The nurse must closely monitor perfusion parameters, record accurate intake and output, obtain serial weights, and monitor laboratory values in the context of the patient's history and clinical presentation.

Children with AKI require insertion of a large-bore venous catheter. If possible, a central venous catheter should be inserted to enable measurement of CVP and provide venous access for blood sampling. An indwelling urinary catheter should be inserted to allow continuous determination of urine volume and to facilitate urine collection for analysis.

Occasionally, the child's urine output may increase after a period of oliguric prerenal failure, only to begin a phase of nonoliguric renal failure. The nurse should monitor the urine specific gravity and osmolality in an attempt to assess renal concentrating abilities.

Nonoliguric renal failure can produce water and salt depletion, because both are lost in the urine. Additional electrolytes such as calcium, potassium, and hydrogen ions may be lost with high urine flow; therefore the child's serum electrolyte and acid-base status should be monitored closely.

Assessment of Systemic Perfusion. The nurse should closely monitor the child's systemic perfusion, because hypovolemia and shock are frequent prerenal causes of AKI in critically ill children (see Preoperative Evaluation of the Renal Transplant Patient in the Renal Transplantation section later in this chapter). The child's mucous membranes and nail beds should be pink, and the extremities should be warm. The child's heart rate, respiratory rate, and blood pressure should be appropriate for age and clinical condition. Peripheral pulses should be readily palpable and the CVP should be 2 to 5 mm Hg.

If the child has pale mucous membranes or nail beds and cool extremities with sluggish capillary refill, cardiac output may be inadequate and systemic and renal perfusion may be compromised. Inadequate cardiac output also results in tachycardia and tachypnea (unless the child's respiratory rate is controlled with mechanical ventilation), diminished intensity of peripheral pulses, metabolic acidosis and oliguria. Hypotension is often a late sign of poor perfusion in children (see "Shock" in Chapter 6).

If clinically significant hypovolemia is present, the child's CVP usually is less than 5 mm Hg. Patients with AKI may require administration of 20 mL/kg boluses of isotonic crystalloid (normal saline or Ringer's lactate); the fluid bolus is repeated (up to three times) based on the patient's response, with careful monitoring to prevent fluid overload.[27] If hypovolemia results from hemorrhage, isotonic crystalloid may be administered initially, but blood products will be required.

If the child's systemic perfusion improves after fluid administration, but urine output does not increase, furosemide (or mannitol [0.2-0.5 g/kg] in rhabdomyolysis) can be prescribed early in the course of AKI in an attempt to convert from oliguric to nonoliguric renal failure; however, this approach has not reduced mortality. Because persistent vasoconstriction is often present in AKI, larger doses of furosemide (e.g., 2-5 mg/kg) should be administered intermittently followed by an infusion of furosemide.[71]

Furosemide should stimulate a urine output of 6 to 10 mL/kg over a 1- to 3-hour period, unless AKI is caused by intrinsic renal damage or postrenal causes. If urine output does not improve, administration of other potentially nephrotoxic diuretic agents should be avoided because they may increase renal damage. In this case, fluid and potassium administration should be limited, and providers should evaluate doses of any drugs excreted by the kidneys and adjust the doses as needed.

Cardiovascular Support. If oliguria is associated with poor systemic perfusion and a high CVP (>5 mm Hg), the renal failure can result from low cardiac output caused by heart (pump) failure. Alternatively, the AKI could be causing hypervolemia with resultant congestive heart failure. It will be helpful to determine the child's baseline cardiovascular function and attempt to restore it.

Because hypoglycemia, hypocalcemia, and acidosis all can depress cardiovascular function, the child's electrolyte and acid-base status should be assessed carefully. In the absence of such disorders, administration of a sympathomimetic inotropic agent may be required.

The drug of choice for oliguria with cardiovascular dysfunction is dopamine, because it dilates the renal vasculature, increasing renal blood flow (20%-40%) and GFR (5%-20%) when it is administered in low (0.5-2 mcg/kg per minute) doses.[20,59] There is no evidence to support the use of low-dose dopamine in the prevention of AKI,[26,95] but it is used once AKI is present. Higher doses of dopamine (>8-10 mcg/kg per minute) should be avoided, because they can produce alpha-adrenergic effects, including renal vasoconstriction and decreased renal blood flow, and can result in decreased urine output.

An additional sympathomimetic drug such as dobutamine (2-20 mcg/kg per minute) may also be administered. If systemic perfusion remains poor, systemic vasodilators such as sodium nitroprusside (0.5-8 mcg/kg per min) or nitroglycerin (0.25-10 mcg/kg per min) may be required (see Management of Shock in Chapter 6).

If urine output does not improve within 1 to 3 hours after the administration of a diuretic, the child is presumed to have AKI and renal parenchymal damage. If hypervolemia is producing cardiovascular dysfunction, hemodialysis or hemofiltration will be required.

Fluid Therapy. When oliguric AKI is present, the child's fluid intake should be restricted to insensible water losses (approximately 300-400 mL/m^2 body surface area per day) plus 24-hour urine output.[71] Too often, repeated boluses of fluid are administered in an unsuccessful attempt to increase urine output, and they produce hypervolemia. Repeated administration of osmotic diuretics also should be avoided once the patient has failed to respond to them, because these agents will increase intravascular volume and serum osmolality.

The child's insensible water losses are increased in the presence of fever (more fluid is lost through evaporation) and during periods of catabolism (more metabolic water is produced). If the child is receiving mechanical ventilation with adequate inspired humidity, water losses through the respiratory tract should be negligible.

During strict fluid regulation, all sources of fluid intake should be calculated, including fluids required to flush monitoring lines and administer medications. Types of fluids administered should be selected based on the child's electrolyte and acid-base balance. If the child develops hypervolemia that produces cardiovascular compromise, hemodialysis or hemofiltration will be required to remove the excess fluid.

Electrolyte and Acid-Base Balance. When AKI is present, the child's electrolyte balance must be monitored closely. Serum electrolytes, BUN, creatinine, albumin, total protein, calcium, magnesium, phosphorus, uric acid, plasma osmolality, colloid osmotic pressure, and arterial blood gases should all be monitored.

Potassium Balance. The child's serum potassium concentration should be assessed frequently, especially if the child develops concurrent acidosis, bleeding, or infection. Potassium administration should be curtailed unless significant hypokalemia is present.

If the child's serum potassium concentration is less than 6.5 mEq/L with no ECG changes, all that may be needed is to stop any source of potassium or drugs that decrease its secretion, and continue to monitor the child. If the serum potassium is between 6.5 and 7.0 mEq/L in the asymptomatic patient and the ECG is normal, sodium polystyrene sulfonate (Kayexalate) can be administered orally, via nasogastric tube or rectally in doses of (1-2 g/kg in sorbitol).

If the serum potassium concentration exceeds 7 mEq/L, or if there are ECG abnormalities (such as peaked T waves, widened QRS complex, bradycardia, heart block, or ventricular arrhythmias), the hyperkalemia must be treated on an urgent basis, using any of the following mechanisms:

1. Intravenous infusion of 10% calcium chloride (0.1-0.2 mL/kg [10-20 mg/kg]) over 1 to 5 minutes, or 10% calcium gluconate (0.5-1.0 mL/kg [50-100 mg/kg]) over 2 to 4 minutes. Give calcium slowly while monitoring the ECG carefully for bradycardia. The administration of calcium is thought to reduce cardiotoxicity of high serum potassium, counteracting the adverse effects of hyperkalemia on neuromuscular membranes.

2. Intravenous infusion of a sodium bicarbonate (1-3 mEq/kg [average of 2.5 mEq/kg] over 30 min will raise the serum pH so that potassium shifts from the vascular and interstitial spaces into cells (in exchange for hydrogen ions that move from the cells). The bicarbonate solution generally is diluted 1:1 with sterile water to reduce osmolality.

   NOTE: The bicarbonate solution should not be mixed with the calcium, because a precipitate will form.

3. Intravenous infusion of concentrated glucose or glucose and insulin (1-2 mL/kg of 25% glucose plus 0.1 units/kg of regular insulin) to enhance intracellular movement of potassium.

   NOTE: A solution may be prepared mixing 6 units of regular insulin with a 25% dextrose solution totaling 100 mL; administration of 1-2 mL/kg of this mixture provides the proper glucose-insulin mix[76] (Box 13-6).

4. Nebulized albuterol (rapid nebulizer or continuous nebulizer of 0.1-0.3 mg/kg) or salbutamol (IV dose of 4-5 mcg/kg over 20 min and repeated after 2 hours)[103]: as a beta-2 adrenergic agonist, albuterol activates the sodium-potassium pump and stimulates the pancreas to secrete insulin; these actions shift potassium into the cells.[81]

5. The previous treatments do not remove potassium from the body; they merely transiently lower the serum potassium concentration by shifting potassium into cells. Potassium must be removed either through the use of sodium polystyrene sulfonate or through hemodialysis or hemofiltration before the serum potassium concentration reaches critical levels.

Phosphorus and Calcium Therapy. Most patients with ARF develop hyperphosphatemia. Although a high phosphate level alone can produce symptoms, hyperphosphatemia usually produces hypocalcemia that can result in neuromuscular or cardiovascular dysfunction. In addition, the calcium and phosphorus can precipitate, forming renal crystals.

The healthcare team should treat significant hyperphosphatemia before the patient develops hypocalcemia or before mild hypocalcemia becomes severe. Severe hyperphosphatemia can be treated only with dialysis or hemofiltration.

Oral phosphate binders will bind ingested phosphate before it is absorbed.[98] Calcium carbonate (Tums) tablets will bind phosphate before absorption. Antacid solutions containing magnesium (e.g., Maalox) are avoided because the magnesium can lower calcium levels. Aluminum hydroxide solutions (Amphojel) are no longer used because aluminum deposition in bone tissue has been reported with prolonged use.

Hypocalcemia should be prevented, because it can depress cardiovascular function and exacerbate cardiac arrhythmias resulting from hyperkalemia. Hypocalcemia is most effectively treated by lowering serum phosphate levels. Significant hypocalcemia (i.e., producing tetany or cardiac arrhythmias) is usually treated with infusions of 10% calcium chloride (20 mg/kg, with a maximum dose of 1 g) or, in infants, with 10% calcium gluconate (60-100 mg/kg, with a maximum dose of 2 g). Administer the calcium slowly to prevent bradycardia.

Because patients with rhabdomyolysis and myoglobinuria tend to deposit calcium in damaged muscle, calcium infusion in children with AKI should be restricted to those children with signs of significant or symptomatic hypocalcemia or to those with severe hyperkalemia. Calcium administration is often ineffective in treating hypocalcemia unless hyperphosphatemia is corrected.

Metabolic Acidosis. The child's arterial blood gases should be monitored frequently to assess the effectiveness of oxygenation and ventilation and to determine the arterial pH. The child's serum lactate should also be monitored. Acidosis must be treated because it will depress enzyme and cellular mitochondrial function and may contribute to nausea, vomiting, hyperkalemia, and cardiovascular dysfunction.

If acidosis is severe despite effective ventilation, administration of sodium bicarbonate will be necessary. Sodium bicarbonate should not be administered in the presence of hypercarbia with respiratory acidosis, because the buffering action of bicarbonate will result in the generation of CO_2 and worsening of the respiratory acidosis.

The typical dose of the sodium bicarbonate is 1 mEq/kg, but a buffering dose also may be determined by the calculated base deficit or the child's bicarbonate or serum CO_2. The formula for calculating the sodium bicarbonate ($NaHCO_3$) dose using the base deficit is as follows[66]:

$$\text{mEq } NaHCO_3 = \text{Base deficit} \times \text{Weight (kg)} \times 0.3$$

Another formula for calculation of the $NaHCO_3$ dose is based on the patient's serum bicarbonate as follows[66]:

$$\text{mEq } NaHCO_3 = (24 - \text{Serum } HCO_3[\text{mEq/L}]) \times \text{Weight (kg)} \times 0.5$$

Sodium bicarbonate 8.4% has a high osmolality; therefore it is diluted to half strength (or 4.2% concentration is given) for administration to neonates and young infants. If possible, the total daily dose of sodium bicarbonate for all patients is limited to 8 mEq/kg, because higher total daily doses are thought to be associated with an increased risk of neurologic

---

Box 13-6	**Administration of Glucose and Insulin to Reduce Critical Hyperkalemia**

Standard dose: 1-2 mL 25% glucose/kg body weight + 0.1 unit regular insulin/kg body weight

A. Standard solution

   Combine: 6 U regular insulin plus 25% dextrose to total 100 mL

   Administer 1-2 mL/kg, **or**

B. Ratio method

   Premature infant: 0.5-1 mL 50% glucose/kg + 1 unit regular insulin/12 g glucose infused *or* 0.5-1 mL 50% glucose/kg + 0.02-0.04 units regular insulin/kg

   Child: 0.5-1 mL 50% glucose/kg + 1 unit regular insulin/ 8 g glucose infused *or* 0.5-1 mL 50% glucose/kg + 0.03-0.04 units regular insulin/kg

   Adult: 0.5-1 mL 50% glucose/kg + 1 unit regular insulin/ 4 g glucose infused *or* 0.5-1 mL 50% glucose/kg + 0.06-0.125 units regular insulin/kg

complications. Because NaHCO$_3$ does contain sodium, its administration may enhance water retention and edema.

Acidosis causes a shift of the potassium into the extracellular compartment, including the vascular space, resulting in an elevation in the serum potassium concentration. As a result, acidosis should be prevented in the patient with AKI, because it will worsen existing hyperkalemia.

Glucose. The infant's serum glucose concentration should be checked frequently with point-of-care testing (e.g., heelstick glucose evaluation) so that hypoglycemia can be detected and treated promptly. When hypoglycemia is present, treatment with a continuous glucose infusion (2-4 mL/kg per hour of 5% dextrose solution or 1-2 mL/kg per hour of 10% dextrose solution) is preferable to intermittent bolus infusion of hypertonic glucose, because repeated bolus therapy can cause intermittent increases in the serum osmolality and contribute to the risk of intracranial hemorrhage.[84] If the serum glucose is extremely low, an initial bolus dose of glucose (2-4 mL/kg of 25% dextrose, diluted for infants and for peripheral infusion) may be necessary to establish an adequate serum glucose concentration. The continuous glucose infusion must, of course, be considered when totaling fluid intake.

Hematologic Complications. Because AKI can produce anemia and coagulopathies, the nurse should look for petechiae, ecchymoses, gastrointestinal bleeding, or other sources of bleeding. A BUN >100 mg/dL increases bleeding time caused by platelet dysfunction.

The healthcare team should evaluate the child's platelet count, prothrombin time, and activated partial thromboplastin time on a regular basis, and administer appropriate blood components as needed (see Chapter 15 for doses of and cautions regarding blood component therapy).

The child's hematocrit should be measured daily, and a sudden fall in the hematocrit should be verified and reported to an on-call provider immediately, because it may indicate the presence of bleeding. Anemia in the patient with AKI can result from compromise in kidney production of erythropoietin factor or from uremic bone marrow suppression, and may also be caused by frequent blood sampling.

Transfusions of packed RBCs should be provided to maintain a satisfactory hematocrit (infants, above 40%; children, above 30%-35%) according to physician (or on-call provider) order and unit policy, with consideration of the child's fluid restriction and volume status. Packed RBCs are preferred to minimize volume and potassium administration. Washed cells should be used if renal transplantation is anticipated.

If bleeding develops, desmopressin or l-deamino-8-arginine vasopressin (DDAVP) will correct uremic platelet dysfunction, although the mechanism of action is unclear. The effects of an intravenous dose of approximately 0.3-0.4 mcg/kg should be apparent within several hours. Side effects are minimal, although fluid retention may be exacerbated by this drug. DDAVP also may be administered prophylactically to patients with uremia to prevent bleeding during surgery.[51]

Gastrointestinal bleeding is a potential complication of AKI resulting from uremic platelet dysfunction, stress, and use of anticoagulant during hemodialysis or hemofiltration

therapy. Ranitidine or other H$_2$ blockers can be used to prevent gastric ulcer formation and associated bleeding.

If the child develops a coagulopathy, the number of venipunctures and injections prescribed should be minimized. If venipuncture is required, apply pressure for 5 to 15 minute, or longer if necessary, to reduce the risk of hematoma.

Infection Control. The child with AKI is often immunologically and nutritionally compromised and usually requires insertion of multiple catheters and tubes for hemodynamic monitoring, urine drainage, or dialysis. In addition, the child is examined frequently every day by many physicians and nurses. These aspects of care all increase the risk of healthcare-acquired infection. It is therefore imperative that every member of the healthcare team adopt flawless hand-washing technique before and after examination of the child to reduce the child's risk of nosocomial infection.

Notify the physician or other provider if the child develops a fever or any localizing signs of infection, such as wound drainage. Blood cultures should be obtained if bacteremia is suspected.

Treatment of Hypertension. When the child with AKI develops hypervolemia, hypertension can result. This hypertension can be exacerbated by the high plasma renin activity that accompanies some renal disorders. If hypertension becomes severe, neurologic complications, such as hypertensive encephalopathy, and cardiovascular compromise can develop. Sodium and water restriction is critical, and diuretic therapy may be of benefit.

Antihypertensives will be prescribed if the infant or child demonstrates severe hypertension or moderate hypertension with symptoms (Box 13-7). The use of angiotensin converting enzyme inhibitors (e.g., captopril) is controversial in patients with AKI, because it can decrease renal blood flow and cause potential ischemic injury.[71,73] The doses of all drugs should be evaluated and adjusted as needed in the presence of reduced GFR (see section, Adjustment of Medication Dosages).

Box 13-7 | **Examples of Drugs Used to Treat Hypertension in Patients with Renal Failure**

Intravenous
- Sodium nitroprusside: begin with infusion of 0.3-0.5 mcg/kg per min, and titrate to a maximum infusion of 8 mcg/kg per min
- Labetalol: 0.25-1 mg/kg per hour—titrate to patient response with a maximum dose of 3 mg/kg per hour
- Hydralazine: 0.1-0.2 mg/kg per dose
- Esmolol: 75-300 mcg/kg per min*

Oral
- Nifedipine: 0.25-0.5 mg/kg PO every 6-8 hours (capsules may be pierced and liquid placed sublingually)
- Hydralazine: 1-3 mg/kg per day, not to exceed 20 mg/dose
- Isradipine: 0.05-0.15 mg/kg per dose maximum dose 5 mg qid
- Propranolol: 0.5-1 mg/kg per day, given in three divided doses

*Vogt BA and Avner ED: Conditions particularly associated with proteinuria. In Kliegman RM, et al, editors: *Nelson textbook of pediatrics*, ed 18. Philadelphia, 2007, WB Saunders.

Table 13-5	Estimated Normal Maintenance Caloric Requirements for Infants and Children

Age	Kcal/kg per 24 hours
0-6 months	90-110
6-12 months	80-100
12-36 months	75-90
4-10 years	65-75
>10 years, male	40-45
>10 years, female	38-30

Nutrient	Percent of total daily calories	
Carbohydrates	40-70	Combined 85-88
Fat	20-50	
Protein	7-15	

Nutrition. If the child can tolerate oral or nasogastric feedings, these should be instituted as soon as possible to prevent excess protein catabolism. If oral or nasogastric feedings are impossible, parenteral alimentation should be instituted within the limits of the child's daily fluid restriction.

Any form of nutrition should provide calories in the form of glucose or essential amino acids to minimize the accumulation of metabolic waste products.[98] The child's daily caloric requirements will total approximately 50% to 75% of normal daily maintenance requirements when AKI is present, because a large portion of the daily maintenance calories are used for basal requirements and growth (Table 13-5).

Adjustment of Medication Dosages. When the child develops renal failure, the healthcare team should reevaluate the doses of all drugs the child is receiving, especially drugs excreted by the kidney. The drug dose can be reduced or the interval between drug doses can be increased in light of the child's reduced GFR. A review of guidelines for drug therapy in renal failure should be consulted to determine the relative portion of renal and nonrenal modes of excretion of specific drugs.[7]

If the rate of nonrenal excretion of a drug and the child's creatinine clearance are known, providers can estimate the daily excretion of the drug, and therefore the daily replacement dose needed. If drug levels are available, they should be used to evaluate drug metabolism and drug replacement requirements.

Dose adjustments should be made carefully for those drugs with potentially toxic metabolites (e.g., partial metabolism of sodium nitroprusside results in thiocyanate and cyanide formation). Drug levels should be assessed frequently in these patients. Even after the dose of a drug has been reduced, the nurse must be alert for evidence of drug toxicity; this requires knowledge of side and toxic effects of each drug that the child is receiving. Of course, if dialysis is instituted, the medication doses will again require adjustment.

Psychosocial Aspects. When the child develops AKI, the child and the family are usually frightened. At the same time that the nurse must provide the most thorough observations and skilled care, the child and family are most in need of reassurance and support. If the child's physical care requires the nurse's undivided attention, the nurse should request assistance from a colleague or additional supportive staff (e.g., chaplain, social worker, patient ombudsman). The child requires explanations and preparation for uncomfortable treatments or procedures (as age appropriate), gentle handling, and soothing verbal and nonverbal interaction. (See Chapter 2 for further information.) Box 13-8 summarizes the care of the child with AKI.

Indications for Dialysis. If the condition of the infant or child with AKI continues to deteriorate despite aggressive medical management, then peritoneal dialysis, hemodialysis, or continuous renal replacement therapy (CRRT) may be required. The indications for dialysis and choices for renal replacement therapy are listed in the following section.

CARE OF THE CHILD DURING DIALYSIS, HEMOPERFUSION, AND HEMOFILTRATION

Dialysis in Children

Dialysis is indicated for the child with AKI when aggressive medical management has failed to control hypervolemia, hypertension, bleeding, hyperkalemia, hyperuricemia, or acidosis. Dialysis also is indicated when uremia produces cardiovascular or neurologic deterioration or when elimination of toxins or poisons is required (Box 13-9).

Both hemodialysis and peritoneal dialysis use osmotic and concentration gradients between the child's blood and the dialysate to reduce the child's intravascular volume and to alter intravascular electrolyte concentrations. The content of the dialysate, or dialysis solution, will determine the specific changes made in the child's volume and electrolyte status.

When peritoneal dialysis is used, a peritoneal catheter is inserted and the dialysate is infused into the peritoneal cavity, so that it comes into contact with the peritoneal membrane. The peritoneal membrane acts as the semipermeable membrane, allowing diffusion of electrolytes and water between the peritoneal capillaries and the dialysate.

In children, peritoneal dialysis removes water and electrolytes from the blood by virtue of the osmotic and electrolyte concentration gradients that exist between the dialysate and the patient's blood (across the peritoneal membrane). Manipulation of the osmolality and electrolyte concentration of the dialysate determines the quantity and speed of fluid movement. Peritoneal dialysis enables fluid removal at a rate slower than hemodialysis, so can avoid the complications created by rapid intravascular and extravascular fluid and electrolyte shifts.

Hemodialysis uses an artificial semipermeable membrane and dialysate located outside the patient's body (i.e., it is extracorporeal). Vascular access for acute hemodialysis can be achieved with single- or double-lumen catheters inserted in the vena cava or upper right arm, using the femoral, internal jugular, or subclavian approach. These catheters can be maintained in place for long periods of time. Chronic hemodialysis in the older child may require placement of an arteriovenous fistula or graft.

If good circulatory access is achieved, hemodialysis is much more efficient than peritoneal dialysis in the child and

Box 13-8   Nursing Care of the Child with Acute Kidney Injury (Acute Renal Failure)

1. Potential Acute Prerenal Failure Related to:
- Poor systemic perfusion
- Inadequate renal perfusion

Expected Patient Outcomes
- Patient will demonstrate effective systemic perfusion.
- Patient will demonstrate normal urine output with good renal concentrating ability (specific gravity greater than 1.005) when urine volume is reduced.
- Patient will demonstrate adequate, but not excessive, intravascular volume.
- Patient will demonstrate normal serum electrolyte concentration (including BUN and creatinine).

Nursing Interventions
- Record urine volume and total fluid intake hourly and notify provider if urine output <1-2 mL/kg per hour or if fluid intake greatly exceeds output.
- Insert and maintain urinary catheter—ensure that catheter is functioning properly. Irrigate per physician (or other on-call provider) order or unit policy if patency is questionable. Maintain aseptic technique when manipulating catheter.
- Ensure that catheter tubing is placed to facilitate gravity drainage of urine.
- Record urine osmolality and specific gravity every 2-4 hours (or per orders or unit policy); notify on-call provider if urine osmolality and specific gravity do not rise when urine volume falls.
- Monitor color of urine; notify on-call provider of cloudy or rusty urine. Cloudy urine can indicate infection or the presence of cell casts in the urine. Rusty urine can indicate hemolysis.
- Assess patient's systemic perfusion: skin should be warm, peripheral pulses should be strong, capillary refill should be brisk, and mucous membranes should be pink. If the skin is cool, peripheral pulses are difficult to palpate, and capillary refill is sluggish, or color is pale or mottled, notify the on-call provider. Monitor urine output; a fall in urine output in the presence of poor systemic perfusion may indicate inadequate renal perfusion, and on-call provider should be notified.
- Support cardiovascular function as needed (and ordered) to maintain urine output greater than 1 mL/kg per hour. Fluid challenge of 20 mL/kg isotonic crystalloid or colloid initially may be ordered to improve systemic perfusion. If systemic perfusion does not improve despite the presence of a CVP greater than 5-10 mm Hg and signs of adequate intravascular volume (see Box 13-11), administration of inotropic agents or vasodilators may be necessary.
- Administer diuretic agents (furosemide [1-2 mg/kg IV] or mannitol [0.25-0.5 g/kg]) as ordered; monitor patient response and notify on-call provider if response is inadequate.
- Obtain urine samples as ordered for laboratory analysis of osmolality, sodium concentration, BUN and creatinine. Simultaneous serum samples must also be obtained.
- If prerenal failure is present, serum BUN will usually begin to rise before serum creatinine.
- When hypovolemia produces prerenal failure, urine sodium content will fall to less than 10 mEq/L (sodium is actively reabsorbed by functioning kidneys in presence of hypovolemia), and urine osmolality will exceed 500 mOsm/L (kidneys conserving water).

- After urine and serum electrolytes are obtained, calculate FE_{Na}

$$FE_{Na} = \left[\frac{(U_{Na}/P_{Na})}{(U_{Cr}/P_{Cr})} \right] \times 100$$

Where
U_{Na} = Urine sodium concentration
P_{Na} = Plasma (serum) sodium concentration
U_{Cr} = Urine creatinine concentration
P_{Cr} = Plasma (serum) creatinine concentration

An FE_{Na} of less than 1% in children and less than 2.5% in neonates is associated with prerenal failure, and an FE_{Na} greater than 1% to 3% is usually associated with intrinsic AKI.

NOTE: This calculation will not provide a valid indicator of the type of AKI present if diuretics, including mannitol, are administered before measuring urine and serum sodium and creatinine, because these drugs will increase urine sodium content regardless of the effectiveness of renal function.

2. Potential Hypervolemia/Fluid Volume Excess Related to:
- Oliguria
- Excessive fluid administration
- Sodium and water retention

Expected Patient Outcomes
- Patient will not demonstrate signs of hypervolemia, including high CVP, hepatomegaly, systemic edema, tachycardia, hypertension, tachypnea or increased requirement for ventilation support, pulmonary edema, high pulmonary artery wedge pressure, full (tense) fontanelle in infants, hyponatremia.
- Patient will not demonstrate excessive weight gain (greater than 50 g/24 hours in infants, greater than 200 g/24 hours in children, greater than 500 g/24 hours in adolescents).

Nursing Interventions
- Measure and record all fluid intake and output hourly; notify on-call provider immediately if urine output falls or positive fluid balance is present.
- Limit fluid intake (as ordered) once AKI is suspected. Typically, fluid intake is restricted to 300-400 mL/m² BSA per day plus urine output if renal failure is present. Minimize fluid used to flush monitoring lines and dilute medications. Closely supervise oral intake, if allowed or tolerated.
- Administer diuretic therapy as ordered. Monitor patient's urine response and monitor electrolyte balance closely.
- Monitor for signs of hypervolemia including tachycardia, high CVP or PAWP, systemic and pulmonary edema and hypertension, possible signs of congestive heart failure.
- Measure child's weight daily or twice daily (as ordered or per unit policy); utilize same scale each time and ensure consistent weighing time. Use bed scales for unstable patients. Notify provider of excessive weight gain.
- Be prepared to assist in initiation of CRRT if clinically significant hypervolemia develops.

3. Potential Electrolyte Imbalance Related to:
- Decreased renal potassium excretion
- Increased renal sodium excretion
- Decreased renal excretion of phosphate, calcium phosphate precipitation and decreased renal activation of vitamin D

Box 13-8 **Nursing Care of the Child with Acute Kidney Injury (Acute Renal Failure)—cont'd**

Expected Patient Outcome
- Patient will demonstrate normal serum electrolytes.

Nursing Interventions
- Monitor patient's serum electrolytes closely; notify on-call provider of abnormal results, including high or rapidly rising potassium concentration.
- Limit potassium intake (as ordered).
- Monitor for clinical signs of hyperkalemia, including peaked T wave, arrhythmias, diarrhea, and muscle weakness. If hyperkalemia is suspected, notify on-call provider, obtain serum sample for measurement of potassium concentration, and prepare to institute emergency measures to reduce serum potassium concentration.
- If significant hyperkalemia is present, administer (as ordered):
  ○ Calcium chloride (10% solution: 20 mg/kg) or calcium gluconate (10% solution: 60-100 mg/kg)
  ○ Sodium bicarbonate: 1 mEq/kg
  ○ Concentrated glucose: 1-2 mL/kg of 25% dextrose *or* glucose plus insulin (0.1 U/kg): combine 6 units regular insulin with 25% Dextrose to total 100 mL; administer 1-2 mL/kg (for further information, see Box 13-6)
  ○ Administer sodium polystyrene sulfonate (Kayexalate) enema as ordered (0.5 g/kg of 20% solution) approximately two to three times per day to reduce serum potassium approximately 1 mEq/L per 24 hours.
- If symptomatic hyperkalemia persists, prepare to assist with initiation of hemofiltration or dialysis.
- Be prepared to support cardiovascular function as needed.
- Monitor serum sodium concentration; notify provider of hyponatremia or hypernatremia.
- Monitor for clinical evidence of hyponatremia, including change in level of consciousness, muscle cramps, anorexia, abnormal reflexes, Cheyne-Stokes respiration, or seizures. Notify on-call provider if these are observed, obtain serum sample to evaluate sodium concentration, and prepare to administer 3% saline if ordered (2-4 mEq/kg).
- Monitor serum calcium concentration; notify physician of reduced total or ionized calcium concentration.
- Monitor for clinical signs of hypocalcemia, including muscle tingling or change in muscle tone, seizures, tetany, positive Chvostek sign (twitching of the side of the face when the facial nerve is tapped in front of the ear), or compromised cardiovascular function. If these signs are observed, notify the on-call provider, draw a serum sample for measurement of total and ionized serum calcium concentrations, and prepare to administer calcium chloride (20 mg/kg of 10% CaCl; use calcium gluconate in infant).
- Administer antacid-phosphate binders (as ordered) to reduce serum phosphate levels.
- Administer vitamin D as ordered to enhance calcium absorption.

4. Potential Metabolic Acidosis Related to:
- Poor systemic perfusion associated with prerenal failure
- Decreased renal ability to excrete hydrogen ions

Expected Patient Outcomes
- Serum pH, serum lactate and serum bicarbonate within normal levels
- Anion gap less than 15 mEq/L

Nursing Interventions
- Monitor arterial blood gases and serum lactate, and notify provider of development of acidosis.
- If metabolic acidosis develops, administer sodium bicarbonate as ordered (1 mEq/kg or mEq dose to correct part or all of the calculated deficit: base deficit × Weight in kg × 0.3).
- Administer sodium bicarbonate only if ventilation is effective or effectively supported.
- Monitor serum potassium concentration, because acidosis will produce a rise in serum potassium concentration.
- Calculate anion gap (AG):

$$AG = ([Na^+] + [K^+]) - ([Cl^-] + [HCO_3^-])$$

Anion gap exceeding 11-14 mEq/L can be associated with metabolic acidosis or alteration in serum potassium, calcium, or magnesium ions.

5. Potential Drug Toxicity Related to:
- Reduced renal excretion of drugs or drug metabolites

Expected Patient Outcomes
- Patient will not demonstrate clinical or laboratory evidence of drug toxicity.

Nursing Interventions
- When renal failure develops, review patient's drug doses and drug administration schedule, and discuss these with on-call provider (doses of drugs excreted by kidneys will be reduced as renal function is reduced).
- Note clinical signs of toxicity of all drugs child receives in the nursing care plan, and monitor for these signs; notify on-call provider of any signs of drug toxicity.

6. Potential Infection, Related to:
- Multiple invasive catheters
- Compromised immune system
- Compromised nutritional intake
- Poor nutritional status

Expected Patient Outcome
- Patient will demonstrate no leukocytosis, fever, or localizing signs of infection, sepsis or septic shock (see Chapter 6).

Nursing Interventions
- Perform meticulous hand washing before and after patient contact; ensure that hand washing is performed by every member of the healthcare team.
- Change all dressings and IV tubing per unit policy.
- Monitor patient temperature and white blood cell count, and notify physician (or on-call provider) of fever, leukocytosis, or leukopenia.
- Assess all skin puncture sites and notify provider of any erythemia, drainage, or fluctuance of wound edges, obtain cultures of urine, skin puncture sites, and blood (as ordered) if infection or sepsis are suspected.
- Monitor appearance of urine and peritoneal dialysis fluid; notify physician of cloudiness and obtain cultures as ordered.
- Administer antibiotics as ordered (check dose in light of compromised renal function).

7. Potential Patient/Family Anxiety Related to:
- Limited understanding of patient condition
- Patient fluid and electrolyte imbalance
- Severity of patient condition

Continued

Box 13-8 Nursing Care of the Child with Acute Kidney Injury (Acute Renal Failure)—cont'd

Expected Patient Outcomes
- Child will be able to cooperate (as age-appropriate) with treatment plan and will not demonstrate any self-destructive behavior.
- Family members will demonstrate understanding of the child's illness, prognosis, and treatment and will be able to participate in the child's care.

Nursing Interventions
- Provide the child (as age-appropriate) and family with consistent explanations and support (see Chapter 2).
- Provide the child with positive reinforcement and encouragement.
- Provide explanations before any treatments are performed, and prepare the child for painful therapy with truthful information.
- Plan activities that will allow the child (as age-appropriate) to demonstrate anger, frustration, or sadness; encourage expression of these feelings if the child is willing to discuss them.

8. Potential Patient Discomfort or Pain Related to:
- Invasive catheters
- Electrolyte imbalances
- Multiple venipunctures, diagnostic studies
- Multiple invasive catheters or treatments
- Neuropathies associated with electrolyte imbalances

Expected Patient Outcomes
- Patient will verbalize (as age-appropriate) or communicate the absence of pain or a decrease in pain.

Nursing Interventions
- Assess patient for evidence of pain, including tachycardia, splinting of abdomen or extremities, facial grimace, tears, expressions of pain.

- Use consistent tool to assess presence, severity, and location of pain; use tool to monitor effectiveness of analgesia provided (see Chapter 5).
- Handle the child gently.

9. Impaired Skin Integrity Related to:
- Uremia

Expected Patient Outcomes
- Patient will demonstrate no skin breakdown.
- Urticaria will not cause patient discomfort.

Nursing Interventions
- Keep skin warm and dry.
- Change patient position frequently.
- Assess skin integrity; apply lotion to areas of irritation.
- Administer antihistamines and apply antipruritic lotions as ordered; monitor effectiveness.

10. Potential Compromise in Nutrition Related to:
- Renal disease

Expected Patient Outcomes
- Patient will demonstrate nutrition adequate to prevent protein catabolism.
- Positive nitrogen balance will be maintained. Patient will not demonstrate weight loss, and weight will be appropriate for age.

Nursing Interventions
- Assess patient's baseline nutritional status.
- Monitor patient's total caloric intake (including oral and IV intake) and calculate patient's nutritional requirements; discuss with provider if patient is receiving inadequate nutrition.
- Monitor for signs of poor nutrition, including decreased albumin, poor skin turgor, delayed wound healing, weight loss, diarrhea, or constipation.
- Obtain order for consultation with dietician.

AKI, Acute kidney injury; *BSA,* body surface area; *BUN,* blood urea nitrogen; *CRRT,* continuous renal replacement therapy; *CVP,* central venous pressure; FE_{Na}, fractional excretion of filtered sodium; *IV,* intravenous.

Box 13-9 Indications for Dialysis in Children

Hypervolemia with congestive heart failure, uncontrolled hypertension, or hypertensive encephalopathy
Deterioration in neurologic status
Bleeding that is unresponsive to blood component therapy
Biochemical alterations (these criteria are not absolute):
- Serum potassium concentration above 6.5-7 mEq/L, despite maximal medical therapy and administration of sodium polystyrene sulfonate exchange resin
- Persistent metabolic acidosis, particularly in the presence of hypervolemia or hyperkalemia

- Serum BUN greater than 125-150 mg/dL
- Serum sodium concentration above 160 mEq/L
- Serum calcium concentration above 12 mg/dL
Acute poisonings or drug toxicity, including ingestion of the following substances:
- Salicylates
- Phenytoin
- Barbiturates
- Heavy metals
- Other poisons

---

adolescent. Hemodialysis with hemoperfusion is especially effective for the removal of poisons after drug overdose. However, good circulatory access can be difficult to obtain in infants or young children. In addition, the volume of the hemodialysis circuit cannot exceed 10% of the child's circulating blood volume unless the circuit is primed with blood before each use. As a result, hemodialysis during infancy should be performed only at institutions experienced in the procedure.

Two additional techniques, hemoperfusion and hemofiltration, can be used to adjust serum water and electrolyte concentrations. These techniques will be discussed in two separate sections, Hemoperfusion and Hemofiltration, below.

Acute Peritoneal Dialysis

When the decision to begin peritoneal dialysis (PD) is made, informed consent is obtained from the parents by the physician. The results of serum chemistries obtained within the previous 8 hours should be available at the bedside, and the child's weight is obtained before dialysis. If the child is small, the predialysis weight should be obtained after the peritoneal catheter is in place and dressings are applied.

There are few contraindications to PD in children. Patient age and size do not constitute any contraindication, because PD has been performed in small neonates. However, neonates with omphalocele, diaphragmatic hernia, or gastroschisis cannot be treated with PD.

Recent abdominal surgery is not a contraindication to PD, provided the patient has no draining abdominal wounds. However, smaller infusion volumes will be required in these patients. Minor abdominal adhesions will not preclude successful PD, although extensive adhesions may prevent successful instillation and removal of the dialysate.

The presence of a vesicostomy or other urinary diversion, polycystic kidneys, colostomy, gastrostomy, or prune-belly syndrome does not preclude the use of PD. Acute renal failure associated with renal transplant rejection can be treated with peritoneal dialysis, provided the allograft has been placed in the extraperitoneal space.

Bedside (Percutaneous) Placement of Peritoneal Catheter

If peritoneal dialysis is expected to be required for a short time (<72 hours), the catheter can be placed percutaneously at the bedside (i.e., not surgically). When bedside placement is planned, all needed equipment is assembled and checked before the procedure (see Box 13-10). Because the incidence of catheter-related infection increases when percutaneously placed catheters remain in place beyond 72 hours, surgical catheter placement (i.e., in the operating suite) is indicated if peritoneal dialysis is expected to be required beyond 3 days.

When the decision for dialysis is first considered, the preparation of the child must begin. The discussion should be appropriate for the child's age and comprehension, and it should involve the physician, family, and nurse. The nurse must attempt to understand the aspects of the procedure that are frightening or confusing to the child and address those points directly. It is important that the parents understand the procedure and support the child throughout the dialysis.

The parents and the nurse must be comfortable with the facts before attempting to discuss them with the child. Often a sedative will be prescribed for the child to reduce pain and anxiety during the procedure.

A surgical preparation of the abdomen is performed, using a surgical skin cleaner, followed by an appropriate scrub. Sterile procedure will be used throughout catheter placement, which requires that the surgeon and any assistants wear gown, gloves, and masks. Local anesthetic is infiltrated along the lower quadrant of the abdominal wall. Before perforation of the abdominal wall, the child's vital signs should be documented for comparison during the procedure.

The 16-gauge polyethylene over-the-needle catheter is joined to the primed dialysate tubing, and the needle and catheter are inserted into the abdomen at the midline. Using the symphysis pubis and the umbilicus as distance markers, the catheter will be inserted one third of the total distance down from the umbilicus. The catheter is joined to the tubing of a warmed and primed bag of dialysate and is advanced into the peritoneal cavity until the drip chamber of the inflow line demonstrates free flow of solution into the abdomen. The inflow should be interrupted temporarily while the inflow line is disconnected and the steel needle is removed from the catheter. The catheter is then advanced into the abdomen (to the hub), the tubing is connected

---

Box 13-10   Equipment Typically Needed for Bedside Placement of Peritoneal Dialysis (PD) Catheter

1. Two pediatric PD catheters with trocars, Y tubing, and a PD tray, dialysate fluid with warmer.
   - A blood warmer and administration coil or warming pad with thermometer is needed.
   - Water baths are inconvenient and introduce risk of contamination, so should not be used. Do not use a microwave oven to warm the fluid, because doing so produces inconsistent heating and a burn risk.
2. Acute PD is accomplished with four or six 2-L bags of dialysate containing either 1.5% glucose or 4.25% glucose. The dialysate must be warmed to body temperature before infusion, to prevent hypothermia. Dialysate bags must be checked for punctures or leaks before use.
3. A patent urinary catheter must be in place. If the child's catheter has been in place for several days, it may be wise to replace it to ensure patency; this ensures the emptying of the bladder and reduces the risk of bladder perforation when the PD catheter is placed.
4. Laboratory results obtained within the previous 8 hours should include hemoglobin, hematocrit, BUN, electrolytes, glucose, phosphorus, uric acid (if appropriate, as in uric acid nephropathy associated with chemotherapy), a PT,

aPTT, and platelet count, as well as a type and cross match for a unit of blood (or packed cells).

5. One thousand units of sodium heparin are added to each 2-L bag of dialysate (500 U/L) unless frank abdominal bleeding is present. Heparin crosses the peritoneal membrane poorly, and its presence in the dialysate will reduce fibrin formation and assist in maintaining peritoneal catheter patency.
6. Two 16-gauge polyethylene over-the-needle catheters and two short sets of extension tubing. Two sets of tubing are used to infuse a volume of solution into the peritoneum to distend the peritoneal space and reduce the risk of bowel perforation when the trocar is inserted.
7. Two small (1-mL) syringes and lidocaine (Xylocaine) without epinephrine.
8. No. 11 blade.
9. Sterile gloves, masks, and gowns.
10. Sterile dressings, tape, surgical skin cleaner, and povidone-iodine solution.
11. Tubes for culture of the peritoneal fluid. The first outflow is cultured, and then cultures of fluid are obtained from every sixth pass

aPTT, Activated partial thromboplastin time; *PD,* periotoneal dialysis; *PT,* prothrombin time.

to the catheter, and a volume of 30 mL/kg is infused into the abdomen to distend it. Occasionally, a volume of up to 50 mL/kg is required to elevate the anterior abdominal wall sufficiently. During fluid infusion, the child's ventilation and perfusion must be monitored closely; infusion should be interrupted if cardiorespiratory distress develops.

When the peritoneal space is judged to be full and the abdominal wall is elevated and tense, the catheter is withdrawn and a small stab wound is made at the site of catheter insertion (without entering the peritoneum). The catheter and trocar are then inserted using steady pressure aimed at the right or left lower quadrant. Once the abdominal wall is penetrated, the catheter will be advanced as the trocar is withdrawn. Easy inflow and outflow of fluid should occur through the catheter.[101]

The catheter will be trimmed to leave only 4 to 6 cm outside the abdominal wall. The catheter should be secured with a silk purse-string suture and water-resistant tape. The outflow tubing is then clamped, and the first warmed exchange dialysate of 20 to 30 mL/kg is infused.

The child's blood pressure, temperature, respiratory rate, and heart rate are assessed and documented every 15 minutes for 1 hour, then every hour once the child's condition is stable. Changes in the child's level of consciousness and activity level should be noted and reported to a physician, because these can indicate serious fluid or electrolyte disturbances.

The dialysate remains in the peritoneal space for 15 to 90 minutes (this may vary), and then the outflow connection is opened and the fluid is drained slowly. All subsequent weights are obtained at the end of the outflow cycle when the peritoneal cavity is empty.

If the dialysate fails to drain easily, the catheter is probably obstructed by omentum. If the problem continues, surgical replacement of the catheter may be required. If the dialysate returns cloudy or consistently bloody, or if diarrhea or polyuria are noted, a physician should be notified immediately; these signs may indicate perforation of the bowel or bladder. The catheter must be removed and replaced, and the patient should be observed closely for evidence of further symptoms.[101]

Surgical Placement of Dialysis Catheter

When the dialysis catheter is placed surgically, a cuffed catheter is used and is inserted at the level of the umbilicus through a small incision in the rectus muscle. The catheter is inserted to the level of the Dacron cuff and is held in place with a peritoneal purse-string suture. Once the catheter is inserted, a small volume of dialysate or normal saline is infused in the catheter to ensure that the site does not leak and that fluid flows easily into and out of the catheter. Finally, the catheter is tunneled under the skin and exits through the skin at a site separate from the catheter entrance into the peritoneal cavity.[3]

Dialysate Solution

Commercially available dialysis solutions contain electrolytes in concentrations similar to that of normal plasma, except that potassium is absent and the concentration of glucose and osmolality vary. The absence of potassium ion creates a concentration gradient for potassium between the dialysate and the capillary vessels of the peritoneum so that potassium moves from the vascular space into the dialysate.

The dialysate is selected by glucose concentration and osmolality; the higher the glucose and osmolality of the dialysate, the greater will be the fluid shift from the vascular space to the dialysate (i.e., more fluid is withdrawn from the child). Commercially available solutions contain 1.5% (15 g glucose/L, osmolality of 347 mOsm/L), 2.5% (25 g glucose/L, osmolality of 398 mOsm/L), and 4.25% glucose (42.5 g glucose/L, osmolality of 486 mOsm/L). Because glucose can move from the dialysate into the vascular space according to a concentration gradient, the child's serum glucose must be monitored closely. In the patient without diabetes, endogenous insulin secretion should prevent hyperglycemia, but insulin should be added to the dialysate of diabetic patients (see "Fluid or Electrolyte Imbalance").

Commercially available dialysates vary in electrolyte concentration (Table 13-6). Some critically ill infants are unable to tolerate lactate in the dialysate, because the lactate may worsen acidosis. Dialysate can be reformulated in the hospital pharmacy, using a sterile hood, to contain bicarbonate instead of lactate (see Table 13-6). When the dialysate contains bicarbonate, calcium must be administered intravenously and cannot be added to the dialysate; it will precipitate with the bicarbonate.

If the serum potassium concentration begins to fall after several dialysis cycles (usually 4-6 cycles are required), a small amount of potassium (typically to a maximum of 4 mEq/L) may be added to the dialysate with a physician or other on-call provider order.

Dialysis Exchange

The initial dialysate volume (inflow or exchange volume) is determined by the method of catheter placement. If the catheter is placed percutaneously at the bedside, initial exchange volumes of 20 to 30 mL/kg are used. If the catheter is placed surgically, smaller initial volumes (15-20 mL/kg) are used to reduce the likelihood of leak around the catheter.[3] Small exchange volumes also may be necessary if respiratory distress is present and the child is breathing spontaneously.[101] Heparin (500 units/L) usually is added to the dialysate for the first 24 hours of dialysis.

Exchange volumes are increased gradually as tolerated to 35 to 50 mL/kg/exchange. These volumes are ideal because they enable the correction of acidosis, electrolyte imbalance, and uremia.

Typically, 2.5% glucose dialysate is utilized for initial exchanges in the uremic child with acidosis and hyperkalemia. If fluid removal is not required, 1.5% glucose dialysate may be utilized. The 4.25% glucose dialysate is used for those patients with hypervolemia requiring fluid removal. The prolonged use of 4.25% glucose dialysate can be associated with hyperglycemia, hyponatremia, and hypovolemia.

For each exchange, dialysate is instilled over 5 minutes with a dwell time of 15 to 90 minutes (this may vary). The drain time varies with the size of the patient and the exchange volume; usually 5 to 10 minutes is sufficient, although drain times of 20 minutes may be required. Peritoneal dialysis is maximally effective during the first 15 to 90 minutes of dwell time. Therefore if maximum fluid removal and correction of hyperkalemia, acidosis, and uremia are required, frequent exchanges (often every 30 minutes) are performed.

Table 13-6 Standard and Modified Peritoneal Dialysis Fluids

	1.5% Dextrose	2.5% Dextrose	4.25% Dextrose
Standard Dialysis Solutions (2-L Volumes)*			
Dextrose in water	15 g/L	25 g/L	42.5 g/L
Sodium	132 mEq/L	132 mEq/L	132 mEq/L
Calcium	3.5 mEq/L	3.5 mEq/L	3.5 mEq/L
Magnesium	0.5-1.5 mEq/L	1.5 mEq/L	1.5 mEq/L
Chloride	102 mEq/L	102 mEq/L	102 mEq/L
Lactate	35-40 mEq/L	35 mEq/L	35 mEq/L
Total osmolality	347 mOsm/L	398 mOsm/L	486 mOsm/L
Approximate pH	5.5	5.5	5.5
Lactate-free Dialysate Solution[†]			
NaCl (0.45%)	896 mL	—	—
NaCl (2.5 mEq/mL)	12 mL	—	—
NaHCO$_3$ (1 mEq/mL)	40 mL	—	—
MgSO$_4$ (10%)	1.8 mL	—	—
50% dextrose/water:	50 mL	—	—
Total volume	999.8 mL	—	—
Electrolyte Content			
Sodium	139 mEq/L	—	—
Chloride	99 mEq/L	—	—
Magnesium	1.5 mEq/L	—	—
Sulfate	1.5 mEq/L	—	—
HCO$_3$	40 mEq/L	—	—
Glucose	25 g	—	—
Calculated osmolality	423 mOsm/L	—	—

*Diamed, Travenol Laboratories. Baxter US, Deerfield, IL
[†]Calcium must be provided intravenously.

Automated peritoneal dialysis cyclers are now available that provide exchange volumes as small as 50 to 100 mL. These cyclers incorporate a heater to warm the dialysate, and they automatically monitor the drain volume or outflow and can calculate the volume of fluid removed from the patient. Audible alarms indicate volume or infusion problems. Because the equipment manipulates the dialysate it can substantially reduce the nursing time needed for each exchange.

Manual peritoneal dialysis requires the use of buretrols or other graduated cylinders to monitor the precise volume of fluid infused and drained. When the exchange volume is small, buretrols can be used to measure both inflow and outflow (drain) volume. Graduated urine collection systems also can be utilized to measure outflow volume. Finally, the serial dialysate drainage bags used for continuous ambulatory peritoneal dialysis also can be utilized to measure the drain volume; clamps are used to direct the draining fluid into a separate bag following each exchange.

The large (2-L) dialysate bags should never be hung so they infuse directly into the child; if a clamp loosens or is inadvertently left open, the entire 2 L volume could be infused into the child's abdomen, causing respiratory distress and possible cardiovascular collapse. The dialysate fluid always should be warmed before use in infants and children to prevent heat loss and reduce discomfort. Room temperature dialysate may be used in adolescents unless it produces discomfort.

For dialysis in infants, exchange volumes will be small and tubing dead space should be minimized. Adult peritoneal dialysis Y tubing sets contain too much dead space for use in infants, so intravenous tubing (containing a Y or a stopcock) can be utilized to direct dialysate flow. Infant peritoneal dialysis circuits are commercially available.

Because dialysis removes fluid from the vascular space, the nurse should assess the child's volume status frequently. Signs of hypovolemia include tachycardia and signs of poor systemic perfusion (such as decreased intensity of pulses, pale mucous membranes, and cool extremities with weak pulses and sluggish capillary refill). The CVP will be low unless heart failure is present. The development of hypotension indicates critical hypovolemia and hypotensive shock.

If edema is present, peritoneal dialysis will not immediately abolish all fluid excess. However, as fluid is removed from the vascular compartment the intravascular proteins and sodium ions (osmolality) will draw water out of the edematous tissues into the vascular space, (where it can then be removed during dialysis).

Calculation of Fluid Balance

During peritoneal dialysis, two patient records of total fluid intake and output must be strictly maintained. One record documents the dialysate infused and the dialysate recovered (drain volume) at the end of each cycle (Fig. 13-9).

The amount of fluid recovered always should equal or exceed the amount infused; this produces a negative fluid balance. If less dialysate is recovered than was infused, the nurse should check for signs of catheter or tubing obstruction (see section, Catheter Dysfunction and Obstruction). If additional dialysate cannot be recovered, the difference between the

Text continues on p. 741

THE CHILDREN'S MEMORIAL HOSPITAL

PERITONEAL DIALYSIS FLOW SHEET

DIAGNOSIS _____

HEIGHT _____

PROCEDURE _____

WEIGHT _____

DATE _____

DATE

FLOOR

PATIENT

HOSP. NO.

BIRTHDATE   SEX

PHYSICIAN

	1	2	3	4	5	6	7	8	9	10	11	12	13	14	15	16	17	18	19	20	21	22	23	24

O · RESPIRATIONS

● · TEMPERATURE

V · SYSTOLIC (RED)

Λ · DIASTOLIC (RED)

X · PULSE

104 — 220
103 — 210 / 200
102 — 190 / 180
101 — 170 / 160
100 — 150 / 140
99 — 130 / 120 / 110
98 — 100
97 — 90 / 80
96 — 70 / 60
95 — 50
94 — 40
93 — 30
92 — 20
91 — 10

MONITOR ARTERIAL PRESSURE

C V P

STUDIES / LABORATORY		1	2	3	4	5	6	7	8	9	10	11	12	13	14	15	16	17	18	19	20	21	22	23	24
Hgb.																									
Hct.																									
Na																									
K																									
Cl																									
BUN																									
CREATININE																									
CALCIUM																									
HCO_3																									

FIG. 13-9 Example of peritoneal dialysis flow chart template. (Courtesy Children's Memorial Hospital, Chicago, IL.)

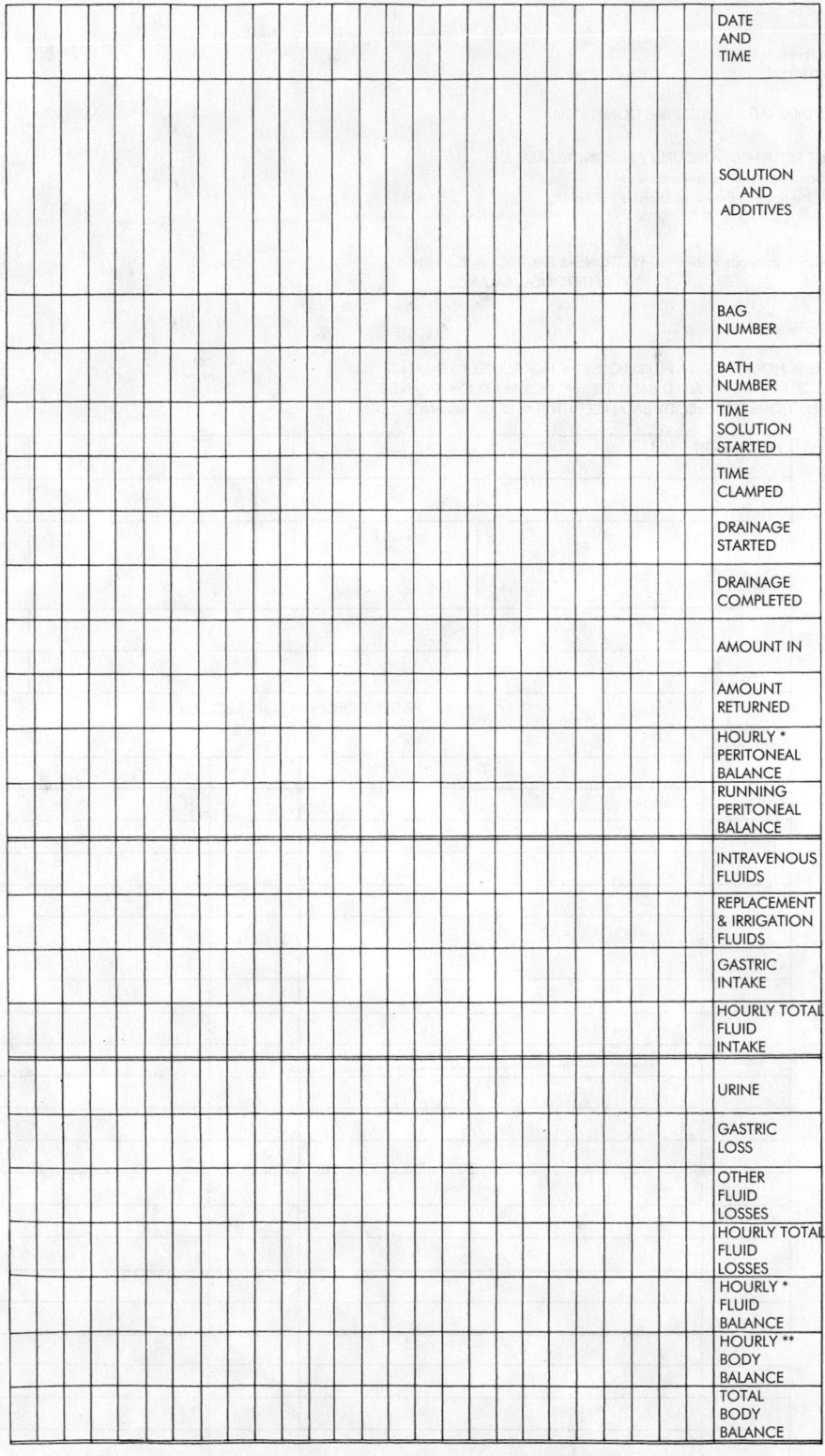

FIG. 13-9, cont'd

Continued

INSTRUCTIONS

Record BAG NUMBER and BATH NUMBER
Record TIME SOLUTION STARTED
Follow Step 4 in Procedure
Record TIME CLAMPED, when DRAINAGE STARTED and COMPLETED

AMOUNT IN MINUS AMOUNT RETURNED = HOURLY PERITONEAL BALANCE
  +(Positive) = Amount of Solution Retained in Peritoneum
  −(Negative) = Amount of Drainage in Excess of Dialysis Solution
      Example: (+75 plus − 75 = 0)

HOURLY PERITONEAL BALANCE + previous RUNNING PERITONEAL BALANCE = RUNNING
                                                    PERITONEAL BALANCE

Record and total all fluids IN for one hour.
Record and total all fluids OUT for one hour.
  HOURLY TOTAL FLUID INTAKE + HOURLY TOTAL FLUID LOSSES = HOURLY FLUID BALANCE
 *HOURLY PERITONEAL BALANCE + * HOURLY FLUID BALANCE = ** HOURLY BODY BALANCE
**HOURLY BODY BALANCE + PREVIOUS TOTAL BODY BALANCE = TOTAL BODY BALANCE

Form #75053
(N-76)

TREATMENTS			

PATIENT OBSERVATION RECORD

Date & Time		Date & Time	

FIG. 13-9, cont'd

amount infused and the amount recovered is recorded as a positive fluid balance, and a physician should be notified.

During the initial cycles of peritoneal dialysis, a larger volume may be recovered than was infused, indicating removal of intravascular fluid. When this occurs, the amount of fluid recovered in excess of the amount infused should be recorded as a negative number, because this represents fluid loss for the child. If significant fluid loss continues, a physician or on-call provider should be notified; it may be necessary to reduce the osmolality of the dialysate to prevent excessive fluid loss and dehydration.

The time and the duration of each infusion, dwell time, and drainage cycle should be recorded. Because maximum solute transfer occurs during the first 30 to 90 minutes the dialysate is in the peritoneal cavity, the dwell time is rarely longer than this. The temperature of the dialysate also should be measured and recorded; this temperature should be as close as possible to 37° C to improve the efficiency of dialysis and to minimize the child's heat loss and discomfort.

The second record of the child's fluid balance includes a total of all sources of fluid intake and output. The net dialysis balance is recorded as part of this total. It is extremely important that this record be carefully maintained, because it will aid in the evaluation of the child's progress and need for modifications in dialysis. When dialysis is begun, drug doses and administration schedules should be adjusted, because many drugs are removed by dialysis.

Potential Complications

Peritonitis. As many as one third of children who receive peritoneal dialysis develop peritonitis. The risk is directly proportional to the duration of the dialysis and is inversely proportional to the child's age. Critically ill patients are especially susceptible to the development of peritonitis. Clinical signs and symptoms of peritonitis during peritoneal dialysis include cloudy return, abdominal pain and tenderness, and leukocytosis. Fever is usually present in children, but young infants may become hypothermic. Paralytic ileus and constipation also may develop.

Because the risk of peritonitis is significant in critically ill patients, a sample of outflow often is obtained on a daily basis and should be obtained whenever peritonitis is suspected. The sample is centrifuged and a Gram stain, cell count, and culture and sensitivity tests are performed. If clinical evidence of peritonitis is present, antibiotics usually are administered as soon as the cultures from the outflow sample and blood are obtained. Cefazolin and gentamicin may be administered into the peritoneal cavity. If the patient is clinically unstable, a single dose of IV vancomycin may be given.[19]

The risk of fungal and bacterial infections is reduced by scrupulous attention to sterile technique during the catheter insertion process and aseptic technique during exchanges. When the outflow collection bag is examined, the bag must not be raised above the level of the bed, because elevation will produce reflux of outflow back into the peritoneal cavity.

Catheter Dysfunction and Obstruction. When dialysate will not flow either into or out of the peritoneal cavity, an external kink or an internal plug is likely to be present in the tubing. If external causes of flow obstruction are eliminated and flow does not resume, a catheter plug is presumed to be present.

A physician (or other on-call provider) can gently irrigate the catheter with normal saline or urokinase, using aseptic technique.[101] Every time a break is made in the dialysis tubing system, the patient's risk of peritonitis increases. Before the dialysis tubing is separated, the connection between the tubing and the catheter must be scrubbed for 5 minutes with a povidone-iodine solution, and clamps are placed on both the catheter and the tubing. The separated ends of the tubing should be wrapped in dry sterile 4 × 4 gauze during separation. Aspiration should not be performed in an attempt to dislodge any plugs, because this may result in catheter occlusion with omentum.

A flat plate radiograph (x-ray film) of the abdomen can be made to confirm the presence of a catheter plug and rule out catheter migration. A solution consisting of three parts 1.5% dialysate and one part Renografin M60 can be infused by gravity or administered by syringe into the catheter at the time the abdominal films are made. This solution will opacify the lumen of the catheter and enable identification and location of plugs.

After catheter manipulation, the dialysis tubing can be reconnected if it is not contaminated during the manipulation. As noted above, the ends should be wrapped in sterile gauze during the manipulation. If the tubing is to be reused, ensure that no fluid leaks out of the system. If a solid column of fluid is maintained in the tubing, air does not enter the tubing and fluid does not drain out of the tubing during catheter manipulation.

With most forms of catheter obstruction, dialysate will flow freely into the peritoneal cavity, but fluid will not drain freely from the peritoneal cavity. Often the catheter floats above the level of the fluid in the peritoneal cavity or becomes wrapped in the omentum. Catheter obstruction also may be caused by constipation, which locks the catheter into a position that restricts drainage. Once the bowel is evacuated, dialysis can proceed. If the child is repositioned or turned from side to side, drainage often can be restored.

Sluggish outflow also can be caused by loops in the dialysis tubing that hang off the edge of the bed. The collection bag and tubing should be repositioned so that the tubing falls straight down from the bed to the collection bag. Any extra tubing should be coiled on the bed to facilitate drainage.

Pain. Almost all patients with new peritoneal catheters complain of pain during the initial dialysis infusions and outflows. The pain experienced upon inflow can be relieved by slowing the rate of infusion or by infusing smaller dialysate volumes.

Pain also can be caused by encasement of the catheter in a false passage; this causes the dialysate to fill only a small area of the peritoneal cavity instead of spreading throughout the peritoneal space. That small area can distend and become painful. If the catheter has been immobilized so that the dialysate flow is directed at the same point in the peritoneal cavity, it usually causes pain in the lateral or posterior peritoneal wall. It may be possible to float the catheter to another position when the abdomen is filled with dialysate. Occasionally, insertion of a new catheter may be necessary. Painful inflow also may be related to extremes of dialysate temperature.

Pain is usually present during dialysate inflow; patients rarely complain of pain only during outflow. Pain at the end of outflow will occur when the abdomen is emptied completely, and it can be abolished by stopping the outflow when a small volume of solution remains in the peritoneal cavity. The presence of this residual solution also diminishes the likelihood of catheter obstruction by omentum. Limiting the outflow time to 5-10 min also should alleviate this problem.

Miscellaneous Complications. Bloody return is a common observation during the initial 24 to 48 hours following catheter implantation. This condition is usually self limiting, and heparin still should be added to the dialysate to prevent the formation of fibrin plugs in the catheter. Heparin will not cross the peritoneal membrane, and it will not affect the patient's coagulation. If the amount of blood in the outflow seems excessive, serial hematocrits can be obtained from the outflow to quantify the amount of blood present. Transfusion may be required if excessive blood loss occurs.

Leaking around the catheter is common when the catheter is placed under urgent conditions at the bedside; it seldom occurs in surgically placed or chronic catheters. Whenever a leak occurs, the nurse should check for overfilling of the abdomen by feeling the tenseness of the abdomen at the end of inflow. The abdomen will feel full, but should not feel rigid. Reassess the catheter insertion wound and tubing to determine whether the catheter is migrating into or out of the peritoneal cavity.

If a leak occurs, weigh and then pack (using aseptic technique) sterile dressings around the catheter and change and weigh them when they become soaked, to measure the volume of the leak. Notify a physician or on-call provider of the leak volume; a smaller volume of dialysate inflow may be ordered.

Fluid leak into the abdominal subcutaneous tissues occasionally develops. The fluid is likely to accumulate in dependent perineal areas. The volume of the subcutaneous leak is usually small and is commonly reabsorbed. If a large volume leaks into closed tissue areas such as the penis or scrotum, it may be necessary to replace the catheter.

Pulmonary Complications. Because peritoneal dialysis results in abdominal fullness, it may compromise diaphragm excursion, resulting in shallow breathing and atelectasis, particularly if the patient is breathing spontaneously. Atelectasis especially in the lower lobes is more likely to develop when the child remains in the supine position.

Assess the child's breath sounds frequently, and constantly evaluate the effectiveness of ventilation. Provide chest physical therapy if areas of atelectasis are noted. If the child is alert and cooperative, encourage the child to cough and take deep breaths or perform inspiratory exercises (e.g., incentive spirometry) to prevent atelectasis. The infant may require other exercises to encourage deep breathing (see Chapter 9). The head of the child's bed should be elevated to facilitate maximal diaphragm excursion and chest expansion.

Fluid or Electrolyte Imbalance. Throughout the dialysis period, the child's electrolyte and acid-base balance should be monitored closely, and electrolyte or acid-base imbalances should be discussed immediately with an on-call provider.

Hypertonic dehydration and hemoconcentration can develop if peritoneal dialysis removes too much water too rapidly; this can result in hypernatremia and can exacerbate hyperkalemia. If dehydration is suspected the nurse should assess the child's level of hydration, heart rate, systemic perfusion, and blood pressure.

If the serum sodium concentration is elevated and the child is dehydrated or hypovolemic, free water may be administered orally, intravenously (with 5% dextrose), or intraperitoneally (using a less concentrated dialysate). The osmolality of the dialysate solution should be reduced for subsequent peritoneal dialysis.

Hypokalemia can develop if a hypokalemic dialysate is used after the serum potassium concentration normalizes. If hypokalemia develops, small doses of potassium can be added to the dialysate, or small doses of potassium chloride can be administered intravenously (0.5-1.0 mEq/kg over several hours). Hypokalemia also can develop if a 4.25% glucose dialysate is used for prolonged periods; the treatment of choice is to change the dialysate solution if the child's condition permits.

Hypoproteinemia can develop if peritoneal dialysis is required for several days, because 0.2 to 8.0 g of protein is lost per liter of outflow. Higher amounts of protein loss occur during episodes of peritonitis. As a result, the child's total protein and albumin should be monitored, and the nurse should assess the child for signs of peripheral edema. If hypoproteinemia develops, administration of amino acids may be needed.

Hyperglycemia can develop if concentrated glucose dialysate is required to eliminate large amounts of free water. The serum glucose concentration (and point of care evaluation of glucose, if available) should be monitored closely, and hyperglycemia or hypoglycemia should be reported to an on-call provider. It may be necessary to reduce the glucose concentration of the dialysate. If the patient has diabetes mellitus, exogenous insulin should be added to the dialysate.

Catheter Removal
The percutaneously placed PD catheter is removed using sterile technique. While one provider withdraws the catheter, a second provider maintains tension on the purse-string stitch that was placed during the catheter insertion. The suture is drawn tight as the catheter is withdrawn. The catheter tip can be sent to the laboratory for culture (per policy). Sterile dressings are placed over the catheterization site. If the dialysis catheter is placed surgically, it must be removed surgically.

Extended Peritoneal Dialysis: Continuous Ambulatory Peritoneal Dialysis and Continuous Cycling Peritoneal Dialysis
Some patients with AKI will require PD for a long period of time (i.e., longer than 5-10 days). In these patients a permanent cuffed peritoneal catheter can be placed surgically for ambulatory peritoneal dialysis.

Method
Continuous Ambulatory Peritoneal Dialysis. Continuous ambulatory peritoneal dialysis (CAPD) is a form of continuous dialysis that does not require bed rest or hospitalization. CAPD uses a surgically placed, cuffed PD catheter and disposable plastic bags of dialysate. Approximately four to five exchanges are performed daily, and each exchange volume totals approximately 30 to 50 mL/kg (or 0.5-2 L total). The exchange time is

approximately 4 to 6 hours, which is much longer than the exchange time during acute peritoneal dialysis.[101] However, during the exchanges the empty dialysate bag is clamped and strapped to the patient's abdomen, and the patient is free to be relatively active. At the end of each exchange period, the empty dialysate bag is placed at a level lower than the patient's abdomen, the drainage tubing is unclamped, and outflow from the patient's abdomen drains into the bag. The bag of outflow is then discarded, and a new disposable dialysate bag is obtained for use in the next exchange.

CAPD will not rapidly correct hypervolemia, acidosis, or hyperkalemia; therefore it is not the dialysis method of choice for acutely ill children. However, CAPD allows excellent regulation of fluid and serum electrolyte concentrations when it is used on a daily basis for the child in stable condition with chronic kidney disease. Children who receive CAPD generally require less frequent blood transfusions than children who receive chronic hemodialysis, and serum urea nitrogen and phosphorus concentrations may be better controlled than with hemodialysis. However, renal osteodystrophy and hyperphosphatemia do occur.[36]

Children receiving CAPD have few dietary restrictions, because their relatively continuous dialysis can remove excess fluid and allow constant regulation of electrolyte and acid-base balance. As a result, children receiving CAPD may be better nourished than those who require intermittent forms of dialysis. Control of hypertension is also excellent when children with renal failure receive CAPD.

Continuous Cycling Peritoneal Dialysis. Continuous peritoneal dialysis may be made less labor intensive with the addition of mechanical cycling to the dialysis process. Continuous cycling peritoneal dialysis (CCPD) provides mechanical (automatic) delivery of a prescribed volume of dialysate at prescribed intervals, with a set indwell time. Drainage of outflow is initiated mechanically, and audible alarms sound if flow problems occur.[72] Current cycling machines are capable of infusing dialysate volumes of 50 to 100 mL.

CCPD is performed most commonly while the child sleeps. The dialysis cycling machine should not require any attention during the night unless an alarm sounds. A small dialysate volume is allowed to remain in the peritoneal cavity during the day, providing continuous dialysis. The child is able to resume school and other normal childhood activities. All exchange bags are hung at the same time when CCPD is begun at night; this can reduce the risk of contamination and peritonitis.[72]

Complications

The most frequent complications associated with CAPD and CCPD are mechanical problems and infection. The mechanical problems are related to cuff erosion and fluid leaks, and the infection problems are related to peritonitis.

The cuffed peritoneal catheter can erode the abdominal wall; this can cause a fluid leak and require catheter replacement. Hernias can develop from subcutaneous fluid leaks around the dialysis incision, and these hernias often require surgical repair.

The incidence of peritonitis among children receiving CAPD and CCPD varies widely in clinical reports, but averages one infection every 14.7 patient months.[36] Many patients also develop local infections around the catheter site.

When selecting patients for CAPD, it is important that the child and the parents are reliable and able to follow the established protocol. Children or families must be taught the dialysis technique, and they should be instructed to contact the CAPD nurse whenever the patient experiences abdominal pain, inflow or outflow occlusion, inflammation of the catheter site, a feeling of weakness or dizziness when standing, hypotension, cloudy outflow, catheter disconnection or contamination, fever, excessive weight gain, edema, or other illness.

Because the dialysate dwells in the peritoneal cavity for a long time and the risk of peritonitis is relatively high in children receiving CAPD and CCPD, hospital protocols often try to minimize the number of personnel providing any in-hospital CAPD or CCPD that the child requires. This action minimizes the child's exposure to people and contaminants and may reduce the risk of peritonitis.

Hemodialysis
Method

Hemodialysis is one of the most efficient artificial methods of removing nitrogenous wastes from the body and of restoring fluid, electrolyte, and acid-base balance. However, pediatric hemodialysis requires the assembly of skilled personnel capable of establishing and maintaining vascular access, recognizing and responding to potential complications of dialysis, and supporting cardiorespiratory function in extremely unstable patients. If urgent dialysis is required and experienced personnel are not available, PD may be provided until the child's condition can be stabilized and the child transported to an appropriate facility.

Indications for pediatric hemodialysis are GFR <15 mL/min per 1.73 m^2 or intractable complications of AKI, even at a higher GFR. GFR is roughly equivalent to the creatinine clearance estimated by the Schwartz formula (see Box 13-5).

Complications of hemodialysis include but are not limited to hypervolemia, hyperkalemia, metabolic acidosis, hyperphosphatemia, hypocalcemia, hypercalcemia, and neurologic dysfunction.[52]

Hemodialysis requires access in an artery, arterialized vessel, or large vein. If chronic hemodialysis is planned, an arteriovenous fistula may be created or a graft may be placed in a large artery. In the critical care unit, vascular access is often achieved with a single- or double-lumen catheter (at least size 6 French) placed through the subclavian vein into the right atrium, or from the femoral vein into the inferior vena cava.[15]

During hemodialysis, blood is withdrawn from the body and pumped at high flow rates to a blood compartment that makes contact with a semipermeable membrane. This blood compartment and semipermeable membrane are immersed in dialysate, which is pumped at rates that exceed blood flow rate by 50%. The dialysate flows in the direction opposite the blood flow.[37]

The dialysate contains a fairly standard concentration of electrolytes, but the potassium concentration usually is determined individually (based on the amount of potassium to be removed). Nitrogenous wastes pass from the blood into the dialysate as the result of a concentration gradient. Free water will move from the blood into the dialysate if the osmolality of the dialysate is greater than the serum osmolality. Free water movement is also enhanced by a positive transmembrane hydrostatic pressure from the blood compartment to the dialysate compartment. This positive pressure can be generated by the blood pump and by manipulation of resistance to blood outflow, although newer dialysis machines automatically generate the transmembrane hydrostatic pressure required to provide the volume of ultrafiltrate prescribed.[37]

The amount of fluid and solute removal from the blood is determined by the flow rates of the blood and dialysate, the surface area and permeability of the membrane, the concentration and osmolality gradients between the dialysate and blood, and the transmembrane pressure gradient. Electrolytes move across the semipermeable membrane as the result of concentration gradients. If the concentration of an electrolyte (e.g., potassium) or other small molecule (e.g., urea) is lower in the dialysate than in the blood, that electrolyte or molecule will move out of the blood and into the dialysate. If the concentration of an electrolyte or other molecule (e.g., glucose) is higher in the dialysate than in the blood, that electrolyte or molecule will move into the blood. Other substances can be removed from the blood as the result of ultrafiltration and solvent drag (the passive movement of solutes as the result of movement of large amounts of water).

Because hemodialysis requires that blood be drawn from and returned to the body, pumps must be present in the dialysis circuit. In addition, the filter and the tubing (the dialysis circuit) must be primed with fluid or blood before the dialysis begins. Because the circulating blood volume of the infant or child is low, extracorporeal movement of a large quantity of blood (e.g., to prime the dialysis circuit) is likely to produce hypovolemia. As a rule, the filling volume of the dialysis circuit should be no greater than the equivalent of 10% of the child's circulating blood volume. If the circuit requires a larger filling volume, the circuit should be primed with colloid (5% albumin or packed RBCs diluted with albumin to a hematocrit of 35%).[37] Few centers have experience in the hemodialysis of infants, and it should not be attempted by inexperienced personnel. In adolescents, the dialysis circuit can be primed with normal saline or 5% albumin.

The dialysate contains glucose, sodium, calcium, and potassium, in concentrations that are specified by the physician. The dialysate usually contains little potassium (0-4 mEq/L) and no urea, so that high concentration gradients between the dialysate and the blood will hasten removal of these solutes from the blood. The presence of glucose in the dialysate at levels of 200 to 250 mg/dL creates a high osmolality in the dialysate, favoring the movement of water from the blood to the dialysate, provided the patient's serum glucose concentration and osmolality are lower than the glucose and osmolality of the dialysate.

The glucose concentration in patients with diabetes mellitus is often higher than 200 to 250 mg/dL. As a result, the osmotic forces will favor free water movement from the dialysate into the patient's blood, exacerbating hypervolemia. This inappropriate fluid movement can be prevented by increasing the pressure gradient across the dialysis filter (creating higher pressure within the blood compartment or generating negative pressure in the dialysate compartment) or by adding albumin to the dialysate.

The high glucose concentration in the dialysate produces a serum glucose of approximately 200 mg/dL during dialysis. This mild hyperglycemia is usually well tolerated in the patients without diabetes mellitus; however, patients with diabetes will require adjustment of insulin dose (particularly long-acting insulin) in anticipation of this period of relatively low serum glucose.

The blood and the dialysate are typically pumped through the circuit in opposite directions. This pumping maximizes the concentration and osmotic gradients between the dialysate and the blood so that dialysis can be accomplished within a short period of time (exchange time of approximately 3-4 hours).

As noted previously, the creation of either positive pressure in the blood compartment or negative pressure in the dialysate compartment or both will increase the rate of fluid removal from the blood. Positive pressure is created in the blood compartment by increasing the resistance to flow on the venous side of the blood circuit. This increase in resistance usually is accomplished by placement of an adjustable clamp on the venous blood line, and the clamp is tightened until the desired pressure in the blood compartment is reached.

Negative pressure can be applied across the filter. This negative pressure draws free water and small particles from the blood, across the semipermeable membrane, and into the ultrafiltrate.

The dialysis nurse and the bedside nurse will be responsible for continuously evaluating the effect of fluid removal on the patient's systemic perfusion. If the patient's clinical condition deteriorates, some adjustment in the rate of fluid removal is often required.

When hemodialysis is initiated, a small amount of heparin is injected into the dialysis catheters and into the dialysis circuit to prevent clot formation in the filter and tubing. Heparin will then be administered at 30-minute to 1-hour intervals or by continuous infusion. The rate of infusion is adjusted based on the activated clotting time (ACT) or the Lee-White clotting time. Heparin dose and adjustment will be determined by dialysis unit policy and procedure. Citrate may be the anticoagulant of choice in hemodialysis therapy, and it is useful in the prevention of heparin-induced thrombocytopenia. Refer to protocols published on-line[17] and in print[69] for additional information.

Complications

Hemodialysis is efficient, but it is extremely expensive and can produce complications that do not develop during PD or hemofiltration. These complications are related largely to hypovolemia and resultant hypotension, fluid shifts (also known as *dysequilibrium*), hypervolemia, bleeding, anemia, infection, or malfunction of the vascular access site. Each of these is discussed in the following sections.

Hypotension and Hypovolemia. Hypotension can develop from removal of a large amount of intravascular water, resulting in hypovolemia, or from circulatory instability.

The patients most at risk for developing hypotensive crises during dialysis are patients with vasomotor instability (including patients with paraplegia or quadriplegia), low cardiac output or myocardial dysfunction, those receiving vasodilators, or those with a history of hypotensive episodes during dialysis.

If the child develops hypotension during dialysis, the dialysis nurse will reduce any transmembrane pressure created across the filter, because this pressure gradient enhances fluid removal from the blood. In addition, the bedside nurse may be required to administer albumin or other volume expanders (per unit policy or physician or on-call provider order), place the patient in modified Trendelenburg position (head flat, feet elevated), or initiate cardiopulmonary resuscitation (as needed).

To avoid hypotension, any existing hypovolemia should be corrected before dialysis is begun. In addition, the patient's blood should be drawn slowly into the circuit so the patient does not experience an acute loss of intravascular volume. If excess intravascular fluid is to be removed during dialysis, venous positive pressure or negative pressure across the filter will be applied very slowly. The dialysis nurse and the bedside nurse are both responsible for monitoring the child's systemic arterial blood pressure and systemic perfusion. Deterioration in clinical status should be reported immediately to a physician or appropriate on-call provider.

Fluid Shifts and Dysequilibrium. If many osmotically active particles such as sodium or urea are removed rapidly from the patient's blood, the patient's serum osmolality will fall quickly. As a result, free water may shift from the intravascular and interstitial spaces to the intracellular compartment, producing cerebral edema. This edema following dialysis has been called *dialysis dysequilibrium syndrome.* The child may complain of severe headaches or may demonstrate nausea, vomiting, confusion, irritability, or seizures.

To reduce the risk of dysequilibrium, solute removal from the blood must be gradual; peritoneal dialysis may initially be performed to gradually reduce the BUN concentration. The efficiency of the hemodialysis can be reduced: the blood flow through the filter can be slowed, the direction of dialysate flow can be changed to the same direction as the blood, or the duration of the dialysis treatment can be shortened.

Intravenous mannitol can be administered slowly to increase serum osmolality and slow the removal of water by dialysis. Mannitol should be administered if evidence of dysequilibrium develops.[64]

Hypervolemia. If too much fluid is administered to the patient during dialysis or if an excessive volume of fluid and blood is transfused to the patient from the circuit at the end of dialysis, the child can develop hypervolemia. This condition can produce significant cardiovascular problems, particularly if the patient has preexisting cardiac disease.

The child can rapidly develop signs of congestive heart failure, including tachycardia, peripheral vasoconstriction, hepatomegaly, periorbital edema, elevated CVP, tachypnea, and increased respiratory effort. If severe hypervolemia is present, the child can develop pulmonary edema or hypertension.

Bleeding and Anemia. Because the child's blood must be anticoagulated during dialysis, bleeding can occur. The child can bleed from wounds or puncture sites or into the brain, pericardium, or abdomen. To reduce the risk of bleeding, regional heparinization may be performed. The heparin is injected into the arterial (or inflow) tubing that carries blood from the patient to the filter. To prevent large heparin infusion to the patient, protamine sulfate is administered into the tubing that is returning blood from the filter to the patient. Protamine sulfate neutralizes heparin, but can produce a coagulopathy or hypotension if it is administered separate from or in excess of heparin, or if the patient inadvertently receives a bolus of protamine.

Bleeding also can occur in patients with renal failure, because uremia is associated with depression of platelet function. If active bleeding is present in a patient with uremia, the most common treatment is the use of desmopressin or l-deamino-8-arginine vasopressin (DDAVP). Although the exact mechanism of action is unknown, desmopressin has been shown to increase release of factor VIII from storage sites, increasing the concentration of factor VIII and minimizing the effects of uremic dysfunctional von Willebrand factor. The dose of DDAVP to treat bleeding with renal failure is approximately 10-fold higher than the dose used for treatment of diabetes insipidus; it ranges from 0.3 to 0.4 mcg/kg intravenously and will improve platelet function within 1 hour after infusion. The effects disappear within 24 hours.[51] DDAVP also can be administered before surgical procedures to reduce the risk of bleeding in patients with uremia.

Patients with renal failure often have anemia. Anemia can result from loss of blood within the dialysis system (through blood leaks, loose connections, clot formation, frequent blood sampling, or dilution of blood with dialysis tubing prime), from hemorrhage, or from the effects of uremia. Red cell lysis also can occur if blood is exposed to a dialysate of significantly higher osmolality. Levels of erythropoietin are low among uremic patients; therefore RBC production and survival are both reduced.

To prevent anemia, blood sampling should be minimized. Whenever blood is drawn, the amount should be recorded in the child's record of intake and output; blood replacement should be considered whenever the blood loss totals 5% to 7% of the child's circulating blood volume (circulating blood volume is approximately 70 to 80 mL/kg in infants and children and 70 mL/kg in adolescents). Because hemodialysis often is accomplished through the use of an arterial access catheter, laboratory sampling of blood can be performed during dialysis. This procedure reduces the number of venipunctures required and allows immediate replacement of the sample amount through the dialysis circuit.

Packed RBCs usually are administered to replace lost blood. Iron therapy will not be effective in the treatment of uremia-induced anemia and can contribute to the development of iron toxicity. Anemia can complicate the care of children with associated cardiovascular disease, because cardiac output must increase to maintain oxygen delivery.

Infection and Febrile Reactions. Patients with renal disease have increased risk of infection resulting from loss of immune proteins in nephrosis, multiple invasive catheters and cannulae, compromised nutritional status, frequent handling by hospital personnel, and frequent transfusions. The risk of infection can be minimized if all healthcare personnel practice strict hand-washing technique and strict asepsis, if the child receives adequate nutrition and if hepatitis and HIV screening is performed by the blood bank (for further discussion of hepatitis see Chapter 14).

The nurse should assess all of the patient's wounds and vascular access sites daily and report any areas of inflammation to an on-call provider. All wounds should be dressed according to unit policy or physician or on-call provider order.

Patients receiving hemodialysis may experience a sudden increase in temperature, known as a *febrile reaction*. This fever may result from an allergic reaction to the filter, from a reaction to blood administered during dialysis, or from systemic seeding from an infected shunt or access site. A preexisting fever suddenly may become manifest when the patient's serum urea, which can act as an antipyretic, is lowered.

When fever develops, the on-call provider can request that blood cultures be obtained from two different collection points; one set of cultures is typically collected from the dialysis tubing by the dialysis nurse after a 3-min povidone-iodine (Betadine) scrub. The second culture usually is obtained from a peripheral vein, although a second culture can be obtained from the dialysis circuit if at least 30 min elapse between samples. Cultures also can be collected from the ultrafiltrate.

If a transfusion reaction is suspected, specimens are collected from the transfusion bag and patient, and they are sent to the laboratory for hemolysis and incompatibility checks (see Chapter 15). If hemolysis is present, the child's serum potassium concentration should be monitored closely, because hyperkalemia can develop. A hematocrit also should be obtained, and a serum sample should be checked for evidence of hemolysis.

Hemodialysis Access

The establishment and maintenance of vascular access in small children is one of the most challenging aspects of pediatric hemodialysis. Dependable, double lumen, cuffed venous catheters are now available and they are the acute and long-term dialysis catheters of choice. If these catheters are placed surgically in the right atrium and infused appropriately with heparin, they can be maintained for a long time. When vascular access is needed, the injection port of the catheter can be used and no skin punctures are required. The care of these catheters is identical to the care of any long-term central venous catheter; meticulous care is required to ensure catheter longevity and minimize the risk of infection. Refer to hospital policies and procedures regarding central venous catheter care (also, Box 22-6).

Arterial access can be provided by a graft. Grafts consist of tubes made of Teflon or polytetrafluoroethylene. The tube is attached to an artery and then looped subcutaneously and connected to a parallel large vein.[15] After surgical placement, time is allowed for the graft to become coated with the patient's endothelial cells (i.e., the graft endothelializes) before it is used for dialysis. Vascular access is achieved by piercing the graft with standard large-bore needles.

Arteriovenous fistulae can still be created in older children to provide vascular access for hemodialysis. The fistula is surgically created in the nondominant arm by connection of the radial artery to the cephalic vein.[15] Soon after the fistula is created, the vein distends and is punctured easily to obtain vascular access. The risk of infection in the fistula is low because no prosthetic material is involved in its construction. However, any arteriovenous shunt will increase venous return to the heart and may precipitate or worsen congestive heart failure.

Continued Problems of Uremia

The patient requiring hemodialysis is still susceptible to complications of uremia. Although dialysis may provide temporary relief of some fluid and electrolyte or acid-base imbalances, anemia, hypertension, infection, osteodystrophy, endocrine imbalance, pruritus, anorexia, nausea, vomiting, fatigue, ulcers, and depression can persist (see section, Chronic Kidney Disease).

Throughout the care of the child with renal failure, the nurse should consult support personnel to assist in the psychosocial care of the child and family. Frequent multidisciplinary conferences and meetings with the social worker, dietician, financial counselor, physicians, and primary nurses will help the family to be aware of the support systems available to them and ensure that communication is optimal among team members and the family. As appropriate, the bedside nurse or case manager should begin to plan for the child's discharge to home or to another unit.

Whenever the critically ill child requires dialysis, the bedside nurse remains responsible for coordinating the care of the child and family. Although a dialysis nurse may be present and responsible for the dialysis procedure and circuit, the bedside nurse still must assess and document the child's fluid balance and systemic perfusion. The dialysis nurse and the bedside nurse should coordinate efforts. It is important to time the administration of medications, blood products, and fluids based on the timing and effectiveness of the dialysis. Both the dialysis nurse and the bedside nurse must provide the child and family with skilled support and compassion.

Hemoperfusion

Definition

Hemoperfusion is a treatment which exposes blood or plasma to an adsorbent material for the removal of toxins, solutes, or other materials. Adsorbent materials used can include charcoal, resin, protein A, synthetic materials, and monoclonal antibodies.[21]

Although hemodialysis is highly efficient at removing water-soluble drugs with low molecular weights (e.g., salicylates, ethanol, methanol, lithium) from the blood, it does not remove protein and lipid-bound substances; therefore it is not effective in the treatment of hypercholesterolemia, hyperbilirubinemia, toxicity associated with fulminant hepatic failure, or ingested toxins. Hemoperfusion is extremely effective in the treatment of these problems.[21] Large molecules such as β_2-microglobulin have been successfully removed by hemoperfusion with lower cardiovascular mortality,[87] and clinical trials are currently underway with new adsorbents that are effective in removing β_2-microglobulin.[21]

Hemoperfusion uses a hemodialysis circuit; however, the blood is passed through a cartridge containing the adsorbent surface, and no dialysate is present. Life-threatening poisonings from theophylline, carbamazepine, phenobarbital, and phenytoin may be an indication for charcoal hemoperfusion.[74] With the use of activated charcoal, substances normally bound by lipid or protein are quickly and effectively removed from the intravascular space. Because hemoperfusion will not remove urea, it is not the treatment of choice for uremia.

Method

In the following discussion, a charcoal filter or cartridge will be used as the example of the adsorbent surface. As noted previously, the vascular access and circuit tubing used for hemoperfusion are often identical to those required for hemodialysis.

The charcoal filter is prepared, and the filter is given a glucose-heparin rinse. Because most commercially available cartridges require a priming volume of 50 to 300 mL, the total hemoperfusion circuit is primed with the equivalent of more than 10% of the circulating volume of a small child. As a result, the circuit usually is primed with blood before initiation of hemoperfusion.[24]

Some anticoagulation must be provided to prevent clot formation in the cartridge. Heparin usually is infused into the inflow tubing, between the patient and the cartridge. To minimize the risk of bleeding, protamine sulfate usually is added to the blood in the circuit beyond the cartridge (i.e., between the cartridge and the patient) to bind the heparin before the blood is returned to the patient.

Approximately 3 hours are required for hemoperfusion. The activated charcoal quickly will become saturated with the drug or substance removed from the blood. Frequently, several cartridges are required to complete one treatment. To determine the amount of toxin binding provided by the cartridge, blood levels of the toxic substance are drawn from the circuit immediately proximal to and distal from the cartridge. If these levels become nearly identical or if clotting is observed in the cartridge, the cartridge should be changed.

Complications

The activated charcoal binds lipid or protein-bound toxins. In addition, it binds glucose, calcium, and platelets; therefore serum concentrations of these substances must be monitored closely during hemoperfusion. Severe thrombocytopenia is the most common complication observed during this procedure.[24]

Occasionally, hemoperfusion effectively removes the toxins from the blood, but rebound toxicity develops several hours later as tissue-bound toxins move into the vascular space. For this reason, serum levels of the toxin should be monitored during the hemoperfusion and at regular intervals for several hours following hemoperfusion.

Bleeding can result from thrombocytopenia or heparinization. Because the half-life of protamine sulfate is shorter than the therapeutic effect of heparin, it may be necessary to administer additional protamine sulfate several hours after hemoperfusion

is performed. During and after the procedure, the child should be observed closely for any evidence of bleeding, and all body secretions should be checked for the presence of blood.

Continuous Renal Replacement Therapy

The history of pediatric continuous renal replacement therapy (pCRRT) is rich with innovation, challenges, and change. In the late 1970s and early 1980s, the care of pediatric patients with AKI requiring renal replacement therapy involved improvised arteriovenous systems. Control of ultrafiltration rates in these systems required vigilant monitoring and frequent adjustment on the effluent side of the extracorporeal system.

Today, continuous renal replacement therapy (CRRT) devices are primarily venovenous and provide compact, efficient, and controlled management of fluid and electrolytes in pediatric patients with AKI. The Prospective Pediatric Continuous Renal Replacement Therapy Registry (ppCRRT Registry) was designed to evaluate clinical and therapeutic aspects of pCRRT in a prospective, observational manner.[39] The ppCRRT Registry is a voluntary, multicenter, collaborative effort designed to evaluate clinical and therapeutic aspects of pCRRT and gather information about best pCCRT practices.[38]

The First Acute Dialysis Quality Initiative Conference examined evidence-based research and published consensus practice guidelines for CRRT in 2002.[61] Complete guidelines are available online at http://www.ccm.pitt.edu/adqi/.[1]

Definition

CRRT performs the work of the kidney through an extracorporeal system designed to run continuously. The patient's blood flows through a filter to remove excess fluid, waste products, and toxins and to establish electrolyte and pH balance before it is returned to the patient. CRRT is similar to hemodialysis, but treatment is continuous rather than intermittent. The continuous aspect of CRRT provides more gradual fluid and electrolyte shifts and enables more tightly calibrated fluid management. CRRT as provided by current technology enables minute-to-minute adjustments in therapy titrated to patient need.

Indications for Continuous Renal Replacement Therapy

In the setting of AKI, the indications for renal replacement therapy are fluid and solute removal. Similar to PD, CRRT provides a gradual fluid and solute removal, but CRRT allows more sensitive fluid control than PD.[101] Comparable to HD, CRRT can treat hypervolemia and electrolyte imbalance but instead of correcting these imbalances over 3 to 4 hours as with HD, CRRT will correct them over 1 day or more. For these reasons, CRRT is a valuable treatment choice in critically ill pediatric patients with AKI who are hemodynamically unstable with signs of multiorgan dysfunction syndrome. In data from the ppCRRT Registry, the most common acute diagnoses in patients receiving CRRT were sepsis and cardiogenic shock, and the most common comorbid conditions were bone marrow transplant and solid organ transplants—primarily the liver.[38,88]

In data from the ppCRRT Registry, immediate indications for CRRT include: fluid overload and electrolyte imbalance, fluid overload only, electrolyte imbalance only, prevention of fluid overload to allow intake, or other indications such as intoxications and inborn errors of metabolism. The combination of fluid overload and electrolyte imbalance was the most frequently encountered indication and had the lowest survival.

Recent experience supports the use of CRRT as a treatment modality for sepsis, not only for the management of fluids and electrolytes but also for the removal of inflammatory mediators of sepsis.[26,28,33] CRRT has been effective after stem cell transplant, for treatment of drug toxicities, in acute solute removal in tumor lysis syndrome with associated hyperkalemia and hyperuricemia and to treat inborn error of metabolism.

Continuous Renal Replacement Therapy Modalities

CRRT is a broad term that encompasses treatment modalities involving an extracorporeal system and water removal by filtration. The treatment modalities include continuous arteriovenous hemofiltration (CAVH) and a variety of modalities provided by continuous venovenous hemofiltration.

The mechanism of solute transport is the distinguishing feature of the CRRT modalities. Solutes are removed by diffusion, convection, or both.

When solute is removed by diffusion, the process is similar to that described in the hemodialysis portion of this chapter. Solutes are removed from the blood through the filter's semipermeable membrane as the result of concentration gradients. Solutes move from the area of high concentration (blood) through the semipermeable membrane into an area of low concentration (i.e., fluid on the opposite side of the membrane).

The second mechanism of solute transport is convection. Solutes in solution are carried with the water across the semipermeable membrane in response to a transmembrane pressure gradient. Convection has been described as "solvent drag": the bulk water flow literally drags the solutes through the semipermeable membrane. In venovenous CCRT, the transmembrane pressure gradient is generated by the speed of the blood pump or blood flow rate (BFR), which transmits a positive hydrostatic pressure inside the blood tubule of the filter. The rate of the effluent pump, or effluent and dialysate pump if dialysis is used, creates a negative pressure in the space surrounding the blood tubules, therefore increasing the transmembrane pressure gradient.

Continuous Arteriovenous Hemofiltration

Definition

CAVH uses an extracorporeal circuit and a small filter that is highly permeable to water and small solutes, but is impermeable to proteins and formed elements of the blood. The filter system is joined to both an arterial and a venous catheter. Passage of arterial blood through the filter results in the formation of an ultrafiltrate of plasma that consists of water and nonprotein bound solutes. The filtered blood is then returned to the patient through the venous catheter.

Because the filter used for CAVH contains no dialysate there are no concentration gradients established across the filter. The volume and content of the ultrafiltrate is determined by the rate of blood flow through the filter (essentially determined by the patient's blood pressure), the permeability of the filter, and the transmembrane pressure. The transmembrane pressure is created largely by the patient's arterial pressure, but it also can be augmented by elevating the patient above the fluid drainage bag. The transmembrane pressure also will be enhanced by the oncotic pressure difference between the patient blood and the ultrafiltrate, which is protein-free with an oncotic pressure of zero.

The volume of ultrafiltrate can also be adjusted through the use of negative pressure generated on one side of the filter by the use of a volume-controlled infusion pump that draws ultrafiltrate at a set hourly rate. The faster the rate set for the volume-controlled pump, the more ultrafiltrate drawn from the blood through the filter every hour. The infusion pump can create resistance to flow if it is adjusted to a relatively slow hourly rate. As a result, resistance to ultrafiltrate production will be created by slow flow through the infusion pump circuit. The use of infusion pumps in this setting is not optimal for neonates and small infants, because the pumps may be inaccurate and might remove fluid at an unreliable rate. For example, the amount of ultrafiltrate could actually be greater than the hourly rate set on the infusion pump.

CAVH can provide effective therapy for the treatment of AKI complicated by hypervolemia or electrolyte or acid-base disturbances. It is particularly useful in patients with extremely limited venous access, in neonates or small infants, and in patients with unstable cardiovascular function or multisystem organ failure who are likely to be intolerant of hemodialysis. This form of renal replacement is not recommended for the rapid treatment of hyperkalemia, because the rate of ultrafiltration is low and potassium removal is slower than with hemodialysis.[19]

CAVH may be used to remove a small but predictable volume of fluid from the vascular space. This procedure is helpful in the management of chronically ill patients with oliguria and hypervolemia (e.g., those with severe congestive heart failure), because excess fluid can be removed and replaced with parenteral fluid that has high nutrient value.

With the appropriate equipment, CAVH systems can be assembled and implemented relatively quickly. CAVH also can provide a useful option when resources are scarce. However, in many critical care areas CAVH has been replaced by venovenous hemofiltration machines with more precise technology to provide safer and more predictable blood flow and precise ultrafiltration.[12,69]

Contraindications

There are few contraindications to the use of CAVH. Active bleeding is a relative contraindication; PD is preferred in such patients. A severe coagulopathy is not a contraindication to the use of CAVH, although the risk of bleeding at the access site is increased.

Method

Preparation for Continuous Arteriovenous Hemofiltration. To begin CAVH, arterial and venous access must be achieved. It is extremely important to catheterize an artery large enough to allow sufficient flow into the filter; the femoral artery is used most frequently, although the umbilical artery may be catheterized in neonates. The femoral and external jugular veins are used most frequently for venous access.

The circuit tubing should contain multiple sampling ports, and it should be primed before use. A heparin infusion system (with appropriate infusion pump) should be joined to the arterial side of the circuit, and stopcocks and tubing should be placed in the circuit to enable bypass of the filter; these stopcocks will be used when the filters are changed. The filter and circuit are prepared, and the prime fluid should be warmed to no more than 37° C.

Many CAVH filters are commercially available, and most use a hollow fiber design. It is preferable to use small filters (20-mL prime volume) designed for use in small children to keep the volume in the circuit as low as possible during treatment. The ideal filter has a short fiber length, a large surface area, and a small priming volume. If the entire extracorporeal circuit must be primed with a volume exceeding 10% of the patient's blood volume, fresh bank blood should be used to prime the circuit.

As noted previously, a volume-controlled infusion pump may be required to enhance or limit the formation of ultrafiltrate. Occasionally, an additional fluid infusion pump and infusion system are prepared to administer fluid to the patient to enable replacement of ultrafiltrate with fluid that differs in solute or nutritional content (Fig. 13-10).

Initiation of Continuous Arteriovenous Hemofiltration. To initiate hemofiltration, the arterial and venous catheters are joined to the filter and drainage system. Clamps are placed on each limb of the circuit. The arterial and venous limbs are unclamped first, while the bypass tubing and the drainage limb remain clamped. The heparin infusion should commence when the vascular lines are unclamped. Once the area in the filter surrounding the blood tubules is filled with the patient's ultrafiltrate, the tubing of the drainage line can be unclamped.

During CAVH, the nurse is responsible for monitoring the volume of ultrafiltrate, which can be regulated with a volume-controlled infusion pump. Periodic sampling of the ultrafiltrate will be performed to monitor the solute content of the filtrate, so that appropriate replacement therapy can be provided.

Regular monitoring of the patient's activated clotting time (ACT) is required during CAVH. The heparin infusion is titrated to maintain an ACT that is approximately 1.5-fold of

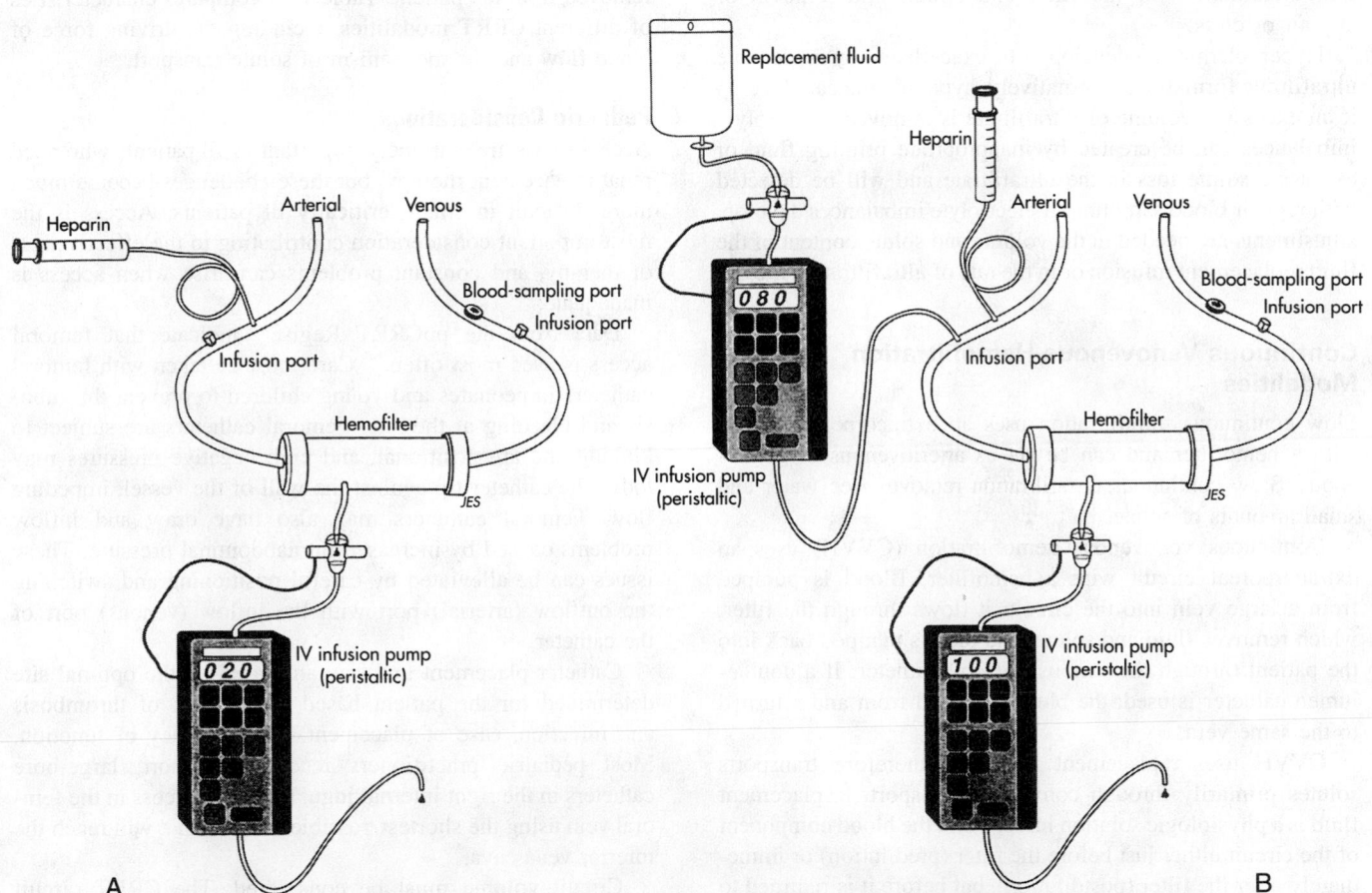

FIG. 13-10 Continuous arteriovenous hemofiltration. **A,** The rate of fluid removal can be controlled if a pediatric volume infusion pump is joined to the hemofilter. The variable resistance generated by the infusion pump will control the hemofilter transmembrane pressure and the filtration rate. **B,** Continuous hemofiltration generally requires infusion of replacement fluid to prevent volume depletion and to control the electrolytes lost through hemofiltration. Use of two pediatric infusion pumps enables controlled removal of fluid and controlled replacement of fluid and electrolytes. (From Stark JE, Hammed J: Continuous hemofiltration and dialysis. In Blumer J, editor: *A practical guide to pediatric intensive care,* ed 3. St Louis, 1990, Mosby-Year Book.)

baseline (maximum, 200 s). The arterial ACT should be no greater than 10% above baseline to prevent bleeding.[2]

The filter should be examined frequently for the presence of clot formation. If clots are observed or ultrafiltrate formation decreases significantly, a physician or on-call provider should be notified and the filter probably should be changed. Filters can be expected to last approximately 12 hours, although the duration varies widely with patient condition.

Hemoglobin and hematocrit and serum chemistries should be monitored on a regular basis per unit protocol. The patient should be weighed once or twice every 24 hours.

Complications. The most common complications during CAVH are bleeding, thromboembolic events, and fluid balance problems. Bleeding occurs when heparinization is excessive, and it should be prevented with careful monitoring of arterial and venous ACTs. Anemia can result from excessive clot formation in the filters; therefore the child's hematocrit should be monitored frequently.

Air is trapped in air chambers, but thrombi entering the system or leaving the filter can embolize to the central venous system. These thrombi can be prevented by scrupulous examination of the filter and circuit and removal of any air or clots.

Hypervolemia can develop or be exacerbated by inadequate ultrafiltrate formation. Alternatively, hypovolemia can develop if an excessive volume of ultrafiltrate is removed. Electrolyte imbalances can be created by inappropriate priming fluid or excessive solute loss in the ultrafiltrate and will be detected with regular blood sampling. If electrolyte imbalances develop, adjustments are needed in the volume and solute content of the fluid replacement infusion or in the rate of ultrafiltrate removal.

Continuous Venovenous Hemofiltration Modalities

Slow continuous ultrafiltration uses an extracorporeal circuit with a hemofilter and can be set as arteriovenous or venovenous. Slow continuous ultrafiltration removes free water and small amounts of solute.

Continuous venovenous hemofiltration (CVVH) uses an extracorporeal circuit with a hemofilter. Blood is pumped from a large vein into the circuit; it flows through the filter, which removes fluid and solute, and then is pumped back into the patient through the venous line and catheter. If a double-lumen catheter is used, the blood is pulled from and returned to the same vein.

CVVH uses replacement fluid and therefore transports solutes primarily through convective transport. Replacement fluid is a physiologic solution infused into the blood component of the circuit either just before the filter (predilution) or immediately after the filter (postdilution), but before it is returned to the patient. The replacement fluid is used to replace large volumes of ultrafiltrate to help maintain the patient's fluid and electrolyte balance. The machine weighs the ultrafiltrate bag and calculates the volume of fluid removed (ultrafiltrate).

Continuous venovenous hemodialysis (CVVHD) uses an extracorporeal circuit with a filter. Blood is pumped from a large vein into the circuit, through the filter, which removes

fluid and solute, and then the blood is pumped back into the patient's venous circulation. Dialysate fluid is pumped into the space surrounding the blood tubules in the filter in the direction opposite the blood flow (countercurrent flow).

Solute removal in CVVHD results from diffusion that is caused by concentration gradients between the blood and dialysate. The ultrafiltration fluid and the dialysate fluid are recovered into the same large effluent bag for disposal. The machine weighs and calculates the actual amount of fluid removed.

Continuous venovenous hemodiafiltration (CVVHDF) uses an extracorporeal system with a filter. Blood is pumped from a large vein into the circuit and through the filter, which removes fluid and solute, and then the blood is pumped back into the patient's venous circulation. CVVHDF uses dialysis fluid and replacement fluid as described previously; therefore solute transport occurs through both diffusion and convective transport mechanisms. In CVVHDF the ultrafiltrate, which includes the replacement fluid volume, and the dialysate are recovered in the same effluent bag. The machine is designed to subtract the dialysate and replacement fluid volumes from the ultrafiltrate volume to calculate the actual volume of fluid removed from the patient. Table 13-7 compares characteristics of different CRRT modalities, including the driving force of blood flow and the mechanism of solute transport.

Pediatric Considerations

Access issues are extremely important in all patients who need renal replacement therapy, but these challenges become much more difficult in small, critically ill patients. Access is the most important consideration contributing to the effectiveness of therapy, and constant problems can arise when access is inadequate.[100]

Data from the ppCRRT Registry indicate that femoral access is used most often.[88] Care must be taken with femoral catheters in neonates and young children to prevent thrombosis and bleeding at the site. Femoral catheters are subject to kinking and are positional, and high negative pressures may lodge the catheter tip against the wall of the vessel, impeding flow. Femoral catheters may also have draw and inflow problems caused by increased intraabdominal pressure. These issues can be alleviated by careful positioning and switching the outflow (arterial) port with the inflow (venous) port of the catheter.

Catheter placement and size are based on the optimal site determined for the patient based on the risk of thrombosis and infection, ease of placement, and adequacy of function. Most pediatric practitioners recommend short, large-bore catheters in the right internal jugular vein or access in the femoral vein using the shortest possible catheter that will reach the inferior vena cava.[16]

Circuit volume must be considered. The CRRT circuit volume can represent a large percentage of the total blood volume in neonates or infants, especially if the patient is hemodynamically unstable as the result of sepsis, shock, or cardiac failure. The guidelines[17,61] recommend a blood prime if the circuit volume represents >10% of the patient's blood volume or if the patient is hemodynamically unstable. It is important to remember that packed RBCs from the blood

Table 13-7 **Continuous Renal Replacement Therapy Nomenclature**

Abbreviation	Definition	Driving Force	Circuit	Ultraf	Sol Transp
		DESCRIPTION			
CAVH	Continuous arteriovenous hemofiltration	BP	A-V	Replaced	Convection
CVVH	Continuous venovenous hemofiltration	Pump	V-V	Replaced	Convection
SCUF	Slow continuous ultrafiltration—form of CAVH or CVVH	BP/Pump	A-V/V-V	Not repl	Small amt
CAVHD	Continuous arteriovenous hemodialysis: dialysate delivered countercurrent to blood flow (1-2 L/hour)	BP	A-V	Not repl	Diffusion
CVVHD	Continuous venovenous hemodialysis: dialysate delivered countercurrent to blood flow (1-2 L/hour)	Pump	V-V	Not repl	Diffusion
CAVHDF	Continuous arteriovenous hemodiafiltration: dialysate delivered countercurrent to blood flow (1-2 L/hour)	BP	A-V	Replaced	Convection Diffusion
CVVHDF	Continuous venovenous hemodiafiltration: dialysate delivered countercurrent to blood flow (1-2 L/hour)	Pump	V-V	Replaced	Convection Diffusion

Adapted from Kellum JA, et al: The first international consensus conference on continuous renal replacement therapy. *Kidney Int* 62:1853-1863. Available at www.nature.com/ki/journal/v62/n5/full/4493298a.html, Accessed September 28, 2011; and Bellomo R, Mehta RL, Ronco C: Nomenclature for continuous renal replacement therapies. *Am J Kid Dis* 28(Suppl. 3):S2-S7, 1996.
A-V, Arteriovenous; *BP,* blood pressure; *Sol Transp,* solute transport mechanism; *Ultraf,* ultrafiltration; *V-V,* venovenous.

bank have high potassium concentration and a hematocrit of approximately 80%; therefore they should be diluted by 50% using either normal saline or albumin before the circuit prime.

Blood priming can cause early clotting and in some filters may cause acute hypotension that is thought to be caused by bradykinin release.[17] If a blood prime is required, several procedures may help maintain hemodynamic stability while connecting the patient to the circuit.

The first procedure prepares the bank blood for infusion into the patient. This procedure, called *zero balance ultrafiltration*,[46] circulates the bank blood through the CRRT circuit to normalize electrolytes and improve the acid-base status of the blood before connecting the circuit to the patient.

A second procedure uses a priming mixture of 75 mL of PRBCs, 75 mL of sodium bicarbonate, and 300 mg of calcium gluconate to be transfused post hemofilter.[17] In a third option, called the *bypass maneuver,* RBCs are administered to the patient at the same rate that the patient's blood is entering the circuit. The heparinized priming solution is discarded as it is displaced by the patient's blood. When the circuit is completely primed with the patient's blood, the venous line of the circuit is attached to the patient and CRRT treatment is begun.[35]

Hypothermia is a significant problem in pediatrics, especially in neonates or small infants, whenever an extracorporeal system is used. Heat loss is related to the blood flow rate (BFR) and the volume of blood in the circuit. Heat loss can be problematic even in children with higher BFR and smaller circuit volume-to-blood volume ratios. All possible measures should be instituted to maintain normothermia. Newer machines incorporate blood warmers. However, if a warmer is not included in the circuit, the nurse should institute some method of providing external warming. Blood warmers can be attached to the patient return line of the circuit to warm the blood just before it is returned to the patient. Potential external warming devices include radiant warmers, body warmers, heating mattresses, and solution heaters.

Most commercially available systems have membrane choices that will meet the patient's needs and the prescribed therapy that is based on those needs. For a list of access catheters see Table 13-8. Table 13-9 lists characteristics of CRRT hemofilters used for children, including priming volume, and Table 13-10 lists machines.

Nutritional considerations in the pediatric patient during CRRT are focused on protein requirements. In critically ill children or in children during the postoperative period, provision of adequate dietary protein is the most important nutritional intervention. Recommended daily amounts of protein to be administered to these children range from 1.5 g/kg for patients with AKI who are not receiving dialysis to 3 to 4 g/kg for patients receiving CRRT.[17] When critical illness is complicated by renal injury or failure, protein loss increases and it is imperative to consider this loss in planning the child's nutritional support. Protein loss in this setting results from increased muscle protein catabolism from insulin resistance, acidosis, and the presence of catabolic hormones and mediators.[68]

CRRT prescription variables include selecting the CRRT modality, the blood flow rate (BFR), the ultrafiltration rate, the dialysate rate, and the replacement fluid rate appropriate for the patient's clinical condition. In pediatric CVVH, a BFR of 4 to 6 mL/kg per minute is used, while attempting to keep the venous return pressure below 200 mm Hg. Dialysate and replacement fluid rates at 2000 mL/1.73 m^2 per hour have historically been used with a minimum rate of 35 mL/kg per hour.[17,100] The available data are insufficient to guide dialysate or replacement fluid rates, and wide variations exist worldwide in dialysis dosing.[78,81,100] Because of the many options available, prescription decisions should be tailored to the needs of the patient.[100]

Contraindications and Indications

As with CAVH, there are few contraindications to venovenous CRRT. It is often the treatment of choice for critically ill pediatric patients who are hemodynamically unstable as a result of

Table 13-8 **Recommended Catheter Sizes and Sites for Pediatric Continuous Renal Replacement Therapy**

Patient Size	Catheter Size and Location	Site of Insertion
Neonate <3-5 kg	Two 5-French single lumen	Femoral, internal jugular vein
	Single 7-French double lumen, 10 cm (Medcomp)	Internal jugular, femoral vein
	Single 7-French double lumen, 13 cm (Cook)	Femoral vein
	Two 7-French umbilical venous catheters	Umbilical vein
Infant or school-aged, 5-20 kg	Single 7-French triple lumen, 16 cm (Arrow)	Internal jugular, subclavian, or femoral vein
	Single 8-French double lumen, 11-16 cm (Arrow, Kendall)	
Infant or school-aged, >20-30 kg	Single 9-French double lumen, 12-15 cm (Medcomp)	Internal jugular, subclavian, or femoral vein
	Single 10-French double lumen, 12-19.5 cm (Mahurkar)	
Pediatric, 30-70 kg	Single 11.5-French double lumen, 12-20 cm (Medcomp, Mahurkar)	Internal jugular, subclavian, or femoral vein
	Single 11.5- or 12-French triple lumen, 12-20 cm (Medcomp, Mahurkar, respectively)	

Data supplied by Cook Critical Care, Bloomington, IN.; Mahurkar catheters are marketed by Kendall Company, Mansfield, MA; Medcomp, Harleysville, PA.; The Kendall Company, Mansfield, MA.
Adapted from McBryde KD, Bunchman TE: Continuous renal replacement therapy. In Wheeler DS, Wong HR and Shanley TP, editors: *Pediatric critical care medicine basic science and clinical evidence*, London, 2007, Springer-Verlag.

Table 13-9 **Hemofilters for Continuous Renal Replacement Therapy in Children**

Company	Hemofilter	Membrane Structure Type	Membrane Type	Membrane Surface (m²)	Priming Volume (mL)
Amicon	Minimiser Plus	MT	PS	0.08	15
	Diafilter 10S	MT	PS	0.20	15
	Diafilter 20S	MT	PS	0.25	38
	Diafilter 30S	MT	PS	0.60	58
Baxter	PHSF 400 gold	MT	PS	0.30	28
	PHSF 700 gold	MT	PS	0.71	53
	PHSF 700 gold	MT	PS	1.25	83
Fresenuis	F-5	MT	PS	1.00	63
	F-6	MT	PS	1.30	82
Gambro	FH 22	MT	C	0.16	11
	FH 66	MT	P	0.60	43
Hospel	Multiflow 60	MT	AN69	0.60	92
	Multiflow 100	MT	AN69	0.90	130
	HF 1000	MT	PAE	1.15	128
	HF 1400	MT	PAE	1.40	186
Renaflo	HF 250	MT	PS	0.25	27
	HF 400	MT	PS	0.30	28
	HF 500	MT	PS	0.50	39

From Butt WW, Skippen PW, Jouvet P: Renal replacement therapies. In Nichols DG, editors: *Rogers' Textbook of Pediatric Intensive Care*, Philadelphia, 2008, Lippincott Williams and Wilkins.
Amicon made by Amicon Corp, Danvers, MA; Baxter, Baxter Healthcare Corporation, Deerfield, IL; Braun, Braun Medical Incorporated, Renal Therapies Division, Bethleham, PA; Edwards Lifesciences, Draper UT: Fresenius, Fresdius Medical Care North America, Waltham, MA; Gambro, Gambro USA, Lakewood, CO; Hospal, Meyzieu, France; Renaflow made by Minntech Corporation, Minneapolis, MN.
AN69, Polyacrylonitrile; *C*, cuprophane; *MT*, microtubule; *P*, polyamine; *PAE*, polyarylethersulfone; *PS*, polysulfone.

shock, sepsis, or poor cardiac function. It is also used in patients after transplant (e.g., liver, bone marrow, stem cell transplant) who are fragile and have a metabolic milieu that does not promote optimal organ function. Even bleeding is not a contraindication to venovenous CRRT.[19] The patient must always be observed for bleeding at catheter sites, and vigilance must be heightened if the patient exhibits severe coagulopathy.

Method

Preparation for Venovenous Continuous Renal Replacement Therapy. When venovenous CRRT is ordered, the first step is to gather all the equipment: the machine, solutions, medications, and the circuit containing the hemofilter (cassette). With the new technology, all steps for inserting the cassette and priming the circuit are illustrated on the screen of the hemofiltration machine. It is imperative to follow each step in

Table 13-10 **Hemofiltration Machines**

Company	Machine	Lines
Edwards Lifesciences	Aquarius	Adult Peds
Gambro	Prismaflex	Adult
	Prisma*	Peds
Baxter	BM 11[†]	Adult
	BM 11a[†]	Peds
	BM 25	
	Accura	
Fresenius	2008	Adult Peds
B. Braun	Diapact	Adult Peds

From Brophy PD, Bunchman TE: *References and overview for hemofiltration in pediatrics and adolescents.* Available at http://www.pcrrt.com/Protocols%20PCRRT%20Zurich.pdf, Accessed January 14, 2010.
Baxter, Baxter Healthcare Corporation, Deerfield, IL; Braun, Braun Medical Incorporated, Renal Therapies Division, Bethleham, PA; Edwards Lifesciences, Draper UT: Fresenius, Fresdius Medical Care North America, Waltham, MA; Gambro, Gambro USA, Lakewood, CO; Hospal, Meyzieu, France.
*Prisma system no longer available, but supported by Gambro.
[†]Blood pump only; need the addition of the BM 14 to make the total of a BM 25 for the blood and ultrafiltration monitor together.

sequence. Do not jump to an "obvious" next step, because this can cause errors in preparation with omission of small but important details.

Initiation of Venovenous Continuous Renal Replacement Therapy. When priming of the circuit is complete, the patient is connected to the circuit. If the priming solution will be infused into the patient upon initiation of treatment, the patient's outflow catheter hub is connected to the red arterial outflow tubing of the circuit, and the venous return tubing is attached to the inflow hub of the patient's catheter.

To avoid infusing the priming solution into the patient when treatment is initiated, connect the outflow (arterial) line to the outflow hub of the patient's catheter, but do not connect the venous return tubing to the patient. As the patient's blood fills the circuit, begin the anticoagulation therapy (per physician order). Collect the priming solution in a sterile bag as it is flushed out of the circuit by the patient's blood. Once the patient's blood fills the circuit up to the venous return line and all of the prime solution has been displaced, stop the machine and attach the venous return tubing to the inflow hub of the patient's catheter, and restart the machine. This method discards the priming solution instead of infusing it into the patient, and prevents infusion of heparin and excess volume into the patient. This technique is especially suited for small patients, patients with poor cardiovascular function, and patients who are unable to handle the excess volume.

When considering priming methods, it is important to determine whether the patient can tolerate initial blood loss into the machine. To mitigate the effects of volume displacement, fluids (normal saline, albumin, packed RBCs) can be administered to the patient via the venous inflow catheter as

priming takes place (similar to the bypass procedure described previously).

When the therapy is started, only the BFR and the anticoagulation therapy should be running. The other flow rates may be kept at zero to allow time to assess the patient's response to the extracorporeal treatment. Assess vital signs (heart rate, respiratory rate, and blood pressure) and systemic perfusion. If the patient is tolerating the procedure well, the flow rates can be adjusted to the prescribed settings. After a patient has received venovenous CRRT for a period of time, the critical care nurse becomes familiar with the patient's tolerance to treatment and can work with the healthcare team to address specific patient needs.

Throughout venovenous CRRT, the nurse assesses the patient's vital signs (including temperature) and systemic perfusion. The catheter insertion site is assessed frequently for bleeding and kinks or any obstruction to flow from the patient and back to the patient. Access for medications, calcium infusion (if using citrate as the anticoagulant), and maintenance fluid must be functional and frequently assessed. If possible, a triple lumen central venous catheter is ideal for performing venovenous CRRT and delivering calcium. The third lumen is used for intravenous administration of medications and fluid.[69]

It is essential to prevent hypothermia in pediatric patients; the patient should be kept normothermic. Cover the child with sufficient blankets, use warming pads or warming mattresses, and use a blood warmer placed as close to the patient's venous return site as possible. Many of the newer machines incorporate blood warmers in the system and they will be needed for most patients. The CRRT treatment may mask the development of fever; fever should be suspected if a patient no longer requires external warming procedures to maintain body temperature.

During the venovenous CRRT procedure the nurse is responsible for monitoring the patient, the machine and the entire circuit. This monitoring includes the catheter insertion site for bleeding, inadvertent clamping of the catheter, or kinks; the pressures of the pull (arterial) side, the filter and the venous return side; the flow rates; the character of the effluent (ultrafiltrate); the blood leak detector; the air chamber or detection site; and the circuit tubing for leaks, kinks, and to ensure proper attachment to the solution or effluent bags. The nurse must respond to each alarm and perform a thorough assessment and a step-by-step troubleshooting procedure to resolve the issue associated with the alarm.

Blood sampling and laboratory studies must be performed as needed (per protocol) to maintain appropriate anticoagulation. If heparin is used, ACT levels are drawn from a blood draw site distal to the filter. The ACT range is generally maintained in the range of 180 to 200 s or approximately 1.5-fold the baseline. If citrate anticoagulation is used, the ionized calcium for the machine should be drawn distal to the filter, and the patient's ionized calcium should be drawn from a separate site, such as the arterial line. Available protocols provide guidelines for the rate of citrate infusion into the outflow tubing and the proportional calcium infusion into the patient. The goal of the protocol is to maintain the patient's ionized calcium at 1.1 to 1.3 mmol/L and the machine's ionized calcium at 0.35 to 0.45 mmol/L.[17,69]

Patient management during CRRT focuses on the effectiveness of the treatment as assessed by the patient's perfusion parameters, fluid status, and serum laboratory values. The monitored laboratory values include serum electrolytes, glucose, ionized and total Ca^{2+}, Mg^{2+}, hemoglobin and hematocrit, pH, albumin, prothrombin time, activated partial thromboplastin time, BUN, and creatinine. Depending on the indication for CRRT, additional laboratory values may be monitored.

Complications. Complications associated with venovenous CRRT in general include bleeding, problems with fluid balance (hypervolemia or hypovolemia), hypothermia, and anemia. Bleeding is a consequence of the severity of illness and the need for optimal CRRT circuit function, which in turn relies on safe and reliable anticoagulation. Anticoagulation must be maintained within narrow parameters.

Careful patient assessment is needed. Support of optimal fluid balance requires monitoring of the patient's perfusion, CVP, meticulous records of intake and output, and close attention to the ultrafiltration rate and serial patient weights. The patient's clinical status is the best guide to treatment adjustments. Anemia can develop from clots formed in the filter or from discontinuing treatment without reinfusing the blood from the circuit back into the patient. The patient's hematocrit should be followed closely.

Anticoagulation therapy can cause specific complications in addition to those listed previously. Heparin therapy can cause systemic bleeding including epistaxis; intracranial, pulmonary, gastrointestinal, bladder and vaginal hemorrhage; and heparin-induced thrombocytopenia. These developments may require a change in anticoagulation therapy or discontinuation of all anticoagulation.[18] Citrate anticoagulation can induce metabolic alkalosis (from the conversion of citrate to bicarbonate) and citrate lock, which is most common in patients with hepatic dysfunction or failure. Citrate lock occurs when citrate is not being cleared either in the filter or by the patient's liver. It is characterized by high serum total calcium and low serum ionized calcium. Treatment of this complication is to stop the citrate and calcium infusion for a designated period of time according to protocol (usually 30 min) and restarting the citrate at 70% of the prior rate.[17]

Brophy et al. published a multicenter evaluation of anticoagulation from ppCRRT Registry data comparing anticoagulation methods, filter life span, and patient complications. They concluded that when both heparin and citrate regional heparinization methods were commonly used, neither resulted in a longer filter life span, and citrate anticoagulation may result a in lower incidence of life-threatening complications.[18]

SPECIFIC DISEASES

Pediatric patients may require critical care for serious complications of primary renal disease such as sepsis, hypovolemia, thromboembolism, and AKI. Of the pediatric patients with failure-level AKI, primary renal diseases such as nephrotic syndrome (NS) and glomerulonephritis account for 7% to 9%.[67] Some of the more common primary renal diseases are discussed in this major part of the chapter.

In general, glomerular diseases have a clinicopathologic presentation that manifests as NS or nephritic syndrome. NS is generally inflammatory in nature, with visceral epithelial cell (podocyte) injury to the glomerular capillary wall from subepithelial immune deposits. NS is addressed as a specific disease in this part.

Nephritic syndrome typically arises from mesangial or subendothelial immune deposits on the glomerular capillary wall. These deposits lead to inflammation of the glomerulus and resultant urine sediment that is said to be *active*, including RBCs, white blood cells, and cellular and granular casts.[57,77] This active urine sediment reflects glomerular injury, inflammation, and cellular proliferation, all of which are hallmarks of this syndrome.[77] Injury to the glomerulus can result from a number of disorders, but immunologic injury is the most common cause. Two major mechanisms of immunologic injury have been described: (1) glomerular deposition of circulating antigen-antibody immune complexes and (2) development of an immune complex by antibody intereaction with an antigen that is part of the glomerular wall environment. Thus, injury of the glomerular endothelium results in an active inflammatory response associated with antibody-mediated binding or immune complex formation and deposition in the subendothelial and mesangial areas.[77]

Pediatric diseases characterized by nephritic syndrome include acute glomerulonephritis, systemic lupus erythematosus (SLE), Henoch-Schonlein purpura nephritis (HSP), and hemolytic uremic syndrome. Information about each of these diseases is summarized separately in this part of the chapter.

Similar to any organ or localized area within an organ, the kidney and the glomerulus respond to injury in a limited manner. To this end, glomerular diseases may manifest with only nephrotic features; they may manifest with dominant nephrotic features, but with some nephritic aspects and vice versa. Table 13-11 outlines this concept of glomerular diseases manifesting features from one or both types of syndromes, but with a dominance of features in one syndrome.[57]

Nephrotic Syndrome

NS is a clinical state characterized by the presence of massive proteinuria (the critical level for diagnosis is in excess of 40 mg/m² per hour or 1 g/m² body surface area per day in children and >3.5 g/day in adults), hypoalbuminemia (<2.5 g/dL), and edema (a common presenting sign). Hypercholesterolemia, hyperlipidemia, and lipiduria are associated complications.[67]

Etiology

NS is primarily a pediatric disease, developing in approximately 2 to 5 in 100,000 children per year.[91] It is 15-fold more common in children than in adults. Although NS can occur at any age, the initial onset of the disease is most often between 2 and 7 years of age. NS is seen approximately twice as often in boys as in girls in this age group.[91]

NS is currently categorized into primary and secondary forms. Primary or idiopathic NS is the most common form of NS in

Table 13-11   Tendencies of Glomerular Diseases to Manifest Nephrotic and Nephritic Features*

Glomerular disease	Nephrotic Features	Nephritic Features
Minimal change glomerulopathy (MCNS or MCD)	++++	−
Membranous glomerulopathy	++++	+
Diabetic glomerulosclerosis	++++	+
Amyloidosis	++++	+
Focal segmental glomerulosclerosis (FSGS)	+++	++
Fibrillary glomerulonephritis	+++	++
Mesangioproliferative glomerulopathy[†]	++	++
Membranoproliferative glomerulonephritis	++	+++
Proliferative glomerulonephritis	++	+++
Acute diffuse proliferative glomerulonephritis	+	++++
Crescentic glomerulonephritis	+	++++

Adapted from Jennette JC and Falk RJ: Glomerular clinicopathologic syndromes. In Greenber A, editor: *Primer on kidney diseases,* ed 4. National Kidney Foundation, Philadelphia, 2005, Elsevier, p. 151.
*Most diseases can manifest both nephrotic and nephritic features, but there is usually the tendency for one to predominate.
†Mesangioproliferative and proliferative glomerulonephritis (focal or diffuse) are structural manifestations of a number of glomerulonephritides, including immunoglobulin A nephropathy and lupus nephritis.
+ through ++++ indicates increasing tendency; −, no nephritic features.

children (90% of cases); the cause remains unclear. Secondary NS is seen less frequently (10% of cases) in children and results from infections, drugs or toxins,[97] systemic diseases, or glomerular disease (e.g., membranous nephropathy, membranoproliferative glomerulonephritis).

Primary Nephrotic Syndrome. There are three distinct histologic variants of primary childhood NS based on findings from light microscopy: (1) minimal change disease (MCD), (2) focal segmental glomerulosclerosis (FSGS), and (3) mesangial proliferation.[97] The histologic typing is important in the diagnosis of NS, because it predicts response to therapy and prognosis. Table 13-12 defines terms and classifications used in renal pathophysiology.

Minimal change nephrotic syndrome (MCNS), also called MCD, represents approximately 85% of primary NS in children. The onset is after 1 year of age and peaks between 2 and 3 years of age; it is unlikely to develop after approximately 7 of age.[97] In MCD, glomeruli are normal or nearly normal when examined by light microscopy, with only a minimal increase in mesangial cells and matrix. The mesangial cells and matrix support the glomerular capillaries. Separation of MCD from other types of primary NS is important because children with MCD are most likely to respond to treatment and have the best long-term prognosis.[91]

FSGS is the second most common histologic subtype of primary NS, seen in approximately 15% of children. The incidence of FSGS has increased in recent years, doubling and tripling in its occurrence, especially in African American populations.[13,67] In FSGS, the glomeruli show mesangial proliferation and "segmental areas of capillary collapse with obliteration of the capillary lumens, entrapment of hyaline material in some capillaries and adhesion of the tuft to Bowman's capsule."[77] Progression to AKI is common. Of note, FSGS may recur in 20% to 30% of patients after initial renal transplantation and in higher percentages after retransplantation.[67]

Approximately 5% of children who develop primary NS have mesangial proliferation characterized by diffuse increase in mesangial cells and matrix on light microscopy. These children have signs and symptoms identical to children with MCNS (MCD); however, only 50% respond to the initial course of steroid treatment.

Secondary Nephrotic Syndrome. NS can also result from secondary renal involvement associated with systemic diseases. The most common causes are infections, drugs or toxins, sickle cell disease, renal vein thrombosis, Hodgkin's disease, systemic lupus erythematosus (SLE), or Henoch-Schonlein purpura.[67]

Congenital Nephrotic Syndrome. Congenital NS is an inherited, autosomal recessive form of NS originally described in Finnish newborns. The diagnosis is generally made within the first 2 months of life. The gene responsible for congenital NS is located on chromosome 19 and encodes nephrin, an important protein in the slit diaphragm of glomerular podocytes. Nephrin is essential for normal glomerular function because it prevents filtration of protein macromolecules.[102]

Congenital NS can cause a large placenta and prematurity. The clinical presentation includes massive proteinuria, edema, abdominal distension, ascites, umbilical hernia, and separation of cranial sutures. These patients do not respond to steroid or immunosuppressive therapy.[67]

Pathophysiology

Primary NS is believed to have immune pathogenesis, although the precise mechanism remains to be elucidated.[91] Primary NS may be related to lymphocyte dysfunction and suppressor cytokines, or lymphocytes may initiate the syndrome. The permeability of the glomerular filtering membrane is increased, with electron microscopy revealing effacement or fusion of foot processes of podocytes (cells forming the outer layer of the glomerular capillary). The foot processes of the podocytes normally interconnect, leaving small filtration slits that normally do not allow filtration of protein.

The increase in glomerular capillary permeability may be related to a change in the electrostatic charge of the glomerular capillary wall by a highly cationic plasma protein. Under

Table 13-12   Renal Pathophysiology: Classifications and Definitions

Term	Definition
Focal	Involves <50% of glomeruli on light microscopy*
Diffuse	Involves >50% of glomeruli on light microscopy
Segmental	Involves part of the glomerular tuft, usually in a focal manner
Global	Involves the entire glomerular tuft; can be seen in either focal or diffuse disease
Membranous	Thickening of the glomerular capillary wall, usually with distinctive basement membrane "spikes"
Proliferative	Increased number of cells in the glomerulus; these cells can be either proliferating glomerular cells or infiltrating circulating inflammatory cells
Exudative	Prominent infiltration of neutrophils; a specific proliferative type
Membranoproliferative	Presence of thickening of the glomerular capillary wall with distinctive double contours or "tram tracks" and proliferative changes in the glomeruli
Crescent	Accumulation of cells (mostly mononuclear cells derived from the circulation and proliferated parietal epithelial cells) within Bowman's space; crescents often compress the capillary tuft and are associated with more severe disease
Glomerulosclerosis	Segmental or global capillary collapse or obsolescence with closure of the capillary lumens; it is presumed that there is little or no filtration across sclerotic areas
Glomerulonephritis	Any condition associated with inflammation in the glomerular tuft
Mesangium	Important component of the glomerulus; glomerular capillary network is attached and organized around the mesangium; consists of mesangial cells and mesangial matrix
Mesangial Cells	Possess properties of smooth muscle cells, surround glomerular capillaries, secrete the extracellular matrix, exhibit phagocytic activity that removes macromolecules from the mesangium, secrete prostaglandins and proinflammatory cytokines
Mesangial Matrix	Network of fibrous and fluid-filled material that is excreted by the mesangial cells; surrounds them and supports them
Podocytes	Tubular epithelial cells of Bowman's capsule that compose the visceral epithelial layer; they have long fingerlike processes called *foot processes* that surround the glomerular capillaries and interdigitate to cover the basement membrane that separates them from the endothelial cells; foot processes are separated by gaps called *filtration slits*
Filtration barrier/membrane	Composed of three layers: fenestrated glomerular endothelial cells, basement membrane, and foot processes of the podocytes
Slit diaphragm	Thin porous diaphragms that bridge the filtration slit between the foot processes of the podocytes; appear as continuous structure viewed on electron microscopy (EM); composed of several proteins: nephrin, podocin, α-actinin 4, and CD2-AP; create the size-selective filter, which impedes filtration of proteins and macromolecules

Based on data from Rennke HG and Denker BM: Pathogenesis of major glomerular and vascular diseases. In Rennke HG, Denker BM, editors: *Renal pathophysiology: the essentials,* ed 2. Philadelphia, 2007, Lippincott Williams and Wilkins; Koeppen BM, Stanton BA: Structure and function of the kidneys. In Koeppen BM, Stanton BA, editors: *Renal physiology,* ed 4. 2007, Mosby-Elsevier.
*This limitation to light microscopy is important, because most glomerular diseases involve almost all the glomeruli if the latter are examined by electron or immunofluorescence microscopy.

normal conditions, the glomerular endothelial cells and basement membrane express negatively charged glycoproteins, and they repel negatively charged proteins. If the charge becomes positive, then large, negatively charged proteins are no longer electrically repelled, and they begin to pass through the glomerular membrane, resulting in severe proteinuria.[102]

Common Elements. The presentation of NS in general reflects noninflammatory injury to the glomerular capillary wall. The common structural finding in all nephrotic conditions is prominent and extensive injury to the glomerular visceral epithelial cells (see Fig. 13-4), resulting in effacement of the foot processes. This damage increases glomerular permeability resulting in massive proteinuria.[77]

Regardless of the type of NS, the proteinuria causes a fall in serum albumin levels and a decrease in intravascular colloid osmotic (oncotic) pressure. This change enhances movement of fluid from the intravascular to the extravascular spaces, producing edema and decreased intravascular volume. The fall in

intravascular volume produces a fall in GFR and stimulates the release of aldosterone and antidiuretic hormone. These hormones produce an increase in sodium and water reabsorption that may temporarily increase intravascular volume, but further reduces intravascular osmolality and encourages further movement of fluid into the tissues. Thus the patient with NS may demonstrate a low or high intravascular volume, determined in part by renin, ADH and aldosterone secretion, and subsequent sodium and water retention.

All patients will demonstrate edema. Generalized edema is likely to develop once the serum albumin concentration falls below 2 g/dL. It is of interest that most studies have failed to document elevated levels of renin, angiotensin, or aldosterone even during times of significant sodium retention. As a result, the precise cause of edema is uncertain and may be associated with all of the preceding responses in addition to diminished atrial natriuretic hormone, activities of inflammatory cytokines, and physical factors within the vasa recti.[91]

Clinical Signs and Symptoms

Periorbital edema is often the first sign noted by parents of children with NS. Initially the eyes are puffy only in the morning and appear normal later in the day. Soon, however, the child develops dependent edema. If the child is ambulatory, the edema will first be apparent in the ankles and feet. It is common for children to be diagnosed with allergies during this time. As the edema becomes more generalized, it will be noted in the abdomen. The development of abdominal distension may accentuate inguinal and umbilical hernias, and labial and scrotal edema may be excessive. Moderate hepatomegaly often is noted. If ascites becomes severe, it may compromise diaphragm excursion and cause respiratory distress.

Generalized edema may also produce diarrhea, vomiting, and anorexia. These gastrointestinal symptoms and the presence of a generalized catabolic state further deplete body protein stores. Malnutrition and loss of muscle mass may become severe, but may not become apparent until the edema resolves. During the edematous phase, fever may be absent despite the presence of infection.

The patient with NS is oliguric; the urine has an acid pH and contains large quantities of protein, so it foams. Urine may be tinted pink or red from microscopic hematuria; it may contain granular and cellular casts and lipid bodies. Severe hypoalbuminemia is generally present among children with NS, and most have albumin levels of less than 2.5 g/dL. Serum complement levels are low in some patients with nephritic syndrome (e.g., membranoproliferative glomerulonephritis or systemic lupus erythematosus nephritis), but are normal in children with MCNS.

Total serum calcium concentration may be falsely low. Because hypoalbuminemia is present, the fraction of the total calcium bound to protein is reduced; therefore serum ionized calcium concentration may be normal. The patient with chronic NS, however, may demonstrate genuine hypocalcemia resulting from loss of vitamin products, including vitamin D. Water retention may contribute to the development of hyponatremia; hyperaldosteronism and poor dietary intake may produce hypokalemia.[10] Approximately one fourth of the children with MCNS demonstrate an increase in serum creatinine and BUN. Children who have focal glomerulosclerosis may demonstrate glycosuria and bicarbonaturia, with only moderate reduction of creatinine clearance.

A secondary anemia may be present and may be severe when significant glomerular disease is associated with renal failure. Because the patient's skin is edematous, the pallor of anemia may be more pronounced. If the child's intravascular volume is reduced, hemoconcentration may maintain the measured hematocrit within normal limits.

The risk of thromboembolism is high among patients with NS. These children demonstrate a hypercoagulability that may be related to increased platelet aggregation and increased levels of beta-thromboglobulin, as well as decreased fibrinolytic activity. As a result, the nurse should monitor for signs of thromboembolic events and minimize venipunctures and use of longdwelling central venous or arterial catheters.

During NS relapse, edema can accumulate rapidly in tissues, depleting the intravascular volume. If this fluid shift from the intravascular space occurs during sodium restriction and diuretic therapy, hypovolemia may result in circulatory collapse.

Children with NS usually develop anorexia and demonstrate growth failure. The administration of steroids and immunosuppressive agents can further compromise the child's growth. In addition, the steroids and immunosuppressive agents increase the child's risk of infection, as does the loss of immune proteins in the urine. Sepsis, especially gram-positive sepsis, frequently occurs among children with NS in relapse.

A renal biopsy is necessary to firmly establish the degree of glomerular damage associated with NS, but it may not be performed as part of the initial workup. Because MCNS is the most common form of NS occurring in children, a 4-week course of corticosteroid therapy abolishes symptoms in approximately 93% of children with NS who are between 1 and 7 years of age.[67]

If the child with NS does not respond to the initial steroid therapy, a renal biopsy is often indicated.[67] The biopsy specimen is examined using both electron and light microscopy techniques. Identification of the degree of glomerular involvement will enable better evaluation of therapy and establishment of prognosis.

Management

Treatment of the child with NS is aimed at restoration or maintenance of adequate circulating blood volume and systemic perfusion, minimization of glomerular damage and maximization of renal function, maintenance of fluid and electrolyte balance, maximization of patient comfort, and prevention of infection. Respiratory function also must be monitored and supported.

If the child with NS has signs of poor systemic perfusion (e.g., tachycardia, cool, clammy extremities, and decreased intensity of peripheral pulses) and intravascular volume depletion (no hepatomegaly, low CVP, small heart silhouette on chest radiograph), then a large-bore central venous catheter should be inserted if one is not already in place. This catheter will enable measurement of CVP and infusion of intravenous fluids. Usually bolus administration of 10 to 20 mL/kg of saline, Ringer's lactate, albumin, or a mixture of saline and albumin (80 mL of saline plus 20 mL of 25% albumin) will reestablish adequate intravascular volume (see "Management of Shock" in Chapter 6). Fluid resuscitation should proceed with care to avoid pulmonary edema, and the healthcare team should be prepared to support ventilation.

The use of albumin may cause rapid fluid shift from the third space into the vascular space. If the child is oliguric, fluid administration probably should be curtailed as soon as intravascular volume is adequate as indicated by a CVP >5 mm Hg, with good systemic perfusion and a heart rate that is appropriate for age and clinical condition.

Once systemic perfusion is acceptable, laboratory studies should be performed, including complete blood count, serum electrolytes, calcium, phosphorus, BUN, creatinine, total protein, albumin, globulin, cholesterol, triglycerides, complement (C_3), and urinalysis. Each time the child voids, the urine should be measured and tested for proteins. The urine specific gravity will be falsely elevated in the presence of proteinuria or with administration of osmotic diuretics. The urine osmolality is the best indicator of renal function, because it reflects renal concentrating ability and is not affected by the presence of large molecules in the urine.

Collection of urine samples from the infant or child with NS may be difficult. Catheterization should be avoided if possible, because it introduces risk of infection. Adhesive urine collection bags can irritate the edematous perineal skin; therefore they should be avoided. Small children may be allowed to void on nonabsorbant surfaces, such as the outside of a disposable diaper, so that some urine can be collected for analysis. Cotton balls may be placed in the diaper to catch the urine; the urine is then squeezed out of the cotton ball into a container to be sent for analysis. The specimen should be labeled as that collected into a cotton ball, because it will not yield reliable cell counts.

The child with NS requires careful measurement of all sources of fluid intake and output. The child's daily weight should be measured using the same scale and technique at the same time of day. Frequent, but rough, estimates of the degree of edema should be made. If ascites is present, the child's abdominal girth should be measured at least once daily.

Usually, children with NS are asymptomatic except for the discomfort caused by edema. Bed rest is necessary only during acute infections or when severe incapacitating edema is present. Because bed rest is associated with problems of large vessel venous stasis, possible decubitus, and possible development of contractures, mobility is encouraged as soon as it is feasible.

Salt restriction, albumin infusion, or diuretics may be necessary to reduce edema. All of these methods of reducing edema, except albumin infusion, can result in intravascular volume depletion, so they should be used with caution. In addition, the hemoconcentration produced by edema and vigorous diuresis can aggravate the hypercoagulability, resulting in increased risk of thromboembolic events.

If a diuretic is prescribed, the nurse should assess the child's systemic perfusion carefully before administering the drug, and then monitor perfusion during and after diuresis. Furosemide is the most commonly used diuretic for children with NS, whether administered by scheduled doses or by infusion[67] (see Table 13-2).

Furosemide (1-2 mg/kg per intravenous dose) may be prescribed; this dose can be increased each time the drug is given until a maximum of 4 to 5 mg/kg every 12 hours is reached. If the patient develops resistance to furosemide, other diuretics such as metolazone, hydrochlorothiazide, and spironolactone (an aldosterone antagonist) can be used.

For maximal diuretic effect, the infusion of salt-poor albumin may be ordered to be followed by intravenous administration of furosemide (1-2 mg/kg) within 30 minutes. The administration of 25% albumin before diuresis will diminish the risk of hypovolemia, and a target albumin level of approximately 2.8 g/dL is considered sufficient to restore intravascular volume and oncotic pressure.[67] The nurse should monitor for signs of hypervolemia after albumin administration, although risks can be reduced by infusing albumin at a slow continuous rate. Signs of hypervolemia include tachycardia, hypertension, and congestive heart failure. The increase in intravascular

volume is usually only transient while the albumin remains in the vascular space.

If the child is between 1 and 7 years of age with a normal complement (C_3) concentration and minimal hematuria, MCNS is likely to be present, and steroid therapy is the treatment of choice. Prednisone is given in a dose of 2 mg/kg per 24 hours, for a maximum total daily dose of 80 mg in divided doses.[65] Proteinuria should disappear within the first 2 weeks of therapy in most children. Once the child responds to the prednisone, the dose can be tapered over a period of several months while the child or parents continue to test the child's urine for proteinuria.

If the child continues to demonstrate proteinuria after 28 days of continuous prednisone therapy, a renal biopsy usually is planned to determine the etiology of the NS. NS that is unresponsive to prednisone may include MCNS or mesangial proliferation or focal glomerulosclerosis.

Treatment of steroid-resistant or relapsed NS may require the use of alkylating agents such as cyclophosphamide or chlorambucil. These drugs can produce alopecia, leukopenia, and increased susceptibility to infection, so careful evaluation and preparation of the child and family is required before such drugs are prescribed. Cyclosporine has become one of the most commonly used drugs for children with steroid-resistant NS (SRNS). More recently, tacrolimus has been used with prednisone to treat SRNS, with a high rate of complete remission reported.[67]

The child will be extremely uncomfortable if severe edema is present. Measures should be taken to avoid friction between adjacent skin surfaces, such as between the inner leg and the scrotum or between the chest and under arm areas. Rolls of cotton can be placed in these areas, or nonperfumed talc or cornstarch can be placed over friction points. Because the skin is extremely fragile, tape or adhesive dressings should be avoided. The bedridden child should be turned frequently to avoid pressure sores over bony prominences.

Resistance to infection is compromised by loss of immune proteins in the urine, poor systemic perfusion, steroid and/or immunosuppressive therapy, poor nutrition, and appetite loss. The nurse and dietician should make every effort to provide the child with small, frequent, nutritious, and appetizing meals.

The development of significant abdominal effusion can increase the risk of peritonitis, causing unexplained fever and ascites. Administration of prophylactic antibiotics usually is not indicated, because it can foster the growth of resistant organisms. The pneumococcal vaccine should be administered to any patient with new onset NS and every 5 years thereafter to reduce the risk of infection.

The mortality rate of NS is low (3% to 7%), and the prognosis for children with MCNS is best if the child has only signs of proteinuria and responds immediately to prednisone therapy. If the child has nonresponsive (i.e., steroid-resistant) or steroid-dependent NS, recovery is less complete, and relapses may occur frequently. If the child is unresponsive to steroids (i.e., has SRNS), immunosuppressive drugs, and alkylating agents, the prognosis is poor because many of these patients (estimated risk >40% within 5 years of diagnosis) develop end-stage renal disease (ESRD). SRNS causes greater than 10% of pediatric ESRD.[67] Severe glomerular sclerosis that is resistant to treatment often is associated with a fulminant and fatal course.

Because the child's illness is often sudden and the prognosis is usually uncertain for several weeks, it is imperative that the child and family receive adequate support and consistent information from all members of the healthcare team.

Acute Glomerulonephritis

Etiology

Acute glomerulonephritis is a significant cause of AKI in pediatric patients and among children who require acute dialysis.[67] Glomerulonephritis can be a primary or secondary disease resulting in glomerular injury leading to hematuria, mild proteinuria, edema, hypertension, and oliguria. The injury to the glomerulus is characterized by glomerular inflammation and cellular proliferation. Nephritogenic forms of streptococcus have been associated with the most common form of glomerulonephritis in children, though other bacterial, viral, parasitic, pharmacologic, and toxic agents have also been implicated.[25]

Pathophysiology

When antibody reacts with circulating antigen that is unrelated to the kidney and forms immune complexes, these complexes are deposited in the glomerulus. The deposits contain immunoglobulins and complement that can be visualized with immunofluorescence microscopy. This deposition stimulates glomerular endothelial proliferation, mesangial proliferation, and invasion of white blood cells. When antibody reacts with antigen located on the glomerular basement membrane, the deposition of immunoglobulin and complement forms crescents.[59,77] These deposits also activate the inflammatory response.

Clinical Signs and Symptoms

The onset of glomerulonephritis is usually abrupt with manifestations of nephritis: azotemia (excess of urea or other nitrogenous wastes), oliguria, edema, hypertension, proteinuria, and active urine sediment.[57] If glomerulonephritis is related to a nephritogenic streptococcal infection, it generally develops in children between the ages of 2 and 12 years, and symptoms develop approximately 7 to 14 days after a group A beta-hemolytic streptococcal pharyngitis or 21 to 40 days after streptococcal skin infection (impetigo).[59] The symptoms are usually self limiting, although prolonged hematuria and proteinuria occasionally occur.

Macroscopic hematuria (excretion of rusty colored urine) is a frequent presenting sign, although microscopic hematuria is occasionally present. The child usually develops systemic edema; periorbital edema may be noted initially, although generalized edema is often present. Proteinuria is present, but is not as severe as that seen with NS.

Hypertension is present in 50% to 60% of children with acute streptococcal glomerulonephritis,[25,67] and it can be severe. Occasionally, hypertensive encephalopathy develops and will be associated with signs of altered level of consciousness, irritability, and increased intracranial pressure.

Signs of hypervolemia may be associated with signs of congestive heart failure, including tachycardia, hepatomegaly, high CVP, tachypnea, and increased respiratory effort.

Radiologic evidence of cardiomegaly and pulmonary edema are often apparent.

The child with glomerulonephritis is often oliguric but rarely anuric. The GFR is reduced, but renal concentrating ability may be normal. The fractional excretion of sodium often is reduced, and sodium and water retention develop (see "Acute Kidney Injury" earlier in this chapter for information regarding fractional excretion of sodium). Hematuria with RBC casts are the characteristic urinalysis findings associated with acute glomerulonephritis and are documented in nearly half of involved patients.[57] A renal biopsy rarely is indicated to confirm the diagnosis of glomerulonephritis.

Changes in the child's serum and urinary electrolyte concentrations often resemble those associated with prerenal failure (see Table 13-4). The creatinine is often normal, but the BUN typically is elevated. The child may demonstrate dilutional hyponatremia, and the serum albumin concentration will be low. Serum hyperkalemia also may develop and produce associated changes in cardiac rhythm (see "Hyperkalemia" earlier in this chapter, and in Chapter 12). A dilutional anemia may also be observed.

Antibodies to streptococcal products (such as antistreptolysin-O) usually can be documented in patients with poststreptococcal glomerulonephritis from pharyngeal infection, but may not be present after a skin infection. The most consistent indicators of a recent streptococcal infection are serum titers of antihyaluronidase and antideoxyribonuclease B (antiDNAase B). High serum immunoglobulin (Ig) G levels and low C_3 levels will be present.[59]

Management

Most children with acute glomerulonephritis will recover completely if complications of renal disease can be prevented.[25] If AKI failure develops, fluid restriction will be required, and treatment of electrolyte and acid-base imbalances will be necessary (see section, Acute Renal Failure and Acute Kidney Injury). In general, treatment is symptomatic and supportive.

Sixty percent of children with acute glomerulonephritis will develop hypertension.[25] The nurse should notify the on-call provider if hypertension develops and perform frequent neurologic examinations to detect any deterioration in the child's level of consciousness. The child with significant hypertension may develop headaches and signs of encephalopathy, including nausea, vomiting, irritability, lethargy, seizures, coma, and increased intracranial pressure. Standard therapies to treat hypertension include sodium restriction and drug therapy including diuretic therapy with furosemide, calcium channel blockers, vasodilators and ACE inhibitors.[25]

Significant hyperkalemia must be treated on an urgent basis to prevent the development of malignant arrhythmias. Administration of calcium, sodium bicarbonate, glucose and insulin, or a sodium polystyrene sulfonate (Kayexalate) enema may be needed (see "Hyperkalemia" in this chapter and in Chapter 12).

If signs of congestive heart failure develop, the child will require treatment with fluid restriction and diuretics. Intravenous inotropic agents and/or vasodilators may be necessary. (See "Management of Shock" in Chapter 6, and "Congestive Heart Failure" in Chapter 8).

Because antibiotic administration does not influence the recovery of children with glomerulonephritis, antibiotic administration is indicated only if the child has positive bacterial cultures.

Systemic Lupus Erythematosus: Renal Involvement

SLE is a chronic inflammatory autoimmune disease affecting multiple systems. The etiology and pathogenesis are incompletely understood, although clinicopathologic studies have enabled classification of the lupus nephritis that results from renal injury (Table 13-13).

Renal disease occurs in 30% to 70% of children with SLE, primarily mediated by deposition of immune complexes in the kidney. Patients with SLE who have clinical manifestations of proteinuria or hematuria, a positive serologic test result for lupus, and other clinical signs typical of SLE are diagnosed with lupus nephritis after a renal biopsy. Children typically present with signs of SLE after 5 years of age, with a peak incidence in late childhood. SLE is highly prevalent in adolescent females, and these adolescents develop nephritis far more frequently than do adults.[29] African American females have a 10-fold higher incidence of SLE than Caucasians.[67]

The clinical findings in class II and some patients with class III lupus nephritis show hematuria and proteinuria of less than 1 g/24 hours (see Table 13-13). These findings are considered the milder forms. The more severe forms of lupus nephritis, represented by most patients in class III and those in class IV, are associated with decreased renal function including AKI and NS. NS is present in 45% to 80% of patients with SLE and renal disease.[67] Class V, the least common form of lupus nephritis, is also associated with NS.

Immunosuppressive treatment involves an induction of prednisone followed by a low steroid taper. For severe forms of the disease, intravenous cyclophosphamide is administered ($500\text{-}1000 \text{ mg/m}^2$) every month for 6 months then every 3 months for 18 months.[25] Combination therapy of prednisone and cyclophosphamide has improved renal survival by 40%.[67]

Henoch-Schonlein Purpura

Henoch-Schonlein purpura (also known as *anaphylactoid purpura*) is a disease of childhood with the greatest incidence between 2 and 8 years of age. It is a disease of unknown etiology manifested by nonthrombocytopenic purpura in the lower extremities and buttocks in addition to pain, joint swelling, and signs of glomerular disease. HSP occurs most frequently in the winter months and often follows an upper respiratory infection. It affects boys more commonly than girls and recurrent episodes may occur.

HSP includes vasculitis with IgA dominant immune deposits affecting small vessels such as capillaries, venules, and arterioles. The areas most commonly affected are the skin, gut, and glomeruli. Active disease is characterized by elevated

---

Table 13-13   World Health Organization Classification of Lupus Nephritis and General Clinical Manifestations

Classification	Histologic Findings*	Clinical Manifestations
Class I	No histologic abnormalities	SLE signs and symptoms
Class II	Mesangial lupus nephritis: mesangial deposits of immunoglobulin and complement	Hematuria, normal renal function, and proteinuria of <1 g/24 hours
II-A	Includes mild mesangial hypercellularity and increased matrix	
II-B	Includes moderate mesangial hypercellularity and increased matrix	
Class III	Focal segmental lupus glomerulonephritis: mesangial deposits in almost all glomeruli and subendothelial deposits; occasional glomeruli show necrosis, crescent formation, and sclerosis	Hematuria, normal renal function and proteinuria of <1 g/24 hours; some have NS, reduced renal function, or AKI failure
Class IV	Diffuse proliferative lupus nephritis: all glomeruli contain significant mesangial and subendothelial deposits of immunoglobulin and complement; capillary walls thickened and demonstrate necrosis, crescent formation and scarring	Most common and severe form; hematuria, NS, reduced renal function or AKI failure; highest risk for progression to end-stage renal disease
Class V	Membranous lupus nephritis: immune complexes deposited on epithelial side of glomerular membrane cause diffuse thickening (spikes on glomerular basement membrane) and granular deposits of IgG and C_3, and linear staining of IgG, IgA, and C_3	Least common form of NS

Data from Davis ID, Avner ED: Membranous glomerulopathy (glomerulonephritis). In Kliegman RM, et al, editors: *Nelson textbook of pediatrics,* ed 18. Philadelphia, 2007, WB Saunders; Davis ID, Avner ED: Membranoproliferative (mesangiocapillary) glomerulonephritis. In Kliegman RM, et al, editors: *Nelson textbook of pediatrics,* ed 18. Philadelphia, 2007, WB Saunders; Davis ID, Avner ED: Glomerulonephritis associated with systemic lupus erythematosus. In Kliegman RM, et al, editors: *Nelson textbook of pediatrics,* ed 18. Philadelphia, 2007, WB Saunders.
*Based on light microscopy, immunofluorescence, and electron microscopic findings.
AKI, Acute kidney injury; C_3, complement; *Ig,* immunoglobulin; *NS,* nephrotic syndrome; *SLE,* systemic lupus erythematosus.

serum concentrations of the cytokines tumor necrosis factor-α and interleukin-6.[25]

Microscopic hematuria and nephritis may be present. The renal biopsy demonstrates antibody-antigen complexes with glomerular fibrin deposition. Patients with the worst prognosis include those who have NS or an AKI associated with oliguria, uremia, and hypertension (see section, Acute Renal Failure and Acute Kidney Injury). Most children will recover with supportive care; there is no specific treatment for this disorder.[77]

Hemolytic-Uremic Syndrome

Etiology

Hemolytic uremic syndrome (HUS) is a thrombotic micro-angiopathic disease involving endothelial damage, which leads to platelet and fibrin deposition in small vessels. It has several etiologies.

HUS is characterized by a triad of symptoms: acute hemolytic anemia, thrombocytopenia, and AKI causing uremia. HUS is classified as postdiarrheal (D+HUS, the typical form) or nondiarrheal (D-HUS, the atypical form). HUS is the most common cause of AKI in children[25,59]; it affects both sexes equally and most cases occur in children younger than 4 years of age. Advances in treatment of the D+HUS have greatly improved prognosis with most children regaining normal renal function.[75]

Pathophysiology

The inciting event most commonly associated with D+HUS is the absorption of verotoxin (also called a *Shiga toxin*) from a form of *Escherichia coli*, known collectively as *Shiga toxin-producing E. coli* (STEC). In North America, the most commonly identified STEC is *E. coli* O157:H7 (also called *E. coli O157*).[41] STEC is transmitted through ingestion of contaminated and undercooked or uncooked beef, or contaminated milk or cheese. Contaminated water, fruits, vegetables, and juices have been implicated less frequently.[75]

The primary site of injury with hemolytic uremic syndrome is the endothelial lining of the small arteries and arterioles, particularly in the kidney. This microangiopathic process results in the intravascular deposition of platelets and fibrin, resulting in partial or complete occlusion of small arterioles and capillaries in the kidney. As erythrocytes and platelets traverse these partially occluded vessels, they are fragmented by mechanical injury from the narrowed vessels and the fibrin strands. RBC fragmentation also results from oxidative damage.[75] The life span of the erythrocytes is reduced, and the damaged erythrocytes are removed from the circulation by the spleen; this results in a severe and often rapidly progressing anemia.

Most patients with HUS also demonstrate thrombocytopenia for 1 to 2 weeks. It is not clear whether this thrombocytopenia results from destruction of platelets, consumption of the platelets, or aggregation of the platelets within the kidney. Platelet survival time is drastically reduced, from a normal survival of 7 to 10 days to approximately 1.5 to 5 days. Platelet antigen has been found in the kidneys of affected patients and HUS patients often demonstrate a thrombocytopathia. In addition, there is evidence of peripheral platelet destruction.

As noted previously, HUS is associated with damage to the glomerular endothelial cells. The cells tend to swell and detach from the glomerular basement membrane, and the space between the cells and the membrane becomes filled with lipid, fibrin strands, platelets, and cell fragments. The glomerular capillary lumen often is occluded by fibrin, thrombi, and platelets. As a result, renal blood flow and GFR can be reduced in a degree proportional to the glomerular injury.

Renal ischemia may produce cortical necrosis, and renal tubular injury also may be seen. Although much of this damage is reversible, recurrences can occur or progressive renal failure can develop.

HUS may involve the gastrointestinal or central nervous systems. Young children often have a mild gastroenteritis that can progress to bloody diarrhea. The development of neurologic symptoms, particularly coma, is associated with a poor prognosis. The patient may develop irritability, seizures, abnormal posturing, hemiparesis, or hypertensive encephalopathy.

In contrast to D+HUS, the presentation of D-HUS (the atypical form) does not include a prodrome of enterocolitis and diarrhea. D-HUS can be genetic, acquired, or idiopathic in origin. Atypical HUS also predominantly affects children, and the glomerular endothelial pathology is similar to that of D+HUS. However, D-HUS has a worse prognosis and a tendency to recur, and a large percentage of the patient's progress to end-stage renal disease.[25] D-HUS is likely to recur even after renal transplant.

Clinical Signs and Symptoms

The appearance of D+HUS closely follows or is coincident with an episode of mild gastroenteritis that may include bloody stools. HUS also may follow upper respiratory infections, urinary tract infections, measles, or varicella.[41] Within 1 to 2 days, the child demonstrates a notable pallor, with purpura, rectal bleeding, or other signs of hemorrhage (e.g., petechiae or ecchymoses).

The child's peripheral blood smear shows fragmented RBCs (a microangiopathic hemolytic anemia), fibrin split products, and a decreased platelet count (thrombocytopenia) seen in 90% of patients. The hemoglobin concentration is typically 5 to 9 g/dL. Within a few days of the onset of anemia, the reticulocyte count will be high. The serum bilirubin level usually is not elevated, although hepatosplenomegaly is often present.

Renal manifestations range from mild insufficiency to AKI. If the child exhibits oliguria or anuria, the serum creatinine, BUN, phosphate, and potassium will be elevated. Hyperkalemia can develop and progress rapidly if gastrointestinal bleeding and gastrointestinal reabsorption of blood products occurs. Congestive heart failure, pulmonary edema, and hypertension can result from decreased renal function, hypervolemia, and increased plasma renin activity.

Examination of the child's urine reveals the presence of fibrin, proteinuria, microscopic or macroscopic hematuria, and urinary cell casts. Evidence of consumptive coagulopathy (decreased levels of fibrinogen, factor V, and factor VIII) is not present.

Most children younger than 2 years demonstrate mild hemolytic anemia and renal involvement, and the course of the disease is short. Mortality has declined to less than 10% as a result of aggressive treatment focused on the support of fluid and electrolyte balance and nutrition, with early dialysis. A small number of patients recover renal function slowly, whereas some will develop chronic renal failure. Recurrence of HUS has been reported after renal transplantation, particularly in patients with D-HUS.[25]

Management

The management of the child with hemolytic uremic syndrome requires assessment and support of fluid and electrolyte balance, administration of RBCs as needed, management of hypertension, and recognition and treatment of neurologic complications. Insensible fluid loss (300-400 mL/m^2 per day) is replaced with 5% dextrose and 0.45% sodium chloride without potassium supplement. Urine output is typically replaced milliliter for milliliter with 0.45% sodium chloride. Furosemide is given intravenously in a dose of 1 to 5 mg/kg every 6 hours to convert oliguric renal failure to the polyuric form, which is ostensibly easier to treat.[75]

Approximately one third to half of children with D+HUS[75] and the majority of those with D-HUS become anuric or develop oliguric renal failure, and fluid and electrolyte therapy must be adjusted accordingly. Renal replacement therapy, usually in the form of PD, may be necessary. If the illness is severe and is complicated by intestinal perforation or severe neurologic symptoms, CVVH is used (see Care of the Child During Dialysis, earlier in this chapter). The healthcare team should review doses and dosing intervals of all drugs that the child is receiving and adjust as needed.

Anemia is treated through careful administration of packed RBCs whenever the child becomes symptomatic or the hematocrit falls below 20%. Frequent transfusions may be required, because the life span of transfused erythrocytes is shortened in the presence of HUS. Only small amounts (3-5 mL/kg) of blood should be administered at any one time if hypervolemia, hypertension, or hyperkalemia are complicating the renal failure. Often transfusions will be planned around the institution of CRRT to manage fluid balance. Fresh packed RBCs are preferable to older bank blood, because the potassium content of fresh blood is low. Administration of leukocyte-poor packed RBCs may be ordered if irreversible renal failure and ultimate renal transplantation are anticipated. Platelet transfusions should be avoided, because they can create further consumptive coagulopathy and microthrombosis.[75]

Hypertension related to hypervolemia should be managed with hemofiltration or dialysis. Pharmacologic agents may be needed (see Box 13-7).[104] Doses and dosing intervals should be adjusted as needed in the presence of renal dysfunction.

The nurse should perform careful neurologic assessments at least every hour. Signs of irritability, lethargy, seizures, posturing, or hemiparesis should be reported immediately. If the child develops signs of neurologic deterioration, refer to Increased Intracranial Pressure in Chapter 11.

If bloody diarrhea persists or the child develops abdominal distension with decreased intestinal motility, provide nothing by mouth and plan to administer caloric requirements through parenteral alimentation. Calories should be provided chiefly with glucose, using less protein than would be provided for patients without renal failure. Maximize caloric intake within the fluid restrictions necessary to prevent hypervolemia.

The parents of the child with hemolytic uremic syndrome will require a great deal of support. They will require reassurance that there was no way they could have known that the child's prodromal illness would lead to serious illness. It is imperative that all members of the healthcare team use consistent terminology and provide a consistent prognosis to minimize confusion.

Chronic Kidney Disease

Etiology

Chronic kidney disease (CKD) is an irreversible, progressive decrease in renal function that leads to ESRD. CKD is defined by the Kidney Disease Outcome Quality Initiative (KDOQI) as either kidney damage or a decreased level of kidney function as measured by the GFR. The criteria for kidney damage (with or without a decrease in GFR) specify damage for 3 months or more as defined by pathologic abnormalities or markers of kidney damage, such as abnormalities in the blood or urine or abnormal imaging tests. The second defining criterion of CKD is a GFR of <60 mL/minute per 1.73 m^2 body surface area (BSA) for 3 or more months with or without kidney damage. Regardless of the etiology of the renal injury, the continued decline in GFR reflects the process of sclerosis and nephron loss, which is irreversible.[22]

The KDOQI has published a classification system for the stages of CKD, with emphasis on early detection and treatment to prevent or delay the progression of the disease. This staging of CKD[22] is as follows:

Stage I: Kidney damage with normal or increased GFR (≥90 mL/minute per 1.73 m^2 BSA)

Stage II: Kidney damage with mild reduction in GFR (60-89 mL/minute per 1.73 m^2 BSA)

Stage III: Moderate reduction in GFR (30-59 mL/minute per 1.73 m^2 BSA)

Stage IV: Severe reduction in GFR (15-29 mL/minute per 1.73 m^2)

Stage V: Kidney failure; GFR < 15 L/minute per 1.73 m^2 BSA

The kidney reserve function is such that more than 50% of renal capacity must be lost before imbalances occur. Although manifestations of renal insufficiency vary, continued dialysis will be necessary for the patient with severe renal insufficiency, whereas the patient with moderate renal impairment typically responds to careful medical and dietary management.

Functional disturbances associated with CKD involve impaired removal of metabolic byproducts as well as fluid excess and electrolyte and acid-base imbalances. Renal dysfunction will affect the growth and formation of bones, RBC formation, and general body growth and will greatly alter the child's daily life.

Pathophysiology

Chronic kidney disease may result from malformation of the renal system, infections, inherited renal disorders, severe trauma, or glomerular disease. The leading causes of CKD in young children are congenital defects, and cystic and hereditary diseases. ESRD from glomerulonephritis, hereditary diseases, and acquired diseases such as HUS are seen in older children.[10]

At stage III, chronic renal disease is associated with moderate reduction in the GFR with or without kidney damage. At this level the serum urea is greater than 20 mg/dL, and serum creatinine is greater than 1.5 mg/dL. (Normal creatinine concentration in infants and small children is approximately 0.3-0.8 mg/dL; the creatinine concentration in larger children and adults is approximately 0.7-1.5 mg/dL.)[40]

Uremia. *Uremia* refers to the cluster of symptoms, clinical signs, and biochemical changes associated with the accumulation of waste products and the fluid and electrolyte imbalances that occur in patients with CRD. These changes can include hypervolemia, electrolyte and acid-base imbalances, anemia, hypertension, renal osteodystrophy, metastatic calcification, and accumulation of uremic toxins.[41]

Sodium and Water Balance. The characteristic feature of early renal insufficiency is a defect in the renal ability to concentrate urine. This defect leads to the production of urine with a fixed osmolality. The patient may maintain a relatively normal serum sodium concentration despite a marked reduction in GFR, because the remaining functioning nephrons handle more sodium. Most patients with chronic renal disease are able to excrete reasonable quantities of sodium and maintain normal serum sodium concentration, provided that acute increases in sodium intake are avoided.

Sodium and water restriction may result in hyponatremia because the diseased kidneys are unable to conserve sodium. The resultant urinary loss of sodium and water can produce volume depletion, further reductions in the GFR, and a greater increase in BUN. Prolonged administration of diuretics also can lead to sodium depletion.

A change in sodium balance is seen in severe ESRD. In these patients, the low GFR is inadequate to excrete sufficient amounts of sodium and water in light of sodium and water intake. Retention of sodium and water produce edema and vascular congestion, often with resultant hypertension, pulmonary edema, and heart failure. These complications often must be treated with dialysis.

Potassium Balance. Because the entire quantity of potassium filtered by the glomerulus is reabsorbed by the proximal tubule, the maintenance of a stable serum potassium concentration requires potassium secretion by the distal tubules. When renal damage is present, undamaged nephrons have the ability to increase potassium secretion. Patients with chronic renal failure and chronically low GFR may generate urine containing a secreted potassium concentration in excess of the amount present in the filtrate. For this reason, it usually is not necessary to restrict dietary potassium until the GFR is at extremely low levels.

The patient with chronic renal insufficiency requires a longer period of time to rid the body of excess potassium.

As a result, acute hyperkalemia can result from the ingestion of a large potassium load, hemolysis, acidosis, or a catabolic state associated with fever. Hypokalemia occasionally develops as a result of a decreased potassium intake or diuretic therapy.

Acidosis. One of the primary functions of the kidney is the excretion of metabolic acids. This function involves three aspects of tubular function: reabsorption of bicarbonate, secretion of ammonium ions, and secretion of titratable acids (acidification of urinary buffers). Patients with chronic renal disease generally develop metabolic acidosis caused by bicarbonate wasting and decreased distal tubule ability to produce ammonia once the GFR decreases by 30% to 40%.[41] Exogenous bicarbonate administration might only increase urinary bicarbonate loss. The rate of ammonia production decreases in proportion to the fall in GFR. The ability of the kidney to form phosphate buffers remains effective until late stages of CKD.[41]

Calcium, Phosphate, and Bone. Patients with CKD have reduced intestinal absorption of calcium. This reduced absorption may result from deficiency in the active form of vitamin D that is produced by the kidney.

When the GFR falls below 25% of normal, the plasma phosphate concentration begins to rise. Under normal conditions, a reciprocal fall in the serum level of ionized calcium follows phosphate retention, because the ionized calcium and phosphate form a precipitate. This lowering of the ionized calcium stimulates release of parathyroid hormone (PTH). PTH normally increases renal excretion of phosphate and promotes bone reabsorption, liberating calcium and phosphate ions. It simultaneously reduces renal phosphate reabsorption. PTH also assists the kidney in the formation of active vitamin D, which increases intestinal calcium absorption and bone reabsorption. The net result of PTH secretion is normally a fall in serum phosphate and a rise in serum ionized calcium, removing the stimulus for PTH secretion.

When renal disease is present, the rise in phosphate concentration results in a fall in serum ionized calcium. The low serum calcium level stimulates PTH release. Because the kidneys are impaired, they are unable to excrete more phosphate and cannot synthesize vitamin D to increase intestinal calcium absorption. The serum calcium remains low, triggering an increase in PTH synthesis and secretion, causing chronic bone reabsorption. This excessive secretion of PTH by the parathyroid is referred to as *secondary hyperparathyroidism,* and it causes renal osteodystrophy (Fig. 13-11).

Anemia. Chronic renal failure affects both RBCs and platelets. RBC production is impaired by a decrease in production of erythropoietin, and the life span of the RBC is shortened by uremia. Although the platelet count is normal, platelet function is reduced (a thrombocytopathia is present).

Uremic Encephalopathy and Neuropathy. The cause of uremic encephalopathy in patients with CKD is unknown. It seems to be related to changes in the fluid and electrolyte

↓ GFR [<30 mL/min; stages 4 and 5 of chronic kidney disease]

⇓

↑ Serum phosphate [Inability of the kidneys to excrete excess dietary phosphate due to the low GFR]

⇓

↓ Vitamin D [Hyperphosphatemia suppresses the hydroxylation of inactive vitamin D in the kidney]

⇓

↓ Serum calcium [Hypocalcemia from decreased intestinal calcium absorption and from calcium precipitation with phosphate]

⇓

↑ PTH synthesis [All 3 of the abnormal conditions above trigger parathyroid hormone synthesis]

⇓

Secondary hyperparathyroidism [Leads to bone disease called renal osteodystrophy]

FIG. 13-11 Advanced concepts: pathophysiology of hyperphosphatemia in chronic kidney disease.

balance, serum osmolality, and accumulation of uremic toxins. Ultimately, these abnormalities can affect the brain cell membrane permeability, the sodium-potassium pump, and the cerebral uptake of glucose.[64]

CKD also can be associated with the development of a peripheral neuropathy. With this neuropathy, demyelination of distal portions of the nerves can occur, resulting in decreased nerve conduction.[31]

Clinical Signs and Symptoms

Patients with CKD often have vague complaints of fatigue, weakness, anorexia, nausea, abdominal pain, and headaches. Growth failure is usually present. Specific signs and symptoms include an initial polyuria and polydipsia, mild edema (especially around the eyes), and oliguria. The child's complexion may be sallow or pale with a faint uremic tint. Skin rashes or arthritis also may be present. The child usually has a history of previous kidney or urologic disease or of an episode of renal injury.

Initial evaluation includes analysis of serum electrolytes, phosphate, pH, bicarbonate, BUN, creatinine, PCO_2 and base deficit or excess, hematocrit, hemoglobin, white cell count, and blood culture. Urine is collected for culture, sediment, pH, osmolality, and sodium. A 24-hour or timed urine collection may be performed to quantify urine volume and creatinine and protein excretion.

The child with CKD usually demonstrates a normal serum sodium and potassium concentration (unless chronic diuretic therapy is provided, and then hypokalemia may be present), a high serum phosphate and low serum calcium concentration, a high BUN, high uric acid, and an elevated serum creatinine concentration. Metabolic acidosis may be present, and serum bicarbonate ion concentration is low. If an infection is present, the child's white blood cell count may be elevated. In addition, the child is usually anemic, with a prolonged bleeding time resulting from thrombocytopathia.

If uremic encephalopathy develops, the child may demonstrate signs of increased intracranial pressure, such as irritability, lethargy, or seizures. If a uremic neuropathy is present, the child may develop muscle cramps, tetany, weakness, or muscle wasting.[64]

Management

The hospitalized child with CKD requires careful fluid and electrolyte therapy. Parents or primary caregivers of children with CKD are often valuable resources regarding the child's food preferences and feeding techniques. The dietician will assist by helping plan menus on an individual basis.

Children with CKD are more susceptible to infections and need careful skin and wound attention. The staff must be extremely careful to use good hand-washing technique before and after examining the child.

Once the child develops any form of renal failure, doses of medications must be adjusted (see section, Adjustment of Medication Dosages in the Management of Acute Renal Injury earlier in this chapter).

Treatment of uremia in children with CKD can be accomplished through dietary restrictions, dialysis, or both. Because protein is essential for normal growth and development in children, dietary protein restriction is generally not recommended.[98]

Indications for dialysis in children with chronic kidney disease include: hypervolemia or congestive heart failure, deterioration in neurologic status, severe bleeding, metastatic calcification as a result of calcium phosphate precipitation, severe hyperkalemia, acidosis, BUN greater than 125 to 150 mg/dL, serum sodium concentration above 160 mEq/L, or serum calcium concentration above 12 mg/dL.

Generally, once the child with CKD is in stable condition, dialysis can be scheduled at relatively regular intervals. Next, hemodialysis or a form of PD can be used to maintain fluid and electrolyte balance (see "Dialysis," earlier in this chapter). Whenever possible, children with CKD are prepared for renal transplantation.

Nutritional support for children with chronic renal failure is extremely challenging. Anorexia is common among patients with CKD, and inadequate ingestion of protein and carbohydrates compounds the severe growth failure associated with the disease. Tube feedings can provide 100% of the recommended dietary allowances for infants (100 Kcal/kg per day) and older children (40-70 Kcal/kg per day) for normal growth (see Chapter 14). However, no catch-up growth can be achieved by providing calories exceeding recommended daily allowances.

Daily protein requirement for children is approximately 2.5 g/kg. The aim should be to provide proteins that are metabolized into useable amino acids—that is, amino acids that do not produce as much nitrogenous wastes. These proteins include: eggs, milk, meat, fish, and foul (listed from lowest to highest in nitrogenous waste production).[98] Patients receiving PD should receive the higher ranges of protein. Meals must be appetizing, and the caloric content of foods should be maximized. For example, if the child enjoys drinking milkshakes, then they should contain protein and caloric supplements so that the child ingests more than milk and ice cream. Regular consultation with a dietician is usually necessary.

Fluid, sodium, and potassium restrictions usually are not required when the patient is receiving PD. If hemodialysis is provided, the need for fluid restrictions is determined by the amount of remaining renal function and urine output present, by the child's volume status, and by the success of fluid removal during dialysis.

If the patient develops mild hyperkalemia, treatment should focus on elimination of the cause of the elevation. If the hyperkalemia is severe, however, and ECG changes develop, urgent treatment with calcium, sodium bicarbonate, glucose plus insulin, sodium polystyrene sulfonate, or dialysis are indicated (see "Hyperkalemia" and "Acute Kidney Injury," this chapter).

It is important to regulate the child's phosphate intake and intestinal absorption. Phosphate binders, especially calcium-based phosphate binders, should be prescribed when phosphate cannot be controlled by dietary restriction.[22] Control of the serum phosphate concentration helps prevent hypocalcemia and hyperparathyroidism and the bone mineral disease that results.

Anemia is often present in children with CKD. The 2007 clinical practice guidelines recommend maintaining the hemoglobin concentration in children with CKD between 11 and 12 g/dL using erythropoietin stimulating agents.[22]

Oral hygiene and skin care are extremely important because urea tends to accumulate in the mouth and on the skin, which can cause odor, irritation, and discomfort. Uremia is usually especially high just before dialysis treatments.

Renal (Kidney) Transplantation

Indications

The major indication for renal transplantation is deterioration in renal function leading to ESRD, requiring chronic dialysis therapy. Children in ESRD have the greatest chance of surviving 5 years with transplantation (93% compared with 79% for hemodialysis and 82% for peritoneal dialysis).[92] Although transplantation is virtually always preferable to dependence on dialysis, the availability of continuous ambulatory peritoneal dialysis and continuous cycled peritoneal dialysis offers tolerable options for support of the child while awaiting transplantation, and they probably offer improved transplantation selection criteria and survival.

Preemptive transplantation (transplantation before dialysis is required) has the benefit of preventing potential complications of dialysis as well as limiting the adverse effects created by complete kidney failure. This strategy is challenging because it requires predicting when kidney failure will become significant, transplanting only when necessary and avoiding dialysis. As stated in the KDOQI Guidelines, "the initiation of dialysis therapy remains a decision informed by clinical art, as well as by science and the constraints of regulation and reimbursement."[22]

If transplantation is considered, the nephrologist, the transplant surgeon, and the nurse transplant coordinator will each discuss with the child (as age-appropriate) and family the type of transplant recommended (cadaver versus living related), and the expected posttransplant care regimen. The child's role in postoperative activities and the immunosuppressive regimen should be discussed before the procedure takes place.

Preparation for Transplantation

Multiple diagnostic studies will be necessary to evaluate the renal transplant recipient (Table 13-14). Because many children with renal disease demonstrate associated anomalies of the urinary tract, a voiding cystourethrogram (VCUG) is performed to ensure that drainage of the urinary system is normal. If abnormalities, such as reflux are detected, they usually are repaired surgically before the child is listed for transplantation.

The child must be free of infection at the time of transplantation. In addition, a social worker interviews the family and determines the support they will require and their ability to comply with the child's posttransplant care requirements. A psychosocial evaluation of the child and family is required by federal law. There should also be a discussion with the family regarding alternative therapies and the option to decline escalation of care. Families will need support for their decisions.

Blood type identification and tissue typing is performed to identify the category of tissue that is most likely to result in successful transplantation. Use of a living donor is preferable to a cadaver donor for long-term outcome. The most important factors in finding a suitable donor have been shown to be ABO blood type compatibility and youth.

Typing of human leukocyte antigens (HLAs) is performed on all potential donors and recipients. These antigens are located on the sixth chromosome, and three pairs of antigens—including A, B, and DR antigens—are present in each patient. Long-term graft survival is best if the transplant recipient and the kidney are HLA-compatible.

Each child receives a haploid or haplotype from each parent; the haploid contains the genetic material from either the sperm or egg (half of the genetic material required). Therefore a biologic parent always shares one haplotype with the child. Siblings may demonstrate identical haplotypes (25% probability), share one haplotype (50% probability), or share no haplotype (25% probability). Transplants from living related donors with identical haplotypes are more successful than all other transplants, because the donor will share identical chromosomal material with the recipient.[94]

Parents and family members of the patient will be tissue typed. Identical twins will, of course, match all six antigens. If a compatible family donor is identified, baseline laboratory studies must be performed, including complete blood count with white cell differential, serum electrolytes, liver and renal function studies, and cytomegalovirus, HIV, and hepatitis B antigen screening. An ECG and chest radiograph also are performed. If the results of all serum studies are acceptable, a renal computed axial tomography scan, renal arteriograms, and psychiatric evaluation are performed. These studies are more extensive than those required of a cadaver donor, because the family member must be assured of adequate renal function even after the donation of one kidney; two functioning structurally normal kidneys must be present in order for one kidney to be donated. The donor must be prepared for surgery and a potentially painful recovery. Laparoscopic kidney donation has minimized the risk to the donor with far quicker recovery time. In addition, the donor and recipient must be prepared for the psychological stress of possible rejection of the transplanted kidney.

A cadaver kidney is obtained when a kidney to be donated is matched with a computerized listing of potential recipients available from the United Network of Organ Sharing and

Table 13-14   **Preoperative Evaluation of the Renal Transplant Patient**

Tissue Typing and General Evaluation	Metabolic Evaluation	Infectious and Immune Evaluation
Recipient		
ABO blood type, tissue type	Bili (total and direct)	Measles, mumps, rubella and
Chest radiograph	Total protein, albumin	Varicella titer
Echocardiogram	Lipid profile, fasting blood sugar	Hepatitis B surface antigen
Stool guaiac × 2	Magnesium	Hepatitis B antibody
Dental evaluation	CBC with differential, platelet count	Hepatitis profile
Ophthalmology evaluation	PT, aPTT, thrombosis evaluation	HIV antibody, VDRL
Urinalysis (UA), urine culture	PTH-N terminal	CMV titer; EBV titer
Voiding cystourethrogram (VCUG) and/or ultrasound	SMA 12, alkaline phosphatase	Herpes titer
Urology evaluation if indicated		PPD
		Immunization records
		Communicable disease history
Donor		
ABO tissue type, initial crossmatch	CBC, SMA 12	CMV titer; EBV titer
History, physical	Renal and liver panel	HIV antibody
ECG, chest radiograph	Lipid panel	Hepatitis B surface antigen
Urine culture, UA	Amylase, lipase	VDRL
Renal CT scan	PT, aPTT, SGOT, SGPT, alkaline phosphatase	Nasopharyngeal culture
Psychiatric evaluation		Peritoneal fluid culture (if peritoneal dialysis patient)
24-hour urine-volume, protein, creatinine	BUN, creatinine, SMA-12, CBC with differential	
Final pretransplant testing immediately before transplant surgery		
Cross-match recipient with donor—if positive, transplant canceled		
Chest radiograph		
Urine analysis, urine culture		

regional organ procurement organizations. This network lists the age; ABO blood type, presence or absence of Rh (rhesus) D-antigen (i.e., Rh⁺ or Rh⁻), and tissue type; antigen sensitivity; time on list; and urgency status of recipients on the network roster. When a kidney is donated, it becomes available to the patient with the highest priority based on time waiting, urgency of condition, tissue matching, percentage of reactive antibody, and age.

The United Network of Organ Sharing agrees that children younger than 18 years have priority on the list. This priority of pediatric over adult transplant recipients was approved because significant deleterious effects of transplant delay on growth and development have been documented in pediatric patients with renal failure. Current policies give pediatric transplant candidates priority for kidneys from donors younger than 35 years.[93] The impetus for this prioritization was an attempt to decrease the need for a second transplant in pediatric patients and to attempt to provide more effective use of organs. In the past, older transplant patients were dying with functioning grafts from younger donors, and children were requiring second transplants after they received initial grafts from older donors.

Kidneys are preferentially allocated locally, then regionally, and then cross-regionally. A cadaver kidney should ideally be transplanted within 24 hours of harvest, because longer preservation times are associated with a higher incidence of acute tubular necrosis and primary nonfunction.

The final step in matching the donated kidney and the recipient is the panel reactive antibody (PRA) which is used to detect antibodies in the recipient to the HLA antigens in the potential donor. The PRA test is reported as a percentage; a high percentage means that the recipient possesses preformed antibodies to the donor cells and will reject the kidney acutely.

If all crossmatches, the PRA test, and assessment of the donor, the donated kidney, and the recipient indicate that the donor is healthy and infection free and the donor and recipient are compatible, the transplant is performed. The procedure lasts approximately 4 hours. In children larger than approximately 20 kg, the new kidney is placed in the retroperitoneal space in the right or left iliac fossa. The renal artery of the donated kidney is sewn to the recipient iliac artery, the donor vein is sewn to the recipient's external iliac vein, and the ureter is implanted into the posterior wall of the recipient bladder. In small children (less than 20 kg), the kidney can be placed in the intraperitoneal space. It is routinely attached to the aorta and vena cava. The dialysis catheter remains in place if kidney function is not immediately observed during surgery, so the dialysis catheter will be available if needed for dialysis postoperatively.

Posttransplant Care

The child usually returns from renal transplantation with a urinary catheter, large-bore peripheral intravenous catheters, and one central venous monitoring catheter. A multilumen central venous catheter will enable simultaneous CVP measurement and intravenous access. The first dose of immunosuppressive agent can be administered preoperatively or intraoperatively.

The goals of posttransplant care include maintenance of effective circulating blood volume, maintenance of systemic and kidney perfusion, and prevention of infection. Fluid balance and daily weight must be monitored closely and reported to the on-call provider. Routine postoperative cardiorespiratory support and psychosocial and family support also will be required.

The transplant surgery and flank incision will create a significant amount of pain postoperatively. Adequate analgesia must be provided (see Chapter 5 for further information).

Fluid Therapy. The child's intravascular volume must be carefully assessed (Box 13-11) and supported throughout posttransplant care, because hypovolemia will result in further compromise of renal function and may contribute to thrombosis of the transplanted graft. Transplanted kidneys are exquisitely sensitive to volume changes and initially lack the ability to protect renal perfusion and GFR if hypovolemia develops. Systemic perfusion, heart rate, CVP, and arterial pressure should be monitored continuously.

The CVP usually is maintained between 5 and 10 mm Hg to ensure the presence of adequate circulating blood volume. The fluid administration rate will total insensible water losses (approximately 300-400 mL/m² body surface area per day) plus urinary losses. One intravenous infusion will consist of 0.45% sodium chloride (occasionally normal saline is alternated with 5% dextrose and 0.45% sodium chloride) and may contain sodium bicarbonate. This fluid replaces urine output (milliliter for milliliter for urine output up to 200 mL/hour) exclusively; the replacement rate is calculated on an hourly or 30-minute basis. The second intravenous infusion is used to administer a glucose-containing solution at a rate designed to replace insensible water losses. Glucose is monitored (including point-of-care testing if available) and is frequently elevated as the result of steroid use; fluid intake is adjusted accordingly.

The CVP will be maintained with intravenous infusion of normal saline and occasional 5% albumin infusion. Care should be taken to maintain the CVP at 5 to 10 mm Hg, but overhydration should be avoided. If the transplanted kidney is healthy and functioning well, an osmotic diuresis usually is observed immediately after surgery; urine output of 100 to 200 mL/hour or more is often observed during the first 24 to 72 hours after transplantation.

Approximately 25% of transplanted kidneys develop acute tubular necrosis,[49] which can result in oliguria and may produce complications of renal failure, including hyperkalemia and acidosis. If ATN develops, fluid restriction will be necessary, and dialysis ultimately may be required. Indications for

---

Box 13-11 **Assessment of Intravascular Volume**

Clinical Signs of Adequate Intravascular Volume
- Adequate systemic perfusion (severe hypovolemia will compromise systemic perfusion)
- Central venous pressure 0-5 mm Hg; no systemic edema
- Pulmonary artery wedge pressure 4-8 mm Hg; no pulmonary edema
- Good skin turgor, round (not tense) fontanelle (in infants)
- Body weight appropriate for age
- Heart rate appropriate for age and clinical condition
- Normal heart size on chest radiograph
- Urine volume approximately 1-2 mL/kg per hour

Laboratory Results Consistent with Adequate Intravascular Volume
- BUN 5-22; serum sodium 135-145 mEq/L, serum osmolality 275-295 mOsm/L
- Hematocrit appropriate for age and condition
- Urine specific gravity less than 1.020

Clinical Signs and Laboratory Results Consistent with Significant Hypovolemia
- Poor systemic perfusion
- Tachycardia
- Oliguria with increased urine specific gravity and osmolality
- Dry mucous membranes, sunken fontanelle
- CVP and pulmonary artery wedge pressure (PAWP) less than 5 mm Hg
- Rise in serum sodium concentration and hematocrit

Clinical Signs and Laboratory Results Consistent with Significant Hypervolemia
- Tachycardia
- Hepatomegaly and systemic edema
- Moist mucous membranes, full and tense fontanelle
- Hypertension
- Clinical and radiographic evidence of pulmonary edema, possible pericardial effusion
- Increased heart size on chest radiograph
- Decrease in serum sodium concentration and hematocrit

BUN, Blood urea nitrogen; *CVP,* central venous pressure.

---

dialysis and treatment of AKI are presented earlier in the chapter (see section, Acute Renal Failure and Acute Kidney Injury).

Accurate documentation of fluid intake and output must be maintained scrupulously, and a physician (or the transplant coordinator or other on-call provider) should be notified of any decrease in urine output. If urine output falls, the urine collection system should be checked for the presence of kinks or clots. With physician (or other on-call provider) order, the urinary drainage system can be entered using aseptic technique, and the urinary catheter can be irrigated gently with sterile solution. If the irrigant does not return through the catheter, the catheter may be obstructed and catheter replacement is required.

Serum electrolytes and urine and serum osmolality should be monitored closely. The child's BUN and creatinine concentrations should approach normal by the third day.

Additional information about postoperative care, and particularly about surgical complications following kidney transplantation, can be found in Chapter 17.

Infection. Strict hand-washing technique and careful surveillance for signs of infection are mandatory in the treatment of the immunocompromised renal transplant patient. All hospital personnel involved in the care of the child, and family members must protect the child from infection, and visitors must be screened carefully for evidence of transmittable disease.

A urinary catheter is required during the postoperative period to avoid tension on the incision site in the bladder; the catheter serves as a potential site of infection. The catheter should be immobilized with secure tape in a position that avoids tension on the catheter. The collection tubing should be coiled on the bed to facilitate gravity drainage and should never be elevated to allow reflux of urine into the bladder. The final portion of the tubing should drain straight down into the collection chamber, without the development of dependent loops.

The child's temperature and white blood cell count should be monitored closely. Any signs of infection should be reported to a physician or other on-call provider immediately, and appropriate cultures of blood and urine should be obtained.

Potential Causes of Renal Failure. After renal transplantation, renal failure can develop as the result of prerenal (e.g., hypovolemia, acute tubular necrosis) or postrenal causes. Prerenal causes of renal failure should be prevented with adequate intravascular fluid therapy and careful monitoring of blood volume and systemic perfusion.

ATN is most likely to occur in a cadaveric kidney that had prolonged cold ischemic time before transplantation. Preprocurement ischemia will also contribute to the development of posttransplant ATN.

If ATN develops, the child will be oliguric or anuric and will be susceptible to all the complications associated with AKI failure. When urine output falls, a fluid challenge of 10 mL/kg of normal saline may initially be provided. In addition, furosemide can be administered to encourage a diuresis.

Hypervolemia, acidosis, and hyperkalemia all require aggressive treatment. Hypervolemia usually produces hypertension and can result in cardiovascular dysfunction and congestive heart failure. Dialysis is indicated for the treatment of congestive heart failure associated with hypervolemia and for a serum potassium concentration exceeding 6.0 to 6.5 mEq/L. Renal function often returns within several days after surgery.

Postrenal causes of post transplant renal failure include obstruction of the newly anastomosed ureter. In addition, urine may leak from the anastomosis into the abdomen. Such a leak will be apparent if a renal scan or ultrasound examination is performed. If such obstruction or leak occurs, placement of a urinary stent, creation of a nephrostomy, or reimplantation of the ureters may be required.[48]

Renal Vascular Complications. Partial or complete obstruction of the renal artery may occur from torsion or kinking of the vessel. Renal artery obstruction usually produces escalating hypertension with oliguria. A renal scan, ultrasound examination with Doppler, or arteriogram enables distinction of arterial obstruction from ATN. Reoperation or balloon angioplasty will be required to relieve the obstruction.

In pediatric transplantation, vascular thrombosis is a potential cause of graft failure. It generally develops in the first 24 to 48 hours, but may develop as late as 7 to 15 days after transplant.[48] If a computed tomography scan or magnetic resonance imaging confirms the presence of the thrombosis, reoperation will be required. For additional information about renal artery stenosis and thrombosis, see "Renal Transplantation, Surgical Complications" in Chapter 17).

Rejection. Despite effective tissue cross-matching, most transplanted kidneys (except those received from identical twins) will be rejected to some degree. Hyperacute rejection begins almost immediately when blood flow to the kidney is established in surgery. Within minutes to hours, circulating preformed antibodies begin destroying the kidney, which must be removed immediately. However, hyperacute renal rejection mediated by preformed or T cell-mediated antibodies is rare.

Acute renal rejection may occur within 2 to 10 days of transplantation, although it may develop within the first 2 months after transplantation. Acute rejection can result in an acute fall in urine output, fever, and tenderness over the graft. This rejection may be identified early, before signs or symptoms are apparent. Leukopenia can also be noted, although it may be associated with excessive immunosuppressive therapy. Additional signs of rejection include hypertension, rising serum creatinine, weight gain, proteinuria, decreased fractional excretion of sodium, evidence of renal tubular acidosis, and abnormal imaging studies.[94]

A renal biopsy will be performed to document the presence of rejection and differentiate it from other causes of renal failure. If rejection continues, removal of the kidney may be necessary, although it is rare to have a rejection episode refractory to treatment.

The immunosuppressive drugs used to prevent rejection vary among transplant centers. New protocols are being devised to limit the use of prednisone to reduce or avoid growth failure and other steroid side effects such as edema, hypertension, central nervous system effects and glucose intolerance.[32] The immunosuppressive agent cyclosporin A was most widely used in the past, but new protocols are being designed to limit its use to prevent nephrotoxity resulting in renal damage, hypertension, and increasing serum creatinine.

Tacrolimus is a drug in the same category as cyclosporine A (both are calcineurin inhibitors), but it is less nephrotoxic and is being used more widely in recent years.[48] Initiation of therapy using either drug is delayed until good function is established in the new kidney (Table 13-15). Additional information about immunosuppressive agents can be found in Chapter 17.

Late Complications
The most common cause of death during the first year after renal transplantation is infection, especially from Epstein-Barr virus (EBV) and cytomegalovirus (CMV). Antibody titers for

Table 13-15 Immunosuppressive Drugs: Category, Mechanism of Action, and Major Side Effects

Category	Mechanism of Action	Major Side Effects
Antibodies: Polyclonal: Atgam and antithymocyte globulin	Target T-lymphocyte surface antigens to inactivate peripheral T-lymphocytes; prevents initiation of the immune response to the allograft	Increased risk of infection, serum sickness
Monoclonal: Muromonab CD-3 (OKT3)	Binds with CD-3 receptor complex on T-cells and renders T-cell receptor incapable of activating the cell	Cytokine release syndrome: fever, capillary leak, and neurologic symptoms
Basiliximab and daclizumab	Target interleukin 2 (IL-2) receptor on activated T-lymphocytes and prevent T-lymphocytes from responding to IL-2	Few if any
Calcineurin Inhibitors: Cyclosporin A and tacrolimus	Inhibits calcineurin phosphatase and reduces IL-2 expression. Disrupts the signal from T-cell receptor to nucleus and prevents T-lymphocyte activation	Increased risk of malignancy, nephrotoxicity (cyclosporine greater than tacrolimus), neurotoxicity, diabetes, hypertension, cardiotoxicity, and hyperlipidemia, hirsutism (cyclosporine), alopecia (Tacrolimus)
Target of Rapamycin Inhibitors: Sirolimus and everolimus	Targets T-lymphocytes and to lesser extent B-lymphocytes by binding with a protein that prevents their proliferation in response to activation	Increased risk of infection (boxed warning issued by FDA), delayed wound healing, lymphoceles, hyperlipidemia, and thrombocytopenia, nephrotoxicity (when combined with calcineurin inhibitors)
Antiproliferative Agent: Mycophenolate mofetil = replacing azathioprine in kidney transplantation*	Blocks T-lymphocyte proliferation by inhibiting its ability to synthesize DNA (selectively inhibits inosine monophosphate dehydrogenase, which interferes with DNA purine synthesis)	Gastrointestinal: diarrhea Hematologic: increased risk of infection, leukopenia
Azathioprine (Imuran)	Prevents proliferation of leukocytes by inhibiting purine synthesis	Hematologic: increased risk of infection and malignancy; leukopenia, thrombocytopenia, anemia
Corticosteroids: Glucocorticoids (prednisone and derivatives)	Anti-inflammatory effects target antigen-presenting cells and inhibit cytokine production; block the production of chemokines that signal immune cells to migrate to area of inflammation and block the migration itself	Growth suppression, glucose intolerance, hypokalemia, alkalosis, edema, hypertension, headache, seizures

Data from Formica RN, Lakkis FG: Kidney transplantation: Management and outcome. In Greenberg A, editor: *Primer on kidney diseases*, ed 4. National Kidney Foundation, Philadelphia, 2005, Elsevier, pp. 547-548. Chapter 69; and Hanevold CD, Wynn JJ, Ortiz LA: Renal Transplantation. In Wheeler DS, Wong HR, Shanley TP, editors: *Pediatric critical care medicine basic science and clinical evidence*, London, 2007, Springer-Verlag London Limited, pp. 1253-1254. Chapter 107.
*Formica RN Jr, Lakkis FG: Kidney transplantation: management and outcome. In Greenberg A, editor: *Primer on kidney disease*, ed 4. National Kidney Foundation, Philadelphia, 2005, Elsevier.

both of these viruses are screened in the donor and recipient before transplantation. Cytomegalovirus can lead to direct graft tissue injury and loss.[94]

Malignancies are another serious complication that can lead to death. Most (up to 73%) result from posttransplantation lymphoproliferative disease caused by Epstein-Barr virus (EBV) infection during aggressive immunosuppressive therapy.[94] Other complications include, but are not limited to, recurrence of glomerular disease in the new kidney, ATN, bleeding, and drug toxicity.[32]

DIAGNOSTIC STUDIES

Most of the tests used to evaluate renal function—including creatinine clearance, fractional excretion of sodium, renal failure index, and urine osmolality—have been discussed in previous sections of this chapter. The formulas for these calculations are included in Box 13-12.

Because many techniques for the clinical evaluation of renal function require an accurately timed collection of a urine specimen, the technique for collection of a 24-hour urine specimen is reviewed briefly here. Whenever timed collection of a urine specimen is planned, the child, family, and nursing staff should have specific instructions about the collection, and these should be documented in the patient's care plan.

A timed urine collection begins when the first urine specimen is collected and discarded. Next, all urine is saved in appropriate containers until the end of the collection period. At the time that the collection is to end, the patient is encouraged to void (or the Foley catheter tubing and urometer are emptied) and the collection container is labeled with the patient's name, hospital number, the time the collection was begun, and the time the collection ended.

It is important that the nurses discuss contingency plans with a physician or other appropriate provider in the event that a portion of the collection is lost or discarded inadvertently. If the continuous collection is interrupted, it may be possible to perform studies on the volume collected over the duration of the study up to the time of the specimen loss (e.g., instead of a 24-hour creatinine clearance study, a 12- or 16-hour study

Box 13-12   Common Formulas Used in Evaluation of Renal Function

Fractional Excretion of Filtered Sodium (FE$_{Na}$)

$$FE_{Na} = \frac{\text{Urine sodium concentration}/\text{Serum sodium concentration}}{\text{Urine creatinine concentration}/\text{Serum creatinine concentration}} \times 100$$

Prerenal azotemia is associated with a FE$_{Na}$ less than 1% (less than <2.5% in neonates), and intrarenal renal failure is associated with a FE$_{Na}$ greater than 2% (greater than 3.5% in neonates). This equation is not valid if recent diuretic therapy has been provided.

Glomerular Filtration Rate (GFR)

$$GFR = \frac{\text{Urine concentration creatinine} \times \text{Volume of urine per minute}}{\text{Plasma concentration of creatinine}}$$

This relationship is not valid in the presence of severe renal dysfunction.

Estimated Creatinine Clearance (eCrCl) using the Schwartz Formula

$$eCrCl\ (mL/min\ per\ 1.73m^2) = K \times Height\ (cm) \div SCr\ (mg/dL)$$

Estimated creatinine clearance in mL/min/m^2 body surface area is equal to K (a constant value that varies with age) times the height in centimeters divided by serum creatinine in mg per deciliter.

Age	K value
<2 years	0.45
2 to <13 years	0.55
13 to <20 years	0.70 for males; 0.55 for females

Estimation of Serum Osmolality

$$2 \times \text{Sodium concentration (mEq/L)} = \underline{\hspace{3cm}}$$

$$+ \frac{\text{Glucose concentration (mg/dL)}}{18} = + \underline{\hspace{3cm}}$$

$$+ \frac{\text{Blood urea nitrogen (mg/dL)}}{2.8} = + \underline{\hspace{3cm}}$$

$$\text{Total serum osmolality (mOsm/L)} = \underline{\hspace{3cm}}$$

$$\text{Normal serum osmolality} = 275 - 295\ mOsm/L.$$

eCrCl, Estimated creatinine clearance; *FE$_{Na}$,* fractional excretion of filtered sodium; *GFR,* glomerular filtration rate; *SCr,* serum creatinine.

may be performed). If estimates of the quantity of lost urine are available, the collection may continue, with special note made of the quantity and timing of specimen loss. Contingency plans should be discussed with the nursing staff and the specimen laboratory before the collection is begun.

The plans should be documented carefully in the nursing care plan so there is no confusion about appropriate response to specimen loss.

Finally, some timed urine collections require the use of specially prepared containers and refrigeration of the urine sample during the collection period. These specifications should be followed strictly, or the study results may be inaccurate.

If the child has acute renal failure and oliguria, it is important to know that urine collections over long periods of time are not necessary to evaluate renal function. Fractional excretion of sodium, creatinine clearance, and urine osmolality usually can be calculated from small quantities of urine. Many of these calculations will, however, require simultaneous collection of blood samples for measurement of serum sodium or creatinine concentrations or serum osmolality.

References

1. ADQI workshop results. http://www.ccm.pitt.edu/adqi/. Accessed February 29, 2012.
2. ADQI II: ARF Research. 1. Defining Acute Renal Failure. Available at http://www.ccm.pitt.edu/adqi/adqi02.html. Accessed February 29, 2012.
3. ADQI Documents IV: Primary Prevention of Acute Renal Failure. Available at http://www.ccm.pitt.edu/adqi/adqi04.html. Accessed February 29, 2012.
4. Akcan-Arikan A, et al: Modified RIFLE criteria in critically ill children with acute kidney injury. *Kidney Int* 71:1028, 2007.
5. Allon M: Disorders of potassium metabolism. In Greenberg A, editor: *Primer on kidney disease,* ed 5, National Kidney Foundation, Philadelphia, 2009, Elsevier.
6. Andreoli SP: Clinical Evaluation and Management. In Avner ED et al., editors: *Pediatric nephrology,* ed 5, Philadelphia, 2004, Lippincott Williams and Wilkins.
7. Aronoff GR, et al: *Drug prescribing in renal failure dosing guidelines for adults and children,* ed 5, Philadelphia, 2007, American College of Physicians.
8. Askenazi OJ, Bunchman TE: Pediatric acute kidney injury: the use of the RIFLE criteria. *Kidney Int* 71:963–964, 2007.
9. Bailey D, et al: Risk factors of acute renal failure in critically ill children: a prospective descriptive epidemiological study. *Pediatr Crit Care Med* 8:29–35, 2007.
10. Ball JW, Bindler RC: *Child health nursing partnering with children and families,* Upper Saddle River, NJ, 2006, Pearson Education.
11. Bellomo R, et al: Acute renal failure—definition, outcome measures, animal models, fluid therapy and information technology needs: the Second International Consensus Conference of the Acute Dialysis Quality Initiative (ADQI) Group. *Crit Care* 8:R204–R212, 2004.
12. Benfield MR, Bunchman TE: Management of acute renal failure. In Avner ED et al., editors: *Pediatric nephrology,* ed 5, Philadelphia, 2004, Lippincott Williams and Wilkins.
13. Birk PE: The not-so-minimal lesions of the idiopathic nephrotic syndrome of childhood. *Kidney Int* 71:284–285, 2007.
14. Breault DT, Majzoub JA: Other abnormalities of arginine vasopressin metabolism and action. In Kliegman RM et al., editors: *Nelson textbook of pediatrics,* ed 18, Philadelphia, 2007, WB Saunders.
15. Breen C, Windt K: Hemodialysis: assist. In Verger JT, Lebet RM, editors: *AACN procedure manual for pediatric acute and critical care,* St Louis, 2008, Saunders.
16. Brophy PD: Access in Pediatric CRRT. Available at http://www.pcrrt.com/pcrrtA2004.html. Accessed September 21, 2010.
17. Brophy PD, Bunchman TE: References and overview for hemofiltration in pediatrics and adolescents. Available at http://www.pcrrt.com/Protocols%20PCRRT%20Zurich.pdf. Accessed September 4, 2009.
18. Brophy PD, Somers MJG, Baum MA: Multi-centre evaluation of anticoagulation in patients receiving continuous renal replacement therapy (CRRT). *Nephrol Dial Transplant* 20:1416–1421, 2005.

19. Butt WW, Skippen PW, Jouvet P: Renal replacement therapies. In Nichols DG, editor: *Roges' textbook of pediatric intensive care*, ed 4, Philadelphia, 2008, Lippincott Williams and Wilkins.
20. Carcillo JA, et al: Shock: an overview. In Wheeler DS, Wong HR, Shanley TP, editors: *Pediatric critical care medicine basic science and clinical evidence*, London, 2007, Springer-Verlag London Limited.
21. Cheung A: Hemodialysis and hemofiltration. In Greenberg A, editor: *Primer on kidney disease*, ed 5, National Kidney Foundation, Philadelphia, 2009, Elsevier.
22. Chronic kidney disease: evaluation, classification, and stratification. Available at http://www.kidney.org/professionals/kdoqi/guidelines.cfm. Accessed July 3, 2008.
23. Coffman TM: Kidney function impairment caused by therapeutic agents. In Greenberg A, editor: *Primer on kidney disease*, ed 5, National Kidney Foundation, Philadelphia, 2009, Elsevier.
24. Dabbagh S, Atiyeh B: Hemoldialysis and hemoperfusion. In Levin DL, Morriss FC, editors: *Essentials of pediatric intensive care*, ed 2, New York, 1997, Churchill Livingston.
25. Davis ID, Avner ED: Glomerular disease. In Kliegman RM et al., editors: *Nelson textbook of pediatrics*, ed 18, Philadelphia, 2007, WB Saunders.
26. Dellinger RP, et al: Surviving sepsis campaign: international guidelines for management of severe sepsis and septic shock: 2008. *Intensive Care Med* 34:17–60, 2008.
27. Devarajan P, Woroniecki RP: Acute tubular necrosis. Available at http://www.emedicine.com/ped/topic28.htm. Accessed March 15, 2008.
28. DiCarlo JV, Alexander SR: Hemofiltration for cytokine-driven illnesses: the mediator delivery hypothesis. *Int J Artif Organs* 28:777–786, 2005.
29. Dooley MA, Nachman PH: Kidney manifestations of systemic lupus erythematosus and rheumatoid arthritis. In Greenberg A, editor: *Primer on kidney disease*, ed 4, National Kidney Foundation, Philadelphia, 2005, Elsevier.
30. Elder JS: Vesicoureteral reflex. In Kliegman RM et al., editors: *Nelson textbook of pediatrics*, ed 18, Philadelphia, 2007, WB Saunders.
31. Ellison DH: Edema and the clinical use of diuretics. In Greenberg A, editor: *Primer on Kidney Disease*, ed 5, National Kidney Foundation, Philadelphia, 2009, Elsevier.
32. Formica RN, Jr, Lakkis FG: Kidney transplantation: management and outcome. In Greenberg A, editor: *Primer on kidney disease*, ed 4, National Kidney Foundation, Philadelphia, 2005, Elsevier.
33. Fortenberry JD, Paden ML: Extracorporeal therapies in the treatment of sepsis: experience and promise. *Semin Pediatr Infect Dis* 17:72–79, 2006.
34. Ganong WF: *Review of medical physiology,* ed 22, New York, 2005, Lange Medical Books-McGraw-Hill.
35. Gardner J: Nursing Issue 13. Available at http://www.pcrrt.com/talks/pcrrtT2006.html. (select Gardner Nursing Issue 13 file on page) Accessed September 28.
36. Gokal R, Hutchinson AJ: Peritoneal dialysis. In Greenberg A, editor: *Primer on kidney disease*, ed 4, National Kidney Foundation, Philadelphia, 2005, Elsevier.
37. Goldstein SL, Jabs K: Hemodialysis. In Avner ED, Harmon WE, Niaudet P, editors: *Pediatric nephrology*, ed 5, Philadelphia, 2004, Lippincott Williams and Wilkins.
38. Goldstein SL, et al: Pediatric patients with multi-organ dysfunction syndrome receiving continuous renal replacement therapy. *Kidney Int* 67:653–658, 2005.
39. Goldstein SL, et al: The prospective pediatric continuous renal replacement therapy (PPCRRT) registry: design, development and data assessed. *Int J Artif Organs* 27:9–14, 2004.
40. Gomez RA, Norwood VF: The kidney in infants and children. In Greenberg A, editor: *Primer on kidney disease*, ed 4, National Kidney Foundation, Philadelphia, 2005, Elsevier.
41. Gray M, Huether S, Forshee B: Alterations of renal and urinary tract function in children. In McCance KL, Huether SE, editors: *Pathophysiology: the biologic basis of disease in adults and children*, ed 5, St Louis, 2006, Elsevier.
42. Greenbaum LA: Electrolyte and acid-base disorders. In Kliegman RM et al., editors: *Nelson textbook of pediatrics*, ed 18, Philadelphia, 2007, WB Saunders.
43. Greenbaum L: Maintenance and replacement fluid. In Kliegman RM et al., editors: *Nelson textbook of pediatrics*, ed 18, Philadelphia, 2007, WB Saunders.
44. Greenberg A: Urinalysis. In Greenberg A, editor: *Primer on kidney disease*, ed 5, National Kidney Foundation, Philadelphia, 2009, Elsevier.
45. Guyton AC: Micturition, diuretics, and kidney disease. In Guyton AC, Hall JE, editors: *Textbook of medical physiology*, ed 9, Philadelphia, 1996, WB Saunders Company.
46. Hackbarth RM, et al: Zero balance ultrafiltration (Z-BUF) in blood primed CRRT circuits achieves electrolyte and acid-base homeostasis prior to patient connection. *Pediatr Nephrol* 20:1328–1333, 2005.
47. Hackbarth RM, Maxvold NJ, Bunchman TE: Acute Renal failure and end-stage renal disease. In Nichols DG, editor: *Rogers' textbook of pediatric intensive care*, ed 4, Philadelphia, 2008, Lippincott Williams and Wilkins.
48. Hanevold CD, Wynn JJ, Ortiz LA: Renal transplantation. In Wheeler DS, Wong HR, Shanley TP, editors: *Pediatric critical care medicine basic science and clinical evidence*, London, 2007, Springer-Verlag London Limited.
49. Harmon WE: Pediatric renal transplantation. In Avner ED, Harmon WE, Niaudet P, editors: *Pediatric nephrology*, ed 5, Philadelphia, 2004, Lippincott Williams and Wilkins.
50. Hauser GJ, Kulick AF: Electrolyte disorders in the pediatric intensive care unit. In Wheeler DS, Wong HR, Shanley TP, editors: *Pediatric critical care medicine basic science and clinical evidence*, London, 2007, Springer-Verlag.
51. Hedges SJ, et al: Evidence-based treatment recommendations for uremic bleeding. *Nat Clin Pract Nephrol* 3:138–153, 2007.
52. Hemodialysis guidelines from the kidney disease outcome quality initiative. Available at http://www.kidney.org/professionals/KDOQI/guideline_upHD_PD_VA/index.htm. Accessed September 22, 2011.
53. Hoste EA, Schurgers M: Epidemiology of acute kidney injury: how big is the problem? *Crit Care Med* 36:S146–S151, 2008.
54. Huether SE: Mechanisms of hormonal regulation. In McCance KL, Huether SE, editors: *Pathophysiology: the biologic basis of disease in adults and children*, ed 5, St Louis, 2006, Elsevier.
55. Huether SE: Structure and function of the renal and urologic systems. In McCance KL, Huether SE, editors: *Pathophysiology: the biologic basis of disease in adults and children*, ed 5, St Louis, 2006, Elsevier.
56. Hus C: Clinical evaluation of kidney function. In Greenberg A, editor: *Primer on kidney disease*, ed 5, National Kidney Foundation, Philadelphia, 2009, Elsevier.
57. Jennette JC, Falk RJ: Glomerular clinicopathologic syndromes. In Greenberg A, editor: *Primer on kidney disease*, ed 5, National Kidney Foundation, Philadelphia, 2009, Elsevier.
58. Jennette CJ, Falk RJ: Kidney involvement in systemic vasculitis. In Greenberg A, editor: *Primer on kidney disease*, ed 5, National Kidney Foundation, Philadelphia, 2009, Elsevier.
59. Jones DP, Chesney RW, Friedman AL: Glomerulotubular dysfunction and acute renal failure. In Fuhrman BP, Zimmerman JJ, editors: *Pediatric critical care*, ed 3, Philadelphia, 2006, Mosby.
60. Kellum JA: Acute kidney injury. *Crit Care Med* 36:S142, 2008.
61. Kellum JA, et al: The first international consensus conference on continuous renal replacement therapy. *Kidney Int* 62:1853–1863, 2002.
62. Koeppen BM, Stanton BA: Glomerular filtration and renal blood flow. In Koeppen BM, Stanton BA eds: *Renal physiology*, ed 4, Philadelphia, 2007, Mosby Elsevier.
63. Koeppen BM, Stanton BA: Regulation of calcium and phosphate homeostasis. In Koeppen BM, Stanton BA, editors: *Renal physiology*, ed 4, Philadelphia, 2007, Mosby Elsevier.
64. Kovalik EC: Endocrine and neurologic manifestations of kidney failure. In Greenberg A, editor: *Primer on kidney disease*, ed 5, National Kidney Foundation, Philadelphia, 2009, Elsevier.
65. Lechner BL, Siegel NJ: Minimal change disease. In Greenberg A, editor: *Primer on kidney disease*, ed 4, National Kidney Foundation, Philadelphia, 2005, Elsevier.
66. Lee C, Robertson J, Shilkofski N: Drug doses. In Robertson J, Shilkofski N, editors: *The Harriet Lane handbook*, ed 17, Philadelphia, 2005, Mosby.

67. Lin J, Smoyer WE: Renal disorders in the pediatric intensive care unit: glomerulonephritis and nephrotic syndrome. In Wheeler DS, Wong HR, Shanley TP, editors: *Pediatric critical care medicine basic science and clinical evidence*, London, 2007, Springer-Verlag.

68. Maxvold NJ: Nutrient Support in Critically Ill Children with ARF. http://www.pcrrt.com/talks/pcrrtT2006.html. Must select Maxvold Norma Nutri from list on page. Accessed September 28, 2011.

69. McBryde KD, Bunchman TE: Continuous renal replacement therapy. In Wheeler DS, Wong HR, Shanley TP, editors: *Pediatric critical care medicine basic science and clinical evidence*, London, 2007, Springer-Verlag.

70. Mehta RL, et al: Acute kidney injury network: report of an initiative to improve outcomes in acute kidney injury. *Crit Care* 11:R31, 2007.

71. Nguyen MT, Bissler JJ: Acute renal failure. In Wheeler DS, Wong HR, Shanley TP, editors: *Pediatric critical care medicine basic science and clinical evidence*, London, 2007, Springer-Verlag.

72. O'Connor P: Peritoneal dialysis: pass management. In Verger JT, Lebet RM, editors: *AACN procedure manual for pediatric acute and critical care*, St Louis, 2008, Saunders.

73. Pinsk MN, Norwood VF: Renal structure and function. In Fuhrman BP, Zimmerman JJ, editors: *Pediatric critical care*, ed 3, Philadelphia, 2006, Mosby-Elsevier.

74. Powers KS, Cholette JM, Abboud P: Toxic exposures: diagnosis and management. In Wheeler DS, Wong HR, Shanley TP, editors: *Pediatric critical care medicine basic science and clinical evidence*, London, 2007, Springer-Verlag.

75. Proulx F, Tesh VL: Renal diseases in the pediatric intensive care unit: thrombotic microangiopathy, hemolytic uremic syndrome, and thrombotic thrombocytopenic purpura. In Wheeler DS, Wong HR, Shanley TP, editors: *Pediatric critical care medicine basic science and clinical evidence*, London, 2007, Springer-Verlag.

76. Quigley R, Alexander SR: Acute renal failure. In Levin DL, Morris FC, editors: *The essentials of pediatric intensive care*, St Louis, 1997, Churchill Livingston.

77. Rennke HG, Denker BM: *Renal pathophysiology: the essentials*, ed 2, Philadelphia, 2007, Lippincott Williams and Wilkins.

78. Ricci Z, Bellomo R, Ronco C: Dose of dialysis in acute renal failure. *Clin J Am Soc Nephrol* 1:380–388, 2006.

79. Roberts KE: *Fluid and electrolyte balance: critical care case studies. Critical Care Nursing Clinics of North America*, Philadelphia, 2005, Elsevier.

80. Robertson J: Blood chemistries and body fluids. In Robertson J, Shilkofski N, editors: *The Harriet Lane handbook*, ed 17, Philadelphia, 2005, Mosby.

81. Ronco C, Zaccari R, Bellomo R: Current worldwide practice of dialysis dose prescription in acute renal failure. *Curr Opin Crit Care* 12:551–556, 2006.

82. Safirstein RL: Pathophysiology of acute renal failure. In Greenberg A, editor: *Primer on kidney disease*, ed 4, National Kidney Foundation, Philadelphia, 2005, Elsevier.

83. Schwartz GJ: Potassium. In Avner ED, Harmon WE, Niaudet P, editors: *Pediatric nephrology*, ed 5, Philadelphia, 2004, Lippincott Williams and Wilkins.

84. Sperling MA: Hypoglycemia. In Kliegman RM et al., editors: *Nelson textbook of pediatrics*, ed 18, Philadelphia, 2007, WB Saunders.

85. Stoll BJ: The newborn infant. In Kliegman RM et al., editors: *Nelson textbook of pediatrics*, ed 18, Philadelphia, 2007, WB Saunders.

86. Stone B: Fluids and electrolytes. In Robertson J, Shilkofski N, editors: *The Harriet Lane handbook*, ed 17, Philadelphia, 2005, Mosby.

87. Suzuki Y, et al: Efficacy of the CTR-001 direct hemoperfusion adsorption column in sepsis. *Crit Care* 12:459, 2008.

88. Symons JM, et al: Demographic characteristics of pediatric continuous renal replacement therapy: a report of the prospective pediatric continuous renal replacement therapy registry. *Clin J Am Soc Nephrol* 2:732–738, 2007.

89. Taketomo C, editor: *Children's Hospital Los Angeles pediatric dosing handbook and formulary*, Hudson OH, 2008-2010, Lexi-Comp.

90. Trachtman H: Sodium and water. In Avner ED, Harmon WE, Niaudet P, editors: *Pediatric nephrology*, ed 5, Philadelphia, 2004, Lippincott Williams and Wilkins.

91. Travis L: Nephrotic syndrome. Available at http://www.emedicine.com/ped/topic1564.htm. Accessed July 2008.

92. *US Renal Data System, USRDS 2007 Annual Data Report: Atlas of Chronic Kidney Disease and End-Stage Renal Disease in the United States: Transplantation*. Bethesda, MD, 2007, National Institutes of Health, National Institute of Diabetes and Digestive and Kidney Diseases. Available at http://www.usrds.org/2007/pdf/07_tx_07.pdf. Accessed September 2009.

93. United Network for Organ Sharing. Policies 3.5. Organ Distribution: Allocation of Deceased Kidneys. Available at www.unos.org/PoliciesandBylaws2/policies/pdfs/policy_7.pdf. Revised June 29, 2011. Accessed September 30, 2011.

94. Urizar RE: Renal transplantation. In Kliegman RM et al., editors: *Nelson textbook of pediatrics*, ed 18, Philadelphia, 2007, WB Saunders.

95. Venkaturaman R: Can we prevent acute kidney injury? *Crit Care Med* 36:S166–S171, 2008.

96. Verbalis J: Hyponatremia and hypoosmolar disorders. In Greenberg A, editor: *Primer on kidney disease*, ed 5, National Kidney Foundation, Philadelphia, 2009, Elsevier.

97. Vogt BA, Avner ED: Conditions particularly associated with proteinuria. In Kliegman RM et al., editors: *Nelson textbook of pediatrics*, ed 18, Philadelphia, 2007, WB Saunders.

98. Vogt BA, Avner ED: Renal failure. In Kliegman RM et al., editors: *Nelson textbook of pediatrics*, ed 18, Philadelphia, 2007, WB Saunders.

99. Vogt BA, Avner ED: Toxic nephropathy. In Kliegman RM et al., editors: *Nelson textbook of pediatrics*, ed 18, Philadelphia, 2007, WB Saunders.

100. Walters S, Porter C, Brophy PD: Dialysis and pediatric acute kidney injury: choice of renal support modality. *Pediatr Nephrol* 24:37–48, 2009.

101. Warady BA, Morgenstern BZ, Alexander SR: Peritoneal dialysis. In Avner ED, Harmon WE, Niaudet P, editors: *Pediatric nephrology*, ed 5, Philadelphia, 2004, Lippincott Williams and Wilkins.

102. Wartiovaara J, et al: Nephrin strands contribute to a porous slit diaphragm scaffold as revealed by electron tomography. *J Clin Invest* 114:1475–1483, 2004.

103. Wood EG, Lynch F: Electrolyte management in pediatric critical illness. In Fuhrman BP, Zimmerman JJ, editors: *Pediatric critical care*, ed 3, Philadelphia, 2006, Mosby.

104. Zaritsky A, Whitby D: Hypertension in the pediatric intensive care unit. In Fuhrman BP, Zimmerman JJ, editors: *Pediatric critical care*, ed 3, Philadelphia, 2006, Mosby.

Gastrointestinal and Nutritional Disorders

14

Sarah A. Martin • Cindy L. Kerr

ⓔvolve Be sure to check out the supplementary content available at http://evolve.elsevier.com/Hazinski.

PEARLS

- Abdominal distension can compromise diaphragm expansion and can lead to respiratory insufficiency.
- A child with significant intraabdominal pathology may have subtle clinical signs, such as somnolence and mental status changes.
- Bilious vomiting with a clinical examination suggestive of an acute abdomen can be a sign of a bowel-threatening pathologic condition (e.g., volvulus) and almost always warrants immediate operative intervention.
- If a child does not recover as expected after gastrointestinal surgery, a technical complication of the procedure should be considered as a cause until it is ruled out.
- Correct placement of a nasogastric or orogastric tube is verified with an abdominal radiograph.
- Enteral feedings should begin as soon as possible, because even small quantities of feedings reduce the risk of infection and promote gut healing.

INTRODUCTION

The pediatric critical care nurse frequently encounters children with gastrointestinal (GI) disorders and nutritional problems. This chapter summarizes fundamental aspects of pediatric GI anatomy, physiology, and pathophysiology and applies them to common GI problems and diagnoses that may require intervention in the critical care unit. This chapter also includes principles governing nutritional assessment and management.

ESSENTIAL ANATOMY AND PHYSIOLOGY

This section summarizes the basic anatomy and physiology of major structures composing the GI tract (Fig. 14-1). See the Chapter 14 Supplement on the Evolve Website for additional information on maturational anatomy and physiology.

Mouth

Chewing begins the breakdown of food by reducing the size of food particles. Tastes on the tongue initiate salivation and stimulate secretion of gastric juices in the stomach. Saliva produced by the salivary glands includes the enzyme ptyalin, which commences digestion of carbohydrates.

Esophagus

Food is propelled from the mouth and oropharynx through the esophagus into the stomach. The esophagus has two layers of striated muscle that produce peristalsis when the fibers are stretched by food entering the esophagus. Peristalsis is an organized sequence of muscle contraction and relaxation that propels ingested material along the entire length of the GI tract.

The distal end of the esophagus includes a muscular sphincter called the *lower esophageal sphincter* (LES); this sphincter relaxes (i.e., opens) as food particles are swept through the lower portion of the esophagus into the stomach. After the food particles have passed into the stomach, the LES resumes its resting tone, creating a barrier between the esophagus and stomach. The LES normally prevents reflux of acidic gastric contents into the esophagus. However, because the LES is functionally immature and frequently incompetent during the first 4 to 6 months of life, young infants may demonstrate gastroesophageal reflux (GER).

Stomach

The stomach is a hollow muscular organ that serves as a temporary reservoir for ingested food, and is the site of the initial phases of protein digestion. Three smooth muscle layers of the stomach mix food with gastric secretions, creating a substance called *chyme*. Two muscular sphincters, the LES at the entrance to the stomach and the pyloric sphincter at the stomach outlet, contract to contain food within the stomach while the food is being churned and mixed with the gastric secretions. These muscle barriers also protect cells of the esophagus and duodenum from caustic stomach acid, which can erode and ulcerate the mucosa.

Specialized cells within the gastric mucosa (called *parietal cells* and *chief cells*) produce mucus, acid, enzymes, hormones, and intrinsic factor. Each of these products has a specific role in digestion.

Secreted mucus forms a protective barrier between the mucosa and the acid and proteolytic enzymes. Acid produced by partial cells creates a gastric pH of 1 to 2 that dissolves food fiber, acts as a bactericide against swallowed organisms, and converts pepsinogen to pepsin. Pepsinogen arises from chief cells. Under the influence of gastric acid, pepsinogen is converted into pepsin, a proteolytic enzyme that continues the breakdown of proteins that was started by gastric acids. Intrinsic factor is a glycoprotein required for vitamin B_{12} absorption.[27]

773

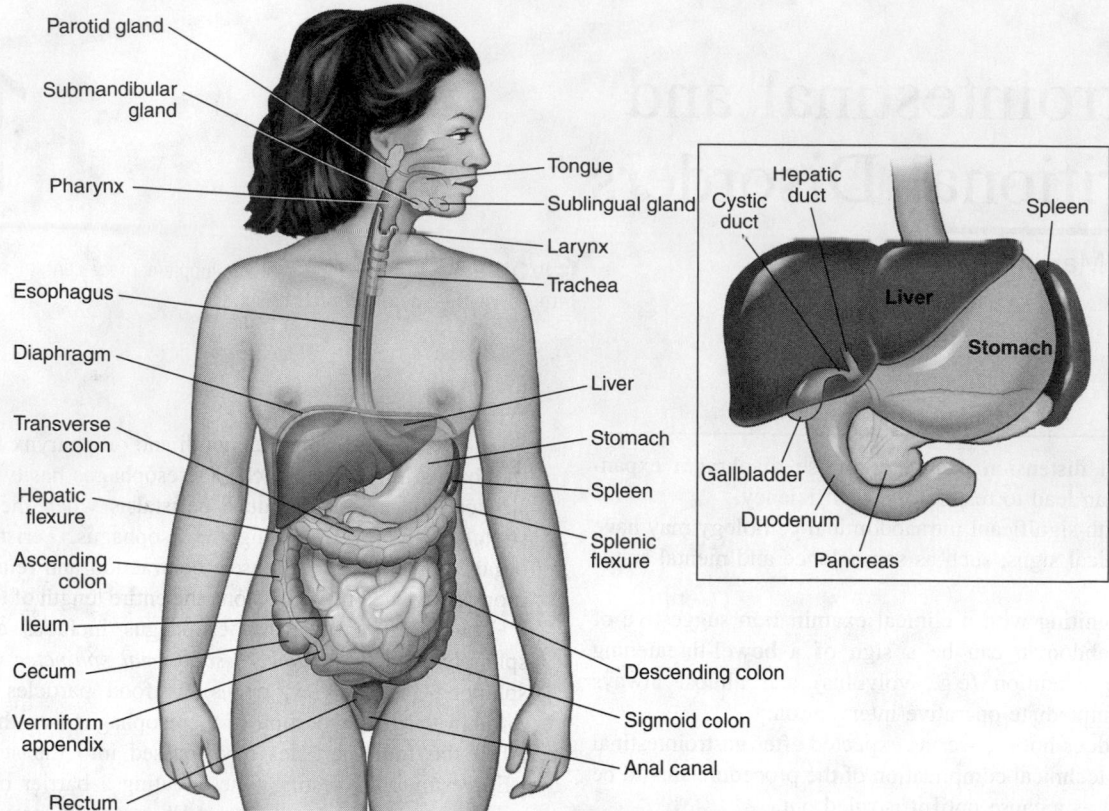

FIG. 14-1 Structure and function of the digestive system. Digestion begins in the mouth with chewing, which breaks down food mechanically and mixes it with saliva. Swallowing propels chewed food through the esophagus to the stomach, where acids and stomach motility liquefy it further. Next the liquefied food enters the small intestine, where secretions of the intestinal walls, liver, gallbladder, and pancreas digest it into absorbable nutrients. Nutrients are absorbed through intestinal walls, and unabsorbed wastes enter the large intestine (colon), where fluids are removed. Solid wastes then enter the rectum and leave the body through the anus. (From Patton KT, Thibodeau GA: *Anatomy and physiology*, ed 7, St Louis, Mosby, 2010.)

Gastric secretions consist predominantly of hydrochloric acid, potassium chloride, and sodium chloride. Stimulated parietal cells dispense these substances into the lumen of the stomach through active transport involving a proton pump. Histamine—H2 type—stimulates the H2 receptors in parietal cells, causing the cells to secrete gastric acid. H2 receptor antagonists inhibit gastric acid secretion by preventing histamine from activating the H2 receptors. Proton pump inhibitor medications inhibit hydrochloric acid directly at the cellular level.

Gastric Emptying

Gastric emptying is affected by stomach content and by external neural and hormone signals. Carbohydrates are emptied from the stomach faster than proteins, and fats require the longest gastric emptying time. Hypertonic and acidic substances empty slowly, and liquids empty faster than solids.

Nervous system control of gastric emptying is predominantly from the vagus nerve, which is part of the parasympathetic nervous system. Hormonal control is vast and works in a variety of ways. The hormones may directly affect smooth muscle contraction and may also stimulate the parietal cells.

Vascular Supply

The blood supply to the stomach, small intestine, and colon constitutes the splanchnic circulation. The three major arterial branches to these structures are the celiac artery, the superior mesenteric artery, and the inferior mesenteric artery. Each is a distinctive branch of the abdominal aorta.

Venous drainage from the stomach, pancreas, small intestine, and colon empties into the portal vein and perfuses the liver. Blood then returns to the heart through the hepatic vein and inferior vena cava. Nearly one fourth of cardiac output is distributed to the splanchnic circulation.

Small Intestine

The small intestine (Fig. 14-2) begins beyond the pylorus of the stomach and is divided into the duodenum (receives enzymes important for digestion), the jejunum (principle absorbing site), and the ileum (the only site for the absorption of vitamin B_{12} and bile acids). Two layers of smooth muscle, an outer longitudinal layer, and an inner thicker circular layer produce peristalsis.

The inner mucosal layer has transverse folds or plicae circulares. This design increases surface area (and absorption) and slows the progression of food, allowing more time for digestion to occur. Villi, which are extensions of the mucosal layer,

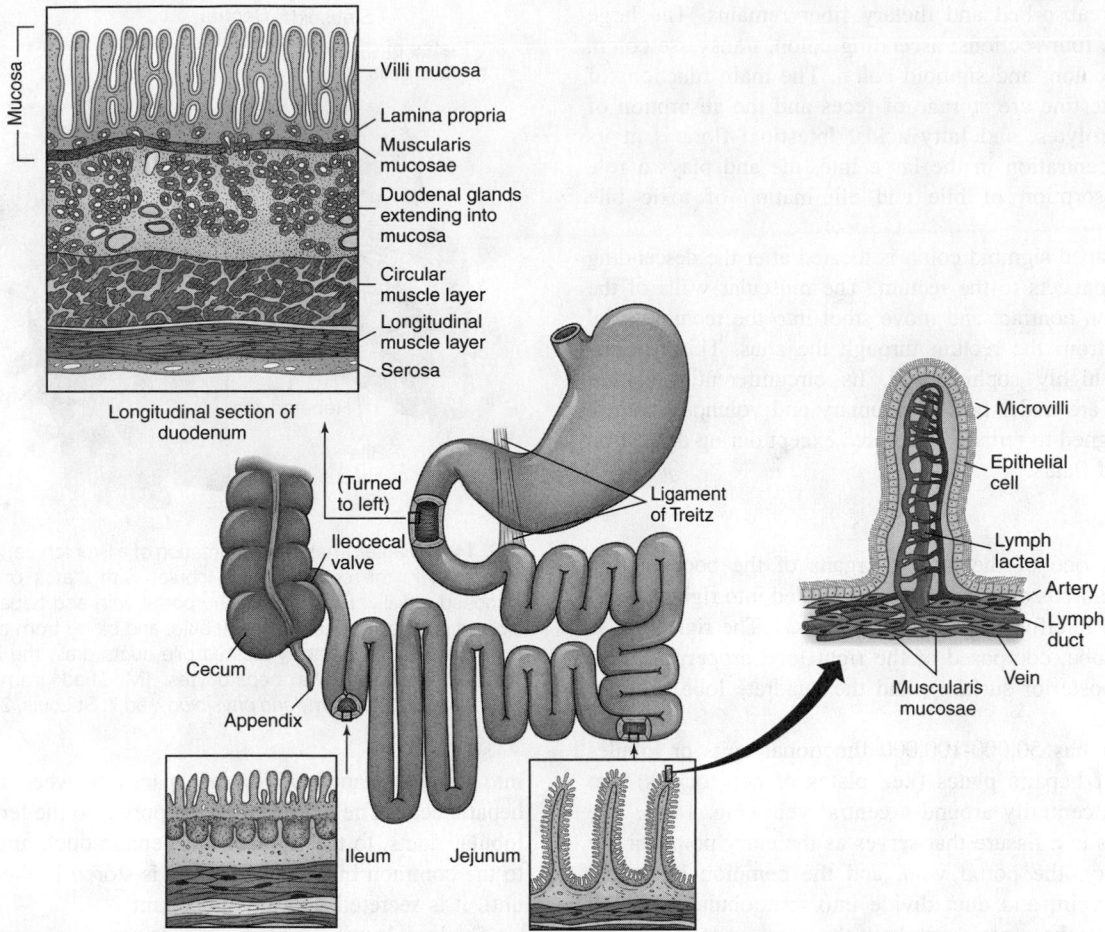

FIG. 14-2 The small intestine. (From McCance KL, Heuther SE, editors: *Pathophysiology: the biologic basis for disease in adults and children*, ed 6, St Louis, 2010, Elsevier.)

cover the mucosal folds as projections. These villi, composed of absorptive columnar cells and mucus-secreting goblet cells, are considered the functional units of the GI tract. Each villus is covered with tiny projections called *microvilli;* together these form the brush border of the intestine. This brush border contains digestive enzymes and contributes to the transfer of nutrients and electrolytes. See the Chapter 14 Supplement, Nutrition section, on the Evolve Website for additional information about the digestion of nutrients.

Epithelial cells in the small intestine have one of the most rapid turnover rates of any cells in the body. Villus cells continuously proliferate to maintain a consistent quantity within the intestinal epithelium. The loss of villi leads to decreased absorptive capacity. The capacity to renew these villi is lower during infancy and can be compromised in malnourished states and by intestinal disorders. Recovery following injury to the intestinal mucosa (e.g., from viral infection or malnutrition) may be prolonged, creating a vicious cycle of impaired intestinal function and persistent malabsorption leading to malnutrition and further compromise of intestinal function.

Duodenum

The duodenum is a portion of the small intestine that extends from the pylorus to the jejunum and transitions from a retroperitoneal structure to an intraperitoneal structure at the ligament of Treitz. Pancreatic and hepatic enzymes (bile) enter the second portion of the duodenum through the sphincter of Oddi. These enzymes work to neutralize acidic chyme and promote digestion. The duodenum is the primary site for absorption of iron, trace metals, and water-soluble vitamins.

Jejunum

The jejunum lies between the duodenum and ileum and comprises approximately half of the small bowel. Ninety percent of nutrients and 50% of water and electrolyte absorption is completed by the jejunum.

Ileum

The ileum connects the small intestine to the colon. Its functions include absorption of vitamin B_{12} and bile salts and completion of any remaining nutrient absorption. The ileocecal valve is situated between the ileum and the colon. This valve delays entry of intestinal contents into the colon and prevents reflux of colon contents back into the small intestine.

Large Intestine

The large intestine consists of the cecum, appendix, sigmoid colon, rectum, and anal canal. By the time food has reached the large intestine, almost all nutrients and 90% of the water have been reabsorbed and dietary fiber remains. The large intestine has four sections: ascending colon, transverse colon, descending colon, and sigmoid colon. The main functions of the large intestine are storage of feces and the absorption of water, electrolytes, and fatty acids. Intestinal flora is at its highest concentration in the large intestine and plays a role in the reabsorption of bile and elimination of toxic bile metabolites.

The S-shaped sigmoid colon is located after the descending colon and connects to the rectum. The muscular walls of the sigmoid colon contract and move stool into the rectum. Stool is expelled from the rectum through the anus. This external opening is highly sophisticated. Its circumferential muscle components are under both involuntary and voluntary control and are designed to remain contracted except during defecation or passing of flatus.

Liver

The liver is one of the largest organs of the body, and it performs hundreds of functions. It is divided into right and left lobes by the falciform ligament (Fig. 14-3). The right lobe is the largest lobe, composed of the right lobe proper, the caudate lobe (posterior surface), and the quadrate lobe (inferior surface).

The liver has 50,000-100,000 functional units or lobules composed of hepatic plates (i.e., plates of hepatocytes) that each radiate centrally around a central vein (Fig. 14-4). The porta hepatis is a fissure that serves as the entry point for the hepatic artery, the portal vein, and the common bile duct. The artery, vein, and duct divide into intralobular branches as they follow the septa throughout the liver.

Nearly three quarters of the blood flow to the liver is supplied by the portal venous system that carries blood from the GI tract that is rich in nutrients to the liver. The remaining 25% of hepatic blood flow is well-oxygenated blood from the hepatic artery.

The hepatobiliary system has many synthetic, metabolic, storage, and removal functions. Bile is composed of bile salts and is made by hepatocytes within the liver. Bile is secreted

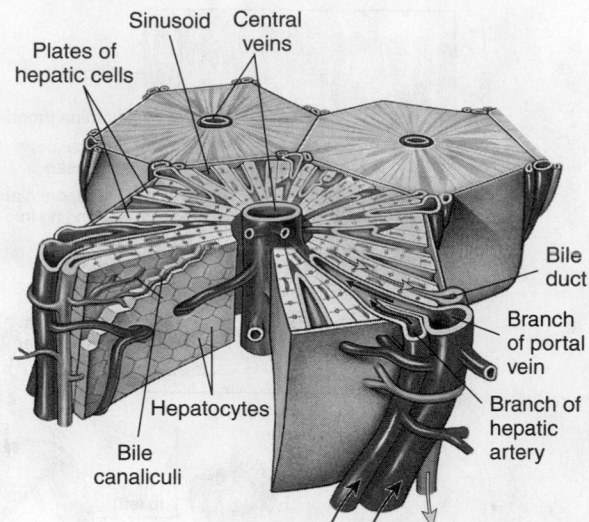

FIG. 14-4 Diagrammatic representation of a liver lobule. A central vein is located in the center of the lobule, with plates of hepatocytes disposed radially. Branches of the portal vein and hepatic artery are located on the periphery of the lobule, and blood from both perfuses the sinusoids. Peripherally located bile ducts drain the bile canaliculi that run between the hepatocytes. (Modified from Patton KT, Thibodeau GA: *Anatomy and physiology*, ed 7, St Louis, 2010, Mosby.)

into the bile canaliculi or the spaces between the rows of hepatic cells. The bile is then transported to the terminal interlobular ducts, to the right or left hepatic duct, and eventually to the common bile duct. The bile is stored in the gallbladder until it is secreted into the duodenum.

The liver is responsible for a wide variety of synthetic, metabolic, and excretory functions. In addition to bile production, liver functions include the synthesis of plasma proteins and clotting factors. The liver synthesizes almost all plasma proteins, including albumin and clotting factors I, II, V, VII, IX, X, and XI. The liver metabolizes carbohydrates, proteins, and lipids. It is the major storage site for glycogen, fat, and fat-soluble vitamins (A, D, E, and K). In addition, the liver deactivates many drugs and waste products, including conversion of ammonia to urea.

FIG. 14-3 Gross structure of the liver. **A,** Anterior view. **B,** Inferior view. (From Patton KT, Thibodeau GA: *Anatomy and physiology*, ed 7, St Louis, 2010, Mosby.)

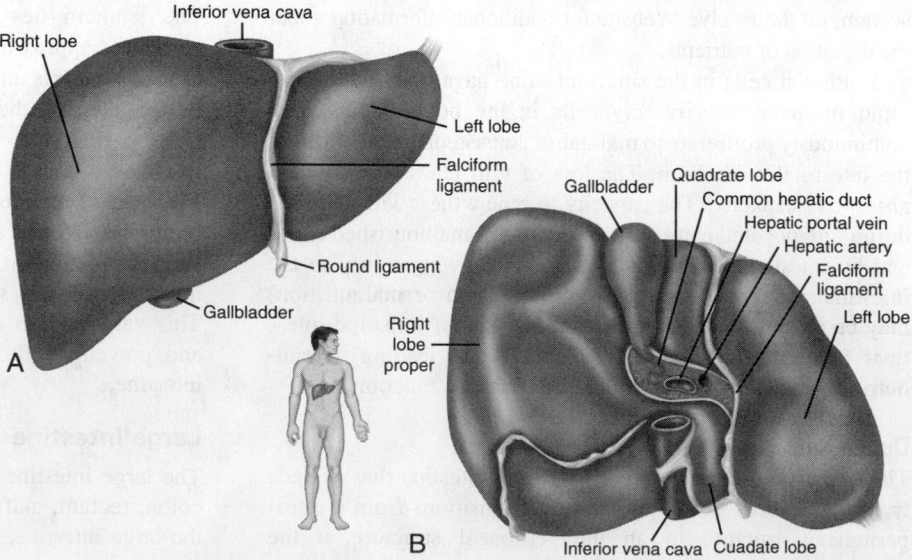

Toxic metabolic waste products from medications and bilirubin are metabolized in the liver through oxidation or conjugation reactions. Metabolic products are then excreted in the bile or urine. Kupffer cells are macrophages that line the sinusoid vessels and serve as the liver's internal immune system; they remove intestinal and foreign bacteria in addition to other toxins.

Gallbladder

The gallbladder is a saclike organ that sits below the liver. Its primary functions are storing and concentrating bile produced by the liver. The right and left hepatic ducts drain from the liver into the common bile duct and then into the cystic duct that empties into the gallbladder. The gallbladder is stimulated to contract by hormones (cholecystokinin and motilin) that are released when fats are present in the duodenum. Gallbladder contraction propels bile down the common bile duct, through the sphincter of Oddi, and into the duodenum.

Pancreas

The pancreas is composed of a head, a body, and a tail. The head is tucked into the curve of the duodenum, and the tail reaches laterally across the midline to the spleen. The pancreas is a retroperitoneal organ and is well protected from most environmental impacts. It functions as both an exocrine and endocrine organ. The working cells of the exocrine pancreas are acini cells; these cells are organized as spheres encompassing small secretory ducts scattered throughout the organ. This series of ducts transports fluid containing the digestive enzymes (proteases, amylase, and lipase) and sodium bicarbonate (pH 7.1-8.2) produced by acini cells to the pancreatic duct.[27] The pancreatic duct runs the length of the organ and then drains into the common bile duct at the ampulla of Vater, ultimately draining into the duodenum through the sphincter of Oddi.

The endocrine pancreas is responsible for production of glucagon and insulin that regulate carbohydrate, fat, and protein metabolism within the body. The islets of Langerhans are scattered throughout the pancreas. These islets have three types of hormone-secreting cells: alpha cells secrete glucagon, beta cells secrete insulin, and delta cells secrete gastrin or somatostatin.

NUTRITION

There is little evidence to identify the best nutritional support of the critically ill child.[30,44] A recent Cochrane review that attempted to assess the impact of enteral and parenteral nutrition (PN) on clinically important outcomes in the critically ill child found only one trial that was relevant to the review question.[30] Appropriate nutritional assessment, determination of energy requirements, and the timing, route, and type of nutritional delivery have yet to be established for seriously ill or injured children in the critical care unit.

Recommended Daily Nutritional Intake

Adequate energy (caloric) intake is necessary for rapid growth and development throughout childhood. During infancy the requirement for energy intake per kilogram is greater than in all other age groups. The average requirements for energy

Table 14-1	Daily Energy Requirements for Infants and Children	
Age	**kcal/kg**
Up to 6 months	90-110
6-12 months	80-100
12-36 months	75-90
4-6 years	65-75
7-10 years	55-75
11-18 years	40-55

intake during infancy and childhood are shown in Table 14-1. Of note, these requirements are for healthy, active infants and children.

It is useful to divide energy requirements into resting energy expenditure (REE) and requirements for growth and physical activity. REE is determined by the basal metabolic rate or the energy consumed for the normal maintenance of cellular energy. Estimates of an ill child's REE by standard equations are unreliable, and indirect calorimetry is not always available to clinicians.[44] Caloric requirements for the hospitalized child may be substantially more or less than the normal daily recommended requirements. Hypermetabolic states, excessive nutrient losses, trauma, burns, and surgery will increase energy requirements, whereas neurologic impairment, reduced activity, and ventilator support can decrease energy needs. Typically, fever increases energy requirements 12% per day for each degree Celsius elevation in temperature above 37° C.

A dietitian should assist in the assessment of the child's nutritional needs. These assessments will require basic anthropometric measurements (including body mass index [BMI] percentile), obtained as the child's clinical status allows. Clinicians are challenged to determine appropriate needs for the obese child (i.e., with a BMI greater than the 85th percentile), and it may be appropriate to determine caloric requirements based on ideal body weight.

Fluid and electrolyte requirements vary as a function of age, weight, and clinical condition. Normal daily fluid and electrolyte requirements are listed in Table 14-2. Any calculation of maintenance fluid requirements should use the formulas only to estimate a baseline. The actual volume of fluid administered to the patient must be tailored to the patient's clinical condition and fluid balance. For additional information about fluid and electrolyte balance, see Chapter 12.

Macronutrient Metabolism and Requirements

Recommended daily requirements of carbohydrate, fat, and protein are summarized in Table 14-3. The percentage of fat required in younger children is usually greater than requirements in older children. Disease states including renal and liver failure may decrease the amount of protein needed.

Carbohydrates

Carbohydrates are consumed as disaccharides, oligosaccharides, and polysaccharides. These are digested, absorbed, and transported through the body primarily as glucose, which is the primary metabolic fuel.

Table 14-2 Formulas for Estimating Daily Maintenance Fluid and Electrolyte Requirements for Children

	Daily Requirements	Hourly Requirements
Fluid Requirements Estimated from Weight*		
Newborn (up to 72 h after birth)	60-100 mL/kg (newborns are born with excess body water)	–
Up to 10 kg	100 mL/kg (can increase up to 150 mL/kg to provide caloric requirements if renal and cardiac function are adequate)	4 mL/kg
11-20 kg	1000 mL for the first 10 kg + 50 mL/kg for each kg over 10 kg	40 mL for first 10 kg + 2 mL/kg for each kg over 10 kg
21-30 kg	1500 mL for the first 20 kg + 25 mL/kg for each kg over 20 kg	60 mL for first 20 kg + 1 mL/kg for each kg over 20 kg
Fluid Requirements Estimated from Body Surface Area (BSA)		
Maintenance	1500 mL/m² BSA	–
Insensible losses	300-400 mL/m² BSA	–
Electrolytes		
Sodium (Na)	2-4 mEq/kg	–
Potassium (K)	1-2 mEq/kg	–
Chloride (Cl)	2-3 mEq/kg	–
Calcium (Ca)	0.5-3 mEq/kg	–
Phosphorous (Phos)	0.5-2 mmol/kg	–
Magnesium (Mg)	0.4-0.9 mEq/kg	–

*The "maintenance" fluids calculated by these formulas must only be used as a starting point to determine the fluid requirements of an individual patient. If intravascular volume is adequate, children with cardiac, pulmonary, or renal failure or increased intracranial pressure should generally receive less than these calculated "maintenance" fluids. The formula utilizing body weight generally results in a generous "maintenance" fluid total.

Table 14-3 Caloric Distribution of Daily Macronutrient Intake

Macronutrient	Percent of Total Calories (%)
Carbohydrates	40-70
Fat	20-50 (40-50 in infants)
Protein	7-15

Fats

A variety of lipids (fats) are consumed in the diet; the highest quantity is in the form of triglycerides. Dietary triglycerides are a major source of energy; they have a higher caloric density than the other macronutrients (i.e., carbohydrates and proteins). Adequate dietary lipids are needed to allow for the absorption of fat-soluble vitamins A, D, E, and K.

Protein

Dietary proteins are necessary for maintaining body proteins and increasing protein mass associated with growth. If dietary protein is inadequate, growth is retarded. Renal and liver disease, cancer, and infections are associated with loss of body proteins.

Enteral Nutrition

Enteral feeding is preferable to parenteral nutrition, because enteral feedings will maintain gut structure and function and will reduce complications and cost. Specific benefits include intestinal trophism and preservation of the gut barrier to minimize bacterial translocation.[38]

Selection of the appropriate formula is based on the patient's age and disease process. Because breast milk is the preferred source of nutrition for infants, nursing mothers should be provided with a breast pump if their infant is unable to breast feed but can be fed enterally. Standard infant formulas are not appropriate for the premature infant (specialty premature formulas should be used) or for children older than 1 year. Specific formulas are available for disease states such as renal failure (NovaSource Renal [Nestlé Nutrition, North America, Minneapolis, MN] or Nepro [Abbott Nutrition, Columbus, OH]) or liver insufficiency (e.g., Pregestimil [Mead Johnson Nutrition, Evansville, IN] for infants, Peptamen Jr. [Nestlé Nutrition, North America, Minneapolis, MN] and PediaSure Peptide [Abbott Nutrition, Columbus, OH] for children). The renal formulas are not designed specifically for children, so they should be used with caution.

If possible, the patient should be encouraged to take nutrition orally; however, for many critically ill children enteral nutrition is provided through a feeding tube. Enteral feedings should be tailored to each patient. When a gastric feeding tube is in place, continuous feedings are often initially provided to achieve goal calories before transitioning to physiologic bolus feedings. Children with significant reflux may benefit from venting of the gastric tube (i.e., leave the tube open to air, with the open end elevated above the level of the stomach).

Postpyloric feeding should be considered for children with delayed gastric emptying and poor intestinal motility who are intolerant to gastric feedings. To prevent dumping syndrome, feedings into the jejunum are administered at a continuous hourly rate.

The practice of aspirating residual liquid and refeeding it is controversial. Although a large volume of residual feeding that remains in the stomach may contribute to inadvertent aspiration,[45] the residual volume that should be considered significant has not been clearly established. Nurses should measure and record the volume of residual feeding and notify the on-call provider according to unit policy or orders. Enteral feeding delivery devices, routes, placement methods, nursing considerations, and complications are summarized in Table 14-4.

Parenteral Nutrition (PN)

When a child is unable to absorb nutrients through the GI tract, or when the child requires a supplement to enteral nutrition, PN is indicated. PN is defined as the administration of nutrients by the intravascular route. PN was first demonstrated as a practical mode of nutritional therapy in the 1960s and is now widely accepted as beneficial for nutritionally compromised children. Some children receive PN in the home setting.

PN may be used over a long period of time to allow a poorly functioning GI tract to rest. PN can also be used for long periods in children with "short gut" and for critically ill children with multiorgan failure when enteral feeding is not possible.

Indications for Parenteral Nutrition

PN is most often is used as a supportive rather than a definitive therapy for infants and children with complex illnesses and structural GI anomalies. Indications for the supportive use of PN in the neonatal period include: congenital GI anomalies requiring extensive resection of the small bowel, intestinal obstruction, and necrotizing enterocolitis. Beyond infancy, indications for PN include: severe malnutrition, acute

Table 14-4 Delivery of Enteral Nutrition

Delivery Routes	Devices	Placement	Nursing Considerations	Complications
NGT	• Sizes: 5 Fr to 10 Fr • Use smallest tube with adequate length • Polyvinyl chloride tube: change every 72 h (they stiffen in the presence of acid) • Polyurethane tube: change every 30 days • Although feeding tubes are the preferred device, decompression tubes can be used with caution (eye ports proximal to the end of the tube may result in delivery of feeding into esophagus, creating risk of aspiration)	• Most common method to determine proper insertion length is to measure from the nose to earlobe to between the xiphoid process and the umbilicus (NEX method) • Clinical methods used to evaluate placement: auscultation over stomach during air injection, initial pH aspirate (should be less than 4; tracheobronchial secretions have a pH of >6), general color and quality of fluid, and bilirubin level)* • Current standard for verifying placement is radiographic confirmation, because other methods may be inaccurate	• Tape tube securely to prevent dislodgement; tape tube in dependent position to minimize pressure on nares • Provide nasal and oral care every 4 h or per hospital policy • Confirm placement before each use • Feed by bolus or continuous infusion • Monitor for signs of feeding intolerance: abdominal distension, emesis, and diarrhea	• Malplacement or migration to lungs, esophagus, and to small intestine • Dislodgement may require repeated insertion and need for additional radiographs • Pressure necrosis or skin breakdown from tube and tape • Tube obstruction • Possible occlusion of nasal passage • Erosion of gastric mucosa and gastric bleeding from hardened distal tube (polyvinyl chloride tubes)
Orogastric tube	• May be appropriate for the neonate (tube in nares may contribute to airway obstruction in these obligatory nose breathers) • See NGT section for devices	• Measurement is the same as with an NGT, except that the measurement begins at the corner of the mouth	• See NGT section	• See NGT section
GT	• Tube devices: Corpak tube (CORPAK MedSystem, Incorporated, Wheeling, IL), MIC (Kimberly Clark, Roswell, Georgia), de Pezzer (Kimberly Clark, Roswell, Georgia), and Malecot (Kimberly Clark, Roswell, Georgia); 3-8 weeks after placement (as per surgeon preference) can be changed to a skin level device	• Percutaneous placement by endoscopy • Surgical placement with either an open or laparoscopic procedure	• Assess the site every 4 h • Site should be cleansed with soap and water every 12-24 h • Feed by bolus or continuous infusion • Monitor for signs of feeding intolerance: abdominal distension, emesis, and diarrhea	• Percutaneous or endoscopic placement is blind with risk of perforation of transverse colon; monitor for signs of acute abdomen after placement • Separation of the stomach from the abdominal wall may produce signs and symptoms of peritonitis • Malposition • Dislodgement

Continued

Table 14-4   Delivery of Enteral Nutrition—cont'd

Delivery Routes	Devices	Placement	Nursing Considerations	Complications
	• Low profile or skin level devices are balloon tubes and mushroom types; these are now preferred devices for surgical placement • Balloon tubes: MIC-KEY (Kimberly Clark, Roswell, Georgia), AMT Mini (Applied Medical Technology, Incorporated, Cleveland, Ohio), and NutriPort (Kendall-Tyco Healthcare Group, Mansfield, MA); kept in place by fluid in balloon (1-2 mL in neonates to 5 mL in older children); tube should be changed every 6 months; most common cause of malfunction is balloon rupture • Mushroom types: Bard Button (Bard Access Systems, Salt Lake City, UT), Ross Stomate (Abbott Laboratories, Abbott Park, IL), and EntriStar (Tyco Healthcare, Mansfield, MA); these tubes are flatter because the one-way valve is in the stomach; these tubes are painful to remove and are changed only once a year; the most common cause of malfunction is valve incompetence		• If a Nissen procedure is performed in conjunction with GT placement, vent feedings for at least 2 weeks	• Wound complications: separation, infection, granulation tissue • Leakage and periostomy skin irritation • Gastric outlet obstruction (will produce signs including abdominal distension, pain, and vomiting)
Transpyloric feeding tube	• Sizes: 5-12 Fr • Tubes can be weighted or nonweighted with or without a stylet	• Placement can be directly beyond pylorus or weighted devices can be inserted into stomach and allowed to pass • Placement should be verified by radiograph, and the external tube distance from the exit point to the end should be measured after radiologic confirmation • Device placement requires specialized skills and should be inserted per hospital policy	• See NGT section • Can use measured external tube length to verify placement; a radiograph should be obtained if placement is in question • Feedings should be administered as continuous infusion • Monitor for signs of feeding intolerance: abdominal distension, emesis, and diarrhea	• Malplacement into lungs, esophagus and stomach • Dislodgement • Occlusion • Gastric or intestinal perforation (will produce signs of an acute abdomen)
Jejunostomy tube	• Sizes: 16 Fr to 24 Fr, with various lengths of the jejunal extension	• Placement should be verified radiologically with fluoroscopy study	• See Transpyloric Feeding Tube section	• See Transpyloric Feeding Tube section

*Ellett MLC et al: Gastric tube placement in children. *Clin Nurs Res* 14:238, 2005; Huffman S et al: Methods to confirm feeding tube placement: application of research in practice. *Pediatr Nurs* 30:10, 2004; Westhus N: Methods to test feeding placement in children. *MCN Am J Matern Child Nurs* 29:282, 2004.
GT, Gastrostomy tube; *NEX*, nose, earlobe, xiphoid process; *NGT*, nasogastric tube.

pancreatitis, fulminant liver failure, inflammatory bowel disease, extensive burns, malabsorption syndromes, refractory anorexia nervosa, and other disorders causing intestinal failure (see the Intestinal Failure section in this chapter).

Parenteral Nutrition Solutions

PN solution consists primarily of glucose (as a source of carbohydrate), amino acids (as a source of protein), and fat emulsions. Dextrose provides 3.4 Kcal/g and constitutes 60% to 70% of the total PN caloric intake. Protein can be administered as Trophamine (recommended for infants younger than 1 year and for children with liver failure), or as Clinisol or Travasol (for children older than 1 year). Protein provides 4 Kcal/g and should constitute 14% to 20% of the total PN caloric intake. Fat emulsions (Intralipid) may be administered as a separate solution to provide a major source of calories (20% solution provides 2 Kcal/mL) and should constitute 30% to 50% of the total PN caloric intake. Providing adequate calories from fat (0.5 g/kg per day) prevents essential fatty acid deficiency states. Electrolytes, vitamins, minerals, and trace elements are added to these solutions to meet the child's known nutritional requirements.

The PN orders are individually tailored to deliver appropriate amounts of fluid, nutrients, and electrolytes. The critically ill child's fluid requirements often change and may differ from estimated maintenance fluid requirements. In addition, it may be necessary to alter electrolyte content based on the child's clinical condition or changes in medications. For example, medications such as furosemide (Lasix) will increase the daily potassium requirements; if the furosemide dose is reduced, the child will require less supplementary potassium.

When PN is initiated, there is gradual titration of additives until goal calories are achieved. The goal calories should be determined by the healthcare provider in consultation with a dietitian or pharmacist.

Nursing Responsibilities

The nurse must closely monitor the child's clinical appearance and fluid and electrolyte balance to prevent and detect complications of PN as soon as possible. This monitoring requires documentation of the quantity and content of the child's fluid intake and output and evaluation of the child's fluid and electrolyte status and daily weight. A sample monitoring schedule for children receiving PN is provided in Table 14-5.

Whenever the child receives concentrated glucose solutions, the nurse must verify that the fluid volume and content are appropriate for the child's estimated daily requirements. Before every new bag of PN solution is infused, the nurse should confirm that the prepared solution is accurate and consistent with the order by checking the solution content against the provider's original order. Reduction in the PN administration rate (e.g., if the intravenous [IV] catheter malfunctions or with the initiation of enteral feedings or feeding advancement) will reduce the child's fluid, glucose, and electrolyte intake unless enteral feedings provide the difference.

Potential complications of PN include electrolyte abnormalities, infection, cholestasis leading to hepatic dysfunction, and hyperlipidemias (with triglyceride administration). In

Table 14-5	Sample Monitoring Schedule for Children Receiving Parenteral Nutrition: Must Be Tailored to Child's Clinical Status
Monitoring	**Frequency**
General and Anthropometric Measurements	
Vital signs	Every 4 hours, or more often as patient condition warrants
Weight	Daily
Strict intake and output	Constant
Caloric intake	Daily
Height	Weekly
Head circumference	Weekly (for children younger than 2 years)
Blood Sampling	
Glucose	Initial + Daily until stable (more often in neonates)
Electrolytes	Initial + Daily until stable
BUN, Creatinine	Initial + Weekly
Ca^{2+}/ionized calcium, PO_4^+, Mg^{2+}	Initial + Weekly (PO_4^+, Mg^{2+} should be checked daily if values not within reference range)
Alkaline phosphatase, AST, ALT	Initial + Weekly
Total and direct bilirubin	Initial + Weekly
Total protein, albumin	Initial + Weekly
Prealbumin	Initiation
Triglycerides, cholesterol	Weekly
Zinc, copper, selenium, manganese, iron	Monthly
Glucose point-of-care testing	When PN is abruptly discontinued, cycled, or if signs or symptoms of hypoglycemia or hyperglycemia suspected
CBC count with differential	When febrile
Blood culture	When febrile

ALT, Alanine aminotransferase; *AST,* aspartate aminotransferase; *BUN,* blood urea nitrogen; Ca^{2+}, calcium; *CBC,* complete blood count; Mg^{2+}, magnesium; *PN,* parenteral nutrition; PO_4^+, phosphorous.

critically ill children, there is an association between hyperglycemia and organ dysfunction.[33]

Because PN solution contains a high concentration of glucose, it provides an excellent medium for bacterial growth. When hanging a new bag of PN solution and tubing, the nurse must use strict aseptic technique to prevent line contamination. Many hospitals require that the entire tubing system (between PN solution and the patient, including infusion pump tubing) be changed every 24 hours to decrease the possibility of significant bacterial growth. The dressing over the catheter insertion site should be changed when it is no longer occlusive (per hospital policy), using sterile technique and an occlusive dressing. The nurse should assess the catheter insertion site for evidence of inflammation (erythema or exudate) and should report any abnormalities to the appropriate provider. Wound exudate should be cultured and sent for gram stain analysis as ordered (or per protocol). Nurses should be careful to follow the healthcare institutional policies and protocols to prevent central venous catheter-associated blood stream infections (see Chapter 22, Box 22-6 for further information).

Monitor the child's temperature at least every 4 hours (or according to hospital PN policy). Blood cultures are typically ordered if the child's temperature rises above 38.5° C or if the child develops signs of infection. The child may be placed on empiric antibiotics until culture results are available. The antibiotics are then adjusted if the culture is positive and the bacterial sensitivities or susceptibilities support a change. Often the catheter is maintained during an attempt to clear an existing infection, because if the child requires long term PN it may be difficult to achieve and maintain venous access. Therefore existing access sites are salvaged if possible.

When PN is initiated, a low glucose concentration and a low rate of infusion are used, and then both are increased gradually so that the child's insulin production can accommodate the glucose load. Once the PN infusion is established, providers should maintain the infusion at a uniform rate as ordered; it should not be decreased or increased, because hypoglycemia or hyperglycemia can result. Once goal calories are achieved, it may be appropriate to stop the PN for increasing time intervals, allowing intervals without the PN. When neonates or children are receiving high dextrose compositions, dosing may need to be decreased and increased (with a gradual decrease in rate of administration before and gradual increase after the off cycle) to prevent hypoglycemia or hyperglycemia. To discontinue PN, the glucose concentration and the rate should be weaned gradually.

When PN infusions are initiated, serum glucose measurements can be performed several times per day. Point-of-care glucose measurements may be performed every 4 to 8 hours in infants if unit or hospital policy allows such testing. The presence of either glucosuria or ketonuria should be reported to an on-call provider, and the child's serum glucose level should be checked. Glucosuria usually indicates the presence of high serum glucose levels that exceed the renal threshold of 150 to 200 mg/dL blood.

If the PN catheter infiltrates or becomes occluded, providers should promptly insert a temporary IV catheter to continue glucose administration and avoid the development of hypoglycemia that could result from a sudden cessation of glucose infusion. Monitor the child closely for clinical evidence of hypoglycemia (e.g., lethargy, irritability, tremors, diaphoresis, tachycardia, headache, vomiting, dizziness, blurred vision) until the PN infusion is resumed. Point-of-care glucose measurements can be obtained from infants to rule out hypoglycemia. An additional source of IV glucose administration may be needed if the PN solution contains a dextrose concentration of greater than the maximum 12.5% dextrose solutions that can be infused peripherally.

Because serum magnesium, phosphate, and calcium levels may fall during PN therapy, providers will monitor the concentration of these elements at least weekly. Trace element deficiencies are more likely to develop with long-term PN therapy or when PN therapy is used in premature infants. The signs and symptoms of copper deficiency include anemia, neutropenia, loss of taste (obviously difficult to assess), and rash. Zinc deficiency can produce an erythematous maculopapular rash (called *acrodermatitis enteropathica*) over the face, trunk, and digits; poor wound healing; hair loss and loss of taste; and a functional ileus.[62] A chromium deficiency can produce a diabetes-like syndrome.[62]

Complications of the PN catheter may also develop. Cardiac arrhythmias can occur if the central venous catheter migrates into the heart, particularly into the right ventricle. Venous thrombosis can develop if a clot is allowed to form at the catheter tip. Superior vena caval thrombosis can complicate PN therapy, particularly in infants who require prolonged PN therapy. An air embolus can be caused by careless coupling of the IV line or stopcock.

Because the central venous PN catheter is inserted into a relatively large vein, a loose or cracked tubing connection can rapidly result in significant loss of blood (i.e., hemorrhage). It is important that the nurse check all tubing and catheter connections at least every hour. Because insertion of a central venous catheter creates risk of significant complications, the nurse must ensure that the catheter is secured in place with no possibility of dislodgement. If catheter misplacement or migration is suspected, a chest radiograph may be needed to verify placement (for further information, see Chapter 10).

Fat emulsions are typically piggybacked into the PN line just before the solution enters the vein. This practice evolved during the initial years of parenteral alimentation using fat emulsions and arose from a concern that prolonged contact between the PN amino acids and the lipids would cause emulsification of the fat and result in the production of fat emboli.

Administration of fat emulsion is contraindicated in neonates with jaundice. Lipid binds with albumin and will displace bilirubin, resulting in an increased risk of hyperbilirubinemia.

Children who receive prolonged PN frequently demonstrate abnormalities in liver function studies (i.e., elevation of the liver enzymes and bilirubin values). Many of these abnormalities are transient and resolve shortly after PN nutrition is discontinued; however, if these abnormalities are noted, the child should be weaned from the PN as clinically appropriate.

Cholestatic jaundice is a serious but incompletely understood complication of PN that is associated with periportal fibrosis, bile duct proliferation, and bile stasis. This complication contributes to morbidity and mortality in younger infants and children with short gut syndrome (SGS) following intestinal resection.[10] The first sign of cholestatic jaundice is elevation in concentrations of liver enzymes (alanine aminotransferase [ALT] and aspartate aminotransferase [AST]).

In addition, the bilirubin will begin to rise and the child may appear jaundiced; cholestasis is defined as a direct bilirubin greater than 2 mg/dL. Risk of cholestatic jaundice can be reduced by cycling and limiting lipid administration to 1 g/kg per day or using alternate day dosing of the fat emulsion. If cholestasis is present, treatment includes administration of ursodeoxycholic acid.

COMMON CLINICAL CONDITIONS

Intestinal Failure

Intestinal failure is the loss of the absorptive function of the intestine, with resulting malabsorption and malnutrition necessitating PN support. Although the terms *intestinal failure* and *short gut syndrome (SGS)* are sometimes used interchangeably, children can have intestinal failure even when they have normal bowel length. Most children afflicted with this disease are diagnosed at less than 1 year of age and are rendered "short gut" when extensive surgical resection of the intestine is required during infancy to treat congenital anomalies or necrotizing enterocolitis (NEC).

With the availability of PN as a form of replacement therapy, many children with intestinal failure survive to adulthood. Multidisciplinary teams (including a nurse practitioner, gastroenterologist, surgeon, dietitian, social worker, and speech therapist) can provide medical and surgical care for intestinal rehabilitation and to promote optimal growth and development in this patient population. Early referrals to such teams should be made for children that are dependent on PN.

Etiology

The etiologies of intestinal failure can be categorized as congenital anomalies with bowel loss or resection (e.g., complicated gastroschisis, malrotation with volvulus, multiple intestinal atresias), postsurgical complications (e.g., NEC, trauma), dysmotility disorders (e.g., chronic intestinal pseudoobstruction, total intestinal Hirschsprung disease), inflammatory bowel disease (e.g., Crohn's disease), and congenital enteropathies (e.g., microvillus inclusion disease, intestinal epithelial dysplasia, secretory diarrhea).

Pathophysiology

Each child with intestinal failure is unique, because there are no absolute criteria for the amount and type of bowel needed to sustain absorption of nutrients for appropriate growth. The normal estimated bowel length at birth is 250 ± 40 cm.[22] After the loss of a bowel segment, the intestine undergoes a process termed *intestinal adaptation*. As a general rule, infants can experience acceptable intestinal function with less than 15 cm of intestine if the ileocecal valve is intact, and with 30 to 45 cm of intestine if the ileocecal valve is absent or does not function.[17] It is unlikely that children with less than 20 cm of remaining bowel will be able to grow and develop with enteral nutrition alone. Intestinal transplantation may offer hope to these patients.

Many children with SGS no longer have a functioning ileocecal valve; this results in more rapid intestinal transit and decreased absorption of nutrients. Small bowel distension results in stasis and bacterial overgrowth. Small bowel bacterial overgrowth can result in bacterial translocation and sepsis that contributes to morbidity and mortality in this patient population. For these reasons, enteral antibiotics, and most recently probiotics (bacteria administered to support healthy intestinal flora), are often prescribed for children with SGS to minimize small bowel bacterial overgrowth.

Intestinal adaptation is characterized by increasing intestinal mass, lengthening of villi, and improved absorption at the epithelial level.[10,22] This process allows for the remaining intestine to compensate for the loss of the bowel by increasing its surface area and functional abilities.[10] Successful adaptation is described as the ability to achieve normal growth, fluid balance, and electrolyte concentration without PN.[53] The time frame required for adaptation is unclear and dependent on the etiology of the SBS and the functional state of the remaining bowel, although adaptation can occur over weeks to months.[10,22] Children have been transitioned to enteral feedings exclusively over periods as long as 8 years. There are a number of metabolic derangements that occur after loss of bowel that are summarized in Table 14-6.

Management

The care of patients with intestinal failure includes complementary medical and surgical interventions with the goals of optimizing oral or enteral diet, PN prescription, treatment of bacterial overgrowth, and use of stool bulking agents. Surgical procedures include bowel lengthening procedures and intestinal transplantation.

In order for the bowel to adapt it must be fed; therefore initiation of early enteral feeding is paramount. Enteral feeding can start with a continuous infusion of nutrition administered through a nasogastric, gastrostomy, or transpyloric feeding tube. Appropriate fluid administration is as important as caloric intake. Many of these children will require 150% to 160% of maintenance fluid to remain hydrated. Once a continuous rate of feeding is tolerated, the time interval can be shortened and feedings can be consolidated if larger volumes are tolerated. Once a consolidated hourly feeding schedule is tolerated, the child can be advanced to bolus feeding.

Table 14-6 Metabolic Derangements and Consequences in Children with Short Gut Syndrome

Derangements	Consequences
Early	
Gastric hypersecretion	Peptic ulceration
Dumping syndrome	Diarrhea, hyperglycemia, reactive hypoglycemia
Rapid intestinal transit	Nutrient malabsorption
High output from enterostomies	Electrolyte disturbances
Late	
Bile and fatty acid malabsorption	Gallstones, steatorrhea
Bowel dilation and stasis	Bacterial overgrowth syndrome, D-lactic acidosis
Anastomotic ulceration	Gastrointestinal bleeding

From Cohran VC and Kocoshis SA: Short bowel. In Baker S, Baker R, David A, editors: *Pediatric nutrition support*, Sudbury, MA, 2007, Jones and Bartlett.

Often 20 Kcal/ounce feedings are initiated and can be advanced to higher caloric density (to as high as 30 Kcal/ounce [1 Kcal/mL]) as tolerated. Usually these children are fed with casein hydrolysate formulas and elementary amino acid-based formulas such as Pregestimil (Mead Johnson, Evansville, IN), EleCare (Abbott Nutrition, Columbus, OH), and Neocate (Nutricia North America, Gaithersburg, MD) in infants and Peptamen Jr (Nestle Nutrition, North America, Minneapolis, MN) and Neocate Jr.(Nutricia North America, Gaithersburg, MD) in older children. These formula types are easier to digest and are less likely to trigger an immune response, so they will enhance bowel adaptation.[10]

The eventual goal of medical and surgical therapy is appropriate growth with enteral intake alone, without the need for PN. Promotion of oral food intake should be encouraged; many of these children will have an oral aversion.

When children are unable to achieve appropriate growth with enteral feedings, they may be considered surgical candidates for procedures to restore normal bowel diameter, lengthen the bowel, or both. The goals of surgical intervention include reducing stasis, improving motility, and increasing the effective mucosal surface area.[29] The most common short bowel procedures are the Bianchi, Kimura, and the serial transverse enteroplasty procedure.

The Bianchi procedure is the oldest procedure and involves a longitudinal incision to create two tubes to lengthen the bowel (Fig. 14-5). The Kimura procedure (Fig. 14-6) is an alternative procedure for patients with SGS and inadequate mesentery who are not candidates for the Bianchi procedure. The serial transverse enteroplasty (STEP) procedure augments bowel length by stapling dilated bowel in a zigzag fashion to achieve more effective bowel surface area (Fig. 14-7).

With advances in surgical techniques and immunosuppressive therapy, intestine transplantation is successful as an isolated procedure and when combined with transplantation of other organs.[54] A major reason for the increased success of intestinal transplantation is the availability of more potent immunosuppressants such as tacrolimus (Prograf). The major limiting factor that prevents widespread use of transplantation is the lack of available organs for transplantation. Because children with less than 15 cm of bowel are not likely to tolerate enteral feeding and thrive, they should be referred to an intestinal rehabilitation and transplant program as soon as possible.

The ideal intestine donor has the same blood type, weighs within 10% of the recipient's body weight, and is close in age to the recipient. All intestine recipients have a stoma to

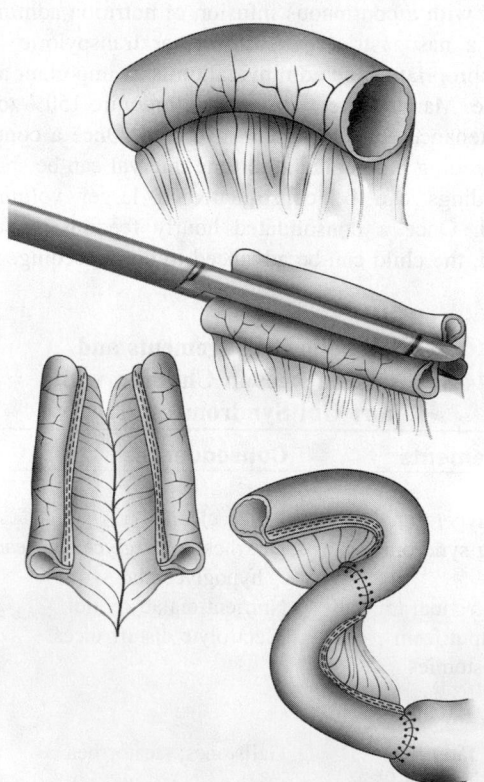

FIG. 14-5 The Bianchi intestinal lengthening procedure. The bowel is divided in a longitudinal plane to create two tubes, which after reanastomosis results in doubling of the intestinal length at the expense of halving the bowel wall circumference. (From Warner BW: Short-bowel syndrome. In Grosfeld JL et al, editors: *Pediatric surgery*, ed 6, Philadelphia, 2006, Mosby.)

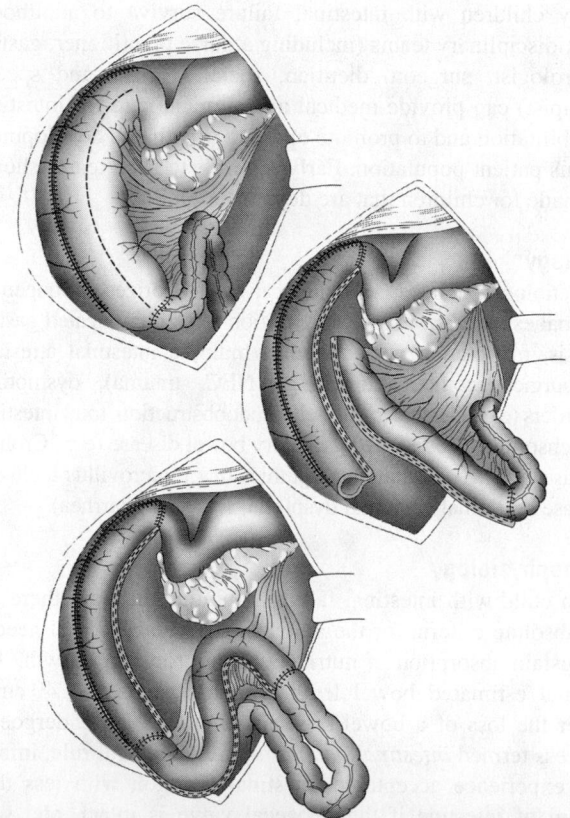

FIG. 14-6 The Iowa (Kimura) intestinal lengthening procedure. The antimesenteric bowel wall is pexed to the undersurface of the abdominal wall. A seromyotomy along the bowel wall and mechanical abrasion of the abdominal wall before pexing promote neovascularization of the antimesenteric bowel, based on the systemic-derived abdominal wall. Several months later, the bowel may be longitudinally divided into two limbs. The first is based on the systemic blood supply to the antimesenteric limb, and the other is based on the mesenteric blood supply. These two limbs are then reapproximated to double the intestinal length. (From Warner BW: Short-bowel syndrome. In Grosfeld JL et al, editors: *Pediatric surgery*, ed 6, Philadelphia, 2006, Mosby.)

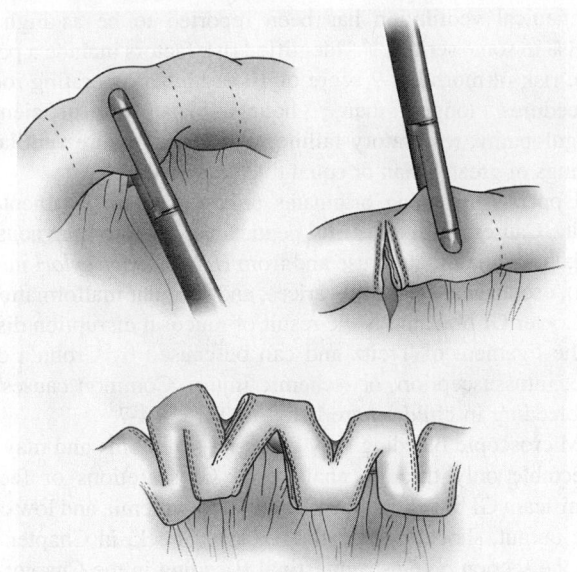

FIG. 14-7 The serial transverse enteroplasty procedure. Multiple fires of an anastomotic stapling device to alternating sides of the bowel wall result in decreased bowel caliber with an increased length of enteral nutrient transit. (From Warner BW: Short-bowel syndrome. In Grosfeld JL et al, editors: *Pediatric surgery*, ed 6, Philadelphia, 2006, Mosby.)

allow for bowel surveillance and access for endoscopy and biopsy. Figure 14-8 shows the technical details of isolated intestine transplant procedure and intestine transplant in combination with other organs.[54]

The priorities of care for patients with liver-intestine failure (so-called "ABCs" of care) in the pediatric critical care unit include aeration, bowel integrity, and caloric or hydration requirements. As with any critical care patient, the nurse will

assess and support the child's airway, breathing, and circulation. Bowel integrity is initially assessed by evaluating the physical appearance of the stoma (normal stoma appears pink and moist) and enteric output. Initially caloric requirements are met with PN. Enteral feedings are initiated as soon as possible after the transplant.

Critical care goals are to support the patient to be hemodynamically stable, with adequate oxygenation and ventilation, free of requirement for mechanical ventilation support. Airway clearance and spontaneous ventilation may be ineffective as a result of the lengthy abdominal surgical procedure (and resultant need for anesthetic administration during the long procedure), visceral edema, and pain. With the postoperative resolution of coagulopathies, aggressive chest physiotherapy is initiated. Intestine recipients generally require mechanical ventilation longer than isolated liver recipients (see Liver Transplantation in Chapter 17), because intestine recipients typically are in poor health before the transplant and often have a precarious fluid balance. Additional challenges include open abdominal wounds and potential need for surgical reexploration for complications such as perforation or bleeding.

Complications of intestine transplant procedures include rejection, infection, and posttransplant lymphoproliferative disease (PTLD). Signs and symptoms of intestinal graft rejection include a pale or dusky stoma, an increase or decrease in enteric output, abdominal pain, and guaiac positive output. Postoperative endoscopic biopsies of the transplanted bowel are made through the child's stoma on a routine and as needed basis. Rejection is not usually a visual finding during endoscopy, and there are no known confirmatory laboratory tests. Endoscopy with biopsy is the gold standard.

Infection is a common complication following intestine transplant. Viral infection is the most threatening infection

Small Bowel Transplantation Surgery

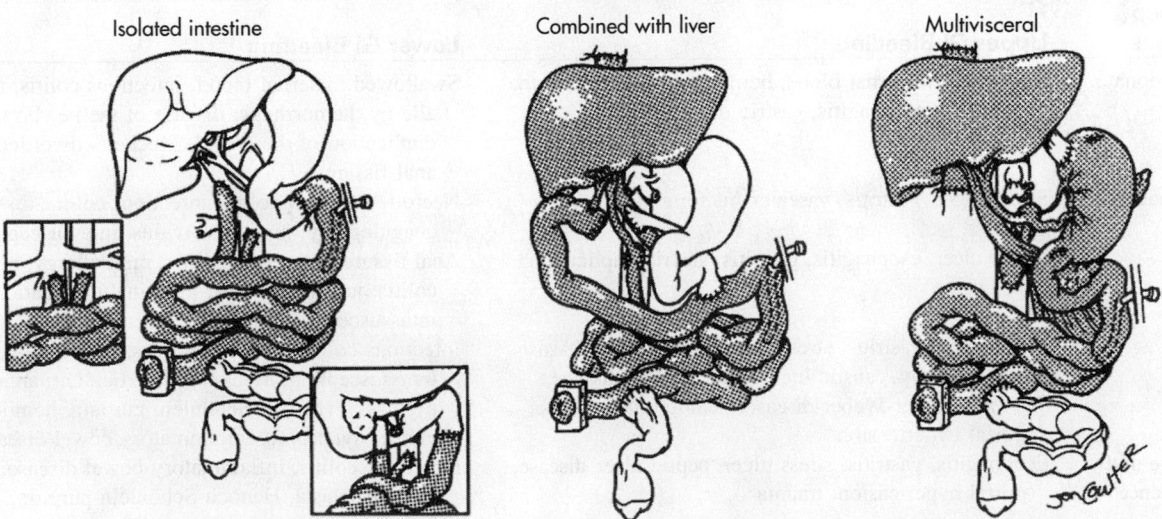

FIG. 14-8 The three basic intestinal transplant procedures (the graft is shaded): Isolated intestine transplant, Intestine transplant combined with liver transplant, and multivisceral transplant. With the isolated intestine transplant, the venous outflow may be to the recipient portal vein (*center*), to the inferior vena cava (*left*), or to the superior mesenteric vein (*right*). (From Reyes JD: Intestinal transplantation. *Semin Pediatr Surg* 15:228-234, 2006.)

for the intestine recipient. Primary infections are typically more serious and occur when the recipient has had no previous exposure to a virus and becomes infected in the posttransplant period. A secondary infection represents reactivation of a previous latent virus.

The most common infecting organisms are cytomegalovirus and Epstein-Barr virus. For the isolated intestine recipient efforts are made to match the recipient and donor cytomegalovirus status. The donor-recipient serology relationship is important because prophylactic therapy is initiated based on viral titers.

Post-transplant lymphoproliferative disorder (PTLD) is one of the most underrated complications of immunosuppression. PTLD is the development of continually proliferating B-lymphocytes, presumably under the influence of Epstein-Barr virus. Diagnosis is made by clinical examination and histologic review. Clinical signs and symptoms include fever, lymphadenopathy, GI symptoms, and weight loss. If the biopsy specimen is diagnostic for PTLD, treatment includes holding or reducing immunosuppression and initiating IV antiviral therapy and immunoglobulin therapy (see Chapter 17 for additional information).

PTLD is a difficult complication to treat following intestine transplantation, because rejection can develop following withdrawal of immunosuppression. Therefore careful titration of immunosuppression is imperative to promote recovery, although the graft may be lost to preserve the child's life.

Gastrointestinal Bleeding

Etiology and Pathophysiology

GI bleeding in children can result from inflammation of the intestine, congenital or acquired visceral or vascular anomalies, trauma, esophageal varices, ulcers, or coagulopathies. The incidence of acquired GI bleeding in critically ill children receiving mechanical ventilation has been reported to be as high as 51.8% in some series.[14,47] Identified risk factors include a pediatric risk of mortality 2 score of 10 or higher, operating room procedures longer than 3 hours, hepatic insufficiency, coagulopathy, respiratory failure, and high-pressure ventilator settings of greater than or equal to 25 cm H_2O.[14,47]

Upper GI bleeding originates proximal to the ligament of Treitz. Causes include gastritis, peptic ulcer disease (from nonsteroidal antiinflammatory use and from *Helicobacter pylori* infection), esophageal or gastric varices, and vascular malformations.

Lower GI bleeding is the result of mucosal disruption distal to the ligament of Treitz and can be caused by Crohn's disease, intussusception, or ischemic injury. Common causes of GI bleeding in children are listed in Table 14-7.

Microscopic bleeding may cause no symptoms and may be detectable only through analysis of GI secretions or feces. Significant GI bleeding may result in hypovolemia and low cardiac output, shock, and death (see also Shock, in Chapter 6). See the section on Gastrointestinal Bleeding in the Chapter 14 Supplement on the Evolve Website for additional information about the pathophysiology of GI hemorrhage.

Clinical Signs and Symptoms

The appearance of the child with GI bleeding varies considerably, and it is affected by the amount and rapidity of blood loss. Usually the child is brought to the provider's office or emergency department for treatment after vomiting blood, passing black, tarry stools (melena), or passing bright red blood per rectum (hematochezia). Bright red vomitus indicates recent or ongoing upper GI hemorrhage, whereas coffee-ground vomitus indicates partial digestion of the blood.

The color and the source of the bleeding often help to identify the location of the bleeding. Bright red vomitus usually results from esophageal or gastric bleeding, and bright red

Table 14-7   Causes of Gastrointestinal Bleeding in Infants and Children

Age Group and Status	Upper GI Bleeding	Lower GI Bleeding
Healthy neonate	Swallowed maternal blood, hemorrhagic disease of the newborn, esophagitis, gastric duplication	Swallowed maternal blood, infectious colitis, milk allergy, hemorrhagic disease of the newborn, duplication of the bowel, Meckel's diverticulum, anal fissure
Sick neonate	Stress ulcer, gastritis, vascular malformations	Necrotizing enterocolitis, infectious colitis, disseminated coagulopathy, midgut volvulus, intussusception
Infancy	Stress ulcer, esophagitis, gastritis, gastric duplication	Anal fissure, infectious colitis, milk allergy, nonspecific colitis, juvenile polyps, intestinal duplication, intussusception, Meckel's diverticulum
Preschool age	Esophagitis, gastritis, stress ulcer, peptic ulcer disease, foreign body, caustic ingestion, vascular disease (Rendu-Osler-Weber disease, hemophilia), trauma, portal hypertension	Infectious colitis, juvenile polyps, anal fissure, intussusception, Meckel's diverticulum, angiodysplasia, Henoch-Schönlein purpura, hemolytic-uremic syndrome, inflammatory bowel disease
School age and adolescence	Esophagitis, gastritis, stress ulcer, peptic ulcer disease, portal hypertension, trauma	Infectious colitis, inflammatory bowel disease, polyps, angiodysplasia, Henoch-Schönlein purpura, hemolytic-uremic syndrome, hemorrhoids, rectal trauma

Data from Arensman RM, Browne M, Madonna MB: Gastrointestinal bleeding. In Grosfeld JL et al, editors: *Pediatric surgery,* ed 6, Philadelphia, 2006, Mosby; Martin SA, Simone S: Gastrointestinal system: In Slota MC, editor: *Core curriculum for pediatric critical care nursing,* ed 2, St Louis, 2006, Mosby-Elsevier. *GI,* Gastrointestinal.

blood in the stool results almost exclusively from rectal bleeding. Maroon, black, or tarry stool often indicates the presence of upper GI bleeding; the color derives from blood that is partially digested during passage through the bowel.

The patient with sudden, significant bleeding is more likely to demonstrate faintness, pallor, tachycardia, thready pulses, diaphoresis, thirst, apprehension, and other signs of acute blood loss. The child with gradual bleeding, however, may experience only weakness and faintness; the child may be aware of passing black stools, but may not know that significant blood loss has occurred.

The child with GI bleeding may have a normal systolic blood pressure, particularly in the recumbent position, despite significant intravascular volume loss and shock. Signs of decreased peripheral perfusion are usually the earliest signs of severe hemorrhage and include tachycardia; cool, pale, mottled skin; decreased peripheral pulses; and oliguria (urine output averaging less than 0.5-1.0 mL/kg per hour despite adequate fluid intake) or anuria.

Arterial constriction makes blood pressure measurement by cuff difficult or inaccurate, because automated oscillometric blood pressure cuffs may provide falsely high readings in the presence of shock with or without hypotension. The arterial waveform displayed from an indwelling arterial line usually is dampened in appearance, with a narrow pulse pressure.

Metabolic acidosis and a rise in serum lactate may be noted. Oxyhemoglobin desaturation may not be present or detected by pulse oximetry, because existing hemoglobin may be saturated with oxygen. The oximeter device may have difficulty detecting a signal if the child's pulses are weak. The nurse should notify an on-call provider immediately of these findings, because the patient's status is critical (see Chapter 6 for more information about recognition and treatment of shock).

Digested blood has a specific odor that may be noted on the patient's breath even before the onset of melena or the first expulsion of hematemesis. This odor is qualitatively the same as that of melena, but it is usually fainter. To detect early evidence of GI bleeding, all GI fluids and stools of patients at risk should be tested for the presence of blood (hemoprotein). The presence of occult blood in gastric fluid may be determined with point-of-care (bedside) testing such as the use of Gastroccult (Beckman Coulter, Brea, CA).

During the first days of life, the Apt test (named for Leonard Apt) may be performed to distinguish between swallowed maternal blood and GI bleeding as a cause of blood in the newborn's stool.[4] The Apt test is performed by placing blood from the neonate on filter paper with 1% sodium hydroxide (a reagent that reacts with fetal hemoglobin).[4] Maternal blood will appear rusty brown, whereas the neonate's blood that contains fetal hemoglobin will remain pink or red.[4] The pink or red color is a positive result, indicative of presence of blood from the neonate.

Management

The three phases of management of the child with GI bleeding are resuscitation, specific diagnosis, and specific treatment. A diagnostic algorithm for upper GI bleeding is presented in Fig. 14-9.

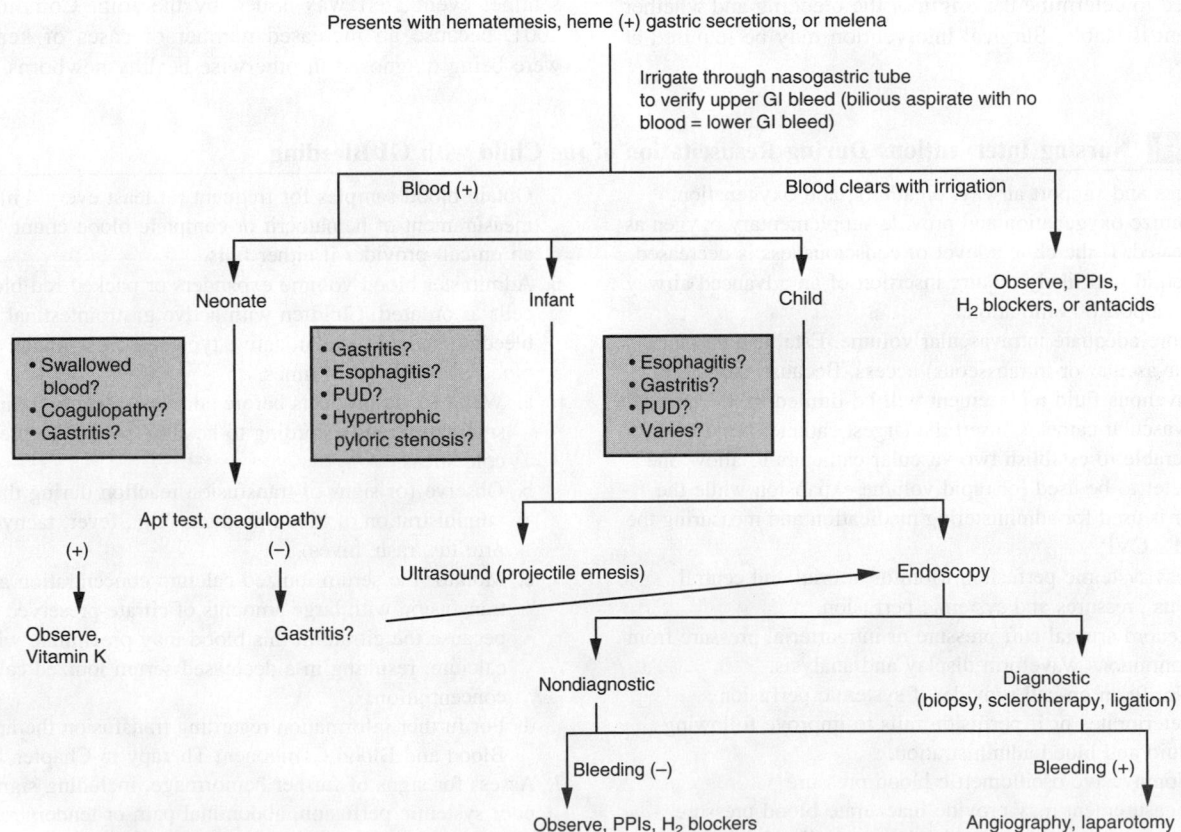

FIG. 14-9 Diagnostic algorithm for upper gastrointestinal (GI) hemorrhage. *PPI,* Proton pump inhibitor; *PUD,* peptic ulcer disease. (From Arensman RM, Browne M, Madonna MB: Gastrointestinal bleeding. In Grosfeld JL, O'Neill JA, Coran AG, Fonkalsrud EW, editors: *Pediatric surgery,* ed 6, Philadelphia, 2006, Mosby.)

During resuscitation and replacement of intravascular volume, nursing observations may help to determine the source of the child's bleeding. If saline lavage through a nasogastric tube reveals grossly bloody or red-tinged aspirate, ongoing upper intestinal bleeding is present. Nursing interventions during resuscitation of the child with GI bleeding are summarized in Box 14-1.

Proton pump inhibitors and histamine-2 receptor antagonists are the most commonly used pharmacologic agents to prevent the development of GI bleeding (Table 14-8). Although only a small number of critically ill children will develop gastric bleeding, the associated morbidity justifies the common practice of prophylaxis.

Upper GI endoscopy is indicated when bleeding is significant. It can be performed in the critical care unit and is the diagnostic procedure of choice. Push endoscopy is one method, and newer diagnostic tools include video capsule endoscopy. For diagnosis of small bowel bleeding, video capsule endoscopy can be a valuable diagnostic tool. A minute endoscope is embedded in a capsule that is swallowed. The capsule is propelled by peristalsis and captures images that are recorded on a hard drive attached to the patient's belt.

Indications for urgent surgical intervention include the development of intestinal perforation (identified by the presence of free air on an abdominal radiograph) or severe hemorrhage unresponsive to blood replacement therapy. If GI bleeding is stopped effectively with medical management and after resuscitation is complete, further studies will be performed to determine the origin of the bleeding and whether the patient is stable. Surgical intervention may be required at that time.

Hyperbilirubinemia
Etiology
Bilirubin is the major byproduct of hemoglobin breakdown. Hyperbilirubinemia is an elevation in the level of total serum bilirubin (TSB); it results from an imbalance between bilirubin production and excretion. An increase in bilirubin production can result from increased red blood cell (RBC) breakdown (such as hemolysis or decreased RBC life span in the neonate), or impaired bilirubin excretion (such as decreased capacity for elimination in the neonate or cholestatic liver disease). This section addresses hyperbilirubinemia in the neonate; hyperbilirubinemia in the older child is included in the liver failure section.

When the neonate's TSB is elevated, the bilirubin can cross the blood-brain barrier, causing acute bilirubin encephalopathy or the chronic form of bilirubin encephalopathy, kernicterus. Kernicterus is a yellow staining and brain tissue damage with degenerative lesions, resulting from central nervous system exposure to high concentrations of unconjugated bilirubin. Hyperbilirubinemia is commonly associated with prematurity, breast feeding, and other factors summarized in Box 14-2.

In the first week of life, it is estimated that approximately 60% of normal newborns will become clinically jaundiced.[42] Newborns are now discharged from the hospital at approximately 24 to 48 hours after birth, before the typical TSB peak at 48 to 96 hours. As a result, hyperbilirubinemia is the most common reason for hospital readmission of the neonate. A sentinel event alert was issued by the Joint Commission in 2001, because an increased number of cases of kernicterus were being diagnosed in otherwise healthy newborns.

Box 14-1   **Nursing Interventions During Resuscitation of the Child with GI Bleeding**

1. Assess and support airway, breathing, and oxygenation. Optimize oxygenation and provide supplementary oxygen as indicated. If the child's level of consciousness is decreased, the child will likely require insertion of an advanced airway and support of ventilation.
2. Restore adequate intravascular volume. Establish vascular (intravascular or intraosseous) access. Because the rate of intravenous fluid replacement will be limited by the size of the vascular catheter, insert the largest catheter possible. It is preferable to establish two vascular catheters to allow one catheter to be used for rapid volume expansion while the other is used for administering medication and measuring the child's CVP.
3. Assess systemic perfusion. Monitor arterial and central venous pressures and systemic perfusion.
   a. Record arterial cuff pressure or intraarterial pressure from continuous waveform display and analysis.
   b. Notify an on-call provider if systemic perfusion deteriorates or if perfusion fails to improve following fluid and blood administration.
   c. Noninvasive oscillometric blood pressure measurement may provide inaccurate blood pressure values if the child is in shock, especially if the child is hypotensive.
4. Insert a urinary catheter to monitor urine output.
5. Obtain blood samples for frequent (at least every 4 h) measurement of hematocrit or complete blood count; notify an on-call provider if either falls.
6. Administer blood volume expanders or packed red blood cells as ordered. Children with active gastrointestinal bleeding should have an active type and cross match with blood available at all times.
   a. Warm blood products before administration to infants and small children (according to hospital policy) to prevent cold stress.
   b. Observe for signs of transfusion reaction during the administration of blood products (e.g., fever, tachycardia, pruritus, rash, hives).
   c. Monitor the serum ionized calcium concentration after transfusion with large amounts of citrate-preserved blood, because the citrate in this blood may precipitate with calcium, resulting in a decreased serum ionized calcium concentration.
   d. For further information regarding transfusion therapy, see Blood and Blood Component Therapy in Chapter 15.
7. Assess for signs of further hemorrhage, including signs of poor systemic perfusion, abdominal pain or tenderness, changes in bowel sounds, hematemesis, or hematochezia.
8. Administer antibleeding pharmacologic agents as prescribed. See Table 14-8 for specific drug information.

Table 14-8 Drugs Used for Prophylaxis and Treatment of Gastrointestinal Bleeding

Drug	Indications for Use	Dose	Side Effects	Nursing Implications
Histamine Type 2 Receptor Antagonist, Decreases Gastric Acid Secretion				
Ranitidine (Zantac)	Treatment of ulcers, GERD, and hypersecretory states, GI tract prophylaxis	Premature and term infants <2 weeks old: 1.5 mg/kg as a loading dose, then 12 hours later 1.5-2 mg/kg per day divided every 12 hours Children ≥1 month to 16 years: 2-4 mg/kg per day divided every 6-8 hours (maximum dose 200 mg/day) Children ≥ 16 years: 50 mg every 6-8 hours	Bradycardia, tachycardia, dizziness, sedation, constipation, nausea, vomiting, thrombocytopenia, elevated serum creatinine	Dose reduction recommended for children with renal impairment Rapid IV administration has been associated with bradycardia
Cimetidine (Tagamet)	Treatment of ulcers, GERD, and hypersecretory states, GI tract prophylaxis	Neonates: 5-10 mg/kg per day in divided doses every 8-12 hours Infants: 10-20 mg/kg per day in divided doses, given every 6-12 hours Children: 20-40 mg/kg per day in divided doses every 6 hours	Bradycardia, hypotension, dizziness, mental confusion, rash, mild diarrhea, nausea, vomiting, neutropenia, elevated ALT, AST, and serum creatinine	Dose reduction recommended for children with renal impairment Use with caution for children with hepatic impairment Rapid IV administration may cause hypotension or cardiac arrhythmias
Famotidine (Pepcid)	Treatment of ulcers, GERD, and hypersecretory states, GI tract prophylaxis	Children 1-12 years old: 1 mg/kg per day divided every 12 hours Children >12 years old: 20 mg every 12 hours	Bradycardia, tachycardia, headache, vertigo, acne, thrombocytopenia, weakness, ototoxicity, elevated BUN and creatinine	Dose reductions recommended in children with renal impairment
Proton Pump Inhibitor, Direct Inhibitor of Hydrochloric Acid Secretion at the Cellular Level				
Pantoprazole (Protonix)	More direct inhibition of acid as compared to other PPIs, GERD, hypersecretory conditions, adjunct to duodenal/peptic ulcer disease, GI tract prophylaxis	Oral: 0.5-1.5 mg/kg per day (limited data) IV: 1-2 mg/kg (limited data)	Chest pain, tachycardia, headache, dizziness, urticaria, hyperglycemia, diarrhea, nausea, thrombocytopenia, ear pain, hematuria, anaphylaxis (IV form)	Long term treatment (>3 years) may lead to malaabsorption of vitamin B_{12} IV therapy should be discontinued as soon as oral therapy is tolerated
Omeprazole (Prilosec)	Severe erosive esophagitis, GERD, peptic ulcer disease	Only oral available Children 1-16 years old: Weight 5-10 kg: 5 mg once daily Weight 10 to ≤20 kg: 10 mg daily Weight >20 kg: 20 mg daily	Chest pain, tachycardia, headache, dizziness, rash, diarrhea, nausea, abdominal pain, agranulocytosis, tinnitus, hematuria, hypersensitivity reactions	Manufacturer recommends mixing capsule in acidic juice (apple or cranberry) for NG administration
Lansoprazole (Prevacid)	Erosive esophagitis, hypersecretory conditions, ulcer disease, GERD, GI tract prophylaxis	Only oral preparation available Infants 3-7 months old: 7.5 mg *bid* or 15 mg once daily Children 1-11 years old: <30 kg: 15 mg once daily for up to 12 weeks Children ≥12 years: 15 mg once daily for ulcer prophylaxis	Diarrhea, angina, hypertension, fatigue, dizziness, rash, hyperglycemia, abdominal pain, agranulocytosis, elevated AST and ALT, tinnitus, proteinuria, hypersensitivity reaction	Dose reduction for severe hepatic impairment; long-term effects not known

Continued

Table 14-8 Drugs Used for Prophylaxis and Treatment of Gastrointestinal Bleeding—cont'd

Drug	Indications for Use	Dose	Side Effects	Nursing Implications
Antacids, Neutralizing Agents with Potency Based on Acid-Neutralizing Capacity				
Maalox, Mylanta	Treatment of peptic ulcer disease, relief of ulcer pain, GI tract prophylaxis	Prophylaxis against GI bleeding Neonates: 1 mL/kg every 4 hours Infants: 2-5 mL/kg every 1-2 hours, titrate dose to keep gastric pH >3.5 Children: 5-15 mL every 1-2 hours, titrate to keep gastric pH >3.5	For magnesium-containing products, diarrhea, hypermagnesemia, and renal insufficiency; for aluminum-containing products, constipation and hypophosphatemia	
Cryoprotective Agents and Toxic Substance Binders, Paste Forms Adhere to Ulcer/Damaged Mucosa				
Sucralfate (Carafate)	Gastric protectant, ulcer treatment	Only oral available Children, dosing not well established; doses of 40-80 mg/kg per day divided every 6 hours have been used	Facial edema, dizziness, sleepiness, rash, constipation, diarrhea, laryngospasm	Administration may alter the absorption of other drugs for up to 2 hours, avoid administration of other enteral medications if possible
Antibleeding Agents				
Vasopressin (Pitressin)	Short acting vasoconstrictor, decreases splanchnic blood flow and portal hypertension, GI hemorrhage	IV continuous infusion, 0.002-0.005 units/kg per minute; maximum dose, 0.01 unit/kg per minute	Circumoral pallor, hypertension, vertigo, fever, water intoxication, abdominal cramps, wheezing, diaphoresis	IV infiltration may lead to localized tissue necrosis Abrupt discontinuation may result in hypotension
Somatostantin analog– Octreotide acetate (Sandostatin)	Decreases splenic blood flow, inhibits gastric acid output GI hemorrhage, intractable diarrhea	Children, 1 mcg/kg bolus, followed by infusion of 1 mcg/kg per hour, taper dose by 50% when no active bleeding; can discontinue when 25% of initial dose	Flushing, edema, chest pain, dizziness, erythema, hepatitis, jaundice, oliguria, shortness of breath	Patients must be monitored for glucose tolerance Dose modification for patients in renal failure

Note: Many of these drugs may affect absorption or levels of other drugs, so check with pharmacist regarding drug interference.
Data from Taketomo CK, Hodding JH, Kraus DM: *Pediatric dosage handbook*, ed 16, Hudson, OH, 2009, Lexi-Comp. Consistent with doses in Custer JW, Rau RE: Formulary. In *The Harriet Lane Handbook*, ed 18, Philadelphia, 2009, Mosby-Elsevier.
ALT, Alanine aminotransferase; *AST*, aspartate aminotransferase; *bid*, twice per day; *BUN*, blood urea nitrogen; *GERD*, gastric esophageal reflux disease; *IV*, intravenous; *NG*, nasogastric; *PPI*, proton pump inhibitor.

Pathophysiology

When RBCs reach the end of their 120-day life span, they normally are sequestered in the spleen. The cells are destroyed, and the heme portion of the hemoglobin molecule is oxidized, and bilirubin is formed. Bilirubin is bound to albumin in the plasma and taken up in the liver, where it is combined with a sugar through the action of the enzyme, bilirubin uridine diphosphate glucuronosyltransferase, making conjugated bilirubin.[11] Conjugated bilirubin is water soluble, it cannot cross the blood-brain barrier, and it is normally excreted in bile (Fig. 14-10). Free bilirubin, called *unconjugated* (indirect) *bilirubin,* is lipid soluble and not water soluble. Because unconjugated bilirubin is thought to diffuse freely into the brain, high concentrations of this form of bilirubin may be neurotoxic and cause kernicterus.

Increased TSB concentrations can result from an elevation in conjugated or unconjugated bilirubin. An elevation in the level of conjugated bilirubin is known as *direct hyperbilirubinemia*. It most commonly results from biliary tree obstruction or liver disease, although it also may occur with metabolic disorders, sepsis, meningitis, or drug reactions.

Elevation of unconjugated bilirubin levels is known as *indirect hyperbilirubinemia*. It most commonly occurs as a result of excessive bilirubin production in the neonatal period. Premature and critically ill neonates bind bilirubin less effectively than do healthy infants, so indirect hyperbilirubinemia is common among premature neonates. In addition, it can result from impaired transport of bilirubin caused by hypoxia, acidosis or the administration of albumin-binding drugs that displace bilirubin from the albumin. Impaired hepatic uptake of bilirubin also may cause indirect hyperbilirubinemia.

Box 14-2	Risk Factors for Hyperbilirubinemia in the Neonate

Factors That Increase Risk

- Jaundice in first 24 h (usually related to hemolysis)
- Visible jaundice before hospital discharge or TSB or TcB level in the high-risk zone
- Hemolytic disease: blood group incompatibility, Rh incompatibility, glucose-6-phosphate dehydrogenase deficiency
- Pyruvate kinase deficiency
- Prematurity (less than 35 weeks' gestation)
- Cephalohematoma or significant bruising
- Asphyxia
- Sibling previously received phototherapy (possible genetic cause)
- Breast feeding
- Ethnicity: East Asian, certain Native American tribes, and Greek ancestry
- Maternal age greater than 25 years
- Macrosomic infants of diabetic mothers
- Male

Other Genetic Causes

- Rotor's syndrome
- Dubin-Johnson syndrome
- Gilbert's disease
- Crigler-Najjar syndrome
- Hereditary spherocytosis

Factors That Decrease Risk

- African American
- Greater than 41 weeks' gestation

Data from American Academy of Pediatrics Subcommittee on Hyperbilirubinemia: Management of hyperbilirubinemia in the newborn infant 35 or more weeks of gestation, *Pediatrics* 114:297, 2004; Watson RL: Hyperbilirubinemia. *Crit Care Nurs Clin N Am* 21:97, 2009.
Rh, Rhesus (factor); *TcB,* transcutaneous bilirubin; *TSB,* total serum bilirubin.

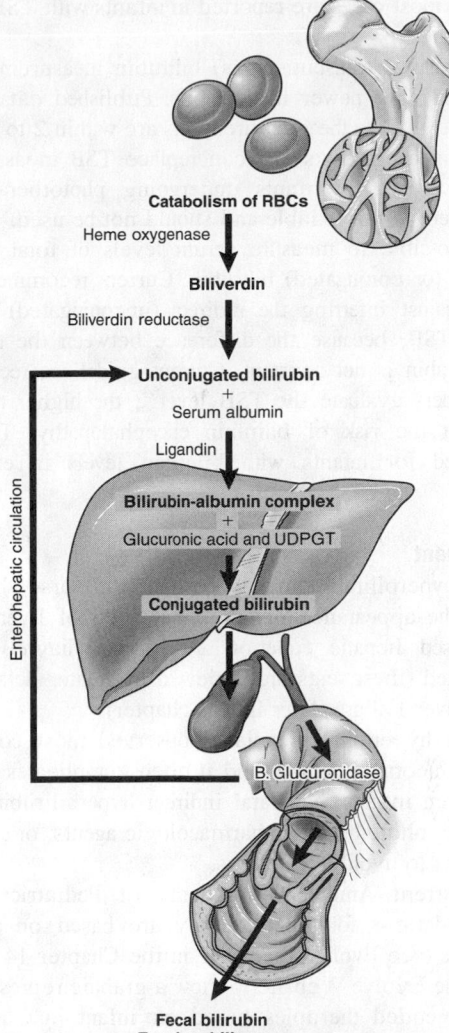

FIG. 14-10 The pathophysiology of neonatal hyperbilirubinemia. (From Colletti JE, et al: An emergency medicine approach to neonatal hyperbilirubinemia. *Emerg Med Clin N Am* 25:1117-1135, 2007.)

Kernicterus is yellow (bilirubin) staining of the basal ganglia in the brain of neonates with severe jaundice. Although the precise mechanisms responsible for the entry of bilirubin into the brain are not known, disruption of the blood brain barrier from increased permeability (e.g., caused by hyperosmolarity or severe asphyxia), prolonged transit time (e.g., caused by increased central venous pressure [CVP]), or increased blood flow (e.g., caused by hypercarbia and acidosis) are thought to be contributory.[63]

Jaundice (icterus) can usually be detected when the child's TSB level exceeds 3.0 to 5.0 mg/dL (normally it is less than 1.5 mg/dL). Jaundice is characterized by the accumulation of yellow pigment in the skin and other tissues. In the skin, the jaundice is apparent with digital blanching. Jaundice is usually evident first in the sclera and then progresses in a cephalocaudal distribution. The urine color may become brown as the result of the urinary excretion of conjugated bilirubin. In addition, the stools may become gray or acholic, indicating the absence of normal fecal elimination of bilirubin.

Clinical signs that the jaundice is pathologic include persistently elevated direct bilirubin level, dark urine, and acholic stools. Infants with these signs should be evaluated for liver disease.

The neurotoxic sequelae of hyperbilirubinemia are the most worrisome, and a grading for acute bilirubin encephalopathy has been proposed. The earliest signs may include alteration in the tone of extensor muscles (hypotonia or hypertonia), retrocollis (backward arching of the neck), opisthotonus (backward arching of the trunk), and a poor suck.[3] The early symptoms may intensify and be accompanied by a shrill cry and unexplained irritability alternating with lethargy.[3] Therapy at this stage may prevent advancement of symptoms. Cessation of feeding, irritability, seizures, and altered mental status are later symptoms of acute bilirubin encephalopathy. The final stage is kernicterus and may be irreversible with the development of cerebral palsy, deafness or hearing loss, and impairment of upward gaze. Kernicterus has a significant mortality (at least 10%) and long-term morbidity (at least

70%), and most cases are reported in infants with TSB greater than 20 mg/dL.[28]

Noninvasive (transcutaneous) bilirubin measurements can be obtained with newer instruments. Published data suggest that in most infants the measurements are within 2 to 3 mg/dL of serum measurements and can replace TSB measurements in most cases.[2] In infants undergoing phototherapy, this measurement is not reliable and should not be used.

It is possible to measure serum levels of total bilirubin and direct (or conjugated) bilirubin. Current recommendations caution against inferring the indirect (unconjugated) bilirubin from the TSB, because the difference between the total and direct bilirubin is not constant. Current guidelines recommend that providers evaluate the TSB level[63]; the higher the TSB, the greater the risk of bilirubin encephalopathy. Treatment is indicated for infants with bilirubin levels in excess of 20 mg/dL.

Management

If direct hyperbilirubinemia is present, the nurse should be alert for the appearance of additional signs of liver disease or decreased hepatic function. Additional diagnostic tests are indicated (these tests are reviewed in greater detail in the section, Liver Failure, later in this chapter).

Indirect hyperbilirubinemia is observed most commonly during the neonatal period, and it often complicates the care of premature infants. Neonatal indirect hyperbilirubinemia is treated with phototherapy, pharmacologic agents, or exchange transfusions to avoid kernicterus.

The current American Academy of Pediatrics (AAP) recommendations for phototherapy are based on age and TSB levels (see Evolve Fig. 14-1 in the Chapter 14 Supplement on the Evolve Website to view a graphic representation of recommended therapies based on infant age and total serum bilirubin concentration). Prophylactic phototherapy is often instituted for neonates weighing less than 1500 g. Although exclusive breast feeding can contribute to high TSB levels, the AAP recommends that breast feeding be continued with 10 to 12 feedings recommended per day, plus administration of supplementary intravenous fluid to treat dehydration.[2]

Phototherapy converts bilirubin to a water-soluble form that can be excreted without glucuronidation. Phototherapy units contain day lights, fluorescent tubes, fiberoptic light, and halogen bulbs. The effectiveness of phototherapy is determined by the type of light, the infant's distance to the light, and the amount of exposed body surface area. Light emitted at a wavelength in the blue-green spectrum of 425 to 495 nm is thought to be most effective because of the optical qualities of bilirubin and the skin. The AAP recommends the use of special blue fluorescent lamps or light-emitting diodes.[41,42]

The infant is unclothed while receiving phototherapy to expose maximum surface area. Remove the diaper if the TSB levels are approaching exchange transfusion level. Place protective eye shields over the infant's closed eyes, because the light can injure the retina. Exposure of body surface area may be enhanced in low-birth weight infants by placing a fiberoptic pad under the infant. Unless serum bilirubin levels are critically elevated, phototherapy should be interrupted briefly several times each day. During these interruptions the eye patches should be removed, and the infant (if condition allows) should be wrapped and held to provide comforting tactile and visual stimulation.

The infant's insensible water loss may be increased during phototherapy, so accurate measurement of fluid intake and output is required and weights should be recorded daily. Discuss evidence of excessive fluid loss or inadequate fluid intake with the responsible provider immediately. Neonates receiving phototherapy often develop diarrhea, which can contribute to fluid loss and nutritional compromise.

The infant receiving phototherapy should be turned frequently, and pressure points should be gently massaged. The phototherapy light must be turned off while blood specimens are obtained. If the blood specimens are exposed to light (especially phototherapy), then the bilirubin may be oxidized, thus altering the measured serum bilirubin levels in the blood samples and rendering them inaccurate.

Long-term sequelae of phototherapy are not known. Known complications include potential disruption of maternal infant bonding and possible eye injuries. Transient skin bronzing can occur in infants with cholestasis, although the cause of this bronzing is not clear.

The duration of phototherapy required is affected by the TSB level, the cause of the hyperbilirubinemia, and the infant's age. For infants readmitted for phototherapy during the first days of life, the treatment is usually discontinued when TSB levels reach 13 to 14 mg/dL. It is not uncommon for infants to experience a rebound increase in TSB level of 1 to 2 mg/dL when the therapy is discontinued.[41]

With the aggressive and early use of phototherapy and pharmacologic intervention, exchange transfusions are not often required. Exchange transfusions are most often used for infants with a hemolytic cause of hyperbilirubinemia. Exchange transfusion should be performed only in a pediatric or neonatal critical care unit with appropriate hemodynamic monitoring and resuscitation capabilities.

Pharmacologic options for treatment of hyperbilirubinemia include the administration of gamma globulin for hemolytic disease, possible use of tin-mesoporphyrin, and reduction of medications that bind albumin, if possible. For infants with isoimmune hemolytic disease, IV gamma globulin should be administered at a dose of 0.5 to 1 g/kg over 2 hours if TSB levels continue to rise despite phototherapy or if the TSB level is within 2 to 3 mg/dL of exchange transfusion levels.

There is some evidence to support administration of a drug that inhibits the production of heme oxygenase (the precursor to bilirubin development) to prevent hyperbilirubinemia. This drug is not yet approved by the U.S. Food and Drug Administration. Drugs that bind with serum albumin (ceftriaxone, sulfonamides, oxacillin, gentamicin, diazepam, furosemide, hydrocortisone, and digoxin) are avoided if possible, because they may displace serum bilirubin from albumin, thereby increasing the concentration of free bilirubin and the risk of bilirubin diffusion across the blood brain barrier.

Portal Hypertension

Etiology

Portal hypertension is an increase in portal venous pressure above 5 to 10 mmHg. It is caused by obstruction to the normal flow of blood through the portal venous system, the liver sinusoids, or the hepatic vein from the mesenteric vascular bed (small and large intestine, stomach, spleen, and pancreas).[61] It may be caused by (1) obstruction of the portal vein or its immediate tributaries (this is a form of extrahepatic or prehepatic portal hypertension), (2) an increase in vascular resistance within the liver that occurs secondary to fibrosis of the liver (this form is called *intrahepatic* or *hepatocellular portal hypertension*), or rarely (3) obstruction of hepatic venous outflow into the inferior vena cava (this is a form of suprahepatic or posthepatic portal hypertension).

Children can develop extrahepatic portal hypertension as a result of thrombosis of the portal vein. Most portal vein thrombosis is idiopathic in origin. It may also be congenital in origin, it may result from the use of umbilical venous catheters during the newborn period, or it may result from a hypercoagulable disease state.

Intrahepatic portal hypertension can complicate any form of chronic liver disease, including neonatal or childhood hepatitis, biliary atresia, congenital hepatic fibrosis, or liver disease secondary to infection or metabolic diseases (e.g., alpha1-antitrypsin deficiency). Suprahepatic portal hypertension may be caused by inferior vena cava (IVC) obstruction, hepatic vein occlusion, thrombosis from Budd-Chiari syndrome, or stenosis of the hepatic vein orifice.[61]

Pathophysiology

Portal venous blood flows into liver sinusoids. Because these sinusoids offer more resistance to blood flow than normal capillaries, pressure in the portal vein is normally higher than the CVP. If flow through the liver is obstructed, pressure in the portal vein and the splenic and mesenteric circulations may increase rapidly.

Anything that obstructs blood flow within the portal venous system, liver, or inferior vena cava can produce portal hypertension. Thrombosis of the portal vein will cause a significant rise in pressure in the portal vein proximal to the clot. Fibrosis of the liver compresses and distorts liver architecture and blood vessels; this will increase the resistance to blood flow through the liver and elevate portal venous pressure. Any obstruction to the flow of blood through the hepatic vein and into the IVC can increase sinusoidal pressure and distend the liver sinusoids with blood. If this obstruction is severe or chronic, resistance to the flow of blood into those sinusoids will increase and portal hypertension will result.

The three major physiologic complications of portal hypertension are: congestion of the splenic and mesenteric circulations, the development of collateral vessels, and sequestration of blood in the splanchnic circulation (the blood vessels from the gut and spleen that normally drain into the portal vein). When portal vein pressure increases, blood flow from the splanchnic circulation is impeded; this results in the pooling of blood in the splanchnic circulation. Because the splanchnic circulation consists of the mesenteric and splenic veins, splenic congestion and enlargement will result.

Hypersplenism and stasis of blood in the spleen cause damage to or sequestration of the formed elements of the blood, producing anemia, thrombocytopenia, and neutropenia. Engorgement of mesenteric vessels may cause mesenteric vein thrombosis or mesenteric infarction.

Impedance to portal blood flow and hypertension in the portal and splanchnic circulation promote the formation of collateral vessels between the systemic and portal circulations and the IVC, or other major central veins (Fig. 14-11). Major collateral vessels form from the portal vein, along the stomach and esophagus to the intercostal veins, in the paraumbilical veins (causing enlarged abdominal wall vessels), and around the rectum and anus (in the hemorrhoidal veins). Submucosal veins of the esophagus often enlarge and form collateral vessels between the portal venous system and vena cava. These enlarged veins often protrude into the esophagus and are known as *esophageal varices*.

Clinical Signs and Symptoms

Splenomegaly is often one of the first clinical signs of portal hypertension in children. Children with portal hypertension may also have ascites, markedly dilated superficial abdominal veins (caput medusae), and hypoalbuminemia.

If esophageal varices are present, sudden, severe esophageal and GI bleeding may occur without warning (see Gastrointestinal Bleeding, earlier in this chapter) with the onset of hematemesis, melena, or hematochezia. The bleeding from esophageal varices can be complicated by high variceal pressure and associated thrombocytopenia, so it may be particularly difficult to control.

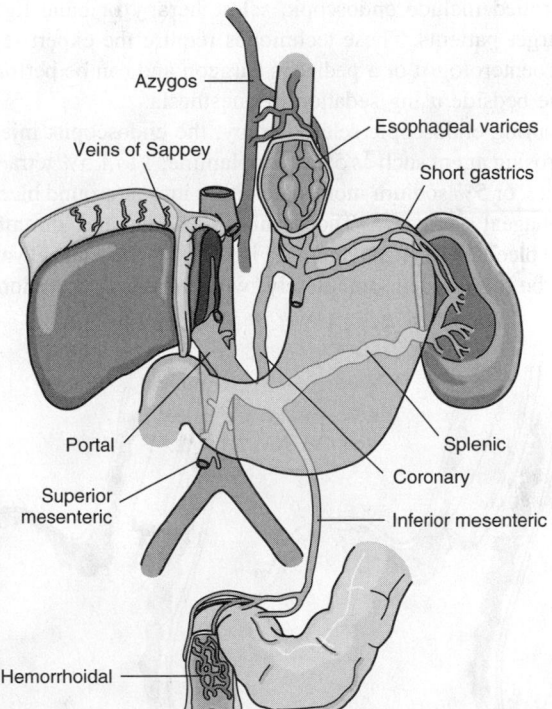

FIG. 14-11 Varices related to portal hypertension. Portal vein, its major tributaries, and the most important shunts (collateral veins) between the portal and caval systems. (From Monahan FD, Sands JK, Neighbors M, Marek JF, Green-Nigro CJ: Hepatic problems. In *Phipps' medical-surgical nursing: health and illness perspectives*, ed 8, St Louis, 2007, Mosby.)

The mortality rate for patients with bleeding esophageal varices was previously high; however, current treatment with vasopressin and somatostatin, correction of coagulopathy, endoscopic sclerotherapy and ligation (banding), and balloon tamponade (with a Sengstaken-Blakemore tube) are generally effective in controlling bleeding in children.[55] Balloon tamponade requires skilled personnel and is reserved for uncontrollable bleeding in larger patients.

The diagnosis of portal hypertension can be confirmed with ultrasound examination and assessment of the splenic or hepatic veins with vascular mapping. In some centers, computed tomography (CT) angiograms are performed to assess the existing vasculature. Liver function tests and a liver biopsy can be performed to determine the cause or extent of the primary disease in children with intrahepatic portal hypertension.

Management

Bleeding from esophageal varices is a life-threatening complication of portal hypertension. The goals of initial management are to maintain intravascular volume and systemic perfusion and to stop active bleeding (Box 14-3). For patients with portal hypertension from intrahepatic causes, there is a higher mortality when the initial bleeding episode is associated with liver dysfunction, malnutrition, and coagulopathy.

If bleeding from esophageal varices persists after correction of coagulopathies and volume resuscitation, a continuous IV infusion of vasopressin or somatostatin analog (octreotide acetate) can be initiated (see Table 14-8).

Alternative therapies for the treatment of bleeding esophageal varices that can be performed once acute bleeding is controlled include endoscopic sclerotherapy or band ligation in larger patients. These techniques require the expertise of a gastroenterologist or a pediatric surgeon and can be performed at the bedside using sedation or anesthesia.

During endoscopic sclerotherapy, the endoscopist injects a sclerosing agent such as 5% ethanolamine, 1 to 1.5% tetradecyl sulfate, or 5% sodium morrhuate either into or around bleeding esophageal varices.[55] The resulting edema and thrombosis stops bleeding in most patients (Fig. 14-12). Esophageal varices can be obliterated completely with repeated injections at

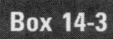

Box 14-3 | **Management of Hemorrhage Associated with Portal Hypertension**

Resuscitation
- Establish intravenous access and appropriate hemodynamic monitoring (e.g., arterial and central venous monitoring).
- Provide isotonic intravenous crystalloid boluses (20 mL/kg and repeat as needed) and blood (10 mL/kg as needed). Warm blood products before administration in infants and young children (or per hospital policy).
- Evaluate systemic perfusion frequently.
- Assess for signs of ongoing hemorrhage (abdominal pain, changes in bowel sounds, hematemesis, or hematochezia).
- Monitor fluid and electrolyte balance.

Diagnosis
- Assess color, location of bleeding.
- Monitor for indications that surgical intervention is required (free air observed on abdominal radiograph, severe hemorrhage unresponsive to blood replacement, or continuing hemodynamic instability). Endoscopy may be performed when the child is stable.

Treatment
- Saline lavage
- Vasopressin or somatostatin infusion
- Endoscopy with sclerotherapy or ligation
- Shunt procedure for patients as appropriate
- Transjugular portasystemic shunt in larger patients

From Lin PW, Stoll BJ: Necrotizing enterocolitis. *Lancet* 368:1271-1283, 2006.

2 to 4-week intervals, thus preventing recurrent episodes of bleeding. Potential complications of this technique include exacerbation of bleeding, esophageal stricture, and esophageal perforation.[43]

A pediatric Sengstaken-Blakemore tube (Fig. 14-13) can be inserted at the onset of the bleeding. Although this tube is usually effective in controlling bleeding, it is used infrequently because the complication rate is high. The tube must be inserted by skilled, experienced personnel, and the child typically requires arterial pressure monitoring and airway

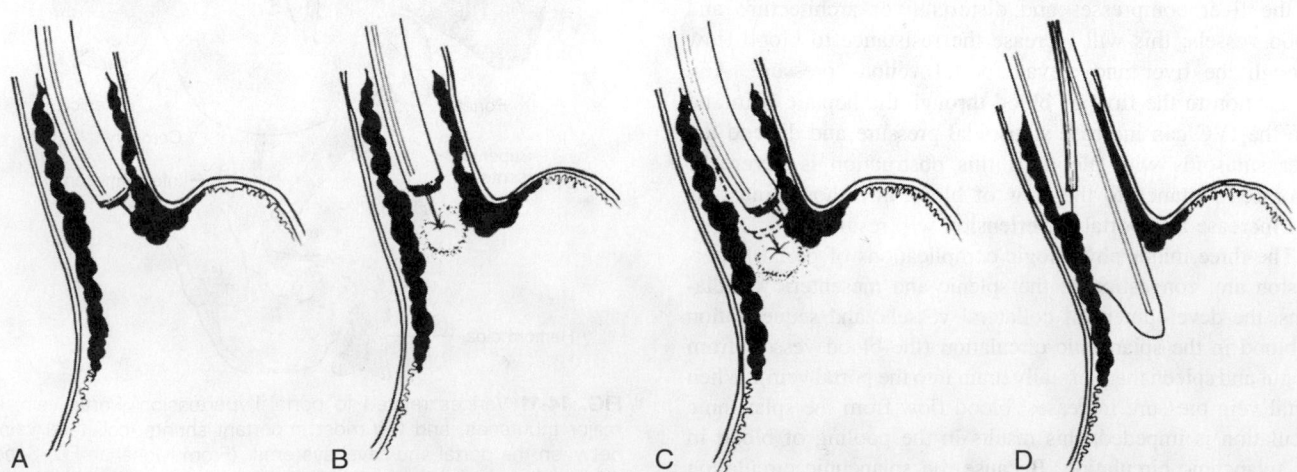

FIG. 14-12 Techniques of injection sclerotherapy. (From Terblanche J, Burroughs AK, Hobbs EKF. Controversies in the management of bleeding esophageal varices. *N Engl J Med* 320:1393-1398, 1989.)

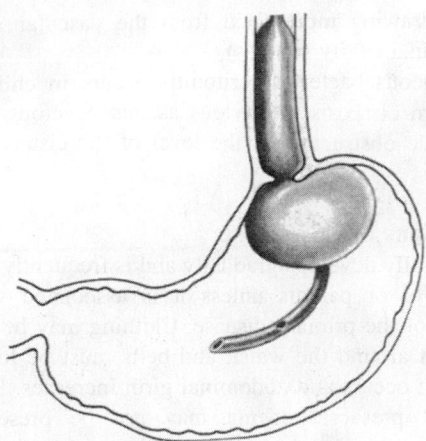

FIG. 14-13 Positioning of a Sengstaken-Blakemore tube. (From Given B, Simmons S: *Gastroenterology in clinical nursing,* ed 4, St Louis, 1984, Mosby.)

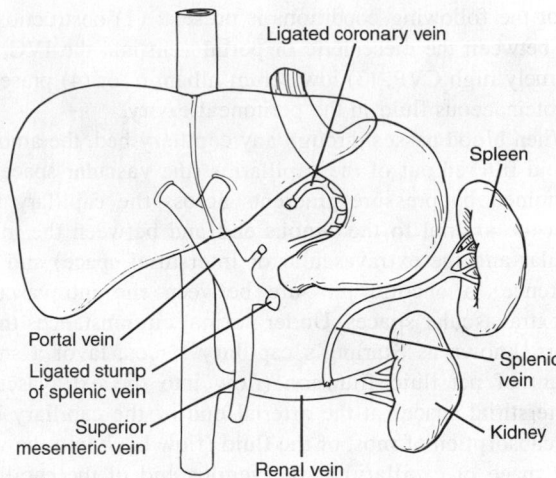

FIG. 14-14 Distal splenorenal shunt. The lesser sac is entered, and the splenic vein is dissected off the interior border of the pancreas, ligating and dividing small pancreatic branches. The left renal vein is then found and mobilized, preserving the gonadal and adrenal branches. The splenic vein is divided close to the confluence with the superior mesenteric artery (SMA) and anastomosed end to side with the left renal vein. The vein should lie in a smooth curve to avoid kinking. The coronary and gastroepiploic veins are ligated and divided. Blood flows from the gastric and esophageal varices via the short gastric veins, across the spleen, and into the splenic vein. The spleen is also decompressed in this fashion while portal flow to the liver is preserved. (From Superina R: Portal hypertension. In Grosfeld JL et al, editors: *Pediatric surgery,* ed 6, St Louis, 2006, Mosby).

control with endotracheal intubation. Complications include pulmonary aspiration, discomfort, and pressure necrosis of the distal esophagus. When a Sengstaken-Blakemore tube is used, bedside providers should constantly monitor the tube function, placement, and integrity. In many instances bleeding reoccurs after the tube is removed. See the Chapter 14 Supplement on the Evolve Website, Portal Hypertension, Management, for additional information on The Sengstaken-Blakemore Tube.

Surgery to decompress the hypertensive portal system may be necessary if life-threatening variceal bleeding recurs, although these procedures are most successful in children who are older than 10 years, when veins are of larger size. These procedures reduce the portal venous pressure by shunting portal blood flow directly into the IVC, bypassing the scarred liver or thrombosed portal vein.

The Rex shunt is an option for surgical correction of extra-hepatic portal vein obstruction. The word *Rex* refers to the anatomic name of the portion of the liver to which the blood is shunted. The Rex shunt uses an autologous vein, most commonly the left jugular vein; this vessel extends from the superior mesenteric vein to the left branch of the portal vein.[13] To prevent clotting of the shunt, heparin is initially provided. When oral intake is tolerated, anticoagulation therapy is transitioned to baby aspirin and dipyridamole (Persantine). The duration of this anticoagulation is variable, and is determined by the size of the child, the size of the graft, and the presence of any hypercoagulable conditions. For further information, readers are referred to websites about this procedure (e.g., http://www.childrens memorial.org/depts/siragusa/transplant-surgery/rex-shunt.aspx)

Additional shunting procedures include the splenorenal shunt and the mesocaval shunt. The most popular shunting procedure performed in children is the distal splenorenal shunt, which results in anastomosis of the splenic vein to the left renal vein (Fig. 14-14). An alternative procedure, the mesocaval shunt, is occasionally performed; it redirects blood from the obstructed mesenteric system to the patent intrahepatic system.

A potential postoperative complication of the shunting procedure is thrombosis of the anastomotic vessel and recurrence of the portal hypertension. The mesocaval shunt diverts some blood from the splanchnic circulation, reducing flow to the liver. As a result, the shunt may reduce liver detoxification of some circulating toxins, such as nitrogenous substances. The nurse must monitor for the development of hepatic encephalopathy (see discussion under Liver Failure later in this chapter).

Nursing interventions during acute episodes of GI bleeding secondary to portal hypertension are summarized earlier in this chapter (see Gastrointestinal Bleeding). Intervention for the treatment of ascites is presented in the following section.

Ascites

Etiology

Ascites is the accumulation of free fluid in the peritoneal cavity. It can result from diffuse inflammation of the peritoneal surface such as occurs with peritonitis, or it can be associated with increased portal capillary pressure resulting from cirrhosis, severe congestive heart failure, or other obstructive vascular conditions. Ascites may also be associated with diseases that result in sodium and water retention with decreased plasma colloid osmotic pressure (e.g., nephrotic syndrome). In children, significant ascites is caused most often by liver disease, severe congestive heart failure, infection, or nephrotic syndrome. Chylous ascites may occur in newborns and may be acquired in older infants and children.

Pathophysiology

Ascites results from the exudation of fluid from the surface of the liver, bowel, or peritoneum. This fluid enters the abdominal cavity instead of the mesenteric or portal venous system if any of the following conditions is present: (1) obstruction to flow between the mesenteric or portal vein and the IVC, (2) extremely high CVP, (3) low serum albumin, or (4) presence of proteinaceous fluid in the peritoneal cavity.

When blood passes through any capillary bed, the amount of fluid filtered out of the capillaries (the vascular space) is determined by pressure gradients across the capillary bed (from the arterial to the venous end and between the intravascular and the extravascular or interstitial space) and the difference in oncotic pressure between the intravascular and extravascular spaces. Under normal circumstances these factors, known as Starling's capillary forces, favor a small amount of net fluid filtration (flow into the extravascular or interstitial space) at the arterial end of the capillary bed and reabsorption of most of the fluid (flow back into the vascular space or capillary) at the venous end of the capillary bed. The slight tendency for fluid to filter out of the capillary as the result of capillary hydrostatic pressure is balanced almost exactly by the oncotic pressure normally exerted by plasma (intravascular) proteins, so that a near equilibrium exists between fluid filtration and reabsorption. A rise in venous hydrostatic pressure, an increase in extravascular (interstitial) oncotic pressure (e.g., caused by leak of protein from the vascular space), or a fall in intravascular oncotic pressure (hypoalbuminemia) can destroy the capillary equilibrium and produce a net loss of fluid from the vascular space to the extravascular space. This net loss of fluid to the extravascular space in the abdominal cavity results in ascites.

When hepatic and portal venous blood flow is obstructed, such as in cirrhosis of the liver, venous capillary and hepatic sinusoidal pressures rise. Initially the veins and sinusoids expand to accommodate larger quantities of blood. Eventually, however, as the capillary hydrostatic pressure rises, fluid begins to exude from the surface of the liver into the peritoneal cavity. Because liver sinusoids are far more permeable than normal capillaries, both fluids and proteins leak into the abdominal cavity. Once a sufficient quantity of proteins is present in the abdominal cavity, the extravascular colloid osmotic (oncotic) pressure rises, drawing more fluid from the vascular space into the abdominal cavity.

Congestive heart failure may produce ascites if the CVP rises sufficiently. Initially, hepatic venous and sinusoidal pressures rise, and the veins and sinusoids expand to accommodate a greater blood volume. This venous congestion causes one of the earliest signs of congestive heart failure in children—hepatomegaly (see Congestive Heart Failure in Chapter 8). If the CVP continues to rise, the liver's storage capacity for blood is exceeded, and fluids and proteins will exude into the abdominal cavity, creating ascites.

Children with nephrotic syndrome or hypoalbuminemia demonstrate a low plasma oncotic pressure. This low oncotic pressure enhances net fluid filtration from the vascular space, even if capillary pressure remains low. Hypoalbuminemia usually produces generalized edema, including ascites.

Peritoneal inflammation results in the formation of protein-rich ascitic fluid. The presence of this fluid in the peritoneal cavity creates an increase in extravascular colloid osmotic pressure, drawing more fluid from the vascular space into the abdominal cavity (ascites).

Spontaneous bacterial peritonitis occurs in children with ascites from cirrhosis.[35] Chylous ascites develops secondary to lymphatic obstruction at the level of the cisterna chyli or above.

Clinical Signs and Symptoms

Ascites usually develops gradually and is frequently unnoticed by the child or parents unless it is associated with other symptoms of the primary disease. Clothing may be perceived as too tight around the waist, and belts must be loosened as weight gain occurs and abdominal girth increases. Peripheral, ankle, and presacral edema may not be present unless hypoalbuminemia develops. If the ascites results from inferior vena caval, portal, or abdominal venous obstruction or a high CVP, superficial abdominal veins will be distended and visible on the surface of the abdomen (caput medusae).

The child's abdomen will be visibly distended. The abdominal girth should be measured every 4 hours, and more often if the patient's condition changes, to allow for monitoring of the severity of the ascites. The abdomen is generally dull to percussion, indicating the presence of fluid. Ascitic fluid will collect in dependent areas of the abdominal cavity, so the location of the area of dullness may change when the patient changes position; this is called *shifting dullness*.

If the child is cooperative and a second observer is present, it may be possible to elicit a fluid wave during palpation of the abdomen. The first observer places a hand firmly on the midline of the child's abdomen. The second observer places one hand along one side of the child's abdomen and, with the second hand, sharply taps the other side of the child's abdomen. If significant amounts of free peritoneal fluid are present, both observers feel a "wave" of fluid transmitted from one side of the abdomen to the other. The first observer's midline hand will rise when the fluid wave passes the midline.

Patients with ascites demonstrate a wide variety of fluid and electrolyte imbalances. Hypoalbuminemia may result from the primary disease or from a loss of protein into the ascitic fluid. Protein synthesis also is decreased if liver function is impaired. If the child has cirrhosis, antidiuretic hormone levels are elevated because the liver does not inactivate the antidiuretic hormone; this causes water retention and may produce a dilutional hyponatremia. In addition, aldosterone is not inactivated by the cirrhotic liver, so both water and sodium retention increase. Hypokalemia may result from aldosterone excess or from potassium loss caused by administered diuretics.

If significant fluid accumulates in the child's abdomen, it can impede diaphragm excursion. The child will demonstrate tachypnea with shallow breaths and may develop atelectasis. Providers should monitor for signs of respiratory distress, because assistance may be needed, using mechanical ventilation.

With the accumulation of large amounts of ascitic fluid, the child may develop a hydrothorax or accumulation of fluid in the thorax. This fluid most commonly enters the right chest, although bilateral hydrothoraces may develop. The child with a hydrothorax demonstrates dyspnea, increased respiratory effort (retractions and nasal flaring), and tachypnea. Breath sounds over the area of fluid usually are decreased, although the observer simply may note a change in the pitch of breath sounds caused by transmission of breath sounds from other areas of the chest through the pleural fluid.

If the ascites is secondary to liver, cardiovascular, or renal disease, then the child will exhibit signs of the primary disease and the ascites. For further information, see the appropriate sections in this chapter (e.g., Liver Failure), in Chapter 8 (Congestive Heart Failure) and in Chapter 13 (Acute Renal Failure).

The child with ascites may be extremely self-conscious about the abdominal distention. These children often complain of a sensation of "fullness" in the abdomen, and they may be anorexic. Nutritional weight loss may be masked by the weight gain produced by ascites.

Management

Ideally, healthcare providers should identify and treat the cause of the ascites before it is severe and produces respiratory compromise. Nurses should carefully measure fluid intake and output for any child at risk for the development of ascites. Weigh the child at the same time of day with the same scale and technique to detect small weight changes. Measure the child's abdominal girth frequently if ascites is developing or worsening.

Strict fluid and possibly sodium restriction are often required in the treatment of severe ascites. Administration of diuretics will necessitate close monitoring of fluid and electrolyte balance. The nurse must carefully monitor systemic perfusion during diuresis to prevent compromise in intravascular volume and systemic perfusion.

If a CVP catheter is placed in the child with an obstruction or compression of the IVC, it is important to know the location of the tip of the catheter in relation to the obstruction or compression. If the catheter tip is distal to the IVC obstruction or compression (e.g., catheter tip located in femoral vein in the child with severe ascites), the IVC pressure measured at that point will not reflect right atrial pressure. If possible, the tip of the catheter should be advanced beyond any area of obstruction (e.g., to the junction of the IVC and right atrium) if the central venous catheter pressure measurements are to be used to evaluate intravascular volume and cardiac preload.

If oral feedings are permitted, hard candy may be given to older children to assuage thirst and provide some glucose intake during periods of fluid restriction. An effort must be made to make meals palatable. Small, frequent feedings usually are better tolerated than infrequent, larger ones because gastric distention increases the sensation of abdominal fullness. If possible, allow the older child to plan disbursement of the restricted fluid intake during the day.

The child may develop lower lobe atelectasis from the pressure of abdominal fluid on the diaphragm and resultant shallow breathing. To prevent atelectasis, encourage the child to sit upright, rather than recline, and to remain as ambulatory as possible. Ambulation and use of incentive spirometry or bubbles may prevent atelectasis; chest physical therapy will be needed if pneumonia or atelectasis develops. If the child develops signs of respiratory distress, elevate the head of the bed to maximize diaphragm movement. Infants can be placed in an infant seat, and older children may prefer to sit at the side of the bed, leaning forward over a bedside table. Use pulse oximetry and titrate oxygen administration during episodes of respiratory distress.

Most cases of chylous ascites resolve without surgical intervention. The goal of treatment is to reduce lymphatic flow. For mild cases, reduce enteral fat intake with or without the use of medium chain triglyceride. Some patients require a period of no enteral intake and PN. In others, the addition of somatostatin will be effective. Palliative procedures to reduce fluid include decompression with paracentesis or placement of an intraabdominal drain and thoracentesis. After paracentesis, monitor the child closely for complications such as hypotension (large shifts of intravascular volume) and bacterial peritonitis.[35] Surgical decompression using a peritoneal-jugular shunt may necessary.

Bowel Obstruction

Etiology

Bowel obstruction can be mechanical or functional in origin, and it can occur anywhere along the length of the GI tract. Mechanical obstruction is a physical barrier that blocks the lumen of the GI tract, so that peristaltic contractions are unable to propel GI contents forward. Four main causes of mechanical bowel obstruction are: (1) congenital GI malformations (e.g., duodenal atresia, annular pancreas), (2) intraluminal obstruction (e.g., foreign body, stool, bezoars [masses of organic or inorganic material—often swallowed material—trapped in the gastrointestinal system]), (3) intramural lesions within the bowel wall (e.g., tumors, Crohn's disease, webs), and (4) extramural causes (e.g., bowel adhesions, hernias, intestinal volvulus).[32]

A functional obstruction, also called an *ileus,* occurs when the motor function or peristalsis of the GI tract is impaired, creating a stasis of bowel contents. Functional obstruction can develop after abdominal surgery (i.e., postoperative ileus) but can be related to sepsis, medications (e.g., opioids), trauma, head injury, pneumonia, and metabolic imbalances.

Clinical Signs and Symptoms

Clinical signs and symptoms vary depending on the location of the obstruction, the type of obstruction (mechanical or functional), and whether the obstruction is complete or partial. Presentation can be acute with signs of peritonitis (e.g., volvulus) or subtle and chronic with incomplete or recurring bouts of obstruction (e.g., intussusception).

When obstruction develops, bowel proximal to the obstruction becomes distended by a collection of air and fluids. Distal bowel collapses from a lack of intraluminal content. Proximal obstructions create a relatively larger amount of bowel collapse, and physical findings can include a scaphoid or sunken abdomen.

An obstruction in the lower GI tract will result in more bowel distention and, consequently, more abdominal distension. Clinical findings include a rounded, distended, and tympanic abdomen with bowel loops that may be visible and palpable. If the bowel obstruction is mechanical, bowel sounds will be present and often are high pitched and tinkling in character, because the peristaltic waves continue to propel contents against the obstruction. Pain is initially mild, but increases in severity and often corresponds with peristalsis.

Functional obstructions are referred to as *the silent abdomen,* because there is lack of peristaltic activity. Pain associated with a functional obstruction is constant and increases in intensity as the bowel becomes further dilated. In cases of obstruction associated with compromised intestinal perfusion such as volvulus, pain results from ischemia and is continuous with escalating intensity.

Obstructions may be complete or partial and intermittent. Complete obstruction stops all progression of bowel contents, but patients will evacuate distal contents before all output ceases. Many patients with complete obstruction will develop bowel ischemia.[46] Patients with partial or intermittent obstructions will pass some air and liquid stool (diarrhea and flatus).

Vomiting is a common symptom of both mechanical and functional bowel obstruction. The character and frequency of vomiting may provide clues to the location of the obstruction. Higher obstructions result in more rapid onset and more frequent episodes of vomiting. With lower obstructions there is more space to accommodate the accumulation of air and fluid, so there is typically a longer time before the onset of vomiting. Vomiting is typically a late sign of a lower obstruction and is preceded by bowel and abdominal distension.

Emesis typically is described as nonbilious (yellow) or bilious (green) in color. Vomiting associated with obstruction proximal to the sphincter of Oddi will more likely be nonbilious, because the expelled fluids have not yet mixed with bile excreted at the sphincter. Bilious emesis usually represents an obstruction occurring beyond the sphincter of Oddi and is regarded as a hallmark sign of a probable surgical emergency that requires rapid investigation and treatment.

Abdominal plain radiographs are the first choice for diagnostic imaging when bowel obstruction is suspected. The normal bowel gas pattern includes a paucity of air in the small bowel, but air is normally visible in the colon and rectum (Fig. 14-15, A). With obstruction, bowel proximal to the obstruction dilates as air and fluid accumulate, causing air fluid levels that are visible in the abdominal plain radiographs (Fig. 14-15, B). The colon and rectum have little or no air, so they may not be visible. The more distal the obstruction, the higher the visible air fluids levels (Fig. 14-15, C). With complete obstruction a paucity of air is visible distal to the obstruction and a cutoff point maybe evident. It is difficult to differentiate between large and small bowel obstruction on the basis of plain abdominal radiographs in infants.

Management

Mechanical obstruction is more likely to require surgical intervention. Functional obstruction is often managed with supportive measures such as bowel rest, nasogastric tube decompression, and pharmacologic interventions (e.g., neostigmine, metoclopramide, naloxone, erythromycin).

Placement of a nasogastric or orogastric tube can create a route for bowel decompression, although recent data calls into question the need for nasogastric decompression in all patients with obstruction. If a tube is inserted, low intermittent suction is often used to remove pooled fluid and air and reduce distension. To maintain fluid balance, the child will likely require additional intravascular fluids (typically isotonic crystalloids) to replace those lost through GI suction.

Bowel obstruction is often associated with dehydration caused by a lack of oral fluid intake and recurrent vomiting. Vomiting expels both fluids and electrolytes, contributing to dehydration and electrolyte imbalance. Distention reduces the ability of the bowel to reabsorb water and electrolytes, further increasing fluid and electrolyte losses. Alkalosis with low chloride and elevated serum bicarbonate is commonly observed with a high obstruction, such as pyloric stenosis.

Abdominal distension can produce respiratory compromise. Increasing intraabdominal pressure compromises diaphragm excursion and can contribute to respiratory distress. Raising the head of the bed can help to maximize diaphragm excursion, decrease the work of breathing, and improve oxygenation and ventilation.

Surgery is often required for the management of bowel obstruction and may be required on an emergent basis to avoid loss of bowel. Emergent surgery is indicated in the setting of complete obstruction (e.g., midgut volvulus, unsuccessful reduction of intussusception, incarcerated hernia) or when the patient demonstrates signs of bowel ischemia and peritonitis. Patients without clinical signs of septic shock, peritonitis, or bowel ischemia can be treated safely with nasogastric decompression and fluid resuscitation before surgical intervention. Partial obstructions can be treated initially with decompression that may resolve the obstruction.[46]

CARE OF THE CHILD AFTER ABDOMINAL SURGERY

Preoperative electrolyte imbalance, dehydration, sepsis, and malnutrition can complicate both perioperative and postoperative care of the child requiring abdominal surgery. These conditions are often exacerbated by general anesthesia and surgical manipulation. It is important to correct electrolyte imbalances and hypovolemia and, when necessary and possible, maximize nutritional status before administering general anesthesia.

Fluid Balance

Maintenance of the child's fluid and electrolyte balance can be challenging. Significant fluid shifts after abdominal surgery can result in the loss of intravascular fluids into nonfunctional compartments (third spacing). Treatment of third spacing includes fluid administration to maintain intravascular volume. As postoperative inflammation or infection decreases, the patient begins to rebound from the third-spacing phenomenon. As the tissues and injured areas heal, fluid in the nonfunctional compartments shifts back into the vascular space. This recovery phase is identified by an increasing diuresis with low urine specific gravity and osmolality.

Postoperative Ileus

Ileus is hypomotility of the GI tract in the absence of a mechanical bowel obstruction. This hypomotility or paralytic state creates a lack of coordinated propulsive action, so food and air do not move through the GI tract. The most common causes of ileus include abdominal surgery, peritonitis, and trauma. The consequences of an ileus are the accumulation

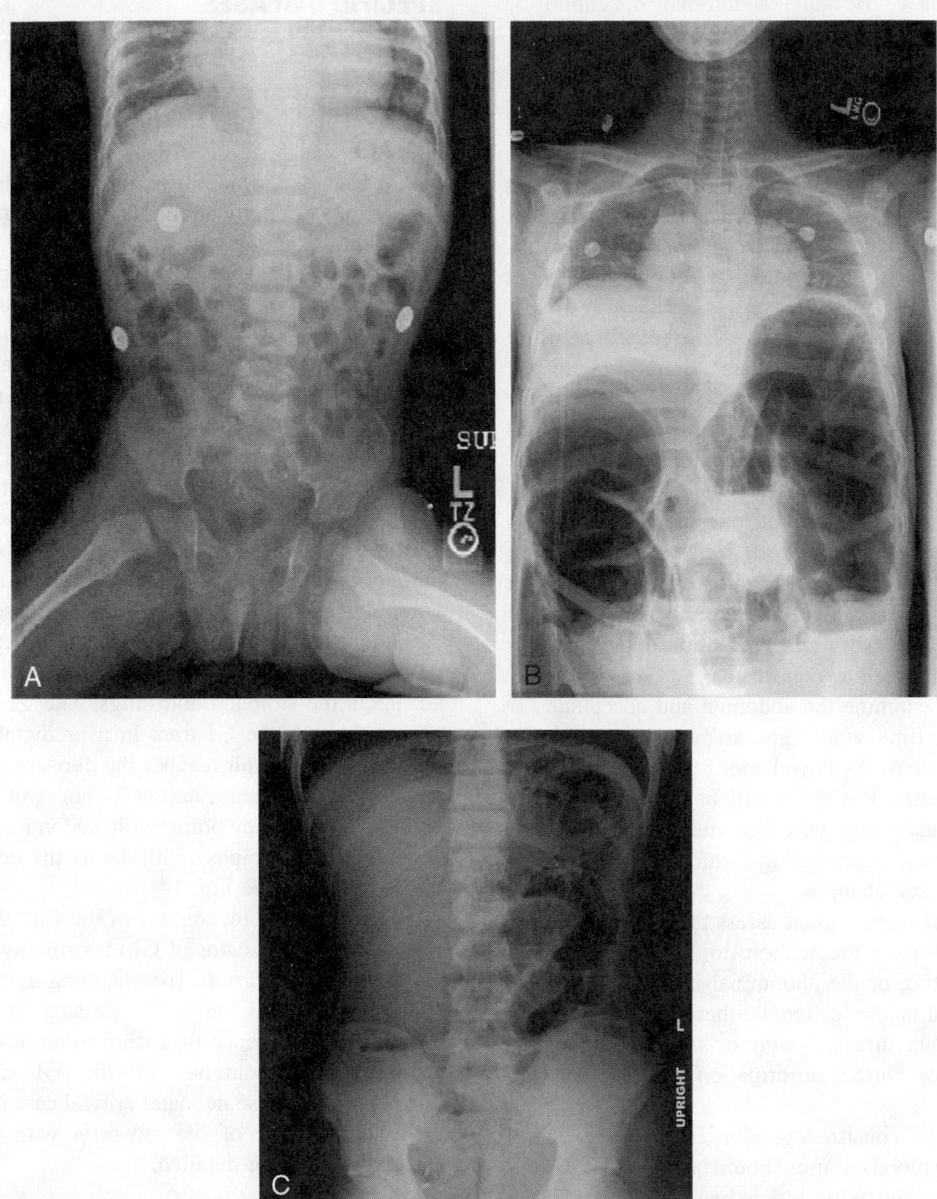

FIG. 14-15 A, Normal gas pattern. Typical caliber of bowel with air seen throughout the intestine, including the rectum. **B,** Bowel obstruction with severely dilated bowel and air fluid levels in the left lower quadrant. The bowel distension extends to below the diaphragm on the left side. **C,** Multiple air fluid levels are present with a paucity of air in the lower abdominal quadrants. This radiograph is consistent with bowel obstruction.

of both air and fluids within the bowel, causing distension. Clinical findings of an ileus include a distended, tympanic abdomen. Pain and discomfort increase as the bowel becomes more distended. Patients require analgesia and are hesitant to move. In addition to the abdominal signs, the compromised diaphragm function can cause increased work of breathing and risk of atelectasis and pneumonia.

Infection

The most common nonsurgical sites of postoperative infection and fever are the respiratory tract, urinary tract, and intravenous catheters. Fever during postoperative days 1 to 3 most likely has a noninfectious cause (e.g., atelectasis). When fever develops after postoperative day 5, the likelihood of an

infectious source (e.g., wound infection) rises. Blood and urine specimens should be sent for culture if a fever develops at this time. If pulmonary symptoms are present, a chest radiograph is obtained. All surgical wounds should be inspected for any signs of infection.

Management

Goals of postoperative nursing care of the child recovering from abdominal surgery include preventing respiratory complications, maintaining the child's fluid and electrolyte balance and nutrition, and preventing and detecting any infection.

During the immediate postoperative period, the nurse should assess and support respiratory function and prevent respiratory compromise. Because abdominal distention or ascites can compromise diaphragm excursion, and abdominal pain or discomfort can contribute further to inadequate ventilation, postoperative mechanical ventilation may be planned after major GI manipulation or resection. If the child is breathing spontaneously, the nurse should encourage the child to cough and breathe deeply. Spirometry and chest physical therapy may be ordered to prevent atelectasis, and adequate analgesia is needed. Early ambulation will supplement these efforts and will promote resumption of bowel function.

The nurse should carefully measure and record all fluid intake and output. Third spacing of fluids should be anticipated postoperatively, and the nurse should monitor for evidence of inadequate intravascular volume (hypovolemia) and poor systemic perfusion. Fluid administration is indicated if intravascular volume is inadequate.

A nasogastric tube can be inserted postoperatively to prevent abdominal distention, discomfort, and excessive tension on the suture line. The nurse should evaluate the total amount of nasogastric drainage every 4 to 8 hours. Typically, half of this fluid loss is replaced with an IV solution determined by the surgeon or other on-call provider.

The nurse should examine the abdomen and auscultate for bowel sounds every time vital signs are assessed. Initially, bowel sounds are absent. As bowel motility resumes, bowel sounds gradually return. The child will begin to pass flatus or stool, and the abdomen will become softer and less distended. Serial measurements of abdominal girth are often useful in infants to track changes.

Postoperatively the nurse should assess the child's pain and administer adequate pain medication to maintain comfort and to prevent splinting of the abdominal incision. Typically an intravenous opioid is administered either as an intermittent bolus or a continuous infusion with or without a patient-controlled mode. For further information about analgesia, see Chapter 5.

Monitor the amount, consistency, odor, and color of wound drainage. Wound and blood cultures should be ordered if wound drainage becomes purulent or the patient becomes febrile. If the wound becomes inflamed, it can be excised and drained.

Peritonitis or GI bleeding can complicate the care of children with preoperative ascites and cirrhosis (see Ascites, Portal Hypertension, and Liver Failure in this chapter). Throughout the child's care, the nurse should monitor the child closely for evidence of abdominal pain or tenderness and check all nasogastric drainage and stools for the presence of blood. Intravenous antibiotics are indicated when peritonitis is present. Broad-spectrum antimicrobials are often ordered initially until specific infecting organisms are identified.

The nurse should carefully explain all procedures and treatments to the child and family and should give the child the opportunity to discuss questions and concerns about therapy. Surgical incisions can be frightening and threatening to the child's body image and sense of body integrity, so the child may require reassurance that the incisions will heal. If the child's condition allows, therapeutic play can offer the child the opportunity to express fears or frustration about the surgery.

SPECIFIC DISEASES

Congenital Gastrointestinal Abnormalities

The most important aspects of the management of congenital GI anomalies are prenatal or early diagnosis, a birth plan to allow for transfer to a tertiary care center, surgical intervention, early enteral feeding, and prevention or treatment of postoperative complications. With the frequent use of prenatal ultrasound examinations, most families are aware of the child's anomalies before birth. This knowledge allows for additional testing, including chromosomal analysis if the identified anomaly (e.g., omphalocele, duodenal obstruction) is associated with chromosomal abnormalities. If surgery is indicated, the parents can meet with a perinatologist, pediatric surgeon, and neonatologist to discuss the child's anticipated prognosis, delivery, and postnatal surgical plan.

One early sign of fetal upper GI obstruction is maternal polyhydramnios—the presence of excessive amniotic fluid during pregnancy. When fetal intestinal obstruction prevents the normal passage and absorption of amniotic fluid, the volume of maternal amniotic fluid increases.

Failure to pass air through the GI tract immediately after birth is an early sign of a GI anomaly. During the first breath, air enters the stomach and lungs. The gastric air normally is passed through the GI tract in a predictable sequence. With the second breath, air reaches the duodenum. At 6 hours of life air reaches the cecum, and at 24 hours of life air reaches the rectum. In most newborns with abdominal obstruction, plain abdominal radiographs (with air as the contrast) will outline the obstruction (see Fig. 14-15).

Failure to pass meconium in the first 24 hours of life is a strong clinical indicator of GI abnormality and is observed in children diagnosed with Hirschsprung disease or cystic fibrosis. Nurses should verify the passing of a meconium stool and report the absence of a stool to an on-call provider.

Congenital anomalies of the GI tract are listed in Table 14-9. Because neonatal critical care is not a focus of this text, nursing care of the newborn with these anomalies is highlighted but not detailed.

Necrotizing Enterocolitis

Etiology

NEC is an acquired disease of unknown origin that develops during the neonatal period. NEC typically occurs in premature low-birth weight newborns (<1500 g), but cases have been described in term babies.[60] Infants with NEC develop necrotic lesions in the GI tract, most commonly in the ileum and colon. The necrosis may be superficial and only detectable microscopically, or it may be transmural and involve both the small and large intestines. Mild disease may be completely reversible, but infants with extensive involvement may not survive or may be rendered as short gut with subsequent intestinal failure following surgical resection of the affected bowel.

A large number of epidemiologic factors have been associated with the development of NEC. The majority (more than 90%) of patients are premature neonates (less than 36 weeks' gestation), who have received enteral nutrition. Newborns with low-flow states, such as patent ductus arteriosus

Table 14-9 **Congenital Gastrointestinal Abnormalities**[39,51]

Disease	Etiology	Pathophysiology	Clinical Signs and Symptoms	Nursing Interventions
Congenital Gastrointestinal Anomalies Associated with Respiratory Distress				
Diaphragmatic hernia	Incomplete formation of diaphragm at week 10 of gestation; left side typically involved	Abnormal opening between abdomen and thorax allows stomach and intestines to enter left chest area; left lung fails to develop and is hypoplastic; heart is displaced to contralateral thorax, so development of right lung may also be compromised	Abdomen appears scaphoid; severe respiratory distress develops, including respiratory failure; heart sounds shifted; right-to-left shunt resulting from pulmonary hypertension	Insert tube to decompress stomach Provide skilled respiratory support; infant may require oscillatory ventilation or ECMO For further information, see Chapters 7 and 9 Monitor arterial blood gases; if evidence of right-to-left shunt, consider use of nitric oxide
Esophageal atresia with or without tracheoesophageal fistula	Abnormal separation of esophagus from the trachea (develops after day 24 of gestation) Associated with VACTERL anomalies	Upper segment of esophagus ends in blind pouch above bifurcation of trachea; fistula between trachea and esophagus may be present (additional fistula to stomach may be present) Multiple variations possible	Respiratory distress Dysphagia Excessive salivation Inability to pass NG tube Radiograph reveals tip of tube in upper mediastinum	Respiratory support IV fluids NPO Place tube in upper esophageal pouch and apply low intermittent suction to keep the pouch empty and reduce risk of aspiration Prone positioning will facilitate emptying of upper pouch Prepare for surgical correction or palliative procedure and possible gastrostomy tube insertion
Congenital Gastrointestinal Anomalies Associated with Obstructive or Bleeding Symptoms				
Malrotation with volvulus (80% of volvulus cases are symptomatic in first month of life)	Lack of rotation and retroperitoneal fixation of the intestines during week 10 of gestation	Malrotation obstructs the duodenum in varying degrees; compression of the superior mesenteric artery can result from severe and prolonged volvulus of the small intestine	Vomiting of bilious material after first 24-48 h of life, Characteristic blood and mucous stools Upper GI shows abnormal rotation of bowel with obstruction of the duodenum	IV fluids NPO Prepare for emergent surgery
Hirschsprung disease	Failure of innervation of GI tract at weeks 5-12 of gestation	Lack of innervation results in lack of peristalsis in the lower GI tract; fecal contents are not eliminated, internal sphincter fails to relax	Newborns: failure to pass meconium within 24-48 h after birth; may develop bilious vomiting and abdominal distention Child: chronic constipation; may develop enterocolitis Barium enema: normal caliber or narrow distal segment with dilation beyond aganglionic segment	Newborn: IV fluids, NG tube, prepare for surgery Child: Prepare for surgery

Continued

Table 14-9   Congenital Gastrointestinal Abnormalities—cont'd

Disease	Etiology	Pathophysiology	Clinical Signs and Symptoms	Nursing Interventions
Intestinal atresias (duodenal, jejunal, and ileal)	Absence of recanalization or vascular injury to the intestine at 8-10 weeks' gestation	Lack of patency of any segment of bowel caused by aborted development of or vascular injury to that area of bowel	*High obstruction* Radiograph: duodenal (double bubble), jejunal (few loops of dilated bowel) Bilious emesis *Low obstruction* Radiograph: obstructed pattern with dilated, air-filled bowel Abdominal distention, vomiting	Measure abdominal girth Note absence or presence of meconium or stools IV fluids NG tube Prepare for surgery
Imperforate anus	Abnormal partitioning between cloaca and urorectal septum at week 8 of gestation; may be part of the VACTERL syndrome	Single membrane covering anus or anal agenesis or atresia Fistula to genitourinary tract may be present	Usually diagnosed by physical examination; although anus absent, meconium may be visible from a mucocutaneous fistula	Low lesions: early repair High lesions: initial colostomy and then later posterior sagittal anorectoplasty

Congenital Gastrointestinal Anomalies Associated with Abdominal Wall

Disease	Etiology	Pathophysiology	Clinical Signs and Symptoms	Nursing Interventions
Omphalocele	Incomplete closure of abdominal wall with failure of GI tract to return to abdominal cavity by 10-11 weeks' gestation; high incidence of additional anomalies	Herniation of abdominal organs (including the intestine and liver) out of the abdomen Organs are covered by a protective sac with umbilical arteries and vein inserted into the apex of the defect; variable in size	Most infants are delivered by cesarean section to avoid rupture of the sac Usually no initial symptoms unless other anomalies present	Stabilize the airway NPO Insert NG tube and attach to low suction Provide IV fluids or PN Calculate caloric intake and discuss with provider if inadequate Maintain neutral thermal environment Keep sac covered with an antibiotic ointment and sterile dressing
Gastroschisis	Etiology not known; 50% of infants are born prematurely	Abdominal wall defect to the right of the umbilicus without a covering; herniation of the small and large intestine; may be associated with intestinal atresia	Temperature instability; dehydration from insensible fluid loss; protein loss; hypoglycemia from increased caloric expenditure; electrolyte disturbances	NPO Insert NG tube and provide low suction Provide IV fluids or PN Calculate caloric intake and discuss with provider if inadequate Maintain neutral thermal environment Keep sac covered with warm sterile saline sponges and cover with plastic bag or wrap or silastic silo Position bowel so that it will remain perfused, notify surgeon of discolorization or if kink suspected Prepare for primary surgical closure or staged reduction (silo is placed with daily manipulation to return the bowel to the abdominal cavity)

Table 14-9 **Congenital Gastrointestinal Abnormalities—cont'd**

Disease	Etiology	Pathophysiology	Clinical Signs and Symptoms	Nursing Interventions
GI Congenital Anomalies Presenting After the Neonatal Period				
Intussusception	Occurs in otherwise healthy children usually before 2 years of age (peak incidence is 5-12 months)	Slipping or telescoping of one intestinal segment into another; this compromises blood supply and intestinal patency (90% ileocolic)	Acute paroxysmal abdominal pain (infant draws knees to chest); vomiting that increases as condition worsens; stools become red (containing blood and mucous) Ultrasound is modality of choice for diagnosis; look for distinct mass in the shape of a donut or target	Provide appropriate IV replacement fluid and electrolytes as ordered Insert NG tube NPO Prepare for water-soluble contrast or air enema reduction Prepare for surgical correction if enema reduction unsuccessful
Meckel's diverticulum	Outpouching of the ileum containing ectopic mucosa	Ulceration of ectopic gastric mucosa leads to painless lower GI bleeding (sometimes large amount)	Bright red or dark red painless rectal bleeding; may result in severe anemia and shock	Observation and treatment necessary for stabilization of hypovolemic shock (see Chapter 6) Prepare for surgical resection of the diverticulum

Data from Louis JP: Essential diagnosis of abdominal emergencies in the first year of life. *Emerg Med Clin North Am* 25:100-1040, 2007; Pierro A, Hall NJ, Chowhury MM: Gastrointestinal surgery in the neonate. *Curr Paedeatr* 16:153-164, 2006; King J, Askin DF: Gastroschisis: etiology, diagnosis, delivery options, and care. *Neonatal Netw* 22: 7-12, 2003.

ECMO, Extracorporeal membrane oxygenation; *GI,* gastrointestinal; *IV,* intravenous; *NG,* nasogastric; *NPO,* nothing by mouth; *PN,* parenteral nutrition; *VACTERL,* vertebral, anal, cardiac, tracheoesophageal, renal, limb anomalies.

or congenital heart disease (especially in infants with left ventricular outflow tract lesions), are at risk.[20,60] NEC can also develop following repair of gastroschisis. Further discussion of the etiology can be found in the Chapter 14 Supplement on the Evolve Website, Specific Diseases, Necrotizing Enterocolitis.

Pathophysiology

The pathophysiology of NEC is poorly understood but includes: intestinal ischemia, distension, colonization by pathogenic bacteria, subsequent bacterial translocation, and intestinal necrosis and perforation. The proposed inciting mechanisms are schematically presented in Fig. 14-16. The initiating injury in NEC is disruption of the intestinal mucosal epithelium; this disruption can result from a variety of mechanisms, most likely hypoxia or an infection. Most cases occur after the second week of life following bacterial colonization of the intestine.[25] See the Chapter 14 Supplement on the Evolve Website, Necrotizing Enterocolitis, for additional information about the role of enteral feeding in the development of NEC.

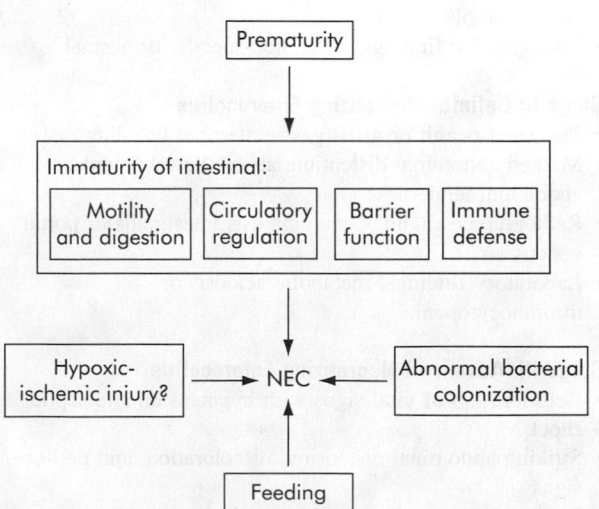

FIG. 14-16 Pathophysiology of necrotizing enterocolitis. (From Lin PW, Stoll BJ: Necrotizing enterocolitis. *Lancet* 368:1271-1283, 2006.)

Pneumatosis intestinalis, a radiologic hallmark of well-established NEC, is the accumulation of extraluminal gas in the submucosal intestinal tissue following the invasion of intestinal bacterial flora. It is postulated that progressive infiltration of the mucosa and bowel wall with gram-negative or gram-positive bacteria leads to more extensive tissue inflammation and destruction from activated neutrophils, producing a vasoconstrictive response, with progression to necrosis, and perforation.[25]

Clinical Signs and Symptoms

The classic clinical presentation of infant NEC includes the symptom group of abdominal tenderness, abdominal distension, hemepositive stools (or other gross or occult signs of GI bleeding), and ileus (decreased bowel sounds and increased gastric residual volume following tube feeding). Abdominal distension is the most commonly observed symptom.[25] Bilious vomiting after feeding also may be noted.

Signs of clinical deterioration in the child with NEC include apnea and bradycardia, lethargy, temperature instability, decreased urine output, further abdominal distension and discoloration of the abdominal wall. The wide range of symptoms in NEC has led to a clinical categorization or Bell's staging of the condition.[6] Symptoms and factors utilized in this staging include the infant's history (and risk factors), nonspecific manifestations of distress, and specific gastrointestinal and radiographic clinical indicators (Box 14-4). Recently, a modification of Bell's staging has been proposed to include histologic findings of each stage.[21]

Box 14-4 **Bell's Staging of Necrotizing Enterocolitis**

Stage I: Suspected Disease
- History of perinatal stress
- Nonspecific systemic manifestations: apnea, bradycardia, lethargy, temperature instability
- Gastrointestinal manifestations: poor feeding, increased residual volumes, emesis, mild distention
- Bloody stools
- Radiographic findings: ileus, non-specific or normal

Stage II: Definite Necrotizing Enterocolitis
- Persistent occult or gross gastrointestinal bleeding
- Marked abdominal distention, absent bowel sounds, abdominal tenderness
- Radiographic findings: pneumatosis intestinalis or portal venous air
- Laboratory findings: metabolic acidosis or thrombocytopenia

Stage III: Advanced Necrotizing Enterocolitis
- Deterioration of vital signs with hypotension and septic shock
- Striking abdominal distension, discoloration, and peritoneal signs
- Radiographic findings: pneumoperitoneum
- Laboratory findings: metabolic and respiratory acidosis, disseminated intravascular coagulopathy

Data from Lin PW, Stoll BJ: Necrotizing enterocolitis. *Lancet* 368:1271, 2006.

Management

Preventative interventions currently under investigation include: antenatal glucocorticoid administration, preferential use of breast milk, use of a standardized feeding regimen, restricting water intake without compromising hydration, and the use of probiotics (i.e., live microorganisms that may confer health benefits when administered in adequate amounts) and immunoglobulin A and arginine supplementation.[37,49,60]

If NEC is identified in its early stages and prompt medical treatment is provided, 30% to 50% of affected infants will improve without surgical intervention.[25] Once the diagnosis of NEC is suggested, enteral feedings are discontinued and a nasogastric or orogastric tube is passed for gastric drainage and decompression. Umbilical artery or venous catheters are discontinued. The infant will require administration of IV fluid therapy, including PN and appropriate IV antibiotics for both gram-negative and gram-positive organisms. Blood, urine, and sputum cultures should be sent before initiation of antibiotic therapy.

During the early stages, nursing interventions include monitoring of vital signs (including blood pressure), measuring abdominal girth and fluid intake and output (including weighing of all stools), evaluating daily weight, and testing all stools for blood.

The nurse must monitor the infant's systemic perfusion closely. Signs of poor systemic perfusion include tachycardia, tachypnea, decreased intensity of peripheral pulses, coolness of extremities, pallor or mottled color, and a urine output of less than 0.5-1.0 mL/kg per hour. Hypotension may be only a late sign of cardiovascular compromise. Infants require aggressive fluid resuscitation (typical bolus volume is 10 mL/kg, repeated as needed), with administration of blood products as needed. Thrombocytopenia may develop secondary to gram-negative sepsis.

The infant with sepsis may develop hypothermia and lethargy rather than fever and irritability. If significant bowel edema or free peritoneal fluid is present, the infant may demonstrate evidence of third spacing of fluid, including signs of hypovolemia (inadequate circulating blood volume as the result of loss of fluid into the bowel wall or peritoneum). Additional signs include tachycardia, decreased intensity of peripheral pulses, hypotension, peripheral vasoconstriction, lactic acidosis, oliguria, and anuria.

Surgical intervention is indicated if the infant demonstrates evidence of intestinal perforation, erythema of the abdominal wall, persistent metabolic acidosis, or clinical deterioration that is unresponsive to vigorous medical management (Box 14-5).[39,51] Surgical options include laparotomy with the resection of the affected bowel and creation of stomas or the placement of a peritoneal drain. See the Chapter 14 Supplement on the Evolve Website, Necrotizing Enterocolitis, for information about treatment with a peritoneal drain.

During surgery, necrotic bowel is resected, although attempts are made to salvage as much viable intestine as possible. A second operation may be performed to maximize the amount of retained bowel (the salvaged intestine is checked again for evidence of viability). The creation of an ileostomy or a jejunostomy permits the minimum possible amount of bowel resection and allows the distal, involved intestine a period of rest. This approach has afforded the highest survival.

These infants often require short-term postoperative mechanical ventilation. Parenteral nutrition (PN) is also necessary until oral feedings are resumed (see sections on Care of the Child after Abdominal Surgery and Parenteral Nutrition, earlier in this chapter).

Postoperative complications include rendering the infant as short gut and the development of intestinal obstruction. Late obstruction can result from stricture, most commonly in the colon (sigmoid colon); it may develop in up to one third of infants undergoing operative intervention and may also develop in infants who are managed medically. Infants rendered as short gut may be candidates for intestinal transplantation (see Intestinal Failure).

Biliary Atresia

Etiology

Biliary atresia (BA) is an inflammatory obstruction of the extrahepatic bile ducts with progressive inflammation of intrahepatic bile ducts. The atresia can involve isolated segments of the bile duct system or the entire biliary tree including the gallbladder. The progressive inflammation leads to fibrosis, with eventual bridging fibrosis and cirrhosis. There are two types of BA: the embryonic (fetal) form and the perinatal or acquired form. The embryonic form is usually associated with other congenital anomalies (e.g., polysplenia, cardiac anomalies, malrotation). Eighty percent of patients with biliary atresia in Western countries have the perinatal or acquired form of the disease, in which infants born with a patent hepatobiliary system develop progressive obstruction.[40] Precipitating factors include viral, toxic, vascular or immune mediators.[40]

Pathophysiology

Obstruction of the biliary tree prevents bile drainage from the liver into the duodenum. The accumulation of bile in the liver causes direct (conjugated) hyperbilirubinemia. Cirrhosis may develop despite early diagnosis and surgical palliation.

Clinical Signs and Symptoms

Infants with BA exhibit persistent jaundice and direct (conjugated) hyperbilirubinemia during the first 2 months of life. Acholic or gray-colored stools indicate a lack of bile drainage in the GI tract, and dark-colored urine indicates increased bilirubin in the urine. In older children, a high serum bilirubin can cause pruritus. If the BA is not diagnosed within approximately the first month of life, signs of progressive liver disease (e.g., malabsorption of fats and fat-soluble vitamins, poor growth, rickets, hypoproteinemia) may develop. Cirrhosis will be associated with signs and symptoms of portal hypertension (see Portal Hypertension, earlier in this chapter).

An ultrasound examination may reveal a small noncontractile gallbladder, or the gallbladder is not visualized.[18] A radionuclide hepatoiminodiacetic scan will detect movement of a radioactive tracer. The injected tracer is filtered by the liver, which adds it to the bile, so that the tracer normally flows through the bile ducts into the gallbladder and finally into the small intestine. In infants with BA there is no detectable excretion of the isotope into the small intestine.[18] A liver biopsy may reveal bile duct proliferation and portal tract fibrosis, which suggest the diagnosis.

Management

Surgical palliation with the Kasai (portoenterostomy procedure) should be planned and discussed with the parents when diagnostic testing is underway, because surgery should be performed as soon as possible after the diagnosis to optimize postsurgical outcome. In the Kasai procedure, the atretic segments are resected, and a segment of jejunum is sewn between the liver and the duodenum to facilitate bile drainage (see Evolve Fig. 14-2 for an illustration of the Kasai procedure in the Chapter 14 Supplement on the Evolve Website). If successful bile drainage can be achieved, the prognosis for these patients is relatively good. The best outcomes are achieved in infants younger than 2 months of age.

When there is significant fibrosis or cirrhosis at the time of operation, the prognosis is poor, even after the Kasai procedure. These patients will demonstrate progressive liver failure postoperatively and will require liver transplantation (see Chapter 17, Overview of Solid Organ Transplantation).

Nursing interventions for the child undergoing a portoenterostomy procedure include postoperative laparotomy care (see Care of the Child after Abdominal Surgery, earlier in this chapter). Postoperative complications include infection (e.g., cholangitis), alteration in fluid and electrolyte balance, portal hypertension, and progression to liver failure. The risk of postoperative liver failure is increased if significant liver damage (scarring) is present at the time of surgery. Additional nursing interventions are those appropriate for the care of the child with liver failure (see Liver Failure, later in this chapter).

Hepatitis

Etiology

Hepatitis, or inflammation of the liver, is most commonly caused by viral illness. Other causes include autoimmune liver disease, toxins, and idiopathic neonatal hepatitis. Six etiologically and immunologically distinct viruses are known to cause hepatitis: hepatitis A, B, C, D, E, and G. Hepatitis that is not type A, B, or type C is referred to as *non-A–non-B–non-C hepatitis* and is a diagnosis of exclusion in fulminant hepatic failure when other serologic markers are negative. Other classifications of hepatitis and common viruses that can cause hepatitis are listed in Box 14-6. Idiopathic neonatal hepatitis is considered a distinct form of hepatitis and is not thought to be caused by a virus, but is a histologic descriptive term of giant cell hepatitis.

Box 14-6   Classification of Hepatitis

- Type A
- Type B
- Type C
- Type D
- Type E
- Type G
- Non-A–non-B, non-C hepatitis
- Other viruses: cytomegalovirus, herpes simplex virus, Epstein-Barr virus, adenovirus, parvovirus
- Neonatal hepatitis
- Autoimmune disease
- Toxins

Hepatitis A. Hepatitis A virus (HAV) is present in the blood and feces during the incubation period and can be carried by persons who never develop the disease. This type of hepatitis is spread by the fecal-oral route, by feces-infected food and water, and by blood-borne infection. Food, water, and milk contaminated by virus-containing feces are typical sources of hepatitis A. Children and younger adults are infected most often with hepatitis A; peak incidence in children occurs in the early school-age period.

Hepatitis A typically begins as an acute illness after an incubation period of 14 to 40 days (average, 30 days). Fever is a common symptom early in the disease, whereas jaundice and prodromes of arthritis and rash are uncommon in children with hepatitis A. Fortunately this disease has little clinical significance and is not known to cause chronic liver disease.

Hepatitis B. Hepatitis B virus (HBV) is transmitted through blood transfusions or other contact with secretions (including saliva, breast milk, vaginal fluids, and semen) and serum containing HBV. In highly endemic areas of the world, children usually contract the virus through vertical transmission (mother to child); however, in the United States and other developed countries horizontal transmission is more common.[58]

This form of hepatitis frequently is preceded by a prodrome of arthritis and rash; fever is less common. The onset of hepatitis B is usually insidious and occurs after an incubation period of 60 to 180 days. When infants and young children are infected, they are at high risk (50% to 90%) to become chronically infected; by comparison, only 10% of infected adults become chronically infected.[58,59]

Hepatitis C. Hepatitis C virus (HCV) is transmitted through blood exposure or transfusion and is less contagious than HBV. In children, vertical transmission at birth (from mother to infant) accounts for most cases.[56] The incubation period lasts 6 to 12 weeks, and RNA of the HCV can usually be detected in the serum 2 weeks after infection.[56]

Hepatitis D. Hepatitis D virus (HDV) occurs only in the presence of HBV. Transmission is the same as for HBV, although vertical transmission is less common. HDV is rare in children born in the United States, because they are

vaccinated for HBV in infancy. Children with HBV who have rapid progression of disease usually have co-infection with HDV.

Hepatitis E. Hepatitis E virus (HEV) is similar to HAV. HEV is uncommon in the United States and is most common in developing countries.

Hepatitis G. Hepatitis G virus (HGV) is the newest strain of hepatitis, and little is known about it. Transmission is thought to be through blood. Often HGV produces no clinical symptoms and has not caused liver failure.

Pathophysiology
Viral hepatitis causes the destruction of liver cells and results in hepatic inflammation, necrosis, and autolysis. Changes occur diffusely throughout the liver, and the liver structure may be distorted. Regeneration of cells begins as soon as damaged ones are removed by phagocytosis. Most patients with nonneonatal forms of hepatitis recover with minimal residual damage. Unfortunately the hepatitis viruses mutate, and reinfection of the host can occur.

Fulminant hepatitis with accompanying hepatic encephalopathy may occur during the course of the viral illness (see Liver Failure, later in this chapter) and chronic hepatitis and cirrhosis may develop with chronic disease (HBV and HCV). An additional concern is that chronically infected patients can develop hepatocellular carcinoma (HCC).

Clinical Signs and Symptoms
The symptoms of viral hepatitis vary depending on the inciting virus. Many children have no apparent signs or symptoms, and the disease is often diagnosed when a child is tested for the disease after a parent is diagnosed with the disease.

General symptoms include flulike symptoms, fever, fatigue, nausea, vomiting, anorexia, abdominal pain (particularly right upper quadrant), diarrhea, and muscle soreness. Jaundice, producing yellow sclera and dark colored urine, is a later symptom that often triggers consultation with a healthcare provider. Jaundiced children will have elevated bilirubin and liver transaminases (AST and ALT).

Hepatitis A. Children with HAV may be asymptomatic, but they are contagious (see Hepatitis and Evolve Fig. 14-3 in the Chapter 14 Supplement on the Evolve Website for more details)

Hepatitis B. Children with HBV are less likely than adults to exhibit symptoms. Chronically infected children are usually asymptomatic unless they develop cirrhosis or hepatocellular carcinoma. In addition to general symptoms, children may develop extrahepatic symptoms including glomerulonephritis, papular acrodermatitis (papular rash of the face, extremities, and trunk), and lymphadenopathy.[58,59] For further information about clinical course of HBV, see Hepatitis and Evolve Fig. 14-4 in the Chapter 14 Supplement on the Evolve Website.

Hepatitis C. Infants infected by vertical transmission are usually asymptomatic.[59]

Laboratory Tests. The hepatitis serologies (antigens and antibodies) are used to diagnose HAV, HBV, HCV, and the disease stage and to identify contaminated units of blood. If the critically ill patient has serologic markers, the nurse should be knowledgeable about implications for the patient's possible disease state and transmission of the infection. A brief summary of the clinical significance of these markers and their interpretation is included in Table 14-10.

Management

All healthcare providers should practice standard precautions when handling any patient's body fluids (e.g., blood, urine, saliva, any wound or fluid drainage) and feces. There is no well-established treatment for the eradication of viral hepatitis. Medical treatment and nursing care is directed toward the relief of discomfort and maintenance of adequate nutrition and hydration.

If the child is eating, it is important to offer small, frequent tasty and nutritious meals. Typically hepatitis requires no dietary restrictions. Special treats, such as milk shakes, can provide fluid and calories without the appearance of a meal; therefore they may be appetizing to a child with anorexia or nausea. Antiemetics may be required if nausea prevents adequate nutrition.

Patients and families should be educated about the contagious nature of the disease and preventative measures. Family members should be vaccinated against HAV and HBV if not previously immunized. If known exposure has occurred, it may be appropriate to administer immunoglobulin preparations for HAV and HBV. Patients should be advised to eliminate exposure to hepatotoxic drugs, including alcohol.

In some affected patients, progression of liver damage occurs and cirrhosis develops; this indicates a poor prognosis for long-term survival without transplantation (see Liver Failure in this chapter and in Chapter 17, Overview of Solid Organ Transplantation).

Hepatitis A. HAV vaccine is available and should be given to children characterized by the following: over 1 year of age, living in areas of the country where infection rates are above the national average (e.g., Arizona, Alaska, Oregon, New Mexico, Utah, Washington, Oklahoma, South Dakota, Idaho, Nevada, California) or in areas with a community outbreak, those attending day care centers that have experienced outbreaks, and those with chronic liver disease with coagulopathies.

For children with HAV, supportive care is indicated. Approximately one third of infected patients will not develop immunity, so reinfection is possible. However, those infected do not develop chronic carrier states or chronic hepatitis.[64]

Hepatitis B. Hepatitis B vaccination is now available, and all children born in the United States after 1992 should be

Table 14-10 Hepatitis Virus Serum Markers and Interpretation

Virus, Virus Component, or Antibody	Abbreviation	Interpretation
Hepatitis A Virus	**HAV**	
Antibody (IgM subclass) directed against HAV	Anti-HAV IgM	Current or recent infection; present for 4-6 months
Antibody (IgG subclass) directed against HAV	Anti-HAV IgG	Confirms past exposure and immunity (resulting from immunization or following an infection)
Hepatitis B Virus	**HBV**	
HBV surface antigen	HBsAg	Indicates infection (either acute or chronic)
Hepatitis Be antigen	HBeAg	Is a derivative of HBsAg that correlates with viral replication and signifies high infectivity; if present beyond 6-8 weeks, suggests chronic carrier or disease
Antibody to HBsAg, subclass IgM (early) and IgG	Anti-HBs	Indicates clinical recovery from HBV infection and immunity
Total antibody to HBV core antigen	Anti-HBc	Indicates active HBV infection (either acute or chronic)
IgM antibody to HBcAg	Anti-HBc IgM	Early index of acute HBV infection, increases during the acute phase then declines (over 4-6 months), not present with chronic HBV
DNA of HBV	HBV DNA	Indicates HBV replication
Hepatitis C Virus	**HCV**	
Antibody to HCV	Anti-HCV	Indicates exposure to HCV
RNA of HCV	HCV RNA	Indicates HCV infection
Hepatitis δ (Delta) Virus	**HDV**	
δ antigen	HDV Ag	Indicates HDV infection
Total antibody to HDV	Anti-HDV	Indicates exposure to the agent (HDV)
RNA of HDV	HDV DNA	Indicates HDV replication

Adapted from Yazigi NA, Balistreri WF: Acute and chronic viral hepatitis. In Suchy FJ, Sokol RJ, Balistreri WF, editors: *Liver disease in children,* ed 2, Philadelphia, 2001, Lippincott Williams and Wilkins.
Ig, Immunoglobulin.

immunized (unless the child received no immunizations). All healthcare workers who may have contact with blood or blood products should be screened for hepatitis and vaccinated against hepatitis B. The need for "boosters" is unclear, and serologies for immunity should be periodically assessed. Prophylactic administration of hepatitis B immune serum globulin is recommended after parenteral exposure to HBV, such as occurs with a needle stick or direct mucous membrane contact, such as an accidental splash.

Current treatment for chronic HBV infection includes administration of lamivudine alone or in combination with interferon.[24,58] Lamivudine inhibits HBV replication and is prescribed for 1 year.[58] The advantage of this therapy is its oral route of administration. Interferon reduces viral replication, so it accelerates seroconversion in those who would have naturally cleared the virus.[58] Interferon is administered subcutaneously for 4 to 6 months.[9] Side effects can be problematic and include flulike symptoms, weight loss, and decreased growth velocity.[58] It is unclear whether interferon alone or in combination with lamivudine is the most effective therapy.

Hepatitis C. There is no vaccine available for HCV. Therapy with pegylated interferon alpha (weekly infusion) and ribavirin have been shown to be most effective in children.[24] Children appear to respond better than adults to treatment, probably because children have a shorter duration of chronic disease.[16]

Liver Failure

Etiology

Liver failure can be acute in children, but it is most often the end stage of chronic liver disease. Liver failure in children with chronic liver disease and disease progression is often termed *pediatric end stage liver disease*. Patients in the late stages of chronic liver failure will begin to demonstrate the complications of acute severe liver failure (e.g., acute encephalopathy). This condition is termed *acute on chronic failure*.

Acute necrosis of a previously normal liver is often termed *fulminant hepatic failure* (FHF). FHF is defined as the development of hepatic encephalopathy within 8 weeks of diagnosis without previous evidence of liver disease.

Acute liver failure (ALF) usually occurs as the result of a toxin exposure, viral illness, or unrecognized diagnoses (e.g., Wilson's disease). Other causes of ALF in previously normal children include idiosyncratic reactions to anesthetics, antibiotics, and chemotherapeutic agents. Ingestion of drugs or toxins such as acetaminophen (as may occur with therapeutic dosing or overdose), pesticides, cleaning compounds, or some plant alkaloids also can produce ALF.

Several causes of liver disease, including hepatitis and BA are addressed elsewhere in this chapter (see Biliary Atresia and Hepatitis sections). Other causes of liver disease in neonates and infants include genetic disorders such as Caroli's disease, tyrosinemia type 1, alpha-1 antitrypsin deficiency, and Alagille syndrome. Reye's syndrome was caused by an abnormal accumulation of fat in the liver and typically presented as a form of ALF. Following a published description of an association between aspirin administration to children with primary varicella or influenza (viral syndrome)

and the development of Reye's syndrome, the use of aspirin in children has been nearly abolished and this disorder is rarely seen.

Wilson's disease is an autosomal recessive disorder that results in excessive accumulation of copper in the liver. Treatment includes administration of D-penicillamine and dietary restriction of copper; however, some patients will exhibit ALF and will require liver transplantation.

Nonalcoholic fatty liver disease has become the most common cause of liver disease in children in developed countries.[34,36] This diagnosis is considered in children with mild to moderate elevation in ALT and AST levels with a body mass index in the 95th percentile or higher. The diagnosis is confirmed by liver biopsy, which reveals the accumulation of droplet fat in the hepatocytes in a child with no alcohol exposure.[36] Treatment goals include identification and treatment of obesity, alleviation of risk factors such as insulin resistance, and avoidance of factors that may worsen the liver disease (e.g., exposure to hepatotoxic drugs and alcohol).[36] There are no standard treatment regimens available, although lipid-lowering drugs, metformin, and vitamin E have been studied.[34,36]

Pathophysiology

The liver performs hundreds of synthetic, metabolic, and excretory functions, including drug detoxification, synthesis of protein and clotting factors, conversion of ammonia to urea, and phagocytosis with Kupffer cells. Liver failure produces both an accumulation of substances normally removed by the liver and a lack of substances normally manufactured by the liver. Although liver functions are fairly well preserved until 80% to 90% of liver function is lost, liver failure can contribute to multiorgan dysfunction. Major organ dysfunction with ALF includes the development of hepatic encephalopathy, coagulopathy, and hepatorenal syndrome.

Hepatic Encephalopathy. There are three major proposed mechanisms for development of this complication: the ammonia hypothesis, the gamma-aminobutyric acid (GABA)-benzodiazepine hypothesis and the false neurotransmitter hypothesis.[15] There is evidence to support each of these theories and some successes and failures in the associated treatment modalities.

The ammonia hypothesis contends that encephalopathy results from hyperammonemia that develops when the liver is no longer able to detoxify ammonia. Ammonia is formed in the GI tract after bacterial and enzymatic breakdown of proteins, including blood. This ammonia is normally absorbed into the splanchnic and portal venous systems, converted to nontoxic urea by the liver, and ultimately excreted by the kidneys. During the development of hepatic encephalopathy, the child's serum ammonia levels are often inversely related to the child's level of consciousness.

According to the GABA hypothesis, hepatic encephalopathy results from a buildup of endogenous benzodiazepines that cause neuroinhibition.[15] The false neurotransmitter hypothesis is based on the observation that branch chain amino acids are increased in liver failure and aromatic amino acids are decreased in liver failure.[15] In FHF, aromatic amino acids in the brain are metabolized to false neurotransmitters. These false transmitters inhibit actual neurotransmitters and disrupt message transmission in the brain.[15] This neurotransmitter dysfunction appears to be secondary to hyperammonemia.

Other theories suggest that toxins such as ammonia and manganese cross the blood-brain barrier and damage nerve cells and astrocytes.[8] Ammonia appears to have a direct toxic effect on the brain, and increased ammonia levels correlate with increasing grades of encephalopathy.

The end result of hepatic encephalopathy is the development of cerebral edema, a major cause of morbidity and mortality in the patient with ALF. This cerebral edema is associated with astrocyte swelling and increased brain water content that can lead to increased intracranial pressure. Although the specific pathophysiology of the cerebral edema has not been established, coma ensues if the process is not reversed in the early stages.

Coagulopathy. The child with liver failure will demonstrate coagulopathies from abnormal production of clotting factors (fibrinogen-factor I, prothrombin-factor II, and factors V, VII, IX, and X), sequelae of splenomegaly, and disseminated intravascular coagulation caused by acceleration of normal clotting. If the child with liver failure has portal hypertension, the resultant hypersplenism can produce thrombocytopenia, anemia, and leukopenia and further increase the child's risk of hemorrhage, particularly from varices.

Renal Failure. Mechanisms of renal failure in the child with liver failure include prerenal azotemia (prerenal failure), hepatorenal syndrome, and acute tubular necrosis. Liver failure can cause decreased renal perfusion and prerenal failure as the result of the extravascular fluid shift caused by ascites, splanchnic sequestration that develops with portal hypertension, or from acute hemorrhage caused by coagulopathy. Any decrease in circulating blood volume will stimulate aldosterone secretion, causing renal retention of sodium and water (see Acute Renal Failure and Acute Kidney Injury in Chapter 13).

Hepatorenal syndrome is the development of renal failure in the patient with advanced liver disease. It is characterized by reduced renal function, abnormal arterial circulation (possible hypotension, decreased renal perfusion, and possible intrarenal vasoconstriction), and increased aldosterone and renin activity with increased circulating vasoconstrictive mediators.

Liver failure produces many alterations in acid-base and electrolyte balance. Chronic hyperaldosteronism increases potassium and magnesium loss in the urine and increases hydrogen ion excretion (the kidneys excrete hydrogen ion in exchange for the sodium that is saved). Increased renal hydrogen ion excretion can produce a mild metabolic alkalosis, which further increases renal potassium loss. Excess renal excretion of hydrogen ion increases the renal production of ammonia, raising serum ammonia levels. Gastrointestinal disturbances, such as diarrhea and vomiting, can result in potassium loss and the development of metabolic acidosis or alkalosis.

Clinical Signs and Symptoms

Signs of chronic liver disease in the child with acute failure include sequelae of portal hypertension with ascites and dilation of superficial abdominal veins (caput medusae),

xanthoma formation, clubbing of the nails, gynecomastia, skin ecchymosis, palmar erythema, and spider angiomas. Jaundice is often present. The child frequently appears malnourished, and scratch marks and scabs may be visible signs of itching triggered by the pruritus.

Early signs of hepatic encephalopathy include poor school performance, forgetfulness and malaise. Neurologic signs of hepatic encephalopathy include tremors, incoordination, muscle twitching, and violent movements. The classic early symptom of hepatic encephalopathy is a peculiar flapping tremor known as *asterixis*. It can be elicited by asking an older child to stretch the arms straight out and dorsiflex the hand. The child will be unable to maintain the hyperextended position of the hand and will develop coarse bursts of twitching movements at the wrist (see Chapter 11 for further information about encephalopathy).

A staging of hepatic encephalopathy is described in Box 14-7, and children with acute failure can progress to stage 4 (coma) in a period as short as 1 or 2 days. Progressive encephalopathy is indicated by a decreased level of consciousness. Cerebral edema can produce increased intracranial pressure (see Chapter 11 for further information regarding the recognition and management of increased intracranial pressure).

Liver failure produces many hematologic, coagulation, and serum chemistry derangements. Both the intrinsic and extrinsic clotting cascades are affected (see Chapter 15). An ominous laboratory constellation for the child with ALF is markedly elevated liver transaminases (>1000 IU/L with a trend to normal values once few functioning hepatocytes remain to release enzymes) with a rising prothrombin time. Decreased production of serum clotting factors by the liver causes a prolonged prothrombin time, manifested by ecchymosis or petechiae and increased bleeding from puncture sites or from mucosal irritation.

The child's serum direct bilirubin, transaminases, alkaline phosphatase, and ammonia level are usually elevated. Serum albumin levels may be normal in the setting of FHF because the half-life of albumin is 21 days; it may be low with acute or chronic disease. Anemia, leukopenia, hypoglycemia, hypokalemia, and hypocalcemia will develop in the presence of significant hepatic necrosis.

Clinical signs of hepatorenal syndrome include abrupt oliguria and azotemia, often without apparent precipitating

---

Box 14-7 Stages of Hepatic Encephalopathy

Stage 1: Mild confusion with periods of depression and euphoria, disrupted sleep
EEG typically normal
Stage 2: Moderate confusion, lethargy
EEG abnormal, with generalized slowing
Stage 3: Marked confusion, incoherent speech, sleeps but is arousable
EEG markedly abnormal
Stage 4: Coma
EEG markedly abnormal

Data from Han MK, Hyzy R: Advances in critical care management of hepatic failure and insufficiency. *Crit Care Med* 2006; 34(Suppl):S235-S241.
EEG, Electroencephalogram.

factors such as infection, sepsis, or shock. Diagnostic criteria in adults include a creatinine greater than 1.5 mg/dL (or 24-hour creatinine clearance less than 40 mL/min); absence of shock, infection, or fluid losses; no improvement in renal function after withdrawal of diuretics and expansion of intravascular volume with plasma expander (adult receives 1.5 L, child receives 20 mL/kg boluses); proteinuria less than 500 mg/day; and no evidence of parenchymal or obstructive renal disease.[23] Additional laboratory findings include a normal urinalysis, hyponatremia (despite the renal retention of sodium, the serum sodium falls because there is relatively greater renal absorption of water), and hypokalemia (see the discussion of Acute Renal Failure and Acute Kidney Injury in Chapter 13).

If the cause of the hepatic failure has not been identified, diagnostic studies will be performed immediately. These studies include extensive toxicology screening (for evidence of alcohol, drug, or chemical ingestion), liver function studies, hepatitis serologies, ultrasound examination to evaluate vessels, and possible liver biopsy (Table 14-11). Although a liver biopsy can be performed in the presence of significant

Table 14-11 **Common Liver Function Tests and Changes with Liver Failure**

Test	Normal Value	Interpretation
Serum Enzymes		
Alkaline phosphatase	Infant, 150-420 units/L 2-10 years, 100-320 units/L	Increases with biliary obstruction and cholestatic hepatitis
γ-Glutamyltransferase	0-3 months 0-120 units/L 3-12 months, male: 5-65 units/L 3-12 months, female: 5-35 units/L 1-15 years.: 0-28 units/L	Increases with biliary obstruction and cholestatic hepatitis
Aspartate aminotransferase	5-40 units/mL	Increases with hepatocellular injury
Alanine aminotransferase (ALT)	5-35 units/mL	Increases with hepatocellular injury
Lactate dehydrogenase	10 days to 24 months: 180-430 units/L; 24 months to 12 years,: 110-295 units/L	Isoenzyme is elevated with hypoxic and primary liver injury
5'-nucleotidase	2-11 units/mL	Increases with increase in alkaline phosphatase
Bilirubin Metabolism		
Serum bilirubin		
Indirect (unconjugated)	<0.8 mg/dL	Increases with hemolysis (lysis of red blood cells)
Direct (conjugated)	Neonate, <0.6 mg/dL Infants/children, <0.2 mg/dL	Increases with hepatocellular injury or obstruction
Total	0-1 days, <8 mg/dL 1-2 days, <12 mg/dL 3-5 days, <12-16 mg/dL Older infant, < 2 mg/dL Adult, 0.3-1.2 mg/dL	Increases with biliary obstruction
Urine bilirubin	0	Increases with biliary obstruction
Urine urobilinogen	0-4 mg/24 h	Increases with hemolysis or shunting of portal blood flow
Serum Proteins		
Albumin	3.5-5.5 gm/dL	Reduced with hepatocellular injury
Globulin	2.5-3.5 gm/dL	Increases with hepatitis
Total	6-7 gm/dL	
Albumin/Globulin (A:G) ratio	1.5:1 to 2.5:1	Ratio reverses with chronic hepatitis or other chronic liver disease
Transferrin	203-380 mcg/dL	Liver damage with decreased values, iron deficiency with increased values
Blood Clotting Functions		
Prothrombin time	11.5-14 s or 90%-100% of control	Increases with chronic liver disease (cirrhosis) or vitamin K deficiency
Activated partial thromboplastin time (aPTT)	30-33 seconds	Increases with severe liver disease or heparin therapy

Data from Huether SE: Structure and function of the digestive system. In McCance KL, Huether SE, editors: *Pathophysiology: the biologic basis for disease in adults and children,* ed 6, St Louis, 2010, Mosby; Custer JW: Blood chemistries and body fluids. In Custer JW, Rau RE, editors: *The Harriet Lane Handbook,* ed 18, St Louis, 2009, Mosby-Elsevier; Values for blood clotting functions from Aquino J: Hematology. In Custer JW, Rau RE, editors: *The Harriet Lane Handbook,* ed 18, St Louis, 2009, Mosby-Elsevier.

coagulopathy, a coagulation profile should be obtained and significant coagulopathy corrected before the biopsy. Viral, bacteriologic, and fungal blood cultures also may be ordered.

Management

All children who are critically ill require planned nursing assessment and support of all body systems. The child with liver failure with multiorgan failure is no exception. Careful monitoring for respiratory cardiac, neurologic, and renal function is often more important than monitoring the child's liver function. The focus of the following information is on clinical assessment and prevention of the complications of liver failure and encephalopathy. Figure 14-17 is an overview of care considerations for the child with end stage liver disease.

The principal problems of the child with liver failure include any or all of the following: alteration in neurologic function, respiratory insufficiency, blood loss, changes in intravascular and interstitial fluid balance, compromised nutritional status, renal dysfunction, electrolyte or acid-base imbalance, increased risk of infection, decreased activity level, and patient and family anxiety.

Until liver function returns, treatment of the child with liver failure is primarily supportive. During the acute phase the most important goal of therapy is the prevention of major complications, such as increased intracranial pressure, respiratory failure, hemorrhage, fluid and electrolyte imbalances, and renal failure. Nutritional support and prevention of the complications of chronic liver failure, such as portal

hypertension, are also important. The presence and severity of associated encephalopathy and intracranial hemorrhage often have the greatest effect on the child's survival.

Encephalopathy. The child with hepatic failure may develop encephalopathy and resultant increased intracranial pressure. The nurse must monitor for early signs of neurologic compromise. Nurses should perform brief but careful neurologic evaluation when recording vital signs. The nurse should evaluate pupil size and constriction to light, and report any pupil sluggishness or inequality to the child's on-call provider. Observe the child's voluntary movements, and immediately report any decreased movement, decreased sensation, abnormal posturing, or asterixis.

A decrease in the child's level of consciousness, such as decreased response to commands or the presence of unusual irritability or lethargy may indicate the development of increased intracranial pressure. If the child's condition allows, ask the child to write his or her name or identify common objects in the room. Record the names of the child's siblings and household pets, because conversation about them may be used to evaluate the child's short- and long-term memory. Whatever the method of evaluation, providers should make the evaluation as consistent as possible to detect changes in responsiveness with examinations over time.

If the child develops stage III or IV encephalopathy, management will be supportive. Endotracheal intubation should be performed whenever there is any question of the child's ability to maintain a patent airway, and mechanical ventilation

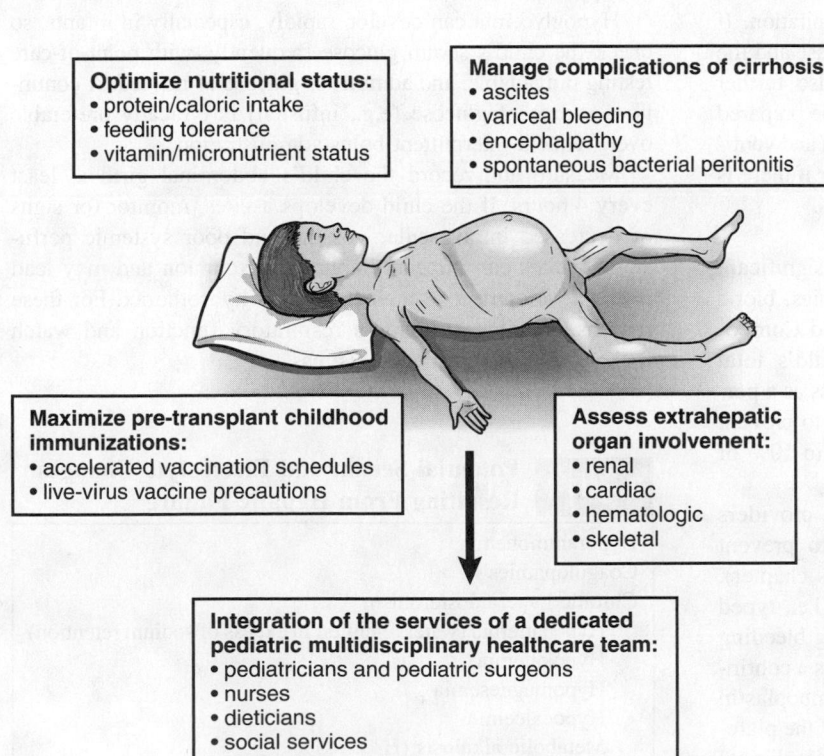

FIG. 14-17 Optimizing care for the child with end-stage liver disease. Critically ill children with end-stage liver disease have multiple complex medical issues that must be addressed adequately to achieve optimal healthy outcomes. (From Leonis MA, Balistreri WF: Evaluation and management of end-stage liver disease in children. *Gastroenterology* 143:1741-1751, 2008.)

Optimize nutritional status:
• protein/caloric intake
• feeding tolerance
• vitamin/micronutrient status

Manage complications of cirrhosis:
• ascites
• variceal bleeding
• encephalpathy
• spontaneous bacterial peritonitis

Maximize pre-transplant childhood immunizations:
• accelerated vaccination schedules
• live-virus vaccine precautions

Assess extrahepatic organ involvement:
• renal
• cardiac
• hematologic
• skeletal

Integration of the services of a dedicated pediatric multidisciplinary healthcare team:
• pediatricians and pediatric surgeons
• nurses
• dieticians
• social services
• psychology
• financial services
• home healthcare
• pediatric hospital setting

is needed if hypoventilation develops. Placement of an ICP monitor may be indicated. The child's arterial carbon dioxide tension should be maintained at approximately normal range. Routine hyperventilation is not indicated and may reduce cerebral blood flow. Provide oxygen if needed to maintain a normal arterial oxygen tension and prevent the development of hypoxemia. The child should be appropriately medicated for pain and agitation.

Because a high serum ammonia concentration can contribute to encephalopathy, attempts are made to reduce ammonia production and absorption. Ammonia is produced in the GI tract during bacterial and enzymatic breakdown of endogenous and exogenous proteins. Administration of nonabsorbable antibiotics (e.g., neomycin, rifaximin) via nasogastric tube will decrease GI bacteria and subsequent ammonia production. Lactulose (1 mL/kg, 3 to 6 times daily) will be administered to acidify colonic content, thus promoting ammonium ion excretion.

If the child develops gastric bleeding related to coagulopathies, gastric blood should be drained to prevent GI blood breakdown and further ammonia production. Prophylactic antacids should be administered via nasogastric tube and intravenous administration of histamine type 2 blockers or sucralfate should be considered (see Gastrointestinal Bleeding, earlier in this chapter).

Mannitol and diuretics can be administered to treat increased intracranial pressure. Maintain the child's serum osmolality at approximately 300 to 310 mOsm/L, and do not allow the serum sodium concentration to rise or fall acutely (see Chapter 11, Increased Intracranial Pressure).

Respiratory Insufficiency. As the child's level of consciousness decreases, the child is at risk for developing hypoventilation, respiratory failure, upper airway obstruction and aspiration. If ascites is present, the child's tidal volume may decrease and the child may develop atelectasis. Hydrothorax can also further compromise respiratory function. Providers should be prepared to insert an advanced airway and support oxygenation and ventilation if the child's respiratory effort is insufficient or if there is any doubt about the child's airway protective reflexes.

Coagulopathies. If the child has any clinical or significant laboratory (i.e., serologic) evidence of coagulopathies, blood components are administered (see Blood and Blood Component Therapies in Chapter 15). Calculate the child's total circulating blood volume and consider any blood loss as a percentage of this blood volume. Consider transfusion to prevent hemodynamic compromise if blood loss totals 7% to 10% of the child's estimated blood volume.

If a severe GI hemorrhage occurs, all bedside providers must be prepared to provide prompt treatment to prevent shock (see Gastrointestinal Bleeding, earlier in this chapter). Blood and blood components should be available (i.e., typed and cross-matched) in the blood bank for use during bleeding episodes. Fresh frozen plasma can be administered as a continuous infusion if the child's activated partial thromboplastin time is elevated, and platelets should be transfused if the platelet count is less than 20,000/mm^3 or the child has clinical evidence of bleeding. Vitamin K can be administered as needed. All efforts must be made to prevent oral, tracheal, and GI trauma during intubation, suctioning, and mouth care.

Fluid and Electrolyte Balance. The child with liver failure can develop fluid shifts and fluid imbalances related to hyperaldosteronism (and increased sodium and water retention), hypoalbuminemia, portal hypertension, and resultant splanchnic sequestration (see Portal Hypertension earlier in this chapter), or hepatorenal syndrome.

Measure all sources of fluid intake and output, and record body weight at least daily. Evaluate the child's level of hydration by assessing the moisture in mucous membranes, the presence of tearing, fullness of the fontanelle (in infants younger than 16 to 18 months), skin turgor, and urine output.

A central venous catheter will provide reliable vascular access and enable more precise evaluation of the child's intravascular volume. The presence of a high CVP is undesirable, because it can contribute to increased intracranial pressure and can increase esophageal variceal pressure and promote bleeding. As a result, when blood component or fluid administration is necessary, the nurse should monitor the child's response and tolerance, including changes in CVP. Diuretics may be prescribed, and the nurse should note the child's response. Notify the child's on-call provider if urine response is inadequate.

For the treatment of renal failure, the child may require hemodialysis or continuous hemofiltration. The goal should be to achieve euvolemia, and to correct electrolyte imbalances (refer to Acute Renal Failure and Acute Kidney Injury in Chapter 13).

Electrolyte and coagulation abnormalities and problems associated with liver failure are listed in Box 14-8. Electrolyte imbalance may result from fluid shifts, hyperaldosteronism, or diuretic therapy. Evaluate the child's serum electrolyte concentrations frequently, and provide electrolyte replacement therapy as needed.

Hypoglycemia can develop rapidly, especially in infants, so check the child's serum glucose frequently, with point-of-care testing if available, and administer glucose as needed. A continuous source of glucose (e.g., infusion) is typically preferable over frequent intermittent bolus administration.

Measure and record the child's abdominal girth at least every 4 hours. If the child develops ascites, monitor for signs of decreased intravascular volume and poor systemic perfusion. Ascites can impede diaphragm excursion and may lead to the development of atelectasis or a hydrothorax. For these reasons, monitor the child's respiratory function and watch for evidence of respiratory distress.

Box 14-8	**Potential Serum and Electrolyte Changes Resulting From Hepatic Failure**

Hyperammonemia
Coagulopathies
Chronic hyperaldosteronism
    Hyponatremia (water retention in excess of sodium retention)
    Hypokalemia
    Hypomagnesemia
    Hypocalcemia
    Metabolic alkalosis (H$^+$ loss)
Hypoglycemia
Azotemia (increased nitrogen wastes, including blood urea
    nitrogen, creatinine)

Nutritional Support. Liver failure can rapidly produce nutritional compromise. Parenteral nutrition will be required if the child is unable to tolerate enteral (oral or tube) feedings. Calculate the child's daily caloric requirements, and consult with the child's on-call provider and a dietician as needed if the child is not receiving adequate nutrition. Vitamin supplementation (especially vitamins A, D, E, and K) is usually necessary.

Additional Supportive Care. If the child is receiving any medications that are normally metabolized by the liver, review the doses of the medications and adjust as necessary (to prevent development of toxic drug levels). Box 14-9 details nursing interventions appropriate for care of the child with hepatic failure (note that it assumes that appropriate diagnostic studies have been performed).

If severe liver failure persists despite supportive therapy, liver transplantation should be considered. Some liver assist devices have been developed for use in children, and clinical trials have demonstrated significant reduction in intracranial pressure; however, currently there are no pediatric devices approved by the U.S. Food and Drug Administration for use in children.

Liver transplantation is challenging in these extremely unstable children, particularly if multiorgan failure is present.

Box 14-9 **Nursing Care of the Child with Liver Failure**

Treatment of liver failure requires problem-oriented supportive care and treatment of metabolic and neurologic complications.

Potential for Depressed Level of Consciousness and Potential for Increased Intracranial Pressure Related to:
- Accumulation of toxic substances
- Hyperammonemia
- Altered amino acid profile and accumulation of possible false neurotransmitters
- Increased neuroinhibitory substances
- Development of cerebral edema
- Fluid and electrolyte imbalances

Alteration in Cerebral Perfusion or Alteration in Thought Processes Related to:
- Hepatic encephalopathy

Expected patient outcomes
- Patient's level of consciousness will improve.
- If patient's level of consciousness and responsiveness deteriorate, the patient's airway will be protected and oxygenation and ventilation will be supported as needed.

Nursing interventions
- Assess patient level of consciousness and neurologic function at regular intervals:
  1. General level of consciousness and responsiveness
  2. Ability to follow commands (ask child to hold up two fingers, wiggle toes, or stick out tongue)
  3. Spontaneous movement and movement in response to central painful stimulus (note quality of movement and any posturing)
  4. Pupil size and response to light
  5. Evidence of cranial nerve function (e.g., cough, gag, blink)
  6. Systemic perfusion, heart rate, and respiratory rate
  7. Spontaneous respiratory effort and oxygenation
- Determine stage of hepatic encephalopathy (see Box 14-7), and report any change (particularly in arousability, speech, irritability, pupil size, and response to light) to a provider immediately.
- Monitor for early signs of encephalopathy, including tremors, lack of coordination, muscle twitching, and flapping tremors (called *asterixis*). These tremors may be elicited if the child is asked to outstretch the arms and dorsiflex the hand; monitor for coarse bursts of twitching at wrist.
- If the child's level of consciousness deteriorates, monitor airway patency and airway protective mechanisms (e.g., cough, gag). Be prepared to assist with emergency intubation and begin mechanical ventilatory support.
- Once signs of increased intracranial pressure are observed, provide standard treatment (as ordered (see Chapter 11).
- Assist in diagnostic studies, including computed tomography to determine presence and severity of cerebral edema, and laboratory studies to monitor hepatic function and causes of hepatic failure.

Potential Respiratory Insufficiency as a Result of:
- Encephalopathy and depressed level of consciousness
- Elevation of diaphragm from ascites
- Deterioration in neurologic function

Expected patient outcomes
- Patient will demonstrate effective systemic arterial oxygenation and carbon dioxide elimination (ventilation).
- Respiratory rate will remain appropriate for age and clinical condition, oxygenation and carbon dioxide elimination will be adequate, and child will not demonstrate increased or inadequate respiratory effort.

Nursing interventions
- Monitor patient's respiratory rate and effort; report any tachypnea and increased respiratory effort to provider immediately.
- If patient is breathing spontaneously, elevate the head of the bed and position the patient comfortably to maximize diaphragm excursion.
- Monitor patient level of consciousness and be prepared to assist with intubation and to provide assisted ventilation if airway protective mechanisms are compromised or respiratory insufficiency develops.
- Monitor pulse oximetry and exhaled (end-tidal) carbon dioxide or arterial blood gases to determine effectiveness of oxygenation and ventilation; notify provider of any deterioration.
- Auscultate breath sounds on a regular basis; notify provider of decreased intensity or change in pitch of breath sounds, which may indicate the development of atelectasis or hydrothorax.
- If mechanical ventilatory support is required, ensure that support is appropriate and that the child's chest expands equally and adequately during positive pressure inspiration.

Continued

Box 14-9 **Nursing Care of the Child with Liver Failure—cont'd**

- Monitor heart rate and systemic perfusion; if a deterioration in clinical appearance is observed, evaluate systemic oxygenation and ventilatory support.
- Maintain emergency intubation (and reintubation) equipment at the bedside.

Potential Hypovolemia Related to:
- Bleeding (especially via esophageal varices)
- Third-spacing of fluid into peritoneal space
- Hypoalbuminemia

Expected patient outcomes
- Patient will maintain adequate intravascular volume as indicated by effective systemic perfusion (warm extremities with brisk capillary refill, good color, strong peripheral pulses, urine output of 1 mL/kg per hour), a central venous pressure of 2-5 mmHg, and appropriate heart rate and blood pressure for age and clinical condition.
- Patient will maintain adequate hemoglobin and hematocrit, and significant acute blood loss will be replaced (per provider order).
- Patient will not demonstrate excessive weight gain associated with edema.

Nursing interventions
- Constantly evaluate systemic perfusion; notify provider of signs of inadequate systemic perfusion, including tachycardia, cool extremities, mottled color, delayed capillary refill, decreased intensity of peripheral pulses, and oliguria. Note that hypotension is usually only a late sign of hypovolemia in children.
- Monitor for signs of dehydration, including dry mucous membranes, poor skin turgor, negative fluid balance, and sunken fontanelle in infants. Notify provider if these signs are observed.
- If esophageal or gastrointestinal bleeding develops, notify provider, estimate quantity, and provide replacement blood products as ordered. Monitor serial hemoglobin and hematocrit, and notify provider of a fall in these variables.
- Calculate daily maintenance fluid requirements and record fluid intake and output. Notify provider of imbalance. Administer crystalloids and colloids as ordered to maintain intravascular volume and support systemic perfusion.
- Record patient weight daily or twice daily. Notify provider of significant weight gain or loss.
- Measure abdominal girth.
- Administer diuretics as ordered and monitor their effectiveness. These drugs are usually avoided unless increased intracranial pressure develops, because they can contribute to acute reduction in intravascular volume.
- Monitor electrolyte balance, and notify provider of signs of hemoconcentration. In general, sodium intake is limited, and potassium supplements must be administered.
- Monitor for signs of hepatorenal syndrome (oliguria and azotemia) caused by reduced renal perfusion. Notify provider of reduction in urine volume, and monitor renal function as needed (e.g., serum-urine creatinine). Low-dose dopamine therapy may be ordered to optimize renal perfusion.
- Assist in abdominal paracentesis as needed.

Potential for Bleeding Related to:
- Coagulopathies
- Esophageal varices

- Frequent administration of blood products
- Potential sepsis

Expected patient outcomes
- Patient will demonstrate no active bleeding. Hemoglobin and hematocrit will remain adequate for age.
- Significant coagulopathies will be detected and effectively treated.

Nursing interventions
- Observe patient closely for evidence of bleeding. Test gastric drainage and stool for evidence of blood, and notify provider of positive results.
- Insert nasogastric tube and institute gastric gravity drainage. Administer nasogastric antacids, intravenous histamine type 2 receptor blockers, and proton pump inhibitors as ordered.
- If esophageal varices are present, institute precautionary measures (e.g., prevent Valsalva maneuver, provide soft diet), and monitor the patient closely for evidence of bleeding. If bleeding develops, monitor the quantity of bleeding and be prepared to provide replacement blood therapy. (Ensure that a patient blood sample has been sent for type and cross-match analysis.) Also see Portal Hypertension elsewhere in this chapter; management of hemorrhage associated with portal hypertension includes:
  1. Resuscitation and replacement of lost blood
  2. Identification of bleeding site
  3. Specific therapy to stop bleeding (e.g., sclerotherapy)
- Monitor results of coagulation studies. Notify provider of coagulopathies and ensure that appropriate blood components are available before invasive procedures. Be alert for the appearance of petechiae or ecchymoses; notify provider if these are observed.
- Avoid injections and minimize venipunctures if possible. Assist with insertion of indwelling arterial line for blood sampling. It may be necessary to administer blood components before catheter insertion to ensure hemostasis during procedure.
- Provide a safe environment for the child.

Potential Infection and Sepsis Related to:
- Impaired liver function
- Multiple invasive catheters
- Compromise in nutritional status

Expected patient outcomes
- Patient will demonstrate no signs of infection, such as fever or hypothermia, localized inflammation, leukocytosis or leukopenia, or positive wound or blood cultures.
- Existing infection will resolve promptly.

Nursing interventions
- Ensure that every member of the healthcare team washes their hands before and after every patient contact.
- Ensure that sterile and aseptic procedures are used for insertion and maintenance of monitoring and treatment catheters (see Box 22-6).
- Change dressings and intravenous tubing and catheters according to unit policy. Maintain occlusive dressings over central venous and intracranial pressure catheter skin entrance sites (per hospital or unit policy).
- Monitor for signs of infection, including localized signs of inflammation, fever or hypothermia, leukocytosis, or

Box 14-9	Nursing Care of the Child with Liver Failure—cont'd

leukopenia. Notify provider of cloudy urine or drainage from wounds or catheter insertion sites. Obtain cultures as ordered or per unit policy.
- Administer antibiotics as ordered.
- If infection is present, monitor for evidence of bacteremia and development of sepsis, including a change in level of consciousness, tachycardia, respiratory alkalosis (if patient is breathing spontaneously), and thrombocytopenia. Notify provider if these signs are observed.

Potential for Poor Nutrition Related to:
- Impaired liver function
- Inadequate nutritional intake
- Increased metabolic requirements
- Impaired gastrointestinal absorption of nutrients

Expected patient outcomes
- Patient will receive sufficient protein and caloric intake to prevent catabolism, but limited enough protein intake to prevent rise in amino acid levels.
- Patient skin turgor and wound healing will remain satisfactory.

Nursing interventions
- Monitor patient's total daily intake of protein; typically, protein intake is limited to approximately 0.5-1.0 g/kg per day.
- Monitor serum albumin; notify provider of hypoalbuminemia.
- Calculate maintenance caloric requirements (see Table 14-3); determine child's caloric intake and notify provider if caloric intake is inadequate.
- Monitor serum glucose concentration; ensure ongoing source of glucose intake and notify provider if hypoglycemia or hyperglycemia develop.
- Consult dietician to optimize the child's nutritional status.

Additional Potential Patient Problems
Patient and family stress and anxiety related to:
- Uncertain patient prognosis
- Painful procedures
Patient and family knowledge deficit related to:
- Patient condition
- Hospital and home therapy required
- Progressive liver dysfunction

However, transplantation affords the child with ALF the greatest chance of survival (see Chapter 17, Overview of Solid Organ Transplantation). Five-year survival for children undergoing liver transplantation for acute liver failure is relatively high (exceeding 70%).[30a,31] For the most recent transplantation survival data, the reader is referred to the National Organ Procurement and Transplantation Website National Data (http://optn.transplant.hrsa.gov/latestData/viewDataReports.asp).

Pancreatitis

Etiology

Pancreatitis in children is relatively rare. Causes are diverse and can be categorized as nonobstructive, obstructive, or inflammatory. Nonobstructive causes predominate and include blunt abdominal trauma, typically caused by bicycle handle bar injuries and motor vehicle crashes. Nonobstructive pancreatitis is also associated with several medications, including didanosine, azathioprine, mercaptopurine, L-asparaginase, and valproic acid.[52]

Up to one third of cases of pancreatitis result from obstructive disorders in the biliary or pancreatic duct, with cholelithiasis being the most common. Cholelithiasis is frequently associated with hemolytic disorders, including spherocytosis, beta-thalassemia, and sickle cell disease. Inflammatory causes of pancreatitis include mumps, ulcerative colitis, mononucleosis, HIV, and cystic fibrosis. Hereditary pancreatitis is another cause of obstructive pancreatitis and is often recurrent.

Pathophysiology

When pancreatic acinar cells are damaged, they release and activate digestive enzymes, triggering an inflammatory process referred to as *autodigestion*. The inflammatory cascade causes edema, ischemia, and necrosis. When the autodigestion-inflammation affects structures surrounding the pancreas, multiorgan failure can result.

Acute pancreatitis refers to a single inflammatory episode. When this process resolves, the pancreas is left with no residual effects. With recurrent episodes, morphologic changes in the pancreas begin to interfere with exocrine and endocrine functions, resulting in chronic pancreatitis.

Clinical Signs and Symptoms

Classic symptoms of pancreatitis in children are abdominal pain, nausea, vomiting, and anorexia. Symptom severity varies from mild abdominal pain to signs and symptoms of severe shock and end organ failure. Abdominal pain is typically the most intense in the epigastrium. Because the pancreas is retroperitoneal, back and flank pain are also common. Movement increases the intensity of the pain, so patients often lie still and are hesitant to move. Eating usually triggers or increases the pain and can induce vomiting that may be bilious. Pain may increase in intensity after vomiting occurs, because vomiting increases intraductal pressures producing further obstruction of pancreatic secretions.

Physical findings may include a bluish discoloration around the umbilicus (Cullen's sign) or in the flanks (Turner's sign), signifying hemorrhagic pancreatitis. Ascites may also be present.

Amylase and lipase are enzymes derived from pancreatic acinar cells; elevated levels aid in the diagnosis of pancreatitis. Amylase levels typically peak approximately 48 hours after the onset of pancreatitis and may remain elevated for as long as 4 days. Amylase levels may be elevated by other more common diseases, but levels typically do not reach those found in pancreatitis. Because amylase is produced by the salivary glands, levels can also increase with head and mouth trauma. Amylase isoenzymes are helpful in separating acute pancreatitis from other diseases that cause a rise in amylase, such as injury to the main salivary gland. Lipase is more specific to pancreatic injury than amylase, and it can remain elevated for as long as 14 days. Serum enzyme levels are diagnostic for pancreatitis if they are at least threefold greater than normal ranges. The severity of the rise of these enzymes does not correlate with the extent of pancreatic injury.

Metabolic complications of acute pancreatitis include lipid abnormalities, hypocalcemia, hyperglycemia and metabolic acidosis.[12] Hypocalcemia is observed in approximately 15% of patients with pancreatitis and develops when extensive fat necrosis occurs. Approximately 25% of patients with acute pancreatitis demonstrate hyperglycemia, because damaged pancreatic tissue releases less insulin than normal. The white blood cell count and differential are frequently normal, whereas the hematocrit reflects hemoconcentration secondary to dehydration.

A variety of radiologic studies are useful for detecting pancreatic abnormalities. Ultrasound examination is often the study of choice to evaluate pancreatic size and contour and to evaluate the progress of pancreatic or biliary obstruction in small, thin subjects. CT scans allow evaluation of the presence and extent of pancreatic necrosis, inflammation, ascites, and gallstones. Magnetic resonance cholangiopancreatography provides more accurate information about duct integrity.

Endoscopic retrograde cholangiopancreatography (ERCP) is both diagnostic and therapeutic, but is also the most invasive of these studies. When a pancreatic duct abnormality is detected during the study, procedures such as a sphincterotomy at the sphincter of Oddi, stent placement, and stone removal can be performed. This study is not advised during the acute phase of pancreatitis, because it may worsen the condition.

Management

The two goals of management of pancreatitis are to minimize causative factors and provide meticulous supportive care. Supportive care includes taking steps to decrease the production of digestive enzymes: the child should receive PN and should receive no enteral feeding (i.e., nothing by mouth or nasogastric tube). Octreotide acetate can be used to suppress GI hormones that stimulate pancreatic secretion.

Because the pain associated with pancreatitis can be severe, parenteral analgesia with narcotics or nonsteroidal antiinflammatory agents is generally required (see Chapter 5). The use of morphine and other opiate derivatives is theoretically less desirable in patients with pancreatitis, because these medications increase spasm of the sphincter of Oddi and may cause additional pain.

Shock is the leading cause of death in patients with acute fulminant pancreatitis.[19] Nurses must closely monitor the child's vital signs, systemic perfusion, and evidence of fluid balance, including CVP and urine output. Fluid shifts can cause severe abdominal distension that hinders diaphragm excursion. Close monitoring of respiratory status (oxygenation, ventilation, aeration, and respiratory effort) is required.

Surgical intervention may be necessary in cases of pancreatic trauma with fracture of the pancreas and disruption of the pancreatic duct. Surgery may also be necessary for patients with familial pancreatitis.

Inflammatory Bowel Disease with Toxic Megacolon

Inflammatory bowel disease (IBD) is a general descriptive term that includes Crohn's disease and ulcerative colitis. Both conditions are chronic, relapsing inflammatory disorders of unknown etiology.

Crohn's disease is an autoimmune disease that can affect any portion of the GI tract from the esophagus to the anus, but most often involves the distal small intestine and colon. Extraintestinal manifestations of Crohn's disease include arthralgias, skin lesions, sclerosing cholangitis, uveitis, and stomatitis.

Ulcerative colitis is a chronic inflammatory disease that affects only the colon and rectum and can involve the entire colon (e.g., pancolitis). The rectum is involved in nearly all cases. Toxic megacolon is a complication of IBD (it is rare with Crohn's disease) that may require admission to the critical care unit, so it is reviewed in detail here.

Etiology and Pathophysiology

Toxic megacolon is a term for acute toxic colitis with dilation of the colon that is often present in patients with ulcerative colitis. It is almost always a complication of pancolitis. Pathologic analysis reveals acute inflammation involving all layers of the colon, with variable amounts of necrosis and degeneration.

Clinical Signs and Symptoms

The diagnosis of megacolon is based on clinical history, physical examination, and radiologic studies. Fever, acute abdominal pain, and abdominal distention are the primary symptoms of toxic megacolon. Other symptoms include rectal bleeding, and vomiting. Because high dose corticosteroids are used for treatment of IBD, fever may not be present.

If bowel perforation occurs, physical findings include abdominal distension, hypoactive bowel sounds, and peritoneal signs (e.g., rebound tenderness, abdominal rigidity, pain with movement). The diagnosis of toxic megacolon is confirmed by the presence of marked dilation (greater than 6 cm) of the colon on a single flat-plate radiograph of the abdomen.

Management

Goals of treatment include: reduction of colon distension, correction of fluid and electrolyte imbalances and treatment of toxemia. Medical management includes discontinuation of oral intake and provision of IV fluids, initiation of nasogastric suction, and administration of systemic antibiotics. Intravenous steroids are administered to patients with IBD.

The child requires PN because oral feeding is contraindicated for several days. Complications of high-dose systemic steroids can develop, including leukocytosis, decreased immunologic defenses and diabetes. Continued steroid administration can cause bone demineralization with resultant-vertebral collapse or aseptic necrosis of the femoral heads. Steroids also cause redistribution of body fat, especially in the face (Cushingoid changes), neck, and posterior shoulder area.

When the child is admitted to the critical care unit with the diagnosis of toxic megacolon, the healthcare team should explain the possibility and details of surgery to both the patient and the family. This ensures that the child and family are prepared if a bowel perforation occurs and the child requires urgent surgical intervention.

If toxic megacolon does not resolve with supportive medical therapy or if bowel perforation occurs, emergency surgery is required. Colectomy with an ileostomy will be performed. The child requiring a colectomy should receive careful preoperative preparation, including explanation and demonstration of ileostomy appliances. This preparation should be given a high priority, even when time is limited before the surgery.

Acute Diarrhea

Acute diarrhea is a sudden change in the frequency and consistency of stools.[5] Because many GI fluids contain large amounts of sodium, chloride, hydrogen, and bicarbonate ions, any significant GI fluid loss can result in dehydration and electrolyte imbalances. The severity and type of dehydration resulting from these conditions will be influenced by the volume and content of any replacement fluids administered.

Etiology

In children, diarrhea is most often the result of a viral or bacterial organism (Table 14-12). Rotavirus is the most common inciting pathogen worldwide in children younger than 5 years.[5,48] Two live oral rotavirus vaccines (Rota Teq, Merck, Sharp and Dohme, Merck Incorporated, Whitehouse, NJ; and Rotarex, GlaxoSmithKline, Research Triangle Park NC), have been approved by the Food and Drug Administration for use in the United States, and current recommendations are to immunize all children for rotavirus starting at 2 months of age.[1,48]

Table 14-12 **Infectious Causes of Acute Diarrhea**

Agents	Pathology	Characteristics	Comments
Viral			
Rotavirus Incubation: 48 h Diagnosis: EIA	Fecal-oral transmission Seven groups (A-G): most group A virus replicates in mature villous epithelial cells of small intestine; leads to (1) imbalance in ratio of intestinal fluid absorption to secretion and (2) malabsorption of complex carbohydrates	Mild to moderate fever Vomiting followed by the onset of watery stools Fever and vomiting generally abate in approximately 2 days but diarrhea persists 5-7 days	Most common cause of diarrhea in children <5 years of age Infants 6-12 months are most vulnerable Peak occurrences in winter months Important cause of nosocomial infections Affects all ages; usually milder in children >3 years of age; immunocompromised children at greater risk for complications
Norwalk-like organisms Incubation: 12-48 h Also called *caliciviruses* Diagnosis: EIA	Fecal-oral; contaminated water Pathology similar to rotavirus: affects villous epithelial cells of small intestine and leads to (1) imbalance in ratio of intestinal fluid absorption to secretion and (2) malabsorption of complex carbohydrates	Abdominal cramps, nausea, vomiting, malaise, low-grade fever, watery diarrhea without blood; duration brief (2-3 days); tends to resemble so-called food poisoning symptoms, with nausea predominating	Affects all ages Multiple strains often named for the location of outbreak (e.g., Norwalk, Sapporo, Snow Mountain, Montgomery)
Bacterial			
Escherichia coli Incubation: 3-4 days Variable depending on strain Diagnosis: Sorbitol MacConkey agar (SMAC agar) positive for blood but fecal leukocytes are absent or rare	*E. coli* strains produce diarrhea as result of enterotoxin production, adherence, or invasion (ETEC) EHEC Enteroaggregative *E. coli*	Watery diarrhea 1-2 days, then severe abdominal cramping and bloody diarrhea Can progress to HUS	Foodborne pathogen Traveler's diarrhea Highest incidence in summer Cause of nursery epidemics Symptomatic treatment Antibiotics may worsen course Antimotility agents and opioids should be avoided

Continued

Table 14-12   Infectious Causes of Acute Diarrhea—cont'd

Agents	Pathology	Characteristics	Comments
Salmonella groups			
Nontyphoidal; gram-negative rods, nonencapsulated nonsporulating Incubation: 6-72 h Diagnosis: gram-stained stool culture	Invasion of mucosa in the small and large intestine; edema of the lamina propria; focal acute inflammation with disruption of the mucosa and micro abscesses	Nausea, vomiting, colicky abdominal pain, bloody diarrhea, fever; symptoms variable, mild to severe May have headache and cerebral manifestations (e.g., drowsiness confusion, meningismus, seizures) Infants may be in afebrile and nontoxic condition May result in life-threatening septicemia and meningitis Nausea and vomiting typically short duration; diarrhea may persist as long as 2-3 weeks Typically shed virus for average of 5 weeks; cases reported up to 1 year	Incidence highest in warm months: July to November Foodborne outbreaks common Usually transmitted person to person, but may transmit via undercooked meats or poultry Poultry and poultry products cause approximately half of cases In children: transmission from pets (e.g., dogs, cats, hamsters, turtles) possible Communicable as long as organisms are excreted Antibiotics not recommended in uncomplicated cases Antimotility agents also not recommended—prolong transit time and carrier state Incidence has decreased over past 10 years
Salmonella typhii			
Produces enteric fever, systemic syndrome Incubation is usually 7-14 days, but could be 3-30 days depending on size of inoculum Diagnosis: positive blood cultures; also sometimes positive stool and urine Late stage: positive bone marrow culture	Bloodstream invasion; after ingestion, organisms attach to microvilli of ileal brush borders and bacteria invade the intestinal epithelium via Peyer's patches Next, they are transported to intestinal lymph nodes and enter bloodstream via thoracic ducts, and circulating organisms reach reticuloendothelial cells causing bacteremia	Manifestations depend on age Abdominal pain, diarrhea, nausea vomiting, high fever, lethargy Must be treated with antibiotics	Incidence is much lower in developed countries; United States has approximately 400 cases per year 65% of US cases acquired via international cases Ingestion of foods or water contaminated with human feces is most common mode of transmission Congenital and intrapartum transmission can occur Three vaccines are available
Shigella groups			
Gram-negative Nonmotile Anaerobic bacilli Incubation: 1-7 days Diagnosis: stool culture loaded with polymorphonuclear leukocytes	Enterotoxins: invades the epithelium with superficial mucosal ulcerations	Patients appear sick Symptoms begin with fever, fatigue, anorexia Crampy abdominal pain precedes watery or bloody diarrhea Symptoms usually subside in 5-10 days	Most cases in children younger than 9 years, with approximately one third of cases in children ages 1-4 weeks Antibiotics shorten illness and lower mortality All patients are at risk for dehydration Acute symptoms may persist for a week or more Antidiarrheal medications not recommended; may predispose to toxic megacolon

Table 14-12 **Infectious Causes of Acute Diarrhea—cont'd**

Agents	Pathology	Characteristics	Comments
Yersinia enterocolitis Incubation period: dose-dependent, 1-3 weeks Diagnosis: stool culture serology; ELISA Patients have leukocytosis; elevated sedimentation rate	Pathology is poorly understood; believed to involve production of enterotoxin	Mucoid diarrhea, sometimes bloody; abdominal pain suggestive of appendicitis; fever, vomiting	Seen more frequently in the winter months Transmitted by pets and food Antibiotics usually do not alter the clinical course in uncomplicated cases; antibiotics should be used in complicated infections and compromised hosts
Campylobacter jejuni Microaerophilic, motile, gram-negative bacilli Incubation period: 1-7 days Ability to cause illness appears dose related Diagnosis by stool culture, sometimes in the blood Commonly found in GI tract of wild or domestic animals	Not fully understood; Possibly (1) adherence to intestinal mucosa by toxin; (2) invasion of the mucosa in the terminal ileum and colon; (3) translocation in which the organisms penetrate the mucosa and replicate in the lamina propria	Fever, abdominal pain, diarrhea, can be bloody; vomiting Watery, profuse, foul-smelling diarrhea Clinically like *Salmonella* or *Shigella* spp. infection Fecal-oral transmission	Most infections in humans relate to consumption of contaminated foods or water, undercooked meats (particularly chicken) Also acquired from contaminated household pets (e.g., dogs, cats, hamsters) Bimodal peaks in infants younger than 1 year and again at 15-29 years Antibiotics do not prolong the carriage of bacteria and may eliminate organism more quickly Erythromycin is the drug of choice Antimotility agents not recommended and tend to prolong symptoms
Vibrio cholerae Gram-negative, motile, curved bacillus living in bodies of salt water Incubation 1-3 days Diagnosis by stool culture	Enters via oral route in contaminated food or water; if it survives acid stomach environment, it travels to the small intestine, adheres to the mucosa, and produces toxin	Onset abrupt; vomiting, watery diarrhea without cramping or tenesmus Dehydration can occur quickly	More prevalent in developing countries Rehydration most important treatment Antibiotics can shorten diarrhea Despite continued efforts still no vaccine
Clostridium difficile Gram-positive anaerobic bacillus Diagnosis by detecting *C. difficile* toxin in stool culture	Produces two important toxins (A and B) Toxin binds to the enterocyte surface receptor resulting in alteration in permeability, protein synthesis, and direct cytotoxicity	Most mild watery diarrhea lasting few days Some prolonged diarrhea and illness May cause pseudomembranous colitis Some individuals are extremely ill with high fever, leukocytosis, hypoalbuminemia	Associated with alteration of normal intestinal flora by antibiotics Adults tend to have more severe symptoms than children Treatment with antibiotics in symptomatic patients—metronidazole Resistant strains have developed Relapse is common

Continued

Table 14-12   Infectious Causes of Acute Diarrhea—cont'd

Agents	Pathology	Characteristics	Comments
Clostridium perfringens Incubation period: 8-24 h; Gram-positive, anaerobic, spore-producing bacilli	Toxins produced in the intestine after ingestion of organism	Acute onset; watery diarrhea, crampy abdominal pain Fever, nausea, and vomiting rare Duration of illness usually 24 h	Transmitted by contaminated food products, most often meats and poultry Usually self-limiting and medical intervention not needed Oral rehydration usually sufficient Antibiotics serve no purpose and should not be used
Clostridium botulinum Incubation period: 12-26 h (range, 6 h to 8 days) Gram-positive, anaerobic, spore-producing bacilli Blood and stool culture should be obtained and transmitted to special laboratory (usually state health department) to detect toxin	Botulism caused by binding of toxin to the neuromuscular junction	Clinical presentation related to age and the strain of the botulism Gastrointestinal: abdominal pain, cramping, and diarrhea Other strains: respiratory, compromise, central nervous system symptoms	Transmitted in contaminated food products Can be acquired via wound infection Treatment involves supportive care and neutralization of the toxin
Staphylococcus spp. Incubation period is generally short, 1-8 h Gram-positive nonmotile, aerobic, or facultative anaerobic bacteria Diagnosis by identifying organism in food, blood, pus, aspirate	Direct tissue invasion and production of toxin	Clinical presentation depends on site of entry In food poisoning, profuse diarrhea, nausea, and vomiting	Gastrointestinal illness transmitted in inadequately cooked or refrigerated foods Self-limiting in gastrointestinal illness Symptomatic treatment

From Wilson D, Hockenberry MJ: *Wong's clinical manual of pediatric nursing*, ed 7, St Louis, 2008, Mosby; Baker RAU, Mondozzi MA, Hockenberry MJ: Infectious causes of acute diarrhea conditions that produce fluid and electrolyte imbalance. In Hockenberry MJ, Wilson D, editors: *Wong's nursing care of infants and children*, ed 8, St Louis, 2007, Mosby-Elsevier.
EHEC, Enterohemorrhagic *E. coli*; *EIA,* enzyme immunoassay; *ELISA,* enzyme-linked immunosorbent assay; *ETEC,* enterotoxigenic-producing; *GI,* gastrointestinal; *HUS,* hemolytic uremic syndrome.

Clostridium difficile is a common cause of antibiotic-associated diarrhea. This gram-positive organism is part of the normal GI bacterial flora, but antibiotics and some other medications and conditions can disrupt normal bacterial flora and allow some organisms to grow unchecked. Hospitalized children at risk for *C. difficile* disease include those receiving antimicrobial agents. Additional conditions that increase risk for this organism include recent abdominal surgery, presence of a feeding tube, and decreased stomach acidity from the administration of histamine type 2 antagonists and proton pump inhibitors.[50] Medications that increase GI motility (e.g., docusate [Colace], polyethylene glycol [MiraLax]) can also cause diarrhea.

Milk intolerance and dietary changes, such as changing formula and introducing new foods, can lead to diarrhea. Often children with failure to thrive are fed with concentrated formulas (up to 30 Kcal/ounce), and they may develop diarrhea from the hyperosmolar formulas and overfeeding. Some disease processes, including inflammatory bowel disease and Hirschsprung disease, may increase risk for colitis that can be life threatening.

Pathophysiology

Acute diarrhea alters the GI tract and can lead to dehydration. Dehydration is present when the total output of all fluids and electrolytes exceeds the total fluid intake. Dehydrated patients are deficient in both fluids and electrolytes. Dehydration is classified according to severity, based on clinical examination, and according to effects on the serum sodium and osmolality (see Dehydration and Hypovolemia in Chapter 12).

Clinical Signs and Symptoms

All children with diarrhea and dehydration will have a history of inadequate fluid intake and excessive fluid loss. The child may be febrile and usually is irritable and looks ill; there may or may not be associated vomiting. Initial clinical signs produced by dehydration can be difficult to separate from those produced by meningitis, because both can include a history of fever and irritability. However, a careful examination will reveal signs of dehydration, including sunken eyes, dry mucous membranes, and a sunken fontanelle in infants. The child will be tachycardic, and signs of compensated or hypotensive shock may be present. For further information, see Shock in Chapter 6 and Dehydration and Hypovolemia in Chapter 12.

The characteristics of the diarrhea stool can vary depending on the pathogen (see Table 14-12). If there is blood or mucous in the stool, stool studies should be obtained. The stool should be sent to identify stool pH, presence of reducing substance, presence of white blood cells, and *C. difficile* toxin and to check for ova and parasites and perform culture and sensitivity studies.

Initial diagnostic studies typically include evaluation of a serum chemistry panel and a complete blood cell count. Once the serum sodium concentration is determined, the estimate of the severity of dehydration (based initially on clinical examination alone) is modified as needed. Often these children have a metabolic acidosis, which may be evident from the low carbon dioxide level on the chemistry panel.

Management

The goals of the treatment of dehydration include restoration and maintenance of intravascular volume and systemic perfusion, and correction of abnormal serum electrolytes. If shock is present a urinary catheter is placed to enable continuous evaluation of urine production. Urine output should average approximately 0.5-1.0 mL/kg per hour. If urine output does not improve despite the presence of adequate systemic perfusion, notify an on-call provider immediately, because renal failure may be present (see Acute Renal Failure and Acute Kidney Injury in Chapter 13).

Treatment of dehydration requires replacement of the fluid deficit and any ongoing losses, and provision of maintenance fluid requirements. Regardless of the type of dehydration present, moderate or severe dehydration requires establishment of reliable vascular (IV or intraosseous) access. Children with mild dehydration may be able to replenish fluid losses with oral rehydration solutions, offered in small increments of 5-30 mL.

The child with moderate to severe dehydration will require IV fluid resuscitation with initial boluses (20 mL/kg) of isotonic crystalloids such as normal saline or Ringer's lactate. Fluid boluses are repeated until systemic perfusion improves, with normalization of vital signs and urine output. Monitor the child's systemic perfusion and continue fluid resuscitation as long as signs of shock are present.

It is important to monitor the child's response throughout therapy. If the shock is corrected and rehydration is successful, systemic perfusion, neurologic function, acid-base and electrolyte balance, and urine output should all improve (for further information, see Shock in Chapter 6 and Dehydration and Hypovolemia in Chapter 12).

Children with diarrhea from a bacterial cause require contact isolation until antibiotic therapy is complete. When diarrhea

has a viral cause, contact isolation is maintained until the symptoms resolve. Contact isolation must be enforced with meticulous attention to hand washing, because most of these organisms are contagious and are a frequent cause of healthcare-acquired infection.

Obtain an accurate weight as soon as possible after admission. This weight measurement can be helpful in determining the severity of dehydration and evaluating the patient's response to therapy. Weight measurements are most reliable if the child is weighed using the same scale and technique at the same time every day. The nurse should carefully record intake and output and notify the on-call provider if the child's urine output is less than the 0.5 to 1 mL/kg hour.

Monitor the child's temperature throughout therapy. Young infants should be resuscitated under a warmer to prevent cold stress. If the infant is profoundly hypothermic, it may be necessary to warm resuscitation fluids before administration.

Treatment becomes supportive as diarrhea resolves. Initially, when stools are frequent and watery, the child receives nothing by mouth and maintenance fluid requirements are provided intravenously. The irritated GI tract requires a period of rest, followed by the gradual resumption of oral feedings with oral electrolyte solutions. Once stool output has decreased and the child is no longer vomiting, clear liquids are offered and enteral feeding can be advanced slowly as tolerated to an age-appropriate diet. If diarrhea resumes during diet advancement, the child should be placed back on a clear diet or the last tolerated intake.

Although the majority of acute diarrhea episodes are caused by viral pathogens, antimicrobial agents are administered for some bacteria or culture-proven parasitic infections. For culture-positive *C. difficile* infection, the causative antibiotic is discontinued if possible, and a 7-day oral course of metronidazole (Flagyl) is provided.[50] Oral vancomycin can also be administered to patients who cannot tolerate metronidazole or any adolescent patients who are breastfeeding or pregnant.[50]

For the child who is experiencing concomitant vomiting and diarrhea, ondansetron (Zofran) can help with symptom control. For children with mild dehydration, the medication can be administered orally in the form of an oral disintegrating tablet; IV administration is recommended for children with moderate or severe dehydration.

DIAGNOSTIC TESTING

Several abdominal imaging options are available for the evaluation of suspected abdominal pathology. The selection of imaging mode is based on patient symptoms, clinical examination findings, and the differential diagnosis. Each type of study has advantages and disadvantages. Three of the most common modalities used for abdominal imaging are abdominal plain films, CT, and ultrasound.

Abdominal Plain Film

Abdominal plain films are frequently the first radiologic images obtained when abdominal pathology is suspected. Abdominal plain films are readily available, noninvasive, inexpensive, require no patient preparation, and can be obtained with portable machines in a timely manner. To review principles of interpretation of radiographs, refer to Chapter 10.

On a plain film, air appears black against a background of white and grey representing bony and soft tissue structures. This color contrast allows assessment of the distribution of air in the GI tract (see Fig. 14-15, A). Anteroposterior (AP) views are generally ordered for abdominal films, with specific positioning options such as spine, upright, and lateral decubitus. These positioning strategies are implemented to assess the distribution of air and fluid that change because of gravity. Free air rises, so when free intraperitoneal air is present it will rise to the highest location within the abdomen. With upright imaging, free intra-abdominal air will be visible just below the diaphragm. When an upright image is not possible because the patient is unstable, the lateral decubitus film is used. When the patient is placed with the left side down (left lateral decubitus), free air will appear as a dark border (air) outlining the light tissue density of the liver. Free fluid in the abdominal cavity will also be affected by gravity and will assume a dependent position.

Air fluid levels refer to a visible demarcation where air and fluid meet. When present, an air fluid level can be diagnostic of a bowel obstruction (see Fig. 14-15, B and C).

Abdominal plain films can serve as a triage tool for further evaluation of patients with an acute condition in the abdomen, especially with perforation of hollow viscera or intestinal obstruction.[26]

Abdominal Computed Tomography

The cross-sectional images, or slices, produced by CT can provide spatial detail and allow better differentiation of soft-tissue densities than do other modes of imaging. These qualities make CT scans extremely useful in patients with complex disease affecting multiple organ systems.

The use of a contrast agent for CT imaging of the abdomen can optimize the imaging and subsequent interpretation. The contrast agent can be administered via IV, oral, or rectal routes, and often studies will use a combination of these options. Decisions regarding the use of a contrast agent are based on the clinical entity to be evaluated. IV contrast outlines vessels to highlight their size, patency, and relationship to intraabdominal organs. When evaluating a tumor or abdominal mass, IV contrast allows visualization of the blood supply feeding the tumor. Oral contrast delineates the small and large bowel from intraabdominal masses and can identify fluid collections such as a perforated appendix. Rectal contrast can be used when pelvic pathology is suspected or for enhanced visualization of the lower GI tract.

There are several important considerations for use of oral contrast. Oral contrast takes time to flow through the GI tract. After administration, bowel opacification takes 60 to 90 min. To achieve maximal benefit, an adequate volume of contrast is needed, and the amount varies by age. In general, a contrast volume of 60 to 90 mL is used for patients younger than 1 month, and up to 1 L of contrast can be used for the adolescent patient. In patients experiencing nausea and vomiting, ingestion of the contrast can be difficult

if not impossible, so administration via a nasogastric tube can be helpful.

If barium-based contrast extravasates outside of the GI lumen (e.g., as in a patient with bowel perforation), it can induce severe intraperitoneal inflammation. If aspirated, contrast can cause severe pneumonia. Diatrizoic acid (Gastrografin), a dilute water-soluble contrast, is used in cases of possible bowel perforation or when there is risk of aspiration. Although Gastrografin is considered safer under these conditions, it does result in low-quality imaging.

IV contrast is iodine-based, so patients with seafood or iodine allergies must be premedicated to avoid an allergic reaction. IV contrast is cleared by the kidneys and requires adequate renal function. The nurse or other providers should verify appropriate blood urea nitrogen and serum creatinine concentration before the contrast injection. A large bore (22-gauge) IV catheter is required for administration of contrast, because power injectors are often used to ensure accurate timing between contrast administration and imaging.[57]

Oral or IV contrast administration can cause delays in obtaining CT images, delaying diagnosis and treatment. Collaboration and coordinated timing with the radiology department is essential.

Patient movement during the study can negatively affect image quality, so sedation is recommended for children younger than 5 years or when patients are unable to cooperate with the procedure. Nothing-by-mouth status is recommended before CT imaging to minimize risks of vomiting the oral contrast. Studies have shown no increase in risk of aspiration when sedation is started after administering oral contrast.[57]

Exposure to ionizing radiation is a serious risk associated with CT imaging. In children, this radiation exposure can increase the risk of cancer.[57] Caution and careful consideration should be taken before radiation exposure. For pediatric patients the dose of radiation can be decreased, because children have less body mass than adults. Studies limited to the specific areas of interest (i.e., pelvic CT versus full abdominal CT) will decrease radiation exposure.

CT technology continues to improve with the advent of multidetector CT scanners. This technology speeds image acquisition and will decrease artifacts associated with patient motion, such as breathing. This technology also maximizes contrast vascular enhancement. High-quality, three-dimensional images can be reconstructed, thus enhancing the diagnostic capabilities of this scanner. One of the biggest advantages for pediatric patients is a shorter scan time, so less sedation is needed.[57]

Abdominal Ultrasound

Ultrasound examination uses reflected sound waves to produce real-time pictures and excellent visualization (i.e., imaging) of the liver, kidneys, gallbladder, spleen, pancreas, and female pelvis.[7] Different tissues (fluid, air, bone) reflect sound waves differently, so transmission and recording of reflected sound waves will produce outlines of structures on the ultrasound screen. Ultrasound with color Doppler capability can be used to evaluate blood flow characteristics and patency of blood vessels. One frequent application of this feature is to rule out the possibility of a deep vein thrombus.

Advantages of ultrasound include: portability, no exposure to ionizing radiation, and minimal if any patient preparation. Limitations of this imaging mode include inconsistent quality of study; quality is highly dependent on the operator. Ultrasound also requires patient cooperation—the patient must remain still and tolerate the compression of sensitive areas. Finally, ultrasound is less sensitive in obese patients and in patients with excessive bowel gas.

References

1. American Academy of Pediatrics Committee on Infectious Disease: Prevention of rotavirus disease: guidelines for use of rotavirus vaccine. *Pediatrics* 119:171, 2007.
2. American Academy of Pediatrics Subcommittee on Hyperbilirubinemia: Management of hyperbilirubinemia in the newborn infant 35 or more weeks of gestation. *Pediatrics* 114:297, 2004.
3. American Academy of Pediatrics Subcommittee on Hyperbilirubinemia: Neonatal jaundice and kernicterus. *Pediatrics* 108:763, 2001.
4. Arensman RM, Browne M, Madonna MB: Gastrointestinal bleeding. In Grosfeld JL et al, editors: *Pediatric surgery*, ed 6, Philadelphia, 2006, Mosby.
5. Baker RAU, Mondozzi MA, Hockenberry MJ: Conditions that produce fluid and electrolyte imbalance. In Hockenberry MJ, Wilson D, editors: *Wong's nursing care of infants and children*, ed 8, St Louis, 2007, Mosby-Elsevier.
6. Bell M, et al: Neonatal necrotizing enterocolitis. Therapeutic decisions based upon clinical staging. *Ann Surg* 187:1–7, 1978.
7. Bloom DA, Siegel MJ: Acute abdominal pain in childhood. In Bluth EI et al, editors: *Ultrasound: a practical approach to clinical problems*, ed 2, New York, 2008, Thieme Medical Publishers.
8. Butterworth RF: Hepatic encephalopathy. *Alcohol Res Health* 27:240, 2003.
9. Chang M: Hepatitis B virus infection. *Semin Fetal Neonatal Med* 12:160, 2007.
10. Cohran VC, Kocoshis SA: Short bowel. In Baker S, Baker R, Davis A, editors: *Pediatric nutrition support*, ed 1, Sudbury, MA, 2007, Jones and Bartlett.
11. Colletti JE, et al: An emergency medicine approach to neonatal hyperbilirubinema. *Emerg Med Clin N Am* 25:1117, 2007.
12. Czako L, et al: Interactions between endocrine and exocrine pancreas and their clinical relevance. *Pancreatology* 9:351, 2009.
13. Dasgupta R, et al: Effectiveness of REX shunt in the treatment of portal hypertension. *J Ped Surg* 41:108, 2006.
14. Deerojanawong J, et al: Incidence and risk factors of upper gastrointestinal bleeding in mechanically ventilated children. *Pediatr Crit Care Med* 10:91, 2009.
15. Faint V: The pathophysiology of hepatic encephalopathy. *Nurs Crit Care* 11:69, 2006.
16. Fischler B: Hepatitis C virus infection. *Semin Fetal Neonatal Med* 12:168, 2007.
17. Fishbein TM, Matsumoto CS: Intestinal replacement therapy: timing and indications for referral of patients to an intestinal rehabilitation and transplant program. *Gastroenterology* 130:S147–S151, 2006.
18. Flanigan LM: Biliary atresia and choledochal cyst. In Brown NT et al, editors: *Nursing care of the pediatric surgical patient*, ed 2, Sudbury, MA, 2007, Jones and Bartlett.
19. Gavaghan M: The pancreas-hermit of the abdomen. *AORN J* 75:1109, 2002.
20. Giannone PJ, et al: Necrotizing enterocolitis in neonates with congenital heart disease. *Life Sci* 82:341, 2008.
21. Gordon PV, et al: Emerging trends in acquired neonatal intestinal disease: is it time to abandon Bell's criteria? *J Perinatol* 27:661, 2007.
22. Goulet O, et al: Irreversible intestinal failure. *J Pediatr Gastroenterol Nutr* 38:250, 2004.
23. Han MK, Hyzy R: Advances in critical care management of hepatic failure and insufficiency. *Crit Care Med* 34:S225, 2006.
24. Heller S, Valencia-Mayoral P: Treatment of viral hepatitis in children. *Arch Med Res* 38:702, 2002.
25. Henry MCW, Moss LR: Current issues in the management of necrotizing enterocolitis. *Semin Perinatol* 28:221, 2004.
26. Hernanz-Schulman M, Spottswood S: Gastrointestinal tract. In Slovis TL, editor: *Caffey's pediatric diagnostic imaging*, ed 2, Philadelphia, 2008, Mosby.
27. Huether SE: Structure and function of the digestive system. In McCance K, Huether SE, editors: *Pathophysiology: the basis for disease in adults and children*, ed 5, St Louis, 2006, Elsevier.
28. Ip S, et al.: An evidence-based review of important issues concerning neonatal hyperbilirubinemia. *Pediatrics* 114:e130, 2004.
29. Iyer KR, Richard M: Surgery for intestinal failure. In Matrese LE, Steiger E, Seidner DL, editors: *Intestinal failure and rehabilitation: a clinical guide*, Boca Raton, FL, 2005, CRC Press.
30. Joffe A, et al.: Nutritional support for critically ill children (review). *Cochrane Database Syst Rev* Apr 15; (2): CD005144, 2009.
30a. Kamath BM, Olthoff KM: Liver transplantation in children: update 2010. *Pediatr Clin North Am* 57(2):401–414, 2010.
31. Kelly DA: Managing acute liver failure. *Current Paediatr* 11:96–101, 2001.
32. Khan AN, Macdonald S, Howat J: Small-bowel obstruction, 2009. Available at http:emedicine.medscape.com/article/374962. Accessed October 3, 2011, Updated July 22, 2001.
33. Kyle UG, et al.: Organ dysfunction is associated with hyperglycemia in critically ill children. *Intens Care Med* 36:312–320, 2010.
34. Lee CK, Jonas MM: Pediatric hepatobiliary disease. *Curr Opin Gastroenterol* 23:306, 2007.
35. Leonis MA, Balistreri WF: Evaluation and management of end-stage liver disease in children. *Gastroenterology* 143:1741, 2008.
36. Lerret SM, Skelton JA: Pediatric nonalcoholic fatty liver disease. *Gastroenterol Nurs* 31:115, 2008.
37. Lin PW, Stoll BJ: Necrotising enterocolitis. *Lancet* 368:1271, 2006.
38. Lopez-Herce J: Gastrointestinal complications in critically ill patient: what differs between adults and children? *Curr Opin Clin Nutr Metab Care* 12:180, 2009.
39. Louie JP: Essential diagnosis of abdominal emergencies in the first year of life. *Emerg Med Clin N Am* 25:1009, 2007.
40. Mack CL, Sokol RJ: Unraveling the pathogenesis and etiology of biliary atresia. *Pediatr Rev* 57:87R, 2005.
41. Maisels MJ: A primer on phototherapy for the jaundiced infant. *Contemp Pediatr* 22:38, 2005.
42. Maisels MJ, McDonagh AF: Phototherapy for neonatal jaundice. *N Eng J Med* 358:920, 2008.
43. Martin SA, Simone S: Gastrointestinal system. In Slota MC, editor: *Core curriculum for pediatric critical care nursing*, ed 2, St Louis, 2006, Elsevier.
44. Mehta NM, Compher,: C A.S.P.E.N. Board of Directors: A.S.P.E.N. clinical guidelines: nutrition support of the critically ill child. *JPEN J Parenter Enteral Nutr* 33:260, 2009.
45. Metheny NA: Residual volume measurement should be retained in enteral feeding protocols. *Am J Crit Care* 17:62, 2008.
46. Moyer MS, Warner B: Surgical disorders. In Kleinman RE, et al, editors: *Walker's pediatric gastrointestinal disease: physiology, diagnosis and management*, ed 5, Ontario, Canada, 2008, B.C. Decker, Incorporated, Hamilton.
47. Nithiwathanapong C, Reungrongrat S, Ukarapol N: Prevalence and risk factors of stress induced gastrointestinal bleeding in critically ill children. *World J Gastrol* 11:6839, 2005.
48. Parez N: Rotavirus gastroenteritis: why to back up the development of new vaccines? *Comp Immun Microbiol Infec Dis* 31:253, 2008.
49. Patole S: Prevention and treatment of necrotizing enterocolitis in preterm neonates. *Early Hum Devel* 83:635, 2007.
50. Pelleschi ME: *Clostridium difficile*-associated disease diagnosis, prevention, treatment, and nursing care. *Crit Care Nurs* 28:27, 2008.
51. Pierro A, Hall NJ, Chowdhury MM: Gastrointestinal surgery in the neonate. *Curr Paedeatr* 16:153, 2006.
52. Pietzak TT, Thomas DW: Pancreatitis in childhood. *Pediatr Rev* 21:406, 2000.
53. Quiros-Tejeira RE, et al: Long-term parenteral nutritional support and intestinal adaptation in children with short bowel syndrome: a 25-year experience. *J Pediatr* 145:157, 2004.
54. Reyes JD: Intestinal transplantation. *Semin Pediart Surg* 15:228, 2006.
55. Ryckman FC, Alonso MH: Causes and management of portal hypertension in the pediatric population. *Clin Liver Dis* 5:789, 2001.
56. Sehgal S, Allen PLJ: Hepatitis C in children. *Pediatr Nurs* 20:409, 2004.
57. Siegel MJ: Practical CT techniques. In Siegel MJ, editor: *Pediatric body CT*, ed 2, Philadelphia, 2008, Lippincott.

58. Sims RJM, Woodgate RL: Managing chronic hepatitis B in children. *J Pediatr Health Care* 22:360, 2008.

59. Slowik MK, Jhaveri R: Hepatitis B and C viruses in infants and young children. *Semin Pediatr Infect Dis* 16:296, 2005.

60. Srinivasan PS, Brandler MD, D'Souza A: Necrotizing enterocolitis. *Clin Perinatol* 35:251, 2008.

61. Superina R: Portal hypertension. In Grosfeld JL et al, editors: *Pediatric surgery*, ed 6, Philadelphia, 2006, Mosby.

62. Teitelbaum DH, Coran AG: Nutritional support. In Grosfeld JL et al, editors: *Pediatric surgery*, ed 6, Philadelphia, 2006, Mosby.

63. Wennberg RP, et al.: Toward understanding kernicterus: a challenge to improve the management of jaundiced newborns. *Pediatrics* 117:474, 2006.

64. Yazigi NA, Balistreri WF: Acute and chronic viral hepatitis. In Suchy FJ, Sokol RJ, Balistreri WF, editors: *Liver disease in children*, ed 2, Philadelphia, 2001, Lippincott Williams and Wilkins.

Hematologic and Oncologic Emergencies Requiring Critical Care

15

Michelle Lynn Burke • Deborah Salani

ⓔvolve Be sure to check out the supplementary content available at http://evolve.elsevier.com/Hazinski.

PEARLS

- Severe anemia associated with a hemoglobin (Hgb) concentration less than 5 g/dL and a hematocrit (Hct) less than 15% is likely to produce congestive heart failure (CHF). Transfuse packed red blood cells (PRBCs) slowly (3 mL/kg per hour).
- Complete bone marrow failure produces a fall in Hgb of approximately 0.7-1 g/dL per day. A more precipitous fall in Hgb is likely to be caused by bleeding or increased red blood cell (RBC) destruction.
- The risk of spontaneous bleeding is increased if the platelet count is less than 20,000/mm^3 and intracranial hemorrhage is more likely once the platelet count is less than 5000/mm^3.
- Rule out intracranial hemorrhage in any child with severe thrombocytopenia and unilateral headache. If hemorrhage is suspected, you will often need to begin to stabilize first; obtain scans and radiographs later.
- Acute tumor lysis syndrome produces hypocalcemia, hyperkalemia, hyperuricemia, and hyperphosphatemia. Disseminated intravascular coagulation (DIC) is also possible.
- An absolute neutrophil count less than 500/mm^3 is associated with a significant risk of infection. Monitor these patients closely for evidence of infection.
- Whenever blood products are administered, label the crossmatch specimen carefully at the bedside and double-check patient and blood product identification (an extra time).

ESSENTIAL ANATOMY AND PHYSIOLOGY

Blood Components

Blood is the fluid that sustains life. This highly specialized body fluid has many functions, including transporting oxygen and nutrition, eliminating waste, acid-base buffering, and maintaining homeostasis. The hematopoietic system consists of the bone marrow, liver, spleen, lymph nodes, and thymus gland.[27] Each of these components plays a specific role in the regulation of blood.

Blood is composed of a liquid phase called *plasma* and a formed or cellular phase. Approximately 90% of plasma consists of water, and the remaining portions are solutes including factors that form clots (e.g., clotting factors, fibrinogen, globulins) and serum that contains electrolytes, hormones, antibodies, nutrients, and other factors. The cellular portion of the blood consists of the formed elements: RBCs, white blood cells (WBCs), and platelets (for an illustration, refer to Evolve Fig. 15-1 in the Chapter 15 Supplement on the Evolve Website).

The body's first hematopoietic stem cell is produced in the yolk sac of the embryo. The fetal liver becomes the site for hematopoiesis at approximately the second month of fetal life. The liver is the main organ producing blood cells from the second to the fifth month of fetal life.[27] At approximately the fourth month, the bone marrow begins producing blood cells and remains the production site throughout life. Bone marrow, one of the largest organs in the body, is located in the cavities of all bones.

Hematopoiesis consists of the production, differentiation, and development of blood cells; it normally occurs in the bone marrow.[27] RBCs, WBCs, and platelets are all thought to arise from multipotential stem cells that inhabit the bone marrow. These stem cells have the ability to differentiate into any of the three cell lines, based on the needs of the body. The process of cell differentiation by the pluripotent stem cell is normally (i.e., in the absence of disease) self regulatory. In children, all bones produce blood cells. When bone growth ceases, often by 18 years old, only the ribs, sternum, vertebrae, and pelvis continue to produce blood cells.[27]

The lymphatic system—the lymph fluid, lymph structures and nodes, spleen, tonsils and thymus—plays an important role in the regulation of blood cells in hematopoiesis. However, the lymphatic system does not produce the blood cells.

The formed elements of the hematopoietic system are the RBCs, WBCs, and platelets. Each has a unique function in the blood. RBCs, also called *erythrocytes,* transport hemoglobin from the lungs to the tissues. Hemoglobin (Hgb) is the iron-containing pigment of RBCs. The hematocrit (Hct), or packed cell volume (PCV), is a measure of the proportion of RBCs present in the blood. As a general rule, the Hct is normally three times the Hgb concentration (in grams per deciliter).

When the Hgb and Hct are abnormally high, this condition is called *polycythemia.* Polycythemia may be present in children with cyanotic congenital heart defects and in newborn infants. A relative polycythemia can be seen in dehydrated patients, but this represents a deficit in intravascular fluid rather than an excess of RBCs.

When the Hgb and Hct are abnormally low, this condition is known as *anemia.* Anemia can result from an acute episode of bleeding or from other causes such as increased destruction of the RBCs or decreased production. When anemia develops gradually it may be asymptomatic, whereas acute (e.g., after hemorrhage) or severe anemia often produce cardiovascular compromise.

825

After RBCs are made in the bone marrow, they normally extrude their nuclei before reaching the peripheral circulation. Nucleated RBCs can be found in the peripheral blood at times of increased RBC production, including the neonatal period. Young, developing RBCs are called *reticulocytes*. A reticulocyte count measures the amount of immature RBCs in the blood and can be helpful in determining the cause of an anemia. As a general rule, the reticulocyte count is high when there is increased RBC destruction, and it is low if the bone marrow is not producing cells.

The life span of normal RBCs is approximately 120 days. Transfused RBCs have a shorter life span, as do RBCs in patients with hematologic disease such as sickle cell anemia and thalassemia.

WBCs, also called *leukocytes,* defend the body against infectious agents. Their main function is to fight infection by migrating to the site of inflammation to assist in defending the body against foreign antigens. There are several different types of WBCs, each with a specific purpose. The differential of a complete blood cell count (CBC) reveals the percentages of neutrophils, lymphocytes, monocytes, and eosinophils. The numeric value of the WBCs is not as important as an evaluation of the absolute neutrophil count (ANC), a more accurate measure of the body's ability to fight infection (see Neutrophils below and formula for ANC calculation in Box 15-1).

A WBC such as the large macrophage or monocyte that has an unsegmented nucleus, is a type of mononuclear cell. Some leukocytes contain granules in their cytoplasm; these cell are called *granulocytes* and are divided according to the shape of their nuclei and the staining of the cytoplasmic granules. Neutrophils are granulocytes with segmented nuclei; these cells also are called *polymorphonuclear leukocytes.* Other granulocytes include eosinophils and basophils. Nongranular leukocytes include the monocytes and lymphocytes, which contain clear cytoplasm. The function of each of these WBCs is discussed briefly as follows.

Lymphocytes are an essential part of the immune system. B lymphocytes produce antibodies (immunoglobulins), which are proteins that recognize and bind to bacteria and speed their destruction. T lymphocytes attack viruses, parasites, and other nonbacterial infections and also mediate the rejection of transplanted tissues. In an analogous fashion, foreign T cells introduced into a host by transfusion or transplantation can attack host tissues, producing graft-versus-host disease. A subset of T lymphocytes, T helper cells, is the primary target of the human immunodeficiency virus.

Neutrophils provide the primary defense against bacterial infections, because they engulf and destroy invading organisms. The ANC is determined from a WBC differential by multiplying the percent of neutrophils plus bands by the total WBC count (Box 15-1 shows an example of ANC calculation). In general, children with an ANC of less than 500/mm^3 have a high risk of developing life-threatening bacterial infections. The risk of infection is particularly high in patients with neutropenia as the result of failure of neutrophil production, rather than those with immune-mediated neutropenia.

Monocytes are large mononuclear WBCs that differentiate into macrophages when they leave the vascular space. Both monocytes and macrophages migrate to areas of infection and inflammation, where they play important roles in phagocytosis of bacteria and debris.

Basophils are polymorphonuclear leukocytes that are located in tissue, usually adjacent to small arterioles. They are similar but not identical to mast cells. Substances released by basophils, such as histamine or arachidonic acid, and their metabolites mediate the inflammatory response.

Eosinophils are leukocytes that resemble neutrophils but contain only two nuclear lobes. These cells contain granules that stain red with Wright's stain and are filled with enzymes. Eosinophils contribute to inflammation, and they migrate to areas where antigen-antibody complexes are forming.

Leukemia is cancer of WBCs in which immature lymphoid or myeloid cells (blasts) fill the bone marrow and replace normal cells. Leukemic cells commonly are found in the peripheral circulation and in the marrow.

Platelets are derived from megakaryocytes. Platelets in a true sense are not actually cells, because they lack cellular structure. The primary function of platelets is hemostasis and vascular repair following injury to a vessel well. When there is a site of injury, the platelets aggregate at the site and quickly develop a plug. The life span of a platelet is approximately 7 to 10 days. At any time, approximately one third of all circulatory platelets can be found normally in the spleen. In normal circumstances, platelets are removed by the liver and spleen in 10 days if not utilized in a clotting reaction.

Clotting Cascade

Normal hemostasis is maintained by a complex balance of procoagulant and anticoagulant factors. Together, these factors provide rapid and localized control of bleeding at sites of injury while preventing the clotting process in unaffected tissues. A simplified scheme of the coagulation process is shown in Evolve Fig. 15-2 in the Chapter 15 Supplement on the Evolve Website.

The activated partial thromboplastin time (aPTT) measures activity of the intrinsic and common pathways. This test is useful when screening for deficiencies of most plasma coagulation factors (V, VIII, IX, X, XI and XII, with the exception of factors VII and XIII. Factors VII and XIII are not evaluated with the aPTT; these factors must be activated by tissue injury (the extrinsic pathway). The aPTT may be prolonged

---

Box 15-1   Calculation of Absolute Neutrophil Count

The ANC is the total number of white blood cells multiplied by the percentage (expressed in decimal form) of neutrophils (segs plus bands) to determine the ANC. Here is a sample calculation:

White blood cells = 1100/mm^3
Segs = 11% = 0.11
Bands = 5% = 0.05

ANC = Percent neutrophils × Total WBCs
= (Percent segs + Percent bands) × Total WBCs
= (0.11 + 0.05) × 1100
= 176

ANC, Absolute neutrophil count.

(abnormal) in patients with coagulation factor deficiencies (e.g., hemophilia, von Willebrand disease), in the presence of circulating inhibitors, and in patients receiving heparin.

The prothrombin time (PT) measures activity of the extrinsic and common pathways; this test is used to screen for deficiencies of factors V, VII, and X and to monitor patients receiving warfarin (Coumadin). Either the PT or aPTT, or both, may be abnormal if DIC is present.

Formation of a normal clot requires the conversion of fibrinogen, a soluble clotting protein, into fibrin through the action of the enzyme thrombin. When fibrinogen is broken down, fibrin monomers are formed and will then polymerize with other fibrin monomers to form the latticework of the clot. The presence of fibrin monomer in the blood indicates that the clotting cascade has been activated and clot formation is occurring.

At the same time that fibrin is formed to create a clot, the fibrinolytic system is activated through factor XII, and clot lysis begins. *Fibrin split products* (FSPs) are released as fibrin is broken down by plasmin during clot breakdown. The presence and quantity of FSPs can be used to monitor the degree of activation of the fibrinolytic system. FSPs are quantified using a blood sample sent to the laboratory in a tube containing thrombin (blood always clots in this tube). A rise in FSPs normally is observed after surgery, trauma, or burns, but also may indicate the development of DIC. FSPs are insoluble, but they normally are cleared by the liver. If liver disease is present, the level of FSPs is likely to be higher than normal.

A D-dimer test can be ordered if DIC is suspected. A positive D-dimer means there is an abnormally high level of FSPs in the body, which is indicative of significant clot formation and breakdown. The D-dimer is abnormally high in the presence of DIC, a deep vein thrombosis, or a pulmonary embolus. The D-dimer does indicate clot formation and breakdown, but does not indicate the cause or identify the location.

The Spleen

The spleen is a large vascular organ located in the left upper quadrant of the abdomen behind the stomach and just beneath the left diaphragm. Splenic blood flow is supplied by the splenic artery, which arises from the abdominal aorta via the celiac trunk. Splenic venous return occurs through the portal vein. The spleen serves as a filter for the blood; its network of red pulp, splenic sinuses, splenic cords, and white pulp removes aged and damaged red cells, platelets, and encapsulated bacteria from the circulation. In addition, the spleen is a site of antibody production.

Lack of normal splenic function can result in the persistence of nuclear remnants within RBCs, called *Howell-Jolly bodies*. If these Howell-Jolly bodies are observed microscopically on a peripheral blood sample, true asplenia or splenic dysfunction (functional asplenia) may be present.

The child with asplenia is at increased risk for the development of infection from encapsulated organisms, such as *Haemophilus influenzae* or *Pneumococcus* species. These infections may cause sepsis and septic shock. Pneumococcal vaccination and antibiotic prophylaxis with penicillin decrease the risk of septicemia in patients with both functional and true asplenia.

A palpable spleen is normal in infants and young children. If the spleen tip descends below the edge of the left costal margin in a child older than 6 months, splenomegaly is present. Hypersplenism is enlargement of the spleen, with resultant entrapment and destruction of normal blood cells and consequent reduction in circulating blood cells.

COMMON CLINICAL CONDITIONS

Acute Anemia

Etiology

Anemia is present when the number of circulating RBCs is reduced, resulting in decreased oxygen-carrying capacity of the blood. Anemia is the most common hematologic condition of infancy and childhood. Most patients with anemia have an underlying disease, so anemia is a symptom rather than a disease. Causes of anemia include acute or chronic blood loss, decreased production of RBCs, splenic sequestration, and hemolysis (Box 15-2).

Pathophysiology

Anemia results from blood loss, decreased RBC production, or increased RBC destruction. The pathophysiology of each is different.

Blood Loss. When a patient experiences acute blood loss, the Hgb and Hct are not initially affected because both plasma and RBCs have been lost. If only crystalloid and colloids are

---

Box 15-2 **Etiology of Severe Anemia**

Blood Loss
- Trauma, surgery
- Bleeding disorders (thrombocytopenia, disseminated intravascular coagulation, hemophilia)
- Occult gastrointestinal loss (ulcers, polyps, gastrointestinal bleeding)

Decreased Production
- Bone marrow replacement (leukemia, other malignancies)
- Bone marrow failure (aplastic anemia)
- Bone marrow suppression (chemotherapy, radiation)
- Transient erythroblastopenia of childhood
- Congenital red cell aplasia (Diamond-Blackfan syndrome)
- Aplastic crisis (sickle cell anemia, hemoglobin sickle cell disease, hereditary spherocytosis)

Splenic Sequestration
- Hypersplenism
- Sickle cell anemia, hemoglobin sickle cell disease

Hemolysis
- Transfusion reaction
- Drug induced
- Autoimmune
- Burns
- Infection
- RBC membrane abnormality (hereditary spherocytosis)
- RBC enzyme abnormality (glucose-6-phosphate dehydrogenase deficiency, pyruvate kinase deficiency
- Toxins (spider bite), hemolytic uremic syndrome
- Hemolytic disease of the newborn (Rh incompatibility)
- Neonatal ABO incompatibility

RBC, Red blood cell.

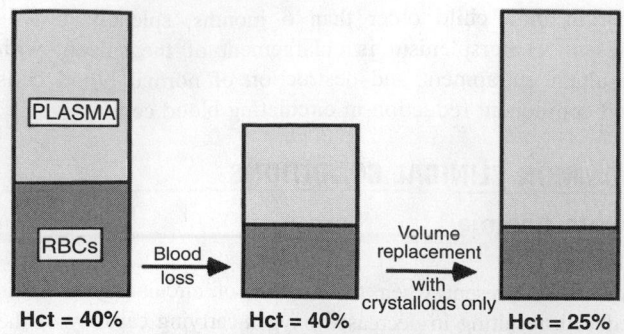

FIG. 15-1 Effects of acute hemorrhage and crystalloid resuscitation on hematocrit. The patient's hematocrit might not decrease initially following hemorrhage, because the loss of red blood cells is proportional to the loss of plasma. However, replacing the whole blood loss with crystalloids only will result in a decreased hematocrit.

used (without blood) for fluid resuscitation, then the Hct will fall because whole blood loss has been replaced with fluid that does not contain RBCs (Fig. 15-1). The patient may remain anemic until blood is administered.

Decreased RBC Production. Patients that have decreased RBC production have a defect or impairment in the bone marrow function; this may be caused by disease or treatment of a disease. Diseases that affect hematopoiesis in the bone marrow include malignancies, autoimmune disorders, hematologic disorders (e.g., transient erythroblastopenia of childhood) and congenital conditions (e.g., RBC aplasia, Diamond-Blackfan syndrome). Treatments that may affect bone marrow production include chemotherapy, radiation therapy, immunosuppressive drugs, and some medications. Whether the decreased RBC production is congenital or acquired, the resulting pathology is the same.

When complete bone marrow failure is present, the Hgb will fall approximately 0.7 to 1 g/dL per day[7]; this usually produces a chronic rather than an acute anemia. If the Hgb or Hct falls precipitously (greater than 1 g/dL per day) in the patient with bone marrow suppression, then hemorrhage or increased RBC destruction is probably present.

Increased RBC Destruction. Hemolysis may be related to the abnormalities in the RBC membranes, RBC corpuscles, enzymes, or Hgb. In addition, there may be immune and idiopathic RBC destruction.

Clinical Signs and Symptoms

The signs and symptoms of anemia will vary based on the acuity and severity of the anemia and the resultant effect on oxygen delivery. Mild anemia can manifest insidiously, and the patient may be asymptomatic because heart rate and cardiac output maintain oxygen delivery. In contrast, if anemia is acute or severe, overt clinical symptoms may be present. If anemia is chronic, the child retains fluid to maintain circulating blood volume and increases heart rate and cardiac output to maintain oxygen delivery. High-cardiac-output congestive heart failure may develop.

An increase in heart rate may be associated with a systolic flow murmur caused by high flow passing through normal valves. Patients often report fatigue, dizziness, lethargy, dyspnea on exertion, headache, and heart palpitations. Physical signs may include pallor and tachycardia.

Signs of congestive heart failure, including tachycardia with a gallop, pulmonary edema, poor peripheral perfusion and hepatosplenomegaly, usually develop once the Hct is less than 15% or the Hgb concentration is less than 5 g/dL.

Anemia from RBC hemolysis often causes jaundice. Splenomegaly will be noted if sequestration of RBCs develops.

Laboratory studies will demonstrate a fall in Hct; the average Hgb concentration varies based on age and gender, so values should be evaluated in light of these characteristics. Anemia can be classified on the basis of the mean corpuscular volume as microcytic if the RBCs are small, normocytic if they are normal, and macrocytic if the RBCs are large. Examination of a peripheral smear of blood enables assessment of RBC morphology (i.e., shape, size, and color). The reticulocyte count is helpful in diagnosing the cause of the anemia; it is decreased in disorders of RBC production and usually elevated in the presence of increased RBC destruction (e.g., a hemolytic process). Laboratory studies will differentiate whether the anemia is of one cell line (RBCs only) or all cell lines (RBCs, WBCs, and platelets).

Management

The management of a patient with anemia is influenced by the severity and cause of the anemia. If the child exhibits congestive heart failure or shock, initial therapy focuses on supporting oxygen delivery and cardiorespiratory function. Once the child's condition is stable, the cause of the anemia must be identified to effectively restore the RBCs.

Management of anemia with severe cardiorespiratory distress (e.g., CHF) includes immediate oxygen administration, insertion of two large-bore venous catheters, or establishment of intraosseous access for blood product and fluid administration. Insertion of an arterial line is recommended to allow continuous blood pressure monitoring. Although phlebotomy should be limited in a child with severe anemia, obtain a CBC with a reticulocyte count, and blood for type and cross match. If shock is present, a venous pH will enable quantification of any acidosis. If possible, a purple-top EDTA (ethylenediamine tetraacetic acid) and a green-top (heparin) tube should be filled for later establishment of the cause of the anemia (e.g., these samples can be used for Hgb electrophoresis, osmotic fragility, or G-6 PD [Glucose-6-phosphate dehydrogenase] deficiency studies).

If chronic anemia is present, the child has retained fluid and albumin to maintain circulating blood volume and has increased cardiac output to maintain oxygen delivery. Transfusion therapy in this patient can produce hypervolemia and precipitate (or worsen) congestive heart failure. Administering PRBCs at the rate of approximately 3 mL/kg per hour should prevent hypervolemia and worsening of CHF. Often a diuretic is administered simultaneously.

If severe CHF or profound compensated anemia is present, a partial exchange transfusion will enable removal of some intravascular volume (which contains a low Hgb and Hct) and replacement with PRBCs (with an Hgb of approximately 18 to 20 g/dL and an Hct of approximately 65% to 70%). This will produce an improvement in oxygen-carrying capacity without expanding the intravascular volume (refer to Blood Component Therapy later in this chapter).

The symptomatic patient with hemolytic anemia caused by intrinsic RBC abnormalities will benefit from RBC transfusions. Because the transfused RBCs are unaffected, they will not be susceptible to hemolysis.

In contrast, immune-mediated hemolytic anemia might not be responsive to transfusions, because the offending antibodies might not distinguish between host and transfused RBCs. The presence of antibodies can preclude crossmatching of blood (in the blood bank) for these patients, using standard Coomb's testing. Therefore virtually every unit of blood administered to the patient may be labeled as *incompatible*. In these patients, in vivo crossmatching is performed: blood is administered, and the patient is monitored closely for evidence of a severe transfusion reaction (see Blood and Blood Component Therapy). In some cases, steroid therapy (prednisone, 2 to 10 mg/kg per day) or splenectomy may be effective in reducing RBC antibody formation and RBC destruction.

Serial monitoring of blood counts is essential to evaluate response to therapy. Patients with some types of anemia, such as decreased production of RBCs, may benefit from the administration of hematopoietic growth factors. Administering growth factors may decrease the need for blood transfusions.

Thrombocytopenia
Etiology and Pathophysiology
Patients with thrombocytopenia have a decrease in circulating platelets. This condition can occur as a result of decreased production of platelets, increased destruction of platelets, or sequestration of platelets in the spleen or liver (Box 15-3). The cause of the thrombocytopenia affects the treatment.

Box 15-3	**Most Common Causes of Thrombocytopenia**

Decreased Production
- Bone marrow failure (aplastic anemia)
- Bone marrow replacement (leukemia, other malignancies)
- Congenital megakaryocytosis
- Bone marrow suppression (chemicals, insecticides, chemotherapy, radiation therapy, chloramphenicol, alcohol)
- Hereditary thrombocytopenia (Alport's syndrome, Fanconi syndrome, Wiskott-Aldrich syndrome)

Increased Destruction
- Bacterial sepsis
- Idiopathic thrombocytopenia purpura
- Disseminated intravascular coagulation
- Thrombotic thrombocytopenic purpura
- Hemolytic uremic syndrome
- Hypersplenism
- Neonatal autoimmune thrombocytopenia
- Toxin (snake venom)
- Drug induced (heparin, quinidine, morphine, sulfonamide derivatives, heroin)

Sequestration
- Sickle cell disease

From Turgeon ML: *Clinical hematology: theory and procedures*, ed 4. Philadelphia, 2005, Lippincott Williams and Wilkins.

Patients with decreased platelet production may have an underlying failure of hematopoiesis in their bone marrow. For example, in leukemia the bone marrow may be overwhelmed with blast cells, which overwhelm and replace the platelet-forming megakaryocytes, decreasing platelet production.

Thrombocytopenic patients with increased platelet destruction may have developed platelet antibodies. This process is immune mediated. The antibodies attach to the patient's platelets, and the platelet-antibody complexes are rapidly removed from the circulation in the liver and spleen. Immune-mediated thrombocytopenia may be triggered by a viral illness, or it may be caused by drugs (e.g., heparin) or by a breakdown in the body's ability to recognize its own antigens (e.g., systemic lupus erythematosus and other collagen vascular diseases).

Clinical Signs and Symptoms
There is no definitive test to determine the etiology of thrombocytopenia. Immune-mediated thrombocytopenia is a diagnosis of exception when other diseases or disorders have been ruled out. Diagnostic procedures include a CBC with evaluation of peripheral smear, coagulation studies, and a reticulated platelet value and platelet function testing. Normal platelet counts range from 150,000 to 400,000/mm^3, and patients with severe thrombocytopenia may have a platelet count of less than 20,000/mm^3. Spontaneous bleeding can occur when the platelet count is less than 20,000/mm^3, and intracranial hemorrhage can occur when the platelet count is below 5000/mm^3.

Reticulated platelets (RPs) are newly synthesized platelets with increased ribonucleic acid content. These new platelets can be identified and quantified, and the RP value can aid in determining the cause of the thrombocytopenia. A decrease in RP value in the patient with thrombocytopenia suggests bone marrow suppression (i.e., platelets are not being made despite a fall in platelet count), whereas a high RP value in a patient with thrombocytopenia suggests immune-mediated thrombocytopenia (i.e., platelets are being made but are not correcting the thrombocytopenia).[21]

The clinical presentation of thrombocytopenia will vary based on the platelet count and the patient's activity level. The most common clinical signs of thrombocytopenia include: easy bruising, petechia, purpura, menorrhagia, and bleeding from mucous membranes such as the nose, mouth, and gastrointestinal tract. More worrisome signs and symptoms of internal bleeding include: hematuria, headache, dizziness, retinal hemorrhages, hematemesis, melena, precipitous decrease in Hgb and Hct levels, and symptoms of a cardiovascular collapse (e.g., tachycardia, hypotension, peripheral vasoconstriction).

Intracranial bleeding is a serious potential complication of thrombocytopenia. Such bleeding may be particularly difficult to diagnose in infants and toddlers, because it can produce vague symptoms such as irritability, fussiness, and poor feeding. In patients with severe thrombocytopenia, nurses must quickly identify and investigate any change in level of consciousness or behavior, severe headache, vision changes, ataxia, slurred speech, complaints of weakness or numbness, and severe vomiting not associated with nausea; these may be signs of intracranial hemorrhage.

Management

The priority for management is to prevent, quickly detect, and treat bleeding episodes. Nurses should test urine, gastric drainage, and stool for the presence of blood, report any positive results, and watch for any signs of frank bleeding. Nurses should handle the patient gently, provide a soft mechanical diet, provide stool softeners, and avoid rectal medications. Intramuscular injections are to be avoided, and prolonged pressure must be applied to any injection or venipuncture sites. Aspirin and other drugs (e.g., some antiinflammatory agents) that inhibit platelet function are contraindicated.

If severe thrombocytopenia is present, nurses should perform neurologic examinations frequently and with any change in patient condition. Unilateral headache is often a sign of intracranial hemorrhage.

Prophylactic platelet transfusion is provided if the platelet count is less than 10,000/mm^3, to reduce the risk of spontaneous intracranial hemorrhage. Although published data indicate no difference in outcomes for patients with leukemia when platelet transfusion thresholds were 10,000/mm^3 or 20,000/mm^3 in the absence of active bleeding, institutional practices vary widely based on local practice guidelines.[28] In general, lower thresholds are used for platelet transfusion for children with conditions such as fever, central nervous system tumors, bleeding, or coagulopathies or those requiring procedures.[2] Patients can safely have "major invasive procedures" such as bone marrow aspirate and biopsies with platelet counts of 50,000/mm^3; the thresholds can vary slightly among institutions.[23,24,28]

It is important to identify the underlying cause of thrombocytopenia to provide appropriate therapy. For patients with decreased platelet production or bone marrow failure, provide supportive care, including administration of platelet transfusions to maintain hemostasis and treatment of the underlying disorder or continuing support until the condition resolves.

Patients with immune-mediated thrombocytopenia typically do not benefit from platelet transfusions, because administered platelets will likely be destroyed by the same mechanism that produced the thrombocytopenia. However, when life-threatening bleeding is present, platelet transfusion is provided. HLA-matched platelet transfusions can increase platelet count more effectively, but will be more challenging to acquire.

Patients with immune-mediated platelet destruction can be treated with high-dose steroids (prednisone, 4 to 8 mg/kg per day), intravenous immune gamma globulin (0.5 to 1 g/kg of immunoglobulin G), or both. Children with exceptionally low platelet counts and acute bleeding require inpatient hospitalization with close observation. Bone marrow aspirate is recommended before initiating high-dose methylprednisolone (30 to 50 mg/kg per day) to treat severe bleeding. These children may also receive a 2- or 3-day course of intravenous immune gamma globulin.[13] Frequent monitoring of laboratory tests may be necessary until the platelet count improves. Monitor the patient closely for signs of bleeding.

When thrombocytopenia is chronic, caretakers and patients (if age-appropriate) should be taught safety precautions, including restriction of high-risk activities and management of common bleeding episodes. Children with chronic thrombocytopenia should wear medical alert jewelry.

Disseminated Intravascular Coagulation

Etiology

Disseminated intravascular coagulation is characterized by the intravascular consumption of platelets and plasma clotting factors.[13] DIC is not a primary disease but a complication of other disease processes.[27] DIC can complicate sepsis, hypoxemia, major trauma with severe tissue injury, malignancy, thrombotic thrombocytopenic purpura, hemolytic uremic syndrome (HUS), extensive burns, and severe viral infections (Box 15-4).

Pathophysiology and Clinical Signs and Symptoms

DIC is characterized by an abnormal coagulation process—the entire clotting mechanism is triggered inappropriately. Unrestrained clotting causes systemic or local formation of fibrin clots. This development of fibrin clots leads to microthrombi and excessive bleeding secondary to the consumption of the platelets and clotting factors. The fibrin clot development triggers the clotting cascade process to break down the clots and fibrin that have been formed. Fibrinolysis results in the development of fibrin degradation products, which in turn will act as anticoagulants and promote more bleeding. Organ injury may be the end result of intravascular clots, which cause microvascular occlusions and anoxia.[20] In addition, when the RBCs flow through obstructed vessels the end result is additional hemolysis that can lead to hemolytic anemia (Fig. 15-2).

The mechanisms producing DIC are not completely understood. Excess activation with subsequent depletion of essential coagulation factors produces unrestrained clotting and consumption of procoagulants, and bleeding results. The final common pathway includes production of thrombin, which converts the soluble clotting protein—fibrinogen—into insoluble fibrin, the major component of normal clots.

Box 15-4   Most Common Causes of Disseminated Intravascular Coagulation

Infection
- Gram-negative bacteria
- Gram-positive bacteria (especially meningococcemia)
- Viruses
- Rickettsiae (especially Rocky Mountain spotted fever)

Shock
- Septic, hypovolemic, cardiogenic, anaphylactic

Trauma
- Head injuries, crush injuries, burns, surgery

Malignancies

Obstetric Problems
- Placental abruption, retained dead fetus, amniotic fluid embolization

Vascular Abnormalities
- Giant hemangiomas (Kasabach-Merritt syndrome)

Venomous Snakebite

Transfusion Reaction

Heat Stroke

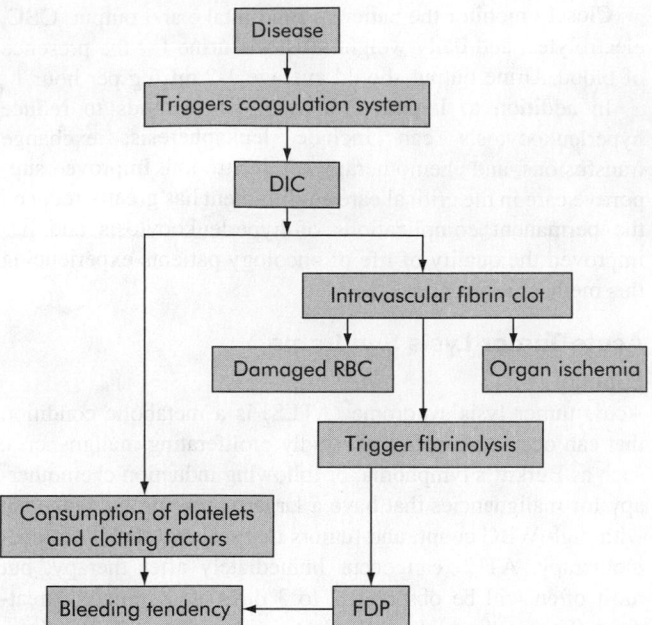

FIG. 15-2 Pathophysiology of disseminated intravascular coagulation. (From Pagana K, Pagana T: *Mosby's manual of diagnostic and laboratory tests*, St Louis, 2006, Mosby-Elsevier.) *DIC*, Disseminated intravascular coagulation; *FDP*, fibrin degradation products.

Microthrombi will be present, and fibrin deposition will occur in the microvasculature. In turn, disseminated deposits of fibrin trap and destroy platelets and RBCs and consume clotting factors, so that a consumptive coagulopathy (synonymous with DIC) results. This process, if unchecked, can result in continuous activation of clotting components and a collapse of normal hemostasis, with resultant widespread bleeding and clotting manifestations. The patient with DIC then demonstrates evidence of both excessive clotting (with a fall in fibrinogen, consumptive coagulopathy, and presence of fibrin monomer) and clot breakdown (with a resultant rise in levels of fibrin degradation products).

If low-fibrin degradation product DIC is present, a predominance of clot formation is present, and embolic vascular obstruction is likely to occur. Renal artery embolization will produce renal failure, and peripheral extremity embolization will result in ischemia and necrosis of digits or extremities.

The clinical signs and symptoms of DIC include: petechia, purpura, ecchymosis, hematomas, prolonged oozing, or bleeding from orifices or minor procedures such as venipuncture sites or incisions. Critically ill patients in the critical care unit may also experience life-threatening thrombotic complications of DIC, such as uncontrolled bleeding, pulmonary embolism, stroke, renal compromise, organ failure, ischemia, and possible gangrene of extremities. Closely monitor the child with DIC to detect changes in perfusion, level of consciousness, organ function, and urine output.

No single test can be used to diagnose DIC. Laboratory abnormalities consistent with the diagnosis of DIC include thrombocytopenia, prolonged PT or activated partial thromboplastin time (aPTT), decreased fibrinogen, elevated fibrin degradation products (fibrin split products), and anemia (Table 15-1). The presence of fibrin monomer indicates that fibrinogen is being broken down by thrombin and that clot is being formed. A rise in fibrin monomer is an early indication of DIC.

Table 15-1	Disseminated Intravascular Coagulation Blood Tests
Test	**Result**
Bleeding time	Prolonged
Platelet count	Decreased
Prothrombin time	Prolonged
Activated partial thromboplastin time	Prolonged
Coagulation factors	I, II, V, VIII, X, and XIII decreased
Fibrin degradation products	Increased
Red blood smear	Damaged red blood cells
Euglobulin lysis time	Normal or prolonged
D-dimer	Increased
Thrombin time	Prolonged
Fibrinopeptide A	Increased
Prothrombin fragment	Increased

Management

The primary goal of management of DIC is identification and treatment of the underlying cause. However, supportive therapy is often needed to reverse existing coagulation abnormalities and to treat shock. The healthcare team will use clinical and laboratory data to monitor the course of the disease and the patient's response to therapy.

Perform frequent and ongoing assessment to detect and treat shock, bleeding, or any compromise in organ perfusion and function. Evaluate tissue perfusion and oxygenation and monitor for bleeding, petechiae, dyspnea, lethargy, pallor, tachycardia, hypotension, headache, dizziness, muscle weakness, and restlessness. When the patient is actively bleeding, the nurse must measure external blood loss, avoid disturbing clots, and control bleeding by applying pressure and ice. The nurse must also monitor for internal bleeding, by checking both the urine and stool for occult blood, and for signs of intraabdominal and intracranial bleeding.

Patients with DIC may require frequent administration of blood or blood components. The overall prognosis for DIC has improved significantly over the last two decades because of advances in critical care, such as prompt recognition of DIC, and improved supportive care such as treatment of shock and antifibrinolytic and blood transfusion therapy.

Heparin can be administered to patients with purpura fulminans (e.g., DIC with necrosis of digits and thromboembolic phenomena). In this case, the fibrin degradation products may be elevated moderately, suggesting that little clot breakdown is occurring, and clot formation predominates. Before heparin therapy is initiated under these conditions, plasma must be administered to restore levels of antithrombin III in order for heparin to provide anticoagulation.

Hyperleukocytosis

Etiology

Hyperleukocytosis is defined as a peripheral WBC count greater than 100,000/mm³. This common oncologic emergency is often a presenting symptom of patients with leukemia, specifically acute myelogenous leukemia and acute lymphoblastic leukemia.

Pathophysiology

As the patient's WBC count increases, so do the complications that may be present. Hyperleukocytosis results in increased blood viscosity, which can in turn obstruct blood vessels, leading to thrombi development in the microcirculation. Patients with acute nonlymphoblastic leukemia (ANLL) may develop sequestration of blast cells in the lungs, producing intrapulmonary shunting. Patients with ANLL are most likely to develop cerebral thromboembolic events, because the myeloblasts readily adhere to one another. All patients with hyperleukocytosis may develop metabolic abnormalities from cell lysis (see Acute Tumor Lysis Syndrome), including hyperkalemia, hyperuricemia, hyperphosphatemia, and hypocalcemia.

Clinical Signs and Symptoms

Patients with hyperleukocytosis often have clinical complications from clumping of the leukemia cells in the lungs and brain,[27] with resultant pulmonary sequestration or cerebral thromboembolic events. Signs and symptoms of pulmonary sequestration include hypoxia, restlessness, agitation, shortness of breath, tachypnea, cyanosis, decreased lung sounds, and increased work of breathing. Respiratory distress will persist despite oxygen administration.

The clumping of the WBCs in the central nervous system and cerebral thromboembolic events (infarct or hemorrhage) can cause blurred vision, headache, decreased level of consciousness, confusion, disorientation, inability to follow commands, and pupil dilation. Stroke or intracranial hemorrhage can produce increased intracranial pressure with decrease in level of consciousness and pupil dilation. Signs of impending cerebral herniation include bradycardia, systolic hypertension and abnormal breathing pattern (possible apnea).

If there is reason to suspect intracranial bleeding or infarct, a neurosurgeon should be consulted. Diagnostic testing can include computed tomography (CT) or magnetic resonance imaging (MRI) if the patient's clinical condition is stable.

Management

Perform frequent pulmonary and neurologic assessment to detect early respiratory or neurologic compromise. Evaluate oxygenation and respiratory effort, and evaluate the patient's ability to follow commands, pupil size, and response to light. Next, immediately investigate any change in level of consciousness or headache (see Increased Intracranial Pressure in Chapter 11). In addition, monitor systemic perfusion and fluid and electrolyte balance.

The initial intervention for patients with an increased WBC count is hyperhydration (approximately 3000 mL/m^2 per day). In general, avoid (or use with caution) fluids containing potassium, because the rapid WBC turnover increases the risk of hyperkalemia.

Uric acid-lowering agents such as oral allopurinol (rasburicase [Elitek]) are given. These drugs assist in reducing the uric acid level and usually prevent the development of hyperuricemic nephropathy (renal failure). For the majority of newly diagnosed oncology patients, oral allopurinol is sufficient as a uric acid lowering agent; the intravenous form is reserved for patients with large tumor burdens and/or for children who are unable to take oral medications.

Closely monitor the patient's fluid intake and output, CBC, electrolytes, and daily weight. Test the urine for the presence of blood. Urine output should average 1-2 mL/kg per hour.

In addition to hyperhydration, other methods to reduce hyperleukocytosis can include leukapheresis, exchange transfusions, and chemotherapy administration. Improved supportive care in the critical care environment has greatly reduced the permanent complications of hyperleukocytosis and has improved the quality of life of oncology patients experiencing this medical emergency.

Acute Tumor Lysis Syndrome

Etiology

Acute tumor lysis syndrome (ATLS) is a metabolic condition that can occur as a result of rapidly proliferating malignancies, such as Burkitt's lymphoma, or following induction chemotherapy for malignancies that have a large tumor burden, leukemia with high WBC count, and tumors that respond rapidly to chemotherapy. ATLS can occur immediately after therapy, but most often will be observed 2 to 3 days after initiating treatment. The syndrome typically lasts approximately 7 days.[4]

One of the key factors in development of ATLS, regardless of the underlying malignancy, is the presence or development of hyperuricemia. As a result, oncology patients at risk for ATLS include those with impaired renal status such as those with dehydration, hyperuricemia, or underlying renal abnormalities.

Pathophysiology

ATLS occurs when there is a rapid breakdown of cells with a release of intracellular contents into the circulation. These metabolites can overwhelm the ability of the kidneys to excrete them, so they accumulate in the blood. Electrolyte abnormalities include hyperuricemia, hyperkalemia, hyperphosphatemia, and hypocalcemia. Hyperuricemia can result in the formation of uric acid crystals in the kidneys and urinary tract, producing renal obstruction and failure.

Destroyed cells release a large amount of potassium, producing hyperkalemia that can rapidly worsen with the development of renal failure (Fig. 15-3). Hyperkalemia is one of the most dangerous electrolyte imbalances, and fatal arrhythmias may occur with potassium levels greater than 7.0 mEq/L. Hyperphosphatemia can cause the formation of calcium phosphate crystals. Similar to uric acid crystals, calcium phosphate crystals can also obstruct the renal tubules compromising renal function. The precipitation of calcium phosphate crystals also may cause a secondary hypocalcemia.

Clinical Signs and Symptoms

Identifying patients at risk for tumor lysis syndrome can assist in prompt recognition and treatment. Hallmark metabolic abnormalities are hyperuricemia, hyperkalemia, hyperphosphatemia, and hypocalcemia. Patients may also develop an elevated blood urea nitrogen (BUN) and creatinine, elevated lactic dehydrogenase (LDH) and elevated WBC. Because the LDH is a marker of cell turnover, a high initial value is suggestive of rapid cell turnover, such as with Burkitt's lymphoma or leukemia; ongoing monitoring of LDH is not typically needed.

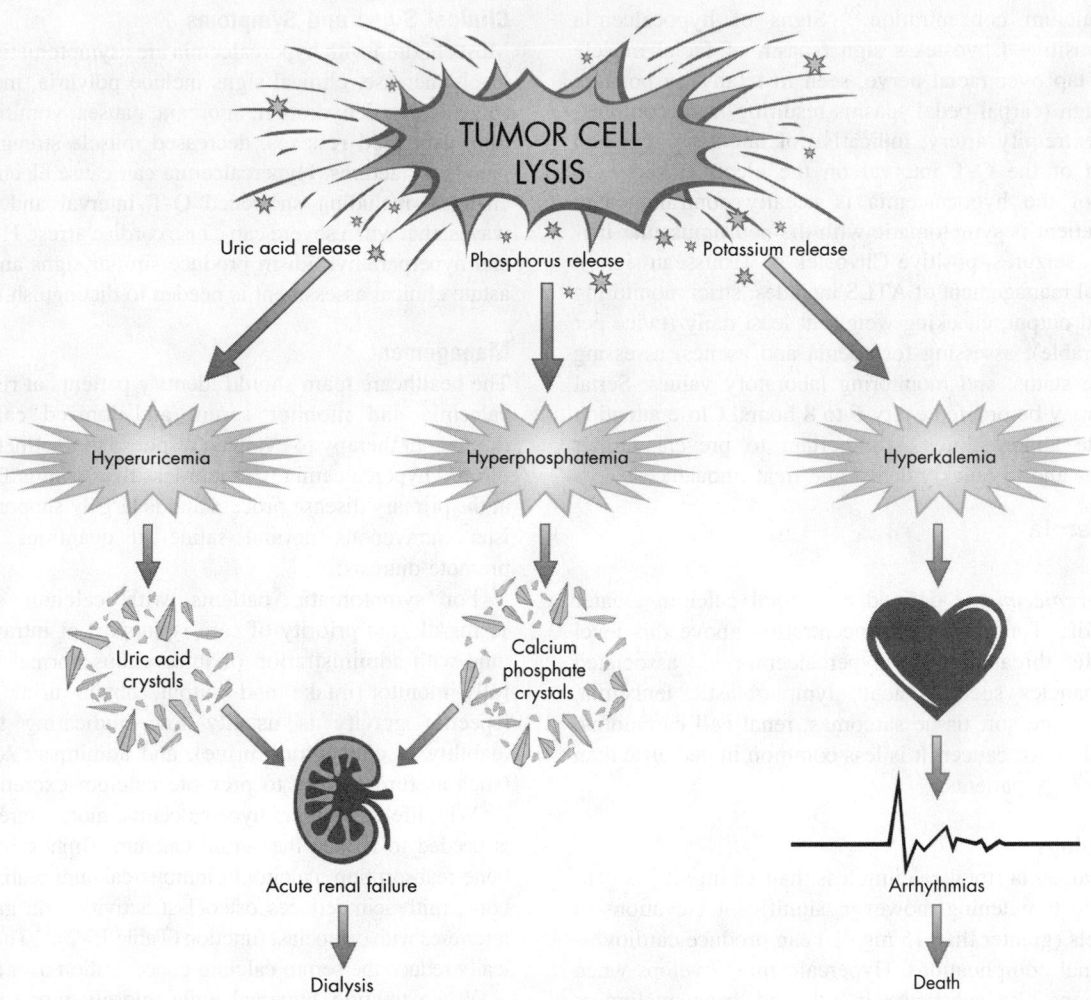

FIG. 15-3 Acute tumor lysis syndrome.

Clinical symptoms include abdominal or flank pain, nausea, vomiting, decreased urine output, edema, muscle cramps, twitching, numbness, tingling, lethargy, and fluid overload. Symptoms can include those of complications of renal failure and signs of hypervolemia, hyperkalemia, and hypocalcemia, such as CHF, cardiac arrhythmias, seizures, and cardiac arrest.

Management

The best treatment for ATLS is identifying patients at risk and instituting therapy to avoid the complications of rapid cell breakdown. Once ATLS is present, nurses should closely monitor the patient's heart rate and rhythm, systemic perfusion, fluid intake and output, CBC, electrolytes, and daily weight.

Uric acid crystal formation can be reduced with intravenous hyperhydration (approximately 3000 mL/m^2 per day). Avoid, or use cautiously, intravenous fluids that contain potassium, because the patient is already at risk for hyperkalemia.

A uric acid-lowering agent such as oral allopurinol (rasburicase) is administered. Allopurinol assists in reducing the uric acid level and usually prevents the development of hyperuricemic nephropathy (renal failure). Currently, the intravenous form of allopurinol is extremely costly; in light of the effectiveness of oral allopurinol (rasburicase) the intravenous form is reserved for children who are unable to take oral medications.

Closely monitor renal function; place a urinary catheter to enable continuous evaluation of urine output. In general, fluids are administered to maintain urine output of at least 2 mL/kg per hour. Test the urine for the presence of blood.

For asymptomatic hyperkalemia, treatment includes diuretics such as furosemide (Lasix) or mannitol or the administration of sodium polystyrene sulfonate (Kayexalate) orally or rectally. The rectal route (i.e., enema) will reduce the serum potassium faster than oral administration, but the oral route will result in a greater reduction over several hours.[12] Symptomatic hyperkalemia requires more aggressive interventions such as calcium, sodium bicarbonate, and insulin and glucose infusion, which shift potassium back into cells. Other interventions for symptomatic hyperkalemia can include peritoneal dialysis, hemodialysis, and continuous venovenous hemofiltration. For additional information about hyperkalemia, see Chapter 12; for additional information about renal failure, see Chapter 13.

Hyperphosphatemia does not produce symptoms, but it will produce hypocalcemia and related symptoms. The phosphate combines with calcium and forms a precipitate in tissues. The serum ionized calcium is considered a more sensitive and reliable indicator of effective calcium concentration than the total calcium concentration.[20] Signs of hypocalcemia include: a positive Chvostek's sign (spasm of facial muscle following a tap over facial nerve, seen in tetany), a positive Trousseau sign (carpal-pedal spasms resulting from compression of an extremity artery, indicative of latent tetany), and prolongation of the Q-T interval on the electrocardiogram. Correction of the hypocalcemia is usually contraindicated unless the patient is symptomatic with the neuromuscular irritability (e.g., seizures, positive Chvostek or Trousseau signs).

Additional management of ATLS includes: strict monitoring of intake and output, checking weight at least daily (twice per day is preferable), assessing for edema and ascites, assessing fluid volume status, and monitoring laboratory values. Serial electrolytes may be ordered every 6 to 8 hours. Close attention to electrolyte abnormalities is important to prevent further complications and to quickly detect and treat imbalances.

Hypercalcemia

Etiology

Severe *hypercalcemia* is defined as a total calcium greater than 15 mg/dL. Total calcium concentration above this level may be life threatening.[14] Hypercalcemia is associated with malignancies such as acute lymphoblastic leukemia, lymphomas, some soft tissue sarcomas, renal cell carcinoma, and lung and breast cancer. It is less common in pediatric than in adult oncology patients.

Pathophysiology

Mild hypercalcemia (total calcium less than 15 mg/dL) is generally not life threatening; however, significant elevations in calcium levels (greater than 15 mg/dL) can produce cardiovascular and renal complications. Hypercalcemia develops when a parathormone-like substance is released from malignant cells. This substance stimulates bone reabsorption and the release of calcium. Hypercalcemia can also result from malignancies causing bone destruction and from decreased renal calcium excretion.[16,20,26]

Hypercalcemia can produce complications similar to hyperparathyroidism, including development of renal stones, osteoporosis, and neuromuscular pain and tingling. Severe hypercalcemia can produce a polyuria-polydipsia syndrome with dehydration. If the polyuria produces dehydration, renal excretion of calcium is reduced; this can exacerbate the hypercalcemia.

Clinical Signs and Symptoms

Most children with hypercalcemia are asymptomatic. As calcium levels increase, clinical signs include polyuria, increased thirst (polydipsia), dehydration, anorexia, nausea, vomiting, constipation, depressed reflexes, decreased muscle strength, and bone pain and fractures. Hypercalcemia can cause electrocardiogram changes, including shortened Q-T interval and depressed T waves, that when severe can cause cardiac arrest. Hypercalcemia and hyperparathyroidism produce similar signs and symptoms; astute clinical assessment is needed to distinguish them.

Management

The healthcare team should identify patients at risk for hypercalcemia and monitor serum and ionized calcium levels throughout therapy to evaluate response to treatment. Treatment of mild hypercalcemia (calcium less than 15 mg/dL) is directed at the primary disease process and is largely supportive. Administer intravenous normal saline in quantities sufficient to promote diuresis.

For symptomatic patients with calcium greater than 15 mg/dL, the priority of care is support of intravascular volume with administration of intravenous normal saline. Carefully monitor intake and output, obtain urine for analysis (specific gravity is usually low, indicating the kidneys' inability to concentrate urine), and administer loop diuretics (such as furosemide) to promote calcium excretion.

With life-threatening hypercalcemia, more aggressive therapy is needed to reduce the serum calcium. Biphosphonate inhibits bone reabsorption, calcitonin inhibits calcium reabsorption from bone, mithracin reduces osteoclast activity, and gallium nitrate interferes with osteoclast function (Table 15-2).[14] These drugs typically reduce the serum calcium concentration over several days.

When treating hypercalcemia, closely monitor the child's urine output, renal function, serum calcium, and phosphate and magnesium levels. Delayed hypokalemia, hypophosphatemia and hypomagnesemia may develop. Renal replacement therapies may be needed if hypercalcemia is complicated by renal failure.

Neutropenia

Etiology and Pathophysiology

Neutropenia is defined as an absolute neutrophil count of less than 1000/mm^3 in infants younger than 1 year and 1500/mm^3 in children older than 1 year.[13] The ANC is the total number of WBCs multiplied by the percentage of neutrophils (segmented

Table 15-2   Medications for Severe Hypercalcemia

Drug	Description and Action	Dose*
Pamidronate	Second-generation biphosphate inhibits bone reabsorption; effective in malignancy-induced hypercalcemia	1 mg/kg, may be repeated once in 24 h
Calcitonin	Hormone that inhibits calcium reabsorption from bone	4 IU/kg body weight, given subcutaneously or intramuscularly
Plicamycin (Mithramycin)	Osteoclast RNA synthesis inhibitor that reduces osteoclast activity	Short infusion of 25 mcg/kg, given over 30 min or longer; dose may be repeated after 48 h
Gallium nitrate	Hydrated gallium salt that interferes with osteoclast function	Continuous infusion of 200 mg/m^2 body surface area per day for a total of 5 days

*Pamidronate dose from Kerdudo C and others: Hypercalcemia and childhood cancer: a 7-year experience. *J Pediatr Hematol Oncol* 27:23-27, 2005. Remaining doses from National Cancer Institute: *Hypercalcemia (PDQ)*. Available at: http://www.cancer.gov/cancerinfo/pdq/supportivecare/hypercalcemia. Accessed January 4, 2012.

BOX 15-5	**National Cancer Institute Neutropenia Grading System**

- Grade 1 (Slight): ANC less than 2000/mm^3
- Grade 2 (Minimal): ANC less than 1500/mm^3
- Grade 3 (Moderate): ANC less than 1000/mm^3
- Grade 4 (Severe): ANC less than 500/mm^3

ANC, Absolute neutrophil count.

neutrophils or segs plus bands). (For calculation, see Box 15-1.) The National Cancer Institute neutropenia grading system developed a classification scale for neutropenia (Box 15-5). The risk of serious bacterial infection increases dramatically when the ANC is less than 500/mm^3.

In addition to the classification of severity, neutropenia can be further classified as acquired or congenital; acquired neutropenia is more common than the congenital form. Acute acquired neutropenia can be caused by an acute transient neutropenia or infections. Viral infections that may cause acquired neutropenia include respiratory syncytial virus, hepatitis A and B, Epstein-Barr virus, measles, rubella, and varicella. Bacterial infections that can cause acquired neutropenia include typhoid, paratyphoid, tuberculosis, and rickettsia infection.[13] Acquired chronic neutropenia can be caused by bone marrow aplasia, bone marrow infiltration, or treatment such as chemotherapy, radiation therapy, or immunosuppressive medications. Bone marrow infiltration leading to neutropenia can result from diseases such as neuroblastoma, lymphoma, or rhabdomyosarcoma.

Congenital neutropenia, or primary neutropenia, is usually profound and is caused by a genetic abnormality. Examples include severe combined immunodeficiency syndrome, Wiskott-Aldrich syndrome, and Kostmann's syndrome. Often these congenital neutropenia disorders are associated with the future development of more serious illnesses, such as myelodysplastic syndromes or acute myelogenous leukemia.

Neutrophils provide the major defense against bacterial invasion, so neutropenia is associated with increased risk of infection. Patients with neutropenia can develop infection or sepsis from organisms in the body. These opportunistic infections may include *Staphylococcus epidermidis, S. aureus, Klebsiella* species, *Escherichia coli,* and *Pseudomonas* species.

Clinical Signs and Symptoms

The child with neutropenia requires a detailed history and physical examination. Carefully assess for signs or symptoms of infection, especially infection of the mouth, skin, ears, and perianal area. Neutropenia produces no symptoms. Because neutrophils play a major role in the inflammatory response, signs of inflammation (e.g., redness, edema, drainage) may be absent from sites of infection. Fever may be the only clinical sign of an infection. Assess for the presence of lymphadenopathy, organomegaly, pallor, bruising, petechia, and other abnormalities. Ask patients about any localized pain or discomfort. Infants and small children may exhibit nonspecific clinical signs and symptoms of infection or sepsis, such as irritability, fussiness, and poor feeding, and can develop a change in level of consciousness.

If fever is present in a child with neutropenia, obtain blood and urine cultures. Additional evaluation as indicated by physical assessment findings often includes a chest radiograph, and cultures of stool, throat culture, cerebral spinal fluid (CSF), and any wounds. Be vigilant while evaluating for potential infections, because this patient population is at high risk for developing life-threatening infections.

If the child has other clinical findings such as pancytopenia (all cell lines depressed) with no known cause, then a bone marrow aspirate may be indicated. The bone marrow aspirate often determines the cause of the neutropenia.

Management

The most important aspect of care for patients with neutropenia is to protect them from potential infections. Every member of the healthcare team should practice strict hand hygiene using both soap and water and alcohol based gels for all contacts with patients with neutropenia. Patients with neutropenia should have limited invasive procedures if possible. In addition, nurses should avoid obtaining rectal temperatures or giving medications via the rectal route.

Treatment of neutropenia is primarily supportive with a focus on evaluating risk for infection and on detecting and treating infection. Patients may be treated with colony-stimulating factors such as granulocyte colony-stimulating factor (GCSF; Neupogen [Amgen]) that stimulate the bone marrow to produce more neutrophils.[13]

Fever, defined as an oral temperature greater than 38° C, in the patient with neutropenia should be treated as a potential medical emergency because the patient may develop septic shock.[9] After cultures are obtained, administer broad-spectrum antibiotics while waiting for culture results; administer antibiotics within 1 hour of the child's first medical contact. Dosing is often adjusted based on reported culture and sensitivity results. Monitor the child's vital signs and appearance to detect clinical signs of sepsis or septic shock, such as hyperthermia, hypothermia, tachycardia, hypotension, and changes in perfusion. Note that children with gram-negative bacteremia may deteriorate after antibiotic administration, because lysis of the gram-negative bacteria results in endotoxemia that can perpetuate the septic cascade.

Treatment of septic shock requires immediate antibiotics, aggressive fluid resuscitation, and hemodynamic support with vasoactive agents. Survival from septic shock has increased dramatically in recent years following appreciation of the need for repeated fluid bolus therapy (often totaling 80 mL/kg or more in the first hour of therapy and 240 mL/kg or more in the first 8 h of therapy) and early vasoactive support. For further information, see Chapter 6, and Fig. 6-8.

Nurses should teach patients with neutropenia the importance of strict handwashing, avoiding crowds and contacts who are ill, meticulous skin and oral care, and a low-microbial diet. Adolescent females with neutropenia should not use tampons, to reduce the risk of toxic shock syndrome. Patients should be aware of signs and symptoms that should be reported to a healthcare provider immediately including fever, pain, inflammation, and changes in level of consciousness.

Spinal Cord Compression
Etiology and Pathophysiology

Spinal cord compression is a neurologic emergency that requires immediate treatment to prevent permanent disability. It is usually attributed to tumor growth near the spinal cord or increased pressure in the spinal column. Tumors most likely to cause spinal cord compression include brain and central nervous system tumors, sarcomas (rhabdomyosarcoma, Ewing's sarcoma, and primitive neuroectodermal tumors), neuroblastomas, and lymphomas.

Clinical Signs and Symptoms

Many patients with spinal cord compression complain of back pain. Other clinical symptoms will be related to the level and degree of cord compression. Motor deficits may include weakness, unsteady gait, paralysis, hyporeflexia, muscle atrophy, and paralysis. Sensory deficits can include the inability to sense pain or changes in temperature, bowel or bladder dysfunction, and paresthesias. A thorough neurologic evaluation with special attention to reflexes and strength will help identify these deficits.

A preliminary spine radiograph is the often the first and most convenient diagnostic test, but it is not definitive. To image the soft tissues involved, a CT scan is definitive, and an MRI study can further delineate the size and location of the tumor. If the patient with suspected spinal cord compression has possible increased intracranial pressure, such as caused by brain tumors with spinal (drop) metastases, then a CT scan should be obtained to rule out increased intracranial pressure before a lumbar puncture is performed to evaluate the cerebral spinal fluid. CSF protein will be elevated in patients with complete spinal cord obstruction.[22]

Management

Children with the diagnosis of cancer and complaints of back pain should be evaluated for a spinal cord compression. Prompt referral to a neurologist and neurosurgeon is needed to provide immediate treatment and prevent permanent neurologic dysfunction. Some patients will require surgical intervention, such as tumor debulking or laminectomy. Medical treatment includes high-dose corticosteroids (dexamethasone 1 to 2 mg/kg), chemotherapy, or emergency radiation (if the tumor is radiosensitive) therapy directed to the tumor site.

Some patients may be candidates for newer treatments such as spinal stereotactic radiosurgery (i.e., stereotactic radiotherapy or CyberKnife [Accuray Incorporated]). These therapies deliver higher radiation directly to the tumor and attempt to preserve surrounding tissue.

Several factors influence the outcome of a spinal cord compression treatment plan. Patients with minimal neurologic involvement have more favorable outcomes than do patients with complete paralysis or other severe neurologic deficits. The importance of prompt assessment and treatment cannot be overstated.

Nursing responsibilities include supportive care measures. The child requires pain management, frequent neurologic assessment, position changes with skin care assessment, and maintenance of bowel and bladder function. Provide explanations to the child and family throughout the child's care.

Obstructive Mediastinal Mass

Etiology

A mediastinal mass is a tumor that may be growing rapidly and thus causing respiratory compromise and airway obstruction. Some mediastinal masses also produce superior vena cava (SVC) obstruction. Childhood cancers most often causing mediastinal mass are non-Hodgkin's lymphoma, Burkitt's lymphoma, T cell lymphoblastic lymphoma or leukemia, neuroblastoma, and sarcomas.[22] The most common cause of mediastinal mass in pediatric oncology is non-Hodgkin's lymphoma.

Pathophysiology

Tumors of the mediastinum can affect the airway structures of the trachea and main bronchus. These tumors often grow rapidly, producing airway compression that progresses rapidly. In addition to respiratory compromise, the mediastinal mass may produce compression or obstruction of the superior vena cava, causing SVC syndrome. SVC compression results in a decreased venous return from the head, neck, and upper chest area to the heart. In some cases, this obstruction may be life-threatening. Often collateral flow through the intercostal veins will aid venous return.

Clinical Signs and Symptoms

Patients with mediastinal airway or vascular compression can be asymptomatic until the compression is critical or the patient receives sedation or anesthesia. Changes in airway tone, chest wall compliance, and respiratory effort that may result from sedation or anesthesia can contribute to collapse or compression of airways and nearby vascular structures, with consequent cardiorespiratory collapse.

Once the patient with mediastinal mass develops symptoms of airway compression, these symptoms typically progress rapidly. The initial clinical symptoms can include mild respiratory distress such as cough, hoarseness, orthopnea, and chest pain. These symptoms can quickly progress to moderate or severe respiratory distress, and the patient may experience wheezing, stridor, dyspnea, increased respiratory effort, and changes in level of consciousness. If the mass produces SVC obstruction, the patient may also develop edema of the face, neck, and upper extremities, cyanosis, or a plethora of upper body and distended neck veins.

A chest radiograph will usually reveal a large mass in the anterior mediastinum and possible tracheal deviation. Be extremely careful during positioning of the child for diagnostic procedures, because the supine position will often exacerbate tumor compression of the airways and increase respiratory distress. A CT or MRI scan may be useful in determining the extent of tracheal compression, but the patient's condition may be too unstable to tolerate the transport to the radiology department or the time or positioning required for the studies (see Fig. 10-24).

Management

Patients with a mediastinal mass require immediate treatment and may deteriorate rapidly as treatment is provided. The goal of treatment is to prevent further respiratory deterioration; the basic principle of management is to keep the patient breathing spontaneously if possible. Emergent tracheal intubation may be required, but will not maintain the airway if the mass compresses the trachea distal to the end of the tube. If such distal compression is present, the airway can be maintained by rigid bronchoscopy. For severe distal airway compression, rapid initiation of extracorporeal membrane oxygenation (ECMO) support may be required (see Chapter 7).

Perform thorough and ongoing assessment of cardiorespiratory function, and support adequate airway, oxygenation, and ventilation. Positioning the child on the side or even the prone position may minimize airway compression. Intubation must be performed by skilled providers and the nurse should be prepared for the need for emergent bronchoscopy or ECMO. Healthcare providers should use extreme caution when administering sedation to the nonintubated patient with a mediastinal mass, because a decrease in the child's respiratory effort and change in muscle tone can result in cardiorespiratory collapse.

A malignant mass is treated with emergent radiation therapy, chemotherapy, steroids, or surgical resection. Tissue diagnosis is desirable to guide treatment, but in emergent situations chemotherapy can be initiated based on a presumed diagnosis. A tissue biopsy can be performed when the patient's clinical condition permits.

Most mediastinal tumors are radiosensitive, so radiation therapy can effectively shrink large mediastinal tumors. However, radiation therapy is usually not a desirable option for pediatric patients with critical airway compromise. If radiation is administered, the patient may initially experience some airway edema, so that symptoms may become worse before they improve. The majority of these masses are associated with the diagnosis of T cell leukemia or a type of lymphoma. Surgery is occasionally needed in select cases.

Syndrome of Inappropriate Antidiuretic Hormone

Syndrome of inappropriate antidiuretic hormone (SIADH) is present when there are high circulating levels of antidiuretic hormone (ADH) in the absence of a physiologic stimulus. SIADH causes an increase in water reabsorption by the kidneys, resulting in a dilutional hyponatremia that can cause cerebral edema, seizures, and increased intracranial pressure. Childhood cancers associated with SIADH include central nervous system tumors, Hodgkin's disease, or non-Hodgkin's lymphoma. Other causes include pulmonary infections and central nervous system trauma. Drugs linked to the development of SIADH include steroids, vincristine, cyclophosphamide, cisplatin, narcotics, anesthetics, and thiazide diuretics.

Patients with SIADH usually exhibit hyponatremia, a decreased urine output, increased urine specific gravity with high urine sodium concentration, adequate intravascular volume, and possible increased weight without noticeable edema. Worrisome signs and symptoms include deterioration in neurologic function and seizures. Management includes fluid restriction, careful monitoring of fluid intake and output and correction of serum electrolytes, and treatment of the underlying cause. See Chapter 12 for more information.

Typhlitis
Etiology and Pathophysiology

Typhlitis is an invasion of bacteria in the intestines, most commonly the cecum, leading to necrotizing colitis. The consequences of the bacterial invasion can range from a mild inflammation to a severe full thickness infarction, which may progress to an acute bowel perforation. The primary organisms

responsible for typhlitis are anaerobes and gram-negative bacilli. Also, *Clostridium difficile* is becoming more prevalent as an etiology of typhlitis. The patient population most at risk is the oncology patient with prolonged neutropenia. In fact, it is the most likely cause of abdominal pain in an oncology patient with prolonged neutropenia. High-risk patients include leukemia patients (e.g., those with acute myelogenous leukemia) on induction therapy or leukemia patients with a high WBC count and patients with infections or mucositis.

Clinical Signs and Symptoms

The patients most at risk should be identified and assessed thoroughly for possible typhlitis. The presenting symptoms are abdominal pain to the right lower quadrant, fever, distended abdomen, diminished or absent bowel sounds versus high pitched bowel sounds, nausea, vomiting, and diarrhea. Patients with neutropenic enterocolitis, typhlitis, or appendicitis may have similar presenting signs and symptoms. To accurately diagnose typhlitis, an ultrasound examination of the abdomen and a CT scan may be necessary. The area of the bowel most often affected is the cecum of the large intestine.

Management

Patients with typhlitis are severely neutropenic, so they are best managed medically. Treatment includes administration of broad-spectrum antibiotics, bowel rest, hydration, nutritional support, pain management, and administration of blood products as needed. Infectious disease specialists are often consulted to assist in antibiotic selection. A surgical evaluation may be necessary if the patient has symptoms of an acute abdomen, including active bleeding despite correction of thrombocytopenia and coagulopathies, free air in abdomen, or overwhelming sepsis.

Additional nursing interventions include administration of intravenous antibiotics, pain management, careful gastrointestinal assessment, and monitoring for signs of an acute abdomen, including auscultation of bowel sounds and measurement of abdominal girth. All healthcare providers should adhere to neutropenic precautions.

Anaphylaxis

Anaphylaxis is an allergic hypersensitivity reaction to a foreign protein or drug that causes a systemic response. This reaction is presented in more detail in the Chapter 15 Supplement on the Evolve Website and in Chapters 6 and 16.

For patients with a known allergy or hypersensitivity reaction, premedications can be prescribed before the exposure to the potential allergen. Medications commonly used for pretreatment are corticosteroids, antihistamines, and antipyretics.[6] Patients with known hypersensitivity responses should wear medical alert jewelry and should have an epinephrine pen readily available.

Hematopoietic Stem Cell Transplantation
Etiology and Indications

Treatment for some hematologic, oncologic, and genetic diseases includes hematopoietic stem cell transplant (HSCT), also referred to as *bone marrow transplantation*. The goal of this therapy is to cure the patient's illness.

Preparation and Procedure

The preparative regimen consists of near-lethal doses of chemotherapy, radiation, or both. This regimen is designed to ablate the defective bone marrow and create space for new healthy cells to populate. In addition, it is an immunosuppressant to reduce the risk of graft rejection and to decrease the risk of graft-versus-host disease.[17] The combination of the patient's illness and conditioning regimen can produce severe complications that require critical care. These patients often experience severe myelosuppression and multisystem failure.

There are three types of HSCT: autologous, allogeneic, and umbilical cord blood. Autologous transplantation uses the patient's own stem cells. These donor stem cells can be harvested through peripheral access or directly from the bone marrow. Patients with solid tumors such as neuroblastoma and brain tumors may be candidates for autologous transplants.

Allogeneic transplantation requires matching of a compatible donor with the recipient's human leukocyte antigens (HLAs). In the optimal allogeneic transplant, six of six HLAs match between the donor and the recipient. The preferred donor is a sibling of the patient; this is termed a *matched related donor*. The best allogeneic transplant is a syngeneic transplant; in this transplant, the donor and recipient are identical twins. In most cases, the allogeneic donor may be a matched unrelated donor who has been identified from the registry of bone marrow donors. Use of an unrelated donor often results in more complications than use of sibling-matched donors.

The third type of HSCT is an umbilical cord blood stem cell transplant obtained from a cord blood bank. A cord blood HSCT is also an allogeneic transplant. These stems cells are obtained in the delivery room after childbirth. Stem cells have only recently become available as a viable type of bone marrow transplantation.[3]

Management

The phases of the bone marrow transplant process are classified as early, immediate, and late. Complications can occur during any phase of the transplant process; see Table 15-3 for complications of the bone transplant process. These patients require numerous admissions to the critical care setting for management of their disease.

BLOOD AND BLOOD COMPONENT THERAPY

Pediatric critical care nurses must be familiar with indications for use of blood products, methods of administration, safety precautions, and appropriate volumes to administer. In addition nurses must be familiar with monitoring needed during transfusion (Table 15-4), and they must be able to detect and manage potential complications and adverse reactions.

Red Blood Cell Transfusion

RBC transfusion is indicated to treat symptomatic anemia and acute blood loss with hypovolemia and to improve oxygen carrying capacity. RBCs are administered in whole blood or as PRBCs.

A general threshold suggesting a need for RBCs transfusion in stable critically ill children is an Hgb concentration of 7 g/dL or less, typically associated with an Hct of 20% to 21% or less. This threshold was evaluated in *stable* children in critical care units[11]; different thresholds may be appropriate for children with severe hypoxemia (including those with cyanotic heart disease), hemodynamic instability, or active blood loss. Children with respiratory disease and cyanotic heart disease may require higher Hgb concentration; these children may require an Hgb concentration greater than 12 g/dL and Hct greater than 35% to maintain oxygen carrying capacity, although such thresholds are determined individually. Other thresholds may be appropriate for children with sickle cell anemia or noncyanotic heart defects.

Whole blood transfusions are typically reserved for patients with major trauma or other critical blood loss. Type O-negative blood can be rapidly infused for any patient, because O-negative blood is considered a universal donor. Most emergency departments that treat trauma patients use a rapid infuser to warm and infuse the blood rapidly.

Obtaining a Type and Crossmatch

Before a transfusion is needed, send a patient blood sample for type and crossmatch. The typing identifies the patient's general blood type (A, B, O, or AB) and whether the patient's blood type is Rh-negative or Rh-positive (Table 15-5). When blood is sent for typing and crossmatch, the patient's blood is crossmatched with donor blood to determine compatibility. To reduce error, hospitals require labeling of the patient blood specimen that is sent for typing at the bedside, and placement of a blood bracelet containing the crossmatch number at the time the blood sample is obtained (Box 15-6). In addition, most facilities require a double check with the patient identification and two signatures to prevent fatal errors associated with incorrect blood typing.

In general, to reduce Rh-sensitization in females, Rh-negative blood and blood products are ideally used for female patients of child-bearing age who are Rh-negative. Rh-positive blood and blood products are used for male patients and for female patients who are beyond child-bearing age. This attention to Rh sensitization can reduce the risk of Rh incompatibility during pregnancy.[24] Patients who receive multiple transfusions can develop antibodies, and additional blood samples may be required to complete the necessary crossmatching.

Blood Product Administration

Blood should be administered only after verifying that the correct blood product is available and that the patient's clinical condition is appropriate to receive a blood transfusion. The nurse must also complete the preassessment process for blood administration and should record baseline patient vital signs, including body temperature. Several clinical conditions may delay the administration of a blood product, including body temperature greater than 101° F (Box 15-7).

A clinical staff member should be designated to remain at the bedside for the first 15 minutes of the transfusion, to detect a severe adverse reaction. During those first 15 minutes, the blood component should be administered slowly. If there are no signs of adverse reaction, the rate of administration can be increased according to the patient's size and tolerance.

Table 15-3 **Complications of Hematopoietic Stem Cell Transplant**

Early Complications (Pretransplant to Engraftment)	
Bone marrow suppression	All cell lines may be depressed; patient may be neutropenic, thrombocytopenic, and anemic; patient will require blood transfusions for support; lab values should be closely monitored
Gastrointestinal toxicities (nausea, vomiting, diarrhea, mucositis)	Gastrointestinal imbalances may result in critical electrolyte abnormalities; mucositis may compromise the airway and is extremely painful
Infections	Related to neutropenia and immunosuppressive agents; must be aggressively treated with appropriate therapy (i.e., antibacterial, antifungal, antiviral, antiprotozoan); can progress to life-threatening sepsis
Skin erythema	Radiation and chemotherapy may alter the skin integrity, resulting in vulnerability of the body's protection
Capillary leak syndrome	Radiation and chemotherapy may cause tissue damage that results in cytokine release, which increases the permeability of cells; clinical symptoms may include systemic and pulmonary edema, fluid retention, and ascites
Acute renal insufficiency	Radiation, chemotherapy, and nephrotoxicity medications may result in decreased renal function; dialysis may be required if toxicity is severe
Hemorrhagic cystitis	The metabolite acrolein from cyclophosphamide-ifosfamide is a known irritant to the bladder and can cause acute bleeding; provide hydration and administer 2-mercaptoethane sufonate sodium (mesna) per protocol or physician orders
Venoocclusive disease	Toxicity to the liver caused by radiation, chemotherapy, and preexisting liver conditions can result in narrowing or fibrosis of the vessels
Seizures	Certain chemotherapy medications (e.g., busulfan) and electrolyte imbalances can predispose the patient to changes in neurologic status
Intermediate Complications (Engraftment to 100 Days)	
Infections	Related to immunosuppressive agents and compromised function of the new bone marrow; must be aggressively treated with appropriate therapy; can progress to life-threatening sepsis
Acute GVHD	An immune-mediated response of the donor T cells that attack the host antigens; the body systems affected are the skin, liver, and gut; initial presentation is a usually a maculopapular rash on the palms and soles that progresses to a generalized rash; diarrhea, abdominal pain, and abnormal liver function tests are other characteristics; degree of severity is based on organ involvement; skin or liver biopsy may be required to confirm diagnosis; treatment consists of immunosuppressive therapy and symptom management
Graft failure	Can result if the complete ablation is not achieved, stem dose is too low, infection occurs, or disease reoccurs; treatment can include an additional infusion of donor cells if available
Interstitial pneumonitis	Can result from infection or damage to the lung tissue from the preparative regime; respiratory status may be compromised; may require ventilatory support
Late Complications (>100 Days)	
Immunosuppression and infections	Immunosuppression is directly related to the extent of infections and the presence of GVHD; patients with GVHD will require additional immunosuppressive agents, which increases their risk for this complication
Chronic GVHD	This autoimmune syndrome is similar to a patient with collagen vascular disease; organs affected may include the skin, mouth, gastrointestinal tract, liver, lungs, eyes, and vaginal mucosa; treatment consists of immunosuppressive therapy; numerous experimental treatments are now available
Endocrine dysfunction	As a result of the preparative regimen, patients may experience thyroid dysfunction, growth and development delays, and gonadal dysfunction
Disease recurrence	Patients with aggressive disease before transplant may experience an increased rate of disease reoccurrence; poor prognosis if this occurs within 1-2 years following transplant
Secondary malignancies	Patients treated with specific cytotoxic drugs, radiation therapy, and immunosuppressants are at increased risk for developing secondary malignancies throughout their lifetime

GVHD, Graft-versus-host disease.

Platelet Transfusions

Indications for the administration of platelets to the patient with thrombocytopenia include bleeding or a platelet count of less than 10,000 to 20,000/mm^3.[24] Prophylactic platelet transfusion is provided if the platelet count is less than 5000/mm^3 to reduce the risk of spontaneous intracranial hemorrhage.

Although published data indicate no difference in outcomes for patients with leukemia whose platelet transfusion thresholds were 10,000/mm^3 or 20,000/mm^3 in the absence of active bleeding, institutional practices vary widely based on local practice guidelines.[28] In general, lower thresholds are used for platelet transfusion for children with conditions

Table 15-4　Transfusion Therapy

Blood Product, Dose	Clinical Indications	Nursing Interventions
Red blood cells (10-15 mL/kg) Acute massive blood loss (10-20 mL/kg)	Hgb <7-8 g/dL in a stable patient with a chronic anemia Hypovolemia due to acute blood loss Evidence of impending heart failure secondary to severe anemia Patients on hypertransfusion regimen for sickle cell disease and history of: • Cerebral vascular accident • Splenic sequestration • Acute chest syndrome • Recurrent priapism • Preoperative preparation for surgery with general anesthesia • Hypoxia Children requiring increased oxygen carrying capacity (i.e., complex congenital heart, intracardiac shunting, severe pulmonary disease-ARDS): • Shock states (decreased BP, increased peripheral vasoconstriction, pallor, cyanosis, diaphoresis, clamminess, mottled skin, increased oxygen requirement, decreased urine output) • Cardiac failure • Respiratory failure requiring significant ventilatory support Postoperative anemia	Verify blood unit and patient Use PPE Monitor vital signs per hospital policy and procedure Monitor Hgb and Hct During infusion, observe for signs of adverse reactions • Mild: fever or allergic reaction • Severe: hemolysis (fever, chills, hemoglobinuria, DIC, renal failure) Blood can only be stored in a designated blood refrigerator
Autologous blood (self-donated blood product)	Presurgical donated blood may be obtained for scheduled procedures when a blood transfusion may be necessary; check with blood bank facilities for time criteria for this type of donation For general surgical procedures the recommended Hgb is 10 g/dL or greater; for orthopedic surgery the recommended Hgb is 11.5 g/dL or greater.	Verify unit and patient and verify with parent that self-donation has occurred Patient identification and administration process is the same as all other blood products Use PPE
Whole blood or PRBC reconstituted with FFP (5-10 mL/kg)	Hypovolemia from acute blood loss nonresponsive to crystalloids • Hct <35% • Hypovolemia from acute massive blood loss (i.e., major trauma) • History of blood loss at delivery or large amount of blood drawn for lab studies (10% blood volume) • Cardiac patients: Hct <40% (structural heart disease, cyanosis, or CHF) Drop in Hgb to <10 g/dL intraoperatively Exchange transfusion	Same nursing actions as for red blood cell infusions: verify unit and patient For major trauma, may transfuse with O-negative blood (the universal donor) until crossmatch is complete Use PPE Use blood warmer and rapid infuser if available During infusion, observe for signs of adverse reactions • Mild: fever or allergic reaction • Severe: hemolysis (fever, chills, hemoglobinuria, DIC, renal failure)
Platelets Platelet pheresis (single donor unit, may be split for small infants and neonates) Random donor (1-8 units per transfusion)	Platelet count <20,000/mm^3 Active bleeding with symptoms of DIC or other significant coagulopathies Platelet count <100,000/mm^3 with planned invasive procedure (i.e., surgical procedure, central line insertion), not including drawing blood, intramuscular injection, or intravenous catheter insertion. Prevention or treatment of bleeding associated with thrombocytopenia (secondary to chemotherapy, radiation, or bone marrow failure) Treatment of patients with severe thrombocytopenia secondary to increased platelet destruction or immune thrombocytopenia associated with complication of severe trauma Massive transfusion with platelet dilution	Verify platelet unit and patient Use PPE Monitor for allergic reaction During infusion, observe for signs of adverse reactions • Mild: fever or allergic reaction • Severe: hemolysis (fever, chills, hemoglobinuria, DIC, renal failure) Hemolysis may develop if sufficient incompatible plasma is present in transfusion

Table 15-4   Transfusion Therapy—cont'd

Blood Product, Dose	Clinical Indications	Nursing Interventions
FFP (10-15 mL/kg)	Replacement for deficiency of factors II, V, VII, IX, X, or XII, protein C, or protein S Bleeding, invasive procedure, or surgery with documented plasma clotting protein deficiency (i.e., liver failure, DIC, septic shock) Prolonged PT and/or aPTT without bleeding Significant intraoperative bleeding (>10% blood volume/hour) in excess of normally anticipated blood loss with high risk of clotting factor deficiency Massive transfusion Therapeutic plasma exchanges Warfarin anticoagulant overdose	Notify blood bank to thaw FFP; must use within 6 h of thawing Verify unit and patient Use PPE Monitor vital signs per hospital policy and procedure Monitor coagulation studies Observe for adverse reactions
Cryoprecipitate (cryo)	Fibrinogen levels <150 mg/dL with active bleeding Bleeding or prophylaxis in von Willebrand disease or in factor VIII deficiency (hemophilia A) unresponsive to or unsuitable for DDAVP or factor VII concentrates Replacement therapy, bleeding, or invasive procedure in patients with factor XIII deficiency Patients with active intraoperative hemorrhage in excess of normally anticipated blood loss who are at risk of clotting factor deficiency	Assess for signs and symptoms of bleeding Use appropriate PPE Monitor vital signs per hospital policy and procedure Monitor coagulation studies Observe for adverse reactions during cryoprecipitate infusions
Granulocytes (WBC transfusion)	Bacterial or fungal sepsis (proven or strongly suspected) unresponsive to antimicrobial therapy Infection (proven or strongly suspected) unresponsive to antimicrobial therapy	Type and crossmatch required for all WBC transfusions Verify unit and patient Premedications may be ordered, such as antihistamines or acetaminophen
Factor VII (90 units/kg)	Treatment of factor VII deficiency Treatment of factor VIII inhibitors Treatment of factor IX inhibitors Idiopathic uncontrolled bleeding	Order in micrograms or milligrams Assess for signs and symptoms of bleeding Use appropriate PPE, even with recombinant product Monitor coagulation studies If undiluted, dilute vial with indicated amount of sterile water and administer intravenously per manufacturer's guidelines
Factor VIII concentrate (10-50 units/kg)	Hemophilia A (factor VIII deficiency) Patient with factor VIII inhibitors Patients with von Willebrand disease	Order in units Check product to determine whether refrigeration is necessary Record expiration date and lot number of product Assess for signs and symptoms of bleeding Use appropriate PPE Monitor coagulation studies
Factor IX concentrate (prothrombin complex; 1 IU/kg)	Treatment of hemophilia B Hemophilia A with factor VIII inhibitors Patients with congenital deficiency of prothrombin, factor VII, and factor X	Order in units Record expiration date and lot number of product Assess for signs and symptoms of bleeding Use appropriate PPE Monitor coagulation studies
IVIG	Congenital or acquired antibody deficiency Immunologic disorders such as idiopathic thrombocytopenia, Kawasaki disease Posttransplant patients (used prophylactically) Newborns with severe bacterial infections	Obtain from pharmacy Record expiration date and lot number of product Use appropriate PPE Monitor vital signs per hospital policy and procedure Start infusion slowly and increase rate; titrate per physician orders During IVIG infusion, observe for adverse reactions such as fever, chills, and headache

From Norville R, Bryant R: In Baggott CR, et al, editors: *Blood component deficiencies in nursing care of the child with cancer*, ed 3. Philadelphia, 2002, WB Saunders, Association of Pediatric Oncology Nurses.
ARDS, Acute respiratory distress syndrome; *BP*, blood pressure; *CHF*, congestive heart failure; *DDAVP*, 1-deamino-8-arginine vasopressin; *DIC*, disseminated intravascular coagulation; *FFP*, fresh frozen plasma; *Hct*, hematocrit; *Hgb*, hemoglobin; *IVIG*, intravenous immunoglobulin; *PPE*, personal protective equipment; *PRBC*, packed red blood cell; *WBC*, white blood cell.

Table 15-5   ABO Compatibilities

Recipient	First Choice Donor	Second Choice Donor	Third Choice Donor
A+	A+	O+, A−	O−
B+	B+	O+, B−	O−
AB+	AB+	AB−, A+, B+	O+, A−, B−, O−
O+	O+	O−	—
A−	A−	O−	A+, O+
B−	B−	O−	B+, O+
AB−	AB−	A−, B−, O−	AB+, A+, B+, O+
O−	O−	O+	—

Box 15-6   Blood Transfusion Safety Measure

At the time the blood sample is collected for crossmatch, the nurse should place a blood bracelet containing the specific identifying number on the patient's extremity at the bedside. This safety measure is designed to ensure that the patient receives the correct blood product that has been crossmatched specifically for the patient. Fatal hemolytic reactions can result from erroneous administration of incorrect blood units. Such errors can be reduced by adherence to this safety measure.

Box 15-7   Checklist for Blood Administration

Before the Transfusion

- Verify physician orders and consent for blood products.
- Obtain a complete set of vital signs including temperature.
- Verify whether there are any orders for pre-medications.
- Obtain blood product (i.e., blood bank, pharmacy, unit blood refrigerator). Check for special instructions such as autologous, leukocyte reduced, or irradiated.
- The transfusion must be started within 30 min after the blood has left the refrigerator.
  ◦ The maximum total infusion time is 4 h; this includes the first 30 min.
  ◦ Transfusion must start immediately to reduce the risk of bacterial contamination and cell lysis.*
  ◦ Most blood banks will not accept blood back after 30 min.
- Follow hospital policy for obtaining, verifying, and transporting blood products obtained from sources outside the critical care unit.
- Ensure accurate patient identification—most commonly name and date of birth. Two appropriate healthcare team members must check all blood products at the patient's bedside per institutional policy.
- Confirm R number (for red and white blood cells) with patient's bracelet and blood product.
- Always use personal protective equipment, including eye shields and gloves.

At Initiation of the Transfusion

- Obtain baseline vital signs, including body temperature.
- Administer the blood product slowly for the first 15 min.

- Designate a clinical staff member to remain with patient for the first 15 min of transfusion to respond in the event of an adverse reaction.

During the Transfusion

- Never infuse any solutions (other than normal saline) through the same catheter with blood.[1]
- Never add any medications to blood.
- Monitor vital signs per the institution's policy and procedures.
- Leave all identification information attached to the blood product until the transfusion is complete.
- Monitor for signs and symptoms of adverse reactions (see the discussion under Transfusion Reactions).

After the Transfusion

- Save the transfusion bag for at least 1 h after transfusion has ended, in the event of an adverse reaction.
- Complete the blood slip as indicated per institution's required information.
- According to the 2006 American Association of Blood Banks guidelines,[1] information to be included in the patient's medical record must include the transfusion order, the type of blood product, the donor unit number, date and time of transfusion, vital signs before and after transfusion, the volume infused, required signatures, and any transfusion adverse events.
- Required documentation should be placed in the medical record and sent to the blood bank for record keeping per American Association of Blood Banks guidelines.

such as fever, central nervous system tumors, bleeding, or coagulopathies or those requiring procedures.[2] According to the American Society of Clinical Oncology, patients can safely have "major invasive procedures" (such as bone marrow aspirate and biopsies) with platelet counts of $50,000/mm^3$,[24] although the threshold varies among institutions.[23,28] Platelet preparations are listed in Box 15-8.

Single-donor plateletpheresis provides the equivalent of approximately 5 to 8 units of random donor platelets. The life span of transfused platelets is approximately 4 days, although several variables can influence their effectiveness. Infections, fever, and coagulopathies can all contribute to decreasing the lifespan of transfused platelets. Rapid turnover of platelets may necessitate more frequent platelet transfusions. Monitoring of bleeding and platelet counts will be required in these clinical conditions.

Platelet products are administered intravenously with varying infusion times; the maximum transfusion interval is 4 hours. If large patients can tolerate the volume, platelets can be administered rapidly (over 20 to 30 minutes). Platelets are typically administered more slowly to infants, children, and patients with fluid restriction.

Platelet transfusions should be used judiciously to prevent alloimmunization to RhD antigens. Ideally, female patients of childbearing age or younger who are Rh-negative should receive platelets from Rh-negative donors, to minimize

*American Association of Blood Banks Standards for Blood Banks and Transfusion Services, ed 24, Bethesda, MD, 2006, American Association of Blood Banks Press.

Box 15-8 **Types of Platelet Preparations**

Random donor platelets are obtained by removing the platelet portion from donated whole blood. This is generally not the preferred product because of the exposure of numerous blood donors or antigens.

Platelet pheresis is obtained from a single donor. These units are preferred for platelet transfusions to decrease patient exposure to multiple donors and donor antigens.

HLA-matched platelets are used specifically for hematology-oncology patients who have developed antibodies as a result of numerous blood product transfusions. The purpose of HLA-matched platelets is to improve the outcome (greater increase in the platelet count) of the platelet transfusion by minimizing platelet destruction.

development of maternal-fetal Rh incompatibility. However, in extreme emergencies the available blood is administered.

Platelet transfusion will not substantially increase the platelet count if the patient has alloimmunization. Essentially these patients become refractory to platelet transfusion. The most common cause of alloimmunization is multiple transfusions. Patients who receive multiple blood products may produce antibodies that attack transfused platelets so that they are destroyed as foreign antigens. When such patients become thrombocytopenic, they may require HLA-matched platelet transfusions that can be more challenging to acquire.

Transfusion Reactions

Critical care nurses must be able to immediately recognize and respond to transfusion reactions. Most reactions occur during the first minutes of a transfusion, although they can occur at any time, including after completion of the transfusion. Reactions can vary from mild (e.g., febrile or allergic) to life-threatening with severe hemolysis, anaphylaxis, and death. Patients who have had multiple transfusions are at higher risk for developing a febrile transfusion reaction.[10] Although general recommendations are provided in Box 15-9, nurses should follow institutional guidelines for management and documentation of transfusion reactions.

Box 15-9 **Treatment of Transfusion Reaction**

- Stop transfusion, keep vein open (administer intravenous fluids per order or protocol).
- Support airway, oxygenation, ventilation, and circulation if compromised.
- Reassess vital signs.
- Notify physician; activate emergency response team, if indicated.
- Treat symptoms per physician order; prepare to administer diphenhydramine, hydrocortisone, and epinephrine if applicable.
- Recheck identification labels.
- Notify blood bank.
- Obtain blood and urine sample if indicated.
- Complete transfusion reaction documentation.
- Follow institutional policies for blood transfusion reactions.

Febrile Nonhemolytic Reaction

Fever is one of the most common adverse reactions observed during transfusion, although its frequency has been reduced with the use of leukocyte-depleted blood products. In some cases, pre-medication with acetaminophen can prevent this type of adverse reaction.

A febrile reaction usually occurs upon initiation or shortly after initiation of a transfusion. Signs and symptoms that can occur during a febrile nonhemolytic transfusion reaction include fever, chills, nausea, vomiting, abdominal cramps, and skin flushing. The reaction can progress to include more serious complications such as hemolysis or anaphylaxis with respiratory failure, hypotension, shock.

Monitor the patient's temperature to identify febrile reactions early and enable prevention or treatment of complications. If the patient develops a febrile reaction, the nurse must immediately stop the transfusion, restart intravenous fluids per physician order or protocol, notify a physician or on-call provider, and closely monitor vital signs and cardiorespiratory function.

Febrile reactions can be caused by bacterial contamination of a unit of blood, because blood products provide an excellent medium for bacterial growth. Bacterial contamination is more common with platelets than other blood products because platelets are stored at room temperature, which allows more bacterial growth than refrigeration.[24] Contamination of products can occur at any phase of the transfusion process, from collection to administration. Guidelines from the American Association of Blood Banks[1] require strict adherence to the completion of all transfusions within 4 hours or less to reduce the risk of contamination and cell lysis. In addition, blood collection centers should function within strict guidelines for screening of potential donors and for collection and storage of blood products.

Hemolytic Reaction

The most serious blood transfusion reaction is an acute hemolytic reaction from ABO blood type incompatibility or mismatch. This acute reaction is a medical emergency produced by rapid destruction of the donor red blood cells by the host antibodies. Signs and symptoms include fever, chills, anxiety, lower back pain, pink or red urine, jaundice, disseminated intravascular coagulation, hypotension, renal failure, and death.

If you suspect a hemolytic reaction, stop the transfusion immediately and administer intravenous fluids per physician or provider orders or per protocol; support airway, breathing, and circulation as needed; evaluate patient vital signs; notify a physician; recheck the patient's identification and compatibility label; and notify the blood bank. Return the unit of blood to the blood bank for re-crossmatching, and obtain blood samples and the first posttransfusion urine sample for urinalysis.

Most hemolytic reactions are from red blood cells. A hemolytic reaction can develop if sufficient incompatible plasma is given during a platelet transfusion.

Allergic Reaction

Another common reaction to transfusion is an allergic reaction triggered by allergens found in the plasma of donor blood. Most of these reactions occur during transfusions in patients who have had a previous exposure to a particular allergen in a blood product. The previous exposure to the allergen stimulated development of antibodies, and the next exposure results in an allergic reaction. The reaction can occur during the next infusion after exposure or during subsequent transfusions.

Symptoms can develop within seconds to hours of the transfusion and include rash, hives, pruritus, swelling of the lips, wheezing, and anxiety. If the patient experiences an allergic reaction, stop the transfusion immediately and restart intravenous fluids per physician order or protocol; assess and support airway, breathing, and circulation; evaluate vital signs; and notify a physician. If the allergic reaction is mild, the transfusion can be restarted after administering an antihistamine such as diphenhydramine (Benadryl). Monitor the patient closely when the transfusion is restarted. In moderate to severe allergic reactions, the patient may require the administration of steroids such as hydrocortisone and possibly epinephrine. The nurse must follow the procedure for transfusion reaction, including documentation and return of the blood product to the blood bank. Future blood transfusions may require prophylaxis with diphenhydramine and hydrocortisone.

Anaphylaxis

In rare cases, an allergic transfusion reaction can progress to life-threatening anaphylaxis, a medical emergency. Patients with immunoglobulin A deficiency may be more susceptible to these reactions. A classic anaphylactic reaction has a sudden onset after administration of only a few milliliters of the blood product. The patient develops bronchospasm, shortness of breath, respiratory distress, and hypotension. The designated staff member at the bedside during the first 15 minutes of the transfusion should be prepared to rapidly identify and respond to these severe adverse reactions. In severe anaphylaxis, stop the transfusion and administer intravenous fluids per physician order or protocol); support airway, oxygenation, ventilation, and circulation as needed; evaluate vital signs; notify a physician; and activate the emergency response system, as appropriate. For further information, see Anaphylaxis earlier in this chapter and in Chapters 6 and 16.

Circulatory Overload

An uncommon transfusion reaction is circulatory overload, also known as transfusion-associated circulatory overload. This complication is caused by rapid administration of a blood transfusion with resulting hypervolemia. At-risk patients include very young patients, patients with impaired cardiac and renal function, and patients with chronic anemia. Clinical signs and symptoms include respiratory distress with pulmonary edema (including dyspnea, rales or crackles, and hypoxemia), distended neck veins, hypertension or hypotension, tachycardia or bradycardia, clammy skin, and peripheral cyanosis. If these symptoms develop, immediately stop the transfusion; support airway, oxygenation, and ventilation and circulation as needed; monitor vital signs; elevate the head of the bed, with the feet in dependent position; and notify a physician (activate the emergency response system if needed). Diuretics may be ordered. Closely monitor cardiorespiratory function and evaluate intake and output.

Transfusion-Related Acute Lung Injury

Transfusion-related acute lung injury (TRALI) is a serious blood transfusion reaction characterized by acute onset of pulmonary edema, a similar clinical picture to acute respiratory distress syndrome. TRALI and clerical error causing mismatched blood transfusion reaction are the most common causes of transfusion-related deaths.[5] TRALI occurs when there is an atypical antigen-antibody reaction caused by human leukocyte antibodies in the donated blood. These donor antibodies are transfused to the patient during the transfusion; they attach to the patient's WBCs and form microaggregates. When the microaggregates circulate to the lungs, they trigger an inflammatory response that causes increased vascular permeability, pulmonary edema, and life-threatening respiratory failure.[10]

Patients experiencing TRALI can develop sudden signs of respiratory distress such as shortness of breath, hypoxia, hypotension, fever, and abnormal breath sounds. This reaction typically occurs within 1 to 2 hours after the transfusion has started, and full blown acute respiratory distress syndrome can develop within 6 hours.[10] For mild cases of TRALI, the patient may respond to oxygen administration (perhaps with bilevel positive airway pressure) and diuretics. In severe cases, patients will also require intubation and mechanical ventilation with positive end-expiratory pressure. If TRALI is suspected, this transfusion reaction is reportable to the FDA.

Transfusions and Jehovah Witnesses

Jehovah Witnesses believe that blood transfusions—even in life-threatening situations—are forbidden by scripture. They also believe that if blood is removed from the body, it cannot be re-infused, such as with the cell-saver technology used in operating rooms. In addition, they believe that self-donation is also prohibited. Further information is available in the Chapter 15 Supplement on the Evolve Website.

If the child requires a life-saving transfusion, physicians can obtain a court order that will enable blood product administration. With the court order, decisions related to the administration of blood and blood products are made by a court-appointed guardian.[15]

If the life of the child is in imminent danger and there is no time to obtain a court order, blood can be administered with a physician order and documentation in the chart of the dire need for the blood transfusion. If this situation occurs, follow hospital policy and notify risk management.

Apheresis

The word *apheresis* is derived from Greek, meaning "to separate or remove." The apheresis procedure involves removing blood from a donor or patient and separating its components. One or more of the components are selectively retained, and the remaining components are recombined and returned to the donor.[18,19] Apheresis is often used in the critical care setting for patients with hematologic, oncologic, and other emergencies.

Intravenous access is required; a double lumen central venous catheter is the preferred route of access. For larger patients, such as adolescents and young adults, two large-bore peripheral venous catheters may be acceptable.

Intermittent flow centrifugation[19] is a form of apheresis that uses a single intravenous access site. Intermittent flow centrifugation is performed in cycles (pull in and pull out): blood is removed with the assistance of a pump and placed in a centrifuge separator for component removal; the needed components are collected for storage, and the remaining product is returned to the patient through the intravenous access. Another method of apheresis is continuous flow centrifugation. In this method blood is withdrawn through one catheter, processed, and returned through a second venous catheter.

All pheresis procedures use anticoagulants in order to prevent blood from clotting. The most common anticoagulants are acid citrate dextrose or heparin.

The apheresis machine is comparable to a dialysis machine, with one line to withdraw blood from the patient and another to return the blood to the patient. The apheresis procedure is often named according to the major component to be extracted: erythrocytapheresis (red cell exchange), plasmapheresis, leukapheresis (stem cell collection or leukodepletion), and platelet pheresis.

Erythrocytapheresis (Red Blood Cell Exchange)

The patient's RBCs are removed from the patient's blood and replaced by donor RBCs that are infused into the patient with the patient's plasma, WBCs, and platelets. This treatment can be used for sickle cell anemia with acute crises, such as acute chest syndrome, cerebral vascular accident, or severe priapism. Other diseases that can benefit from an RBC exchange include erythrocytosis polycythemia vera and severe malaria.[19]

Plasmapheresis

Plasma may contain components such as circulating immune complexes, antibodies, inflammatory mediators, lipoproteins, protein-bound toxins, and platelet aggregating factors that can contribute to inflammation and disease. With plasmapheresis, plasma alone is extracted from the patient's blood and replaced by donor plasma or a plasma substitute that is infused with the patient's own blood components. Plasmapheresis may be helpful for patients with HUS, autoimmune hemolytic anemia, thrombotic thrombocytopenic purpura, meningococcemia, toxic ingestion, Guillain-Barré syndrome, and systemic lupus erythematosus.

Leukapheresis (Stem Cell Collection or Leukodepletion)

Leukapheresis for a stem cell collection harvests hematopoietic progenitor cells (identified by markers on the white cell called a CD34 antigen) for autologous or allogenic hematopoietic stem cell transplant. Several sessions may be required to collect an appropriate amount of CD34 targeted cells. Hematopoietic growth factors can be administered before the leukapheresis to improve the yield of stem cells. After collection, these cells are cryopreserved for future use; they will be reinfused at a later date, after the preparative regimen has ablated the patient's bone marrow.

Leukapheresis can also be used to remove excess WBCs in the circulation when patients have high WBC counts (e.g., newly diagnosed patients with T cell lymphomas and patients with acute or chronic leukemias) at risk for acute complications. The patient's clinical condition, WBC counts, and renal status will determine the need for this type of pheresis, although leukapheresis is commonly used for patients with WBC counts of $100,000/mm^3$ and greater.

WBC transfusions may be administered to severely neutropenic oncology patients who are septic and unresponsive to traditional therapy. This type of treatment modality is controversial and often a method of last resort.

Adverse Effects of Apheresis

During the apheresis process, there is potential for adverse effects. Table 15-6 summarizes potential complications of apheresis.

SPECIFIC DISEASES

Sickle Cell Disease

Etiology

Sickle cell anemia is one of the most common genetic hematologic conditions in children. The disease is transmitted by an autosomal recessive pattern of inheritance; both parents

Table 15-6 Complications of Apheresis

Complication	Nursing Intervention
Air embolism	Closely monitor connection sites and tubing
	Prime line with normal saline or compatible fluid
Citrate toxicity	Monitor for signs and symptoms (numbness and tingling around mouth)
	Decrease re-infusion rate to diminish symptoms
Hypocalcemia	Verify ionized calcium before pheresis, correct abnormalities
	Monitor ionized calcium concentration hourly during pheresis (or per physician orders)
	Consider calcium infusion if clinical condition indicates
Hypotension	Have fluids available in case of rapid onset of hypotension
	May need to increase rate of vasopressors
Hypothermia	Monitor body temperature frequently to prevent or promptly treat hypothermia
	Use blood warmer on pheresis machine
	Keep patient warm with blankets, external warmers, or both
Infection	Strict hand washing
	Maintain sterile technique with all invasive lines.
Risk for bleeding	Monitor coagulation profile before prior to pheresis therapy
	Platelet or other blood products such as clotting factors may be required during the procedure
Transfusion reaction	Use leukodepleted, irradiated blood products if indicated
	Monitor for transfusion reactions from the replacement products; follow the transfusion reaction protocol if this occurs
	Consider administration of an antihistamine for patients receiving multiple treatments
Thrombus	Obtain platelet count before catheter placement and be aware when possible transfusion of platelets is necessary
	Flush vigorously with normal saline per hospital policy

are carriers of the sickle cell gene (For more information, see Evolve Fig. 15-4 in the Chapter 15 Supplement on the Evolve Website).[13,27]

Patients with sickle cell disease are homozygous for the sickle cell gene; this means that both genes are abnormal.[27] Patients with sickle cell trait are heterozygous for the sickle cell gene; these patients are generally asymptomatic because they possess one sickle and one normal gene.

Pathophysiology

In sickle cell disease, the patient has inherited two copies of the gene for an abnormal Hgb protein, called *Hgb S*. Hgb S has a single amino acid substitution of valine for glutamine that makes the protein polymerize upon desaturation (i.e., loss of oxygen). The RBC is more susceptible to deformity, causing it to assume the characteristic sickle shape when the Hgb loses oxygen. The higher the percentage of Hgb S in the circulating blood, the more likely the RBCs are to "sickle" during periods of decreased oxygenation.

Sickled RBCs have reduced flexibility and tend to be "sticky" so that they will adhere more readily to the blood vessel walls and to each other, causing occlusion of small vessels and tissue ischemia. Sickled RBCs are more fragile (i.e., they readily hemolyze) so turnover of RBCs is more rapid, causing chronic anemia.[19] These changes in RBC morphology compromise microvascular blood flow and tissue oxygenation that can lead to ischemia and infarcts, in a cycle of hypoxia and RBC sickling called a *vasoocclusive crisis.*

Sickle cell vasoocclusive crises can involve the central nervous system, bone, lungs or other visceral organs. Sickled cells have the tendency to clump and can cause splenic sequestration (RBC trapping within the spleen that causes sudden anemia, hypotension, and shock), functional asplenia (loss of splenic function from chronic occlusion of splenic vessels), cerebral vascular accident, acute chest syndrome, avascular necrosis of the femoral head, leg ulcers, priapism, hand-foot syndrome (dactylitis), and chronic organ damage.

Complications of hemolysis include anemia, cholelithiasis (gallstones), jaundice, and retarded growth and sexual maturation. The complications that may require critical care are the occurrence of acute chest syndrome, cerebral vascular accident, and priapism (painful and continuous erection of the penis).

The definitive diagnostic test for sickle cell disease or trait is Hgb electrophoresis.[19] This test measures the various types and percentages of Hgb present.

Clinical Signs and Symptoms

The signs and symptoms associated with sickle cell anemia largely result from microvascular occlusions created by the sickled red blood cells; these may be diffuse and may result in organ or tissue ischemia or infarct. Children with sickle cell anemia may also have clinical manifestations of anemia, including weakness, pallor, and fatigue. Patients with sickle cell disease have decreased Hgb and Hct and an elevated reticulocyte count.

Vasoocclusive crises requiring critical care include the complications noted above, acute chest syndrome, cerebral

vascular accident and priapism. These conditions are medical emergencies and treatment must be provided immediately to prevent permanent disability or death. Pain associated with vasoocclusive crises may be severe.

Acute Chest Syndrome. Acute chest syndrome can cause the sudden onset of respiratory distress, characterized by dyspnea, tachypnea, cough, fever, arterial oxygen desaturation (oxyhemoglobin saturation less than 90%), hypoxemia, and confusion. The chest radiograph may show increased infiltrates and pleural effusion. Clinical signs may be difficult to distinguish from pneumonia. With acute chest syndrome, onset and deterioration may be more sudden, and the radiograph often reveals multilobar infiltrates. Mortality is high.[27]

Cerebrovascular Accident (Stroke). Signs of cerebral vascular accident include the sudden onset of neurologic changes such as sudden confusion, trouble speaking or change in motor function. Patients may demonstrate a deterioration in level of consciousness, motor weakness, severe headache (sometimes unilateral), visual changes, or seizures. The diagnosis of a cerebral vascular accident is confirmed by cerebral angiography or a CT scan; these tests are typically performed once the patient's condition is stable, often after treatment is initiated.

Priapism. Priapism is persistent erection caused by trapping of blood in the network of spaces in the penis. Under normal conditions, the arteries contract and blood drains from the penis and the erection subsides. If the blood is trapped and RBCs begin to sickle, the tissue of the penis may become ischemic and gangrene can result.

Splenic Sequestration Crisis. Splenic sequestration crisis occurs in young children with sickle cell anemia who have not yet lost splenic function; the cause is unknown. RBC trapping in the spleen leads to sudden anemia, hypotension, and shock. A massively enlarged spleen can be palpated readily on physical examination.

Management

Excellent outpatient care of patients with sickle cell anemia may reduce the frequency of many of the complications of the disease. This care includes promoting adequate hydration and avoiding conditions that can contribute to Hgb desaturation (e.g., change in altitude, strenuous exercise) or decreased blood flow (e.g., shock, infection).

At times of crisis, provide immediate hydration with intravenous crystalloids (normal saline or oral re-hydration if tolerated); typically fluids are administered at a rate of 1.5 times maintenance requirements. Adequate hydration promotes hemodilution, increasing blood flow and decreasing risk of microvascular occlusion and tissue ischemia. If the child with splenic sequestration exhibits hypovolemic shock, provide PRBC transfusion to restore intravascular volume and RBC mass. Ultimately, splenectomy may be required.

RBC exchange is used for severe crises, to reduce the concentration of Hgb S. Generally the goal is to reduce the concentration of Hgb S to less than 30%, although this goal is tailored to the patient and the patient's clinical condition. Pain control is essential, ideally with a combination of both pharmacologic and nonpharmacologic therapies (see Chapter 5); intravenous narcotic administration may be needed. It is helpful to determine the pain control measures that have worked previously.

Assess and support respiratory status and oxygenation. Monitor for signs and symptoms of respiratory distress, auscultate lung sounds (decreased and abnormal breath sounds may indicate complications such as effusion, pulmonary infarct, pneumonia, or edema), evaluate respiratory rate and effort, perform continuous monitoring of oxyhemoglobin saturation, and monitor color and perfusion. Administer oxygen as needed to maintain oxyhemoglobin saturation above 92% to 93%. Inform the medical team immediately of any abnormal findings. Pneumonia and pulmonary infarcts occur more often in this patient population.

Hypertransfusion can be provided for patients who have experienced severe complications, such as a stroke and acute chest syndrome, to prevent further episodes. The patient receives monthly scheduled PRBC transfusions to keep the Hgb S level below 30% (may be tailored to the patient). Hematopoietic stem cell transplant may be performed to cure the sickle cell anemia (see Hematopoietic Stem Cell Transplantation earlier in chapter).

Hemophilia

Etiology. Hemophilia is a recessive hereditary bleeding disorder; it is X-linked, so it primarily affects males.[13] In rare cases, a female may be afflicted with hemophilia if both X chromosomes are defective.

Pathophysiology

This group of bleeding disorders is characterized by a deficiency of either factor VIII or IX that results in the inability to form a clot at a site of injury. Hemophilia A, also known as *classic hemophilia,* is characterized by a deficiency of factor VIII. Hemophilia B, also known as *Christmas disease,* is a deficiency of factor IX.[25] Children with hemophilia have prolonged bleeding.

Hemophilia is classified as mild, moderate, or severe; the severity of the bleeding disorder is directly related to the degree of factor deficiency (Table 15-7). The child with a significant factor deficiency will experience more bleeding episodes than the child with mild deficiency. Bleeding is not faster in these patients; bleeding is prolonged and causes the clinical manifestations and risks of complications such as intracranial bleeding, hemorrhage, and hemarthrosis.

Clinical Signs and Symptoms

The most obvious sign of a bleeding disorder is persistent oozing, associated with small lacerations or minor procedures. Infant males may be diagnosed after prolonged bleeding after circumcision; the older child may exhibit bleeding after a dental procedure or tooth loss (Table 15-8). Other potential clinical signs and symptoms of factor deficiency include pain, swelling, bleeding into a joint after injury, bleeding from the mouth or nose, and menorrhagia. Life-threatening bleeding events for hemophiliacs include head injury, neck and throat

	Percentage of Factor	
Type	**VIII/IX (%)**	**Type of Hemorrhage**
Severe	<1	Spontaneous: hemarthroses and deep soft-tissue hemorrhages
Moderate	1-5	Gross bleeding following mild to moderate trauma; some hemarthroses; rare spontaneous hemorrhage
Mild	5-25	Severe hemorrhage only after moderate to severe trauma or surgery
High-risk carrier females	Variable	Gynecologic and obstetric hemorrhage common; other symptoms depend on plasma factor level

Table 15-7 Relationship of Factor Levels to Severity of Clinical Manifestations of Hemophilia A and B

From Lanzkowsky P: *Manual of pediatric hematology and oncology,* ed 4. Philadelphia, 2005, Elsevier, p. 311.

bleeding, an acute abdomen, and bleeding into the iliopsoas muscle near the femoral artery.

Patients with bleeding disorders who develop any head, neck, or torso injury must be evaluated immediately, because bleeding in these areas can be life threatening. When treating life-threatening bleeding, the first and most important step is to stop the bleeding; the diagnostic analysis is completed after replacement factors are initiated.[25]

Common laboratory tests include aPTT and PT; both will be elevated (prolonged). The most important test is the direct assay of plasma factor activity level for hemophilia A and B.[8]

Management

For any patient with active bleeding, the first priority is to control or stop the bleeding. After bleeding is controlled, patients with hemophilia should receive replacement factor products. The appropriate type and dose of factor products is determined by the location or body part affected and the type of hemophilia present. For example, a patient with factor VIII deficiency with minor trauma can be managed with replacement factor VIII products to raise the factor activity levels to 20% to 40%; this level should provide adequate hemostasis in most circumstances. To control life-threatening (e.g., head injury) bleeding in the same patient requires administration of replacement factors to raise the factor activity levels to 100%. The aPTT should normalize after factor VIII transfusion.

Some patients with hemophilia may benefit from factor prophylaxis to prevent complications and bleeding episodes. Patient treatment plans are individualized, but typically call for infusions three times per week for patients with hemophilia A and infusions twice per week for patients with hemophilia B.[25]

Rarely, patients with hemophilia can develop inhibitors to coagulation proteins after receiving numerous (more than

Table 15-8 Incidence of Severity and Clinical Manifestations of Hemophilia

Variable	TYPE (SEVERITY) OF HEMOPHILIA		
	Severe	Moderate	Mild
Incidence			
Hemophilia A (%)	70	15	15
Hemophilia B (%)	50	30	20
Bleeding Manifestations			
Age of onset (year)	≤1	1-2	2 to adulthood
Neonatal hemorrhage following circumcision	Common	Common	None
Neonatal intracranial hemorrhage	Occasionally	Rare	Rare
Muscle or joint hemorrhage	Spontaneous	Following minor trauma	Following trauma
CNS hemorrhage	High risk	Moderate risk	Rare
Postsurgical hemorrhage	Common	Common	Rare
Oral hemorrhage	Common	Common	Rare

From Lanzkowsky P: *Manual of pediatric hematology and oncology,* ed 4. Philadelphia, 2005, Elsevier, p. 312.
CNS, Central nervous system.

20 to 30) doses of replacement factor products.[8] You should suspect development of inhibitors in patients who have continued prolongation of the aPTT despite receiving 100% of corrective dose of factor products. If the patient develops inhibitors, changes in or additions to the treatment regimen may be necessary to provide adequate replacement factors.

Nursing priorities for the child with hemophilia include control of bleeding, timely administration of factor products, monitoring of laboratory values, and supportive measures including treatment of pain. Patient and family teaching should focus on safety, injury prevention, and avoiding high-risk activities. Patients should also be instructed to wear medical alert jewelry, avoid nonsteroidal antiinflammatory drugs, and intramuscular injections. Finally, for women of childbearing age with a family history of hemophilia, genetic counseling is recommended.

Hemolytic Uremic Syndrome

Hemolytic uremic syndrome is an uncommon renal disease that is seen most often in children younger than 5 years. The causative agent is usually *Escherichia coli* O157:H7,[27] and the dominant clinical feature of this disease is acute renal failure. These patients generally have a prodromal illness, such as acute gastroenteritis or an upper respiratory illness. Most cases of HUS present with bloody diarrhea and gastric symptoms. These patients have a history of consumption of undercooked meat, specifically ground beef. Other possible sources of *E. coli* infection include unpasteurized milk or juices, alfalfa sprouts, lettuce, and drinking or swimming in water contaminated with sewage.

The clinical signs of HUS itself can include the acute onset of purpura, irritability, lethargy, marked pallor, oliguria, hemolysis, and eventual renal failure. Diagnosis is usually confirmed by the clinical features of anemia, thrombocytopenia, and renal failure. The renal failure is characterized by an elevated blood urea nitrogen and creatinine, proteinuria, hematuria, and casts in urine. A CBC often reveals a decrease in Hgb and Hct and an increase in reticulocyte count, indicative of HUS. Management of HUS in young children may differ slightly than for older adolescents and adults. Generally, young children will recover with only hemodialysis support

and minimal complications. The older adolescent and adult with HUS should be managed with apheresis (plasma exchange) and hemodialysis. Most patients with HUS recover without long-term sequelae, although a potential long term complication may be the development of chronic renal failure (for further information, see Chapter 13).

COMMON DIAGNOSTIC TESTS

Lumbar Puncture

A lumbar puncture—also known as a *spinal tap*—may be performed to obtain cerebrospinal fluid to identify a neurologic illness or a central nervous system infection or malignancy. It also provides information about the pressure and composition of the cerebrospinal fluid. This test is completed under sterile conditions. Contraindications include bleeding disorders, anticoagulant therapy, very low platelet count and, in some patients, increased intracranial pressure. If increased intracranial pressure is suspected, a CT scan is performed before the procedure.

Procedure

The patient is positioned in the side with the head flexed (chin to chest) and the knees drawn; this position opens the intravertebral spaces. Alternatively, patients can be positioned sitting upright, with the buttocks placed on the edge of the procedure table with the head flexed (chin to chest). Nurses will need to assist the child in maintaining proper position (Fig. 15-4).

Often, pediatric patients will be sedated for this procedure (see Chapter 5). If the patient is not sedated, a topical anesthetic is applied to the puncture site and additional local anesthetic may be used.

This procedure is always performed under sterile conditions. The nurse assists the practitioner with obtaining appropriate supplies and in positioning the patient.

Following sterile preparation and administration of local anesthetic, an appropriately sized spinal needle with stylet is inserted through the skin and into the intervertebral space at the midline, between the third and fourth or the fourth and fifth lumbar vertebrae. The spinal needle is then inserted

remain flat to promote even distribution of chemotherapy throughout the CSF.

The CSF specimen is sent to the laboratory to determine WBC count, protein and glucose values (see Table 11-11) and, if appropriate, for cytologic examination for cancer cells and cultures for possible infections. CSF is examined for color and presence of blood. Normal CSF is clear and colorless.

Bone Marrow Aspirate and Biopsy

Bone marrow aspirate or biopsy is a common diagnostic procedure to examine the hematopoietic system. This procedure is often performed to evaluate the function and quality of the marrow. Bone marrow examination will reveal the number, size, and shape of the formed elements (RBCs, WBCs, and platelets) in the various stages of development.

A bone marrow aspirate is more common than a bone marrow biopsy, and it is performed by aspirating liquid marrow through a hollow needle into a syringe. A bone marrow biopsy is obtained by coring out a small piece of bone using a hollow needle.

Possible contraindications to this procedure include coagulation disorders. General anesthesia or moderate sedation may be used during this painful procedure.

Procedure

Both of these procedures are performed under sterile conditions, and both use large bore needles that contain stylets. After the site is prepared and appropriate local or systemic analgesia is provided, the needle is inserted through the soft tissue of the skin, into the outer layer of the pelvic bone, and into the marrow cavity. The most common site used is the posterior superior iliac crest. Alternative collection sites include the anterior iliac crest, proximal tibia, and sternum. Once the needle is inside the marrow, the stylet is removed and a syringe is attached to obtain specimens. A portion of these specimens is often placed on slides for microscopic examination.[20] When the procedure is complete, the bone marrow needle is removed and a dressing is applied. If the patient has a low platelet count, less than $50,000/mm^3$, then a pressure dressing is recommended.

If an inadequate specimen is obtained with a bone marrow aspirate (often referred to as a *dry tap*), then a bone marrow biopsy is required for diagnostic purposes. The specimen may indicate little cellular activity or that the bone marrow is packed with abnormal cells, such as in leukemia.

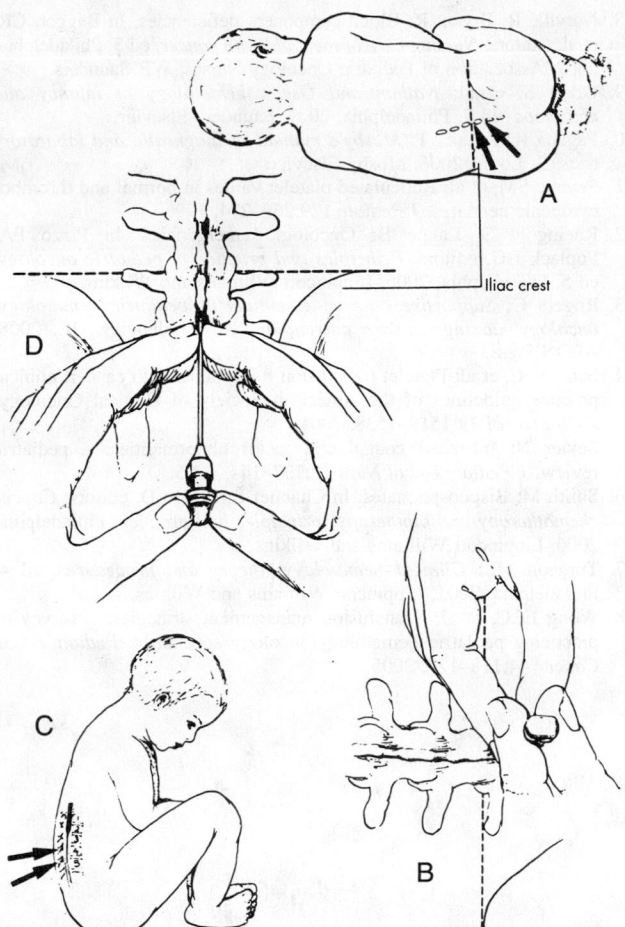

FIG. 15-4 Lumbar puncture. (A) The infant or child is usually restrained firmly in the lateral decubitus position, with the spine maximally flexed. The iliac crest is palpated to identify the level of the interspaces between the third and fourth or fourth and fifth lumbar vertebrae. (B) Using sterile technique, and following application of local anesthetic, insert the needle with bevel up, stabilizing the needle with the fingers of both hands. (C) The child may also be restrained in a sitting position for the lumbar puncture. The iliac crest is still palpable. (D) The needle should be advanced slowly into the intervertebral space. (From Fleisher G, Ludwig S: *Textbook of pediatric emergency medicine*, ed 2. Baltimore, 1988, Williams and Wilkins.)

through the dura and into the subarachnoid space. The stylet is removed and, if indicated, the opening CSF pressure is measured with a manometer. A pressure measurement of 20 cm of water or greater is considered abnormal and is suggestive of increased intracranial pressure.[20] The appropriate collection tubes are placed under the needle to collect the cerebral spinal fluid. Providers should describe the color and clarity (or opacity) of the fluid in the chart. For cancer patients who require intrathecal therapy, the appropriate volume of CSF is removed and the chemotherapy is administered.

When the procedure is complete, the spinal needle is removed and an adhesive dressing (typically an adhesive bandage strip) is applied to site. The postprocedure care includes observing the site for any CSF leak and instructing the patient to lie flat for a minimum of 30 minutes to prevent headache. If intrathecal medication is administered, the patient should

References

1. American Association of Blood Banks Standards for Blood Banks and Transfusion Services, ed 24, Bethesda, MD, 2006, American Association of Blood Banks Press.
2. Beutler E: Platelet transfusions: the 20,000/μL trigger. *Blood* 81:1411–1413, 1993.
3. Bollard CM, Krance RA, Heslop HE: Hematopoietic stem cell transplantation in pediatric oncology. In Pizzo PA,, Poplack DG, editors: *Principles and practice of pediatric oncology*, ed 5, Philadelphia, 2006, Lippincott Williams and Wilkins.
4. Cairo MS, Bishop M: Tumor lysis syndrome: new therapeutic strategies and classification. *Br J Haematol* 127:3–11, 2004.
5. Department of Health and Human Services: *Transfusion related acute lung injury (TRALI)*. FDA Patient Safety Newsletter. *http://www.fda.gov/BiologicsBloodVaccines/SafetyAvailability/BloodSafety/ucm095556.htm*. October 2001.
6. Gobel B: Chemotherapy induced hypersensitivity reactions. *Oncol Nurs Forum* 32:1027–1055, 2005.

7. Hastings C, Lubin B, Feusner J: Hematologic supportive care for children with cancer. Chapter 40. In Pizzo PA, Poplack DG, editors: *Principles and practice of pediatric oncology*, ed 5, Philadelphia, 2006, Lippincott Williams and Wilkins.

8. Hillman RS, Ault KA, Leporrier M, Rinder HM: *Hematology in clinical practice*, ed 4, New York, 2005, McGraw Hill.

9. Khilnani P: *Practical approach to pediatric intensive care,* New York, 2005, Oxford University Press.

10. Knippen M: Transfusion-related acute lung injury. *Am J Nurs* 6:61–64, 2006.

11. Lacroix J, et al: Transfusion strategies for patients in pediatric intensive care units. *N Engl J Med* 356:1609–1619, 2007.

12. Lacy CF et al., editors: *Lexi-Comp's drug information handbook: a comprehensive resource for clinicians and all healthcare professionals*, ed 18, Hudson, OH, 2009, Lexi-Comp.

13. Lanzkowsky P: *Manual of pediatric hematology and oncology*, ed 4, Philadelphia, 2005, Elsevier.

14. Leyland-Jones B: Treating cancer-related Hypercalcemia with gallium nitrate. *J Support Oncol* 2:509–520, 2004.

15. Linnard-Palmar L, Kools S: Parents' refusal of medical treatment based on religious and/or cultural beliefs: the law, ethical principles and clinical implications. *J Pediatr Nurs* 19:351–356, 2004.

16. National Cancer Institute: Hypercalcemia (PDQ). Available at http://www.cancer.gov/cancerinfo/pdq/supportivecare/hypercalcemia. Accessed January 21, 2009.

17. Norville R: *Hematopoietic stem cell transplantation in essentials of pediatric hematology/oncology nursing: a core curriculum*, ed 3, Glenview, IL, 2008, APON Press.

18. Norville R, Bryant R: Blood component deficiencies. In Baggott CR, et al., editors: *Nursing care of the child with cancer*, ed 3, Philadelphia, 2002, Association of Pediatric Oncology Nurses; WB Saunders.

19. Orkin S, et al: *Nathan and Oski's hematology of infancy and childhood*, ed 7, Philadelphia, 2009, Saunders-Elsevier.

20. Pagana K, Pagana T: *Mosby's manual of diagnostic and laboratory tests,* St Louis, 2006, Mosby-Elsevier.

21. Peterec SM, et al: Reticulated platelet values in normal and thrombocytopenic neonates. *J Pediatr* 129:269–274, 1996.

22. Rheingold S, Lange B: Oncologic emergencies. In Pizzo PA, Poplack DG, editors: *Principles and practice of pediatric oncology*, ed 5, Philadelphia, 2006, Lippincott Williams and Wilkins.

23. Rogers C: *Supportive care in essentials of pediatric hematology/oncology nursing: a core curriculum*, ed 3, Glenview, IL, 2008, APON Press.

24. Schiffer C, et al: Platelet transfusion for patients with cancer: clinical practice guidelines of the American Society of Clinical Oncology. *J Clin Oncol* 19:1519–1538, 2001.

25. Sevier N: Inherited coagulation factor abnormalities: a pediatric review. *J Pediatr Oncol Nurs* 22:137–144, 2005.

26. Smith M: Bisphosphonates. In Chabner B, Longo D, editors: *Cancer chemotherapy and biotherapy: principles and practice*, Philadelphia, 2006, Lippincott Williams and Wilkins.

27. Turgeon ML: *Clinical hematology: theory and procedures,* ed 4, Philadelphia, 2005, Lippincott Williams and Wilkins.

28. Wong ECC, et al: Transfusion management strategies: a survey of practicing pediatric hematology/oncology specialists. *Pediatr Blood Cancer* 44:118–127, 2005.

Immunology and Infectious Disorders

16

Kathryn E. Roberts • Susan E. Coffin

PEARLS

- The critically ill child may have immune compromise and is at risk for a variety of healthcare-acquired infections. The critical care nurse must be alert for evidence of inflammation and infection and signs of developing sepsis.
- It is likely that adherence to prevention measures can reduce risk of healthcare-acquired infections such as catheter-related bloodstream infections, ventilator-associated pneumonia, and urinary tract infections.
- Children with septic shock require early and aggressive fluid resuscitation, vasoactive support, early antibiotic therapy, and support of organ system function.

ANATOMY AND PHYSIOLOGY: IMMUNOLOGY

Immunology Overview

The human immune system is comprised of multiple components that play complementary roles in maintaining health. The innate immune system is often referred to as the *first line of defense* and includes natural barriers, such as intact skin, and cellular components, such as granulocytes. Defects in the innate immune system provide an opportunity for invasion and infection from a wide variety of pathogens. For example, breaches in skin integrity associated with invasive medical devices provide one of the most common immune defects of critically ill children.

The adaptive or acquired immune system is characterized by cellular and soluble factors that provide protection against specific pathogens. Examples include antibodies that are specific for a surface protein on an organism, or cytotoxic T-lymphocytes that can attack a specific virus. Typically, adaptive immune responses arise after exposure to either natural infection or vaccination. However, adaptive immunity can be passively provided in select circumstances, such as the infusion of botulinum toxin immunoglobulin for children with infant botulism.

Developmental Considerations

At the time of birth, a neonate is considered to be fundamentally immunocompromised for several reasons.[14] First, although infants born at term have passively acquired immunity from maternal antibodies that were transferred transplacentally before birth, the titers of these antibodies quickly wane, leaving the infant without immunity to most specific pathogens.

Until exposure to common pathogens by natural infection or immunization, infants lack durable organism-specific immunity. In addition, the function of specific components of the immune system does not mature until approximately 2 years of age. Until that time, infants are unable to make a robust antibody response to pathogens that have polysaccharide molecules on their surface. This developmental defect explains why the incidence of invasive pneumococcal infection, an organism with a polysaccharide coat, is relatively high in young children.

The transfer of maternal antibodies during fetal life occurs chiefly in the last trimester of gestation. The premature infant, born before the last trimester, lacks those transfused maternal antibodies, and therefore has a higher risk of infection, especially during the first months of life.

Infectious Disease Overview

Infection is a common cause and can be a common complication of critical illness in hospitalized children.[45] Common community-acquired infections such as bacterial pneumonia and viral infections can lead to life-threatening illnesses in both immunocompetent and immunocompromised children. Local and systemic complications of community-acquired infections include respiratory failure, shock, and renal insufficiency. Critically ill children are also at high risk of healthcare-acquired infections including catheter-associated bloodstream infections, ventilator-associated pneumonia, and surgical site infections. These infections can be caused by viruses, bacteria, or fungal organisms.

Colonization and Infection

At birth, a neonate is normally essentially sterile. Within hours, however, bacteria from both the environment and people who handle the infant are transferred onto and begin to grow on the baby's skin and mucous membranes.[20] These bacteria are typically referred to as *colonizing flora*. The predominant colonizing organisms vary with anatomic site. For example, skin organisms such as *Staphylococcus epidermidis* can be found on almost all keratinized skin. In contrast, anaerobic and gram-negative organisms are typically found only in the intestinal tract. Colonizing flora typically do not cause inflammation or invasive infection. Many infections, however, do arise from the patient's colonizing flora, often when a medical device breaches the integrity of skin or mucous membranes or when skin or mucous membranes become inflamed.

COMMON CLINICAL CONDITIONS

Immunodeficiency Versus Immunosuppression

Immunodeficiency is a permanent state of impaired immune function. It is typically genetic or congenital in nature. *Immunosuppression* is typically a temporary state of impaired immune function. It may be intentional (e.g., pharmacologic suppression in the transplant population) or unintentional (e.g., retroviral infections). *Immunocompromise* (or impaired immune function) results from both immunodeficiency and immunosuppression.

Allergic Reactions and Anaphylaxis

Etiology

Allergic or "hypersensitivity" reactions occur when the body mounts an exaggerated or inappropriate immune response to a substance perceived as foreign, resulting in local or general tissue damage. Such reactions are usually classified by severity and involvement,[1] as in types I to IV (Table 16-1).

Anaphylaxis is an allergic hypersensitivity reaction to a foreign protein or drug that causes a systemic response. Exposure to the antigen may be oral or intravenous, or through inhalation or via direct contact. The anaphylactic reaction can occur within seconds or minutes after exposure.[42]

Reactions can range from mild itching and hives to life-threatening airway obstruction, hypotension, and cardiovascular collapse. Generally, the more the rapid the development of the reaction, the more severe will be the adverse reaction.

Pathophysiology

Clinical signs and symptoms usually appear within seconds to minutes of exposure to an antigen. They are caused by the action of numerous inflammatory mediators, including histamine and histamine-like substances on surrounding tissues and blood vessels. These mediators cause significant changes in capillary permeability that lead to facial edema, airway edema, and bronchoconstriction as well as vasodilation, hypotension, and possible circulatory collapse. Constriction of airway smooth muscle tissues results in wheezing, crackles, stridor, and progressive respiratory distress. Erythema and pruritus may also be seen as the result of an influx of eosinophils. Mortality from anaphylaxis results from complications of bronchospasm and airway compromise or profound hypotension.

Any medication has the potential to cause an allergic reaction, although some agents are more commonly associated with anaphylaxis than others. Agents with a higher potential for causing anaphylactic reactions include antibiotics (e.g., penicillin or sulfa drugs), chemotherapy agents (e.g., Asparaginase or Etoposide), antifungal agents, biotherapy agents (e.g., monoclonal antibodies), blood products, immunoglobins, radiologic contrast media, latex products, and food.

Clinical Signs and Symptoms

Signs and symptoms of hypersensitivity or anaphylaxis can develop within seconds or minutes after exposure. Patients often initially describe a sense of impending doom, accompanied by pruritus and flushing. This can evolve rapidly into other clinical manifestations of hypersensitivity (Table 16-2).

Table 16-1   Hypersensitivity Reactions

Type	Description	Example
Type I (anaphylactic reaction)	Triggered in response to an exposure to an environmental antigen Mediated by IgE antibodies that bind to specific receptors on the surface of mast cells and basophils Results in the release of a host of mediators to produce a classic anaphylactic response	Anaphylaxis Asthma Allergic rhinitis, hay fever
Type II (tissue specific hypersensitivity)	Triggered by the presence of an antigen found only on a cell or tissue Mediated by antibody (usually IgM, but also IgG) through two different mechanisms (complement and Fc receptors on phagocytes) Results in the destruction of the antibody-coated cell with consequences dependent on the cell or body that is destroyed (e.g., RBC, WBC, or platelet)	ABO incompatibility Rh incompatibility Drug-induced thrombocytopenia
Type III (immune complex reaction)	Triggered by the formation of antigen-antibody complexes that activate the complement cascade Immune complexes are formed in the circulation and are later deposited in blood vessels or healthy tissue. Multiple forms of the response exist depending on the type and location of the antigen Results in local edema and neutrophil attraction, and thus degradative lysosomal enzymes resulting in tissue injury	Serum sickness Glomerulonephritis
Type IV (delayed hypersensitivity)	Triggered by the recognition of an antigen mediated by activated T lymphocytes and release of lymphokines, which then stimulate the macrophage to phagocytize foreign invaders and some normal tissue Results in a delayed onset. Does not have an antibody component; this response is strictly a cellular reaction	Contact sensitivities such as poison ivy and dermatitis Tuberculin reactions Graft rejection

From Roberts KE, Brinker D, Murante B. Hematology and immunology. In Slota M, editor: *Core curriculum for pediatric critical care nursing*, ed 2. Philadelphia, 2006, Saunders Elsevier, p. 597.
RBC, Red blood cell; *WBC*, white blood cell.

Table 16-2	Clinical Manifestations of Hypersensitivity Reactions
Organ System	**Clinical Manifestation(s)**
Cutaneous/ocular	Flushing, urticaria, angioedema, cutaneous and/or conjunctival pruritus, warmth, and swelling
Respiratory	Nasal congestion, rhinorrhea, throat tightness, wheezing, shortness of breath, cough, hoarseness
Cardiovascular	Dizziness, weakness, syncope, chest pain, palpitations
Gastrointestinal	Dysphagia, nausea, vomiting, diarrhea, bloating, cramps
Neurologic	Headache, dizziness, blurred vision, and seizure (very rare and often associated with hypotension)
Other	Metallic taste, feeling of impending doom

Data from Linzer JF: Pediatrics, anaphylaxis. 2008. Emedicine, http://emedicine.medscape.com/article/799744-overview.

Once the clinical manifestations of the reaction become systemic, anaphylaxis is present. Mild symptoms include irritability, coughing, anxiety, disorientation, erythema, hives, and itching. Severe symptoms include dyspnea; cyanosis; difficulty speaking; swelling of the tongue, face, and airways; intense coughing; chest tightness; wheezing; stridor; laryngospasm; seizures; sense of impending doom; hypotension; and cardiorespiratory arrest.[23]

Management

When a patient develops signs of a severe hypersensitivity reaction or anaphylaxis, immediately stop the causative infusion or remove the offending agent (if known) and call for assistance (i.e., activate emergency response and notify a physician). Support the patient's airway, oxygenation, and ventilation and circulation as necessary and initiate cardiopulmonary resuscitation if needed. Healthcare providers should always be prepared for further patient deterioration, particularly if symptoms develop soon after the exposure.

Evaluation of airway and breathing includes assessment of oxygenation and ventilation. Administer supplementary oxygen as needed. In extreme cases, intubation and mechanical ventilation will be required. In patients with laryngeal or tracheal edema, an emergent tracheostomy may be needed.

Establish vascular access, ideally with two large-bore vascular catheters and be prepared to administer fluid boluses (to treat relative hypovolemia resulting from vasodilation and increased capillary permeability) and vasoactive support (e.g., an epinephrine infusion) to restore and maintain adequate blood pressure and systemic perfusion. (For further information, please refer to Chapter 6.)

Epinephrine 1:1000 is administered intramuscularly in the prehospital setting, but is administered intravenously (if arrest has occurred or is imminent, it can be administered by intraosseous route) in the hospital setting. Additional vasoactive medications such as norepinephrine may also be required to maintain blood pressure and systemic perfusion.

Medications typically used to treat anaphylactic reactions include oxygen, IM epinephrine (an infusion may be needed for refractory hypotension), diphenhydramine (and possibly an H_2-blocker antihistamine), albuterol nebulizer, and methylprednisolone.[10,23] Antihistamines are administered to antagonize the effects of histamine. Bronchodilators relax bronchial smooth muscles. Corticosteroids are antiinflammatory agents to enhance the effects of bronchodilators. (For further information, please refer to Chapter 6.)

Skin testing may help identify patients who may experience a hypersensitivity reaction with a known high-risk agent. Patients are given a small intradermal test dose of the agent and are monitored for at least 20 minutes.[17] Emergency equipment and medications should be readily available. Patients receiving medications or agents with a higher risk of producing anaphylactic reaction and those with a history of anaphylaxis should be identified and monitored appropriately.

When a patient has a known allergy or hypersensitivity reaction to a drug, premedications may be prescribed before the agent is administered. Medications commonly used for pretreatment are corticosteroids, antihistamines, and antipyretics.[17] Patients with known hypersensitivity responses should wear medical alert jewelry and should have an anaphylaxis kit (epinephrine autoinjector pen) readily available.

Systemic Inflammatory Response Syndrome (SIRS)

Etiology

In 1992, the American College of Chest Physicians (ACCP) and the Society of Critical Care Medicine (SCCM) introduced definitions[3] for systemic inflammatory response syndrome (SIRS), sepsis, severe sepsis, septic shock, and multiple organ dysfunction syndrome (MODS).

SIRS is a state of inflammatory/immune activation. SIRS is present when the adult patient demonstrates two or more of the following variables[3,8a]:

- Altered temperature: fever of more than 38° C rectal or less than 36° C rectal
- Tachycardia (age related)
- Tachypnea (age related) or a $PaCO_2$ less than 32 mm Hg
- Abnormal white blood cell count: greater than 12,000/mm^3 or less than 4000/mm^3 or greater than 10% bands

SIRS is nonspecific and can be caused by a number of diverse clinical conditions (Table 16-3), including ischemia, inflammation, trauma, infection, or a combination of several insults. SIRS does not always occur as a result of infection. A number of underlying conditions may predispose patients to infections with specific pathogens and the development of SIRS (Table 16-4).

Pathophysiology

Inflammation is the body's response to nonspecific insults that arise from chemical, traumatic, or infectious stimuli. The inflammatory cascade is a complex process that involves humoral and cellular responses and complement, and cytokine cascades. This inflammatory response, regardless of cause, generally has the same pathophysiologic properties; minor differences are caused by the inciting factor.

Table 16-3	Infectious and Noninfectious Causes of SIRS
Infectious Causes	**Noninfectious Causes**
Bacterial sepsis	Autoimmune disorders
Burn wound infections	Burns
Candidiasis	Chemical aspiration
Cellulitis	Dehydration
Cholecystitis	Erythema multiforme
Community-acquired	(Stevens-Johnson
pneumonia	syndrome)
Infective endocarditis	Hemorrhagic shock
Influenza	Intestinal perforation
Intraabdominal infections	Pancreatitis
Meningitis	Surgical procedures
Healthcare-acquired pneumonia	Transfusion reactions
Pyelonephritis	Upper gastrointestinal
Toxic shock syndrome	bleeding
Urinary tract infections	Vasculitis

From Burdette SD, et al: *Systemic inflammatory response syndrome.* Emedicine, http://emedicine.medscape.com/article/168943-overview. Updated July 20, 2010. Accessed April 27, 2011.

Trauma, inflammation, or infection leads to the activation of the inflammatory cascade. The proinflammatory interleukins either function directly on tissue or work via secondary mediators to activate the coagulation cascade, the complement cascade, and the release of nitric oxide, platelet-activating factor, prostaglandins, and leukotrienes. Activation of the white blood cells leads to secretion of tumor necrosis factor-alpha (TNF-α), a proinflammatory mediator (TNF derived its name from the fact that it causes hemorrhagic necrosis of tumors). Messenger RNA for TNF is normally present in tissues throughout the body, and levels of TNF rise early in the inflammatory process, leading to further vasodilation, capillary leak, and release or activation of additional cytokines (vasoactive peptides), including platelet-activating factor and many interleukins. The complement cascade is designed to coat invading organisms, making them vulnerable to phagocytosis. Activation of the complement cascade includes activation of the coagulation cascade (described further in the following paragraphs and later section, Sepsis and Septic Shock).

Numerous proinflammatory polypeptides are found within the complement cascade. Two of these, protein complements C3a and C5a, contribute directly to the release of additional cytokines, causing vasodilatation and increasing vascular permeability. Prostaglandins and leukotrienes incite endothelial damage, leading to multiorgan system failure (MOSF).

More than 15 years ago, Bone[4] described the relationship between these complex inflammatory interactions. He described SIRS and MOSF as a five-stage process (Table 16-5). His definitions remain very helpful today.

The relationship between inflammation and coagulation directly affects the potential clinical progression of SIRS. Interleukin-1 (IL-1) and TNF-α directly affect endothelial surfaces, leading to the expression of tissue factor. Tissue factor initiates the production of thrombin, thereby promoting coagulation; tissue factor is also a proinflammatory mediator. Fibrinolysis is impaired by IL-1 and TNF-α through production of plasminogen activator inhibitor-1.

Proinflammatory cytokines also disrupt the naturally occurring antiinflammatory mediators, antithrombin, and activated protein-C (APC). If unchecked, this coagulation cascade leads to complications of microvascular thrombosis, including organ dysfunction. The complement system also plays a role in the coagulation cascade. Infection-related procoagulant activity is generally more severe than that produced by trauma.

The cumulative effect of this inflammatory cascade is an unbalanced state with inflammation and coagulation. To counteract the acute inflammatory response, the body is equipped to reverse this process via a counter-inflammatory response syndrome (CARS). Co-morbidities and other factors can influence a patient's ability to respond appropriately. The balance of SIRS and CARS determines a patient's prognosis after an

Table 16-4	Predisposing Conditions/Risk Factors for Development of SIRS
Acquired immunodeficiency syndrome (AIDS)	Predisposes to SIRS from both typical and unusual pathogens, particularly pneumococcus
Hemoglobin SS (Sickle Cell) disease	400-Fold increased risk of sepsis caused by pneumococcus and *Salmonella,* among other pathogens
Congenital heart disease (with few exceptions)	Risk for endocarditis (see Endocarditis in Chapter 8) and SIRS
Genitourinary anomalies	May increase the risk of urosepsis
Significant burns	Risk of SIRS, caused by skin flora and nosocomial gram-negative pathogens in particular
Splenic dysfunction or absence, as well as complement, immunoglobulin, and properdin deficiency	Predispose to infection from encapsulated organisms and resulting sepsis
Hematologic and solid-organ malignancies (before or during treatment)	Increased risk for SIRS from many organisms
Hospitalization (particularly if prolonged, in the critical care unit, or with invasive devices)	Increased risk of SIRS; prolonged stay and invasive devices increase risk of infection
Indwelling devices or prosthetic material and other breaches in barrier protective function	Increased risk of SIRS

Modified from Burdette SD, et al: *Systemic inflammatory response syndrome.* Emedicine, http://emedicine.medscape.com/article/168943-overview. Updated July 20, 2010. Accessed April 27, 2011.

Table 16-5 Bone's Five Stages of SIRS and Multiple Organ System Failure (MOSF)

Stage 1	• Begins at a site of local injury or infection • Proinflammatory mediators are released locally to promote wound healing and combat foreign organisms or antigens • Antiinflammatory mediators are released to downregulate this process if the original insult is small and the patient is healthy, homeostasis will be quickly restored
Stage 2	• Occurs if local defense mechanisms are insufficient to correct the local injury or eliminate the local infection • Proinflammatory mediators are released into the systemic circulation and recruit additional cells to the local area of injury • Systemic release of antiinflammatory mediators follows under normal circumstances, these mediators ameliorate the proinflammatory reaction and restore homeostasis
Stage 3	• Occurs if the systemic release of proinflammatory mediators is massive or if the antiinflammatory reaction is insufficient to permit downregulation • Most patients have symptoms of the systemic inflammatory response syndrome (SIRS) and evidence of the multiple organ system failure (MOSF) • Excessive systemic levels of antiinflammatory mediators develop as a response to a massive proinflammatory response
Stage 4	• Compensatory antiinflammatory response syndrome (CARS) • Marked immunosuppression; at increased risk for infection • If the body can reestablish homeostasis after stage 3 or 4, the patient may survive
Stage 5	• Final stage of MOSF • The balance between proinflammatory and antiinflammatory mediators has been lost • Some patients may have persistent, massive inflammation • Others may have ongoing immunosuppression and secondary infections • Others may oscillate between periods of inflammation and immunosuppression

From Bone RC: Immunologic dissonance: a continuing evolution in our understanding of the systemic inflammatory response syndrome (SIRS) and the multiple organ dysfunction syndrome (MODS). *Ann Intern Med* 125(8):680-687, 1998.

insult. Some researchers believe that, because of CARS, many of the new medications meant to inhibit the proinflammatory mediators may lead to deleterious immunosuppression.[4]

If SIRS is identified and reversed early, the subsequent inflammatory cascade can often be avoided or mitigated. However, in some situations, the cascade continues because the insult or the resultant host inflammatory response is too great. This damage can trigger cardiovascular dysfunction (increased cardiac output, peripheral vasodilation, maldistribution of blood flow, and impaired oxygen utilization), with resultant shock and a hypermetabolic state (i.e., warm shock).

If SIRS continues to progress, cardiac output may fall, peripheral vascular resistance may increase, and shunting of blood may ensue (i.e., cold shock). This results in development of tissue hypoxia, end-organ dysfunction, metabolic acidosis, end-organ injury and/or failure, and can be fatal.[35]

Clinical Signs and Symptoms

Fever is the most common presenting symptom of children with SIRS. Fever is one component of the triad of hyperthermia (or hypothermia), tachypnea, and tachycardia that typifies the earliest, mildest manifestation of SIRS. The international consensus terminology defines SIRS in children as present when the patient demonstrates two or more of the following (see details in Box 16-1)[18]:

• Alteration in temperature: fever of more than 38° C rectal or temperature less than 36° C rectal
• Alteration in heart rate (age related): tachycardia or bradycardia (in infants)
• Tachypnea (age related) or a $PaCO_2$ less than 32 mm Hg
• Abnormal white blood cell count (greater than 12,000/mm³ or less than 4000/mm³ or greater than 10% bands)

Box 16-1 Pediatric Signs of Sepsis/Systemic Inflammatory Response Syndrome

Manifested by two or more of the following four criteria:

Alteration in temperature (fever above 38.5° C or less than 36° C)
    Requires 0.5° C elevation higher fever than adult level of 38° C
    Consider support required by warming device

Tachycardia OR bradycardia in infant less than 1 year old
    Tachycardia:
        Mean heart rate more than 2 standard deviations (SD) above normal for age in absence of external stimulus, chronic drugs, or painful stimuli OR
        Otherwise unexplained persistent elevation over a 0.5- to 4-h time period
    Bradycardia:
        Mean heart rate less than the 10th percentile for age in absence of external vagal stimulus, ß-blocker drugs, or congenital heart disease
        Persistent depression over a 0.5-h time period

Tachypnea
    Mean respiratory rate more than 2 SD above normal for age OR
    Mechanical ventilation for an acute process not related to underlying neuromuscular disease or the receipt of general anesthesia

Leukocyte count elevated or depressed for age (not secondary to chemotherapy-induced leukopenia) *or more than 10% immature neutrophils*

Modified from Goldstein B, et al: International pediatric sepsis consensus conference. *Pediatr Crit Care Med* 6(1):5, 2005.
SD, Standard deviations.

Management

Treatment of SIRS is focused on treating the inciting cause. Empiric antibiotics are not administered routinely to all patients. Indications for empiric antimicrobial therapy include suspected or diagnosed infectious etiology, hemodynamic instability, neutropenia, and asplenia.[8a] Broad spectrum antibiotics are initiated when there is concern for an infectious cause but no definitive infection has been diagnosed.

Drotrecogin alpha, a recombinant form of human recombinant activated protein C (APC), reduces microvascular dysfunction by reducing inflammation and coagulation and increasing fibrinolysis. It has been hypothesized that APC may be beneficial in the management of SIRS. However, the supporting evidence to date is limited. In the prospective, randomized multicenter controlled PROWESS trial,[2] mortality was reduced by 28% in adult patients with severe sepsis who received APC. Patients who received APC also demonstrated significantly more bleeding than control patients. However, a Cochrane meta-analysis of adult trials[25] involving over 4000 patients (including some children who were not randomized) did not find overall evidence of improved survival when APC was administered; a multicenter pediatric study was halted because excessive bleeding occurred when children received APC.

APC currently has no role in the routine management of SIRS unless the presentation is consistent with septic shock. Although APC may be considered in the management of severe septic shock in adolescents and adults (see section, Sepsis and Septic Shock), it is not routinely used in pediatric patients.

Fluid resuscitation should be initiated in those patients who exhibit signs of hypovolemia and hypovolemic shock (see section, Sepsis and Septic Shock and Chapter 6). All patients require establishment of adequate intravenous access. Administer isotonic fluids boluses (typically 20 mL/kg boluses; smaller volumes may be used in children with poor myocardial function) as needed to treat shock and monitor hemodynamic status closely.[22,33] If signs of shock are present, antibiotics, aggressive fluid resuscitation and vasoactive support should be provided within the first hour after the onset of symptoms (see section, Sepsis and Septic Shock and Chapter 6).[5]

Assess and support adequate oxygenation and ventilation. The oxyhemoglobin saturation in the superior vena cava ($S_{CV}O_2$) allows tracking of the balance between oxygen delivery and oxygen use; therapy should be titrated to maintain this $S_{CV}O_2$ 70% or higher.[5] Patients with increased oxygen requirement should receive supplementary oxygen. Intubation and mechanical ventilation may be required in some patients.

Sepsis and Septic Shock
Etiology

The term *sepsis* is often used to refer to a broad spectrum of pathophysiologic and clinical derangements ranging from initial infection and bacteremia to SIRS, generalized sepsis, severe sepsis, septic shock, and refractory septic shock. *Sepsis* is the systemic response to infection and is defined as the presence of SIRS in addition to a documented or presumed infection.[15] *Severe sepsis* is defined as sepsis plus sepsis-induced MOSF or tissue hypoperfusion or insufficient end-organ perfusion.[15,43]

Septic shock is defined as sepsis criteria plus persistent hypotension despite the administration of 20 mL/kg of crystalloid or colloid plus an inotrope/vasopressor requirement, a Glasgow coma score less than 15 in the absence of CNS disease, arterial lactate greater than 1.6 mmol/L (verify laboratory normal), or urine output less than 1 m/kg per hour for two consecutive hours with a urinary catheter in place.[43] Septic shock is addressed in greater detail in Chapter 6.

Pathophysiology

Sepsis is a complex clinical disorder that results from three potential factors that interact with one another, leading to severe sepsis and potentially to septic shock. First, an infecting pathogen can cause direct injury to the tissues, which results in the development of MOSF. Second, sepsis may develop as a secondary response to an excessive host inflammatory response. Third, sepsis may involve a failure of counter regulatory mechanisms.[43] The end result of sepsis is dysregulation of the inflammatory cascades leading to endothelial injury, coagulation and fibrinolytic abnormalities, microcirculatory disturbances, myocardial depression, organ dysfunction, and increased susceptibility to healthcare-acquired infections.[39]

Clinical Signs and Symptoms

The most common clinical manifestations of sepsis include fever or hypothermia, tachycardia, tachypnea, leukocytosis or leucopenia, thrombocytopenia, and change in mental status. Fever is often the first clinical manifestation that alerts practitioners to the possibility of an infection.

Hypotension is a late sign of septic shock. Diastolic blood pressure begins to fall as sepsis produces a decrease in vascular tone. Systolic blood pressure is typically maintained for a longer period of time and only falls once a significant compromise in hemodynamic status has occurred. Clinical diagnosis is made in children with a suspected infection manifested by hypothermia or hyperthermia, and clinical signs of inadequate tissue perfusion. Hypotension is not necessary for a clinical diagnosis of septic shock. However, the presence of hypotension in a child with a clinical suspicion of infection is confirmatory for septic shock.[5]

Management

The management of pediatric sepsis and septic shock is targeted at maintaining cardiopulmonary stability and preventing or correcting metabolic abnormalities.[21] The 2007 update to the ACCM guidelines for the hemodynamic support of pediatric and neonatal patients with septic shock[5] emphasizes the importance of early antibiotics and aggressive fluid resuscitation and use of vasoactive agents among other age-specific therapies to achieve time-sensitive goals (Fig. 16-1).

NURSING CARE MEASURES TO REDUCE RISK OF INFECTION

Infection Control: Basic Principles

Hospitals and healthcare systems now recognize the importance of protecting the critically ill child from developing healthcare-acquired infections (HAIs). HAIs are a serious

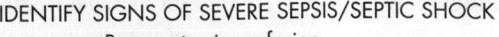

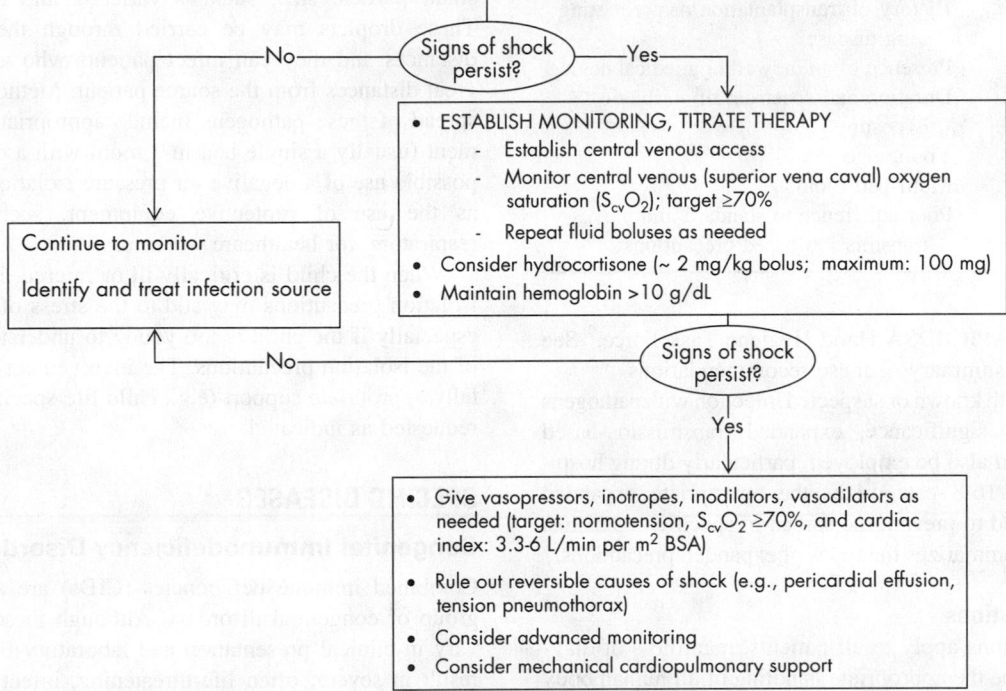

IDENTIFY SIGNS OF SEVERE SEPSIS/SEPTIC SHOCK
- Poor systemic perfusion
- Change in mental status, responsiveness
- Possible hypotension

Give oxygen; monitor and support airway and ventilation
Begin resuscitation and treat infection
  Immediate:
  - Establish IV/IO access
  - Give 20 mL/kg isotonic crystalloid bolus; reassess, repeat as needed
  - Correct hypoglycemia, hypocalcemia
  Within first hour:
  - Give antibiotics
  - Repeat fluid boluses as needed, monitor for evidence of myocardial failure (respiratory distress, rales, hepatomegaly)
    - Give up to 3-4 boluses (or more) as needed to treat shock
    - Give isotonic crystalloid, colloid, or combination
  - Begin vasoactive therapy (via perpheral catheter, if necessary) if shock persists
  - Transfer to pediatric critical care unit as soon as possible

Signs of shock persist? — No / Yes

ESTABLISH MONITORING, TITRATE THERAPY
- Establish central venous access
- Monitor central venous (superior vena caval) oxygen saturation ($S_{cv}O_2$); target ≥70%
- Repeat fluid boluses as needed
- Consider hydrocortisone (~ 2 mg/kg bolus; maximum: 100 mg)
- Maintain hemoglobin >10 g/dL

Continue to monitor
Identify and treat infection source

Signs of shock persist? — No / Yes

- Give vasopressors, inotropes, inodilators, vasodilators as needed (target: normotension, $S_{cv}O_2$ ≥70%, and cardiac index: 3.3-6 L/min per m² BSA)
- Rule out reversible causes of shock (e.g., pericardial effusion, tension pneumothorax)
- Consider advanced monitoring
- Consider mechanical cardiopulmonary support

FIG. 16-1 Suggestions for hemodynamic support in pediatric septic shock. Based on recommendations of Brierley J, Carcillo JA, Choong K, Cornell T, et al: Clinical practice parameters for hemodynamic support of pediatric and neonatal septic shock: 2007 update from the American College of Critical Care Medicine. *Crit Care Med* 37:666–688, 2009. *BP*, Blood pressure; *CI*, cardiac index; *SVRI*, systemic vascular resistance index.

problem for hospitalized children; they contribute to increased morbidity, mortality, and cost of care.[11] For example, investigators have demonstrated that catheter-associated bloodstream infections have an attributable mortality of 10% to 35%, can prolong hospitalization by an average of 7 days, and increase hospital costs up to $39,000 per episode.[45] New technologies are under investigation to attempt to reduce the incidence of these infections. Approaches include use of antiseptic- or antibiotic-impregnated catheters, use of maximal sterile barrier during placement of catheters, and consistent use of effective skin disinfectants (i.e., chlorhexidine gluconate/70% isopropyl alcohol). Risk factors for HAI in critically ill children are highlighted in Table 16-6.

Using Standard and Expanded Precautions to Prevent Disease Transmission (SC)

One of the most important aspects of infection prevention and control is the prevention of microorganism transmission between patients and between healthcare workers and patients. Standard precautions should be used for every patient encounter,[37] regardless of the setting in which care is being delivered.

Hand hygiene is one of the most basic, yet most important strategies in infection prevention and control by healthcare providers. And yet, healthcare providers continue to struggle to comply with the Recommendations of the 2002 Healthcare Infection Control Practices Advisory Committee and the

Table 16-6	Risk Factors for Healthcare-Acquired Infections
Type of Infection	**Risk Factors**
Catheter-related bloodstream infection	Arterial catheter Multiple venous catheters Transport out of the critical care unit (e.g., to operating room or radiology) Genetic syndrome
Ventilator-associated pneumonia	Invasive ventilation Reintubation Genetic syndrome Immunodeficiency Aspiration of oropharyngeal or gastric secretions
Surgical site infection	Malnutrition Steroid use Inappropriate perioperative antibiotic prophylaxis Placement of prosthetic material or device
Multidrug resistant organism (MDRO) infection	History of transplantation or preexisting lung disease Presence of an indwelling medical device Duration and spectrum of antibiotic exposure
Viral infection	Young age Multi-bed room Poor adherence to standard and transmission-based precautions

HICPAC/SHEA/APIC/IDSA Hand Hygiene Task Force.[9] See Table 16-7 for a summary of these recommendations.

For patients with known or suspected infection with pathogens of epidemiologic significance, expanded transmission-based precautions should also be employed, particularly during hospitalization. Table 16-8 categorizes the appropriate expanded precautions needed to prevent the spread of specific organisms, and Table 16-9 summarizes the types of expanded precautions.

Standard Precautions

Standard precautions apply to all patients, regardless of diagnosis, and describe the appropriate handling of all human body substances, including blood, secretions, excretions (except sweat), non-intact skin, and mucous membranes. These precautions presume that all patients may have unidentified blood-borne pathogens such as HIV, or Hepatitis B or C virus.

Implementation of these precautions includes: (1) hand hygiene; (2) gloves when at risk of exposure to blood, body fluids, or mucus membranes; (3) masks, eye protection, and face shields when there is a risk of splashes or sprays of blood or body substances; and (4) gowns when soiling of clothing is possible as the result of either direct contact or splashing or spray of body substances.

Contact Precautions

Contact is the most common mode of transmission of potentially pathogenic organisms within the hospital setting. The pathogens in this category include many viruses and bacteria that can live for variable lengths of time on the hands of healthcare workers or inanimate objects. The most important actions to prevent this mode of transmission are the use of gloves and nonsterile gowns when in contact with the patient or the patient care environment. To interrupt patient-to-patient transmission, healthcare providers must change gowns and gloves between patients and perform hand hygiene before and after every patient contact.

Droplet Precautions

Pathogens in this category are usually spread by larger droplets expelled from the respiratory tract by the infected person. Because the droplets are large in size, transmission usually only occurs when the source patient is relatively close to a healthcare worker or another susceptible patient. Thus, droplet precautions focus on protecting the healthcare workers and other patients by the use of masks by anyone who will be within three feet of a source patient.

Airborne Precautions

This category of infections involves organisms with very small particle size, such as varicella and measles viruses. These droplets may be carried through the air over long distances and they can infect patients who are positioned at great distances from the source patient. Methods used to limit spread of these pathogens include appropriate patient placement (usually a single bed in a room with a closed door, and possible use of a negative air pressure isolation room) as well as the use of protective equipment, such as masks or respirators, for healthcare workers.

When the child is critically ill or injured, infection control isolation precautions may add to the stress of hospitalization, especially if the child is too young to understand the purpose of the isolation precautions. The involvement of developmentally appropriate support (e.g., child life specialists) should be requested as indicated.

SPECIFIC DISEASES

Congenital Immunodeficiency Disorders

Combined immune deficiencies (CIDs) are a heterogeneous group of congenital disorders. Although these disorders may vary in clinical presentation and laboratory findings, they all result in severe, often life-threatening, infections because of the body's inability to mount a normal, protective immune response to infections involving bacteria, viruses, and fungi. Without prompt and aggressive therapy, these disorders generally are fatal in the first 2 years of life.

Severe Combined Immunodeficiency Disorder (SCID)

Etiology

Severe combined immunodeficiency disorder (SCID) is a rare combined B- and T-lymphocyte disorder. Estimations of incidence range from 1:70,000 to 1:1,000,000 live births, but may be as frequent as 1:35,000.[27,44] The majority of cases are inherited in an X-linked or autosomal recessive pattern. SCID is fatal if untreated and is considered a pediatric emergency. In most cases survival requires expeditious stem cell transplantation.

Table 16-7 Hand Hygiene for Healthcare Workers

Indications for hand washing and/or hand antisepsis	• Wash hands before and after every patient contact.
	  ◦ When hands are visibly dirty or contaminated with proteinaceous material or are visibly soiled with blood or other body fluids, wash hands with either a non-antimicrobial soap and water or an antimicrobial soap and water.
	  ◦ If hands are not visibly soiled, use an alcohol-based hand rub for routinely decontaminating hands OR wash hands with an antimicrobial soap and water in the following clinical situations:
	    ▪ Before having direct contact with patients
	    ▪ Before donning sterile gloves
	    ▪ When inserting a central intravascular catheter
	    ▪ Before inserting indwelling urinary catheters, peripheral vascular catheters, or other invasive devices that do not require a surgical procedure
	    ▪ After contact with a patient's intact skin (e.g., when taking a pulse or blood pressure, and lifting a patient)
	    ▪ After contact with body fluids or excretions, mucous membranes, nonintact skin, and wound dressings if hands are not visibly soiled
	    ▪ If moving from a contaminated-body site to a clean-body site during patient care
	    ▪ After contact with inanimate objects (including medical equipment) in the immediate vicinity of the patient
	    ▪ After removing gloves
	• Before eating and after using a restroom, wash hands with a non-antimicrobial soap and water or with an antimicrobial soap and water.
	• Consider antimicrobial-impregnated wipes (i.e., towelettes) as an alternative to washing hands with non-antimicrobial soap and water. Because they are not as effective as alcohol-based hand rubs or washing hands with an antimicrobial soap and water for reducing bacterial counts on the hands of healthcare workers, they are not a substitute for using an alcohol-based hand rub or antimicrobial soap.
	• Wash hands with non-antimicrobial soap and water or with antimicrobial soap and water if there is risk of exposure to *Bacillus anthracis* (suspected or proven). The physical action of washing and rinsing hands under such circumstances is recommended because alcohols, chlorhexidine, iodophors, and other antiseptic agents have poor activity against spores.
	• No recommendation can be made regarding the routine use of non-alcohol-based hand rubs for hand hygiene in healthcare settings.

Hand hygiene technique	• When decontaminating hands with an alcohol-based hand rub, apply product to palm of one hand and rub hands together, covering all surfaces of hands and fingers, until hands are dry. ◦ Follow the manufacturer's recommendations regarding the volume of product to use. • When washing hands with soap and water, wet hands first with water, apply an amount of product recommended by the manufacturer to hands, and rub hands together vigorously for at least 15 seconds, covering all surfaces of the hands and fingers. Rinse hands with water and dry thoroughly with a disposable towel. Use towel to turn off the faucet. • Avoid using hot water, because repeated exposure to hot water may increase the risk of dermatitis. • Liquid, bar, leaflet, or powdered forms of plain soap are acceptable when washing hands with a non-antimicrobial soap and water. When bar soap is used, soap racks that facilitate drainage and small bars of soap are recommended. • Multiple-use cloth towels of the hanging or roll type are not recommended for use in healthcare settings.
Surgical hand antisepsis	• Remove rings, watches, and bracelets before beginning the surgical hand scrub. • Remove debris from underneath fingernails using a nail cleaner under running water. • Surgical hand antisepsis using either an antimicrobial soap or an alcohol-based hand rub with persistent activity is recommended before donning sterile gloves when performing surgical procedures. • When performing surgical hand antisepsis using an antimicrobial soap, scrub hands and forearms for the length of time recommended by the manufacturer, usually 2-6 min. Long scrub times (e.g., 10 min) are not necessary. • When using an alcohol-based surgical hand-scrub product with persistent activity, follow the manufacturer's instructions. • Before applying the alcohol solution, prewash hands and forearms with a non-antimicrobial soap and dry hands and forearms completely. • After application of the alcohol-based product as recommended, allow hands and forearms to dry thoroughly before donning sterile gloves.
Selection of hand hygiene agents	• Provide personnel with efficacious hand-hygiene products that have low irritancy potential, particularly when these products are used multiple times per shift. • This recommendation applies to products used for hand antisepsis before and after patient care in clinical areas and to products used for surgical hand antisepsis by surgical personnel. • To maximize acceptance of hand-hygiene products by healthcare workers, solicit input from these employees regarding the feel, fragrance, and skin tolerance of any products under consideration. • The cost of hand hygiene products should not be the primary factor influencing product selection.

Table 16-7 Hand Hygiene for Healthcare Workers—cont'd

	• When selecting non-antimicrobial soaps, antimicrobial soaps, or alcohol-based hand rubs, solicit information from manufacturers regarding any known interactions between products used to clean hands, skin care products, and the types of gloves used in the institution. • Before making purchasing decisions, evaluate the dispenser systems of various product manufacturers or distributors to ensure that dispensers function adequately and deliver an appropriate volume of product. • Do not add soap to a partially empty soap dispenser. This practice of "topping off" dispensers can lead to bacterial contamination of soap.
Skin care	• Provide healthcare workers with hand lotions or creams to minimize the occurrence of irritant contact dermatitis associated with hand antisepsis or handwashing. • Solicit information from manufacturers regarding any effects that hand lotions, creams, or alcohol-based hand antiseptics may have on the persistent effects of antimicrobial soaps used in the institution.
Other aspects	• Do not wear artificial fingernails or extenders when having direct contact with patients at high risk (e.g., those in critical care units or operating rooms). • Keep tips of natural nails less than 1/4-inch long. • Wear gloves when contact with blood or other potentially infectious materials, mucous membranes, and nonintact skin could occur. • Remove gloves after caring for a patient. Do not wear the same pair of gloves for the care of more than one patient, and do not wash gloves between uses with different patients. • Change gloves during patient care if moving from a contaminated body site to a clean body site • No recommendation can be made regarding wearing rings in healthcare settings. This remains an unresolved issue.
Healthcare worker educational and motivational programs	• As part of an overall program to improve hand hygiene practices of healthcare workers, educate personnel regarding the types of patient-care activities that can result in hand contamination, and the advantages and disadvantages of various methods used to clean their hands. • Monitor healthcare workers' adherence with recommended hand-hygiene practices and provide personnel with information regarding their performance. • Encourage patients and their families to remind healthcare workers to decontaminate their hands.
Administrative measures	• Make improved hand-hygiene adherence an institutional priority, and provide appropriate administrative support and financial resources. • Implement a multidisciplinary program designed to improve adherence of healthcare personnel to recommended hand-hygiene practices. • As part of a multidisciplinary program to improve hand-hygiene adherence, provide healthcare workers with a readily accessible alcohol-based hand rub product. • To improve hand-hygiene adherence among personnel who work in areas where high workloads and high intensity of patient care are anticipated, make an alcohol-based hand rub available at the entrance to the patient's room or at the bedside, in other convenient locations, and in individual pocket-sized containers to be carried by healthcare workers. • Store supplies of alcohol-based hand rubs in cabinets or areas approved for flammable materials.

Adapted from Centers for Disease Control and Prevention: Guideline for hand hygiene in health-care settings: Recommendations of the Healthcare Infection Control Practices Advisory Committee and the HICPAC/SHEA/APIC/IDSA Hand Hygiene Task Force. *MMWR* 51(RR-16):32-34, 2002.

Table 16-8 Modes of Organism Transmission and Isolation Precautions

Mode of Transmission	Isolation Precaution
Standard • Applicable to all body fluids except sweat. • All patients should be considered as potentially infected with a blood-borne pathogen.	• Hand hygiene before and after contact with patient or patient care environment • Gloves when touching blood, body fluids, or contaminated items • Masks and/or eye protection if spray or splash is possible • Gowns if spray or splash is possible (to prevent soiling of clothing and protect skin)
Contact • Direct (host-to-host) • Indirect (with intermediary contaminated object)	• Private room, if available; if not, cohort patients • Gloves and gowns • Hand hygiene after glove and gown removal
Droplet • Large respiratory droplets are inoculated directly onto mucosal surfaces (e.g., mouth, nose)	• Private room, if available; if not, cohort patients or place minimum 3 feet away from other patients • Masks within 3 feet of patient
Airborne • Infection may be spread by aerosolization of small (≤ 5 micrometer) droplets that may be suspended for prolonged periods in the air	• Private room in hospital • Negative air-pressure ventilation with 6-12 air changes/hour • Masks (for TB, N-95 respirator masks)

Table 16-9	Isolation Precautions for Specific Infections

Isolation Precautions	Clinical Example
Standard	• All patient care
Airborne	• Tuberculosis • Varicella zoster • Measles
Droplet	• Adenovirus • Influenza • Meningococcal disease • *Mycoplasma pneumoniae* • Parvovirus B19 • Pertussis • *Streptococcus pyogenes* pharyngitis or pneumonia (untreated)
Contact	• Abscess or cellulitis • *Clostridium difficile* colitis • Enteroviruses • Herpes simplex virus (mucocutaneous) • Parainfluenza • RSV • Rotavirus • Multi-drug resistant bacteria

Pathophysiology

SCID occurs as the result of mutations in 1 of 10 known genes.[36] There are many variants of the disorder ranging from partial to almost complete loss of T-lymphocyte function. X-linked SCID is the most common form. Other forms of SCID usually follow an autosomal recessive inheritance pattern or are the result of spontaneous mutations. One of these other forms is linked to a deficiency of the enzyme adenosine deaminase (ADA). B and T lymphocytes produce chemicals that can accumulate to toxic levels within these cells. Normally, these cells produce an enzyme (ADA) that destroys the excess toxins. When this vital "detoxifying enzyme" is missing, these toxins accumulate, "poisoning" the B and T lymphocytes.

Clinical Signs and Symptoms

SCID is characterized by multiple severe or recurrent illnesses such as dermatitis, otitis media, and diarrhea.[36] Infection is not present at birth, because the infant is protected from bacterial infections by transplacental delivery of maternal IgG antibody. However, signs and symptoms of infection develop soon after birth with the majority of cases presenting in patients less than 3 months of age.[36]

Infants with SCID frequently develop a severe skin rash with red, peeling skin during the first few weeks of life. This rash may resemble eczema, but is more diffuse and typically does not respond to topical corticosteroids. Superinfection of the skin with *Staphylococcus aureus* is often seen.

Infections are characteristic in terms of severity, recurrence (persistent in nature), type of organism, and location. Common sites of infection include the respiratory tract, mucous membranes, liver, GI tract, and blood. Bacterial infections such as otitis media, pneumonia, and skin infections develop

frequently. Infants have recurrent mucocutaneous infections with *Candida* that is resistant to therapy. This candidal esophagitis can result in poor feeding and poor weight gain. Chronic diarrhea responds weakly to alterations in diet and may become life threatening.

Recurrent, severe, and sometimes fatal infections occur with common viruses such as adenovirus, parainfluenza, and varicella. Opportunistic infections including *Pneumocystis carinii* pneumonia (PCP) and cytomegalovirus (CMV) are the hallmarks of a T-cell immune defect. Their presence should immediately prompt investigation for an underlying immune defect. In children with SCID, PCP infection is frequently fatal.

Management

Early immune reconstitution offers the best chance of long-term survival. Bone marrow or stem cell transplantation can be performed within the first 3 months of life, with reported survival as high as 97%.[7] Donors may be human leukocyte antigen-identical siblings, cord blood units, or matched unrelated donors identified through the national registries or haploidentical parents. Bone marrow transplantation (BMT) using stem cells obtained from a related, HLA-identical donor (RID) is the optimal treatment for patients with SCID. In the absence of a RID, HLA-mismatched related donors (MMRDs) are often used. However, compared with RIDs, use of MMRDs for BMT is associated with reduced survival and inferior long-term immune reconstitution. Grunebaum and co-workers[19] found that use of HLA-matched unrelated donors (MUDs) had an 80% cure rate for SCID and are associated with long-term robust immune reconstitution. They suggest that this mode of treatment may be an important therapeutic alternative for patients with SCID when a RID is not available.

Before transplantation, supportive care is essential. This includes prophylaxis against PCP pneumonia with trimethoprim-sulfamethoxazole and administration of intravenous gamma-globulin. Infants with SCID may have severe, sometimes fatal reactions after vaccination with live vaccines (e.g., for measles-mumps-rubella or varicella). As a result, these live vaccines are contraindicated for all children with SCID.

When transfusion is required, CMV-negative, leuko-depleted, irradiated blood products are administered. The development of graft-versus-host disease has been described in infants with SCID after a blood transfusion. Because more than half of SCIDs are caused by an X-linked defect, genetic counseling is important for parents and siblings to determine their carrier status.

Diarrhea may result from persistent infection, rotavirus, *Giardia lamblia*, or malabsorption. The use of an elemental formula may be helpful to reduce the diarrhea. If there is severe weight loss or failure to thrive, parenteral nutrition may be necessary.

Meningitis

Bacterial meningitis is a life-threatening illness that results from bacterial infection of the meninges. Following the neonatal period, the three most common organisms that cause acute bacterial meningitis are *Streptococcus pneumoniae*, *Neisseria meningitidis,* and *Haemophilus influenzae* type b (Hib). With the routine use of Hib, conjugate pneumococcal, and conjugate meningococcal vaccines in the United States, the incidence of meningitis has decreased significantly.[13] See Chapter 11 for a complete discussion of the etiology, pathophysiology, clinical signs and symptoms, and management of meningitis.

Meningococcemia

Etiology

Meningococcemia is a rare but frequently devastating condition. It primarily affects children and is the leading cause of bacterial meningitis in the United States. *N. meningitidis* (the meningococcus) is an encapsulated gram-negative diplococcus that causes infections with a broad spectrum of clinical involvement and severity of symptoms, including meningitis, sepsis, conjunctivitis, pericarditis, epiglottitis, pneumonia, and arthritis. Meningitis, sepsis, or a combination of the two is most frequently seen in the pediatric critical care unit.

Pathophysiology

N. meningitidis is transmitted from person to person via direct contact with infected droplets of respiratory secretions. Carriers are often asymptomatic at the time of transmission. Immunity to *N. meningitidis* is thought to be acquired through intermittent nasal carriage of meningococci and antigenic cross-reaction with enteric flora during the first two decades of life.[16] Once the bacteria colonize and cross the nasal mucosa, disease symptoms often appear within 10 days.

The virulence or severity of meningococcemia is related to the release of endotoxin. The endotoxin of meningococcus is structurally different from that of other gram-negative bacteria.[34] Levels of endotoxin correlate with the severity of illness and may be 50- to 100-fold that occurring with other gram-negative infections.

The clinical manifestations of meningococcemia result from capillary leak, myocardial failure, coagulopathy, and metabolic derangement. These processes work together to produce a state of multisystem organ failure that typically causes cardiorespiratory dysfunction and, frequently, renal, neurologic, and gastrointestinal dysfunction.[30]

In the first 2 to 4 days after onset of illness, there is a massive increase in vascular permeability with resulting capillary leak. Initially, the body compensates through normal homeostatic mechanisms, including vasoconstriction. As the capillary leak continues, hypovolemia develops. This hypovolemia leads to decreased venous return and cardiac output. Vasodilation and maldistribution of blood flow contribute to inadequate tissue perfusion, tissue hypoxia, and lactic acidosis, and may produce cell death and organ dysfunction. For additional information, see Chapter 6.

Hypovolemia and maldistribution of blood flow are primary causes of cardiovascular collapse, although they may be further complicated by development of myocardial dysfunction. Myocarditis, pericarditis, or direct bacterial invasion of the heart may contribute to this cardiac dysfunction.

Patients with meningococcemia often present with disseminated intravascular coagulation (DIC). The combination of microvascular thrombosis and bleeding (caused by initiation of the clotting cascade) is particularly challenging to manage. DIC, in combination with the described hypoxia and hypovolemia, can cause significant end-organ damage. Waterhouse-Friderichsen syndrome (massive adrenal hemorrhage) can complicate meningococcemia and may further exacerbate cardiovascular collapse. See Chapter 15 for additional information about DIC.

Clinical Signs and Symptoms

The clinical manifestations of meningococcal disease can be extremely variable, ranging from the typical signs of meningitis to full-blown septic shock (Table 16-10). In cases of severe meningococcemia, the disease may progress extremely quickly, with death occurring within a few hours of the onset of symptoms. The classic petechial rash is considered to be pathognomic for meningococcemia. However, up to 20% of children with this disorder have no rash or petechiae at presentation.[26]

Management

Antibiotic therapy is the only definitive treatment for meningococcemia and should be initiated as soon as the diagnosis is made. The sequelae of this disease may be devastating, but *N. meningitidis* itself is relatively easy to eradicate. A blood culture should be obtained before initiation of antibiotic therapy but should *not* delay treatment. In a stable patient, a lumbar puncture may be performed. However, it may be deferred in those who are considered unstable or are exhibiting signs of increased intracranial pressure. Recommended antibiotic therapy may include cefotaxime, ceftriaxone, or penicillin G.[28,32,41] Doses vary based on the patient's clinical condition (i.e., presence or absence of associated meningitis).

Table 16-10	Clinical Manifestations of Meningococcemia
System	**Clinical Manifestations**
Neurologic/ neuromuscular	Headache
	Photophobia
	Lethargy
	Neck stiffness
	±Brudzinski sign
	±Kernig sign
	Seizures
	Myalgia
Cardiovascular	Tachycardia
	Bradycardia
	Hypotension
	Cool extremities
	Diminished peripheral pulses
	Delayed capillary refill time
Respiratory	Tachypnea
GI	Vomiting
	Abdominal pain
Skin	Rash (may be erythematous initially and then progress to petechiae and purpura)

Further management is aimed at restoring adequate oxygen and substrate delivery to the tissues. This is achieved through aggressive fluid resuscitation to replete intravascular volume, correction of DIC, and optimization of oxygenation and ventilation. Patients with meningococcemia may require as much as 80 mL/kg of crystalloid during the first hour of therapy and 240 mL/kg or more during the first 8 hours of therapy. This fluid is administered in boluses of 20 mL/kg per Pediatric Advanced Life Support (PALS) guidelines.[10,22,33] The child's hemodynamic and cardiovascular status should be reassessed after each intervention. If shock persists after initial volume therapy, inotropic support is recommended, and should be instituted within the first hour of therapy, even if this requires administration via peripheral venous access. Epinephrine and dopamine may be used to improve myocardial contractility and enhance vasoconstriction.

After initial resuscitation and stabilization, afterload reducing agents such as milrinone are often needed. Arterial and central venous catheters should be placed to allow for close monitoring of hemodynamic status and response to interventions. Insertion of a central venous catheter should not delay administration of fluid boluses and vasoactive support; both can be initiated through large-bore peripheral venous catheters until a central venous catheter is placed. For additional information about management of septic shock, see Chapter 6.

Administration of corticosteroids in the pediatric patient with meningococcemia is controversial. In those patients who are at risk for adrenal insufficiency (those with chronic steroid use, recent steroid use, purpura fulminans, or hypothalamic, pituitary, or adrenal disease) or those with persistent hypotension after adequate volume resuscitation and initiation of inotropic support, it may be prudent to administer hydrocortisone.[28] However, the safety and efficacy of stress-dose steroids as adjunctive therapy for pediatric septic shock have not been established.[46] Glucocorticoid administration does add potential risks, including anti-anabolic effects, attenuated immunity, depressed wound healing, calcium mobilization, impaired insulin action, and associated hyperglycemia and possible alteration in brain development.[46]

Correction of DIC is essential to prevent complications such as intracranial bleeding, GI hemorrhage, and bleeding into skin lesions. Fresh-frozen plasma, platelets, cryoprecipitate, and factor VII are administered as indicated to correct specific deficiencies. Packed red blood cells are administered to restore hemoglobin concentration and improve oxygen carrying capacity. For additional information about management of DIC, see Chapter 15.

Optimizing oxygenation and ventilation typically requires the use of supplementary oxygen and mechanical ventilation. The patient with depressed level of consciousness may require endotracheal intubation to establish a patent airway and reduce risk of aspiration. If increased capillary permeability produces pulmonary edema, noninvasive positive pressure ventilation (e.g., bi-level positive airway pressure) or ventilation with positive end-expiratory pressure will be needed. For additional information, see Chapter 9.

Treatment of septic shock is presented in more detail in Chapter 6.

Colonization with Multidrug Resistant Organisms

Over the past decade, antibiotic resistant organisms have emerged as a growing problem for patients with community- or healthcare-acquired infections.[40] Some organisms carry genetic elements that confer resistance to multiple classes of antibiotics. These multidrug-resistant organisms (MDRO) can easily colonize hospitalized patients and are a common cause of invasive infection in critically ill children.

MDRO can be easily transmitted through direct or indirect contact. Because at any one time, several critically ill patients may harbor MDRO species, healthcare providers must be especially vigilant to use hand hygiene and contact precautions, and appropriate expanded precautions (as indicated) for patients known to be colonized or infected with MDRO.

Infections Associated with Medical Devices or the Gastrointestinal Tract

Medical devices are among the greatest risk factors for healthcare-acquired infection (see Table 16-6).[45] Central venous catheters, urinary catheters, and endotracheal tubes all provide portals of entry that permit organisms to migrate from the skin and mucous membranes to sterile body sites (Box 16-2). Implantable devices can also disrupt host defenses and provide a site sequestered from the surveillance of the immune system where bacteria can flourish. Box 16-3 lists common organisms related to medical devices.

The risk of device-related infections can be reduced by several important preventive measures.[38] First, devices should only be used when they are essential to patient care. Strict aseptic technique must be observed during insertion or manipulation

---

Box 16-2 **Routes of Infection of Medical Devices**

Inoculation at the time of insertion of the device
- Endogenous flora of the host
- Environmental flora

Inoculation during manipulation of the device
- Breaks in aseptic technique

Hematogenous seeding
- Transient bacteremia
- Nonintact mucous membranes or gastrointestinal tract

Extension of local infection

Box 16-3 **Infectious Organisms Found in Infected Medical Devices**

Most common
- Coagulase-negative staphylococci
- *Staphylococcus aureus*
- Other skin flora

Common
- Gram-negative enteric bacilli
- Environmental organisms
- *Candida* spp., especially *C. albicans* and *C. glabrata*

Occasional
- Other fungi
- Nontuberculous mycobacteria

of a device. In addition, limiting the frequency of device manipulation reduces the likelihood of contamination. Finally, temporary devices should be removed as soon as they are no longer needed. Although the use of antimicrobial prophylaxis at the time of insertion is commonplace, the efficacy of such measures for many devices has not been established.

Recent advances in materials used for catheters and prosthetic devices have decreased rates of infection. The use of central venous catheters impregnated with antiseptics has been shown to reduce the incidence of both catheter colonization and catheter-related bloodstream infection in adult patients. However, few efficacy studies of these devices have been performed in children.

Central Venous Catheter Infections

Catheter-associated bloodstream infections are among the most common healthcare-acquired infection in hospitalized children. Catheter-associated infections include localized infection at the site of catheter entry, phlebitis, or bloodstream infection.

Evidence-based practices that are associated with a reduced risk of catheter-associated infections include: (1) use of maximal sterile barrier precautions (e.g., cap, mask, sterile gown, sterile gloves, and large sterile drape) during catheter placement; (2) use of 2-3% chlorhexidine gluconate/70% isopropyl alcohol or other appropriate antiseptic agents to prepare the skin before placement or during routine care of the catheter; (3) prompt removal of catheters as soon as they are no longer required; and (4) strict adherence to appropriate hand hygiene practices.[29] For additional information, see Box 22-6.

In studies performed in adult critical care units, antiseptic impregnated catheters have been associated with reduced rates of catheter associated bloodstream infection[8b,10b] (Box 16-4). Studies performed in children have described delayed time to infection but not reduced infection rate associated with use of antibiotic-impregnated catheters.[10a]

Complications of catheter-related infection include sepsis and septic shock, endocarditis, septic thrombophlebitis, and metastatic infection with seeding of bone and organs (lung, kidneys, liver, spleen, brain, and skin). The prognosis for patients with a catheter-related infection is influenced by factors related to the pathogen, host, and therapy. If the infection is promptly identified and appropriate antimicrobial therapy is instituted, there can be a high rate of cure and salvage of the catheter. Delayed recognition or therapy for an infection is associated with increased morbidity and mortality. Overall, fatality rates for central catheter bacteremia are 10% to 25%, with rates as high as 50% in critically ill patients.

Urinary Tract Infections

Experts estimate that catheter-associated urinary tract infections are the most common device-associated infection among hospitalized patients, although the burden of disease is likely greater in adult, as compared with pediatric patients. Inappropriate and prolonged use of urinary catheters has been found in as many as 50% of patients who develop a catheter-associated urinary tract infection. Important strategies to prevent urinary catheter infections are: (1) limiting catheterization to those for whom it is medically necessary; (2) attention to

---

Box 16-4	**Prevention of Vascular Catheter-Associated Infections**

General
Avoid unnecessary catheter insertion
Evaluate necessity of catheter daily

Catheter Insertion
Use chlorhexidine for skin antisepsis
Adhere to strict aseptic technique
Use maximal barrier precautions

Catheter Care
Minimize manipulation of and breaks into catheters
Perform hand hygiene before handling catheter
Vigorously disinfect hub prior to accessing catheter
Change catheter hubs every 72 h or earlier if soiled or malfunctioning

Catheter Selection
Select a catheter with the fewest lumens needed for management of the patient
Consider use of antiseptic- or antimicrobial-coated central catheters and silver-impregnated, collagen-cuffed catheters when infection rates remain high despite other measures (e.g., maximal barrier precautions)
For long-term (>30 days) access in children older than 4 years, consider peripherally inserted central catheters or tunneled or totally implantable devices

Stopcocks
Cover all openings
Minimize use

Monitoring Devices (Transducers, etc.)
Sterilize if being reused; avoid contamination during use

---

strict aseptic technique during catheter insertion; and (3) removal of the catheter as soon as possible.[24] Catheters are commonly left in place for too long; one study of adult medical inpatients revealed that clinicians were unaware that their patients had a catheter 28% of the time.[34a]

Ventilator-Associated Pneumonia (VAP)

An endotracheal tube provides an ideal portal of entry for the many organisms colonizing the oropharynx to migrate into the lower respiratory tract. The tube itself is an ideal substrate for the formation of biofilm. Pediatric patients appear to have lower risk of ventilator-associated pneumonia than adults, likely because they have fewer co-morbid conditions such as chronic heart or lung disease or immunosuppressing conditions. However, pediatric critical care clinicians have embraced strategies to reduce the risk of VAP, including whenever possible: (1) the use of noninvasive ventilation; (2) the avoidance of nasotracheal intubation; (3) the use of in-line suctioning to prevent the aspiration of pooled tracheal sections; and (4) the elevation of the head of the bed at 45 degrees from horizontal, especially for patients receiving enteral nutrition.[12] Additional information is included in Box 22-7.

Clostridium difficile Colitis

In both children and adults, the most important cause of healthcare-acquired gastrointestinal disease is *C. difficile*. The epidemiology of *C. difficile* colitis is complex and somewhat confusing in the pediatric population.[6] Up to 50% of healthy neonates may be colonized with toxigenic forms of *C. difficile*. After the age of 2 years, colonization rates decrease to adult levels of less than 5%, although higher levels are seen in hospitalized patients with or without exposure to antimicrobial agents.

Clinically apparent disease occurs when the microbial ecology of the gut is upset, for example, when a patient is undergoing antimicrobial therapy. With the decline of normal intestinal flora, *C. difficile* proliferates and elaborates potent toxins A and B, which lead to secretory diarrhea and inflammatory colitis. The major risk factor for pseudomembranous colitis is exposure to antimicrobial agents. Other risk factors include underlying gastrointestinal disease, bowel stasis, and anatomic obstructions.

Symptoms of *C. difficile* colitis typically begin 4 days (range, 1 to 21 days) after initiation of antimicrobial therapy. Associated signs and symptoms include fever, cramping abdominal pain, distension, nausea, and vomiting. Typically, hematochezia does not occur. Although symptoms often resolve when antibiotics are discontinued, oral metronidazole or vancomycin are typically given to critically ill children with *C. difficile* colitis.

DIAGNOSTIC TESTS

The most common diagnostic tests performed to evaluate critically ill children with a potential immune disorder or infectious process are hematology studies (including evaluation of hemoglobin and hematocrit) and evaluation of the white blood cell (WBC) count and differential. For quick reference, normal results of these and other common studies are listed in Tables 16-11 to 16-13.

Table 16-11 Diagnostic Tests: Hematology Values

Age	Hgb (g/dL)	Hct (%)	RBC (mill/mm³)	Plts ($\times 10^3$/mm³)
0-3 days	15-20	45-61	4-5.9	250-450
1-2 weeks	12.5-18.5	39-57	3.6-5.5	250-450
1-6 months	10-13	29-42	3.1-4.3	300-700
7 months-2 years	10.5-13	33-38	3.7-4.9	250-600
2-5 years	11.5-13	34-39	3.9-5	250-500
5-8 years	11.5-14.5	35-42	4-4.9	250-550
13-18 years	12-15.2	36-47	4.5-5.1	150-450
Adult male	13.5-16.5	41-50	4.5-5.5	150-450
Adult female	12-15	36-44	4-4.9	150-450

Data from Pediatric Drug Lookup: Normal laboratory values for children. http://www.pediatriccareonline.org/pco/ub/view/Pediatric-Drug-Lookup/153930/0/Normal_Laboratory_Values_for_Children.%202010. Updated March 21, 2011. Accessed April 27, 2011.
Hct, Hematocrit; *Hgb,* hemoglobin; *Plts,* platelets; *RBC,* red blood cells.

Table 16-12 Diagnostic Tests: White Blood Cell (WBC) Count and Differential

Age	WBC ($\times 10^3$/mm³)	Bands	Segs	Lymphs	Monos	Eosinophils	Basophils	Atypical Lymphs	No. of NRBCs
0-3 days	9-35	10-18	32-62	19-29	5-7	0-2	0-1	0-8	0-2
1-2 weeks	5-20	6-14	14-34	36-45	6-10	0-2	0-1	0-8	0
1-6 months	6-17.5	4-12	13-33	41-71	4-7	0-3	0-1	0-8	0
7 months-2 years	6-17	5-11	15-35	45-76	3-6	0-3	0-1	0-8	0
2-5 years	5.5-15.5	5-11	23-45	35-65	3-6	0-3	0-1	0-8	0
5-8 years	5-14.5	5-11	32-54	28-48	3-6	0-3	0-1	0-8	0
13-18 years	4.5-13	5-11	34-64	25-45	3-6	0-3	0-1	0-8	0
Adults	4.5-11	5-11	35-66	24-44	3-6	0-3	0-1	0-8	0

Shift to the left: indicates predominantly immature neutrophils (bands); seen in overwhelming infection or use of colony stimulating factors

Shift to the right: indicates an increased number of mature neutrophils (polys or segs);seen in patients with vitamin B_{12} deficiency, folate deficiency

Absolute neutrophil count (ANC) (normal: 1500-7200/mm³)
ANC<1000: moderate risk for infection
ANC <500: high risk for infection

Absolute lymphocyte count (ALC) (normal: varies with age)
<15-10% of differential WBC count is considered abnormal

Data from Pediatric Drug Lookup: Normal laboratory values for children. http://www.pediatriccareonline.org/pco/ub/view/Pediatric-Drug-Lookup/153930/0/Normal_Laboratory_Values_for_Children.%202010. Updated March 21, 2011. Accessed April 27, 2011.
Bands, Band neutrophils; *Lymphs,* lymphocytes; *Monos,* monocytes; *Segs,* segmented neutrophils; *WBC,* white blood cell.

Table 16-13 Other Diagnostic Studies

Diagnostic Test	Normal Values	Comments
Erythrocyte sedimentation rate (ESR) (Westergren)	Child: 0-20 mm/hour Adult male: 0-15 mm/hour Adult female: 0-20 mm/hour	Nonspecific indicator of acute inflammatory response Measures the amount of RBCs that settle in 1 hour
Reticulocyte count	Newborns: 2-6% Children: 0-2.8% Adults: 0.5-1.5%	
C-reactive protein (CRP)	<6 mg/dL	Increase within 6-8 h of onset of infection or injury CRP is produced by the liver during periods of inflammation

Data from Pediatric Drug Lookup: Normal laboratory values for children. http://www.pediatriccareonline.org/pco/ub/view/Pediatric-Drug-Lookup/153930/0/Normal_Laboratory_Values_for_Children.%202010. Updated March 21, 2011. Accessed April 27, 2011.

References

1. Baines PB, Hart CA: Severe meningococcal disease in childhood. *Br J Anesthes* 90(1):72–83, 2003.
2. Bernard GR, et al: Recombinant human protein C Worldwide Evaluation in Severe Sepsis (PROWESS) study group, Efficacy and safety of recombinant human activated protein C for severe sepsis. *NEJM* 344(10):699–709, 2001.
3. Bone RC, et al: Definitions for sepsis and organ failure and guidelines for the use of innovative therapies in sepsis, the ACCP/SCCM Consensus Conference Committee. *Chest* 101:1644–1655, 1992.
4. Bone RC: Immunologic dissonance: a continuing evolution in our understanding of the systemic inflammatory response syndrome (SIRS) and the multiple organ dysfunction syndrome (MODS). *Ann Intern Med* 125:680–777, 1996.
5. Brierley J, et al: Clinical practice parameters for hemodynamic support of pediatric and neonatal septic shock: 2007 update from the American College of Critical Care Medicine. *Crit Care Med* 37 (2):666–681, 2009.
6. Bryant K, McDonald LC: *Clostridium difficile* infections in children. *Pediatr Infect Dis J* 28:145–146, 2009.
7. Buckley RH: Molecular defects in human severe combined immunodeficiency and approaches to immune reconstitution. *Annu Rev Immunol* 55:625–656, 2004.
8. (a)Burdette SD, et al: *Systemic inflammatory response syndrome*, 2011: Emedicine http://emedicine.medscape.com/article/168943-overview. Page updated July 20, 2010. Accessed April 26, (b) Casey AL, Elliott TS: Prevention of central venous catheter-related infection: update. *Br J Nurs* 19(2):78, 80, 82, 2011.
9. Centers for Disease Control and Prevention: Guideline for Hand Hygiene in Health-Care Settings: Recommendations of the Healthcare Infection Control Practices Advisory Committee and the HICPAC/SHEA/APIC/IDSA Hand Hygiene Task Force. *MMWR* 51(No. RR-16):32–34, 2002.
10. Chameides L, Samson R, Schexnayder S, Hazinski MF, editors: *Part 10: management of shock*. Pediatric Advanced Life Support Provider Manual, Dallas, 2011, American Heart Association.
10a. Chelliah A, Heydon KH, Zaoutis TE, et al: Observational trial of antibiotic-coated central venous catheters in critically ill pediatric patients. *Pediatr Infect Dis J* 26:816–820, 2007.
10b. Cicalini S, Palmieri F, Petrosillo N: Clinical review: New technologies for prevention of intravascular catheter-related infections. *Crit Care* 8(3):157–162, 2007. Published online 2003 September 29. doi: 10.1186/cc2380.
11. Coffin SE, Zaoutis TE: Healthcare-associated infections. In Long S, Pickering L, Prober C, editors: *Principles and practice of pediatric infectious diseases*, ed 3. Philadelphia, 2008, Churchill Livingstone.
12. Coffin SE, et al: Strategies to prevent ventilator-associated pneumonia in acute care hospitals. *Infect Cont Hosp Epidemiol* 29:S31–S40, 2008.
13. Cohn AC: Immunizations in the United States: a rite of passage. *Pediatr Clin North Am* 52:669–693, 2005.
14. de la Morena M: Immunologic development and susceptibility to infection. In Long S, Pickering L, Prober C, editors: *Principles and practice of pediatric infectious diseases*, ed 3. Philadelphia, 2008, Churchill Livingstone.
15. Dellinger RP, et al: Surviving sepsis campaign: international guidelines for management of severe sepsis and septic shock. *CCM* 36(1):296–327, 2008.
16. Faust MA, Cathie K, Levin M: *Meningococcal infections*. Emedicine. http://emedicine.medscape.com/article/966333-overview. Updated July 20, 2010. Accessed April 27, 2011.
17. Gobel B: Chemotherapy induced hypersensitivity reactions. *Oncol Nursing Forum* 32(5):1027–1055, 2005.
18. Goldstein B, et al: International pediatric sepsis consensus conference: definitions for sepsis and organ dysfunction in pediatrics. *Pediatr Crit Care Med* 6:2–8, 2005.
19. Grunebaum E, et al: Bone marrow transplantation for severe combined immune deficiency. *JAMA* 295(5):508–518, 2006 2006.
20. Hunstad DA, St. Geme JW: Mechanisms of pediatric bacterial disease. In Bergelson JA, editor: *Pediatric infectious disease requisites*, ed 1. Philadelphia, 2008, Mosby.
21. Khilnani P, Deopujari S, Carcillo J: Recent advances in sepsis and septic shock. *Ind J Pediatr* 75:821–830, 2008.
22. Kleinman M, et al: Part 14, pediatric advanced life support in 2010 American heart association guidelines for cardiopulmonary resuscitation and emergency cardiovascular care. *Circulation* 122:S876–S908, 2010.
23. Linzer JF: *Pediatrics, anaphylaxis*, Emedicine, http://emedicine.medscape.com/article/799744-overview, 2008. Accessed January 15, 2012.
24. Lo E, et al: Strategies to prevent catheter-associated urinary tract infections in acute care hospitals. *Infect Cont Hosp Epidemiol* 29:901–994, 2008.
25. Marti-Carvajal A, Salanti G, Cardona AF: Human recombinant activated protein C for severe sepsis. *Cochrane Database Sys Rev* (1): CD004388, 2008.
26. Marzouk O, et al: Features and outcomes in meningococcal disease presenting with maculopapular rash. *Arch Dis Child* 66:485–487, 1991.
27. McGhee SA, Stiehm ER, McCabe ERB: Potential costs and benefits of newborn screening for severe combined immunodeficiency. *J Pediatr* 147:603-608.
28. Milonovich L: Meningococcemia: epidemiology, pathophysiology and management. *J Pediatr Healthcare* 21:75–80, 2006.
29. O'Grady NP, et al: Guidelines for the prevention of intravascular catheter-related infections. *Clin Infect Dis* 35:1281–1307, 2009.
30. Pathan N, Faust SN, Levin M: Pathophysiology of meningococcal meningitis and septicaemia. *Arch Dis Child* 88(7):601–607, 2003.
31. Pediatric Drug Lookup: Normal laboratory values for children. http://www.pediatriccareonline.org/pco/ub/view/Pediatric-Drug-Lookup/153930/0/Normal_Laboratory_Values_for_Children.%202010. Updated March 21, 2011. Accessed April 27, 2011.
32. Pollard AJ, et al: Emergency management of meningococcal disease: eight years on. *Arch Dis Child* 92:283–286, 2007.
33. Ralston M et al., editors: *Pediatric advanced life support provider manual*, Dallas, 2006, American Heart Association.
34. Rosenstein NE, et al: Medical progress: meningococcal disease. *NEJM* 344:1378–1388, 2001.
34a. Saint S, Wiese J, Amory JK, et al: Are physicians aware of which of their patients have indwelling urinary catheters? *Am J Med* 109:476–480, 2000.
35. Santhanam S, Tolan RW: *Sepsis*. Emedicine. http://emedicine.medscape.com/article/972559-overview. Updated April 25, 2011. Accessed April 27, 2011.

36. Schwartz RA, Sinha S: *Severe combined immunodeficiency*. Emedicine. http://emedicine.medscape.com/article/888072, 2010. Updated September 29, 2010. Accessed April 27.

37. Siegel JD, Grossman L: Pediatric infection prevention and control. In Long S, Pickering L, Prober C, editors: *Principles and practice of pediatric infectious diseases*, ed 3. Philadelphia, 2008, Churchill Livingstone.

38. Siegel JD, et al: *Preventing transmission of infectious agents in healthcare settings*. http://www.cdc.gov/hicpac/2007IP/2007isolation-Precautions.html.

39. Skippen P, et al: Sepsis and septic shock: progress and future considerations. *Ind J Pediatr* 75:599–607, 2008.

40. Stockwell JA: Nosocomial infections in pediatric intensive care unit. *Ped Crit Care Med* 8:S21–S37, 2007.

41. Thielen U, et al: Management of invasive meningococcal disease in children and young people: summary of SIGN guidelines. *BMJ* 336:1367–1370, 2008.

42. Venes D, Taber CW, editors: *Taber's cyclopedic medical dictionary*. ed 20. Philadelphia, 2005, Davis.

43. Wong H: Sepsis/inflammatory response syndrome. In Conway E, editor: *Pediatric multiprofessional critical care review*, Des Plaines, IL, 2006, Society of Critical Care Medicine.

44. Yee A, et al: Severe combined immunodeficiency: a national surveillance study. *Pediatr Allergy Immunol* 19:298–302, 2008.

45. Zaoutis TE, Coffin SE: Clinical syndromes of device-associated infections. In Long S, Pickering L, Prober C, editors: *Principles and practice of pediatric infectious diseases*, ed 3. Philadelphia, 2008, Churchill Livingstone.

46. Zimmerman JJ: A history of adjunctive glucocorticoid treatment for pediatric sepsis: moving beyond steroid pulp fiction toward evidence-based medicine. *Pediatr Crit Care Med* 8(6):530–539, 2007.

Overview of Solid Organ Transplantation

17

John B. Pietsch

HISTORY

History of Solid Organ Transplantation

Early attempts at solid organ transplantation were unsuccessful for many reasons. There was insufficient development of basic surgical techniques and methods for organ preservation, and also inadequate knowledge of the immune system and tissue rejection.

In the early 1950s steroids were used to suppress rejection, and this resulted in some successful kidney transplants. In 1954, Dr Joseph Murray[21] performed the first truly successful kidney transplant between identical twins. Although human liver transplantation was attempted by Starzl in 1963,[32] it was not successful until 1967. Also in 1967, the first successful human heart transplant was performed by Christiaan Barnard on a 55-year-old man who survived 18 days.

It wasn't until the mid-1970s that the development of more effective immunosuppression resulted in substantial improvement in transplantation survival. The first successful pediatric heart transplant was performed in 1984. The 4-year-old recipient received a second heart transplant in 1989 and is currently alive and well.

Evolution of Immunosuppression

In the late 1950s, kidney transplantation with nonidentical twins was attempted, with pretreatment of 10 recipients using sublethal total body irradiation. Nine of the ten recipients died within a month. Death was caused by the effects of radiation and not allograft failure.

In the 1960s, the development of tissue typing and drugs such as 6-mercaptopurine and azathioprine resulted in improved transplantation outcomes. Combinations of irradiation, splenectomy, thymectomy, high-dose corticosteroids, and azathioprine were used in attempts to overcome rejection. However, this combination therapy was associated with a remarkably high rate of opportunistic and often multiple bacterial, fungal, viral, and protozoal infections. Many of the infections were undetected and untreated before death.

In the late 1960s through the 1990s, as knowledge of the immune system evolved and more effective antibacterial and antiviral drugs were developed, results of transplantation again improved. Therapy targeting specific immunoregulatory sites became possible. The first polyclonal antilymphocyte globulin was used in 1967. Cyclosporin, a calcineurin inhibitor, became available in the 1980s. This drug, in combination with azathioprine and steroids, has been credited with a dramatic improvement in transplant graft survival.

In 1994, the next advance in transplantation came with the introduction of mycophenolate mofetil (MMF) and tacrolimus (another calcineurin inhibitor). Tacrolimus has gradually supplanted cyclosporine in many posttransplant protocols, because tacrolimus has been associated with lower rates of steroid-resistant acute rejection than cyclosporin.[20] In contrast, MMF quickly and almost universally replaced azathioprine in posttransplant protocols.[20,22]

There are three stages of immunosuppressive therapies: induction, maintenance, and antirejection therapy. *Induction immunosuppression* therapy refers to all medications given in intensified doses immediately after transplantation for the purpose of preventing acute rejection. Although the drugs may be continued after discharge for the first 30 days after transplant, they are usually not used long term for immunosuppression maintenance.

Maintenance immunosuppression therapy includes all immunomodulation medications given before, during, or after the transplant with the intention of maintaining them long term. *Antirejection immunosuppression* therapy includes all immunosuppressive medication administered for the purpose of treating an acute rejection episode during the initial posttransplant period or during a specific follow-up period, usually as long as 30 days after the diagnosis of acute rejection.

A combination of biologic agents (Table 17-1) and immunosuppressants (Table 17-2) are used to prevent and treat rejection. Because immunosuppressive regiments vary from institution to institution, providers should consult their institutional protocols and the institutional pharmacy to verify drugs and dosing regimens used.

PEDIATRIC HEART TRANSPLANTATION

Kelly Lankin

Overview

As of 2011, approximately 5437 pediatric heart transplants have been performed in the United States for recipients to the age of 17,[24] and many more have been performed worldwide.[7] Pediatric patients less than 17 years of age comprise approximately 10% of all heart transplant recipients.[24]

Heart transplantation is now an acceptable therapy for end-stage heart failure in infants, children, and adolescents (see,

Table 17-1 Biologic Agent

Biological Agent	Mechanism of Action	Toxicity
Antithymocyte globulin	Depletes lymphocytes	Increases risk of infection
Corticosteroid	Suppresses eicosanoid production: Increases TGF expression	Increases risk of infection and malignancy
IL-2 antibody	Selectively blocks IL-2 receptors on T helper cells	Increases risk of malignancy
Muromonab CD3 (OKT3)	Targets CD3 receptor complex on T cells Depletes T lymphocytes	Increases risk of infection
Alemtuzumab	Targets CD52 on T cells, B cells, and NK cells causing depletion	Increases risk of infection
Rituximab	Binds CD20 and B cells	Increases risk of infection
Belatacept	Binds to T cells and prevents their activation, preventing CD28 signaling	

CD: Cluster of differentiation or cluster of designation (numerical nomenclature that identifies white blood cell surface molecules that affect cell signaling and other functions).

Table 17-2 Immunosuppressants

Immunosuppressant	Dose*	Mechanism of Action	Toxicity
Azathioprine	Initial: 2-5 mg/kg/dose (PO/IV) once daily Maintenance: 1-3 mg/kg/dose once daily	Inhibits purine nucleotide synthesis, which interferes with DNA synthesis	Increases risk of infection and malignancy
Mycophenolate, mycophenolate mofetil (MMF)	*Note: Check cautions and instructions for administration before use (e.g., do not open or crush capsules, administer on empty stomach 1 hour before meals, etc.). Tablets, capsules, and suspension should not be used interchangeably with delayed-release tablet.* MMF: 600 mg/m^2 body surface area per dose, PO, given twice daily (maximum daily dose: 2 g) Mycophenolate delayed-release tablet: 400 mg/m^2 body surface area per dose, PO, given twice daily (maximum dose: 720 mg)	Selectively inhibits inosine monophosphate dehydrogenase—interferes with DNA purine synthesis	Increases risk of infection
Sirolimus	Children ≥13 years and less than 40 kg: • Loading dose: 3 mg/m^2 orally† (on day 1) • Maintenance dose: 1 mg/m^2 orally,† divided every 12 h or once daily; Children ≥13 years and more than 40 kg: • Loading dose: 6 mg orally* (on day 1) • Maintenance dose: 2 mg orally,* once daily NOTE: Titrate maintenance dose to achieve target trough level 6-15 ng/mL.	Rescue agent for acute and chronic rejection. Blocks B- and T-cell proliferation by blocking pathway between IL-2 receptor and nucleus; synergistic with cyclosporine	Increases risk of infection (boxed warning issued by FDA) and hyperlipidemia
Cyclosporin A	IV Dose: • Initial: 5-6 mg/kg per dose, administered 4-12 hours before organ transplantation • Maintenance: 2-10 mg/kg per day, in divided doses every 8-24 hour; switch to oral route as soon as possible	Inhibits calcineurin phosphatase and reduces IL-2 expression	Increases risk of malignancy, nephrotoxicity, cardiotoxicity, and hyperlipidemia

Table 17-2 Immunosuppressants—cont'd

Immunosuppressant	Dose	Mechanism of Action	Toxicity
	Oral Dose: • Initial: 14-18 mg/kg per dose, administered 4-12 hour before organ transplantation • Maintenance: 5-15 mg/kg per day divided every 12-24 hours postoperatively; tapered to 3-10 mg/kg per day.		
Tacrolimus	Oral dose: 0.15-0.4 mg/kg per day (liver transplant: 0.15-0.2 mg/kg per day), divided every 12 hours IV: 0.03-0.15 mg/kg per day, given in continuous infusion.	Inhibits calcineurin phosphatase and reduces IL-2 expression	Increases risk of malignancy, nephrotoxicity, cardiotoxicity, and hyperlipidemia

*All doses consistent with the following source: Taketomo CK, Hodding JH, Kraus DM: *Pediatric dosage handbook*, ed 15, Hudson, OH, 2008, Lexi-Comp.
[†]Tablets and oral solution of sirolimus are absorbed differently; therefore, they are not bioequivalent. Providers are advised to check with their institutional pharmacy and transplant protocols to verify dose.

also, Chapter 8). One-year patient survival is 83% to 90%, with 5-year survival of 71% to 77%.[24] The graft survival is somewhat lower than patient survival (82%-89% 1-year and 68%-75% 5-year graft survival), with some children requiring retransplantation.[24] Unfortunately, about 20% of children and about 30% of infants less than 6 months of age who are waiting for a heart transplant die before receiving a heart.

Timing is crucial when listing a patient for a heart transplant, and the risks and benefits of transplantation must be evaluated in light of the limited donor pool. Bridge to transplant therapies such as extracorporeal membrane oxygenation (ECMO) and ventricular assist devices (VADs) are commonly needed for short- or long-term support (see Chapter 7). A recent review has demonstrated improved survival using the Berlin heart.[16]

Immediate Postoperative Care

After cardiac transplants, all patients are monitored in the critical care unit. Patients are usually intubated and receive mechanical ventilation for at least 24 hours. Antibiotics are usually continued until chest tubes and monitoring lines are removed. Daily chest radiographs are performed to verify endotracheal tube depth of insertion and monitor for evidence of pneumothorax, atelectasis, or pleural effusions, and to evaluate heart size and chest tube placement.

Close postoperative observation and cardiopulmonary support are needed to ensure adequate graft function and minimize risk of graft failure. Because hypoxia and metabolic acidosis can cause pulmonary vasoconstriction and worsen right heart failure, monitoring and therapy are planned to avoid both.

Pulse oximetry is monitored continuously to detect changes in arterial oxygenation and central venous oxygen saturation ($S_{CV}O_2$) is monitored frequently to evaluate the balance between oxygen delivery and utilization. Arterial blood gas analysis is performed on a scheduled basis and as needed to ensure that systemic arterial oxygenation, carbon dioxide tension, pH, and serum lactate are appropriate.

Hemodynamic status is also closely monitored, including continuous display and recording of heart rate and rhythm and intraarterial pressure, and at least hourly recording of central venous pressure. If a pulmonary artery catheter is in place, then pulmonary artery (PA) pressure, PA wedge pressure, and mixed venous oxygen saturation are monitored. Pulmonary artery pressure monitoring is helpful in determining the severity of pulmonary hypertension and response to therapy, particularly during administration and weaning of inotropes and vasodilators (including inhaled nitric oxide). The pulmonary artery wedge pressure will rise in the presence of left ventricular dysfunction, and the mixed venous oxygen saturation reflects the balance of systemic oxygen delivery with tissue oxygen consumption.

If a PA catheter is not in place, evaluation of the balance between oxygen delivery and consumption is accomplished through frequent evaluation of central venous oxygen saturation ($S_{CV}O_2$), typically drawn from a central venous catheter placed in the superior vena cava. The difference between arterial and central venous oxygen saturation is typically 30% if cardiac output is adequate (for further information, see Chapter 6, Clinical Recognition and Management of Shock, Use of Central Venous Oxygen Saturation). If arterial oxygen content is stable, a fall in $S_{CV}O_2$ indicates either a fall in cardiac output or an increase in tissue oxygen consumption. If a central venous catheter is not in place, a venous sample can be drawn simultaneously with an arterial blood gas sample to assess arterial and venous oxygen saturations and evaluate the balance of oxygen delivery and consumption.

Laboratory tests evaluated on a frequent basis include: complete blood count with differential, basic metabolic panel, ionized calcium, magnesium, coagulation panel, and liver function tests. Serum electrolytes are monitored frequently because electrolyte imbalances can cause cardiac arrhythmias in the postoperative period.

Viral surveillance is common before the transplant and weekly during the acute postoperative period. Bacterial cultures are also performed as needed when fever occurs beyond 48 hours postoperatively.

Both perioperative and immediate postoperative management focus on optimizing allograft function. Challenges to the function of a newly transplanted heart include: denervation, graft ischemia, and acclimation to the recipient's hemodynamics.[7] The newly transplanted heart has a relatively fixed stroke volume; therefore, an increased heart rate is necessary to augment cardiac output. The heart rate can be increased through administration of inotropes or with atrial pacing.

Systolic function of the transplanted heart typically recovers rapidly, despite the ischemic insult that occurs between harvest and transplant. By comparison, the diastolic function may require weeks to recover and may respond to administration of low-dose inotropes in the early postoperative period. If the ischemic time was short and the recipient's pulmonary vascular resistance (PVR) is low, only short-term inotropic therapy is likely to be needed after the transplant.

The transplanted heart is no longer innervated by sympathetic nervous system fibers, and the vagal effects on the heart are blunted. Therefore, if sympathetic nervous system stimulation is needed, the child should receive exogenous catecholamines. Sympathomimetics that stimulate alpha-2 and beta-receptors are likely to be more effective than those that stimulate alpha-1 (innervated) receptors. For this reason, dobutamine is likely to produce more significant effects on heart rate and contractility than dopamine.

The most common postoperative complications include: pulmonary hypertension, acute allograft dysfunction, arrhythmias, vasodilatory heart failure, renal dysfunction, and hypertension. These complications are presented in more detail in the text that immediately follows.

Pulmonary Hypertension and Right Ventricular Failure

Most patients experience some degree of elevation in PVR before transplantation, and postoperative elevation in PVR can affect the transplanted heart function. Right heart failure often develops after 24 hours and typically lasts 3 to 5 days. Signs of right heart failure include a high right atrial or central venous pressure and hepatomegaly. Severe right heart failure may compromise cardiac output and systemic perfusion.

Several measures can be taken to reduce pulmonary vascular resistance and decrease right ventricular afterload, including the administration of milrinone, prostaglandin, prostacyclin, nitroprusside, and inhaled nitric oxide. Milrinone is often used because it has both vasodilatory properties (that can reduce pulmonary and systemic vascular resistance) and inotropic effects.[1] Alveolar hypoxia and acidosis should be avoided, because these conditions can exacerbate pulmonary artery constriction, worsening right ventricular failure (for further information, see section, Pulmonary Hypertension in Chapter 8). Some patients with significant elevation in PVR benefit from administration of neuromuscular blockers with sedation (see Chapter 5) and controlled mechanical ventilation for 24 to 48 hours posttransplant.

Treatment of right ventricular failure is largely supportive and includes judicious fluid administration to maximize right ventricular preload, and inotropic support to improve contractility. In rare instances, right heart failure may be so severe that extracorporeal membrane oxygenation (ECMO) is required to support the circulation (see Chapter 7).[1] Hemodynamic monitoring and serial echocardiograms will be used to monitor right ventricular function, particularly in response to therapy and during weaning of therapy.

Acute Allograft Dysfunction

Acute allograft dysfunction poses a significant clinical problem that accounts for approximately 30% of early posttransplant deaths. The causes include ischemia-reperfusion injury, problems with preservation, prolonged ischemic time, and unrecognized or underappreciated donor heart dysfunction.[7] Allograft dysfunction may be detected even during the operative procedure with intraoperative transesophageal echocardiography (TEE).

A 12-lead electrocardiogram (ECG) is performed shortly after arrival from the operating room and daily after transplantation, because ECG changes may signify early rejection or graft dysfunction. Dobutamine and milrinone infusions are usually adequate to support lesser degrees of allograft dysfunction. On rare occasions, the recipient requires use of a ventricular assist device or ECMO until heart function improves (see Chapter 7).

Arrhythmias

The incidence of tachyarrhythmias after pediatric heart transplantation is about 15%, similar to that reported after adult cardiac transplantation.[5] Most tachyarrhythmias resolve after a relatively brief period of medical treatment (see Arrhythmias in Chapter 8), and recurrence is uncommon.[19] Although ectopic atrial tachycardia is more common in children than adults, it appears to be well tolerated in the younger age group.[5] Atrial flutter tends to be associated with cardiac rejection, and atrial fibrillation is associated with a poor clinical outcome.[5]

Bradycardia, although not common, can result from sinus node dysfunction and typically requires pacemaker therapy. Because vagal (cholinergic) effects on the transplanted heart are blunted, administration of atropine (an anticholinergic) may not produce a significant rise in heart rate. Adrenergic drugs are likely to be more effective than an anticholinergic in increasing heart rate.

Vasodilatory Hypotension

Vasodilatory hypotension can result from several factors after cardiac transplantation. Loss of vascular tone after heart transplant can be caused by the use of drugs, including angiotensin-converting-enzyme (ACE) inhibitors, amiodarone, and inodilators (e.g., milrinone). Vasodilation can also be caused by a systemic inflammatory response from inflammatory cytokine activation following cardiopulmonary bypass.[7] In addition, vasodilation can result from a baroreflex-mediated depletion of arginine vasopressin (AVP). Treatment of vasodilatory hypotension requires the use of vasopressors (catecholamines).

Renal Dysfunction and Hypertension

Urine output, central venous pressure, and serum blood urea nitrogen (BUN) and creatinine are monitored closely after transplantation. Renal dysfunction can result from decreased renal perfusion associated with prolonged aortic cross-clamp time, as well as from thromboemboli or perioperative hypotension. The introduction of calcineurin inhibitors for immunosuppression (see Table 17-2) can suppress renal function further.

The corticosteroids given for posttransplant immunosuppression can cause fluid retention. Administration of diuretics is often useful to eliminate excess intravascular fluid that can be overloading the transplanted heart. In rare cases, temporary dialysis may be initiated until the return of renal function.

Hypertension is common during the early and late postoperative periods, and is often a side effect of medications. Pediatric patients typically require antihypertensive therapy after heart transplantation. Calcium channel antagonists, angiotensin-converting enzyme inhibitors, and diuretics are all acceptable first-line treatments in children with hypertension after cardiac transplantation.[27] Individual patient blood pressure profiles and evaluation of drug tolerance and responsiveness are needed to determine optimal drug choice and dosing.

Posttransplant Immunosuppression

The survival of the transplanted heart relies heavily on immunosuppressive therapy. Ideally the goal of immunosuppression is to manipulate the immune response to promote tolerance to the foreign antigens, without rendering the recipient vulnerable to infection.[1]

Induction immunosuppression is started in the perioperative period. Many institutions begin administration of calcineurin inhibitors, such as cyclosporine or tacrolimus, before the start of the transplant surgery. High-dose corticosteroids are given intraoperatively and continued for 48 hours; they are then either discontinued or tapered to a low-dose maintenance regimen.[1]

Additional immunosuppressive medications may be given postoperatively in the form of polyclonal antibodies such as antithymocyte globulin (ATG). The *maintenance* immunosuppressive regimen uses the "triple therapy" approach: a calcineurin inhibitor (cyclosporine or tacrolimus), mycophenolate mofetil (MMF), and corticosteroids (see Tables 17-1 and 17-2).

Rejection

Most pediatric heart transplant recipients experience at least one rejection episode during their lives, with a majority of these occurring during the first 3 months after transplantation.[7] Clinical evaluation of rejection is important but can be misleading, especially in the pediatric population, because the inflammatory response associated with an infection can mimic the presentation of rejection.[1] Clinical signs of rejection can include vague signs such as fatigue, irritability, gastrointestinal problems (e.g., vomiting, diarrhea, or poor feeding), or the development of specific cardiovascular signs such as heart failure, low cardiac output, or arrhythmias.

Cellular rejection, often referred to as T-cell-mediated rejection, is most common and is characterized by an infiltration of the heart by lymphocytes. The treatment options include optimizing current immunosuppressive therapy plus the administration of high-dose corticosteroids for mild cases of rejection and antithymocyte globulin (ATG) or muromonab CD-3 (OKT3) for severe cases of rejection (see Table 17-1).

Humoral- or antibody-mediated rejection occurs when donor-specific antibodies attack the transplanted allograft. This type of rejection is B-cell mediated and is associated with a higher rate of graft loss, development of transplant vasculopathy, and decreased long-term survival.[7] Treatment for humoral rejection includes the use of high-dose corticosteroids, ATG, cyclophosphamide, and plasmapheresis.

Although the most effective way to detect rejection is through an endomyocardial biopsy (see Fig. 8-72), studies are underway to develop less invasive methods for rejection surveillance. Biohumoral markers such as B-type natriuretic peptide (BNP) and vascular endothelial growth factors (VEGF) are currently being studied as markers for rejection. Elevated BNP levels at 1 year or more posttransplant are associated with worse graft survival in pediatric heart transplant patients.[28]

Summary

Pediatric critical care nurses play an important role in the assessment and management of infants and children after cardiac transplantation. As noted, very subtle changes in the patient clinical presentation can indicate significant problems, such as acute rejection. Nurses are able to detect subtle and early changes in patient status, and provide both physical care and the psychosocial support that are so crucial during the early posttransplantation phases. Discharge planning and patient and family education can have a substantial impact on patient and family compliance and long-term success of transplantation.

Although late complications and long-term effects of immunosuppressive therapy are ongoing challenges for clinicians caring for pediatric patients after heart transplants, enormous progress has been made during the past 20 years to improve survival and functional outcome of these patients. Pediatric heart transplant recipients are often able to lead relatively normal lifestyles, although they do require daily medications and chronic medical surveillance. Incremental changes and refinements in therapy continue as researchers and clinicians strive to improve longevity and quality of life in the pediatric heart recipient.

PEDIATRIC LIVER TRANSPLANTATION

The first human liver transplant was performed by Starzl in 1963.[32] Since that time, graft and recipient survival and functional outcomes have steadily improved as the result of advances in immunosuppression and improved surgical techniques. There are now approximately 100 liver transplant centers in the United States, and about 250 pediatric liver transplantations are performed each year.[24] Pediatric patients comprise approximately 9% of all liver transplant recipients.[24]

For the interested clinician, additional information about pediatric liver transplantation is contained in the Chapter 17 Supplement on the Evolve Website. The US Department of Health and Human Services maintains an Organ Procurement website with valuable information, including a numerical scale used for allocation of livers for transplantation (for a link to this website, see the Chapter 17 Supplement on the Evolve Website). Additional recommended readings are also provided (see Recommended Reading: Liver Transplantation in the Chapter 17 Supplement on the Evolve Website).

Immediate Postoperative Care

After liver transplant surgery, patients are cared for in a pediatric critical care unit. Because the transplant procedure and associated anesthesia are long, support with mechanical ventilation is typically planned for 24 to 48 hours. The length of stay in the pediatric critical care unit varies from several days to many weeks.

Immediately following liver transplantation, patients typically return to the critical care unit with multiple catheters and tubes in place (central venous and arterial catheters, urinary catheters, and nasogastric tubes). Careful monitoring of vital signs and urine output are always required, and administration of blood products may be needed. Laboratory studies, including sampling for arterial blood gas analysis, hematocrit, coagulation studies, liver function tests, and analysis of serum electrolytes, are performed frequently.

Graft function is confirmed biochemically if there is evidence of hepatic synthetic and metabolic function (e.g., correcting prothrombin time, reversal of acidosis). Alternatively, the lack of graft functional recovery can be evident in the first hours after transplantation, with findings such as a high serum lactate or prolonged prothrombin or activated partial thromboplastin time (aPTT), or if the patient fails to awaken despite suspension of sedation.

Failure of graft functional recovery is an extremely serious complication that must be treated aggressively and immediately by infusing prostaglandin E1, adopting the necessary measures to prevent brain edema (e.g., mannitol, oxygenation and ventilation), and addressing the effects of the liver failure by infusing plasma and glucose.[31] Failure of a graft in the absence of vascular compromise (primary nonfunction) requires retransplantation in almost all cases, with the outcome best in patients with the shortest duration of liver failure before retransplantation. The incidence of primary nonfunction in pediatric patients is 5% to 10%.[8,31]

Posttransplant Immunosuppression

Currently, most liver transplantation centers use a tacrolimus-based regimen, combined with corticosteroid therapy with or without adjunctive agents (see Tables 17-1 and 17-2).[26] Cyclosporine and tacrolimus share certain acute and long-term side effects while having some that are unique to each agent. The most important side effect of these immunosuppressives is nephrotoxicity, which acutely results from vasoconstriction of the afferent renal arterioles; this nephrotoxicity is usually reversible. These drugs can also produce a more chronic nephrotoxicity marked by tubular atrophy, interstitial fibrosis, and glomerulosclerosis. The chronic nephrotoxicity is variably reversible, depending on the degree of disease. To minimize acute toxicity and to allow lower tacrolimus levels, especially in patients with pretransplant renal insufficiency, a purine antimetabolite mycophenolate mofetil (MMF) can be used as an adjunctive agent.[20,22]

Treatment of acute rejection uses a high-dose methylprednisolone bolus, but unresponsive cases may require use of antibody therapy (e.g., OKT-3).[8] Acute rejection accounts for less than 3% of overall patient and graft loss.[20] However, treatment of acute rejection is an important risk factor for the development of cytomegalovirus and Epstein-Barr virus (EBV) infections in children. The EBV, in turn, is a risk factor for the development of posttransplant lymphoproliferative disorder.[13] Therefore, it is necessary to achieve a balance between adequate immunosuppression to prevent acute rejection and avoiding excessive immunosuppression to reduce the risks of toxicity and other complications.

Chronic rejection is a common cause of late graft loss in children, whereas disease recurrence is uncommon. Chronic rejection may result from a number of factors that share a final common pathway of graft injury. The hallmark of chronic rejection is the intrahepatic loss of bile ducts, which has been termed *vanishing bile duct syndrome*, based on the histologic appearance noted on biopsy. Rejection is suspected by the presence of progressive jaundice and a rising serum alkaline phosphatase level. Currently, there is no prophylactic or therapeutic agent available to treat chronic rejection. The only accepted treatment when decompensated graft failure occurs is retransplantation.

Long-term immunosuppression protocols focus on sustaining graft acceptance while limiting morbidity. Transplant centers have reported successful withdrawal of immunosuppression in patients who still achieved prolonged graft survival. Long-term clinical experience with steroid use has documented a host of adverse effects including hypertension, malignancy, and infections.[31] In addition to age and growth deficit at the time of transplantation, two other major factors affecting growth after transplantation include allograft function and steroid therapy.[20]

Complications of Liver Transplantation

Complications of liver transplantation include the following:
- Hepatic artery thrombosis
- Biliary complications
- Infection
- Nephrotoxicity
- Central nervous system toxicity
- Lymphoproliferative disorders
- Psychosocial stress

These complications are addressed separately in the following.

Hepatic Artery and Portal Vein Thrombosis

Major vascular complications include hepatic artery thrombosis, portal vein thrombosis, and vena caval thrombosis or stenosis. Intravenous low-dose unfractionated heparin with or without low-molecular-weight dextran is routinely used for prophylaxis to prevent vascular thromboses. Early vascular complications are usually technical in nature; by comparison, immunologic and infectious (e.g., cytomegalovirus) causes have been ascribed to those occurring months after transplantation.

Hepatic artery thrombosis is the most common vascular complication, with an incidence that varies from 5% to 18% depending on patient age and type of graft.[8,23,31] Hepatic artery thrombosis occurring in the first week after liver transplantation is commonly associated with graft nonfunction and biliary necrosis or leak. Graft nonfunction produces acute liver failure, rising bilirubin, and mental status deterioration. Biliary leaks can develop when ischemia from the arterial thrombotic event produces disruption of the anastomosis. Duplex ultrasonography and computed tomography or conventional angiography are accepted means of diagnosis.

Hepatic artery thromboses occurring later after the transplant may not affect graft function immediately but can produce biliary complications. These include intrahepatic biliary abscesses, biliary anastomotic stricture, and sclerosing cholangitis with sepsis, all of which lead to significant morbidity. If diagnosed sufficiently soon after the development of the thrombosis, some patients can be managed by thrombectomy and surgical revision. Others require urgent retransplantation. Late hepatic artery thrombosis with preserved graft function can be managed by radiologic interventional techniques, with later retransplantation (i.e., remote from the time of the initial transplant procedure).

Thrombosis of the portal vein occurs in 2% to 4% of pediatric liver transplant procedures and is often associated with loss of the graft.[23] If interventional radiology techniques are unsuccessful, prompt retransplantation is required for patient salvage.

Patients with late portal vein thrombosis usually present with recurrent variceal bleeding or ascites and can be managed medically, endoscopically, or surgically with either shunting or retransplantation. Vena caval or hepatic vein thrombosis or stenosis occurs in 3% to 6% of pediatric liver transplant patients and is usually best managed with balloon dilation in an interventional radiology unit.[23]

Biliary Complications

Biliary complications are the most frequent technical complication after liver transplantation. Bile leaks and anastomotic strictures account for most notable biliary problems encountered in the postoperative period. Biliary complications may result from hepatic artery thrombosis; in some series, 70% of patients with hepatic artery thrombosis have concurrent biliary complications.[18] Biliary complications may also be associated with prolonged preservation time, ischemia, or surgical technique.

Early biliary leaks are usually best handled by reoperation. Strictures (either anastomotic or intrahepatic) can frequently be managed nonoperatively with tube drainage, stent placement, or both.

Infection

Infections after liver transplantation follow a rather consistent time course. In the early postoperative period, bacterial infections are most common. After approximately 2 weeks, fungal infections are the increasing concern. Beginning about 6 weeks after the transplant and for the remainder of the patient's life, viral infections dominate the infectious disease concerns.[4,25]

Given the known time course of causes of likely infection, most patients are given prophylactic antibiotics, antifungals, and antiviral medications from the time of the transplant. The antibiotics and antifungals are usually stopped within the first days to weeks after transplant, if no signs of bacterial or fungal infections are present. Antiviral medications are usually given for the first several months after transplantation.

The most frequent viral infections in liver transplant recipients are cytomegalovirus (CMV), Epstein-Barr virus (EBV), adenovirus, and respiratory syncytial virus (RSV). Epstein-Barr virus is an especially important virus to identify in this population, because increased levels of EBV in the transplant recipient can lead to posttransplant lymphoproliferative disease (PTLD).[4,13,25] Lymphoproliferative disorders are summarized in a section that follows (see section, Lymphoproliferative Disorders).

A major challenge in posttransplant management is preventing viral illness secondary to immunosuppression. Antiviral prophylaxis with ganciclovir has been proved to be valuable against CMV infections. Cytomegalovirus hyperimmune globulin may also be somewhat protective against EBV. Detection is paramount in ameliorating the negative effects of EBV- and CMV-associated illness. The use of polymerase chain reaction (PCR) for this purpose has been particularly useful.[25,34]

Nephrotoxicity

Although calcineurin inhibitors (e.g., tacrolimus and cyclosporine) are integral to posttransplant care, these drugs have a negative effect on kidney function. This phenomenon is dose related.

Histologic examination from kidney specimens of patients receiving calcineurin inhibitors shows chronic progressive interstitial fibrosis. Importantly, creatinine levels have not been shown to be a good indicator of renal function. A rise in serum creatinine concentration occurs only after a 50% reduction of glomerular filtration rate (GFR). Thus, ongoing monitoring of urine output, fluid balance, and renal function is essential.

Central Nervous System Toxicity

The use of tacrolimus as an immunosuppressant has been shown to induce seizures. This CNS toxicity has been attributed directly to elevated serum concentration of tacrolimus.[2] As a result, when tacrolimus is initially administered, serum concentration is closely monitored.

Lymphoproliferative Disorders

Immunosuppression has led to the development of cancers in transplant recipients. For some tumor types, the incidence is 100 times more frequent among transplant recipients than in the general population. Skin cancers account for most of the newly diagnosed cases.

An important tumor recognized to result from immunosuppression is posttransplant lymphoproliferative disease (PTLD). Posttransplant lymphoproliferative disease is most common during the first 2 years following transplantation. This disease process has been attributed to EBV secondary to drug regimens that inhibit immune surveillance.[13] Epstein-Barr virus-related PTLD plays a major role in morbidity and mortality among pediatric transplant recipients.

Posttransplant lymphoproliferative disease affects 6% to 20% of posttransplant patients.[8] Treatments for PTLD are largely centered on reducing the level of immunosuppression. Novel therapies involving the use of rituximab, a monoclonal antibody against CD20, may also prove beneficial.[2,8,13]

Psychosocial Stress

A unique set of psychosocial risk factors may be present among pediatric liver transplant recipients, leading to poor adherence to medication regimens and subsequent graft dysfunction.[20] Risk factors for poor compliance include inflicted trauma (intentional injury), single-parent households, substance abuse, and the patient dropping out of school. A formal assessment of these risk factors must be performed to identify them and assess and modify their impact on patient compliance with postsurgical treatment.[10,17]

PEDIATRIC KIDNEY TRANSPLANTATION

History

In 1954, Dr. Joseph Murray performed a successful kidney transplant between identical twins, thus skirting the problems of immune compatibility.[9] Several transplants between twins followed. However, the possibility of kidney transplantation for patients with renal failure who did not have a twin donor remained unrealized.[15,21] In the early 1960s, Calne demonstrated that a derivative of 6-mercaptopurine (azathioprine) increased the success of experimental kidney transplantation in dogs.[3] Human use of azathioprine followed, and long-term graft survival from nonidentical donor kidneys became a possibility.

The success of kidney transplantation increased significantly when Goodwin and Starzl added prednisolone to azathioprine immunosuppression.[33] Encouraged by this success, transplant centers began performing nonidentical living donor kidney transplantation.

Terasaki reported a marked decrease in early allograft failure from hyperacute rejection when a crossmatch between donor lymphocytes and recipient serum was performed.[35] A negative crossmatch (no reaction against donor lymphocytes when incubated with recipient serum) indicated that no antibody directed against the donor's organ was present in the recipient.

Kidney transplantation has now become the primary method of treating end-stage renal disease (ESRD) in the pediatric population (see Chapter 13). During the past decade, survival following kidney transplantation has improved in all pediatric age groups. This improvement is particularly noteworthy in children younger than 2 years of age who previously had the worst outcomes; these children now have outcomes that equal the outcomes of any age group.[9,29] Recent reports demonstrate that the youngest recipients now have the longest transplant half-lives of all recipients; this is especially true if the pediatric recipient receives an adult kidney that functions immediately.[12] These improvements likely reflect better donor selection, improvement in surgical techniques, better immunosuppression agents, and a better understanding of immunosuppression management in children.

Although the current short-term success of kidney transplantation in the pediatric population is encouraging, it is also important to realize that long-term graft survival in the adolescent group (ages 11-17 years) is relatively poor.[12] The reasons for this significant rate of graft loss are speculative, but noncompliance likely plays a significant role.[20,29] Regardless of the cause, improving the long-term outcomes in this patient population represents one of the most significant challenges in pediatric transplantation.

Immediate Postoperative Care

To monitor and replace urine output on an hourly basis, patients are often admitted to the critical care unit for 1 to 2 days after renal transplantation. For some smaller children, mechanical ventilation is planned for 24 hours postoperatively; these patients will all be admitted to the critical care unit. If careful monitoring of fluid and electrolyte balance can be accomplished on a surgical acute care unit, larger children can be admitted to an area specializing in the care of renal transplant patients.

Careful attention to detail in the postoperative period is essential to the care of the child after renal transplant. Special care must be directed to monitoring and maintaining the child's fluid and electrolyte balance.

Many children are polyuric before transplant, and this obligate urine loss will continue in the immediate postoperative period. Intravenous fluids are administered, with administration rate adjusted in light of urine output as well as insensible losses. The composition of intravenous solutions is adjusted as needed, based on measurement of serum electrolytes at regular intervals. Serum sodium, potassium, and calcium levels are monitored closely and replaced as necessary.

Heart rate, blood pressure, and central venous pressure are carefully monitored. No single parameter alone is entirely reliable in assessing intravascular volume, and some variables may not reflect the true status of the patient.

Urine output is a critical indicator of graft function. However, urine volume must be evaluated in light of the patient's pretransplant renal function in combination with evaluation of the posttransplant graft function and the patient's volume status. For patients who were oliguric or anephric (i.e., underwent nephrectomy) before transplantation, if the graft functions immediately, improved urine output posttransplant will be an excellent indicator of graft function. If the patient had high urine output renal failure before transplant, a high posttransplant urine volume may mask delayed graft function.

Oliguria should be carefully evaluated; the urinary catheter may require flushing with small amounts of sterile saline. The volume status of the patient should also be carefully assessed. A fluid bolus followed by evaluation of urine output is usually warranted, both as a diagnostic test and as a therapeutic intervention. An ultrasound with Doppler study may be helpful to confirm adequate arterial flow to the graft and adequate venous outflow. In addition, the ultrasound will reveal any evidence of fluid or blood around the kidney, and will allow assessment for possible ureteral obstruction.

In patients with oliguria who appear to have adequate intravascular volume and hemodynamic stability, a dose of diuretic may be given to monitor response. It is important to administer diuretics carefully, because sudden massive urine output can cause significant intravascular volume depletion, with resulting decrease in renal perfusion. If the patient is massively volume overloaded or has significant electrolyte abnormalities, dialysis or continuous venovenous hemofiltration (CVVH) may be indicated (see Chapter 13).

Hypertension can be problematic after renal transplantation. The volume loading associated with the renal transplant procedure, as well as the use of calcineurin inhibitors for immunosuppression, can result in significant hypertension. The hypertension can be severe and require aggressive therapy to prevent seizures and other sequelae.[20]

Enteral feedings are usually begun at a slow rate shortly after surgery if an extraperitoneal approach is used for the transplantation. Most children can leave the hospital within 5 to 7 days after transplantation, assuming graft function is adequate, the child is able to eat, and the family is familiar with the immunosuppression regimen.

Posttransplant Immunosuppression

Over the past several decades, significant advances have been made in our understanding of the immune response, and several new immunosuppressive agents have been introduced into clinical care. There are now several posttransplant immunosuppressive regimens available, but all require a balance between prevention of rejection and prevention of unwanted side effects associated with immunosuppression.[12,29]

Some transplant centers use a standard protocol for all renal transplant recipients, whereas other centers individualize the regimen for each patient. Immunosuppressive agents are used for induction, maintenance, and treatment of rejection episodes (see Tables 17-1 and 17-2).

Complications of Kidney Transplantation

Surgical Complications

Lymphocele. A lymphocele is an accumulation of lymphatic fluid around the kidney. Lymphoceles occur in 1% to 10% of pediatric renal transplant recipients.[20] Because this complication is known to occur, some transplant surgeons prefer to place transplanted kidneys within the peritoneal cavity to allow lymph fluid to be reabsorbed by the peritoneum. Lymphoceles can produce fullness over the allograft, pain, or decreasing renal function. Large lymphoceles can compress the pelvis and ureter of the transplanted kidney and cause urinary obstruction. They can also cause venous obstruction.

Ultrasonography is the optimal means of imaging a lymphocele. A lymphocele appears as a fluid collection adjacent to the kidney transplant. If the diagnosis is in question, the fluid collection can be aspirated under sterile conditions using ultrasonographic guidance. Analyze fluid thus removed for creatinine level (high in urine leak, low in lymphocele), lipids (high in lymphocele, low in urine leak), and cell count (high lymphocyte count in lymphocele, low count in urine leak) to establish the diagnosis.

Treatment options include laparoscopic drainage with creation of a peritoneal window (communicating tract between the perinephric fluid collection and the peritoneum) and open creation of a peritoneal window. Laparoscopic surgery is currently the preferred method of treatment.

Wound Infection. With the use of lower doses and more rapid tapering of steroid therapy in kidney transplantation, the risk of wound infection is decreasing. Children with augmented bladders or complete diversion of the urine (e.g., ileal conduit) are at increased risk of wound infection after transplantation.[14] Signs of wound infection include swelling, erythema, or purulent drainage from the incision, usually within days of transplantation.

Imaging studies are usually not needed to make the diagnosis. However, a febrile patient with wound tenderness or erythema should undergo ultrasonography or CT scan of the pelvis or abdomen to detect potentially infected perinephric fluid. Prompt surgical drainage and administration of parenteral antibiotics are required.

Thrombosis. One of the most devastating complications of transplantation, thrombosis (either of the renal artery or the renal vein) occurs in 0.5% to 3% of kidney transplants.[6] Thrombosis should be suspected in any patient who demonstrates a sudden decrease in urine production after transplantation. Thrombosis may also produce a persistently elevated serum creatinine despite an adequate urine volume.

Thrombosis is readily diagnosed with the assistance of color Doppler ultrasonography. If a prompt diagnosis is made, emergency exploration will be performed to remove the thrombus, flush the kidney, and reconstruct the affected vascular anastomosis. However, once the clotting cascade is initiated in a transplanted kidney, the probability of salvage by surgery is low.

Renal Artery Stenosis. Obstruction of arterial inflow to a transplanted kidney occurs in 1% to 23% of kidney transplants.[6] Renal artery stenosis should be suspected in patients who develop hypertension that is difficult to control, and appropriate evaluation should be performed. Renal artery stenosis can result from the transplantation surgery, causing constriction at the point of anastomosis, from kinking of the renal artery, or segmental hypertrophy of the intima of the renal artery or a branch thereof.

Cyclosporine causes an increase in tone of the smooth muscles of the efferent arteriole of the kidney. This commonly results in hypertension after transplantation. However, when multiple antihypertensive medications are required to control blood pressure or when controlling hypertension is impossible, the patient should be evaluated for renal artery stenosis.

Although ultrasonography may demonstrate a narrowing in the renal artery or decreased velocity of arterial flow, it is not sufficiently sensitive to confirm the diagnosis of renal artery stenosis. Digital subtraction angiography is the most sensitive diagnostic test. Three-dimensional CT scanning has also been used in making the diagnosis. Treatment options include balloon angioplasty (highest success rate with the lowest risk of complications) or open surgical revascularization.

Urologic Complications

Urologic problems are the most common surgical complications after pediatric kidney transplantation. These complications occur in approximately 7% to 13% of all kidney transplant patients.[30]

Obstruction. Obstruction of urine drainage may be caused by faulty surgical technique or ischemia of the distal ureter. It most often occurs at the point where the ureter is anastomosed to the bladder. Kidneys from young donors (<6 years of age) are at increased risk of ureteral ischemia because of the more tenuous blood supply present in these young children. Suspect obstruction in a recipient with hydronephrosis on posttransplantation ultrasonography, decreasing urine output, or if the expected drop in serum creatinine fails to occur.

Ultrasonography is the best method of diagnosing obstruction. When the diagnosis is in question, percutaneous antegrade pyelography and a pressure-flow study (Whitaker test) is indicated.[36] Treatment options include balloon dilation or open surgical revision of the ureterovesical anastomosis. When obstruction is found in the recipient of a kidney from a pediatric donor, it may be preferable to proceed with open surgical revision. Occasionally, in such cases, complete loss of the ureter may be observed. When this occurs, anastomosis of the native ureter to the transplant kidney pelvis may be possible.

Urine Leak. A breakdown in the anastomosis of the ureter to the bladder results in leak of urine into the perinephric space. This can result from a technical failure or from ischemia of the distal ureter. Ischemic necrosis is more common in recipients of kidneys from pediatric (<6 years of age) donors. A urine leak may manifest as a leak of fluid from the incision, a perinephric fluid collection observed on ultrasonography, or a failure of the serum creatinine to decrease as expected after transplantation.

When significant drainage from the incision follows kidney transplantation, send a sample of the fluid for creatinine measurement. A high creatinine level (two times the serum creatinine) differentiates urine leak from other causes of perinephric fluid collections such as lymphocele or hematoma. If the volume of the leak is small, temporary diversion of urine with a nephrostomy tube and Foley catheter may be successful. A high-volume leak and persistent leak are treated with open surgical repair.

Use of cadaver allografts from infants is associated with an increased risk of ureteral complications (stenosis and leakage) because of the tenuous blood supply of infant ureters. Flechner et al. used a novel adaptation to the technique of en bloc infant kidney transplantation, harvesting the trigone and adjacent tissues intact and transplanting this entire segment, as a patch, onto the recipient bladder.[11]

SUMMARY

Optimal outcome after solid organ transplantation in children requires careful patient selection, surgical technique, early postoperative care, and long-term follow-up and immunosuppression. Postoperative care of these patients requires careful assessment of patient cardiorespiratory and graft function, and immediate detection and treatment of surgical complications, including graft failure, infection and rejection.

The use of immunosuppressive therapy requires a careful balance to maintain adequate immunosuppression and maximize graft survival while minimizing short- and long-term complications. The pediatric transplant recipient and family require skilled physical, immunologic, and psychosocial support.

References

1. Boucek MM, et al: Pediatric heart transplantation. In Allen JD, Driscoll DJ, Shaddy RE, Feltes TF, editors: *Moss & Adam's heart disease in infants, children, & adolescents*, 7th ed, Philadelphia, 2008, Lippincott Williams & Wilkins.
2. Bucuvalas JC, Ryckman FC: Long-term outcome after liver transplantation in children. *Pediatr Transplant* 6(1):30–36, 2002 [Medline].
3. Calne RY, Alexandre GP, Murray JE: A study of the effects of drugs in prolonging survival of homologous renal transplants in dogs. *Ann NY Acad Sci* 99:743–761, 1962 [Medline].
4. Chang FY, et al: Fever in liver transplant recipients: changing spectrum of etiologic agents. *Clin Infect Dis* 26(1):59–65, 1998 [Medline].
5. Collins KK, et al: Atrial tachyarrhythmias and permanent pacing after pediatric heart transplantation. *J Heart Lung Transplant* 22 (10):1126–1133, 2003.
6. Dimitroulis D, et al: Vascular complications in renal transplantation: a single-center experience in 1367 renal transplantations and review of the literature. *Transplant Proc* 41(5):1609–1614, 2009.
7. Edwards NM, Chen JM, Mazzeo PA: *Cardiac transplantation.* Totowa, NJ, 2004, Humana Press.
8. Evrard V, et al: Impact of surgical and immunological parameters in pediatric liver transplantation: a multivariate analysis in 500 consecutive recipients of primary grafts. *Ann Surg* 239(2):272–280, 2004 [Medline].
9. Filler G, Huang SH: Progress in pediatric kidney transplantation. *Ther Drug Monit* 32(3):250–252, 2010.
10. Fine RN, et al: Pediatric transplantation of the kidney, liver and heart: summary report. *Pediatr Transplant* 8(1):75–86, 2004 [Medline].
11. Flechner SM, et al: Use of the donor bladder trigone to facilitate pediatric en bloc kidney transplantation. *Pediatr Transplant* 15(1):53–57, 2011 [Medline].
12. Gulati A, Sarwal MM: Pediatric renal transplantation: an overview and update. *Curr Opin Pediatr* 22(2):189–196, 2010.
13. Guthery SL, et al: Determination of risk factors for Epstein-Barr virus-associated posttransplant lymphoproliferative disorder in pediatric liver transplant recipients using objective case ascertainment. *Transplantation* 75(7):987–993, 2003 [Medline].
14. Hatch DA, et al: Kidney transplantation in children with urinary diversion or bladder augmentation. *J Urol* 165(6 Pt 2):2265–2268, 2001 [Medline]
15. Hume DM, et al: Experiences with renal homotransplantation in the human: report of nine cases. *J Clin Invest* 34(2):327–382, 1955 [Medline].
16. Imamura M, et al: Bridge to cardiac transplant in children: berlin heart versus extracorporeal membrane oxygenation. *Ann Thorac Surg* 87:1894–1901, 2009.
17. Kamath BM, Olthoff KM: Liver transplantation in children: update 2010. *Pediatr Clin North Am* 57(2):401–414, 2010.
18. Kling K, Lau H, Colombani P: Biliary complications of living related pediatric liver transplant patients. *Pediatr Transplant* 8(2):178–184, 2004 [Medline].
19. LaPage MJ, Rhee EK, Canter CE: Tachyarrhythmias after pediatric heart transplantation. *J Heart Lung Transplant* 29(3):273–277, 2010. Epub Sept 26, 2009.
20. La Rosa C, Jorge Valuarte H, Meyers KEC: Outcomes in pediatric solid-organ transplantation. *Pediatr Transplant* 15:128–141, 2011.
21. Murray JE, Merrill JP, Harrison JH: Kidney transplantation between seven pairs of identical twins. *Ann Surg* 148(3):343–359, 1958 [Medline].
22. Nobili V, et al: Mycophenolate mofetil in pediatric liver transplant patients with renal dysfunction: preliminary data. *Pediatr Transplant* 7(6):454–457, 2003 [Medline].
23. Ooi CY, et al: Thrombotic events after pediatric liver transplantation. *Pediatr Transplant* 14(4):476–482, 2010. Epub October 22, 2009.
24. Organ Procurement and Transplantation Network. National Data Reports. OPTN. Available at http://optn.transplant.hrsa.gov/latestData/viewDataReports.asp Accessed 09.05.11.
25. Paya CV, et al: Risk factors for cytomegalovirus and severe bacterial infections following liver transplantation: a prospective multivariate time-dependent analysis. *J Hepatol* 18(2):185–195, 1993 [Medline].
26. Reding R: Tacrolimus in pediatric liver transplantation. *Pediatr Transplant* 6(6):447–451, 2002 [Medline].
27. Roche SL, O'sullivan JJ, Kantor PF: Hypertension after pediatric cardiac transplantation: detection, etiology, implications and management. *Pediatric Transplantation* 14(2):159–168, 2010. Epub July 16, 2009.
28. Rossano JW, et al: B-type natriuretic peptide levels late after transplant predict graft survival in pediatric heart transplant patients. *J Heart Lung Transplant* 29(3):385–386, 2010. Epub September 26, 2009.
29. Shapiro R, Sarwal M: Pediatric kidney transplantation. *Pediatr Clin North Am* 57(2):393–400, 2010.
30. Shoskas DA, et al: Urologic complications in 1,000 consecutive renal transplant recipients. *J Urol* 153:18–21, 1995.
31. Spada M, et al: Pediatric liver transplantation. *World J Gastroenterol* 15(6):648–674, 2009.
32. Starzl TE, et al: Homotransplantation of the liver in humans. *Surg Gynecol Obstet* 117:659–676, 1963 [Medline].
33. Starzl TE, Marchioro TL, Waddell WR: The reversal of rejection in human renal homografts with subsequent development of homograft tolerance. *Surg Gynecol Obstet* 117:385–395, 1963 [Medline].
34. Takada Y, Tanaka K: Living related liver transplantation. *Transplant Proc* 36(2 Suppl.):271S–273S, 2004 [Medline].
35. Terasaki PI, et al: Serotyping for homotransplantation. V. Evaluation of a matching scheme. *Transplantation* 4(6):688–699, 1966 [Medline].
36. Whitaker RH: Clinical assessment of pelvic and ureteral function. *Urology* 12(2):146–150, 1978 [Medline].

18

Toxicology and Poisonings

Anthony J. Scalzo •
Carolyn M. Blume-Odom

PEARLS

- The "ABCDE" primary assessment (Airway, Breathing, Circulation, Disability, Exposure) similar to that used to evaluate and stabilize trauma victims, is a useful tool to assess and stabilize poisoned patients.
- During stabilization of the patient with poisoning or overdose, general principles of pediatric advanced life support (PALS) apply. Focus should begin with support of airway, oxygenation, ventilation and circulation.
- Advanced life support for all poisoned patients includes meticulous attention to maintaining a patent airway and adequate oxygenation, ventilation, and circulation. Children with overdoses of some drugs may require modified resuscitation therapies or sequences.
- The critical care nurse should carefully analyze the ECG for changes that may be caused by tricyclic antidepressants (TCAs), calcium channel blockers, and beta (β)-blockers. Such changes include a widened QRS complex, prolonged corrected QT interval (QT_c), bradycardia, sino-atrial (SA) and atrioventricular (AV) nodal conduction delays, ventricular tachycardia (VT), ventricular fibrillation (VF), and asystole.
- Adjustments in the bolus volume used for fluid resuscitation may be necessary for children who ingest drugs that affect myocardial contractility or drugs that may contribute to the development of noncardiogenic pulmonary edema. In these patients boluses of 5 to 10 or 10 to 15 mL/kg may be used instead of the traditional 20 mL/kg bolus. In general, fluid boluses can be administered over 5 to 20 minutes, but when myocardial contractility is compromised or pulmonary edema is present, the bolus is typically administered over about 10 to 20 minutes. Reassess the patient carefully between boluses, be prepared to support oxygenation and ventilation (with possible continuous positive airway pressure), and repeat the bolus as needed.

SCOPE OF THE PROBLEM

Poisonings and toxic exposures resulting in injury or death are significant problems for pediatric emergency and critical care. In 2009, approximately 1.6 million poisonings occurred in children 19 years of age or younger.[26] From 1995 to 2005, poisoning accounted for 1.2 million emergency department visits.[120] The average annual rate of poisoning-related visits was disproportionately higher among children under 5 years of age than among children in older age categories.[107] Poisonings and drug overdoses are the most common toxicities that result in admission to pediatric critical care units.[107] Figure 18-1 illustrates the burden of poisoning in the United States.

Toxic exposure can complicate resuscitation priorities and support. In unusual cases of poisoning or when life-threatening complications are anticipated, the American College of Emergency Physicians (ACEP) and American Academy of Clinical Toxicology (AACT) recommend consultation with a medical toxicologist or certified regional poison information center and transfer to a poison treatment center.[2,7] Dedicated poison treatment centers can provide diagnostic and treatment services beyond those available in most hospitals. Poisoned children with life-threatening complications should ideally receive care at a children's hospital or Emergency Department Approved for Pediatrics (EDAP) facility.

This chapter provides an overview of the general approach to the poisoned patient. It highlights the epidemiology, clinical recognition, and management of five major types of poisonings and overdose: cocaine, calcium channel blockers, β-adrenergic blockers, opioids, and TCAs. It is consistent with the detailed recommendations contained in the Toxicology chapter of the American Heart Association (AHA) 2002 Pediatric Advanced Life Support (PALS) Provider Manual,[61] developed by Scalzo, Hazinski, et al. In addition, the recommendations are consistent

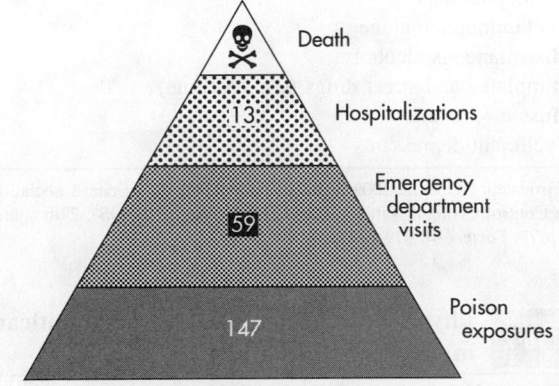

FIG. 18-1 Relationship of the number of poison exposures to Emergency Department visits, hospitalizations, and deaths caused by poisoning. (From Centers for Disease Control and Prevention and National Center for Health Statistics, National Vital Statistics System, 1995; National Hospital Discharge Survey, 1995; National Hospital Ambulatory Medical Care Surveys, 1993-1996; and Toxic Exposure Surveillance System, 1995.)

with those in the Pediatric Advanced Life Support section of the 2010 AHA Guidelines for Cardiopulmonary Resuscitation and Emergency Cardiovascular Care.[79]

GENERAL APPROACH TO THE POISONED PATIENT

Life-threatening morbidity associated with poisoning may manifest as respiratory depression, seizures, depressed level of consciousness, hypotension and cardiac arrhythmias. The ten top exposures causing death are listed in Box 18-1.

The initial approach in toxicologic emergencies is to follow basic principles of PALS: assess and rapidly support the airway, oxygenation, ventilation, and circulation (i.e., the ABCs of airway, breathing, and circulation). The provider should perform an ABCDE primary assessment to detect life-threatening manifestations of the poisoning. The nurse will provide ongoing support of the ABCs in the critical care setting while the secondary and tertiary evaluations (detailed assessment, including laboratory studies and diagnostic imaging) are conducted.

Subsequent priorities for the support of airway, oxygenation, and ventilation include reversing the effects of the toxin (when possible) and preventing further absorption of the agent. When available, the patient history may provide important information. A list of drugs and chemicals in the home may offer clues to identify an unknown toxin and is an important part of the general assessment of suspected poisoning.

In addition to a thorough history and assessment of drugs and toxic chemicals in the child's environment, physical findings beyond those detected by the primary and secondary assessments may have particular value and diagnostic significance for the patient with a toxic exposure (Box 18-2).

Box 18-1 Ten Top Exposures Causing Deaths in 2009

- Sedatives/hypnotics/antipsychotics
- Cardiovascular drugs (i.e., calcium channel blockers and β-blockers)
- Opioids
- Acetaminophen in combination with narcotic analgesics (e.g., opioids)
- Antidepressants
- Acetaminophen alone
- Miscellaneous alcohols
- Stimulants and street drugs (e.g., cocaine)
- Muscle relaxants
- Cyclic antidepressants

From Bronstein AC, et al: 2009 Annual Report of the American Association of Poison Control Centers' National Poison Data System (NPDS): 27th annual report. *Clin Toxicol* 48:979-1178, 2010.

Box 18-2 Physical Findings of Diagnostic Significance in the Poisoned Patient

- Changes in heart rate or rhythm
- Pupil size and response to light
- Changes in skin temperature and moisture
- Changes in mental status
- Seizures
- Presence or absence of bowel sounds

The characteristic clinical manifestations of a specific poisoning or toxin are termed a *toxidrome*. Examples of toxidromes include: (1) the clinical constellation of tachycardia, mydriasis, diaphoresis, seizures, and the presence of bowel sounds suggests the sympathomimetic toxidrome (e.g., cocaine); (2) the combination of tachycardia, mydriasis, dry skin, seizures, and absent bowel sounds is consistent with the anticholinergic toxidrome (e.g., atropine).[61] Recognition of common toxidromes can be vital to efficient resuscitation, supportive care, decontamination, and administration of antidotes.

Regardless of the type of toxin, protection of the airway is of fundamental importance in the management of any poisoning. Elective endotracheal intubation in a poisoned patient should be considered earlier than in a patient without a history of toxin exposure because poisoned patients are at high risk for development of sudden or progressive respiratory failure. Many toxins cause respiratory failure by depression of respiratory drive, hypoperfusion of the central nervous system (CNS), or direct toxic effects on the CNS or pulmonary systems. Toxins can affect oxygenation by causing alveolar hypoventilation (e.g., opiate intoxication)[54] or direct pulmonary toxicity (e.g., TCAs).[41] Table 18-1 lists potential mechanisms and toxic agents that cause decreased oxygenation in the poisoned patient.

During initial examination, the poisoned patient may be conscious, but confused or combative. Some patients may be effectively supported with bag-mask (manual) ventilation. Bag-mask

Table 18-1 Potential Mechanisms of Decreased Oxygenation in Poisoning

Mechanism	Examples of Toxic Etiology
Alveolar hypoventilation (hypercarbia with normal alveolar-arterial oxygen difference)	Opiates, tricyclic antidepressants, benzodiazepines, barbiturates, and clonidine
Ventilation-perfusion mismatch (includes acute respiratory distress syndrome)	Direct pulmonary toxicity (e.g., tricyclic antidepressants, calcium channel blockers, or inhaled hydrocarbons) or secondary injury resulting from decreased level of consciousness and aspiration of gastric contents, or pulmonary embolism (complication of chronic IV drug abuse)
Intrapulmonary shunting	Pneumothorax caused by cocaine, by internal jugular injections of heroin by drug abusers, and by iron intoxication
Diffusion abnormality	Chlorine, chloramine, and ammonia gas inhalation
Decrease in alveolar oxygen content	Simple asphyxiants: carbon dioxide, methane, inhalants (e.g., propane, butane, fluorocarbons), and nitrogen oxides

Modified from Hazinski MF, et al: Toxicology. In *PALS provider manual.* Dallas, 2002, American Heart Association, p. 307.

ventilation, however, is often complicated by vomiting and aspiration, particularly if the poisoned patient has a full stomach or is receiving gastric decontamination. If the patient requires intubation, sedation and neuromuscular blockade may be indicated to facilitate mechanical ventilation.

When the poisoned patient does require intubation and mechanical ventilation, several factors must be carefully considered regarding the selection of sedative and neuromuscular blocking agents. These considerations include the patient's cardiovascular function, the effects of the toxin involved, and possible interactions of sedatives or neuromuscular blocking agents with the toxin. As an example, organophosphate insecticides inhibit acetylcholinesterase and plasma cholinesterase enzymes; this inhibition could dangerously prolong the half-life of the neuromuscular blockade agent, succinylcholine, and its properties.

Nondepolarizing neuromuscular blocking agents, such as vecuronium and rocuronium, are most useful for the intubation of poisoned patients. They have minimal cardiovascular side effects, rapid onset, and a relatively short duration of action (see also Chapter 5). The use of short-acting sedatives, in conjunction with short-acting neuromuscular blocking agents, enables rapid and efficient repeat assessment of a patient's mental status. Such assessments are particularly important in the management of patients with status epilepticus.[61]

If the poisoned patient demonstrates effective spontaneous breathing and can maintain airway patency, consider placing the patient in a recovery position. The left lateral decubitus position reduces absorption of ingested substances[154] as well as the risk for aspiration.

Gastrointestinal Decontamination

If airway patency cannot be maintained, the patient should receive *nothing by mouth* (i.e., maintain NPO status) during transport and initial observation. This approach will reduce the likelihood of aspiration if mental status deteriorates.

If a patent airway can be maintained in a poisoned patient, gastrointestinal decontamination may be considered. It is important to note that gastrointestinal decontamination has not been shown to improve outcome[35,153] as defined by morbidity, mortality, cost, or length of hospital stay.[84] In addition to achieving skill in administering gastrointestinal decontamination, critical care nurses should understand the inherent risks and benefits.

Administration of oral fluids for dilution purposes is of no proven benefit in most poisonings. In instances of acid ingestion, limited animal data suggests that oral dilution with water or milk as a demulcent may be helpful.[67]

Administration of syrup of ipecac is not recommended by the American Academy of Pediatrics for the treatment of poisonings.[5,84] When applicable, recommended gastric decontamination basically consists of activated charcoal and rarely gastric lavage.

Activated Charcoal

Activated charcoal adsorbs many drugs as well as some other compounds.[38] Although there is no evidence that administration of activated charcoal improves clinical outcome,[35] it is often considered when children present to emergency care very soon after toxic ingestion. Caution is advised to limit the use of activated charcoal in children less than 6 months

of age because they have a high risk of aspiration. Activated charcoal reduces the mean bioavailability of the drugs by approximately 69% when it is given within 30 minutes after drug or toxin ingestion; however, the bioavailability of drugs is only reduced by half that amount when activated charcoal is given an hour or more after ingestion.[34,35]

Most toxicologists and poison centers do not recommend prehospital administration of activated charcoal, although emergency department administration of activated charcoal may be useful in the treatment of some poisonings, particularly if the ingestion has occurred within 1 hour of presentation. There are insufficient data to either support or exclude the use of activated charcoal at greater than 1 hour after an ingestion.[34,35]

The optimal dose of activated charcoal has not been established in controlled human trials. The AACT and the European Association of Poisons Centres and Clinical Toxicologists have developed consensus oral dose recommendations for activated charcoal (Box 18-3).[34,35]

Repeated doses of activated charcoal can be administered to treat certain specific ingestions,[3] but there is no evidence that multi-dose administration is superior to a single dose.[45] Use of multiple dose activated charcoal is not recommended if the toxic agent slows gastrointestinal motility (e.g., TCAs, calcium channel blockers, and opiates), because the activated charcoal can contribute to regurgitation and aspiration or can become impacted, leading to intestinal perforation.[56]

Contraindications to the administration of activated charcoal include an unprotected airway, ingestion of volatile substances (e.g., hydrocarbons) and anatomic anomalies of the gastrointestinal tract. Administration of activated charcoal may lead to regurgitation and aspiration, hence placement of an endotracheal tube before administration of activated charcoal may reduce but not reliably prevent aspiration.[114]

Gastric Lavage

Although emergency personnel have used gastric lavage for years, there is no convincing evidence that it improves clinical outcome.[153] Like activated charcoal, gastric lavage increases the risk of aspiration.[78,138,152] In addition, complications of lavage tube placement include hypoxia,[151] tension pneumothorax and charcoal-containing empyema,[71] and esophageal[9] and gastrointestinal perforation.[102] For these reasons, gastric lavage is only indicated in a patient who presents soon after ingestion of some life-threatening toxins (Box 18-4).

Antidotes

Following the assessment and support of airway, oxygenation, ventilation, and circulation, the critical care nurse may need to administer a specific antidotal therapy. Use of true antidotes as defined by the International Programme for Chemical Safety (IPCS) is relatively infrequent in pediatric poisonings, with the exception of naloxone, which is a classic antidote that

Box 18-3	Oral Doses of Aqueous Activated Charcoal (without cathartic)[34,35]
Children up to 1 year of age: 1 g/kg	
Children 1-12 years of age: 25-50 g	
Adolescents and adults: 25-100 g	

Box 18-4	Key Issues in Gastrointestinal Decontamination

- Sudden changes in level of consciousness and respiratory depression may develop in poisoned pediatric patients. For this reason, support the ABCs and establish and maintain a patent airway before administering gastrointestinal decontamination. Alert patients may be able to maintain their airways, whereas others will require intubation.
- Syrup of ipecac is **not** recommended for any of the five types of poisoning discussed in this chapter.
- If activated charcoal is indicated, administer it early after ingestion because it is most effective within 1 h of ingestion.
- Gastric lavage is **not** a routine intervention; its effectiveness is limited in poisoned patients. Lavage may be considered for asymptomatic patients who present early (usually within 60 min or less) after ingestion of some life-threatening toxins.
- Whole bowel irrigation may be beneficial in select poisonings, but further research is needed.

Table 18-2   Common Antidotes for Common Poisons

Poison	Antidote(s)
Acetaminophen	N-acetylcysteine (NAC)
Organophosphate and Carbamate Insecticides, Nerve Agents	Atropine Pralidoxime (2-PAM); (not usually required with Carbamate Insecticides)
Iron	Deferoxamine
Digoxin	Digoxin Immune Fab
Mercury	Dimercaprol (BAL)
Benzodiazepines	Flumazenil (not recommended for overdose but may be used to reverse procedural sedation)
Methanol, ethylene glycol	Fomepizole
Cyanide	Hydroxocobalamin (preferred) Cyanide Antidote Package • Amyl nitrite (adjunctive therapy for inhalation) • Sodium nitrite • Sodium thiosulfate
Opioids	Naloxone
Lead	Succimer (DMSA)

effectively reverses opiate toxicity. The IPCS classifies naloxone as an A1 agent (i.e., A: should be available within 30 min or less; 1: effectiveness is well documented).[70,132] A list of other antidotes is included in Table 18-2.

MANAGEMENT OF SPECIFIC POISONINGS

Many poisonings, particularly in adolescents, may be comprised of multiple agents ("polypharmacy" overdoses). Critical care nurses caring for the poisoned patient should be prepared to assist in the management of multiple complications related to more than one toxic agent. A careful history, physical examination, and drug screens may offer clues to potential toxins.

The following section highlights epidemiology, pathophysiology, clinical manifestations, and management of five common poisoning entities.

Cocaine

Epidemiology, Pathophysiology, and Clinical Manifestations

Cocaine has complex pharmacologic effects, and the route of administration and the form of cocaine involved can affect the onset, duration, and magnitude of the clinical signs and symptoms and potential complications.[14] Cocaine is absorbed from all mucous membranes, from the gastrointestinal tract (most common route in pediatric unintentional exposure), and the genitourinary tract.[55,61]

Cocaine binds to the reuptake pump in presynaptic nerves, blocking the uptake of norepinephrine, dopamine, epinephrine, and serotonin from the synaptic cleft. This action leads to local accumulation of these neurotransmitters (Fig. 18-2), which produces both peripheral and CNS effects.[61]

The accumulation of norepinephrine and epinephrine at β-adrenergic receptors results in tachycardia, increased myocardial contractility, tremor, diaphoresis, and mydriasis. Tachycardia increases myocardial oxygen demand while reducing the time for diastolic filling and for coronary perfusion (particularly of the left ventricle).[87] Accumulation of neurotransmitters at peripheral α-adrenergic receptors results in vasoconstriction and hypertension. The peripheral endothelial nitric oxide system can also be impaired, leading to further vasoconstriction.[113]

Centrally mediated dopaminergic effects of cocaine include mood elevation and movement disorders. Centrally mediated stimulation of serotonin (i.e., 5-hydroxytryptamine or 5-HT) receptors results in exhilaration, hallucinations, and hyperthermia. Stimulation of peripheral 5-HT receptors also results in coronary artery vasospasm that can lead to acute coronary syndrome (ACS) and myocardial infarction. In addition, cocaine stimulates both platelet aggregation[62] and increases in circulating epinephrine; these effects can lead to secondary platelet activation and coronary occlusion.[73]

In adults, the most frequent cause of cocaine-induced hospitalization is ACS, caused by coronary vasoconstriction and platelet aggregation with resulting myocardial ischemia, chest discomfort and possible infarction.[24,65,87] Although ACS is a rare complication in children, it has been reported, particularly when ethanol and cocaine are combined.[164] Concurrent use of cocaine and ethanol precipitates the formation of the cocaine metabolite, cocaethylene, which increases the cardiotoxic and neurotoxic effects of either substance alone.[48] Although myocardial infarction in the neonate with a structurally normal heart and coronary arteries is rare, its association with maternal cocaine abuse has been reported.[28]

Cocaine-induced ACS can lead to myocardial ischemia and subsequent infarction and complications such as ventricular arrhythmias, congestive heart failure, and death.[61,65] Cocaine-induced ACS is diagnosed by ECG changes characteristic of myocardial ischemia; infarction has occurred if serum troponin levels are elevated. In addition to ischemia-induced arrhythmias, cocaine also disturbs cardiac electrophysiology by altering sodium and potassium channel conduction and may induce

CENTRAL NERVOUS SYSTEM SYNAPSE

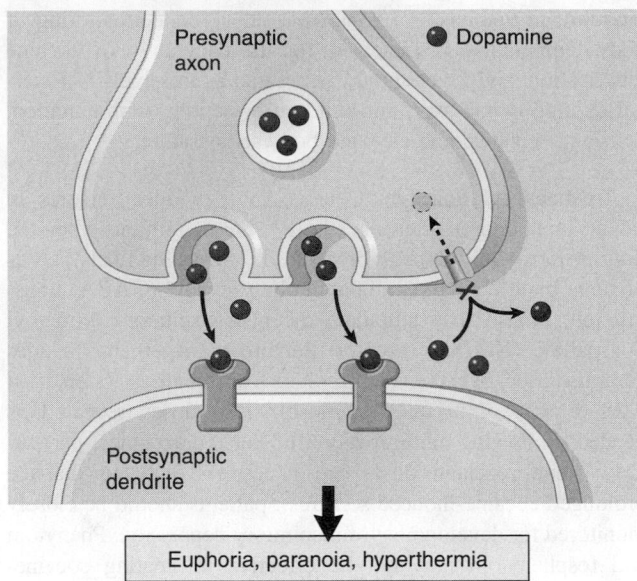

Euphoria, paranoia, hyperthermia

SYMPATHETIC NEURON–TARGET CELL INTERFACE

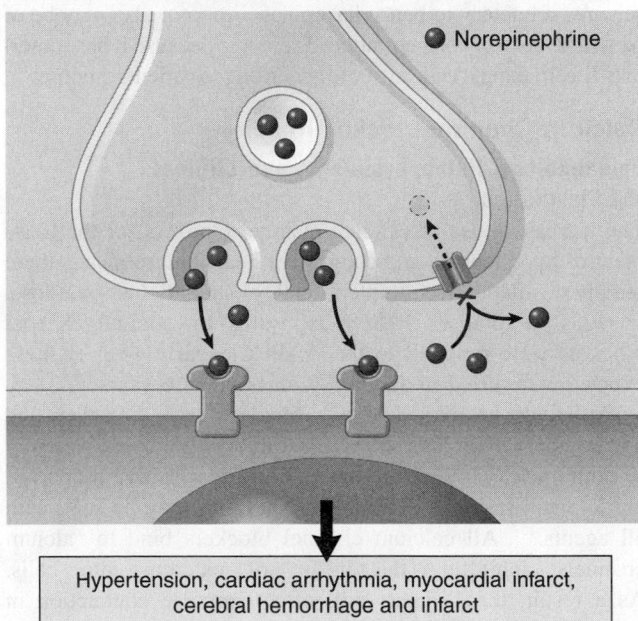

Hypertension, cardiac arrhythmia, myocardial infarct, cerebral hemorrhage and infarct

FIG. 18-2 Effect of cocaine on presynaptic nerves. Cocaine blocks the uptake of norepinephrine, dopamine, epinephrine, and serotonin from the synaptic cleft. This action leads to local accumulation of these neurotransmitters, which produces adrenergic, dopaminergic, and serotonin effects on the peripheral and central nervous systems. (From Kumar V, et al, editors. *Robbins basic pathology,* ed 8. 2007, Elsevier.)

wide-complex arrhythmias, VT, and VF, including torsades de pointes.[13,14,81,127]

Children who ingest cocaine can present with multiple medical complications including altered sensorium, seizures, tachycardia, shock, and cardiovascular compromise. Cocaine affects the CNS, cardiovascular system, and respiratory system in a common three-phase pattern of early stimulation, advanced stimulation, and then depression. These phases can occur in rapid succession, with death taking place within minutes after a significant exposure.

Crack cocaine is the most potent form of the drug. Crack is also the form that small children may likely ingest. Ingestion of a small "rock" of crack cocaine by a child may result in toxic manifestations, whereas ingestion of the same amount by an adult is unlikely to produce toxicity.

Infants can be exposed to cocaine in breast milk,[166] and infants or children may experience passive inhalation of vapors from adults smoking crack cocaine.[63,116] The presence of the cocaine metabolite benzoylecgonine in the urine of children who are otherwise medically stable may reflect passive inhalation; it does not necessarily indicate poisoning or intentional cocaine administration.[63] This situation raises legitimate concern for the well-being of such children, because deaths have been linked to passive inhalation of crack cocaine smoke.[112]

Because cocaine is rapidly metabolized, serum levels generally are of little use and often do not correlate with clinical findings.[19] Table 18-3 summarizes the pharmacokinetics and pharmacodynamics of cocaine hydrochloride.

Management

General Care. Initial treatment of cocaine toxicity consists of oxygen administration, continuous ECG monitoring, and administration of a benzodiazepine (e.g., diazepam or lorazepam).[42,61] This care is summarized in Box 18-5.

Benzodiazepine administration is the mainstay of cocaine toxicity treatment because it offers both anticonvulsant and CNS-depressant effects, and it reduces heart rate and systemic arterial pressure.[42] Benzodiazepines also appear to attenuate the toxic myocardial effects of cocaine.[87] In contrast, phenothiazines and butyrophenones (e.g., haloperidol) provide no benefit and may be harmful to patients with cocaine toxidrome. β-Blockers are contraindicated in cocaine intoxication because their use has been associated with increased blood pressure, coronary vasospasm and fatal myocardial infarction.[79]

Because cocaine is a sodium channel blocker, sodium bicarbonate in a dose of 1 to 2 mEq/kg may be effective in the treatment of cocaine-associated ventricular arrhythmias.[61,79] In an experimental model of cocaine-induced ECG changes, sodium bicarbonate significantly reduced the prolonged PR

Table 18-3 **Pharmacokinetics and Pharmacodynamics of Cocaine Hydrochloride**

Route	Onset of Symptoms	Peak Effects	Peak Plasma Levels	Duration	Half-Life
Intranasal	5 min	20 min	20-60 min	≥30 min	16-87 min
Intravenous	2 min	5-10 min	3-5 min	30 min	54 min
Oral			50-90 min		48-78 min
Topical to mucous membranes	1 min	5 min	15-120 min	≥30 min	

From Hazinski MF, et al: Toxicology. In *PALS provider manual,* Dallas, 2002, American Heart Association.

| Box 18-5 | Recognition and Management of Cocaine Toxicity |

Clinical Signs and Problems
Altered sensorium
Seizures
Tachycardia
Shock
Cardiovascular compromise

Management
Administer oxygen.
Provide continuous ECG monitoring; observe for and treat ventricular arrhythmias (for arrhythmias secondary to infarction, consider lidocaine).
Administer a benzodiazepine.
Treat hyperthermia aggressively.
For ACS, consider nitroglycerin, a benzodiazepine, and phentolamine.
Consider administration of sodium bicarbonate (1-2 mEq/kg).
Consider administration of aspirin and heparin.

Do not administer β-blockers

and QT intervals and reduced the QRS duration.[127] Sodium bicarbonate also may be effective in treating the cocaine-associated acidemia that is thought to contribute to intraventricular conduction delays (prolonged QRS interval), arrhythmias, and depressed myocardial contractility.[156]

Lidocaine administration may be considered for patients with ventricular arrhythmias associated with cocaine-induced myocardial infarction that are refractory to other treatments.[79] The effectiveness of lidocaine in this patient population has not been well established. Because of the fact that lidocaine inhibits fast sodium channels, it has been shown to potentiate cocaine toxicity in animals,[43] although this effect has not been documented in humans. Cocaine and lidocaine together also may have additive effects that increase the likelihood of seizure activity.[142,168]

The effectiveness of epinephrine in the treatment of cocaine-induced circulatory failure is questionable.[111] Epinephrine may exacerbate cocaine-induced arrhythmias and should not be administered for ventricular arrhythmias. If VF or pulseless VT develop, epinephrine is used to increase coronary perfusion pressure during cardiopulmonary resuscitation (CPR).[61]

Treatment of ACS. In addition to benzodiazepines, the administration of nitroglycerin, morphine, and supplementary oxygen may be used to treat ACS. Aspirin and heparin may be simultaneously administered in an attempt to reverse the platelet-activating effects of cocaine and the biochemical manifestations of a procoagulant state; however, this treatment has not been evaluated in clinical trials. Morphine should be used with caution, particularly if blood pressure or myocardial function is unstable.

Treatment of Hyperthermia. The CNS manifestations of cocaine intoxication often include loss of thermoregulation with resulting hyperthermia. High ambient temperature has been

associated with a significant increase in mortality from cocaine overdose in humans.[104,105] As a result, vigilant monitoring of body temperature is indicated for all patients with cocaine intoxication, and fever should be treated aggressively.[79] External cooling is necessary for children presenting with agitation, delirium, seizures, and elevated body temperature.

Treatment of Seizures. Cocaine may produce seizures in infants and children after ingestion,[37,46] and in infants when the drug is transmitted through breast milk.[33] Cocaine likely causes seizures by affecting gamma aminobutyric acid (GABA) transmission; it also may stimulate the neuroexcitatory N-methyl D-aspartate (NMDA) receptor. Seizure management includes administration of a benzodiazepine. Lorazepam is often used (0.05-0.1 mg/kg, up to 2 mg/dose), with doses repeated as needed. Following administration of benzodiazepines, particularly when repeated doses are necessary (e.g., to manage prolonged cocaine-induced seizures), patients should be closely monitored for development of respiratory depression. Phenytoin and fosphenytoin may not be effective in treating cocaine-induced seizures because they lack an effect on the $GABA_A$ receptor.[159] Phenobarbital is recommended for the treatment of seizures refractory to benzodiazepines. Propofol also may be of benefit to control cocaine-induced seizures because it has a short half-life, making it easy to titrate according to patient response.[159]

Calcium Channel Blocker Toxicity
Epidemiology, Pathophysiology, and Clinical Manifestations
The increasing use of calcium channel blockers for the treatment of hypertension and congestive heart failure makes them readily available for unintentional or intentional overdose. In 2009, a total of 10,868 exposures to calcium channel blockers were reported to the AAPCC; nearly 14% of these exposures occurred in children younger than 6 years.[26]

Although calcium channel blockers can be classified according to their effects on the myocardium and vascular smooth muscle, in cases of overdose these selective properties are lost and serious cardiovascular toxicity may be seen with all agents.[134] All calcium channel blockers bind to calcium channels, inhibiting the influx of calcium into cells. As a result, these agents will affect impulse conduction in slow-channel-dependent tissue such as the sinoatrial (SA) and AV nodes, coupling of myocardial excitation-contraction, and vascular smooth muscle tone.

The life-threatening clinical manifestations of calcium channel toxicity include bradyarrhythmias (caused by inhibition of pacemaker cells) and hypotension (caused by vasodilation and impaired cardiac contractility).[115,134] Electrocardiographic changes can include a prolonged PR interval, inverted P waves, AV dissociation, AV block,[1] ST segment changes, low-amplitude T waves, sinus arrest, and asystole. Cerebral hypoperfusion can cause altered mental status (e.g., syncope, seizures, and coma).

The lung and gastrointestinal system are affected directly or indirectly by calcium channel blocker poisoning. Pulmonary complications include cardiogenic and noncardiogenic pulmonary edema,[69,90] which will necessitate cautious fluid resuscitation and early support of ventilation.

Gastrointestinal complications include hypomotility, ileus,[49] and constipation; these effects may be secondary to the inhibition of gastrointestinal motility hormone release.[135] Patients with calcium channel blocker overdose often have absent or greatly diminished bowel sounds. Use of activated charcoal or whole-bowel irrigation may not be appropriate for these patients.

Careful serial assessment of bowel sounds should be performed if any form of gastrointestinal decontamination is being considered, particularly if the patient has ingested sustained-release products. Some experts advocate whole-bowel irrigation for patients who ingest sustained-release products to prevent further absorption,[148] but controlled trials have not been performed to determine the effectiveness of whole bowel irrigation after calcium channel blocker overdose.[4]

Management

General Care. Although the supportive and specific therapies discussed in this section can be very effective in children, third-degree atrioventricular (AV) block with cardiac arrest[161] and death have been reported.[39,89] As a result, providers should monitor the patient closely and be prepared to institute resuscitation. Onset of symptoms may be immediate or delayed for up to 12 to 16 hours, especially when a sustained-release preparation has been ingested.[145,157]

The initial approach to therapy for calcium channel blocker overdose is to support oxygenation and ventilation, provide continuous ECG monitoring, and carefully monitor and support cardiovascular function and systemic perfusion (Box 18-6). All patients with a significant overdose require close monitoring of blood pressure because severe myocardial dysfunction and hypotension may develop. Continuous intra-arterial blood pressure monitoring should be considered for symptomatic patients.

If hypotension develops in cases of mild intoxication, administration of normal saline boluses may restore blood pressure. To prevent pulmonary edema and worsening of myocardial dysfunction, limit fluid boluses to 5 to 10 mL/kg, administer the boluses over 10 to 20 minutes, and reassess after each bolus for evidence of fluid overload. With more severe calcium channel blocker intoxication, the hypotension may be refractory to fluid administration.

Calcium is often infused to treat calcium channel blocker overdose (to overcome the channel blockade), but the effectiveness of this therapy varies.[15,68,134] Calcium chloride is generally recommended because it results in greater elevation of the ionized calcium concentration,[25] but it should be administered through a central venous catheter because infiltration causes severe tissue injury. The optimal dose of calcium for treatment of calcium channel blocker overdose has not been established. Typically, a dose of 20 mg/kg (0.2 mL/kg) of 10% calcium chloride is given over 5 to 10 minutes, followed by an infusion of 20 to 50 mg/kg per hour.[86] Adolescents may require additional calcium. Serum ionized calcium should be closely monitored to prevent hypercalcemia.[143] If central venous access is not available, calcium gluconate should be administered by peripheral venous catheter[79] (typical dose: 100 mg/kg).

High-dose norepinephrine or epinephrine has been reported to be effective for treatment of hypotension (vasopressor effects) or bradycardia (chronotropic effects) associated with severe calcium channel blocker toxicity.[121,131,148] These drugs should be carefully titrated to the desired hemodynamic effect.

Two small case series[21,170] suggest that hyperinsulinemia euglycemia therapy (HIET) may be beneficial in calcium channel blocker toxicity. Some clinicians advocate using HIET early in the management of severe calcium channel blocker overdose,[58,93,110,123] as it enhances myocardial glucose uptake and metabolism, and has positive inotropic properties. Maximal efficacy may be obtained when HIET is administered in conjunction with IV calcium and vasopressors early in the course of serious calcium channel blocker overdose when insulin resistance is high.[57] Presumably, the beneficial effects result from better myocardial glucose utilization through

---

Box 18-6 **Recognition and Management of Calcium Channel Blocker Toxicity**

Clinical Signs
Heart block and bradyarrhythmias (including progression to cardiac arrest)
Hypotension, poor systemic perfusion
Altered mental status, seizures

Management
Support airway, oxygenation, and ventilation.
Establish continuous ECG monitoring; consider intra-arterial pressure monitoring.
Support blood pressure and systemic perfusion as needed (administer small fluid boluses [5-10 mL/kg], vasopressors, inotropes).
Treat bradycardia as needed with chronotropic drugs (e.g., epinephrine).
Calcium chloride (central line infusion): 20 mg/kg of 10% solution over 5-10 min, followed by infusion of 20-50 mg/kg per hour); monitor serum ionized calcium. If only peripheral IV access available, administer calcium gluconate.

Consider early administration of:
HIET (hyperinsulinemia euglycemia therapy):
- Administer glucose bolus of 0.5 g/kg.
- Administer insulin loading dose of 1 unit/kg.
- Establish continuous glucose infusion of 0.5 g/kg per hour; adjust according to serum glucose concentration (maintain approximately 100-200 mg/dL).
- Establish continuous insulin infusion of 0.5-1 unit/kg per hour (or higher as required).
- Follow potassium levels closely to avoid hypokalemia.
Glucagon:
- Adolescents and adults: Administer 5-10 mg over several minutes, followed by infusion of 1-5 mg/hour or higher if needed.
- Younger children: Administer 0.05-0.1 mg/kg up to 1 mg, followed by continuous infusion of 0.05-0.1 mg/kg per hour up to a maximum adult dose.
Sodium bicarbonate: 1 mEq/kg
Consider mechanical support of cardiopulmonary function (see Chapter 7).

activation of pyruvate dehydrogenase and subsequent production of adenosine triphosphate through aerobic metabolism.

Precise dosing[11,57,128] recommendations for HIET are unavailable. Using a central venous line, administer a loading dose of glucose (0.5 g/kg). The loading dose of glucose is followed by a continuous infusion at a rate of 0.5 g/kg per hour, adjusted accordingly. After the glucose bolus, an insulin bolus of 1 unit/kg of regular insulin is administered, followed by an insulin drip of 0.5-1 unit/kg per hour. Severely poisoned patients may require more than 1 unit of insulin/kg per hour. but careful attention to avoid hypoglycemia is imperative. Serum glucose concentration must be closely monitored, and it is often necessary to administer higher doses of glucose if high doses of insulin are required. The target range for glucose administration is to maintain the serum glucose concentration between 100 and 200 mg/dL by titration. Patients should be closely monitored for hypokalemia during HIET because potassium moves intracellularly with glucose. Potassium administration may be required.

Glucagon may be beneficial in the treatment of myocardial toxicity caused by calcium channel blocker overdose.[1,126,171] Glucagon increases serum glucose concentration and causes a transient release of intracellular calcium. It has both positive chronotropic and inotropic effects, thereby increasing heart rate and contractility. In adults and adolescents, an initial bolus of 5 to 10 mg can be administered over several minutes, and repeated as needed. The initial bolus may be followed by a continuous glucagon infusion of 1 to 5 mg/hour or more in an adult.[12,76,,93] In younger children, bolus doses of 0.05 to 0.1 mg/kg up to a total dose of 1 mg or higher may be indicated. The range for continuous infusion of glucagon in children is 0.05 to 0.1 mg/kg per hour up to the typical adult dose of about 1-5 mg/hour.[8,12]

There is insufficient evidence to recommend for or against the use of sodium bicarbonate in the treatment of calcium channel blocker toxicity.[79]

Treatment of Cardiac Arrest. Cardiac arrest caused by calcium channel blocker overdose requires traditional management with high-quality CPR and epinephrine. Cardiac pacing and extracorporeal membrane oxygenation (ECMO) also may be useful.[66] Mechanical cardiopulmonary support (e.g., ECMO, left ventricular assist device, intra-aortic balloon pumping) can also be effective (see Chapters 6 and 7). Aggressive resuscitation may be warranted in cases of calcium channel blocker overdose because recovery has been reported after prolonged verapamil-induced pulseless arrest.[47,158] Calcium channel blockers may have some neuroprotective effects.

β-Adrenergic Blocker Toxicity

Epidemiology, Pathophysiology, and Clinical Manifestations

β-Adrenergic antagonists or β-blockers are widely prescribed and are responsible for a large number of poisonings every year. Intentional overdose by adolescents may result in severe intoxication. In 2009 a total of 22,135 ingestions of β-blockers were reported to the AAPCC, with nearly 15% of these exposures occurring in children younger than 6 years of age.[26] Another retrospective review of data over an 11-year period

showed more than 50,000 β-blocker exposures; overdoses of these agents accounted for 2.5% of all poison-related fatalities.[101] A cohort study of 280 β-blocker exposures found that propranolol was the most commonly ingested β-blocker and the drug most frequently responsible for cardiovascular toxicity.[100]

β-adrenergic blockers compete with the sympathetic neurotransmitters, norepinephrine and epinephrine, at the β-adrenergic receptor site. These β-adrenergic receptors are located in cardiac, renal, liver tissue and in the smooth muscle cells of blood vessels, the trachea, the airway and the gastrointestinal tract.

β-blockade decreases intracellular cyclic adenosine monophosphate (cAMP), with resultant decrease in the metabolic, chronotropic, and inotropic activities of the heart and decreased vasoconstriction in blood vessels. A low intracellular cAMP concentration also decreases release of calcium from intracellular stores,[76,163] producing bradycardia and conduction disturbances (e.g., sinus pauses, prolonged PR interval, various degrees of heart block, intraventricular conduction defects, and prolonged QRS interval). Arrhythmias including torsades de pointes,[10] VF, and in rare cases, asystole[149] may occur with severe poisoning. Hypotension paired with bradycardia, and various degrees of heart block are also common clinical manifestations of β-blocker toxicity.[76]

In addition to the cardiovascular effects, altered mental status, seizures, and coma may develop in cases of β-blocker toxicity. Altered mental status is particularly likely with agents that have high lipid solubility (e.g., propranolol) because these agents readily cross the blood-brain barrier.[40,76] The CNS effects of β-blocker toxicity are direct effects separate from the effects of cerebral hypoperfusion that develop secondary to systemic hypotension. CNS toxicity may occur in the absence of clinical cardiac symptoms.[98]

Metabolic disturbances associated with β-blocker toxicity, such as hypoglycemia, are especially common in children and may contribute to a decreased level of consciousness. In addition, bronchospasm and increased airway resistance may contribute to airway compromise. Patients with β-blocker toxicity likely will require management of hypoglycemia and support of airway, oxygenation, and ventilation, in addition to circulatory support.

Management

General Care. The initial approach to treatment of β-blocker overdose includes supporting adequate oxygenation and ventilation, assessing perfusion, establishing vascular access, and treating shock if present. Continuous ECG monitoring and frequent clinical reassessments are important (Box 18-7).

To overcome β-adrenergic blockade, high-dose epinephrine infusions may be effective.[79,160] Other high-dose adrenergic agents (e.g., norepinephrine, dobutamine, isoproterenol, and dopamine) have been used successfully.[72,92,144] Phosphodiesterase inhibitors such as inamrinone (formerly amrinone)[82] or milrinone also can be used to improve myocardial contractility.

Limited experimental data[76,171] and case reports[92,160] suggest that glucagon may be beneficial in the treatment of β-adrenergic blocker overdose. In adults and adolescents, infusion of 5 to 10 mg of glucagon (administered over several minutes) followed

Box 18-7 **Recognition and Management of β-Blocker Toxicity**

Clinical Signs

Heart block and bradyarrhythmias (including prolonged QRS and QT intervals)

Decreased myocardial function and vasodilation, hypotension, poor systemic perfusion

Bronchospasm

Hypoglycemia

Altered mental status, seizures

Decreased gastrointestinal motility

Management

Support airway, oxygenation, and ventilation.

Establish continuous ECG monitoring; consider intra-arterial pressure monitoring.

Support blood pressure (epinephrine infusion at high doses may be required) and systemic perfusion (consider inotropes and inodilator).

Administer small fluid boluses; titrate to patient response.

Glucagon:
- Adolescents and adults: Administer 5-10 mg over several minutes, followed by infusion of 1-5 mg/hour or higher if needed.
- Younger children: Administer 0.05-0.1 mg/kg up to 1 mg, followed by continuous infusion of 0.05-0.1 mg/kg per hour up to a maximum adult dose.

HIET (hyperinsulinemia euglycemia therapy):
- Administer glucose bolus of 0.5 g/kg.
- Administer insulin loading dose of 1 unit/kg.
- Establish continuous glucose infusion of 0.5 g/kg per hour, adjust according to serum glucose concentration (maintain approximately 100-200 mg/dL).
- Establish continuous insulin infusion of 0.5-1 unit/kg per hour (or higher as required).
- Follow potassium levels closely to avoid hypokalemia.

Consider calcium if unresponsive to glucagon and HIET.

Consider mechanical support of cardiopulmonary function (see Chapter 7).

---

by an IV infusion of 1-5 mg/hour or higher may be used.[79] In younger children, bolus doses of 0.05 to 0.1 mg/kg up to 5 mg may be needed. In lieu of glucagon, HIET (hyperinsulinemia euglycemia therapy) also may be useful in the treatment of β-adrenergic blocker overdose (see doses in Box 18-7).

β-adrenergic blockade reduces cytoplasmic calcium concentration. Limited animal data[99] and limited case reports[23,129] suggest that calcium administration may be beneficial[144] if glucagon and catecholamines are ineffective.[79] Consider the administration of calcium to patients with β-blocker poisoning unresponsive to catecholamines and glucagon. In cases of intraventricular conduction delay (i.e., prolonged QRS interval), sodium bicarbonate[44,141] (in addition to therapy with glucagon[12,76] or HIET),[110,125] catecholamines,[76] and calcium[122] may be given.

Nonpharmacologic Therapies. Nonpharmacologic therapies such as cardiac pacing[75] and extracorporeal circulation[109] may be successful in β-blocker overdose when other modalities and pharmacologic therapies fail. Children suspected of ingesting massive amounts of β-blockers or who manifest early signs of impending cardiovascular collapse may benefit from transport to a tertiary care pediatric center capable of providing these advanced therapies (see Chapters 6, 7 and 8).

Opioid Toxicity

Epidemiology, Pathophysiology, and Clinical Manifestations

Exposures related to opiates account for a large number of cases reported to poison centers and presenting to emergency departments. In 2009 a total of 88,609 exposures to opiates (either alone or in combination with other analgesics) were reported to the AAPCC.[26] This number does not include heroin overdoses managed by EMS and emergency departments. According to 2009 NPDS statistics, opioids accounted for the third largest number of poison related fatalities.[26] Opiate exposures and deaths have increased in many communities

in the United States.[31,50,53] Toxicity and overdose from opiates and opioids can occur with pediatric procedural sedation.[54] Published reviews of procedural sedation and analgesia for children highlight the need for providers to be familiar with the sedative agents used and reversal agents such as naloxone.[18,83,139]

Narcotic overdose in children may occur from a number of different opioids (e.g., morphine, codeine, hydrocodone, oxycodone, hydromorphone, meperidine, pentazocine, and propoxyphene) and sources (i.e., intentional overdose, recreational use, and ingestion by small children). Abuse of the synthetic agent oxycodone as a recreational drug has recently increased among adolescents. Over-the-counter agents such as dextromethorphan, the d-isomer of the opiate agonist levorphanol, have been abused by adolescents, resulting in overdose deaths.[119] Butorphanol nasal spray also may be available for abuse or accidental ingestion by children. A controlled-release form of oxycodone (i.e., OxyContin) is available in dosage strengths of up to 160 mg; this preparation can contribute to serious and prolonged opioid toxicity in instances of overdose and abuse.

Methadone is prescribed for chronic pain, but it is more commonly used to prevent withdrawal symptoms in patients recovering from opiate addiction. Its widespread use puts children at risk for inadvertent exposure.[27,94] Because methadone has a long half-life and active metabolites, the patient with methadone overdose is usually admitted for monitoring and observation. Similar to opiates, clonidine (a centrally-acting imidazoline α2-receptor agonist) may cause respiratory depression, miosis, and coma. Clonidine has a prolonged effect, so patients require intensive monitoring.

Whenever a child is admitted with coma or respiratory depression of unknown cause, providers should consider the possibility of opiate overdose. These drugs are commonly used in both intentional abuse and Munchausen syndrome by proxy.[32,108]

Rapid urine immunoassays may detect opiates, but these tests can produce both false-negative and false-positive results. As an example, screening immunoassays often do not detect methadone, but more comprehensive assays will detect it.[16] Whenever child maltreatment is suspected, qualitative screens such as urine immunoassays are insufficient for medicolegal purposes. In these situations, samples should be sent with documented chain of custody to a reference laboratory for analysis using advanced techniques.

Many opiates (e.g., codeine, hydrocodone, oxycodone, and propoxyphene), are often formulated in combination with acetaminophen or aspirin. When children present with symptoms or history of overdose with opiates, providers must assess for additional toxicities related to acetaminophen or aspirin.

Some opioids are available in transdermal patches that are formulated to release the opioid at a relatively slow rate; however, the patches themselves contain very large total amounts of the drug. Ingestion of a small amount of fentanyl from a fentanyl patch can produce severe toxicity in a child because of the potency of this opioid. The fentanyl on transdermal patches also can be inhaled. In one case severe toxicity developed within seconds after the patient heated a fentanyl patch and inhaled the vapors.[103]

Heroin may be inhaled, ingested, or injected. Heroin accounts for very few unintentional exposures in children, but it may be abused by adolescents.[136] Heroin overdose is a major problem in most urban emergency departments.

Narcotics produce CNS depression and may cause hypoventilation, apnea, and respiratory failure. Respiration is controlled principally through brain respiratory centers in the medulla with peripheral input from chemoreceptors and other sources. Opioids produce inhibition at the chemoreceptors through mu opioid receptors and in the medulla through mu and delta receptors.

Although children may present with respiratory failure caused by ingestion of only one opiate or opioid, adolescents often mix these agents with alcohol and other substances. Glutamate is the major excitatory neurotransmitter and GABA is the major inhibitory neurotransmitter contributing to control of respiration. Both benzodiazepines and alcohol facilitate the inhibitory effect of GABA; alcohol also decreases the excitatory effect of glutamate.[162] As a result, the combination of benzodiazepines and alcohol can produce significant respiratory depression that is usually evident early after ingestion and may require support with mechanical ventilation.[146]

Severe opiate intoxication may cause cardiovascular symptoms such as hypotension, tachycardia or bradycardia, arrhythmias, circulatory collapse, and cardiac arrest. Noncardiogenic pulmonary edema may occur with heroin overdose.[146]

Decreased gastrointestinal motility is common with opioid overdose, presumably caused by peripheral opioid receptor effects.[30,118] Delayed gastric emptying may cause "cyclical" coma. The first phase of drug absorption results in a decreased level of consciousness. This phase is followed by some metabolism of the drug, so the patient begins to awaken. Further delayed absorption of the drug may cause another decrease in level of consciousness. This inconsistency in level of consciousness generally precludes administration of activated charcoal unless preceded by endotracheal intubation. Seizures may occur with the opiate meperidine,[59,85] further complicating management.

Management

General Care. Therapy for opiate or opioid toxicity should begin with assessment and support of the airway, oxygenation, and ventilation. If significant respiratory depression or respiratory failure is present, provide immediate bag-mask ventilation with oxygen. Endotracheal intubation with mechanical ventilation may be required.[79]

Naloxone is the antidote of choice for treatment of severe opiate or opioid toxicity. In the presence of the opiate toxidrome, characterized by coma, depressed respirations, and miosis (pinpoint pupils), naloxone administration should be considered once adequate ventilation has been established (Box 18-8).[61]

Naloxone has been used for more than 20 years.[6,74] Although patients generally tolerate naloxone well,[147,169] adverse reactions, including ventricular arrhythmias, acute pulmonary edema,[133] asystole, and seizures, may occur.[124] The opioid and adrenergic systems are interrelated; opioid antagonists stimulate sympathetic nervous system activity.[77] In addition, hypercapnia stimulates the sympathetic nervous system. Thus, administration of naloxone (an opioid antagonist) in the presence of significant hypercapnia from respiratory depression can produce substantial adrenergic stimulation with possible tachycardia, increased blood pressure, acute pulmonary edema, arrhythmias, seizures, and even cardiac arrest.[79] Effective ventilation to normalize the partial pressure of CO_2 ($PaCO_2$) should be established *before* administration of naloxone to reduce potential adrenergic stimulation and attendant toxic effects of naloxone administration.[79]

For treatment of the adverse effects of opiate overdose, the recommended naloxone dose is 0.1 mg/kg by IV or intraosseous (IO) route; for children 5 years of age and older (or larger than 20 kg), administer up to 2 mg in a single dose.[6] To avoid the sudden hemodynamic effects of opioid reversal, repeated doses of 0.01 to 0.03 mg/kg may be indicated. Very low doses (0.001-0.005 mg/kg [1-5 mcg/kg]) can be used to reverse respiratory depression caused by therapeutic doses of opiates.[79]

Box 18-8	Recognition and Management of Opioid Toxicity

Clinical Signs

Respiratory depression, apnea

Bradycardia, circulatory collapse

Decreased level of consciousness including coma and cyclical coma

Delayed gastric emptying

Management

Establish patent airway, support oxygenation and ventilation. Give Naloxone:

- Less than 5 years (or 20 kg or less): 0.1 mg/kg IV/IO
- 5 years or older (or more than 20 kg): Up to 2 mg IV/IO
- In suspected narcotic addiction, use low initial doses (e.g., 0.01 mg/kg, up to 0.4 mg in a single dose; repeat as needed) to avoid withdrawal symptoms.
- For treatment of respiratory depression associated with therapeutic opioid use as in procedural sedation: 0.001-0.005 mg/kg (1-5 mcg/kg), repeat as needed.
- After initial dose, consider infusion, particularly for significant overdose or overdose with long-acting formulations.

To treat respiratory depression in patients with suspected narcotic addiction, many toxicologists use low initial doses of naloxone (e.g., 0.01 mg/kg, up to 0.4 mg in a single dose; repeat as needed) to avoid withdrawal symptoms such as vomiting with the attendant risks of aspiration and agitation. The concept of "go low and go slow" is most appropriate in these patients.

The half-life of naloxone is much shorter than the half-life of opiates. Following the initial doses of naloxone, a continuous infusion may be needed to reverse the toxic effects of opiate poisoning.[150] Continuous infusion of naloxone also may be necessary to treat poisoning from some long-acting opioids such as methadone, continuous release oxycodone, and diphenoxylate. Naloxone may also be administered intramuscularly, subcutaneously, or through the endotracheal tube, but use of these routes may delay its onset of action, particularly if perfusion is poor.

TCAs and Other Sodium Channel Blocking Agents

Epidemiology, Pathophysiology, and Clinical Manifestations

Despite the introduction of safer treatment options for depression, tricyclic (cyclic) antidepressant toxicity continues to be a leading cause of morbidity and mortality. In 2009 a total of 102,792 ingestions involving an antidepressant and 79 total deaths caused by cyclic antidepressants were reported to the AAPCC.[26] In children, TCAs are currently used to treat depression, attention deficit hyperactivity syndrome, migraine headaches, neuropathic pain, cyclic vomiting syndrome, nocturnal enuresis, and sleep disturbances, making them readily available to children for toxic ingestion.

TCAs typically are considered within the broader context of sodium channel blocking toxins, but when taken in overdose TCAs are also potassium channel blockers. The combined sodium and potassium channel blocking effects of TCAs may cause repolarization abnormalities and prolongation of the QT interval. Seizures can develop as the result of TCA blockade of the neuroinhibitory gamma aminobutyric acid ($GABA_A$) chloride channel.[36,91]

Although full therapeutic effects of TCAs may take up to 2 weeks or longer to develop, toxic effects typically appear within 4 hours of ingestion. Experts have yet to agree on a distinct and well-recognized toxidrome for TCAs. Principle symptoms of TCA overdose are: depressed level of consciousness, seizures, life-threatening arrhythmias, and sometimes acidosis. A helpful mnemonic to remember these symptoms is "Three Cs and an A," corresponding to *C*oma, *C*onvulsions, *C*ardiac arrhythmias, and *A*cidosis (sometimes). The clinical features of TCA overdose arise from four major sources: anticholinergic effects, excessive blockade of norepinephrine reuptake at the postganglionic synapse, direct sodium channel blockade, and quinidine-like effects on the myocardium.

Symptoms of early CNS stimulation may be the first signs of TCA toxicity. These symptoms likely result from the anticholinergic effects of the TCA, characterized by agitation, irritability, confusion, delirium, hallucinations, choreoathetosis (irregular, uncontrolled random movements, flowing from one part of the body to another), hyperactivity, seizures, and hyperpyrexia.[61,155] Sinus tachycardia, hypertension, and supraventricular tachycardia may be observed early after ingestion and likely are related

to excessive norepinephrine. Catecholamine depletion soon develops because norepinephrine reuptake into neurons is inhibited and the released norepinephrine is metabolized by catechol-O-methyltransferase and monoamine oxidase.[61]

With serious intoxication, cardiac rhythm disturbances result from prolongation of the action potential. This inhibition delays intraventricular conduction, causing QRS prolongation[167] with QRS duration often exceeding 100 ms.[52,60] The presence of these ECG abnormalities may be predictive of seizures as well as ventricular arrhythmias.[20,52,60] Predictors of severe toxicity are an R wave in lead aVR equal to or greater than 3 mm or an R wave to S wave ratio in lead aVR equal to or greater than 0.7 (Fig. 18-3).[96,97] TCA toxicity also is associated with preterminal sinus bradycardia and heart block with junctional or ventricular (wide-complex) escape rhythms.[81]

TCA overdose also may cause direct pulmonary toxicity. In addition, noncardiogenic pulmonary edema and acute lung injury in the setting of TCA overdose have been reported.[137,172] The combined cardiac and respiratory manifestations of TCA overdose may precipitate cardiorespiratory arrest.

Other sodium channel blockers with toxicity similar to that of TCAs include β-adrenergic blockers (particularly propranolol and sotalol), procainamide, quinidine, local anesthetics (e.g., lidocaine), carbamazepine, type IC antiarrhythmics (e.g., flecainide and encainide), and cocaine.[81] A common antihistamine, diphenhydramine, also can produce prominent sodium channel blocker effects resulting in wide-complex tachyarrhythmias with significant overdoses.[117]

Management

General Care. If there is no specific history of TCA exposure but an overdose is suspected based on symptoms of the TCA toxidrome (i.e., coma, convulsions, cardiac arrhythmias, and sometimes acidosis) and ECG changes, a number of bedside rapid urine immunoassays are available to screen for TCAs.[140] For both suspected and known sodium channel blocker toxicity of any type, establishment of a patent airway and assessment and support of adequate oxygenation and ventilation are priorities; early endotracheal intubation should be considered.

Poison centers traditionally have recommended gastric lavage for TCA overdose, but there is no clear evidence that it is effective. If a patient ingests a potentially life-threatening amount of a TCA and presents asymptomatic within an hour of ingestion, lavage may be considered.[152]

Treatment of TCAs and other sodium channel blocker toxicants requires continuous ECG monitoring and treatment of arrhythmias with sodium bicarbonate (Box 18-9).[22,79] Sodium bicarbonate raises the sodium concentration, which helps

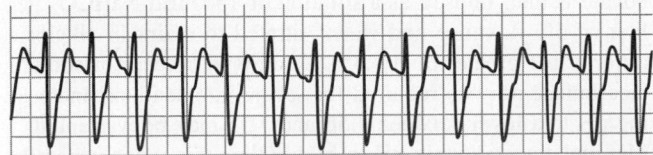

FIG. 18-3 Sinus tachycardia with wide QRS complex in child with tricyclic antidepressant overdose. The QT interval is prolonged. Rhythm strip courtesy of Stephen M. Schexnayder, Little Rock, Arkansas.

Box 18-9 **Recognition and Management of Tricyclic Antidepressant Toxicity**

Clinical Presentation

Three Cs and an A

Coma

Convulsions

Cardiac arrhythmias

Acidosis (sometimes)

Early symptoms

Signs of CNS stimulation: agitation, irritability, confusion, delirium, hallucinations, choreoathetosis, hyperactivity, seizures, and hyperpyrexia

Cardiovascular signs: sinus tachycardia, hypertension, and supraventricular tachycardia

Management

General Management

Protect the airway (consider early intubation).

Maintain adequate oxygenation and ventilation.

Provide continuous ECG monitoring.

Treat arrhythmias with sodium bicarbonate: 1-2 mEq/kg IV/IO boluses until arterial pH is 7.45 or higher (or 7.50-7.55 for severe poisoning).

Follow boluses with IV/IO sodium bicarbonate infusion (150 mEq NaHCO₃/L solution); titrate to maintain alkalosis.

Administer small normal saline boluses (10 mL/kg each) in addition to sodium bicarbonate as needed to support systemic perfusion; monitor for pulmonary edema.

Administer vasopressors (e.g., epinephrine, norepinephrine) to maintain adequate vascular tone and blood pressure (high doses may be required).

Consider ECMO and cardiopulmonary bypass if vasopressors are insufficient to maintain blood pressure.

Seizure Management

Support airway, oxygenation, and ventilation.

Give benzodiazepines. If refractory, give phenobarbital.

Correct acid-base disturbances.

Do *not* use phenytoin or fosphenytoin

---

overcome the sodium channel blockade. The creation of alkalosis appears to contribute to the therapeutic effect by increasing protein binding of the TCA, thus reducing the amount of free drug available to cause toxicity. Administration of sodium bicarbonate should produce narrowing of the QRS complex, shortening of the QT interval, and increased myocardial contractility.[61] These actions typically suppress ventricular arrhythmias, increase blood pressure, and improve systemic perfusion.[64,106]

Sodium bicarbonate is administered in 1 to 2 mEq/kg boluses until the arterial pH is 7.45 or higher. Sodium bicarbonate is then infused as a solution of 150 mEq NaHCO₃ per liter of 5% dextrose and water, titrated to maintain alkalosis (arterial pH greater than 7.45). Additional boluses of sodium bicarbonate may be required for severe intoxications; increasing pH to a level between 7.50 and 7.55 may be warranted.[79] Manipulating systemic pH to higher than this range generally is not recommended because of the risk of excessive alkalosis.[81,95] Support of normal ventilation is recommended while the pH is increased with sodium bicarbonate administration.

Although hyperventilation-induced alkalosis reportedly improves cardiac conduction,[17] the effectiveness of respiratory alkalosis for TCA overdose has not been established.[106]

If ventricular arrhythmias caused by a TCA or other sodium channel blocker toxicant do not respond to sodium bicarbonate administration, consider lidocaine administration.[51,61,79] Providers should be aware that many antiarrhythmics may worsen cardiovascular problems, including arrhythmias. Class I_A (quinidine, procainamide) and Class I_C (flecainide, propafenone) antiarrhythmics are contraindicated because they may exacerbate cardiac toxicity.[95] Class III antiarrhythmics (amiodarone, sotalol) should not be administered because they prolong the QT interval.[95]

Treatment of Hypotension. If hypotension caused by TCA, or other sodium channel blocker toxicant is present, administer small normal saline boluses (5-10 mL/kg each), in addition to sodium bicarbonate.[22,79,130] Cautious administration of intravenous fluid is essential because antidepressants and other sodium channel blocking drugs have myocardial depressant effects, and excessive or rapid intravenous fluid administration may contribute to myocardial failure and pulmonary edema.

Because TCAs block reuptake of norepinephrine at the neuromuscular junction, overdose can cause catecholamine depletion that contributes to vasodilation and hypotension. Vasopressors such as norepinephrine or epinephrine may be needed to maintain adequate vascular tone and blood pressure.[61,79,80] Pure β-adrenergic agonists (e.g., dobutamine and isoproterenol) generally are not used because they may cause further vasodilation and hypotension. Furthermore, administration of dopamine may not result in sufficient vasoconstriction to correct hypotension unless given in high doses (i.e., greater than 20 mcg/kg per minute).[155]

If high-dose vasopressors are insufficient to maintain blood pressure, ECMO and cardiopulmonary bypass may be effective,[88,165] but these therapies require rapid availability of equipment and trained personnel.[79] Early identification of at-risk patients is important to enable possible referral to a facility capable of providing these therapies.

Treatment of Seizures. Benzodiazepines (e.g., lorazepam or diazepam) are indicated to treat seizures caused by TCA or other sodium channel blocker agents. In addition, patients require careful support of the airway, oxygenation, and ventilation and correction of acid-base imbalances. Phenobarbital is recommended for the treatment of seizures refractory to benzodiazepines. Phenytoin and fosphenytoin are ***not*** recommended to treat seizures, because they lack a subreceptor on the GABA_A chloride channel that is partially blocked by the TCAs. As a result, these drugs will not help restore the brain equilibrium and stop the seizures. In addition, phenytoin and fosphenytoin may have pro-arrhythmic effects in patients with TCA toxicity.[29]

ADVANCED CONCEPTS

The advanced practitioner will be able to identify common toxidromes and anticipate the development of complications related to poisoning. Advanced concepts in the care of the patient with toxicologic problems are listed in Box 18-10.

| Box 18-10 | **Advanced Practice Concepts: Toxicology** |

- Several toxins and drugs (e.g., tricyclic antidepressants, β-blockers, and cocaine) have sodium channel blocking properties and effects on cell membrane stability that predispose children to ventricular arrhythmias. These arrhythmias may respond to administration of sodium bicarbonate.
- Specific antidotes that are not used routinely in cardiopulmonary resuscitation may be useful in certain types of drug overdose:
  - Sodium bicarbonate for sodium channel blocking agents, including tricyclic antidepressants and cocaine
  - Calcium chloride for β-adrenergic overdose (more controversial and less uniformly efficacious than when used for calcium channel blocker overdose)
  - HIET for calcium channel blocker and β-blocker overdoses
  - Glucagon for calcium channel and β-blocker overdose
  - Naloxone for opiate intoxication

References

1. Adams BD, Browne WT: Amlodipine overdose causes prolonged calcium channel blocker toxicity. *Am J Emerg Med* 16:527–528, 1998.
2. American Academy of Clinical Toxicology: Facility assessment guidelines for regional toxicology treatment centers. *J Toxicol Clin Toxicol* 31:211–217, 1993.
3. American Academy of Clinical Toxicology and European Association of Poisons Centres and Clinical Toxicologists: Position statement and practice guidelines on the use of multi-dose activated charcoal in the treatment of acute poisoning. *J Toxicol Clin Toxicol* 37(6):731–751, 1999.
4. American Academy of Clinical Toxicology and European Association of Poison Centres and Clinical Toxicologists: Position paper: whole bowel irrigation. *J Toxicol Clin Toxicol* 42(6):843–854, 2004.
5. American Academy of Clinical Toxicology and European Association of Poisons Centres and Clinical Toxicologists: Position Paper: Ipecac Syrup. *J Toxicol Clin Toxicol* 42(2):133–143, 2004.
6. American Academy of Pediatrics Committee on Drugs: Naloxone dosage and route of administration for infants and children: addendum to emergency drug doses for infants and children. *Pediatrics* 86:484–485, 1990.
7. American College of Emergency Physicians: Poison information and treatment systems. *Ann Emerg Med* 37:370, 2001.
8. Arroyo AM, Kao LW: Calcium channel blocker toxicity. *Ped Emerg Care* 25(8):532–538, 2009.
9. Askenasi R, et al: Esophageal perforation: an unusual complication of gastric lavage. *Ann Emerg Med* 13:146, 1984.
10. Assimes TL, Malcolm I: Torsade de pointes with sotalol overdose treated successfully with lidocaine. *Can J Cardiol* 14:753–756, 1998.
11. Azendour H, et al: Severe amlodipine intoxication treated by hyperinsulinemia-euglycemic therapy. *J Emerg Med* 38(1):33–35, 2010.
12. Bailey B: Glucagon in β-blocker and calcium channel blocker overdoses: a systemic review. *J Toxicol Clin Toxicol* 41(5):595–602, 2003.
13. Bauman J, DiDomenic R: Cocaine-induced channelopathies: emerging evidence. *J Cardiovasc Pharmacol Ther* 7:195–202, 2002.
14. Bauman JL, Grawe JJ, Winecoff AP, et al: Cocaine-related sudden cardiac death: a hypothesis correlating basic science and clinical observations. *J Clin Pharmacol* 34:902–911, 1994.
15. Belson MG, Gorman SE, Sullivan K, Geller RJ: Calcium channel blocker ingestions in children. *Am J Emerg Med* 18:581–586, 2000.
16. Belson MG, Simon HK: Utility of comprehensive toxicologic screens in children. *Am J Emerg Med* 17:221–224, 1999.
17. Bessen HA, Niemann JT: Improvement of cardiac conduction after hyperventilation in tricyclic antidepressant overdose. *J Toxicol Clin Toxicol* 23:537–546, 1985.
18. Bhatt M, et al: Consensus-based recommendations for standardizing terminology and reporting adverse events for emergency department procedural sedation and analgesia in children. *Ann Emerg Med* 53 (4):426–435, 2009.
19. Blaho K, et al: Blood cocaine and metabolite concentrations, clinical findings, and outcome of patients presenting to an ED. *Am J Emerg Med* 18:593–598, 2000.
20. Boehnert MT, Lovejoy FH, Jr.: Value of the QRS duration versus the serum drug level in predicting seizures and ventricular arrhythmias after an acute overdose of tricyclic antidepressants. *N Engl J Med* 313:474–479, 1985.
21. Boyer EW, Shannon M: Treatment of calcium-channel-blocker intoxication with insulin infusion. *N Engl J Med* 344:1721–1722, 2001.
22. Bradberry SM, et al: Management of the cardiovascular complications of tricyclic antidepressant poisoning: role of sodium bicarbonate. *Toxicol Rev* 24(3):195–204, 2005.
23. Brimacombe JR, Scully M, Swainston R: Propranolol overdose—a dramatic response to calcium chloride. *Med J Aust* 155:267–268, 1991.
24. Brody SL, Slovis CM, Wrenn KD: Cocaine-related medical problems: consecutive series of 233 patients. *Am J Med* 88:325–331, 1990.
25. Broner CW, Stidham GL, Westenkirchner DF, Watson DC: A prospective, randomized, double-blind comparison of calcium chloride and calcium gluconate therapies for hypocalcemia in critically ill children. *J Pediatr* 117:986–989, 1990.
26. Bronstein AC, et al: 2009 Annual Report of the American Association of Poison Control Centers' National Poison Data System (NPDS): 27th annual report. *Clin Toxicol* 48:979–1178, 2010.
27. Brooks DE, Roberge RJ, Spear A: Clinical nuances of pediatric methadone intoxication. *Vet Hum Toxicol* 41:388–390, 1999.
28. Bulbul ZR, Rosenthal DN, Kleinman CS: Myocardial infarction in the perinatal period secondary to maternal cocaine abuse: a case report and literature review. *Arch Pediatr Adolesc Med* 148:1092–1096, 1994.
29. Callaham M, Schumaker H, Pentel P: Phenytoin prophylaxis of cardiotoxicity in experimental amitriptyline poisoning. *J Pharmacol Exp Ther* 245:216–220, 1988.
30. Camilleri M: Opioid-induced constipation: challenges and therapeutic opportunities. *Am J Gastroenterol* 106(5):835–842, 2011.
31. Centers for Disease Control and Prevention: Unintentional opiate overdose deaths—King County, Washington, 1990-1999. *MMWR* 49:636–640, 2000.
32. Centers for Disease Control and Prevention: Emergency department visits involving nonmedical use of selected prescription drugs—United States, 2004-2008. *MMWR* 59(23):705–709, 2010.
33. Chaney NE, Franke J, Wadlington WB: Cocaine convulsions in a breast-feeding baby. *J Pediatr* 112:134–135, 1988.
34. Chyka PA, Seger D, et al: American Academy of Clinical Toxicology; European Association of Poisons Centres and Clinical Toxicologists: Position statement: single-dose activated charcoal. *J Toxicol Clin Toxicol* 35:721–741, 1997.
35. Chyka PA, et al: Position paper: single-dose activated charcoal. *Clin Toxicol (Phila)* 43(2):61–87, 2005.
36. Citak A, et al: Seizures associated with poisoning in children: tricyclic antidepressant intoxication. *Pediatr Int* 48(6):582–585, 2006.
37. Conway EEJ, Mezey AP, Powers K: Status epilepticus following the oral ingestion of cocaine in an infant. *Pediatr Emerg Care* 6:189–190, 1990.
38. Cooney DO: *Activated charcoal in medicinal applications,* New York, 1995, Marcel Dekker.
39. Cosbey SH, Carson DJ: A fatal case of amlodipine poisoning. *J Anal Toxicol* 21:221–222, 1997.
40. Cruickshank JM, et al: (-Adrenoreceptor-blocking agents and the blood-brain barrier. *Clin Sci* 59(Suppl. 6):453s–455s, 1980.
41. Dahlin KL, et al: Acute lung failure induced by tricyclic antidepressants. *Toxicol Appl Pharmacol* 146:309–316, 1997.
42. Derlet RW, Albertson TE: Diazepam in the prevention of seizures and death in cocaine-intoxicated rats. *Ann Emerg Med* 18:542–546, 1989.
43. Derlet RW, Albertson TE, Tharratt RS: Lidocaine potentiation of cocaine toxicity. *Ann Emerg Med* 20:135–138, 1991.
44. Donovan KD, Gerace RV, Dreyer JF: Acebutolol-induced ventricular tachycardia reversed with sodium bicarbonate. *J Toxicol Clin Toxicol* 37:481–484, 1999.

45. Eddleston M, et al: Multiple-dose activated charcoal in acute self-poisoning: a randomised controlled trial. *Lancet* 371(9612):579–587, 2008.

46. Ernst AA, Sanders WM: Unexpected cocaine intoxication presenting as seizures in children. *Ann Emerg Med* 18:774–777, 1989.

47. Evans JS, Oram MP: Neurological recovery after prolonged verapamil-induced cardiac arrest. *Anaesth Intensive Care* 27:653–655, 1999.

48. Farooq MU, Bhatt A, Patel M: Neurotoxic and cardiotoxic effects of cocaine and ethanol. *J Med Toxicol* 5(3):134–138, 2009.

49. Fauville JP, et al: Severe diltiazem poisoning with intestinal pseudo-obstruction: case report and toxicological data. *J Toxicol Clin Toxicol* 33:273–277, 1995.

50. Fingerhut LA, Cox CS: Poisoning mortality, 1985-1995. [published correction appears in Public Health Rep 113:380, 1998] *Public Health Rep* 113:218–233, 1998.

51. Foianini A, Joseph Wiegand T, Benowitz N: What is the role of lidocaine or phenytoin in tricyclic antidepressant-induced cardiotoxicity? *Clin Toxicol (Phila)* 48(4):325–330, 2010.

52. Foulke GE: Identifying toxicity risk early after antidepressant overdose. *Am J Emerg Med* 13:123–126, 1995.

53. Friedman LS: Real-time surveillance of illicit drug overdoses using poison center data. *Clin Toxicol (Phila)* 47(6):573–579, 2009.

54. Gill AM, et al: Opiate-induced respiratory depression in pediatric patients. *Ann Pharmacother* 30:125–129, 1996.

55. Goldfrank LR, Hoffman RS: The cardiovascular effects of cocaine. *Ann Emerg Med* 20:165–175, 1991.

56. Gomez HF, et al: Charcoal stercolith with intestinal perforation in a patient treated for amitriptyline ingestion. *J Emerg Med* 12(1):57–60, 1994.

57. Greene SL, et al: Relative safety of hyperinsulinemia/euglycemia therapy in the management of calcium channel blocker overdose: a prospective observational study. *Intensive Care Med* 33(11):2019–2024, 2007.

58. Hadjipavlou G, Hafeez A, Messer B, Hughes T: Management of lercanidipine overdose with hyperinsulinaemic euglycaemia therapy: case report. *Scand J Trauma, Resusc Emerg Med* 19:8, 2011.

59. Hagmeyer KO, Mauro LS, Mauro VF: Meperidine-related seizures associated with patient-controlled analgesia pumps. *Ann Pharmacother* 27:29–32, 1993.

60. Harrigan RA, Brady WJ: ECG abnormalities in tricyclic antidepressant ingestion. *Am J Emerg Med* 17:387–393, 1999.

61. Hazinski MF, et al: Toxicology. In: *PALS provider manual*, Dallas, 2002, American Heart Association.

62. Heesch CM, et al: Cocaine activates platelets and increases the formation of circulating platelet containing microaggregates in humans. *Heart* 83:688–695, 2000.

63. Heidemann SM, Goetting MG: Passive inhalation of cocaine by infants. *Henry Ford Hosp Med J* 38:252–254, 1990.

64. Hoffman JR, et al: Effect of hypertonic sodium bicarbonate in the treatment of moderate-to-severe cyclic antidepressant overdose. *Am J Emerg Med* 11:336–341, 1993.

65. Hollander JE, et al: Prospective multicenter evaluation of cocaine-associated chest pain. Cocaine Associated Chest Pain (COCHPA) Study Group. *Acad Emerg Med* 1:330–339, 1994.

66. Holzer M, et al: Successful resuscitation of a verapamil-intoxicated patient with percutaneous cardiopulmonary bypass. *Crit Care Med* 27:2818–2823, 1999.

67. Homan CS, et al: Thermal characteristics of neutralization therapy and water dilution for strong acid ingestion: an in-vivo canine model. *Acad Energ Med* 5(4):286–292, 1998.

68. Horowitz BZ, Rhee KJ: Massive verapamil ingestion: a report of two cases and a review of the literature. *Am J Emerg Med* 7:624–631, 1989.

69. Humbert VH, Jr., Munn NJ, Hawkins RF: Noncardiogenic pulmonary edema complicating massive diltiazem overdose. *Chest* 99:258–259, 1991.

70. Jacobsen D, Haines JA: The relative efficacy of antidotes: the IPCS evaluation series. International Programme on Chemical Safety. *Arch Toxicol Suppl* 19:305–310, 1997.

71. Justiniani FR, Hippalgaonkar R, Martinez LO: Charcoal-containing empyema complicating treatment for overdose. *Chest* 87:404–405, 1985.

72. Kalman S, Berg S, Lisander B: Combined overdose with verapamil and atenolol: treatment with high doses of adrenergic agonists. *Acta Anaesthesiol Scand* 42:379–382, 1998.

73. Karch SB: Cardiac arrest in cocaine users. *Am J Emerg Med* 14:79–81, 1996.

74. Kattwinkel J, et al: An advisory statement from the Pediatric Working Group of the International Liaison Committee on Resuscitation. *Pediatrics* 103:e56, 1999.

75. Kenyon CJ, et al: Successful resuscitation using external cardiac pacing in beta adrenergic antagonist-induced bradyasystolic arrest. *Ann Emerg Med* 17:711–713, 1988.

76. Kerns W: Management of β-adrenergic blocker and calcium channel antagonist toxicity. *Emerg Med Clin N Am* 25(2):309–331, 2007.

77. Kienbaum P, et al: Profound increase in epinephrine concentration in plasma and cardiovascular stimulation after mu-opioid receptor blockade in opioid-addicted patients during barbiturate-induced anesthesia for acute detoxification. *Anesthesiology* 88:1154–1161, 1998.

78. Klasner AE, Luke DA, Scalzo AJ: Pediatric orogastric and nasogastric tubes: a new formula evaluated. *Ann Emerg Med* 39(3):268–272, 2002.

79. Kleinman ME, et al: Part 14: Pediatric advanced life support. 2010 American Heart Association Guidelines for Cardiopulmonary Resuscitation and Emergency Cardiovascular Care. *Circulation* 122:S876–S908, 2010.

80. Knudsen K, Abrahamsson J: Effects of epinephrine, norepinephrine, magnesium sulfate, and milrinone on survival and the occurrence of arrhythmias in amitriptyline poisoning in the rat. *Crit Care Med* 22:1851–1855, 1994.

81. Kolecki PF, Curry SC: Poisoning by sodium channel blocking agents. *Crit Care Clin* 13:829–848, 1997.

82. Kollef MH: Labetalol overdose successfully treated with amrinone and α-adrenergic receptor agonists. *Chest* 105:626–627, 1994.

83. Krauss B, Green SM: Sedation and analgesia for procedures in children. *N Engl J Med* 342:938–945, 2000.

84. Krenzelok E, Vale A: Position statements: gut decontamination. American Academy of Clinical Toxicology; European Association of Poisons Centres and Clinical Toxicologists. *J Toxicol Clin Toxicol* 35:695–786, 1997.

85. Kyff JV, Rice TL: Meperidine-associated seizures in a child. *Clin Pharm* 9:337–338, 1990.

86. Lam YM, Tse HF, Lau CP: Continuous calcium chloride infusion for massive nifedipine overdose. *Chest* 119(4):1280–1282, 2001.

87. Lange RA, Hillis LD: Cardiovascular complications of cocaine use. *N Engl J Med* 345:351–358, 2001.

88. Larkin GL, Graeber GM, Hollingsed MJ: Experimental amitriptyline poisoning: treatment of severe cardiovascular toxicity with cardiopulmonary bypass. *Ann Emerg Med* 23:480–486, 1994.

89. Lee DC: Fatal nifedipine ingestions in children. *J Emerg Med* 19:359–361, 2000.

90. Leesar MA, et al: Noncardiogenic pulmonary edema complicating massive verapamil overdose. *Chest* 105:606–607, 1994.

91. Lester L, McLaughlin S: SALT: a case for sodium channel blockade toxidrome and the mnemonic SALT. *Ann Emerg Med* 5:214, 2008.

92. Lewis M, et al: Survival following massive overdose of adrenergic blocking agents (acebutolol and labetalol). *Eur Heart J* 4:328–332, 1983.

93. Lheureux PE, et al: Bench-to-bedside review: hyperinsulinaemia/euglyceamia therapy in the management of overdose of calcium channel blockers. *Crit Care* 10(3):212, 2006.

94. Li L, Levine BE, Smialek JE: Fatal methadone poisoning in children: Maryland 1992-1996. *Subst Use Misuse* 35:1141–1148, 2000.

95. Liebelt EL: Targeted management strategies for cardiovascular toxicity from tricyclic antidepressant overdose: the pivotal role for alkalinization and sodium loading. *Pediatr Emerg Care* 14:293–298, 1998.

96. Liebelt EL, Francis PD, Woolf AD: ECG lead aVR versus QRS interval in predicting seizures and arrhythmias in acute tricyclic antidepressant toxicity. *Ann Emerg Med* 26:195–201, 1995.

97. Liebelt EL, Ulrich A, Francis PD, Woolf A: Serial electrocardiogram changes in acute tricyclic antidepressant overdoses. *Crit Care Med* 25:1721–1726, 1997.

98. Lifshitz M, Zucker N, Zalzstein E: Acute dilated cardiomyopathy and central nervous system toxicity following propranolol intoxication. *Pediatr Emerg Care* 15:262–263, 1999.

99. Love JN, Hanfling D, Howell JM: Hemodynamic effects of calcium chloride in a canine model of acute propranolol intoxication. *Ann Emerg Med* 28(1):1–6, 1996.

100. Love JN, Howell JM, Litovitz TL, et al: Acute beta blocker overdose: factors associated with the development of cardiovascular morbidity. *J Toxicol Clin Toxicol* 38:275–281, 2000.

101. Love JN, Litovitz TL, Howell JM, Clancy C: Characterization of fatal beta blocker ingestion: a review of the American Association of Poison Control Centers data from 1985 to 1995. *J Toxicol Clin Toxicol* 35:353–359, 1997.

102. Mariani PJ, Pook N: Gastrointestinal tract perforation with charcoal peritoneum complicating orogastric intubation and lavage. *Ann Emerg Med* 22:606–609, 1993.

103. Marquardt KA, Tharratt RS: Inhalation abuse of fentanyl patch. *J Toxicol Clin Toxicol* 32:72–75, 1994.

104. Martinez M, Devenport L, Saussy J, Martinez J: Drug-associated heat stroke. *South Med J* 95(8):799–802, 2002.

105. Marzuk PM, et al: Ambient temperature and mortality from unintentional cocaine overdose. *JAMA* 279:1795–1800, 1998.

106. McCabe JL, et al: Experimental tricyclic antidepressant toxicity: a randomized, controlled comparison of hypertonic saline solution, sodium bicarbonate, and hyperventilation. *Ann Emerg Med* 32 (pt 1):329–333, 1998.

107. McCaig LF, Burt CW: Poisoning-related visits to emergency departments in the United States, 1993-1996. *J Toxicol Clin Toxicol* 37:817–826, 1999.

108. McClure RJ, et al: Epidemiology of Munchausen syndrome by proxy, non-accidental poisoning, and non-accidental suffocation. *Arch Dis Child* 75:57–61, 1996.

109. McVey FK, Corke CF: Extracorporeal circulation in the management of massive propranolol overdose. *Anaesthesia* 46:744–746, 1991.

110. Mégarbane B, Karyo S, Baud FJ: The role of insulin and glucose (hyperinsulinaemia/euglycaemia) therapy in acute calcium channel antagonist and beta-blocker poisoning. *Toxicol Rev* 23(4):215–222, 2004.

111. Mets B, Jamdar S, Landry D: The role of catecholamines in cocaine toxicity: a model for cocaine "sudden death." *Life Sci* 59(24):2021–2031, 1996.

112. Mirchandani HG, et al: Passive inhalation of free-base cocaine ('crack') smoke by infants. *Arch Pathol Lab Med* 115:494–498, 1991.

113. Mo W, et al: Role of nitric oxide in cocaine-induced acute hypertension. *Am J Hypertens* 11:708–714, 1998.

114. Moll J, et al: Incidence of aspiration pneumonia in intubated patients receiving activated charcoal. *J Emerg Med* 17:279–283, 1999.

115. Moser LR, Smythe MA, Tisdale JE: The use of calcium salts in the prevention and management of verapamil-induced hypotension. *Ann Pharmacother* 34:622–629, 2000.

116. Mott SH, Packer RJ, Soldin SJ: Neurologic manifestations of cocaine exposure in childhood. *Pediatrics* 93:557–560, 1994.

117. Mullins ME, Pinnick RV, Terhes JM: Life-threatening diphenhydramine overdose treated with charcoal hemoperfusion and hemodialysis. *Ann Emerg Med* 33:104–107, 1999.

118. Murphy DB, et al: Opioid-induced delay in gastric emptying: a peripheral mechanism in humans. *Anesthesiology* 87:765–770, 1997.

119. Murray S, Brewerton T: Abuse of over-the-counter dextromethorphan by teenagers. *South Med J* 86:1151–1153, 1993.

120. Newar FW, Niska RW, Xu J: National Hospital Ambulatory Medical Care Survey: 2005; Emergency Department Summary. *Adv Data* 29 (386):1–32, 2007.

121. Oe H, Taniura T, Ohgitani N: A case of severe verapamil overdose. *Jpn Circ J* 62:72–76, 1998.

122. O'Grady J, Anderson S, Pringle D: Successful treatment of severe atenolol overdose with calcium chloride. *CJEM* 3(3):224–227, 2001.

123. Ortiz-Múnoz L, Rodriguez-Ospina LF, Figueroa-Gonzalez M: Hyperinsulinemic-euglycemic therapy for intoxication with calcium channel blockers. *Bol Assoc Med P R* 97(3 Pt 2):182–189, 2005.

124. Osterwalder JJ: Naloxone—for intoxications with intravenous heroin and heroin mixtures—harmless or hazardous? A prospective clinical study. *J Toxicol Clin Toxicol* 34:409–416, 1996.

125. Page C, Hacket LP, Isbister GK: The use of high-dose insulin-glucose euglycemia in beta-blocker overdose: a case report. *J Med Toxicol* 5(3):139–143, 2009.

126. Papadopoulos J, O'Neil MG: Utilization of a glucagon infusion in the management of a massive nifedipine overdose. *J Emerg Med* 18:453–455, 2000.

127. Parker RB, et al: Comparative effects of sodium bicarbonate and sodium chloride on reversing cocaine-induced changes in the electrocardiogram. *J Cardiovasc Pharmacol* 34:864–869, 1999.

128. Patel NP, Pugh ME, Goldberg S, Eiger G: Hyperinsulinemic euglycemia therapy for verapamil poisoning: case report. *Am J Crit Care* 16(5):520, 518–520, 519, 2007.

129. Pertoldi F, D'Orlando L, Mercante WP: Electromechanical dissociation 48 hours after atenolol overdose: usefulness of calcium chloride. *Ann Emerg Med* 31:777–781, 1998.

130. Pierog JE, et al: Tricyclic antidepressant toxicity treated with massive sodium bicarbonate. *Am J Emerg Med* 27(9):1168.e3–e7, 2009.

131. Proano L, Chiang WK, Wang RY: Calcium channel blocker overdose. *Am J Emerg Med* 13:444–450, 1995.

132. Pronczuk de Garbino J, et al: Evaluation of antidotes: activities of the International Programme on Chemical Safety. *J Toxicol Clin Toxicol* 35:333–343, 1997.

133. Prough DS, et al: Acute pulmonary edema in healthy teenagers following conservative doses of intravenous naloxone. *Anesthesiology* 60:485–486, 1984.

134. Ramoska EA, et al: A one-year evaluation of calcium channel blocker overdoses: toxicity and treatment. *Ann Emerg Med* 22:196–200, 1993.

135. Ray JM, Squires PE, et al: L-type calcium channels regulate gastrin release from human antral G cells. *Am J Physiol* 273:G281–G288, 1997.

136. Remskar M, et al: Profound circulatory shock following heroin overdose. *Resuscitation* 38:51–53, 1998.

137. Roy TM, et al: Pulmonary complications after tricyclic antidepressant overdose. *Chest* 96:852–856, 1989.

138. Scalzo AJ, Tominack RL, Thompson MW: Malposition of pediatric gastric lavage tubes demonstrated radiographically. *J Emerg Med* 10:581–586, 1992.

139. Scherrer PD: Safe and sound: pediatric procedural sedation and analgesia. *Minn Med* 94(3):43–47, 2011.

140. Schwartz JG, Hurd IL, Carnahan JJ: Determination of tricyclic antidepressants for ED analysis. *Am J Emerg Med* 12:513–516, 1994.

141. Shanker UR, Webb J, Kotze A: Sodium bicarbonate to treat massive beta blocker overdose. *Emerg Med J* 20(4):393, 2003.

142. Shih RD, et al: Clinical safety of lidocaine in patients with cocaine-associated myocardial infarction. *Ann Emerg Med* 26:702–706, 1995.

143. Sims MT, Stevenson FT: A fatal case of iatrogenic hypercalcemia after calcium channel blocker overdose. *J Med Toxicol* 4(1):25–29, 2008.

144. Snook CP, Sigvaldason K, Kristinsson J: Severe atenolol and diltiazem overdose. *J Toxicol Clin Toxicol* 38:661–665, 2000.

145. Spiller HA, et al: Delayed onset of cardiac arrhythmias from sustained-release verapamil. *Ann Emerg Med* 20:201–203, 1991.

146. Sporer KA, Dorn E: Heroin-related noncardiogenic pulmonary edema: a case series. *Chest* 120:1628–1632, 2001.

147. Sporer KA, Firestone J, Isaacs SM: Out-of-hospital treatment of opioid overdoses in an urban setting. *Acad Emerg Med* 3:660–667, 1996.

148. Stanek EJ, Nelson CE, DeNofrio D: Amlodipine overdose. *Ann Pharmacother* 31:853–856, 1997.

149. Stinson J, Walsh M, Feely J: Ventricular asystole and overdose with atenolol. *BMJ* 305:693, 1992.

150. Tenenbein M: Continuous naloxone infusion for opiate poisoning in infancy. *J Pediatr* 105:645–648, 1984.

151. Thompson AM, Robins JB, Prescott LF: Changes in cardiorespiratory function during gastric lavage for drug overdose. *Hum Toxicol* 6:215–218, 1987.

152. Vale JA: Position statement: gastric lavage. American Academy of Clinical Toxicology; European Association of Poisons Centres and Clinical Toxicologists. *J Toxicol Clin Toxicol* 35:711–719, 1997.

153. Vale JA, Kulig K: American Academy of Clinical Toxicology and European Association of Poisons Centres and Clinical Toxicologists: Position paper: gastric lavage. *J Toxicol Clin Toxicol* 42(7):933–943, 2004.

154. Vance MV, Selden BS, Clark RF: Optimal patient position for transport and initial management of toxic ingestions. *Ann Emerg Med* 21:243–246, 1992.

155. Walsh DM: Cyclic antidepressant overdose in children: a proposed treatment protocol. *Pediatr Emerg Care* 2:28–35, 1986.

156. Wang RY: pH-dependent cocaine-induced cardiotoxicity. *Am J Emerg Med* 17:364–369, 1999.

157. Watling SM, et al: Verapamil overdose: case report and review of the literature. *Ann Pharmacother* 26:1373–1378, 1992.

158. Waxman AB, White KP, Trawick DR: Electromechanical dissociation following verapamil and propranolol ingestion: a physiologic profile. *Cardiology* 99:478–481, 1997.

159. Weigand T: Phenytoin is not successful in preventing cocaine-induced seizures: a response to the article, "Cocaine body packing in pregnancy." *Ann Emerg Med* 49(4):543–544, 2007.

160. Weinstein RS: Recognition and management of poisoning with β-adrenergic blocking agents. *Ann Emerg Med* 13:1123–1131, 1984.

161. Wells TG, et al: Nifedipine poisoning in a child. *Pediatrics* 86:91–94, 1990.

162. White JM, Irvine RJ: Mechanisms of fatal opioid overdose. *Addiction* 94:961–972, 1999.

163. Whitehurst VE, et al: Reversal of propranolol blockade of adrenergic receptors and related toxicity with drugs that increase cyclic AMP. *Proc Soc Exp Biol Med* 221:382–385, 1999.

164. Williams JJ, Restieaux NJ, Low CJ: Myocardial infarction in young people with normal coronary arteries. *Heart* 79:191–194, 1998.

165. Williams JM, et al: Extracorporeal circulation in the management of severe tricyclic antidepressant overdose. *Am J Emerg Med* 12:456–458, 1994.

166. Winecker RE, et al: Detection of cocaine and its metabolites in breast milk. *J Forensic Sci* 46:1221–1223, 2001.

167. Wolfe TR, Caravati EM, Rollins DE: Terminal 40-ms frontal plane QRS axis as a marker for tricyclic antidepressant overdose. *Ann Emerg Med* 18:348–351, 1989.

168. Ye JH, et al: Cocaine and lidocaine have additive inhibitory effects on the GABA A current of acutely dissociated hippocampal pyramidal neurons. *Brain Res* 821:26–32, 1999.

169. Yealy DM, et al: The safety of prehospital naloxone administration by paramedics. *Ann Emerg Med* 19:902–905, 1990.

170. Yuan TH, et al: Insulin-glucose as adjunctive therapy for severe calcium channel antagonist poisoning. *J Toxicol Clin Toxicol* 37:463–474, 1999.

171. Zaritsky AL, Horowitz M, Chernow B: Glucagon antagonism of calcium channel blocker-induced myocardial dysfunction. *Crit Care Med* 16:246–251, 1988.

172. Zuckerman GB, Conway EE, Jr, : Pulmonary complications following tricyclic antidepressant overdose in an adolescent. *Ann Pharmacother* 27:572–574, 1993.

Pediatric Trauma

19

Alisha Armstrong • Purnima Unni •
John B. Pietsch

eVolve Be sure to check out the supplementary content available at
http://evolve.elsevier.com/Hazinski.

PEARLS

- Differences between adult and pediatric trauma care relate directly to the differences in physiology, anatomy, and mechanism of injury. The care of victims of all ages requires the same fundamental sequences of assessment and care (primary and secondary ABCDE surveys), but slight differences in their application.
- The most common serious complications of pediatric trauma are problems with airway and breathing rather than bleeding and shock, because the most serious pediatric trauma is blunt trauma involving the head.

INTRODUCTION

Trauma is the leading cause of pediatric mortality and morbidity in the United States,[7] and it is a common reason for admission to a pediatric critical care unit (PCCU). Managing the child with multisystem trauma requires specific knowledge, precise management, and keen attention to detail.[1,59] This chapter reviews essential aspects of nursing care of the pediatric trauma victim. Chapters 2, 3, 6, 9 and 11 contain additional helpful information.

EPIDEMIOLOGY AND INCIDENCE OF PEDIATRIC TRAUMA

Frequency of Injuries

Although often preventable, injury continues to be the leading cause of death and disability for children older than 1 year.[3,17] Nearly 3000 children 0 to 14 years old die every year as the result of injuries—more deaths than all diseases combined.[45,47] Leading causes of injury death are falls, motor vehicle crashes, burn injuries, pedestrian injuries, and drowning.[45,47] For additional information, see Epidemiology and Incidence of Pediatric Trauma in the Chapter 19 Supplement on the Evolve Website.

Intentional (Inflicted) Versus Unintentional Injuries

Injuries in the child can be categorized as either intentional or unintentional.[19] Intentional injuries are inflicted injuries (i.e., child abuse) or injuries that result from neglect (see Intentional Injuries/Inflicted Trauma, later in the chapter). Unintentional injuries, such as many burns, drowning, and traffic-related injuries are often preventable.

Eighty to ninety percent of life-threatening pediatric trauma is blunt injury, resulting from motor vehicle-related causes and falls[4,7]; approximately half of motor vehicle-related injuries and fatalities are thought to be preventable with the use of age-appropriate safety restraints.[27,60] Children can also sustain motor vehicle-related injuries as pedestrians or on bicycles. Although bicycle riding is a common childhood activity, it can be dangerous. The most severe head injuries are sustained when children who are not wearing bicycle helmets collide with motor vehicles.[48,50,68] When a child is in a bicycle crash, a helmet will likely decrease the severity of head injuries.[27]

Role of Nurses and Healthcare Providers in Injury Prevention

Prevention of unintentional injuries requires an understanding of risk factors at each child's developmental stage, and knowledge of risk-reducing actions.[15,46,70] Nurses should use every "teachable moment" with families to increase parental awareness[49] of the risk of unintentional injuries and to promote the use of appropriate safety equipment. A teachable moment can occur during encounters such as a well-child checkup or a parent visit to the school,[20,35,60] but is probably not present when the child is in the PCCU after an injury occurred. Nurses will need to select the best opportunities and methods to teach injury prevention strategies. See the Chapter 19 Supplement on the Evolve Website, for information about injury prevention.

PHYSIOLOGIC DIFFERENCES AFFECTING MANIFESTATION AND TREATMENT OF INJURIES

Airway and Ventilation

Larynx and Advanced Airways

The larynx in infants and children is smaller and is more anterior and cephalad than the larynx in adults. Intubation of children is difficult and should not be attempted by inexperienced practitioners (see Chapter 9). Unless the injured child has upper airway injury, edema, or obstruction, bag-mask ventilation usually provides adequate short-term oxygenation and ventilation. However, if the duration of transport is long, continued bag-mask ventilation is suboptimal, and skilled personnel should insert an advanced airway before transport.

The laryngeal mask airway (LMA) is an acceptable advanced airway when used by experienced providers for

895

supporting a comatose patient.[16] The LMA can be inserted blindly and, when properly positioned, isolates the trachea and produces less gastric distension than bag-mask ventilation. The LMA cannot be inserted in a patient with a cough or gag reflex.

The correct endotracheal tube size is determined by the size and configuration of the child's larynx. The vocal cords are the narrowest portion of the adult larynx; in general the proper size of an adult endotracheal tube is the largest that can pass through the vocal cords.

In children younger than approximately 8 years, the narrowest portion of the larynx is in the subglottic area at the level of the cricoid cartilage, a circular cartilage with no membranous portion (C-shaped cartilages are present in the rest of the trachea, with the ends of the C-shaped cartilage connected by membrane). Endotracheal tube size for the child must be evaluated carefully, because a tube can readily pass through a child's vocal cords but be too large in the subglottic area. If the tube is too large, then it can produce complications such as subglottic stenosis. The tube is likely the proper size if an air leak is present when a positive inflation pressure of 25 cm H_2O is provided.

Either cuffed or uncuffed endotracheal tubes may be used in children, and cuffed tubes may be more appropriate if the child's lung compliance is low (e.g., as following a pulmonary contusion) or if the child has high airway resistance or a large glottic air leak. If a cuffed tube is used, the cuff inflation pressure must be monitored and maintained at the pressure recommended by the manufacturer (typically less than 20-25 cm H_2O).[9a,38a]

Providers can determine approximate airway equipment sizes (including endotracheal tubes) using a color-coded, length-based tape (e.g., a Broselow Pediatric Emergency Tape; Armstrong Medical Industries, Lincolnshire, IL).[54] A table containing these approximate sizes is included on the inside back cover of this book.

Chest Wall

The chest wall of infants and children is highly compliant, so rib fractures occur in only approximately one third of children with blunt thoracic trauma.[13] The child may sustain significant intrathoracic injuries, yet may not have rib fractures.[3] If a rib fracture is present, it suggests that major thoracic trauma has occurred involving substantial force and energy transfer,[13] and the trauma team should suspect that underlying organs including the liver, spleen, and lungs may be injured. Upper rib injuries are associated most commonly with pulmonary and major vessel injuries, whereas lower rib fractures typically are associated with liver, spleen, lung, and kidney injury.[44]

Because the ribs are relatively compliant in young children, the child's chest should expand outward easily during positive-pressure ventilation. A unilateral reduction in chest expansion during positive pressure ventilation can result from endotracheal tube migration into a mainstem bronchus or from a unilateral pneumothorax, hemothorax, pleural effusion, or atelectasis.

The chest wall of the child is thin, and breath sounds are transmitted easily through the chest wall. When auscultation is performed over an area of atelectasis or fluid accumulation

(e.g., a hemothorax), the nurse may note a change in pitch rather than a decrease in the intensity of breath sounds. For this reason, nurses must perform thorough auscultation and compare breath sounds heard over one side and one part of the chest to those heard over the other side and other parts of the chest.

Respiratory Muscles

During early childhood, the intercostal muscles are capable of only stabilizing the chest wall; they cannot elevate the chest wall to initiate inspiration. Therefore the infant or young child relies on diaphragm excursion for effective ventilation. Anything that impedes diaphragm movement can impair ventilation.

The child in respiratory distress frequently swallows air during spontaneous ventilation, and bag-mask ventilation can produce gastric distension. Gastric distension may compromise ventilation by restricting movement of the left hemidiaphragm; insertion of an orogastric or nasogastric tube may be required.

Cardiovascular Function and Circulating Blood Volume

Cardiac Output and Heart Rate

Children require a higher cardiac output per kilogram of body weight than do adults, because a child's oxygen consumption and metabolic rate are higher than an adult's. In infants and young children, cardiac output is primarily dependent on an adequate heart rate to maintain cardiac output; changes in stroke volume have less effect on cardiac output. Bradycardia is, therefore, often associated with a fall in cardiac output. Bradycardia is an ominous clinical finding in a pediatric trauma victim, usually indicating the presence of hypoxia or impending cardiopulmonary arrest. Tachycardia may be a nonspecific sign of distress, common in the frightened or injured child. However, tachycardia may also be a sign of significant volume loss, such as with hemorrhage. Hypotension is typically only a late sign of shock in children.

Circulating Blood Volume

Although a child's circulating blood volume is large per kilogram body weight (80-85 mL/kg in newborns, 75-80 mL/kg in infants, 70-75 mL/kg in children, and 65-70 mL/kg in adolescents and adults), children have a smaller absolute circulating blood volume and cardiac output than adults. Consequently, small amounts of blood loss can produce significant reductions in the child's circulating blood volume and can compromise systemic perfusion.

A useful way to determine the significance of blood loss in a child is to estimate the child's total blood volume (TBV) and a 10% blood loss (an amount likely to require transfusion). For example, a 4-kg baby has a TBV of about 320 mL (4 kg × 80 mL/kg), so a 10% blood loss would be 32 mL. A 10-kg infant has a TBV of about 750 mL (10 kg × 75 mL/kg), so a 10% blood loss would be approximately 75 mL. A 30-kg child has a TBV of about 2,250 mL (30 kg × 75 mL/kg), so a 10% blood loss would be approximately 225 mL. A 10% blood loss is approximately 8 mL/kg for infants and 7.5 mL/kg for children. If the child's weight is unknown, a color-coded

Broselow tape will allow estimation of weight. A useful formula for estimating weight in children 1 to 10 years of age is:

$$\text{Approximate weight (kg)} = (2 \times \text{Age[y]}) + 8$$

Tachycardia is an early sign of hemorrhage in children. Significant hemorrhage (10%-15% of circulating blood volume) will produce signs of poor systemic perfusion (e.g., mottled color, cool extremities, delayed capillary refill, thready peripheral pulses). Because the child can initially compensate for blood loss by increasing the heart rate and systemic vascular resistance, hypotension often does not develop unless the child acutely loses 20% to 25% or more of circulating blood volume.[54]

Neurologic Function

The morbidity and mortality of pediatric head injury is lower than the morbidity and mortality of similar head injury in adults. Many children who survive head injury recover completely; however, severe head injury can be fatal or produce long-term disability.

Neurologic Assessment

Although widely used, the Glasgow Coma Scale (GCS) may not be ideal for pediatric use for several reasons. It has not been validated in children, and it requires a cooperative child who is verbal and able to follow directions. If the child is preverbal or intubated, the verbal component of the GCS cannot be used.

The child's level of consciousness and responsiveness will provide clues to the severity of the injuries. If the child is appropriately frightened and crying for parents and the child recognizes and responds to the parents, that child is presumed to be relatively alert and oriented. Irritability may be an early sign of neurologic deterioration or hypoxia, so an irritable child requires careful evaluation. Finally, if the child fails to respond to parents and is unresponsive to painful stimuli, neurologic compromise is present and urgent evaluation and support are needed.

Spinal Cord Injury

Many children with spinal cord injury have ligamentous injury with no evidence of vertebral fracture or other radiographic abnormalities on routine (anteroposterior and lateral) spine radiographs or CT scan.[42a] These children have spinal cord injury without radiographic abnormality (SCIWORA), and many of these patients develop permanent neurologic injury.[3,23]

Nurses should carefully assess movement and sensation in all extremities on admission and at frequent intervals throughout the child's hospitalization (see Chapter 11). The mechanism of injury should increase the index of suspicion of spinal cord injury. For example, a child wearing a lap belt without a shoulder strap who presents with abrasions or contusions on the lower abdomen may have an acute flexion injury of the lower spine (with or without a Chance fracture). Data from the National Trauma Data Bank[51] indicates that 66% of cervical spine injuries in children younger than 3 years are caused by motor vehicle crashes, and only 15% are from falls. In the National Trauma Data Bank, cervical spine injuries were present in approximately 2.3% of all children less than 3 years of age injured in motor vehicle crashes.[51] However, cervical spine injuries in children younger than 3 years were still relatively uncommon.[51]

Thermoregulation

Children have large surface area-to-volume ratios, so they lose more heat to the environment through evaporation, conduction, and convection than do adults. An injured child may experience a rapid fall in body temperature from exposure to a cold environment, submersion in cold water, or from evaporative losses when resuscitated in the out-of-hospital setting. Hypothermia, in turn, complicates resuscitation. Cold stress can be exacerbated by exposure in a cool emergency department (ED) or computed tomography (CT) scan room.

Every effort must be made to keep the injured child warm. Warm blankets and warming lights should be used if needed. In general, patient warming and rewarming should be performed with careful monitoring to prevent hyperthermia.

It may be necessary to warm intravenous (IV) fluids before they are administered to the child. Because microwave ovens warm fluids inconsistently, they should not be used to warm IV fluids.

Cold stress produces vasoconstriction that can mask the severity of blood loss; as the child is warmed, peripheral vasodilation may result in development or worsening of hypotension. Providers should anticipate the need for administration of additional fluid or blood during rewarming.

Fluid Administration

Rate

To control and accurately tally the total fluid administration rate, it is important to record all sources of fluid intake and output and administer all fluids by syringe or volume-controlled infusion pump. Adequate shock resuscitation is required for the trauma patient with hemorrhage, but excessive fluid administration should be avoided, particularly for the child with traumatic brain injury (it can be associated with free water retention in excess of sodium, a fall in serum sodium and cerebral edema) or the child with penetrating injury in the prehospital setting (it can increase blood pressure and increase hemorrhage). Fluid is not withheld from the hypovolemic patient; on the other hand, if the child is euvolemic (i.e., has adequate intravascular volume), excessive fluid administration may be harmful and should be avoided.

Vascular Access

It may be difficult to establish and maintain vascular access in the child with poor systemic perfusion. If vascular access can be achieved, providers should insert two large-bore venous catheters to enable effective volume administration.

If IV access cannot be achieved, intraosseous (IO) access is established; this route of access can be used for emergency fluid resuscitation and drug administration in patients of all ages.[14] IO needles can be placed in the proximal or distal tibia or distal femur. Other placement options include the radius, ulna, pelvis, clavicle, and calcaneus. Medications and drugs can be given intraosseously until suitable venous access is achieved. Fluid may be delivered by infusion pump into an IO catheter, and bolus infusions can be provided through a syringe, an infusion pump, or a pressure bag (inflated up to 300 mm Hg). IO fluid boluses in children may be given as rapidly as 20 mL/kg over 5 min.

INITIAL STABILIZATION OF THE PEDIATRIC TRAUMA PATIENT

Field Triage and Scoring

Scoring systems have been developed to quantify injury severity and predict patient outcome. These scoring systems also provide objective criteria to determine the need to transfer the trauma victim to a pediatric trauma center. As a result the transport team must select an accepted triage scoring system and use it consistently.

The trauma score (TS) is designed for scoring injury severity in the field; it uses the GCS score and the scoring of four additional physiologic parameters: systolic blood pressure, capillary refill, respiratory rate, and respiratory effort. Each category is scored and then totalled.[10]

The revised trauma score (RTS) was created to identify patients for triage to a trauma center.[11] It requires evaluation of fewer physiologic parameters than the TS. To calculate the RTS, the provider assigns a coded value to the GCS score, the systolic blood pressure, and the respiratory rate and then adds these three values together (Table 19-1). A weighted version of the RTS is a predictor of mortality; an RTS of less than four is correlated with a probability of survival of less than 60%, and should prompt consideration for transfer to a trauma center.[2]

The pediatric trauma score (PTS) was developed to better identify the manifestations of injuries in children and better quantify their severity. The PTS evaluates the following six parameters: (1) patient size, (2) airway stability, (3) systolic blood pressure, (4) mental status, (5) wounds, and (6) skeletal injuries (Table 19-2).

In the PTS, large size and optimum status result in a score of 2 for each parameter; extremely small size or systemic dysfunction results in a score of −1 for each parameter. The highest possible score is a 12 and the lowest possible score is a −6.[67] Children with a PTS totaling 8 or less have the highest potential for preventable mortality and morbidity, and they should be transported to a facility with the resources necessary to provide optimal pediatric care (e.g., a pediatric trauma center).[67]

The PTS is a conservative scoring system and will result in the triage of some children who have only moderate injuries; however, conservative triage is generally thought to be appropriate for injured children. The PTS has not been shown to be consistently superior to the RTS, so many centers continue to use the RTS for the triage of children and with good results. Because vital signs (e.g., particularly blood pressures) are often not evaluated in the field,[22,38] a simple scoring system that uses fewer vital signs (e.g., the RTS) can be used more consistently than one requiring evaluation of heart rate and respiratory rate in addition to blood pressure (i.e., the PTS).

In 2006, the National College of Surgeons Committee on Trauma convened a panel of national experts on trauma field triage to develop consensus trauma triage criteria for adults and children based on physiologic criteria (GCS score, systolic blood pressure, and respiratory rate), anatomy of the injury (e.g., penetrating trauma to the head, neck, or torso; flail chest; two or more long bone fractures; amputation; pelvic fractures; open or depressed skull fractures), the mechanism of injury (e.g., falls of 10 feet [3.048 m], or a distance of more than twice or threefold the child's height, high risk auto crashes, motor vehicle vs. pedestrian crashes, motorcycle crashes), special patient or system considerations (e.g., children should be preferentially triaged to pediatric trauma centers; patients with associated anticoagulation or bleeding disorders; the EMS provider judges transport is indicated[59]), and protocols.

The criteria contained in the National College of Surgeons Committee on Trauma guidelines are included in Box 19-1. A detailed explanation of these guidelines was published by the Centers for Disease Control and Prevention in 2009.[56] A link to this publication is available in Triage of Injured Patients in the Chapter 19 Supplement on the Evolve Website.

Table 19-1 Revised Trauma Score*

GCS Score[†]	Systolic BP (mmHg)	RR (Breaths/min)	Coded Value
13-15	>89	10-29	4
9-12	76-89	>29	3
6-8	50-75	6-9	2
4-5	1-49	1-5	1
3	0	0	0

From Champion HR, et al: A revision of the trauma score. *J Trauma* 29:623-629, 1989.

*Revised trauma score (RTS) = GCS Coded Value + Systolic BP Coded Value + RR Coded Value. A weighted version of the RTS (0.9368 GCS + 0.7326 SBP + 0.2908 RR) is predictive of potential mortality.
[†]Refer to Table 19-7 (Glasgow Coma Scale) later in this chapter.
BP, Blood pressure; *GCS*, glasgow coma scale; *RR*, respiratory rate.

Table 19-2 Pediatric Trauma Score

| PTS Component | CATEGORY | | |
	+2	+1	−1
Size	≥20 kg	10-20 kg	<10 kg
Airway	Normal	Maintainable	Not maintainable
Systolic blood pressure	>90 mm Hg	90-50 mm Hg	<50 mm Hg
Central nervous system	Awake	Obtunded, history of LOC	Coma, decerebrate
Open wound	None	Minor	Major, penetrating
Skeletal	None	Closed fracture	Open or multiple fractures

From Tepas JJ, et al: The pediatric trauma score as a predictor of injury severity in injured children. *J Pediatr Surg* 22:14, 1987.
LOC, Loss of consciousness.

Box 19-1 | **Indications for Transport of a Pediatric Trauma Victim To A Level I Trauma Center or a Pediatric Critical Care Unit**

Physical and Physiologic Findings

- Shock unresponsive to one bolus (defined as hypotension, with systolic BP less than 60 mm Hg in infants and less than 90 mm Hg in children) or associated with persistent prolonged capillary refill (systolic BP less than 90 mm Hg is contained in the NCS-Committee On Trauma Expert Panel Guidelines for transfer*)
- Clinical evidence of altered level of consciousness (GCS score less than 14*); coma is an absolute indication for transfer
- Respiratory rate less than 10/min or greater than 29/min*
- Any cardiac arrhythmias (including bradycardia)
- Diffuse abdominal tenderness following trauma
- Anticipated need for mechanical ventilation

Types and Anatomy of Injuries

- Virtually any penetrating injury of the head, thorax, abdomen, neck or extremities proximal to the elbow and knee*
- Unstable chest wall (flail chest)*
- Two or more proximal long bone fractures*
- Crushed, degloved, or mangled extremity*
- Amputation proximal to the wrist or ankle*
- Pelvic fractures*
- Open or depressed skull fracture*
- Paralysis*

- Gunshot wound to the trunk
- Orbital or facial fractures

Mechanism of Injury and Evidence of High-Energy Impact

- Fall from height greater than 10 feet (3.048 m) or a distance of twice or three-fold the child's height*
- Intrusion into vehicle greater than 1 foot (0.3 m) into passenger space or 1.5 feet (0.46 m) on any side*
- Ejection*
- Death in same passenger compartment*
- Vehicle telemetry data consistent with high risk of injury*
- Motor vehicle versus pedestrian or bicyclist thrown or run over or with significant (greater than 20 mph) impact*
- Motorcycle crash greater than 20 mph*

Special Patient or System Considerations

- Anticoagulation or bleeding disorder*
- Burns*
- Time-sensitive extremity injury*
- End-stage renal disease requiring dialysis*
- Pregnancy greater than 20 weeks' gestation*
- EMS provider judgment*
- Suspected child abuse

Modified from PCCC Transport Criteria, Harbor-UCLA Medical Center, Los Angeles, 1990; and Sasser SM, et al: Guidelines for field triage of injured patients: Recommendations of the National Expert Panel on Field Triage. *Morbidity and Mortality Weekly Report* 2009; 58 (RRO1):1-35.
*These criteria are consistent with the 2006 National Expert Panel recommendations, detailed by Sasser, et al.
BP, Blood pressure; *EMS,* emergency medical services; *GCS,* glasgow coma scale.

MANAGEMENT OF THE PEDIATRIC TRAUMA VICTIM IN THE EMERGENCY DEPARTMENT

Team Approach to Management

Optimal trauma care requires organization of resources and personnel. The trauma team should have protocols in place that designate responsibilities for initial assessment and management of the injured child to specific members of the trauma team. Team composition can vary among institutions based on the number and skill level of personnel, but intervention priorities remain the same.

Emergency Department Stabilization and Transfer

The amount of care provided in the ED will be determined by the child's clinical status and the distance between the ED and the definitive treatment center. Preferably, the child with major trauma will be transported from the ED directly to the PCCU in the same hospital. In this case, the time in the ED will be short. If the PCCU is located in a separate hospital, a more thorough evaluation should be performed in the ED to detect and stabilize major occult injuries before transfer. This evaluation requires a delicate balance between taking time to perform adequate evaluation and stabilization and the need to avoid excessive delay in transferring the child to the (definitive) trauma center. The child always should be stabilized before extensive diagnostic studies, such as CT scans, are performed. The radiology department is not the optimal location for the initiation of resuscitation.

General indications for transfer of the critically ill child to a trauma center with a PCCU include multisystem trauma, shock requiring multiple transfusions or vasoactive drug therapy, head injury accompanied by alteration in level of consciousness, multiple long bone fractures, rib fractures in the young child, penetrating injuries, traumatic amputations, significant burns, and anticipated need for prolonged mechanical ventilation (see Box 19-1).[56]

INITIAL SURVEY, RESUSCITATION, AND STABILIZATION

The initial evaluation and stabilization (primary and secondary surveys) of the pediatric trauma victim are performed in the field and then repeated as needed in the ED. By the time the child arrives in the PCCU, the child should have a perfusing rhythm, an advanced airway (with confirmation of correct placement) and vascular access. However, if major trauma is present and the child is extremely unstable, resuscitation may continue in the PCCU.

The admitting critical care unit or the acute care unit admitting team should carefully assess the child to verify that cardiopulmonary function is adequate. In effect, they are performing a tertiary survey, repeating the primary and secondary surveys in a more thorough and methodical manner to ensure that the child is responding to therapy and that no injuries were missed. If the child is deteriorating, resuscitation is provided, and the primary and secondary surveys begin again.

The following information may apply to care in the ED, the acute care unit, or the PCCU. For further information regarding cardiopulmonary resuscitation in children, refer to Chapter 6.

Airway

Positioning, Jaw Thrust

The first priority of stabilization and management is to establish a patent airway. The tongue of the infant and small child is large relative to the size of the oral cavity and posterior pharynx. When the patient is unconscious, the tongue can fall into the posterior pharynx, causing obstruction.[54] The sniffing position (head tilt, chin lift) usually opens the airway; however, this procedure should be performed as the initial airway maneuver only if cervical spine injury has been ruled out.

If the injured child is unconscious or if the child's mechanism of injury or presentation suggests potential cervical spine injury, the cervical spine is stabilized at the same time the airway is opened. In these children, the "jaw thrust" should be used to relieve airway obstruction; the provider holds the head and neck steady while providing gentle forward-upward pressure at the angle of the mandible to open the airway.[2] For some trauma victims, such as those with isolated injury of an extremity, a cervical spine injury is unlikely and no such precautions are needed. If the airway can't be opened with a jaw thrust, a chin lift with a slight head tilt may be needed, because an adequate airway must be established.[9a,38a]

If the child arrives with a cervical collar in place, the trauma team must assess suitability of the collar size and fit. The child's neck should be neither flexed nor extended.

Suctioning

Relatively small amounts of foreign matter in the child's hypopharynx can obstruct the airway. As a part of initial stabilization, providers should suction the airway to eliminate obstruction such as blood, mucus, loose teeth, or vomitus. Neonates and young infants are obligate nose breathers. In these infants, gentle nasal suctioning or opening of the airway may be the only intervention required to stimulate spontaneous ventilation.[2]

Airway Obstruction

Rare causes of airway obstruction include clothes-line injuries that cause penetrating or crushing injury to the larynx or trachea. When airway manipulation causes air hunger and providers cannot deliver adequate ventilation with positioning and a bag-mask device, intubation or a surgical airway will be needed.

Airway obstruction can also result from supraglottic edema associated with chemical or thermal burns. Treatment is supportive, and intubation will be required until the edema resolves. Intubation should be accomplished before severe airway obstruction develops.

Spine Stabilization

Spinal cord injuries are less common in children than in adults. When these injuries occur in children, they are generally associated with motor vehicle-related crashes, falls, and inflicted head trauma and can result in injuries of the upper or lower cervical spine (Fig. 19-1).[4]

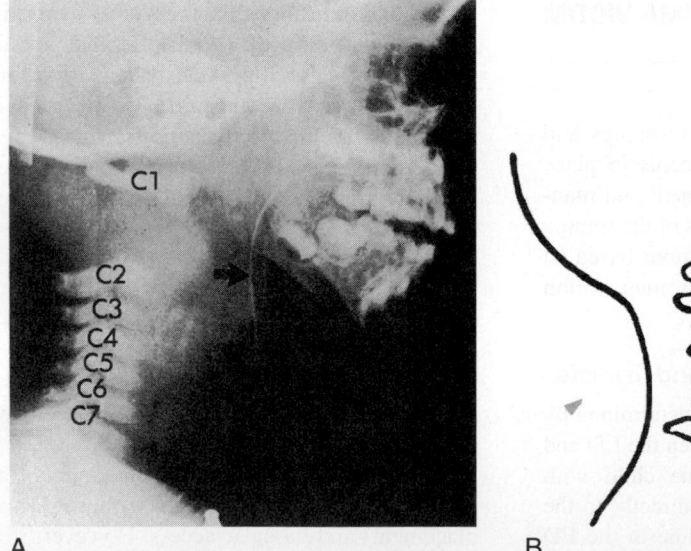
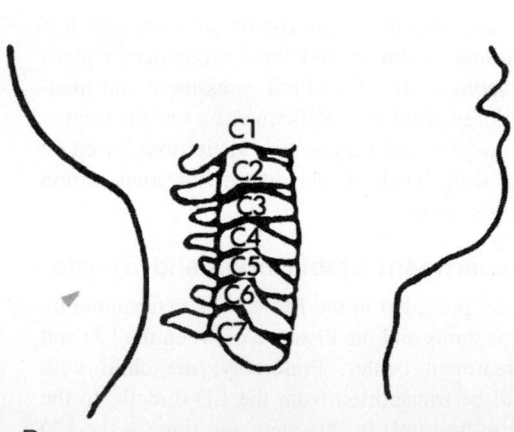

A   B

FIG. 19-1 Cervical spine injury. Lateral cervical spine radiograph indicating cervical spine injury. **A,** Cervical spine radiograph of a toddler demonstrating wide separation between the first and second cervical vertebrae, consistent with complete cervical spine injury at the level of C1 to C2. Note the anterior displacement of the nasogastric tube (*arrow*) indicating anterior displacement of the esophagus (which should lie just anterior to the vertebrae) caused by edema at the site of the spinal cord injury. This child was intubated, but the endotracheal tube is not visible because it is not radiopaque. **B,** Normal anatomy of the cervical spine in a toddler. Note the horizontal articulation of the vertebrae, which increases the mobility of the upper cervical spine in this age group. (A. Radiograph courtesy of John B. Pietsch, Nashville, TN. B. Illustration from Riviello JJ, et al: Delayed cervical central cord syndrome after trivial trauma. *Pediatr Emerg Care* 6:116, 1990. Williams and Wilkins.)

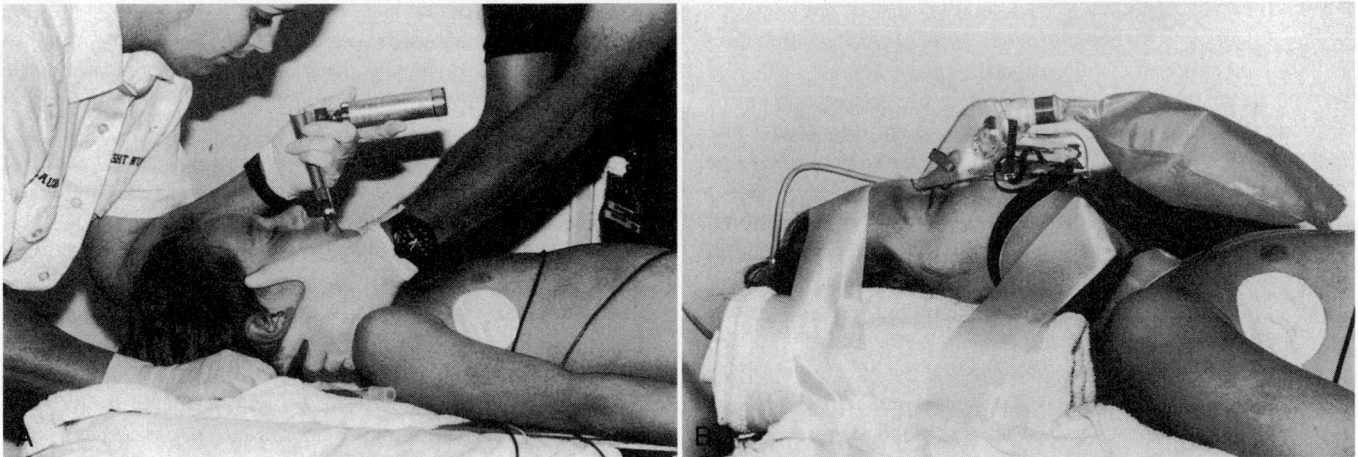

FIG. 19-2 Cervical spine manual stabilization and immobilization. **A,** Preparation for intubation using a second person to stabilize cervical spine. This two-person technique may be necessary if a hard cervical collar of appropriate size is not available. No traction or force should be applied to the cervical spine, but movement is prevented. **B,** With a hard cervical collar in place, the patient's torso is taped or strapped to the board, then the patient's head and neck (with collar) are secured to the backboard. Linen rolls are used to prevent lateral movement of the head.

Spine stabilization and then immobilization is indicated after motor vehicle crashes, after pedestrian-related crashes, after crashes in which the child was unrestrained, for any unconscious trauma victim (because it is difficult to ascertain the extent of injury), and for any major trauma associated with head injury.[2] Manual stabilization is provided initially, and then a device is used to immobilize the cervical spine during transport and initial evaluation (Fig. 19-2).

There are many acceptable methods for immobilizing the cervical spine. A semirigid collar (e.g., an extrication collar) immobilizes the cervical spine, but these collars are not recommended for use in children younger than 4 years.[5] Foam collars can be applied easily and are available in small sizes, but they often provide no protection against head and neck movement. If an excessively large collar is applied, flexion of the neck may cause airway obstruction or hyperextension of the neck can result in the very movement and possible injury that the collar is designed to prevent.

Cervical spine immobilization in children requires a combination of a cervical collar (of the appropriate size) with a rigid spine board. The child's head is supported in a neutral position on the board, using a board with head well or pads under the torso, and, foam blocks and straps. Towel rolls, and tape should be used to secure the torso and the head (see Fig. 19-2).[3,25,29]

If the mechanism of injury suggests thoracic spine trauma, providers should avoid any flexion or torsion of the torso. If lap belt injuries are suspected (see Secondary Survey, Abdomen), providers should prevent movement of the lumbar spine until further examination.[55] The child should be log-rolled whenever turning is required until an injury to the spine is ruled out (i.e., the spine is cleared). If the child is sufficiently stable, the provider should evaluate and document movement and sensation of all extremities.

Airway Management

Oropharyngeal and nasopharyngeal airways can help to maintain a patent upper airway. Oral airways are reserved for the child with absent cough and gag reflex. Oral airways must be sized appropriately, because airways that are too small can push the tongue back into the oropharynx and those that are too long can obstruct the pharynx.[54] The length of the airway should equal the distance from the mouth to the angle of the mandible. Nasal airways can be inserted in the alert child or the unresponsive child who has no facial trauma; they may facilitate suctioning.

Intubation

Intubation may be necessary to maintain a patent airway and prevent anticipated deterioration. Indications for intubation of the pediatric trauma victim (Box 19-2) include: (1) inability to ventilate the child's lungs adequately using a bag-mask device, (2) need for prolonged airway control and prevention of aspiration, (3) severe head injury (in anticipation of a need for controlled ventilation and oxygenation), (4) flail chest, (5) severe facial burns, and (6) shock unresponsive to volume infusion.[2,54]

When the child has inhalation injuries, trauma to the head and neck, or facial burns, elective intubation is performed in anticipation of the development of progressive airway

---

Box 19-2 | **Indications for Intubation in the Pediatric Trauma Victim**

- Respiratory arrest, apnea
- Significant respiratory distress
- Hypoventilation
- Hypoxemia despite oxygen therapy
- Respiratory acidosis
- Signs of airway obstruction: stridor, increased work of breathing; suprasternal, supraclavicular retractions
- Injuries associated with potential airway obstruction (e.g., inhalation injuries, crushing facial or neck injuries)
- Head injury or signs of increased intracranial pressure
- Thoracic injury (rib fractures, pulmonary contusion, flail chest, penetrating injuries)
- Anticipation of need for mechanical ventilation support

obstruction. The trauma team should not wait for signs of severe respiratory distress to develop, because the intubation is then likely to be far more difficult.

The nurse must be able to select intubation equipment of appropriate size. Formulas, tables, or a length-based tape that indicates the equipment sizes (i.e., the Broselow tape—see inside back cover) may be used (Table 19-3).[54]

In the past, only uncuffed tubes were used for children younger than 8 years, because there was concern that cuffed tubes could produce subglottic tracheal injury.[2] However, for some children (e.g., those with noncompliant lungs, high airway resistance or large glottic air leak), the use of a cuffed tube may be preferable to an uncuffed tube, particularly if the child requires ventilation with high inspiratory pressure or maintenance of positive end-expiratory pressure.[9a,38a] Slightly different formulas are used to determine the internal diameter of a cuffed versus an uncuffed tube (see Table 19-3).

Gastric distension increases the risk of vomiting and aspiration, can stimulate a vasovagal reflex and bradycardia, compromises diaphragm movement, and can mimic or mask symptoms of abdominal injury. If gastric distension develops, providers should remove air through an orogastric tube. If the patient has craniofacial trauma with maxillofacial or basilar skull fracture, an orogastric tube is used for gastric decompression rather than a nasogastric tube. Case reports have documented intracranial migration of nasogastric tubes if they are inserted blindly.[4,18]

Sedation and administration of neuromuscular blockers are advisable before intubation of a conscious trauma victim, particularly if the child is struggling or has a full stomach. Rapid sequence intubation (also known as *drug assisted intubation*) is designed to reduce stimulation of gag reflex (and the associated risk of vomiting and aspiration) when the child has a full stomach or when the time of the last meal cannot be determined (for further information about rapid sequence intubation, see Chapter 9 and Box 9-11).

Oral intubation is preferred over nasotracheal intubation. Nasotracheal intubation is not performed if cervical spine injury is suspected, because nasotracheal intubation will likely require excessive cervical spine manipulation. In addition, nasotracheal intubation is avoided if the child has maxillofacial injury and a dural tear, because the tracheal tube may be inserted intracranially and produces the added complication of introducing bacteria through the dura.

As soon as the endotracheal tube is inserted, providers should verify correct tube position using both clinical evaluation (including auscultation and visual assessment of chest expansion and monitoring of heart rate and oxyhemoglobin saturation) and a confirmation device (e.g., exhaled CO_2 detector, ideally with continuous capnography). If the tube is in the proper position, chest expansion should be visible and equal bilaterally during positive pressure ventilation, and bilateral breath sounds should be equal and adequate. In addition, the child's oxyhemoglobin saturation (assessed via pulse oximetry) should improve.

Because breath sounds can be transmitted easily through the thin chest wall of the infant or child, as well as into the abdomen, use of a device to confirm tracheal tube placement is particularly important for children. If the child has a perfusing rhythm, an exhaled CO_2 detector (a colorimetric device or capnograph) can be used. If, after six positive-pressure breaths, CO_2 is detected in exhaled air using a colorimetric device or if a CO_2 waveform is documented via capnography, and the clinical exam documents breath sounds and chest expansion, tracheal tube placement is confirmed. If the child has a perfusing rhythm and CO_2 is not detected in exhaled air, the tube is not in the trachea; providers should remove it and provide bag-mask ventilation until another tube can be inserted.

Once the clinical and device confirmation have verified tube placement, a chest radiograph ultimately is performed to confirm depth of tube insertion. The chest x-ray cannot, however, confirm tube placement in the trachea.

Cricothyrotomy and Tracheostomy

If positioning of the child, bag-mask ventilation, and intubation do not relieve airway obstruction and providers cannot deliver adequate ventilation, then injury to the larynx or trachea is likely to be present. Needle cricothyrotomy, although

Table 19-3   Endotracheal and Tracheostomy Tube Sizes

Age	Cuffed* or Uncuffed[†] Internal Diameter (mm)	Laryngoscope Blade	Oral Length (cm)[‡]	Nasal Length (cm)	Tracheostomy (Internal Diameter in mm)	Suction Catheter (in French Sizes)
Premature	2.5-3.0	0 straight	8	11	4-5	5½ - 6
Newborn	3.0-3.5	1 straight	8.5-10	13	4-5	6-8
6 months	3.5-4.0	1 straight	10.5-12	15	5.5	6-8
18 months	4.0-4.5	1 straight	12-13.5	16	6.0	8-10
24 months	4.5-5.5	1 straight	13.5-14	17	6-7	10
2-4 years	5.0-6.0	1 straight	15	18	6-7	10-12
4-7 years	5.5-6.5	2 straight or 2 curved	16	19	7.0	12
7-10 years	6.0-7.0	2 straight or 2 curved	17-19.5	21	8.0	12-14
10-12 years	6.5-7.5	3 straight	20-21	22-25	9.0	14

*Formula for estimation of *uncuffed* endotracheal tube: (Age [years] ÷ 4) + 4 = Internal diameter (mm).
[†]Formula for estimation of *cuffed* endotracheal tube: (Age [years] ÷ 4) + 3.5 = Internal diameter (mm).
[‡]Formula for estimation of depth of tube insertion: Tube internal diameter (mm) × 3 = Insertion at the lip (cm).

rarely necessary in the child, should be considered at this time.[54] This procedure is challenging because it can be difficult to identify landmarks in the short neck of an infant or young child, and the needle is difficult to secure once it is inserted.

Although needle cricothyrotomy can provide short-term oxygenation, it will not allow sufficient air movement to produce effective ventilation (i.e., CO_2 elimination). Even large-bore catheters are unlikely to provide adequate ventilation.

Emergency tracheostomy is rarely necessary and should be reserved for times when intubation attempts by experienced practitioners fail to establish an adequate airway and satisfactory oxygenation. Emergency tracheostomy is a difficult procedure in conscious children, has a high complication rate, and should be performed only by experienced physicians.

Ongoing Airway Assessment

The nurse and members of the trauma team should evaluate the child's respiratory rate, effort, and effectiveness every few minutes during acute management. Providers must be able to recognize signs of airway obstruction in the intubated child as well as in the child without an advanced airway. Signs in the unintubated child include changes in responsiveness, change in respiratory rate and depth, nasal flaring, retractions, grunting, wheezing, stridor, and changes in the inspiratory/expiratory ratio. Inspiration is typically prolonged when upper airway obstruction is present, and exhalation is typically prolonged when lower airway obstruction is present. Diaphoresis and tachycardia are nonspecific signs of distress. Hypoxemia may be only a late sign of airway obstruction in the child who is breathing spontaneously, and it may be noted only when fatigue develops and respiratory arrest is imminent.

If the intubated child's condition suddenly deteriorates, the bedside nurse should provide bag-mask ventilation and quickly assess tube position and patency, and assess for complications such as a pneumothorax. The mnemonic *D-O-P-E* can be used to recall the causes of sudden deterioration in the child with an advanced airway: tube *d*isplacement, tube *o*bstruction, *p*neumothorax, and *e*quipment failure.[9a,38a] If the tube is no longer in the trachea, the nurse should remove it and provide bag-mask ventilation as needed until reintubation can be accomplished.

Breathing
Oxygen Administration

In general, providers should initially administer 100% oxygen by nonrebreathing face mask at 10 to 12 L/minute to all victims of major trauma. Use of 100% oxygen is important in the treatment of shock or central nervous system injury, when cardiac output and distribution of blood flow to the brain and tissues may be inadequate.

Assessment of Ventilation and Oxygenation

The team should continuously assess the child's respiratory rate and effort, ventilation, and response to oxygen administration. Apnea, gasping, and cyanosis despite oxygen therapy

---

Box 19-3 Signs of Respiratory Failure and Need for Mechanical Ventilation

- Severe respiratory distress, including grunting, retractions
- Hypoxemia despite oxygen therapy
- Hypercarbia, particularly if $PaCO_2$ rising rapidly
- Acidosis
- Rising alveolar-arterial oxygen difference (A-a DO_2)
- Late signs:
  - Decreased air movement
  - Apnea or gasping
  - Bradycardia

---

indicate the need for positive pressure ventilation (Box 19-3). The pulse oximeter and exhaled CO_2 detectors are useful adjuncts to clinical assessment; they enable continuous evaluation of oxyhemoglobin saturation, CO_2 elimination, and response to therapy.

As a general guide when a perfusing rhythm is present, infants require a spontaneous or assisted ventilation rate of at least 20/min, preschool-aged children require a minimum ventilation rate of 15/min, and school-aged children require a ventilation rate of at least 12/min to produce sufficient oxygenation and ventilation. Faster spontaneous respiratory rates are common in the presence of pain, fear, hemorrhage, or respiratory distress.[2]

Life-Threatening Thoracic Injuries

Not all thoracic injuries are immediately recognizable, and not all injuries are immediately life threatening. It is important to note that these complications often can be identified on the basis of clinical findings. When thoracic injuries or their complications (e.g., tension pneumothorax, severe hemorrhage) are life threatening and produce typical signs and symptoms, treatment should be initiated before a radiograph is obtained.

Injuries to the lung parenchyma or accumulation of intrathoracic air or fluid can impair oxygenation and ventilation and can produce cardiorespiratory failure. Injuries may be internal, external, or both. Common life-threatening thoracic injuries include tension pneumothorax, open pneumothorax (sucking chest wound), massive hemothorax, and cardiac tamponade. Additional injuries that are potentially life threatening include pneumothorax, tracheobronchial injuries, and pulmonary contusion. Fortunately, injuries resulting from penetrating trauma are relatively uncommon in children.[7]

Pneumothorax

Pneumothorax is a common complication of thoracic injury in children.[13] Most injuries result from blunt chest trauma and are not associated with rib fractures. The child with pneumothorax may be asymptomatic or exhibit dyspnea, chest pain, and severe respiratory distress.[44] Symptomatic children demonstrate hypoxemia, asymmetric chest wall movement, and decreased breath sounds or altered pitch of breath sounds on the involved side; this altered pitch may be difficult to identify in the small child because referred breath sounds from other parts of the chest may be heard over the pneumothorax.

Tension Pneumothorax

Tension pneumothorax develops from progressive air entry into the pleural space from the lung or airways; this air accumulation elevates intrapleural pressure, compresses the lung, and can compromise cardiovascular function. The lung on the side of the tension pneumothorax is partially collapsed, and severe hypoxemia develops (Fig. 19-3; see Fig. 10-7). Breath sounds and chest expansion on the side of the pneumothorax are decreased or absent.

A tension pneumothorax shifts the mediastinum away from the affected side. This shift reduces venous return to the heart and decreases cardiac output; neck vein distension may be observed. In addition, the point of maximal impulse and the trachea shift away from the tension pneumothorax,[4] although the tracheal shift may be difficult to appreciate in infants and children. The resultant decrease in cardiac output and oxygen delivery are life threatening. The mediastinal shift can result in compression of the contralateral lung, further compromising oxygenation and ventilation.

A tension pneumothorax requires immediate needle decompression followed by tube thoracostomy. Needle decompression should be performed on the basis of clinical examination, and providers should not delay therapy to obtain a chest radiograph. A simple pneumothorax is treated with chest tube insertion.

To perform needle decompression, insert a large-bore (13, 16, or 18 gauge) angiocatheter on the affected side, into the second intercostal space at the midclavicular line.[54] The diagnosis of tension pneumothorax is confirmed when needle or tube thoracostomy results in evidence of air evacuation and immediate improvement in the patient's condition. After initial air evacuation, the provider can use a stopcock to prevent entrainment of air into the chest. The provider can also attach the angiocatheter to tubing with the tubing tip placed 2 to 3 cm below the surface of a bottle of sterile water; this maintains an underwater seal until a chest tube is inserted.

Chest tubes are inserted to treat pneumothorax and hemothorax. Appropriate chest tube size is based on the age of the child (Table 19-4), and sizes can be predicted from length-based (e.g., Broselow) resuscitation tapes. Before the chest tube is inserted, the skin is prepared with a povidone iodine or chlorhexidine scrub, and the provider administers local anesthetic (e.g., lidocaine). A small stab wound is made in the skin and subcutaneous tissue along the long axis of the rib, in the fifth or sixth intercostal space at the midaxillary line. A curved hemostat followed by the chest tube is advanced through the chest wall and pleura, into the chest cavity (see Evolve Fig. 19-1 in the Chapter 19 Supplement on the Evolve Website for an illustration of chest tube insertion).

Sucking Chest Wounds

Sucking chest wounds result from penetrating trauma. These wounds allow air to move into and out of the pleural space, making a sucking noise.[58] Treatment is immediate application of an occlusive dressing (e.g., Opsite [Smith and Nephew, Memphis, TN] or Vaseline gauze [Kendall, division of Covidien, Norwalk, CT]).

Once an open pneumothorax is sealed, the child will likely require chest tube insertion and treatment of the underlying lung injury (e.g., mechanical ventilation for treatment of a

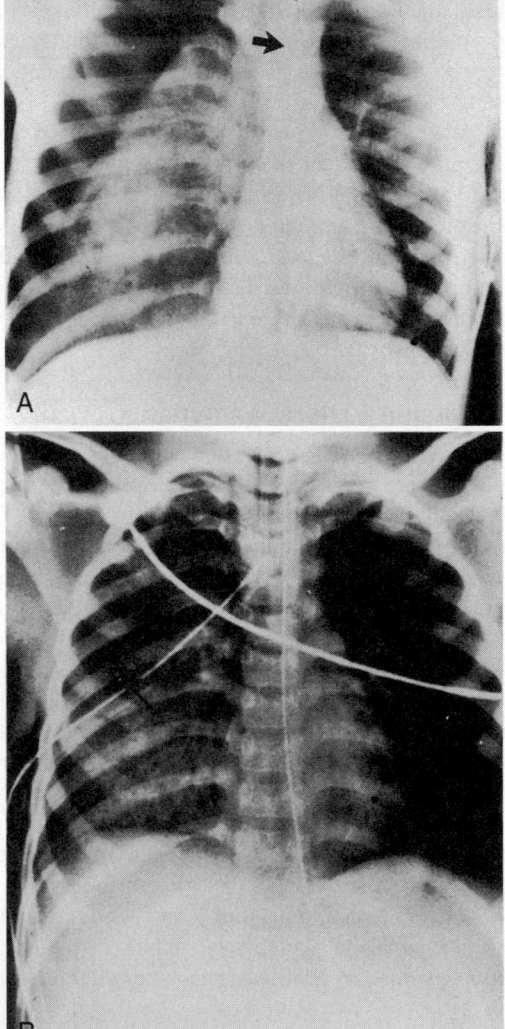

FIG. 19-3 Chest radiograph showing tension pneumothorax. **A,** Right tension pneumothorax produces displacement of the mediastinum to the patient's left side *(arrow)*. Note the absence of rib fractures. This injury was sustained when the rear wheels of a car ran over the child's right chest, and the tension pneumothorax was apparent on clinical examination. **B,** Reexpansion of the right lung is apparent after insertion of a chest tube. The mediastinum has shifted back to the midline. Opacification of the right lung is consistent with pulmonary contusion. The child is intubated and a nasogastric tube is in place. Note that the chest radiograph did not and should not delay thoracostomy. (Chest radiographs courtesy of James Betts, Oakland, CA.)

Table 19-4 Pediatric Chest Tube Sizes

Age	Chest Tube Size (French)
Full-term neonate (6 months)	10-12
Older infant (6-18 months)	12-14
Toddler (1-3 years)	14-16
Young school age (4-7 years)	16-20
Older school age (8-12 years)	20-24
Adolescent	24-32

pulmonary contusion). Continuous observation is required to identify development of a pneumothorax.[58] If the child has an advanced airway and is receiving positive pressure ventilation, a chest tube should be inserted.

Hemothorax

A hemothorax is the accumulation of blood in the pleural cavity. The severity of symptoms produced by the hemothorax is determined by the extent and rapidity of blood loss and by the presence of associated injuries (i.e., lung or great vessel tears).[44] If the child is asymptomatic, the most effective immediate therapy is the placement of an IV catheter to replace ongoing blood loss, followed by placement of a chest tube to evacuate accumulated blood. Providers should monitor the child's systemic perfusion and replace ongoing blood loss as needed.

If the child has significant hemorrhage and hemothorax, the child will demonstrate signs of poor systemic perfusion and respiratory compromise. In cases of large hemothorax, rapid blood replacement will be required. Significant ongoing hemorrhage (i.e., significant volume of blood loss via chest tube) may indicate rupture of a large thoracic vessel or lung laceration, and urgent exploratory thoracotomy is indicated.[13]

Cardiac Tamponade

Cardiac tamponade results from the accumulation of a significant amount of blood in the pericardial sac. Tamponade develops when sufficient blood or fluid (as little as 25-50 mL) accumulates to compress the heart and compromise both venous return to the heart and cardiac output.

Cardiac tamponade is a form of obstructive shock. Classic clinical signs include persistent hypotension, distension of neck veins, muffled heart sounds, and pulsus paradoxus (a fall in systolic arterial pressure of 8-10 mm Hg or more during spontaneous inspiration). However, these signs are virtually impossible to appreciate in patient with tachypnea and hypotension. The presence of a cardiac tamponade can be confirmed by echocardiography and, more recently, with the use of ultrasonography (e.g., emergency ultrasound or focused assessment with sonography for trauma [FAST]); fluid in the pericardium (i.e., hemopericardium) will appear black against the gray heart muscle.[42]

When tamponade is present, the tamponade must be evacuated by pericardiocentesis. Administration of autologous blood and fluid boluses may initially help support cardiac output. A pericardial drain can be placed or an emergency thoracotomy can be performed for pericardial decompression and immediate repair of the associated cardiac injury.[4,13]

To perform pericardiocentesis, the chest is cleaned and a needle is inserted in the left subxyphoid region. While constant negative pressure is applied, the needle is aimed superiorly and posteriorly. Once blood or fluid enters the barrel of the syringe, the needle is likely in the pericardium. At this point, the needle or catheter is held in place and blood is aspirated to decompress the pericardium.[4]

If neither a FAST scan nor ultrasonography is available, pericardiocentesis may be accomplished using an 18-gauge metal spinal needle joined to an alligator clamp (i.e., the alligator clamp is joined to the base of the needle) to allow simultaneous needle insertion and monitoring of the electrocardiogram (ECG). The alligator clamp is then joined to the electrode of an ECG recorder (see Evolve Fig. 19-2 in the Chapter 19 Supplement on the Evolve Website for an illustration of this technique).

Flail Chest

As noted previously, rib fractures are present in one third or less of children with blunt trauma. Rib fractures indicate injury associated with substantial force and energy transfer.[3,13] When three or more contiguous ribs are fractured at two points, typically in the back,[44] flail chest can develop.

Flail chest is characterized by a portion of the chest wall that moves paradoxically with changes in intrathoracic pressure; it typically is drawn inward when the child inspires spontaneously and moves outward during exhalation. Flail chest will increase work of breathing and decrease effective tidal volume. Treatment of flail chest requires positive pressure ventilation; plans should be made to provide mechanical ventilation and analgesia until the segment no longer moves paradoxically with spontaneous inspiration.

Whenever rib fractures are present, providers should closely assess and monitor the child for evidence of underlying organ injury (e.g., liver, spleen, lung).[13,44] Patients with flail chest always have associated pulmonary contusions, the primary cause of the hypoxia associated with this condition.

Diaphragm Rupture

Rupture of the diaphragm (usually the left diaphragm) is a relatively uncommon complication of blunt trauma in children. It will produce significant respiratory distress if the trauma victim is breathing spontaneously, because when spontaneous inspiration occurs the diaphragm is drawn up into the chest. Because it is difficult to generate adequate tidal volume, the child will develop increased respiratory effort, atelectasis, and increased work of breathing.

Diaphragm rupture may be impossible to detect once positive pressure ventilation is instituted. Occasionally, herniation of abdominal contents into the chest will occur, and these will be apparent on the chest radiograph or CT scan; an inserted nasogastric tube may be visible in the left chest.[13,44] Surgical repair through an abdominal or thoracic approach will be required.

Pulmonary Contusion

A pulmonary contusion is a bruise on the lung resulting from lung parenchymal injury. Although a pulmonary contusion can be asymptomatic and diagnosed only on CT scan, it can cause respiratory compromise following major blunt chest trauma.[13,44] A significant pulmonary contusion will cause hypoxemia, and opacification is visible on a chest radiograph or CT scan (see Figs. 19-3, B and 19-4).

An associated hemothorax typically suggests the presence of a more severe lung injury. Treatment includes supplementary oxygen and may require positive-pressure ventilation with oxygen support and positive end-expiratory pressure.

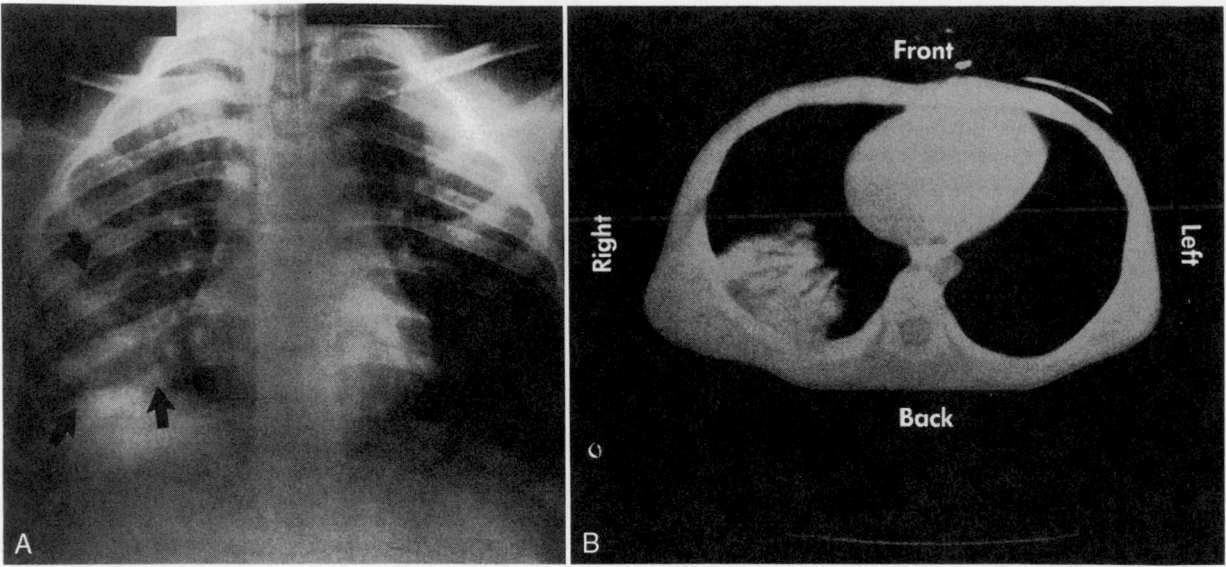

FIG. 19-4 Pulmonary contusion on chest radiograph and computed tomography (CT) scan. **A,** Chest radiograph. Note the increased opacification in the patient's right lower lung fields (*arrows*). Note the absence of rib fractures. **B,** CT scan from the same patient demonstrating opacification (white contusion is visible in the dark air density) of the right lower lung. The trachea is not visible in mediastinum, so opacification is below the area of bifurcation of the trachea into bronchi. This CT view is shot from below the area of contusion with a view in the cephalad direction. The patient's right chest appears on the left side of this image, and the patient's left chest is visible on the right side of this image. The front of the patient is the top of this image, and the patient's back is at the bottom of this image; thus, the patient's heart is anterior (visible as a white oval) and vertebral column is posterior.

Circulation

Assessment and support of circulation includes: (1) assessment of systemic perfusion, including assessment for signs of hemorrhage; (2) control of external bleeding; and (3) treatment of hypovolemia and any other causes of inadequate systemic perfusion. The nurse should monitor the child's heart rate and assess systemic perfusion frequently.

Cardiovascular compromise in the trauma patient generally is caused by hypovolemia, but it may also be caused by hypoxia or severe head injury. Even if effective cardiovascular function is present on arrival in the hospital, the trauma team should assess and reassess systemic perfusion to detect any signs of deterioration. These signs may be subtle in the child and include: tachycardia; weak peripheral pulses, mottled skin; cool, pale extremities; delayed capillary refill; and unusual irritability or lethargy (Box 19-4).

Box 19-4 | **Signs of Poor Systemic Perfusion in the Pediatric Trauma Patient**

- Tachycardia, tachypnea
- Cool skin
- Delayed capillary refill
- Diminished intensity of pulses
- Irritability, then lethargy with diminished pain response
- Oliguria
- Metabolic (lactic) acidosis
- *Late signs:*
  ○ Hypotension
  ○ Bradycardia

If the child has an ineffective or absent pulse in a central artery (e.g., carotid, femoral), or the infant has no brachial pulse, cardiopulmonary resuscitation is needed (see Chapter 6). Additional indications for the initiation of chest compressions include symptomatic bradycardia (a heart rate less than 60/min associated with signs of poor systemic perfusion) that is unresponsive to adequate oxygenation and ventilation.[26,54]

The most common terminal (prearrest) cardiac rhythm in pediatric patients is a bradycardia that deteriorates to an agonal rhythm or asystole. Ventricular tachycardia and ventricular fibrillation are less common in children than in adults. For further information regarding cardiopulmonary resuscitation in children, see Chapter 6. Survival following prehospital cardiac arrest and cardiovascular collapse in pediatric victims of blunt trauma is poor.[26] To prevent arrest, providers must detect and treat signs of airway compromise, respiratory failure, and shock.

Recognition of Hypovolemia

As blood volume is depleted, the child's blood pressure initially remains unchanged, because systemic vascular resistance increases proportionately.[54] The pediatric trauma victim typically does not develop hypotension until approximately 30% of blood volume has been lost.[2,13,25,54] This ability to compensate for blood loss with vasoconstriction and redistribution of blood flow means that signs of hemorrhage may be insidious in the child and vital signs alone may not identify evolving shock.[2]

The most consistent signs of hemorrhage will include tachycardia, alteration in responsiveness, peripheral vasoconstriction,

Table 19-5 Systemic Responses to Blood Loss in Pediatric Patients

System	Mild Blood Volume Loss (Less Than 30%)	Moderate Blood Volume Loss (30%-45%)	Severe Blood Volume Loss (More Than 45%)
Cardiovascular	Increased heart rate; weak, thready peripheral pulses; normal systolic blood pressure (80-90 + 2 × age in years); normal pulse pressure	Markedly increased heart rate; weak, thready central pulses; absent peripheral pulses; low normal systolic blood pressure (70-80 + 2 × age in years); narrowed pulse pressure	Tachycardia followed by bradycardia; very weak or absent central pulses; absent peripheral pulses; hypotension (systolic blood pressure <70 + 2 × age in years); widened pulse pressure (or undetectable diastolic blood pressure)
Central Nervous System	Anxious; irritable; confused	Lethargic; dulled response to pain*	Comatose
Skin	Cool, mottled; prolonged capillary refill	Cyanotic; markedly prolonged capillary refill	Pale and cold
Urine Output†	Low to very low	Minimal	None

From American College of Surgeons, Committee on Trauma, Advanced Trauma Life Support for Doctors. *Extremes of Age: Pediatric. ATLS Student Course Material*, ed 8, Chicago, 2008, American College of Surgeons.
*The child's dulled response to pain with this degree of blood loss (30%-45%) may be indicated by a decreased response to IV catheter insertion.
†After initial decompression by urinary catheter. Low normal is 2 mL/kg per hour (infant), 1.5 mL/kg per hour (younger child), 1 mL/kg per hour (older child), and 0.5 mL/kg per hour (adolescent). Intravenous contrast can falsely elevate urinary output.

thready pulses, and diminished pulse pressure.[4,54] Hypotension is a late and ominous sign of cardiovascular compromise.[54] Clinical findings can be used to classify the severity of the hemorrhage and to estimate the volume of blood loss (Table 19-5).

Initial blood pressure measurement is useful in identifying frank hypotension, and it is used as a baseline for identifying trends in the patient's condition. Accurate blood pressure measurements require the use of an appropriately sized cuff (with a non-invasive measurement system) or an intraarterial catheter joined to a properly zeroed, leveled, and calibrated fluid-filled monitoring system. Intraarterial monitoring should be established early when severe trauma is present, because it provides access for blood gas and other blood sampling and enables continuous evaluation of the patient's blood pressure and response to therapy.

Noninvasive oscillometric blood pressure measurements may provide falsely high blood pressure measurements in the hypotensive patient.[38a] Such measurements are less reliable than intraarterial measurements in an unstable child.

Control of External Bleeding

The most efficient method of controlling external hemorrhage is the application of simple direct pressure over the bleeding site. Additional measures can include pressure over a proximal portion of the related artery and, if an extremity is involved, elevation of the extremity. Even when an artery has been severed, these procedures are generally the only interventions required until definitive surgery is performed. In the rare instance when direct pressure fails to control the bleeding, the use of a hemostat or tourniquet may be required.

Vascular Access

Vascular access can be obtained through percutaneous peripheral venous cannulation, percutaneous central venous (e.g., the femoral, external jugular, internal jugular, or subclavian vein) access, the IO route, or venous cutdown. Any of these routes will provide effective vascular access for fluid, blood, and drug administration.

It is often difficult to establish IV access in the small child, particularly if hypovolemia and poor systemic perfusion are present. If providers are unable to establish peripheral vascular access and the child is in shock, they should establish IO access. If a catheter with a small-bore lumen is in place, that catheter is used for fluid administration while attempts are made to insert a second catheter. Inserting one large-bore venous catheter may be acceptable initially if the child does not have hemorrhage or shock; however, insertion of two large-bore catheters is optimal. Note the child's response to insertion of an IV catheter as part of the evaluation of the child's neurologic function.

IO access is a suitable alternative to rapid peripheral venous cannulation for administration of crystalloid, colloid, blood, and drugs for the child in shock. IO needles provide access to the marrow cavity of a long bone in an uninjured extremity and are safe and effective, and they require less time to establish than venous cut downs.[3,9a,38a,54,61] Drugs administered by the IO route reach the heart in approximately the same time as drugs given by central venous access.

IO access can be established in the anterior tibia 1 to 3 cm below the tibial tuberosity[54] or in the inferior third of the femur, 3 cm above the external condyle, anterior to the midline.[3] Bone marrow needles are preferred for this procedure. Occasionally, marrow will obstruct the flow of fluids through the needle, and the use of a pressure infusion device may be required to increase the rate of fluid administration.[54]

Central venous cannulation enables rapid fluid administration and assessment and continuous monitoring of central venous pressure. However, central venous cannulation should be performed only by personnel trained in these procedures. Ultrasound guidance may be helpful.[42]

The jugular approach to the superior vena cava may be difficult to achieve in the small child during bag-mask ventilation or resuscitation, or when spinal injury is suspected. However, the subclavian or supraclavicular route may introduce complications such as pneumothorax and subclavian artery puncture.

The femoral vein can be used to gain access to the inferior vena cava. The advantage of the femoral vein approach is the distance from the major sites of activity during resuscitative efforts; however, some physicians prefer to cannulate other smaller vessels.[54]

Management of Shock

Even a small volume of blood loss can be significant for the child, because the child's blood volume is much smaller than that of the adult. Estimate the child's circulating blood volume on admission (75-80 mL/kg for infants, 70-75 mL/kg for children, and 65-70 mL/kg for adolescents), and consider all blood lost as a percentage of the child's circulating blood volume. A 10% blood loss (8 mL/kg for infants, 7.5 mL/kg for children and 6.5-7 mL/kg for adolescents) is significant, and providers should consider blood administration (see Cardiovascular Function and Circulating Blood Volume).

Treatment of Hypovolemia

Fluid resuscitation begins with a bolus of isotonic crystalloid solution (lactated Ringer's solution or normal saline) administered in boluses of 20 mL/kg over 5 to 20 minutes.[2,54] If the child has signs of substantial blood loss or shock, the bolus should be administered as quickly as possible, typically over 5 to 10 minutes. The patient with trauma and hemorrhage also will require blood administration. Typically one bolus of packed red blood cells (RBCs) is administered after every two to three boluses of isotonic crystalloid (Fig. 19-5).

Boluses (10-20 mL/kg) of type O, Rh-negative packed RBCs can be administered when type-specific blood is not available; type-specific whole blood can be administered if packed RBCs are not available. Rh-negative blood is typically reserved for young females and females of reproductive age, to reduce the incidence of Rh sensitization. Rh-positive blood can be used in prepubescent females if there is no alternative, although this predisposes them to developing antibodies that can complicate future pregnancies. Either Rh-positive or Rh-negative blood may be administered to males.

Both isotonic crystalloids and colloids are used for intravascular volume resuscitation, and a larger quantity of fluid will be administered than the estimated volume lost. As a result of the distribution and effects of IV crystalloids and colloids, usually a crystalloid-to-colloid ratio of 3:1 is administered to produce the same effects (the "3 to 1 rule"). Although both crystalloids and colloids are ultimately distributed throughout the extracellular space, colloids remain in the vascular space for a longer period of time and may enable restoration of circulating blood volume with fewer boluses. However, there is no evidence that colloids are superior to crystalloids for volume resuscitation.

If the blood pressure, capillary refill, and quality of peripheral pulses remain poor and tachycardia persists despite the administration of two or three fluid boluses, then substantial hemorrhage has likely occurred or a continuing source of blood loss is present.[31] Surgical exploration should be considered if the child's condition is still unstable despite administration of two boluses of packed RBCs (in addition to the isotonic crystalloids). Abdominal bleeding can result from a solid organ or major vessel injury, and the trauma team should look for occult retroperitoneal or pelvic bleeding.[13] Additional causes of shock that is unresponsive to initial fluid resuscitation include cardiac tamponade, tension pneumothorax (discussed previously), and neurogenic shock.

Disability: Neurologic Function

Rapid neurologic evaluation is an essential component of the primary survey of the injured child. The initial neurologic examination consists of an assessment of pupil size and response to light, evaluation of responsiveness (GCS score or modified GCS score) and voluntary movement and sensation, and (in the infant) palpation of the fontanelle.

Signs of increased intracranial pressure include: deterioration in level of consciousness, pupil dilation (unilateral or bilateral), lack of response to a central painful stimulus, and, in the infant, a firm fontanelle. Late signs of increased intracranial pressure (often associated with impending brainstem herniation) include bradycardia, systolic hypertension with widening pulse pressure, and altered respiratory pattern, such as apnea (see Box 19-5).

Effective cerebral resuscitation in the pediatric trauma victim requires adequate shock resuscitation; cerebral perfusion will not be optimal if shock is present. The trauma team should provide shock resuscitation until systemic perfusion is

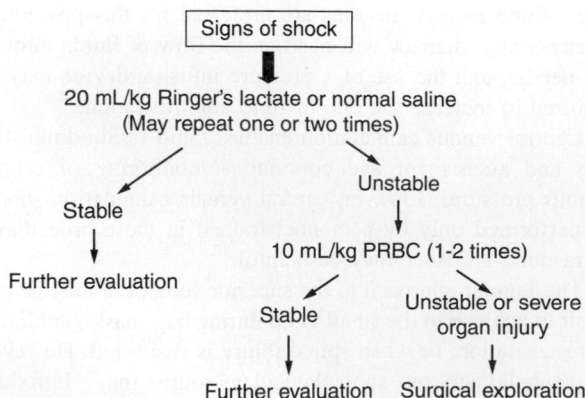

FIG. 19-5 Trauma fluid resuscitation.

| Box 19-5 | Signs of Increased Intracranial Pressure in Children |

- Change in level of consciousness
- Irritability, then lethargy
- Confusion, disorientation
- Decreased responsiveness (decreased eye contact, decreased response to parents or pain)
- Reduced ability to follow commands (hold up two fingers, wiggle toes, stick out tongue)
- Pupil dilation with decreased response to light
- Reduced spontaneous movement or deterioration in motor function or reflexive posturing
- Decorticate posturing, followed by decerebrate posturing and flaccid response to pain
- Cushing reflex or triad (bradycardia, systolic hypertension with widening pulse pressure, and altered respiratory pattern, such as apnea) may occur only as a late sign

effective. If signs of impending herniation develop (i.e., bradycardia, systolic hypertension, and altered respiratory pattern), it may be helpful to provide mild hyperventilation to reduce carbon dioxide levels and, thus, cerebral blood flow as a temporary emergency measure. Hyperventilation is not routinely performed unless signs of impending herniation are present. IV mannitol (0.25-0.5 g/kg) is given to shift water from the cellular to the extracellular (including intravascular) space; this rapidly decreases blood viscosity, leading to an increase in cerebral blood flow and tissue oxygen delivery. Hypertonic saline (3%-23.5%) may also be administered to produce an osmotic diuresis and improve cerebral perfusion; it may have other additional benefits. For further information, see Management of Increased Intracranial Pressure in Chapter 11.

Status epilepticus is uncommon, but must be identified and treated aggressively in the patient with increased intracranial pressure, because continuous seizures will increase cerebral metabolic oxygen consumption and will cause cerebral ischemia. Intermittent seizures will increase intracranial pressure transiently and are treated with diazepam (0.25 mg/kg).[2] A prophylactic anticonvulsant (i.e., phenytoin) is typically administered for 1 week to infants and children with moderate or severe head injury (GCS less than 12) who are thought to be at high risk for seizures.

Infants rarely lose a significant percentage of blood volume from intracranial hemorrhage, but bleeding from scalp wounds in infants or children can result in significant blood loss. After initial resuscitative efforts and treatment of the scalp wounds, persistent signs of shock are likely explained by other causes.

Exposure

Once the child's condition is hemodynamically stable, the trauma team should remove the child's clothes to inspect the entire body for injuries. Infants and small children can rapidly become hypothermic during transport and during resuscitation in cool rooms. Warm blankets or a radiant warming device should be available for all pediatric trauma victims. Throughout initial resuscitation and stabilization, the nurse should closely monitor the child's skin and core body temperature.

Fever will increase metabolic rate and can contribute to worse outcome following resuscitation.[9a,38a] Therefore, it is important to prevent or promptly treat fever.

SECONDARY SURVEY: "HEAD-TO-TOE" ASSESSMENT

The secondary assessment begins as soon as all aspects of the primary survey and resuscitation have been completed. The first goal of the secondary survey is evaluation of the patient response to the initial resuscitative effort; this requires frequent assessment of systemic perfusion. If the child fails to respond to volume resuscitation or deteriorates after the initial response, additional injuries may be present or surgical exploration may be needed.

Another goal of the secondary assessment is to perform a systematic evaluation of each area of the body. This head-to-toe assessment is designed to identify hidden injuries or injuries that were not detected during the primary assessment.

Head

The most common head injury in children is closed head injury.[58] Closed head trauma is not always immediately recognizable. For this reason, the mechanism of injury and the initial response to therapy (or lack of response) should provide a high index of suspicion. The first priority of management is to maintain cerebral perfusion and treat increased intracranial pressure by performing intubation and providing adequate ventilation, oxygenation, shock resuscitation, osmotic diuresis, and analgesia and sedation if needed. Early identification of increased intracranial pressure is essential to reduce morbidity and mortality.

It is important to palpate the entire head carefully to identify fractures or wounds. In addition, the nose and ears are examined carefully for blood or cerebrospinal fluid drainage, which is indicative of maxillofacial fracture or basilar skull fracture with dural tear. If clear fluid drains from the nose or the ears, it should be tested for the presence of glucose; the presence of glucose suggests that the fluid is cerebrospinal fluid. An ocular examination should be performed to identify papilledema or lateralizing extraocular muscle paresis or eye injury.

Providers should evaluate cranial nerve function when possible and immediately report any absence of cranial nerve function to the trauma surgeon or the trauma team leader. The nurse can often correlate patient neurologic function with the site of central nervous system injury through careful assessment of signs of cranial nerve function and evaluation of any abnormal posturing or respiratory patterns (Table 19-6).

A CT scan will provide important information about the extent and severity of the head injury and potential causes of further deterioration, such as intraparenchymal, subdural, or epidural hemorrhage (Fig. 19-6). In addition, it will provide information about the need for surgical intervention. If a CT scan is performed to evaluate a head injury, the scan should include the upper cervical spine.[23] Magnetic resonance imaging (MRI) has been used more often in recent years because it provides better detail of head injuries and may be more useful to predict outcome (see the following discussion under Neck and Spine).[24]

Brain injury causes the release of biomarkers that can be measured in the blood, cerebral spinal fluid, and extracellular brain fluid. These biomarkers include inflammatory mediators (e.g., interleukins, tumor necrosis factor), nerve growth factor, and adhesion molecules to proteins. Monitoring levels of biomarkers may be useful in evaluating the severity of brain injury and response to therapy and in predicting outcome.[6,24]

The trauma team and especially the bedside nurse should frequently assess the patient's mental status. The use of a standardized scoring system will enable quantification of the patient's progress and responsiveness and trends in the patient's condition. The GCS or the modified (pediatric) GCS[36] will be helpful (Table 19-7). Frequent assessments are needed to detect subtle signs of deterioration.

Occasionally children with diffuse cerebral injury will demonstrate sudden deterioration several hours after injury; such deterioration must be immediately detected and treated. For further information regarding the assessment and management

Table 19-6 Relationship Between Anatomic Site of Injury, Level of Consciousness, Abnormal Pupil Response, Respiratory Patterns and Motor Responses

Level of CNS Lesion	Level of Consciousness	Pupil Size and Reactivity	Oculocephalic and Oculovestibular Reflexes	Respiratory Pattern	Motor Responses
Thalamus	Lethargy, stupor	Small, reactive	Increased or decreased	Cheyne-Stokes*	Normal posture, tone slightly increased
Midbrain	Coma	Midposition, fixed	Absent	Central neurogenic hyperventilation†	Decorticate,‡ tone markedly increased
Pons	Coma	Pinpoint	Absent	Eupnea§ or apneustic‖ breathing	Decerebrate,¶ flaccid
Medulla	Coma	Small, reactive	Present	Ataxic breathing	No posturing, flaccid

From Morriss FC: Altered states of consciousness. In Levin DL, Morriss FC, Moore GC: *A practical guide to pediatric intensive care*, ed 2, St Louis, 1984, The CV Mosby Co.

*Cheyne-Stokes respiration: type of regular periodic breathing characterized by crescendo-decrescendo breaths interspersed with periods of apnea.
†Central neurogenic hyperventilation: hyperventilation with forced inspiration and expiration.
‡Decorticate posturing: upper extremities flexed against chest, lower extremities extended.
§Eupnea: normal breathing.
‖Apneustic breathing: pattern of breathing in which there is cessation of respiration in inspiratory position, usually rhythmical.
¶Decerebrate posturing: arms and legs extended with arms internally rotated, neck extended.

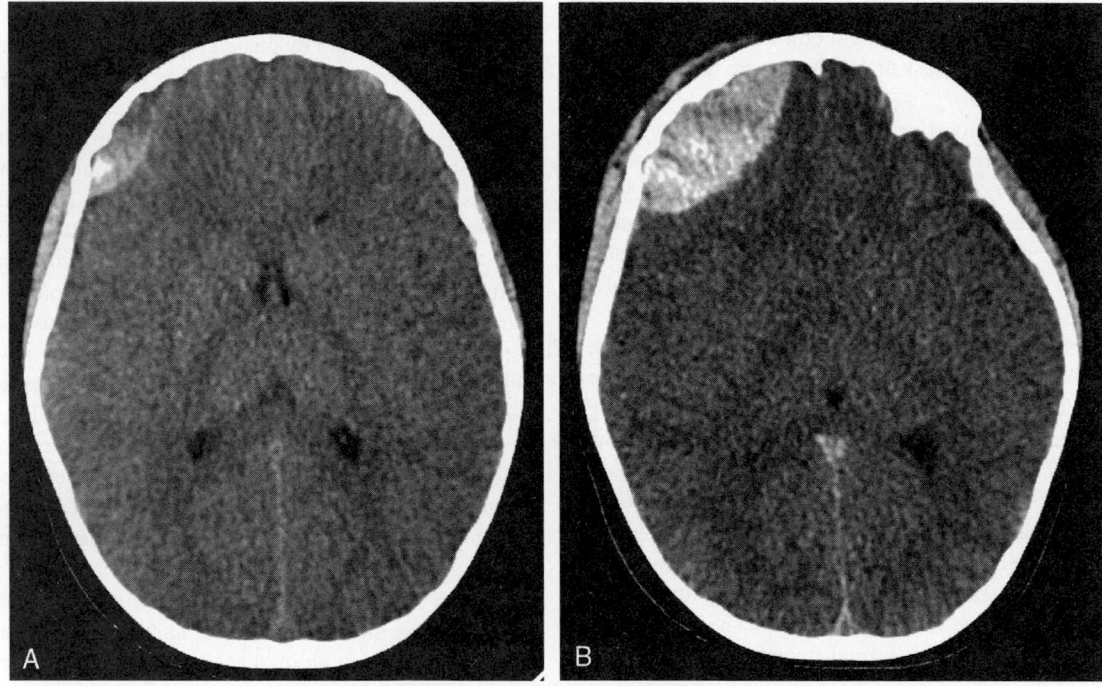

FIG. 19-6 Epidural hematoma in two CT scans taken 2 hours apart. These two images show the rapid progression of an epidural hematoma. **A,** This first scan was taken soon after the child's arrival in the emergency department. The epidural hematoma (blood) is visible as a white density in the patient's right temporal area (visible on the top left side of this image). The lateral ventricles and third ventricles are partially visible as dark densities at the midline and on either side of the midline of this image. **B,** This second scan was obtained 2 hours later when the child's level of consciousness deteriorated. The child's right pupil dilated and reacted sluggishly to light. The image is at the same level as image **A** and now shows a much larger epidural hematoma (white density on patient's right side). The lateral ventricles and third ventricle are almost completely obliterated as the result of compression from the expanding epidural hematoma. This child required urgent surgical intervention. (Images courtesy of Thomas Abramo, Nashville, TN.)

of the child with head injury and increased intracranial pressure, see Chapter 11.

If spine trauma is suspected, hypotension persists, and hypovolemia and pericardial tamponade have been ruled out, then neurogenic shock may be present. Neurogenic shock results from a spinal cord injury that produces loss of autonomic (sympathetic nervous system) tone and results in vasodilation and hypotension (see below).[25]

The most consistent indicators of poor prognosis following closed head injury in children include flaccid paralysis and

Table 19-7 Modified Glasgow Coma Scale for Infants and Children

	Child	Infant	Score
Eye opening	Spontaneous	Spontaneous	4
	To verbal stimuli	To verbal stimuli	3
	To pain only	To pain only	2
	No response	No response	1
Verbal response	Oriented, appropriate	Coos and babbles	5
	Confused	Irritable cries	4
	Inappropriate words	Cries to pain	3
	Incomprehensible words or nonspecific sounds	Moans to pain	2
	No response	No response	1
Motor response	Obeys commands (e.g., child holds up two fingers, wiggles toes or sticks out tongue)*	Moves spontaneously and purposefully	6
	Localizes painful stimulus (e.g., child reaches for hand that is rubbing sternum or pinching trapezius)*	Withdraws to touch	5
	Withdraws in response to pain (e.g., child adducts each extremity when medial aspect is pinched)*	Withdraws in response to pain	4
	Flexion in response to pain (i.e., decorticate posturing when sternum rubbed or trapezius muscle pinched)*	Decorticate posturing (abnormal flexion) in response to pain	3
	Extension in response to pain (i.e., decerebrate posturing when sternum rubbed or trapezius muscle pinched)*	Decerebrate posturing (abnormal extension) in response to pain	2
	No response (flaccid)	No response (flaccid)	1
TOTAL			**3-15**

Modified from Tasker RC: Head and spinal cord trauma. In Nichols DG, editor: *Rodgers' textbook of pediatric intensive care*, 4th ed, Philadelphia, 2008, Lippincott Williams & Wilkins; Originally proposed in Morray JP, et al: Coma scale for use in brain-injured children. *Crit Care Med* 12:1018, 1984.
*Additions in parentheses were added to scale by the Chapter 11 authors (LM Milonovich, V Eichler) and editor (MF Hazinski).

fixed, dilated pupils despite the restoration of satisfactory perfusion. Other poor prognostic indicators include the development of diabetes insipidus at or soon after admission (often indicates cessation of pituitary function), cardiovascular instability unrelated to hemorrhage, and disseminated intravascular coagulation. Brain injury results in the release of fibrinogen; severe head injury can result in substantial fibrinogen release and disseminated intravascular coagulation.[3] Concentrations of some combinations of biomarkers of brain injury may predict poor outcome from head trauma, although research in this area continues to evolve.[6,24]

If a devastating neurologic injury is present and brain death is diagnosed or imminent, the family should be asked about organ donation. The request should be made in accordance with local protocols, which can vary by jurisdiction. For further information, see Brain Death in Chapter 11; see also Chapter 3.

Neck and Spine

If the child has a mechanism of injury that is likely to cause spine injury or if the child has head or neck trauma, then providers should immobilize the cervical and thoracic spine as a precautionary measure. Once the child's condition has been stabilized, further evaluation is warranted to determine whether spinal cord injury can be ruled out.

If the child has a mechanism of injury that is consistent with possible spinal cord injury, has neurologic signs of spinal cord injury, or is comatose or hypotensive without neurologic signs, then the extrication collar should remain in place until spinal cord injury is ruled out; this requires a combination of clinical assessment, cervical spine radiographs, CT scan, and possibly an MRI (Fig. 19-7).[23]

It is difficult to rule out cervical spinal cord injury solely on the basis of anteroposterior and lateral radiographs and CT scans, because many children experience spinal cord injuries that are not associated with abnormalities in standard radiographs and CT scans.[3,23,42a] Historically, a complete radiographic cervical spine series includes anteroposterior and lateral cervical spine radiographs and oblique and odontoid views.[32,69]

In adults, the CT scan has largely replaced radiographs for evaluation of the cervical spine, particularly in obtunded patients,[33] but similar comparison data have not been published for children.[23] Cervical spine subluxation or vertebral fracture can be identified with CT scan, and the combination of spine radiographs and limited CT scan of the occiput to the third cervical spine can increase identification of cervical spine injuries in obtunded or young children.[21,23]

In many centers, a screening trauma CT scan ("traumagram") can be performed in less than 10 minutes. This screening scan consists of a CT of the head, neck, chest, abdomen, and pelvis using a rapid scanner that requires no repositioning of the child or transport to different rooms in the radiology department. MRI also can be helpful, but is not feasible in the evaluation of the patient in an unstable condition; it will be performed if clinical findings suggest the presence of a cervical spine injury.

If the child is awake and oriented, the presence of neck or back pain is suggestive of vertebral injury.[23,69] The National Emergency X-Radiography Utilization Study Group

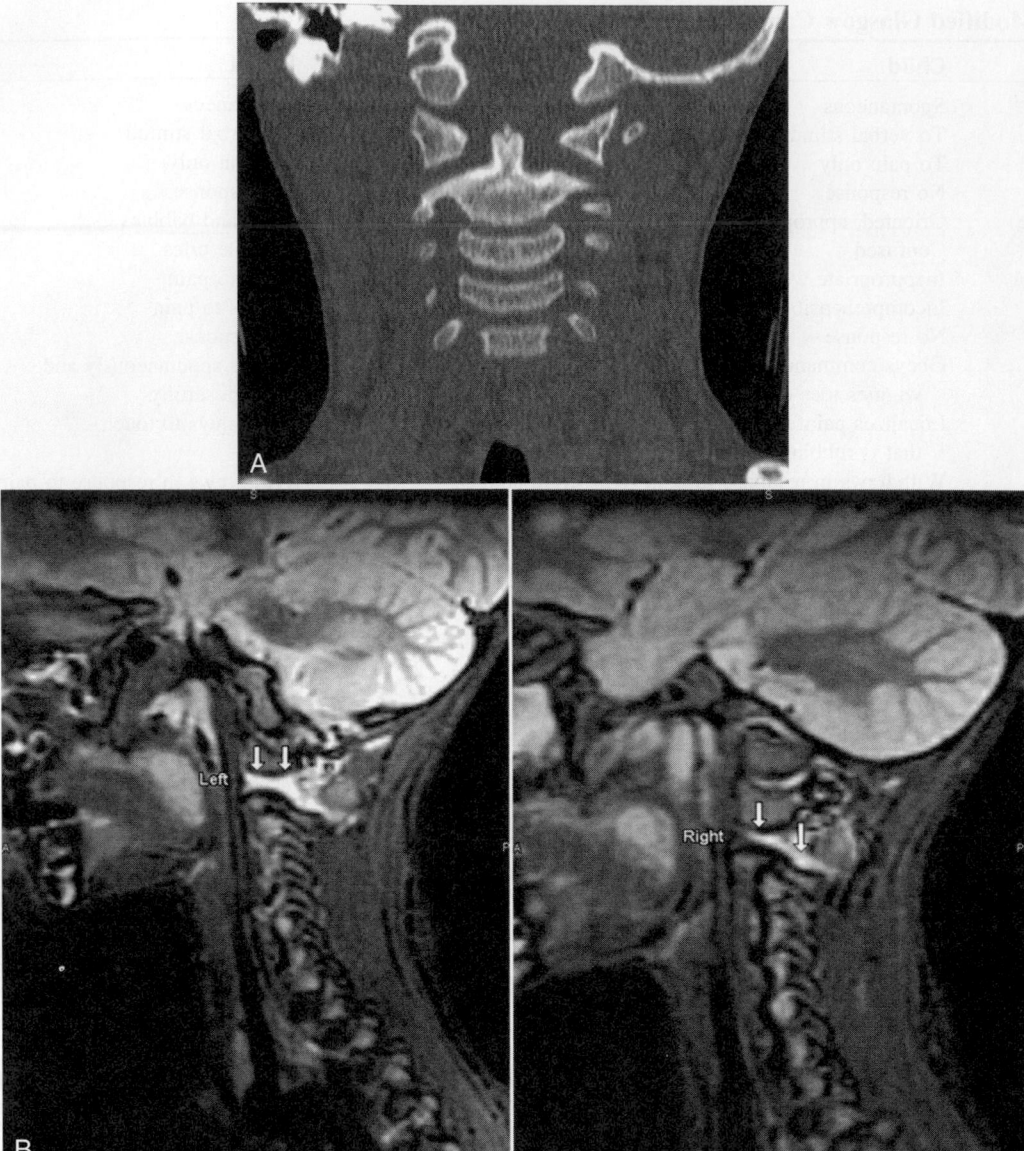

FIG. 19-7 Computed tomography (CT) and magnetic resonance image (MRI) to detect cervical spine injury in a child. **A,** Coronal CT from a 4-year-old girl who was an unrestrained passenger in a motor vehicle crash shows widening of the bilateral atlantoaxial joints. **B,** Sagittal MRI short T1-weighted inversion recovery images show signal changes within the bilateral atlantoaxial joints (*arrows*) and within the right occipitoatlantal joint (*arrows*). MRI confirmed that the transverse ligament was intact (not shown). (From Gore PA, Chang S, Theodore N: Cervical spine injuries in children: attention to radiographic differences and stability compared to those in the adult patient. *Semin Pediatr Neurol* 16:42-58, 2009.)

developed a decision instrument of clinical criteria to rule out cervical spine injuries in patients with blunt trauma (Box 19-6)[32] that performed well in a multicenter trial involving more than 3000 children. However, the study authors recommended caution in interpreting the results because there were fewer than 90 infants and toddlers in the study.[69]

At some trauma centers, the extrication collar is left in place until the child is sufficiently awake to respond when providers check for tenderness during movement. If the child remains comatose for a long time, the cervical spine is screened using an MRI, and the collar is removed if the MRI is interpreted as normal. The child with no tenderness plus a normal MRI or a normal neurologic examination is unlikely

to have a cervical spine injury and so is unlikely to produce a secondary injury with spontaneous movement.

If clinical findings or the mechanism of injury suggest the likelihood of a lower spine injury, then thoracic, lumbar, and sacral spinal films and CT scan are indicated. Lap belt bruising should raise the possibility of a Chance fracture, caused by flexion against the lap belt with resultant distraction injury to the lumbar spine (see Abdomen, below).

Chest

As noted previously, children have softer, more compliant rib cages than do adults. Therefore rib fractures are relatively uncommon, occurring in one third or less of children with blunt trauma.

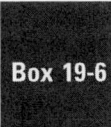

Box 19-6

Clinical Criteria to Help Rule Out Cervical Spine Injury in Children: Modified National Emergency X-Radiography Utilization Study Group (NEXUS) Criteria[23,32,69]

If *all five* of the following clinical indicators are met, the likelihood of cervical spine injury in the child with blunt trauma is low. These criteria were shown to be valid in a multicenter study of nearly 3000 injured children 2-18 years old.[69] Use caution in application for infants and toddlers (few infants and toddlers were evaluated in the multicenter study).
1. Absence of tenderness at the posterior midline of the cervical spine
2. Absence of neurologic abnormality (e.g., focal neurologic deficits)
3. Absence of altered level of consciousness or intubation
4. Absence of intoxication
5. Absence of clinically apparent pain that might distract the patient from the pain of cervical spine injury (i.e., absence of distracting injury or pain)

Additional criteria: ability to communicate verbally[23]

Severe intrathoracic injury may be present despite the absence of rib or sternal fractures or other manifestations of abnormality on external examination.[3,13] However, thorough chest inspection and palpation should reveal obvious signs of injury. The nurse may note chest asymmetry associated with respiratory effort or caused by rib fractures. Careful auscultation should identify localized alteration in the intensity or pitch of breath sounds; pulmonary edema may cause crackles and hypoxemia.

Chest radiographs, including anteroposterior and lateral films, should be performed on any child with severe injury to the chest or torso.[13] CT scans may provide additional information and detail, particularly to evaluate airway abnormalities and fluid collections. A pulmonary contusion will produce localized opacification of the lung (see Fig. 19-4) and increased density on the CT scan.

Although rare, cardiac contusions may be present in any child with a history of blunt thoracic trauma. Clinical signs include chest pain, arrhythmias, and myocardial dysfunction. The child may have a new murmur or evidence of congestive heart failure, including systemic and pulmonary edema and a gallop rhythm. The diagnosis is made by evaluating cardiac isoenzymes, a 12-lead ECG, and an echocardiogram.[4]

The cardiac troponin complex consists of three troponins (C, I, and T) that are involved in the interaction of the actin and myosin filaments in cardiac muscle.[37] These troponins are normally present only in cardiac muscle, and their levels will rise with cardiac necrosis (death of heart muscle) and myocardial injury. In adults, concentrations of troponins I and T are monitored to determine the presence of an acute coronary syndrome; elevation of troponins I and T can be more sensitive indicators of myocardial injury than elevation of the creatinine kinase myocardial band (CK-MB).[37] Although troponin concentrations are normally negligible in children, they are often elevated after cardiac contusion. It is important to note that not all children with cardiac contusion

demonstrate elevation of troponins, and troponins may be elevated by conditions other than cardiac contusions.[30]

ECG signs of a cardiac contusion may include atrial or ventricular arrhythmias (uncommon) or S-T segment depression or elevation, which may be confused with myocardial ischemia. The echocardiogram may detect abnormalities of contraction and wall motion.

Treatment of cardiac contusion is primarily supportive and includes careful fluid titration to optimize cardiac preload, support of myocardial function with inotropes (e.g., dobutamine), and manipulation of afterload (e.g., using vasodilators or vasopressors). Providers should be alert for the sudden development of arrhythmias such as ventricular tachycardia or fibrillation, and they should be prepared to treat them.

Abdomen

Hemorrhage from thoracoabdominal injuries is a leading cause of traumatic death in pediatric victims, as are head injury and complications of airway and ventilation.[4,54a] Children do not often have penetrating abdominal injuries; blunt abdominal trauma accounts for the vast majority of pediatric abdominal injuries.

Providers should examine the child carefully to identify both overt and subtle signs of intraabdominal injuries. Fifteen percent of injured children with negative abdominal examinations are subsequently found to have significant intraabdominal injuries, even in the presence of normal mental status and vital signs.[4,13]

Signs of abdominal hemorrhage are difficult to detect in the comatose patient or one with spinal cord injury and loss of abdominal sensation. In these patients, additional evaluation and diagnostic studies are needed. Emergency ultrasound and FAST are now the diagnostic tools of choice for unstable (particularly those who are obtunded) patients, because they can be performed at the bedside as often as necessary, without radiation exposure or the need to transport the patient. With these devices, free fluid or blood (i.e., hemoperitoneum) appears black against the gray of organs.[42] FAST scans have a higher specificity (i.e., when fluid is observed, the child has intraabdominal bleeding) than sensitivity (i.e., children can have organ injury without detection of free fluid or blood in the abdomen). Therefore FAST is often used in conjunction with the CT scan to detect intraabdominal bleeding in children with trauma and hypotension.[42]

A CT scan will usually reveal the presence of significant injury (see below). As noted above, a screening trauma CT scan can be performed in many medical centers in less than 10 min. The CT series includes scans of the head, neck, chest, abdomen, and pelvis using a rapid scanner that requires no repositioning of the child or transport to different rooms in the radiology department. Peritoneal lavage is rarely used in children because it is not as accurate as the use of FAST or a CT scan. In addition, it will create a painful site that complicates later assessment of abdominal tenderness.[4]

Injuries resulting from improperly positioned lap belts frequently produce abdominal ecchymosis and bruising (Fig. 19-8). If the lap belt was positioned across the lower abdomen and not over the pelvis, the bruising may indicate the possibility of intestinal and lumbar spine injury (Fig. 19-9).[55,66]

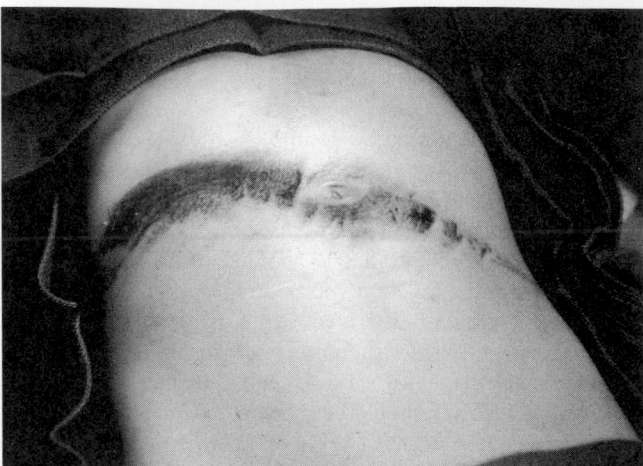

FIG. 19-8 Lap belt contusion. This contusion should raise suspicion of abdominal injury and lumbar spine injury (Chance fracture). This child had a small intestinal injury and a Chance fracture with resulting paraplegia. (Courtesy John B. Pietsch, Nashville, TN.)

Any visible bruising on the abdomen should raise the suspicion of an intraabdominal injury.[43] The bruise itself makes it more difficult to examine the conscious child, because the bruise will cause abdominal wall tenderness that is difficult to distinguish from tenderness associated with intraabdominal injury. Pain itself may be difficult to evaluate. The severity of pain does not necessarily correlate with the severity of abdominal injury.

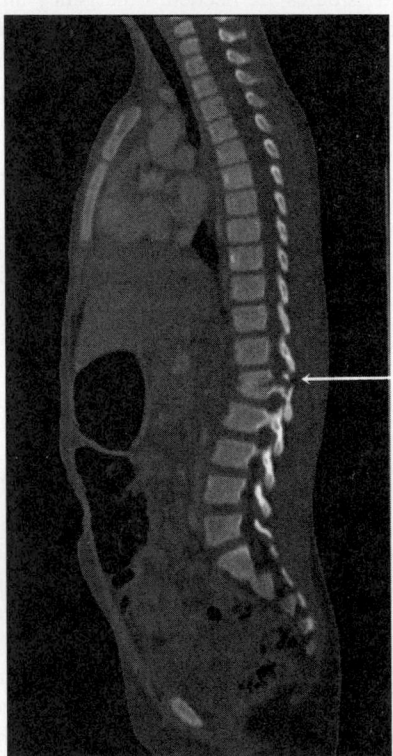

FIG. 19-9 Chance fracture of first lumbar vertebra. This fracture resulted from hyperflexion of the child over a lap belt during a high-speed automobile collision. (Courtesy John B. Pietsch, Nashville, TN.)

Progressive abdominal distension is one of the first signs of major abdominal injury, so measurement of the abdominal girth, especially in infants and young children, may be helpful. Pain and abdominal distension will reduce the child's effective tidal volume and ventilation, altering the child's respiratory rate, respiratory effort, and chest expansion (Box 19-7). Unilateral splinting of respirations with or without evidence of rib fracture is an indication for liver and spleen scans.[58] Additional high-risk variables, in addition to abdominal tenderness and systolic hypotension, found to be sensitive for radiographically confirmed intraabdominal injury in children after blunt torso trauma include: femur fracture, elevated liver enzymes, microscopic hematuria, and an initial hematocrit less than 30% (see Box 19-7); however, these variables were not specific for intraabdominal injury.[34]

Signs of splenic or hepatic injury include tachycardia, hypotension, and abdominal tenderness. The splenic injury will be apparent on a CT scan (Fig. 19-10). Splenic injury can cause a positive Kehr's sign (referred pain to the left shoulder during compression of the left upper quadrant) and leukocytosis.[13]

Box 19-7	**Physical Findings Suggestive of Abdominal Injury**

Physical Signs
- Rapid, shallow breathing
- Abdominal tenderness (high-risk variable*)
- Flank or abdominal mass, contusion, or wound
- Increasing abdominal girth
- Blood in the urethral meatus, hematuria (NOTE: Microscopic hematuria with more than five RBCs per high-powered field is high-risk variable*)
- Inability to void
- Genital swelling or discoloration
- Referred shoulder pain with upper abdominal palpation:
  ∘ Right shoulder pain—hepatic injury
  ∘ Left shoulder pain—splenic injury
- Systolic hypotension (high-risk variable*)

Injuries Frequently Associated with Abdominal Injury
- Fractured lower ribs
- Penetrating trauma to the lower chest
- Pelvic fracture
- Multisystem trauma sustained during motor vehicle accident
- Femur fracture (high-risk variable*)

Laboratory Results
- Elevated serum transaminases may indicate hepatic injury (high-risk variable*):
  ∘ Serum alanine aminotransferase greater than 125 U/L
  ∘ Serum aspartate aminotransferase greater than 200 U/L
- Elevated serum amylase (pancreatic, small bowel injury)
- Leukocytosis (may be nonspecific sign of stress or splenic trauma)
- Initial hematocrit less than 30% (high-risk variable*)

*Six "high-risk" variables in children with blunt torso trauma were found to be sensitive for radiographically-confirmed intra-abdominal trauma but not very specific for such trauma.

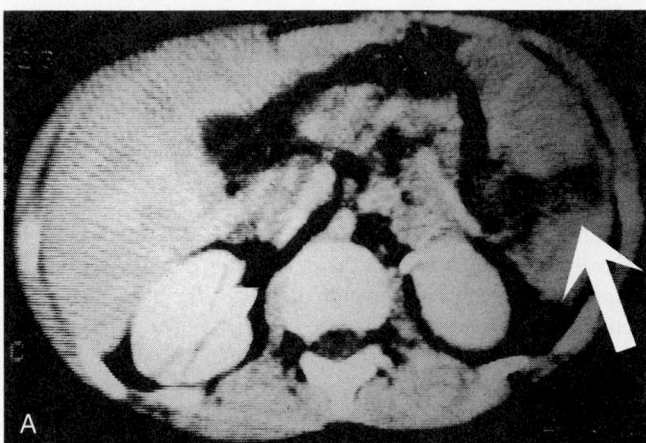

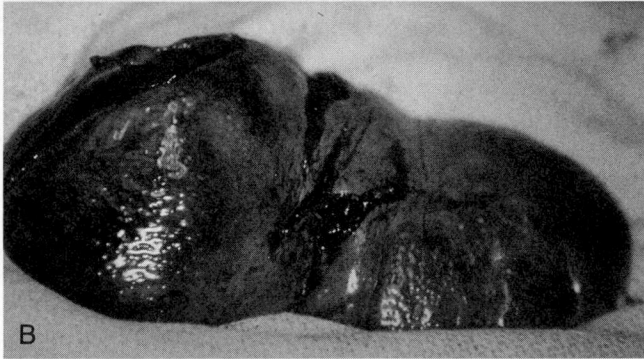

FIG. 19-10 Splenic injury. **A,** Computed tomography scan reveals splenic laceration visible on the patient's left side (*white arrow* on right side of the image). As in all CT scans, the view is from below and the patient's right side is on the left of this image and the patient's left side is on the right side of the image. The front of the patient's abdomen is at the top of the image and the patient's back is at the bottom of the image. **B,** Spleen after splenectomy in the operating room. Three large lacerations are visible, and a large contusion causes discoloration seen on the left side of the photograph. (Courtesy John B. Pietsch, Nashville, TN.)

Hepatic trauma (Fig. 19-11) can cause referred right shoulder pain instead of Kehr's sign or left shoulder pain.[13] Most significant hepatic injury will result in elevation of the serum transaminases (aspartate aminotransferase greater than 200 International Units/L and alanine aminotransferase greater than 125 International Units/L).[28]

Further evaluation for abdominal injury includes a thorough rectal examination to rule out the presence of blood within the rectum, to assess sphincter tone, and to ensure that there has been no disruption of the lower urinary tract. Absence of sphincter tone can indicate spinal cord injury.

The pediatric patient with a history of blunt trauma requires close observation. The nurse should obtain frequent vital signs and must be able to recognize signs of pain and subtle signs of deterioration in systemic perfusion. If the patient's condition is unstable, continuous nursing care and medical supervision is necessary during all phases of transport and testing. Notify the physician or other on-call provider immediately if the patient's condition deteriorates. Appropriate resuscitation equipment should always be readily available. Occasionally, a follow-up CT scan is useful if the initial scan is not diagnostic and the child is not improving (e.g., the child may have intestinal injury).

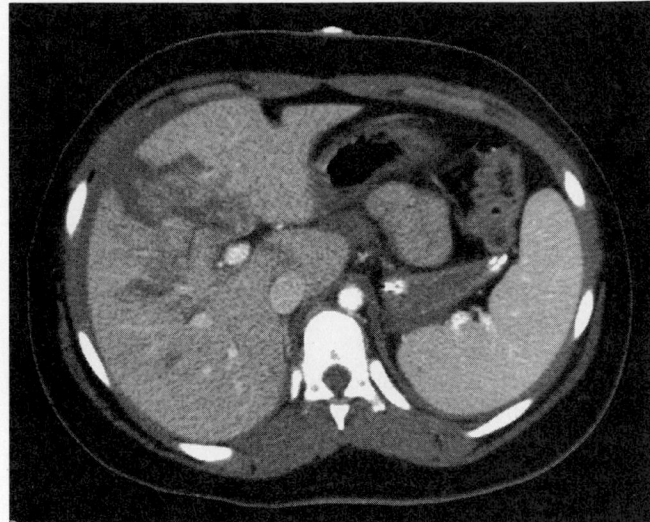

FIG. 19-11 Computed tomography scan image of liver laceration showing disruption of the capsule of the right lobe. Bleeding from the liver injury (dark gray density) extends from the liver injury to the surface of the liver, separating the liver from the abdominal wall. As in all CT scans, the view is from below and the patient's right side is on the left of this image and the patient's left side is on the right of the image. The front of the patient's abdomen is at the top of the image and the patient's back is at the bottom of the image. (Courtesy Thomas Abramo, Nashville, TN.)

Conservative management of splenic, hepatic, or renal contusions and lacerations includes supportive care and close observation in a PCCU. Typically, bleeding from such lacerations has ceased by the time the child arrives at the hospital, and these organs often will heal without intervention.[4] If conservative management is provided, the child's systemic perfusion must be monitored closely.

Surgical intervention is required in the presence of ongoing hemorrhage, hemodynamic instability (including the need for excessive fluid administration to maintain blood pressure and perfusion), hollow viscous perforation, or catastrophic organ injury.[31] In hemodynamically stable patients, surgical exploration can be accomplished through laprascopy.[64]

When surgical intervention is required, the injured organ is often repaired rather than removed (see Evolve Fig. 19-3, A and B in the Chapter 19 Supplement on the Evolve Website for color surgical photographs of splenic injury and lap belt injury to the intestine). Removal of the injured spleen, liver lobe, or kidney usually is required only for devastating injury or if the organ is separated from its vascular supply.

Genitourinary Trauma

Genitourinary trauma is seldom life threatening. However, injured children are more prone to renal injuries than injured adults, because the kidneys are less well protected by muscle, ribs, and fat. Hematuria, abdominal pain, and flank hematomas are all signs of renal injury.[13] The presence of threadlike clots in the urethra is a pathognomonic finding indicative of renal injury, and the amount of hematuria correlates well with the severity of renal trauma.[62]

Although insertion of a urinary catheter is routine during trauma resuscitation, a catheter should not be inserted in the trauma victim if frank blood is observed in the urinary meatus.

Such blood often is caused by urethral disruption and is a contraindication to urinary catheter insertion.[41] The presence of blood in the urinary meatus indicates the need for a retrograde urethrogram and urologic consultation.[8a] Severe renal injury with separation of the kidney from the urethra may not be associated with hematuria; these patients will demonstrate evidence of extravasation of urine that will be detected by a CT scan.

Bladder rupture should be suspected if any degree of hematuria is detected in the child with a pelvic fracture. A cystogram is indicated to rule out bladder injury.[8a]

Extremities

Extremities should be observed for tenderness, deformity, swelling, pallor, coolness, and decreased peripheral pulses. Subtle fractures can be missed during initial resuscitative management, but they should be detected during the secondary survey.

Long bone fractures and pelvic fractures can produce significant blood loss, especially in older children. When a pelvic fracture is suspected, the trauma team should assess the integrity of other structures within the pelvis, including the urethra, bladder, and pelvic vessels. Disruption of pelvic vessels can cause rapid and severe blood loss.[4]

Compartment Syndrome

Compartment syndrome occurs when external forces compress an area of muscle, or when bleeding or edema increase pressure within the compartment that is created by sheaths of fascia surrounding the muscle bundle and related nerves and vessels. As the pressure within the compartment rises, vascular supply to the muscle and tissue is compromised and ischemic and nerve damage may develop.[52]

Although compartment syndrome is uncommon in children, it may complicate any skeletomuscular injury; the tissues most often involved following trauma are the lower legs and the forearms. Compartment syndrome may also develop following a burn injury.

Signs of compartment syndrome include pain that worsens with movement, edema, altered movement and sensation, and decreased perfusion (cooling of the extremity with decreased intensity of the pulses); these can be recalled by considering the "five P's": *p*ain, *p*allor, *p*ulselessness, *p*aresthesia, and *p*aralysis.[4,52] A sixth *P* can be added—*p*uffiness.[63] Specific clinical findings associated with involvement of the major compartments are listed in Table 19-8. A physician or other on-call provider should be notified immediately if signs of compartment syndrome develop, because urgent surgical intervention may be needed.

Bedside Doppler ultrasound examination can be used to evaluate blood flow. If the pressure in the compartment is measured, a pressure exceeding 40 cm H_2O is considered an indication for surgical intervention (i.e., fasciotomy), but normal pressures and pressure thresholds are not well established in children.[60]

Treatment of compartment syndrome requires surgical release of the restriction surrounding the muscle. A fasciotomy is performed and the area is left open, but covered with a sterile dressing, and may require later skin grafting (see, also, Chapter 20).[52]

Skin

During initial stabilization of the trauma victim, visibility of some areas of skin will be compromised by pressure dressings. Once the primary survey and stabilization have been accomplished, the undressed pediatric patient should be examined carefully for the presence of other injuries, including contusions and burns. If burns are present, the trauma team should plan fluid resuscitation based on the estimated burn depth and extent. For information about burns, refer to Chapter 20.

Most fire-related deaths result from smoke inhalation, and the most common cause of death during the first hour after burn injury is respiratory failure.[2] A history of closed space confinement should lead to evaluation for the presence of carbon monoxide poisoning. The child should be inspected for

Table 19-8 Clinical Signs and Symptoms Associated with Compartment Syndrome

Compartment	Location of Sensory Changes	Painful Passive Movement	Weakened Movement	Location of Pain or Tenseness
Lower Leg				
Anterior	First web space	Toe extension	Toe flexion	Along lateral side of anterior tibia
Lateral	Dorsum (top) of foot	Foot eversion	Foot inversion	Lateral lower leg
Superficial posterior	None	Foot plantar flexion	Foot dorsiflexion	Calf
Deep posterior	Sole of foot	Toe flexion	Toe extension	Deep calf—palpable between Achilles tendon and medial malleoli
Forearm				
Volar	Volar (palmar) aspect of fingers	Wrist and finger flexion	Wrist and finger extension	Volar forearm
Dorsal	None	Wrist and finger extension	Wrist and finger flexion	Dorsal forearm
Hand				
Intraosseous	None	Finger adduction and abduction	Finger adduction and abduction	Between metacarpals on dorsum of hand

From Proehl JA: Compartment syndrome. *J Emerg Nurs* 14:283, 1988.

(1) singed eyebrows and nose hair, (2) dark sputum, (3) carbon deposits and inflammatory changes in the mouth, (4) cyanosis and dyspnea, and (5) altered level of consciousness. Initial treatment includes oxygen administration and close observation for deteriorating respiratory status. Note that carboxyhemoglobin is not detected by a pulse oximeter, so pulse oximetry will be falsely high in the presence of carbon monoxide poisoning (see Pulmonary Injuries in Chapter 20).

HISTORY

Once the patient's condition is stable, providers should ask the parent and (as age appropriate) the patient about the child's medical history, including allergies, past illnesses, and current medications. Additional information required includes events leading up to the injury, mechanism of injury, status at the scene, location and degree of pain, last meal, and changes in patient status during initial stabilization and transport.

The Advisory Committee on Immunization Practices recommends administering a tetanus booster every 10 years. Clean, minor wounds do not require prophylaxis unless the patient has not received tetanus toxoid in more than 10 years or the history is unknown.[39] If the wound is tetanus prone, prophylaxis is recommended if the tetanus toxoid was administered longer than 5 years before the injury. The Surgical Infection Society recommends administration of 25 IU tetanus prophylaxis if the wound is tetanus prone (e.g., from a bite) and if the patient is elderly, immunocompromised, or has not completed the tetanus vaccination regimen. For children a dose of 4 IU/kg is recommended.[35]

INTENTIONAL INJURIES/INFLICTED TRAUMA

Definition and Epidemiology

Intentional injuries are inflicted injuries (e.g., child abuse) or injuries that occur as a result of neglect. In the United States it is estimated that 1% or more of all children are abused or neglected, and approximately 4000 children die annually as victims of abuse.[57]

The term *child abuse* applies to any maltreatment of a child, including infliction of physical injuries, sexual exploitation, infliction of emotional pain, or neglect. Child abuse usually is not a random, isolated act of violence, but rather a pattern of maladjusted behavior. The three components of the child abuse syndrome include the maladjusted adult, the vulnerable child, and the presence of situational stressors.[65] For more information, refer to Intentional Injury/Inflicted Trauma; Definition and Epidemiology in the Chapter 19 Supplement on the Evolve Website.

History of Injuries Suggesting Intentional Injuries (Inflicted Trauma)

It is estimated that as many as 10% of children younger than 5 years who are seen in EDs with traumatic injuries have inflicted injuries.[57] Healthcare workers must be vigilant in attempting to detect evidence of abuse and are obligated to report suspected abuse to the local child protective agency.[9]

Explanations for traumatic injuries that should be questioned include unknown injury, implausible sequence of events, self-inflicted injury, or sibling-inflicted injury. Any injury followed by a delay in seeking medical care is suspicious. Finally, when a child or a spouse names an adult as the cause of the injuries, the accusation usually is true.[57]

Characteristics of Injuries Suggestive of Intentional Injury

Implausible injuries are those that are inconsistent with the history. For example, if a child allegedly sustained multiple bruises when falling down the stairs, bruises will most likely be located over bony prominences; bruises will rarely appear over soft tissues. If a head injury occurs when the child falls out of bed, usually a single lump is present, and the skull is not fractured. Although small linear skull fractures may occur with minor falls, loss of consciousness and multiple bruises are inconsistent with a simple fall.[57]

Suspicious bruises are located on the buttocks, inside of the child's legs, over the cheeks or flanks, near the upper lip or inside of the mouth, and around the neck. Any bruises or lacerations near the genitals should be examined carefully and investigated. Bilateral black eyes, retinal hemorrhages, detached retina, and traumatic cataracts usually are inflicted injuries.

The marks of injury can be characteristic of the method or instrument of injury. Human hand marks often can be identified, and bite marks can be used to confirm the identity of the abuser. Marks from belt buckles or hair brushes may be identifiable.

Inflicted burns may be splash burns, hot water immersion burns, or branding. Inflicted splash burns may be difficult to distinguish from unintentional burns. Hot water immersion burns usually have circumscribed borders. If the hands or feet are immersed, the burns may resemble the areas covered by gloves or socks, respectively. If the child's buttocks are dunked in the water, a characteristic V burn will be associated with the water level on the back and thighs. Irregular margins consistent with splashing or movement by the child will be notably absent, indicating that the child was held in the water. Branding burns usually will reflect the shape of the hot object, which may include a pan, a hot radiator, a cigarette tip, or a cigarette lighter.

Subdural hematomas are among the most common results of inflicted head injury in children. Many subdural hematomas are associated with skull fracture, and some may be associated with retinal hemorrhage (the shaken baby syndrome). Scalp bruises and traumatic alopecia also may be observed in these victims.[57]

Inflicted head trauma[12] (formerly called *shaken baby syndrome*) is the term used to encompass the spectrum of inflicted head injuries, including associated cerebral, spinal, and cranial injuries and their complications. The trauma can result from the combination of vigorous shaking of the child associated with the application of force (e.g., the child is shaken and struck or is shaken while being held against a mattress in bed). However, injuries can also result from blunt head trauma and may be associated with spinal cord injury or hypoxia.[12] These injuries include the primary injury as well as secondary injuries such as hypoxia, ischemia, increased intracranial pressure, and long-term complications including seizures, developmental delay, and other disabilities.[12]

Signs of inflicted head trauma include retinal hemorrhages and subarachnoid hemorrhage documented by cerebrospinal fluid examination and a CT scan. Additional injuries include brainstem and spinal cord hematoma, subdural hematoma or cerebral contusion, and spinal cord injuries.[12]

Intentional injuries should also be considered if the child has shock that does not respond to conventional therapy. For example, if the child exhibits shock and has a history of vomiting and diarrhea or a nonspecific history, and the child's perfusion and level of consciousness do not improve with adequate hydration, then other causes of shock should be considered, such as intraabdominal injury (Fig. 19-12).

Responsibilities of the Healthcare Team

The first priority in the care of the abused child is providing necessary resuscitation and support of cardiopulmonary function. In addition, the child must be protected from further abuse, and both the child and the family must receive compassionate emotional support. The parents may not have injured the child, but they are likely to feel guilty that they left the child in the care of someone who hurt the child.

The trauma team should carefully document the size, shape, and color of all injuries, but the recording should not interfere with or delay the resuscitation. If possible, color photographs of the child should be taken as soon as possible after the child's arrival, but this should not delay the institution of appropriate care.

A thorough examination is required to identify all current injuries and evidence of healed injuries. A skeletal series of radiographs and possibly a bone scan will be performed to

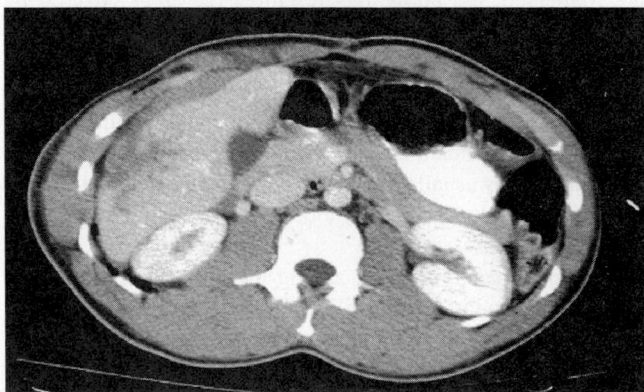

FIG. 19-12 Inflicted liver laceration. This standard computed tomography (CT) scan was obtained in a 21-month-old infant who was brought to the ED with a history of vomiting and diarrhea. He also had unusual bruising to his abdomen and abdominal distension. A standard abdominal CT with contrast confirmed the presence of liver and pancreatic injuries. The CT scan provides an image similar to that achieved by looking up at a cross-section of the abdomen, with the child's liver on the patient's right (but on the left side of this image). The front of the child's abdomen is depicted at the top of the image, and the child's back is depicted at the bottom of the image. The contrast appears white in the kidneys and the aorta. The dark grey, irregular shape on the outer edge of the liver is the liver laceration; the lighter grey density is the liver itself. Additional views of the abdominal CT scan demonstrated free fluid in the abdomen and a linear pancreatic defect consistent with a pancreatic laceration. (Image courtesy of Cristina Estrada, Nashville, TN.)

identify healed fractures. Levels of biologic markers of head injury can be determined from blood or cerebral spinal fluid and can assist in the identification of head injury when inflicted trauma is suggested in the child without neurologic symptoms.[6] These markers can also be useful for monitoring the child's response to therapy and for predicting outcome of the head injury.[24]

Suspected abuse must be reported to the local child protective service agency, and nurses must be familiar with the hospital policy and the sequence. The child abuse team is often the first and best contact and can advise the nurse and the entire team regarding documentation. The report to the local child protective service agency ultimately must be in writing, although an initial telephone contact may be acceptable. The child protective agency usually will arrange that temporary custody of the child be awarded to the hospital or to the state. The healthcare team must be aware of this custody information, because the child's custodian must provide permission for any elective surgery or procedures for the duration of the custody order.

If a child abuse team is present in the hospital, they should be consulted about the proper recording of injuries and documentation of parental statements. This team also is experienced in examining abused children and frequently will identify additional injuries that may be related to abuse.[40]

TRANSITION FROM THE PEDIATRIC CRITICAL CARE UNIT AFTER INJURIES

The transition from the PCCU to an acute care unit may be stressful for the patient, family, and pediatric nurses. The patient and family generally have established a relationship with the PCCU staff that started at a time when the family mobilized defenses against feelings of helplessness and anger about the child's injuries. As the child's condition improves, the family's defenses may be dropped. Because it may still be uncomfortable for the family to express feelings of anger toward the child, they may instead redirect them toward the new staff.[53]

PCCU nurses can help to ease the transition to the acute care unit. The family and child probably became accustomed to the continuous care the child received in the PCCU. Obviously, the child is improving if discharge from the PCCU to an acute care unit is planned, but it may be frightening to the parents to lose the continuous presence of a nurse at the bedside. PCCU nurses who are involved with the family should emphasize that the care the family can give the child is of increasing importance to the child's recovery and that the decreased acuity of nursing and medical care indicates improvement in their child's condition.

LONG-TERM FOLLOW-UP

Relatively few pediatric trauma patients require inpatient treatment at a rehabilitation center. Most pediatric trauma victims are discharged to their homes and require minimal follow-up, usually one or two return outpatient visits. Some children require home health nurses, physical or occupational therapy, or outpatient services provided by either the acute-care or rehabilitation facility.[8]

The full effects of a head injury may not be apparent during hospitalization. In fact, many deficits related to a child's injury may be detected only after the child resumes activities of daily living. It is important that injured children receive regular follow-up examinations and evaluations. Telephone calls can be used to determine how well a child is recovering.

References

1. American Academy of Pediatrics: Management of pediatric trauma policy statement. *Pediatrics* 121:849–859, 2008.
2. American Academy of Pediatrics and American College of Emergency Physicians: Pediatric trauma. In *APLS: the pediatric emergency medicine resource*, ed 4, Sudbury, MA, 2006, Jones and Bartlett.
3. American College of Surgeons, Committee on Trauma. Advanced Trauma Life Support for Doctors. In *Extremes of Age: pediatric trauma*, ed 7, Chicago, 2004, American College of Surgeons, pp. 242–261.
4. Baird JS, Cooper A: Multiple trauma. In Nichols DG, editors: *Rogers' textbook of pediatric intensive care*, ed 4, Philadelphia, 2008, Lippincott, Williams and Wilkins.
5. Barkin R, Rosen P, editors: Spinal cord injuries. In *Emergency pediatrics*, ed 3, Mosby, 1990, St Louis.
6. Berger RP, et al: Multiplex assessment of serum biomarker concentrations in well appearing children with inflicted traumatic brain injury. *Pediatr Res* 65:97–102, 2009.
7. Borse NN, et al: *CDC childhood injury report: patterns of unintentional injuries among 0-19 year olds in the United States, 2000-2006*, Atlanta GA, 2008, Centers for Disease Control and Prevention, National Center for Injury Prevention and Control.
8. Brogan DR: Rehabilitation service needs: physicians perceptions and referrals. *Arch Phys Med Rehabil* 62:215, 1981, 1981.
8a. Brown RL, Garcia VF: Genitourinary trauma. In O'Neill J, Grossfeld JL, Coran AG, Fonkalsrud EW, editors: *Grossfeld: pediatric surgery*, ed 6, Mosby, 2006, Saint Louis, an imprint of Elsevier.
9. Carroll CA, Haase CC: The function of protective services in child abuse and neglect. In Heifer RE, Kempe RS, editors: *The battered child*, ed 4, Chicago, 1987, University of Chicago Press.
9a. Chameides L, Samson S, Schexnayder S, Hazinski MF, editors: *Pediatric advanced life support provider manual*, Dallas, 2011, American Heart Association.
10. Champion HR, Sacco WJ, Carnazzo AJ, et al: Trauma score. *Crit Care Med* 9:672, 1981.
11. Champion HR, Sacco WJ, Copes WS, et al: A revision of the Trauma Score. *J Trauma* 29:623–629, 1989.
12. Christian CW, Block R, Committee on Child Abuse and Neglect; American Academy of Pediatrics: Abusive head trauma in infants and children. *J Pediatrics* 123:1409–1411, 2009.
13. Cooper A, et al: Mortality and truncal injury: the pediatric perspective. *J Pediatr Surg* 29:33–38, 1994.
14. DeBoer S, et al: Intraosseous infusion: not just for kids anymore. *EMS Magazine*; March 2005.
15. Dowd MD, Bull M: Emergency medicine and injury prevention: meeting at the intersection. *Clin Ped Emerg Med* 4:83, 2003.
16. Emergency Cardiovascular Care Committee and American Heart Association: 2005 Guidelines for cardiopulmonary resuscitation and emergency cardiovascular care, Part 12: Pediatric advanced life support. *Circulation* 112:IV167–IV187, 2005.
17. Finkelstein EA, Corso PS, Miller TR: *Incidence and economic burden of injuries in the United States,* New York, 2006, Oxford University Press.
18. Fletcher SA, et al: The successful surgical removal of intracranial nasogastric tubes. *J Trauma* 27:948, 1987.
19. Garbarino J: Preventing childhood injury: developmental and mental health issues. *Am J Orthopsychiatry* 58:1, 1988.
20. Gardner HG: Office-based counseling for unintentional injury prevention. *Pediatrics* 119:202, 2008.
21. Garton HJ, Hammer MR: Detection of pediatric cervical spine injury. *Neurosurgery* 62:700–708, 2008.
22. Gausche M, Henderson DP, Seidel JP: Vital signs as part of the prehospital assessment of the pediatric patient: a survey of paramedics. *Ann Emerg Med* 19:173, 1990.
23. Gore PA, Chang S, Theodore N: Cervical spine injuries in children: attention to radiographic differences and stability compared to those in the adult patient. *Semin Pediatr Neurol* 16:42–58, 2009.
24. Guerguerian AM, Lo M, Hutchinson JS: Clinical management and functional neuromonitoring in traumatic brain injury in children. *Curr Opin Pediatr* 21:737–744, 2009.
25. Harris B, et al: The crucial hour. *Pediatr Ann* 16:4, 1987.
26. Hazinski MF, et al: Outcome of cardiovascular collapse in pediatric blunt trauma. *Ann Emerg Med* 201:1229–1235, 1994.
27. Hazinski MF, et al: Pediatric injury prevention. *Ann Emerg Med* 22:456, 1993.
28. Hennes HM, et al: Elevated liver transaminase levels in children with blunt abdominal trauma: a predictor of liver injury. *Pediatrics* 86:87, 1990.
29. Herzenberg JE, et al: Emergency transport and positioning of young children who have an injury of the cervical spine: the standard backboard may be hazardous. *J Bone Joint Surg Am* 71:15, 1989.
30. Hirsch R, et al: Cardiac troponin I in pediatrics: normal values and potential use in the assessment of cardiac injury. *J Pediatrics* 130:872–897, 1997.
31. Hoelzer DF, et al: Selection and nonoperative management of pediatric blunt trauma patients: the role of quantitative crystalloid resuscitation and abdominal ultrasonography. *J Trauma* 26:57, 1986.
32. Hoffman JR, et al: Validity of a set of clinical criteria to rule out injury to the cervical spine in patients with blunt trauma. *N Engl J Med* 343:94–99, 2000.
33. Holmes JF, Akkinepalli R: Computed tomography versus plain radiography to screen for cervical spine injury: a meta-analysis. *J Trauma* 58:902–905, 2005.
34. Holmes JF, et al: Validation of a prediction rule for the identification of children with intra-abdominal injuries after blunt torso trauma. *Ann Emerg Med* 54:528–533, 2009.
35. Howdieshell TR, Heffernan D, Dipiro JT: Surgical infection society guidelines for vaccination after traumatic injury. *Surg Infect* 7:275–291, 2006.
36. James H, Anas N, Perkin RM: *Brain insults in infants and children,* New York, 1985, Grune and Stratton.
37. Kanaan UB, Chiang VW: Cardiac troponins in pediatrics. *Pediatr Emerg Care* 20:323–329, 2004.
38. Kaufman CR, et al: Evaluation of the pediatric trauma score. *J Am Med Assoc* 263:69, 1990.
38a. Kleinman ME, Chameides L, Schexnayder SM, Samson RA, Hazinski MF, Atkins DL, Berg MD, de Caen AR, Fink EL, Freid EB, Hickey RW, Marino BS, Nadkarni VM, Proctor LT, Qureshi FA, Sartorelli K, Topjian A, van der Jagt EW, Zaritsky AL: Part 14: pediatric advanced life support: 2010 American Heart Association guidelines for cardiopulmonary resuscitation and emergency cardiovascular care. *Circulation* 122(18 Suppl 3):S876–S908, 2010.
39. Kretzinger K, et al: Preventing tetanus, diphtheria and pertussis among adults: use of tetanus toxoid, reduced diphtheria toxoid and acellular pertussis vaccine. *Morbid Mortal Weekly Rep* 55(R17):1–33, 2006.
40. Krugman R: The assessment process of a child protection team. In Heifer RE, Kempe RS, editors: *The battered child*, ed 4, Chicago, 1987, The University of Chicago Press.
41. Kuppermann N, et al: Identification of children at very low risk of clinically-important brain injuries after head trauma: a prospective cohort study. *Lancet* 374:1127, 2009.
42. Levy JA, Noble VE: Bedside ultrasound in pediatric emergency medicine. *Pediatrics* 121:e1401–e.1412, 2008, 2008.
42a. Luerssen TG: Central nervous system injuries. In O'Neill J, Grossfeld JL, Coran AG, Fonkalsrud EW, editors: *Grossfeld: Pediatric surgery*, ed 6, St Louis, 2006, Mosby.
43. Lutz N, et al: Incidence and clinical significance of abdominal wall bruising in restrained children involved in motor vehicle crashes. *J Pediatr Surg* 39:972, 2004.
44. McDevitt BE, Foltin GL, Cooper A, Thoracic trauma. In Baren JM et al, editors. *Pediatric emergency medicine*, Philadelphia, 2008, WB Saunders.
45. Nance ML, Carr BG, Branas CC: Access to pediatric trauma care in the United States. *Arch Pediatr Adolesc Med* 163:512, 2009.
46. Nansel TR, et al: Preventing unintentional pediatric injuries: a tailored intervention for parents and providers. *Health Educ Res* 23:656, 2008.
47. Nathans AB, Fantus RJ: *National Trauma Data Bank—Pediatric Report, version 8,* Chicago, 2008, American College Of Surgeons.
48. National Safe Kids Campaign: *Bicycle injury fact sheet,* Washington DC, 2004, National Safe Kids Campaign.
49. Nelson CS, Wissow LS, Cheng TL: Effectiveness of anticipatory guidance: Recent developments. *Curr Opin Pediatr* 15:630, 2003.

50. Ortega HW, Shields BJ, Smith GA: Bicycle attitudes regarding bicycle safety-related injuries to children and parental. *Clin Pediatr* 43:251, 2004.

51. Polk-Williams A, et al: Cervical spine injury in young children: a national trauma data bank review. *J Pediatr Surg* 43:1718–1721, 2008.

52. Proehl JA: Compartment syndrome. *J Emerg Nurs* 14:283, 1988.

53. Ragiel CA: The Impact of critical injury on patient, family, and clinical systems. *Crit Care Q* 7:73, 1984.

54. Ralston M, et al: *PALS provider manual*, Dallas, 2006, American Heart Association.

54a. Ramenofsky M: Pediatric abdominal trauma. *Pediatr Ann* 16:4, 1987, 1987.

55. Reid AB, Letts RM, Black GB: Pediatric Chance fractures: association with intra-abdominal injuries and seatbelt use. *J Trauma* 30:384, 1990.

56. Sasser SM, et al: Guidelines for field triage of injured patients: recommendations of the National Expert Panel on Field Triage. *Morbidity and Mortality Weekly Report* 58(RRO1):1–35, 2009.

57. Schmitt BD: The child with nonaccidental trauma. In Heifer RE, Kempe RS, editors: *The battered child*, ed 4, Chicago, 1987, The University of Chicago Press.

58. Seidel J, Henderson D: *Prehospital care of pediatric injuries,* Los Angeles County, Torrance, CA, 1987, Harbor UCLA Medical Center.

59. Seidel JS, et al: Emergency medical services and the pediatric patient: are needs being met? *Pediatrics* 5:769, 1984.

60. Shadgun B, et al: Diagnostic techniques in acute compartment syndrome of the leg. *J Orthop Trauma* 22:581–587, 2008.

61. Spivey WHL: Intraosseous infusions. *J Pediatr* 111:639, 1987.

62. Stalker HP, Kaufman RA, Stedje K: The significance of hematuria in children after blunt abdominal trauma. *AJR Am J Roentgenol* 154:569, 1990.

63. Strange JM, Kelly PM: Musculoskeletal injuries. In Cardona VD, et al, editors: *Trauma nursing: from resuscitation through rehabilitation*, Philadelphia, 1988, WB Saunders.

64. Streck CJ, Lobe TE, Pietsch JB, Lovvorn HN, 3rd: Laparoscopic repair of traumatic bowel injury in children. *J Pediatr Surgery* 41 (11):1864–1869, 2006.

65. Steele B: Psychodynamic factors in child abuse. In Heifer RE, Kempe RS, editors: *The battered child*, ed 4, Chicago, 1987, The University of Chicago Press.

66. Stylianos S, Harris BH: Seatbelt use and patterns of central nervous system injury in children. *Pediatr Emerg Care* 6:4, 1990.

67. Tepas JJ: Update on pediatric trauma: severity scores. In *Report of the Ninety-Seventh Ross Conference on Pediatric Research: Emergency Medical Services for Children, Columbus*, 1989, Ross Laboratories, Inc.

68. Thompson RS, Rivara FP, Thompson DC: A case-control study of the effectiveness of bicycle safety helmets. *N Engl J Med* 320:1361, 1989.

69. Viccellio P, Simon H, Pressman BD, et al: A prospective multicenter study of cervical spine injury in children. *Pediatrics* 108:E20, 2001.

70. Zuckerman BS, Duby JC: Developmental approach to injury prevention. *Pediatr Clin North Am* 32:1, 1985.

Care of the Child with Burns

20

John B. Pietsch • Dai H. Chung

PEARLS

- Intentional injury (child abuse) should be considered and ruled out as a cause of burns and scalds in children.
- Burns are painful; therefore analgesia should be provided and supplemented as needed before burn care.
- Formulas developed to estimate burn size in adults should not be used to calculate the burn surface area and fluid resuscitation requirements for children.
- Children with large burns should receive nursing and medical care in units with nurses and physicians who have pediatric expertise. Strong consideration should be given to transfer of a child to a pediatric critical care unit when large burns or complicating factors, such as smoke inhalation, are present.

INTRODUCTION

The incidence of pediatric burn injuries has declined as a result of preventive measures and legislation. However, more than 1 million burn injuries still occur each year in the United States. Although most of these burn injuries are minor, each year in the United States approximately 45,000 patients suffer moderate to severe burns that require hospitalization. Of these cases, 67% are young males, and 40% are children younger than 15 years.[31a] Burns are the second leading cause of unintentional death in children younger than 5 years. It is estimated that the number of serious disabilities from burns is triple the number of deaths. Three fourths of these burns are thought to be preventable.[22]

Eighty-five percent of thermal injuries in children occur at home, usually in the kitchen or bathroom. Infants and toddlers are injured most frequently by scald burns (Table 20-1),[1] whereas contact burns become more common once the infant is crawling or walking. Flame burns are seen in children 2 to 4 years of age and older and are the most common cause of burn injury in children 5 to 18 years of age. Electrical and chemical burns are uncommon in children and can be lethal if they are severe.[128]

Inflicted injury is an additional cause of thermal injury in infants and children. These injuries often have a typical pattern of delayed presentation for medical care, bilateral symmetry of the burn, or a stocking or glove distribution.

The purpose of this chapter is to discuss the normal functions of the skin and the pathophysiologic changes that occur as a result of a burn injury. The management of thermal injuries, complications of burns and burn therapy, and nursing interventions in the care of the child with burns will be presented.

ESSENTIAL ANATOMY AND PHYSIOLOGY

The skin is the largest organ of the body, amounting to 4 to 5 square feet in the child. Children have larger skin surface area to volume ratios than adults. As a consequence, the child has relatively greater daily fluid requirement and evaporative water loss per kilogram of body weight.

The skin is composed of three layers: epidermis, dermis, and subcutaneous tissues (Fig. 20-1). The epidermis is a superficial layer of stratified epithelial tissue that is composed of five microscopic levels of maturing cells. The epidermis is thinner in infants than in older children, and its thickness also varies over parts of the body. This layer is constantly shed to the environment, so that it regenerates continually. After a superficial burn, the epidermis will regenerate because portions of the epidermal appendages are present.

The dermis layer is thicker than the epidermis and composes the bulk of the skin; it consists of connective tissue containing nerve endings, blood vessels, hair follicles, the lymph spaces, and the sebaceous and sweat glands. When the entire layer of dermis is burned, all epithelial elements are destroyed, and the skin cannot heal or regenerate spontaneously.

The subcutaneous tissue, located below the dermis, contains collagen and adipose tissue. This layer can be damaged by deep burns that leave bones, tendons, and muscles exposed. In third-degree burns, eschar (thick, coagulated particles from destroyed dermis) attaches to this subcutaneous layer and may be difficult to remove.

Functions of the Skin

The skin has multiple functions. It provides a protective barrier, and it assists in the maintenance of fluid and electrolyte balance and thermoregulation. In addition, the skin is an excretory and a sensory organ. The skin also participates in vitamin D production and determines appearance. All these functions are threatened after a burn.

When the skin is intact, it forms a protective barrier against bacteria and pathogenic organisms; disruption of this barrier leaves the patient vulnerable to infection. The skin also limits evaporative fluid losses. When a burn occurs, the transmission

Table 20-1 Epidemiology of Pediatric Burns

Age	Scald (%)	Flame (%)	Contact (%)	Electrical (%)	Chemical (%)
1-23 months	72	10	15	2	1
2-4 years	54	23	20	2	1
5-12 years	30	63	5	1	1
13-18 years	19	70	5	4	2

Compiled and modified from East MK, et al: Epidemiology of burns in children. In Carvajal HF, Parks DH, editors: *Burns in children: pediatric burn management*, Chicago, 1988, Year Book Medical Publishers; O'Neill JA: Burns in children. In Artz CP, Moncrief JA, Pruitt BA, editors: *Burns: a team approach*, Philadelphia, 1979, WB Saunders; Chung DH, Sanford AP, Herndon DN: Burns. In O'Neill J, Grossfeld JL, Coran AG, Fonkalsrud EW, editors: *Grossfeld: Pediatric surgery*, ed 6, St Louis, 2006, Mosby.

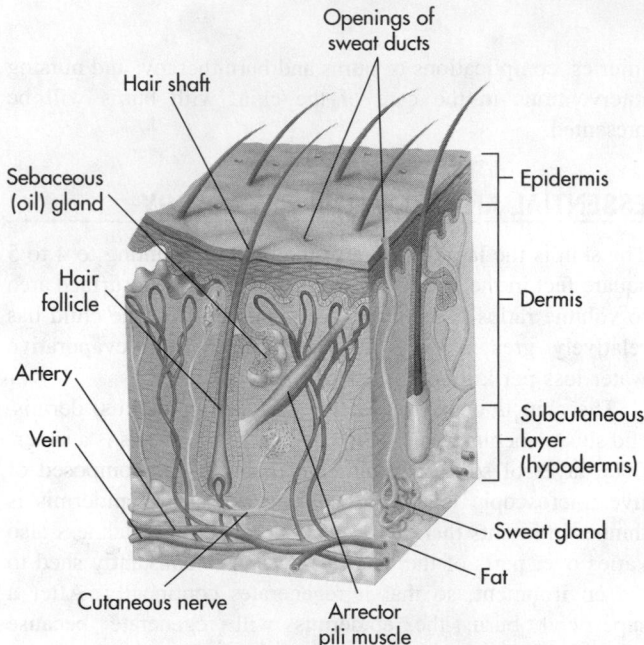

FIG. 20-1 Anatomy of the skin. (From Thibodeau GA, Patton KT: *Anatomy and physiology*, ed 5, St Louis, 2003, Mosby.)

of water vapor to the environment will increase; this evaporative water loss is proportional to the extent and depth of injury in burns affecting up to 50% of body surface area, and then it plateaus.

A third function of the skin is temperature control. Normally, body temperature can be maintained despite a mild reduction in the environmental temperature, because blood flow to the skin is reduced and the subcutaneous fat provides insulation. When the skin is burned, heat loss to the environment is significant, and body temperature (particularly in small children) may decrease.

The skin functions as an excretory organ when perspiration occurs. When deep burns are present, sweat glands are destroyed and this ability is lost. The skin also functions as the largest sensory organ of the body. Receptors located in the skin enable detection of pain and pressure. When moderate burns are present, nerve endings are exposed to the surface, which is extremely painful; deep burns destroy nerve endings, and sensation is lost.

A sixth function of the skin is the production of vitamin D, which is essential for bone growth. Vitamin D is absorbed by the skin and promotes calcium and phosphate deposition in bones. This function is compromised in second-degree

burns, and completely lost in third-degree burns. The skin also determines physical appearance and identity. The alteration in appearance caused by a burn can be extremely stressful.

Severity and Classification of Injury
Depth of Burn
The severity of the burn injury is determined by estimating the depth and extent of the injury. The degree of tissue destruction is affected by the burning agent, its temperature, and the duration of exposure to the heat source. Healthy skin can tolerate brief exposure to temperatures up to 40° C (104° F) without injury, but higher temperatures will produce burns. Severity of the injury increases as the temperature and duration of contact increase.[180]

Significant variations in skin thickness throughout the body also influence the depth of the burn. Where the epithelium is thin (such as over the ears, genitalia, medial portions of upper extremities, and in very young patients), even a brief exposure to a heat source can result in a full-thickness injury.

Classically, description of burn injury refers to the three concentric zones of tissue damage.[143,180] The central area of the burn wound, called the zone of coagulation, is injured most severely and is characterized by coagulation necrosis. The zone of stasis is an area of direct but milder injury, which can be damaged further if ischemia develops.[232] The zone of hyperemia is the area of tissue most peripheral to the initial burn and is injured only minimally.

A second method of burn classification describes the specific depth of injury (Table 20-2). A first-degree burn involves the top portion of the epidermis and does not extend into the dermis layer (Fig. 20-2). The burn area is characterized by erythema, mild edema, pain, and blanching with pressure. There is no vesicle formation. First-degree burns (e.g., sunburn) heal spontaneously without scarring in 7 to 10 days.

A second-degree burn (i.e., a partial thickness burn) involves the entire epidermis and part of the dermis layer of the skin. These burns can be classified further as *superficial partial thickness* or *deep partial thickness*, depending on the amount of dermis injured. Superficial second-degree burns are limited to the papillary dermis and are typically erythematous and painful with blisters. These burns spontaneously reepithelialize in 10 to 14 days from retained epidermal structures and may leave only slight skin discoloration. Deep second-degree burns extend into the reticular layer of the dermis. The deep epidermal appendages allow some of these wounds to heal slowly over several weeks, often with significant scarring.

A full-thickness, or third-degree burn, encompasses the entire epidermis and dermis layers. The wound surface, called

Table 20-2 **Characteristics of Burn Injury**

Depth	Appearance	Healing	Scarring	Examples
Superficial (first degree)	Erythema, mild edema and pain, blanches with pressure	3-7 days	No	Sunburn, flash burn
Partial thickness (second degree)	Pink to red, moist, moderate edema, extremely painful, vesicles	14-21 days	Variable	Scald, flame, brief contact with hot objects
Full thickness (third degree)	Waxy-white to black, dry, leathery, thrombosed vessels, edema, painless	Requires grafting	Yes	Flame, scald, prolonged contact with hot objects, electrical source, chemical
Fourth degree	Dry, leathery, black, painless; possibly exposed bones, tendons, or muscles	Requires grafting, flaps, or amputation	Yes	Prolonged contact with flame, chemical

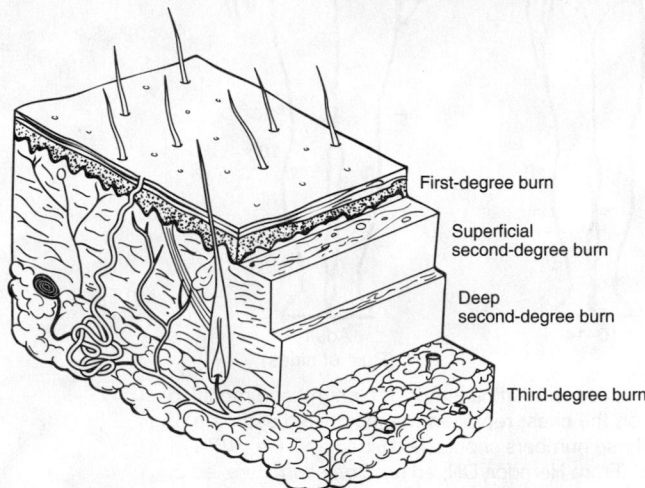

First-degree burn

Superficial second-degree burn

Deep second-degree burn

Third-degree burn

FIG. 20-2 Classification of burn depth. First-degree burns involve the epidermis, second-degree burns involve the epidermis and dermis, and third-degree burns penetrate to the subcutaneous tissue. From Garner WL: Thermal burns. In Achauer BM, Eriksson E, editors: *Plastic surgery: indications, operations, and outcomes*, St Louis, 2000, Mosby.

eschar, will appear dry and leathery, with a waxy-white or black color produced by particles from destroyed dermis. Thrombosed vessels may be seen beneath the surface of the burn. The patient with a third-degree burn experiences little or no pain, because the nerve endings in the dermis layer have been destroyed. This type of burn will require surgical repair. Fourth-degree burns, typically resulting from profound thermal or electrical injury, involve organs beneath the layers of the skin, such as muscle and bone.

An accurate and rapid determination of burn depth is vital to the proper management of burn injuries. In particular, the distinction between superficial and deep dermal burns is critical, because it dictates whether the burn can be managed without surgical procedures. Unfortunately, the determination of whether an apparent deep dermal burn will heal in 3 weeks is approximately 50% accurate, even when made by an experienced surgeon. Early excision and grafting provide better results than nonoperative therapy for such indeterminate burns.

Extent of Injury

A variety of methods have been developed for determination of the extent of any burn injury, but most involve expression of the burn as a percent of the total body surface area (TBSA) involved. Accurate calculation of the surface area of the burn is required to estimate fluid losses and fluid requirements.

A rapid method of calculating burn area in adolescents and adults, developed in the 1940s by Pulaski and Tennison,[174a] is called the *rule of nines* (Fig. 20-3).[1] In the rule of nines, each upper extremity and the head constitute 9% of the TBSA, and the lower extremities and the anterior and posterior trunks are each 18% of TBSA. The perineum, genitalia, and neck comprise the remaining 1% of the TBSA. A quick estimate of burn size can also be obtained by using the patient's palm to represent 1% of TBSA and transposing that measurement to estimate the wound size.

Use of the rule of nines can be misleading in children because the child's body proportions differ from those in adolescents and adults. In children, the head and neck constitute a relatively larger portion of the TBSA, and the lower extremities constitute a smaller portion. For example, an infant's head constitutes 19% of TBSA, compared with 9% in an adult. Thus, a modified rule of nines, based on the anthropomorphic differences of infancy and childhood, is generally used to assess pediatric burn size (see Fig. 20-3). Clinical criteria can also be used to estimate the percentage of TBSA burned, based on the patient's age and the body part burned (see Classification of Burns).

Another widely used method of determining the extent of pediatric burn injury is the Lund and Browder method (Fig. 20-4). This method allows for changes in body surface area as the average-sized child grows.[119]

Computer-generated estimates of burn injury size are available. Such programs are gaining in popularity, because they can provide estimates of fluid requirements and drug doses.

Factors Influencing Severity of Burn

To appreciate the significance of a burn, other factors in addition to the depth and extent of the injury must be considered. The age and underlying clinical condition of the child and the location of the injury also must be evaluated. Complications related to fluid resuscitation and organ system failure are most common in children younger than 2 years. Children with underlying organ system failure also will be less tolerant of fluid shifts associated with the burn and fluid resuscitation.

The location of the burn can have a significant effect on morbidity and mortality. A thermal injury to the face, hands, or feet can result in serious sequelae, particularly loss of function. Burns of the face may be associated with severe edema

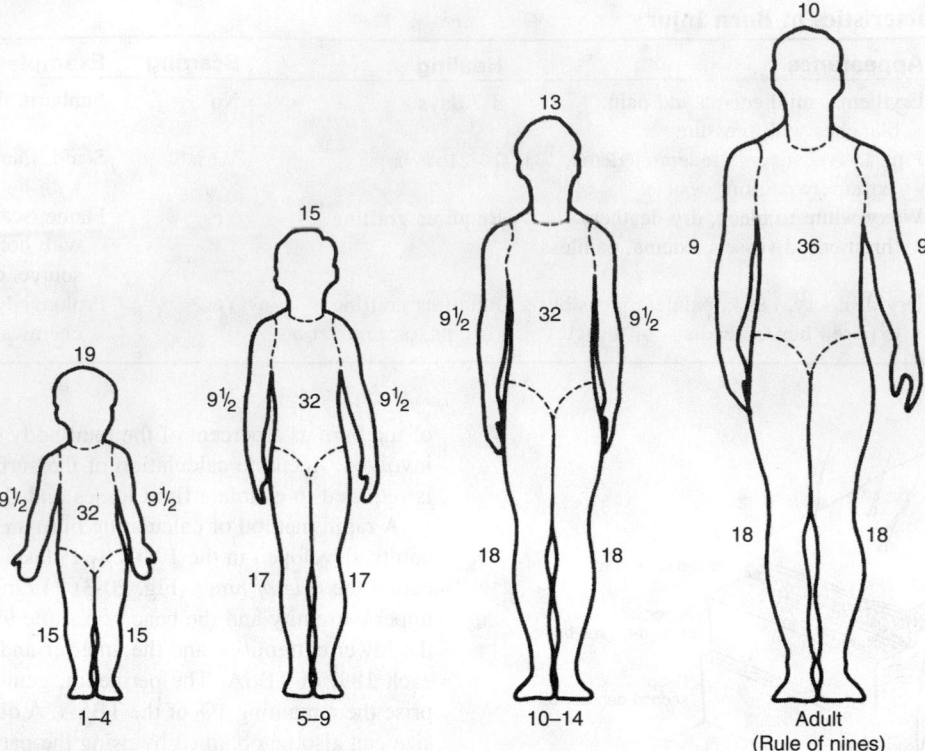

FIG. 20-3 Estimation of extent of burn injury: rule of nines applied to adult patient (see far right) and modified rule of nines for pediatric patients. Note that the numbers on the chest represent the combined estimate of total body surface area (TBSA) of the chest plus the back. These numbers should be divided by 2 (i.e., 16% of TBSA) to estimate the TBSA of either the front or the back. (From Herndon DN, editor: *Total burn care*, ed 2, Philadelphia, 2002, WB Saunders.)

and airway occlusion. Skin over the ears and perineum is relatively thin, so injuries sustained in these areas can result in a full-thickness injury.

Full-thickness circumferential burns to the extremities produce a constricting eschar, which can result in vascular compromise to the distal tissues, including nerves. Accumulation of tissue edema beneath the nonelastic eschar impedes venous outflow, resulting in a compartment syndrome and eventually affecting arterial flow. When distal pulses are absent on palpation or Doppler examination and a central circulation problem has been ruled out, an escharotomy is performed to avoid vascular compromise of the limb tissues.

Classification of Burns
After providing first aid and initiating appropriate fluid resuscitation, providers should consider transferring the patient to a tertiary burn center. Burn units with experienced multidisciplinary teams are best prepared to treat patients with major burns. In addition to physicians and nurses, respiratory and rehabilitation therapists play a critical role in managing acute burns. Any patient who sustains a major burn injury, as defined by the American Burn Association (Box 20-1), should be transferred to a nearby burn center for further care.

Pathophysiology of a Burn
Pathophysiologic changes resulting from a thermal injury can affect all organs and systems of the body. The severity of the injury determines the significance of the changes.

Local Circulatory Destruction
Immediately after the burn, major circulatory destruction occurs at the burn site. The severity of the damage depends on the extent of the burn injury and might not be immediately apparent.

The vessels supplying the burned skin are occluded, and there is reduction in or cessation of blood flow through the arteries and veins. Release of vasoactive substances (especially histamine) from injured cells will produce vasoconstriction,[143] and peripheral vessel thrombosis ultimately may occur. The reduction in skin perfusion can produce tissue necrosis and increase the depth of the burn.

When a partial thickness burn is present, rapid restoration of arterial and venous circulation is observed within 24 to 48 hours. Cellular necrosis beyond the immediate area of the burn is prevented, and reepithelialization occurs from viable dermal elements. When a full-thickness burn is present, progressive tissue necrosis occurs over 3 to 4 weeks, because blood vessels in the dermis have been destroyed. This destruction ceases only after new vessels (the neovasculature) arise from underlying tissue.

Capillary Permeability (Third-Spacing) Period
When the child sustains a major burn, normal fluid homeostasis is altered, and intravascular volume and cardiac output will be affected. The first 12 to 36 hours after a burn are characterized by fluid shift from the intravascular to the

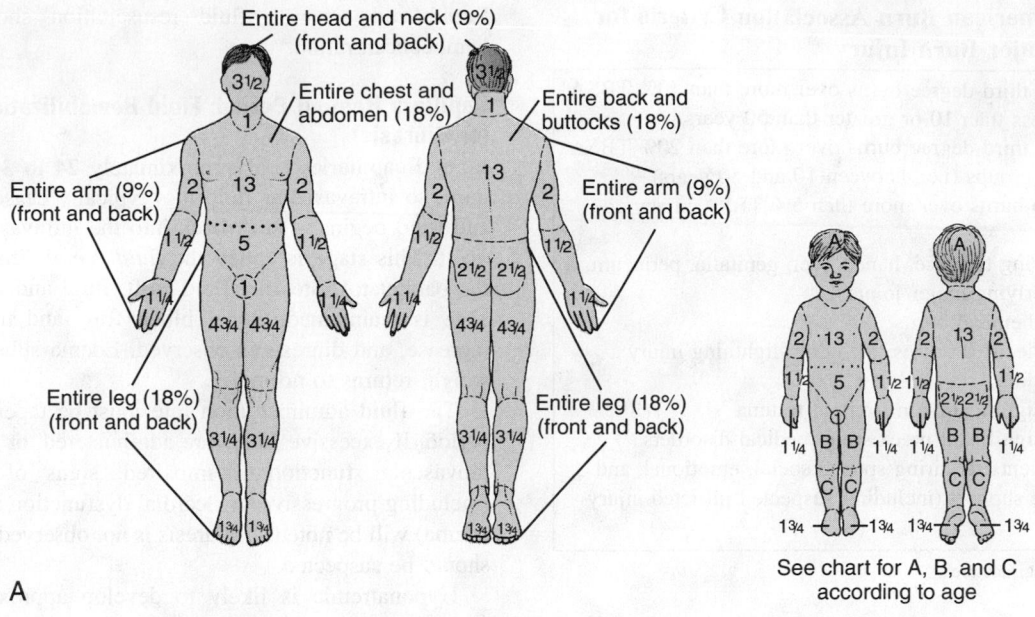

Entire head and neck (9%)
(front and back)

Entire chest and
abdomen (18%)

Entire back and
buttocks (18%)

Entire arm (9%)
(front and back)

Entire arm (9%)
(front and back)

Entire leg (18%)
(front and back)

Entire leg (18%)
(front and back)

A

See chart for A, B, and C
according to age

AGE	Birth-1 yr	1-4 yr	5-9 yr	10-14 yr	15 yr	Adult
Head	19	17	13	11	9	7
Neck	2					
Ant trunk	13					
Post trunk	13					
R buttock	2½					
L buttock	2½					
Genitalia	1					
R U arm	4					
L U arm	4					
R L arm	3					
L L arm	3					
R hand	2½	6½	8	8½	9	9½
L hand	2½	6½	8	8½	9	9½
R thigh	5½	5	5½	6	6½	7
L thigh	5½	5	5½	6	6½	7
R leg	5					
L leg	5					
R foot	3½					
L foot	3½					

B   BODY AREA

FIG. 20-4 A, The Lund and Browder charts are somewhat more accurate than the rule of nines in estimating the total body surface area (TBSA) burned. **B,** The proportion of TBSA of individual areas, according to age. Compared with adults, children have larger heads and smaller legs. Other areas are relatively equivalent throughout life. The adult rule of nines is not accurate for determining the percentage of TBSA burned in children. (From Bethel CA, Mazzeo AS: Burn care procedures. In Roberts JR, editor: *Clinical procedures in emergency medicine*, ed 5, Philadelphia, 2009, WB Saunders.)

interstitial space as a result of increased capillary permeability. This fluid shift is known as *third-spacing* of fluid, because the fluid is located in neither the intravascular nor the intracellular space—it is in a third space, in this case it moves to the surface of the burn and to the interstitial space. With third spacing of fluid, a significant volume of fluid is unavailable to the circulation to support cardiac output and systemic perfusion. Third-spacing is most significant during the first 12 hours after a burn.

Normally, intravascular proteins remain in the vascular space, because they are too large to escape through capillary pores. The increased capillary permeability associated with a thermal injury allows intravascular proteins and fluid to escape

the vascular space. The amount of fluid shift that occurs is determined by the extent and severity of the burn injury. Burns affecting 15% or less of the TBSA produce minor fluid shifts, whereas large burns not only result in fluid loss from the surface of the burn, the burn affects capillary permeability in noninjured tissues, resulting in a major loss of intravascular fluid. If the intravascular fluid loss is not replenished, hypovolemia will result in compromise of systemic perfusion.

As protein rich fluids, electrolytes, and plasma escape into the interstitial space, peripheral edema develops. Movement of proteins into the interstitial space will increase tissue colloid osmotic pressure, enhancing the intravascular-to-interstitial fluid shift.[136]

American Burn Association Criteria for Major Burn Injury

- Second- and third-degree burns over more than 10% TBSA in patients less than 10 or greater than 50 years
- Second- and third-degree burns over more than 20% TBSA in other age groups (i.e., between 10 and 50 years)
- Third-degree burns over more than 5% TBSA in any age group
- Burns involving the face, hands, feet, genitalia, perineum, and skin overlying major joints
- Significant chemical burns
- Significant electrical burns, including lightning injury
- Inhalation injury
- Burns with significant concomitant trauma
- Burns with significant preexisting medical disorders
- Burns in patients requiring special social, emotional, and rehabilitative support (including suspected inflicted injury and neglect)

TBSA, Total body surface area.

Pulmonary capillary permeability is typically normal unless severe inhalation injury is present or fluid administration is excessive. When pulmonary edema develops, it is often temporary, because pulmonary lymph flow often increases proportionately and rapidly eliminates the pulmonary interstitial fluid.

Fluid lost from the vascular space is relatively isotonic; therefore if it is replaced with isotonic or hypertonic fluids, electrolyte balance should be maintained. Dilutional hyponatremia, hypocalcemia, and hypomagnesemia are seen occasionally,[213] particularly if antidiuretic hormone secretion is significant (antidiuretic hormone secretion causes water retention in excess of sodium—see Chapter 12). It is rarely necessary to replace these electrolytes if isotonic fluids are administered; however, electrolyte balance should be monitored closely. Hypotonic fluids (e.g., 5% dextrose and water or 5% dextrose and 0.45% sodium chloride) should not be administered during this period.

Potassium is released from injured cells into the extracellular fluid. For this reason, supplementary potassium chloride may not be required in resuscitation fluids. If fluid resuscitation is inadequate, or renal failure develops, hyperkalemia may be problematic.

The concentration of base bicarbonate in the extracellular fluid decreases after a burn, and fixed acids are released from the injured tissues into the extracellular fluid, including the plasma. These acids normally are excreted by the kidney and buffered by respiratory compensation. If fluid resuscitation is inadequate, or respiratory function is compromised, the patient may develop metabolic acidosis. Young infants are less able to compensate for significant metabolic acidosis, because the infant kidneys are unable to excrete large quantities of acids or absorb large quantities of bicarbonate.[179]

During the third-spacing period, hemoconcentration develops and the viscosity of the blood increases. This hemoconcentration can produce sluggish blood flow through small vessels and platelet and leukocyte accumulation in capillaries. Red blood cell (RBC) destruction also is enhanced.

Rapid and accurate fluid resuscitation should minimize hemoconcentration.

Capillary Healing Period: Fluid Remobilization (or Diuresis)

Injured capillaries heal approximately 24 to 36 hours after a burn, so intravascular fluid loss typically ceases at this time, and fluid begins to shift back into the intravascular compartment. This stage is called the *fluid remobilization period.* If the patient tolerates the fluid shift, fluid and electrolyte balance is maintained. Renal blood flow and urine formation increase, and diuresis is observed. Edema subsides and body weight returns to normal.

The fluid administration rate must be tapered during this period. If excessive fluids are administered, or if renal or cardiovascular function is impaired, signs of hypervolemia (including progressive myocardial dysfunction and pulmonary edema) will be noted. If diuresis is not observed, renal damage should be suspected.

Hyponatremia is likely to develop approximately 24 to 36 hours after a burn, because renal sodium excretion is enhanced during diuresis. Normal serum sodium concentration should be restored approximately 72 to 96 hours after the burn. Hypokalemia may be observed as potassium returns to the intracellular compartment. The serum potassium concentration should be monitored closely, and potassium supplementation may be required.

Anemia frequently develops as a result of hemodilution and, to a lesser extent, from enhanced RBC destruction. As much as 10% of the patient's erythrocytes may be destroyed immediately after a burn, but transfusion is rarely necessary.

Cardiovascular Dysfunction

Cardiac output falls after a burn as the result of decreased intravascular volume and the development of myocardial dysfunction.[123] Myocardial dysfunction after a burn is not explained entirely by intravascular fluid loss. Within 30 minutes after a large burn (i.e., 50% or more of TBSA), cardiac output may decrease to 30% of preburn levels and may remain depressed for 18 to 36 hours. Cardiac output returns to normal levels long before plasma volume has been restored completely.[47]

The fall in cardiac output after a burn has been attributed to the presence of circulating myocardial depressant factor or the development of a catecholamine (stress induced) increase in systemic and pulmonary vascular resistances and increased ventricular afterload.[229] Treatment of low cardiac output requires supportive care; the efficacy of vasoactive (inotropic) drug therapy in the treatment of this cause of myocardial dysfunction has not been determined.

Immediately after a burn, catecholamine secretion can produce an increase in systemic and pulmonary vascular resistances. Although vasoconstriction may help to maintain mean arterial pressure in the face of a fall in cardiac output and extravascular fluid shifts, it also may contribute to increased ventricular afterload and increased ventricular work. The relative significance of this vasoconstriction in pediatric patients is unknown.

In general, treatment of inadequate cardiovascular function requires support of maximal oxygen delivery (including support of oxygenation, ventilation, and cardiac output) with titration of intravenous volume administration. The effectiveness of vasoactive agents for children with significant burns has not been studied (refer to discussion of shock in Chapter 6).

Cardiac output may increase to high levels (as much as 300% of normal values) about 36 or more hours after a burn. Increased metabolic rate and anemia contribute to this hyperdynamic state.

Pulmonary Injuries

Respiratory insufficiency can result from the inhalation of superheated air, steam, toxic fumes, or smoke, and it is a major cause of morbidity and mortality in burned children.[94,97,126,146,197] This respiratory failure may result from airway edema or obstruction or from microcirculatory changes and increased capillary permeability. Pulmonary edema can result from inhalation injuries, excessive volume administration during resuscitation, or sepsis.

Inhalation of smoke, steam or other irritants will produce upper airway edema, erythema, and blistering. Progressive edema can cause upper airway obstruction. Ciliated epithelial cells may be damaged during inhalation, so that foreign particles can enter the bronchi. The damaged mucosal layer may slough 48 to 72 hours after a burn, producing acute airway obstruction.[30,94]

Damage to the pulmonary parenchyma can result from an inhalation injury and can complicate shock and fluid resuscitation (see Respiratory Failure, later in this chapter and Acute Respiratory Distress Syndrome in Chapter 9). Increased alveolar capillary membrane permeability will produce pulmonary edema with resultant intrapulmonary shunting and hypoxemia, decreased lung compliance, and increased work of breathing.[118]

Carbon Monoxide Poisoning. Carbon monoxide (CO) is produced in almost every fire, and CO poisoning can cause immediate death during the fire or death during the first 12 hours after a burn. CO has much higher affinity for hemoglobin than does oxygen; as a result, it will bind tightly with hemoglobin, forming carboxyhemoglobin (COHb). Each gram of hemoglobin bound to CO is unable to carry oxygen, so impaired oxygen transport, decreased oxygen delivery, tissue hypoxia, and metabolic acidosis will result if CO levels are high. COHb levels greater than 40% usually produce significant tissue and organ ischemia and dysfunction, and levels greater than 60% are usually fatal.[78,216]

It is important to note that pulse oximeters will not reflect the severity of CO poisoning because they do not recognize CoHb. As a result, the pulse oximeter will indicate only the saturation of normal hemoglobin. If CO poisoning is suspected, the child's oxyhemoglobin saturation must be measured by cooximeter.

Gastrointestinal Dysfunction

When cardiac output falls after a burn, blood flow is diverted from the liver, kidney, and gastrointestinal circulations to maintain blood flow to the brain and heart. This decrease in gastrointestinal perfusion results in impaired gastrointestinal motility. Severe compromise in motility results in further

reduction in blood flow, so severe gastrointestinal ischemia can develop.

Gastrointestinal ischemia can increase the permeability of gastrointestinal mucosa to gram-negative bacteria and endotoxins. As a result, translocation of gram-negative bacteria or endotoxin can occur and may precipitate gram-negative sepsis (see Septic Shock in Chapter 6, and Septic Shock: Mediators of the Septic Cascade in the Chapter 6 Supplement on the Evolve Website).

When gastrointestinal motility is reduced, mucosal secretions and gases can accumulate in the intestine and stomach, causing severe abdominal distension. Gastrointestinal perfusion and motility should return to normal when hypovolemia is corrected and cardiac output is restored.

Curling's ulcer, or acute ulcerative gastroduodenal disease, may develop after a burn. The etiology of this condition is unknown, but it relates to compromised gastrointestinal perfusion and resultant mucosal damage. The mucous membrane ordinarily prevents autodigestion, because it acts as a barrier to the absorption of hydrogen ions that are secreted into the gastric lumen. An alteration in gastric mucosal function can compromise this barrier and increase the production of hydrogen ions, so that gastric and duodenal ulcerations may develop.

The incidence of Curling's ulcer is unknown, because it typically is diagnosed at autopsy. Superficial gastric and duodenal mucosal changes are common in children with major burns,[67] but ulcer prophylaxis has ensured that clinically significant bleeding and ulceration are still relatively uncommon.

Gastrointestinal ulceration may produce pain, hemorrhage, or perforation. Gastric suction and stool samples should be tested for the presence of blood (heme protein), and the use of antacids or sucralfate (a hydrogen ion diffusion barrier) should be considered.[131] Administration of histamine receptor antagonists (e.g., cimetidine or ranitidine) is controversial, because the morbidity of these drugs may be higher than the risk of stress ulceration. Severe pneumonias may result from aspiration of gastric bacteria that can flourish after these drugs are administered. The gastric pH should be maintained at 3.5 to 5.0 (see Chapter 14).

Metabolic Changes

The patient with a burn is in a hypermetabolic state, with high oxygen consumption and caloric requirements. Metabolic rate reaches its peak at double (or more) normal values approximately 4 to 12 days after a burn.[5b] Catecholamine secretion activates the stress response, and heat production and substrate mobilization will result in protein and fat catabolism, increased urinary nitrogen losses, and rapid utilization of glucose and calories.[70] An increased metabolic rate continues until after the burn is healed or covered by graft.

Central thermoregulation is altered at this time, and the hypermetabolic condition often produces a low-grade fever.[205] In contrast, heat loss and a fall in body temperature may be observed in the very young child with an extensive burn.

Because a burn is a major body stress, muscle protein catabolism increases to provide amino acids for gluconeogenesis and fuel sources for local tissue needs.[69] Insufficient protein administration and nutrition will result in a marked catabolic state (negative nitrogen balance) and major muscle loss. Large amounts of urea in the urine indicate increased nitrogen loss.[218]

Thermal injury and hypermetabolism result in increased serum free fatty acids. Hydrolysis of stored triglycerides is accelerated, and catecholamine secretion stimulates mobilization of fat stores. Hypoalbuminemia results from increased protein loss at the burn surface and can, in turn, reduce fatty acid transport.[75]

Compromise in Immune Function

A thermal injury destroys the protective barrier of the skin, creating an open wound. The burn activates the inflammatory response, but may compromise immune function, leaving the patient at risk for infection.

After a burn, several circulating immunosuppressive substances are present. Nonspecific suppressor T cells compromise lymphocyte response for approximately 48 hours.[154] Leukocyte phagocytosis is reduced, and the reticuloendothelial system is often depressed.[220] Burn toxin, a high-molecular-weight protein, is thought to contribute to postburn immunosuppression. The patient's immune function may be compromised further by the application of topical antimicrobial agents and the insertion and contamination of intravascular catheters.

A burn activates the complement system. This system consists of a series of circulating proteins that are present in an inactive form. Some of these proteins coat invading organisms, rendering them susceptible to phagocytosis. In addition, the complement system participates in the coagulation cascade.

Infection or injury can activate the complement system, resulting in a normal inflammatory response.[88] Extensive burns result in a decrease in serum complement levels and a potential reduction in the inflammatory response during infection (see Septic Shock in Chapter 6, and Septic Shock: Mediators of the Septic Cascade in the Chapter 6 Supplement on the Evolve Website).

COMMON CLINICAL CONDITIONS

Care of the child with burns requires support of cardiorespiratory function, prevention of infection, and preparation of the burn surface for healing or grafting. In addition, potential complications of the burn and its treatment must be prevented. An overview of this nursing care is provided in the nursing care plan (Box 20-2), and the major potential patient problems are reviewed in the following discussion.

Inadequate Intravascular Volume and Cardiac Output: Third-Spacing Phase

Etiology and Pathophysiology

The child with burns loses a large amount of fluid from the burn surface itself. In addition, increased capillary permeability produces third-spacing of fluid. Significant unreplaced intravascular volume loss will result in a fall in cardiac output and a compromise in systemic perfusion.

The magnitude of the intravascular volume deficit will depend on the depth and surface area of the injury and the time elapsed before adequate fluid resuscitation.[28] In general,

deeper and larger (15% or more of TBSA) burns are associated with more significant fluid shifts and circulatory complications.

Clinical Signs and Symptoms

After a significant burn, intravascular volume loss will eventually produce signs of hypovolemia (Box 20-3). Children often do not exhibit significant signs of hypovolemia, including hypotension until more than 25% of the circulating volume is depleted and complete cardiovascular collapse is imminent.

Tachycardia reflects a compensatory response to hypovolemia, but caution is needed to avoid overinterpreting this finding, because reflex tachycardia from postinjury catecholamine response is common. A lethargic child with tachycardia plus decreased capillary refill and cool, clammy extremities needs prompt attention, because shock is likely to be present.

Significant hypovolemia will compromise systemic perfusion and may produce shock. Such hypovolemia will produce tachycardia, prolonged capillary refill time, and cold extremities. Anuria is often present. The development of a metabolic acidosis (i.e., fall in arterial pH, rise in serum lactate) indicates critical compromise in tissue perfusion. The young infant in shock often will demonstrate temperature instability and hypoglycemia. Hypotension may develop only as a late sign of shock.[47]

Following the stress of the burn, antidiuretic hormone secretion is enhanced, so urine volume usually is reduced even if fluid resuscitation is adequate. Hour-to-hour fluctuations in urine volume are common during this time.

Interstitial fluid accumulation can produce diffuse peripheral (systemic) edema. Such edema will be most severe in dependent areas. If pulmonary edema develops, it will produce intrapulmonary shunting. The resultant hypoxemia will be detected with pulse oximetry or arterial blood gases. Tachypnea, nasal flaring, and retractions will indicate decreased lung compliance and increased work of breathing. Crackles may be heard, and pulmonary edema also will be noted on a chest radiograph. If the child is intubated, frothy secretions may be suctioned from the tube.

Management

Initiation of Therapy. Adequate fluid resuscitation and replacement in a severely burned child is critical to ensure survival. Initial fluid resuscitation is designed to restore adequate intravascular volume and maintain effective tissue and organ perfusion. In addition, electrolyte and acid-base balance must be maintained, and excessive fluid administration must be avoided.

Repeated bolus administration of isotonic fluid (20 mL/kg administered over 5 to 20 minutes) may be necessary until systemic perfusion and urine output are restored. Next, the volume and content of the fluid deficit is calculated (based on the child's body surface area and the size of the burn), and maintenance fluid requirements are estimated.

If the burn totals less than 15% TBSA, it may be possible to replace the deficit by providing oral fluids, including protein supplements, milk products, and clear liquids. Throughout fluid administration, the effectiveness of the child's perfusion

Box 20-2 Nursing Care of the Child with Thermal Injuries

Inadequate Cardiac Output and Tissue Perfusion (Alteration in Tissue Perfusion) Related to: Extravascular Fluid Shift and Relative Hypovolemia, Inadequate or Delayed Fluid Resuscitation, Constriction of Eschar

Expected Patient Outcome

Patient will demonstrate adequate tissue perfusion as evidenced by:

- Persistence or return of peripheral pulses
- Brisk capillary refill, warm extremities with no evidence of compartment syndrome (see Chapter 19)
- Pink mucous membranes, nail beds
- Effective cardiac output and organ perfusion
- Absence of metabolic acidosis
- Urine volume averaging 1 mL/kg per hour or more

Nursing Activities

- Constantly assess fluid balance, systemic perfusion. Monitor for signs of hypovolemic shock, including: tachycardia, oliguria, cool skin and cool extremities, weak peripheral pulses, altered level of consciousness, negative fluid balance, low central venous or pulmonary artery wedge pressure, development of lactic acidosis, and absence of hepatomegaly (by clinical examination) and of cardiomegaly (on chest radiograph).
- Calculate fluid replacement requirements and discuss inadequate fluid administration or excessive fluid losses with the on-call provider immediately.
- Administer fluid boluses and maintenance fluids as needed to restore adequate intravascular volume and systemic perfusion and to replace ongoing fluid losses.
- Assess perfusion and appearance of and movement and sensation in extremities and digits.
  - Report decreased or absent peripheral pulses, delayed capillary refill, edema, cyanosis, or cool extremities or digits to the on-call provider immediately.
  - Assess blood flow to extremities using Doppler; if Doppler indicates low flow to extremities, monitoring of compartment pressures may be ordered (see Chapter 19).
- Assist with escharotomies or fasciotomies on arms, legs, and chest as needed.
- Perform passive and active range-of-motion exercises to extremities as ordered.
- Position patient carefully to prevent compromised blood flow to extremities.

Potential Hypovolemia or Inadequate Fluid Volume Related to: Fluid Loss Through Evaporation from Burn Surface, Increased Capillary Permeability and Extravascular Fluid Shift, Inadequate Fluid Administration, Excessive Fluid Losses Through Fever, Diarrhea

Expected Patient Outcomes

- Patient will demonstrate adequate intravascular volume as evidenced by: effective systemic perfusion, balanced fluid intake and output (with consideration of fluid loss from surface of burn), urine volume of 1 mL/kg per hour, electrolyte balance, central venous pressure or pulmonary artery wedge pressure of approximately 2 to 5 mm Hg (or higher as needed to maintain adequate systemic perfusion), normal arterial pH, and normal serum lactate.

- Patient will demonstrate no signs of hemoconcentration or dehydration, such as dry mucous membranes, poor skin turgor, increase in serum electrolyte concentration and hematocrit, sunken fontanelle (in infants), and oliguria with increased urine specific gravity.

Nursing Activities

- Monitor patient systemic perfusion: signs of hypovolemia include signs of poor systemic perfusion associated with a low central venous pressure or pulmonary artery wedge pressure, small heart size on chest radiograph, and absence of hepatomegaly. Report these findings to the on-call provider immediately.
- Monitor for signs of dehydration, including: sunken fontanelle in infants, dry mucous membranes, poor skin turgor, evidence of weight loss, rise in serum electrolyte concentration, and increase in hematocrit. Report findings to the on-call provider.
- Monitor urine output and fluid balance every hour; report oliguria or negative fluid balance to the on-call provider (consider fluid loss through burn).
- Titrate fluid administration as needed (and with physician or other provider order) to maintain systemic perfusion.
- Monitor heart size and evidence of pulmonary edema on chest radiograph; discuss these findings with on-call provider.
- Monitor electrolyte balance, serum albumin, and hematocrit.
- Obtain daily weights, report them to the on-call provider, and discuss changes in fluid requirements.

Potential Hypervolemia or Fluid Volume Excess Related to: Excessive Fluid Administration and Renal Failure

Expected Patient Outcomes

- Patient will demonstrate no evidence of hypervolemia, such as signs of congestive heart failure, pulmonary edema, or hemodilution.
- Patient will maintain electrolyte balance.

Nursing Activities

- Monitor systemic perfusion and fluid balance; report signs of congestive heart failure (tachycardia, tachypnea, periorbital edema, hepatomegaly, increased respiratory effort, cardiomegaly, and oliguria), excessive weight gain, or positive fluid balance to the on-call provider (note that most patients will demonstrate weight gain following fluid resuscitation after a burn).
- Assess for evidence of pulmonary edema, including crackles and increased respiratory effort; be prepared to support oxygenation and ventilation as needed.
- Palpate liver margin; report the presence or progression of hepatomegaly to the on-call provider.
- Monitor electrolyte balance; report a fall in electrolyte concentration or hematocrit to the on-call provider.
- Administer diuretic as ordered.

Potential Airway Obstruction Related to: Airway Inflammation, Pulmonary Interstitial Edema, Reduced Ciliary Function Following Inhalation Injury, Altered Level of Consciousness

Expected Patient Outcomes

- Patient will demonstrate patent airway as demonstrated by: normal spontaneous respiratory rate and effort, adequate depth

Continued

Box 20-2 **Nursing Care of the Child with Thermal Injuries—cont'd**

of respirations and air movement, effective oxygenation and carbon dioxide removal (per arterial blood gases, pulse oximetry and exhaled carbon dioxide tension [$P_{ET}CO_2$]), and absence of crackles and stridor
- If patient develops airway obstruction, intubation and appropriate support will be provided immediately.

Nursing Activities
- Monitor patient respiratory rate, effort, and air movement. Notify on-call provider of signs of airway obstruction, including tachypnea, retractions, nasal flaring, stridor, or weak cry. Be prepared to assist with emergency intubation as needed. Resuscitation bag and mask with oxygen source should be available at the bedside.
- Note that the diagnosis of respiratory failure from airway obstruction is a clinical diagnosis and can be present despite normal arterial blood gases and pulse oximetry. Hypoxemia and hypercarbia will only be late signs of airway obstruction, and intubation should be accomplished before these develop.
- Monitor for evidence of inhalation injury, including singed nasal hairs, excessive secretions, progressive respiratory distress; report these findings to the on-call provider immediately.
- Provide oxygen therapy as needed and monitor the effect on systemic oxygenation, including pulse oximetry and arterial blood gases.
- Perform tracheal suctioning as needed to maintain a clear upper airway.
- Encourage the alert patient (as age-appropriate) to take deep breaths and cough as needed to clear the airway.
- Insert oral or nasal airway as needed (and ordered by on-call provider).
- Position child to maintain airway patency (particularly important if level of consciousness is impaired).
- Assess patient responsiveness; discuss elective intubation if the patient is obtunded or demonstrates decreased response to stimulation
- Relieve pain and discomfort as needed.
- Assist with escharotomies of the chest as needed.

Hypoxemia, Hypoxia and Impaired Gas Exchange Related to: Airway Obstruction, Inhalation Injury, Pulmonary Edema, Acute Respiratory Distress Syndrome, Carbon Monoxide Poisoning, Impaired Level of Consciousness
Expected Patient Outcomes
- Patient will demonstrate adequate respiratory function as evidenced by: appropriate respiratory rate, depth and effort; patent airway; normal arterial blood gases; COHb level less than 10%; absence of crackles or pulmonary edema on chest radiograph.
- If patient demonstrates hypoxemia despite oxygen therapy, or ineffective ventilation, support of airway, oxygenation, and ventilation will be provided,
- Patient will remain alert and oriented with adequate respiratory rate and effort.

Nursing Activities
- Monitor respiratory rate and effort, and notify a provider of development of respiratory distress.

- Monitor pulse oximetry, exhaled carbon dioxide ($P_{ET}CO_2$), and arterial blood gases; notify a provider of any development of hypoxemia or hypercarbia.
- Monitor for evidence of inhalation injury, including headache, dizziness, confusion, flushed appearance (late finding), visual disturbance, seizures, and metabolic acidosis. Report these findings to the on-call provider immediately.
  ○ If inhalation injury and carbon monoxide poisoning are suspected, obtained blood gas specimen for qualification of COHb level; notify on-call provider of result (COHb levels greater than 10% can be associated with significant compromise of oxygen delivery).
  ○ Severe carbon monoxide poisoning may be present despite a normal oxyhemoglobin saturation as measured by pulse oximetry, because the pulse oximeter does not recognize COHb. To determine actual hemoglobin saturation, the hemoglobin saturation must be measured using a cooximeter in the blood gas laboratory.
- Administer oxygen as ordered, and monitor the patient's response.
- Be prepared to assist with non-invasive positive-pressure ventilation, hyperbaric oxygen therapy or intubation and mechanical ventilation as needed. Ensure that emergency equipment is readily available.

Pain Related to Burn, Multiple Invasive or Painful Catheters, and Painful Dressing Changes and Procedures
Expected Patient Outcomes
- Patient will demonstrate no pain, as evidenced by verbal reports of pain (as age-appropriate), facial expression, crying or whining, and increased heart rate and blood pressure.
- Patient will demonstrate relaxed body position, relaxed facial expression, ability to sleep when undisturbed, and appropriate heart rate and blood pressure for age and clinical condition.
- Patient will indicate reduction or elimination of pain as indicated and quantified using consistent pain assessment tools (see Chapter 5).

Nursing Activities
- Assess nature, location, quality, and intensity of pain every hour and as needed using consistent pain assessment tool (see Chapter 5).
- Monitor patient closely for nonverbal evidence of pain, including: restlessness, guarding of burned areas, wrinkled brow, clenched fingers, reluctance to move, facial pallor or flushing, diaphoresis, tachycardia or hypertension, pupil dilation.
- Assess analgesic administration and discuss modification of analgesic dose, schedule, or type with a physician or other on-call provider if pain persists.
- Administer analgesics as ordered and evaluate effectiveness; if continuous infusion medications are ordered, ensure that bolus administration of the drug is used to initiate infusion therapy and achieve therapeutic drug levels. Bolus therapy may also be required if dose of drug is increased (see Chapter 5). Ensure adequate analgesia before painful procedures.
- Identify factors that aggravate or alleviate pain and modify patient support accordingly.
- Assist with nonpharmacologic methods of pain relief.
- Ensure uninterrupted periods of rest.

Box 20-2   Nursing Care of the Child with Thermal Injuries—cont'd

Potential Burn Wound Infection or Septic Shock Related to: Open Wound, Presence of Multiple Invasive Catheters, Compromise in Immune Function

Expected Patient Outcomes

- Patient will demonstrate no signs of infection, including fever or hypothermia, leukocytosis or leukopenia, wound erythema, wound drainage, or positive blood cultures.
- If infection develops, it will be promptly treated with antibiotics and the patient will be closely monitored for evidence of sepsis.
- Burn wound and graft sites will heal within appropriate interval.

Nursing Activities

- Assess wound appearance for evidence of local signs of infection, including: erythema; change in color, appearance, odor, or amount of wound drainage; change in color of wound to black or dark brown, progression of burn to full thickness injury; sloughing of graft or wound breakdown after closure.
- Monitor patient temperature and white blood cell count and differential; notify the on-call provider of changes.
- Obtain blood cultures as ordered.
- Administer antibiotics as ordered (precisely on time) and monitor for side effects.
- Ensure strict aseptic technique during all invasive procedures; ensure clean technique during all noninvasive procedures including wound care.
- Maintain closed delivery system for all intravenous lines.
- Ensure good hand-washing technique by all members of the healthcare team before and after patient contact.
- Monitor the patient closely for signs of sepsis, including fever, hypothermia, tachycardia, tachypnea, alteration in responsiveness, leukocytosis, leukopenia, metabolic acidosis, evidence of organ system dysfunction (e.g., oliguria, diarrhea or vomiting, abdominal distension, elevation in liver transaminases), evidence of relative hypovolemia (and increased intravascular fluid requirements to maintain perfusion), and signs of septic shock (sepsis plus cardiovascular and one other organ system failure). See Boxes 6-2 and 6-3.

Potential Temperature Instability Related to Heat Loss Through Burn Surface

Expected Patient Outcomes

- Patient will maintain normal body temperature with absence of shivering and chills.
- Patient skin temperature will remain normal and extremities will be warm to the touch.

Nursing Activities

- Monitor body temperature hourly initially, then every 2 to 4 hours when the patient's condition is stable.

- Monitor for signs of cold stress, including shivering or chills, or tachycardia, tachypnea and hypoxemia in young infant.
- Use a heat shield, over bed warmer, or warming blanket as needed to maintain the patient's body temperature.
- Keep ambient air warm, and prevent any room draft.
- Use warmed (not hot) solution during burn care.
- Perform burn care under a heat shield or overbed warmer for infants or young children and as needed for older children.
- Minimize patient exposure during treatments or wound care (e.g., perform burn care on one extremity at a time, and redress that extremity before the next extremity is unwrapped).
- Consider warming of intravenous fluids and blood products; warming should be performed according to hospital policy for infants and young children.

Potential for Inadequate Nutrition Related to: Excessive Caloric Requirements, Inadequate Caloric Intake, Altered Metabolism

Expected Patient Outcome

- Patient will demonstrate adequate nutritional status as evidenced by no weight loss, good wound healing and skin turgor, absence of nausea and vomiting, adequate recorded caloric intake.

Nursing Activities

- Calculate the patient's caloric and protein needs and notify the on-call provider if these are not being met. Monitor patient tolerance of tube, oral, or parenteral feedings. Ensure appropriate distribution of calories within protein, fat, and carbohydrates.
- Begin enteral feedings as ordered; notify a provider of feeding intolerance (including abdominal distension, vomiting, diarrhea, increased residual volume after gastric feeding, reflux). For additional information, see Chapter 14.
- Implement measures to reduce nausea and vomiting as needed, including position changes and administering an antiemetic.
- Ensure adequate oral intake when tolerated; calculate caloric intake and ensure provision of multiple opportunities to eat a wide variety of appetizing foods.
  ◦ Determine the child's preferences and encourage the parents to bring the child's favorite foods.
  ◦ Allow adequate time for meals uninterrupted by treatments or examinations.
- Obtain daily weight; notify a provider of weight loss or failure to gain weight.
- Obtain consultation with dietician as needed. Evaluate oxygen and caloric expenditure using calorimetry as needed.

Additional Potential Problems

- Fear and anxiety
- Potential alteration in self-concept

COHb, Carboxyhemoglobin.

is closely monitored, and urine volume and fluid balance must be evaluated regularly.

Intravenous Access and Monitoring. When the burn totals 15% or more of TBSA, intravenous therapy will be mandatory to restore intravascular volume and maintain fluid and electrolyte balance. Major peripheral veins should be cannulated

using large-bore catheters. A urinary catheter should be inserted to enable continuous monitoring of urine output.

Whenever a major burn is present or systemic perfusion is compromised significantly, insertion of a central venous catheter (into the subclavian, internal jugular, or femoral vein) should be considered to provide reliable, large-bore venous access. Use of a multilumen central venous catheter will

Clinical Signs Observed During Third-Spacing Period

Signs of Hypovolemia
- Peripheral vasoconstriction, diminished pulses
- Tachycardia
- Oliguria, increased urine specific gravity
- Low central venous pressure, pulmonary artery pressure
- Sunken fontanelle
- Metabolic (lactic) acidosis

Evidence of Edema
- Periorbital, extremity edema
- Respiratory distress
- Weight gain

provide two or more ports to facilitate fluid administration and central venous pressure (CVP) monitoring. Any central venous catheter must be inserted under strict sterile conditions and cared for using strict aseptic technique (see Chapter 21 and Box 22-6).

Determination of Fluid Requirements. A variety of formulas have been developed to assist in determining fluid losses and requirements in patients with burns (Table 20-3). Many formulas, however, have been designed for use in adult patients and are based solely on body weight and percentage of TBSA burned. Use of these adult formulas will result in inadequate pediatric fluid resuscitation.[62,135]

The most popular formula for use in adolescent and adult patients with burns is the Parkland (by Baxter) formula.[10] Modification of the Parkland formula for children provides for crystalloid administration during the first 24 hours of therapy. The volume administered during this time is based on the burn surface area (4 mL/kg per percent of TBSA burned) plus

maintenance fluid requirements (1500 mL/m^2 BSA).[215] Half of this calculated fluid is administered during the first 8 hours of therapy, and the remaining half is administered during the next 16 hours of therapy.

The child's fluid resuscitation requirements should be based on body surface area rather than weight. Because children have a greater body surface area in relation to weight, weight-based formulas can underestimate the fluid requirements of children with minor burns and may grossly overestimate the fluid requirements of those with extensive burns.[79] TBSA can be rapidly estimated from height and weight using standard nomograms (see inside back cover of this text).

The Galveston formula[26] (developed by Carvajal at the Shriners Hospital for Children in Galveston, Texas) provides 5000 mL/m^2 BSA burned plus 2000 mL/m^2 BSA of lactated Ringer's solution given over the first 24 hours after the injury, with half the volume administered during the first 8 hours and the remaining half over the next 16 hours. The Carvajal formula[26] recommends crystalloid and colloid administration based on the absolute surface area of the child's burn, plus generous maintenance fluid administration.

The formula selected for burn resuscitation usually is based on physician preference or burn unit protocols. Any fluid resuscitation formula, however, should serve only as a guide for initiation of therapy. Ongoing assessment of systemic perfusion, intravascular volume status, and fluid and electrolyte balance should be used to modify therapy.

Selection of Fluid Content. There is continued debate regarding the relative benefits of crystalloid versus colloid administration during burn resuscitation.[27,42,51,176] Proponents of crystalloids advocate the use of isotonic or hypertonic crystalloids because they are physiologic, inexpensive, and readily available.

Table 20-3 **Recommendations for Fluid Administration Rate for Patients with Burns**

Reference*	Fluid administration	Solution	Rate of Administration
Cope and Moore (1947)	150 mL per percent of BSA burned every 24 h + maintenance fluid	½ colloid and ½ crystalloid D$_5$W given as maintenance	½ given in first 8 h; ½ given in subsequent 16 h
Evans et al (1952)	2 mL/kg per percent of BSA burned every 24 h + 2000 mL/day maintenance fluid	½ colloid and ½ crystalloid D$_5$W given as maintenance	½ given in first 8 h; ½ given in subsequent 16 h
Brooke, developed by Reiss et al (1953)	2 mL/kg per percent of BSA burned + 2000 mL/day maintenance fluid	¼ colloid and ¾ crystalloid D$_5$W given as maintenance	½ given in first 8 h; ½ given in subsequent 16 h
Eagle (1956)	30 mL per percent of BSA burned + 10% of body weight (kg) every 48 h	Crystalloid with 20 g albumin per liter	Divided equally over 48 h
Batchelor (1961)	1-5 mL/kg per percent of BSA burned every 24 h	Colloid and blood only	Individualized
Parkland by Baxter and Shires (1968)	4 mL/kg per percent of BSA burned every 24 h	Crystalloid only	½ given in first 8 h; ½ given in subsequent 16 h
Monafo (1970, 1984)	None	Crystalloid (hypertonic saline: Na$^+$ = 250 mEq/L)	Adjust to maintain urine output of 30 mL/h
Modified Parkland	4 mL/kg per percent of BSA burned + 15 mL/m^2 of BSA	Crystalloid only	½ given in first 8 h; ½ given in subsequent 16 h
Galveston, by Carvajel (1975)	5000 mL/m^2 BSA burned + 2000 mL/m^2 BSA every 24 h	Crystalloid with 12.5 g serum albumin per liter	½ given in first 8 h; ½ given in subsequent 16 h

*Based on data from References 8,10,26,37,56,59,89,123,140,141,177,185,202,185,215.
BSA, Body surface area; *D$_5$W*, 5% dextrose in water.

Critics of crystalloid administration note that immediately after administration, isotonic crystalloids will equilibrate between the intravascular and interstitial spaces, and only a fraction of administered intravenous crystalloids will remain in the vascular space.[178] Therefore, large quantities of crystalloids generally are required to restore intravascular volume. In addition, the fluid that moves into the interstitial space may contribute to worsening systemic edema. Pulmonary interstitial water usually does not increase substantially during this time, because pulmonary capillary permeability remains normal unless significant inhalation injury occurs. In addition, lymph flow is usually proportional to the amount of pulmonary interstitial water movement.

Colloid resuscitation may restore intravascular volume and pressure more efficiently than will crystalloid administration. If capillary permeability is normal, administered colloids will remain in the vascular space for several hours, exerting oncotic pressure. This oncotic pressure will increase intravascular volume and maintain intravascular osmolality, so that continued fluid shift from the vascular space is less likely. Because colloids are thought to diffuse more slowly into the interstitial space, colloid resuscitated patients may develop less edema than crystalloid-resuscitated patients.[163] Adequate fluid resuscitation should be possible with relatively small volumes of colloids,[86,201] so that the patient receives a small volume and salt load.

Critics of colloid administration note that membrane permeability is not normal in patients immediately after burns, and proteins may move from the vascular to the interstitial space during the first 24 hours after a burn.[9] Movement of administered colloids into the interstitial space can increase interstitial oncotic pressure, enhancing the fluid shift from the intravascular space into the interstitial space.

Colloid administration during the first day after a burn was avoided in the past, based on the fear that it would increase the severity of third-spacing of fluid.[182] However, the validity of this criticism has been challenged during the last decade. Although albumin may leave the vascular space, an equal amount of albumin may be returned to the vascular space by lymphatics approximately 8 hours or more after a burn. Therefore many institutions have successfully added small amounts of colloids to their early burn resuscitation protocols.

In general, adequate resuscitation can be provided if isotonic crystalloids are administered in sufficient quantity.[48] Lactated Ringer's (LR) solution, an isotonic crystalloid, is the most widely used solution for burn resuscitation. The composition of LR's solution closely mimics extracellular (including intravascular) fluid composition (Table 20-4); therefore

LR's solution is ideal for replenishing intravascular water and electrolytes. In addition, LR's solution contains lactate, which is metabolized to bicarbonate, so it will buffer mild acidosis. Lactated Ringer's solution is inexpensive, readily available, and effective in the treatment of nonhemorrhagic hypovolemia.

Normal saline (0.9% sodium chloride) can be used as an alternative to lactated Ringer's solution for isotonic crystalloid resuscitation. Because normal saline contains no potassium, use of normal saline may be ideal for the patient with hyperkalemia or renal failure. Potassium chloride (20-40 mEq/L) is usually added to normal saline if renal function is adequate and the child's serum potassium is acceptable. Normal saline does not contain lactate or other buffers.

During fluid resuscitation, the child's systemic perfusion and urine output must be monitored closely. These parameters should improve if fluid administration is adequate (Table 20-5). The serum hemoglobin concentration, electrolyte balance, and acid-base status (including serum lactate) must also be monitored closely.

Because only a portion of administered isotonic crystalloids will remain in the vascular space, generous crystalloid administration is needed to restore effective or adequate intravascular volume. Systemic edema should be anticipated, because some of the administered volume moves into the interstitial space. It is important to note that the development of such edema does not indicate that fluid resuscitation is adequate; titration of fluid administration should be based on assessment of perfusion and intravascular volume status.

Pulmonary edema usually is not problematic during early burn resuscitation. However, because respiratory failure can develop for a variety of reasons, the patient's respiratory function must be monitored closely, and appropriate support (with intubation, mechanical ventilatory support, and positive end expiratory pressure) must be provided as needed.

Hypotonic crystalloids should not be used for fluid resuscitation, because such fluid will tend to lower intravascular sodium concentration and osmolality and enhance the fluid shift from the vascular space. Hypoosmolality will worsen systemic edema and may contribute to the development of cerebral edema. Furthermore, the fluids will not assist in the restoration of intravascular volume.

Hypertonic saline resuscitation can be beneficial in treating burn-induced shock.[16,17,64,84] This process maintains intravascular volume more effectively because it induces movement of free water from the interstitial to the intravascular space, thus decreasing generalized tissue edema. However, hypertonic saline is not widely used because of the potential risk of

Table 20-4 Composition of Resuscitation Solutions

Solution	Tonicity	ELECTROLYTE COMPOSITION (mEq/L)				
		Na[4]	K[4]	Ca[4]	Cl-	Lactate*
Lactated Ringer's	Isotonic	130	4	3	109	28
Normal saline	Isotonic	154	0	0	154	0
1.5% Hypertonic saline	Hypertonic	250	0	0	150	100
Normal extracellular fluid		142	5	5	103	26

*Metabolized to bicarbonate.

Table 20-5 **Clinical Responses to Fluid Resuscitation in Burned Patients**

Parameter	Desirable Response (Fluid Resuscitation Adequate)	Undesirable Response (Fluid Administration Inadequate)
Urine output	1 mL/kg per hour (up to 30 kg, then 25-30 mL/h)	<1 mL/kg per hour (for children above 30 kg, less than 25 mL/h)
Specific gravity	1.010-1.025	>1.025
Weight	Preburn level	10% less than preburn level
Blood pressure	Normal for age or high*	Low for age*
Pulse	Normal for age*	Normal or high*
Level of consciousness	Alert, clear, and lucid	Lethargic and stuporous
Hematocrit	35%-45%	48%-55%
Serum sodium	135-145 mEq/L	>150 mEq/L
Blood urea nitrogen	5-20 mg/dL	>25 mg/dL
Creatinine	0.8-1.4 mg/dL	>2.0 mg/dL
Osmolality (serum)	275-295 mOsm/L	>300 mOsm/L
Urine sodium	60-100 mEq/L	≤40 mEq/L
Blood pH	7.20-7.50	<7.20
Serum lactate	Venous: 0.5-2.2 mmol/L Arterial: 0.5-1.6 mmol/L	>4 mmol/L
Peripheral circulation	Brisk capillary refill; normal color in unburned areas	Cyanosis; prolonged capillary refill
Central venous pressure (CVP)	4-8 mmHg	<2-4 mmHg
Pulmonary artery pressure (PAP)	Systolic, 20-30 mmHg Diastolic, 5-15 mmHg	Systolic, <20 mmHg Diastolic, <5 mmHg
Cardiac index	3.0-4.5 L/min per m² BSA	<3.0 L/min per m² BSA

*See normal blood pressure and heart rate ranges for age in Tables 1-1 and 1-3 (and on pages inside front cover).
BSA, Body surface area.

hypernatremia, hyperosmolarity, renal failure, and alkalosis.[98,173,222] Some favor the use of a modified hypertonic solution—adding an ampule of sodium bicarbonate to each liter of lactated Ringer's solution during the first 24 hours of resuscitation.[19]

Routine Care. Regardless of the type of resuscitation fluid being used, the nurse must closely monitor the patient's response to volume resuscitation (see Table 20-5). Adequate systemic perfusion, demonstrated by warm extremities, brisk capillary refill, strong peripheral pulses, and adequate (1-2 mL/kg body weight per hour) urine volume should be observed.

The child's level of consciousness should be appropriate for clinical condition. Irritability may be an early sign of cardiovascular or neurologic deterioration,[150] and lethargy or decreased response to painful stimulation is abnormal and requires investigation.

Tachycardia may continue despite adequate fluid resuscitation, but it should not be extreme, and the blood pressure should be appropriate for age. Extreme tachycardia, thready peripheral pulses, hypotension, and metabolic acidosis indicate serious compromise in cardiac output and systemic perfusion, as well as a probable urgent need for volume administration.

During fluid resuscitation, the nurse should be alert for the development of pulmonary edema, and the team should have a plan for a sequence of appropriate respiratory support. Elective intubation should be performed before decompensation occurs (see Respiratory Failure in this chapter and Chapter 9).

Urine volume should be recorded every hour, and urine specific gravity should be determined every 2 to 4 hours.

Frequency of assessment of serum electrolytes, hematocrit, and blood gases during the first hours of therapy will be determined by patient condition; hourly evaluation may be required for the patient in unstable condition.

Pulse oximetry should be used for continuous monitoring of arterial oxyhemoglobin saturation. Additional monitoring, including the use of near-infrared spectroscopy (NIRS) and monitoring of exhaled carbon dioxide ($P_{ET}CO_2$) should be used based on unit protocols.

During fluid resuscitation of the infant, the serum glucose concentration should be monitored closely. Young infants may rapidly develop hypoglycemia during stress, so it is necessary to provide a continuous source of glucose intake and monitor point-of-care (e.g., bedside) or intravascular glucose concentration frequently.

Once the child's condition is stable, hematocrit, hemoglobin, blood urea nitrogen (BUN), creatinine, electrolytes, glucose, serum osmolality, and urine sodium are monitored daily—more often if abnormalities are present. The hematocrit and BUN often rise immediately after a burn, but sustained and significant increase in these values usually suggests the need for further volume administration. An increase in the serum creatinine often indicates the presence of renal failure.

The urine sodium may also be monitored. Normal urinary excretion of sodium is approximately 60 to 100 mEq/L. A low urine sodium (less than 40 mEq/L) usually results from aldosterone secretion in the presence of inadequate intravascular volume[123] and indicates the need for further volume administration.

The rate, content, and function of each fluid infusion system should be checked hourly, and each infusion site should be examined. Intravenous tubing must be changed using strict aseptic technique. Intravenous catheters must be taped or sutured securely, so that kinking or dislodgement is impossible.

The child's daily weight without dressings should be recorded accurately using the same scale or method at the same time each day. The child's weight immediately after the burn should be used as the baseline weight. If the child is not weighed until fluid resuscitation is underway, estimation of the preburn weight should be made after an interview with the parents. During this period, the child's weight typically will increase by 10% to 20% or more.

Evaluation of Therapy. There is no single parameter that will indicate effectiveness of postburn resuscitation. Systemic perfusion and neurologic function must be maintained at satisfactory levels. Mean arterial pressure should be appropriate for age. Whereas hypotension certainly indicates cardiovascular compromise and the need for further resuscitation, a normal mean arterial pressure may be present despite significant hypovolemia and shock. Acidosis should be absent or mild and improving if resuscitation is effective.

Urine volume and CVP should also be monitored closely, but they will fluctuate significantly during resuscitation. It is usually advisable to evaluate the average urine volume over 2-hour periods to better monitor fluid balance and adjust fluid administration. Low urine volume usually indicates the need for additional fluid administration. Diuretic therapy should not be provided during the initial phase of standard burn resuscitation, because it may contribute to intravascular volume depletion. Mannitol administration may be necessary after severe electrical injuries to enhance clearance of myoglobin.

Increased fluid administration is probably necessary if inadequate systemic perfusion and continuing acidosis are associated with a low CVP. Vasoactive drug therapy will not improve systemic perfusion produced by hypovolemia. Poor systemic perfusion and extreme acidosis despite adequate fluid administration indicate severe shock and are associated with a high mortality (see Shock in Chapter 6).

Hypervolemia: Fluid Mobilization Phase
Etiology and Pathophysiology
Approximately 24 to 48 hours after a burn, capillary healing results in the restoration of normal capillary permeability, and fluid begins to shift back into the vascular space from the interstitial space. Hypervolemia is the problem most likely to be encountered during this period.

Clinical Signs and Symptoms
As fluid returns to the vascular space, the patient's peripheral edema should subside, and evidence of pulmonary edema (on chest radiograph and by pulmonary function) should disappear. Reduction in pulmonary interstitial fluid may be difficult to appreciate if the patient has sustained significant inhalation injury or if acute respiratory distress syndrome (ARDS) has developed. Urine volume should increase significantly, and the child's weight should begin to decrease toward the baseline (preburn) weight (Box 20-4).

Hyponatremia may persist as the result of increased renal sodium excretion. Potassium will shift back into the cells,

---

Box 20-4	**Clinical Signs Observed During Fluid Mobilization Period**

Signs of Hypervolemia
- Increased central venous pressure
- Increased urine volume, fall in specific gravity

Resolving Edema
- Decreased peripheral edema
- Improved respiratory function, unless acute respiratory distress syndrome is present
- Fall in body weight to baseline

Electrolyte Abnormalities
- Decreased sodium concentration, potassium concentration, hematocrit, blood urea nitrogen, and creatinine concentration

---

and urinary potassium loss is increased, so hypokalemia is usually noted.[28] Finally the hematocrit falls as the result of hemodilution and increased destruction of RBCs.

Management
This phase of burn care requires continued monitoring of systemic perfusion and fluid and electrolyte balance. The volume and content of intravenous fluid provided must be appropriate for the changes in intravascular volume and electrolyte balance that are occurring.

Fluid and Electrolyte Therapy. Fluid loss during this period will consist of continued evaporative water losses from the burn surface and basal metabolic (insensible) water losses (Box 20-5). Evaporative water losses become significant approximately 24 hours after the burn, and they may be as high as 2000 mL/day in the child. Because fluid lost by evaporation is predominantly water, replacement with 5% dextrose and 0.45% sodium chloride solution is provided.

Hypokalemia is more likely to develop if dextrose-containing intravenous fluids are used, because such fluids will enhance intracellular movement of potassium. Supplementary potassium administration should be planned to maintain normal serum potassium concentration.

Colloids are often administered to maintain intravascular oncotic pressure and enhance the interstitial-to-intravascular fluid shift. Usually a volume of colloid equivalent to 20% of the circulating blood volume is administered over 24 hours.

Box 20-5	**Fluid Requirements 24-48 h after Burn Injury**

Maintenance fluid* = Basal fluid requirements + Evaporative water loss
- Basal fluid per hour = $(1500 \text{ mL} \times \text{m}^2 \text{ BSA}) \div 24$
- Evaporative water loss per hour = $(35 + \% \text{ burn}) \text{ m}^2 \text{ BSA}$
Colloid = 20% of circulating blood volume
- mL/hour = $0.20 \times (70^† \text{ mL/kg} \times \text{kg body weight})/24$

*Given as 5% dextrose in water or D_5W/0.45% sodium chloride.
†Adjust to mL/kg blood volume for age
BSA, Body surface area; *kg,* body weight in kilograms; % burn is the estimated percent of body surface area that is burned (see Fig. 20-3 and 20-4).

Blood administration may be necessary if significant anemia develops. The hematocrit should be maintained at approximately 25% to 30%, using whole blood or packed RBCs. Administration of 10 mL/kg of packed RBCs will increase the hematocrit by approximately 10 percentage points (e.g., from 25% to 35%). This volume should be administered over 3 to 4 hours, and patient tolerance of the volume should be assessed constantly during the transfusion. A diuretic may be administered immediately before the transfusion to prevent hypervolemia (for further information regarding transfusion therapy, see Chapter 15).

Routine Care. Continuous evaluation of systemic perfusion is required. Color, peripheral perfusion, oxygenation, and level of consciousness should remain excellent. A mild tachycardia may continue. Urine volume should exceed 1 to 2 mL/kg body weight per hour with a specific gravity of less than 1.020 as intravascular volume is restored.

Urine volume should be totaled hourly, and urine specific gravity should be recorded every 2 hours. Assessment of fluid balance should be made at these times. A urine specific gravity greater than 1.025 usually indicates the need for additional fluid administration.

The child's hematocrit, hemoglobin, BUN, creatinine, electrolytes, glucose, serum osmolality, and urine sodium should continue to be monitored. A fall in hemoglobin, hematocrit, and serum sodium and osmolality typically are observed during this phase of therapy. A rise in serum BUN and creatinine may indicate renal dysfunction. The urine sodium may rise (above the normal 60-100 mEq/L) as renal sodium excretion increases.

The content, infusion rate, and infusion system for each intravenous line should be checked at least every hour. The infusion site also should be checked hourly, and the catheter and tubing should be secured to prevent dislodgement or kinking. The tubing must be changed using strict aseptic technique.

The child's daily weight should be recorded accurately, and weight changes should be evaluated. The child's weight typically falls during this time; it may return to near baseline values by the sixth day after the burn.

Evaluation of Therapy. If cardiorespiratory function remains adequate, systemic perfusion should continue to improve. If hypervolemia is present, the child will demonstrate high CVP, and hepatomegaly and pulmonary edema may develop or persist (Table 20-6).

If cardiovascular dysfunction is associated with the hypervolemia, poor systemic perfusion will be noted in addition to the signs of pulmonary and systemic edema, and oliguria may be present. Ventricular dilation and reduced contractility will be apparent on echocardiography. In these patients, diuretic therapy and support of cardiovascular function should be intensified, and vasoactive drug therapy probably is necessary. See Chapters 6 and 8 for further information about management of shock and congestive heart failure.

If urine volume does not improve and the serum BUN and creatinine rise during this time, renal failure may be present. See Chapter 13 for information regarding management of renal failure.[198,211]

Table 20-6 Clinical Parameters Indicating Hypervolemia During Fluid Resuscitation 24-48 h after Burn Injury

Parameter*	Signs of Hypervolemia
Urine output	>2 mL/kg per hour
Specific gravity	<1.010
Weight	≥20% above preburn level
Blood pressure	Elevated[†]
Heart rate	Normal or high[†]
Level of consciousness	Can be alert or lethargic
Hematocrit	25-30%
Serum sodium	<130 mEq/L
Blood urea nitrogen	<5 mg/dL
Creatinine	<0.5 mg/dL
Osmolality	<250 mOsm/L
Urine sodium	≥100-120 mEq/L
Blood pH	>7.50
Peripheral circulation	Bounding peripheral pulses
Central venous pressure	>10 mmHg
Pulmonary artery pressure PAP	Systolic, >30 mmHg Diastolic, >15 mmHg
Cardiac index	>8.0 L/min per m² BSA

*See Box 20-4 for desirable responses.
[†]See normal blood pressure and heart rate values for age in Tables 1-1 and 1-3 and on pages inside front cover.
BSA, Body surface area.

Respiratory Failure

Etiology

Respiratory failure in the burn patient may be the result of inhalation of toxic substances, airway edema, or increased capillary permeability pulmonary edema. These pulmonary insults will produce the problems of airway obstruction or of acute respiratory failure with permeability pulmonary edema (i.e., ARDS). CO poisoning will compromise oxygen delivery. These problems will be discussed briefly here; see Chapter 9 for a more detailed discussion of respiratory failure and ARDS.

Pathophysiology

Inhalation of smoke, hot gas, and combustion products can produce oropharyngeal edema and injury to the ciliated mucosal epithelial layer of the trachea. Edema and airway obstruction usually are evident during the first 24 hours after the burn. If the mucosal layer is injured severely, it may slough 48 to 72 hours after the burn, causing acute airway obstruction.[94]

Permeability pulmonary edema and ARDS result from damage to the pulmonary alveolar capillary membrane.[183] This damage allows both proteins and fluids to move from the vascular space into the interstitium of the lung, causing pulmonary edema. This edema produces intrapulmonary shunting, hypoxemia, decreased pulmonary compliance, and increased work of breathing.[118]

Following the thermal injury, leukocytes and platelets accumulate in the small vessels of the lungs, obstructing some pulmonary arteries. This obstruction may compromise pulmonary blood flow or result in development of increased pulmonary vascular resistance, with resultant increase in right ventricular afterload.

The insult of the burn, inhalation injury, resulting shock, and fluid resuscitation all can contribute to the development of ARDS. Other pathologic mechanisms may contribute to the progression of pulmonary injury, including production of arachidonic acid metabolites and release of vasoactive substances. However, the most common cause of postburn pulmonary capillary injury, pulmonary edema, and respiratory failure is the development of sepsis (see Septic Shock in Chapters 6 and 16, and Septic Shock, Mediators of the Septic Cascade, in the Chapter 6 Supplement on the Evolve Website).

CO injury or chemical injury may result from inhalation of smoke or other products of combustion. CO binds readily with hemoglobin, so the hemoglobin it binds is not available to carry oxygen.[82] Small amounts of inhaled CO can substantially reduce hemoglobin oxygen-carrying capacity and tissue oxygen delivery. Progressive tissue hypoxia and acidosis will result in tissue and organ (including neurologic) dysfunction.

Inhalation of other products of combustion can produce pharyngeal or tracheobronchial edema or ulceration, with a resultant risk of airway obstruction. In addition, the inhaled substances can decrease ciliary action or produce bronchorrhea, bronchospasm, airway ulceration, or pulmonary edema (Table 20-7).

Clinical Signs and Symptoms

Respiratory symptoms will be determined by the location of the burn and the quantity and type of gas inhaled. Inhalation injuries can produce respiratory failure over time (Table 20-8).

Burns of the face and neck and severe inhalation injuries typically produce edema and upper airway obstruction during the first 8 hours after a burn. CO poisoning also will be apparent during this time.

Respiratory failure with permeability pulmonary edema usually does not develop until approximately 8 to 48 hours or more after a burn. Children with burns are at risk for the development of secondary infections, particularly pneumonia, which usually develop approximately 5 days or more after the burn.

Airway Obstruction. The child with airway obstruction will demonstrate tachypnea, nasal flaring, and retractions. Upper airway obstruction will produce drooling and stridor with prolonged inspiratory time. Lower airway obstruction will produce wheezing and prolonged expiratory time. If a significant increase in respiratory effort is noted within the first

hours after a burn, severe airway obstruction is probably present and will likely increase in severity over the course of the first 8 hours following the burn. If evidence of respiratory fatigue (including irritability or decreased responsiveness, severe retractions, or slowing of respiratory rate), hypoxemia, or hypercarbia is observed, respiratory arrest is probably imminent and urgent support of airway, oxygenation and ventilation is needed.

Acute Respiratory Distress Syndrome. The first signs of respiratory failure related to increased capillary permeability pulmonary edema (i.e., ARDS) usually include tachypnea and hypocapnia, with a resultant respiratory alkalosis. Although the chest radiograph may initially be normal, reticular infiltrates indicative of interstitial pulmonary edema are often apparent within 8 hours of the inhalation, the burn, or the development of sepsis.

Within 24 to 96 hours after the pulmonary insult, the child with ARDS will demonstrate clinical evidence of significant pulmonary edema and decreased pulmonary compliance (tachypnea with increased respiratory effort). Crackles often are noted on clinical examination. Arterial blood gases or pulse oximetry will demonstrate hypoxemia, which is not relieved by supplementary oxygen administration.[184]

Carbon Monoxide Poisoning. CO poisoning should be suspected in any child who has been burned in a fire involving

---

Table 20-8 Clinical Stages of Inhalation Injury

Stage	Onset (Hours After Burn)	Characteristics
Ventilatory insufficiency	0-8	Bronchospasm and alveolar damage
Pulmonary edema	8-48	Edema of upper or lower airways and pulmonary interstitial edema, hypoxemia and decreased lung compliance
Bronchopneumonia	≥72	Bronchorrhea, pneumonia, decrease in ciliary and mucosal activity

---

Table 20-7 Toxic Products and Clinical Symptoms Produced from Burning Substances

Substances	Toxic Products	Clinical Symptoms
Polyvinylchloride	Hydrogen chloride, phosgene	Dyspnea, burning mucous membranes, lightheadedness, laryngeal and pulmonary edema
Wood, cotton, paper	Acetaldehyde, formaldehyde, acrolein, acetic acid, methane	Decrease in ciliary action, decrease in macrophage activity, pulmonary edema
Polyurethane foam	Isocyanate, hydrogen cyanide	Dyspnea, lightheadedness, confusion, dizziness, unconsciousness
Wool, silk	Ammonia, sulfur dioxide, hydrogen sulfide	Bronchorrhea, bronchospasm, ulceration, pulmonary edema, hoarseness, stridor, dyspnea
Nylon	Ammonia, hydrogen cyanide	Dyspnea, dizziness, bronchospasm, pulmonary edema, unconsciousness
Teflon	Octafluoroisobutylene	Dyspnea, wheezing, pulmonary edema

wood or furniture. The presence of carbonaceous material in the sputum will confirm the inhalation of smoke and possible CO poisoning.

CO poisoning will produce a fall in measured hemoglobin saturation if a cooximeter (e.g., Corning IL282 or Corning 2500; Corning, N.Y.) is used for blood-gas analysis. The hemoglobin saturation obtained by pulse oximetry can be normal despite significant CO poisoning, because the COHb is not recognized as functioning hemoglobin by the oximeter. If the hemoglobin saturation from a blood gas sample is calculated based on the child's arterial oxygen tension and pH, a normal saturation may be derived despite progressive hypoxemia.[43] Dissolved oxygen in the arterial blood may produce a normal arterial oxygen tension, even in the presence of significant compromise in arterial oxygen content and tissue oxygenation. For these reasons the arterial oxyhemoglobin saturation should be measured with a cooximeter.

To determine the presence and severity of CO poisoning, COHb levels should also be determined, and the hemoglobin saturation should be measured. In addition, the child's arterial pH and serum lactate should be closely monitored, because they will reflect the severity of tissue hypoxia. COHb levels begin to fall within hours of CO exposure; therefore low COHb levels may be obtained in the child with severe CO poisoning if blood sampling is delayed.

Mild CO poisoning will produce headache and shortness of breath, but CO toxicity will result in cardiorespiratory distress, coma, severe metabolic acidosis, and multisystem organ failure (Table 20-9). Significant CO toxicity produces vasodilation and a characteristic cherry red color in the mucous membranes and cheeks. Late neurologic dysfunction following CO inhalation has been reported in children and includes headache, personality and behavioral changes, memory loss, and poor school performance; this dysfunction is thought to result from hypoxic injury to the cerebral cortex.[112]

Management

Inhalation injury should be suspected in any burn victim with evidence of oral burns, singed nasal hairs, pharyngeal ulceration, carbonaceous material in the nose or mouth, congestion, or a high-pitched cough.[188] Tachypnea, dyspnea, stridor, wheezing, cough, and increased respiratory secretions indicate

Table 20-9	Relationship Between Blood Carboxyhemoglobin Levels and Clinical Signs and Symptoms

CoHb Level (%)	Symptoms
<10	None
10-20	Mild headache, dyspnea, visual changes, confusion
20-40	Dizziness, shortness of breath, nausea and vomiting, irritability, weakness, ringing in the ears, hypotension, tachycardia
40-60	Hallucinations, confusion, coma, cardiopulmonary instability, arrhythmias
>60	Usually fatal

COHb, Carboxyhemoglobin.

development of significant airway obstruction. Resultant hypoxia may produce changes in color and responsiveness.

Because inhalation injury may be present, the child with burns and respiratory distress should receive 100% inspired oxygen concentration and must be monitored closely. Intubation equipment should be readily available, and intubation should be accomplished on an elective basis for any child with evidence of severe airway obstruction or inhalation injury. Mechanical ventilation support must be planned whenever deterioration in respiratory effort or function is detected and before it becomes severe.

Airway Obstruction. Specific signs of airway obstruction and the need for intubation include the development of severe respiratory distress or failure, fatigue, or inability to cry forcefully or speak. Hypoxia will be only a very late sign of critical airway obstruction and often indicates that respiratory arrest is imminent. Succinylcholine should not be used for intubation of burn patients, because it may produce potassium release from muscles and severe hyperkalemia (particularly 48 or more hours after a burn).

Occasionally, severe upper airway edema makes intubation difficult, and a tracheostomy may be necessary. However, early elective intubation, rather than late emergency intubation may preclude the need for tracheostomy and its potential complications.[132]

Maintenance of proper tube placement is essential for the child with critical airway obstruction. If severe facial burns are present, facial tape cannot be used to secure the endotracheal tube. Twill tape can be wrapped around the neck and the endotracheal tube to secure the tube. The twill tape should be placed above one ear and under the other ear to minimize nasal distortion.[2] Commercial tube holders may also be used.

Sedation or pharmacologic paralysis (with analgesia) may be necessary to maintain endotracheal tube position until edema subsides. For unknown reasons, patients with extensive burns usually are resistant to all but extremely high doses of nondepolarizing neuromuscular blocking agents.

Acute Respiratory Distress Syndrome. If the child develops permeability pulmonary edema and ARDS, then intubation and mechanical ventilation will be required.[184] Mechanical ventilation support must be skilled, and high inspired oxygen concentration and titrated positive end-expiratory pressure (PEEP) may be required to achieve optimal oxygen delivery.

PEEP effectively reduces intrapulmonary shunting because it expands atelectatic areas of the lung and improves functional residual capacity.[188] In addition, PEEP probably moves edema fluid to harmless areas of the lung.

Titration of PEEP is designed to ensure maximal oxygen delivery—optimal arterial oxygen content without significant depression of cardiac output. Ideally, titration of PEEP will enable reduction of potentially harmful levels of inspired oxygen and will improve arterial oxygen content and lung compliance. However, it is important to note that high levels of PEEP may produce barotrauma, which can be as harmful to the lung as high levels of inspired oxygen. High PEEP can also reduce systemic venous return and cardiac output, with resultant reduction in oxygen delivery. Therefore the levels of inspired oxygen and PEEP should be the lowest levels consistent with satisfactory oxygen delivery and end organ function. For further information about the management of ARDS, see Acute Respiratory Distress Syndrome in Chapter 9.

Carbon Monoxide Poisoning. The only widely accepted treatment for CO poisoning is administration of 100% oxygen. A high concentration of inspired oxygen will break the CO hemoglobin bond, and hyperoxemia will reduce the half-life of CO. Monitor COHb levels; they typically begin to fall 45 to 60 minutes after CO exposure, and reach normal within 8 to 12 hours. High inspired oxygen should be provided until the COHb level falls to less than 5% to 10% of total hemoglobin.

The child may survive the initial CO exposure, but die from progressive hypoxic cerebral edema 48 to 72 hours after exposure. During this time, careful neurologic assessment should be performed. Signs of increased intracranial pressure include: deterioration in level of consciousness (progressive irritability, then lethargy), decreased spontaneous movement or reduced movement in response to pain, inability to follow commands, and pupil dilation with decreased response to light. Bradycardia, systolic hypertension, and altered respiratory pattern (with possible apnea) may be only late signs of increased intracranial pressure, when cerebral herniation is imminent.

Unfortunately, the development of increased intracranial pressure following cerebral hypoxia is usually a sign of devastating neurologic insult, which is typically unresponsive to conventional therapy for increased intracranial pressure. For further information regarding assessment and management of increased intracranial pressure, see Chapter 11.

Use of hyperbaric oxygen (HBO) has been advocated as a treatment for CO poisoning,[78,234] although its efficacy has not been studied in controlled clinical trials. Brief (30-90-minute) periods in HBO (at 2.5-3.0 times atmospheric pressure) will approximately double the amount of dissolved oxygen present in the blood, so oxygen delivery will improve. In addition, HBO therapy displaces CO from hemoglobin, myoglobin, and cells; this reduces the half-life of carboxyhemoglobin to approximately 20 to 30 minutes, compared with approximately 5 to 6 hours in room air and 80 to 90 minutes in 100% oxygen. HBO therapy also results in rapid removal of CO from intracellular cytochromes, so effects of cellular hypoxia may be halted.[216]

HBO therapy is performed in designated HBO units. If the child's condition is unstable, a multiplace chamber must be used to allow constant attendance by physicians and nurses. HBO is used most frequently for treating patients with isolated CO poisoning, particularly if COHb levels are high (exceeding 25%-30%). HBO therapy may be effective even after COHb levels have returned to normal. Several pediatric case reports have noted promising results of this therapy.[78]

If evidence of inhalation injury is present, elective intubation should be performed before evidence of respiratory function deterioration develops. Humidification of inspired air and suctioning will facilitate removal of airway secretions, but bronchoscopy may be necessary to confirm the diagnosis and to remove carbonaceous material or sloughed epithelium.

Evaluation of Therapy. If airway patency is maintained and inhalation injury is mild, the child should demonstrate effective, spontaneous respiratory effort throughout care. If significant hypoxemia or increased work of breathing is observed, increasing levels of respiratory support (increased inspired oxygen concentrations, intubation, mechanical ventilation, and titration of PEEP) must be provided until oxygen delivery is acceptable.

If burns are extensive, respiratory function is likely to deteriorate during the first days of hospitalization. As a result, continuous assessment of respiratory function and evaluation of the effectiveness of mechanical ventilation support is mandatory. If high concentrations of inspired oxygen and PEEP are required to maintain oxygenation, severe parenchymal injury is probably present, and prolonged mechanical ventilation support may be required (refer to Chapter 9 for treatment of ARDS).

Late deterioration in respiratory function most likely is caused by secondary pneumonia. Appropriate mechanical ventilation support and antibiotic therapy will be required.

Pain
Etiology and Pathophysiology
The child with a burn will experience pain from tissue destruction, exposure of nerve endings, painful debridement and dressing changes, and psychological effects of the injury. Second-degree burns typically hurt continuously, as the result of release of enzymes and proteins in the area of the burn itself. Although nerve endings are destroyed with a third-degree burn, manipulation of the wound or surrounding tissue and exposure of the fascia to air can be extremely painful. There may be little correlation between the size of the burn injury or anatomic location and the intensity of pain.

Debridement of the burn wound can be extremely painful, particularly if enzymatic agents are used. Active and passive range-of-motion exercises, splinting, and positioning will be painful if they involve burned extremities. Finally, insertion of intravenous and monitoring catheters, intubation, suctioning, and phlebotomy also will be painful.

Pruritus is a common complaint following burns. The itching sensation may develop from injured nerves or from healing tissue, and it can be extremely uncomfortable.

Clinical Signs and Symptoms
Virtually all burn patients will be uncomfortable and in pain during the early days of therapy. The conscious and alert child older than preschool age may be able to quantify and localize pain and discomfort, whereas the preverbal, frightened, or disoriented child may not. The nurse should look for nonverbal signs of pain, including tachycardia, facial grimace, pupil dilation, hypertension, diaphoresis, and irritability.

If the child is awake and responsive, assessment tools such as the Eland Color Tool, the Hester Poker Chips, or the Beyers "Oucher" may be used to quantify and perhaps localize pain. These assessment tools are discussed in Chapter 5 (see also Evolve Fig. 5-1 in the Chapter 5 Supplement on the Evolve Website).

Management
Critically ill children often receive inadequate analgesia. The child with a burn injury probably will be in pain throughout the first days of hospitalization. Continuous analgesics should

be provided, and plans should be made to ensure provision of supplementary analgesia during dressing changes and other potentially painful treatments.

If continuous infusion narcotics are provided, the dose may simply be increased during the dressing changes or painful manipulation and decreased when painful stimuli are reduced. If intermittent analgesia is provided, additional medication must be administered at a time sufficiently before the painful event, so effective analgesia is achieved during the procedure. If intermittent analgesics are administered, they should be administered around the clock during the first days after a burn.

Morphine and morphine derivatives frequently are administered to patients with burns. Psychotropic drugs often are administered with morphine to produce amnesia and potentiate the analgesic effect. If the child is breathing spontaneously, it is especially important to monitor the child's respiratory effort, because morphine may depress respiratory function. In addition, significant vasodilation and possible hypotension should be anticipated. High doses of narcotics may produce constipation.

Subanesthetic doses of fentanyl, ketamine, or nitrous oxide also may provide effective analgesia with amnesia for the pediatric patient with a burn. The analgesic and hypnotic effects of ketamine have made it popular in burn units. However, this drug can produce hallucinations, hypertension, and laryngospasm.

A variety of narcotic and psychotropic drugs are currently available to provide analgesia and amnesia. The potential complications of the drugs should not preclude their use. Instead, the nurse and physician should be familiar with the drugs used, anticipate the complications, and monitor the patient accordingly. The goal of therapy is to provide effective analgesia with minimal side effects (see Chapter 5).

Antihistamines frequently are prescribed to relieve pruritus. These drugs may produce tachycardia and drowsiness. Nonpharmacologic methods of pain relief, including imagery, relaxation techniques, transcutaneous nerve stimulation, and hypnosis also may provide effective pain relief under appropriate conditions. These methods are discussed further in Chapter 5.

Potential Infection, Sepsis, and Septic Shock

Etiology
After a burn, the child is at risk for infection from the burn wound itself, from postburn immunosuppression, and through invasive monitoring and therapy equipment. Despite the recent advances in the care of burned children, infection remains the leading cause of post burn morbidity and mortality.[45]

Pathophysiology
Normal Inflammatory Response. The burn wound is the most common site of infection in patients with burns who develop sepsis. For infection to occur, a microorganism must colonize the wound and survive local conditions at the site of entry,[153] then the organism or its toxins must disseminate into the surrounding tissue.

Once the organism enters the body, it triggers a local inflammatory response that includes vasodilation and increased capillary permeability (for further information, see Septic Shock in Chapters 6 and 16, and Septic Shock: Mediators of the Septic Cascade in the Chapter 6 Supplement on the Evolve Website). The inflammatory response is designed to deliver white blood cells (WBCs; particularly the neutrophils) to the area of infection. The organism also may be ingested by macrophages or eliminated by circulating neutrophils.

The complement system is a network of serum proteins that normally are present in the inactive form; activation of any of the complement proteins will result in activation of a series of proteins in a cascading fashion. The complement proteins contribute to the inflammatory process and immunity when they bind with invading organisms, facilitating phagocytosis in a process called opsonization.[88] In addition, activation of the complement system results in stimulation of the clotting cascade and may result in changes in vascular tone and alteration in platelet function.

Enzymes and granules released by macrophages and WBCs will also contribute to the inflammatory response and destruction of the organism.[45,221] A specific immune response may be initiated by the lymphocytes to enable the development of immunity.

If the organism is not destroyed at the tissue level, it may enter the blood stream; at this point, bacteremia is present (if the organism is a fungus, fungemia is present; if the organism is a virus, viremia is present). As blood passes through lymph tissue, specific antibodies and lymphocytes may combat the infection.[203] The success of the response to an invading organism will depend on the virulence of the organism itself and the strength of the body's lymphocyte and immune response.[223]

Effects of Thermal Injury. Thermal injury activates the body's inflammatory response and creates changes in immune function. The ability of the body to fight infection is compromised by decreased neutrophil phagocytosis, alteration in complement function, circulation of burn generated toxins, suppression of lymphocyte function, and administration of antimicrobial agents (especially tetracycline).[157,159] The extent of postburn immunosuppression depends on a variety of factors, including the severity of the burn, the patient's nutritional status, and the patient's hormonal balance.

Neutrophil phagocytic function is typically normal immediately after a burn. However, approximately 5 or more days after the burn, phagocytic function may be normal, depressed, or increased.[46,80] Because neutrophils provide the first-line response to infection, neutrophil depression can significantly increase the patient's risk of infection.

Circulating immunosuppressive substances are present in patients with burns. These substances appear within 24 hours of injury and may persist until the wound is closed.[152] The origin of these suppressors is not known, although substances secreted from WBC granules or membranes have been implicated.[4,5a,36,53,87,154,160,209] Burn toxin, a high-molecular-weight protein, is known to contribute to postburn immunosuppression.[108,109,158]

The complement system may be activated after a burn; this can produce blood pressure instability, fever, peripheral vasodilation with increased capillary permeability, changes in leukocyte function, coagulopathies, and microcirculatory

| Box 20-6 | Signs of Possible Burn Wound Infection |

- Conversion of partial-thickness to full-thickness injury
- Hemorrhagic discoloration or ulceration of healthy skin at the burn margins
- Erythematous, modular lesions in unburned skin and vesicular lesions in healed skin
- Edema of healthy skin surrounding the burn wound
- Pale, boggy, dry, or crusted granulation tissue
- Sloughing of grafts and wound breakdown after closure
- Odor

| Box 20-7 | Signs of Sepsis in the Child with Burns: Clinical Findings* |

Signs of systemic inflammatory response (two or more of the following four)
- Altered temperature (fever, hypothermia, or temperature instability)
- Tachycardia (or bradycardia in infants)
- Tachypnea (or requirements for increased support with mechanical ventilation)
- Altered white blood cell count (leukocytosis, leukopenia, or greater than 10% bands)

Plus Suspected infection

*Signs of septic shock include the clinical findings plus signs of dysfunction in the cardiovascular system (e.g., hypotension, poor perfusion, lactic acidosis) plus one other organ failure (see Boxes 6-2 and 6-3).

obstruction.[220] The complement system also may be dysfunctional after a thermal injury.

Immediately after a burn, lymphocyte response to antigen usually is depressed.[156] This depression lasts approximately 48 hours and may compromise the patient's immune response.

Clinical Signs and Symptoms

General Findings. Burn wound sepsis is the most serious complication of burn injury and is defined as a bacterial count of greater than 10^5 organisms per gram of tissue associated with invasion of viable tissue beneath the eschar.[194] Infections and sepsis also may be caused by other organisms, including *Candida* species, other fungi,[49,208] or viruses.

Signs of possible local burn wound infection are listed in Box 20-6; they include a change in wound appearance or drainage, vesicular or coloration changes in the skin surrounding the burn, and the presence of a distinctive odor. If any of these changes are noted, burn wound infection should be suspected, and a wound biopsy should be performed.[189]

Signs of sepsis in the burned child are listed in Box 20-7 and include alteration in neurologic, gastrointestinal, and skin perfusion, subtle changes in vital signs (including unexplained tachycardia and early tachypnea or the need for increased oxygen or mechanical ventilation support), alteration in temperature (fever or hypothermia) and alteration in WBCs.[165] Clinical and laboratory evidence of end organ dysfunction (e.g., lactic acidosis, oliguria, disseminated intravascular coagulation) will be observed when septic shock develops (see, also, Boxes 6-2 and 6-3).

Initially the child with sepsis may demonstrate peripheral vasodilation with increased capillary permeability similar to that seen during the third-spacing phase following a burn.

Increased fluid administration suddenly may be necessary to maintain systemic perfusion, and systemic and pulmonary edema may develop. In addition, laboratory findings may indicate nonspecific signs of stress, including hyperglycemia (or hypoglycemia in infants), early disseminated intravascular coagulation (particularly thrombocytopenia), and metabolic acidosis. Leukocytosis or leukopenia may develop. When septic shock develops, cardiovascular dysfunction (e.g., hypotension and signs of poor perfusion, such as lactic acidosis) and other organ failure will develop (see Septic Shock in Chapter 6 and Box 6-3).

There is no single laboratory or clinical finding that confirms the presence of sepsis.[2a] A wound biopsy will aid in identifying an infecting organism and its sensitivities, and histologic examination will determine whether bacterial invasion of healthy tissue has occurred.[189] In addition, sepsis caused by gram-positive, gram-negative, and fungal infections can produce characteristic clinical findings. The characteristics of potential infections and resulting sepsis are summarized briefly here (Table 20-10).

Gram-Positive Infections and Sepsis. Group A streptococcus is a gram-positive, highly transmissible pathogen. Gram-positive infection typically develops during the first week after a burn and also may invade freshly grafted wounds and donor sites, potentially causing graft loss and conversion of donor sites to full-thickness injuries.

This infection is characterized by wound erythema, pain, induration, and swelling. The erythema may extend from the

Table 20-10 Clinical Signs and Symptoms of Gram-Positive, Gram-Negative and Fungal Sepsis in Burned Patients

Clinical Signs	Gram-Positive	Gram-Negative	Fungal
Onset	Insidious, 2-6 days	Rapid, 12-36 h	Delayed
Sensorium	Severe disorientation and lethargy	Mild disorientation	Mild disorientation
Ileus	Severe	Severe	Mild
Diarrhea	Rare	Severe	Occasional
Temperature	Fever	Hypothermia (especially in infants or those with Pseudomonas) or high fever	Fever
Hypotension	Late	Early	Late
White count	Neutrophilia	Neutropenia	Neutrophilia
Platelets	Normal	Low	Low

margin of the burn wound, indicating streptococcus invasion of normal tissue.[124]

Staphylococcus aureus and *Staphylococcus epidermidis* are also gram-positive organisms; they are easily transmitted by contact or airborne routes. These infections usually have an insidious course, and 2 to 5 days may elapse between the onset of signs of infection and the development of sepsis. Staph wound infections are characterized by microabscesses, tissue necrosis, and increased exudate,[29] and they may cause graft loss. Staph sepsis will produce high fever and leukocytosis, and a gastrointestinal ileus is often present.

Gram-Negative Infections and Sepsis. *Pseudomonas aeruginosa* is an opportunistic gram-negative organism that rarely causes infection in healthy individuals. Because it grows well in moist, open wounds, it frequently invades immunosuppressed patients with burns. This infection results in a green, foul-smelling wound discharge over a 2- to 3-day period. The eschar may become dry with a green exudate, often progressing to patchy areas of necrosis. Occasionally, when *Pseudomonas* species sepsis is present, a spidery lesion (ecthyma gangrenosum) develops in healthy tissue. The patient with a *Pseudomonas* species infection often has hypothermia with a depressed WBC count. A paralytic ileus may develop.

Other gram-negative organisms, including *Escherichia coli, Klebsiella, Proteus, Enterobacter,* and *Providencia* species have been observed with increasing frequency in burn units. These infections usually colonize the wound from the patient's own flora and produce infection when other organisms are eliminated by antibiotic therapy.[3] Translocation of gram-negative bacteria or endotoxin from the patient's own gastrointestinal tract can also contribute to the development of gram negative sepsis.

Fungal Infections and Sepsis. *Candida albicans,* a fungal infection, most frequently develops in patients with extensive burns after prolonged broad-spectrum antibiotic therapy. The antibiotics suppress the child's normal bacterial flora, so that susceptibility to fungal infection increases. If a *Candida* species infection develops on a granulating wound, the wound becomes dry and flat with a yellow or orange color. A wound biopsy will be necessary to confirm the diagnosis. Systemic candidiasis is a common complication.

Management

Prevention. The most important actions to prevent burn infection are good hand-washing technique and the use of topical antimicrobials. In burn units, cross-contamination (infection spreading from patient to healthcare workers to patient) will occur if healthcare workers fail to wash hands before and after patient contact. Burn care should always be performed using strict clean or aseptic technique, with clean gown, gloves, mask, and hat (or according to unit policy). In addition, strict aseptic technique must be practiced during catheter and intravenous tubing changes, and sterile technique during procedures.

Topical antimicrobial agents are applied to prevent colonization of the wound. In addition, providing early and adequate nutrition will help maintain adequate immune function.

Some physicians advocate excising the burn eschar within 72 hours of injury to reduce the possibility of burn wound sepsis.[61,137,196] Early excision is thought to be effective, because it enables early closure of the wound (with biologic dressings or grafting), eliminates the potential source of immunosuppressive factors, stops the consumption of immune defense factors, reduces the length of hospital stay (see Management of Escharotomy), and provides better functional and cosmetic results.

Care of an Infected Wound. Once a burn wound infection develops, appropriate antimicrobial agents are provided. In addition, the wound is extensively debrided, and topical antimicrobial agents and systemic antibiotics are administered in an attempt to gain bacteriologic control of the wound.

Aggressive debridement of devitalized and infected tissue can eliminate the source of bacteria and produce marked improvement in patient condition. Following debridement, continuous monitoring is required to detect reappearance of infection.

Once the infectious organism is identified, careful adherence to hospital and Centers for Disease Control (CDC) infection precautions is mandatory. Caution is required to prevent contamination of noninfected areas with soiled dressings or wash solutions.

Application of topical antibiotics will reduce the bacteria present in the wound and may prevent bacterial invasion of healthy tissue. During use of topical antibiotics, the wound appearance must be monitored closely to detect the development of secondary infections.

Treatment of Sepsis. Once sepsis is suspected, blood cultures are obtained and systemic antibiotics are administered. In addition, providers should closely monitor for the development of shock and provide shock resuscitation and support of cardiopulmonary function and oxygen delivery when indicated.

Initially, broad-spectrum antibiotics are prescribed until results of blood cultures and sensitivity studies are available; more specific antibiotics are then used. If aminoglycoside antibiotics are administered, peak and trough levels are monitored to ensure effective blood concentrations (see Chapter 4).

Occasionally, antibiotics may be injected or infused into the wound itself in an attempt to eliminate the infection at its site.[142,174] This therapy is controversial, however, because it may increase the formation of resistant organisms.

Detailed discussion of the treatment of septic shock is included in Chapter 6 (see Fig. 6-8). Aggressive fluid resuscitation (with administration of bolus therapy) is indicated; typically three or four boluses of 20 mL/kg are administered in the first hour after the development of signs of septic shock, unless signs of heart failure (e.g., hepatomegaly, pulmonary edema, and respiratory distress) suggestive of myocarditis develop. Beta-adrenergic and vasoactive drug support should be initiated if shock persists, and support of the airway, oxygenation, and ventilation are required.

Evaluation of Therapy. Throughout therapy the burn wounds should be inspected to determine progress in healing.[150] When sepsis is present, intravenous catheters should be changed every 72 hours, and more often if sites appear inflamed. Routine culture of catheter tips was shown to have no demonstrable benefit,[190] because these tips often are contaminated during removal. However, if catheter infection is suspected, tip culture may aid in confirmation of the diagnosis. Meticulous catheter care should be performed at least every 24 to 48 hours, using aseptic technique per unit policy (See Box 22-6).

Nutritional Compromise

Etiology

The body's response to the stress of a burn injury is characterized by a hyperdynamic state with a pronounced increase in energy and caloric demands. If nutritional intake does not increase to meet these demands, impaired wound healing, decreased resistance to infection, and loss of lean body mass will result.

Basal metabolic rate increases when burns total 15% or more of TBSA. The metabolic rate increases as soon as fluid resuscitation is complete and peaks between days 4 and 12 after the burn injury. The metabolic rate will remain elevated until the burn is covered by graft or is completely healed.

Pathophysiology

Metabolic Rate and Oxygen Consumption. After a burn, catecholamine secretion in response to stress will stimulate metabolic rate, oxygen consumption, heat production, and substrate mobilization.[70] When a major burn is present, the basal metabolic rate may be twofold higher than normal. The actual metabolic rate can be determined by measuring the exchange of respiratory gases and calculating heat production from oxygen consumption and carbon dioxide production (see Indirect Calorimetry, later in this section).[206]

Oxygen consumption increases when the metabolic rate increases. However, this increase in oxygen consumption varies in different tissue beds after a burn. Despite the fact that blood flow to the burn wound is enhanced,[73] the burn uses little or no oxygen for its metabolic processes. As a result, anaerobic burn metabolism can produce localized metabolic acidosis. Visceral oxygen consumption increases markedly with a burn injury, whereas peripheral oxygen uptake remains a fixed percentage of total aerobic metabolism.[206]

A 1 to 2° C elevation in skin and core temperature frequently is observed immediately after a burn, as the result of increased heat production. Central thermoregulation is altered at this time to maintain this higher temperature. The child is usually asymptomatic, with a mild elevation in body temperature.

Glucose and Fat Metabolism. Hyperglycemia is observed after a burn, resulting from accelerated gluconeogenesis, reduced insulin levels, and abnormal glucose utilization. Hepatic gluconeogenesis is stimulated by catecholamine release, and the quantity of glucose made is directly related to the extent of the injury.[207]

Glucose utilization is not uniform throughout the body after a burn. The net glucose flux across healthy tissues and skeletal muscles is low, whereas glucose uptake by burned tissue is extremely high. In addition, injured tissues release large quantities of bacteria, which consume most of the available glucose.[206] Renal glucose consumption is also elevated,

whereas central nervous system glucose consumption remains normal.

Exogenous glucose from intravenous fluids is not utilized appropriately at this time, so serum glucose concentration often remains elevated long after glucose administration. Hepatic gluconeogenesis will continue despite exogenous glucose administration.[226]

Major thermal injury and hypermetabolism produce an increase in serum free fatty acids. Hydrolysis of stored triglycerides is accelerated, and mobilization of fat stores is stimulated by catecholamine secretion and elevated glucagon levels.[25] Postburn hypoalbuminemia also contributes to the elevation in free fatty acids,[75] because the serum albumin is not available to transport free fatty acids across cell membranes. Albumin administration at this time may help reduce serum free fatty acids.

Negative Nitrogen Balance. A thermal injury results in the breakdown of protein from skeletal muscle in burned and unburned areas.[218] This muscle breakdown provides amino acids for gluconeogenesis and fuel sources for local tissue needs.[69] If protein intake and synthesis do not increase and protein breakdown from skeletal muscle continues, a marked negative nitrogen balance ensues and nitrogen is excreted with urea in the urine. Urinary nitrogen loss is related primarily to the metabolic rate of the child, but is also affected by the child's nutritional status and muscle mass.

Approximately 20% of daily nitrogen losses occur from the surface of the burn wound itself. If appropriate nutrition is not provided, lean body mass and total body weight may decrease as much as 30%. Such massive protein loss will result in accelerated tissue destruction, delayed wound healing, graft failure, and increased susceptibility to infection.

Clinical Signs and Symptoms

Physical Assessment of Nutritional Status. A variety of parameters must be examined to determine the child's nutritional status (Table 20-11). However, these standard parameters do not allow for the effects of a large burn and its therapy on metabolic rate, so the child's nutritional support must be evaluated constantly.

Anthropometric measurements include daily weight, triceps skin fold, and middle upper arm circumference.[33] The most useful of these measurements is the daily weight.

Laboratory analysis of serum (visceral) proteins and lymphocyte counts, and calculations made from urine creatinine clearance and urea also can be used to evaluate nutritional status. However, each measurement or calculation has its limitations and will be useful only for evaluating changes in patient body mass or fat stores. It is imperative that the measurements be obtained under identical conditions each time and that several parameters be used to determine the effectiveness of nutritional therapy.

If the critical care unit bed does not allow immediate determination of the child's weight, the child should be weighed as soon as possible after the burn injury to determine a baseline weight. Once fluid resuscitation and fluid accumulation have occurred, the child's weight will increase significantly. Daily weight measurements should be recorded. The daily weight should be

Table 20-11 Nutritional Assessment Parameters

Nutritional Parameters	Normal	Mild Deficit	Severe Deficit
Weight loss	No loss	Loss of 2%	Loss of 5%
Tricep skinfolds	>90% of normal	80-90% of normal	$\leq$50% of normal
Middle upper arm circumference	>90% of normal	80-90% of normal	$\leq$50% of normal
Serum albumin (g/dL)	4-5 g/dL	3.0-3.5 g/dL	$\leq$2.5 g/dL
Serum transferrin (mg/dL)	200	160-180	$\leq$120
Nitrogen balance	>2	0	$\leq$-3
Total lymphocyte count	>2000 cells/mm^3	1500-1800 cells/mm^3	$\leq$800 cells/mm^3
Creatinine height index	>90% of normal	80-90% of normal	$\leq$70% of normal

From Cohn KH, Blackburn GL: Nutritional assessment: clinical and biometric measurements of hospital patients at risk. *J Med Assoc GA* 71:27, 1982.

obtained using the same process or scale at the same time of day, without dressings or splints, if possible. All catheters and tubing should be factored into the weight or elevated off the scale, so they do not influence weight measurement.

Daily weights should be recorded on a weight chart. A weight change of 10% or more is significant and requires evaluation of caloric and fluid intake. Weight loss of 5% or more of baseline body weight usually indicates inadequate nutritional support.[206] A weight gain can indicate fluid retention, early sepsis, or muscle or fat accumulation. Changes in weight will most accurately reflect nutritional status late after a burn, once edema has disappeared.

Laboratory Evaluation of Nutritional Status. Laboratory evaluation of nutritional status can be an extremely helpful adjunct to the clinical assessment.

Protein Levels. Visceral proteins (e.g., transferrin, albumin, retinol binding protein, thyroxin binding prealbumin) are essential for wound healing, host defense, substrate transport, and many enzyme functions in the body.[104,206] The serum concentrations of these proteins can fall abruptly after a burn as the result of depletion of body fat reserves and skeletal muscle protein.[13]

Serum transferrin is one of the most reliable indicators of visceral protein status and malnutrition because it has a short half-life.[33] A serum transferrin concentration less than 120 mg/dL is consistent with protein depletion[230] and is associated with an increased risk of bacteremia in burn patients.[105,145,161]

Serum albumin concentration is measured frequently, but this protein has a long half-life. In addition, it can be increased by exogenous albumin administration and so may fail to reflect acute changes in nutritional status. The serum albumin level usually does fall within a few days of a burn injury, as a result of albumin movement from the vascular to the interstitial space.[144,155]

Nitrogen Balance. Estimates of nitrogen balance can be used to reflect the rate of body protein synthesis and breakdown. This estimation requires measurement of urine urea nitrogen and estimation of dietary nitrogen intake:

$$\text{Nitrogen balance} = \text{Nitrogen intake} - (\text{Urine urea nitrogen} + 4\,\text{g})^{147}$$

If the child has a large burn, nonurinary nitrogen losses also must be estimated; this requires the use of a multiple

regression equation based on measured urinary urea nitrogen, the age of the child, and the percentage of TBSA burned. A complete 24-hour urine collection for urine urea is fundamental to each of these calculations.[11]

Creatinine Height Index. The creatinine height index is calculated from a 24-hour urine collection. Urinary creatinine excretion and the creatinine height index will decrease when the lean body mass decreases during periods of malnutrition.[144] Results may be inaccurate if the child is receiving tobramycin sulfate, narcotics, ascorbic acid, or dietary creatinine, because these substances will alter urinary creatinine.

Calorie Count. An accurate and comprehensive record of the child's daily caloric intake is a relatively simple method of evaluating the child's nutritional status. All food, beverages, and parenteral nutrition the child receives are recorded by the bedside nurse. The caloric content of the intake can then be calculated by a nurse or dietician.

Determining Nutritional Requirements. The child's nutritional requirements are determined by the amount of calories, nitrogen, and protein needed for normal homeostasis, plus those needed during burn-induced catabolism and healing of the burn wound.[218] Initial estimate of nutritional requirements is made at the time of admission. A variety of equations are available to determine nutritional requirements; all pediatric equations use the child's age, body weight or body surface area (see BSA nomogram on inside back cover of this text), and the percent of TBSA burned. Nutritional requirement equations developed for use in adult patients are not suitable for use in pediatric patients.[40,85,117]

The most popular pediatric formula for determining nutritional needs of children with burns is the Polk formula (Box 20-8); it provides for basal metabolic requirements plus additional calories based on the percent of the child's body surface area burned.[74] Alternative formulas calculate basal metabolic requirements based on the child's body surface area with additional fluid requirements based on burn surface area.[96] Use of body surface area provides a more accurate estimation of caloric requirements than those based on weight alone.

Regardless of the type of formula used, any calculation of nutritional requirements should serve only to provide a baseline estimate of nutritional needs. Nutritional therapy must then be individualized after consideration of the child's

Box 20-8	Formulas for Determining Daily Nutritional Requirement of Children with Burns[74,96]

Polk Formula

(60 kcal × Body weight in kg) + (35 kcal × Percent of TBSA burned)

Carvajal Formula (per day)

$(1800 \text{ kcal/m}^2 \text{ BSA}) + (2200 \text{ kcal/m}^2 \text{ BSA burned})$

BSA, Body surface area; *TBSA,* total body surface area.

preburn nutritional status, associated injuries and therapy, and the child's weight gain and nutritional progress.

Additional Nutritional Requirements. High protein intake will be required after a burn to replace protein lost as a result of the increased metabolic rate, through the burn wound itself, and from tissue breakdown and infection. Protein intake can be calculated based on urinary nitrogen excretion, because 1 g of urinary nitrogen represents the loss of 30 g of lean body tissue, or 6.25 g of protein.[70] An estimate of protein requirements also can be made from the child's weight (3 g protein required per kilogram body weight) plus percent of TBSA burned (1 g protein required per 1% of TBSA burned). Serum protein measurements are unreliable as parameters to guide protein replacement.[5]

Approximately 20% to 30% of the child's total caloric intake should be in the form of proteins, and approximately 50% to 60% of total calories should be administered as carbohydrates. Fats should constitute approximately 5% to 15% of nonprotein caloric intake.[138] It is now thought that W-3 fatty acids, such as those derived from fish oil, are the most desirable form of fat supplement.[76] Excessive carbohydrate intake can result in hyperglycemia,[12] and excessive fat intake can result in immunosuppression, hyperlipidemia, and hepatic dysfunction.[207,209]

Vitamin and mineral supplementation is necessary, although specific requirements after a burn injury have not been determined. Fat-soluble vitamins (A, D, E, and K) are stored in fat deposits and are depleted during prolonged feeding without supplementation. Water-soluble vitamins (B and C) are not stored in large quantities, so they also are depleted rapidly. Although vitamin and mineral deficiency can impair healing,[99] excessive vitamin administration also may be toxic.[52,225] National Academy of Science[34] and American Medical Association[6] recommendations should be followed until more specific information is known about vitamin and mineral requirements after a burn.

Indirect Calorimetry. Indirect calorimetry has only recently been used to determine caloric requirements in children.[102,193] This technique determines kilocalories of energy expenditure based on the measurement of oxygen consumption (VO_2) and carbon dioxide production (VCO_2).[200] An accurate weight measurement is also required.

Although calorimetry is often performed when the child is at rest, more accurate caloric requirements are calculated from measurements performed during typical periods in the child's day. Particularly stressful procedures (e.g., dressing changes, suctioning) should not be performed for 30 min before calorimetry.

The child must be intubated if he or she is unable to cooperate and follow directions. If the child is intubated, the ventilator circuit is connected to the calorimetry circuit (e.g., Waters Instruments, Rochester, MN or Sensormedics, San Diego, CA). Air leaks around the endotracheal tube must be eliminated for accurate results; this may require temporary replacement of the child's tube with a cuffed tube or a larger tube.

If the child is breathing spontaneously, the child inspires and exhales into the calorimetry circuit through a mouthpiece or face mask. If the mouthpiece is used, a nose clip is placed to prevent inadvertent nasal breathing.

The amount of oxygen consumed and carbon dioxide produced is determined by the difference in concentration of these gases between inspiration and exhalation.[117] Energy expenditure is calculated by means of standard equations.[23] Anything that interferes with gas exchange in the lungs (e.g., pneumothorax) or gas conduction to the calorimetry circuit will produce inaccurate results.

Measurements obtained during calorimetry also can be used to calculate the respiratory quotient (RQ). RQ is the ratio of oxygen consumption to carbon dioxide production, and it is useful in assessing energy expenditure. The RQ will vary with the adequacy of feeding and the type of fuel used as energy. An RQ of 0.70 is seen in starvation, and an RQ greater than 1.0 suggests that overfeeding has occurred, with resultant pure carbohydrate metabolism and fat synthesis.[192]

The use of indirect calorimetry still requires refinement. Because oxygen consumption can vary significantly throughout the day as the result of activity, pain, and change in temperature, all measurements must be performed under identical conditions. In addition, calculated allowances (available from the manufacturer) for activity are not accurate for pediatric patients.[200] Calorimetry does not measure nitrogen balance, so it is usually necessary to continue to monitor urinary nitrogen excretion.

Management

Nutritional therapy requires identification of nutritional needs, reduction of net nitrogen losses, promotion of protein repletion, provision of adequate nutrients, and assessment of the effectiveness of therapy. When burns are extensive, it may be difficult to provide high caloric intake on a daily basis. Some form of feeding supplementation almost certainly will be necessary after large burns, because caloric requirements are high, and the child may develop loss of appetite.[127]

Oral Feeding. Although oral feeding is the preferred route of nutrition, only children with uncomplicated burns totaling 15% or less of TBSA can be expected to ingest sufficient calories by this route. To maximize effectiveness of oral feeding, every attempt must be made to maximize the quantity and content of the child's caloric intake. The child's likes and dislikes must be noted, and favorite foods must be available at all times on the unit.[224] When the child is thirsty, high-calorie liquids, including fruit juices, fortified milk drinks, and commercial oral feeding preparations, should be offered instead of water. Commercial nitrogen and caloric supplements should be added to food and beverages to optimize intake. Mealtimes should be made special, and strenuous activity and therapy should not be scheduled immediately before or after eating.

Tube or Enteral Feeding. Whenever possible, the child's gut should be used for feeding. Oral and gastric feeding preserve gut mucosal mass and maintain digestive enzyme control.[218] Tube feeding may be used to supplement oral intake, if the child is unable to ingest at least 75% of caloric requirements.[164] Tube feedings should be planned for any child with burns in excess of 15% of TBSA. Feeding should begin as soon as possible after the burn, because delayed feedings are associated with loss of mucosal mass, elevated catabolic hormones, increased metabolic rate, and decreased feeding tolerance.[54,139] Enteral feeding may prevent or minimize translocation of gram-negative bacteria and endotoxin across the gastrointestinal mucosa.[63]

Continuous tube feedings usually are required to provide maximal caloric intake. Nasogastric feeding may be provided as long as active bowel sounds are present, usually within 48 to 72 hours after a burn injury. Nasoduodenal feeding can begin immediately after a burn, even if bowel sounds are absent, so this method of feeding has recently become popular.[76,77,107] Intravenous albumin administration may help to maintain serum albumin soon after a burn until the child demonstrates ability to tolerate tube feeding.

A nasogastric or nasoduodenal tube should be small (8-10 French), soft, and pliable. A Silastic catheter (e.g., Frederick-Miller tube, Cook, and Dobbhoff) is preferred, because it can remain in place for a month or longer. If a nasoduodenal tube is inserted, fluoroscopy is recommended to ensure proper placement. A nasogastric tube should also be placed to allow the detection of residual feeding or displacement of the duodenal tube into the stomach.

Tube feeding should be started with a small volume of formula, and the hourly feeding volume is increased gradually as tolerated every 4 to 8 hours. The head of the child's bed should be elevated to reduce the risk of regurgitation. Infusion pumps should be used to ensure consistent feeding volume and rate. Intermittent bolus feedings should be avoided, because they are associated with a higher incidence of gastric cramping, diarrhea, gastric distension, regurgitation, and aspiration.[95,99]

Ultimately, tube feeding should contain 1 to 2 calories/mL, with protein, fats, carbohydrates, vitamins, and minerals. Modular feedings have recently become popular, because they allow adjustment of the quantity of specific nutrients according to patient need and because they are thought to reduce the incidence of diarrhea.

Commercial tube feedings designed for adults are inappropriate for use in young infants, because they contain amounts of protein that are excessive for immature kidneys.[76] Infant formulas such as Similac (Abbott, Abbott Park, IL) or Enfamil (Mead Johnson Nutrition, Glenview, IL) are preferred. Caloric content of these formulas can be increased gradually from 20 calories/ounce to 24-27 calories/ounce as tolerated, using commercial feeding supplements if needed.

Isotonic commercial tube feeding preparations (such as Isocal [Mead Johnson Nutrition, Glenview, IL] and Osmolite [Abbott, Abbott Park, IL]) can be used for children older than 1 year; they may be enriched with additional protein (e.g., whey or Pro-mix) to provide additional protein caloric intake.[172] High-nitrogen content formulas, including Isocal HN, have been developed to meet the high nitrogen needs of burn and trauma patients.

Daily multivitamin and mineral supplements including ascorbic acid and zinc sulfate should be administered. Administration of intravenous or enteral glutamine may reduce translocation of gram-negative bacteria across gastrointestinal mucosa during parenteral nutrition. The efficacy of this therapy is under evaluation.[63]

Potential complications of tube feeding include gastric distension, aspiration, respiratory infection, nausea, vomiting, and diarrhea. Abdominal girth should be measured hourly when feedings are initiated or increased and every 2 to 4 hours during feeding. If gastric distension develops, regurgitation and aspiration may occur.

Gastric residual volume should be checked every 4 hours and again as needed. If residual volume during gastric feeding equals more than half of the previous 2-hour feeding, reduction in feeding volume or concentration may be required. If residual gastric volume is present during duodenal feeding, the duodenal tube may have slipped into the stomach, and it must be repositioned.

Diarrhea may develop during tube feeding. It can be caused by excessive feeding volume or a rapid increase in feeding concentration. Other potential causes of diarrhea that should be considered include infection, hypoalbuminemia, lactose intolerance, and inappropriate formula. If diarrhea develops, temporary reduction in the volume of feeding or administration of antidiarrheal agents (e.g., paregoric, loperamide, lomotil) may be necessary. Alteration in the protein content of the formula also may be needed to reduce diarrhea. A variety of formulas (e.g., Reabilan, Clintec Nutrition Company, Deerfield, IL) are available that contain small peptides that can be absorbed more efficiently in the intestine. In addition, these peptide formulas can enhance fluid reabsorption from the gut, so that diarrhea is reduced.

Once the child begins to tolerate oral feeding, he or she can be weaned gradually from tube feeding. When oral intake begins, it is helpful to interrupt the tube feeding for a few hours before meals, so that the child feels hungry before eating. The tube should not be removed until the child has demonstrated adequate oral intake.

Parenteral Feeding. Parenteral alimentation will be required if adequate caloric intake through tube feeding cannot be ensured; it may be used to supplement tube feeding and caloric intake, or as the sole means of nutritional support. Parenteral alimentation should be considered if the child requires more than 3000 calories/day (or 3000 kCal/day).

The term *hyperalimentation* should not be applied to parenteral alimentation. This form of feeding is not better (or *hyper*) when compared with oral or tube feeding. In fact, parenteral feeding is more expensive, with less effective utilization of nutrients, and presents a higher risk of infection than does oral or tube feeding. If parenteral alimentation is begun, daily assessment of the child's nutritional status and requirements must be performed, and the alimentation content or volume should be modified accordingly.

Parenteral alimentation generally is provided through a central venous catheter so that maximum glucose and protein concentration can be delivered. Peripheral alimentation is used only for supplementary feeding because the maximum glucose concentration tolerated through a peripheral venous catheter will be 12.5% dextrose.

Central venous alimentation solutions consist of 20% to 25% dextrose and 25% crystalline amino acids. This solution normally provides approximately 7 g of protein (4 kCal/g) and 800 to 1000 kCal/L. Water- and fat-soluble vitamins, trace elements, and electrolytes must be added to the solution. Lipid solutions (e.g., INTRALIPID 10% or INTRALIPID 20%, Baxter Healthcare Corporation, Clintec Nutrition Division, Deerfield, IL) usually are infused during parenteral alimentation to provide fat calories (9 kCal/g, or 1.1 kCal/mL of 10% lipid solution).

Because hypertonic glucose is an excellent growth medium, strict aseptic technique must be maintained when changing alimentation tubing and catheter entrance site dressings. Ideally, parenteral alimentation catheters should be used only for alimentation and not for drug administration or blood sampling. Potential complications of parenteral alimentation include metabolic imbalance and sepsis.[134] For further information regarding parenteral alimentation, see Chapter 14.

Temperature Instability
Etiology and Pathophysiology
A burn injury destroys skin, subcutaneous tissue, and blood vessels; therefore the child's ability to regulate heat loss is compromised. In addition, room temperature fluid used during fluid resuscitation and burn care may contribute to further loss of body heat. Finally, the burned child has a high metabolic rate, so heat production is increased after a burn. The child's core body temperature may be 1 to 2° C higher than normal after a burn.

The young infant cannot shiver to generate heat to maintain body temperature. Therefore if the young infant develops cold stress, brown fat is broken down in a process called nonshivering thermogenesis. This process increases oxygen consumption. Brown fat will not regenerate if nutrition is compromised.

Clinical Signs and Symptoms
Core temperature should be approximately 38° C. Signs of cold stress include shivering and chills, peripheral vasoconstriction, and tachycardia. If cold stress continues, ultimately, core body temperature will fall, and cardiovascular instability (including arrhythmias) may be observed.

Management
The infant with burns should be placed under a warmer with a servo control device. A warmer should be used during burn dressing changes for any young child and for patients with large burns. Core body temperature should be monitored continually or frequently—at least every hour during initial care, then every 1 to 2 hours as dictated by the patient's condition.

Blood should be warmed in a water bath heated to 37.5 to 40.5° C prior to administration. A microwave oven should not be used to warm fluids, because it will result in uneven heating and may lyse proteins contained in the fluids. Solutions used for wound care also are typically warmed in baths heated to 37.5 to 40.5° C.[186] Follow unit protocols.

The child should be covered unless a radiant warmer is used. Environmental temperature should be controlled at approximately 27 to 30° C (80-86° F), and drafts should be eliminated.

Potential Skin and Joint Contractures
Etiology and Pathophysiology
Skin or joint contractures may develop after a burn. Collagen formation and contraction begin before the burn wound is healed and continue until the scars are fully mature.

Collagen gradually develops on the surface of the burn wound and continues to develop after healing of the open areas and after grafting is complete. In this collagen layer, many fibroblasts gradually proliferate and attach to surrounding tissue. The fibroblasts progressively contract, causing the collagen fibers to disrupt the normal parallel layers and to form a wave pattern.[199] Eventually, the collagen bundles take on a supercoiled appearance, and collagen nodules develop[115]; this can lead to joint and skin contractures.

Clinical Signs and Symptoms
Contractures will impair movement of extremities and joints. Joint edema and pain can contribute to deformity and immobility, so the movement of edematous extremities should be particularly monitored.

Difficulty in moving extremities through passive range-of-motion indicates the need for reevaluation of the physical therapy regimen and a probable need for more frequent range-of-motion exercises. Apparent or expressed patient discomfort during routine care also will identify potential mobility problems.

Management
Rehabilitation must begin during the acute phase of burn care.[71] The child in pain will assume a position of comfort, which is generally a position of flexion of the extremities. If appropriate positioning and exercises are not provided, contractures will develop. Therapeutic positioning of extremities is needed, and splinting of extremities should be accomplished when the child's condition stabilizes.

Positioning. If the anterior neck is burned, the use of pillows should be avoided, and the child's neck should be kept straight or slightly extended. Doughnut pillows placed under the head or linen rolls placed under the shoulders work well. Because this position will facilitate aspiration if vomiting occurs, the child must be monitored closely.

Hands should be splinted in the position of function, with the wrist dorsiflexed at 45 degrees or neutral, according to the physical therapist's preference. Burns in the area of the axillae frequently result in severe contractures. When axillary burns are present, the arms should be positioned at 90-degree angles from the body.[60]

The foot should be positioned at a 90-degree angle from the leg, avoiding both dorsiflexion and plantar flexion. If the feet are not burned, the use of high-topped athletic shoes will facilitate proper positioning. Splints or footboards also may be used. Knees should remain extended, and hips should not be flexed.[199]

Traction, splints, and dressings can be used to maintain appropriate positioning during the acute phase. Active and passive range-of-motion exercises are imperative to avoid the development of joint stiffness and contractures.

Evaluation of Therapy. Constant and thorough assessment of joint function and range of motion is needed to identify any signs of contraction and prevent contracture development. Interruption of the program may be necessary during grafting procedures, but it is imperative that it be resumed as soon as possible after graft stabilization.[38,39,55,83,116,133,166,195]

Psychosocial Challenges
Etiology and Pathophysiology
The general emphasis on burn care for the hospitalized child focuses on the physical aspects, including survival and maintenance of optimal function. Although the physical interventions are critical, the psychological care is equally important, and psychosocial support must be provided for the child and family throughout hospitalization.

A major burn is viewed as a crisis in the life of the child and the family—it is a sudden, traumatic event that alters their lives. The child's response to injury is influenced by the child's age, culture, socioeconomic background, coping skills, body image, family support systems, and previous experience with injury and pain.[187,210] Every child will respond differently and must be treated as an individual while coping strategies are assessed and supported.

The effect of the burn injury begins immediately.[106] The acute stress of pain, hospital procedures, disruption of body chemistry, strange people, and separation from family begins to mold the child's perception and response.[1]

Clinical Signs and Symptoms
The child's behavioral response to the burn must be interpreted in light of the emotional impact of the burn trauma, rather than in terms of normal behavior for age. The child may demonstrate withdrawal, manipulation, anger, depression, or sleep disturbances. The child will be frightened by the hospital environment, procedures, and strangers. Regression frequently is observed in school-aged children and adolescents.[111]

During the acute phase of injury, the family is usually distraught and concerned only with the child's survival. Their behavior should be viewed as crisis behavior, and they may require assistance in determining priorities of action.

Management
Parents should be allowed to visit continuously and to assist with some comforting aspects of care; this will reassure the child and family by allowing the parents to continue to nurture the child in a special way.[111] By minimizing or eliminating separation from the parents, the child will be better able to focus on interaction with the environment and coping with the burn injury and its treatment.

Consistent caretakers will help to alleviate anxieties and fears of both the child and family. The child will become familiar with the personality and routines of the nurse and will begin to tolerate procedures better and interact more with the environment. The nurse will be better able to interpret the child's verbal and nonverbal cues. Finally, the family will receive consistent information and be able to participate in a consistent schedule for the child.

The child should be allowed to participate in care whenever possible. The child's feeling of powerlessness may be reduced if the child is allowed to make age-appropriate choices about some aspects of care (e.g., which arm dressing will be changed first or sequence of bath and meals).[103]

Psychosocial consultations should be arranged with social workers and mental health specialists as soon as possible. These professionals can provide consistent support for the child and family after the child is transferred from the unit and from the hospital.

A burn injury may have permanent psychosocial consequences for the child and family. The nurse will play a pivotal role in shaping the response of the child and family to the burn. For more comprehensive references regarding psychosocial care, see Chapters 2 and 3.[14,15,18,31,32,66,120,110,127,129,149,204,214]

BURN CARE
Burn wound care begins at the scene of the burn (i.e., the prehospital phase) and continues through the emergency department to the pediatric critical care unit or burn facility. Many of the procedures and dressing techniques used for wound care are similar throughout the course of treatment.

The burn wound facilitates bacterial access that can result in infection, sepsis, and death. Thorough assessments during and between dressing changes are necessary to ensure rapid detection of localized infection and to allow appropriate modifications of therapy.

Prehospital Care
At the scene of the burn injury, the burning process must be stopped. The child should be rolled on the ground to smother any remaining flames. All material in contact with the flame, including clothes, socks, and shoes, and all metal objects, should be removed. These materials may be extremely hot, causing additional burns. Metal objects, including rings, watches, and belt buckles, tend to retain heat and may cause deep burns in the areas of contact. Room temperature water (not ice) may be placed on the child to decrease tissue temperature and slow the burning process. However, the child should not remain covered with water, because it reduces the child's body temperature and may produce shivering. Absolutely no oils should be placed on the burn surface.

Once burning clothing has been removed, the child should be wrapped in clean blankets to maintain body temperature. At this stage of injury, the burned areas are considered sterile and do not constitute a major threat to survival. Once the burn has been covered, no further wound care is required until the child arrives in the critical care or burn unit.

Initial Burn Care

Wound care should begin after the child has received adequate fluid resuscitation and systemic perfusion is acceptable (see Shock in Chapter 6). Wound care is designed to: (1) protect the patient from infection, (2) remove nonviable tissue, (3) clean the wound surface, (4) prepare the area for healing and grafting, and (5) provide patient comfort. Burn care can be performed in a treatment room or at the bedside, but bedside care is most practical if the child is seriously ill and requires mechanical ventilation. Appropriate analgesia must be provided (see Chapter 5).

When beginning burn care, the wound should be examined thoroughly. This evaluation includes assessment of the extent and depth of injury, as well as examination of the color and appearance of the wound and the color and perfusion of surrounding tissue. The amount of pain present will help to determine the depth of injury; full-thickness burns will not be painful.

Broken blisters and loose, necrotic tissue should be debrided with forceps and scissors, a washcloth, or a gauze sponge. All loose tissue must be removed because the moist environment will harbor bacteria.

The management of intact blisters depends on their size, location, and appearance.[181] Blisters located on the palms of the hands or soles of the feet should be left intact; the blisters serve as a protective barrier that assists with wound healing and reepithelialization. The blister fluid will be absorbed in 5 or 6 days, and attenuated epidermis and keratinized skin will remain, leaving a bright pink, healed epidermis underneath.[58] The blister promotes rapid healing with minimal scarring or pain.

Management of intact blisters located on mobile, flexible creases is controversial, but they should be broken and debrided. These blisters usually break spontaneously, and they will harbor bacteria and serve as an open wound until they are debrided.

The burn area should be washed thoroughly but gently with mild soap or detergent and water, one to three times per day. The areas then are rinsed with water or normal saline at room temperature. Firm washing or scrubbing should be avoided, because it is no more effective than gentle cleansing and can be extremely painful for the child. In fact, gentle technique probably will be more effective, because the child will be more cooperative.

Clean washcloths or gauze sponges are recommended for burn cleansing. Gowns or aprons, head coverings, and masks should be worn for all dressing changes. Nonsterile gloves can be used without increased risk of infection.[191] Boxes of nonsterile gloves should not, however, be kept for use with different patients, because contamination may occur.

Management of Escharotomy

Burned tissue can become rigid, producing a tourniquet effect on edematous tissue. Circumferential burns of the extremities may produce arterial compression and result in the compromise of extremity perfusion and ischemia, with resultant necrosis. Such compression ischemia can resemble compartment syndrome, which results from fascial constriction of muscle arterial circulation.

Clinical signs of vascular compromise include cyanosis, delayed capillary refill, cooling of extremities, and loss of sensation. These clinical signs indicate the need for an escharotomy.

If arterial compromise to the involved extremity is suspected, tissue pressure measurements are performed. These measurements will provide more information than Doppler assessment of pulses. A wick catheter is inserted under sterile conditions into a muscular compartment beneath the eschar, and the catheter then is connected to a fluid-filled monitoring system, including a pressure transducer and monitor. Measurements are performed in both an anterior and a posterior compartment of the extremity. If tissue or compartment pressure exceeds 30 mm Hg, blood flow to the tissues will be compromised,[114] and an escharotomy should be performed.

An escharotomy is an incision into the burn eschar (with electrocautery, scalpel, or enzyme) to relieve pressure and improve circulation. The incision is extended into the subcutaneous tissue, breaking the tourniquet effect of the eschar and allowing edematous tissue to bulge through the incision.[100] Incisions are made carefully to avoid nerves and blood vessels. The procedure may be performed without anesthesia, because nerve endings to the eschar have been destroyed. If the child is awake and frightened, sedation, local anesthesia, or intravenous hypnotics (see Chapter 5) may be required. If tissue pressure measurements remain high after the escharotomy, a fasciotomy is performed. A fasciotomy is an incision extending through the subcutaneous tissue and the fascia.

Thick eschar surrounding the chest and upper abdomen may limit spontaneous ventilation, producing signs of respiratory distress, including hypoxemia, irritability, tachypnea, and possible carbon dioxide retention. The tourniquet effect on the chest can be relieved by bilateral longitudinal escharotomy incisions along the anterior axillary line, with a transverse incision along the costal margins. An additional vertical midsternal incision may be required. If the escharotomy incisions are effective, the child's oxygenation and ventilation should improve.

Escharotomy and fasciotomy surfaces generally are covered. Antimicrobial ointment may be applied immediately after hemostasis is achieved, or normal saline soaks may be applied for 24 hours, followed by antimicrobial ointment. These sites will require grafting at a later time.

Topical Antibiotic Agents

Topical antibiotics are applied to burn wounds to prevent bacterial colonization of the wounds.[125] These agents restrict the bacterial population of the wound until the child's immune system recovers sufficiently to destroy the bacteria or until the wound is closed surgically. No topical agent will sterilize the wound; bacterial growth can only be diminished. Furthermore, if the burn wound is extensive (60% or more of TBSA), infection often will develop despite these agents. For this reason, major burns usually are treated with early excision and grafting.

Topical agents can mask signs of infection; therefore in unusual cases, burn wound biopsies may be necessary to detect invasive infections at an early stage.[162] Bacterial counts of 10,000 or more organisms per gram of tissue indicate impending burn wound infection; counts exceeding 100,000 organisms per gram of tissue indicate bacterial invasion.

The ideal topical agent should be bactericidal or bacteriostatic against the most common burn infections, should penetrate burn eschar actively, should lack local or systemic toxicity and significant side effects, should be painless and easy to apply, should prevent desiccation and allow reepithelialization, should not injure viable tissue, and should be inexpensive.[151] No one topical agent meets all these requirements. As a result, several topical agents commonly are used, and the most popular are presented in Table 20-12. The agent selected for unit use will depend on specific wound care policies and typical unit pathogens and their sensitivities. Effectiveness of the agent used will be demonstrated by a low or decreased incidence of burn wound infections and sepsis. Silver sulfadiazine is used most frequently.

Silver Sulfadiazine

Silver sulfadiazine is the most popular topical antimicrobial agent available.[219] It is effective against gram-negative and gram-positive organisms as well as yeast. The silver ion produces ultrastructural changes in bacterial cell membranes and cell walls and also binds to bacterial DNA to kill bacteria and prevent its replication.[162,202]

Prophylactic silver sulfadiazine application can delay gram-negative colonization of wounds for 10 to 14 days. However, when large burns are present, resistant gram-negative bacilli will develop rapidly.

Silver sulfadiazine is applied liberally to a wound after it has been washed and debrided. A layer $1/18$ to $1/16$ inch in thickness is applied ("buttered") with a clean, gloved hand.[186] Although the area can be left open, pediatric burn wounds generally are covered with gauze, so that the medication is not transferred onto linens. Because this drug may produce eye or nasal irritation,[81] it should be applied to the face with caution.

Although silver sulfadiazine is stable for up to 48 hours, burn dressings usually are changed every 8 to 24 hours. Each time burn care is performed, the sulfadiazine is removed completely (use of normal saline may be most effective) before fresh cream is applied, to prevent buildup of dried cream.

Silver sulfadiazine does not cause electrolyte imbalances or metabolic acidosis. It is nontoxic under occlusive dressings, and it produces few side effects. Burning after application has been reported by some patients. This drug should not be administered to children with sulfonamide sensitivities.

Silver sulfadiazine does not penetrate eschar as well as other topical agents. In addition, it may produce rash and itching if it comes in contact with unburned areas. Temporary, mild leukopenia has been reported,[167] but this may be the result of the burn rather than the ointment.[24,212,217,231] The child's WBC count should be monitored daily; it generally returns to normal within 72 to 96 hours, even if the drug is continued.

Other Wound Care Modalities

A variety of wound care techniques and materials are currently available. The type of material and modality used will depend on unit protocols, efficacy of the material, product availability, and physician preference. Biologic dressings, including homograft, artificial skin, autologous cultured epithelium, and synthetic dressings are discussed in the following sections. Refer to Table 20-13 for a more comprehensive list of wound care modalities.

Biological Dressings

The term *biological dressings* refers to any natural or synthetic material that can be applied to an open burn wound to facilitate healing or prepare the wound for grafting. The most effective biologic dressings will adhere quickly to the burn surface and hasten healing; they will also provide a water and thermal barrier while remaining permeable to vapor and gas.[148] The dressing should control bacterial growth and facilitate debridement of the wound; it should be painless, readily available, and inexpensive. As with topical antibiotics, no single biologic dressing possesses all these characteristics. As a result, the selection of dressings will be determined by the balance of desirable and undesirable characteristics, availability, and surgeon preference.

Biobrane (UDL Laboratories Inc., Mylan, Rockford, IL) is a thin, synthetic material composed of an inner layer of nylon coated with porcine collagen and an outer layer of rubberized silicone. It is pervious to air but not fluids and is available in simple sheets or preshaped gloves.[113] After placement on clean, fresh, superficial second-degree burn wounds using Steri-strips and bandages, the Biobrane dressing dries, becoming adherent to burn wounds within 24 to 48 hours. Once the dressing is adherent, the covered areas are kept open to air and examined closely for the first few days to detect any signs and symptoms of infection. As epithelialization occurs beneath the Biobrane, the sheet is easily peeled off the wound. If serous fluid accumulates beneath the Biobrane, sterile needle aspiration can preserve its use. However, if foul-smelling exudate is detected, the Biobrane should be removed and topical antimicrobial dressings applied.

Opsite (Smith and Nephew, Memphis, TN) or Tegaderm (3M, St. Paul, MN) can also be used to cover superficial second-degree burn wounds. Commonly used as postoperative dressings in surgical patients, both are relatively inexpensive, are easy to apply, and provide an impervious barrier to the environment. Their transparent nature allows easy monitoring of covered second-degree burn wounds. Despite lacking any special biologic factors (e.g., collagen and growth factors) to enhance wound healing, they promote a spontaneous reepithelialization process.

Biobrane and Opsite are preferred to topical antimicrobial dressings when dealing with small, superficial second-degree burn wounds, especially in outpatient settings, to avoid the pain associated with dressing changes. Another option is TransCyte (Advanced BioHealing, Incorporated, Westport, CT), which is composed of human fibroblasts that are then cultured on the nylon mesh of Biobrane.

Synthetic and biologic dressings are also available to provide coverage for full-thickness burn wounds. Integra (Integra LifeSciences Corporation, Plainsboro, NJ), made of a collagen matrix with an outer silicone sheet, is a synthetic dermal substitute for the treatment of full-thickness burn wounds. After the collagen matrix engrafts into the wound in approximately 2 weeks, the outer silicone layer is replaced with epidermal autografts.[72] Epidermal donor sites heal rapidly without

Table 20-12   Topical Antimicrobial Agents*

Agent	Gram Negative	Gram Positive	Yeast	Duration	Toxic Effects	Side Effects	Comments
Silver sulfadiazine	Yes	Yes	Yes	Stable for 48 h; change dressing every 8-12 h	Rare	Burning, rash, itching when applied; leukopenia (also a result of the burn)	Is not effective for *Pseudomonas* species; painless on application; resistance may develop in large burns; do not apply if child has sulfonamide sensitivity
Mafenide acetate	Yes	Yes	No	Apply every 8-12 h	Metabolic acidosis, mafenide sensitivity-induced pseudochondritis	Burning or stinging on application; allergic reaction	Penetrates eschar well, so use on deep burns (e.g., electrical); should not be the first-line prophylactic agent
Nitrofurazone	Yes	Yes	No	Apply every 8-12 h	Rare	Dermatitis	Especially good against *Staphylococcus aureus*, but not against *Pseudomonas* species; painless upon application; use on fresh grafts or on open wounds if sulfa allergy
Silver nitrate 0.5% solution	Yes	Yes	Yes	Change dressings every 12 h and wet every 2 h	Rare	Methemoglobinemia, hyponatremia, hypocalcemia, hypokalemia, hypomagnesemia, decreased serum osmolality	If *Enterobacter cloacae* on wound, silver nitrate is converted to nitrite and is absorbed through the wound, causing methemoglobinemia; causes leaching of electrolytes from child into dressing; do not allow wound to dry, because the concentration of silver nitrate will increase, damaging granulation tissue; does not penetrate burn wound, so use in second-degree burns; stains wound a blackish-grey color
Povidone iodine	Yes	Yes	Yes	—	Metabolic acidosis, Increased T$_3$ (triiodothyronine) and T$_4$ (thyroxine) levels	Extremely painful because of acidity; allergic reactions, cellulitis	Protein binding of iodine in open wound results in decreased antimicrobial effect
Gentamicin sulfate 0.1% cream	Poor	Poor	No	Apply every 6-12 h	Ototoxicity, nephrotoxicity	Mild skin irritations	Readily absorbed when applied to open wounds; painless when applied; monitor serum levels
Polymyxin B, bacitracin	Yes	Yes	Poor	Apply every 2-8 h	Urticaria, burning and inflammation	Rare	Used on superficial burns; does not penetrate eschar; painless upon application
Cerium nitrate, silver sulfadiazine	Yes	Yes	Yes	—	Rare	Leukopenia, methemoglobinemia	Minimal systemic absorption

*Based on data from references 24,81,122,167,169,170,186,202,219,231,233.

Table 20-13   Alternative Wound Care Modalities

Agent	Description	Duration	Advantages	Disadvantages	Comments
Travase	Enzymatic debriding agent that removes necrotic tissue by proteolytic action	Can change dressings 2-3 times per day	Toxic effect is rare	Burning sensation when applied to large areas; may produce bleeding of thrombosed vessels near wound surface	Should not be applied to more than 15% of TBSA at one time; use in conjunction with antibiotic cream (e.g., silver sulfadiazine, mafenide acetate, gentamicin sulfate)
Wet-to-dry dressing	Application of gauze dressings moist with antibacterial or physiologic solution; gauze is allowed to dry and then removed from wound without rewetting; necrotic debris and eschar are removed	Change every 4-8 hours and wet every 2-4 hours	Toxic effect is rare	Bleeding and pain during removal	Allows fine debridement of clean, granulating wounds; analgesia required with dressing changes as removal is painful; remove dressing gently to not damage viable tissue
Homograft	Cadaver skin removed from deceased donor (usually > 14 years of age)	Can remain in place 14-21 days	Serves as temporary skin substitute until autografts are available; controls bacterial proliferation	Very expensive; low risk of HIV or other transmissible disease	Skin must be stored in a preservative and frozen until use; cannot be used if donor has history of hepatitis or other infectious or malignant diseases
Heterograft (xenograft)	Skin from animal, most commonly porcine	May need to be changed every 24 hours initially, then left on for 72 hours	Can be applied to partial- or full-thickness wounds	Does not control bacterial proliferation; causes fever from antigenic reaction	Provides temporary wound coverage; change dressing frequently until it firmly adheres to the wound bed
Amniotic membrane	Thin outer layer from amniotic sac	Disintegrates in 48 hours	Large size; low cost; readily available; immediately adheres to burn wound when applied to full-thickness wounds; prevents bacterial growth; decreases pain; increases mobility	Very fragile; requires frequent changes because it disintegrates in 48 h; reduces evaporative water loss by only 15%; risk of HIV or other transmissible disease (including hepatitis)	Effective dressing over partial-thickness burn until epithelialization takes place; must be applied smoothly; most frequently used on full-thickness excised wounds
Artificial skin	Two-layer membrane composed of silastic epidermis and of bovine hide chondroitin-6 sulfate from shark cartilage	—	Excellent take; no rejection; improved cosmesis	Presently, limited availability; transplanted dermis may shear easily from neodermis; infection can lead to loss of entire graft	Fibrinous structure formed from collagen matrix of artificial dermis slowly biodegraded and replaced with neodermis
Autologous cultured epithelium	Small skin biopsy of patient taken and epidermal cells are cultured to produce epithelial sheets that can be grafted	—	Use in extensive burns with limited donor sites	Length of time to grow sheets is prolonged; sheets are extremely fragile	Biopsy specimen of 2 cm² can be expanded to provide epithelial sheets to cover the entire body
Epidermal growth factor	Polypeptide that stimulates RNA, DNA, and protein synthesis	—	Limited clinical trials have demonstrated improvement in rate of regeneration of dermis at donor sites	Further trials in children needed	This protein is added to antimicrobial cream and applied with routine burn care

Based on data from references 20,21,41,65,68,84,101,121,175,231.
TBSA, Total body surface area.

significant morbidity, and Integra-covered wounds scar less; however, they are susceptible to wound infection and must be monitored carefully.[7]

AlloDerm (LifeCell Corporation, Branchburg, NJ) is another dermal substitute with decellularized preserved cadaver dermis. These synthetic dermal substitutes have tremendous potential for minimizing scar contractures and improving cosmetic and functional outcome.

Temporary wound coverage can be achieved using biologic dressings, such as xenografts from swine and allografts from cadaver donors. Particularly useful when dealing with large TBSA burns, biologic dressings can provide immunologic and barrier functions of normal skin. The areas of xenograft and allograft are eventually rejected by the immune system and sloughed off, leaving healthy recipient beds for subsequent autografts. Although extremely rare, the transmission of viral diseases from allograft is a potential concern.

Silver-impregnated wound dressings can be an option for use throughout burn wound management. Early in management, these dressings can be used to cover exposed skin, decrease bacterial colonization at the wound surface, and decrease frequency of dressing changes with a resultant decrease in pain and need for analgesics, and increase in comfort and quality of life for the burned child. Reducing discomfort during dressing changes is an important part of burn care and contributes to a patient's overall well-being. Most silver-impregnated dressings offer immediate and sustained effective antimicrobial protection against a broad range of pathogens. Examples of these dressings are Mepilex Ag and Melgisorb Ag (Molnlycke Healthcare, Norcross, GA), Acticoat (Smith and Nephew, St. Petersburg, FL), and Aquacel Ag (ConvaTec, Skillman, NJ). These dressings should be used only with physician order and according to product specifications, and they are usually used in conjunction with surgical interventions.

Autologous Cultured Epithelium

Epithelial sheets now can be produced from cultures of epidermal cells obtained from small skin biopsies. These sheets can then be grafted to generate a permanent epidermal surface.[35,64,84]

Epithelial sheets are especially useful for the child with extensive burns when available donor sites are inadequate to provide wound coverage. Within 3 to 4 weeks, a biopsy specimen of 2 cm^2 can be expanded to provide an epithelial sheet sufficient to cover the entire body surface. Currently, the 2- to 3-week growth period is too long to enable timely coverage of the burn, and the sheets are highly fragile. However, further development of the culture technique should enable improved use of this dressing.[19,68]

Epidermal Growth Factor

Epidermal growth factor is a polypeptide that stimulates RNA, DNA, and protein synthesis in a variety of cells. Accelerated regeneration of the epidermis has been observed after applying this growth factor to partial-thickness burns and graft donor sites on animals.

Initial clinical studies of partial-thickness donor sites in adult patients demonstrated accelerated epidermal regeneration when epidermal growth factor was added to conventional antimicrobial cream.[20] Further clinical studies in children will be required to determine the effects and potential complications of epidermal growth factor on burn surfaces, donor sites, and other wounds, but initial results are promising.[101]

Surgical Intervention
Excision and Grafting

Early excision with skin grafting has been shown to decrease operative blood loss and length of hospital stay and ultimately improve the overall survival of burn patients.[61,90–93] Typically, tangential excision of a full-thickness burn wound is performed within 3 days of injury, after relative hemodynamic stability has been achieved.[137]

The accurate determination of burn depth is vital to proper management. In particular, distinguishing between superficial and deep thermal burns is critical, because this dictates whether the burn wound can be treated with dressing changes alone or with surgical excision.

Eschar is sequentially shaved using a powered dermatome (e.g., made by Zimmer, Wiltshire, UK) or knife blades (e.g., Watson or Weck surgical blades) until a viable tissue plane is achieved. Early excision of eschar (usually less than 24 hours after the burn injury) generally decreases operative blood loss, because vasoconstrictive substances, such as thromboxane and catecholamines are active. Once the burn wound becomes hyperemic, approximately 48 hours after injury, bleeding during excision of the eschar can be excessive. Tourniquets and subcutaneous injections of epinephrine-containing solution can lessen the blood loss, but these techniques may hinder the surgeon's ability to differentiate viable from nonviable tissue.[130] A topical hemostatic agent such as thrombin can also be used, but it is expensive and not very effective against excessive bleeding from open wounds. In patients with deep full-thickness burns, electrocautery is used to rapidly excise eschar with minimal blood loss. More importantly, the earlier the excision, the less is the expected blood loss in burns greater than 30% of TBSA.[50] With scald burns, it is more difficult to assess the burn depth initially; therefore such burns require a more conservative approach, with delayed excision.

Ideally the excised burn wound is covered with autografts. Burns wounds less than 20% to 30% of TBSA can be closed at one operation with split-thickness autografts. Split-thickness autografts are harvested using dermatomes, and donor sites are dressed with petroleum-based gauze, such as Xeroform (Xerofoam petroleum gauze by Kendall, division of Covidien, Norwalk, CT) or Scarlet Red (white petrolatum, lanolin and olive oil on fine mesh gauze [Kendall, division of Covidien, Norwalk, CT]). Opsite (Smith and Nephew, Memphis, TN) can also be used to cover donor sites. Sheet autografts are preferred for a better long-term aesthetic outcome, but narrowly meshed autografts (1:1 or 2:1) have the advantages of limiting the total surface area of donor harvest and allowing better drainage of fluid at the grafted sites.

With massive burns, the closure of burn wounds is achieved by a combination of widely meshed autografts (4:1 to 6:1) with allograft (2:1) overlay. Repeated grafting is required for large burns, with sequential harvesting of split-thickness autograft from limited donor sites until the entire burn wound is closed. As the meshed autografts heal, allografts slough off, but the formation of significant scar is a major disadvantage of this technique.[171] Therefore the use of widely meshed graft is avoided for the face and hands. A full-thickness graft that includes both dermal and epidermal components provides the best outcome in wound coverage, with diminished contracture and better pigment match.[227] However, its use is generally limited to small areas, because there is a lack of abundant full-thickness donor skin available.

Care of Excision Sites. If grafting is performed later on the day of excision, bleeding must be stopped before grafting occurs. Gauze soaked with 1/10,000 strength epinephrine in normal saline, thrombin, or Neo-Synephrine (or other vasoconstrictor or coagulant) is applied over the newly exposed tissue to stop bleeding. Extremities are wrapped with elastic bandages and elevated above the level of the heart; they may be suspended from intravenous poles as long as care is taken to avoid nerve stretch injuries (especially of the brachial plexus). Pressure is applied to dressings over the trunk. The dressings are removed with saline irrigation after 10 to 15 minutes. Any remaining bleeding vessels are cauterized, and grafting can be performed.

If grafting is not performed immediately after excision, the newly exposed dermis, subcutaneous fat, or fascial layer must be kept moist until grafting occurs. Layers of gauze are placed over the tissue, and irrigation catheters are placed between layers of gauze. The entire irrigation dressing is covered with an elastic bandage to keep the dressing intact and to reduce bleeding. Normal saline or an antimicrobial solution is flushed through the catheters every 2 to 4 hours and as needed to keep the gauze moist.

Donor Sites. Patient donor sites should resemble the area to receive the graft, so that hair growth and skin texture will conform to that surrounding the wound.[44] Ideally, the donor sites should be covered by clothing or regrowth of hair, so that any scarring will not be visible. The scalp is an excellent donor site for children, because the head has a large available surface area and hair growth will cover the donor site. Small burns can also be covered with skin removed from the anterior or lateral surfaces of the upper thighs and lower abdomen.

The donor skin is removed using a power-driven dermatome. A full-thickness skin graft consists of the entire donor epithelium and dermis. This type of graft generally is used for reconstruction. Because the graft is thick (0.035 inches or more), the donor site also must be grafted or closed primarily, or it will not heal spontaneously.

A *split thickness skin graft* (STSG) consists of only the epithelium and part of the dermis. If the graft will be placed as a sheet, only a thin (0.004-0.008 inch) graft will be required. If the donor skin will be meshed (to expand the area covered), a thicker (0.010-0.020 inch) graft will be removed. If a mesh is created from donor skin, the surface covered can be expanded to 1.5 to 9 times the size of the original donor area through use of a Tanner mesher. However, the greater the expansion of the donor skin, the more fragile the skin mesh. Generally, expansions of 1.5 to 3 times are preferred. The STSG donor site can heal by epithelialization and contraction.

Postoperatively, the split-thickness donor site should be treated as a partial thickness burn injury.[57] A wide variety of care modalities have been used with comparable results. The site may be covered with dry or antimicrobial-permeated gauze, polyurethane, or a silver sulfadiazine dressing. Gauze is left in place for 2 to 3 weeks, until it naturally separates from the site as the area heals. This technique is relatively simple for the nurse, but is usually uncomfortable for the child, because the gauze tends to pull as it dries and mobility at the donor site is compromised.

If a polyurethane dressing is applied without wrinkles or gaps, it can remain in place for 10 to 14 days. If the donor site is covered with silver sulfadiazine, dressing changes should be performed two or three times per day.

With proper care, the donor site should heal quickly. Complications at the site include hypertrophic scarring, pigmentation, and blistering. The donor site also may become infected or separate. Application of elastic bandages can prevent or minimize hypertrophic scarring and blistering.

Postoperative Care. Once the donor skin is obtained and prepared, it is placed over the clean, granulating burn surface and secured. Staples usually are used to secure the graft, and they can be reinforced with sutures or steri-strips.

The grafted skin must remain in constant contact with the tissue bed to receive nutrients and oxygen supply. Once the graft is applied, a fibrin layer forms between the granulating bed and the graft. Capillary action allows absorption of serum from the bed into the graft during the first days after grafting. Capillary buds then form a fine network of vascular channels to the fibrin layer,[228] and blood flow to the graft is present within 3 days. Complete capillary ingrowth will be established approximately 7 to 10 days after grafting. It is imperative that the graft be secure (e.g., by wrapped dressings), without stress or shear forces applied during this time, to ensure delivery of nutrients to the graft and to prevent the disruption of the fragile capillary network.

Expanded (mesh) grafts are used most commonly because they cling to the recipient bed more easily than do sheet grafts. Epithelial tissue will grow between the interstices of the expanded graft to provide full coverage. In addition, expanded grafts heal by contraction.

Postoperatively, an occlusive dressing usually is applied to an expanded graft, and moist occlusive dressings are usually preferred. Fine mesh gauze soaked in normal saline or antimicrobial solution is applied over the fresh graft, and these are covered with dry gauze. Catheters can be incorporated into the gauze dressings to allow irrigation every 2 to 4 hours. The entire dressing is secured with an elastic bandage to stabilize the dressing and maintain graft position.

Splints should be applied if needed to prevent movement of and tension on the graft site. The dressing is changed 48 to 96 hours after surgery, and the site is inspected. Clean dressings are then applied and changed daily for 2 to 4 days. Dressings are discontinued if the graft is healing well by the sixth postoperative day. A lubricating cream can be applied to keep the graft moist and to prevent cracking.

Sheet grafts are used most frequently over the face and hands, because they provide the best cosmetic results. Sheet grafts also retain moisture, so they are used over exposed arteries, veins, or nerves. In addition, they are usually placed over joints or areas of flexion creases to limit graft contraction.

Sheet grafts are usually left open to the air, without dressings, for the first days after surgery. Serum and exudate that accumulate under the graft must be evacuated, or the graft may fail.[168] The serum may be allowed to seep from under the surface of the graft via small slices in the graft (similar to the small slices on a pie crust). Alternatively, the serum may be aspirated or expressed. Serum aspiration is accomplished with a needle and syringe. To express the serum, a sterile cotton applicator is rolled gently over the sheet graft from the center of the graft toward the nearest incision. The rolling technique should only be performed over a small amount of tissue, without application of pressure, because extensive or firm rolling might interrupt capillary development and blood flow to the graft.

All graft sites must be monitored closely for evidence of erythema, purulent drainage, odor, or sloughing. Folliculitis and pruritus may also develop under skin grafts.

Often, the child is fitted with special elastic (compression) garments to minimize scar formation. All necessary measurements should be recorded as soon wounds are healed so that the garments are available for use before the child is discharged.

Skin grafts speed healing and reduce scarring for children with burns. However, multiple grafting procedures are frequently necessary to complete the burn repair. During this time, children will require extensive rehabilitation and psychosocial support to help them return successfully to a normal life and to cope with changes in appearance resulting from the injury.

ACKNOWLEDGMENTS

The 1992 edition of this chapter was written by Denise Sadowski. Her chapter provided an excellent foundation for this revised chapter and her contribution is gratefully acknowledged.

References

1. Aatoon A, Remensnyder JP: Burns in children. In Boswick JA, editor: *The art and science of burn care*, Rockville, MD, 1987, Aspen Publishers.
2. Adolfson L, Halebian P, Shires GT: Fixation of nasotracheal tubes based on blood supply to the nasal alae (abstract). *American Burn Association Abstracts of 16th Annual Meeting*, San Francisco; 1984, p. 73.
2a. Alexander JW: The body's response to infection. In Artz CP, Moncrief JA, Pmitt BA, editors: *Burns: a team approach*, Philadelphia, 1979, WB Saunders Co.
3. Alexander JW: The role of infection in the burn patient. In Boswick JA, editor: *The art and science of burn care*, Rockville, MD, 1987, Aspen Publishers.
4. Alexander JW, Stinnett JD, Ogle CK: Alterations in neutrophil function. In Ninnemann JL, editor: *The immune consequences of thermal injury*, Baltimore, 1981, Williams and Wilkins.
5. Alexander JW, et al: Beneficial effects of aggressive protein feeding in severely burned children. *Ann Surg* 192:505.
5a. Arturson MG: Arachidonic acid metabolism and prostaglandin activity following burn injury. In Ninnemann JL, editor: *Traumatic injury: infection and other immunologic sequelae*, Baltimore, 1983, University Park Press.
5b. Aulick LH, Wilmore DW: Hypermetabolism in trauma. In Girardier L, Stock MS, editors: *Mammalian thermogenesis*, London, 1983, Chapman & Hall.
6. American Medical Association, Department of Foods and Nutrition: Guidelines for essential trace element preparations for parenteral use. *J Am Med Assoc* 241:2051, 1979.
7. Barret JP, et al: Cost-efficacy of cultured epidermal autografts in massive pediatric burns. *Ann Surg* 231:869, 2000.
8. Batchelor ADR, Kirk J, Sutherland AB: Treatment of shock in the burned child. *Lancet* 1:123, 1961.
9. Baxter CR: Controversies in the resuscitation of burn shock. *Curr Concepts Thermal Care* 5:5, 1982.
10. Baxter CR, Shires GT: Physiological response to crystalloid resuscitation of severe burns. *Ann NY Acad Sci* 150:874, 1968.
11. Bell SJ, et al: Prediction of total urinary nitrogen from urea nitrogen in burned patients. *J Am Diet Assoc* 85:1100, 1985.
12. Bessey PQ, Wilmore DW: *Metabolic and nutrition support for trauma and burn patients, Nutrition Symposium,* West Virginia, 1982, Mead Johnson Nutritional Division.
13. Blackburn GL, Harvey KB: Nutritional assessment as a routine in clinical medicine. *Postgrad Med* 71:46, 1982.
14. Blakeney P, et al: Long-term psychosocial adjustment following burn injury. *J Burn Care Rehabil* 9:661, 1988.
15. Boswick JA: Emotional problems in burn patients. In Boswick JA, editor: *The art and science of burn care*, Rockville, MD, 1987, Aspen Publishers.
16. Bowser-Wallace BH, Caldwell FT: Fluid requirements of severely burned children up to3 years old: hypertonic lactated saline versus Ringer's lactate-colloid. *Burns Incl Therm Inj* 12(8):549–555, 1986.
17. Bowser-Wallace BH, Caldwell FT: The effect of resuscitation with hypertonic versus hypotonic versus colloid on the wound and urine fluid and electrolyte losses in severely burned children. *J Trauma* 23:916, 1983.
18. Brill N, et al: Caring for chronically ill children: an innovative approach for care. *Child Health Care* 16:105, 1987.
19. Brown A, Barot L: Biological dressings and skin substitutes. *Clin Plast Surg* 13:69, 1986.
20. Brown GL, et al: Enhancement of wound healing by topical treatment with epidermal growth factor. *N Engl J Med* 321:76, 1989.
21. Burke JF, et al: Successful use of physiologically acceptable artificial skin in the treatment of extensive burn injury. *Ann Surg* 199:413, 1981.
22. Safe Kids Campaign: *Burn injury fact sheet,* Washington, DC, 2004, National Safe Kids Campaign.
23. Burszstein S, et al: Utilization of protein, carbohydrate and fat in fasting and post absorptive subjects. *Am J Clin Nutr* 33:998, 1980.
24. Caffee HH, Bingham HG: Leukopenia and silver sulfadiazine. *J Trauma* 22:586, 1982.
25. Carpentiera YA, et al: Effects of hypercaloric glucose infusion on lipid metabolism in injury and sepsis. *J Trauma* 19:649, 1979.
26. Carvajal HF: Acute management of burns in children. *South Med J* 68:129, 1975.
27. Carvajal HF: Management of severely burned patients: sorting out the controversies. *Emer Med Rep* 6:89, 1985.
28. Carvajal HF: Resuscitation of the burned child. In Carvajal HF, Parks DH, editors: *Burns in children: pediatric burn management*, Chicago, 1988, Year Book Medical Publishers.
29. Carvajal HF: Septicemia and septic shock. In Carvajal HF, Parks DH, editors: *Burns in children: pediatric burn management*, Chicago, 1988, Year Book Medical Publishers.
30. Charnock EL, Meehan JJ: Postburn respiratory injuries in children. *Pediatr Clin North Am* 27:666, 1980.
31. Chedekel DS: The psychologist's role in comprehensive burn care. In Bernstein NR, Robson MC, editors: *Comprehensive approaches to the burned patient*, New York, 1983, Medical Examination Publishing.
31a. Chung DH, Sanford AP, Herndon DN: Burns. In O'Neill J, Grossfeld JL, Coran AG, Fonkalsrud EW, editors: *Grossfeld: pediatric surgery*, ed 6, St Louis, 2006, Mosby.
32. Clarke AM: Thermal injuries: the case of the whole child. *J Trauma* 20:823, 1980.
33. Cohn KH, Blackburn GL: Nutritional assessment: clinical and biometric measurements of hospital patients at risk. *J Med Assoc Ga* 71:27, 1982.
34. Committee on Dietary Allowances: *Recommended dietary allowances,* Washington, DC, 1980, National Academy of Science.

35. Compton CC, et al: Skin regenerated from cultured epithelial autografts on full-thickness burn wounds from 6 days to 5 years after grafting. *Lab Invest* 60:600, 1989.

36. Constantian MB: Association of sepsis with an immunosuppressive polypeptide in the serum of burn patients. *Ann Surg* 188:209, 1978.

37. Cope O, Moore FD: The redistribution of body water and the fluid therapy of the burn patient. *Ann Surg* 126:1010, 1947.

38. Covey MH: Occupational therapy. In Boswick JA, editor: *The art and science of burn care*, Rockville, MD, 1987, Aspen Publishers.

39. Covey MH, et al: Efficacy of continuous passive motion (CPM) devices with hand burns. *J Burn Care Rehabil* 9:397, 1988.

40. Curreri PW, et al: Dietary requirements of patients with major burns. *J Am Diet Assoc* 65:415, 1974.

41. Cuzzell JZ: Wound care forum: artful solutions to chronic problems. *Am J Nurs* 85:162, 1985.

42. Dahn MS, et al: Negative inotropic effect of albumin resuscitation for shock. *Surgery* 86:235, 1979.

43. Dailey MA: Carbon monoxide poisoning. *J Emerg Nurs* 15:120, 1989.

44. David JA: *Wound management: a comprehensive guide to dressing and healing,* London, 1986, Martin Dunitz.

45. Deitch EA: Immunologic considerations in the burned child. In Carvajal HF, Parks DH, editors: *Burns in children: pediatric burn management*, Chicago, 1988, Year Book Medical Publishers.

46. Deitch EA, Gelder F, McDonald JC: Sequential prospective analysis of the nonspecific host-defense system after thermal injury. *Arch Surg* 119:83, 1984.

47. Demling RH: Fluid replacement in burned patients. *Surg Clin North Am* 67:15, 1987.

48. Demling RH: Fluid resuscitation. In Boswick JA, editor: *The art and science of burn care*, Rockville, MD, 1987, Aspen Publishers.

49. Desai MH, Herdon DN, Abston S: Candida infection in massively burned patients. *J Trauma* 27:1186, 1987.

50. Desai MH, et al: Early burn wound excision significantly reduces blood loss. *Ann Surg* 211:753, 1990.

51. Dingeldein GP: Fluid and electrolyte therapy in the burn patient. In Salisbury RE, Newmann NM, Dingeldein GP, editors: *Manual of burn therapeutics: an interdisciplinary approach*, Boston, 1983, Little Brown.

52. DiPalma JR, Ritchie DM: Vitamin toxicity. *Ann Rev Pharmacol Toxicol* 17:133, 1977.

53. Dobke M, et al: Autoimmune effects of thermal injury. In Ninnemann JL, editor: *The immune consequences of thermal injury*, Baltimore, 1981, Williams and Wilkins.

54. Dominioni L, et al: Prevention of severe post-burn hypermetabolism and catabolism by immediate intragastric feedings. *J Burn Care Rehabil* 5:106, 1984.

55. Duncan CE, Cathcart ME: A multi-disciplinary model for burn rehabilitation. *J Burn Care Rehabil* 9:191, 1988.

56. Eagle JF: Parenteral fluid therapy of burns during the first 48 hours. *NY J Med* 56:1613, 1956.

57. Engeman SA: The burned patient: perioperative nursing care. *AORN J* 10:36, 1984.

58. Ersek RA, et al: A report of the simple two-step system for scalds. *Bull Burn Inj* 5:46, 1988.

59. Evans EI, et al: Fluid and electrolyte requirements in severe burns. *Ann Surg* 135:804, 1952.

60. Fader P: Preserving function and minimizing deformities: the role of the occupational therapist. In Carvajal HF, Parks DH, editors: *Burns in children: pediatric burn management*, Chicago, 1988, Year Book Medical Publishers.

61. Fidler JP: Debridement and grafting of full-thickness burns. In Hummel RP, editor: *Clinical burn therapy: a management and prevention guide*, Boston, 1982, John Wright Publishing.

62. Fimberg L: Interrelationships between electrolyte physiology, growth and development. In Fimberg L, Kravath RE, Fleischman AR, editors: *Water and electrolytes in pediatrics*, Philadelphia, 1982, WB Saunders.

63. Fink MP: Gastrointestinal mucosal injury in experimental models of shock, trauma, and sepsis. *Crit Care Med* 19:627, 1991.

64. Flores JB, et al: Use of cultured human epidermal keratinocytes for allografting burns and conditions for temporary banking of the cultured allografts. *Burns* 16:3, 1990.

65. Frank DH, et al: Comparison of biobrane, porcine, and human allograft as biologic dressings for burn wounds. *J Burn Care Rehabil* 4:186, 1983.

66. Friedman JK, Shapiro J, Plon L: Psychosocial treatment and pain control. In Archauer BM, editor: *Management of the burn patient*, Los Altos, Calif, 1987, Appleton and Lange.

67. Fuchs GJ, Gleason WA: Gastrointestinal complications in burned children. In Carvajal HF, Parks DH, editors: *Burns in children: pediatric burn management*, Chicago, 1988, Year Book Medical Publishers.

68. Gallico G, et al: Permanent coverage of large burn wounds with autologous cultured human epithelium. *N Engl J Med* 311:448, 1984.

69. Gamelli RL: Nutritional problems of the acute and chronic burn patient. *Arch Dermatol* 124:756, 1988.

70. Giel LC: Nutrition. In Archauer BM, editor: *Management of the burned patient*, Los Altos, CA, 1987, Appleton and Lange.

71. Gillespie RW, Halpern M: Rehabilitation services. In Smith DJ, editor: *Symposium: reconstruction and rehabilitation*, Seattle, 1988, American Burn Association.

72. Goodenough RD, Molnar JA, Burke JF: Changes in burn wound closure. In Ninnemann JL, editor: *Traumatic injury, infection and other immunologic sequelae*, Baltimore, 1983, University Park Press.

73. Goodwin CW: Metabolism and nutrition in the thermally injured patient. *Crit Care Clin* 1:97, 1985.

74. Gordon MD: Nursing care of the burned child. In Artz CP, Moncrief JA, Pruitt BA, editors: *Burns: a team approach*, Philadelphia, 1979, WB Saunders.

75. Gottschlich MM, Alexander JW: Fat kinetics and recommended dietary intake in burns. *J Parenter Enter Nutr* 11:80, 1987.

76. Gottschlich MM, Warden GD, Alexander JW: Dietary regimens for the burned pediatric patient. In Herdon DN, editor: *Nutrition and metabolism symposium*, Chicago, 1986, American Burn Association.

77. Gottschlich MM, et al: Therapeutic effects of modular tube feeding recipe in pediatric burn patients. *Proc Am Burn Assoc* 18:84, 1986.

78. Gozal D, et al: Accidental carbon monoxide poisoning; emphasis on hyperbaric oxygen treatment. *Clin Pediatr* 24:132, 1985.

79. Graves TA, et al: Fluid resuscitation of infants and children with massive thermal injury. *J Trauma* 28:1656, 1988.

80. Grogan JB: Altered neutrophil phagocytic function in burn patients. *J Trauma* 16:734, 1976.

81. Guzzett PC, Holihan JA: Burns. In Eichelberger MR, Pratsch GL, editors: *Pediatric trauma care*, Rockville, MD, 1985, Aspen Publishers.

82. Halpern J: Chronic occult carbon monoxide poisoning. *J Emerg Nurs* 15:107, 1989.

83. Hanson NN: Practice and planning in physical therapy. In Berstein NR, Robson MC, editors: *Comprehensive approaches to the burned patient*, New York, 1983, Medical Examination Publishing.

84. Harmel RP, Vane DW, King DR: Burn care in children: special considerations. *Clin Plast Surg* 13:95, 1986.

85. Harris JA, Benedict FG: *A biometric study of basal metabolism in man*, Washington, 1919, Carnegie Institute of Washington, publication 279.

86. Hauser CJ, et al: Oxygen transport response to colloids and crystalloids in critically ill surgical patients. *Surg Gynecol Obstet* 150:811, 1980.

87. Heggers JP, Robson MC: Prostaglandins and thromboxanes. In Ninnemann JL, editor: *Traumatic injury, infection and other immunologic sequelae*, Baltimore, 1983, University Park Press.

88. Heideman M: Complement activation by thermal injury and its possible consequences for immune defense. In Ninnemann JL, editor: *The immune consequences of thermal injury*, Baltimore, 1981, Williams & Wilkins.

89. Heimbach DM: American Burn Association 1988 presidential address "we can see so far because..."*J Burn Care Rehabil* 9:340, 1988.

90. Heimbach DM, Engrav LH: Burn wound excision. *Curr Concepts Trauma Care* 4:14, 1981.

91. Heimbach DM, Engrav LH: *Surgical management of the burn wound*, New York, 1984, Raven Press.

92. Herndon DN, et al: Determinants of mortality in pediatric patients with greater than 70% full-thickness total body surface area thermal injury treated by early total excision and grafting. *J Trauma* 27:208, 1987.

93. Herndon DN, Parks DH: Comparison of serial debridement and autografting and early massive excision with cadaver skin overlay in the treatment of large burns in children. *J Trauma* 26:149, 1986.

94. Herndon DN, et al: Incidence, mortality, pathogens and treatment of pulmonary injury. *J Burn Care Rehabil* 7:185, 1986.

95. Hiebert JM, et al: Comparison of continuous versus intermittent tube feedings in adult burn patients. *J Parenter Enter Nutr* 5:73, 1981.

96. Hildreth M, Carvajal HF: Caloric requirements in burned children: a simple formula to estimate daily caloric requirements. *J Burn Care Rehabil* 3:7880, 1982.

97. Horovitx JH: Heat and smoke injuries of the airway. In Carvajal HF, Parks DH, editors: *Burns in children: pediatric burn management*, Chicago, 1988, Year Book Medical Publishers.

98. Huang PP, et al: Hypertonic sodium resuscitation is associated with renal failure and death. *Ann Surg* 221:543, 1995.

99. Huggins BM, Dingeldein GP: Nutritional support in thermal injuries. In Salisbury RE, Newman NM, Dingeldein GP, editors: *Manual of burn therapeutics: an interdisciplinary approach*, Boston, 1983, Little Brown.

100. Hummel RP: Curling's ulcer and other complications. In Hummel RP, editor: *Clinical burn therapy: a management and prevention guide*, Boston, 1982, John Wright Publishing.

101. Hunt TK, La Van FB: Enhancement of wound healing by growth factors. *N Engl J Med* 321:111, 1989.

102. Ireton CS, et al: Do changes in burn size affect measured energy expenditure? *J Burn Care Rehabil* 6:419, 1985.

103. Jansen MT, et al: Meeting psychosocial and developmental needs of children during prolonged intensive care unit hospitalization. *Child Health Care* 18:91, 1989.

104. Jeejeebhoy KN: Protein nutrition in clinical practice. *Brit Med Bul* 37:11, 1981.

105. Jensen JG, et al: Nutritional assessment indications of post-burn complications. *J Am Diet Assoc* 85:68, 1985.

106. Kibbee E: Life after severe burns in children. *J Burn Care Rehabil* 2:44, 1981.

107. Kravitz M: Nutritional needs of burn patients. In Herdon DN, editor: *Nutrition and metabolism symposium*, Chicago, 1986, American Burn Association.

108. Kremer B, et al: Burn toxin. In Ninnemann JL, editor: *The immune consequences of thermal injury*, Baltimore, 1981, Williams and Wilkins.

109. Kremer B, et al: The present status of research in burn toxins. *Int Care Med* 7:77, 1981.

110. Knudson-Cooper MS: Adjustment to visible stigma: the case of the severely burned. *Soc Sci Med* 15-B:31, 1981.

111. Knudson-Cooper MS, Thomas CM: Psychosocial care for severely burned children. In Carvajal HF, Parks DH, editors: *Burns in children: pediatric burn management*, Chicago, 1988, Year Book Medical Publishers.

112. Lacey DJ: Neurologic sequelae of acute carbon monoxide intoxication. *Am J Dis Child* 135:145, 1981.

113. Lal S, et al: Biobrane improves wound healing in burned children without increased risk of infection. *Shock* 14:314, 2000.

114. Larson M, Leigh J, Wilson LR: Detecting compartment syndrome using continuous pressure monitoring. *Focus Crit Care* 13:51, 1986.

115. Law EJ: Minimizing burn scar and contracture. In Hummel RP, editor: *Clinical burn therapy: a management and prevention guide*, Boston, 1982, John Wright Publishing.

116. Linares HA: Hypertrophic healing: controversies and etiopathogenic review. In Carvajal HF, Parks DH, editors: *Burns in children: pediatric burn management*, Chicago, 1988, Year Book Medical Publishers.

117. Long CL, et al: Metabolic response to injury and illness: estimation of energy and protein needs from indirect calorimetry and nitrogen balance. *J Parenter Enter Nutr* 3:452, 1979.

118. Lough M, Doershuk C, Stern R: *Pediatric respiratory therapy,* Chicago, 1985, Year Book Medical Publishers, Inc.

119. Lund CC, Browder NC: The estimation of areas of burns. *Surg Gynecol Obstet* 79:352, 1944.

120. Luther S, Price JH: Burns and their psychologic effect on children. *J School Health* 51:419, 1981.

121. Luterman A: Artificial skin. In Warden GD, editor: *Wound healing symposium*, Washington, DC, 1987, American Burn Association.

122. MacMillan BG: Infections following burn injury. *Surg Clin North Am* 60:185, 1980.

123. MacMillan BG: Initial replacement therapy. In Hummel RP, editor: *Clinical burn therapy: a management and prevention guide*, Boston, 1982, John Wright Publishing.

124. MacMillan BG: The problem of infection in burns. In Hummel RP, editor: *Clinical burn therapy: a management and prevention guide*, Boston, 1982, John Wright Publishing Co, Inc.

125. MacMillan BG: Wound management. In Wagner MM, editor: *Care of the burn-injured patient: multidisciplinary involvement*, Boston, 1981, PSG Publishing.

126. Madden MR, Finkelstein JL, Goodwin CW: Respiratory care of the burn patient. *Clin Plast Surg* 13:29, 1986.

127. Magrath HL: Nursing pediatric burns from a growth and development perspective. In Wagner MM, editor: *Care of the burn-injured patient: multidisciplinary involvement*, Boston, 1981, PSG Publishing.

128. Mancusi-Ungaro HR: Chemical burns in children. In Carvajal HF, Parks DH, editors: *Burns in children: pediatric burn management*, Chicago, 1988, Year Book Medical Publishers.

129. Mannon JM: *Caring for the burned,* Springfield, Ill, 1985, Charles C Thomas.

130. Marano MA, et al: Tourniquet technique for reduced blood loss and wound assessment during excisions of burn wounds of the extremity. *Surg Gynecol Obstet* 171:249, 1990.

131. Martyn JA: Cimetidine and/or antacid for the control of gastric acidity in pediatric burn patients. *Crit Care Med* 13:1, 1985.

132. Maschinot N, et al: Laryngotracheal stenosis as a complication of upper-airway thermal injury in children: two cases. *Resp Care* 32:785, 1987.

133. McDonald K, Johnson B, Prasad JK: Collaborative physical therapy for a 4-month old infant. *J Burn Care Rehabil* 9:193, 1988.

134. Mechanic HF, Dunn LT: Nutritional support for the burn patient. *Dim Crit Care Nurs* 5:20, 1986.

135. Merrell SW, et al: Fluid resuscitation in thermally injured children. *AM J Surg* 152:664–669, 1986.

136. Metheny NM: *Fluid and electrolyte balance, nursing considerations,* Philadelphia, 1987, JB Lippincott Co.

137. Moberg AW, et al: The comparative advantages of early tangential excision and grafting (TEG) in burn wound management. *Plast Surg Forum* 109:197, 1982.

138. Mochizuki H, et al: Optimal lipid content for enteral diets following thermal injury. *J Parenter Enter Nutr* 8:638, 1984.

139. Mochizuki H, et al: Mechanism of prevention of post burn hypermetabolism and catabolism by early enteral feedings. *Ann Surg* 200:297, 1984.

140. Monafo WW: The treatment of burn shock by the intravenous and oral administration of hypertonic lactated saline solution. *J Trauma* 10:575, 1970.

141. Monafo WW, Chuntrasakul C, Ayvazian VH: Hypertonic sodium solutions in the treatment of burn shock. *Am J Surg* 126:778, 1973.

142. Monafo WW, Salisbury RE, Dimick AR: The perils of sepsis. *Emerg Med* 15:47, 1983.

143. Moncrief JA: The body's response to heat. In Artz CP, Moncrief JA, Pruitt BA, editors: *Burns: a team approach*, Philadelphia, 1979, WB Saunders.

144. Morath MA, et al: Interpretation of nutritional parameters in burn patients. *J Burn Care Rehabil* 4:361, 1983.

145. Morath MA, Miller SF, Finley RK: Nutritional indicators of post burn bacteremic sepsis. *J Parenter Enter Nutr* 5:488, 1981.

146. Mosley S: Inhalation injury: a review of the literature. *Heart Lung* 17:3, 1988.

147. Murphy M, Bell SJ: Assessment of nutritional status in burn patients. *J Burn Care Rehabil* 9:432, 1988.

148. Nahas LF, Swartz BL: Use of semipermeable polyurethane membrane for skin graft dressing. *Plast Reconstr Surg* 67:791, 1981.

149. Nelson M: Identifying the emotional needs of the hospitalized child. *MCN Am J Matern Child Nurs* 6:181, 1981.

150. Newman NM: Monitoring the burn patient. In Salisbury RE, Newman NM, Dingeldein GP, editors: *Manual of burn therapeutics: an interdisciplinary approach*, Boston, 1983, Little Brown.

151. Newman NM: Nursing procedures. In Salisbury RE, Newman NM, Dingeldein GP, editors: *Manual of burn therapeutics: an interdisciplinary approach*, Boston, 1983, Little Brown.

152. Ninnemann JL: Immune depression in burn and trauma patients: the role of circulating suppressors. In Ninnemann JL, editor: *Traumatic injury, infection and other immunologic sequelae*, Baltimore, 1983, University Park Press.

153. Ninnemann JL: Immunologic defenses against infection: alterations following thermal injuries. *J Burn Care Rehabil* 3:355, 1982.

154. Ninnemann JL, Condie JT, Stein MD: Lymphocyte response following thermal injury: the effect of circulating immunosuppressive substances. *J Burn Care Rehabil* 2:196, 1981.

155. Ninnemann JL, Fischer JC, Wachtel TL: Effect of thermal injury and subsequent therapy on serum protein concentrations. *Burns* 6:165, 1980.

156. Ninnemann JL, Fischer JC, Wachtel TL: Thermal injury associated immunosuppression: occurrence and in vitro blocking effect of post recovery serum. *J Immunol* 122:1736, 1979.

157. Ninnemann JL, Stein MD: Induction of suppressor cells by burn treatment with povidone-iodine. *J Burn Care Rehabil* 1:12, 1980.

158. Ninnemann JL, Stein MD: Suppression of in vitro lymphocyte response by "burn toxin" isolates from thermally injured skin. *Immunol Lett* 2:339, 1981.

159. Ninnemann JL, Stein MD: Suppressor cell induction by povidone-iodine: in vitro demonstration of a consequence of clinical burn treatment with Betadine. *J Immunol* 126:1905, 1981.

160. Ninnemann JL, Stockland AE, Condie JT: Induction of prostaglandin synthesis dependent suppressor cells by endotoxin: occurrence in patients with thermal injuries. *J Clin Immunol* 3:142, 1983.

161. Ogle CK, Alexander JW, MacMillan BG: The relationship of bacteremia to levels of transferrin, albumin and total serum protein in burn patient. *Burns* 8:32, 1981.

162. O'Neill JA: Burns in children. In Artz CP, Moncrief JA, Pruitt BA, editors: *Burns: a team approach*, Philadelphia, 1979, WB Saunders.

163. O'Neill JA: Fluid resuscitation in the burned child: a reappraisal. *J Pediatr Surg* 17:604, 1982.

164. O'Neill JA, Roeber J: Burn care protocals: nutritional support. *J Burn Care Rehabil* 7:351, 1986.

165. Parish RA, et al: Fever as a predictor of infection in burned children. *J Trauma* 27:69, 1987.

166. Parrott M, et al: Structured exercise circuit program for burn patients. *J Burn Care Rehabil* 9:666, 1988.

167. Pegg SP: The role of drugs in management of burns. *Drugs* 24:256, 1982.

168. Pensler JM, Mulliker JB: Skin grafts: to mesh or not to mesh. *Contemp Surg* 32:45, 1988.

169. Perry AW, et al: Mafenide-induced pseudochondritis. *J Burn Care Rehabil* 9:145, 1988.

170. Peterson HD: Topical antibacterials. In Boswick JA, editor: *The art and science of burn care*, Rockville, MD, 1987, Aspen Publishers, Inc.

171. Petry JJ, Wortham KA: Contraction of wounds covered by meshed and non-meshed split thickness graft. *Brit J Plast Surg* 39:478, 1986.

172. Prokop-Oliet M, et al: Whey protein supplementation of complete tube feeding in the nutritional support of thermally injured patients. *Proc Am Burn Assoc* 15:37, 1983.

173. Prough DS, et al: Effects on intracranial pressure of resuscitation from hemorrhagic shock with hypertonic saline versus lactated Ringer's solution. *Crit Care Med* 13:407, 1985.

174. Pruitt BA: Burn infection prophylaxis today: an overview. In Alexander JW, Munster AM, Pruitt BA, editors: *Applied immunology: severe burns and trauma*, Berkeley, CA, 1983, Cutter Biological.

174a. Pulaski GR, Tennison AC: Estimation of the amount of burned surface area. *J Am Med Assoc* 103:34–38.

175. Quinby WC, et al: Clinical trials of amniotic membranes in burn wound care. *Plast Reconstr Surg* 70:711, 1982.

176. Rackow EC: Fluid resuscitation in circulatory shock: a comparison of the cardiorespiratory effects of albumin, hetastarch and saline solutions in patients with hypovolemic and septic shock. *Crit Care Med* 11:839, 1983.

177. Reiss E, et al: Fluid and electrolyte balance in burns. *J Am Med Assoc* 152:1309, 1953.

178. Rice V: Shock management: fluid volume replacement. *Crit Care Nurse* 4:69, 1984.

179. Robillard JE, et al: Renal hemodynamics and functional adjustments to postnatal life. *Semin Perinatol* 12:143, 1988.

180. Robson MC, Heggers JA: Pathophysiology of the burn wound. In Carvajal HF, Parks DH, editors: *Burns in children: pediatric burn management*, Chicago, 1988, Year Book Medical Publishers, Inc.

181. Rockwell WB, Ehlich P: Should burn blister fluid be evacuated? *J Burn Care Rehabil* 11:93–95, 1990.

182. Ross AD, Angarar DM: Colloids versus crystalloids: a continuing controversy. *Drug Intell Clin Pharm* 18:202, 1984.

183. Royall JA, Levin DL: Adult respiratory distress syndrome in pediatric patients. I. Clinical aspects, pathophysiology, pathology and mechanisms of lung injury. *J Pediatr* 112:169, 1988.

184. Royall JA, Levin DL: Adult respiratory distress syndrome in pediatric patients. II. Management. *J Pediatr* 112:335, 1988.

185. Rubin WD, Mani MM, Hiebert JM: Fluid resuscitation of the thermally injured patient. *Clin Plast Surg* 13:9, 1986.

186. Sadowski DA: Burn wound care: silver sulfadiazine application. *J Burn Care Rehabil* 8:429, 1987.

187. Sadowski DA: Fears expressed by burned children during the first eighteen months after injury, master's thesis, 1984, University of Cincinnati.

188. Sadowski DA: Smoke inhalation/carbon monoxide poisoning. In Sommers MS, editor: *Difficult diagnosis in critical care nursing*, Rockville, MD, 1988, Aspen Publishers.

189. Sadowski DA, Kishman M: Monitoring burn wounds for infection. *J Burn Care Rehabil* 8:568, 1987.

190. Sadowski DA, et al: The value of culturing central line catheter tips in thermally injured patients. *J Burn Care Rehabil* 9:66, 1988.

191. Sadowski DA, et al: Use of nonsterile gloves for routine noninvasive procedures in thermally injured patients. *J Burn Care Rehabil* 9:613, 1988.

192. Saffle JR, Young E: Energy requirements in thermal injury. In Herdon DN, editor: *Nutrition and metabolism symposium*, Chicago, 1986, American Burn Association.

193. Saffle JR, et al: Use of indirect calorimetry in the nutritional management of burned patients. *J Trauma* 25:32, 1985.

194. Salisbury RE: Wound care. In Salisbury RE, Newman NM, Dingeldein GP, editors: *Manual of burn therapeutics: an interdisciplinary approach*, Boston, 1983, Little Brown.

195. Salisbury RE, Petro JA: Rehabilitation of burn patients. In Boswick JA, editor: *The art and science of burn care*, Rockville, MD, 1987, Aspen Publishers.

196. Sandove AM, et al: Early excision: a financial assessment. *J Burn Care Rehabil* 6:442, 1985.

197. Sataloff D, Sataloff R: Tracheostomy and inhalation injury. *Head Neck Surg* 6:1024, 1984.

198. Schnares RH, et al: Plasma exchange for failure of early resuscitation in thermal injuries. *J Burn Care Rehabil* 7:230, 1986.

199. Schneider RM, Simonton-Thorne S: Treatment of joints and scars. In Achauer BM, editor: *Management of the burn patient*, Los Altos, CA, 1987, Appleton and Lange.

200. Sehune J, Goede M, Silverstein P: Comparison of energy expenditure measurement techniques in severely burned patients. *J Burn Care Rehabil* 8:366, 1987.

201. Shoemaker WC, et al: Fluid therapy in emergency resuscitation: clinical evaluation of colloid and crystalloid. *Crit Care Med* 9:367, 1981.

202. *Silvadene Cream, Product monograph*, Kansas City, 1983, Marion Laboratories, Inc.

203. Smith SL: Physiology of the immune system. *Crit Care Q* 9:7, 1986.

204. Soloman JR: Care and needs in a children's burn unit. In Rickham PP, Hecker WC, Preirot J, editors: *Progress in pediatric surgery*, Baltimore, 1981, Urban and Schwarzenberg.

205. Souba WW, Bessey PQ: Nutritional support of the trauma patient. *Infect Surg* 3:727, 1984.

206. Souba WW, Schindler BA, Carvajal HF: Nutrition and metabolism. In Carvajal HF, Parks DH, editors: *Burns in children: pediatric burn management*, Chicago, 1988, Year Book Medical Publishers.

207. Souba WW, Wilmore DW: Gut-liver interaction during accelerated gluconeogenesis. *Arch Surg* 120:66, 1985.

208. Spevor MJ, Pruitt BA: Candidiasis in the burned patient. *J Trauma* 21:237, 1981.

209. Stein MD, Ninnemann JL: Interferon production in patients with thermal injuries. *Immunol Lett* 2:207, 1981.

210. Stoddard FJ: Body image development in the burned child. *J Am Acad Child Psychol* 21:502, 1982.

211. Stratta RJ, et al: Plasma exchange therapy during burn shock. *Curr Surg* 40:429, 1983.

212. Thomson PD, et al: Leukopenia in acute thermal injuries: evidence against topical silver sulfadiazine as the caustic agent. *J Burn Care Rehabil* 10:418, 1989.

213. Thorton JW: Resuscitation. In Archauer BM, editor: *Management of the burn patient*, Los Altos, CA, 1987, Appleton and Lange.

214. Tse AM, Perez-Woods C, Opie ND: Children's admissions to the intensive care unit: parent's attitudes and expectations of outcomes. *Child Health Care* 16:68, 1987.

215. Uchiyama N, German J: Pediatric considerations. In Archauer BM, editor: *Management of the burned patient*, Los Altos, CA, 1987, Appleton and Lange.

216. VanHoesen KB, et al: Should hyperbaric oxygen be used to treat the pregnant patient for acute carbon monoxide poisoning? A case report and literature review. *J Am Med Assoc* 261:1039, 1989.

217. Vigness RM, Frey CS, Long JM: Acute leukopenia in burn patients treated with silver sulfadiazine and cimetidine. *Proc Am Burn Assoc* 13, 1981.

218. Wachtel TL: Nutritional support of the burn patient. In Boswick JA, editor: *The art and science of burn care*, Rockville, MD, 1987, Aspen Publishers.

219. Wachtel TL: Topical antimicrobials. In Carvajal HF, Parks DH, editors: *Burns in children: pediatric burn management*, Chicago, 1988, Year Book Medical Publishers.

220. Warden GD: Immunologic response to burn injury. In Boswick JA, editor: *The art and science of burn care*, Rockville, MD, 1987, Aspen Publishers.

221. Warden GD: Immunology. In Achauer BM, editor: *Management of the burned patient*, Los Altos, CA, 1987, Appleton and Lange.

222. Warden GD: Fluid resuscitation and early management. In: Herndon DN, editor: *Total burn care*, Philadelphia, 1996, WB Saunders, pp. 53.

223. Warden GD, Ninnemann JL: The immune consequences of thermal injury: an overview. In Ninnemann JL, editor: *The immune consequences of thermal injury*, Baltimore, 1981, Williams and Wilkins.

224. White S, Kampler G: Dietary noncompliance in pediatric patients in the burn unit. *J Burn Care Rehabil* 11:167, 1990.

225. Winter SL, Boyer JL: Hepatic toxicity from large doses of vitamin B3 (nicotinamide). *N Engl J Med* 289:1180, 1973.

226. Wolfe RR, et al: Response of protein and urea-kinetics in burn patients to different levels of protein intake. *Ann Surg* 197:163, 1983.

227. Wooldridge M, Surveyer JA: Skin grafting for full-thickness burn injury. *AJN* 80:2000, 1980.

228. Yannas IV, Burke JF: Design of artificial skin; basic design principles. *J Biomed Mater Res* 14:65, 1980.

229. Yarbrough DR: Pathophysiology of the burn wound. In Wagner MM, editor: *Care of the burn-injured patient*, Boston, 1981, PSG Publishing.

230. Young ME: Malnutrition and wound healing. *Heart Lung* 17:60, 1988.

231. Zamierowski DA, et al: Leukopenia in acute thermal injury: Is silver sulfadiazine responsible? *Proc Am Burn Assoc* 9:118, 1977.

232. Zawacki BE: The local effects of burn injury. In Boswick JA, editor: *The art and science of burn care*, Rockville, MD, 1987, Aspen Publishers.

233. Zawacki BE: Topical antimicrobial therapy using 0.5% aqueous silver nitrate solution. In Warden GD, editor: *Wound healing symposium*, 19, 1987, American Burn Association.

234. Zeller WP, et al: Accidental carbon monoxide poisoning. *Clin Pediatr* 23:694, 1984.

Bioinstrumentation: Principles and Techniques

21

PEARLS

- Monitoring and support systems provide valuable information and assistance in managing patient care, but the focus should always be on the patient and family as a first priority.
- Assess the patient's clinical condition before troubleshooting instruments.
- There are many physical characteristics of children that influence the development, use, size, and accuracy of biomedical instruments.
- No single measurement will be as valuable as the evaluation of trends in measurements over time.
- Not all instruments are necessarily valuable or precise.
- ECG waveforms indicate myocardial *electrical* activity and not the effectiveness of myocardial mechanical function.
- Respiratory monitoring is an invaluable resource to detect cardiopulmonary insufficiency and allow intervention before the development of cardiopulmonary failure.
- The use of mechanical ventilation does not ensure that the child's ventilation is effective. The child's clinical condition is the ultimate indicator of the effectiveness of mechanical ventilation.
- Multimodal monitoring, incorporating several neurologic monitoring parameters, may yield valuable information about the patient's overall clinical status.

OVERVIEW OF PEDIATRIC BIOINSTRUMENTATION

Margaret C. Slota

Bioinstrumentation in the pediatric critical care unit continues to increase in sophistication, paralleling the rapid growth and increasing complexity of pediatric critical care. Currently, a wide variety of instrumentation is available, and can be tailored to the needs of infants and children. The equipment discussed in this chapter is categorized according to the body system for which it is used.

This chapter describes the principles of bioinstrumentation, necessary equipment, specific uses, hazards of devices employed in the care of critically ill children, and troubleshooting techniques. As a first priority, the nurse should always assess the patient's clinical condition before proceeding to troubleshoot the instruments.

Instrumentation may be used to monitor, measure, or support a patient. Monitoring devices can measure patient physiologic parameters and can give warning or advise the clinician of the status of the parameters. Measuring devices regulate components that are administered to the patient, such as intravenous fluids. Patient support systems, such as ventilators, may both monitor and measure while they provide vital support.

For the sake of brevity, types of equipment described in this chapter are called *monitoring devices*. These devices may be subdivided further into two types: those considered *invasive,* which break the normal physiologic barriers (e.g., the skin) and those considered *noninvasive,* which do not break the physiologic barriers and, in some instances, do not even touch the patient.

Not all instruments are necessarily valuable or precise. The value of each device is affected by the skill of the clinicians and biomedical engineers working with the equipment. Karselis[87] maintains that the primary purpose of an instrument is to "extend the range and/or sensitivities of man's faculties" and, as such, should do so "with speed, reproducibility, reliability, and cost effectiveness."

Characteristics of Children that Affect Bioinstrumentation

Although the characteristics of the child that can affect selection and reliability of bioinstrumentation vary with the type of device, there are several key characteristics that must be considered during bioinstrumentation. Key characteristics include the child's body size, cardiovascular structure and function, pulmonary anatomy and physiology, neurologic development and function, metabolic rate, fluid requirements, and immunologic immaturity.

Body Size

Children are obviously smaller than adults. However, children have increased total body surface area in proportion to body mass, which causes higher heat and fluid loss per kilogram body weight than in the adult. Devices requiring exposure of the child to ambient air (e.g., overbed warmers) can increase fluid or heat loss. Compared with adults, infants and children have less absolute surface area available for application of skin electrodes or other contact devices, and this small available surface influences the design and use of some instruments.

Cardiovascular Structure and Function

Several features of the child's cardiovascular system influence the use of biomedical devices:

- Children have small arteries and veins for cannulation. Multiple lumen catheters in smaller sizes may be difficult to keep patent, influencing the choice of catheter and the nursing care required.

- The resting heart rate of the infant and small child is higher than that of the adult. As a result, when tachycardia develops the heart rate may be extremely high, making it difficult to evaluate the cardiac rhythm. A flexible but sensitive cardiac monitor is required that will accurately document changes in the child's heart rate or rhythm, and avoid introduction of errors from movement and other artifacts.
- The major compensatory mechanism for the child with cardiovascular dysfunction is tachycardia. The relatively small stroke volume of the young child is generally near the maximum that can be achieved by the child's small ventricle, so although stroke volume can increase slightly during periods of stress, the major mechanism for increasing cardiac output is an increase in heart rate. If the heart rate falls below normal, cardiac output typically falls. Thus, the child's cardiac output is much more dependent on heart rate than on stroke volume.
- Pulmonary artery wedge pressure may be elevated artificially by the child's rapid heart rate.
- The child has a relatively low systolic, diastolic, and mean arterial blood pressure compared with the adult; these low pressures must be measured accurately by monitoring devices. Quantitatively small changes in blood pressure can indicate qualitatively significant changes in the child's cardiovascular function.
- The technique used to determine cardiac output (CO) by thermodilution may be influenced by the child's limited tolerance of excessive fluid administration. Thermodilution CO calculations are performed in the adult using several 5-10 cc injections that will likely exceed a child's fluid requirements. Therefore the CO computer must be capable of calculating CO based on smaller injectate volumes with an acceptable potential error.

Pulmonary Anatomy and Physiology

The entire respiratory tract of an infant or small child is smaller than that of the adult. In addition, immaturity of components of the respiratory system will affect monitors and supportive devices. Specific considerations include:

- The upper airway of the child is smaller than that of the adult. Therefore, endotracheal and tracheostomy tubes used for children must be smaller. In the past, the tubes used in children were uncuffed. In recent years, evidence has accumulated that cuffed tubes may be as safe as uncuffed tubes and use of cuffed tubes in the operating suite allows more accurate selection of tube size.[92]
- The small tidal volumes, rapid respiratory rates, and short inspiratory times of children require mechanical ventilators that are able to deliver small tidal volumes accurately in short inspiratory times and at low pressures.
- The major compensatory mechanism for the child with respiratory distress is tachypnea. Respiratory monitoring equipment must be capable of accurately measuring rapid respiratory rates, even when tidal volume is low and chest movement is minimal.
- The infant's small airway closing pressure may be greater than atmospheric pressure, so there may be an increased tendency for alveolar collapse unless continuous positive airway pressure (CPAP) or positive end-expiratory pressure

(PEEP) can be provided by pediatric respiratory assist devices.
- The infant's chest wall is very compliant and provides little resistance to expansion during positive pressure ventilation, so visible chest rise should be observed during positive pressure ventilation. However, inadvertent hyperventilation and barotrauma may occur during hand or mechanical ventilation if excessive volume or pressure is provided.
- Although effective inspiratory inflation pressures are the same in normal patients of all ages, the force required to generate inspiratory pressure decreases with decreasing patient age because the lungs are small. Therefore, unless the inspiratory pressure is monitored closely, pneumothorax may be produced during hand ventilation or ventilation with high inspiratory pressure.
- Respiratory work normally accounts for 2% to 6% of the child's total oxygen consumption. When the infant develops respiratory distress, this requirement may be as high as 25% to 30% of the total oxygen consumption.
- A rapid respiratory rate produces increased heat and water loss through the respiratory system. Therefore all respiratory assist devices must heat and humidify inspired air.

Neurologic Development and Function

The infant's skull is thin and fontanelles are present. These characteristics influence the types of intracranial pressure monitoring devices used during infancy.

The critically ill child is typically frightened and uncooperative and is often unable to understand the reasons for monitoring or therapy. Movement artifact can cause interruption or distortion of instrument function or measurements; therefore monitoring devices must be able to differentiate between movement artifact and abnormalities in the child's clinical status.

Metabolic Rate

The child has a higher metabolic rate than the adult and therefore requires greater daily caloric intake per kilogram of body weight. Numerically small changes in the child's caloric intake may create significant changes in nutritional status, including the ability to heal.

Rapid heat loss or inadequate cardiac output, especially in the infant or young child may result in temperature instability. Constant temperature monitoring is required. The infant's oxygen consumption may increase significantly with changes in the ambient temperature.

Fluid Requirements

Infants and small children have a greater proportion of body weight as total body water and extracellular water than older children or adults, yet their absolute fluid requirements are small. Careful attention always must be given to the amounts and types of oral and parenteral fluids that the child receives.

Devices used to regulate the child's IV fluid administration rate and measure urine output must be calibrated in small units. Infusion pumps must be factory tested and clinically evaluated to ensure that they are able to accurately deliver specific fluid volumes and include appropriate alarms.

Immunologic Immaturity

The risk of healthcare-acquired infection is increased among critically ill children when invasive monitoring is performed. Invasive catheters should be used only when clearly indicated and they should be removed as soon as possible. Each child requires close observation for evidence of infection.

General Problems During Monitoring

Although complications and recommendations for each major equipment category are listed at the end of each major section, the following comments are relevant to all types of monitoring equipment. There are three common challenges in critical care units when electrical or mechanical equipment is used:

- *Specialized knowledge is required.* The nurse must understand the principles and components of each piece of equipment used to understand its usefulness and hazards. If the nurse is unfamiliar with any equipment, the nurse must immediately obtain instructions in use and troubleshooting of the device.

  Equipment is continuously being improved and upgraded and, consequently, this impacts interactive software and electronic medical record systems as well. The continuous improvements provide a challenge for ensuring that all staff are competent in the use of the current models of devices.

- *Many alarm systems are in use simultaneously.* The number of monitoring devices in use and subsequently the number of audible alarms sounding in the critical care unit are increasing dramatically. The sheer numbers of alarms may result in "alarm fatigue,"[65] in which clinicians may disable, silence, or ignore alarms when the number, variety, and sounds of the alarms become overwhelming. In addition, alarms may be turned off or malfunction without the knowledge of the bedside nurse. This may allow a problem to progress to a critical state before detection.

  If an alarm fails, the nurse is responsible for the consequences that may follow. All alarm settings and functions must be checked at least at the beginning and end of every shift and whenever vital signs are evaluated.

- *Equipment introduces risk of infection.* Contamination is more likely when invasive equipment is used, but it can also occur with noninvasive equipment.

Instrument Theory and Safety

Most electrical or mechanical monitoring systems include a sensor, a transducer, an amplifier, meters and alarms (Fig. 21-1). The nurse must interact with the patient and monitor at the point at which the device senses the physiologic signal and converts it to an electrical signal. The nurse also can adjust the amplifier and meter with tools such as the "gain" on an ECG monitor. The monitor alarm systems must be adjusted manually to fit the patient's needs.

Filters that eliminate electrical interference and grounding devices that protect both the patient and nurse from electrical shock are essential components of a monitoring system. All of these elements of bioinstrumentation are discussed in subsequent sections of this chapter.

Definition of Terms

Several terms are used to describe the common properties of electrical energy. The application of these terms to equipment function may be clarified by using the biologic correlate of an electrical system—the cardiovascular (hydraulic) system.[87]

Current. Electrical current is the flow of electrons past a given point[147]; electricity is always in motion. Current reflects the number of electrons (negatively charged ions) flowing through a conducting substance per unit of time.

Electrons move from an area of high electron concentration to an area of low electron concentration. In electrolyte solutions (e.g., water), ions move toward ions of the opposite charge. The current flow that is produced by ion movement is measured in amperes (amps). The analog of current in the cardiovascular system is "flow."

Voltage. Voltage is the unit of potential difference in charge between two points (i.e., "gradient" or "potential"). Electrons carry a negative charge. An imbalance in electron concentration between two points creates a negative charge at one point and a positive charge (or less-negative charge) at a second point. This imbalance will create a flow of electrons from the negative to the positive point (see the example immediately below). The analog of voltage in the cardiovascular system is pressure.

Flow of Electrons with Change in Voltage

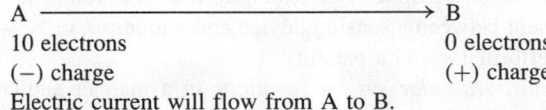

A ————————————————→ B
10 electrons   0 electrons
(−) charge   (+) charge
Electric current will flow from A to B.

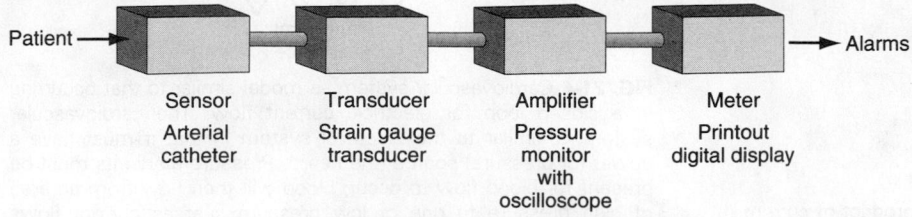

Patient → Sensor | Transducer | Amplifier | Meter → Alarms

Sensor	Transducer	Amplifier	Meter
Arterial catheter	Strain gauge transducer	Pressure monitor with oscilloscope	Printout digital display

FIG. 21-1 Components of monitoring systems. Most instruments used to monitor critically ill patients require a sensor, a transducer, an amplifier, and a meter. In hemodynamic monitoring systems, the *sensor* is the vascular catheter that provides access to the vascular pressure signal; the pulsatile vascular signal is converted to an electrical signal by a *transducer*; an *amplifier* in the monitor enhances the signal, and the digital display and oscilloscope function as the *meter*.

Resistance. The opposition to the flow of electrons or electrical current inherent in any material is called *resistance*. The amount of resistance provided in any material is determined by the conducting property of that material. For example, silver conducts a flow of current with greater ease than glass; therefore glass provides a higher resistance to current flow than silver. The unit of measure for resistance is the ohm.

Pure water is a poor conductor, but water may contain impurities such as salt, acid, and solvents, which turn water and other wet substances into better conductors. Wood, for example, usually stops the flow of electricity; but when saturated with water, wood becomes a conductor.

The relationship among these three terms—current (I), voltage (E), and resistance (R)—is described in the equation that follows and is also illustrated in Fig. 21-2.[87]

Ohm's Law

$$\begin{array}{ccccc} \text{Voltage} & = & \text{Current} & \times & \text{Resistance} \\ E & = & I & \times & R \end{array}$$

Power. Electrical power is the amount of work performed per unit of time; it is measured in watts. The rate at which the current flows (amperes [amps]) and the strength or power of flow (voltage) equals the wattage.[147] The total amount of power in a circuit at any time is expressed in watts. When current flows through a conductor, a certain amount of energy is dissipated into the environment as heat or light (e.g., in a light bulb). The rate of energy dissipation is determined by resistance (R) and current (I). The power (P) generated can then be calculated.[87]

Relationship of Power, Current, and Resistance

$$\begin{array}{ccccc} \text{Power} & = & \text{Current}^2 & \times & \text{Resistance} \\ P & = & I^2 & \times & R \end{array}$$

Application of Terms

Electrical theory explains the properties of electrical energy or power, incorporating several important principles[87]:
- Flow occurs because of electrical voltage gradients (high to low).
- There must be a current source to sustain power (voltage).
- There must be a closed electrical circuit (or loop) for current flow to be possible. For example, a closed loop must be present between a sensing device and a monitor, or between a defibrillator and a patient.

The *cardiovascular system* functions in a manner similar to that described by the electrical principles in the preceding list.

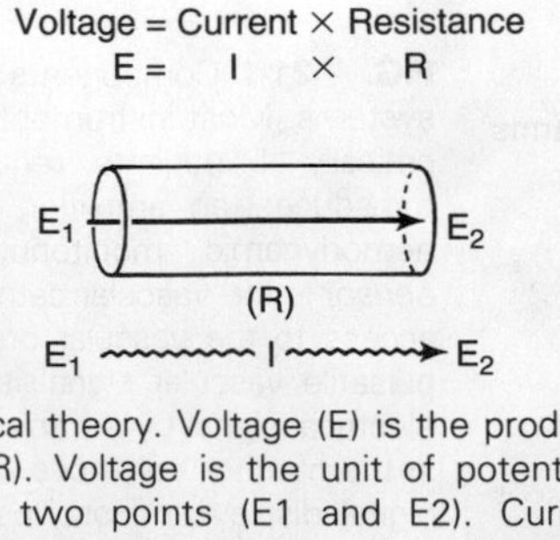

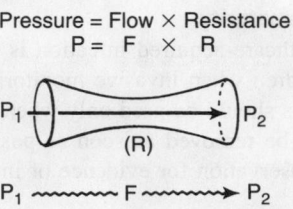

$$\begin{array}{ccccc} \text{Voltage} & = & \text{Current} & \times & \text{Resistance} \\ E & = & I & \times & R \end{array}$$

FIG. 21-2 Electrical theory. Voltage (E) is the product of current (I) and resistance (R). Voltage is the unit of potential difference in charge between two points (E1 and E2). Current flow (I) is determined by voltage and resistance within the material.

FIG. 21-3 Pressure, flow, and resistance. Ohm's law can be applied to the cardiovascular system. Pressure (P) is the product of blood flow (F) and resistance (R). Resistance is determined primarily by the radius of the vessels or chambers through which the blood flows.

Comprehension of cardiovascular physiology requires knowledge of the properties flow (F), pressure (P), and resistance (R), and of their relationship (Fig. 21-3).

Poiseuille's Law

$$\begin{array}{ccccc} \text{Pressure} & = & \text{Flow} & \times & \text{Resistance} \\ P & = & F & \times & R \end{array}$$

There are several important similarities between electrical theory and the cardiovascular system.
- There must be a voltage (or pressure) gradient between one point in the system and another for flow to occur. The direction of flow is from an area of high electron concentration to an area of low electron concentration or from an area of high pressure to one of lower pressure.
- There must be an electron pump or current source to sustain power or voltage. In the cardiovascular system the pump is the heart.
- The system must be a closed circuit or loop if the flow is to be sustained (Fig. 21-4).

Power in the cardiovascular system is generated by the heart and represents the amount of work accomplished by a

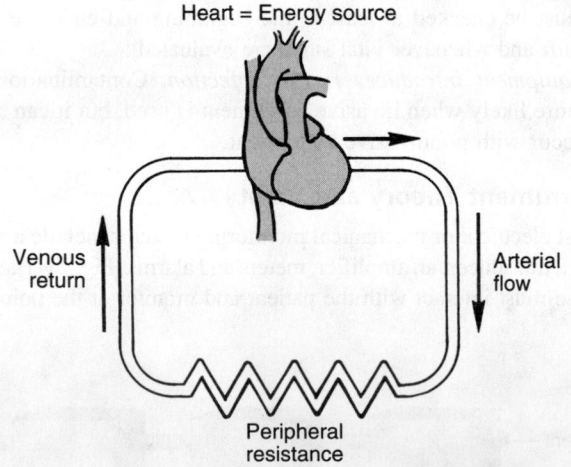

FIG. 21-4 Cardiovascular system as model similar to that occurring in a closed loop for electrical current flow. The cardiovascular system is similar to the electrical system in that it must have a power (or pressure) source (the heart). Pressure gradients must be present for blood flow to occur; blood will then flow from an area of high pressure to one of low pressure, just as current flows from an area of high electron concentration to one of low electron concentration. Finally, the system must remain a closed loop for flow to be sustained.

ventricle over a given unit of time. This power may be calculated as the stroke work index or ventricular ejection fraction.

Electrical Hazards in the Pediatric Critical Care Unit

In healthcare facilities, it is important to prevent establishment of conductive paths from patients to grounded objects.[127] Conductive paths may be established though instrumentation, electrically conductive surfaces, or inadvertently. For example, damaged electrical cords can lead to possible shock or electrocution. A flexible electrical cord may be damaged by door or window edges, staples and fasteners, rolling equipment, or aging.

Hospital staff and patients can be exposed to electrical hazards that create risk of electric shock, electrocution, fires, and explosions.[176] Electrical hazards are more likely when there is a lack of routine maintenance or surveillance of electrical equipment, misuse of the equipment, or a lack of understanding of the equipment and/or its controls. Oxygen-enriched atmospheres and water may also contribute to hazardous conditions.

Electric shock can produce effects that range from slight tingling to immediate cardiac arrest depending on the amount of current, the current's path through the body, the duration of contact with the current, and the frequency of the current. The risk of electrical hazard is increased as the number of instruments increases. Controlling or preventing hazards requires raising the resistance of the conductive circuit or insulating surfaces that could become energized or a combination of both approaches.[127]

The Electrically Sensitive Patient

Some patients are vulnerable to electrical injuries by virtue of the instrumentation used to monitor them. Patients with externalized direct conductive paths to the heart may be electrocuted at very low current levels.[127] They are at risk for macroshock or microshock phenomenon.

Macroshock. Although electrical systems are typically defined by their voltage and resistance, it is current that is the dimension of physiologic significance. Current directed at the body can deliver either a macroshock or microshock depending on the route of transmission.

Macroshock refers to application of current to the outside of the body (direct skin contact). If a current is passed through a human from limb to limb, only 0.5 A (500 mA) are required to produce ventricular fibrillation. Two defenses are present to protect the body from transmission of current:

• Skin resistance in a dry state provides up to 1 million ohms of resistance. This alone would protect a person from an otherwise fatal shock when contact is made with a 120-volt line.
• Diffusion of current, which normally occurs as current passes through body tissue, reduces current density. Therefore the myocardium receives only a portion of the total current delivered to the body.

Microshock. A *microshock* is a small amount of current that may produce significant injury because it has a direct path of entry to the myocardium, such as through a pacemaker wire or intracardiac catheter. A microshock with as little current as 200 mA may produce ventricular fibrillation if it is directed through pacemaker wires (Table 21-1). In comparison, the threshold for ventricular fibrillation applied to the skin is documented at 500 mA or 2500 times the current required for microshock to occur. Therefore a patient with intracardiac catheters is especially vulnerable to microshock because the small amount of current required to produce fibrillation is imperceptible to the care provider.

Current Leak. In a critical care unit setting, current leak from electrical equipment creates a major risk of macroshock or microshock. Current leak does not necessarily result from equipment malfunction, but it occurs naturally when current flows between two electrical conductors that are insulated from one another (e.g., between the internal electronics of an ECG monitor and its chassis). The current will seek a path of least resistance; if a patient is in contact with one electrical device, the current will be conducted through the patient (Fig. 21-5). Therefore, patients should be protected from contact with line-powered equipment.

Grounding. *Grounding* is a protective mechanism built into electrical circuits. A ground is simply a means of conducting electrical current to the earth or some other object connected to the earth. Earth has zero voltage, so the voltage drop to

Table 21-1 Physiologic Effects of Current Leakage

Current	Effect with Skin Contact	Comments
200 microamps (0.2 mA)	No perception	If current contacts intracardiac catheters, it may cause ventricular fibrillation.
1-10 mA (0.001-0.01 A)	Tingling sensations	Tingling when touching an electrical device indicates an impending hazard. Unplug the instrument and have it checked immediately.
100-500 mA (0.1-0.5 A)	"Can't let go" phenomenon	Do not touch victim or instrument. Unplug device if possible. Push the victim out of contact with the device using a broom or folded blanket or throw your body against the victim, moving him or her away from the device.
500-1500 mA (0.5-1.5 A)	Ventricular fibrillation	See comment for 100-500 mA. Note that these victims must receive immediate cardiopulmonary resuscitation.

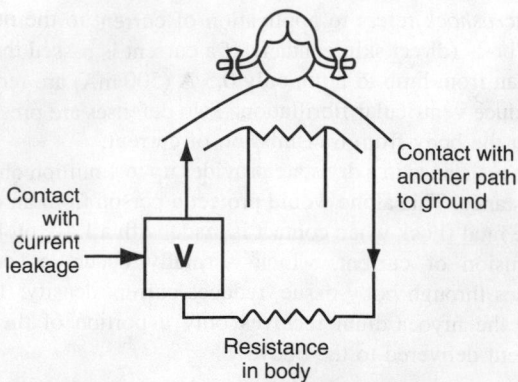

FIG. 21-5 Current leak. Ungrounded equipment may create an electrical hazard for the patient. The patient can become part of a closed loop between a faulty piece of electrical equipment (with current leak) and the ground or another person or object.

earth provides an inherent safety feature for grounded circuits. Current always travels along the path of least resistance, and if a connection to the ground is available it provides the path of least resistance (Fig. 21-6).

There are several methods of grounding used in the critical care environment. They include circuit and system grounding,

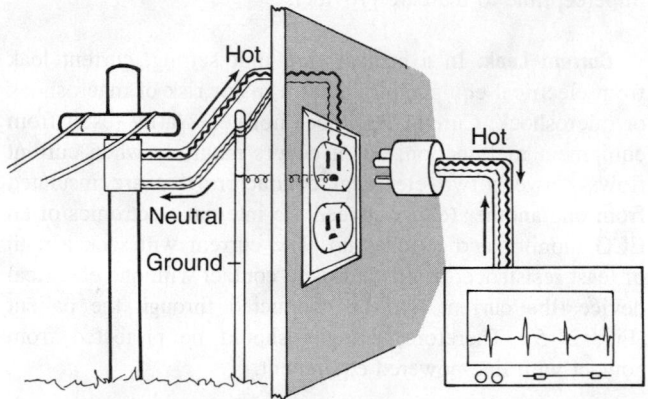

FIG. 21-6 Grounding. Current flows through a "hot" wire to the instrument and returns through a "neutral" or "cold" wire. A third "ground" wire is added as a safety mechanism and provides a low-resistance path for stray current. If there is current leak in the instrument chassis or a fracture in the neutral wire, current will flow to the ground.

equipment grounding, and "isolated" system grounding. Circuit and system grounding are accomplished by the grounding of major power distribution transformers that service entire areas with electrical power. When an individual piece of equipment is grounded, all metal parts of the equipment are connected with a common wire to the ground.

In contrast, an *isolated system* commonly is created in critical care units and operating rooms. In an isolated system, grounding is provided by a special transformer, leaving the equipment "isolated" so that the current flows only from one isolated line to another (Fig. 21-7). In a perfectly isolated system, one could touch a water faucet (ground) with one hand and touch either of the two isolated lines without receiving a shock. This isolated system offers a great advantage over the power systems but is more difficult to construct.[87]

Electrical Safety

Standards for electrical safety in each hospital are based on the principles of electrical theory and current electrical code.[127] Best practices include inspection and labeling of biomedical equipment when it arrives at the hospital plus routinely scheduled equipment inspections and maintenance. Daily instrument surveillance by care providers will prevent many equipment problems. Nurses should always be cognizant of potential safety hazards and they are responsible for preventative safety efforts.

1. Be alert to potential electrical hazards and inspect equipment and cords throughout the course of providing care. Use only equipment in good working condition that is labeled appropriately and inspected on schedule. All users require training before operating new or unfamiliar equipment.

   Visually inspect all equipment cords and plugs and flexible cord sets before use, looking for external defects and for evidence of possible internal damage. Look for breaks in cord insulation, loose or frayed parts, broken prongs, loose plugs that fall out of the wall outlet easily, crushed outer jackets, or warning lights indicating internal malfunction.

2. Note inspection dates posted on equipment by the hospital biomedical engineers and notify the engineers of expired inspection dates. If clinical equipment is found to be damaged, it should be deenergized, tagged, and removed from the area when portable. The Safe Medical Devices

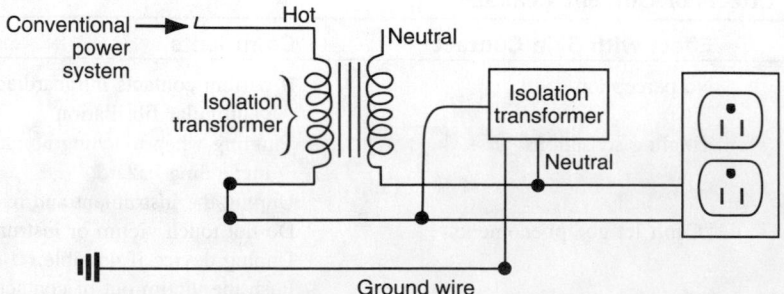

FIG. 21-7 Isolated system. An "isolated" grounding system can be created by directing current from a conventional power system into an isolation transformer. Current then enters an instrument through a "hot" wire and exits by the neutral wire to the transformer. Note that both sides of the circuit are isolated from ground. The isolation transformer represents the lowest potential in the system, so that any stray current from the instrument will flow readily to the transformer (rather than through the ground wire).

Act requires reporting of medical devices believed to have caused or contributed to serious injury or death.[152]

3. Always use three-prong (grounded) plugs. Electricity is delivered through one of the wires in an electric cord—the live or hot wire. The other two wires are the neutral and ground wires. The ground wire is the longer round prong on the electric plug.

   Unless a ground wire is present, there exists a possibility of current leak or a short circuit between the "hot" wire and the equipment housing that may cause conduction of current through the patient to another grounded source. A similar problem will occur if a two-pronged extension cord is used as an adapter between the patient monitor and the wall or if a "cheater plug" (three-pronged to two-pronged) adapter is used.

   Plug three-pronged cords only into three-pronged outlets. Never remove the third prong from three-pronged cords. It is a safety feature designed to reduce the risk of shock.

4. Avoid using extension cords because they provide greater length of conduction material and the possibility of a current leak.[39] Extension cords are often placed on the floor, where they may be crushed by rolling beds or machines.

   Protect all cords from damage. Prevent ECG cables from becoming caught in side rails or bed mechanisms.

5. Make sure that any equipment leads connected to the patient are insulated and isolated from possible contact with stray current or a "hot" wire.

6. Do not allow any conductive liquids to come into contact with intracardiac wires (e.g., pacemaker wires) or catheters, because current leak may be conducted directly to cardiac tissue or through the heart and catheter to the grounded monitor.

7. Avoid 60-cycle (60-Hertz) interference. When two conductive surfaces (e.g., the human body and a monitor) are close to each other, they hold and transmit alternating current (AC) between them and can transmit current to other conductive surfaces. This is termed *capacitance;* the property of "holding" electrical energy. This capacitance between the patient and the monitor system, which is typically surrounded by other conductors (e.g., apnea monitors or IV pumps), produces a "fuzzy" baseline tracing on the ECG and can be minimized or dispersed by several methods:

   - Position ECG leads near one another to avoid exposure of individual leads to environmental capacitance.
   - Apply electrodes carefully to decrease skin resistance caused by oils and loose skin cells; scrub the skin with alcohol and dry it with gauze before electrode application.
   - Move the ground (or reference) electrode to a point closer to other electrodes.
   - Change all electrode wires and patches if interference continues.
   - Change the cable if electrical interference persists.

8. Recognize special precautions for patients who have invasive intracardiac catheters or pacing wires. Be certain that these catheters and wires are not in direct contact with electrical equipment (e.g., ECG leads) to avoid microshock.

9. Pay particular attention to patients who are in high humidity environments (e.g., receiving humidified air via a face tent) if invasive catheters (e.g., central venous catheters) are in place. Water is an electrolyte solution that will conduct current.

10. Do not place any instruments on metal carts or shelves or near water. Water and metal are highly conductive materials that may conduct stray current.

11. Try to avoid touching both the patient and an electrical device simultaneously because you may provide a path for conduction of stray current from the device to the patient. The nurse should never touch two electrical devices simultaneously; if there is a current leak, the nurse becomes the path from the broken instrument to the ground (Fig. 21-8).

12. Minimize the effect of static electricity. Static electricity built up on the surface of an object may discharge to a person, generally resulting in a small shock. However, static electricity shocks can be much more serious in the presence of nearby flammable or combustible substances, creating the potential for explosion.

13. Always use grounded equipment. Stray current from defective equipment will follow the path of least resistance leading to ground. If your body is between a live wire and the ground, electricity will travel through you. Electric currents flow between parts of the body or through the body to a ground or the earth by whatever path possible.

14. Hospital policies regarding the use of electrical devices should be clear and accessible. Generally, biomedical departments must approve, inspect, and label all electrical items brought into the hospital (including any items that patients and families bring from home).

   All electrical equipment used in the hospital must be approved for safety by the Underwriters Laboratory (UL) or another OSHA-approved body. These approvals and inspections ensure that powered equipment meets hospital standards, is compatible with existing equipment, and that service contracts meet the needs of the hospital.[131]

   Biomedical personnel should be familiar resources for the nursing staff. They will ensure that critical care unit equipment is safe for both patients and staff.

15. Safety signs or symbols, such as accident prevention placards, are used where necessary to warn employees about potential electrical hazards. Barricades may be necessary to prevent or limit employee or visitor access to hazardous areas.

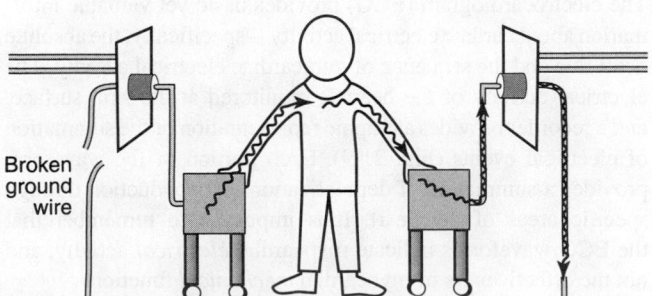

FIG. 21-8 Electrical safety. The healthcare provider should never touch two pieces of electrical equipment at the same time. If the ground wire of one unit is fractured, any stray current may flow through the provider to the other (functioning) ground wire.

In summary, use of high technology electrical equipment creates the potential for electrical shock hazards in the healthcare environment. Staff should be very aware of electrical safety and preventative procedures for their own protection and patient protection.

Exposure to electric shock and explosions is possible because of damaged electrical cords and the lack of routine maintenance to electrical equipment. All electrical equipment used in the hospital should be approved for safety by Underwriters Laboratory (UL) or another OSHA-approved body. Staff should be properly trained on the safe use and application of electrical equipment.

CARDIOVASCULAR MONITORING AND SUPPORT

Cardiovascular Monitoring

Patricia Ann E. Schlosser

The practice of cardiovascular monitoring, as an integral part of cardiovascular care, should be evidence-based. Models for evidenced-based care [61,64,145,156,168] provide a framework to evaluate outcomes and use goal-oriented therapies. The American Association of Critical-Care Nurses (AACN) has updated their level of evidence structure to provide resources for nursing staff.[12]

Technology is being developed that will provide noninvasive and accurate assessment of tissue perfusion with the goal of creating monitors that will detect compromise in tissue perfusion. This will enable therapy adjustments to improve neurodevelopmental outcomes, preserve myocardial function, and prevent end-organ damage. Some research has been reported in these areas[79] for pediatric patients with congenital heart disease; other areas have yet to be studied in prospective, randomized controlled studies.[78]

Cardiovascular monitoring is the most common type of pediatric and neonatal critical care bioinstrumentation. Cardiovascular monitoring includes electrocardiograms; vascular monitoring; pacemakers; pulse oximetry monitors for arterial, mixed venous, and systemic venous oxygen saturations; lactate trend monitors; cerebral oximetry; defibrillators; external emergency pacing; and new technology in cardiac assist devices.

The nurse must be familiar with cardiovascular physiology and pathophysiology to interpret the measurements or trended data derived and must be able to correlate these measurements with changes in the patient's clinical appearance. The current bioinstrumentation trend is toward noninvasive technology.

Electrocardiogram

The electrocardiogram (ECG) provides basic yet valuable information about cardiac electrical activity—specifically, the absolute heart rate and the sequence of intracardiac electrical activity. The electrical activity of the heart is monitored at the skin surface, and a recorder provides a graphic representation of the summation of electrical events (Fig. 21-9). Each portion of the waveform provides a summation of depolarization and conduction through specific areas of the heart. It is important to remember that the ECG waveforms indicate myocardial *electrical* activity, and not the effectiveness of myocardial *mechanical* function.

When ECG monitoring is performed, adhesive electrodes are placed on the surface of the body. When two electrodes are used as reference points to evaluate cardiac electrical activity, a *bipolar lead* has been created.

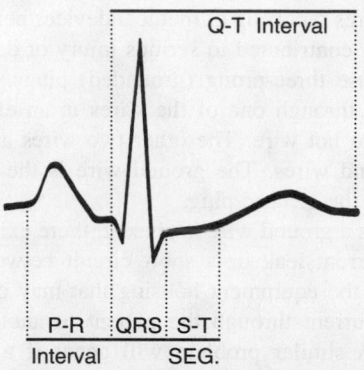

FIG. 21-9 ECG tracing. The P wave represents atrial depolarization, and the P-R interval represents the time needed for conduction of the impulse through the atria (and the junctional tissue) to the ventricles. The QRS complex represents ventricular depolarization, and the Q-T interval represents the entire cycle of ventricular depolarization and repolarization.

Electrodes. Most pediatric electrocardiographic monitors use the "floating" adhesive electrodes, which are manufactured in a variety of sizes. Each electrode rides on a layer of conductive jelly. To ensure stable contact and minimize impedance, the skin at the electrode site is cleaned before placement. Association of Women's Health, Obstetric and Neonatal Nursing (AWHONN) skin care guidelines should be followed when using products for high-risk, low birth weight, or premature infants.[109]

ECG Electrode Placement. Wireless technology allows bidirectional data flow (communication) for monitoring, display, analysis, alarm detection, operator alerts, data storage, and permanent recording of trended data. Monitors are equipped with cables that allow: (1) a three- or five-lead monitoring system, (2) use of limb leads, and (3) a 12-lead capability using a cable with the four limb leads plus a fifth lead for precordial monitoring. Bedside ECG monitoring requires only the placement of three electrodes in a three-lead system to obtain the recording of leads I, II, and III (Fig. 21-10).

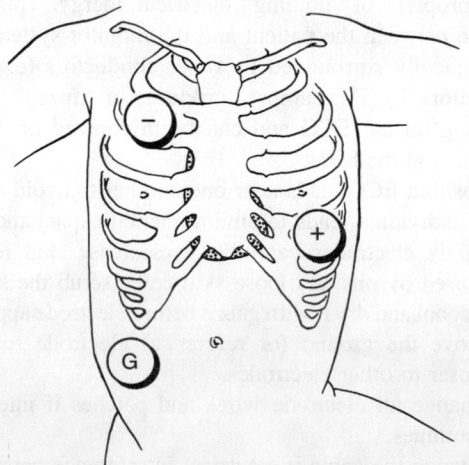

FIG. 21-10 ECG, lead II. The negative (white) electrode is placed on the right upper sternal border, and the positive (black) electrode is placed on the left shoulder or near the apex of the heart (on the left chest, below the nipple). The ground electrode can be placed in a convenient location, but electrical interference will be minimized if the ground is placed near the other electrodes.

A three-lead ECG uses three electrodes: one electrode is specified as negative (−), one as positive (+), and one serves as a ground. It is important to apply the electrodes correctly to enable accurate interpretation of the ECG signals.

A universal color coding system for identification of leads is used by most ECG manufacturers: The negative lead is white, the positive lead is black, and the ground is either red or green. The negative (−) white electrode, designated on some models as "RA" (right arm) should be *superior* to the heart; in leads I and II it should be placed on the right side and in lead III on the left side. The positive (+) black lead is designated usually as "LA" (left arm) or "LL" (left leg), indicating the potential positions of the (+) electrode. For five lead monitoring, the first choice is V6 when V1 cannot be used and the third option is lead III.

The "direction" of the ECG signal between the two electrodes will always flow from the (−) to (+) electrode in the *normal* heart; therefore the lead II monitoring placement most closely parallels the direction of depolarization from the sinoatrial node to the ventricular Purkinje fibers. The lead II ECG in the *normal* child should demonstrate upright P, QRS, and T waves (see Fig. 21-9). Deviations indicate either incorrect lead placement or abnormal myocardial electrical activity.

Limb-lead ECG monitoring is used for obtaining recordings of each of the six limb leads, including the major leads (I, II, III) and three additional leads, designated AVR, AVL, and AVF. These limb leads lie in the frontal plane of dimension, and they reflect the direction of movement of the electrical current that flows from the negative to the positive myocardial cells (Fig. 21-11). Each of the six leads captures a recording of the conduction from a different vantage point. Limb leads are used with an open chest postoperatively.

Digital signals and ECG monitoring filtering are used to reduce artifacts that will detract from waveform quality and cause false alarms. These systems can isolate the impact of broadband interference.

Recordings made from *precordial leads* allow qualification and quantification of cardiac electrical activity on the sagittal plane. Observations and measurements of the speed and voltage of ventricular depolarization and repolarization can provide information about chamber hypertrophy, myocardial ischemia, or infarction (Fig. 21-12).

The use of a *modified chest lead (MCL)* is a variation in standard electrode placement that may be useful in the identification of aberrant rhythms and blocks. The MCL sites produce a *simulated precordial lead* tracing; for example, MCL_1 approximates V_1. In the modified chest lead, the negative electrode is placed near the outer part of the left clavicle, and the ground is placed on the right shoulder. The positive lead can be placed at the fourth intercostal space (ICS) on the right sternal border (RSB), or at the fourth ICS at the left sternal border (LSB) for MCL_1 or MCL_2 leads, respectively (Fig. 21-13).

Pacing pulse detection is available for pacing-dependent patient safety. The technology with bidirectional cellular wireless transceiver takes data from monitoring inputs and

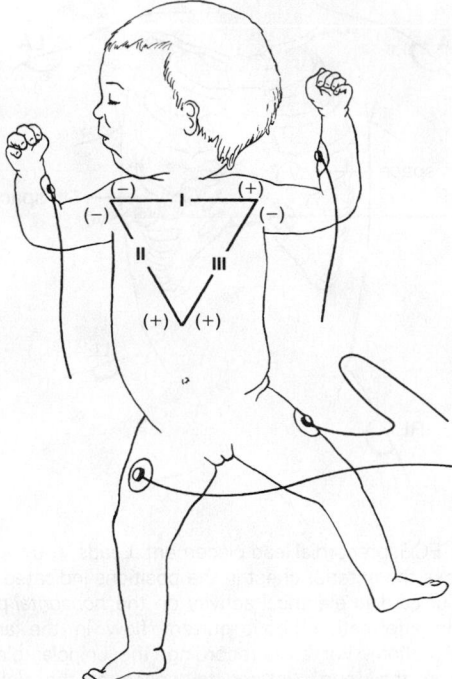

FIG. 21-11 ECG, limb lead placement. A six-lead ECG recording may be accomplished by placing limb leads on all four extremities; this enables assessment of cardiac electrical activity on the *frontal* plane (enabling evaluation of current flow in the anterior, superior, right, or left direction). The triangular symbol, Einthoven's triangle, is formed by the axes of the three bipolar limb leads. During use of the limb leads, Leads I, II, III, aVR, aVL, and aVF are recorded. The ECG unit automatically will adjust the polarity of each limb electrode during recording, so that in aVR, the right arm is the (+) electrode, in aVL, the left arm is the (+) electrode, and in aVF, a leg electrode is (+). If lead I is designated, the left arm electrode is positive, but if lead III is designated, the left arm electrode is negative.

transmits data wirelessly to cell phone-based access points (e.g., Phillips Instrument Technology, www.medical.philips.com).

Telemetry. The choice of electrocardiographic bedside monitors is vast. Monitors are capable of displaying and recording several parameters simultaneously, including the ECG, arterial and venous pressures, respiratory rate, oxyhemoglobin saturation via pulse oximetry (SpO_2), and noninvasive blood pressure. The child's temperature can be monitored via thermistors in indwelling urinary catheters. This can be particularly helpful for continuous monitoring of temperature during therapeutic hypothermia (e.g., treatment of patients with junctional ectopic tachycardia in the immediate postoperative period or following return of spontaneous circulation after cardiac arrest).

Telemetry is essential for patients requiring continuous vasoactive or other essential infusions. Baseline weight and a pediatric code card/form are completed for every patient in a neonatal and pediatric setting. Guidelines for change of shift

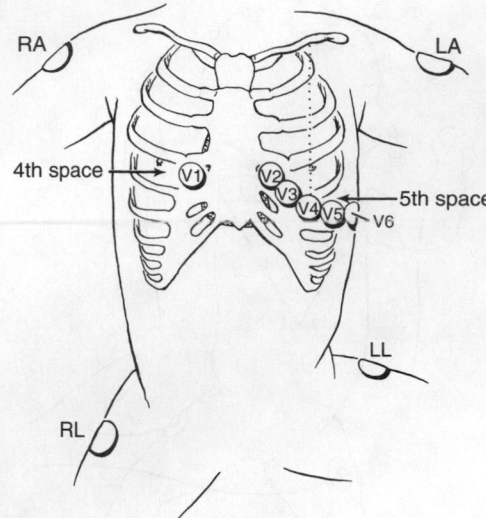

FIG. 21-12 ECG, precordial lead placement. Leads V₁ through V₆ are placed across the anterior chest in the positions indicated to enable evaluation of cardiac electrical activity on the *horizontal* plane (this will provide information about current flow in the anterior or posterior direction). For a V₁ recording, the unipolar electrode is positioned in the fourth intercostal space at the right sternal border. When the precordial leads are recorded, each position (V₁ through V₆) is used sequentially as the positive electrode. Leads V₁ and V₂ provide information about right ventricular conduction, and leads V₅ and V₆ provide information about left ventricular conduction.

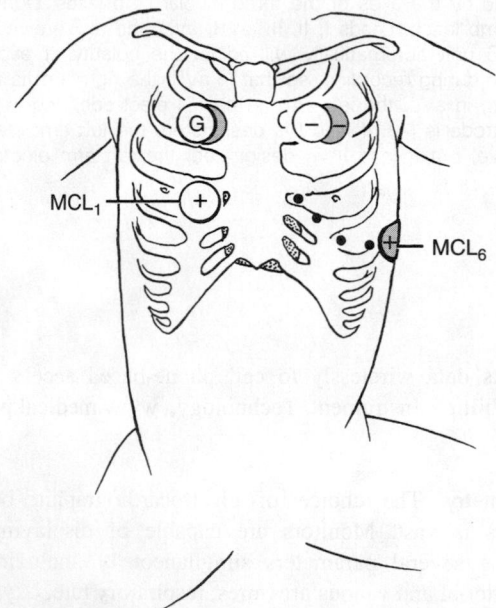

FIG. 21-13 MCL ECG lead placement. The electrode placement for modified chest leads MCL₁ and MCL₆ is illustrated here. Any of the precordial-lead positions can be used to obtain a related modified chest-lead recording.

communications include "line reconciliation"—verification of placement and function of all infusion and drainage catheters and pacing wires.

Electromagnetic interference (EMI) elimination to patient care equipment is guided by clinical engineering expertise in

maintaining a database of frequencies currently used in hospital settings. In highly instrumented settings such as critical care, emergency department, and diagnostic imaging, most clinical equipment is designed to be shielded from unwanted radio emissions.

ECG Monitoring System Components. An ECG monitoring system consists of sensors (electrodes), an amplifier and filter, a digital display (including tachometer), and a recorder. The quality of the monitor is determined by the quality and characteristics of each of these components.

Filtering Units. Digitized ECG and SpO₂ signals detect and analyze for arrhythmias and display alarm conditions. Filters help to minimize interference such as muscle artifact and 60-cycle interference.

Gain Units. "Gain" indicates the degree of amplification of the ECG signal that occurs when the signal passes through the amplifier. This gain determines the size of the P wave and QRS complex. The ability of the tachometer to sense signals for rate computation is affected by the amplitude of electrical signals and the gain setting. The ability of the monitor to sense voltage also may be altered by electrode placement and cardiac pathology.

Diagnostic ECG recordings are often performed with *fixed gain* recorders because they record true voltage without interference or alteration. As a result changes in observed amplitude of the ECG recorded with "fixed gain" recorders are usually clinically significant.

Automatic gain mechanisms adjust the amplitude of the ECG complex internally to maintain consistent amplitude for the screen display or printout. Other monitors have a gain control to enable the operator to adjust the amplitude of the ECG complex. This is necessary for continuous monitoring because the monitor also must count the child's heart rate.

To calculate heart rate, the R-R interval is typically measured (see Display and Recording Units, below). To recognize the R wave, monitors are programmed to sense a QRS complex of a predetermined standard slope. If the intrinsic voltage of the child's QRS complex is low, it is possible that the tachometer may not sense the R wave and the heart rate will not be calculated accurately. In this case, the nurse can adjust the gain or change lead placement so that each QRS complex is recognized by the tachometer.

Alarms. Alarm limits should be displayed at the bedside monitor and at the central station. High and low alarm limits must be established and verified during each work shift for each parameter being monitored. Alarms also should be checked before the nurse leaves the bedside for any reason, or if the nurse must participate in a procedure. The parameters for the alarms used are based on patient severity of illness and hospital policy.

Display and Recording Units. There is a choice of display units with the capability of audible alarms as well as alarm pagers or phones with recording units. Some basic components and options required in the care of critically ill children are reviewed here.

A trigger point—either the QRS complex or T wave—is used to compute the heart rate from the calculated R-R or T-T interval. The device recognizes each complex with the same slope and amplitude as a standard or programmed QRS or T-wave signal. Signals such as pacer spikes or artifact should be ignored by the monitor.

Many monitors compute the heart rate by averaging the QRS frequency over 3 to 4 seconds. The normal beat-to-beat variation in the child's heart rate (sinus arrhythmia) will cause inaccuracies in the heart rate displayed by the monitor if the QRS frequency is averaged during a time when the heart rate is unusually rapid or slow.

Ideally the displayed digital heart rate will be unaffected by a pacemaker impulse, so that a low heart rate alarm will still sound if the pacemaker fails to capture (depolarize) the ventricle (i.e., the pacer spike is not followed by ventricular depolarization) or the ventricle fails to respond to a paced impulse. Some new monitors are programmed to sense only an impulse with the same QRS slope that has been calculated from a sample strip stored in memory.

Monitors are also able to determine the heart rate from the arterial pulse. This is necessary during pacemaker therapy, or when an artifact is producing inaccuracy in the displayed heart rate. This feature typically must be activated by the clinician.

Digital Meter. Digital displays provide a continuous, visual, numeric display of the heart rate and are now standard for precise, instantaneous evaluation of heart rate. There is usually a 2- to 5-second lag through the amplifier between the signal and the display. As the nurse is auscultating the child's heart rate, this discrepancy may be apparent. The auscultated rate should be recorded as the more current and accurate heart rate.

The presence of a digital heart rate display does not eliminate the need for direct assessment of the heart rate and evaluation of peripheral pulses and systemic perfusion at regular intervals. Electromechanical dissociation or pacer impulses may produce regular detectable electrical depolarization despite inadequate (or absent) ventricular function.

Full disclosure allows review of data from the previous 24 hours and enables review of alarms and tracings and trended data in relation to changes in patient condition. This is an important option in a pediatric critical care unit because unexpected arrhythmias are relatively common. Ideally, the "frozen" or stored strip occupies only half of the screen or a channel below or above the continuous ECG display so that "real-time" ECG monitoring and display can continue while a rhythm strip is retained on display.

Trace Speed. The trace speed is the rate (measured in millimeters per second) that the electrocardiographic pattern moves across the screen or recording paper. This may vary from 1 to 100 mm/second; the standard trace speed is 25 mm/second. It is desirable to have the option of at least two trace speeds on every monitor—the 25-mm sweep and a faster sweep, such as a 50-mm sweep. The faster sweep expands the waveform, so the P waves and other signals may be identified more readily (Fig. 21-14).

Paper Recorders. Paper recorders are recording units that permanently inscribe the patient's ECG using a coated, light beam, or ink stylus. In a critical care unit, such recording should be available to document ECG variations for future analysis and reference.

A central recorder, automatically triggered by alarms or "manually" triggered from either the bedside or central station, is more economical than individual bedside recorders. A central recorder must possess a memory so that the waveforms from several monitors may be stored and printed sequentially if simultaneous alarms occur. Any pediatric critical care unit recording system also should be capable of labeling each strip with date, time, and patient bed.

Some recorders have an automatic or a manual delay mechanism that stores the ECG in memory for 9 to 18 seconds and records from memory rather than "real-time." As a result, the ECG recorded is that which occurred several seconds before the recording was initiated. This delay is necessary to allow time for activation of a recording when an abnormal ECG waveform is observed. The recorded strip will then include waveforms immediately before and after the abnormality.

Guidelines for Recording a Rhythm Strip. Whenever a rhythm strip is obtained, the recording must be standardized. The following guidelines will help to optimize the quality of the tracing.

1. Use standard trace speed (25 mm/second), and standard sensitivity (set at 1). The sensitivity device allows the clinician to compare the patient's signal voltage with the internal standard. At a standard sensitivity setting, a 1 millivolt (1 mV) signal produces a 10-mm deflection on the ECG recording paper (Fig. 21-15).
2. Depress the 1-mV standard marker; this should produce a deflection exactly 10 small boxes (two large boxes) high. This standard marker should be displayed as each lead is recorded. If the 1-mV marker does not produce exactly a 10-mm deflection, adjust the sensitivity control setting or gain until it does.

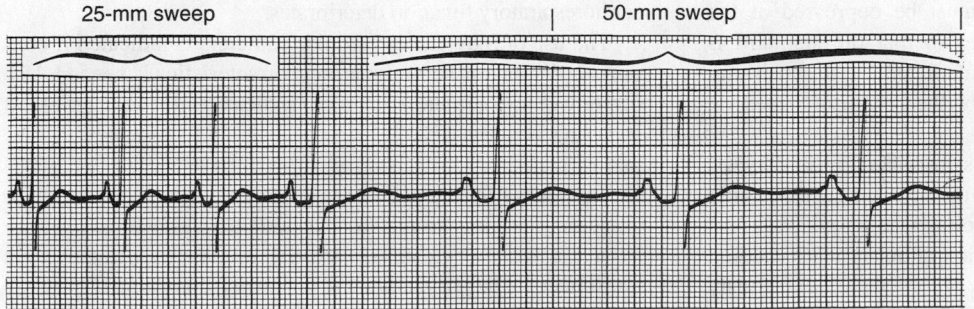

25-mm sweep | 50-mm sweep

FIG. 21-14 Sweep speed on ECG. The same electrocardiogram is recorded here using two different paper speeds of 25 mm/second (standard) and 50 mm/second. Note how clearly the P waves are identified at the faster paper speed (50 mm/second); however, this nonstandard speed distorts the waveforms, and results in misinterpretation of heart rate and intervals unless it is known to be the faster paper speed.

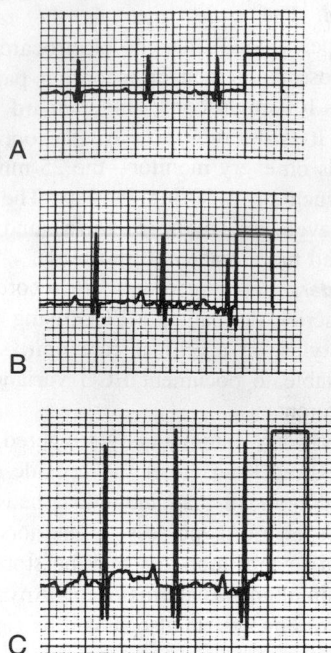

FIG. 21-15 Standardization of ECG voltage with 1 mV marker. Before recording an electrocardiogram or rhythm strip, it is important that the nurse indicate the gain of the ECG by providing a 1-mV signal at the beginning or end of the tracing. **A,** An ECG recorded at ½-standard means that the image is half the normal height; the 1-mV marker will produce only a 5-mm deflection. **B,** Standard ECG recordings are made at 1 standard; this means that the 1-mV signal will create a square wave deflection *exactly* 10 mm high. **C,** If a 2 standard gain is used, the same signal will be doubled in height; the 1-mV marker produces a 20-mm deflection on the ECG. Bedside recordings should be made at the standard gain unless another gain is specifically requested.

3. For accurate representation of the overall ECG, include at least 10 to 12 QRS complexes in the rhythm strip. Each QRS complex should be completely visible on the strip; the complexes should not run off the edge of the paper.

4. If the entire QRS complex does not fit on the paper or a change in the QRS voltage is noted, adjust the sensitivity setting to record a smaller or larger image. If the sensitivity is set at ½, the recorded complexes will be half of the size produced at standard sensitivity. At a sensitivity of ½, a 1-mV impulse creates only a 5-mm deflection on the strip recording. On the other hand, if the sensitivity is set at 2, a 1-mV impulse creates a 20-mm deflection on the strip recording, so the recorded complexes are twice as large as they would be at standard sensitivity.

   The 1-mV standard marker must be depressed at the beginning of each strip recording so that the standard is known when QRS voltage is calculated. If a sensitivity other than standard is used, write the sensitivity used on the strip itself.

5. Inspect the quality of the images inscribed by the stylus. Extremely light or heavy lines must be avoided to be able to appreciate subtle changes in voltage.

6. It is helpful to have access to a multichannel recording device so that the ECG may be recorded simultaneously with other physiologic data. In addition, the ECG may be recorded from multiple leads.

7. Using current technology, intervals can be calculated and stored electronically (online) without paper recordings.

Troubleshooting Sources of Error. The nurse is accountable for the accuracy and safety of the ECG monitoring system. Sources of error must be identified and rectified. Potential sources of error include mechanical noise, electrical noise, biologic variations, and movement artifact.

Mechanical Noise. This artifact results from vibration of the monitor or physical impact. To avoid this, monitors should be mounted permanently above the bed, out of the patient's reach.

Electrical Noise. This artifact results from failure of the monitor to reject outside artifact (resulting from a poor filter or 60-cycle interference), so a "fuzzy" tracing is produced. Electrical "noise" may be alleviated by a change in placement of the electrodes or the electrode patches, or movement of the electrode wires and cables. Grounding of equipment is based on manufacturer and biomedical engineering institutional policy.

Biologic Variations. Interrupted waveform transmission may occur as a result of physiologic changes, such as severe edema or changes in patient position. The nurse must test various lead placements and adjust the sensitivity control on the monitor. The cable itself may pull the electrode away from the chest wall.

A common source of patient interference is shivering, which produces muscle artifact. The problem is usually self-limited in nature.

Movement Artifact. Because patient movement cannot be eliminated in pediatrics, a certain amount of movement artifact must be expected. However, inadequate ECG monitoring should not be tolerated for long periods of time, particularly if a child is at risk for the development of cardiac arrhythmias.

If voluntary movement in the awake child creates movement artifact, the nurse must combine ingenuity with distractions to achieve optimal monitoring. Consulting child life specialists to use play, reading games, art, music, and diversion and parental support can help the child to cope in the pediatric critical care unit.

Vascular Pressure Monitoring

Critically ill pediatric patients frequently demonstrate fluctuations in vascular pressures that may precede or accompany the development of life-threatening crises. These fluctuations may be the result of arrhythmias, altered systemic or pulmonary vascular resistance, or alterations in cardiopulmonary function. Systemic arterial pressure may be the last variable to change as the child's cardiorespiratory function deteriorates.

The use of indwelling vascular catheters is indicated if continuous display of hemodynamic characteristics is needed. Use of indwelling catheters is also indicated if frequent blood sampling is necessary.

Transducer Systems. Direct measurement of intracardiac or vascular pressures requires a system that transmits pressure from the heart or from an arterial or venous catheter to a transducer. The transducer transforms mechanical energy (i.e., pulsatile waves transmitted through the fluid-filled system) into an electrical signal that is transmitted to a monitor.

Most current transducers are disposable and incorporate a microchip as the sensor. In addition, some brands include a calibration stopcock or orifice attached to a port, and most enable continuous irrigation of the catheter during monitoring. For pediatric use, a system should ideally allow a maximum continuous infusion of 1 to 3 mL/hour as a catheter flush.

When vascular monitoring catheters are inserted, the nurse must assist in the initial catheter placement, ensure accuracy of measurement and calibration of the transducer, and maintain catheter patency and sterility of the system. Current technology allows autocalibration options. A square wave test is one method of verifying transducer accuracy.[179]

Once the catheter is in place, the nurse must be certain that it is maintained in the appropriate position (e.g., location relative to the heart or other measured chamber or vessel). In addition, the nurse must ensure that the skin entrance site is protected, and that the catheter and transducer system are functioning properly.

The components of a fluid-filled vascular pressure monitoring system include the monitor, transducer, a source for continuous infusion, ports for access, low compliance tubing, and a device to enable simultaneous pressure monitoring and continuous fluid infusion.

Components of a Fluid-Filled Vascular Monitoring System.
Fluid-filled monitoring systems, whether used for monitoring of vascular, intracardiac, or intracranial pressure, all have the same basic components. These include: monitor and transducer, infusion system, and display.

Variations of the hemodynamic monitoring system may be required to enable large or rapid volume infusions and minimize blood loss and fluid administration during blood sampling. These variations require special tubing and stopcock configurations.

Monitor and Transducer. The monitor and transducer are the fundamental components of any hemodynamic monitoring system. Sometimes a monitor may be purchased from one manufacturer and a transducer from another, because the desired specifications of each may not be met by a single company. Thus, before purchase and use, nurses should be involved to ensure that the selected devices are compatible and meet the patient care and unit needs.

Continuous Infusion Systems. An intravascular fluid flush must be administered to maintain catheter patency and prevent blood back up into the monitoring system. A high-pressure bag or volume infusion pump may provide this flush. If the source of the infusion fluid is a plastic IV container (bag), it is enclosed in a high-pressure bag and joined to a flow-limiting device. The infusion pressure, indicated by a gauge attached to the pressure bag, must be greater than the vascular pressure being monitored. Such a system is not optimal for pediatric use because it does not allow verification of the hourly rate of fluid administration.

A continuous infusion device (pump) allows constant IV infusion and simultaneous monitoring without signal distortion. In addition, the device ensures delivery of fluid at a specified rate. If the infusion rate is low (1 to 3 mL/hour), the pressure generated by the infusion pump should not interfere with the pressure measurement. A continuous heparin flush maintains catheter patency better than intermittent irrigation.[68,84]

Pediatric Monitoring Systems. Limitation of fluid intake is necessary in the care of critically ill children. Many children cannot tolerate the total fluid administered if a standard infusion device provides 3 mL/hour to flush each monitoring catheter. In addition, if the device is flushed by a pressurized bag of fluids, malfunction of the one-way valve in the flow-limiting infusion device or frequent flushing of the catheter can allow delivery of excessive volumes of fluid.

As an alternative, a syringe or other infusion pump may be used in place of the high-pressure bag (Fig. 21-16). Smart pumps can accurately deliver fluid at very low continuous infusion rates. The quantity of fluid injected hourly and with flushes can be verified readily by marking the infusion syringe. A 1 mL/hour infusion rate generally maintains catheter patency if pressures less than 60 mm Hg are present in the system. However, for most arterial lines it will be necessary to infuse 2 mL/hour to ensure continued catheter patency.

Intermittent Monitoring Systems. Some vascular monitoring systems, such as those used for monitoring central venous

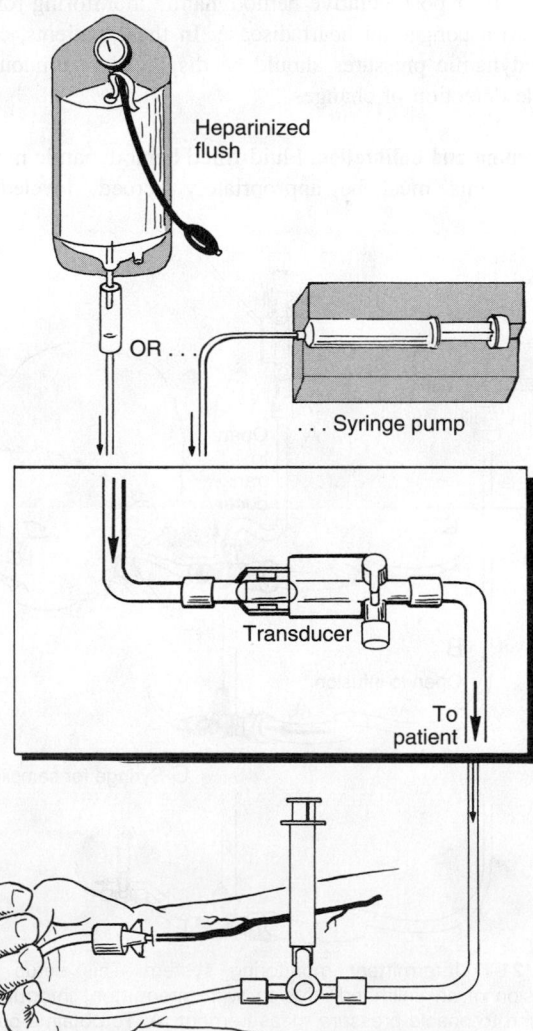

Heparinized flush

OR . . .

. . . Syringe pump

Transducer

To patient

FIG. 21-16 Continuous infusion system. The infusion may be provided through a high-pressure bag and flow-limiting device or through a volume infusion pump with flow-limiting device. Either system allows continuous infusion and monitoring of the vascular pressure.

pressure (CVP), may be prepared using both an IV infusion system and transducer system joined at a stopcock. With this configuration, a constant infusion valve is not used. The vascular catheter is used primarily for IV infusion of fluids or drugs, and pressure measurements are obtained intermittently by turning the stopcock. When measurements are obtained, the stopcock is turned so that the infusion is interrupted and the stopcock port is open between the patient and the transducer (Fig. 21-17).

Intermittent measurement systems are *not* used with arterial catheters or pulmonary artery catheters. The arterial wave form must be continuously monitored and displayed to enable detection of any backflow or other problems in neonates and pediatric patients. The pulmonary artery waveform must be monitored and displayed constantly, because undetected pulmonary catheter migration may result in pulmonary arterial occlusion or rupture. Waveforms of left atrial catheters must be continually displayed and monitored because significant morbidity can result from air or thromboemboli in left atrium.

In general, intermittent monitoring systems are typically not used for postoperative hemodynamic monitoring for children with congenital heart disease. In these patients, critical hemodynamic pressures should be displayed continuously to enable detection of changes.

Zeroing and Calibration. Fluid-filled hemodynamic monitoring systems must be appropriately zeroed, leveled, and

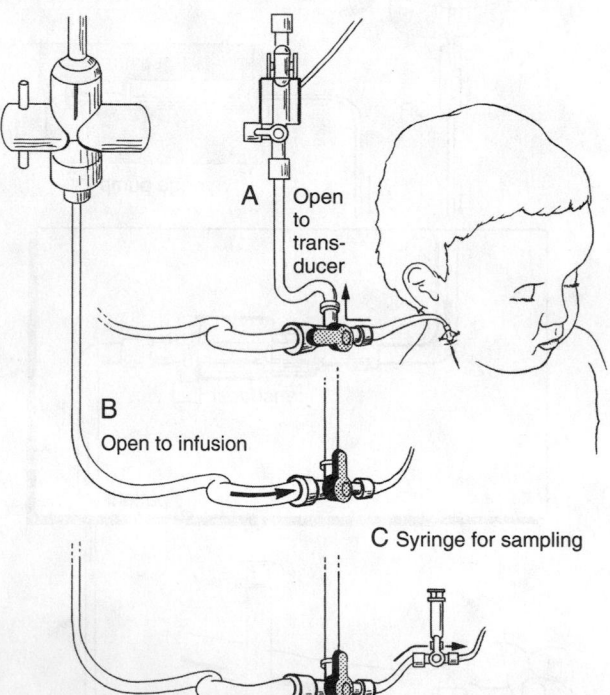

FIG. 21-17 Intermittent monitoring system. This setup allows provision of an unlimited infusion with intermittent interruption of infusion to enable pressure measurement. **A,** To obtain a pressure measurement the stopcock is turned "off" to the infusion, and "open" to the transducer. **B,** To provide infusion the stopcock is turned "off" to the transducer and "open" to the infusion. **C,** An additional proximal syringe and stopcock may be inserted in the line to enable blood sampling and zeroing and calibration of the transducer.

calibrated. Processes of zeroing, leveling, and calibration are described in this section.

Zeroing and Leveling of Transducer. To ensure that hemodynamic measurements are accurate and trends in measured variables can be identified over time, a consistent zero reference point must be used by everyone performing the measurements. The purpose of zeroing the system is to negate the atmospheric pressure, so that the measured vascular pressure is isolated. Leveling is critical, because if the transducer is at a different level from the point being measured, the measured pressure will be influenced by hydrostatic pressure created by the height of the column of fluid between the measured vessel or cavity and the transducer.

Atmospheric pressure exerts a certain weight (e.g., a force of 760 mm Hg at sea level) that is relative to altitude. Physiologic measurements (e.g., central venous pressure) can be isolated by placing the transducer at the designated zero reference point, opening the transducer system to air, and adjusting the display system to read zero. Once the transducer is zeroed, the height relationship of the transducer and the zero reference point must remain the same. If the transducer is zeroed at the level of the right atrium (see *phlebostatic axis*, below), the head of the patient bed may be elevated up to 45 degrees, and intracardiac and central venous pressure measurements will remain accurate as long as the relationship between the zero reference point and the manometer or transducer is consistent.[179]

The zero reference point is determined relative to the source of the pressure being measured. Leveling is important to prevent the addition of hydrostatic pressure to the intracardiac or great vessel pressure being measured. A column of water 1.36 cm high in the tubing will generate a hydrostatic pressure of 1 mm Hg; a column of water 27.2 cm high will create a pressure of 20 mm Hg.

If the transducer is placed *below* the measured pressure source, the pressure detected by the transducer will be falsely high because it detects the pressure generated by the cardiac chamber or great vessel, as well as the hydrostatic pressure created by the column of water in the tubing between the pressure source and the transducer. If the transducer is placed *above* the zero reference point, the transducer will detect a pressure that is lower than the intracardiac or great vessel pressure because the intracardiac or great vessel pressure will have to lift the fluid in the tubing.

If an intracardiac pressure is monitored, the zero reference point is the right atrium. The landmarks used to identify the right atrium are referred to as the *phlebostatic axis*; this is the typical reference point for all cardiovascular measurements. Level the transducer at the phlebostatic axis as follows:

- Using the midclavicle as a guide, locate the fourth intercostal space and follow this space across the chest wall to the midaxillary (or anterior axillary) line (per unit policy). As an alternative, the intersection of the nipple line and midaxillary (or anterior axillary) line may be used.
- Align this site with the CVP transducer whenever cardiac measurements are performed. This reference approximately corresponds with the level of the right atrium.
- Note that whenever the patient's position is changed the measurement system must be releveled because the position of the phlebostatic axis has changed. It has been well

documented that reliable measurements may be made with different patient positions, and with the head of the bed elevated up to 45 degrees, as long as the relationship between the zero point of the measurement system and the patient's right atrium remain consistent.

Transducer Calibration. Transducer calibration is a separate procedure that may be needed before hemodynamic pressure measurements are initiated. Nurses should know how to verify transducer calibration, if there is any question of transducer malfunction.

- Assemble the transducer and flush the system with appropriate irrigation fluid (often normal saline).[84] Join and flush a 12 to 24-inch segment of noncompliant tubing to the "zeroing" stopcock (this is the calibration tubing).
- Select the appropriate monitoring scale.
- Zero the transducer and monitor to the phlebostatic axis.
- Close the "zeroing" stopcock between the zero reference point and the transducer, and open the stopcock between the transducer and the calibration tubing. Begin recording the pressure waveform. Elevate the open end of the calibration tubing about 27.2 cm above the zero reference point: the transducer should detect a 20 mm Hg pressure.
- Return the catheter or tubing tip to the phlebostatic axis to recheck the zero (the transducer should reflect a pressure of 0).
- Depress the graphic calibration signal on the printing pressure display. The pressure recording should reflect both the mechanical (20 mm Hg) calibration and electronic calibration.

Monitor Calibration. The transducer and the monitor require calibration before measurements are made. Most monitors have built-in calibration mechanisms that should be checked before pressure monitoring is initiated. The procedure for *monitor* calibration includes the following (or follow manufacturer's recommendation or unit policy):

- After the readout stabilizes, adjust the pressure readout value to the appropriate standard for the vascular or chamber pressure being calibrated (e.g., the highest gain, 100 or 200 mm Hg is usually the preset value).
- Release the "cal" button and the readout should return to zero.
- Ensure that the waveform is calibrated with the digital display.

Noninvasive Blood Pressure Monitoring
Kate Amond

Indirect blood pressure measurement in infants and children is an essential part of cardiovascular assessment. There are four methods of indirect blood pressure measurement: auscultatory (with a mercury sphygmomanometer), palpatory, ultrasonic, and automated oscillometric.

In the past, auscultation was the preferred technique because normal values found in blood pressure tables are based on this method.[128] This method was often used in the ambulatory setting. However, in recent years, the auscultation method has largely been replaced by the automated oscillometric method. The auscultatory method is often difficult to perform in small infants and children because the heart rate may be extremely rapid and arterial pressures are normally low (by adult standards). In the seriously ill child, the quality of the child's pulses may be diminished and Korotkoff sounds may be faint,

so cuff pressure may not correlate well with intraarterial pressure. In addition, the amount of fat tissue in the arms and legs of children is greater than in adults, which diminishes the intensity of Korotkoff sounds during auscultation of cuff pressures.

Palpation of blood pressure using a cuff is imprecise and provides only an approximate systolic arterial pressure. Ultrasonic measurement requires positioning of a transducer over the brachial artery using conductive jelly. The ultrasound method determines only the systolic pressure.

The automated oscillometric method is based on the principle that pulsatile blood flow through a vessel produces oscillation of the arterial wall. This oscillation is transmitted to a cuff placed over the artery. The cuff is inflated automatically to a preset pressure value, and then is allowed to deflate slowly. As the cuff deflates and the cuff pressure decreases, there is a predictable change in the magnitude of the oscillations at the points of systole, diastole, and mean pressure. The oscillometric devices have automatic deflation patterns, typically ranging from 2 to 7 mm Hg/second in a stepwise fashion. Automated blood pressure monitors may be set to automatically evaluate the blood pressure at set intervals (e.g., every 5 minutes). Alarms may be set to signal low or high systolic, diastolic, or mean pressures.

In pediatrics, automated blood pressure measurement is recommended in situations in which frequent BP readings are necessary, such as in the critical care unit and the care of newborns and young infants when auscultation can be challenging.[128,163] Automated blood pressure monitoring has become one of the most common methods of obtaining blood pressures in children because it is convenient and easy to use. Automated BP measurements eliminate many of the potential problems of auscultation, including deflation of the cuff too quickly, inability to hear soft Korotkoff sounds, rounding of numbers, and observer bias.[128]

Automated blood pressure measurements may be inaccurate, particularly when a patient is crying, having a seizure, or agitated. Some studies have documented the accuracy of the automated technique when used in normotensive children.[41,153] However, they can be inaccurate in the presence of abnormal blood pressures and abnormal vascular tone, such as in the patient with shock or extreme hypertension.[35a] The devices typically overestimate blood pressure in the hypotensive child and underestimate blood pressure when severe hypertension is present.[142]

The right arm is the preferred site for measuring blood pressure in children. Standardized tables are based on right arm measurements, and a false low reading may occur from the left arm if children have coarctation of the aorta or other aortic abnormalities.[128] However, the nurse should avoid taking a blood pressure in an arm with compromised circulation, intraarterial catheter, intravenous catheters, arteriovenous fistula, and peripherally inserted central catheters (PICC).[153] Therefore if any of these conditions is present in the right arm, it may be necessary to perform the blood pressure measurement using the left arm.

Correct measurement of blood pressure in children requires use of a cuff that is of the appropriate size. If the cuff is too small, the blood pressure obtained could be artificially high. If the cuff is too large, the blood pressure detected will be falsely low.[117] The cuff should have a bladder width that is approximately 40% of the circumference of the mid-upper arm. The cuff bladder should extend over at least 50% to 75% of the length of the upper arm (from the axilla to the anticubital fossa).[35a,117,128,142]

Arterial Pressure Monitoring
Kate Amond

Indications. Critically ill pediatric patients frequently demonstrate fluctuations in blood pressure that may precede or accompany the development of life-threatening crises. These fluctuations may result from arrhythmias, changes in fluid balance, altered systemic vascular resistance, changes in pulmonary vascular resistance, or alterations in cardiac output or pulmonary function.

The use of indwelling arterial catheters is indicated if continuous display of blood pressure is desired or frequent blood sampling is necessary. Indwelling arterial catheters may be used to closely monitor blood pressure in cases of shock, vasoactive drug therapy, major surgeries, or labile blood pressures. Indwelling arterial lines may also be used when frequent arterial blood samples are needed to monitor oxygenation and acid-base status, such as in patients with respiratory failure.[15,37] Intermittent venous or arterial sampling may be difficult in a child because adipose tissue obscures small vessels or the child is unable to cooperate during arterial or venous puncture. Venipuncture can also be a painful procedure for a pediatric patient, so placement of an arterial or central venous catheter may be considered whenever frequent blood sampling is necessary.

Risks. Complications associated with indwelling arterial catheters vary with the site and duration of catheterization, the age and size of the child, and the technique of insertion (cut down versus percutaneous).[15,143] Risks include infection, thrombosis, embolism, bleeding, ischemia, vasospasm, bruising, and pain.[15] The greatest risks are associated with arterial cut downs and prolonged duration of catheterization.

Common Insertion Sites. The most common site for an indwelling arterial catheter is the radial artery. Other sites that may be used include femoral, ulnar, dorsalis pedis, posterior tibial, brachial, axillary, and (in neonates) umbilical arteries.

Continuous Infusion Systems. An intravascular fluid flush must be provided to maintain catheter patency and to prevent blood back up into the arterial monitoring system. This flush may be provided by a high-pressure bag or volume infusion pump (see Fig. 21-16).

A continuous infusion device within the disposable transducer module allows for continuous (flush) infusion and simultaneous monitoring without signal distortion. The device contains a one-way valve through which the fluid is infused, so the transducer is shielded from pressure generated by the continuous infusion device. If the infusion rate is low (1 to 3 mL/hour), the pressure generated by an infusion pressure bag or volume infusion pump should not interfere with the pressure measurements.

Pressure Bag. The pressure bag infusion system consists of a cover that fits over a bag of intravenous fluid, a bulb, a clamp, and a pressure gauge. A bag of intravenous fluid is inserted into the cover, and the bulb is used to inflate the cover, creating pressure on the bag and in the system. Once the pressure gauge indicates that the desired pressure is created, the clamp is used to maintain the pressure. The infusion pressure in the bag must be greater than the vascular pressure being monitored.

This pressure bag system may not be optimal for small pediatric patients or neonates because it does not allow verification of the volume of fluid administered each hour. The hand flush "pigtail" contained in some devices allows rapid infusion of a large volume of fluid at a very rapid rate during manual irrigation. Frequent manual flushes with this device may cause fluid overload in the small child and trauma to the catheterized vessel.

Infusion Pump. Limitation of fluid intake is necessary in the care of critically ill children. Many children cannot tolerate the total volume of fluid administered if a standard infusion device provides 3 mL/hour through each monitoring catheter, and additional fluid is administered using the manual pigtail flush, particularly if this flush is provided from a reservoir of fluid contained in a pressure bag.

A syringe or any other infusion pump may be used in place of the high pressure bag to provide continuous flush to the vascular monitoring system. The quantity of fluid injected hourly and with flushes can be verified readily by the use of smart infusion pump technology, or other volume-controlled infusion pump. A 1-mL/hour infusion rate generally maintains catheter patency if the neonate's blood pressure is less than 60 mm Hg. However, for vascular monitoring devices used in most infants and children, it will be necessary to infuse at least 2 mL/h to ensure continued catheter patency.

There is currently insufficient evidence to identify an ideal administration rate for arterial lines for the pediatric population in general, largely because the population includes such a wide range of sizes. When selecting the appropriate infusion system, considerations should include patient size, catheter size, fluid status of patient, other intravenous infusion rates, and institutional policy.

IV Tubing. Low compliance ("high pressure" or "arterial" tubing) will prevent loss of the pressure signal from tubing expansion. Invalid (usually low) measurements or back flow of blood may result if standard, compliant intravenous tubing is used. The shortest practical length of tubing (2 to 3 feet or less) should be used to minimize distortion of pressures.

Heparin. Arterial pressure monitoring catheters maintained with heparinized flush solutions have a significantly greater probability of remaining patent over time than catheters maintained with nonheparinized flush solutions.[6,107] Clinical studies support a heparin concentration of 1 unit/mL.[123,160,186] For patients who have a contraindication to heparin, citrate flush solution may be an acceptable alternative.[37]

Over the years, there has been concern about the use of heparin in critical care units and heparin-induced thrombocytopenia (HIT). However, in a recent study with critically ill adult patients the use of heparin in normal saline as a continuous flush for an arterial catheter did not reduce platelet counts.[70] More studies are needed with pediatric patients.

Papaverine. Papaverine is a nonspecific smooth muscle relaxant that can produce nonspecific arteriolar dilation.[74] Papaverine has been shown to prolong the patency of peripheral arterial catheters in neonates.[67] Studies have shown differing results in the incidence of complications with its use in preterm infants and neonates. More studies are needed with large sample sizes to further evaluate effectiveness in older infants and children. Institutional policies guiding papaverine use should be followed.

Blood Sampling. Arterial catheters are typically used for frequent blood sampling, so providers should monitor the total volume of blood drawn. A child's circulating blood volume is quantitatively less than that of an adult, averaging approximately 70 to 80 mL/kg of body weight. When frequent blood sampling is necessary, the sample size should be recorded and totaled. When the blood loss exceeds 10% of estimated blood volume, an evaluation of hematocrit is needed.[186] The use of microtainer collection tubes is helpful because they reduce the volume of blood needed for laboratory studies.

When drawing blood from an indwelling arterial (or any vascular) catheter, an initial amount of blood plus fluid (in the tubing) must be withdrawn to ensure that the sample sent to the laboratory will be a representative patient blood sample that will provide accurate test results, undiluted by the fluid in the tubing. Samples for coagulation studies that are obtained through a heparinized catheter and flush system can provide accurate results if adequate volume of "waste" (fluid plus blood) is withdrawn to clear the catheter, tubing and sampling port of heparinized fluid before obtaining the blood sample. The volume of the "waste" fluid should be about twice the volume of the catheter and the volume in the tubing between the catheter hub and the sampling port, which is generally approximately 2 mL.[56]

A stopcock should be placed in the tubing at a location close to the catheter insertion site to facilitate blood sampling and reduce the quantity of waste fluid that must be drawn. A variety of blood sampling techniques can be used when drawing laboratory tests from arterial catheters. Closed reservoir sampling systems have become commercially available in recent years.

Two Stopcock Method. One method for drawing blood for laboratory tests from an indwelling arterial catheter is a two stopcock method (illustrated in Fig. 21-18). This method minimizes both blood loss and additional fluid administration.

To avoid excessive blood lost as discard or part of the waste volume, many institutions are supporting the practice of reinfusing the waste fluid and blood back into the patient after blood samples are obtained from an arterial catheter. This technique is especially useful for pediatric patients who require frequent blood sampling or patients with increased severity of illness. To minimize infusion into the arterial catheter and the theoretical risk of embolism, it may be preferable to reinfuse the waste fluid into a venous catheter. If the initial waste fluid is returned into the arterial catheter and whenever the arterial catheter is flushed, the fluid should be infused very slowly (at a rate less than 1 mL/second) to reduce the theoretical risk of arterial irritation and embolization of any partially clotted material in the waste fluid.[56]

After any blood sampling, only gentle irrigation of the catheter and tubing should be performed. Forceful irrigation of arterial catheters may produce arterial spasm or irritation and may result in retrograde arterial (and possibly aortic) flow.

Closed Blood Draw Systems. A reservoir system is a closed blood draw system that connects to an arterial line and allows blood to be drawn back into a reservoir. Such a system shifts the heparin-containing waste fluid into the reservoir and allows an uncontaminated blood sample to be drawn from a sample port. Once a sample is obtained, the blood in the reservoir is returned to the patient. This system prevents blood loss by giving the patient the waste fluid back instead of discarding it.[137]

When used and changed according to the Centers for Disease Control guidelines, these closed blood draw systems (so-called blood conservation devices) do not harbor organisms in the critical care setting. "Blood conservation devices can be used as part of a comprehensive blood conservation program in the critical care setting without undue concern for exacerbating infectious processes."[137]

Waveform Characteristics. The normal arterial pressure is represented by a waveform that reflects systole, aortic valve closure, and diastole. The systolic pressure is the peak of the initial upstroke of the waveform, occurring just after the QRS complex of the ECG. The dicrotic notch is thought to represent the closure of the aortic valve (Fig. 21-19). The down stroke after the dicrotic notch is associated with ventricular diastole.

Valuable information may be gained from analysis of the arterial waveform, as well as from the absolute systolic and diastolic pressures. The normal arterial waveform should have a sharp upstroke, a clear dicrotic notch, and a definite end-diastole.

Mechanical causes of altered arterial waveform include a dampened tracing, which is caused by partial occlusion of the catheter or other loss of signal conduction (e.g., loose tubing connection or air in the tubing), or catheter "fling," which is caused by the tip of the catheter "flinging" inside the vessel. See Table 21-2 for troubleshooting.

Zeroing. To ensure that hemodynamic measurements are accurate, a consistent zero reference point must be used by everyone performing the measurements. The purpose of defining the zero reference point is to negate the atmospheric pressure and hydrostatic pressure, so the measured vascular pressure is isolated.

Atmospheric pressure exerts a certain weight (a force of 760 mm Hg at sea level) that is relative to altitude. Physiologic measurements can be isolated by placing the transducer system at the zero reference point, opening the system to air and adjusting the display system to read zero. The zero reference point is determined relative to the source of the pressure being measured. If an intracardiac pressure is monitored, the zero reference point is the right atrium. The landmarks used to identify the right atrium are referred to as the phlebostatic axis. Leveling of the transducer at the phlebostatic axis is accomplished as follows:
• Using the midclavicle as a guide, locate the fourth intercostal space and follow this space across the chest wall to the

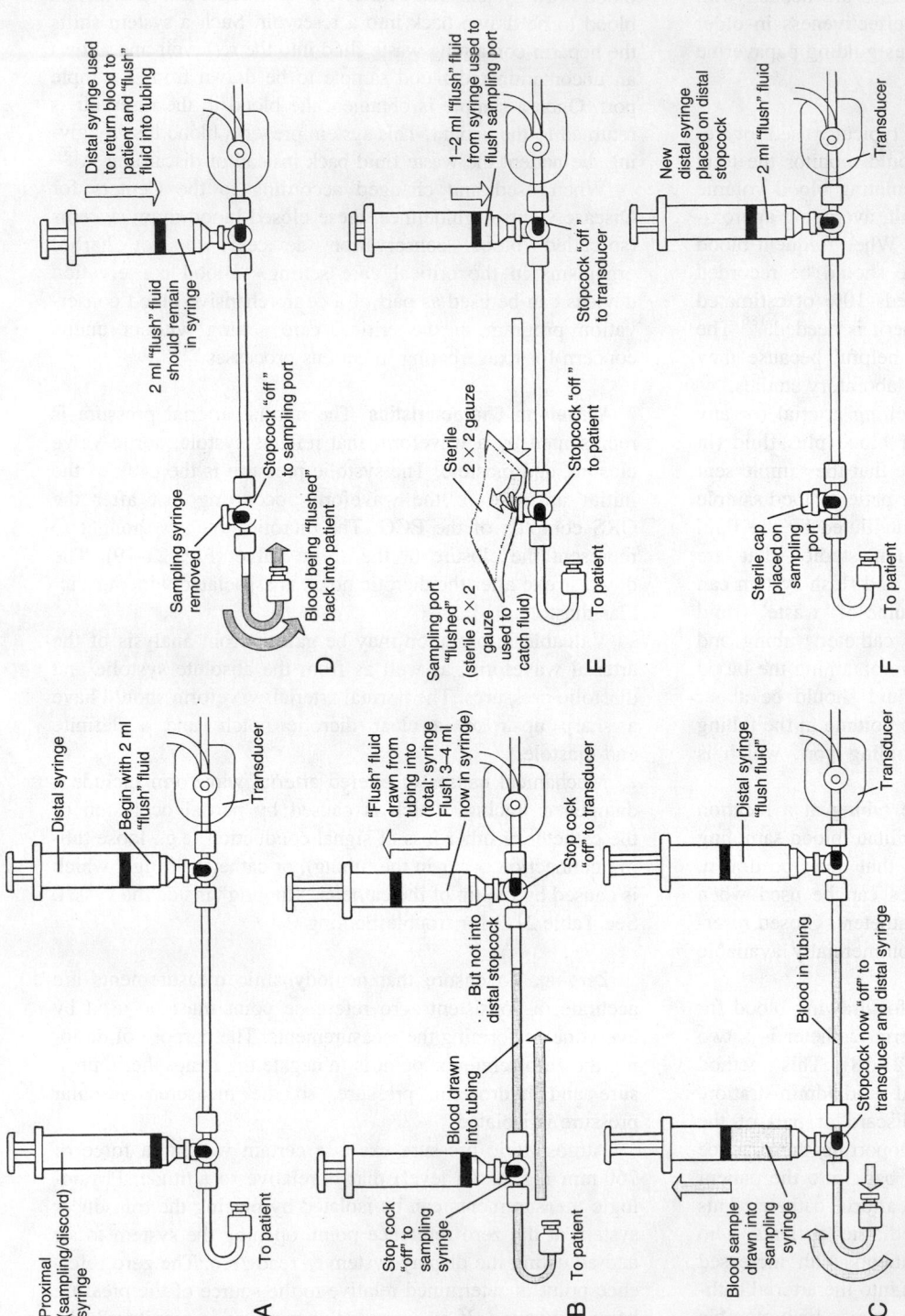

FIG. 21-18 Two-stopcock blood sampling. **A,** Initial arrangement of tubing and syringes. Begin with exactly 2 mL of irrigation fluid in distal syringe (near transducer). **B,** Turn distal stopcock "off" to the transducer and "open" to the catheter, and aspirate until patient blood is drawn into the tubing but not into the distal syringe or stopcock. **C,** Turn proximal stopcock "off" to the transducer and distal syringe, and draw blood sample into proximal syringe (after discarding initial 0.1 mL). **D,** Turn proximal stopcock "off" to the sampling port and "open" between the distal syringe and the patient. Flush irrigation fluid from distal syringe into the tubing and patient until blood is cleared from the tubing. Exactly 2 mL of irrigation fluid should remain in the distal syringe (that is the amount in the syringe before the blood sampling, so the patient has received no net fluid administration). **E,** Turn proximal stopcock "off" to the catheter and "open" between the sampling port and transducer, and use the remaining fluid from the distal syringe to clear blood from the proximal sampling port. This flushes any blood from the tubing. **F,** Turn proximal stopcock "off" to the sampling port and cap it. Turn distal stopcock "off" to the syringe port and attach new irrigation syringe (containing 2 mL of irrigation fluid). Waveform should be visible on the monitor. (From Hazinski MF: Hemodynamic monitoring of children. In Daily EK, Schroeder JS, editors: *Techniques in bedside hemodynamic monitoring,* ed 4, St Louis, 1989, Mosby.)

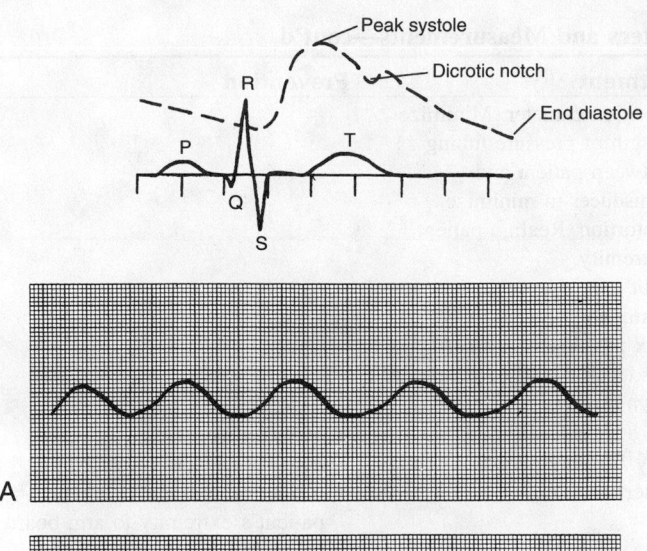

FIG. 21-19 Arterial waveform. The arterial waveform is shown in relation to the ECG cycle. When the waveform is dampened (**A**) the dicrotic notch is no longer visible. If catheter "fling" is present (**B**) an artificial elevation in the peak systolic pressure is noted.

midaxillary (or anterior axillary) line. Alternatively, the intersection of the nipple line with the midaxillary (or anterior axillary) line can be used (follow unit protocol).

• Align this site with the zero point on the transducer whenever measurements are performed. This reference should correspond to the level of the right atrium.

Note that whenever the patient's position is changed the measurement system must be releveled because the position of the phlebostatic axis has changed. It has been well documented that the measurements may be made with the patient in different positions (e.g., flat, head of bed elevated up to 45 degrees) as long as the relationship between the zero reference point and the transducer remain consistent. Zeroing should be performed at standard intervals based on institutional or equipment guidelines.

Nursing Considerations. There are many nursing considerations when caring for a pediatric patient with an arterial catheter. It is the responsibility of the nurse to ensure that the arterial catheter and monitoring system are working properly and maintaining a good waveform. Also, it is important to monitor the insertion site for signs or symptoms of infection, verify patency, maintain a sterile and occlusive dressing, and ensure that all tubing is free of air bubbles. The use of a chlorhexidine gluconate-impregnated sponge in intravenous catheter dressings may reduce catheter-related infections.[17]

Recent recommendations suggest that arterial catheters should not be replaced on a routine basis.[37] Transducers, the

Table 21-2 **Troubleshooting Problems with Arterial Catheters and Measurements***

Problem	Causes	Treatment	Prevention
"Dampened" tracing	Occlusion of catheter tip (by clot or particulate matter) Note that an early indication of a clot may be the inability to aspirate blood (in the presence of continued ability to irrigate catheter).	Attempt to aspirate clot. Use 2 mL of heparinized flush and lightly "bounce" plunger to loosen clot. Never forcefully flush catheter if there is significant resistance to flushing.	Ensure constant flush infusion (flush device may malfunction). Check pressure management system for leaks. Be sure flush solution is heparinized with 1 unit heparin/mL fluid (or per unit policy). Use only noncompliant tubing for transducer system.
	Bleed back caused by patient's pressure exceeding the flush pressure (usually related to loose connections or inadequate irrigation rate or deflation of infusion pressure bag)	Check all connections at regular intervals. Observe flush device for delivery of desired flow rate (if using a high-pressure bag.) Check gauge frequently to ensure that adequate pressure is maintained.	Assess tubing connections at regular intervals. Catheter and tubing should not be concealed by bed linen, because continuous visualization is necessary. Persistent bleed back may require new system set up.
	Catheter tip against vessel wall	Reposition by rotating or withdrawing catheter. Reposition patient or catheterized extremity.	Check dressing and tape frequently and secure tape so that catheter cannot be moved or rotated.
	Clots or bubbles in pressure tubing or transducer	Flush entire system with stopcock port closed to patient. Determine if entire flush system needs changing.	Examine entire system at least every 2 hours for cracks and bubbles and to ensure tight connections.

Continued

Table 21-2   Troubleshooting Problems with Arterial Catheters and Measurements—cont'd

Problem	Causes	Treatment	Prevention
Abnormally high or low readings	Catheter "fling"	Reposition catheter. Minimize length of pressure tubing between patient and transducer to minimize distortion. Realign patient extremity. Use of a dampener device may eliminate "fling."	
Change in position of transducer relative to patient zero reference point		Check position of patient. Transducer should be at level of right atrium. Rezero transducer.	Zero as indicated.
Bleeding at puncture site	Migration or dislodgement of catheter	Apply firm pressure to catheter insertion site.	Secure catheter. If catheter is located in extremity, mount patient's extremity to arm board to minimize extremity and catheter movement.
	Enlarged puncture in artery caused by motion of catheter within artery	Check stability of catheter. Remove all tape/dressing and inspect. Determine if stitch around catheter is required. Check pulse/capillary refill distal to catheter to ensure adequate extremity perfusion.	As above
No waveform visible on monitor	Incorrect scale (see also "dampened" tracing)	Check monitor to see whether scale is inappropriately high or low.	Anticipate the expected pressure ranges when setting up system and use the appropriate scale or use the optimize function.
	Damaged transducer	Use a new transducer or troubleshoot monitor.	When in doubt, palpate pulses and check intraarterial pressure against a cuff pressure.
	Stopcocks turned to wrong position	Ensure all stopcocks are in correct position.	
Cuff pressure differs from direct arterial pressure measurement (arterial measurement is usually 5-10 mm Hg higher)[†]	Hypotension (intra-arterial pressure is more accurate if catheter patent and system correctly zeroed, leveled, and calibrated)	See Chapter 6 for treatment of low cardiac output.	Ensure that cuff size is appropriate (See Chapter 6).
	Low cardiac output or increased systemic resistance may cause Korotkoff sounds to be more difficult to hear; therefore cuff pressures may be misleading	Observe waveform. Clear tracing indicates reliability of signal.	Verify zero of transducer.

*The nurse must first evaluate the patient's clinical condition (including blood pressure cuff measurements) before proceeding to troubleshoot the instruments.
[†]Direct intraarterial pressure measurement is generally a more accurate representation of blood pressure and should be the preferred measurement. The discrepancy between the two, however, may provide a qualitative reflection of the systemic vascular resistance. Markedly increased resistance may cause a wide discrepancy between the cuff and intraarterial pressure measurements.

associated tubing, continuous flush solution, and the device should be replaced at 96-hour intervals[37] or by institution policy.

It is important to ensure stability of the catheter and tubing so that the risk of bleeding or dislodgement remains low. Depending on placement technique, some arterial catheters are sutured in place, and others are kept stable by the use of a stabilization device, such as the Bard StatLock (Bard Medical, Covington, GA). In infants or other patients who are active, the use of an arm board for stabilization may be helpful for radial or pedal arterial lines. High-risk pressure catheters, such as PA and arterial catheters always should be joined to a transducer.

It is considered good practice to check the intraarterial pressure against a cuff blood pressure measurement, but agreement between the two is not a criterion for evaluating accuracy of the intraarterial pressure device. If the transducer is zeroed and leveled appropriately and the monitoring system is prepared correctly (with all connections tight and bubbles eliminated), and the catheter is patent, the intraarterial pressure should be considered the most accurate pressure measurement.

As noted, when hypotension is present, a noninvasive oscillometric blood pressure device may overestimate blood pressure, reporting falsely high blood pressure, with resulting disparity between the cuff pressure and the intraarterial pressure. The noninvasive measurement may underestimate the blood pressure when severe hypertension is present. In such cases, the intraarterial pressure measurement is the more accurate measurement.

Artifact may also cause some disparity between the noninvasive cuff measurement and the intraarterial measurement. The intraarterial measurement may appear to be slightly higher than the cuff pressure; and when the intraarterial measurement is taken from a vessel more distal to the heart, such a disparity is artifactual. The difference in pressure is caused by "reflections" of blood flow as it travels distally, bouncing off the vessel bifurcations.

Vasomotor changes or vascular obstruction also may cause a wide or inverse disparity between the cuff pressure and the intraarterial measurement. Further, the cuff pressure is determined by the quality of the Korotkoff sounds (for auscultated cuff pressure) and cuff vibrations (for oscillometric cuff measurements), which are diminished or lost in low cardiac output states and are increased in the presence of mild to moderate vasoconstriction. Therefore, as with any other physiologic measurement, the clinical appearance of the child always should be considered during the interpretation of hemodynamic measurements. Troubleshooting of arterial lines is outlined in Table 21-2.

Central Venous Pressure (CVP) Monitoring
Patricia Ann E. Schlosser

Indications. Indications for central venous pressure (CVP) catheterization in children include: (a) monitoring of right atrial pressure for the purpose of assessing blood volume and venous return, evaluating right ventricular function, or obtaining indirect information about the pulmonary vascular system; (b) infusion of vasoactive drugs; (c) infusion of hypertonic solutions; (d) rapid infusion of large volumes of fluid; and (e) venous access for blood sampling or monitoring central venous oxygen saturation ($S_{CV}O_2$). Pediatric central venous catheter care bundling uses an evidence based approach to reduce infection risk in infants and children[121] (see Chapter 22, Box 22-6).

Insertion and Measurement. CVP catheters may be inserted percutaneously or by cut down through several sites. The subclavian, femoral, and external jugular veins usually are preferred sites for catheterization (Figs. 21-20 and 21-21).

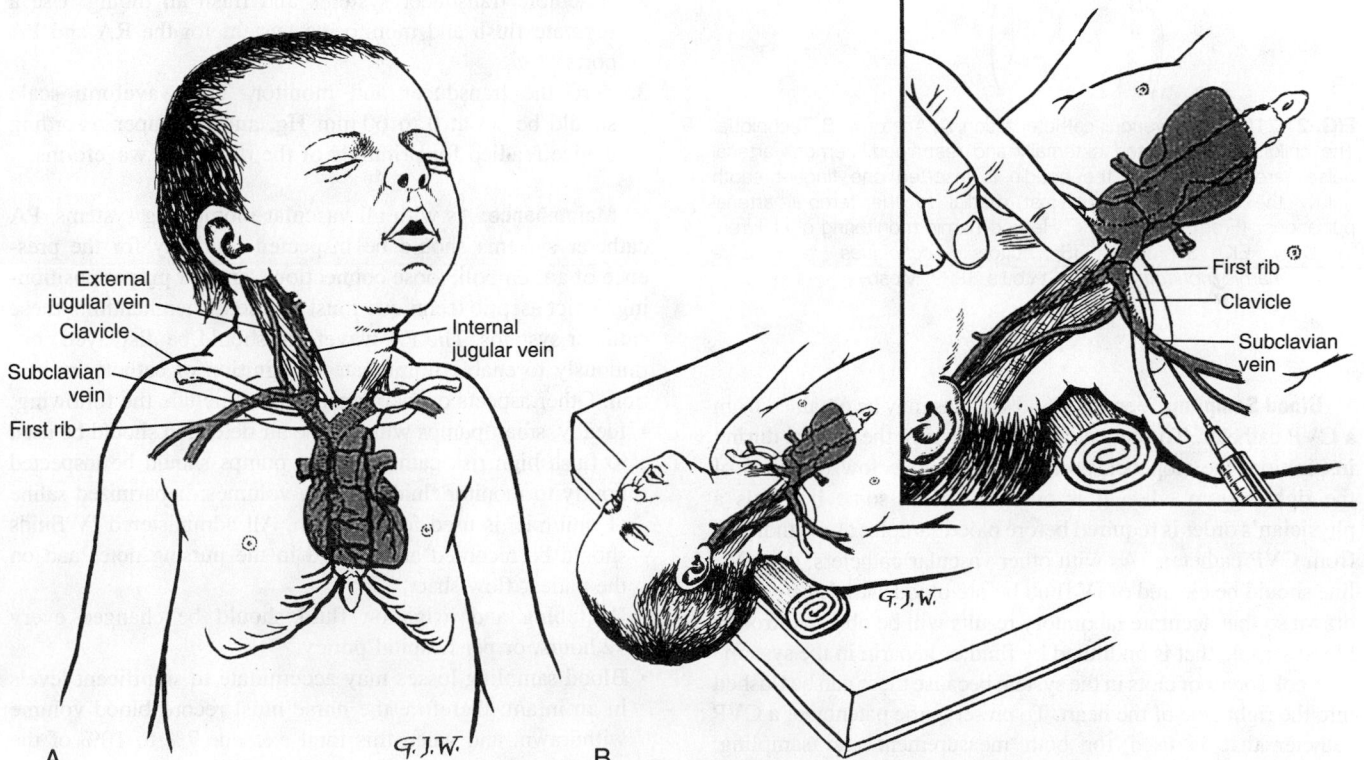

External jugular vein
Clavicle
Subclavian vein
First rib
Internal jugular vein

First rib
Clavicle
Subclavian vein

A   B

FIG. 21-20 Subclavian vein catheterization. **A,** Anatomy. **B,** Technique. The subclavian vein is cannulated at the point where it passes under the clavicle. The clinician's index finger is placed in the suprasternal notch and a needle is inserted under the clavicle at the distal margin of the medial third of the clavicle, with the needle pointing toward the suprasternal notch. Reproduced with permission from Hazinski MF: Hemodynamic monitoring of children. (In Daily EK, Schroeder JS, editors: *Techniques in bedside hemodynamic monitoring*, ed 4, St Louis, 1989, Mosby.)

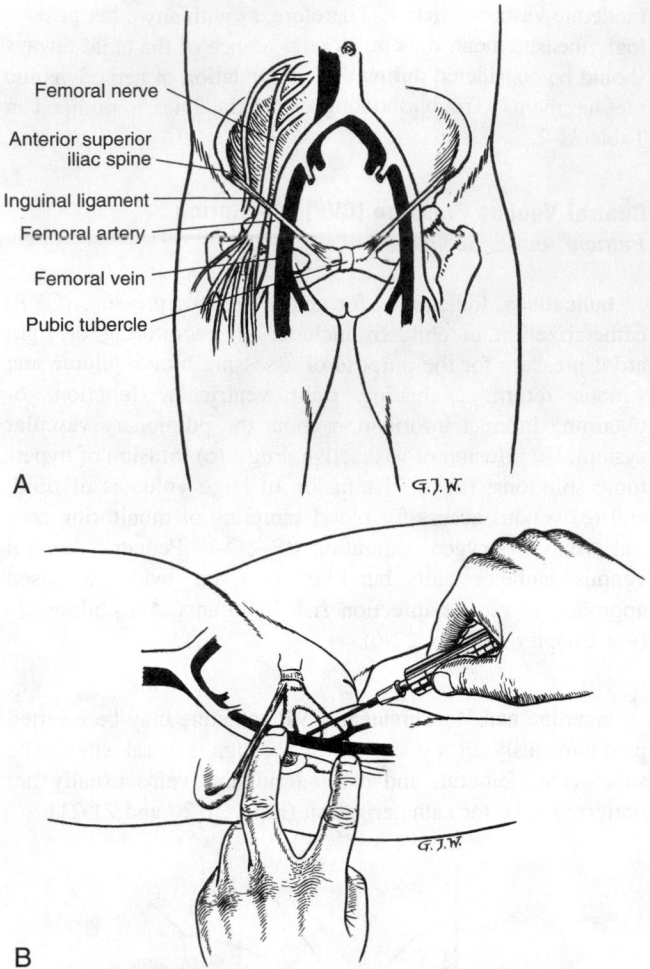

Femoral nerve

Anterior superior iliac spine

Inguinal ligament

Femoral artery

Femoral vein

Pubic tubercle

A

B

FIG. 21-21 Femoral venous catheterization. **A,** Anatomy. **B,** Technique. The child's leg is rotated externally and restrained. Femoral arterial pulses are located, and the needle is inserted one finger-breadth below the inguinal ligament, just medial to the femoral arterial pulsations. (From Hazinski MF: Hemodynamic monitoring of children. In Daily EK, Schroeder JS, editors: *Techniques in bedside hemodynamic monitoring*, ed 4, St Louis, 1989, Mosby.)

Blood Sampling. Venous blood samples may be obtained from a CVP catheter. To prevent air from entering the system during inspiration, the stopcock port must be held below the level of the right atrium when it is open to air. In some hospitals a physician's order is required before blood samples are withdrawn from CVP catheters. As with other vascular catheters, the CVP line should be cleared of IV fluid before blood samples are withdrawn so that accurate laboratory results will be obtained from a blood sample that is undiluted by fluid or heparin in the system.

Look for air or clots in the system because these can be flushed into the right side of the heart. To preserve the patency of a CVP catheter that is used for both measurement and sampling, heparinization of the system is preferred. Troubleshooting of intravascular catheters is outlined in Table 21-3.

Pulmonary Artery Pressure Monitoring

Pulmonary artery catheters in children allow direct measurement of pulmonary artery pressure to diagnose and manage postoperative pulmonary hypertension. The pulmonary artery end-diastolic pressure may be monitored to evaluate left ventricular function.

Indications. Placement of a PA catheter is useful for the diagnosis and management of cardiopulmonary failure that is refractory to standard support of oxygenation and ventilation, fluid therapy, and pharmacologic support. The right atrial port allows assessment of the right atrial and right ventricular end-diastolic pressure (RVEDP). In the presence of abnormal pulmonary vascular resistance or isolated right- or left-ventricular dysfunction, a more direct method of evaluating left ventricular end-diastolic pressure (LVEDP) is necessary.

The contraindications for use of a PA catheter include any conditions in which the potential *benefits* derived from the measurements or calculations are outweighed by the anticipated *risks* of catheter insertion.

Insertion. The PA catheter may be inserted percutaneously or through a cut down site, or it may be placed into the heart in the operating suite. Although fluoroscopy can be used to guide the passage of the catheter, the procedure is performed most often at the bedside using waveform analysis to determine catheter position as the catheter passes from a central vein through the right atrium and ventricle and into the pulmonary artery (Fig. 21-22). The equipment and steps for insertion of a PA catheter include the following:

1. Apply ECG leads and obtain a stable tracing.
2. Assemble transducer systems and flush all tubing. Use a separate flush and monitoring system for the RA and PA ports.
3. Zero the transducer and monitor. The waveform scale should be set at 0 to 60 mm Hg, and the paper recording device readied for printouts of the displayed waveforms.

Maintenance. As with all vascular monitoring systems, PA catheter systems should be inspected routinely for the presence of air, emboli, loose connections, and for proper positioning. Strict aseptic technique must be used when handling these catheter systems. The PA waveform should be displayed continuously to enable immediate recognition of catheter migration. Other aspects of maintenance care include the following:

• Ideally, smart pumps with in-line air detection should be used to flush high risk catheters. The pumps should be inspected hourly to monitor fluid infusion volumes; heparinized saline (1 unit/mL) is used for the flush. All administered IV fluids should be recorded and totaled in the nursing notes and on the patient flow sheet.

• IV tubing and irrigation fluid should be changed every 72 hours, or per hospital policy.

• Blood sampling losses may accumulate to significant levels in an infant; therefore the nurse must record blood volume withdrawn, and when this total exceeds 7% to 10% of the child's estimated blood volume, notify and discuss with the physician or on-call provider. The nurse also should be aware of the child's most recent hematocrit measurement.

• High- and low-pressure alarms should be set for the measurements obtained through the RA and PA ports, to notify the nurse of tubing disconnections (low pressure) or lumen occlusion.

Table 21-3 **Troubleshooting Intravascular Lines**

Problem	Cause	Intervention
Damped waveform	Clot at catheter tip	1. Attempt to aspirate clots (always discard this blood); irrigate catheter gently—never forcibly. 2. Manually flush catheter and tubing after each blood sample. 3. Recheck connections and observe and ensure that flush flow rate is adequate. 4. Always use noncompliant tubing for system.
	Bubble in line	1. Attempt to tap tubing and move bubble to aspiration port or stopcock. 2. Flush system carefully with stopcock off to patient. Never flush PA catheter when balloon is inflated. 3. Use clear transducer and connections when possible to improve visualization of bubbles.
	Kinked catheter or tubing	1. Inspect system for external kinks. 2. Straighten extremity. 3. Loop excess external tubing and tape securely. 4. Be aware of insertion route to anticipate possible sites of angulation.
	Faulty transducer	1. Zero and calibrate every 2-4 h (or per hospital policy). 2. Avoid bumping or dropping transducer or cable. 3. Calibrate transducer with known mercury or water pressure (or per policy). 4. Change transducer if problem does not resolve.
	Catheter tip lodged against vessel wall	1. Rotate catheter (if PA catheter, do so with balloon uninflated and with physician's order) or catheterized extrenity. 2. Withdraw catheter 1 cm with physician's order, observing waveform during process to detect catheter tip location. 3. Identify PA catheter migration by change in waveform (from PA to damped PAW waveform).
	Compliant tubing	1. Ensure that noncompliant tubing is present through entire length of system.
Damped PAWP or "overwedged"	Migration of PA catheter	1. Catheter position should be in zone III below left atrium. 2. Risk of migration can be reduced by maintaining adequate LA volume and reduced mean airway pressure. 3. Forward migration may occur with looping of catheter in RA or RV or inadequate security at insertion site; chest x-ray is necessary to confirm looping.
	Balloon overinflation	1. Use only the volume of air required to produce a wedge tracing; if this volume is significantly less than previously, PA migration should be suspected.
Significant change in waveform or pressure	Actual change in hemodynamic status	1. Always assess patient first.
	Change in transducer position with incorrect zero reference	1. Rezero transducer. 2. Elevate head of bed no more than 45 degrees. 3. Confirm that zero reference leveled at consistent point (level of right atrium).
	Faulty transducer	1. Calibrate transducer with mercury or water pressure (follow unit policy).
	Air or particles in system	1. Check tubing for obvious bubbles. 2. With stopcock off to patient, flush tubing.
	Migration of catheter tip	(See migration of PA catheter above, in damped PAWP).
No pressure	Power off	1. Check power.
	Loose or open connection	1. Check and tighten or close all connections and ports. 2. Check all cables and jacks for firm connections.
	Gain setting too low	1. Ensure that gain setting is appropriate for the pressure monitored.
	Improper pressure scale	1. Ensure that the scale is appropriate for pressure monitored.
	Faulty transducer	1. Verify accuracy with water or mercury pressure devices (or per policy).
Arrhythmias	Catheter tip inappropriately positioned in RA, RV, or outflow tracts	1. Immediately assess waveform appearance to identify catheter tip migration—if this is apparent, the arrhythmias can be managed initially with catheter reposition (for PA catheter, partially inflate balloon and observe for flotation of tip by change in waveform); withdrawal or insertion of catheter is to be done only with physician's order. 2. If arrhythmias are not eliminated, or if catheter tip is in proper position, arrhythmias should be managed according to hospital unit policy.

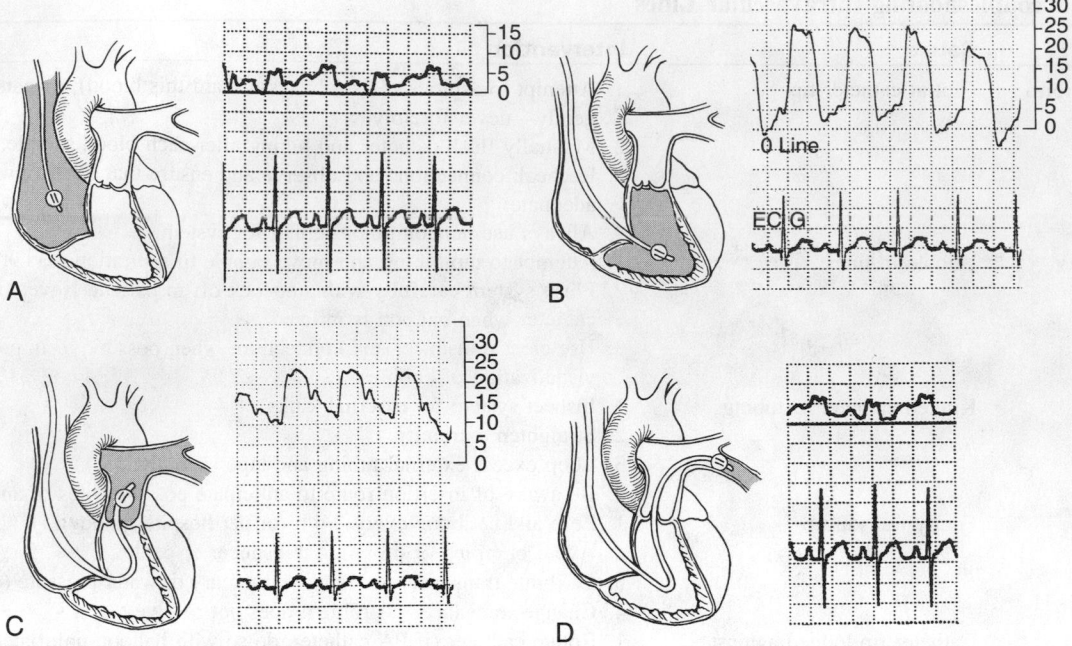

FIG. 21-22 Pulmonary artery catheter insertion. Waveforms observed during insertion of PA catheter. During the insertion procedure, the location of the catheter tip is determined by the pressure measurements and waveforms displayed. **A,** Catheter tip in the right atrium. Mean pressure (RAP) approximately 0 to 5 mm Hg. **B,** Catheter tip in the right ventricle. Systolic pressure approximately 25 to 30 mm Hg, end-diastolic pressure approximately 5 mm Hg (RVEDP = RAP). **C,** Catheter tip in the pulmonary artery. Systolic pressure approximately 25 to 30 mm Hg (equal to RV systolic pressure), and end-diastolic pressure approximately 4 to 8 mm Hg. **D,** Balloon inflated to obtain pulmonary artery wedge (PAW) measurement. Mean pressure is normally approximately 4 to 8 mm Hg (equal to the pulmonary artery end-diastolic pressure if pulmonary vascular resistance is normal).

• In small pediatric pulmonary artery catheters, the pulmonary artery lumen is *very* small and will readily become occluded by clot, fibrin, or crystals from intravenous fluids. As a result, the PA lumen should be used for infusion of drugs only as a last resort.

Measurements with PA Catheter. Because the pulmonary artery catheter contains a right atrial and pulmonary artery port, pressure measurements may be obtained from both sites. Fluid infusion can occur through the catheter sheath or the right atrium.

Right Atrial Pressure. The RA pressure reflects right ventricular end-diastolic pressure (RVEDP) unless tricuspid valve disease is present. The mean pressure typically is recorded by the nurse, although the waveform usually includes an *a* wave, a *v* wave, and a c wave, as does the waveform for the LA pressure (see Fig. 21-23). Normal RA, RV, PA and PAWP pressures are shown in Table 21-4.

Pulmonary Artery Pressure. The PA pressure reflects the systolic pressure generated by the right ventricle and the waveform resembles a systemic arterial waveform. Pressure measurements displayed include the PA systolic, end-diastolic, and mean pressures, and all three should be routinely recorded. Normal PA pressures are shown in Table 21-4.

Normally, the peak pulmonary artery systolic pressure is equal to right ventricular systolic pressure. If pulmonary vascular resistance is normal, the pulmonary artery end-diastolic

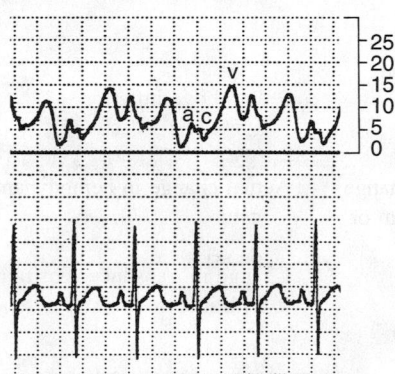

FIG. 21-23 Left atrial pressure tracing. This waveform is identical in appearance to both the right atrial and the pulmonary artery wedge waveforms in the normal patient (assuming proper placement of the pulmonary artery catheter).

Table 21-4   Normal Pediatric Intracardiac Pressures

	Newborn (mm Hg)	Child (mm Hg)
RA	0-4	0-4
RV	50/3	30/3
PA	50/30 (M: 40)	30/8 (M: 15)
PAWP	4-8	4-8

M, Mean; *PA,* pulmonary artery; *PAWP,* pulmonary artery wedge pressure; *RA,* right atrial; *RV,* right ventricular.

pressure will equal pulmonary artery wedge pressure. If pulmonary vascular resistance is elevated, the pulmonary artery end-diastolic pressure will be higher than the pulmonary artery wedge pressure. Thus, as soon as the balloon is inflated, the nurse will know if pulmonary vascular resistance is elevated.

If the PA catheter tip is appropriately placed in a dependent, posterior segment of the lung, the PAWP typically reflects left atrial pressure. However, in cases of extreme tachycardia, pulmonary venous constriction, or pulmonary venous obstruction the PAWP will be higher than the left atrial pressure.

The following steps should be used to obtain a PAWP measurement:

1. Perform or verify transducer calibration, zeroing and leveling before every measurement.
2. The supine position is generally not mandatory for PA or PAWP measurements. The head of the bed, however, should not be elevated more than 45 degrees, and the transducer must be zeroed and leveled at the phlebostatic axis with position changes.
   a. If the patient with respiratory failure demonstrates significant changes in alveolar oxygenation (with possible alteration in pulmonary vascular resistance and cardiac output) with changes in position, wedge pressure measurements should be made with the patient in a consistent position (e.g., supine with head of bed elevated to 15 degrees or 30 degrees) for all measurements.
   b. A graphic recording device should be available for recording the waveform tracings and deriving pressure measurements from them.
3. Gently inflate the PA balloon until a wedge pressure is obtained. Use no more air than the recommended balloon volume.
4. Be careful to avoid introduction of any air or clots into PA catheter, especially with infants or children who have intracardiac (particularly right-to-left) shunts, to prevent pulmonary and possibly cerebral emboli.

Sources of error in PA measurements include mechanical problems such as a faulty transducer or monitor and inaccurate zero reference point. Physiologic alterations also may cause elevation in the PAWP. Mechanical errors may include inappropriate transducer level, air in line, clot formation at the catheter tip, balloon rupture, and loose connections.

Complications of PA Catheterization. Complications of PA catheterization in children include all potential complications of central venous catheter insertion (e.g., bleeding and pneumothorax) and the potential complications of an invasive catheter (e.g., infection). Additional complications unique to the PA catheter include arrhythmias, knotting of the catheter, pulmonary infarction, pulmonary artery rupture, and pulmonary embolism. Infection and complications unique to the PA catheter are reviewed separately in this section.

Infections. Infections are more likely to occur in critically ill children when invasive monitoring is used, and the initial infections most often occur at the skin puncture site. Thrombus formation on the catheter may render the patient more susceptible to thrombotic endocarditis. Full barrier precautions and universal protocol before insertion, and assessment of the insertion site during dressing changes should minimize the risk of infection. Nurses should follow evidence-based unit protocols to reduce risk of central venous catheter-related bloodstream infections (see Box 22-6).

Arrhythmias. Ventricular arrhythmias may occur during catheter insertion as the catheter passes through the right ventricle. After catheter placement, the catheter tip may slip back into the right ventricle, causing arrhythmias. If arrhythmias develop, notify a physician or on-call provider immediately.

Definitive treatment for the arrhythmia is immediate repositioning of the catheter. Lidocaine may be administered (1 mg/kg IV dose). If the catheter is placed in an extremity, that extremity may be repositioned in an attempt to move the catheter tip until repositioning can be accomplished.

Knotting of the Catheter. Knotting may occur during insertion or as the result of migration of the catheter. It is most common in the presence of an enlarged RA or RV. The waveform may be unchanged in the presence of a knot unless the catheter is kinked, occluding the lumen and thus causing a dampened waveform.

If knotting is observed on chest radiograph, a physician may attempt catheter withdrawal under fluoroscopy (a "snare" catheter may be used). However, if the catheter remains knotted within the heart or PA, surgical removal (with use of cardiopulmonary bypass) may be required. The knotted catheter in the right ventricle may cause ventricular arrhythmias, requiring treatment with lidocaine.

Pulmonary Infarction. An infarction may occur at the time of catheter insertion or anytime during the monitoring period, particularly if the catheter migrates into a more peripheral pulmonary vessel and occludes it for extended periods. If the PA tracing spontaneously becomes a PAWP tracing (or a "dampened" tracing) the catheter should be withdrawn approximately 1 cm with physician or on-call provider order (or by the nurse if written hospital protocols allow). The nurse also should aspirate the pulmonary catheter to check for clots (discard the aspirate), and then gently flush the pulmonary port to ensure that a dampened signal is not caused by obstruction. Note that a rapid flush, which may be performed in adults, is not recommended for children because such a flush may damage the intima of the pulmonary vessel.

A pulmonary infarction may be asymptomatic or may cause hypoxemia, pleural pain, dyspnea, syncope, or total consolidation of the lung field on the chest radiograph. The physician or on-call provider must be notified immediately if pulmonary infarction is suspected or if the catheter remains in the wedge position despite maneuvers to dislodge it.

Pulmonary Artery Rupture. This complication is infrequent but can be fatal. Therefore the nurse should be aware of the conditions associated with the highest risk of pulmonary artery rupture:

- During PA catheter insertion with use of a guide wire (the wire can perforate the PA wall)
- Following distal migration of the catheter tip with rupture occurring before balloon inflation
- As the result of inflation of the balloon with an excessive volume of air (the volume used to inflate the balloon should be only that required to produce a PAWP tracing up to a *maximum* of the recommended balloon volume)

- During forceful, manual flush of the PA lumen, especially if the catheter is wedged in a PAWP position.
- The presence of pulmonary hypertension may predispose a patient to PA rupture because the PA tissue is friable and the high PA pressure tends to force the catheter to migrate distally. If the patient exhibits high PAP, the physician should be consulted before the balloon is inflated.

A patient with PA rupture usually demonstrates dramatic clinical changes, including hemoptysis, pulmonary congestion, coughing, and cardiopulmonary instability (including hypotension). Immediate emergency medical care is required.

Pulmonary Embolism. Although this is not a frequent problem with current catheters, thrombi may form on the balloon and the catheter shaft. Although critically ill patients are generally more susceptible to the development of thromboemboli because they have decreased activity and may have decreased pulmonary blood flow, pulmonary embolism is an uncommon complication in children. The patient with pulmonary embolism may exhibit pleuritic pain, cough, hemoptysis, substernal chest pain, syncope, shock, and death.

Intracardiac Catheters

Catheters may be placed directly into chambers of the heart or into the main pulmonary artery (RA, LA, PA) through tiny needle punctures made in these locations during cardiovascular surgery. Each monitoring line is inserted through the chest wall (while the chest is open) and then directly into the heart or vessel. Although the principles for care and maintenance of each catheter are the same as those described for the pulmonary artery catheter, a brief discussion of each is presented here.

Left Atrial Catheter. The LA catheter allows direct measurement of left atrial and left ventricular end-diastolic (filling) pressure and indirect assessment of left ventricular compliance (rise in LVEDP with volume administration). Pulmonary vascular resistance (a component of right ventricular afterload) may be calculated using the LA pressure if the cardiac output and mean pulmonary artery pressure are known.

If the child has a competent mitral valve and normal pulmonary vascular resistance, the PA end-diastolic pressure and the PAWP (obtained with a balloon-tipped pulmonary artery catheter) should equal the mean LA pressure (LAP). If the child has increased pulmonary vascular resistance, pulmonary artery end-diastolic pressure will be higher than PAWP or LAP. If pulmonary venous obstruction is present, the PAWP will *not* reflect the LAP. In such children, direct measurement of LAP (with an LA catheter) is the only means of measuring left ventricular end-diastolic pressure. The normal appearance of the LA waveform is the same as the configuration of the right atrial waveform (Fig. 21-23).

LA catheters generally are inserted during open heart surgery if left ventricular function requires monitoring. There are several important points to remember when caring for a child with an LA catheter:

1. The infusion system should be prepared using a standard transducer monitoring system. Air must be scrupulously eliminated, because any air infused into the LA catheter can cause a cerebral embolus (stroke) or other systemic embolus.

2. Throughout the time the LA catheter is in place, the entire tubing system should be constantly monitored for air bubbles, using smart pump technology with air detection inline if available. If air or other emboli are detected in the system, the stopcock port nearest the patient should be closed immediately (off to the patient) and the air should be evacuated before the stopcock is again opened between the patient and the system.

3. The catheter should *never* be used to infuse medications or supplementary fluids of any kind. It exists solely for LA measurements, so the only fluids entering the catheter should be irrigant fluids to maintain catheter patency.

4. If "dampening" of the waveform occurs the nurse may attempt to aspirate the line, but the *LA line should not be flushed without a physician's (or appropriate on-call provider's) order*. If such an order is provided the nurse should always aspirate the line before it is flushed, and the aspirated fluid (1 to 2 mL) should be discarded because it may contain emboli. Irrigation may push an air or blood embolus into the coronary vessels or cerebral vessels, resulting in cerebral or coronary embolus and infarction.

Right Atrial Catheter. The RA catheter provides the same data as a central venous pressure catheter or the RA port of a pulmonary artery catheter. It is used for right atrial pressure measurements, as a port for thermodilution cardiac output injection, and as a large-bore central venous catheter for infusion of fluids and medications. The configuration of the RA waveform should be the same as that obtained from the RA port of the pulmonary artery catheter.

If a child has an intracardiac septal defect, great care must be exercised to avoid infusion of any air or other thrombotic material through the RA line. Such material may cross to the left side of the heart (particularly if forceful irrigation is used) and enter either the coronary or cerebral vessels, resulting in myocardial or cerebral emboli, ischemia, or infarction.

The RA catheter may be used for injection of medication or fluid because the catheter tip is located in the right atrium where there is a larger volume and faster flow of blood than in peripheral veins. Because the RA pressure is low, RA catheters typically remain patent with continuous flush infusion rates as low as 1 mL/hour.

Pulmonary Artery Catheter. A catheter inserted directly into the main pulmonary artery during open heart surgery will enable measurement of systolic, diastolic, and mean pulmonary artery pressures. Additionally, some catheters contain thermistors for determination of cardiac output. The PA waveform should be the same as that obtained with a balloon-tipped pulmonary artery catheter. However, these catheters usually do not possess a balloon tip and so cannot measure PAWP.

PA catheters inserted during surgery require the same care as a catheter that is placed percutaneously. Extra care is required to maintain catheter patency and prevent trauma to the pulmonary artery. Because the catheter is placed into a small pulmonary vessel with high flow and moderately low pressure (lower pressure than in a peripheral arterial line), a relatively slow continuous infusion rate (1 to 2 mL/hour) should maintain catheter patency.

If pulmonary arterial blood is sampled frequently (to determine mixed venous oxygen tension), the pulmonary vessel intima may be traumatized by frequent aspiration and irrigation. To minimize intimal damage, flush very gently from the port that is furthest from the catheter and use the two-stopcock system for blood sampling (see Fig. 21-18).

Central Venous Catheter Care

Central venous catheter care should include barrier precautions during catheter insertion,[121] chlorhexidine, use of a Biopatch (except for premature low birth weight infants), and rigorous review of hospital-acquired infection in real time by the pediatric critical care unit, infection control, and infectious disease teams (see Box 22-6).

Evaluation of Cardiac Output and Tissue Perfusion

Fick and Thermodilution Cardiac Output Calculation

The calculation of cardiac output enables assessment of myocardial function and allows calculation of derived variables such as vascular resistance or ventricular work indices[134] (Table 21-5). Cardiac output is defined as the volume of blood ejected by the heart per unit of time (L/minute). Cardiac index corrects CO for body size and is defined as the cardiac output/ m^2 body surface area (L/minute per m^2).

Methods for determining CO include calculation with the Fick equation or use of an indicator method employing dye or a thermal indicator. According to the Fick equation (refer to Box 8-6), cardiac output is the ratio of consumption of oxygen to the arteriovenous difference in the content of oxygen. A fall in mixed venous oxygen saturation, with a constant arterial saturation and hemoglobin concentration, suggests increased tissue oxygen consumption or a fall in cardiac output.

The Fick equation

$$\text{Fick Cardiac output} = \frac{\text{oxygen consumption}}{\text{arterial oxygen content}^* - \text{mixed venous oxygen content}^\dagger}$$

* Arterial oxygen content = oxygen bound to hemoglobin in arterial blood + dissolved oxygen in arterial blood
† Mixed venous oxygen content = oxygen bound to hemoglobin in mixed venous blood + dissolved oxygen in mixed venous blood

The thermodilution method for calculating CO is used infrequently in the pediatric critical care unit, because the catheters are difficult to insert. In the thermodilution method, a known quantity of cold (typically iced) solution is injected into the right atrium. As it passes through the right ventricle, it mixes with blood at body temperature, cooling that volume of blood. When right ventricular blood and injectate are ejected into the pulmonary artery (PA), a PA thermistor measures the change in temperature of the blood and plots this change over time. The data are integrated into a time temperature curve and the area under the curve is computed to derive the CO measurement in L/minute.

The area under the thermodilution time-temperature curve is *inversely proportional to the flow rate of the blood*. When the cardiac output is high the flow rate is rapid and the magnitude of the temperature change in the blood will be small and the change will last only a short time; therefore the area under the curve is small. If the CO is low, the injectate produces a greater temperature change in the pulmonary artery, and the change will be sustained for a long period of time; therefore the area under the curve is large (Fig. 21-24).

Pulse Contour Cardiac Output Calculation

Pulse contour intermittent and continuous cardiac output (PiCCO) monitoring is possible using a femoral or axillary arterial catheter and a central venous catheter. Algorithms use pulse contour analysis combined with intermittent thermodilution calculations. The arterial waveform contours are analyzed to

Table 21-5 Derived Hemodynamic Values Using Cardiac Output Determinations

Parameter	Formula	Normal Range	Unit
Cardiac index (CI)	CI = CO/BSA	3.0-4.5	L/min/m²
Stroke volume index (SVI)	SVI = CI/HR	30-60	mL/m²
Systemic vascular resistance index (SVRI)	SVRI = [(MAP−CVP)/CI] × 80	800-1600	dyne-sec/cm⁵/m²
	or		
	(MAP−CVP)/CI	15-20	Wood Units
Pulmonary vascular resistance index (PVRI)	PVRI = [(MPAP−PAWP/CI] × 80	80-240	dyne-sec/cm⁵/m²
	or		
	(MPAP−PAWP)/CI	0-3	Wood Units
Left ventricular stroke work index (LVSWI)	LVSWI = SI × MAP × 0.0136	56 ± 6	g-m/m²
Left cardiac work index (LCWI)	LCWI = CI × MAP × 0.0136	4.0 ± 0.4	kg-m/m²
Right ventricular stroke work index (RVSWI)	RVSWI = SI × MPAP × 0.0136	6.0 ± 0.9	g-m/m²
Right cardiac work index (RCWI)	RCWI = CI × MPAP × 0.0136	0.5 ± 0.06	kg-m/m²

From Katz RW, Pollack M, Weibley R: Pulmonary artery catheterization in pediatric intensive care. *Adv Pediatr* 30:169, 1984.
BSA, Body surface area (m2); *CO*, cardiac output; *CVP*, central venous pressure (mm Hg); *HR*, heart rate (per minute); *MAP*, mean arterial pressure (mm Hg); *MPAP*, mean pulmonary arterial pressure (mm Hg); *PAWP*, pulmonary artery wedge pressure; *SI*, stroke index.

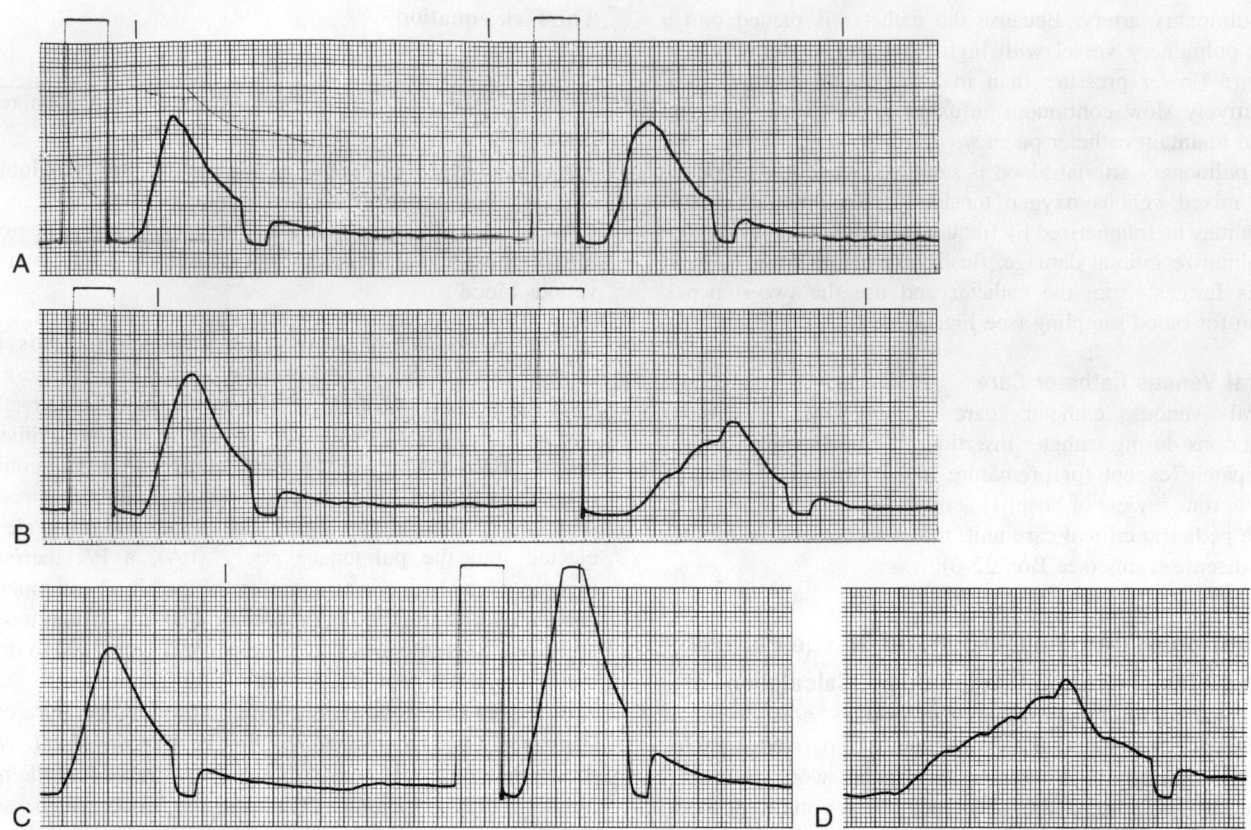

FIG. 21-24 Thermodilution cardiac output injection curves. **A,** Identical curves, consistent with excellent injection technique. **B,** Inconsistent injection technique (second injection is uneven and too slow) that resulted in widely discrepant cardiac output calculations. **C,** Inconsistent injection volume. Second injection utilized 5 mL instead of 3 mL (computer calibration constant set for 3-mL injection), so 5-mL injection provided falsely low cardiac output calculation. **D,** Excessively slow and uneven injection. (From Hazinski MF: Hemodynamic monitoring of children. In Daily EK, Schroeder JS, editors: *Techniques in bedside hemodynamic monitoring,* ed 4, St Louis, 1989, Mosby.)

assess stroke volume and thereby cardiac index (CI). In a pediatric validation study, the PiCCO system provided continuous measurement of CI without the need to perform thermodilution injections with every calculation.[52]

Ultrasound Dilution Cardiac Output Calculations

Cardiac output and blood volume can be calculated from a form of ultrasound dilution. This technology uses a computer and arterial and venous sensors attached to a specialized extracorporeal tubing loop that is placed between an indwelling central venous catheter and an arterial catheter. A small bolus (0.5 to 1.0 mL/kg) of isotonic saline is injected into the central venous catheter to create a dilution curve. The saline dilutes the total blood protein concentration and alters blood velocity detected by the arterial sensor in the extracorporeal loop. The change in blood velocity over time can be graphed, resulting in a dilution curve that is similar to that created during thermodilution cardiac output calculations.

In addition to calculating the cardiac output and index, the ultrasound dilution computer calculates stroke volume index, active circulating volume, systemic vascular resistance, and ejection fraction. This technology has been validated in neonates and children.[94]

Noninvasive Calculation of Cardiac Output

A variety of noninvasive methods to evaluate cardiac output have emerged in recent years. Electrical cardiometry uses four adhesive electrodes placed on an infant's forehead, neck, chest, and leg to evaluate thoracic electrical bioimpedance. The ratio of applied current and measured voltage equals the bioimpedance which is recorded over time. A recent study in children with congenital heart defects found that the cardiometry-derived cardiac output calculation correlated well with a direct Fick cardiac output calculation.[129] Although the absolute cardiac output derived by this method may underestimate the actual cardiac output,[155] the device can be useful for trending cardiac output when correlated with other clinical assessment.

Esophageal Doppler studies of blood flow velocity in the descending aorta have been available for many years and pediatric probes are now available. In the past, the higher heart rates in children compromised reliability of this technique of cardiac output evaluation. Fairly reliable cardiac output calculations have recently been reported in children,[155] although this method of cardiac output evaluation is very operator-dependent.[1]

Partial rebreathing of carbon dioxide may be used to provide continuous cardiac output calculations in patients during mechanical ventilation. This noninvasive cardiac output (NICO) system can be used in children with low tidal volumes, but is not as accurate in patients with small body surface area. In addition, partial rebreathing of carbon dioxide can increase the serum CO_2, making this an unsuitable method of monitoring cardiac output in children with pulmonary hypertension or increased intracranial pressure.

Systemic Venous Oxygen Saturation ($S_{CV}O_2$) Monitoring

Mixed venous and central venous (specifically superior vena caval [SVC]) oxygen saturations are increasingly being used as indirect, but clinically useful variables that can reflect trends in systemic oxygen delivery and cardiac output.[59] Such trending may be useful in the presence of shock.

Mixed or central venous oxygen saturation monitoring may also be useful in the presence of intracardiac or extracardiac shunting, such as in neonatal staged palliation for hypoplastic left heart syndrome (HLHS). However, it is important to remember that in such patients, the central and mixed venous oxygen saturations will be affected not only by cardiac output, but also by the direction and magnitude of shunting and the degree of mixing of pulmonary and systemic venous blood.[115] Lower $S_{CV}O_2$ and wider arteriovenous difference have been correlated with worse early survival, the need for ECMO, and neurodevelopmental morbidity in infants with HLHS (see Hypoplastic Left Heart Syndrome in Chapter 8).[59,79]

Central venous oxygen saturation can be measured through the use of pediatric catheters of 4.0 to 5.5 French that calculate the oxyhemoglobin saturation through reflective spectrophotometry. One optical fiber at the distal end of the catheter emits light that is reflected by passing red blood cells; reflected light is captured by a second optical fiber. The amount of light reflected varies based on the relative concentrations of oxygenated (saturated) and desaturated hemoglobin. The reflected light is used to calculate the percent total hemoglobin that is saturated with oxygen.[110]

Continuous Central Venous Oximetry

There are limited data regarding the use of continuous central venous oximetry using spectroscopy (light reflected from hemoglobin). Mixed venous oximetry requires a pulmonary artery catheter and its associated risks. Trended data from nearinfrared spectroscopy (NIRS) may be helpful in highlighting changes in tissue oxygenation that trend with the central venous oxygen saturation.[110,144]

Near-Infrared Spectroscopy (NIRS)

Near-infrared spectroscopy (NIRS) is a noninvasive optical technique to monitor brain tissue oxygenation.[78] It can also be used for monitoring oxygenation of other tissues.[53] Most devices use two to four wavelengths of near-infrared light at 700 to 1000 nm. Commercially available devices determine the concentrations of oxyhemoglobin and desaturated hemoglobin to determine cerebral oxygen saturation.[9]

The cerebral oximeter electrode is placed on the forehead below the hairline. It contains two light-emitting diodes and light receivers that will detect light reflected from both shallow and deep tissue. A computer is able to discount the shallow light reflection, to allow evaluation of light reflection from the hemoglobin in deeper tissue (i.e., the brain). NIRS

monitoring has wide interpatient variability but is used to trend cerebral and other tissue oxygenation in the pediatric critical care unit setting.[97]

Temporary Pacemakers

Pacemaker therapy is indicated for children who have or have a significant potential for developing atrioventricular (AV) conduction block or arrhythmias that may cause low cardiac output. Most commonly the risk of arrhythmias follows cardiovascular surgery.[167]

Arrhythmias that impact cardiac output include sinus bradycardia, complete A-V block, sinus node dysfunction, junctional ectopic tachycardia, atrial tachycardia, and cardiac arrest. These arrhythmias may require high rate burst overdrive pacing and support before permanent pacemaker placement. Pacing also may be required for complications after invasive procedures, such as cardiac catheterization or central venous catheter placement in patients with previous bundle branch block.[151]

Temporary atrial wires may be used for diagnostics postoperatively with atrial electrocardiograms (ECGs),[179] or for diagnosis of congenital, familial, or idiopathic arrhythmias. Patients with denervated hearts after orthotopic heart transplantation may also require pacing.

This discussion is limited to the use of temporary external pacemakers and transcutaneous pacing.

Function and Nomenclature

Most pacemakers sense the patient's intrinsic electrical activity and provide an electrical stimulus to produce myocardial depolarization when the patient's intrinsic conduction system is dysfunctional. Therefore, most external pulse generators are capable of both *sensing* intrinsic myocardial electrical events and *delivering* a specified amount of current to the heart (Table 21-6).

The function of current pacemakers is described in a threeletter classification system. The code system indicates the chamber that is *paced,* the chamber that is *sensed,* and the *mode of pacemaker response* to sensed intrinsic activity.[51]

- The chamber(s) paced: can be dual, atrium, or ventricle (indicated by the letter D, A, or V, respectively)
- The chamber(s) sensed: can be dual, atrium, ventricle, or none (indicated by the letter D, A, V, or O, respectively)
- The mode of pacemaker response: can be dual (both atrial triggered and ventricular inhibition), inhibited, triggered, or none (D, I, T, or O, respectively)

Table 21-6	NASPE/BPEG Generic Code Applied to Temporary Pacing	
I **Chamber(s)** **Paced**	**II** **Chamber(s)** **Sensed**	**III** **Mode(s) of** **Response**
V = Ventricle	V = Ventricle	I = Inhibited
A = Atrium	A = Atrium	T = Triggered
D = Dual	D = Dual	D = Dual trigger/ inhibit
O = None	O = None	O = None

From The revised NASPE/BPEG generic code. *Pacing Clin Electrophysiol* 25:260-264, 2002.

For example, a DVI pacemaker provides dual atrial and ventricular pacing, ventricular sensing, and is inhibited by intrinsic ventricular activity (within the minimum set rate). A VVI pacing system paces the ventricle, senses intrinsic ventricular activity, and is inhibited by sensed intrinsic ventricular activity. A DDD pacing system paces the atria and the ventricles, senses both atrial and ventricular intrinsic activity and can be both triggered and, in the case of the ventricles, inhibited by intrinsic activity. Most commonly, temporary pediatric pacing uses VVI, DDD, or AAI pacing.

Pacemaker Unit and Leads

The pacemaker unit (pulse generator) is the energy source that has terminals for pacemaker wire connections. One ground (+) and one output (−) terminal exist for each chamber. Temporary external pacemaker wires may be placed on the epicardium through a thoracotomy incision or the wires may be placed transvenously through guided insertion of specialized pacemaker catheters. Transvenous catheters tend to be very stiff and difficult to manipulate, so their use is limited in very small infants.

Pacing Options

Single Chamber Temporary Pacing (VVI or AAI Modes). Temporary epicardial or transvenous leads placed in an atrium or, more commonly, in a ventricle allow both "fixed rate" and "demand" pacing. The fixed rate mode delivers an impulse at a predetermined rate regardless of intrinsic myocardial activity. When fixed rate mode is desired, the sensitivity must be turned to the lowest level to avoid any sensing of the patient's intrinsic electrical activity.

The demand mode senses the patient's intrinsic activity and only delivers an electrical stimulus if no intrinsic electrical activity is sensed within a predetermined interval, based on the preset demand heart rate (and possibly the preset atrioventricular [AV] interval). Sensitivity must be adjusted to ensure that the unit senses intrinsic activity. Typically these pulse generators operate with bipolar leads: one pacing wire (−) and another ground (+) wire for each chamber.

Atrioventricular Sequential Pacing (DDD Mode). In some patients, particularly those with poor myocardial function, preservation of atrial-ventricular synchrony is vital. Such synchrony requires a pulse generator that is capable of pacing both the atria and the ventricles in sequence. Two bipolar channels, one each for the atrium and the ventricle, are used with either epicardial or endocardial (transvenous placement) leads.

The pulse generator has the capability of "sensing" intrinsic atrial and ventricular electrical activity, and "pacing" both the atria and the ventricles. Adjustment in pulse amplitude is possible (0.1 to 20 mA) for both atrial and ventricular output. The A-V interval, which is associated with the P-R interval on the ECG, is manually established with the typical choices between 0 and 300 ms, or 0 and 0.300 second.

Once the leads are placed, a variety of pacing modes can be established (Fig. 21-25):

1. Single chamber pacing (either atria or ventricle) in fixed rate mode (VOO or AOO)

2. Single chamber pacing (either atrial or ventricular) in a demand mode (VVI or AVI)
3. Dual chamber pacing, fixed rate (DOO)
4. Dual chamber pacing, demand rate (DVI)
5. Dual chamber A-V sequential pacing (DDD), P wave synchronous rate response

Temporary Demand Pacemaker Controls and Indicators

For a pacemaker to operate correctly, both the "sensing" mechanisms and "output stimulus" control must be set for each patient. Additional adjustments allow determination of ventricular rate, duration of stimulation (pulse width), and A-V intervals.

Sensitivity Control and Threshold. The *sensitivity control* adjusts the responsiveness of the pacemaker to the patient's intrinsic cardiac electrical activity. The sensitivity can be adjusted between 0.5 and 20 mV (corresponding to the size of patient electrical signal that will be sensed consistently by the pacemaker).

When the control is set fully counterclockwise (to 10 mV in the atrium and 20 mV or "ASYNCH" in the ventricle), the pacemaker is virtually insensitive to the patient's intrinsic rhythm. The pacemaker will provide an electrical stimulus at a set rate (asynchronous mode) regardless of the intrinsic rate. As the sensitivity control is turned clockwise toward 0.4 mV, the pacemaker becomes more sensitive to the intrinsic cardiac activity and is more easily inhibited by smaller intrinsic electrical signals.

Temporary A-V sequential pacemaker models include an atrial sensing mechanism. However, if pacing produces a large voltage, the A-V pacer may sense the atrial pacing spike as an R wave and alter the timing of the ventricular pacer stimulus. Therefore inspect the ECG for evidence of abnormally large P waves when adjusting the ventricular sensitivity control.

The *sensitivity threshold* is the point at which the pacemaker consistently senses every intrinsic patient R- or P-wave signal. It represents the minimum intrinsic electrical signal that will consistently inhibit pacer firing. Once this point is determined, it is prudent to adjust the sensitivity control in a clockwise direction to a point slightly smaller than the threshold to ensure optimum sensitivity to the patient's intrinsic rhythm.

Output Threshold and Control. The *output control* adjusts the amount of current delivered to the epicardium or endocardium by the pacemaker generator. The unit of selected current flow is milliamperes (mA).

The current can be adjusted between 0.1 and 20 mA, as needed to produce myocardial depolarization. The *stimulation threshold* is the minimum pacemaker current necessary to consistently "capture" (produce depolarization of) the paced chamber. Variables that determine this threshold include resistance to the current through the wires (which increases with duration of pacing), the placement of the pacer wire on epicardium or endocardium and the contact point, and the chamber being paced.

The pacer wires must be intact, with a tight connection to the terminal. The electrode tip of the pacer wire must be

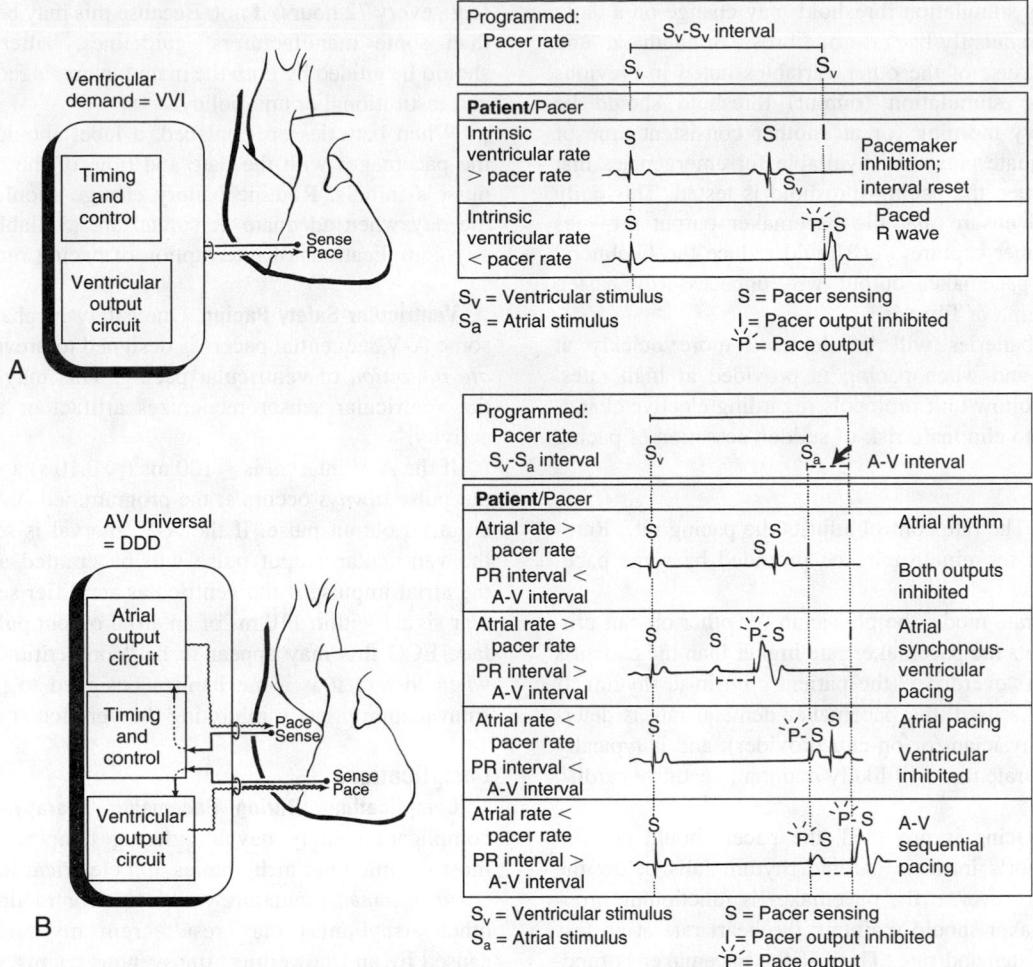

FIG. 21-25 Pacemaker modes: VVI and DDD Modes. This three-letter coding system uses three letters to indicate the chamber paced (atrial, ventricular, or dual atrial and ventricular pacing), the chamber sensed (A, V, or D), and the pacer response to intrinsic electrical activity (it is inhibited or triggered). **A,** VVI pacing is ventricular-demand pacing. The ventricular (S_v-S_v) interval is determined by the preset ventricular demand rate (e.g., if the demand rate is 60, the S_v-S_v interval is 1 second). If intrinsic ventricular activity is sensed within that interval, the pacemaker is inhibited (intrinsic ventricular rate > pacer rate). If no intrinsic ventricular activity is sensed within that interval, the pacemaker provides a ventricular stimulus (intrinsic ventricular rate < pacer rate) **B,** DDD pacing provides true atrioventricular sequential pacing, because it is capable of sensing both intrinsic atrial and ventricular activity. The S_v-S_v interval again is determined by the set ventricular demand rate, and the S_a timing is determined by the set A-V interval. If, within the S_v-S_a interval, patient intrinsic atrial electrical activity is sensed, the pacer waits the set A-V interval; if intrinsic ventricular electrical activity is sensed, both atrial and ventricular outputs are inhibited (atrial rate > pacer rate, and PR interval is < set A-V interval). If an intrinsic atrial impulse is sensed but *not* followed by an intrinsic ventricular impulse within the set A-V interval, a ventricular paced impulse is provided (atrial rate > pacer rate, P-R interval > A-V interval); in this case, ventricular pacing has been provided in synchrony with the patient's atrial activity. If no atrial activity is sensed within the S_v-S_a interval, an atrial impulse is provided. If the atrial impulse is followed by intrinsic ventricular electrical activity within the preset A-V interval, the ventricular pacer output is inhibited (atrial rate < pacer rate, PR interval < A-V interval); in this case, atrial pacing alone is provided. If the atrial impulse is *not* followed by intrinsic ventricular electrical activity within the set A-V interval, a ventricular impulse is provided (atrial rate < pacer rate, P-R interval > A-V interval); in this case, synchronized atrial and ventricular pacing have been provided. (Redrawn and modified from illustrations of pacemaker modes from Medtronic product handbooks, San Antonio, TX.)

implanted near excitable tissue. In general, epicardial thresholds are usually higher than endocardial thresholds and atrial thresholds are higher than ventricular thresholds. Other variables that affect thresholds include oxygenation, pH, electrolyte balance, and the availability of metabolic substrates. With abnormalities of any of these, stimulation thresholds generally will be increased.

With prolonged pacing, inflammation and ultimately fibrosis can develop at the point of contact between the lead and the epicardium or endocardium, so a larger stimulus (i.e., higher mA output) may be required to capture the chamber over time. Steroid-impregnated epicardial leads may reduce fibrosis surrounding these leads and minimize the need for higher stimulus strength over time.

The patient's stimulation threshold may change on a daily basis or more frequently because of fibrosis or edema around the leads or because of the other variables noted in previous paragraphs. The stimulation (output) threshold should be determined every morning (or at another consistent time of day), with adequate personnel available for emergencies that may develop when the pacing threshold is tested. This daily assessment will ensure that the pacemaker output provides consistent chamber capture, yet should reduce the likelihood that excessive pacemaker output will unnecessarily hasten the onset of edema or fibrosis.

Pacemaker batteries will be depleted more quickly at higher outputs and when pacing is provided at high rates. Nurses should follow unit protocols regarding elective changing of batteries to eliminate risk of sudden cessation of pacing function.

Rate Control. The rate control adjusts the pacing rate. Rates up to 800 impulses/minute may be provided by some pacemaker models.

In the fixed rate mode, the physician (or other on-call provider) usually sets the pacemaker rate higher than the patient's intrinsic rate, to "overdrive" the patient's intrinsic rhythm. If demand pacing is used, the pacemaker demand rate is determined by the physician (or on-call provider), and is typically the lowest heart rate that will likely maintain adequate cardiac output.

If demand pacing is provided, the pacer should not fire unless the patient's intrinsic cardiac rhythm falls below the demand rate. However, if the pacemaker is functioning properly, the pacemaker should maintain the heart rate at no less than the pacing demand rate. Thus, if the pacemaker is functioning correctly in the demand mode, *the patient's heart rate should never be less than the pacemaker demand rate.*

Pulse Width. Some pacemaker units allow adjustment of the pulse duration—the length of time the pacemaker current is delivered to stimulate myocardial depolarization. If the myocardial threshold is rising, causing failure to capture, an increased pulse width may produce effective capture and avoid the need to increase the current. This will improve ventricular capture, decrease the focal injury to the myocardium, and improve battery longevity.

A-V Interval. This control is used during DVI and DDD pacing and determines the duration of time between atrial and ventricular depolarization. The settings range from 20 to 300 ms. This interval is approximately equal to the P-R interval on the ECG.

Visual Indicators.
Sense-Pace Indicator. Pacemakers usually have a gauge or light that indicates whether the pacemaker is *sensing* patient P or R waves, or generating an electrical impulse *(pacing)*.

Batteries. A gauge or light on the pacemaker unit indicates low battery voltage. Because low battery voltage causes pacemaker malfunction, in many clinical settings the batteries are replaced at more frequent intervals (e.g., every 24 hours) if the patient is pacemaker dependent and at less frequent intervals

(e.g., every 72 hours) if not. Because this may be more frequent than some manufacturers' guidelines, battery replacement should be guided by both the manufacturer's recommendations and institutional or unit policy.

When batteries are replaced, a label should be placed on the pacemaker with the date and time of the change and the nurse's initials. Routine battery change should occur during the day when adequate personnel are available to deal with any complications of interruption of pacing function.

Ventricular Safety Pacing. One safety mechanism built into some A-V sequential pacers is designed to prevent *inappropriate inhibition* of ventricular pacing. This may occur because the ventricular sensor recognizes artifact or atrial electrical activity.

If the A-V interval is ≤ 100 ms (≤ 0.10 s) a ventricular output pulse *always* occurs at the programmed A-V interval after an atrial output pulse. If the A-V interval is set at > 125 ms, the ventricular output pulse will be emitted at 110 ms after the atrial impulse if the ventricular amplifier senses a ventricular signal within 110 ms of an atrial output pulse. On the surface ECG this may appear to be "competition" (Fig. 21-26), when in fact it is a mechanism designed to prevent artifact from inappropriately inhibiting the ventricular pacer.

Complications
Complications During Pacemaker Therapy. A variety of complications may develop during temporary pacing. The most common are arrhythmias and electrical hazards.

Arrhythmias. Premature ventricular contractions (PVCs) and other arrhythmias may result from myocardial irritability caused by an (indwelling) transvenous pacing wire. Additionally, if a pacemaker stimulus occurs during the "vulnerable period" (the Q-T interval), ventricular tachycardia or ventricular fibrillation may result.

If pacing is discontinued abruptly, a period of asystole may be present until the patient's intrinsic pacemaker resumes activity. In general, the higher the pacemaker rate, the longer will be the potential period of asystole if the pacing is discontinued abruptly. If the pacemaker must be turned off during pacing, it is advisable to reduce the pacemaker rate gradually before turning the unit off, to allow the patient's intrinsic pacemaker time to recover and begin to fire. The patient's systemic perfusion and blood pressure must be monitored closely as the pacemaker rate is reduced.

Electrical Hazards. Exposed wire leads can provide low-resistance pathways for transmission of otherwise harmless electrical current directly to the heart. Stray current also may interfere with pacemaker function or inhibit pacemaker activity.

Many pacemakers have built-in shielding, and with the use of bipolar leads most external interference will not affect pacemaker operation. If interference is too strong (e.g., during electrocautery), the pacemaker output can be suppressed.

Electrical shocks may occur at the skin site of wire insertion if the milliamp output of the pacer is too high. Hiccups may result if pacer output is too high or the pacemaker stimulates the diaphragm directly. Defective leads and continuously high output may shorten lead life. Pacemaker wire fracture also may occur.

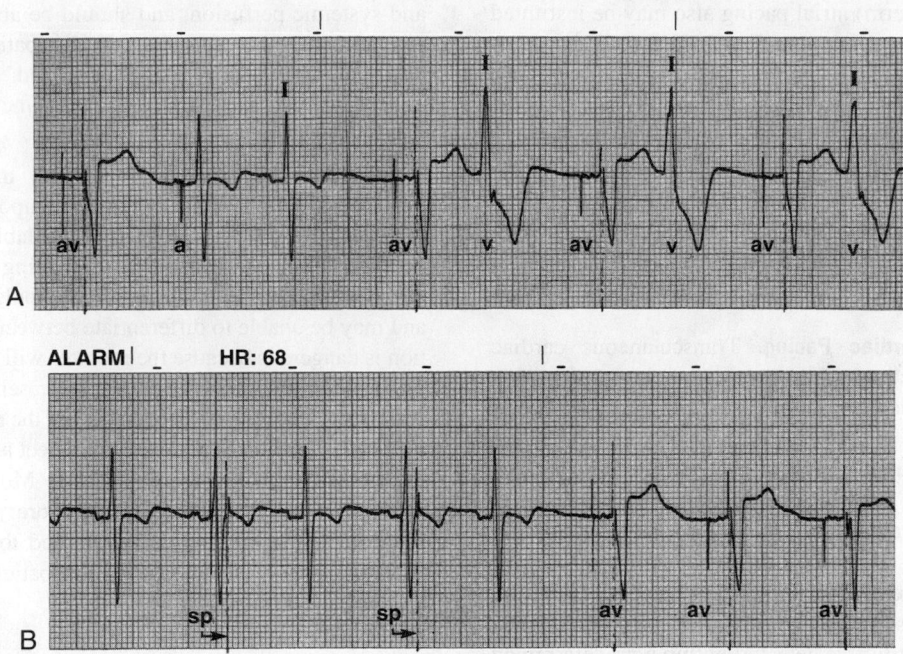

FIG. 21-26 Ventricular safety pacing. This safety feature is designed to prevent inappropriate inhibition of ventricular pacing by artifact or atrial impulses. If the set A-V interval is *less than or equal to 100 ms* (P-R interval of ≤ 0.10 s), a ventricular output impulse *always* will occur at the programmed AV interval (100 ms) following an atrial output pulse. If the programmed A-V interval is *125 ms* (0.125 s) *or greater,* a ventricular impulse is emitted at an A-V interval of 110 ms if the ventricular amplifier senses intrinsic electrical activity within 110 ms of an atrial output pulse. **A,** AV interval is 125 ms. Occasional atrial pacing only occurs (a) when intrinsic ventricular depolarization follows atrial paced impulse within 125 ms. A-V sequential pacing (av) only occurs if intrinsic ventricular activity does not occur within 125 ms of atrial pacing impulse. Note that the pacemaker is inhibited (I) entirely when intrinsic ventricular activity occurs at a rate faster than the preset ventricular demand rate, and premature ventricular contractions (V) inhibit the DVI pacemaker. **B,** Ventricular safety pacing (SP) is observed when intrinsic ventricular electrical activity occurs within 110 ms of the paced atrial impulse. Although it appears that the pacemaker has failed to sense patient ventricular activity, this is a safety feature to prevent failure of ventricular pacing from artifact or sensing of the atrial impulse. Note that, with normal A-V sequential pacing (AV), the A-V interval is 125 ms, but the A-V interval with ventricular safety pacing is 110 ms—this allows recognition of the safety pacing and rules out pacer malfunction.

Exposure to magnetic resonance imaging (MRI) may cause alteration in pacemaker function because of the effect of the magnetic field on the pulse generator. It is advisable to either stop the pacemaker or put it in an asynchronous mode during MRI. Consult the pacemaker manufacturer for device-specific recommendations.

Complications of Lead Insertion. Transvenous and epicardial lead insertion can cause complications.

Transvenous Lead Placement. Complications that may develop during the insertion of transvenous pacer wires include hemorrhage, cardiac perforation, air embolism, and erratic pacemaker function. Perforation of the right ventricle may result (usually within the first 48 hours) when a transvenous wire is used. Pulmonary emboli may be caused by dislodged thrombi at the tip of transvenous pacer wires anytime during pacing. Infection may occur at the insertion site.

Epicardial Lead Placement. Epicardial leads require a surgical approach (thoracotomy) that may be complicated by pneumothorax or a pneumomediastinum with resulting tamponade. Pacemaker function may be erratic if lead placement is not optimal.

Emergency Pacing

Emergency Invasive Pacing. To establish emergency invasive pacing, transthoracic, transvenous, or esophageal pacing wires may be implanted. The *transthoracic method* requires insertion of a needle through the anterior chest wall to the epicardium. The pacer wire is then inserted through the needle to the epicardium. The transthoracic wires can be inserted quickly, but the needle insertion may produce ventricular arrhythmias or puncture.

To insert *transvenous* leads, a catheter is placed in the brachial, femoral, or jugular vein, and then a guide wire is passed through the catheter to the superior or inferior vena cava. A pacing catheter is then threaded over the guide wire and advanced into the right ventricle. Transvenous wires are difficult to place in small vessels. Balloon-tipped, flow-directed pulmonary artery catheters that contain pacer wires are available but experience in children is limited. Whenever transvenous pacing is provided, a second subcutaneous wire also should be placed to serve as a ground. If the pacemaker wire is passed through a vessel in the child's extremity, the extremity should be restrained because the wire may become dislodged if the extremity is moved often.

Temporary (short-term) atrial pacing also may be instituted using *esophageal* pacing catheters. Esophageal pacing is typically performed for diagnostic purposes, for atrial pacing, or to terminate supraventricular tachycardia. The esophageal pacer stimulates the left atrium, so it is only useful for atrial pacing in the absence of AV block. The esophageal pacing catheter is inserted through the nose into the pharynx and ultimately into the lower esophagus. This form of pacing can cause discomfort, so adequate sedation and analgesia is recommended if possible. Esophageal pacing is not used for long-term pacing.

Transcutaneous Cardiac Pacing. Transcutaneous cardiac pacing (TCP) is a method of emergency noninvasive pacing that uses electrode pads to transmit electrical impulses through the anterior and posterior chest. Because the adhesive skin pads can be placed quickly, pacing can be instituted rapidly, obviating the need for surgical intervention or fluoroscopy.

A commercially available pacemaker unit, especially designed for transcutaneous application, functions as a VVI pacemaker, sensing events from the surface electrocardiogram. It delivers a 40-ms pulse (with a current of 20 to 140 mA) when no intrinsic cardiac activity is detected within a predetermined interval. The current is delivered through skin pads, which are applied in an anteroposterior (AP) position (i.e., over and behind the heart). The unit can provide asynchronous and demand pacing modes, ECG display, and adjustable settings for pacing and current outputs.

The indications for transcutaneous cardiac pacing in children are

- Cardioversion to terminate supraventricular tachycardia
- As a backup during permanent pacemaker reprogramming for pacer-dependent children (asystole can occur with reprogramming and the TCP would therefore be available immediately)
- Severe, symptomatic bradycardia

Mechanical capture must be confirmed with the presence of a palpable pulse corresponding to the paced rhythm, or with improvement in blood pressure and perfusion. Factors that may influence mechanical capture are hypoxemia, acidosis, and pleural or pericardial effusion.[167]

No complications have been reported with transcutaneous pacing. Erythema usually develops under the pads, but should disappear within minutes after pad removal. If the patient is conscious during pacing, moderate discomfort has been reported. This discomfort appears to be related to two factors. The first is that conscious patients might require a large pad size to decrease current density (so current flow is felt over a larger area), and the second is that skeletal muscle contractions may occur. Sedation and analgesia are advisable during pacing of conscious patients to minimize discomfort.

Defibrillation During Temporary Pacing. If the patient requires defibrillation, the pacemaker should first be turned off. If time allows, the wires also should be disconnected from their terminals.

Nursing Considerations

Throughout the care of the child with an external pacemaker, the nurse should assess effectiveness of myocardial function and systemic perfusion, and should be able to recognize inadequate pacemaker function. If the patient deteriorates, the nurse should support the patient and also be prepared to quickly troubleshoot the pacemaker function.

ECG and Pulse Monitoring. ECG monitoring should be provided for all patients requiring temporary external pacing. A strip chart recorder also must be available. The patient's *pulse rate* must also be monitored closely during pacing. Some cardiac monitors will sense the pacemaker impulse as a QRS complex and may be unable to differentiate between the two. This condition is dangerous because the monitor will continue to recognize and count pacer spikes even in the presence of asystole. If the pulse rate is monitored closely, even if the monitor fails to recognize loss of capture, the nurse will detect a fall in pulse rate.

A pulse oximeter (see Respiratory Monitoring in this chapter) is extremely useful during temporary pacemaker therapy. Some ECG monitors are programmed to count the heart rate from the arterial waveform, so the patient's pulse is counted rather than pacer spikes.

Pacemaker Settings and Documentation. The pacemaker settings—rate, mode, and output—should be checked against the physician (or other care provider) orders, and documented according to unit policy. Additionally, the sensitivity threshold must be checked every 8 to 24 hours per hospital policy or physician's order. If the child is pacer dependent, pacemaker function should be checked hourly, and the critical care nurse should observe for competition, failure to capture, or pacemaker failure (Table 21-7).

A spare battery and pacemaker generator should be readily available. A rhythm strip should be saved in the nurses' notes at least every 8 hours to verify proper pacemaker function.

Pacemaker equipment must be used safely. The wires and pacemaker should be covered with material to protect them from moisture (especially during baths) and stray current leak. Gloves should be worn during handling of wires to prevent any microshocks. The wires near the insertion site should be secured to prevent inadvertent dislodgement. The wire and cable connection at the pacer terminals should be checked to verify that the wires are held securely by the pacemaker cable.

The pacemaker unit and wires must be protected from patient interference. The external pacer unit should always have a childproof cover so that the responsive child will be unable to change the pacer settings.

If pacer malfunction occurs and all connections are verified and the pacer generator appears to be functioning, a chest radiograph may be required to determine if wire fractures or fraying have occurred.

Defibrillation and Cardioversion

Patricia Ann E. Schlosser and Kate Amond

Defibrillation

Defibrillation is the delivery of a shock to depolarize the entire myocardium and interrupt disorganized electrical activity (i.e., ventricular fibrillation [VF] or pulseless ventricular tachycardia [VT]) to allow an organized electrical activity to return.

Table 21-7 **Troubleshooting Pacemaker Malfunctions**

Observation	Causes	Intervention
Competition: Pacemaker spikes are observed throughout the ECG, unrelated to patient QRS complex; intrinsic heart rate approximates pacemaker demand rate	A. Wire dislodgement or fracture, loose connections, or faulty lead/cable	1. Verify lead integrity (from insertion site to pacemaker). 2. Inspect terminal connections of leads to pacemaker unit; verify tight contact.
	B. Patient's rate is nearly identical to the pacer rate	1. Either increase the pacer rate (to overdrive the patient's rhythm) or decrease the pacer rate to allow distinction of the patient's intrinsic electrical activity from the pacemaker impulses (physician's order required).
	C. Pacemaker failure to sense	1. Sensitivity setting (threshold) is too low to enable pacemaker inhibition by intrinsic activity; increase the sensitivity until consistent sensing occurs or competition ceases.
Failure to capture: Pacing artifact (pacing spikes) not consistently followed by evidence of chamber depolarization	A. Battery failure	1. For pacer-dependent patients an additional pacer generator should be immediately available at all times; a quick switch of generators may be necessary. 2. Battery life indicator should be checked routinely; if battery strength doubtful, change battery.
	B. Lead fracture, loose lead connections, or faulty lead/cable	1. Check external connections. 2. Verify lead placement with physician (or other on-call provider); if both leads are placed in cardiac tissue, switch the bipolar wires in their terminals; if the lead fracture is confined to one wire, this switch may enable the intact lead to function as the pacing lead in the (−) terminal, and the fractured lead will serve as the ground; note that the fractured lead should be secured to an electrode plate with tape, then taped to the skin or placed subcutaneously by the physician. 3. If consistent capture cannot be produced by lead rearrangement, a diagnostic atrial electrogram may be required to determine bipolar lead integrity. Lead replacement may be necessary. 4. Change cable between pacer and leads.
	C. Inhibition of pacer stimulus	1. May occur when the pacer is inhibited by external electrical interference, such as electrocautery, razors, radios, diathermy units. If electrical devices must be used, it may be necessary to set pacer generator in asynchronous mode to provide consistent pacing.
	D. Inadequate pacer output	1. Increase output of pacer. 2. Note that high-amplitude atrial pacing may inhibit ventricular pacer; adjust the atrial output control to decrease the current, but still maintain atrial capture.
Failure to capture: Artifact present	A. Faulty lead placement (or lead displacement), loose connection, or faulty lead/cable	1. Epicardial leads are rarely displaced but a subcutaneous ground lead or transvenous lead may dislodge with movement. 2. If transvenous pacing in place, turn patient on left side to promote contact between transvenous lead and apex of right ventricle. 3. Repositioning of transvenous leads may be accomplished by a physician or other on-call

Continued

Table 21-7   **Troubleshooting Pacemaker Malfunctions—cont'd**

Observation	Causes	Intervention
		provider. Displaced epicardial leads require replacement by a surgeon.
		4. For a pacer-dependent patient, standby pacer generators and transvenous pacing catheter insertion tray should always be immediately available.
		5. Twelve-lead ECG, epicardiograms, and chest x-ray may be required.
	B. Increased myocardial threshold	1. Fibrosis or ischemia at the wire site can increase the stimulation threshold. Increase the pacer output by 1-2 mA or until capture is observed. If loss of capture occurs at high output (20 mA), lead displacement may be present.
		2. Note that with epicardial wires, increased stimulation thresholds often exceed the capability of temporary generators within 7-10 days.
Failure to sense: Pacemaker spikes follow patient QRS complex	A. Faulty lead placement, loose connection, or faulty lead/cable	1. Change cables between patient and leads.
		2. Notify physician or other on-call provider; repositioning of lead may be required.
		3. Safeguard against competition by adjusting pacemaker demand rate to higher or lower than patient's intrinsic heart rate (and optimal systemic perfusion).
	B. Sensitivity too low	1. Adjust pacer sensitivity in a clockwise direction until appropriate sensing occurs.
	C. Fibrosis at wire-tip causing impaired sensing	1. Increase pacemaker sensitivity.
		2. Lead should be repositioned or replaced by physician.
	D. Low battery	1. Change batteries.
Oversensing: Pacemaker inhibited inappropriately; "sensing" indicator documents that pacer is sensing in absence of appropriate intrinsic electrical activity	A. Pacemaker sensitivity too high	1. Pacemaker is "sensing" artifact that occurs at a rate faster than the set demand ventricular rate. If this occurs, patient's intrinsic rate may fall below the pacemaker demand rate.
		2. Turn the sensitivity control counterclockwise toward "asynchronous" until inhibition ceases or pacing rate increases.
	B. Circuit failure within pacemaker	1. Replace the pacemaker unit.

Defibrillation has occurred if the shock eliminates the disorganized electrical activity for 5 seconds. After elimination of the disorganized activity, return of spontaneous rhythm must occur and ultimately result in return of a perfusing rhythm, called return of spontaneous circulation (ROSC). Cardiopulmonary resuscitation (CPR) should be provided until a defibrillator is available and immediately after shock delivery until it is time to recheck the rhythm or ROSC occurs.

As noted above, defibrillation is indicated in cases of VF or pulseless VT. Defibrillation is achieved using adhesive patches or through the use of two metal-plated contacts (paddles) that are placed externally on the chest wall or in some cases, directly on the heart.

When cardiac arrest is caused by a shockable rhythm (ventricular tachycardia or ventricular fibrillation), early CPR plus early defibrillation is consistently associated with a greater likelihood of survival. In the prehospital setting, automated

external defibrillator (AED) programs facilitate early CPR and early defibrillation by trained first responders and have been shown to improve survival from out-of-hospital VF cardiac arrest. AEDs are computerized devices that analyze a cardiac rhythm to determine if a shock is needed, and provide audio and voice prompts to enable those who are not trained in rhythm interpretation to deliver a shock.[63]

In the hospital setting, many defibrillators that are located in inpatient units have manual mode, or automated external defibrillator (AED) mode. In the critical care setting, defibrillation is typically performed in manual mode, eliminating the time it takes for the AED to interpret the rhythm.[191]

When cardiac arrest is associated with a shockable rhythm, prompt CPR and defibrillation are needed for the infant, the child and the adult. Although AEDs can be used for infants, manual defibrillators are preferred to enable dose adjustment. When AEDs are used for infants or children less than 8 years of age, a pediatric attenuator (typically a pad-cable system, although a key may be used) should be used, if available, to reduce the dose delivered. If during AED use a pediatric attenuator is not available, the adult pads and dose should be used because prompt CPR and early shock delivery are necessary for survival from VF or VT cardiac arrest.

Pads and Paddles. When AED pads are used, the "child" pads are used for infants and children and adult pads are used for any patients 8 years of age (about 25 kg) or older. The AED pads are applied as illustrated on the pad package. Typically, a sternoapical position is used (one pad is applied to the patient's right upper sternal border and the other pad is applied lateral to the patient's left nipple, between the nipple and left axilla). However, some AEDs pad packages will illustrate an anterior-posterior adhesive pad placement. The pads should not touch or overlap.

For manual defibrillation, the shock may be delivered through paddles or adhesive electrode pads. If adhesive pads are used for manual defibrillation, the pads selected should generally be the largest size that will fit completely on the chest without touching each other, but users should follow the size recommendations and placement illustrated on the pad package. Adhesive pads have contact gel surface as part of the pads.

Defibrillator paddles are selected based on weight and age. Pediatric-sized paddles should be used when the child is less than 10 kg or less than 1 year old. The adult-sized paddles should be used if the patient is 10 kg or greater or 1 year old or greater. Electrode cream is applied to the paddles before they are placed on the patient's chest (sonographic gel or saline-soaked gauze should not be used), to ensure good contact between the paddles and the chest.

For manual defibrillation the paddles and pads are placed so the heart is between them. The sternoapical position is often used: one pad or paddle is placed on the patient's upper right chest along the patient's right upper sternal border. The other pad/paddle is generally placed lateral to the left nipple in the anterior axillary line. Ensure that the pads/paddles do not touch or overlap.

An alternative pad placement is the anterior-posterior position, placing one pad on the anterior chest and one on the posterior chest. This method is preferred if the patient has a small chest or when only large pads are available for a smaller patient.

Modification of pad placement may be necessary based on the patient's underlying condition or the presence of implanted devices or transdermal patches. In patients with dextrocardia, position the pads/paddles in a mirror image of the standard placement. In patients with implanted devices or transdermal patches, the pads should not be placed directly over the device or the transdermal patch.,[63,54] If time allows, remove the transdermal patch and quickly wipe the medication off the chest.

When using a defibrillator in manual mode, it is the responsibility of the provider to interpret the heart rhythm to determine if a shock is indicated, to charge the device to the appropriate dose, to "clear" the victim before a shock is delivered and deliver the shock. If a shock is indicated, Pediatric Advanced Life Support (PALS) guidelines should be followed:

- Initial dose of 2 to 4 J/kg (for ease of teaching, 2 J/kg is typically used).
- Second dose of 4 J/kg

- Subsequent doses should be 4 J/kg or higher (maximum of 10 J/kg).[92]

Defibrillators deliver energy in a variety of waveforms that are characterized as monophasic or biphasic. Most defibrillators made before the mid-1990s are monophasic devices. All defibrillators manufactured today are biphasic defibrillators that reverse current polarity of the delivered shock 5 to 10 ms after discharge begins.[140] Biphasic waveforms defibrillate more effectively (i.e., they are more likely to eliminate VF with one shock) and at lower energies than monophasic waveforms; however, monophasic waveforms are still highly effective in most situations.[140]

Factors Determining Effectiveness of Attempted Defibrillation

A variety of factors can influence the effectiveness of the defibrillation attempt. These factors include the electrode size and contact, the conductive surface, the chest wall impedance, and myocardial acidosis and ischemia. The time between the last compression and shock delivery also can influence shock effectiveness.[50,103]

Electrodes. Electrodes must be in good position and pad/paddle size must be correct. If using adhesive pads or electrodes, they must completely adhere to the chest to be effective. In adolescent males with chest hair, the chest can be shaved to improve adherence.

Conductive Gel. When adhesive pads are used, a conductive surface is present on the adhesive pad, so no additional conductive gel is needed. When paddles are used, the conductive substance must be placed on the paddles or chest wall to facilitate the transfer of electricity during external defibrillation and preserve skin intactness. Saline-soaked gauze or sonographic gel should not be used.[92,140]

The provider should not allow the conductive gel to create a bridge between the paddles; if such a bridge is present, the current may travel from paddle to paddle, bypassing the heart. The paddles should not touch one another.

Chest (Transthoracic) Impedance. Successful defibrillation may be prevented by chest impedance. Impedance is determined by energy level, electrode size, electrode to skin interface, phase of ventilation (energy can dissipate to the lungs), and thoracic structure.[140] Chest impedance (resistance) to electrical current decreases with successive countershocks. If the same energy output from the defibrillator is maintained, the current delivered to the patient will increase slightly with each defibrillator discharge. The greatest increase in current delivery occurs with the second impulse.

The American Heart Association PALS guidelines recommend a manual defibrillator dose of 4 J/kg for the second defibrillation attempt, and a dose of 4 J/kg or higher for subsequent attempts. The AHA recommends a maximum manual pediatric defibrillation dose of 10 J/kg.[92]

Integration of CPR with Shock Delivery and Optimal Defibrillation. Studies have shown that if the interval between the last compression and shock delivery is 10 seconds or less, the shock is highly likely to eliminate VF. For every additional 10 seconds that elapse between the last compression and shock delivery, the shock effectiveness decreases substantially.[50] As a result, it is very important for the resuscitation team to practice coordination of CPR and shock delivery, to minimize interruptions in chest compressions overall and minimize the interval between the last compression and shock delivery.[103]

Even when shock delivery successfully eliminates the shockable rhythm, the myocardium will be unable to generate a perfusing rhythm for seconds or minutes. CPR, beginning with chest compressions should resume immediately after shock delivery.

An ischemic or acidotic myocardium will be difficult to defibrillate (i.e., it is difficult for the shock to eliminate VF). The patient should be adequately oxygenated and ventilated, and high-quality CPR must be performed. To provide high-quality CPR, providers should compress to an adequate depth (at least one-third the anterior-posterior dimension of the infant or child chest, about 1½ inches for the infant and about 2 inches for the child), with a rate of at least 100/minute, allowing complete chest recoil after each compression, minimizing interruptions in chest compressions, and avoiding excessive ventilation). High-quality CPR should optimize blood flow during resuscitation.

Synchronized Cardioversion

Cardioversion delivers a shock timed to coincide with the patient's intrinsic R wave. It is indicated to terminate tachyarrhythmias such as those involved in a reentrant circuit, atrial fibrillation, atrial flutter and atrial tachycardia, and monomorphic ventricular tachycardia.[140] Cardioversion is not effective for treatment of junctional tachycardia or ectopic or multifocal atrial tachycardia because these rhythms have an automatic focus that results from spontaneous depolarization of local cells.[103] In fact, shock delivery to patients with these automatic rhythms may well increase the tachycardia.

Cardioversion is performed using a defibrillator/cardioverter to deliver a lower dose than the dose used for defibrillation. The synchronized low-dose shock should convert a harmful tachyarrhythmia, such as ventricular tachycardia with pulses, supraventricular tachycardia (SVT), atrial flutter, or atrial fibrillation to a more normal rhythm.[92] To provide synchronized cardioversion, the patient's ECG signal must be sensed by the defibrillator unit. This can be accomplished using the defibrillator pads (ensure they are sticking well to the patient's chest), or ECG leads linked to the defibrillator. The defibrillator must be in synchronized mode and the patient's ECG should be recorded during the cardioversion attempt.

Synchronized cardioversion is administered through adhesive patches or handheld paddles. When the defibrillator unit senses the ECG signal adequately, the defibrillator will display a signal that marks the R wave on the display, indicating readiness for cardioversion. If there is inadequate sensing of the patient R wave, the defibrillator will not discharge.[92,140]

The energy select control enables selection of the energy dose for cardioversion. For pediatric purposes, energy selection must be available in small increments at the low energy levels to allow selection of the lowest but most effective defibrillator energy level for a small patient. The initial energy level recommended by the American Heart Association for

defibrillation of children is 0.5 to 1 J/kg, with the second dose typically increased to 2 J/kg if the first energy is not effective. Pediatric Advanced Life Support guidelines should be followed when cardioversion is performed.[92,103]

Cardioversion can be elective or emergent. In unstable tachyarrhythmias when cardiovascular compromise produces signs such as hypotension or poor perfusion, cardioversion should be delivered immediately by a skilled provider. If possible, provide sedation before shock delivery, but do not delay cardioversion in such emergencies.

Vagal maneuvers stimulate vagal activity and can terminate tachyarrhythmias. In unstable tachyarrhythmias, vagal maneuvers should only be attempted while other arrangements are made for medication management or electrical cardioversion. When the tachyarrhythmia is stable (i.e., not producing shock or other signs of severe compromise in perfusion), vagal maneuvers should be attempted before other interventions.

The vagal maneuvers that are appropriate for use in children depends on the age of the child and the child's ability to cooperate. The most effective vagal maneuver for infants and children is applying ice to the face. A bag or glove may be filled with ice (and a small amount of water) and placed on the patient's face for about 10 to 15 seconds. Ensure that the bag of ice does not cover the patient's nose or mouth. If this maneuver works, the rhythm should convert to a normal sinus rhythm in a matter of seconds.

An older child can be asked to bear down as if having a bowel movement, blow through an obstructed straw, or hold his or her breath while ice is put to the face. For optimum safety and monitoring, the patient should be connected to an ECG monitor when vagal maneuvers are used to attempt cardioversion.[92]

Circulatory Assist Devices

Ventricular Assist Device (VAD)
Nancy A. Pike

Ventricular assist devices (VAD) have been used over the last three decades for temporary support of the failing heart.[73,150] The primary goal of VAD therapy is either to allow myocardial recovery or to act as a "bridge to transplant" when medical therapy has failed.[18] Potential indications for pediatric VAD support include severe ventricular failure producing a "shocklike state" or the progression of multiorgan failure resulting from acute fulminant myocarditis, cardiomyopathy, postcardiotomy failure, posttransplantation graft failure, and end-stage congenital heart disease.

The VAD is a heart pump that can be used to support the right ventricle (right ventricular assist device [RVAD]), the left ventricle (left ventricular assist device [LVAD]), or both ventricles (biventricular assist device [BiVAD]). Most VADs have three major components: a pump (located inside or outside the body), a control system, and an energy source (either battery or compressed air, as seen in pneumatic devices). The VADs most commonly used in pediatrics are extracorporeal (outside of the body) and are connected to inflow and outflow cannulae.

The VAD pumps can be further subdivided into *continuous flow* (nonpulsatile) and *pulsatile* pumps. The most common continuous flow VAD is the centrifugal Bio-Medicus Bio-Pump

(Medtronic, Inc., Eden Prairie, MN) (see Figure 7-3 and Fig. 21-27). The Bio-Pump uses two magnetically coupled, polycarbonate rotator cones that spin to create centrifugal force along a vertical axis.[33] The pump output is proportional to revolutions per minute (rpm) and is adjusted according to the venous return or preload. This pump produces a continuous, nonpulsatile arterial blood flow to the body at a mean pressure.

The pulsatile VADs contain a reservoir. Blood is ejected by the pump either electronically through movement of pusher plates or with compressed air movement of the bladder (Fig. 21-28). These devices propel blood in synchrony with the patient's ventricular ejection, producing pulsatile arterial blood flow to the body.

The selection of VAD type is influenced by the indication for the device, the duration of support anticipated, the size of the patient, and the devices available (see Table 7-3 for information about devices used in children). The continuous flow

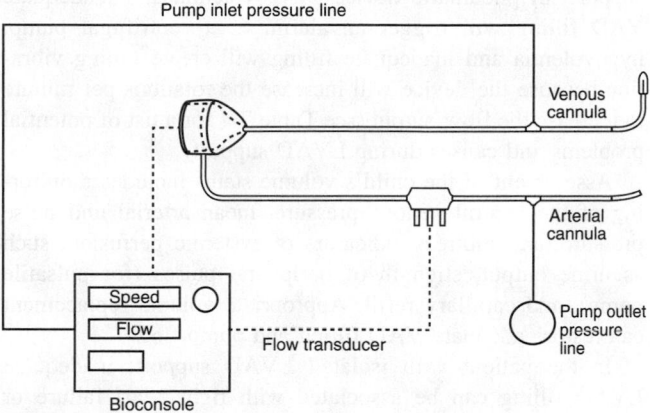

FIG. 21-27 Schematic of centrifugal pump. (Redrawn from an illustration of the centrifugal VAD pump by Medtronic, Minneapolis, Minnesota.)

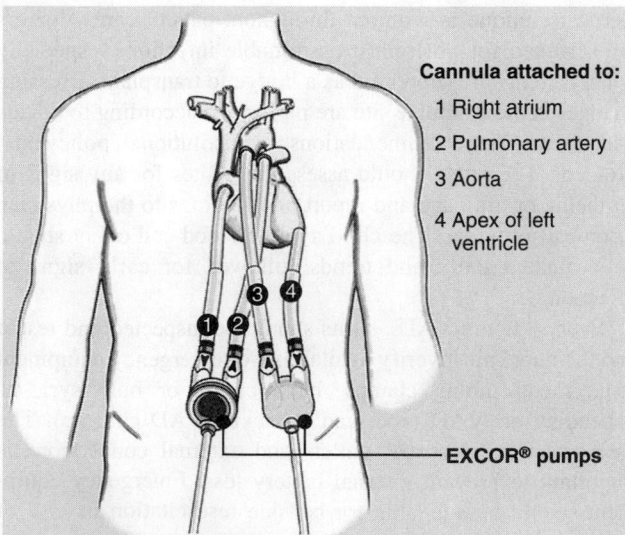

FIG. 21-28 Extracorporeal pneumatic biventricular assist device. (Redrawn from an illustration of the Berlin EXCOR by Berlin Heart, Berlin, Germany.)

or centrifugal VADs are generally used to provide more short-term support and the pulsatile devices are typically considered for long-term support.[33]

Physiologic Effects of VAD Support. All VADs are preload dependent, which means the amount of blood returning to the heart is the amount of blood pumped to the body. The VAD is sensitive to impedance to flow, so hypertension and mechanical obstruction must be corrected.

The LVAD and RVAD allow blood to bypass the failing ventricle. The pumps decompress the ventricle, decrease myocardial work, and reduce oxygen demand while maintaining adequate systemic perfusion to sustain end-organ function. VAD support has been shown to improve myocardial contractility and recovery of ventricular function during support.[47]

Clinical Applications. The VAD cannulae are placed through direct visualization of the mediastinal vessels. When an LVAD is used, the inflow cannula (carrying blood from the patient to the pump) is inserted into either the left atrium or the left ventricle. The outflow cannula (carrying blood from the pump to the patient) is inserted in the ascending aorta. When an RVAD is used, the inflow cannula is inserted in either the right atrium or right ventricle and the outflow cannula is inserted into the pulmonary artery.

If the VAD support is serving as a bridge to recovery, the inflow cannula is often connected to the patient's atrium. This cannulation is technically easier and spares the ventricle further injury. However, ventricular cannulation enables higher flow rates, so ventricular cannulation is used when VAD support is used as a bridge to transplant, because ventricular injury is not a concern.

The inflow and outflow cannulae are brought through skin incisions. When the pneumatic device is used for long-term support the mediastinum is closed. The external pump is connected, deaired, and circulatory assistance is initiated. Centrifugal VAD cannulae are brought through an open mediastinum, which remains open for short-term support.

The VAD console and energy source vary depending on the VAD type. Most pneumatic consoles display both left and right heart support, pump rate in beats per minute, systolic pressure, diastolic (or fill) pressure, and vacuum drive pressure. Flow rates depend on preload and the size of the external pump. An infant-sized pump (preload of 12 or 15 mL) provides flows averaging 0.5-1.3 L/minute, and a child-sized pump (preload of 25 or 30 mL) provides average flows of 1.3-3.3 L/minute.[16,58]

During long-term use, the external pump size can be changed to accommodate the child's growth and increased stroke volume. The consoles also have backup units in case of malfunction. These backup units can be automatically or manually converted depending on the device. In addition, the consoles can be operated by external electrical power as well as internal batteries.

The console of the centrifugal pump displays the speed and blood flow rate; both are manually adjusted by the operator. The VAD is initiated at minimum flow and quickly increased to a flow rate of 150 mL/kg per minute. Once the child is stable, flow is reduced to 70% of the calculated cardiac output.[85] Inlet and outlet pressure monitors are also used to guide pump speed and prevent tubing collapse. External electrical power and internal batteries operate the console if transport is needed.

The duration of VAD support depends on myocardial recovery associated with postcardiotomy or acute myocarditis. Ventricular recovery is monitored by both clinical and echocardiographic parameters. Support can be required for a few weeks to years if awaiting heart transplantation.

The removal of the VAD can be performed at the bedside in children with an open chest (those who have required only a short duration of support). Removal occurs in the operating suite if a redo sternotomy incision is needed for removal.

Potential Complications. The potential benefits of VAD therapy must be weighed against the potential risks. These risks include bleeding requiring reoperation, cerebral emboli (thrombus or air), hemolysis, infection, and mechanical failure. Bleeding and embolism are the most common complications after VAD insertion. Mild to moderate bleeding is common and most often caused by the required anticoagulation, a coagulopathy, or surgical bleeding. Excessive bleeding requiring massive transfusions often results in pulmonary and multiorgan dysfunction and can be fatal.

Neurologic events such as intracranial hemorrhage and cerebral emboli can result in significant long-term neurologic deficits. Cerebral emboli and stroke have multifactorial causes and the risk is compounded by smaller pump sizes, use of lower VAD flows when using larger adult equipment, and challenges of anticoagulation in children.[85] The current use of heparin coated circuits may potentially reduce the occurrence of cerebral embolism related to thrombus formation in the smaller pump sizes with lower flow rates. Hemolysis or destruction of red blood cells can also occur from prolonged or turbulent blood flow through the device.

Children are at high risk for hospital-acquired infections during VAD support. The most common infections reported are from surgical sites.[33] The VAD external cannulae skin sites remain sites of potential infection until the tissue has closed from granulation. Mechanical failure of the pump or console is rare but can occur related to the internal battery or external power failure.

Nursing Considerations. The critical care nurse should understand the physiology of VAD support, and must be familiar with device components and VAD function.[44] In pulsatile pumps, the nurse should verify complete VAD emptying and filling by documenting pressures noted on the device console and through visual inspection every hour. The VAD external pump and drive lines should also be examined hourly for air, thrombus, or tubing stress fractures. If thrombus is noted in the pump or external cannulae, a physician should be notified immediately.

Because cerebral emboli are among the most common complications during VAD support, it is imperative that the nurse perform frequent neurologic assessments. These assessments can be challenging when the patient is sedated during support. Neurologic complications may manifest more as cardiovascular instability, such as changes in heart rate and blood pressure.

The nurse is responsible for ensuring appropriate anticoagulation by following the activated partial thromboplastin time (aPTT) or other anticoagulation parameters (e.g., platelet function assays, antithrombin III levels, or activated clotting times [ACTs]), according to institutional protocols or device recommendations (see Chapter 7). Frequent observation for signs of external and internal bleeding is required to prevent volume loss and unrecognized hemorrhage and preventable neurologic complications.

When stable, the children on long-term pneumatic VAD support can be transitioned from a heparin infusion to oral anticoagulation agents according to the device manufacturer's recommendations and institutional protocols. Additional information about nursing care of the child with a VAD is provided in Box 7-3.

During the initiation of VAD support, the most common cause of inadequate flow is hypovolemia. It is important to monitor for signs of hypovolemia during VAD initiation and support. In pneumatic devices, hypovolemia and inadequate VAD filling will trigger an alarm. In a centrifugal pump, hypovolemia and inadequate filling will create tubing vibration because the device will increase the rotations per minute to increase the flow output (see Table 7-4 for a list of potential problems and causes during LVAD support).

Assessment of the child's volume status includes monitoring of the central venous pressure, mean arterial and pulse pressure, and indirect indicators of systemic perfusion, such as urine output, strength of peripheral pulses (for pulsatile pump), and capillary refill. Appropriate volume replacement can restore adequate VAD filling and pump flow.

In the patient with isolated LVAD support, inadequate LVAD filling can be associated with right heart failure or increased pulmonary vascular resistance with resultant decreased right ventricular output and pulmonary venous return. Right heart failure should be considered if these signs are observed in the presence of adequate vascular volume.

The risk of infection during VAD support is especially high if thoracic cannulation is performed. Meticulous aseptic and sterile technique is required throughout patient care. Visitors are screened for potential transmittable infections, especially when patients are supported as a bridge to transplant. Dressing changes at the cannulae site are performed according to device manufacturer's recommendations or institutional policy and protocol. The nurse should assess these sites for any signs of erythema or drainage and report any findings to the physician or on-call provider. The child's white blood cell count should be evaluated daily and trends followed for early signs of infection.

Every 8 hours VAD alarms should be inspected and tested and the nurse must verify availability of emergency equipment (e.g., metal tubing clamps, hand crank, or bulb syringes depending on VAD type, and a backup VAD console). The assessment of electrical outlets and external connections is important to prevent internal battery loss. Emergency equipment should be available for bedside resuscitation in case of pump malfunction or loss of power.

The child with a VAD that is serving as a bridge to transplant will require adequate nutritional support, emotional support, and physical rehabilitation. Early extubation, ambulation, and removal of invasive lines have been documented to improve outcomes and minimize postoperative complications after pneumatic VAD insertion.[33] For additional information about nursing care of the child with a VAD, see Chapter 7, including the Nursing Care Plan in Box 7-3.

The Intraaortic Balloon Pump (IABP)

The intraaortic balloon pump (IABP) is well-established in adults for treatment of acute low cardiac output syndrome and cardiogenic shock after myocardial infarction or cardiac surgery.[38] The IABP is not used commonly in children because of the widespread availability of extracorporeal membrane oxygenation (ECMO) and left ventricular assist devices at most pediatric cardiovascular surgery centers.[38,83,139]

The IABP can provide temporary left ventricular support in children when maximum pharmacologic support fails to result in adequate cardiac output after intracardiac surgery, cardiomyopathy, myocarditis, or severe sepsis. However, its use in infants and small children remains limited because it is difficult to insert the catheters and difficult to synchronize the device with the small child's rapid heart rate.[38,71,83,139]

The IABP balloon is placed in the aorta through a right femoral artery cut down. A side arm sheath is placed through the skin to the artery, and the balloon catheter is passed through the sheath into the femoral artery and passed retrograde into the descending aorta, so the tip lies just distal to (approximately 2 cm below) the left subclavian artery and the balloon is above the branches of the renal and mesenteric arteries (Fig. 21-29). The standard balloon volume in children ranges from 2.5 to 20 mL. (The adult volume is 40 mL.)[71]

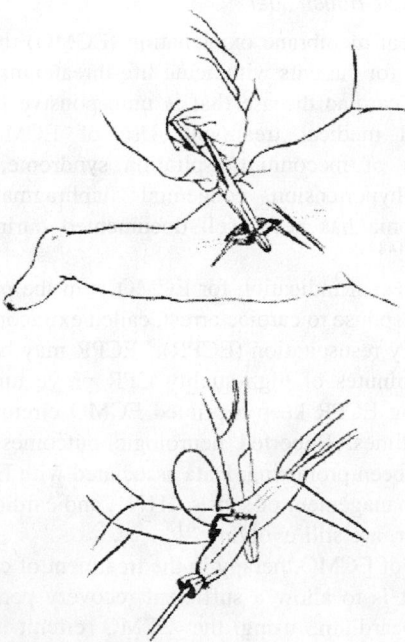

FIG. 21-29 Operative technique for insertion of femoral artery sheath for insertion of intraaortic balloon pumping catheter. The common femoral artery is isolated through a vertical groin incision. The balloon catheter is inserted through a sidearm graft of polytetrafluoroethylene. This graft is sewn to a longitudinal arteriotomy in the femoral artery. (From Pinckney KA, Minich LL, Tani LY, et al: Current results with intraaortic balloon pumping in infants and children. *Ann Thorac Surg* 73:887-891, 2002.)

Physiologic Effects of IABP Counterpulsation. IABP counterpulsation should augment perfusion during diastole and reduce left ventricular afterload. Diastolic augmentation is achieved by balloon inflation during diastole—the balloon displaces blood volume equal to the balloon volume retrograde into the aortic root, to augment coronary artery perfusion and antegrade into the systemic vessels to augment diastolic perfusion.

Afterload reduction is accomplished by balloon deflation just before ventricular ejection. This produces an acute decrease in intraaortic volume and pressure so that resistance to left ventricular ejection decreases. Less left ventricular work is required to eject blood into an area of low blood volume and low pressure, so the efficiency of the left ventricle is improved.

Pediatric Considerations. The challenges with counterpulsation in children relate to their small size, aortic distensibility, and rapid heart rates. IABP insertion is more technically challenging in small pediatric vessels. In addition, balloon size and length of the aorta are not always predictable based on the child's size. If the balloon is too long it may occlude the renal and mesenteric arteries, theoretically producing renal or mesenteric ischemia.

Children exhibit greater aortic compliance than adults, and this may diminish the degree of diastolic augmentation achieved during IABP therapy, because balloon inflation may stretch the aorta more than it provides counterpulsation. In children, afterload reduction, rather than diastolic augmentation, has been shown to be the primary method of circulatory assistance provided during IABP therapy in children.[38]

The child's heart rate is much faster than that of an adult. As a result, the balloon inflation and deflation must be rapid enough during short diastolic and systolic intervals. The standard method of balloon pump timing is "triggering" from the R wave of the electrocardiogram (ECG) or the dicrotic notch on the arterial waveform. Triggering from the ECG and arterial waveform is limited when the heart rate exceeds 150 to 160/minute, or when there is a narrow pulse pressure or potential dampened waveform in low cardiac output; these conditions are common to the critically ill child. For these reasons, the ECG and arterial waveform are used as rough guidelines for adjusting IABP timing in pediatrics. Some centers have reported using M-mode echocardiography to periodically check proper balloon inflation and deflation.[139]

Potential Complications. Complications reported during pediatric IABP therapy include limb ischemia, thrombocytopenia, thromboembolic events, infection, balloon rupture, vessel perforation or aortic dissection, and mesenteric, renal, or cerebral ischemia.[38,71,139] The most frequent pediatric complication of IABP therapy is limb ischemia or circulatory insufficiency in the catheterized limb. This circulatory insufficiency produces a decreased arterial pulse, cool skin, and pallor.

Thrombocytopenia (50% reduction in platelet count) frequently develops during IABP therapy because platelets are deposited on the surface of the balloon. Emboli from the balloon or catheter can develop if the IABP is dormant for longer than 15 minutes, because blood becomes trapped in the folds of the deflated balloon, prompting the formation of clots. If the IABP is dormant for longer than 15 minutes, manual inflation and deflation are required every 5 minutes until the problem is resolved. Of greatest concern is a cerebral embolism; thorough neurologic assessment is warranted at regular intervals.

Rare complications of IABP therapy in children include balloon rupture with possible resultant gas (carbon dioxide or helium) embolism. Blood observed in the driveline or tubing can indicate balloon rupture. The on-call physician should be notified immediately of possible balloon rupture and the nurse should prepare for IABP removal.

Infection or bleeding at the insertion site may develop but is rarely reported. Renal and mesenteric ischemia are also rare but have been reported as possibly related to balloon occlusion of the splanchnic arteries.[38] Renal ischemia will produce oliguria and mesenteric ischemia may produce decreased bowel sounds, abdominal distension and tenderness, and guaiac-positive stool.

Nursing Considerations. The pediatric nurse should be knowledgeable about the purpose and physiologic effect of IABP support, ensure proper console function, and know how to make adjustments to improving timing of balloon inflation and deflation. Every 4 to 8 hours (determined by institutional protocol), a rhythm strip and recording of the arterial pressure waveform should be saved in the patient record to enable comparison of the assisted and unassisted pulse to assess diastolic augmentation at the correct ratio (e.g., 1:2).[71]

In assessing timing of balloon inflation, the peak of diastolic augmentation should be higher than the peak of the unassisted systole. As the balloon deflates just before systole, the pressure in the aorta drops. The assisted aortic end-diastolic pressure should be lower than the unassisted aortic end-diastolic pressure. Because the balloon reduces afterload, the peak of the assisted systole should be lower than the peak of the unassisted systole (see Fig. 21-30 and Figure 7-5).

During IABP therapy, the nurse must vigilantly monitor for signs of the following complications: catheterized limb

ischemia, significant fall in platelet count, emboli (gas or particulate matter), aortic injury, hemolysis, and infection. Flexion of the catheterized limb must be avoided to prevent kinking of the catheter and improper balloon function. This may require the use of a leg splint, restraints, or sedation. While the balloon pump is in place, the patient is turned by log rolling and care should be maintained to prevent skin breakdown.

Strict aseptic technique must be practiced to avoid possible sources of contamination and infection. A urinary catheter should be placed to monitor hourly urine output, but also to reduce the risk of urine contamination at the IABP catheter insertion site. Dressing changes at the insertion site should be performed daily, with signs of erythema or drainage reported to the physician or on-call provider. The white blood cell count should be evaluated daily and combined with patient assessment for signs of infection.

Balloon placement should be evaluated by a daily chest radiograph. The balloon is positioned so it is above the renal artery and distal to (approximately 2 cm below) the origin of the left subclavian artery. Among centers providing pediatric IABP therapy, routine anticoagulation practice includes a heparin infusion to maintain an activated partial thromboplastin time (aPTT) of 40 to 60 seconds.[71,83] The nurse is responsible for ensuring that proper anticoagulation is maintained and monitoring for signs of heparin-induced bleeding.

Daily blood sampling is performed to monitor cardiac enzymes, complete blood count with differential, electrolytes, and blood gas analysis as indicated. Additional information about IABP therapy is included in Chapter 7.

Extracorporeal Membrane Oxygenation
Linda Nylander-Housholder

Extracorporeal membrane oxygenation (ECMO) therapy may be indicated for patients with acute life-threatening reversible lung and/or cardiac disease that is unresponsive to maximal conventional medical treatment. Use of ECMO for the management of meconium aspiration syndrome, persistent pulmonary hypertension, congenital diaphragmatic hernia, and pneumonia has been well documented during the last decade.[14,66,148]

A more recent indication for ECMO is in the provision of support in response to cardiac arrest, called extracorporeal cardiopulmonary resuscitation (ECPR).[5] ECPR may be indicated if 5 to 10 minutes of high-quality CPR prove unsuccessful. Centers using ECPR keep a primed ECMO circuit ready for use at all times. Reported neurologic outcomes following ECPR have been promising. Data associated with ECMO support in the management of sepsis, H1N1, and cardiogenic failure, however, are still evolving.[4,13]

The goal of ECMO therapy in the treatment of cardiac failure or arrest is to allow a sufficient recovery period for the failing myocardium, using the ECMO circuit to provide oxygenation and maintain systemic perfusion. In children with severe respiratory failure, an oxygenation index (OI) greater than 40 (in neonates an OI greater than 35) and worsening respiratory failure despite maximal mechanical support of oxygenation and ventilation is a common indication for ECMO support. Some centers use an alveolar-arterial oxygen content difference (AaDO$_2$) greater than 600 for between 4

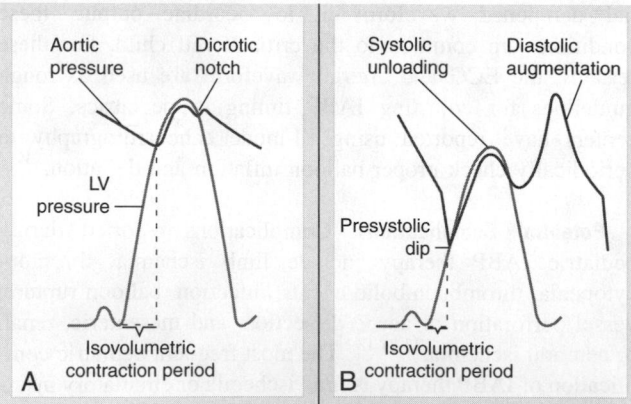

FIG. 21-30 Left ventricular and aortic pressure curves. **A,** Normal curve. **B,** With counterpulsation from intraaortic balloon pump. The balloon inflates rapidly at the beginning of diastole, just after aortic valve closure or at the dicrotic notch, timed with the ECG. Balloon inflation augments the aortic diastolic pressure (see diastolic augmentation), so diastolic pressure may be higher than systolic pressure. Rapid balloon deflation (see presystolic dip) just before ventricular ejection augments ventricular ejection. (From Cercek B, Shah PK: Complications of acute myocardial infarction. In Crawford MH, editor: *Cardiology*, ed 3, St Louis, 2009, Mosby.)

and 12 hours (at sea level) as an indication (see Box 7-1). These criteria have been used to predict probable mortality with medical management and describe possible indications for the use of ECMO. However, lack of standardized patient classification criteria and failure to define standards for maximal medical therapy worldwide have made evaluation of ECMO therapy difficult.

Physiologic Effects of ECMO Therapy. ECMO is a cardiopulmonary bypass device that uses a diffusion membrane oxygenator or a hollow-fiber oxygenator.[4,66,124,148,192] Blood is circulated through the oxygenator by a roller or centrifugal pump at flow rates of approximately 100 to 120 mL/kg per minute (for full support). Roller pumps use compression and displacement to circulate blood as rollers travel the length of the raceway tubing within the pump head. The use of centrifugal pumps has increased in recent years because they are not dependent on gravity to achieve venous flow, cause less hemolysis, and have fewer mechanical complications than the roller pump.

A semipermeable diffusion membrane facilitates oxygen diffusion using a fresh flow of oxygen into the gas compartment of the oxygenator unit; carbon dioxide is removed simultaneously. Entry ports in the circuit allow for the administration of heparin, blood products, or medications, and the withdrawal of blood for laboratory sampling, as well the addition of hemofiltration, continuous arteriovenous hemodilution (CAVHD) or apheresis as deemed by patient need.

A heat exchanger inline or incorporated into the oxygenator maintains appropriate blood temperature. Systemic anticoagulation with heparin is necessary to prevent clot formation within the circuit; the activated clotting times usually are maintained between 200 to 240 seconds (refer to institutional protocols) through titration of heparin administration. Heparin-bonded circuits have the potential to decrease or eliminate the need for systemic anticoagulation.

Clinical Applications. A cannula placed in either the right internal jugular vein or the femoral vein diverts patient venous blood to the ECMO circuit. Oxygenated patient blood is returned to the body through a vein or artery.

When ECMO is used to support cardiac and/or respiratory function, a *venoarterial* (VA) circuit is used and oxygenated blood is frequently returned to the patient through a cannula into the right common carotid artery with the tip of the cannula advanced to the innominate artery. This arterial flow provides antegrade perfusion of the body and retrograde perfusion of the aortic arch vessels and coronary arteries. The femoral artery and vein may be used for VA ECMO cannulation in adolescent and adult patients. With this venoarterial cannulation and full flow, the heart and lungs are bypassed.

A disadvantage of the VA configuration is that the high flow returning to the aorta may increase resistance to left ventricular ejection. In the presence of severe ventricular dysfunction, this increase in left ventricular afterload may cause left ventricular function to deteriorate further. The concomitant use of the intraaortic balloon pump has been proposed to diminish left ventricular afterload, but extensive experience has not been reported.

If myocardial function is good and ECMO will be used to improve oxygenation only, *venovenous* (VV) ECMO may be used. Venous blood is drained to the ECMO device and oxygenated blood is returned to the patient through the femoral or other large central vein.

Two venous cannulae or a double-lumen single venous cannula may be used depending on the child's size. The oxygenated blood then is pumped by the patient's heart through the pulmonary and systemic circulations. Because the venous circulation is used for both drainage and return of blood, some recirculation into the ECMO device may occur. Clinicians can monitor recirculation by comparing the mixed venous oxygenation saturation (SvO_2) with the arterial oxygen saturation (SaO_2). A higher than normal SvO_2 and low SaO_2 may indicate excessive recirculation, requiring adjustment of the blood flow rate or cannula placement.

If ECMO support is provided following cardiovascular surgery, cannulation of mediastinal vessels (e.g., vena cavae or right atrial appendage and aorta for venoarterial ECMO) will be performed, because large cannulae can be placed through the median sternotomy to facilitate maximal ECMO flow rates. In these postoperative patients, EMCO will be discontinued in the operating suite to enable sterile closure of the cannulae insertion sites and the mediastinal incision.

Typically, ECMO perfusion is initiated at low flow rates and gradually increased until near-physiologic levels of blood flow and cardiac output are achieved. Once the desired flow rate is achieved, mechanical ventilation and vasoactive support can be decreased and/or discontinued.

ECMO circuit blood flow is continuous and nonpulsatile; therefore, as ECMO flow increases, the patient's intrinsic cardiac output decreases and the systemic arterial pressure waveform is dampened. Although 100% ECMO flow is possible, usually approximately 80% of the cardiac output is diverted to the ECMO circuit for optimal support. ECMO flow rates used in pediatrics vary related to the normal cardiac output, ranging from 100 mL/kg per minute for infants to 50 mL/kg per minute for adults. Total cardiac output is then equal to the ECMO pump flow rate plus endogenous cardiac output.

During ECMO support the arterial pressure waveform is dampened and pulse pressure is about 10 to 15 mm Hg, but arterial oxygen tension (PaO_2), hemoglobin saturation, and oxygen delivery are maintained at adequate levels. Monitoring of oxygen saturation in the venous side of the circuit allows assessment of SvO_2; an SvO_2 of 70% to 75% indicates adequate oxygen delivery from the ECMO circuit.

The necessary duration of ECMO therapy for cardiac assist is not well defined; several reports indicate a mean duration of approximately 24 to 48 hours. Use of echocardiographic information and clinical assessment of organ system recovery should guide the decision to wean ECMO support. Withdrawal of ECMO may be accomplished slowly, shifting the physiologic burden back to the heart and lungs, or it may be accomplished abruptly. Generally, when ECMO flow rates are reduced to approximately 25% of the estimated cardiac output (to 20 mL/kg per minute) with acceptable patient perfusion, bypass is temporarily discontinued by clamping off the circuit.

If the patient tolerates discontinuation of the ECMO for 1 to 3 hours, the cannulae are removed. When a sternal approach has been used, closure of the sternum may be delayed a day or more to ensure that cardiopulmonary function is effective without ECMO and to allow access to residual bleeding sites after decannulation.

Nursing Considerations. The insertion of cannulae and the initiation of ECMO generally are performed by a specialized surgical team in the critical care unit. As ECMO is initiated and optimal flow rates are achieved, the child's arterial waveform will dampen; this occurs because the perfusion provided by the ECMO unit usually is continuous and nonpulsatile. There should be no change in the ECG because the cardiac conduction system is not affected by ECMO.

When the child receives full ECMO support, mechanical ventilation support is adjusted to low pressure physiologic settings (low pressure, low FiO_2, low positive end-expiratory pressure [PEEP], low respiratory rate) to allow for lung rest. Pharmacologic support of cardiovascular function is decreased and/or discontinued as tolerated once ECMO flow rates are optimal. Generally, administration of neuromuscular blocking agents is avoided to enable ongoing assessment of neurologic function. However, analgesics should be administered and sedation is often provided (see Chapter 5 for additional information).

At the initiation of ECMO, the mean arterial pressure frequently decreases secondary to hemodilution of catecholamines by the prime and from release of vasoactive inflammatory substances. Poor perfusion will be reflected by decreasing venous oxyhemoglobin saturation and falling pH. The treatment of poor perfusion often requires an increase in ECMO flow.

Heparinization may be necessary to prevent clotting in the ECMO circuit. The platelet count will fall and may remain low for up to 4 days after termination of ECMO. The patients' activated clotting time (ACT), antithrombin III levels, platelets, PT/aPTT and international normalized ratio (INR) values, anti-Xa heparin activity, and thromboelastography (TEG) may require monitoring and management during therapy.

Heparin administration, blood product, and factor replacement are based on individual patient needs. Platelet infusions are often required to maintain platelet counts greater than 50,000 to 70,000/mm^3.[56]

Diligent observation for bleeding and prevention of unnecessary invasive therapy is imperative. The nurse should try to avoid any procedure that may produce bleeding such as heel sticks, venipunctures or injections, insertion of a nasogastric tube, or urinary catheter or rectal probe insertion. A gastric tube should be placed (before initiation of bypass) to enable detection of gastric bleeding and administer antacids.

The most devastating hemorrhagic complication during ECMO therapy is intracranial bleeding, which occurs most often in neonates less than 35 weeks of age. Serial head ultrasounds can be valuable tools in the diagnosis and evaluation of intracranial bleeding in neonates. The potential risk of intracranial hemorrhage is still present in older children, however, and the detection and evaluation of intracranial hemorrhage requires performance of thorough neurologic assessments at regular intervals.

Another potential neurologic complication is the occurrence of air emboli. Air may enter the circuit through any loose connection, IV administration system, dislodged cannulae, or excessive gas pressure across the membrane. Air emboli often

can be prevented if precautionary measures are employed during ECMO therapy. If there is any disruption of the circuit or if air detected in the arterial cannula, the cannula should be clamped immediately (see Table 7-2 for Troubleshooting of the ECMO Circuit). Clamps are kept at the bedside for this purpose. Whenever ECMO therapy is interrupted, full ventilatory support and vasoactive medications should be provided immediately to maintain oxygenation and perfusion.

The risk of infection during ECMO therapy is significant and is especially high if thoracic cannulation (rather than peripheral cannulation) is performed. Clinical signs of infection such as elevated temperature may not be present because the child's temperature is controlled by the ECMO circuit. Surveillance blood cultures are used to detect potential infection.

Good hand washing practice, mandatory during the care of *any* patient, is essential during ECMO therapy. Visitors and hospital personnel should be screened for the presence of transmittable infections before they are allowed to approach the patient's bedside. Dressing changes at the cannulae insertion sites are performed aseptically according to institutional protocols.

When the child is weaned from ECMO the nurse should be prepared to provide additional mechanical ventilation and cardiovascular support. After decannulation, bleeding may occur from the entry sites; this must be observed, quantified, reported, and managed appropriately. The nurse also should watch for evidence of infection, particularly at the cannulae insertion sites (see Box 7-3).

Complications. The potential benefits of ECMO therapy must be weighed against known and potential risks. Risks include hemorrhage, sepsis, cerebral thromboembolic events, and neurologic deficits associated with cannulation of the major arterial vessels (particularly the carotid artery).

Mechanical complications associated with the membrane oxygenator have been reported in as many as 20% of patients, but this complication may be preventable (see Table 7-2). Significant complications (10% to 20%) have been reported in all ECMO studies, but *direct* causation attributable to ECMO alone is difficult to separate from the effects of the underlying illness. Before evaluation of ECMO (or any mechanical support device) can be accomplished, well-defined standards of medical support for children in cardiopulmonary failure must be established. Controlled, randomized studies of the efficacy of ECMO therapy are underway.

Some neonates who receive ECMO therapy demonstrate neurologic deficits during long-term followup. Because the carotid artery used for venoarterial cannulation is usually ligated (tied off) after ECMO is discontinued, there is concern that neurologic deficits may be related to sacrifice of this artery. However, no relationship has yet been established between carotid ligation and presence, location, or severity of post-ECMO neurologic deficits.

Chest Tubes and Chest Tube Drainage Systems
Patricia Ann E. Schlosser

Chest tubes are inserted for evacuating air, fluid, chyle, or blood from the pleural, pericardial, or mediastinal spaces. Closed chest suction is intended to remove air and fluid from the thoracic cavity and facilitate the re-expansion of the lung after surgery, trauma, and spontaneous pneumothorax. This section discusses the principles of chest tubes and drainage systems that are used for infants and children, and the important information needed by clinicians.

Principles of Chest Tube Drainage

Disposable closed chest drainage systems consist of three functionally different but connected chambers (an underwater seal, a collection chamber and a suction chamber) in a single plastic unit that includes one inlet and one outlet. The inlet is connected by clear plastic tubing to the patient's chest tube. The outlet is connected to sterile tubing that is, in turn, connected to the suction device. Double drainage systems are available for two chest tubes.

The chest tube is joined to a 2-cm underwater seal. Intrapleural pressure is subatmospheric, so if the chest tube drains directly into a collection chamber (instead of the underwater seal) spontaneous inspiration would pull air and fluid from the collection chamber toward or even into the pleural space. The underwater seal serves as a one-way valve: fluid and air can drain out of the chest, but the resistance created by the 2 cm of water prevents atmospheric air from entering the pleural space.

The collection chamber is connected to, but in a chamber separate from the underwater seal. The separation enables maintenance of a consistent underwater seal (2 cm H_2O) that does not increase as drainage accumulates. The drainage chamber typically has 1-mL markings on the front surface. In addition, the front surface adjacent to the collection chamber can be marked at intervals to provide visual indicators of the drainage level at timed observations.

In order for drainage to occur from the chest, a pressure gradient must be created from the pleural space to the drainage system collection chamber; the pressure in the collection chamber must be lower than the pressure in the pleural space. Although this gradient can be established through the use of gravity (i.e., the collection chamber must be lower than the chest), drainage and evacuation of air is enhanced by applying suction to the system.

The amount of suction applied to the system can be regulated by suction applied to a column of water in the suction chamber, or it may be adjusted using a dial. If a column of water is used, the suction chamber is filled to the prescribed level. The height of the column of water determines the suction applied to the chest drainage system; application of sufficient suction to cause air to gently bubble through the column of water in the suction chamber will create a suction force equal to the cm height of the column of water (i.e., cm H_2O pressure). The degree of bubbling does not change the amount of suction applied. Some systems use a dial gauge rather than a fluid-filled suction chamber to provide a selection dial and visual indication of the suction applied to the system.

During chest drainage, documentation of the presence or absence of an air leak is essential. In addition, it is important to document the volume and consistency (typically described as serosanguineous fluid, blood, or chyle) of any fluid drained.

An air leak is caused by extravasation of air into lung parenchyma and the pleural space by rupture of small saccules; air escapes into the interstitial space and migrates via the neurovascular and peribronchial channels toward the hilum of the lung. The free air can then enter the pleural, pericardial, or mediastinal spaces. If an air leak is present, air bubbles will be observed passing from the patient side of the underwater seal through the water in the underwater seal compartment; in some chest drainage systems, an indicator will note the presence of the air leak. As long as a significant air leak is present, the chest tube must remain in place.

Chest Drainage Equipment and Nursing Management

Placement of the Chest Tube. Before chest tube insertion, a universal protocol should be followed.[130] This protocol includes preprocedure verification, site marking, and taking an active time out to verify the five elements that must be correct: patient, procedure, site, position, and equipment, and documenting this verification.

Chest tubes may be placed by a thoracostomy with a trocar or using a closed hemostat. A modified pigtail catheter is now available from several manufacturers; this catheter is placed using the modified Seldinger technique: a needle is inserted, a guide wire is passed through the needle (and the needle is withdrawn), then the catheter is slid over the guide wire into the chest (and the wire is removed). Neonates with coagulopathy, such as ECMO patients, are ideal candidates for pigtail catheter insertion.[35]

During chest tube insertion, local anesthetizing agents are used. In addition, if the patient is responsive and time and the patient's condition allow, narcotics are generally administered in conjunction with sedation (see Chapter 5).

It is important to assess the patient's response to chest tube insertion. This assessment includes auscultation of heart and breath sounds, evaluation of chest wall excursion and equality, palpation of point of maximal impulse, evaluation of pulses, and assessment of overall respiratory status, pulse oximetry, serum lactate (or arterial blood gases, as appropriate), and tissue perfusion.

A chest x-ray is performed before and after the procedure to document patient response, proper tube location and evacuation of any pneumothorax or visible hemothorax or pleural effusion.[179]

Preparation and Use of the Chest Drainage System. The choice of chest drainage system is determined by the physiologic and clinical needs of the infant and child.[161] Providers must be familiar with the operation of each device used.

If the drainage system is initiated in the operating suite, the system is handled by the scrub nurse as a sterile unit. The water seal chamber is filled to the 2-cm mark, using sterile water. The patient chest tube is connected to the rubber tube that provides an inlet at the top of the drainage system. Once this connection is made, the water seal is established. When the unit is positioned below chest level, drainage occurs by gravity and the water seal prevents atmospheric air from entering the pleural space. Connections (especially between the chest tube and the drainage system) must be secured using a banding gun. The chest drainage system should be secured to the side of the bed or to the floor to prevent tipping and loss of water seal.

Occlusive dressings should be applied to the site of chest tube insertion. Application of petroleum jelly gauze (e.g., Vaseline gauze, Kendall, division of Covidien, Norwalk, CT) and antibiotic ointment are not recommended while the drain is in place, because they may contribute to maceration of the skin. In addition, antibiotics are unnecessary for this application.

Postoperatively, a suction of -15 to -20 cm H_2O is typically applied to the chest drainage system. As noted previously, this suction is created by filling the suction chamber to a height of 15 to 20 cm and joining the outlet port of this suction chamber to a suction device. This suction facilitates drainage of the chest cavity and reexpansion of the lung, if needed.

If bubbling in the water seal chamber is observed, it is important to verify that all connections in the system are tight, including the site of the chest tube insertion into the chest. If bubbling in the water seal chamber is present despite tight connections throughout the system, a pleural air leak is likely to be present.

Both the hourly and the cumulative total of chest drainage are noted in the healthcare record, typically as hourly drainage/cumulative drainage. In the postoperative or trauma patient, chest tube bleeding greater than 3 mL/kg per hour for three consecutive hours or chest tube drainage of greater than 5 mL/kg per hour for 1 hour (or 7.5 mL/kg for children and 8 mL/kg for infants) should be the parameter for notification of a physician or other on-call provider.

Milking or "stripping" of chest tubes is not routinely performed because it can cause negative pressure (suction) of -300 to -400 cm H_2O, which is potentially damaging to tissues. If substantial drainage occurs, the nurse should tap the side of the tubing to promote drainage and to help propel any clots down the tubing and into the collection system.

Pain control and telemetry monitoring of heart rate, respiratory rate, pulse oximetry, and blood pressure are important adjuncts to chest drainage. Recommendations for troubleshooting the chest drainage system are listed in Table 21-8.

Chest Tube Removal. A review of the literature about chest tube removal pain and its management identified two pediatric studies.[30,31] In these studies, most patients experienced moderate to severe pain during chest tube removal, even with administration of narcotics and local anesthetics. Morphine alone may not provide effective pain relief for chest drain removal.[30,31] Future research is needed to determine the efficacy of a multimodal approach to pain control during chest tube removal in children, including use of nonsteroidal antiinflammatory drugs (NSAIDs), local anesthetics, and inhalation agents.[69,149]

When the chest tube is discontinued, petroleum jelly gauze should be placed with an occlusive dressing over the chest tube insertion site. The time and date of the application of the dressing should be written on the dressing and documented in the patient care record.

Table 21-8 Troubleshooting Chest Tubes

Problem	Cause/Intervention
I. Absence of bubbling in suction control (if unit bubbling is normally present) A. Water seal is normal or B. Intermittent, silent bubbling in water seal	Caused by an interruption in suction tubing; check system for: 1. Kink in suction tubing 2. Leak in system distal to water seal 3. Disconnected or compressed suction tubing 4. Malfunctioning unit (replace)
II. Continuous noisy or turbulent bubbling in water seal	A leak is present in the system proximal to the water seal. Check all connections immediately; if leak is not apparent, then: 1. Clamp tube at insertion site and observe water seal for cessation of bubbling; in this case, leak is probably caused by patient air leak in pleural space—unclamp tubing immediately. 2. If bubbling does not stop with clamp at insertion site, reclamp every few inches along tubing down to the unit in an attempt to isolate site of air leak. The point of the air leak is just above (proximal to) that point where clamping eliminates water seal bubbling. 3. Notify on-call provider for unresolved distress or if change of tubing is required.
III. Absence of bubbling or fluctuation in water seal	1. This may be normal if there is little or no air in intrapleural space. 2. With brief tube obstruction, fluid in the suction control chamber may bubble. 3. Partial or complete obstruction of tube within chest may be present; this may lead to accumulation of blood or air (hemo- or pneumothorax). Perform the following actions: a. Check for kinking or compression in patient tubing b. Gently milk chest tube; if clot is successfully removed, fluctuations should resume in water seal c. If condition persists, notify on-call provider, who may elect to apply direct suction in the chest tube to remove clot.
IV. Decrease in chest tube drainage	1. Check for dependent loops in chest tube and drain these loops. 2. Milk tube and reposition tubing; add suction with physician order. 3. Patient condition may be resolving.

It is important to monitor the patient's response to chest tube removal. This assessment includes auscultation of heart and breath sounds, evaluation of chest wall excursion and equality, palpation of point of maximal impulse, evaluation of pulses, and assessment of overall respiratory status, pulse oximetry, serum lactate (or arterial blood gases, as appropriate), and tissue perfusion.

RESPIRATORY MONITORING AND SUPPORT

Bradley A. Kuch

Respiratory Monitoring Devices

Respiratory monitoring, particularly in combination with clinical assessment skills, is invaluable for detecting and documenting cardiopulmonary insufficiency and for guiding intervention. Ideally, such monitoring assists in the detection of cardiopulmonary insufficiency before the development of cardiopulmonary failure or arrest.

As biomedical technology continues to advance, so does the ability to monitor subtle physiologic changes in respiratory function. For these instruments to be used effectively, the clinician must be familiar with their basic principles of operation and must be able to couple use of these instruments with careful clinical observation.

Impedance Pneumography

Impedance pneumography detects chest wall movement by recording changes in resistance (impedance) across an electrical field that result from variations in thoracic volume. Chest wall impedance is measured by placing an electrode on each side of the patient's chest. Many bedside cardiac monitors include filters enabling simultaneous ECG and respiratory monitoring.[45,162]

When the child's respiratory rate is monitored, a high and low rate alarm must be set. In addition to high and low respiratory rate alarms, most monitors have an apnea alarm, with thresholds that can be set at 10-, 15-, or 20-second intervals. If there is a high incidence of false-positive alarms, the bedside nurse should evaluate and adjust electrode placement until placement provides maximum sensitivity to both ECG and respiratory patterns; this should reduce the number of false apnea alarms.

The most significant limitation of impedance pneumography is that *all* chest movement is sensed, whether or not the movement is producing effective ventilation.[162] If airway obstruction develops, struggling respiratory movements will continue to be detected by the monitor, even if ventilation (air movement) is ineffective. If a child's respiratory function is poor, the nurse should not rely on this monitor to determine respiratory rate, and it should never be used to reflect effectiveness of ventilation.

Spirometry

Measurement of lung volume is accomplished by the use of spirometers. Spirometry has become more popular in the pediatric population as advancements in microprocessor technology have allowed for more accurate measurement of small lung volumes and enabled a greater variety of available bedside tests.[23]

Spirometry may be performed in the intubated patient if a cuffed tube is used or if there is minimal air leak around an uncuffed tube. If the patient is not intubated, a mouthpiece may be used if the child can maintain a tight mouth seal around the mouthpiece. However, patient inability to cooperate remains a significant limitation to spirometry in children less than 8 years of age. In this younger age group, patients may be unable or unwilling to make a tight seal around the mouthpiece or provide maximal effort during spirometry testing. These behaviors may result in misleading volume measurements.

A simple manometer or pressure gauge that can read both positive and negative pressures of -150 to $+100$ or $+150$ mm Hg is required for these measurements. School-age children should be able to generate at least -30 mm Hg pressure during inspiration and at least $+30$ mm Hg during expiration.

In the pediatric critical care setting, spirometry may be used to measure spontaneous exhaled tidal volumes of intubated children or the vital capacity of children with restrictive lung disease. Vital capacity is defined as the maximum amount of gas that can be expired after full inspiration (deep breath) and is easily measured with a respirometer. Forced vital capacity may be measured to assess pulmonary reserve.

Other useful bedside spirometry tests include minute ventilation (tidal volume with each breath multiplied by the respiratory rate), peak expiratory flow rate, and maximum inspiratory pressure, also known as negative inspiratory force (NIF).

To measure the peak expiratory flow rate, the child is instructed to give his or her best maximum expiratory effort, exerted after a deep inhalation. A peak expiratory flow rate (PEF) is the maximum flow rate measured during forceful exhalation following a maximum inhalation. The PEF decreases when there is resistance in central airways, and it is a helpful indicator of airway constriction in patients with asthma.

The negative inspiratory force is the maximum negative pressure generated by the respiratory muscles at the patient's peak inspiratory force. It can be measured in children who are school age or older and capable of following directions. To measure the negative inspiratory pressure, the child is instructed to give his or her best maximum inspiratory effort after an exhalation to a near residual volume. Inspiratory force must be at least -20 to -25 cm H_2O (15 to 18 mm Hg) to generate a sufficient cough and clear secretions.

These volumes are presented in more detail in Chapter 9, Essential Anatomy and Physiology—Lung Volumes.

Noninvasive Transcutaneous Blood Gas Monitoring

Transcutaneous measurement of oxygen ($P_{tc}O_2$) and carbon dioxide ($P_{tc}CO_2$) tension provide the clinician with a tool for immediate and continuous assessment of tissue respiration—delivery of oxygen and removal of carbon dioxide. Transcutaneous monitoring is a noninvasive means of assessing the tissue oxygen and carbon dioxide tension, yielding more information about oxygen transport and carbon dioxide elimination than the patient's arterial oxygen tension (PaO_2), pulse oximetry or cardiac index alone.

It is important to note that transcutaneous monitoring provides information regarding the gas tension of the tissue, and not the arterial blood gas tension. When the patient is hemodynamically stable, the arterial blood gas tensions and transcutaneous (tissue) measurements correlate well. However, frequently the $P_{tc}O_2$ is lower than the PaO_2 and the $P_{tc}CO_2$ is slightly higher than the $PaCO_2$.[170,171] This is caused by metabolism at the tissue level consuming oxygen and producing CO_2.

Instrumentation

Transcutaneous Oxygen Monitoring. The $P_{tc}O_2$ is measured by a heated electrode *(Clark electrode)* that is placed on the skin surface. The heat increases the capillary blood flow to the area, thus "arterializing" blood flow under the electrode. The sensor then measures oxygen tension at the skin surface itself; this oxygen tension should reflect the underlying tissue PO_2.[170,171,183] The heat ranges of the electrodes vary (most commonly between 40° C and 45° C), but the typical temperature generated is approximately 44° C.

Transcutaneous Carbon Dioxide Monitoring. Transcutaneous carbon dioxide ($P_{tc}CO_2$) measurements can be obtained using a pH electrode (Stow-Severinghaus electrode), infrared electrode, a mass spectrometer, or gas chromatography. To discuss each of these types of electrodes in detail is beyond the scope of this chapter. For more information regarding these electrodes, the reader is referred to Martin Tobin's *Principles and Practice of Intensive Care Monitoring.*[171]

Measurement of skin-surface or transcutaneous carbon dioxide tension (monitoring) may be a useful adjunct to the nursing care of children with acute or chronic respiratory disease. Several studies have verified high correlations between the $P_{tc}CO_2$ and the $PaCO_2$ in children, with a predictable gradient between the two.[21,60,76,190] Increased gradients may be caused by three of the following conditions: (1) tissue CO_2 production is increased by the heat from the electrode; (2) heating the capillary blood beneath the sensor elevates the CO_2 (anaerobic temperature coefficient); and (3) a countercurrent CO_2 exchange mechanism in the dermal loop maintains a higher PCO_2 at the tip of the loop (where the sensor lies).[170,171]

Consistently good correlations between $PaCO_2$ and $P_{tc}CO_2$ make transcutaneous carbon dioxide monitoring a valuable tool in the pediatric critical care setting. Correlation studies have demonstrated that although the $P_{tc}CO_2$ will be 9 to 23 mm Hg higher than the $PaCO_2$,[98] the relationship between the two remains relatively constant. With application to an individual patient, the nurse should note the difference between $PaCO_2$ and $P_{tc}CO_2$ to enable detection of trends in the patient's $PaCO_2$. With this difference established, the number of necessary arterial blood samples is reduced, and continuous monitoring of trends in CO_2 elimination are possible during procedures and changes in therapy.

The CO_2 electrode is reliable even in the presence of hypotension and decreased cardiac output (i.e., shock regardless of etiology).[21,22,60,76,98] Limitations of $P_{tc}CO_2$ monitoring include delayed measurement, inaccurate measurement, thermal injury, need for repeated calibration and site change, cost, and altered skin perfusion.

Clinical Applications.

A high correlation between PaO_2 and $P_{tc}O_2$ has been verified by many studies,[34,48,101,172,175,185] particularly when the range of PaO_2 is 30 to 100 torr. In fact,

brief periods of hypoxemia that are reflected by a fall in $P_{tc}O_2$ may not be detected by intermittent PaO_2 sampling. These episodes are frequently associated with nursing interventions, such as turning of the patient, vital sign measurement, dressing changes, suctioning, and chest physiotherapy.

Thick skin reduces the accuracy of the $P_{tc}O_2$ because fewer deep capillaries are present beneath the sensor site. In addition, thicker skin offers more resistance to oxygen diffusion than thinner skin, and it has higher oxygen consumption; thus the $P_{tc}O_2$ over thick skin will be lower than the PaO_2. For this reason, the transcutaneous electrodes should not be applied over areas of thickened skin, such as calluses or the soles of the feet.

The $P_{tc}O_2$ electrode also should be placed on the trunk rather than over extremities because extremity perfusion will be influenced more readily by temperature and cardiac output. The patient should never be positioned on top of a sensor because this may decrease local blood flow.

The relationship among $P_{tc}O_2$, PaO_2, and cardiac output have been documented in a somewhat predictive pattern: the $P_{tc}O_2$ correlates linearly with the PaO_2 when the cardiac output is greater than 65% of normal.[172,173,174,175] Tremper[175] reports a high correlation between the PaO_2 and $P_{tc}O_2$ levels when the cardiac index is greater than 1.54 L/minute per m^2 BSA. If cardiac output is compromised significantly (<65% of normal), the $P_{tc}O_2$ will be less than 80% of the PaO_2. This poor correlation reflects a compromise in tissue perfusion and often is observed during episodes of low cardiac output or shock even before the PaO_2 falls.[174,175]

Nursing Considerations.

Erythematous marks may develop at the electrode site, resulting from heat produced by the electrodes. Although these marks may disturb the family and staff, actual blisters (second-degree burns) seldom develop if the electrodes are changed as recommended by the manufacturer.

The schedule for rotation of electrode sites on the skin surface should be strictly maintained and documented. The erythematous marks caused by an electrode may last for hours or days following electrode removal, but rarely leave scars. Many studies recommend a maximum of a 3- to 4-hour interval for each electrode location,[183] but the nurse should check the manufacturer's recommendation for each electrode used.

Accurate transcutaneous monitoring requires meticulous electrode and machine calibration. The nurse should be especially aware of the following:

1. Unit calibration and skin warming time vary from 7 to 25 minutes each time the electrode is moved. The nurse should consult the device operator's manual for manufacturer's recommendations applicable to each specific unit.

2. The correlation between PaO_2 and $P_{tc}O_2$ should be determined if changes in the patient's clinical condition are observed.

3. The electrodes must be replaced and moved to a new location on the child's trunk or extremities at regular intervals to avoid skin irritation and compromise in electrode performance from heat-induced edema or other tissue changes at the electrode site. Microelectrodes heated to 44° C may require changing only every 6 hours, whereas large cathode electrodes require repositioning every 2 to 3 hours (check manufacturer's recommendations).

4. The nurse should recognize electrical drift and/or other sources of machine error.
5. Alarm systems (for low or high $P_{tc}O_2$) should be established and verified at regular intervals.
6. The procedures for troubleshooting problems with the monitor should be available in the unit.

In some hospital units, nurses are required to obtain an arterial sample for blood gas analysis after every electrode change, to compare the child's arterial blood gas values with transcutaneous values. As noted, the nurse must be knowledgeable about the procedure for machine calibration and maintenance (consult operator's manual and unit protocols) and must also be able to recognize electrical drift and/or mechanical error.

Maintenance should include frequent observation of the fluid space in the sensor. Gain or loss of fluid results in an erroneous $P_{tc}CO_2$ measurement. Each nurse must be familiar with interpretation of measurements, procedures for troubleshooting, and setting of alarm systems.

Noninvasive Blood Gas Monitoring: Pulse Oximetry

Oxygen saturation of hemoglobin (oxyhemoglobin saturation) in arterial blood may be monitored continuously using a pulse oximeter. The pulse oximeter is the monitor of choice for noninvasive monitoring of oxygenation, and the accuracy of these monitors has been demonstrated in children over a wide range of clinical conditions.[29,42,136,157,158,159] The response time of the oximeter is shorter than that of the transcutaneous oxygen monitors. The oximeter does not require calibration, and there are virtually no risks to the patient.

Mode of Operation. An instrument probe, housed in a clip or on an adhesive strip, may be placed on the finger, toe, foot, hand, or ear lobe. In the probe are two light-emitting diodes that emit red and infrared light through the tissue to a photodetector (Fig. 21-31). The red light absorption will be inversely related to the amount of saturated hemoglobin (i.e., hemoglobin that is bound to oxygen) passing through the tissue. Well saturated hemoglobin absorbs little red light and desaturated hemoglobin (i.e., hemoglobin not bound to oxygen) absorbs a large amount of red light.

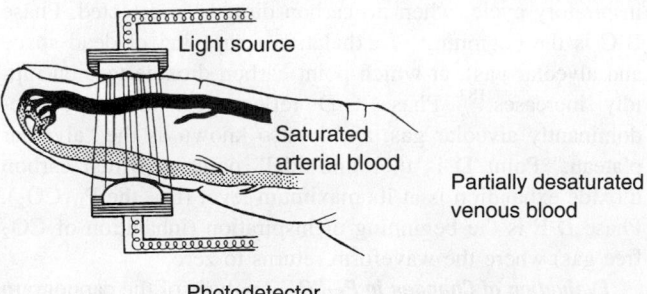

FIG. 21-31 Pulse oximeter. Two light-emitting diodes (light sources) transmit a red and an infrared light through the pulsatile tissue bed. The photodetector must be placed directly across the pulsatile tissue bed from the light source. Oxygenated (saturated) and deoxygenated (desaturated) hemoglobin absorb red and infrared light differently, and the hemoglobin saturation (percent of total hemoglobin that is oxygenated) is related inversely to the amount of red light absorbed.

Because the probe is placed over a pulsatile tissue bed, the pulse oximeter unit computes a pulse rate, and can signal the strength of the pulse. However, patient movement can produce artifact that significantly affects the accuracy of the pulse measurement. A difference between the pulse rate displayed by the pulse oximeter and the heart rate detected by the cardiac monitor should prompt an immediate evaluation of the patient and the patient's systemic perfusion.

Pulse oximeters require pulsatile blood flow to operate properly. These monitors generally provide accurate results over a wide range of clinical conditions (including hypotension, low cardiac output, and hypothermia).[29,42,72,100,157,173,177,183] However, the response time in the presence of hypoxemia varies widely from instrument to instrument. Some units may fail to reflect acute, severe hypoxemia and may overestimate the hemoglobin saturation. This tendency may be observed more frequently with finger probes than with ear probes.[100,158]

Most oximeters provide a *low signal* alert, which may indicate diminished pulse intensity under the probe. Accuracy of the measured O_2 saturation is not necessarily altered by low pulse intensity,[100] but the low signal alert should prompt evaluation of the patient and the patient's systemic perfusion.

The pulse oximeter may be a useful adjunct to cardiovascular monitoring. It enables monitoring of the pulse in an ischemic limb and reflects changes in pulse rate in unstable patients and in patients during pacemaker support.

Pulse oximeters are not reliable in the presence of methemoglobinemia and carbon monoxide poisoning, because the effect of these hemoglobins on light absorption is not factored into the calculation of hemoglobin saturation. As a result, when these conditions are present, the pulse oximeter will display a falsely high hemoglobin saturation, reflecting only the percent saturation of the child's normal hemoglobin, rather than the saturation of the child's total hemoglobin.

Troubleshooting During Pulse Oximetry. Several operator-controlled variables may cause a poor signal (and resulting alarm), including the presence of ambient light and movement artifact. To eliminate ambient light, the monitored area can be wrapped loosely with an opaque material such as gauze. The nail bed should be clean before sensor application.[36,77,189]

Movement artifact is difficult to control in pediatric patients. Ear clip sensors are often the least likely to be disturbed with movement. However, if movement artifact is a significant problem the oximeter may be placed on a restrained extremity. In addition, application of a disposable sensor on the hand or foot may result in less movement artifact than that occurring with placement over a finger or toe. Occasionally, the patient may require sedation (with physician input and order).

Neonatal studies suggest that attachment of the probe to the patient before it is attached to the device may shorten the time required to obtain an initial signal.[132] The nurse must be familiar with the rapidity of signal response required for the pulse oximetry devices used in the critical care unit.

Noninvasive Capnometry: End-Tidal Carbon Dioxide Monitoring ($P_{ET}CO_2$)

Instrumentation. The exhaled carbon dioxide is the tension (in mm Hg) or partial pressure of carbon dioxide in expired (exhaled) gas. The highest exhaled carbon dioxide tension is present at the end of the expiration; this end-tidal CO_2 or $P_{ET}CO_2$ is also known as the end-expiratory CO_2. The $P_{ET}CO_2$ normally trends with the patient's arterial carbon dioxide tension.

The continuous measurement of the $P_{ET}CO_2$ by infrared spectroscopy is called capnometry. Capnography includes a display (graph) of the waveform of the carbon dioxide tension throughout inspiration and exhalation and the monitor typically provides a digital display of the $P_{ET}CO_2$. Analysis of the capnogram is discussed in the section that follows (see Clinical Applications of Capnography).

End-tidal CO_2 monitors can now be purchased as part of a mechanical ventilation system or as separate monitors. Capnometry can also be performed via nasal cannula during spontaneous breathing.[170a]

The infrared CO_2 analyzer consists of three components: an inferred radiation source, a gas sampling chamber, and a detector. Carbon dioxide absorbs infrared radiation of specific wavelengths, so as the infrared rays are passed through expiratory gas, a detector then registers the intensity of the radiation in the gas (and conversely, the absorption of infrared radiation) to determine the tension or partial pressure of CO_2.[171] This analyzer therefore enables evaluation of alveolar ventilation and CO_2 elimination.

Two types of $P_{ET}CO_2$ monitoring methods are used clinically—mainstream and sidestream analyzers. In mainstream analyzers the detector module is placed in the ventilator circuit at the proximal end of the endotracheal tube, in line with the expired gas flow; this placement allows for rapid response to changes in $P_{ET}CO_2$. However, the mainstream module can be affected easily by condensation and mucus, and requires frequent cleaning of the sensor module.

In sidestream modules a low flow (50 to 150 mL per minute) vacuum aspirates a small sample of expired gas to the analysis module located in the monitor. This sampling method is also affected by condensation and mucus, which can occlude the sampling line. Sidestream technology has also been found to be relatively inaccurate at small tidal volumes, increased I:E ratios, and high resistance states.[95,106]

The presence (but not the tension) of CO_2 in exhaled gas can be detected through use of a colorimetric device attached to the proximal end of an endotracheal tube (or between an endotracheal tube and a resuscitation bag or mechanical ventilation system). Colorimetric CO_2 detection devices change color (typically from purple to yellow, but the color change may vary from device to device) when CO_2 is present in the gas flowing through the device. Typically the color change develops within about 6 breaths, and the color will change permanently after several minutes or hours of use. These devices are considered qualitative (i.e., indicating presence or absence of CO_2) rather than quantitative devices, and are not discussed further in this chapter (see Chapter 9 for additional information).

Clinical Applications of Capnography. The correct use of a $P_{ET}CO_2$ device requires an understanding of the patient's alveolar-arterial (A-a) CO_2 gradient. In addition, the $P_{ET}CO_2$ must be evaluated in conjunction with the clinical examination.

Relationship Between Arterial and End-Tidal CO₂ Tension. Normally there is no significant difference between arterial and alveolar (or end-tidal) CO_2 tension, because carbon dioxide in pulmonary capillaries normally diffuses freely into the alveoli to be exhaled and measured as $P_{ET}CO_2$. Thus, the normal difference between the $P_{ET}CO_2$ and the arterial CO_2 tension is 2 to 5 mm Hg or less.[165,183] This small difference results from mixing of CO_2-containing alveolar gas with exhaled gas devoid of CO_2 from anatomic dead space. This high correlation has been documented even in neonates,[120] particularly if they receive muscle relaxants during mechanical ventilation.

The $P_{ET}CO_2$ will be nearly identical to the patient's arterial CO_2 tension ($PaCO_2$) only if there is a normal (very low) alveolar-arterial carbon dioxide (A-aCO_2) gradient and no alveolar dead space. If a large A-aCO_2 gradient or a large amount of alveolar dead space is present, the $P_{ET}CO_2$ will not equal the $PaCO_2$. For example, if there is impairment of CO_2 diffusion from the blood into the alveoli, such as in the neonate with respiratory distress syndrome or the child with acute respiratory distress syndrome,[120,183] the difference between the $P_{ET}CO_2$ and the arterial CO_2 tension increases. However, changes in the $P_{ET}CO_2$ accurately reflect trends in the child's $PaCO_2$, even if a significant lung disease is present.

Any time the $PaCO_2$-to-$P_{ET}CO_2$ gradient increases, dead space ventilation has increased. Increased dead space ventilation occurs any time pulmonary perfusion decreases relative to alveolar ventilation. Conditions causing increased dead space ventilation include pulmonary vascular disease or increased pulmonary vascular resistance, pulmonary embolus, decreased right ventricular output (e.g., shock or cardiac arrest), and excessive PEEP. A sudden decrease in the $P_{ET}CO_2$ to zero could indicate extubation, ETT obstruction, esophageal intubation, or a disruption or leak in the system

The $P_{ET}CO_2$ will not correlate with the $PaCO_2$ if the child is breathing rapidly and shallowly or hyperpnea is present. Such alterations in respiratory patterns will result in sampling error and poor correlation between $P_{ET}CO_2$ and $PaCO_2$.[95,106,171]

Analysis of Capnograph. The waveform that is displayed by variations in exhaled CO_2 throughout the respiratory cycle is known as a capnogram. To use the capnogram, the clinician must first be familiar with a normal $P_{ET}CO_2$ waveform (Fig. 21-32).[183]

A capnogram is divided into four phases. Phase A-B is the inspiratory cycle, when no carbon dioxide is detected. Phase B-C is the beginning of exhalation (emptying of dead space and alveolar gas), at which point carbon dioxide tension rapidly increases.[183] Phase C-D reflects exhalation of predominantly alveolar gas, and is also known as the "alveolar plateau." Point D is the "end-tidal" point at which carbon dioxide exhalation is at its maximum level (i.e., the $P_{ET}CO_2$). Phase D-E is the beginning of inspiration (inhalation of CO_2 free gas) where the waveform returns to zero.

Evaluation of Changes in P_ET_CO₂. Analysis of the capnogram and trends in the $P_{ET}CO_2$ may enable detection of improvement or deterioration in ventilation, increase in dead space, a fall in cardiac output and ET tube displacement. It can enable detection of an obstructed airway, and/or the return of diaphragm function in the paralyzed patient.[183] If the $P_{ET}CO_2$ and the $PaCO_2$ fall together, the patient's ventilation has improved; if both rise, the patient's ventilation is reduced.

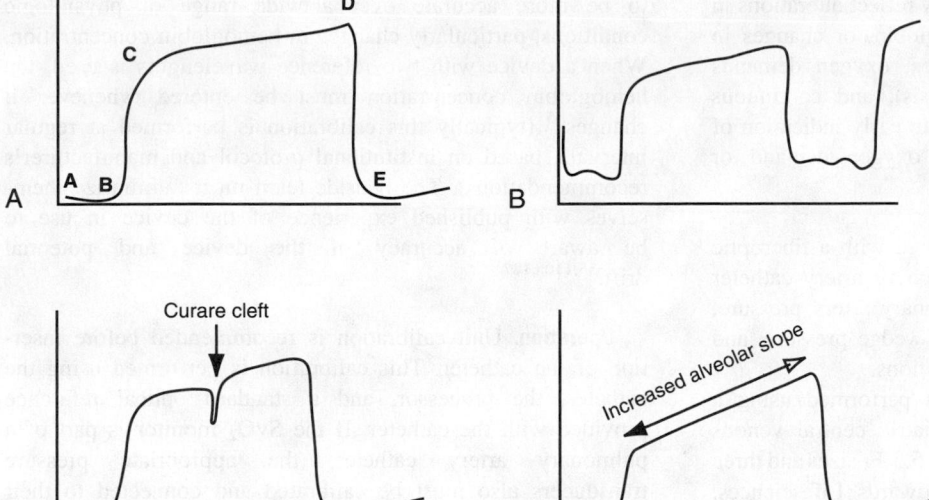

FIG. 21-32 Capnogram phases. **A,** Normal capnogram illustrating each phase of exhalation (see text, Analysis of Capnograph). **B,** Rebreathing capnogram: Inspiratory level does not return to zero. **C,** Curare cleft: Cleft in the alveolar plateau indicates a return of diaphragmatic activity in a patient receiving neuromuscular blockade. **D,** Increased alveolar plateau slope is representative of small airway obstruction (e.g., asthma, bronchiolitis).

As noted, if the $P_{ET}CO_2$ falls and the $PaCO_2$ rises, dead space has been added to the system (areas are ventilated that are not perfused). This condition can develop if the lung is overdistended with PEEP. The $P_{ET}CO_2$ can fall without a rise in the $PaCO_2$ when cardiac output falls, and pulmonary blood flow and delivery of CO_2 to the lungs decreases. The $P_{ET}CO_2$ will fall to near zero with spontaneous extubation. For additional information about $P_{ET}CO_2$ monitoring in the child with pulmonary disorders, see Chapter 9.

Recently capnography has been used to monitor resuscitation quality during cardiac arrest in intubated patients. When cardiac output is very low during attempted resuscitation, little blood flow is delivered to the lungs, so little carbon dioxide is detected in exhaled gases. When blood flow improves during attempted resuscitation, blood flow to the lungs improves and the $P_{ET}CO_2$ rises. The $P_{ET}CO_2$ rises abruptly when there is return of spontaneous circulation (see Chapter 6).

Nursing Considerations. When capnometry is in use, the nurse must be able to calibrate the instrument and must be aware of the relationship between the patient's alveolar (or end-tidal) and arterial CO_2 tensions. The nurse must be able to correlate $P_{ET}CO_2$ values with the clinical status of the patient and must be aware of sources of instrument error.

The absolute $P_{ET}CO_2$ at any one time is usually not as important as the trends documented by this equipment, although a sudden fall in $P_{ET}CO_2$ in an intubated patient should prompt immediate suspicion of spontaneous extubation (see Fig. 9-21). The $P_{ET}CO_2$ should be compared with either a venous or arterial PCO_2 to ensure that the two correlate. In addition, it is critical to verify effectiveness of oxygenation and ventilation through careful clinical assesment.[183]

Invasive Arterial Oximetry

Arterial oximetry is an invasive method of continuously monitoring arterial oxygen saturation. This method of oximetry uses an intraarterial electrode threaded through to the tip of an arterial catheter.

Clinical trials have demonstrated the accuracy of the polarographic electrode, although a high incidence of electrode failure has been reported.[55] LeSoeuf[101] reported moderately high correlations between the indwelling oximeter and the oxyhemoglobin saturation reported by a $P_{tc}O_2$-measuring device. However, the arterial oximetry was not compared with oxygen saturation measured by direct blood sampling and measurement using a co-oximeter.

Clinical Applications. Arterial oximetry allows direct, continuous measurement of oxygen saturation, which is preferable to intermittent measurement. The indwelling electrode does not require frequent repositioning (e.g., as is necessary with transcutaneous oxygen monitoring).

The disadvantages of arterial oximetry are related to vascular effects of a foreign body and the potential for inaccurate results. The catheter may lodge against the arterial wall, producing arterial spasm. Fibrin clots may form at the catheter tip, resulting in inaccurate readings and risk of embolism. Hemodilution (particularly a hematocrit <30%) may result in erroneous oxygen saturation calculations. Finally, electrode failure has been reported.

Use of the arterial oximeter may be limited in pediatric patients because they have small vessel size. The risks of infection, thromboembolic events, and other potential complications of the indwelling arterial oximeter have not been documented in pediatric patients. Currently, arterial oximetry is not performed frequently in children because further research is required to verify its effectiveness.

Invasive Mixed Venous Oxygen Saturation Monitoring

Continuous monitoring of mixed venous oxygen saturation (SvO_2) in pediatric patients is possible with a fiberoptic pulmonary artery catheter. The central venous oxygen saturation ($S_{CV}O_2$), typically obtained from the superior vena cava, approximates the mixed venous oxygen saturation (typically the $S_{CV}O_2$ is about 2% to 3% higher than the SvO_2), and is often used as a surrogate for the mixed venous oxygen saturation. The $S_{CV}O_2$ can be monitored with a fiberoptic central venous catheter.

Changes in the SvO_2 (and $S_{CV}O_2$) may reflect alterations in cardiac output, oxygen delivery, hemoglobin, or changes in oxygen consumption. In some instances, oxygen demands are changing continually (as with sepsis), and continuous SvO_2 ($S_{CV}O_2$) monitoring may provide an early indication of decreased oxygen delivery, increased oxygen demand or decreased oxygen utilization.

Description. The SvO_2 can be monitored with a fiberoptic 5-French, 5-lumen balloon-tipped pulmonary artery catheter that also enables measurement of pulmonary artery pressure, central venous pressure, and pulmonary wedge pressure, and for thermodilution cardiac output calculations.

Continuous monitoring of $S_{CV}O_2$ is performed using a fiberoptic central venous catheter. Pediatric central venous oximetry catheters are available in 4.5 and 5.5-Fr sizes and three different lengths (Edwards PediaSat, Edwards Lifesciences, Irvine, CA).[110a]

The hemoglobin saturation is determined by spectrophotometric *reflection*. The catheter port used for SvO_2 monitoring is connected to an optical module, which transmits a narrow band width (wavelength) of light to the tip of the fiberoptic catheter. This light will be *reflected* by saturated (oxygenated) hemoglobin differently than by desaturated hemoglobin (i.e., hemoglobin not bound to oxygen).

The light emitted by the catheter is reflected by the hemoglobin and transmitted back via a separate fiberoptic filament to the module (Fig. 21-33). The microprocessor analyzes the amount of light transmitted and reflected and averages the signal over 2 to 3 seconds. A tandem recorder trends the SvO_2 on a graph recording. A light intensity indicator (at the tip of the catheter) is also recorded and monitored; changes in the light intensity may indicate a change in catheter position, inadequate blood flow, or damage to the fiber optics.[19,62,81]

Two different reflection spectrophotometry processor units are available: a three-wavelength and a two-wavelength device. The three reference wavelength processor is thought to be more accurate over a wide range of physiologic conditions, particularly changes in hemoglobin concentration. When a device with two reference wavelengths is used, the hemoglobin concentration must be entered whenever it changes[55] (typically this calibration is performed at regular intervals, based on institutional protocol and manufacturer's recommendations). The bedside team must familiarize themselves with published experience of the device in use to be aware of accuracy of the device and potential drift.[55,110a,187]

Operation. Unit calibration is recommended before insertion of the catheter. This calibration is performed using the catheter, the processor, and a standard optical reference provided with the catheter. If the SvO_2 monitor is part of a pulmonary artery catheter, the appropriate pressure transducers also must be calibrated and connected to their respective monitoring systems and catheter ports before the catheter is placed.

Insertion into the central vein is accomplished using a standard Seldinger technique. Pressure waveforms and SvO_2 readings are monitored during insertion to guide catheter placement.

If the fiberoptic is contained in a pulmonary artery catheter, placement is correct when the pulmonary catheter is correctly positioned. If the tip of the pulmonary artery catheter is advanced too far into a pulmonary artery, a falsely high SvO_2 will be calculated, reflecting the proximity of the fiberoptic to blood that is oxygenated by surrounding alveoli.[154]

Recalibration after insertion should be performed according to manufacturer's recommendation: a mixed venous blood sample is sent for laboratory measurement of the oxygen saturation using a co-oximeter (i.e., not a calculated saturation). Simultaneous with the blood sampling, the nurse should document the mixed venous oxygen saturation displayed by the device. Once the laboratory analysis of the blood sample is complete, the device should be recalibrated based on the laboratory measurement.

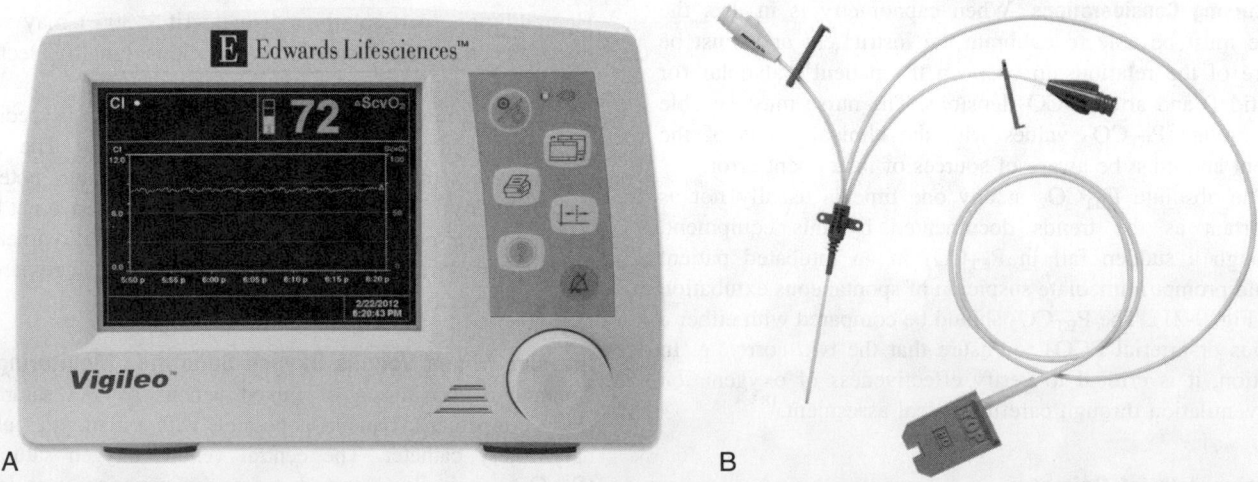

FIG. 21-33 **A,** Continuous central venous oxygen saturation ($S_{CV}O_2$) microprocessor/monitor and **B,** multilumen central venous catheter. The fiberoptic catheter contains filaments that transmit red light to and from the blood. The light is *reflected* by circulating hemoglobin and transmitted via a second optical fiber to the microprocessor, where the hemoglobin saturation is determined. Catheters are available in 3 lengths. (Vigileo monitor and PediaSat catheter photograph courtesy of Edwards Lifesciences, Irvine, California.)

Clinical Applications. The normal mixed venous oxygen saturation is usually between 65% and 75%. A rise in SvO_2 reflects one of four conditions: (1) increased oxygen delivery, caused by a rise in cardiac output, or an increase in arterial oxygen content; (2) reduced oxygen consumption, as observed with hypothermia, neuromuscular blockade, and anesthesia; (3) the presence of a left-to-right intracardiac shunt; or (4) mechanical interference from the measuring unit (e.g., a wedged catheter).

The SvO_2 may fall for the following reasons: (1) decreased oxygen delivery, resulting from decreased cardiac output, hypoxemia associated with pulmonary dysfunction, or anemia, or (2) increased oxygen consumption caused by shivering, seizures, hyperthermia, sepsis, or agitation. The SvO_2 will track with changes in cardiac output, but there are other factors, such as oxygen demand and oxygenation of blood in the lungs, that influence the SvO_2.

The SvO_2-monitoring system has been used in adult patients since 1981, and its efficacy has been documented in a variety of physiologic conditions.[19,55,62,81,93,122,146,154,187] The enthusiasm for its use in adult patients is based on its accuracy and reliability as well as its ability to reflect changes in cardiac output and arterial oxygenation instantly and continuously.

The use of venous fiberoptic oximetric catheters has been successful in the management of pediatric patients following surgery for congenital heart disease and for pediatric patients with septic shock. Muller and co-workers described the use of a 2-French fiberoptic probe that is introduced through a single-lumen central venous catheter in a series of three infants who underwent a stage 1 Norwood procedure.[126] The fiberoptic probe was inserted approximately 2.5 cm beyond the central venous catheter tip, allowing for continuous central venous oximetry ($S_{CV}O_2$). The group found good correlation between the fiberoptic $S_{CV}O_2$ and laboratory SvO_2 evaluated by co-oximeter ($r = 0.912$. 95% CI: 0.716-0.975).[126] However, they reported that the fiberoptic probe was less accurate in conditions of very low saturation ($<40\%$).

More recently, de Oliveira reported that goal-directed resuscitation using the end point of a superior vena caval oxygen saturation ($ScvO_2$) $\geq 70\%$ significantly improved the outcome of pediatric patients with septic shock (28-day mortality 11.8% vs. 39.2%).[43] Since 2006, pediatric $S_{CV}O_2$ catheters have been approved by the Food and Drug Administration for use in children in the United States.

Disadvantages. Changes in the calculated SvO_2 (or $S_{CV}O_2$— in this section they are used interchangeably) are not always indicative of changes in patient condition. The high incidence of artifact during continuous SvO_2 monitoring seems to be linked to the fact that SvO_2 determination is dependent on *reflected* light. As rapid blood flow passes the catheter tip, consistent light reflection may not occur. Faulty connections, fiberoptic fracture, occlusion of the catheter tip by emboli, and wedging of the tip against the vessel wall also may produce inaccurate SvO_2 readings.[122,154]

Whenever a fall in SvO_2 is noted, the patient's oxygenation and systemic perfusion must be assessed. Clinical evaluation always should be used to confirm any changes associated with deterioration in the SvO_2. The function of the monitor should be assessed only after the patient's condition is evaluated.

Factors reducing the accuracy of fiberoptic SvO_2 monitoring include lack of in-vitro and *in vivo* calibration, lack of intensity calibration during insertion, bent or broken optics, catheter tip close to or facing the vessel wall, increased carboxyhemoglobin or methemoglobin, and extreme hypoxemia ($<40\%$).[171]

The limited variety of available sizes of the fiberoptic catheters prevents its use in very small children. Although the 2- to 4-French SvO_2 fiberoptic catheter can be used in infants and for central vein oximetry, these small fiberoptic catheters do not enable other hemodynamic measurements and calculations (e.g., CO, PAWP, vascular resistances) that are possible with a pulmonary artery catheter with fiberoptic and thermistor. With the availability of the pediatric fiberoptic central venous catheter more experience is being gained with continuous monitoring of central venous oxygen saturation as a surrogate for the mixed venous oxygen saturation in critically ill children.[110a] More data about its reliability and effectiveness is anticipated.

Esophageal Pressure Monitoring

Esophageal pressure (P_{es}) monitoring provides important information regarding intrathoracic pressure during mechanical ventilation. It yields an indirect measurement of pleural pressure, providing information regarding the distending pressure of the lung and chest wall. Evaluation of P_{es} also allows for division of the respiratory system's resistance and compliance into pulmonary and chest wall components.

A change in P_{es} (ΔP_{es}) as well as P_{es} swings reflect the level of patient effort during spontaneous and supported mechanical breaths; these values can be used to calculate the work of breathing imposed by the lung and ventilator circuit. The P_{es} may also be useful in determining optimal PEEP in patients with acute lung injury/acute respiratory distress syndrome (ALI/ARDS).

In a randomized controlled trial, Talmor and colleagues reported that a "ventilator strategy using esophageal pressures to estimate the transpulmonary pressure significantly improves oxygenation and compliance" in patients with ALI/ARDS.[20,166] They demonstrated improved PaO_2:FiO_2 ratios, respiratory system compliance, and dead space to tidal volume ratio (V_d/V_t) when the PEEP was set to keep the transpulmonary pressure greater than 0 cm H_2O guided by P_{es} monitoring.[20,166]

Instrumentation. Esophageal pressure is measured using an air-containing balloon that is sealed in a catheter connected to a pressure transducer. The catheter is inserted into the thoracic esophagus. A change in pressure imposed on the balloon is conveyed via the catheter to the pressure transducer, and the pressure is displayed on the monitor or ventilator.

Catheter dimensions range from an internal diameter of 1 to 1.2 mm (for use in newborns and smaller children) to an internal diameter of 1.4 to 1.7 mm (for use in large children and adults). Adequate balloon volume is essential for accurate detection of the P_{es}.[20,171] Typically, a balloon volume of 0.5 mL is sufficient; however, the range of gas volume should be determined from the catheter packaging; the packaging indicates the clinical situations in which more or less volume may be indicated.[171]

The balloon is positioned by passing an empty balloon catheter into the stomach via the nares or mouth. A volume of 0.5 mL of air is then injected into the system and the catheter is attached to the pressure transducer.[171] A positive pressure swing indicates that the balloon is in the stomach. The catheter is then withdrawn until a negative pressure deflection is identified on the monitor, indicating the balloon is in the thoracic esophagus. The catheter is then pulled back an additional 5 to 10 cm, which positions the entire balloon in the esophagus.

The final position of the balloon in the mid- and lower esophagus can be verified by chest radiograph.[20] Correct position of the balloon can be validated by using the "occlusion test," which is accomplished by having the patient take a spontaneous breath against a closed airway while observing the ΔP_{es} and change of pressure at the airway opening (ΔP_{AO}).[171] If the balloon is in correct position, the clinician will find near unity between the ΔP_{es} and ΔP_{AO} throughout the inspiratory cycle.[171]

Clinical Applications. Esophageal pressure monitoring has a wide range of clinical applications. As noted, P_{es} is beneficial in determining the patient's work of breathing imposed by underlying lung disease and the addition of the ventilator circuit. Evaluation of the work of breathing allows adjustment of mechanical support to decrease the patient's metabolic demands and/or identify if the patient is ready for extubation.

In addition to work of breathing assessment, P_{es} monitoring provides information regarding respiratory muscle function. More specifically, monitoring of the P_{es} in conjunction with gastric pressure monitoring enables calculation of diaphragm force-generation, relatively isolated from intercostal and other accessory muscles, and from elastic recoil of the chest wall. Some authors have suggested that isolated diaphragm function should be assessed using P_{es} measurement in patients with suspected diaphragm weakness or paralysis.[20]

Esophageal pressure measurement may be beneficial in any clinical situation characterized by decreased lung compliance.[20,166,171] If poor respiratory system compliance is determined to be caused by chest wall edema, low lung compliance, or abdominal compartment syndrome, the clinician may be better able to titrate PEEP without causing lung trauma.

Nursing Considerations. The bedside nurse must be able to assess the catheter position and document depth and position at the insertion location, as well as P_{es} measurements. The catheter must be secured at the nares without causing tissue breakdown around the nares or mouth.

Oxygen Administration Systems

Supplementary oxygen is commonly used in the pediatric critical care unit. Although oxygen may be administered in a variety of ways, it must always be treated as a drug, with accurate administration and documentation of the dose and careful assessment and documentation of patient response.

The appropriate device for delivery of supplementary oxygen is determined by the patient's age, size, and inspiratory flow rate (tidal volume in mL/sec), and the fraction of inspired oxygen (FiO_2) needed. The method for estimation of inspiratory flow rate is summarized in Box 21-1. Oxygen delivery devices can be divided into two classes: variable-performance oxygen delivery devices (low flow devices) and fixed-performance oxygen delivery devices (high-flow devices).

Low flow (variable-performance) devices are unable to deliver an oxygen flow rate sufficient to supply the patient's inspiratory flow rate. As a result, when the child inspires, room air is entrained with the supplementary oxygen and the FiO_2 varies with the patient's respiratory rate and tidal volume.[183]

High flow (fixed-performance devices) can deliver an oxygen flow rate that meets or exceeds the patient's

---

Box 21-1	**General Principles for Estimation of Required Oxygen Inspiratory Flow Rate**

1. 60 seconds/min ÷ respiratory rate = time of one respiratory cycle in seconds (s)
2. Multiply time of one respiratory cycle (in seconds) × inspiratory fraction (the portion of the respiratory cycle required for inspiration—typically 0.5, but may be 0.3 in children with asthma and long exhalation) = inspiratory time (in second[s])
3. Divide tidal volume (V_T) in mL (typically 4-6 mL/kg) per breath by the inspiratory time (in seconds) = inspiratory flow in mL/s

Note: For convenience, multiply inspiratory flow in mL/s by 60 s/min to compare with gas flow rate in mL/min (and divide mL/min by 1000 to obtain L/min to compare to gas flow rate)

Examples

Example 1: 4 kg Infant

Would a 2 L/min oxygen flow through nasal cannula provide high or low flow and low FiO_2 for a 4 kg infant?

The infant's normal V_t is 20 mL (using 5 mL/kg). This example uses a typical respiratory rate of 60/min with an inspiratory portion of 0.5/breath.

1. 60 s/min ÷ 60/min = respiratory cycle of 1 s
2. 1 s × 0.5 = 0.5 s/breath
3. 20 mL/breath ÷ 0.5 s = 40 mL/s inspiratory flow (× 60 s/min = 2400 mL/min = 2.4 L/min)

A nasal cannula delivering a flow of 2 L/min gives a flow rate that would almost meet the inspired flow rate of a 4 kg infant, and thus the infant's inspired FiO_2 would be fairly high.

Example 2: 20 kg preschooler

Would a 2 L/min oxygen flow through nasal cannula provide relatively high or low flow and low FiO_2 for a 20 kg preschooler? A 4 year old, 20 kg child's normal tidal volume (V_T) is 100 mL.

1. 60 s/min ÷ 30/min = respiratory cycle of 2 s
2. 2 s × 0.35 = 0.7 s inspiratory time
3. 100 mL/breath ÷ 0.7 s = 142 mL/s (× 60 s/min = 8571 mL/min = 8.6 L/min)

The preschooler is breathing at a slower rate than the infant, so the preschooler's inspiratory time is slightly longer (here estimated at 0.7 s for each breath). Mean inspiratory flow rate is ~142 mL/s or 8571 mL/min (8.6 L/min), well higher than the delivered oxygen flow 2 L/min. The preschooler will entrain much more room air so the inspired FiO_2 is low.

Courtesy of Mary Fran Hazinski, Arno Zaritsky, and Stephen S. Schexnayder.

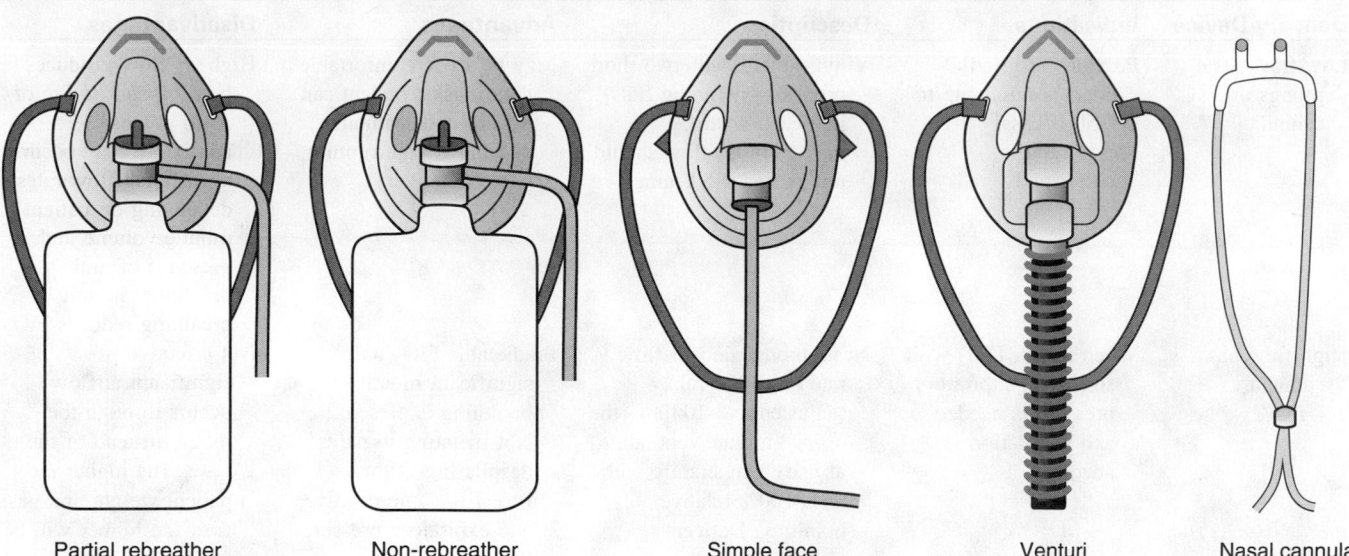

| Partial rebreather | Non-rebreather | Simple face | Venturi | Nasal cannula |

FIG. 21-34 Oxygen administration systems.

inspiratory flow rate. As a result, a high FiO_2 can be consistently delivered. Fig. 21-34 and Table 21-9 describe types of oxygen delivery systems and their advantages and disadvantages.

The nurse caring for the child receiving supplementary oxygen must monitor and record the type of oxygen delivery device, the set liter flow (in liters per minute), the FiO_2, and the child's response to therapy.

Nursing Considerations

The bedside nurse should assess the patient and the oxygen delivery system:

1. Analyze the fraction of inspired oxygen (FiO_2) frequently—many hospitals require continuous or hourly analysis. If O_2 drift is a problem, continuous analysis of the inspired oxygen concentration is usually indicated. Table 21-10 provides a formula for calculation of inspired oxygen concentrations.

2. Monitor patient oxygenation through pulse oximetry and, as needed, obtain an arterial blood gas analysis (the gold standard) to evaluate effectiveness of oxygen therapy. The nurse and the physician should determine the desired frequency of blood gas analysis. Invasive or noninvasive evaluation of oxygenation should be performed 15 to 20 minutes after any change in FiO_2.

3. Observe for changes in respiratory rate, effort, and/or skin color of the patient with any changes to the oxygen delivery device or FiO_2. Document these observations and notify the physician or on-call provider of any clinical changes.

4. Ensure that the inspired oxygen is humidified and warmed unless otherwise directed by the physician or on-call provider.

5. Ensure that any tubing in the O_2 delivery system is changed daily to minimize the risk of tubing contamination and healthcare acquired infection.

6. Keep infants and children dry when humidified oxygen is provided by head hood or face tent. Frequent clothing and

linen changes may be necessary. Monitor the child's temperature closely if heated or cooled aerosol is used.

7. Assess for potential complications of oxygen therapy.[28,183]

   a. Respiratory depression may occasionally occur in some children with chronic lung disease, specifically if the child's respiratory drive occurs as a result of hypoxia rather than hypercarbia.

   b. Absorption atelectasis may develop if an inspired oxygen concentration of 100% (FiO_2 of 1.00) is administered for extended periods of time. If the alveoli become filled with oxygen, alveolar nitrogen subsequently is washed out. As oxygen is absorbed from the alveoli, atelectasis can develop.[28,183]

   c. Substernal pain may develop in patients who receive high inspired oxygen concentration. The mechanism is not well understood but may be related to tracheitis.[28]

   d. Oxygen toxicity can result from high inspired oxygen concentrations (FiO_2 greater than 0.6), particularly if coupled with positive pressure ventilation. It can produce endothelial and alveolar epithelial damage that may produce fibrotic scarring and chronic lung disease. Inspired oxygen concentrations and the duration of oxygen exposure associated with oxygen toxicity have not been established. Individual susceptibility makes it impossible to determine safe or toxic levels of oxygen support. Therefore the child with respiratory distress should receive only as much supplementary oxygen as is needed to ensure satisfactory oxygen delivery. Inadequate or excessive inspired oxygen concentration must be avoided.

   e. Retinopathy of prematurity (ROP) occurs predominantly in extremely premature neonates. In its most severe form, ROP may progress to retrolental fibroplasia (RLF) with retinal detachment and blindness. The etiology of ROP is complex and still poorly understood. Factors such as respiratory failure, hypoxia, hypercarbia, inadequate nutrition, extreme prematurity, and high levels of inspired oxygen have been implicated. In the modern era, severe ROP is rare in infants beyond 30 weeks gestation.[28,183]

Table 21-9 Oxygen Delivery Systems

Delivery Device	Indications	Description	Advantages	Disadvantages
Low-flow nasal prongs or cannula	Provides inspired O_2 concentrations up to 0.50 if nasal breathing is performed	Vinyl catheter with two short prongs—one prong fits into each nostril; maximum O_2 flow should not exceed 4-5 L/min	May be more comfortable than masks; patient can eat and talk without altering or interrupting oxygen delivery	High O_2 flow produces burning and drying of nasal mucosa; admixture may occur at different flow rates depending on patient's minute volume and presence of oral breathing; mouth breathing reduces FiO_2
High-flow nasal cannula (HFNC)	When higher FiO_2 with some end-expiratory pressure is needed and ventilation is adequate	Nasal prongs deliver flow rate of 1-40 L/min (adjusted to 8-10 times the normal minute ventilation) at body temperature with 95%-100% relative humidity. Delivers predictable FiO_2 with oxygen titrated from blender	Predictable FiO_2 unless significant mouth breathing is present. Not irritating to nares despite high flow. Provides some positive end-expiratory pressure if flow rates are 20 L/min or higher.	Not effective if significant airflow occurs through the mouth instead of the nose. The higher the patient weight and gas flow the higher will be the positive pressure created throughout the respiratory cycle.
Head hood	Useful for infant or small child	Clear Lucite or plexiglass box or clear plastic framed box placed over patient's head; sufficient gas flow (7-12 L/min) is necessary to maintain inspired O_2 concentrations and flush CO_2 from hood; FiO_2 of >0.90 may be provided	Provides easy visibility of and access to patient; allows quick recovery time of FiO_2; can be used in isolettes, cribs, or open warmers; FiO_2 may be continuously monitored with an O_2 sensor	If humidified aerosol produces "rain-out" in hood, assessment of child is compromised; cool mist may produce cold stress; extremely moist environment may cause skin irritation
Aerosol mask (connected to aerosol generator)	Useful for children who require an FiO_2 > 0.40	Vinyl face mask fits over nose; open ports on side of mask allow exhalation of CO_2; sufficient flow of gas must enter mask to prevent accumulation of CO_2 and entrainment of room air; can be used to deliver almost any FiO_2 (see disadvantages)	Fairly comfortable for older children unless patient is struggling	Masks in general have the following disadvantages: Patient may entrain room air through side ports if gas flow into mask does not exceed peak inspiratory flow; child cannot eat or drink without interruption of O_2 delivery; vomiting with a mask in place may cause airway obstruction or aspiration
Partial rebreather mask	Useful as above; an FiO_2 of 0.60 or greater may be achieved; the smaller the child's tidal volume, the higher the FiO_2 that can be achieved	Face mask with reservoir bag attached; two valves are used—first valve, between the mask and bag, allows one-way gas flow from bag into the mask and prevents exhaled gas from flowing back into the bag; second valve, located at exhalation ports, opens during exhalation but closes during inspiration to prevent entrainment of room air—O_2 flow rate must be determined by patient's minute ventilation	Can deliver high FiO_2 concentrations in small children	As above; FiO_2 may be variable; it may not be easy to see through mask, and undetected vomiting can cause airway obstruction or aspiration

Table 21-9   Oxygen Delivery Systems—cont'd

Delivery Device	Indications	Description	Advantages	Disadvantages
Non-rebreathing mask	Useful as above; also useful for patients who require high FiO_2	A reservoir bag is added to mask; three valves are used (one between mask and bag, one on each side of mask); O_2 is directed into the bag and the child inhales gas from bag; oxygen and gas flow must be adjusted so that bag does not collapse during inspiration by more than a third of its volume	Can deliver an FiO_2 of 0.90 or more if mask fits snugly and oxygen flow is adjusted so bag never collapses by more than 1/3 during inspiration	If mask fits snugly, kinking of O_2 source tubing or disconnection of O_2 source will result in inadequate gas delivery to patient; it may not be easy to see through mask, and undetected vomiting can cause airway obstruction or aspiration
Venturi mask (high air-flow O_2 enrichment)	Useful when precise inspired oxygen concentration must be delivered	Vinyl face mask and attached wide-bore cone containing an inner "jet" orifice; diameter of inner orifice through which O_2 flows may be altered to increase or decrease inspired O_2 concentration; air entrainment occurs on either side of this jet orifice to provide dilution (blending) of O_2; high FiO_2 may not be attainable without additional oxygen source	Delivers a precise O_2 concentration; only rarely will FiO_2 delivered exceed intended delivery	Air entrainment ports can be occluded by bed linen, gowns, or patient position changes; patient can neither eat nor talk while wearing mask; it may not be easy to see through mask, and undetected vomiting can cause airway obstruction or aspiration

Table 21-10   Examples of Oxygen and Air Flow Rates* Required to Blend Specific Inspired Oxygen Concentrations

Total Flow	Desired FiO_2	O_2 (LPM)[†]	Air (LPM)
20 LPM	0.25	1.25	18.75
	0.35	3.75	16.25
	0.45	6.25	13.75
	0.6	10.0	10.0
	0.8	15.0	5.0
15 LPM	0.25	0.95	14.0
	0.35	2.8	12.2
	0.45	4.7	10.3
	0.6	7.5	7.5
	0.8	11.25	3.75
10 LPM	0.25	0.6	9.4
	0.35	1.9	8.1
	0.45	3.1	6.9
	0.6	5.0	5.0
	0.8	7.5	2.5

*Formula for calculating flow rates: O_2 flow = total flow $\times$ (FiO_2 − 0.21)/0.8.
[†]LPM = liters per minute.

Mechanical Ventilation

Assisted ventilation is indicated for patients who are unable to maintain adequate oxygenation or eliminate carbon dioxide, or who develop refractory circulatory failure. These patients generally exhibit clinical signs of respiratory failure or shock.

Mechanical ventilation is based on the properties of normal pulmonary function. During inspiration, alveolar pressure must be significantly lower (normal breathing or negative pressure ventilation) or greater (positive pressure ventilation) than atmospheric pressure. This is accomplished in two ways:
(1) By making atmospheric pressure or pressure surrounding the chest more negative
(2) By increasing alveolar pressure via delivery of gas under positive pressure.

These inspiratory mechanisms describe the two major forms of mechanical ventilatory assistance: *negative pressure ventilation* and *positive pressure ventilation*.

Negative Pressure Ventilation

Negative pressure ventilation is a relatively uncommon mode of ventilatory support that creates a negative (with respect to airway opening pressure) extrathoracic pressure, so the child's chest expands, causing inspiration. Because negative pressure ventilation is provided without the need for insertion of an artificial airway (e.g., endotracheal tube), it is a form of non-invasive ventilation.

Description. A tank or shell surrounds the thorax; negative pressure is created around the thorax by a vacuum. The negative pressure "pulls" the thoracic cage outward, thereby increasing intrathoracic volume and reducing intrathoracic pressure. A pressure gradient is then present between the mouth and the intrathoracic space (where the pressure is now approximately -10 to -15 cm H_2O), so air flows into the alveoli. Exhalation occurs passively when the vacuum cycles off.[183]

In order to generate the subatmospheric pressure around the thorax, the shell must seal around the arms, neck and lower abdomen. This required proper fit. If diapers are used, they should be secured outside (below) the shell.

Clinical Applications. Negative pressure ventilation may be used for support of children with chronic respiratory failure secondary to neuromuscular disease, such as the child with phrenic nerve injury or muscular dystrophy. The child's lung tissue must allow normal gas diffusion (i.e., pulmonary interstitial disease cannot be present), and the child must be able to maintain a patent airway (with an effective cough reflex).

An advantage of this form of ventilation is that endotracheal intubation is not required. Supplementary oxygen may be administered by nasal prongs or face mask.

Advantages and Disadvantages. There are some distinct disadvantages to negative pressure ventilation, which limits its use. The tanks are cumbersome for the patient and caretakers and they render the child virtually immobile. "Shell" devices must be fitted precisely to the child's thorax to obtain a good seal. Even if the tank fits properly, it is frequently difficult to achieve a good seal around the arms, neck, and abdomen. Air leaks diminish the effectiveness of the machine, thus reducing chest expansion and alveolar ventilation.

Exaggerated dilation of the thoracic great vessels and diminished cardiac output have been reported during negative pressure ventilation. In addition, venous pooling may develop in the legs.

In spite of the challenges during use, negative pressure ventilators may be extremely useful in the care of chronically ill ventilator-dependent patients. This form of ventilation support may be particularly useful for home ventilator therapy because the devices are relatively easy to operate and do not require an advanced (invasive) airway. With practice, the child is able to talk during negative pressure ventilation.[28]

Nursing Considerations. As with all other devices, the nurse must be knowledgeable about the operation of a negative pressure ventilator. At all times a resuscitation bag and mask with an O_2 source should be available to provide manual ventilation in case of machine malfunction.

The child's heart rate, blood pressure and systemic perfusion must be closely monitored when instituting negative pressure ventilation and whenever the ventilator is adjusted. It is also important to monitor the patient closely for signs of venous dilation and signs of hypovolemia (potentially caused by venous pooling outside of the thorax).

If the child will be discharged home with this ventilator, a teaching program must be implemented for the family in the hospital. The parents must be able to provide bag-mask ventilation and troubleshoot common problems with the ventilator.

Positive Pressure Ventilation

Positive pressure ventilation is achieved by delivery of a gas (oxygen/air mixture) to the patient's proximal airway. Positive pressure ventilation changes the normal pressures during the respiratory cycle, because gas is delivered to the alveoli under positive pressure, creating *positive* (rather than negative) pressure during inspiration. Expiration occurs passively.

Description. Ventilators may be classified according to the mechanism that terminates inspiration. However, most new ventilators use a combination of cycling mechanisms and a variety of ventilation characteristics.

Volume-cycled ventilators are preset to deliver a specific tidal volume during inspiration. Once this volume is delivered, inspiration stops, allowing for passive exhalation. *Pressure-cycled* ventilators use a preset peak inspiratory pressure (PIP) at which inspiration is terminated; gas is delivered until the peak pressure is achieved without regard to the volume delivered. *Time-cycled* ventilators, most commonly used in the neonatal/infant population, are preset to allow a specific inspiratory time; gas will be delivered until that time is reached, without regard for the volume delivered or the peak pressure produced.[88,183]

Changes in the child's pulmonary resistance and compliance will affect the tidal volume that is actually delivered to the lung. For this reason, close attention to exhaled volume is required. Some centers measure the patient's effective tidal volume (Vt_{eff}) to ensure that an acceptable tidal volume is delivered. Most ventilators available today are capable of real-time measurements of Vt_{eff}. Effective tidal volume is defined as the actual volume (mL) of gas being delivered to the lung per kilogram (kg) of ideal body weight; it is measured in mL/kg. The most accurate measurements are obtained at the patient wye (the connector that joins the inspiratory and expiratory limbs of a two-limb circuit to the patient's airway); measurement at this point alleviates the need to calculate the compliance factor of the ventilator circuit.[32] Depending on the level of PEEP and underlying pathology, acceptable values of Vt_{eff} range from 5 to 8 mL/kg.[183]

The Vt_{eff} may be calculated using pressure measurements obtained by the ventilator, with correction for tubing compliance (i.e., the circuit compliance factor). Calculation is performed as follows:

Calculation of Effective Tidal Volume Using Ventilator Values (*Values Measured at the Ventilator, not from the patient wye*)

$$Vt_{eff} = V_T \text{ set} - [(P_{plateau} - PEEP^*) \times \text{circuit compliance factor}^\dagger]$$

* The greater the difference between the $P_{Plateau}$ and level of PEEP or change in pressure (ΔP), the greater the volume lost in the ventilator circuit.[183]

† The circuit compliance factor is available from the ventilator circuit manufacturer and varies according to the circuit diameter.

Most newer-generation pediatric ventilators have incorporated flow-sensing devices or *pneumotachographs* at the patient's wye to more accurately determine inhaled and exhaled volumes.[32] Monitoring respiratory volumes at the patient's airway removes the inaccuracy resulting from the aforementioned volume loss related to the circuit tubing compliance.[32]

Most pediatric patients requiring mechanical ventilation in the critical care unit are placed on positive pressure ventilators. Selection of the appropriate ventilator should be based on the following factors:[46,88,183]

1. *Size of the child and minute ventilation requirement.* The ventilator maximum and minimum flow rates must be appropriate for the patient.
2. *Lung compliance.* If the patient requires high inspiratory pressures (>40 cm H_2O), a pressure-cycled ventilator may be preferable to a volume-cycled ventilator.
3. *Rapidly changing lung compliance.* Optimum ventilation of the patient at risk for rapid or frequent changes in compliance may be most effective using a volume-cycled ventilator (or a combination volume/time cycle).
4. *Chest wall stability.* If a child has an unstable chest wall (e.g., with flail chest or a median sternotomy incision), volume-cycled ventilators may be most appropriate.

Characteristics of an Ideal Pediatric Ventilator. The categories in Box 21-2 represent three groups of criteria for selection of the ideal ventilator for pediatric use. See Table 21-11 for more detail regarding each alarm.

Frequently, ventilators with the widest possible clinical application are more practical to purchase than a large number of ventilators with very specific applications. The information in Box 21-2 and Table 21-11 should be considered when selecting ventilators for use with critically ill children, as well as selection of a specific mechanical ventilator for a particular patient.

Clinical Applications. Many of the newer-generation ventilators are capable of providing mechanical support across all or most patient populations. The incorporation of microprocessors into newer-generation ventilators has enabled this wide range of use.

Manufacturer's specifications and recommendations and hospital clinical trials should facilitate the selection of the ventilator(s) that can best serve each patient (e.g., the patient size limit for use of neonatal ventilators is generally 8-15 kg body weight). The clinical condition of the patient will determine the ventilator functions needed to provide optimal ventilation.

Nursing Considerations. Throughout mechanical ventilatory support, the bedside nurse is responsible for assessing effectiveness of ventilation. *The use of mechanical ventilation does not ensure that the child is ventilated effectively.* The ventilator settings must be evaluated constantly in light of the child's clinical appearance.

When ventilator function is in doubt, the child should be ventilated manually with a hand-resuscitator bag. Table 21-11 offers a troubleshooting guide for use when problems arise during mechanical ventilation. It is intended to address *equipment* (rather than patient) problems. For more information, see Chapter 9, Positive Pressure Mechanical Ventilation and the section, Nursing Care of the Child During Mechanical Ventilation).

High-Frequency Ventilation (HFV)

An alternative mode of ventilatory support is *high-frequency ventilation (HFV)*. High-frequency ventilation uses a mean airway pressure (map) and rapid respiratory rates (60 to 3600/minutes) to recruit atelectatic regions of the lung. The tidal volumes used are close to anatomic dead space, so this form of ventilatory support does not create risk of volutrauma that can occur with administration of higher tidal volumes. Simply put, HFV allows for higher end-expiratory pressures with lower peak inspiratory pressures.

HFV is used for infants and children with acute lung injury when conventional ventilation has failed. A metaanalysis of HFV versus conventional ventilation in premature neonates

Text continues on p. 1023

Box 21-2 **Characteristics of an Ideal Pediatric Ventilator**

Specifications
- Volume, pressure or time cycled; mixed modes of ventilation
- Assist/control, control, CPAP (continuous positive airway pressure), PSV (pressure support ventilation), SIMV (synchronized intermittent mandatory ventilation)
- Tidal volume range of 20-450 mL/breath (minute ventilation of 0.4-6 L/min)
- Respiratory rate of 1-100/min (high-frequency ventilation capability is also desirable)
- Variable inspiratory flow of 0.5-40 L/min
- Variable inspiratory/expiratory flow ratios
- Adjustable peak inspiratory pressure of 10-80 cm H_2O
- Adequate humidification
- Provision for PEEP/CPAP with minimal adjustments

Alarms
- High and low pressure
- Apnea

- Loss of PEEP
- Power failure/disconnect
- Loss of air/O_2
- High temperature
- Failure to cycle
- Output jacks to allow ventilator alarms to be connected to a remote alarm in nursing station

Visual Indicators
- Proximal airway pressure (patent airway)
- Proximal airway temperature (patent airway)
- FiO_2 (high and low)
- Inspiratory/expiratory times
- Inspiratory to expiratory ratio
- Flow rate (L/min)
- Tidal volume
- Minute ventilation

Table 21-11   **Mechanical Ventilators Alarms and Associated Clinical Events**

Ventilator Alarm	Causes	Associated Patient Observation	Treatment
High Peak Pressure Alarm	Pneumothorax	Tachycardia Tachypnea Respiratory distress Hypoxemia Hypercarbia Pulsus paradoxus Unilateral chest expansion Unequal breath sounds	Manually provide ventilation (with a bag), assessing bilateral breath sounds and symmetry of chest expansion; watch for improvement in color with manual ventilation If arterial line is in place, observe for pulsus paradoxus on the monitor consistent with tension pneumothorax Order immediate chest radiograph and call physician or other on-call provider if no improvement occurs per unit policy. Do not await chest radiograph to eliminate tension pneumothorax (with needle thoracostomy). Transilluminate infant's chest for free air Prepare for chest tube insertion or needle aspiration of air
	Bronchospasm	Tachycardia Tachypnea Wheezing Respiratory distress Hypoxemia Hypercarbia Ramping on capnogram	Notify physician or other on-call provider Consider the administration of an inhaled bronchodilator Evaluate pulse oximetry and exhaled carbon dioxide tension Obtain an arterial blood gas to check for the presence of severe hypercarbia Consider adjusting ventilator settings to ensure complete lung emptying
	Delivery of excessive tidal volume (V_T) or development of decreased lung compliance	Tachycardia Tachypnea Respiratory distress Hypoxemia Hypercarbia Ventilator asynchrony Coughing	Provide manual ventilation (with bag device) and reassess patient thoroughly. Recheck ventilator settings and validate inspiratory time, flow rate, tidal volume, etc. Notify physician or other on-call provider if clinical status does not improve when patient is manually ventilated or if deterioration occurs when child is placed back on ventilator; call provider to re-evaluate ventilator settings. Check pulse oximetry and exhaled carbon dioxide tension. Obtain arterial blood gases per physician order or unit policy.
	ET tube obstruction	Tachycardia Tachypnea Respiratory distress Hypoxemia Hypercarbia Ventilator asynchrony Paradoxical chest/abdominal movement	Provide manual ventilation and suction advanced airway. Assess chest expansion, lung aeration, and lung compliance—evaluate for "DOPE": • **Displaced ET tube** • **Obstructed ET tube** • **Pneumothorax** • **Equipment failure**

Table 21-11 **Mechanical Ventilators Alarms and Associated Clinical Events—cont'd**

Ventilator Alarm	Causes	Associated Patient Observation	Treatment
			If the following are present: • Diminished breath sounds • Child does not improve with suctioning of the tube and manual ventilation • Chest excursion is diminished • Pneumothorax is not suspected Consider removing ET tube and providing bag-mask ventilation and replacing ET tube (by appropriate provider). Notify physician or other on-call provider immediately.
	Ventilator tubing/ET tube is kinked or obstructed	Tachycardia Tachypnea Respiratory distress Hypoxemia Hypercarbia Ventilator asynchrony Paradoxical chest/abdominal movement	Provide manual ventilation (with bag device). Evaluate ET tube for kinking of ventilator circuit including compression of ET tube/artificial airway. Check all tubing for water collection and/or other obstruction.
	Inadequate humidity or irritation of airways	Tachycardia Tachypnea Coughing Gagging on the ET tube	Provide manual ventilation (with bag device). Assess patient; if other, more serious problems are ruled out (e.g., extubation), check ventilator settings and humidification system. Verify function of humidification system.
	Patient anxiety	Tachycardia Tachypnea Respiratory distress Hypoxemia Hypercarbia Ventilator asynchrony Paradoxical chest/abdominal movement	Provide manual ventilation. Reassess patient, including assessment of pulse oximetry, exhaled CO_2 and arterial blood gases. Reassure patient. Verify function of humidification system. With older children, use of picture boards, alphabet boards, or grease boards for writing may increase the child's ability to communicate, thus alleviating some anxiety. Sedation may be necessary if oxygenation and ventilation are adequate. Consider ventilation in IMV mode (may be better tolerated).
Low Peak Inspiratory Pressure Alarm	Altered ventilator settings Patient disconnected from the ventilator or a large leak within the ventilator circuit Inadvertent extubation Leak around ET tube, improper ET tube size, inadequate cuff inflation, or malpositioned ET tube	Tachycardia Tachypnea Respiratory distress Hypoxemia Hypercarbia Decreased $P_{ET}CO_2$ Diminished breath sounds Audible leak around ET tube	Provide manual ventilation (with bag device). Assess respiratory status, including chest movement, aeration, and lung compliance; observe for leak around ET tube during peak inspiration; check ET tube cuff pressure. Evaluate pulse oximetry and $P_{ET}CO_2$.

Continued

Table 21-11 **Mechanical Ventilators Alarms and Associated Clinical Events—cont'd**

Ventilator Alarm	Causes	Associated Patient Observation	Treatment
			Check ventilator system for flow rate, peak inspiratory pressure setting, I:E ratio, tidal volume provided by ventilator, sensitivity, and adequate humidification. Call physician or other on-call provider if patient has not improved with manual ventilation. Consider obtaining arterial blood gases (and, possibly, chest radiograph) if patient does not immediately improve with manual bag ventilation.
High Tidal Volume Alarm	Delivery of V_T greater then set threshold Improved lung compliance	Hypocarbia Low $P_{ET}CO_2$ Respiratory alkalosis Improved patient condition—color pink, chest excursion improved, breath sounds clearer	Provide manual ventilation; adjust the ventilator to provide ordered V_T. Consider adjusting alarms if V_T is within safe limits. Discuss with physician (or other on-call provider) possible initiation of weaning from mechanical ventilation.
Low Tidal Volume Alarm	Altered ventilator settings, including decreased volume, flow rate, PIP limit, and I:E ratio (see pneumothorax above) Patient disconnected from the ventilator or a large leak within the ventilator circuit Inadvertent extubation Leak around ET tube, improper ET tube size, inadequate cuff inflation, or malpositioned ET tube	Tachycardia Tachypnea Respiratory distress Hypoxemia Hypercarbia Unequal breath sounds	Provide manual ventilation (with bag device); assess respiratory status as described above. Notify physician of observed abnormalities or changes in patient's condition. Evaluate ventilator system. Check all ventilator settings.
Low PEEP Alarm	Inadvertent change in PEEP/CPAP settings Patient disconnected from the ventilator or a large leak within the ventilator circuit Inadvertent extubation Patient's intrinsic inspiratory pressure may be strong enough to override the PEEP with each breath	Tachycardia Tachypnea Respiratory distress Hypoxemia Hypercarbia Diminished breath sounds	Check all ventilator settings and ventilator system. Reassess patient and note respiratory rate, chest excursion, aeration, and breath sounds; check pulse oximetry and exhaled CO_2. Consider increasing gas flow rate to maintain level of PEEP (if PEEP is too low).
High PEEP Alarm	Alarm set below the ordered level of PEEP Occurrence of auto PEEP		Provide manual ventilation (with bag device). Assess patient chest excursion, lung aeration, and color; notify physician (or other on-call provider) of deterioration in clinical condition. Evaluate pulse oximetry (for evidence of hypoxemia) and exhaled CO_2 (for "alveolar ramping"). Check all ventilator settings including flow rate, respiratory rate, and tidal volume. Consider a chest x-ray for hyperinflation.

Table 21-11 **Mechanical Ventilators Alarms and Associated Clinical Events—cont'd**

Ventilator Alarm	Causes	Associated Patient Observation	Treatment
I:E Ratio Alarm (frequently associated with high-pressure alarm)	Inadequate inspiratory flow provided by ventilator Inadvertent change of ventilator settings Inappropriate ventilator sensitivity to patient's respiratory effort Increased airway secretions Subtle leaks in system	Patient may be combative or anxious Tachycardia Tachypnea Respiratory distress Hypoxemia Hypercarbia Diminished breath sounds Clinical condition may or may not change	Provide manual ventilation (with bag device). Assess patient chest excursion, lung aeration, and color; notify physician of deterioration in clinical condition. Evaluate pulse oximetry and exhaled CO_2. Check all ventilator settings including flow rate, respiratory rate, and tidal volume. Suction ET tube. Obtain arterial blood gases.
High FiO_2 Alarm	O_2 analyzer error/Blender error O_2 source error O_2 reservoir leak	Patient may or may not exhibit clinical changes, e.g., in color, respiratory rate, general mental alertness, increase in PaO_2 or oxy-Hgb saturation	If patient has deteriorated, provide manual ventilation with bag device and ensure tube patency. Calibrate O_2 analyzer. Check O_2 systems and correct dysfunction.
Low FiO_2 Alarm	O_2 analyzer error/Blender error O_2 source error O_2 reservoir leak	Patient may or may not exhibit clinical changes, e.g., in color, respiratory rate, general mental alertness, decrease in PaO_2 or oxy-Hgb saturation	If patient has deteriorated, provide manual ventilation (with bag device) and ensure tube patency. Check pulse oximetry. Calibrate O_2 analyzer. Check O_2 systems and correct dysfunction.
High or Low Inspired Gas Temperature	Addition of cold water to humidifier Thermostat failure Altered thermostat settings	Patient's temperature may be increased or decreased Patient may be agitated	Check temperature of patient and treat accordingly. Wait for humidifier water to warm if child can tolerate the delay.

concluded that the use of HFV did not reduce chronic lung disease or mortality in this patient group.[27] With studies including only a small number of pediatric patients, a recent Cochrane analysis concluded that HFV did not improve outcome when compared with conventional mechanical ventilation.[72a]

There are two basic types of high-frequency ventilators—the oscillator and jet ventilator. Each is presented briefly here. For additional information, see Chapter 9.

High-Frequency Oscillatory Ventilation (HFOV). High-frequency oscillatory ventilation (HFOV) employs a piston moving at extremely high frequencies (about 180 to 1500 cycles/minute) to create positive and negative pressure swings. Oscillatory ventilation does not produce bulk gas delivery. It uses a continuous gas flow to eliminate CO_2 and deliver oxygen to the lung's ventilatory units.

In a controlled randomized multicenter NIH trial,[75] HFOV offered no advantages over conventional ventilators in the treatment of neonatal respiratory failure. In this study the incidence of bronchopulmonary dysplasia was similar to conventional ventilation, and mortality rates were equal in both groups.

A randomized, crossover trial of HFOV versus conventional mechanical ventilation in 70 critically ill children with ARDS was published in 1994 by Arnold et al[12a] Children treated with HFOV demonstrated improved oxygenation and decreased use of supplementary oxygen 30 days later.

High-Frequency Jet Ventilation (HFJV). The typical HFJV uses an oxygen source and a high-pressure source to deliver gas through a small-bore injector cannula that extends into the endotracheal (ET) tube. This system allows delivery of relatively large tidal volumes at relatively low peak airway pressures. A flow interrupter adjusts the frequency and relative inspiratory time. Valve devices applied to the expiratory limb of the circuit allow the application of PEEP. A continuous infusion of saline into the path of the jet humidifies inspired air. Often a conventional ventilator is used in tandem as the gas and oxygen source for the HFJV unit.

HFJV is used most often used as a rescue therapy for patients with respiratory failure unresponsive to conventional ventilation, as evidenced by rising inspiratory pressures, persistent hypoxemia, and hypercarbia despite maximal conventional ventilatory support. In recent years high frequency jet ventilation (HFJV) has become less widely used than HFOV.

Mechanisms of Gas Exchange with High Frequency Ventilation. The mechanisms of gas exchange during high-frequency ventilation are not well understood. As previously mentioned, bulk gas flow is not a major mechanism of gas exchange during HFV. Some gas exchange probably occurs simply because of nonhomogeneous alveolar filling and pressures.[183] Other explanations include gas exchange resulting from turbulent mixing of gas molecules ("augmented dispersion"), gas convection, and diffusion.

Multiple mechanisms are probably involved in gas exchange during high-frequency ventilation.[183] Ultimately, the effectiveness of these mechanisms must be determined by the evaluation of the patient's response to support.

Nursing Considerations During High Frequency Ventilation. High-frequency respiratory support is very different from conventional mechanical ventilation. The nurse must be familiar with the principles of operation, assessment of effectiveness of ventilation, and the potential complications of the technique.

The assessment of the infant or child on HFV differs from conventional ventilation in the following ways:

1. The *clinical progress of the patient is the ultimate indicator of the effectiveness of ventilatory support*. Progress is determined through evaluation of the patient's general appearance, color, and blood gases.
2. The chest will not rise during HFV, but may instead appear to be fluttering or vibrating, often referred to as "chest wiggle."[183]
3. During auscultation of breath sounds, "inspiratory" air movement is difficult to identify; the quality of the breath sounds is peculiar to the patient on HFV. Breath sounds have been described as resembling a continuous loud jack hammer and are very high pitched. Low-pitched breath sounds may, in fact, indicate poor ventilation or pneumothorax.
4. Auscultation of the heart rate is nearly impossible; some physicians instruct the nurse to *briefly* place the HFV on standby to assess heart tones. Without the ability to easily auscultate heart tones or blood pressure, the nurse relies on evaluation of color, perfusion, pulses, pulse oximetry, and invasive monitoring for cardiovascular assessment.
5. Assessment of quantity and consistency of secretions obtained from suctioning is critical. Changes in the quantity or consistency of secretions frequently indicates the need for adjustment of the humidification system. A change in secretion quantity or consistency also may herald the development of necrotizing tracheobronchitis. Water particles should be visible traveling down the jet tube; these particles help prevent the development of mucous plugs.[86]

Complications of High-Frequency Ventilation. Many of the potential complications of HFV are identical to the complications of conventional mechanical ventilation, but the *development* of the complication may be more difficult to detect during HFV than during positive pressure ventilation.

1. *Pneumothorax:* The risk of pneumothorax in patients receiving HFV is the same as with conventional ventilation. Pneumothorax may be difficult to recognize during HFV because breath sounds are difficult to evaluate. Clinical signs of pneumothorax may be acute, including severe respiratory distress, cyanosis, hypoxemia, and hypotension. Transillumination and chest radiography are used to confirm the diagnosis.
2. *Tenacious secretions:* Secretions tend to become very thick, and mucous plugs may develop,[86] producing airway obstruction. It may be difficult to achieve adequate humidification. Suctioning should be performed with instillation of saline.[86]
3. *Gas trapping:* Gas trapping often occurs with HFV and causes carbon dioxide retention and decreased compliance. Gas trapping is most likely to occur when high tidal volumes and short expiratory times are used.[183] The optimal HFV settings to minimize air trapping have not been determined.

Endotracheal Tubes

Endotracheal (ET) intubation may be necessary to establish or maintain a patent airway or to facilitate mechanical ventilatory support. Elective intubation is always preferable to intubation under emergency conditions.

Endotracheal Tube Characteristics and Sizes

Shape of the Tube. Some ET tubes are curved sharply to enable rapid intubation to the point of curvature. These tubes should not be used for more than a few hours, because it is difficult to pass a suction catheter beyond the curvature of the tube. Tubes with sharp curvature are designed for orotracheal use, so they can be very difficult to place nasotracheally.

Position Markings. A radiopaque line should be present along the length of the ET tube to allow radiographic verification of the tube's position. In addition, markings should be present at 1-cm intervals on the tube. Such markings allow the nurse to verify appropriate depth of insertion regularly so that tube displacement is detected immediately.

The depth of the tube insertion at the patient lips or nares should be recorded in the patient record and nursing care plan. The nurse should check the depth of insertion whenever the tube is retaped, when vital signs are obtained or if the patient deteriorates suddenly.

Cuffed Versus Uncuffed Tubes. In the past, uncuffed ET tubes were generally used for infants and children less than 8 years of age, because the cricoid diameter of a child is quite narrow and was thought to provide a natural seal around the tube. However, evidence published in recent years has demonstrated that the use of *cuffed* tubes during in-hospital care of young children produces no higher incidence of complications than the use of uncuffed tubes.[92]

Cuffed tubes may reduce the incidence of aspiration, and cuffed tubes may be preferable to uncuffed tubes in some patients (i.e., those with poor lung compliance, high airway resistance, or a large glottic air leak), provided the endotracheal tube size, position and cuff inflation pressure is monitored.[92] The cuff inflation pressure is maintained according to manufacturer specifications, typically at 20 to 25 cm H_2O.[92]

Endotracheal Tube Size Selection. The diameter of the child's trachea is smallest at the level of the cricoid cartilage; therefore an ET tube may pass easily through the vocal cords yet be too large at the level of the cricoid cartilage. The ET tube size is appropriate if a small, audible air leak is present when inspiratory pressure of approximately 20- to 30-cm H_2O is provided. This small leak indicates that the tube is probably small enough to avoid excessive pressure on the trachea below the level of the vocal cords.

If the tube is too large, an air leak is not detected even at positive pressure of more than 25 to 30 cm H_2O. A tube that is too large can cause injury to the trachea.

If the tube is too small, an air leak is detectable at even low (<10 to 15 cm H_2O) inspiratory pressures. If the tube is too small and allows a substantial air leak, it may be impossible to provide adequate oxygenation or ventilation through the ET tube.[92]

The child's *body length* provides the best parameter for estimation of appropriate ET tube size.[142] The relationship between body length and proper ET tube size has been used in the development of the Broselow resuscitation tape, which enables determination of appropriate endotracheal tube sizes, resuscitation equipment sizes, and drug dosages using the child's body length (see Figure 1-1).[3,108]

Several formulas enable estimation of ET tube size from age in children. The most popular formulas for estimation of uncuffed and cuffed tube sizes for children 1 to 10 years of age are:[92]

- Uncuffed ETT (internal diameter [I.D.] in mm) = (age/4) + 4
- Cuffed ETT (internal diameter [I.D.] in mm) = (age/4) + 3.5

These formulas provide a relatively accurate estimate of ET tube size (within 0.5 mm) in most children 1 to 10 years of age. Additional guidelines for estimation of proper ET tube size include the approximation of the size of the patient's little finger or the equivalent of the size of the child's nares.

Essential equipment for endotracheal intubation trays is listed in Table 21-12. Suggestions for intubation equipment size according to the child's age in years are listed in the table.

Resuscitation Bags for Hand Ventilation

A variety of manual resuscitator bags are available, each with distinctive features. In general, there are two main types of bags: the self-inflating bag and the non–self-inflating (gas-inflating or so-called "anesthesia") bag. The self-inflating bag does not require gas flow to provide manual ventilation; the non-self-inflating bag does require gas flow for use.

Self-inflating Bags

Self-inflating bags may be used with or without an oxygen source. The natural recoil of the bag causes the bag to reinflate after it is compressed, whether or not the bag is connected to an oxygen (or other gas) source.

If the bag is connected to an oxygen source and a reservoir bag, 100% oxygen can be delivered to the patient, because

Table 21-12	Essential Equipment for Endotracheal Intubation

ESSENTIAL EQUIPMENT FOR INTUBATION

Laryngoscope handle (2)	Suction catheter to fit
Curved and straight	endotracheal tube
laryngoscope blades	Tonsil suction (Yankauer tube)
Endotracheal tubes (three	Foam donut head rest
sizes)	Oropharyngeal airways
Stylet	Magill forceps or Kolodny
Bag and Mask	hemostats
Oxygen source	1-inch tape
Suction set-up	Benzoin

GUIDELINES FOR PEDIATRIC ENDOTRACHEAL TUBE SIZES

Age/Size	mm Internal Diameter*
Premature newborn	
1000 g	2.5
1000-1500 g	3.0
1500-2500 g	3.5
Full-term Newborns	3.5-4.0
6-12 months	4.0-4.5
1-2 years	4.5
4 years	5.0
6 years	5.5
8 years	6.0
10 years	6.5
Greater than 12 years	
Female	6.5-8.0
Male	7.5-8.0

From Czervinske MP, Barnhart SL: *Perinatal and pediatric respiratory care*, St Louis, 2003, Saunders.

*An ET tube size 0.5 mm larger and one 0.5 mm size smaller than predicted size should be immediately available to accommodate unexpected anatomical deviations.

Note: Intubation should be attempted by an experienced or closely-supervised clinician with resuscitation equipment immediately available.

even when the bag recoils, only oxygen is drawn into the bag and administered to the patient. If oxygen is joined to the bag without a reservoir, when the bag recoils room air can be drawn into (entrained into) the bag so it mixes with the oxygen; as a result the patient receives a mix of room air and oxygen.

The 0.5-L bag is generally appropriate for ventilation of infants through preschool-age children; the 1-L bags are used for children up to 8 to 10 years of age. The larger (i.e., 1.5 L) bags may be used for adolescents and adults.[183]

Clinical Use. Self-inflating resuscitation bags are particularly useful for resuscitation carts because they can be used without oxygen flow, if needed. If used during resuscitation, delivery of a high concentration of oxygen is typically needed, so the bag should include a reservoir and should be attached to oxygen flow as soon as possible. Self-inflating bags require less skill to use than non-self inflating bags.

These bags are also useful for patient transport, when it is frequently impossible to predict how much air/oxygen to carry. If the oxygen source is exhausted, the self-inflating bags still enable effective ventilation of the patient with room air until additional oxygen is obtained.

When the bag is used for ventilation through an ET tube, a pressure gauge should be used, joined to the bag (with a Y connector if necessary). This enables monitoring of peak inspiratory pressures delivered.

Most bags have a pop-off valve to prevent delivery of high pressures. These valves are not precise and it may be necessary to inactivate the pop-off valve to deliver adequate bag-mask ventilation during emergencies.

The bags typically contain a valve near the adaptor where the bag can be joined to the ET tube or a mask. Unless a low-resistance valve is present, the valve opens only when the bag is squeezed (to deliver breaths to the patient) and it closes while the bag recoils and refills with air. An adjustable PEEP valve can be added to maintain positive end-expiratory pressure.

Advantages. The advantages of self-inflating bags include ease of operation (operation of valves is not needed to deliver gas flow) and ability to operate without an oxygen or gas source.

Disadvantages. There are several disadvantages to the use of self-inflating bags. A reservoir must be added to the bag to enable provision of a FiO_2 greater than 0.60.

If an inspiratory pop-off valve is present in older bags (set at 40 mm Hg to prevent the delivery of high inflation pressures), the pop-off valve may prevent delivery of adequate tidal volume during bag-mask ventilation, particularly if there is low airway or lung compliance.

The operator must be familiar with appropriate manual ventilation technique. Because these bags have thicker walls than nonself-inflating bags, it is more difficult for the operator to assess the compliance of the patient's lungs during bag-mask or bag-tube ventilation. A quick, snapping motion on inspiration should be avoided because this technique creates excessive inspiratory pressure that will open the pop-off valve (if one is present) and result in loss of tidal volume (i.e., air flow delivered to the patient).

Gas flow does not occur during spontaneous patient inspiration unless a low-resistance valve is present in the bag to allow the patient to draw in gas from the bag between manually delivered breaths. In many models a valve between the mask-adapter and the bag is opened only by the force of bag compression, so gas flow (and delivery of supplementary oxygen through the bag) during spontaneous ventilation is impossible.

The volume delivered during manual ventilation may be variable and depends on the speed and force of bag compression (and recoil) and patient lung compliance. The oxygen concentration delivered to the patient can also vary widely; if a reservoir is attached to the bag an FiO_2 of 1.00 (100% oxygen) may be reliably delivered.

Non–Self-inflating Bags

Non–self-inflating resuscitation bags are collapsed at rest. They inflate (and reinflate after each breath delivered) only if a continuous gas source is available. The gas flow to the bag must equal at least three to five times the patient's minute ventilation requirements to adequately fill the bag between breaths.

Clinical Use. The non-self-inflating bag ("anesthesia bag") is used in patients with advanced airways; it is not used for mask ventilation. This bag is very useful for assisting respiratory efforts of spontaneously breathing patients, but can also be used for those with no spontaneous respiratory effort.

The operator can deliver a relatively consistent tidal volume to patients who have decreased lung compliance. If the patient is breathing spontaneously, the patient can receive gas flow from the bag between delivered breaths.

Advantages. There are many advantages of this type of resuscitation bag. A FiO_2 of 1.0 can be provided without the addition of a reservoir bag. The bag and adaptor itself contain no internal valves that might dysfunction. During ventilation the provider can easily assess the patient's lung compliance because the walls of the bag are not thick and there are no valves between the bag and the patient's endotracheal tube/airway.

As noted previously, patients can breathe spontaneously and receive a continuous flow of oxygen even when the bag is not squeezed. A CPAP/PEEP valve (that provides resistance to exit of gas from the bag) and a pressure gauge easily can be added to the system.

Disadvantages. The use of this bag requires much greater skill than the use of the self-inflating bag. The use of the bag is best learned in a controlled environment. The operator must be able to monitor the patient and the patient's chest rise while ensuring that gas flow into and out of the bag is adequate.

The provider must be able to adjust gas flow into the bag so the bag will quickly reinflate between delivered breaths yet avoid delivery of high inspiratory pressure to the patient. If gas flow to the bag is insufficient, it will be impossible to deliver an adequate tidal volume and respiratory rate.

The risk of pneumothorax is significant when this bag is used by an inexperienced operator. If the gas flow to the bag is too high in light of the patient's minute ventilation, or if the PEEP valve is adjusted incorrectly, the bag may quickly become distended and ventilation may be delivered at a high pressure. Finally the bag requires a continuous flow of gas, which may be a problem during field resuscitations, such as transports.

NEUROLOGIC MONITORING DEVICES

Jodi E. Mullen

Neurologic monitoring devices are used in the pediatric critical care unit to measure intracranial pressure (ICP) and enable drainage of cerebrospinal fluid (CSF), to monitor cerebral oxygenation, or for evaluating cerebral electroencephalographic (EEG) activity. Multimodal monitoring incorporates several neurologic monitoring parameters to evaluate the patient, and may yield additional information about the patient's overall clinical status.

As with the use of any monitoring or support device, it is imperative that the nurse be familiar with the monitoring technique or device itself, interpretation of values provided, and troubleshooting of the system. No one measurement will be as valuable as evaluation of trends in the measurements over time. As a result, the bedside nurse must ensure that measurements are performed consistently so that errors may be eliminated or standardized.

Invasive Intracranial Pressure (ICP) Monitoring

Invasive monitoring of intracranial pressure (ICP) is often a valuable adjunct to the care of the child with head injury, mass lesions, or metabolic encephalopathy. Measurement of ICP is also used in calculation of the cerebral perfusion pressure (CPP), and can provide indirect information about cerebral compliance and autoregulation. Intracranial pressure monitoring is especially useful when a patient is comatose or heavily sedated and clinical evaluation of neurologic function is difficult.

Common methods of ICP monitoring include intraventricular monitoring using a fluid-filled system, and advanced technologies that use fiberoptics or microchip sensors. An extraventricular drain (EVD) set can be coupled with an ICP monitoring system to enable cerebrospinal fluid (CSF) drainage as a therapeutic intervention. Intraventricular monitoring using a fluid-filled system has long been considered the definitive method of ICP monitoring.[2]

Fiberoptic and microchip devices can be implanted in the intraventricular and intraparenchymal compartments, and the epidural, subdural, and subarachnoid spaces. Although these systems allow flexibility of monitoring location with accuracy that is comparable to the fluid-filled system, a separate monitoring unit supplied by the manufacturer is needed, which adds to the cost as compared to ventriculostomy catheters.

A subarachnoid bolt or screw may also be used to enable monitoring of ICP. Table 21-13 provides a comparison of the advantages and disadvantages of some ICP monitoring systems.

Intraventricular Monitoring and Extraventricular Drain Systems

A ventriculostomy is the creation of a hole in a ventricle, to enable ICP monitoring or drainage of CSF. Typically, a catheter is inserted into a lateral ventricle and the catheter is joined to a fluid-filled system to monitor intracranial pressure. An external ventricular drain (EVD) system is used to drain CSF. The advantages of this ventricular monitoring and drainage system include the direct ICP measurements and the ability to drain CSF during management of increased intracranial pressure.[7,104,114]

Description. A ventriculostomy catheter is introduced into one of the lateral ventricles, usually on the patient's nondominant side. A twist drill is used to create a burr hole through which the catheter is advanced. Once the ventricle is reached the catheter may be tunneled through the scalp via a separate incision or sutured to the scalp at the insertion site. The catheter is then joined to an external fluid-filled monitoring system (with transducer) and to a stopcock and a closed, sterile drip chamber and receptacle for CSF collection.

External ventricular drainage systems include tubing between the catheter and the drip chamber, a stopcock, a drip chamber with a one-way valve, and a collection bag (Fig. 21-35). Many systems contain a built-in level indicator

Table 21-13 **Comparison of Intracranial Pressure Monitoring Systems**

Device	Advantages	Disadvantages
Intraventricular catheter with extraventricular drain (EVD)	• Gold standard for ICP measurement • Can drain and sample CSF • Can set drip chamber at specific height (e.g., 15 cm) above ventricles so CSF will drain if ICP exceeds equivalent cm of water pressure (e.g., 15 cm H_2O or 11.2 mm Hg) • Inexpensive in comparison to other systems	• Invasive • Technically difficult to access ventricle in some patient situations • Catheter occlusion may develop • Transducer must be releveled when patient position changes • Risk of infection • System must be changed if drip chamber filter gets wet
Fiberoptic probe/microchip sensor	• Flexibility in placement location • Accurate with movement of patient position • Calibrated before insertion • Minimal drift • Easily transported • Less risk of infection	• Cannot be recalibrated after insertion • Fragile and prone to breakage • More expensive in comparison to other systems • Cannot drain or sample CSF unless an external ventricular drain set is also in use
Subarachnoid bolt/screw	• Easily placed • Does not enter the brain • Possible lower infection risk	• Catheter can become occluded by blood or tissue • Transducer must be releveled when patient position changes • May not be accurate with elevated ICP readings • May be difficult to place in young infants • Cannot drain or sample CSF

CSF, Cerebrospinal fluid; *ICP,* intracranial pressure.

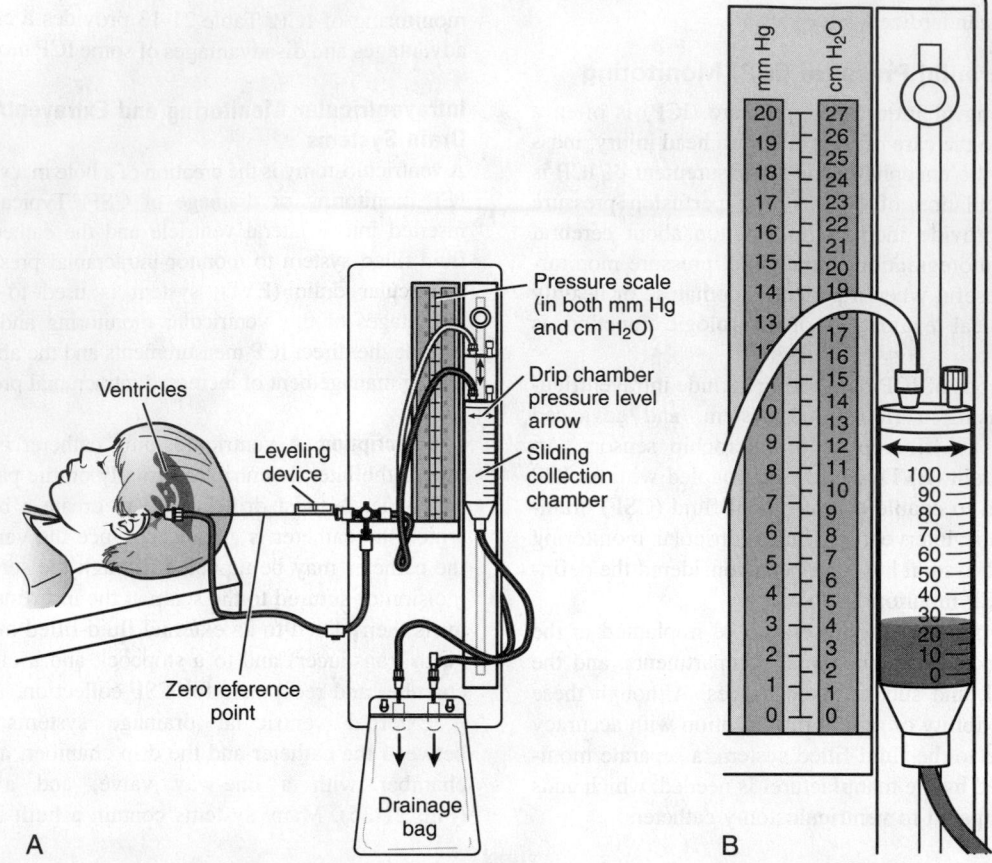

FIG. 21-35 Intraventricular intracranial pressure (ICP) monitoring system with an external ventricular drainage system for controlled drainage of cerebrospinal fluid. **A,** The system consists of an intraventricular catheter joined by tubing to a drainage system with adjustable height and a drainage bag. The system also typically has a stopcock, an injection sampling port, and a clamp. The zero reference point for the system is typically between the outer canthus of the eye and the external auditory canal (see leveling device placed at that level). **B,** The drip chamber pressure level (horizontal arrow) is placed a prescribed height (in cm) above this zero reference point. The drainage stopcock can allow continuous drainage or be turned to allow only intermittent drainage when the child's ICP exceeds a prescribed threshold. If the system is functioning and the stopcock is turned to drainage, CSF will drain from the child's ventricle into the collection chamber and ultimately into the drainage bag once the patient's ICP is sufficiently high. If the drip chamber is placed 27.2 cm (rounded to 27 cm) above the child's ventricles, drainage should occur if the child's ICP equals 27.2 cm H_2O or 20 mm Hg (1.36 cm H_2O pressure = 1 mm Hg pressure; 27.2 cm H_2O pressure = 20 mm Hg pressure). (Redrawn and modified from Owen A: *Clinical guideline: external ventricular drainage.* Great Ormond Street Hospital for Sick Children, Institute of Children's Health and University College of London, Revised, September, 2009.)

to facilitate leveling of the transducer with the patient's lateral ventricles (typically the external auditory canal is used as a landmark); the lateral ventricles are considered the zero reference point of the system.

The flow of CSF to the collection unit is regulated by the height of the drip chamber above the ventricles; this height (in centimeters) creates resistance to CSF drainage equivalent to centimeters of water pressure. For every 1.36 cm the drip chamber is elevated above the ventricle, 1 mm Hg intraventricular/intracranial pressure is required to produce drainage of CSF into the chamber.

Typically the system and stopcocks are arranged to allow automatic drainage once the ICP reaches a pressure specified by the physician (or on-call provider). For CSF drainage to occur, the pressure in the ventricles must exceed the pressure created by the column of water between the ventricle and the drip chamber (1.36 cm H_2O pressure = 1 mm Hg) in the collection system. If the drip chamber is placed 27.2 cm above

the ventricle, resistance to CSF drainage is equal to 27.2 cm H_2O pressure, or 20 mm Hg pressure. When intracranial pressure exceeds 27.2 cm H_2O (or 20 mm Hg), if the stopcock is set to allow drainage between the ventricle and the drip chamber, CSF will flow into the collection system.

If the system is set to allow continuous CSF drainage, the measured ICP will never exceed the pressure equivalent to the centimeters (of water) that the drip chamber is elevated above the ventricles. Some providers may request that some or all ICP measurements be obtained with the drainage briefly interrupted (i.e., the stopcock is temporarily open only between the transducer and the ventricle). Such measurements may be requested if there is any deterioration in the patient's clinical status. Once the isolated ICP measurement is obtained, the stopcock is again opened to the drip chamber as well as between the transducer and the catheter.

If intermittent drainage is preferred, the stopcock is typically closed between the ventricle and the drip chamber (i.e., "off" to drainage) for most periods, and the stopcock is only opened to allow drainage at times specified by the physician or on-call provider. If such intermittent drainage is provided, the ICP may continue to rise and CSF drainage won't occur unless the stopcock is turned to allow drainage from the ventricle into the drip chamber.

The external transducer is secured to a fixed reference point, as ordered by the physician or on-call provider. Usually the transducer is leveled at the lateral ventricle; the landmark used is typically the external auditory meatus.[102] Some centers use the outer canthus of the eye and others use the midpoint of the imaginary line between outer canthus of the eye and the external auditory meatus. While any of these points is acceptable, it is essential that a single leveling point is established, and every practitioner must use the identical zero reference point. Use of the same zero reference point enables identification of changes over time.

Risks and Complications of Intraventricular Monitoring and Drainage.
The need for a ventriculostomy is weighed against the potential complications or difficulties. Use of an intraventricular catheter creates the risk of infection.[113] The system should always be closed and sterile technique must be used if it is necessary to enter the system. Opening the system to sample CSF or rezero and flush the system (not the ventricular catheter) can increase the risk of infection.[112]

Care of the insertion site varies with institution policy, but observation of the site, maintenance of the integrity of the dressing, and immediate reporting of redness or drainage are routine nursing responsibilities. If a catheter infection is suspected, the catheter is removed and appropriate antibiotic therapy initiated. If ICP monitoring is still required, another catheter may be placed in the opposite lateral ventricle. There are commercially available EVD catheters with antibiotic-coated tips that may reduce infection rates, but their routine use in clinical practice requires more research.[24]

When the catheter is passed through brain tissue, there is a risk of interrupting blood vessels. Although the reported incidence is low, resulting hemorrhage may be considered clinically insignificant, and may not be reported in the literature.[113] In one pediatric study, hemorrhagic complications were detected more often with the use of external ventricular drainage systems as compared with fiberoptic monitoring.[8] In an effort to prevent hemorrhage, coagulopathies should also be corrected before the placement of any device.[113]

Blood or brain tissue can obstruct the tip of the catheter any time during catheter use. Obstruction also may occur from compression of the ventricles by cerebral swelling. Additionally, the catheter can migrate or be misplaced or become displaced during use. The external tubing can also become kinked or can remain inadvertently clamped. If CSF drainage decreases or is lower than expected, obstruction or misplacement should be suspected. The pressure tracing may also become dampened or eliminated. The cause of obstruction and location of the catheter tip can be determined by means of a computed tomography (CT) scan.

The flow of CSF is caused by a pressure gradient between the ventricles and the drip chamber. The flow chamber should not be placed below the zero reference point, because that could cause excessive drainage with resulting collapse of the ventricles. Ventricular collapse can result in lateral or upward

brain herniation or tearing of bridging veins as the brain tissue is pulled from the dura. Subdural or subarachnoid hemorrhage can result.

During periods of high volume CSF drainage, the child may develop hyponatremia because CSF sodium is unavailable for reabsorption and is lost in the external drain. It may be necessary to replace the CSF drainage with an equivalent volume of intravenous saline solution to maintain euvolemia and adequate serum sodium concentration.

If the system drip chamber is placed too high in relation to the zero reference point (e.g., as a result of patient movement or inadvertent movement of the drainage point), it will create too much resistance to drainage. As a result, CSF drainage will be inhibited until the ICP is high enough to overcome the resistance created by the fluid column between the ventricle and the drip chamber. This increase in ICP could be detrimental.

Maintenance and Nursing Considerations.
The nurse must monitor the patient and the system closely to detect clinical changes, ensure accuracy of ICP measurements, and prevent complications. Whenever the patient deteriorates clinically, the nurse should assess the patient, check the monitoring and drainage system, and notify a physician or on-call provider immediately. If the ICP measurement or drainage changes acutely, the nurse should assess the patient first and then check the system.

Establishing the Monitoring and Drainage System. Once the ventriculostomy is in place, the transducer is leveled and secured at the zero reference point (the lateral ventricles). The drip chamber, with pressure level indicator, is positioned at the prescribed height in relation to the patient's lateral ventricles. The monitoring system is zeroed to atmospheric pressure, and then opened between the transducer and the ventricle. If ordered, the stopcock is turned so it is also open to drain.

If the system is to be used for continuous drainage, the stopcocks and clamps are placed in the open position, and CSF drainage will automatically occur when the ICP increases sufficiently to overcome the resistance provided by the height of the column of fluid in the collection system. For example, if the chamber is placed at 15 cm above the patient's ventricle, CSF drainage will occur whenever the ICP exceeds 11 mm Hg (15 cm $\div$ 1.36 cm/mm Hg pressure = 11.02 mm Hg). As a rule, the chamber is positioned so that CSF drainage occurs as needed to keep the ICP at a reasonable level.

As noted previously, if the drainage system is functioning properly, the ICP should never exceed the pressure equivalent to the cm H_2O pressure or resistance created by elevation of the drip chamber above the ventricle; venting of the CSF should prevent such rises. If the ICP does exceed the pressure within the collection system, obstruction of CSF drainage is probably present and the on-call provider should be notified immediately.

When the CSF is drained continuously, it is difficult to determine the severity of increases in intracranial volume and pressure that would occur in the absence of the drainage system. However, if CSF drainage is continuous or if it increases in amount, intracranial volume must be high or rising. To monitor the patient's intracranial pressure intermittently, drainage may be interrupted briefly with the stopcock turned off to drainage. The ICP and CPP are quickly measured and recorded, and then the stopcock is turned back to allow ongoing drainage. This procedure is generally performed at routine intervals as ordered (e.g., every 1 to 2 hours).

As noted in the preceding Description section, the ventriculostomy drainage (or extraventricular drain) system can also be used for intermittent CSF drainage. In this case, the practitioner specifies the location of the drip chamber, and specifies that the drainage stopcock is typically to be turned off to drainage but opened to allow drainage only if the patient's ICP reaches a specified value (usually 20 to 25 mm Hg). Whenever such drainage occurs, the patient's ICP will fall to the level equivalent to the pressure within the collection system, and the drainage stopcock should then be turned off to drainage. If frequent CSF drainage is required, the nurse should notify the physician or on-call provider.

Nursing Care and Maintenance of the System. As noted in the first paragraph of this Maintenance and Nursing Considerations section, the nurse should assess the patient and verify patient status before troubleshooting the equipment whenever the patient deteriorates, the measured ICP rises or if a problem develops the system. Report signs of patient deterioration immediately to the physician or on-call provider.

Carefully inspect the system at regular intervals to verify integrity of the system, confirming that clamps and stopcocks are appropriately opened or closed as ordered. Monitor the volume of CSF drainage and notify the physician or on-call provider if the CSF drainage volume varies from the expected.

Nursing documentation should include the characteristics and amount of drainage, the condition of the drainage system (open vs. clamped), and the appearance of the insertion site and dressing. The ICP and CPP are documented at frequent, regular intervals along with changes in ICP associated with patient care activities, such as suctioning. It is important to record the patient's tolerance of maintenance activities and any unexpected responses.

Inspect the dressing and tissue around the ventriculostomy at regular intervals. The dressing around the insertion site must remain clean and dry. Report signs of catheter site inflammation and any signs of potential infection (e.g., fever, leukocytosis) to a physician or on-call provider immediately. The risk of infection increases the longer a ventriculostomy remains in place.[113]

The CSF in the drip chamber should be emptied into the CSF drainage bag when the drip chamber is approximately two-thirds full. The fluid level in the chamber must be well below the level of the drip chamber where the filter is positioned. If fluid fills the chamber or the filter becomes wet, drainage can be obstructed and it will be necessary to replace the entire system.

The CSF drainage bag should be changed when it is approximately three-fourths full. Use personal protective equipment as appropriate for this procedure and dispose of the bag according to hospital biohazard procedures.

To move a patient or reposition the head:

1. Follow the practitioner's order for repositioning the patient or moving the patient out of bed.
2. Clamp the system and observe the patient's tolerance of the clamped drain during the process of moving.
3. Reposition or ambulate patient as ordered.

4. Re-level the transducer (and zero reference point for the system) at the level of the ventricle and the drip chamber at the appropriate height, at the level ordered by the practitioner.
5. Unclamp the system; observe and document the initial volume of fluid that drains.

If obstruction of the ventricular catheter is suspected, a physician (or other on-call provider) should be notified. The physician may gently attempt to instill a small amount of sterile saline into the catheter. As a rule, the catheter is not aspirated, because this can cause hemorrhage.

Fiberoptic and Microchip ICP Transducers

Description. Both the fiberoptic and the microchip ICP transducer can be used to monitor ICP. Either device may be placed in the lateral ventricles, the brain parenchyma, or the subdural, subarachnoid, or epidural space.

The fiberoptic monitoring device transmits light along a fiber (the optical fiber, or fiberoptic, contained in the catheter) to the tip of the catheter and transmits reflected light back to the base unit. A pressure transducer is located near the catheter tip. The mechanical diaphragm of the transducer moves with changes in pressure, and the movement will change the intensity of the light reflected off the diaphragm. The light refraction is then analyzed to derive a pressure reading that is displayed digitally on the ICP monitoring unit display (Fig. 21-36). The fiberoptic catheters must be zeroed before

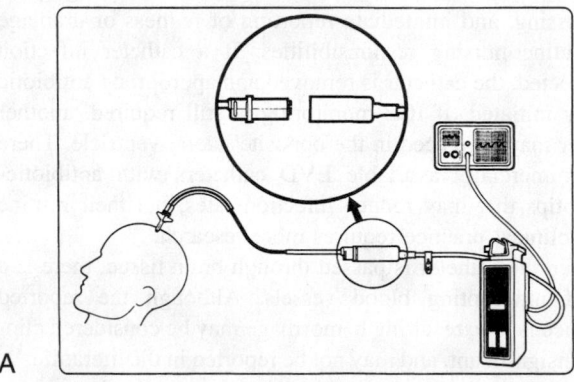

A

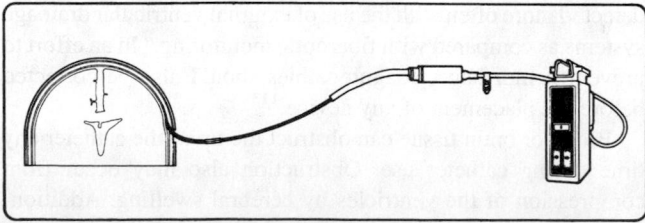

B

FIG. 21-36 Camino fiberoptic intracranial pressure-monitoring system. The fiberoptic catheter is joined to an amplifier-connector, and it transmits signals to the Camino module. The module displays digital ICP pressure measurement, but must be joined to a bedside monitor to display a waveform and provide audible high-pressure alarms. **A,** Camino monitoring system with intraparenchymal or intradural monitoring. Inset shows connection of catheter and monitor cable—at this connection, zeroing of the catheter is performed *before insertion.* **B,** Camino monitoring system for epidural monitoring. (Redrawn from illustrations of fiberoptic intracranial pressure-monitoring system by Integra Camino, San Diego, California.)

insertion; they are calibrated at the factory and cannot be recalibrated after insertion.

The microchip transducer has a pressure sensor at the tip. A change in pressure moves the position of this sensor and causes changes in electrical resistance; these changes are transformed and displayed as ICP measurements. The microchip transducers must be zeroed before insertion; they are calibrated at the factory and cannot be recalibrated after insertion.

Both fiberoptic and microchip ICP monitoring catheters can be coupled with a conventional bedside monitor for waveform display, paper recording, and generation of audible pressure alarms. The portable pressure monitoring unit must be calibrated at regular intervals with the bedside monitor digital display; note that this calibration is not the same as zeroing and calibration of the ICP transducer system (as discussed in the next paragraphs).

The advantages of the fiberoptic and microchip transducers over other systems are accuracy, versatility, small size, and minimal maintenance requirements. Because the transducers are located very near the tip of the catheter, leveling of the transducer to an anatomic reference point is unnecessary. As a result, valid pressure measurements are obtained even with frequent change in patient position.

This system is not dependent on transmission of pressure through a fluid-filled segment of tubing; artifact from air bubbles or particles does not occur. Zeroing is necessary only once before insertion and catheter calibration is performed at the factory. Catheters are also available to enable simultaneous ICP monitoring and CSF drainage (Fig. 21-37), as well as brain temperature monitoring.

Risks and Complications. The fiberoptic and microchip catheters require careful handling to avoid damage; the catheter must be replaced if it is damaged. Drifting of the zero reference point may be observed and can increase daily for as long as the catheter is in use.[113] Manufacturer's recommendations should be followed regarding catheter replacement when monitoring is required for longer than 5 days.

Infection remains a potential problem with any ICP monitoring device. However, because there is no fluid incorporated in these devices, the incidence of infection may be lower than with fluid-filled monitoring systems. As with any invasive

monitoring system, however, attention should be given to ensuring sterile technique during insertion, and aseptic technique during catheter and tubing care.

Complications associated with fiberoptic or microchip ICP monitoring are similar to those described previously for ICP monitoring and ventricular drainage. These include hemorrhage and obstruction, migration, and misplacement.

Maintenance and Nursing Considerations. These catheters are fragile. Care must be taken to avoid any tension on or compression of the catheter. All providers who care for patients with a fiberoptic or microchip ICP catheter must be extremely careful during handling of the patient and catheter. Damage to the light fibers of a fiberoptic catheter can occur readily. At regular intervals, the nurse should assess the security of the catheter at the insertion site.

The catheter must be inserted under sterile conditions and maintained with aseptic technique. The dressing around the insertion site must remain clean and dry. The risk of infection increases the longer a catheter remains in place.[113]

These catheters are zeroed before insertion; once the catheter is inserted, the zero is never adjusted. However, the calibration of the bedside monitor should be checked according to the manufacturer's recommendations, to ensure correlation between the ICP monitor and bedside monitor.

If the patient requires transfer to another location, ICP monitoring may be continued during transfer because the portable monitoring unit contains a rechargeable battery. If ICP monitoring is not performed during patient transfer and the catheter is disconnected, the ICP monitor will not lose calibration and the catheter transducer tip does not lose its zero reference point. However, once the ICP monitoring unit is reconnected to a bedside monitor, the bedside monitor must be recalibrated with the ICP monitor.

If a ventriculostomy drainage system is used, nursing documentation should include the characteristics and amount of drainage. The condition of the drainage system (open vs. clamped), and the appearance of the insertion site and dressing are also documented.

The ICP and CPP are documented at frequent, regular intervals along with changes in ICP associated with patient care activities, such as suctioning. The patient's tolerance of maintenance activities and any unexpected responses or deterioration are reported to a physician or other on-call provider.

ICP Monitoring with a Subarachnoid Bolt or Screw

Description. Another alternative method of ICP measurement is the use of a conventional fluid-filled transducer tubing system connected to the subarachnoid space with either a catheter or subarachnoid bolt or screw, respectively (Fig. 21-38). The transducer and tubing preparation is similar to that used for other fluid-filled monitoring systems; in these neurologic monitoring systems, however, a flush solution and continuous flow device are not used.

A short, direct segment of tubing from the bolt (or catheter) is joined to a transducer. Care must be taken to prime the transducer system with preservative-free saline to eliminate all bubbles before joining the system to the bolt or catheter.

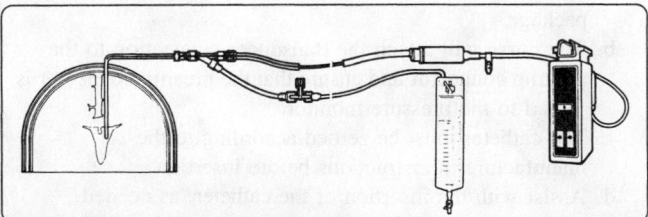

FIG. 21-37 Camino intraventricular monitoring catheter with cerebrospinal fluid drainage system. The sheath of the intraventricular catheter provides a Y connection to a CSF drainage system. Drainage may be accomplished intermittently or continuously, with simultaneous pressure monitoring. The height of the drainage chamber above the ventricles will determine the ease of CSF drainage. (Redrawn from illustrations of intraventricular monitoring catheter with cerebrospinal fluid drainage system by Integra Camino, San Diego, California.)

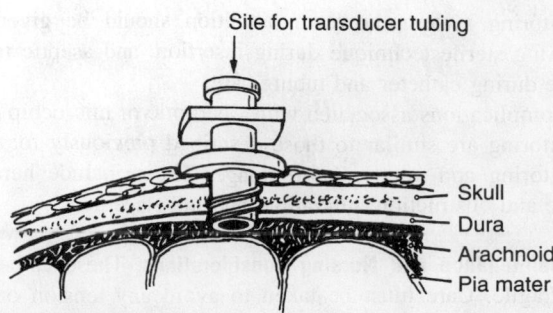

Site for transducer tubing

Skull
Dura
Arachnoid
Pia mater

FIG. 21-38 Subarachnoid bolt. The bolt may be placed in the frontal area through a burr hole. To monitor pressure using a fluid-filled monitoring system, a short piece of (flushed) noncompliant tubing is used to join the bolt to a transducer. A fiberoptic catheter also can be placed for subarachnoid pressure monitoring.

Advantages and Disadvantages. The advantages of using a subarachnoid bolt or screw include ease of insertion, minimal risk of brain tissue injury, and its improved accuracy in the presence of central edema, when the lateral ventricles may be compressed and difficult to catheterize.[10,114]

A disadvantage to the bolt is that it can become occluded with blood clots, tissue, or debris, which can dampen the ICP waveform and cause erroneous results.[10,114] This system may not be accurate when the ICP is elevated (the very condition it is designed to monitor).[182] As with other devices that enter the skull, infection, leak of CSF, and hemorrhage can occur.[10,102] Subarachnoid bolts or screws are difficult to place in infants because of the pliability of the infant skull.

Maintenance and Nursing Considerations. Nursing care and maintenance of the system are similar to other ICP monitoring devices and include evaluating and documenting the integrity of the system, and taking precautions to prevent infection.

ICP Monitoring Equipment Preparation and Insertion

The steps for preparing a fluid-filled system or a fiberoptic or microchip transducer with its associated ICP monitor vary depending on the device, and the nurse should follow the manufacturer's guidelines. Box 21-3 lists the standard equipment and steps for inserting an ICP monitor.

The procedure should always be explained to the patient and family, as appropriate, and informed consent obtained. The child should be appropriately monitored and the nurse should ensure that adequate analgesic and sedative medications are administered.

Box 21-3 **Intracranial Pressure Monitoring Equipment: Preparation and Insertion**

1. Assemble the required equipment:
   a. Sterile gloves, surgical gowns, towels, and drapes
   b. Surgical caps and masks with protective eyewear
   c. Hair clippers
   d. Antiseptic scrub solution
   e. Local anesthetic and syringe with needle
   f. Cranial access kit, as supplied by the manufacturer
   g. Hand drill with appropriate drill bit
   h. Surgical blade
   i. Suture
   j. Supplies for sterile dressing
2. Fluid-filled system
   a. Catheter
   b. Pressure tubing and external strain gauge transducer with bedside monitor cable
   c. Preservative-free saline solution
   d. External ventricular drainage set, if required
3. Fiberoptic or microchip system
   a. Catheter
   b. ICP monitor supplied by manufacturer
   c. Preamp connector cable, supplied with monitor
   d. Cable to join ICP monitor to bedside monitor
4. Insertion site will be clipped, prepared, and draped with sterile towels and/or drapes.
5. Sterile technique is used to make an incision that is extended to the bone.
6. A drill hole is then made through the outer and inner tables of the skull. If the catheter is placed in the subarachnoid space or parenchyma, a bolt is placed in the skull to secure the catheter. Otherwise, the catheter is sutured in place and a sterile dressing is applied.
7. Fluid-filled system:

a. Prepare the drainage system transducer and tubing and EVD set, if using, and flush with preservative-free saline solution.
   b. Assist with the insertion of the ventricular catheter, as needed.
   c. Connect the transducer tubing to the ICP catheter.
   d. Before joining the ventricular catheter to the external ventricular drainage system, check to ensure that the clamp from the drip chamber to the collection bag is closed.
   e. Mount the system on an IV pole with the zero reference point at the level of the patient's ventricle.
   f. Adjust the drainage collection chamber until it is positioned at the specified height above the patient's ventricles.
   g. Observe for CSF flow into the drip chamber.
   h. Zero the bedside monitor and position the system's stopcock to measure ICP.
8. Fiberoptic or microchip system:
   a. The practitioner will remove the catheter from the sterile package.
   b. The nurse will attach the transducer connection to the preamp connector and ensure that the preamp connector is joined to the pressure monitor.
   c. The catheter must be zeroed according to the manufacturer's instructions before insertion.
   d. Assist with the insertion of the catheter, as needed.
   e. If a ventriculostomy drainage system is to be used it should be joined to the ventricular catheter at the Y connection or via stopcock.
   f. The pressure monitor should be joined by a cable to the bedside monitor. The bedside monitor must also be calibrated with the pressure monitor as per the manufacturer's instructions.

EVD, External ventricular device; *ICP,* intracranial pressure.

Brain Oxygen Monitoring

Early detection of cerebral hypoxia and ischemia in the injured brain is important for preventing secondary brain injury and associated morbidity and mortality. Brain oxygen monitoring enables continuous assessment of brain oxygenation and evaluation of the effect of clinical interventions designed to improve brain oxygenation.[80,138,141]

Neurologic monitoring of brain oxygen includes measurement of regional cerebral oxygenation and measurement of more global cerebral oxygenation. These systems can be used separately or together.

Brain Tissue Oxygen Monitoring

Description. Brain tissue oxygen monitoring catheters continuously measure the partial pressure of oxygen in local brain tissue ($PbtO_2$); the $PbtO_2$, in turn, reflects the net balance of cerebral oxygen supply and cellular oxygen consumption.[111] This advanced technology has led to a better understanding of the impact that low oxygen states have on the injured brain.[105]

The brain tissue oxygen monitoring system consists of a triple lumen probe that is inserted via a burr hole into the parenchyma of the brain. When detailed information on cerebral oxygenation in an injured area is desired, the device is placed on the affected side of the brain, in the penumbra area (ischemic but viable tissue surrounding an infarcted or injured area). The probe may also be placed in the nonaffected hemisphere for a reflection of more global cerebral oxygenation.

The tip of the flexible microcatheter contains a polarographic Clark-type electrode. Oxygen diffuses from the cerebral tissue through the polyethylene-coated catheter wall and into an inner electrolyte chamber where the partial pressure of oxygen is converted to a current between a cathode and an anode.[82,118] The amount of current generated is proportional to the $PbtO_2$ and is displayed in mm Hg.[82]

After insertion, the probe is connected by an electrical cable to the monitoring system supplied by the manufacturer. Depending on the monitor selected, the screen displays $PbtO_2$, brain tissue temperature, and ICP.

Advantages, Disadvantages, and Contraindications. The advantage of using this system over conventional ICP monitoring is that it enables the practitioner to evaluate cerebral oxygen delivery and demand in the brain. This can allow the practitioner to identify levels of brain tissue oxygen that may be associated with secondary brain injury, identify and correct conditions associated with reduced cerebral tissue oxygenation, and plan treatment interventions more specifically aimed at improving the oxygenation of the brain.[99,188]

As with any intracranial monitoring system, there is a risk of infection, hematoma, and displacement of the probe. After insertion of the monitor probe, it can take up to 2 hours for the $PbtO_2$ to equilibrate after the microtrauma of the insertion procedure.[181] The practitioner must be aware of this delay in measurements when making clinical decisions based on these parameters. Technical care should be taken in handling these catheters because they can be inadvertently dislodged, misplaced, or broken.

Contraindications to using this system include uncorrected coagulopathy and an infection at the insertion site.[181]

Maintenance and Nursing Considerations. The insertion supplies for the brain oxygen monitor are similar to those needed for inserting a fiberoptic ICP monitor (see Box 21-3). Follow the manufacturer's directions for assisting with inserting the probe, and calibrating and setting up the monitoring system.

After setup is complete and the probe's external ends are attached to the brain tissue oxygen monitor, a cable can be used to connect the brain oxygen monitor with the patient's bedside monitor so that values are displayed and alarm parameters can be set.

After insertion, the nurse should evaluate the insertion site frequently and maintain the sterile dressing. The $PbtO_2$, brain temperature, and ICP values should be assessed and documented routinely as part of the patient's overall assessment, and when there is a change in clinical status or a clinical intervention. When the child must be transported, the probes are gently disconnected from the bedside monitor at the patient end using gentle pulling; the probe device should not be twisted.[181]

Jugular Venous Oxygen Saturation Monitoring

Description. Most of the cerebral venous circulation drains into the external jugular veins, where oxygen saturation can be monitored by spectrophotometry. Because the oxygen saturation in the jugular vein reflects the oxygen remaining after cerebral perfusion and oxygen extraction has occurred, trends in jugular venous oxygen saturation (SjO_2) reflect the balance of global cerebral oxygen delivery to consumption and can be used to evaluate the effectiveness of therapies.

The SjO_2 is used in conjunction with other monitored parameters such as ICP and CPP to evaluate and manage patients with cerebral ischemia. Continuous measurements are obtained via a fiberoptic catheter that is placed retrograde into the internal jugular vein. The catheter is threaded over an introducer and advanced until it sits in the jugular venous bulb.[89] Although either the right or left jugular vein can be used, the right internal jugular vein is usually cannulated because it drains a greater proportion of blood from the sagittal sinus.[180]

The monitoring system uses wavelengths of light (two or three wavelengths, depending on the manufacturer). The light is emitted from the tip of the catheter and then reflected light is detected by a photosensor and transmitted to the base unit. A microprocessor determines the reflection of the different wavelengths of light and because oxygenated hemoglobin (hemoglobin saturated with oxygen) reflects light differently than desaturated hemoglobin, the relative reflection of light allows estimation of the relative percent of hemoglobin in the jugular vein that is saturated with oxygen. The percentage of the oxygenated hemoglobin in the total hemoglobin is expressed as SjO_2.[26]

Advantages, Disadvantages, and Contraindications. A fall in the SjO_2 will identify cerebral ischemia more specifically than ICP monitoring or evaluation of the CPP. However, a decreased SjO_2 represents more global ischemia rather than a particular area of local injury.

One disadvantage of this monitoring system for pediatric patients is catheter size. Because the catheter may impede venous drainage or cause obstruction of the internal jugular vein, continuous SjO_2 monitoring is usually not attempted for children younger than 8 years of age or those who weigh less than 30 kg.[180]

Potential complications include hematoma formation, venous thrombosis, infection, and the potential for catheter-associated bloodstream infection. The catheter can also become clogged with debris, resulting in false readings.

Continuous SjO_2 monitoring is contraindicated in the patient with an infection at the insertion site (in the neck), neck trauma, impaired venous drainage, or jugular venous occlusion or malformation. This monitoring may not be appropriate for the patient with coagulopathy, brain stem or cervical spine injury, or tracheostomy.[164]

Maintenance and Nursing Considerations. Insertion supplies include sterile garb for those involved in the insertion procedure, skin antiseptic and local anesthetic, pressure transducer tubing, the catheter, and the oximetric monitor. Prepare the oximetric monitor according to the manufacturer's instructions.

After the catheter is placed, it is flushed, attached to a continuous flush solution, and attached to the monitoring system. Only flush solution should infuse into the catheter. An occlusive, sterile dressing is applied over the insertion site.

Follow the manufacturer's instructions for obtaining a jugular venous blood gas for calibration of and correlation with the oximetric monitor.[89] The nurse should aspirate the blood calibration specimens from the catheter at a rate of 1 to 2 mL/minute (i.e., very slowly).[114,164] This technique ensures accuracy of the measurements by avoiding contamination of the sample from extracranial blood that also drains into the jugular vein; such contamination could result in falsely high oxygen saturation in the blood calibration specimen.

The nurse should record or store the SjO_2 readings hourly and the insertion site, catheter integrity, and stability should be assessed hourly. Inaccurate measurements can result when the child's head or neck is rotated because the catheter can become improperly positioned within the jugular vein. Slightly repositioning the patient's head or the catheter may help the nurse determine if a desaturation reading is accurate or is a result of catheter misplacement.

Follow the manufacturer's recommendations for calibration of the device and recalibrate the device whenever there is concern about the accuracy of the readings. Accuracy can be affected by the hemoglobin concentration, systemic arterial oxygen saturation, core body temperature, and serum CO_2 levels.[164]

Complications of continuous SjO_2 monitoring include potential infection, pneumothorax, nerve injury, thrombosis, and carotid artery puncture.[114,178] To reduce the risk of infection, strict sterile technique must be used during insertion and aseptic technique used when manipulating the catheter.

Transcranial Cerebral Oximetry Monitoring

Description. Transcranial cerebral oximetry, also known as near-infrared spectroscopy (NIRS), is a technique used for observing changes in regional cerebral oxygenation (rSO_2).

Sensors contained in adhesive electrodes are placed (noninvasively) on the patient's forehead and light waves of near-infrared wavelength penetrate the scalp, skull, and brain tissue to a depth of a few centimeters. The light waves are then absorbed differentially by oxygenated and deoxygenated hemoglobin, so analysis of light absorption can enable estimate of the cerebral tissue oxygen saturation.

The system measures light waves that are absorbed or scattered back to two electrode detectors. The device is able to identify the difference between light reflected from shallow tissue (i.e., the skull) and that reflected from tissue under the skull to identify the deeper tissue light reflection. The percent of the total hemoglobin that is oxygenated is calculated and displayed on the monitor as a numerical value.[26,169]

Advantages, Disadvantages, and Contraindications. The NIRS monitoring system provides real-time continuous monitoring of tissue oxygenation. This oxygenation can be used to evaluate the effect of interventions on tissue oxygenation. The technology is not dependent on the patient's pulse, blood pressure, or temperature, so it can be used in a variety of clinical situations.

A disadvantage to this technology is that brain swelling can affect the accuracy and reliability of NIRS.[25] Additionally, the light waves only penetrate a few centimeters and cannot be used to determine rSO_2 measurements beyond that depth.

The accuracy of the measurements is affected by cerebral infarction, extraaxial hematomas, and extracranial blood.[26] This monitoring technology may not be used when bandages cover the forehead where the sensors must be placed.

Maintenance and Nursing Considerations. A separate transcranial cerebral oxygen monitor must be supplied by the manufacturer. It displays both the rSO_2 value and a graphic trend of the value over time. Small pediatric sensors are available and should be used for children less than 40 kg body weight. Because the skull of a child is much thinner than the skull of an adult, the algorithm for detecting the pediatric rSO_2 is different than the algorithm used in adults.[26,169]

The nurse should follow the manufacturer's instructions for applying the disposable sensors to the frontal temporal area of the forehead (to the left and right of midline) and attaching them to the NIRS monitor. The sensors are not placed on the scalp.

The nurse should note the baseline rSO_2 value. Rather than comparing a given result with an absolute range of normal values, the continuous rSO_2 readings are most useful for evaluating trends and changes from the patient's baseline.[26] The rSO_2 is not a stand-alone value, and the nurse should incorporate the reading with other data collected from the patient's neurologic assessment and other monitoring devices.[169]

Transcranial Doppler Ultrasonography (TCD)

Description. The measurement of cerebral blood flow is important whenever the patient at risk for cerebral ischemia and infarction, particularly risk of cerebral vasospasm and vessel occlusion. Transcranial Doppler ultrasonography (TCD) is a noninvasive method for evaluating cerebral blood flow velocity through the cranium.

A 2-MHz ultrasound probe is held to a thin area of the skull, usually above the zygomatic arch, and velocity signals are displayed as pulsatile waveforms that can be recorded.[180] The measurement is performed by a trained technologist and then interpreted by a radiologist.

Advantages and Disadvantages. TCD is portable and does not require patient transport. The measurement technique is usually performed intermittently, because extended monitoring is hampered by difficulty in maintaining the ultrasound probe in position over a long period of time.[91] Patient movement can affect the accuracy of the study results.

Maintenance and Nursing Considerations. The nurse should anticipate that the measurement of cerebral blood flow via TCD will be performed intermittently, usually daily. It will be combined with other technologic monitoring for determining the patient's overall cerebral oxygenation and neurologic status.[184]

EEG Monitoring

Continuous EEG Monitoring

Description. The electroencephalogram (EEG) is used most frequently to monitor critically ill patients with intracranial hypertension or refractory status epilepticus, or those at risk for secondary ischemia after brain injury. Electrodes are placed on the scalp and head to detect neuronal electrical impulses; these impulses are recorded and the graphic recording is the EEG. The EEG waveform reflects the physiologic state of the cerebral tissue and is an indication of the cerebral metabolic state.[114]

Advantages and Disadvantages. Continuous cerebral EEG monitoring (cEEG) is useful for unconscious patients, those in status epilepticus, and those in a coma, including barbiturate-induced coma; it is also useful for evaluation of the patient receiving neuromuscular blockade. Many critically ill patients may require neuromuscular blockade for several reasons, such as ventilator management; therefore the cEEG can offer more sensitive detection of localized seizure activity in these patients and allows prompt treatment of status epilepticus.[96] Continuous EEG can be combined with other multimodality brain monitoring, allowing the clinician to identify when the brain is at risk for injury and intervene before there is permanent damage.[57]

The EEG electrodes must be placed by a trained technologist, who must be available to reapply any electrodes that loosen during patient transport, movement, or care. Electrical interference from equipment in the critical care environment and patient movement can interfere with the EEG recording.

Maintenance and Nursing Considerations. The nurse will prepare the patient and assist with the placement of EEG electrodes, as needed. Electrodes should not be placed over areas of skin breakdown. Before electrode placement, the skin should be prepared with soap and water or alcohol. Because a loose or misplaced electrode will impact the EEG waveform, the nurse should be vigilant in assessing electrode placement and wires while performing patient care.

Bispectral Index

Description. The bispectral index (BIS) is a processed EEG parameter that is used to monitor the patient's response to sedatives and anesthetic agents.[135] Data are obtained from a single electrode strip that is placed across the patient's forehead. Brain activity in this localized area is reflected in the BIS value, a derived parameter reported on a 0 to 100 linear scale.[11] A value of zero indicates no brain activity, whereas an awake and interactive patient will have a BIS value near 100.

Advantages and Disadvantages. When it is difficult to assess the child's neurologic status or level of sedation, the BIS, in conjunction with other neurologic monitoring technologies, can provide useful information. This technology is beneficial for the patient who is placed in a drug-induced (e.g., pentobarbital) coma for ICP management.

BIS data can be tracked over time and can provide real-time feedback about the patient's response to interventions. Muscle activity from the patient's face and forehead can cause signal artifact and interfere with the BIS data reliability. The BIS should not be considered a stand-alone monitoring technology, but should be used in combination with other monitoring strategies to augment the clinical assessment.

Maintenance and Nursing Considerations. A separate BIS monitor must be supplied by the manufacturer. It displays both the BIS value and a graphic trend of the value over time. Follow the manufacturer's instructions for applying the disposable sensor to the patient's forehead. The nurse should monitor clinical signs of neurologic function (e.g., the Glasgow Coma Scale Score, Table 11-6 or inside back cover) and record the BIS value on a regular basis and in response to therapeutic interventions, including titration of sedatives and administration of neuromuscular blocking agents.

THERMOREGULATION DEVICES

Monitoring of environmental and patient temperature in the pediatric critical care unit is extremely important. Small children have a large body surface area in proportion to their body mass and may lose heat very rapidly by conduction, convection, and radiation. Cold stress can cause increased oxygen consumption, which may compromise the cardiorespiratory function of the critically ill child.

Temperature-Sensing Devices

The assessment of temperature is one of the oldest evaluative tools in medicine; the patient's temperature can provide information about the severity and nature of illness. Core body temperature has been the most accepted form of temperature measurement, and can be derived from a variety of anatomic locations including the rectum, esophagus, bladder, brain, or pulmonary artery. If measurement of temperature from a core body area is not feasible, alternative locations include oral, axillary, temporal artery, and tympanic membrane.

In selection of temperature measurement devices for the pediatric critical care setting, safety, speed of measurement, accuracy, and convenience are important considerations. Guidelines for temperature measurement in critically ill adult patients recommend using core measurements when possible, followed by oral or tympanic membrane measurement, and lastly axillary or temporal artery measurement only when other methods are not available.[133]

Although no guidelines exist for temperature monitoring in pediatric critical care patients, the site selected to monitor the pediatric patient's temperature should be determined by the need for precise measurement and by the patient's age and physiologic status. After one site is elected for monitoring, it should be used consistently for ongoing measurements so that trends can be identified over time.[116]

Measurement by Heat Absorption

Thermoresistive thermometers, or thermistor tips, contain heavy metals that respond to changes in electrical resistance with small changes in temperature. A microchip inside the thermometer measures this resistance, and then converts it into a measurement of temperature. The temperature reading is displayed digitally in degrees Celsius or Fahrenheit. Standard electronic digital thermometers use this technology.

Thermoresistive thermometers have a rapid response time, which may be an important consideration in pediatrics and critical care. Although most thermistors record the standard range of temperatures, some are available for recording lower temperatures. Such thermometers should be acquired by a critical care unit for use with hypothermic patients.

Measurement by Sensing Heat Radiation: Tympanic Membrane Thermometers

The tympanic membrane temperature probe consists of an otoscope-like probe covered with a disposable plastic speculum. The probe and cover are attached to a probe handle that houses the infrared sensing electronics. This thermometer uses infrared radiation and a thermopile detector at the tip of the instrument to measure the tympanic temperature inside the ear.

There is debate about the reliability of tympanic thermometry to detect fever in pediatric patients. Although less accurate than direct measurements of core temperature,[125] the tympanic temperature measurement is thought to be semiequivalent to core temperature because the tympanic membrane receives its blood supply from the same vasculature that supplies the hypothalamus.[40]

Procedure. The speculum probe is positioned in the ear canal by pulling the ear lobe down and back for children less than 3 years of age, and up and back for older children.[179] The probe should fit snugly but not be painful. To initiate measurement, a scan button is depressed.

The sensor receives emitted infrared energy that is fed through an analog to a digital converter. The resultant temperature is displayed within seconds and can be displayed in either Celsius or Fahrenheit degrees. After use the disposable speculum probe cover is removed.

Advantages and Disadvantages. This method of temperature assessment is convenient and rapid. Additionally, there is

relatively low potential for cross-contamination because the probe covers are disposable. Young children may be extremely frightened of an instrument that enters any orifice, including the ear.

The presence of otitis media may result in inaccurate readings. Tympanic temperature measurements can also be affected by the user's positioning of the device during measurement and the size of the child's ear canal.[40]

Measurement by Sensing Heat Radiation: Temporal Artery Thermometers

Description. Using infrared technology, the temporal artery thermometer captures the heat energy from the skin overlying the temporal artery, just below the skin on the forehead. A hand-held infrared scanner is used and provides an estimate of core body temperature using two sensors and an algorithm that incorporates a factor compensating for measured ambient temperature.[90]

Procedure for Use. To obtain a temporal artery temperature reading, the scanner is placed on the skin at the center of the patient's forehead. Begin the measurement by pressing and holding the scan button. Sweep the sensor located at the head of the thermometer horizontally across the forehead to the hairline. While still holding down the scan button, remove the sensor briefly from the skin and place it behind the earlobe to touch the skin overlying the mastoid process. Release the scan button for the digital temperature measurement to display. The skin tap is used to control for evaporative cooling of the forehead that occurs if the patient is sweating. If the temperature at the mastoid is greater than the measurement over the temporal artery, the temperature at the mastoid is displayed.

Advantages and Disadvantages. Temporal artery temperature measurement is rapid and noninvasive. It can be performed quickly and may not disturb the child. The instrument is easy to clean and relatively inexpensive. However, the accuracy of this method of temperature measurement has been debated and the clinician should select the method most appropriate for each patient care situation.[90,133]

Maintenance of Neutral Thermal Environment: Warming Devices

An essential aspect of caring for any critically ill patient is ensuring normal body temperature, which minimizes metabolic stress. Body temperature is affected by both heat production and heat loss. Heat loss may occur through any one of four mechanisms: evaporation, convection, conduction, or radiation. When selecting warming devices, each of these sources of heat transfer must be considered in relation to the device.

Risks of All Warming Devices

The most serious complication of any warming device is overheating, which can cause hyperthermia and increased oxygen consumption. Overheating may produce skin burns, particularly in a patient with poor circulation. The caregiver's impression of the temperature output of the device (i.e., the sensation of heat on the caregiver's hand) should not be used to estimate the amount of heat reaching the patient.

Insensible water loss can be a significant problem and can be exaggerated with concomitant use of phototherapy lights. Additional fluid administration may be required to replace the additional insensible water loss. Also, daily weights and fluid and electrolyte balance should be monitored (see Chapter 12).

Warming/Cooling Blankets

Description. Warming blankets use either forced air or convection to warm the patient. Forced air efficiently transfers heat to the patient by circulating hot air through a "blanket" that covers the patient.

Circulating warm water mattresses raise the patient's temperature and reduce conductive heat losses. The mattress is placed under the patient and warmed water circulates through the mattress.

A water mattress can also be used as cooling device: cool water is circulated through the mattress and conductive cooling lowers the patient's body temperature. Various manufacturers supply the heating or cooling unit and disposable blankets or mattresses.

Advantages and Disadvantages. Devices vary by manufacturer and they heat or cool based on a preset target body temperature. Many include a patient temperature probe and a servo-controlled mechanism to maintain a selected patient temperature.

There is an increased risk of burns when using a circulating water mattress with the child who is cold and peripherally vasoconstricted. The vasoconstricted child has decreased surface capillaries to dissipate heat.

Cooling blankets are not always well tolerated by patients and the blankets can cause thermal injuries to the skin. External cooling can result in reflex shivering and vasoconstriction as the body attempts to generate heat and counteract the cooling process. Shivering increases the patient's temperature, causes discomfort, and increases metabolic demands.

Maintenance and Nursing Considerations. The manufacturer's instructions should be followed for the setup, application, and safety management of any patient heating or cooling device. The nurse should monitor the patient's temperature and response to therapy, and assess the effectiveness of rewarming or cooling interventions. If substantial heat output of a device is necessary to maintain the child's skin temperature, the child's cardiac output may be inadequate.

Closed Infant Warmers (Incubators)

Description. The closed infant warmer is a useful bed for infants who require maintenance of a controlled thermal environment. Air in the closed incubator is warmed and recirculated.

Temperature in the closed infant warmer can be set manually or by a servo control that regulates the thermal environment in the incubator in response to the infant's skin temperature. The servo control mechanism operates by presetting a desired skin temperature; the heating element within the incubator adjusts the environmental temperature automatically. The use of a servo control device should prevent wide fluctuations in environmental temperature and will conserve the infant's energy.

Advantages and Disadvantages. In addition to providing heat, the closed infant warmer minimizes convective heat loss. Ambient humidity of about 40% is maintained in the incubator without the use of additional water. This is an advantage because the water can be a site for bacterial growth.

Access to the infant for general care occurs through portholes, which limit access to the infant in a critical situation. Heat loss can occur when the incubator is opened and can result from radiant heat transfer if the walls of the incubator are subjected to a cool environmental temperature (e.g., near an air conditioning vent or in an area with drafts, near windows, or near outside walls).

Nursing Considerations. When operating the closed warmer in servo control, place the skin temperature probe on the infant's abdomen away from bony areas.[119] The infant should not lie on top of the probe.

The portholes of the isolette should be used to gain access to the patient; the door of the incubator should not be opened for routine care. If the infant must be exposed for procedures, a portable radiant warmer should be placed over the infant. Because the incubator impedes access to the infant, critically ill patients with numerous invasive monitoring lines may benefit from being placed in an open bed with a radiant warmer.

Open Radiant Warming Beds

Description. When infants and other critically ill patients require close monitoring, quick access, and temperature control, the use of open radiant warmers with servo control provide the most effective method of temperature regulation. The radiant warmer consists of electrically heated elements placed over the patient's bed to emit radiant heat above the patient. The heating elements can be obtained as part of a system with an infant bed or as a separate unit that can be placed over a bed.

Skin probes can be used to enable servo control heat regulation. Manual mode can be used to control the heat output, but the patient's temperature must be monitored closely to avoid wide temperature swings.

Advantages and Disadvantages. Quick access to the patient is facilitated by the use of over bed warmers. Unobstructed visibility allows continuous observation of the patient and of all equipment surrounding and attached to the patient. The servo control device usually includes alarms for high and low temperature as well as for indication of continuous or prolonged heating.

Disadvantages to the open warmer include heat loss by convection if the room is drafty and increased insensible water loss that may be as high as twice the normal rate. Assessment of hydration must be performed with even greater vigilance than usual when an overbed warmer is used, and fluid intake adjusted as appropriate.

Maintenance and Nursing Considerations. Whenever radiant warmers are used, the nurse must monitor the patient's core and skin temperature. The servo mode is safer for continuous thermal support and the manual mode should only be used for short-term warming.[49] The skin temperature probe should be placed on the infant's abdomen away from bony areas[119] and the infant should not lie on top of the probe.[49] A rectal temperature probe should not be used for warmer control because the skin can be burned before normal core temperature is reached.

Risks of All Warming Devices

The most serious complication of any warming device is overheating, which can cause hyperthermia and increased oxygen consumption. Overheating may produce skin burns, particularly in a patient with poor circulation. The caregiver's hand sense of temperature should not be used to estimate the amount of heat reaching the patient.

Insensible water loss can be a significant problem and can be exaggerated with concomitant use of some phototherapy lights. Extra fluid replacement may be required to compensate for increased insensible water loss. Also, daily weights and fluid and electrolyte concentrations should be monitored.

CONCLUSION

This chapter has attempted to provide principles for the selection and use of the most common biomedical instruments employed in the critical care unit. In the final analysis, monitoring and support systems are a routine and vital part of nursing care, but the application of these devices should surpass operational principles and focus on accuracy and contribution to patient care.

The critical care nurse is expected not only to master the principles of operation for the various bioinstrumentation devices, but more importantly, to manage the information derived from these systems. Accountability for machine performance and data analysis are important in patient care. If effective, the instrumentation should *support* patient care rather than detract from it.

ACKNOWLEDGMENTS

We acknowledge the following for their support and review of the cardiovascular section: Jayme Frank, Thomas B. Brazelton, Lester T. Proctor, and American Family Children's Hospital, University of Wisconsin at Madison.

References

1. Absi MA, Lutterman J, Wetzel GT: Noninvasive cardiac output monitoring in the pediatric cardiac intensive care unit. *Curr Opin Cardiol* 25:77–79, 2010.
2. Adelson PD, Bratton SL, Carney NA, et al: Guidelines for the acute medical management of severe traumatic brain injury in infants, children, and adolescents. Chapter 7. Intracranial pressure monitoring technology. *Pediatr Crit Care Med* 4:S28–S30, 2003.
3. Agarwal S, Swanson S, Murphy A, et al: Comparing the utility of a standard pediatric resuscitation cart with a pediatric resuscitation cart based on the Broselow tape: a randomized, controlled, crossover trial involving simulated resuscitation scenarios. *Pediatrics* 116 (3):326–333, 2005.
4. Agati S, Ciccarello G, Fachile N, et al: DIDECMO: a new polymethylpentene oxygenator for pediatric extracorporeal membrane oxygenation. *ASAIO J* 52(5):509–512, 2006.
5. Alsoufi B, Al-Radi OO, Nazer RI, et al: Survival outcomes after rescue extracorporeal cardiopulmonary resuscitation in pediatric patients with refractory cardiac arrest. *J Thorac Cardiovasc Surg* 134 (4):952–959, 2007.
6. American Association of Critical Care Nurses: Evaluation of the effects of heparinized and nonheparinized flush solutions on the patency of arterial pressure monitoring lines: the AACN thunder project. *Am J Crit Care* 2(1):3–15, 1993.
7. American Association of Neuroscience Nurses: *Guide to the care of the patient with intracranial pressure monitoring,* Chicago, 2005, AANN.
8. Anderson RCE, Kan P, Klimo P, et al: Complications of intracranial pressure monitoring in children with head trauma. *J Neurosurg Pediatr* 101:53–58, 2004.
9. Andropoulos DB, Stayer SA, Diaz LK, et al: Neurological monitoring for congenital heart surgery. *Anesth Analg* 99(5):1365–1375, 2004.
10. Arbour R: Intracranial hypertension: monitoring and nursing assessment. *Crit Care Nurse* 24:19–32, 2004.
11. Arbour R: Electroencephalograph-derived monitoring. In Littlejohns LR, Bader MK, editors: *AACN-AANN protocols for practice: monitoring technologies in critically ill neuroscience patients,* Sudbury, MA, 2009, Jones & Bartlett.
12. Armola RR, Bourgault AM, Halm MA, et al: AACN levels of evidence: what's new? *Crit Care Nurse* 29(4):70–73, 2009.
12a. Arnold JH, Hanson JH, Toro-Figuero LO, Gutierrez J, Berens RJ, Anglin DL: Prospective, randomized comparison of high-frequency oscillatory ventilation and conventional mechanical ventilation in pediatric respiratory failure. *Crit Care Med* 22(10):1530–1539, 1994.
13. Australia & New Zealand ECMO influenza investigators, Davies A (chair): Extracorporeal membrane oxygenation for 2009 influenza A (H1N1) acute respiratory distress syndrome. *JAMA* 302(17), 2009.
14. Bahrami KR, Van Meurs KP: ECMO for neonatal respiratory failure. *Semin Perinatol* 29(1):15–23, 2005.
15. Bajaj L: *Measurement of arterial blood gases and arterial catheterization in children,* UpToDate. Version 17.2 DBE8E6A10D-998, 2009.
16. Baldwin JT, Borovetz HS, Duncan BW, et al: The national heart, lung, and blood institute pediatric circulatory support program. *Circulation* 113:147–155, 2006.
17. Band JD, Gaynes R: *Prevention of intravascular catheter related infections,* UpToDate. Version 17.2 BFF9EF5E22-998, 2009.
18. Bastardi HJ, Naftel DC, Webber SA, et al: Ventricular assist devices as a bridge to heart transplant in children. *J Cardiovasc Nurs* 23 (1):25–29, 2008.
19. Baulig W, Dullenkopf A, Kobler A, et al: Accuracy of continuous central venous oxygen saturation monitoring in patients undergoing cardiac surgery. *J Clin Monit Comput* 22(3):183–188, 2008.
20. Benditt JO: Esophageal and gastric pressure measurements. *Respir Care* 50(1):68–75, 2005.
21. Bendjelid K, Schutz N, Stotz M, et al: Transcutaneous PCO₂ monitoring in critically ill adults: clinical evaluation of a new sensor. *Crit Care Med* 33(10):2203–2206, 2005.
22. Bernet-Buettiker V, Ugarte MJ, Frey B, et al: Evaluation of a new combined transcutaneous measurement of PCO₂/pulse oximetry saturation ear sensor in newborn patients. *Pediatr* 115(1):e64–e68, 2005.
23. Beydon N: Pulmonary function testing in young children. *Paediatr Respir Rev* 10(4):208–213, 2009.
24. Bhatia A, Gupta AK: Neuromonitoring in the intensive care unit. I. Intracranial pressure and cerebral blood flow monitoring. *Intensive Care Med* 33:1263–1271, 2007a.
25. Bhatia A, Gupta AK: Neuromonitoring in the intensive care unit. II. Cerebral oxygenation monitoring and microdialysis. *Intensive Care Med* 33:1322–1328, 2007b.
26. Blissitt PA: Brain oxygen monitoring. In Littlejohns LR, Bader MK, editors: *AACN-AANN protocols for practice: monitoring technologies in critically ill neuroscience patients,* Sudbury, MA, 2009, Jones & Bartlett.
27. Bollen CW, Uiterwaal CS, van Vught AJ: Cumulative metaanalysis of high-frequency versus conventional ventilation in premature neonate. *Intensive Care Med* 33(4):680–688, 2007.

28. Bower LK, Barnhart SL, Betit P, et al: AARC Guidelines: neonatal and pediatric O_2 delivery. *Respir Care* 47(6):707–716, 2002.

29. Boxer RA, et al: Noninvasive pulse oximetry in children with cyanotic congenital heart disease. *Crit Care Med* 15:1062, 1987.

30. Bruce E, Franck L, Howard RF: The efficacy of morphine and entonox analgesia during chest drain removal in children. *Pediatr Anesth* 16(3):302–308, 2006.

31. Bruce EA, Howard RF, Franck LS: Chest drain removal pain and its management: a literature review. *J Clin Nurs* 15(2):145–154, 2006.

32. Cannon ML, Cornell J, Tripp-Hammel DS, et al: Tidal volumes for ventilated infants should be determined with a pnuemotachometer placed at the endotracheal tube. *Am J Respir Crit Care Med* 162 (6):2109–2112, 2000.

33. Carberry KE, Gunter KS, Germmato CJ, et al: Mechanical circulatory support for the pediatric patient. *Crit Care Nurs Q* 30(2):121–142, 2007.

34. Carter R, Banham SW: Use of transcutaneous oxygen and carbon dioxide tensions for assessing indices of gas exchange during exercise testing. *Respir Med* 94:350–355, 2000.

35. Cates LA: Pigtail catheters used in the treatment of pneumothoraces in the neonate. *Adv Neonatal Care* 9(1):7–16, 2009.

35a. Chameides L, Samson RA, Schexnayder SM, Hazinski MF, editors: *Pediatric advanced life support provider manual*, Dallas, 2011, American Heart Association.

36. Cicek SH, Gumus S, Deniz O, et al: Effect of nail polish and henna on oxygen saturation determined by pulse oximetry in healthy young adult female, *Emerg Med J*, 2010.

37. Clermont G, Theodore A: *Arterial catheterization*, UpToDate. Version 17.2, 2009.

38. Collison SP, Dager SK: The role of the Intra-aortic balloon pump in supporting children with acute cardiac failure. *Postgrad Med J* 83:308–311, 2007.

39. Consumer Product Safety Commission: *Extension cords fact sheet: CPSC document #16.* http://www.cpsc.gov/cpscpub/pubs/16.html Accessed September 11, 2007.

40. Craig JV, Lancaster GA, Taylor S, et al: Infrared ear thermometry compared with rectal thermometry in children: a systemic review. *Lancet* 360:603–609, 2002.

41. Cua CL, Thomas K, Zurakowski D, et al: A comparison of the vasotrac with invasive arterial blood pressure monitoring in children after pediatric cardiac surgery. *Anesth Analg* 100(5):1289–1294, 2005.

42. Deckardt R, Steward D: Noninvasive arterial hemoglobin oxygen saturation versus transcutaneous oxygen tension monitoring in the preterm infant. *Crit Care Med* 12(11):935, 1984.

43. de Oliveira CF, de Oliveira DS, Gottschald AF, et al: ACCM/PALS haemodynamic support guidelines for paediatric septic shock: an outcomes comparison with and without monitoring central venous oxygen saturation. *Intensive Care Med* 34:1065–1075, 2008.

44. Dickerson HA, Chang AC: Perioperative management of ventricular assist devices in children and adolescents. *Semin Thorac Cardiovasc Surg Pediatr Card Surg Annu*, 128–139, 2006.

45. Di Fiore JM: Neonatal cardiopulmonary monitoring techniques. *Semin Neonatol* 9(3):195, 2004.

46. Donn SM, Sinha SK: Advanced neonatal ventilation. In Kurjak A, Chervenak FA, editors: *Textbook of perinatal medicine*, Andover, UK, 2006, Informa Healthcare.

47. Duncan BW: Mechanical circulatory support for infants and children with cardiac disease. *Ann Thorac Surg* 73:1670–1677, 2002.

48. Eberhard P: The design, use, and results of transcutaneous carbon dioxide analysis: current and future direction. *Anesth Analg* 105: S48–S52, 2007.

49. ECRI Institute: *Infant radiant warmers can burn: use with care*, ECRI Institute, 2009, available at http://mdsr.ecri.org/summary/detail.aspx? doc_id=8263. Accessed 11/29/09.

50. Edelson DP, Abella BS, Kramer-Johansen J, et al: Effects of compression depth and pre-shock pauses predict defibrillation failure during cardiac arrest. *Resuscitation* 71:137–145, 2006.

51. Epstein AE, DiMarco JP, Ellenbogen KA, et al: ACC/AHA/HRS 2008 guidelines for device-based therapy of cardiac rhythm abnormalities: a report of the American College of Cardiology/American Heart Association Task Force on Practice Guidelines (writing committee to revise the ACC/AHA/NASPE 2002 guideline update for implantation of cardiac pacemakers and antiarrhythmia devices) developed in collaboration with the American Association for Thoracic Surgery and Society of Thoracic Surgeons. *J Am J Cardiol* 51(21):e1–e62, 2008.

52. Fakler U, Pauli C, Balling G, et al: Cardiac index monitoring by pulse contour analysis and thermodilution after pediatric cardiac surgery. *J Thorac Cardiovasc Surg* 133(1):224–228, 2007.

53. Felix DE, Munro HM, DeCampli WM: Near infrared spectroscopy used to detect preoperative aortic obstruction. *Pediatr Anesth* 17 (6):598–599, 2007.

54. Field JM, Hazinski MF (co-editors), et al: Part 1: executive summary: 2010 American Heart Association Guidelines for Cardiopulmonary Resuscitation and Emergency Cardiovascular Care. *Circulation* 122 (suppl 3):S640–S656, 2010.

55. Finer NN: Newer trends in continuous monitoring of critically ill infants and children. *Pediatr Clin North Am* 27(3):553, 1980.

56. Fowler RA, Rizoli SB, Levin PD, Smith T: Blood conservation for critically ill patients. *Crit Care Clin* 20(2):313–324, 2004.

57. Friedman D, Classen J, Hirsch LJ: Continuous electroencephalogram monitoring in the intensive care unit. *Anesth Analg* 109:506–523, 2009.

58. Fuchs A, Netz H: Ventricular assist devices in pediatrics. *Images Paediatr Cardiol* 9:24–54, 2002.

59. Fullerton DA, St Cyr JA: Mixed venous oxygen saturation in the diagnosis of cardiac tamponade. *J Cardiac Surg* 23(2):180–181, 2008.

60. Gancel P-E, Roupie E, Guittet L, et al: Accuracy of a transcutaneous carbon dioxide pressure monitoring device in emergency room patients with acute respiratory failure. *Intensive Care Med* 37 (2):348–351, 2011.

61. Gawlinski ADNS, Rutledge D: Selecting a model for evidence-based practice changes: a practical approach. *AACN Adv Crit Care* 19 (3):291–300, 2008.

62. Gettinger A, DeTraglia M, Glass D: In vivo comparison of two mixed venous saturation catheters. *Anesthesiology* 66:373, 1987.

63. Gold LS, Rear TD, Eisenberg MS: *Automated external defibrillators.* UpToDate November 24, 2010: Accessed at http://www.uptodate.com/contents/automated-external-defibrillators.

64. Gordon MBSN, Bartruff LMSN, Gordon SMSN, et al: How fast is too fast? A practice change in umbilical arterial catheter blood sampling using the Iowa model for evidence-based practice. *Adv Neonatal Care* 8(4):198–207, 2008.

65. Graham KC, Cvach M: Monitor alarm fatigue: standardizing use of physiological monitors and decreasing nuisance alarms. *Am J Crit Care* 19(1), 2010.

66. Gravlee G, Davis R, Stammers A, Ungerleider R: *Cardiopulmonary bypass: principles and practice,* ed 3, Philadelphia, 2007, Lippincott Williams & Wilkins.

67. Griffin MP, Siadaty MS: Papaverine prolongs patency of peripheral arterial catheters in neonates. *J Pediatr* 146(1):62–65, 2005.

68. Hadaway L: Technology of flushing vascular access devices. *J Infus Nurs* 29(3):129–145, 2006.

69. Haddad F, Zeeni C, Yazigi A, Madi-Jebara S: Multimodal analgesia for chest tube removal after cardiac surgery. *J Cardiothorac Vasc Anesth* 20(5):760–761, 2006.

70. Hall KF, Bennetts TM, Whitta RK, et al: Effect of heparin in arterial line flushing solutions on platelet count: a randomised double-blind study. *Crit Care Resusc: J Aust Acad Crit Care Med* 8(4):294–296, 2006.

71. Hawkin JA, Minich LL: Intraaortic balloon counterpulsation for children with cardiac disease. In Duncan BW, editor: *Mechanical support for cardiac and respiratory failure in pediatric patients*, New York, 2001, Marcel Dekker.

72. Hay WW, Jr, Rodden DJ, Collins SM, et al: Reliability of conventional and new pulse oximetry in neonatal patients. *J Perinatol* 22 (5):360, 2002.

72a. Henderson-Smart DJ, et al: Elective high frequency oscillatory ventilation versus conventional ventilation for acute pulmonary dysfunction in preterm infants. *Cochrane Database Syst Rev* (3):CD000104, 2007.

73. Hetzer R, Stiller B: Ventricular assist device for children. *Nat Clin Pract Cardiovasc Med* 3(7):377–386, 2006.

74. Heulitt MJ, Farrington EA, O'Shea TM, et al: Double-blind, randomized, controlled trial of papaverine-containing infusions to prevent failure of arterial catheters in pediatric patients. *Crit Care Med* 21(6):825–829, 1993.

75. Hi Fi Study Group: High frequency oscillatory ventilation compared with conventional mechanical ventilation in the treatment of respiratory failure. *NEJM* 320(2):88, 1989.

76. Hillier SC, Schamberger MS: Transcutaneous and end-tidal carbon dioxide analysis: complimentary monitoring strategies. *J Intensive Care Med* 20:307–309, 2005.

77. Hinkelbein J, Genzwuerker HV, Sogi R, et al: Effect of nail polish on oxygen saturation determined by pulse oximetry in critically ill patients. *Resuscitation* 72(1):82–91, 2007.

78. Hirsch JC, Charpie JR, Ohye RG, Gurney JG: Near-infrared spectroscopy: what we know and what we need to know: a systematic review of the congenital heart disease literature. *J Thorac Cardiovasc Surg* 137(1):154–159.e12, 2009.

79. Hoffman GM, Stuth EA, Jaquiss RD, et al: Changes in cerebral and somatic oxygenation during stage 1 palliation of hypoplastic left heart syndrome using continuous regional cerebral perfusion. *J Thorac Cardiovasc Surg* 127(1):223–233, 2004.

80. Horvath R, Shore S, Schultz SE, et al: Cerebral and somatic oxygen saturation decrease after delayed sternal closure in children after cardiac surgery. *J Thorac Cardiovasc Surg* 139(4):894–900, 2010.

81. Huber D, Osthaus WA, Optenhofel J, et al: Continuous monitoring of central venous oxygen saturation in neonates and small infants: in vitro evaluation of two different oximetry catheters. *Pediatr Anesth* 17:1257–1261, 2006.

82. Integra Neurosciences: *Licox IMC directions for use,* Plainsboro, NJ, 2004, Integra Neurosciences.

83. Kalavrouziotis G, Karunaratne A, Raja S: Intraaortic balloon pumping in children undergoing cardiac surgery: an update on the Liverpool experience. *J Thorac Cardiovasc Surg* 131:1382–1389, 2006.

84. Kannan A: Heparinised saline or normal saline? *J Periop Pract* 18 (10):440–441, 2008.

85. Karl TR, Horton SB: Centrifugal pump ventricular assist device in pediatric cardiac surgery. In Duncan BW, editor: *Mechanical support for cardiac and respiratory failure in pediatric patients,* New York, 2001, Marcel Dekker.

86. Karp T, et al: High frequency jet ventilation: a neonatal nursing perspective. *Neonatal Network* 4(10):42, 1986.

87. Karselis TC: *Descriptive medical electronics and instrumentation,* Thorofare, NJ, 1973, Slack.

88. Keszler M: State of the art in conventional mechanical ventilation. *J Perinatol* 29(4):262, 2009.

89. Kidd KC, Criddle L: Using jugular venous catheters in patients with traumatic brain injury. *Crit Care Nurs* 21:16–22, 2001.

90. Kirk D, Rainey T, Vail A, et al: Infra-red thermometry: the reliability of tympanic and temporal artery readings for predicting brain temperature after severe traumatic brain injury. *Crit Care* 13:R81, 2009.

91. Kirkness C: Cerebral blood flow monitoring. In Littlejohns LR, Bader MK, editors: *AACN-AANN protocols for practice: monitoring technologies in critically ill neuroscience patients,* Sudbury, MA, 2009, Jones & Bartlett.

92. Kleinman M, Chameides L, Schexnayder SM, et al: Part 14: pediatric advanced life support; 2010 American Heart Association Guidelines for Cardiopulmonary Resuscitation and Emergency Cardiovascular Care. *Circulation* 122:S876–S908, 2010.

93. Kotake Y, Yamada T, Nagata H, et al: Can mixed venous hemoglobin oxygen saturation be estimated using a NICO monitor? *Anesth Analg* 109(1):119–123, 2009.

94. Krivitski NM, Kislukhin VV, Thuramalla NV: Theory and in-vitro validation of a new extracorporeal AV loop approach for hemodynamic assessment in pediatric and neonatal ICU patients. *Pediatr Crit Care Med* 9(4):423–428, 2008.

95. Kuch BA, Saville A, Vehovic W, et al: Accuracy of the sidestream vs. mainstream end tidal capnography: a Bland-Altman analysis. *54th International Respiratory Congress, Anaheim, CA,* 2008.

96. Kurtz P, Hanafy KA, Claassen J: Continuous EEG monitoring: is it ready for prime time? *Curr Opin Crit Care* 15:99–109, 2009.

97. Kussman BDBC, Wypij D, DiNardo JA, et al: Cerebral oximetry during infant cardiac surgery: evaluation and relationship to early postoperative outcome. *Anesth Analg* 108(4):1122–1131, 2009.

98. Lacerenza S, De Carolis MP, Fusco FP, et al: An evaluation of a new combined SpO2/PtcCO2 sensor in very low birth weight infants. *Anesth Analg* 107:125–129, 2008.

99. Lang EW, Mulvey JM, Mudaliar Y, et al: Direct cerebral oxygenation monitoring: a systematic review of recent publications. *Neurosurg Rev* 30:99–107, 2007.

100. Lawson D, et al: Blood flow limits and pulse oximeter signal detection. *Anesthesiology* 67(4):599, 1987.

101. LeSouef PN, et al: Comparison of transcutaneous oxygen tension with arterial oxygen tension in newborn infants with severe respiratory illnesses. *Pediatrics* 62(4):692, 1978.

102. Leeper B, Lovasik D: Cerebrospinal drainage systems: external ventricular and lumbar drains. In Littlejohns LR, Bader MK, editors: *AACN-AANN protocols for practice: monitoring technologies in critically ill neuroscience patients,* Sudbury, MA, 2009, Jones & Bartlett.

103. Link MS, Atlins DL, Passman RS, et al: Part 6: electrical therapies, automated external defibrillators, defibrillation, cardioversion, and pacing, 2010 American Heart Association Guidelines for Cardiopulmonary Resuscitation and Emergency Cardiovascular Care. *Circulation* 122:S706–S719, 2010.

104. Littlejohns LR, Bader M: Guidelines for the management of severe head injury: clinical application and changes in practice. *Crit Care Nurse* 21:48–65, 2001.

105. Littlejohns LR, Bader MK, March K: Brain tissue oxygen monitoring in severe brain injury. I. *Crit Care Nurse* 23:17–25, 2003.

106. Lopez E, Grabar S, Barbier A, et al: Detection of carbon dioxide thresholds using low-flow sidestream capnography in ventilated preterm infants. *Intensive Care Med* 35:1942, 2009.

107. Lopez-Briz E, Ruiz-Garcia V: Heparina frente a cloruro sodico 0,9% para mantener permeables los cateteres venosos centrales. Una revision sistematica. *Farm Hosp* 29(4):258–264, 2005.

108. Lubitz DS, et al: A rapid method for estimating weight and resuscitation drug dosages from length in the pediatric age group. *Ann Emerg Med* 17:576, 1988.

109. Lund CH, Osborne JW, Kuller J, et al: Neonatal skin care: clinical outcomes of the AWHONN/NANN evidence-based clinical practice guideline. *JOGNN* 30(1):41–51, 2001.

110. Maar SP: Searching for the holy grail: a review of markers of tissue perfusion in pediatric critical care. *Pediatr Emerg Care* 24 (12):883–887, 2008.

110a. Mahajan A, et al: An experimental and clinical evaluation of a novel central venous catheter with integrated oximetry for pediatric patients undergoing cardiac surgery: Pediatric Central Venous Oximetry. *Anest Anal* 105(6):1598–1604, 2007.

111. Maloney-Wilensky E, Gracias V, Itkin A, et al: Brain tissue oxygen and outcome after severe traumatic brain injury: a systematic review. *Crit Care Med* 37:2057–2063, 2009.

112. March K: Intracranial pressure monitoring and assessing intracranial compliance in brain injury. *Crit Care Nurs Clin North Am* 12:429–436, 2000.

113. March K, Madden L: Intracranial pressure management. In Littlejohns LR, Bader MK, editors: *AACN-AANN protocols for practice: monitoring technologies in critically ill neuroscience patients,* Sudbury, MA, 2009, Jones & Bartlett.

114. March K, Wellwood J, Arbour R: Technology. In Bader MK, Littlejohns LR, editors: *AANN core curriculum for neuroscience nursing,* ed 4, Philadelphia, 2004, Saunders.

115. Martin J, Shekerdemian LS: The monitoring of venous saturations of oxygen in children with congenitally malformed hearts. *Cardiol Young* 19(1):34–39, 2009.

116. Martin SA, Klein AM: Can there be a standard for temperature measurement in the pediatric intensive care unit? *AACN Clin Issues* 15:254–266, 2004.

117. Mattoo T: Definition and diagnosis of hypertension in children and adolescents. *Pediatrics* 104(3):30, 2009.

118. Mazzeo AT, Bullock R: Monitoring brain tissue oxymetry: will it change management of critically ill neurologic patients? *J Neurol Sci* 261:1–9, 2007.

119. McGrath JM: Neonatal thermoregulation. In Verger JT, Lebet RM, editors: *AACN procedure manual for pediatric acute and critical care,* St Louis, 2008, Saunders Elsevier.

120. McSwain SD, Hamel DS, Smith PB, et al: End-tidal and arterial carbon dioxide measurements correlate across all levels of physiologic dead space. *Respir Care* 55(3):288–293, 2010.

121. Miller-Hoover S, Small L: Research evidence review and appraisal: pediatric central venous catheter care bundling. *Pediatr Nurs* 35 (3):191–201, 2009.

122. Mohseni-Bod H, Frndova H, Gaitaro R, et al: Evaluation of a new pediatric continuous oximetry catheter. *Pediatr Crit Care* 12(5):1, 2011.

123. Mok E, Kwong TK, Chan MF: A randomized controlled trial for maintaining peripheral intravenous lock in children. *Int J Nurs Pract* 13(1):33–45, 2007.

124. Monggero L, Beck J, editors: *On bypass: advanced perfusion techniques,* Totowa, NJ, 2008, Humana Press.

125. Moran JL, Peter JV, Solomon PJ, et al: Tympanic temperature measurements: are they reliable in the critically ill? *A clinical study of measures of agreement. Crit Care Med* 35:155–164, 2007.

126. Muller M, Lohr T, Scholz S, et al: Continous SvO_2 measurement infants undergoing congenital heart surgery: first clinical experiences with a new fiberoptic probe. *Pediatr Anesth* 17:51–55, 2007.

127. National Electrical Code Series 2011: *NFPA 70,* Quincy, MA, 2010, National Fire Protection Association.

128. National High Blood Pressure Education Program Working Group: The fourth report on the diagnosis, evaluation, and treatment of high blood pressure in children and adolescents. *Pediatrics* 114 (2):556–576, 2004.

129. Norozi K, Beck C, Osthaus WA, et al: Electrical velocimetry for measuring cardiac output in children with congenital heart disease. *Br J Anaesth* 100:88–94, 2008.

130. Norton E: Implementing the universal protocol hospital-wide. *AORN* 85(6):1187–1197, 2007.

131. Occupational Safety & Health Administration: Regulations (Standards). OSHA Standard 1910 Subpart S-Electrical-General. http://www.osha.gov/. Accessed September 10, 2007.

132. O'Donnell CP, Kamlin CO, Davis PG, Morley CJ: Feasibility of and delay in obtaining pulse oximetry during neonatal resuscitation. *J Pediatr* 147(5):698–699, 2005.

133. O'Grady NP, Barie PS, Bartlett JG, et al: Guidelines for evaluation of new fever in critically ill adult patients: 2008 update from the American College of Critical Care Medicine and the Infectious Diseases Society of America. *Crit Care Med* 36:1330–1349, 2008.

134. Olsen BS, Kocis KC: Measuring cardiac output in critically ill infants and children: are we still "talking the talk" or can we now "walk the walk"? *Pediatr Crit Care Med* 9(4):449–450, 2008.

135. Olson DM, Chioffi SM, Macy GE, et al: Potential benefits of bispectral index monitoring in critical care. *Crit Care Nurs* 23:45–52, 2003.

136. Palve H, Vivori A: Pulse oximetry during low cardiac output and hypothermia states immediately after open heart surgery. *Crit Care Med* 17(1):66, 1989.

137. Peruzzi WT, Noskin GA, Moen SG, et al: Microbial contamination of blood conservation devices during routine use in the critical care setting: results of a prospective, randomized trial. *Crit Care Med* 24 (7):1157–1162, 1996.

138. Phelps HM, Mahle WT, Kim D, et al: Postoperative cerebral oxygenation in hypoplastic left heart syndrome after the Norwood procedure. *Ann Thorac Surg* 87(5):1490–1494, 2009.

139. Pinkney KA, Minich LL, Tani LY, et al: Current results with intraaortic balloon pumping in infants and children. *Ann Thorac Surg* 73:887–891, 2002.

140. Podrid PJ: *Basic principles and technique of cardioversion and defibrillation,* UpToDate, 2009.

141. Rais-Bahrami K, Rivera O, Short BL: Validation of a noninvasive neonatal optical cerebral oximeter in veno-venous ECMO patients with a cephalad catheter (original article, technical report). *J Perinatol* 26:628–635, 2006.

142. Ralston M, Hazinski M, Zaritsky AL, et al: *Pediatric advanced life support course guide,* Dallas, 2006, American Heart Association.

143. Ramasethu J: Complications of vascular catheters in the neonatal intensive care unit. *Clin Perinatol* 35(1):199–222, 2008.

144. Ranucci M, Isgro G, De la Torre T, et al: Near-infrared spectroscopy correlates with continuous superior vena cava oxygen saturation in pediatric cardiac surgery patients. *Paediatr Anaesth* 18 (12):1163–1169, 2008.

145. Reavy K, Tavernier S: Nurses reclaiming ownership of their practice: implementation of an evidence-based practice model and process. *J Cont Educ Nurs* 39(4):166–172, 2008.

146. Reinhart K, Kuhn HJ, Hartog C, et al: Continuous central venous and pulmonary artery oxygen saturation monitoring in the critically ill. *Intensive Care Med* 30:1572–1578, 2004.

147. Richter HP, Schwan WC, Hartwell FP: *Wiring simplified,* ed 42, Minneapolis, 2008, Park Publishing Inc.

148. Rodriguez-Cruz E, Walters H: Extracorporeal membrane oxygenation. *eMedicine,* 2006.

149. Rosen DA, Morris JL, Rosen KR, et al: Analgesia for pediatric thoracostomy tube removal. *Anesth Analg* 90 (5):1025–1028, 2000.

150. Rosenthal D, Bernstein D: Pediatric mechanical circulatory support. *Editorial. Circulation* 113:2266–2268, 2006.

151. Rozner MA, Trankina M: Cardiac pacing and defibrillation. In Kaplan JA, editor: *Essentials of cardiac anesthesia,* Philadelphia, 2008, Saunders.

152. Safe Medical Device Act of 1990: *The library of congress— Thomas home,* http://thomas.loc.gov/cgi-bin/bdquery/z?d101: HR03095:@@@D&summ2=1&%7CTOM:/bss/d101query.html% 7C Accessed March 5, 2012.

153. Schell KA: Evidence-based practice: noninvasive blood pressure measurement in children. *Pediatr Nurs* 32(3):263–267, 2006.

154. Schroeder JS, Daily EK: *Techniques in bedside hemodynamic monitoring,* ed 3, St Louis, 1989, Mosby.

155. Schubert S, Schmitz T, Weiss M, et al: Continuous non-invasive techniques to determine cardiac output in children after cardiac surgery: evaluation of transesophageal Doppler and electric velocimetry. *J Clin Monit Comput* 22:299–307, 2008.

156. Schulman CS: Strategies for starting a successful evidence-based practice program. *AACN Adv Crit Care* 19(3):301–311, 2008.

157. Secker C, Spiers P: Accuracy of pulse oximetry in patients with low systemic vascular resistance. *Anaesthesia* 52(2):127–130, 1997.

158. Sendak M, Harris A, Donham R: Use of pulse oximetry to assess arterial oxygen saturation during newborn resuscitation. *Crit Care Med* 14(8):739, 1986.

159. Sendelbach DM, Jackson GL, Lai SS, et al: Pulse oximetry screening at 4 hours of age to detect critical congenital heart defects. *Pediatrics* 122(4):e815–e820, 2008.

160. Shah PS, Ng E, Sinha AK: Heparin for prolonging peripheral intravenous catheter use in neonates. *Cochrane Database Syst Rev (Online)* (4):CD002774, 2005.

161. Shalli S, Saeed D, Fukamachi K, et al: Chest tube selection in cardiac and thoracic surgery: a survey of chest tube-related complications and their management. *J Cardiac Surg* 24(5): 503–509, 2009.

162. Sittig SE: *Transitional technology from NICU to home,* AARC Times, 2000, pp 37.

163. Stebor ADP: Basic principles of noninvasive blood pressure measurement in infants. *Advanc Neonatal Care* 5(5):252–261, 2005.

164. Stevens WJ: Multimodal monitoring: head injury management using $S_{JV}O_2$ and LICOX. *J Neurosci Nurs* 36:332–339, 2004.

165. Sullivan KJ, Kisson N, Goodwin SR, et al: End-tidal carbon dioxide monitoring in pediatric emergencies. *Pediatr Emerg Care* 21 (5):327–332, 2005.

166. Talmor D, Sarge T, Malhotra A, et al: Mechanical ventilation guided by esophageal pressure in acute lung injury. *NEJM* 359 (20):2095–2104, 2008.

167. Timothy BC, Rodeman BJCS: Temporary pacemakers in critically ill patients: assessment and management strategies. *AACN* 15 (3):305–325, 2005.

168. Titler MG, Everett LQ: Sustain an infrastructure to support EBP. *Nurs Mgmt* 37(9):14–16, 2006.

169. Tobias JD: Cerebral oxygenation monitoring: near-infrared spectroscopy. *Expert Rev Med Devices* 3:235–243, 2006.

170. Tobias JD: Transcutanous carbon dioxide monitoring in infants and children. *Paediatr Anaesth* 19(5):434–444, 2009.

170a. Tobias JD, Flanagan JF, Wheeler TJ, Garrett JS, Burney C: Noninvasive monitoring of end-tidal CO_2 via nasal cannulas in spontaneously breathing children during the perioperative period. *Crit Care Med* 22 (11):1805–1808, 1994.

171. Tobin MJ: *Principles and practice of intensive care monitoring,* New York, 1998, McGraw-Hill.

172. Tremper KK, Shoemaker WC: Transcutaneous PO_2 monitoring useful in adults, too. *Crit Care Monit* 1(1):1, 1981.

173. Tremper KK, Shoemaker WC: Transcutaneous oxygen monitoring of critically ill adults, with and without low flow shock. *Crit Care Med* 9(10):706, 1981.

174. Tremper KK, Waxman K, Bowman R, et al: Continuous transcutaneous O_2 monitoring during respiratory failure, cardiac decompensation, cardiac arrest and CPR. *Crit Care Med* 8(7):377, 1980.

175. Tremper KK, Waxman K, Shoemaker WC: Effects of hypoxia and shock on transcutaneous $P_{tc}O_2$ values in dogs. *Crit Care Med* 1 (12):526, 1981.

176. U.S. Department of Labor: *Electrical hazards. Hospital eTool— HealthCare wide hazards module.* http://www.osha.gov/SLTC/etools/ hospital/hazards/electrical/electrical.html. Accessed September 12, 2007.

177. Van de Louw A, Cracco C, Cerf C, et al: Accuracy of pulse oximetry in the intensive care unit. *Intensive Care Med* 27:1606–1613, 2001.

178. Velasco AJ: Jugular venous saturation monitoring: insertion assist, monitoring, and care. In Verger JT, Lebet RM, editors: *AACN procedure manual for pediatric acute and critical care*, St Louis, 2008, Saunders Elsevier.

179. Verger JT, Lebet RM, editors: *AACN procedure manual for pediatric acute and critical care*, St Louis, 2008, Saunders Elsevier.

180. Vernon-Levett P: Neurologic system. In Slota MC, editor: *Core curriculum for pediatric critical care nursing*, ed 2, St Louis, 2006, Saunders Elsevier.

181. Wallis WH: Cerebral tissue oxygenation monitoring: insertion assist, monitoring, and care. In Verger JT, Lebet RM, editors: *AACN procedure manual for pediatric acute and critical care*, St Louis, 2008, Saunders Elsevier.

182. Wallis WH, Marcoux KK: Intracranial pressure monitoring. In Verger JT, Lebet RM, editors: *AACN procedure manual for pediatric acute and critical care*, St Louis, 2010, Saunders Elsevier.

183. Walsh B, Czervinske M, DiBlasi R: *Perinatal and pediatric respiratory care*, ed 3, St Louis, 2010, Saunders Elsevier.

184. Wartenberg KE, Schmidt JM, Mayer SA: Multimodality monitoring in neurocritical care. *Crit Care Clin* 23:507–538, 2007.

185. Weaver LK: Transcutaneous oxygen and carbon dioxide tension compared to arterial blood gases in normals. *Respir Care* 52(1):1490–1496, 2007.

186. Webster HP, Chellis MJP: Physiologic monitoring of infants and children. *AACN* 4(1):180–196, 1993.

187. White K: Completing the hemodynamic picture, SvO_2. *Heart Lung* 14(3):272, 1985.

188. Wilensky EM, Bloom S, Leichter D, et al: Brain tissue oxygen practice guidelines using the LICOX CMP monitoring system. *J Neurosci Nurs* 37:278–288, 2005.

189. Wilson BJ, Cowan HJ, Lord JA, et al: The accuracy of pulse oximetry in emergency department patients with severe sepsis and septic shock; a retrospective cohort study, *BMC Emerg Med* 10:9, 2010.

190. Wilson J, Russo P, Russo J, et al: Noninvasive monitoring of carbon dioxide in infants and children with congenital heart disease: end-tidal versus transcutaneous techniques. *J Intensive Care Med* 20:291–295, 2005.

190a. Wunsch J, Mapstone J: High-frequency ventilation versus conventional ventilation for treatment of acute lung injury and acute respiratory distress syndrome. *Cochrane Database Syst Rev* 1: CD004085, 2004.

191. Yamamoto T, Takayama M, Sato N, et al: Inappropriate analyses of automated external defibrillators used during in-hospital ventricular fibrillation. *Circ J Official J Jpn Circ Soc* 72(4):679–681, 2008.

192. Zwischenberger JB, Bartlett R: *ECMO extracorporeal cardiopulmonary support in critical care*, ed 3, Ann Arbor, MI, 2005, Extracorporeal Life Support Organization.

Fundamentals of Patient Safety and Quality Improvement

22

Tara Trimarchi

PEARLS

- Following the documentation of patient death and complication rate related to medical errors and preventable complications, it is now clear that an essential component of healthcare delivery is improving the safety and quality of healthcare.
- Healthcare improvement efforts prevent iatrogenic injury and maximize positive patient outcomes by incorporating the psychology of human behavior, evidence-based standards of care, and performance measurement into clinical processes and systems.
- "High-reliability" organizations have low patient morbidity and mortality, a low rate of error and complications, and they continuously learn from the analysis of potential system flaws and actual adverse events. The staff of high reliability organizations raise concerns and make decisions to support safety practices and standardize processes, and there is leadership support for this approach.
- Pediatric critical care is highly vulnerable to errors and adverse patient events, so pediatric critical care nurses must be particularly vigilant in promoting a safe work environment, and compliance with medication safety, prevention of healthcare-acquired infections, and other evidence-based methods to improve patient care outcomes.

OVERVIEW OF PATIENT SAFETY AND HEALTHCARE QUALITY IMPROVEMENT

Healthcare professionals practice with the intention of promoting the well-being of their patients. Yet despite the dedication, intelligence, and education of healthcare professionals, encounters often fall short of providing safe and high-quality care. The discipline of healthcare improvement has grown out of mounting evidence that many patients are inadvertently harmed by the care that is intended to make them well and that patient outcomes are denigrated by suboptimal care delivery systems.[51,56] Healthcare improvement efforts prevent iatrogenic injury and maximize positive patient outcomes by incorporating the psychology of human behavior, evidence-based standards of care, and performance measurement into clinical processes and systems. Although patient safety and quality improvement programs may be considered the domain of managers and administrators, the ultimate responsibility to deliver safe and high quality care falls squarely on front-line clinicians. Pediatric critical care nurses must understand childhood diseases and their treatment, but also must know when, how, and why their work might fail to meet the needs of patients, and they must have the tools to make care safer and more effective.

Institute of Medicine Reports: The Case for Improving Healthcare Safety and Quality

In 1999, the Institute of Medicine (IOM) report *To Err is Human: Building a Safer Health System* estimated that 100,000 people die every year in the United States as the result of preventable errors made by healthcare professionals.[51] The statistics presented in this study ranked medical errors as the eighth leading cause of death and demonstrated that more people die because of medical errors than from motor vehicle crashes, breast cancer, or AIDS.[7,18,51] The report attributed 7000 of the deaths to medication errors and estimated the annual cost of errors at $17 billion to $29 billion.[51]

The *To Err is Human* report exposed the inadequacies of healthcare systems, focused attention on patient safety, and fostered programs dedicated to measuring and improving performance. Table 22-1 outlines the recommendations for healthcare improvement that were presented in the *To Err is Human* report and endorsed by the IOM's Quality of Health Care in America Committee. In a follow-up to the *To Err is Human* report, in 2001 the IOM published *Crossing the Quality Chasm: A New Health System for the 21st Century,* to more fully address quality problems related to patient-family satisfaction, treatment disparities, and resource accessibility.[21,64,65] *Crossing the Quality Chasm* defines the ideal twenty-first century healthcare system as one that is safe, effective, patient-centered, timely, efficient, and equitable. Table 22-2 defines the six aims set forth by the IOM and highlights the recommendations of the *Crossing the Quality Chasm* report for achieving the ideal healthcare system.

Through the implementation of the IOM recommendations and the work of organizations that have evolved to improve the safety and quality of healthcare (see the table in the Chapter 22 Supplement on the Evolve Website for a list of organizations and their focuses and websites), individual institutions have demonstrated incremental improvement in care. As late as 2005, however, national statistics had not improved substantially.[2,56] Furthermore, the data compiled in 1999 may have underestimated deficiencies in patient safety.[56] For example, the Centers for Disease Control and Prevention (CDC) data subsequent to the *To Err is Human* report suggest that healthcare-acquired blood stream infections may account for as many as 90,000 deaths every year.[19,56] In light of these

Table 22-1	The Institute of Medicine Quality of Health Care in America Committee's Recommendations for Health Care Improvement	

Tier	Goal	Action
Leadership and knowledge	Establish national leadership, research, tools, and protocols to enhance patient safety knowledge	Development of a Center for Patient Safety within the Agency for Healthcare Research and Quality
Identifying and learning from errors	Identify and learn through errors via mandatory and voluntary reporting efforts with an emphasis on using information to make systems safer	Development of reporting standards by the National Forum for Health Care Quality Measurement and Reporting and analysis of the data by the Center for Patient Safety Requirement for state departments of health to report adverse events Designation of federal funding for the development of reporting systems Creation of legislation to extend peer review protections to data related to patient safety and quality improvement
Setting performance standards and expectations	Raise the standard and expectations for the improvement of safety through the actions of oversight organizations, professional organizations, and group purchasers	Inclusion of patient safety indicators in performance standards Implementation of patient safety programs by regulators and accreditors, public and private healthcare purchasers and health professional licensing, certifying and credentialing agencies Development of patient safety committees within professional societies Increased post-marketing monitoring of drugs by the U.S. Food and Drug Administration
Implementing safety systems in healthcare organizations	Create safe systems within healthcare organizations by implementing safe practices at the delivery level	Incorporation of patient safety programs, with executive sponsorship, into all healthcare institutions Adoption of safe medication practices by all healthcare institutions

From Kohn KT, Corrigan JM, Donaldson MS: *To err is human: building a safer healthcare system*, Washington, DC, 1999, National Academy Press; National Academy of Sciences: *To err is human: building a safer healthcare system executive summary*. Available at http://www.nap.edu. Accessed October 8, 2011.

Table 22-2	Institute of Medicine Six Aims for Improvement of Health Care Systems	

Aim	Definition	Recommendations for Achieving the Six Quality Aims
Safe	Avoid injuries to patients from care that was intended to help them.	• Designate federal funding to healthcare quality improvement initiatives.
Effective	Provide services that are based on scientific knowledge to all who could benefit and refrain from providing services to those who are not likely to benefit.	• Reduce illogical variability in treatment between individual clinicians and institutions and promote the use of evidence-based practices.
Patient-centered	Provide care that is respectful of and responsive to individual patient preferences, needs and values and ensures that patient values guide all clinical decisions.	• Increase transparency of information regarding the performance of healthcare institutions. • Allow patients to access to their own medical records and clinical knowledge.
Timely	Reduce wait time and harmful delays for those who both receive and give care.	• Implement mechanisms for active communication and exchange of information among healthcare providers.
Efficient	Avoid waste such as wasteful use of supplies, ideas and energy.	• Create an information technology infrastructure that eliminates the need for handwritten documentation of care.
Equitable	Provide care that does not vary in quality because of personal characteristics such as gender, ethnicity, geographic location and socio-economic status.	• Align payment policies with quality improvement. • Prepare the workforce to understand and implement quality improvement aims.

From Committee on Quality Health Care in America and Institute of Medicine: *Crossing the quality chasm: a new health system for the 21st century*. Washington, DC, 2001, National Academy Press; National Academy of Sciences: *Crossing the quality chasm: a new health system for the 21st century executive summary*, 2003. Available at http://www.nap.edu. Accessed October 8, 2011.

projections, it is clear that an essential component of contemporary healthcare delivery is improving the safety and quality of healthcare for patients of all ages.

To be successful, improvement efforts must be evidence based. To build an evidence-based foundation, the healthcare improvement movement uses clinical outcome research to identify practices that promote positive patient outcomes. To effectively implement best practices, the discipline adopts improvement theories and methods from businesses such as the automotive, nuclear energy, and aviation industries. Refer to the Chapter 22 Supplement on the Evolve Website for a history of quality improvement.

Human Error

Refer to the Chapter 22 Supplement on the Evolve Website for a history of the industry-based theories of human error. Error theorists recommend a systems approach to improving workplace performance. Extrapolated from successful programs in the nuclear power and aviation industries, a systems approach to preventing human error starts with the notion that people are intrinsically fallible. In addition, it encourages error-proofing the systems in which people work. In a systems approach to error-proofing, layers of defensive interventions that respond to failure-prone human behaviors are used to prevent or trap errors before they cause harm. Often referred to as the *Swiss Cheese Model* (Fig. 22-1), Reason's system theory[79] illustrates that despite layers of defense, it is possible for holes in the safeguards to align in such a way that an error passes through the system. The model proposes that to be maximally effective, multiple defensive layers are necessary to reduce the likelihood that the holes will align and allow the system to fail. In environments such as critical care units, layers of defense are often technologic, such as redundant monitor alarms that sound at the bedside and at a central monitoring station and may also alert staff via a visual cue, such as a flashing light.[79]

Reason notes that errors in systems are caused by either "active failures" or "latent conditions."[79] In healthcare, an active failure is an unsafe act performed by a professional who is in direct contact with a patient. A latent condition is a flaw in the design of the care delivery system and its layers of defense. In keeping with the Swiss Cheese Model, patient safety is promoted by barriers to both the active failures of professionals and the latent conditions of a system. Successful error prevention only adds defensive layers and minimizes the number of potential failures that exist in the system. A common approach to prospectively analyzing a system for potential failures is failure mode effect analysis (FMEA). Root cause analysis (RCA) is a technique for assigning a cause to errors that have actually occurred. The methodologies for FMEA and RCA are described later in this chapter. Such preoccupation with errors, their cause, and their prevention is a key characteristic of safe and high reliability industries.[79]

High Reliability Organizations

Reliability is the rate at which a system produces a desired effect without failure.[80] High reliability organizations perform well in hazardous situations that depend on technology and human interactions.[114] (Refer to the Chapter 22 Supplement on the Evolve Website for information about the study of nuclear power and aviation accidents.) By understanding the interplay between the technical and human causes of accidents, the nuclear power and aviation industries have significantly improved the safety of their practices and are now considered high reliability organizations. Regardless of the industry, all high reliability organizations share the following characteristics:

- Preoccupation with failure
- Commitment to resilience
- Deference to expertise rather than status
- Attention to process and systems
- Reluctance to simplify[114]

Box 22-1 lists the characteristics of high reliability organizations. In addition to a high rate of positive patient outcomes and a low rate of error and complications, evidence of reliability in a healthcare organization includes continual learning from the analysis of potential system flaws and actual

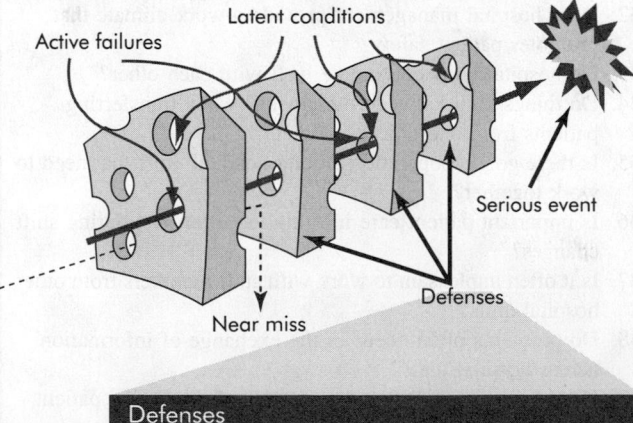

FIG. 22-1 The Swiss Cheese Model of Errors: holes in layers of defense allow errors to pass through a system. (Adapted from Reason JT: *Human error*, New York, 1991, Cambridge University Press.)

Box 22-1 **Characteristics of High Reliability Organizations**

Preoccupation with Failure
- Proactive surveillance for potential failures (failure mode effects analysis)
- Immediate investigation of actual failures (root cause analysis)
- Performance status is transparent to employees and the public

Commitment to Resilience
- Ability to learn from experience and constantly improve

Deference to Expertise
- Flat organizational hierarchy
- Ability of staff of any level to raise concerns or make recommendations
- Willingness to shift decision making from executives to clinical experts

Sensitivity to Operations and Attention to Process and Systems
- Focus on error-proofing the systems and process in which people work
- Nonpunitive, system-focused approaches to failure management

Reluctance to Simplify
- Maintenance of critical steps in a process at all times
- No cuts in steps to save time or money

adverse events, the ability of staff at any level to raise concerns and make decisions that are within the scope of their expertise, standardization of processes, and leadership support for safety practices.[16,60,77]

Culture of Safety

The ability of a healthcare system to be highly reliable hinges on its underlying organizational culture and leadership support for a culture of safety. To fully support a culture of safety, leadership must prioritize and build consensus on the importance of safety and quality improvement goals and must remove barriers and conflicts of interest to achieving these goals. Leadership can also promote a culture of safety by using nonpunitive approaches to investigating errors and by promoting transparency for the purpose of learning from adverse events.[37,92] Evidence that a culture of safety exists in an organization includes sufficient staff and resources, a flat organizational hierarchy, open dialogue about problems

without fear of repercussion, clear lines of communication and effective intradisciplinary and interdisciplinary teamwork.[63,72] The Agency for Healthcare Research and Quality provides a survey that can be used to assess the culture of safety in a hospital[3] (Box 22-2).

Crew Resource Management

Effective teamwork and communication are key features of the safety culture in high reliability organizations. Initially developed by the National Aeronautics and Space Administration Aerospace Human Factors Research Division to train flight crews, crew resource management (CRM), is essential for the effective functioning of multidisciplinary healthcare teams (Box 22-3). CRM includes team training via simulations and interactive group briefings that focus on the development of behaviors critical to decision making and performance in high-risk and high-stress environments that depend on technology, process, and interpersonal communication.[72] The

---

Box 22-2 Agency for Healthcare Research and Quality Hospital Survey Questions on Patient Safety Culture

1. Do people support one another in this unit?
2. Do we have sufficient staff to handle the workload?
3. When a lot of work needs to be done quickly, do we work together as a team to get the work done?
4. Do people treat each other with respect?
5. Do staff members in this unit work longer hours than is best for patient care?
6. Are we are actively doing things to improve patient safety?
7. Do we use more agency or temporary staff than is best for patient care?
8. Do staff believe that their mistakes are held against them?
9. Do mistakes lead to positive changes here?
10. Is it just by chance that more serious mistakes don't happen around here?
11. When one area in this unit gets really busy, do others help out?
12. When an event is reported, does it seem as though the person is being written up, not the problem?
13. After we make changes to improve patient safety, do we evaluate their effectiveness?
14. Do we work in "crisis mode" trying to do too much, too quickly?
15. Is patient safety ever sacrificed to get more work done?
16. Do staff members worry that mistakes they make are kept in their personnel file?
17. Do we have patient safety problems in this unit?
18. Are our procedures and systems good at preventing errors?
19. Does my supervisor or manager say a good word when they see a job done according to established patient safety procedures?
20. Does my supervisor or manager seriously consider staff suggestions for improving patient safety?
21. Whenever pressure builds, does my supervisor or manager wants us to work faster, even if it means taking shortcuts?
22. Does my supervisor or manager overlook patient safety problems that happen repeatedly?

23. Are we are given feedback about changes put into place based on event reports?
24. Will staff members freely speak up if they see something that may negatively affect patient care?
25. Are we are informed about errors that happen in this unit?
26. Do staff members feel free to question the decisions or actions of those with more authority?
27. Do staff members discuss ways to prevent errors from happening again?
28. Are staff members afraid to ask questions when something does not seem right?
29. When a mistake is made, but is caught and corrected before affecting the patient, how often is this reported?
30. When a mistake is made, but has no potential to harm the patient, how often is this reported?
31. When a mistake is made that could harm the patient, but does not, how often is this reported?
32. Does hospital management provide a work climate that promotes patient safety?
33. Do hospital units coordinate well with each other?
34. Do things "fall between the cracks" when transferring patients from one unit to another?
35. Is there good cooperation among hospital units that need to work together?
36. Is important patient care information often lost during shift changes?
37. Is it often unpleasant to work with staff members from other hospital units?
38. Do problems often occur in the exchange of information across hospital units?
39. Do the actions of hospital management show that patient safety is a top priority?
40. Does hospital management seem interested in patient safety only after an adverse event happens?
41. Do hospital units work well together to provide the best care for patients?
42. Are shift changes problematic for patients in this hospital?

Adapted from *Patient Safety culture surveys*, Rockville, MD, 2009, Agency for Healthcare Research and Quality. Available at http://www.ahrq.gov/qual/patientsafetyculture/. Accessed October 1, 2009.

ultimate goal of CRM is a "shared mental model" that aligns all team members to the goals and the strategies for any team activity.[96] Behaviors taught to team members via CRM include:

- Conducting structured inquiries and briefings
- Assertion
- Workload distribution and delegation
- Conflict resolution

In addition to teaching these core behaviors, CRM provides team members with the opportunity to develop technical proficiency and to practice avoiding and trapping errors and mitigating their consequences, and it helps participants appreciate the effects of stress, fatigue, and work overload on performance. Serial performance appraisal of team members is also an important component of CRM programs.[72,96]

Healthcare team training programs have gained acceptance over the past 10 years, and performance of labor and delivery, surgical, and anesthesia teams have demonstrated the positive effects of CRM.[30,59,69] The Joint Commission concluded that communication failures contribute to more than half of all errors.[40] In response, the Joint Commission and other patient safety interest groups have mandated the use of the structured

---

Box 22-3 — Crew Resource Management: Core Components of Teamwork Training

Situational Awareness
- Development of a shared mental model of the goals and strategies for achieving the goals of an activity

Problem Identification and Communication
- Use of structured communication methods to effectively communicate critical information

Decision Making
- Generation of solutions through anticipation of events, actions and their consequences via open dialogue

Workload Distribution
- Thoughtful delegation of tasks to avoid overloading any one team member

Time and Resource Management
- Appropriate use of team members' skill and knowledge with sensitivity to the timing of actions

Conflict Resolution
- Building consensus through active listening and mutual respect among team members and continued commitment to the shared goals

Proficiency
- Reinforcing the knowledge and psychomotor skills needed to make decisions and perform tasks and to avoid and trap errors

Performance Appraisal
- Serial, nonpunitive evaluation of the technical and behavioral competence of all team members with the intent of building capability

---

inquiries and briefings that are central to CRM. Examples of such mandated CRM methods include the performance of "universal protocol" or "time-out" to confirm the correct patient, procedure, and site before invasive interventions, and the use of standardized templates or scripts for hand-off communication between caregivers.[12,40,41,70,84,95]

An appreciation for the importance of CRM has also expanded the use of simulation in healthcare. In critical care settings, the tradition of simulating resuscitations has taken new direction and is now used to teach delegation and communication skills and to reinforce clinical decision-making algorithms and procedural techniques.[29,69] Simulation, which was once a tool reserved for advanced life support and crisis resource management training (such as learning to manage a difficult airway), can be used to develop virtually any aspect of critical care team performance, including noncrisis activities such as daily rounds.[40,69]

HEALTHCARE IMPROVEMENT METHODOLOGY

Model for Improvement

Theories of quality improvement and human error provide a foundation for programs in patient safety and quality improvement, but healthcare teams also need practical methods for orchestrating improvement initiatives. Developed by Associates in Process Improvement, the Model for Improvement (Fig. 22-2) is widely considered an appropriate quality improvement method for healthcare.[104] The Model for Improvement is a two-step process consisting of (1) answering questions to define the improvement opportunity and (2) conducting plan-do-study-act (PDSA) cycles to test interventions that are hoped to improve performance.[24,44,54,104]

To successfully improve a process, it is necessary to define the problems associated with the current state, describe the

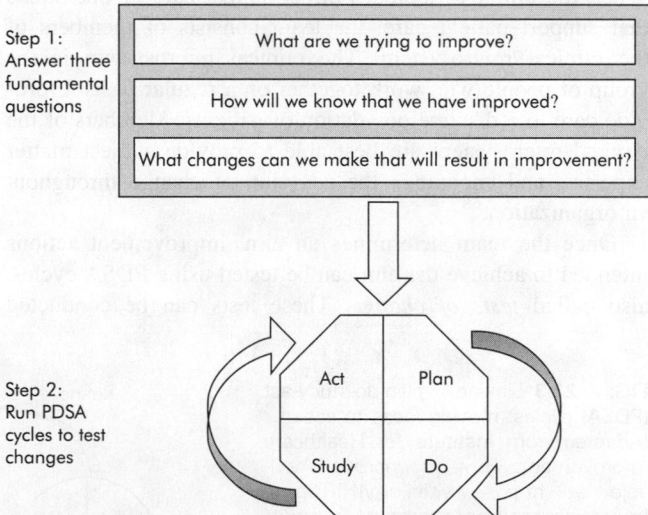

FIG. 22-2 The model for improvement. (Adapted from Institute for Healthcare Improvement: *How to improve.* Available at http://www.ihi.org/IHI/Topics/Improvement/ImprovementMethods/HowToImprove. Accessed April 25, 2008; Langley GJ, et al: *The improvement guide: a practical approach to enhancing organizational performance*, San Francisco, 1996, Jossey-Bass.)

ideal future state, and assign interventions (called *improvement actions* or *changes*) to produce the ideal future state. To identify these elements of an improvement effort, the first step of the Model for Improvement requires answering the following questions:

- What are we trying to improve?
- How will we know that a change is an improvement?
- What changes can we make that will result in improvement?

Answering these three fundamental questions leads to the development of an aim for the initiative. The aim of an improvement initiative must be time specific and measurable, and it must articulate the specific population and scope that will be affected by the effort. An example of a quality improvement aim is: central line-related blood stream infections in patients receiving care in the pediatric critical care unit will be reduced to one infection per 1000 line days (or fewer) within 6 months.

Although the need for improvement may come from external sources such as hospital administration or a regulatory agency, a team of healthcare providers who work within the targeted process or system should be assembled to create the aim, identify improvement actions, and then perform the improvement effort. To comprehensively represent all stakeholders, a typical quality improvement team is composed of the following:

- Sponsors and champions: support and remove barriers to improvement and promote a culture of safety; they are often members of upper management or executive administrators
- Leaders: manage the team and the project and organize the work
- Members: determine the course or action and perform improvement actions or changes; they are subject matter experts
- Facilitators: help the team work together effectively; they are external to the issue

When the initiative includes direct patient care or operations that support patient care, the team consists of members of the clinical microsystem. The clinical microsystem is the group of people who work together on a regular basis to provide care to a discrete population of patients. Members of the clinical microsystem are best able to provide subject matter expertise and encourage the adoption of change throughout an organization.[68]

Once the team determines an aim, improvement actions intended to achieve the aim can be tested using PDSA cycles, also called *tests of change*. These tests can be conducted repeatedly to refine an improvement action. A single PDSA cycle consists of:

- Planning the improvement action, including the measures and data collection process
- Doing or performing the improvement action, as a test or small scale trial, and collecting performance data
- Studying the outcome of the test and using the data to uncover what did and did not work
- Acting on the information learned from the test to plan next steps

When an improvement effort requires multiple improvement interventions, each intervention can be tested via a separate PDSA cycle. All the related PDSA cycles are then linked to create a package of interventions that have been proven to foster improvement (Fig. 22-3). Effective improvement actions can then be spread beyond the initial test setting and population. The use of PDSA cycles to test and refine improvement actions can help to overcome an organization's natural resistance to change.[24,44,54,105]

Performance Measurement

Measures must be developed to identify opportunities for improvement, to test changes, and to continually monitor an organization's performance. A measure is a quantitative indicator of performance. There are three types of improvement measures:

- Outcome measures: measure the end result, overall performance, or outcome of an improvement effort
- Process measures: measure the rate of use and performance of a process within a comprehensive improvement effort
- Balancing measures: measure the consequences of the planned changes associated with the improvement effort[44,54,104]

The goal of reducing the incidence of central line-associated blood stream infections can be used to illustrate the three types of performance measures. The following are sample measures for a central line-associated blood stream infection improvement project:

- The outcome measure is the rate of infection.
- The process measures are the rates of use of recommended practices, such as rate of compliance with conducting and documenting a daily review for continued line necessity. An additional related process measure may also be the time to remove central lines.
- Assuming that the peripheral venous access would be used more often if central lines are removed quickly as a result of daily line necessity reviews, an appropriate balancing measure for the project is the rate of peripheral line complications, such as infiltration.

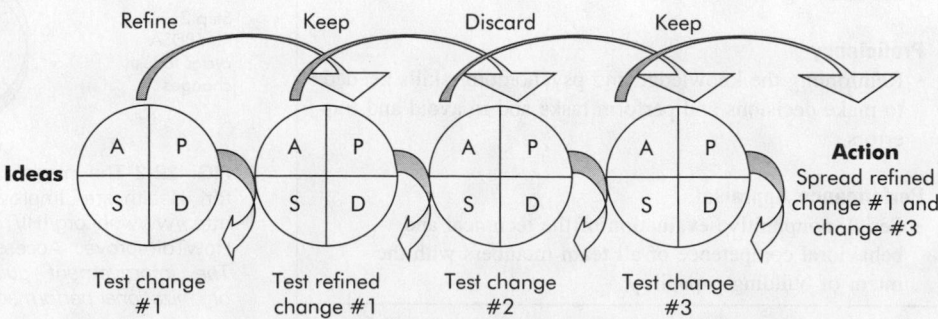

FIG. 22-3 Linking plan-do-study-act (PDSA) cycles: moving ideas to action. (Adapted from Institute for Healthcare Improvement: *How to improve.* Available at http://www.ihi.org/IHI/Topics/Improvement/ImprovementMethods/HowToImprove. Accessed April 25, 2008; Langley GJ, et al: *The improvement guide: a practical approach to enhancing organizational performance,* San Francisco, 1996, Jossey-Bass.)

To analyze performance patterns represented by data, it is helpful to graphically display and apply statistics to the data. Run charts and control charts, which plot data over time, are two essential improvement tools. Refer to Evolve Figs. 22-1 and 22-2 in the Chapter 22 Supplement on the Evolve Website for examples of such charts.

Failure Mode and Effects Analysis

Before the Model for Improvement can be used to manage performance, opportunities for improvement must be identified. As mentioned earlier, high reliability organizations are preoccupied with failure and proactively analyze processes and systems for potential failures, even before failures occur. An FMEA is a tool for prospective analysis of healthcare system vulnerabilities, called *failure modes*. Steps to a healthcare FMEA:

1. Graphically depict a process using a flow diagram (e.g., see Evolve Fig. 22-3 in the Chapter 22 Supplement on the Evolve Website).
2. Analyze each step in the process for potential failure modes, the causes of the failure modes and their effects.
3. Assign a risk priority number (RPN) to each failure mode, based on its likelihood to occur, ability to be detected and trapped before an adverse event results, and the severity of the consequences if it does cause an adverse event.
4. Identify and prioritize the failure modes based on their RPN.
5. Propose actions to prevent the failure modes.
6. Implement the actions to prevent the failure modes (the Model for Improvement may be used to do so).

Table 22-3 provides a sample documentation grid and RPN calculation tool for conducting an FMEA. An FMEA can be used to identify new improvement projects or as a tool to further understand special cause variation demonstrated in the data generated by an existing improvement project. An improvement team that includes all key stakeholders, including members of the clinical microsystem, should be used to conduct FMEAs.[43]

The Institute for Safe Medication Practices has strongly encouraged the use of FMEA, and it has been shown to improve medication safety.[81,91,115] In response to the overwhelming evidence that the technique contributes to patient safety, the Joint Commission mandates that healthcare organizations perform at least one FMEA per year.[33]

Incident Reporting

Healthcare organizations should use tools, such as FMEA, to anticipate and prevent failures before they occur. However when a failure takes place, incident reporting becomes central to the safety and quality improvement effort. Colonel John C. Flanagan, the Director of the Division of Aviation Psychology, developed the critical incident technique for military training in 1954. The critical incident technique was a structured incident reporting process that included the use of personnel directly involved in a failed process to create, at the time of discovery, a qualitative narrative of the event. Flanagan's work also established common terminology for incident reporting that has been adapted for use in healthcare (Table 22-4).[28,51,109] Healthcare incident reporting is the

Table 22-4 Healthcare Incident Definitions

Term	Definition
Adverse event	An injury that was caused by medical management rather than by a patient's underlying disease
Medical error	The failure of a planned action to be completed as intended or to achieve its intended goal or the use of the wrong action to achieve a goal
Serious error	An error that causes permanent injury or transient but potentially life-threatening harm
Minor error	An error that causes harm that is neither permanent nor potentially life threatening
Near miss	An error that could have caused harm, but did not because of timely intervention or chance
Sentinel event	An unexpected occurrence involving death or serious physical or psychological injury, or the risk thereof

Adapted from Garbutt J, et al: Reporting and disclosing medical errors: pediatricians' attitudes and behaviors. *Arch Pediatr Adolesc Med* 161:179-185, 2007; Joint Commission: *Sentinel events.* Available at http://www.jointcommission.org/SentinelEvents. Accessed April 25, 2008; Kohn KT, Corrigan JM, Donaldson MS: *To err is human: building a safer healthcare system.* Washington, DC, 1999, National Academy Press.

Table 22-3 Sample Failure Modes and Effects Analysis Tool

Step in the Process	Failure Mode	Failure Causes	Failure Effects	Likelihood of Occurrence	Likelihood of Detection	Severity	Risk Priority Number	Actions to Prevent Failure
Identified on the flow diagram	What can go wrong during this step?	Why does this failure happen?	What would be the outcome of this failure?	Scale 1-10 10 = very likely to occur	Scale 1-10 10 = very unlikely to detect	Scale 1-10 10 = most severe effect	RPN*	
1								
2								
3								
4								
5								

Adapted from Institute for Healthcare Improvement: *Failure modes and effects analysis tool*, 2004, Institute for Healthcare Improvement. Available at http://www.ihi.org/ihi/workspace/tools/fmea. Accessed April 25, 2008.
*RPN = Likelihood of occurrence × Likelihood of detection × Severity

process by which a clinician documents adverse events, medical errors, and near-miss events, including deviations from standard procedures that could have resulted in an adverse event or error, in real time and at the point of care. Incident reports may also require clinicians to assign a perceived cause and severity grade to the event.[31,42,55,109]

Since 1975, the U.S. Food and Drug Administration has mandated the reporting of blood transfusion reactions, and in 1995 the Joint Commission mandated reporting of all other adverse events, errors, and near misses as part of the Sentinel Event Policy. The hallmark IOM report *To Err is Human* called for the enhancement of voluntary and mandatory incident reporting systems in individual organizations and for public disclosure. Furthermore, and as noted previously, documenting incidents is an important characteristic of High Reliability Organizations.[55,109] Despite a keen focus on incident reporting, however, there are many barriers to the use of incident reports by healthcare providers.[31,97] In a 2004 survey by Taylor et al,[97] 34% of pediatricians and pediatric nurses surveyed indicated that they reported fewer than 20% of their own medical errors, and approximately 33% of those surveyed indicated that they reported fewer than 40% of the errors committed by their colleagues. Other studies have indicated incident reporting rates as low as 10%.[51] Barriers to incident reporting can be inadequacies of reporting systems, organizational culture, or the attitudes or knowledge deficits of healthcare professionals (see Barriers to Incident Reporting in the Chapter 22 Supplement on the Evolve Website for examples).

Despite the barriers to incident reporting, pediatric healthcare providers indicate a willingness to report if and when appropriate and an interest in understanding incidents to improve care.[31] Facilitating the use of incident reports is a key improvement effort of all hospitals. Effective strategies to improve incident reporting rates include:

- Dedicate the reporting system for the sole purpose of capturing clinical incidents.
- Identify the incident reporting system as a *safety reporting system* to emphasize its ultimate purpose.
- Allow anonymous reporting.
- Include cues for clinicians about what constitutes an incident and categories of incidents on the reporting tool.
- Make the incident reporting widely accessible in the clinical environment.
- Make a secure mechanism for submitting incident reports widely accessible in the clinical environment.
- Automate the reporting system.
- Apply a consistently nonpunitive response to reported incidents and positive recognition of clinicians who report.
- Continually provide feedback to clinicians about the improvement actions taken in response to reported incidents and trends in incidents.[42,98,100]

All hospitals should implement a system that provides timely information to front-line clinical leadership about the occurrence of and trends in incidents. Electronic incident reporting systems help to accomplish this goal.[98,100] Continual feedback to clinicians about the improvement actions taken in response to incident reports is also essential to increasing reporting rates and to building a culture of transparency and learning. Often a reported event will undergo an extensive, systematic

evaluation, such as an RCA, that will generate a new improvement initiative for the clinical microsystem.

Root Cause Analysis

Performing an RCA of actual adverse patient events, like FMEA and incident reporting, is a characteristic of a high reliability organization and is mandated by the Joint Commission, as well as by many state regulated incident reporting programs. Reporting programs, which are often public, typically require an RCA of a "sentinel event" or an "unexpected occurrence involving death or serious physical or psychological injury, or the risk thereof."[46] The goal of an RCA is to identify the factors that contributed to an adverse patient event in order to safeguard the system from the same event occurring again. Although an RCA may identify multiple system vulnerabilities, the emphasis of the exercise is to assign and understand the causes of the failure that resulted in death or serious morbidity or the potential for such.[26] Steps for conducting an RCA include:

1. Describe the incident, include the use of a flow-diagram to illustrate the processes in which the incident occurred.
2. Compare the steps of the process that resulted in the event to the usual process used to carry out the activity.
3. Identify the human factor and other factors that contributed to the event (see Box 22-4 for categories of causes of failures and rules for assigning cause; also see Evolve Fig. 22-4 in the Chapter 22 Supplement on the Evolve Website).
4. Propose improvements to the process or system that will prevent the event from recurring.
5. Implement the actions to prevent the event from recurring; the Model for Improvement may be used.[9,15,26,106]

To be effective, the approach to conducting an RCA should be consistent from one event to the next. RCA should be conducted by representatives of all stakeholders in the system in which an event occurred, including members of the

---

Box 22-4	**Root Cause Analysis: Assigning Cause to Adverse Patient Events to Improve Systems**

Categories of Causes for Adverse Patient Events
- Human Factors
  - Communication
  - Training
  - Fatigue
  - Scheduling
- Environment and Equipment
- Policies and Procedures
- Failure or Absence of Barriers

Rules for Assigning Cause
- Clearly show the cause-and-effect relationship
- Do not assign a quality or use a negative descriptor when identifying a cause (e.g., do not use inadequate communication or poorly written policy)
- Identify a preceding cause for each human error
- Identify a preceding cause for each procedural deviation
- Assign failure to act only when there was a preexisting duty to act

Adapted from the Veterans Administration National Center for Patient Safety: *Root cause analysis.* Available at http://www.va.gov/NCPS/CogAids/Triage/index.html?8. Accessed April 25, 2008.

clinical microsystem. To provide an objective analysis of the event, one or more members of the organization who sit outside the system under examination may also be included. In addition, a neutral facilitator should assist with the organization of the RCA and moderate related discussions and debates.[9,15,107]

OPPORTUNITIES FOR IMPROVEMENT IN PEDIATRIC CRITICAL CARE

Environment of Care

Pediatric critical care is highly vulnerable to errors and adverse patient events.[61,85] The needs of critically ill children are complex and heterogeneous, the systems for providing care to critically ill children are tightly coupled, and the work of critical care providers is psychologically stressful and physically exhausting. Accidents related to technology, including dislodgement of invasive catheters and airways and ineffective use of monitoring alarms by staff, are prevalent in critical care, and gaps in care continuity and cognitive biases are particularly problematic when fast-paced decision making is needed.[61,102,103] Elements of the critical care physical environment, such as open layouts and excessive noise, produce interruptions and distractions during care delivery. These elements are also known to impede patient safety in pediatric critical care units.[61] In a study that applied an aviation "sterile cockpit" approach to critical operations, medication errors were reduced when interruptions experienced by the nurse during medication administration were minimized.[61,74] Furthermore, the general effects of fatigue on clinician performance are applicable, if not amplified, in pediatric critical care, where on-call physicians have little time to sleep and nurses frequently work extended shifts. The documented effects of sleep deprivation include a 36% increase in medication and diagnostic errors and a 30% increase in surgical procedure times.[53,61] Similarly, research has shown that nurses are twofold to threefold more likely to make an error after working more than 12.5 consecutive hours.[61,82,87] A 2006 study conducted by the American Association of Critical-Care Nurses reported that 44% of critical care nurses are routinely scheduled to work shifts longer than 12.5 hours and that during a 1-month period, only 13% of nurses left work at the end of their assigned shift and 61% worked 10 or more overtime shifts.[61,87] The ideal hospital environment culture of safety includes leadership support, teamwork, learning from mistakes, work hour restrictions, work load distribution, appropriate physical space, and decision support aids that are readily available at the point of care.[37,73]

Improving the hospital work environment is clearly pertinent to nursing. Leape et al[56] reported that as many as 86% of harmful errors are intercepted by nurses before they reach patients. Several studies have shown that when patient-to-nurse ratios increase and when nurses spend less time with patients, there is an increase in complications such as infection, gastrointestinal bleeding, and cardiac arrest, as well as extended length of hospital stay.[52,67,78] Aiken et al[4,5] have published hallmark research that correlates low nursing education level and high patient-to-nurse ratio with increased patient mortality rates and increased failure to rescue patients

who are experiencing physiologic instability resulting from an unexpected complication. Aiken et al estimated that for every patient receiving care beyond an assignment of four patients there is a 7% increase in the risk of a patient dying within 30 days after discharge.[5] These statistics are particularly daunting in light of the estimated 29% to 40% nursing shortages predicted by the year 2020.[37]

In response to evidence that nursing care plays a pivotal role in patients' outcomes, the IOM Committee for the Work Environment of Nurses and Patient Safety published a manual titled *Keeping Patients Safe: Transforming the Work Environments of Nurses*. The manual, intended to be a companion to the IOM report *To Err is Human*, provides a blueprint for the ideal work environment for nurses.[73] The blueprint builds on research that demonstrates the effects of nursing education, management, staffing, work hours and processes, and the ergonomics of the work space. In addition, the blueprint links the development of a safe work environment with the evolution of a learning organization—that is, an organization that is willing to adapt over time to best meet the needs of its clients.[37,38,73] The requirements set forth by the IOM for a safe and effective work environment for nurses include an organizational commitment to patient safety, effective and evidence-based management and leadership, interdisciplinary collaboration, adequate staffing and work hour restrictions, workplace design that facilitates safe care, decision support aids at the point of care, and opportunities for ongoing learning.

Failure to Rescue

The ultimate outcome of a healthy work environment is the prevention of failure-to-rescue events. Failure to rescue is any event during which a clinician is unable, because of a complication of care or a condition that was not present on admission, to save a hospitalized patient's life.[4] To recognize and intervene early when a life-threatening complication occurs, nurses use surveillance such as clinical assessment for signs and symptoms of physiologic instability, and environmental safety checks, such as verifying the settings of monitor alarms.[4] A workforce and work environment that support surveillance, recognition, and early intervention by nurses are the backbone for rapid response teams (RRTs). RRTs are hospital-based teams of critical care providers who are available to assess, provide consultation, and assist with the care of a patient whose status is deteriorating prior to the need for resuscitation for cardiopulmonary arrest.[116] RRTs have been successfully implemented in pediatric hospitals and have been shown to reduce the rate of cardiopulmonary arrests that occur outside of critical care units and reduce patient mortality. The use of RRTs is strongly encouraged by the Joint Commission and other patient safety interest groups.[48,88,90,116]

Role for Information Technology

There is great promise that evolving information technology will enable safe environments of care. Electronic health record (EHR) and computerized provider order entry (CPOE) systems offer benefits to clinicians, including expanded access to patients' health information, particularly during and after transitions of care, and decision support such as drug-allergy interaction checking and dose calculation.[99,112] By offering identification and tracking applications, electronic information systems can also enhance patient identification and patient flow.[76] Furthermore, electronic capture of clinical information facilitates data mining for clinical research and measurement of performance. The IOM, the Joint Commission, the Center for Medicare and Medicaid Services, the Institute for Safe Medication Practices (ISMP), public interest groups, and many private insurers include electronic information systems in their healthcare improvement requirements and pay-for-performance plans.[6,34]

It is important to note that there are risks associated with EHR and CPOE systems. Because EHR and CPOE systems require changes in routine clinical operations and processes, it will be important to verify that clinical workflow is safe and effective after implementation. Other risks include lack of information security, alert fatigue, downtime, inefficiency,

and the evolution of new types of medical errors, such as keystroke mistakes.[11,110,112]

In addition to the generic risks of clinical information systems, there is national concern that commercially available EHR and CPOE systems do not accommodate the unique needs of pediatric healthcare.[6,89,93,110,112] The Joint Commission mandated that information system vendors develop functionality to help prevent pediatric medication errors,[46,47] and the American Academy of Pediatrics has developed position statements on pediatric requirements for clinical information technology.[6,93] Table 22-5 outlines the pediatric-specific requirements for maximal safety and effectiveness of EHR and CPOE systems.

Additional technologies, such as bar code identification systems and programmable infusion pumps, also have the potential to improve patient safety in pediatric critical care units. Despite somewhat conflicting evidence in the literature, it appears that bar code technology reduces medication

Table 22-5 Requirements for Safe and Effective Pediatric Electronic Information Systems

Requirement	Electronic Health Record	Computerized Provider Order Entry and Prescribing
Immunizations	Ability to record immunization data and link to state immunization registries Ability to print an immunization record for families	Immunization decision support with reminders regarding immunization schedules and electronic entry of immunization orders
Growth documentation and tracking	Automated growth charts with alerts when children fall outside of growth parameters for age, including gestational and adjusted age for premature infants Ability to document gestational age Accommodation of normative values that change specific to the child's age (e.g., vital sign norms)	Weight displays on all order screens Reminders to document a patient's weight Stopping functions that prevent providers from ordering medications without a weight entry in the system
Medication management	Presence of medication lists and the ability to view medication history and a medication administration record Electronic medication administration record with decision support prompts for nurses	Dosing by body weight or body mass index Dose range checking Rounding to safe and convenient doses Age-based (including gestational age) dosing decision support Indication-based dosing decision support Drug allergy checking, drug-drug interaction checking, drug-food interaction checking, and duplicate medication alerts
Patient identification	Availability of two patient identifiers on all screens and printed reports Mechanism for newborn infant identification before a name or Social Security number has been assigned Ability to store prenatal data for an identified fetus and connect this data with the patient after birth, without relying on maternal identifiers Ability to change an infant's name Ability to assign unknown or ambiguous sex	Availability of two patient identifiers on all order screens and printed copies of orders
Privacy	Ability to flag and limit access to protected information, including adolescent health issues as dictated by state laws Ability to accurately and confidentially identify foster and custodial care	Ability to flag and limit access to orders reflecting protected information, including adolescent health issues as dictated by state laws (e.g., pregnancy test)

Adapted from American Academy of Pediatrics Council on Clinical Information Technology, Gerstle RS: Electronic prescribing systems in pediatrics: the rationale and functionality requirements. *Pediatrics* 119:1229-1231, 2007; Joint Commission: Preventing pediatric medication errors. *Sentinel Event Alert, 39,* April 2008. Available at http://www.jointcommission.org/SentinelEvents/SentinelEventAlert/sea_39.htm. Accessed April 25, 2008; Spooner SA: Council on Clinical Information Technology, American Academy of Pediatrics. Special requirements of electronic health record systems in pediatrics. *Pediatrics* 119:631-637, 2007.

administration and lab labeling errors[20,35,62] and that programmable or "smart" infusion pumps reduce duplicate infusion and infusion rate errors.[71] Additional research is needed to determine the most appropriate uses and the true effects of such technologies.[20,58]

Common Pediatric Critical Care Unit Improvement Opportunities

There are unique impediments to improving patient safety in pediatric critical care. Many of the safety and quality improvement efforts launched by regulatory and public interest groups primarily focus on adult populations and may not match the safety risks specific to critically ill children.[85] In light of the high risk for iatrogenic complications and the special needs of sick children, pediatric nurses and physicians must identify the key safety and quality indicators for pediatric critical care.[85] A number of professional organizations, such as the National Initiative for Children's Health Care Quality (NICHQ), the Child Health Corporation of America (CHCA), and related work groups have been formed to define and prioritize pediatric specific safety and quality initiatives and measures. Box 22-5 lists targeted pediatric safety and quality issues; it can be used by pediatric critical care providers to develop their own unit-specific improvement goals. Medication safety and healthcare-acquired infections are the two most consistent themes of all proposed pediatric safety and quality improvement programs.

Pediatric Medication Errors and Adverse Drug Events

Medication errors and adverse drug events (ADE) are the largest subset of medical errors occurring in hospitals.[36,51] A medication error is an error in drug ordering, transcribing, dispensing, administering, or monitoring. An ADE is an injury from a medication that is either unexpected or caused by inappropriate use of the medication or that results from lack of

---

| Box 22-5 | **Common Opportunities for Clinical Improvement in Pediatric Critical Care** |

- Compliance with hand hygiene
- Medication safety
- High-risk medication management
  - Implementation and enhancement of computerized provider order entry
  - Medication reconciliation
- Prevention of healthcare-acquired infections
  - Central line-associated blood stream infections
  - Ventilator associated pneumonia
  - Surgical site infection
  - Surviving severe sepsis
- Prevention of falls
- Prevention of skin breakdown
- Venous thromboembolism prophylaxis
- Unplanned readmission rates
- Patient flow efficiency (admission through discharge)
- Pain assessment
- Implementation of rapid response teams
- Implementation and enhancement of electronic health records
- Asthma care planning across the continuum of care

---

administration of a necessary medication. A potential ADE is an error that had the potential to result in significant injury, but was deflected before drug administration or did not produce the adverse consequence.[8] Children, particularly children younger than 2 years, are up to threefold more likely than adults to experience a drug error or ADE.[39,49,50,57,113] Approximately 3% of all hospitalized children experience an ADE, and 4% of the occurrences are classified as harmful.[36] As many as 28% of medication errors and ADEs are preventable.[13]

There are many reasons why children experience more drug errors and ADEs than adults. Children are often incapable of questioning the appropriateness of a medication. In addition, calculations of drug dose are complicated by weight- or body surface area-based doses and by complex or incomplete information about drug pharmacokinetics and pharmacodynamics in children.[36,39,49,50] The rate of pediatric medication errors and ADEs increases with extended length of stay, and it is higher in units that care for a complex mix of patients and in critical care units.[36,39,49] The drugs most commonly associated with pediatric medication errors and ADEs are analgesics, sedatives, anticoagulants, antimicrobials, antineoplastic agents, corticosteroids, insulin, and vasoactive drugs. In addition, errors are commonly made with intravenous fluid and electrolyte therapy.[36,39,49] For additional information about pharmacokinetics and drug monitoring in children, see Chapter 4.

In general, medication errors and ADEs are more frequently associated with intravenous drugs than with other routes of administration.[36] More than 75% of pediatric medication errors and ADEs are associated with prescribing, and improper dose is reported as the most common type of prescribing error.[36,39,49] Approximately 4% of dose prescribing errors are attributed to a missing or inaccurate patient weight.[49]

The second most common pediatric ADE is failure to administer a necessary medication, with antimicrobial agents being the drugs most frequently omitted.[36] Omissions of medication are often associated with shift changes and transfers between units,[36] and as many as 30% of all medication plans are incomplete or inaccurate at the time of discharge.[105] Frequent failures in medication management during periods of patient transition have led to the regulatory mandate for medication reconciliation, in which planned medications are compared and deliberate actions to continue or discontinue drugs on the list are documented before and after transitioning care.[75,86,105] Additional nursing errors have been reported related to improper infusion rates and errors in pump programming in pediatric critical care units.[36]

In light of the statistics, decreasing the incidence of pediatric medication errors and ADEs is an important safety improvement effort common to all pediatric critical care units. Strategies for improvement include:

- Using CPOE and electronic medication administration records[32,110,112] (see Chapter 23)
- Providing immediate access to patient medical history, allergies, and relevant laboratory data at the time of medication order entry and administration
- Having a unit-based pharmacist actively participate in the care of patients

- Restricting access to drugs until orders are checked and profiled by pharmacists
- Reconciling medications when patients transition between settings
- Standardizing drug concentrations, particularly for continuous medication infusions
- Using unit-dosed dispensing
- Storing medications in patient-specific storage bins
- Identifying and specially managing high-risk medications
- Removing concentrated electrolytes from nursing units
- Using two patient identifiers and potential bar-code identification before every drug administration
- Prohibiting the use of error-prone medication abbreviations
- Prohibiting the use of trailing zeros and encouraging the use of leading zeros
- Using verbal orders for medications only in urgent or emergent situations; when necessary, verbal orders should be written down and read back to the prescribing clinician
- Using tall-man letters to identify look-a-like or sound-a-like medications and separately storing look-a-like or sound-a-like medications
- Implementing vigilant monitoring protocols for patients receiving analgesics and sedatives [13,22,36,83,111–113]

Healthcare-Acquired Infections

Prevention of healthcare-acquired infections is a common focus of safety improvement efforts. The National Nosocomial Infections Surveillance System (NNIS) is a voluntary reporting system that integrates with the CDC to capture data about healthcare-acquired infections in the U.S. Research using NNIS data has shown that bloodstream infections are the most common type of healthcare-acquired infection in children and that 91% of bloodstream infections are associated with central venous catheters.[66,94] Indwelling airways and urinary catheters also contribute to healthcare-acquired infections. Most (95%) healthcare-acquired pneumonia occurs in children who are receiving mechanical ventilation, and 77% of urinary tract infections are associated with indwelling bladder catheters.[66,94,101] NNIS data and related research have also identified the following risk factors for all types of pediatric healthcare-acquired infections:

- Young age, particularly less than 1 year
- Immunosuppression, caused by underlying disease or immunosuppressant drugs
- Chronic disease
- Presence of invasive devices, including central venous catheters, bladder catheters, and endotracheal tubes
- History of antibiotic use
- Medical diagnosis, except for cardiac and neurosurgical diagnoses
- Use of critical care services[17,66,94,101]

Healthcare-acquired infections increase length of stay and contribute significantly to patient morbidity and mortality, and thus are the target of improvement efforts launched by the Joint Commission and the Institute for Health Care Improvement, as well as by the Pediatric Affinity Group, a pediatric critical care consortium sponsored by the NICHQ and CHCA.[94] Collectively these organizations have focused on preventing the two types of infection most pertinent to

pediatric critical care: central line-associated blood stream infections and ventilator-associated pneumonia.[56,94,108]

Preventing Central Line-Associated Blood Stream Infections. Because critically ill children are often dependent on vascular access for monitoring and for fluid, blood product, and medication administration, catheter line-associated blood stream infections are a significant patient safety risk in pediatric critical care units. In pediatric critical care units more than 90% of blood stream infections are associated with central venous catheters; most are caused by skin bacterial flora such as coagulase-negative staphylococcus.[94,101] Mortality from central line-related blood stream infections can be as high as 18%.[10] Substantial reduction in central line-associated blood stream infections is possible through focused quality improvement efforts such as the application of the Institute for Healthcare Improvement's (IHI) Central Line Bundle of recommended practices and the related Pediatric Affinity Group recommended "change package" of interventions proven to reduce blood stream infections.[1,14,108]

Practices to reduce the incidence of central line-associated blood stream infections include:

- Hand hygiene
- Maximal barrier precautions
- Chlorhexidine skin antisepsis
- Optimal catheter site selection
- Daily review of line necessity

The Central Line Bundle recommended by the IHI is described further in Box 22-6.

Ventilator-Associated Pneumonia. Along with central line-associated blood stream infections, the IHI and the NICHQ-CHCA Pediatric Affinity Group identify ventilator-associated pneumonia (VAP) as a critical patient safety improvement effort for pediatric critical care units.[23,94,108] VAP is defined as pneumonia that evolves at least 48 h after endotracheal intubation and the start of mechanical ventilation. Approximately 5.1% of children receiving mechanical ventilation develop VAP.[27] Risk factors for VAP in children include antibiotic administration, underlying chronic condition, gastroesophageal reflux, supine position, presence of a nasogastric tube, immobility, and surgery of the head, neck, or upper abdomen.[23,94] The criteria for diagnosing VAP in children were adapted by Curley et al in 2006 from CDC criteria and include[23]:

- Mechanical ventilation for more than 48 h, fever ($\geq 38°$ C), and leukopenia (< 4000 white blood cells [WBCs] per mm^3) or leukocytosis ($\geq 12,000$ WBCs/mm^3) with no other recognized source
- Any two or more of the following:
  ○ New onset purulent sputum
  ○ New or worsening cough, dyspnea, or tachypnea
  ○ Crackles or bronchial breath sounds
  ○ Worsening gas exchange and two or more serial chest radiographs with at least one of the following findings: new or progressive and persistent infiltrate, consolidation, or cavitation

There are additional customized criteria for children younger than 1 year, between 1 and 12 years old, 13 years or older,

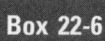

Box 22-6 **Practices to Reduce the Incidence of Central Line-Associated Blood Stream Infections, Adapted from the Institute for Health Care Improvement Central Line Bundle***

Hand Hygiene

As with all healthcare-acquired infection prevention programs, conscious hand hygiene including use of a soap and water or alcohol based hand rub

- Before and after inserting and handling catheter insertion site
- Before and after touching catheter insertion site
- Touch only before antisepsis for placement or with aseptic technique
- Before and after inserting, replacing, accessing, repairing, or dressing a CVC
- When hands are obviously soiled or contaminated
- Between patients
- Before donning gloves and after removing gloves
- After using bathroom

Maximal Barrier Precautions

Use of maximal barrier precautions including use of cap, mask, sterile gown, sterile gloves, and sterile drape

- Use a central line checklist that includes barrier precautions
- Keep equipment, including barriers, stocked in a central line cart that is readily accessible
- Prevent unnecessary interruption of barriers to get supplies
- Create a culture in which clinicians remind each other to maintain precautions

Chlorhexidine Skin Antisepsis for Children Older Than 2 Months

Prepare skin for line insertion with a solution of 2% chlorhexidine, 70% isopropyl alcohol

- When using stick applicator, friction scrub back and forth for 30 seconds
- Allow antiseptic to dry for approximately 2 minutes

Optimal Catheter Site Selection

Select most optimal site for insertion

- In adults the subclavian vein is the preferred site except for patients with high bleeding risk
- In children, when subclavian access is not feasible, the femoral vein is the preferred site
- Avoid using the jugular vein, because it is associated with increased incidence of infection[25]

Daily Review of Line Necessity

- Prompt removal of unnecessary lines
- Incorporate the line review into preexisting multidisciplinary rounds
- Include assessment of line and consideration of removal on a daily goal sheet
- Record time and date of line placement in an accessible place

Adapted from the Institute for Healthcare Improvement: 5 Million lives campaign: how-to guide—prevent central line infections. Copyright 2007, Institute for Healthcare Improvement. Available at: http://www.ihi.org/explore/CentralLineInfection/Pages/default.aspx. Accessed October 8, 2011.[45]
*Note that the Central Line Bundle was developed for adult critical care patients, with supporting evidence from that population.

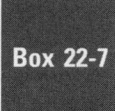

Box 22-7 **Practices to Reduce the Incidence of VAP, Adapted from the Institute for Health Care Improvement VAP Bundle and the CHCA-NICHQ Pediatric Affinity Group *Getting to Zero Campaign***

Bundle

- Head of bed elevated to 35 to 45 degrees
- Daily assessment of extubation readiness
- Daily holiday from sedation
- Peptic ulcer prophylaxis
- Deep vein thrombosis prophylaxis

Additional Care

- Provide oral hygiene (using chlorhexidine if patient is older than 2 months)
- Use in-line suction catheters or single use only open suction catheter systems and store suction devices in a clean environment
- Drain ventilator circuit away from patient every 2-4 h
- Change ventilator circuits and in-line suction catheters only when malfunctioning or visibly soiled
- Perform hand hygiene before and after handling circuit

Adapted from Curley MA, et al: Tailoring the Institute for Health Care Improvement 100,000 Lives Campaign to pediatric settings: the example of ventilator-associated pneumonia. *Pediatr Clin North Am* 53:1231-1251, 2006; Stockwell JA: Nosocomial infections in the pediatric intensive care unit: affecting the impact on safety and outcome. *Pediatr Crit Care Med* 8(Suppl 2): S21-S37, 2007.
CHCA, Child health corporation of America; *NICHQ,* national initiative for children's health care quality; *VAP,* ventilator-associated pneumonia.

and for immunocompromised children.[23] Interventions to prevent VAP have also been extrapolated from adult research and initiatives. They include:

- Elevating the head of the bed to 35 to 45 degrees
- Daily assessment of extubation readiness
- Daily holiday from sedation
- Peptic ulcer prophylaxis
- Venous thromboembolism (deep vein thrombosis) prophylaxis

The effect of daily sedation holidays in children and the appropriateness of venous thromboembolism prophylaxis have not been studied as well in children and should be enacted only after thoughtful consideration and an analysis of the risks and benefits.[23] The IHI and Pediatric Affinity Group recommendations for the prevention of VAP are more fully described in Box 22-7.

CONCLUSION

Errors in healthcare contribute to increased patient morbidity and mortality and increased costs of care. Healthcare organizations must develop systems that ensure the safety and quality of healthcare delivery, and every pediatric critical care nurse should contribute to improving the safety and quality of that care. This chapter and the additional information available in the Chapter 22 Supplement on the Evolve Website provide the tools for establishing programs and processes of quality improvement.

References

1. Aboelela SW, Stone PW, Larson EL: Effectiveness of bundled behavioural interventions to control healthcare-associated infections: a systematic review of the literature. *J Hosp Infect* 66:101–108, 2007.
2. Agency for Healthcare Research and Quality: *National healthcare quality report,* Rockville, MD, 2004, U.S. Department of Health & Human Services.
3. AHRQ Hospital Survey on Patient Safety Culture: Available at http://www.ahrq.gov/qual/hospculture. Accessed on April 25, 2008.
4. Aiken LH, et al: Educational levels of hospital nurses and surgical patient mortality. *J Am Med Assoc* 290:1617–1623, 2003.
5. Aiken LH, et al: Hospital nurse staffing and patient mortality, nurse burnout, and job dissatisfaction. *J Am Med Assoc* 288:1987–1993, 2002.
6. American Academy of Pediatrics Council on Clinical Information Technology, Gerstle RS, Lehmann CU: Electronic prescribing systems in pediatrics: the rationale and functionality requirements. *Pediatrics* 119(6):1229–1231, 2007.
7. American Hospital Association: Chicago, 1999, Hospital statistics.
8. American Society of Health System Pharmacists: Suggested definitions and relationships among medication misadventures, medication errors, adverse drug events, and adverse drug reactions. *Am J Health Syst Pharm* 55(2):165–166, 1998.
9. Apostolakis G, Barach P: Reporting and preventing medical mishaps: safety lessons learned from nuclear power. In Youngberg BJ, Hatlie M, editors: *The patient safety handbook,* ed 1, Boston, 2004, Jones and Bartlett, pp. 205–224.
10. Armenian SH, Singh J, Arrieta AC: Risk factors for mortality resulting from bloodstream infections in a pediatric intensive care unit. *Pediatr Infect Dis J* 24(4):309–314, 2005.
11. Ash JS, et al: The extent and importance of unintended consequences related to computerized provider order entry. *J Am Med Informat Assoc* 14(4):415–423, 2007.
12. Backster A, et al: Transforming the surgical "time-out" into a comprehensive "preparatory pause." *J Card Surg* 22(5):410–416, 2007.
13. Buckley MS, et al: Direct observation approach for detecting medication errors and adverse drug events in a pediatric intensive care unit. *Pediatr Crit Care Med* 8:145–152, 2007.
14. Byrnes MC, Coopersmith CM: Prevention of catheter-related blood stream infection. *Curr Opin Crit Care* 13(4):411–415, 2007.
15. Canadian Root Cause Analysis Framework: A Tool for Identifying and Addressing the Root Causes of Critical Incidents in Healthcare. Available at http://www.patientsafetyinstitute.ca/English/toolsResources/rca/Pages/default.aspx. Accessed October 8, 2011.
16. Carroll JS, Rudolph JW: Design of high reliability organizations in health care. *Qual Saf Health Care* 15(Suppl 1):i4–i9, 2006.
17. Cavalcante SS, et al: Risk factors for developing nosocomial infections among pediatric patients. *Pediatr Infect Dis J* 25(5):438–445, 2006.
18. Centers for Disease Control and Prevention (National Center for Health Statistics: Births and deaths: preliminary data for 1998. *Natl Vital Stat Rep* 47(25):6, 1999.
19. Centers for Disease Control and Prevention: Monitoring hospital acquired infections to promote patient safety—United States, 1990-1999. *Morbidity & Mortality Weekly Report* 49:149–153, 2000.
20. Cochran GL, et al: Errors prevented by and associated with bar-code medication administration systems. *Joint Comm J Qual Patient Saf* 33(5):293–301, 245, 2007.
21. Committee on Quality Health Care in America, Institute of Medicine: *Crossing the quality chasm: a new health system for the 21st century,* Washington, DC, 2001, National Academy Press.
22. Conroy S, et al: Interventions to reduce dosing errors in children: a systematic review of the literature. *Drug Saf* 30(12):1111–1125, 2007.
23. Curley MA, et al: Tailoring the Institute for Health Care Improvement 100,000 Lives Campaign to pediatric settings: the example of ventilator-associated pneumonia. *Pediatr Clin North Am* 53(6):1231–1251, 2006.
24. Deming WE: *The new economics for industry, government, education,* ed 2, Cambridge, MA, 2000, MIT Press.
25. Deshpande KS, et al: The incidence of infectious complications of central venous catheters at the subclavian, internal jugular, and femoral sites in an intensive care unit population. *Crit Care Med* 33 (1):13–20, 2005; discussion 234-235.

26. Duwe B, Fuchs BD, Hansen-Flaschen J: Failure mode and effects analysis application to critical care medicine. *Crit Care Clin* 21(1):21–30, vii, 2005.
27. Elward AM, Warren DK, Fraser VJ: Ventilator-associated pneumonia in pediatric intensive care unit patients: risk factors and outcomes. *Pediatrics* 109(5):758–764, 2002.
28. Flanagan J: The critical incident technique. *Psychol Bull* 51:327–385, 1954.
29. Flin R, Maran N: Identifying and training non-technical skills for teams in acute medicine. *Qual Saf Health Care* 13(Suppl 1):i80–i84, 2004.
30. France DJ, et al: An observational analysis of surgical team compliance with perioperative safety practices after crew resource management training. *Am J Surg* 195(4):546–553, 2008.
31. Garbutt J, et al: Reporting and disclosing medical errors: pediatricians' attitudes and behaviors. *Arch Pediatr Adolesc Med* 161(2):179–185, 2007.
32. Gerstle RS, Lehmann CU, American Academy of Pediatrics Council on Clinical Information Technology: Electronic prescribing systems in pediatrics: the rationale and functionality requirements. *Pediatrics* 119(6):e1413–e1422, 2007.
33. Grissinger M, Rich D: JCAHO: meeting the standards for patient safety. Joint Commission on Accreditation of Healthcare Organizations. *J Am Pharmaceut Assoc* 42(5 Suppl 1):S54–S55, 2002.
34. Hackbarth G, Milgate K: Using quality incentives to drive physician adoption of health information technology. *Health Aff* 24 (1):1147–1149, 2005.
35. Hayden RT, et al: Computer-assisted bar-coding system significantly reduces clinical laboratory specimen identification errors in a pediatric oncology hospital. *J Pediatr* 152(2):219–224, 2008.
36. Hicks RW, Becker SC, Cousins DD: Harmful medication errors in children: a 5-year analysis of data from the USP's MEDMARX program. *J Pediatr Nurs* 21(4):290–298, 2006.
37. Hinshaw AS: Navigating the perfect storm: balancing a culture of safety with workforce challenges. *Nurs Res* 57(Suppl 1):S4–S10, 2008.
38. Holden J: How can we improve the nursing work? *Matern Child Nurs* 1(31):34–38, 2006.
39. Holdsworth MT, et al: Incidence and impact of adverse drug events in pediatric inpatients. *Arch Pediatr Adolesc Med* 157(1):60–65, 2003.
40. Hunt EA, et al: Simulation: translation to improved team performance. *Anesthesiol Clin* 25(2):301–319, 2007.
41. Hunter JG: Extend the universal protocol, not just the surgical time out. *J Am Coll Surg* 205(4):e4–e5, 2007.
42. Iedema R, et al: Narrativizing errors of care: critical incident reporting in clinical practice. *Soc Sci Med* 62:134–144, 2006.
43. Institute for Healthcare Improvement: *Failure modes and effects analysis tool.* Available at http://www.ihi.org/knowledge/Pages/Tools/FailureModesandEffectsAnalysisTool.aspx. Accessed October 8, 2011.
44. Institute for Healthcare Improvement: *How to improve.* Available at http://www.ihi.org/IHI/Topics/Improvement/ImprovementMethods/HowToImprove. Accessed April 25, 2008.
45. Institute for Healthcare Improvement: *5 Million lives campaign: how-to guide: prevent central line infections.* Copyright 2007 Institute for Healthcare Improvement. Available at http://www.ihi.org/NR/rdonlyres/0AD706AA-0E76-457B-A4B0-78C31A5172D8/0/CentralLineInfectionsHowtoGuide.doc. Accessed April 25, 2008.
46. Joint Commission: *Sentinel Events.* Available at http://www.jointcommission.org/SentinelEvents. Accessed April 25, 2008.
47. Joint Commission: Preventing pediatric medication errors. *Sentinel Event Alert* 39, April 2008. Available at http://www.jointcommission.org/SentinelEvents/SentinelEventAlert/sea_39.htm. Accessed April 25, 2008.
48. Jolley J, et al: Rapid response teams: do they make a difference? *Dimens Crit Care Nurs* 26(6):253–260, 2007.
49. Kaushal R, et al: Medication errors and adverse drug events in pediatric inpatients. *J Am Med Assoc* 285(16):2114–2120, 2001.
50. Kaushal R, et al: Pediatric medication errors: what do we know? What gaps remain? *Ambul Pediatr* 4(1):73–81, 2004.
51. Kohn KT, Corrigan JM, Donaldson MS: *To err is human: building a safer healthcare System,* Washington, DC, 1999, National Academy Press.
52. Kovner C, et al: Nurse staffing and postsurgical adverse events: an analysis of administrative data from a sample of U.S. hospitals, 1990-1996. *Health Serv Res* 37(3):611–629, 2002.

53. Landrigan CP, et al: Effect of reducing interns' work hours on serious medical errors in intensive care units. *New Engl J Med* 351 (18):1838–1848, 2004.

54. Langley GJ, et al: *The improvement guide: a practical approach to enhancing organizational performance,* San Francisco, CA, 1996, Jossey-Bass.

55. Le Duff F, et al: Monitoring incident report in the healthcare process to improve quality in hospitals. *Int J Med Informat* 74(2–4):111–117, 2005.

56. Leape LL, Berwick DM: Five years after to err is human: what have we learned? *J Am Med Assoc* 293(19):2384–2390, 2005.

57. Leape LL, et al: Systems analysis of adverse drug events. *J Am Med Assoc* 274(1):35–43, 2005.

58. McDonald CJ: Computerization can create safety hazards: a bar-coding near miss. *Ann Intern Med* 144(7):510–516, 2006.

59. McGreevy JM, Otten TD: Briefing and debriefing in the operating room using fighter pilot crew resource management. *J Am Coll Surg* 205(1):169–176, 2007.

60. McKeon LM, Oswaks JD, Cunningham PD: Safeguarding patients: complexity science, high reliability organizations, and implications for team training in healthcare. *Clin Nurse Spec* 20(6):298–304, 2006.

61. Montgomery VL: Effect of fatigue, workload, and environment on patient safety in the pediatric intensive care unit. *Pediatr Crit Care Med* 8(Suppl 2):S11–S16, 2007.

62. Mulder D: Minimizing mistakes. Beloit Memorial Hospital is focused on bedside bar coding to help eliminate medication errors. *Healthc Informat* 24(9):52–53, 2007.

63. Nance JJ: Admitting imperfection: revelations from the cockpit for the world of medicine. In Youngberg BJ, Hatlie M, editors: *The patient safety handbook,* ed 1, Boston, 2004, Jones and Bartlett, pp. 187–203.

64. National Academy of Sciences: *To err is human: building a safer healthcare system executive summary,* 2003. Available at http://www.nap.edu. Accessed April 25, 2008.

65. National Academy of Sciences: *Crossing the quality chasm: a new health system for the 21st century executive summary,* 2003. Available at http://www.nap.edu. Accessed April 25, 2008.

66. National Nosocomial Infections Surveillance System: National Nosocomial Infections Surveillance (NNIS) System Report, data summary from January 1992 through June 2004, issued October 2004. *Am J Infect Contr* 32(8):470–485, 2004.

67. Needleman J, et al: Nurse-staffing levels and the quality of care in hospitals. *New Engl J Med* 346(22):1715–1722, 2002.

68. Nelson EC, et al: Microsystems in health care: Part 1. Learning from high-performing front-line clinical units. [see comment]. *Joint Comm J Qual Improv* 28(9):472–493, 2002.

69. Nishisaki A, Keren R, Nadkarni V: Does simulation improve patient safety? Self-efficacy, competence, operational performance, and patient safety. *Anesthesiol Clin* 25(2):225–236, 2007.

70. Norton E: Implementing the universal protocol hospital-wide. *AORN J* 85(6):1187–1197, 2007.

71. Nuckols TK, et al: Programmable infusion pumps in ICUs: an analysis of corresponding adverse drug events. *J Gen Intern Med* 23 (Suppl 1):41–45, 2008.

72. Oriol MD: Crew resource management: applications in healthcare organizations. *J Nurs Admin* 36(9):402–406, 2006.

73. Page A, editor: *Keeping patients safe: transforming the work environments of nurses,* Washington, DC, 2004, National Academies Press.

74. Pape TM: Applying airline safety practices to medication administration. *MEDSURG Nurs* 12(2):77–93, 2003; quiz 94.

75. Poole DL, et al: Medication reconciliation: a necessity in promoting a safe hospital discharge. *J Healthc Qual* 28(3):12–19, 2006.

76. Prince SB, Herrin DM: The role of information technology in healthcare communications, efficiency, and patient safety: application and results. *J Nurs Admin* 37(4):184–187, 2007.

77. Pronovost PJ, et al: Creating high reliability in health care organizations. *Health Serv Res* 41(4 Pt 2):1599–1617, 2006.

78. Pronovost PJ, et al: Intensive care unit nurse staffing and the risk for complications after abdominal aortic surgery. *Effect Clin Pract* 4 (5):199–206, 2001.

79. Reason JT: Human error: models and management. *Br Med J* 320:768–770, 2000.

80. Resar RK: Making noncatastrophic health care processes reliable: learning to walk before running in creating high-reliability organizations. *Health Serv Res* 41(4 Pt 2):1677–1689, 2006.

81. Robinson DL, Heigham M, Clark J: Using Failure Mode and Effects Analysis for safe administration of chemotherapy to hospitalized children with cancer. *Joint Comm J Qual Patient Saf* 32(3):161–166, 2006.

82. Rogers AE, et al: The working hours of hospital staff nurses and patient safety. *Health Aff* 23(4):202–212, 2004.

83. Roman N: Innovative solutions: standardized concentrations facilitate the use of continuous infusions for pediatric intensive care unit nurses at a community hospital. *Dimens Crit Care Nurs* 24(6):275–278, 2005.

84. Sandlin D: Improving patient safety by implementing a standardized and consistent approach to hand-off communication. *J Perianesth Nurs* 22(4):289–292, 2007.

85. Scanlon MC, Mistry KP, Jeffries HE: Determining pediatric intensive care unit quality indicators for measuring pediatric intensive care unit safety. *Pediatr Crit Care Med* 8(Suppl 2):S3–S10, 2007.

86. Schwarz M, Wyskiel R: Medication reconciliation: developing and implementing a program. *Crit Care Nurs Clin North Am* 18 (4):503–507, 2006.

87. Scott LD, et al: Effects of critical care nurses' work hours on vigilance and patients' safety. *Am J Crit Care* 15(1):30–37, 2006.

88. Sebat F, et al: Effect of a rapid response system for patients in shock on time to treatment and mortality during 5 years. *Crit Care Med* 35 (11):2568–2575, 2007.

89. Shamliyan TA, et al: Just what the doctor ordered. Review of the evidence of the impact of computerized physician order entry system on medication errors. *Health Serv Res* 43(1 Pt 1):32–53, 2008.

90. Sharek PJ, et al: Effect of a rapid response team on hospital-wide mortality and code rates outside the ICU in a Children's Hospital. *J Am Med Assoc* 298(19):2267–2274, 2007.

91. Sheridan-Leos N, Schulmeister L, Hartranft S: Failure mode and effect analysis: a technique to prevent chemotherapy errors. *Clin J Oncol Nurs* 10(3):393–398, 2006.

92. Singer S, et al: Workforce perceptions of hospital safety culture: development and validation of the patient safety climate in healthcare organizations survey. *Health Serv Res* 42(5):1999–2021, 2007.

93. Spooner SA, Council on Clinical Information Technology, American Academy of Pediatrics: Special requirements of electronic health record systems in pediatrics. *Pediatrics* 119(3):631–637, 2007.

94. Stockwell JA: Nosocomial infections in the pediatric intensive care unit: affecting the impact on safety and outcome. *Pediatr Crit Care Med* 8(2 Suppl):S21–S37, 2007.

95. Sullivan EE: Hand-off communication. *J Perianesth Nurs* 22(4):275–279, 2007.

96. Sundar E, et al: Crew resource management and team training. *Anesthesiol Clin* 25(2):283–300, 2007.

97. Taylor JA, et al: Use of incident reports by physicians and nurses to document medical errors in pediatric patients. *Pediatrics* 114 (3):729–735, 2004.

98. Taylor JA, et al: Evaluation of an anonymous system to report medical errors in pediatric inpatients. *J Hosp Med (Online)* 2 (4):226–233, 2007.

99. Taylor JA, et al: Medication administration variances before and after implementation of computerized physician order entry in a neonatal intensive care unit. *Pediatrics* 121(1):123–128, 2008.

100. Tepfers A, Louie H, Drouillard M: Developing an electronic incident report: experiences of a multi-site teaching hospital. *Healthc Q* 10(2):117–122, 2007.

101. Urrea M, et al: Prospective incidence study of nosocomial infections in a pediatric intensive care unit. *Pediatr Infect Dis J* 22(6):490–494, 2003.

102. Valentin A, Bion J: How safe is my intensive care unit? An overview of error causation and prevention. *Curr Opin Crit Care* 13(6):697–702, 2007.

103. Valentin A, et al: Research Group on Quality Improvement of European Society of Intensive Care Medicine, Sentinel Events Evaluation Study Investigators:: Patient safety in intensive care: results from the multinational Sentinel Events Evaluation (SEE) study. *Intensive Care Med* 32(10):1591–1598, 2006.

104. Varkey P, et al: Multidisciplinary approach to inpatient medication reconciliation in an academic setting. *Am J Health Syst Pharm* 64(8):850–854, 2007.

105. Varkey P, Reller MK, Resar RK: Basics of quality improvement in healthcare. *Mayo Clinic Proc* 82(6):735–739, 2007.

106. Veterans Administration National Center for Patient Safety 1: *Root cause analysis.* Available at http://www.va.gov/NCPS/rca.html. Accessed April 25, 2008.

107. Veterans Administration National Center for Patient Safety 2: Root cause analysis. Available at http://www.va.gov/NCPS/CogAids/Triage/index.html?8. Accessed April 25, 2008.

108. Wachter RM, Pronovosta PJ: The 100,000 Lives Campaign: a scientific and policy review. *Joint Comm J Qual Patient Saf* 32(11):621–627, 2006.

109. Wald H, Shojania KG: Incident reporting. Agency for Health Care Research & Quality: *Making health care safer: a critical analysis of patient safety practices*, Rockville, MD, 2001, AHRQ, pp. 41–51.

110. Walsh KE, et al: Medication errors related to computerized order entry for children. *Pediatrics* 118(5):1872–1879, 2006.

111. Walsh KE, Kaushal R, Chessare JB: How to avoid paediatric medication errors: a user's guide to the literature. *Arch Dis Child* 90(7):698–702, 2005.

112. Walsh KE, et al: Effect of computer order entry on prevention of serious medication errors in hospitalized children. *Pediatrics* 121(3):e421–e427, 2008.

113. Wang JK, et al: Prevention of pediatric medication errors by hospital pharmacists and the potential benefit of computerized physician order entry. *Pediatrics* 119(1):e77–85, 2007.

114. Weick K, Sutcliff K: *Managing the unexpected: assuring high performance in and age of complexity,* San Francisco, 2001, Jossey-Bass.

115. Wetterneck TB, et al: Using failure mode and effects analysis to plan implementation of smart i.v. pump technology. *Am J Health Syst Pharm* 63(16):1528–1538, 2006.

116. Zenker P, et al: Implementation and impact of a rapid response team in a children's hospital. *Joint Comm J Qual Patient Saf* 33 (7):418–425, 2007.

Clinical Informatics

23

Neal R. Patel

PEARLS

- Clinical information technology (IT) involves a dynamic set of interactions that all have to be managed effectively. The categories of people, process, and technology each introduce different challenges and factors that must be addressed for successful IT implementation and adoption.
- To achieve maximal beneficial effects, clinical IT must provide clinicians with the right amount of data in the appropriate context to help them make good clinical decisions.
- The use of IT to enforce compliance and adherence to policies and regulations must be balanced with clinical utility and minimal distractions.
- Effective use of clinical IT tools can markedly improve patient safety and clinical workflow.
- Clinical, administrative, and IT leaders need to develop a shared vision and governance model to deploy and maintain clinical IT systems.

INTRODUCTION

The past two decades have seen significant advances in medical and nursing care for critically ill infants and children. These advances have stemmed from increased research and clinical experience as well as better appreciation for the appropriate use of technology to monitor and deliver state of the art medical care. The incorporation of microprocessors has revolutionized bedside critical care nursing. From networked monitors to ventilators to infusion pumps, many technologic advances have been incorporated into the routine workflow at the bedside.

Information technology is the latest set of tools for the critical care setting. Traditionally, IT was relegated to the administrative tasks of managing and processing transactions for hospital departments. These systems included those used to process and track patient census, billing, the laboratory system, materials management, and pharmacy. Whereas the functions of these systems are essential to the delivery of medical care, these systems were not directly involved at the point of care. Recent efforts have now focused on better use of computerized systems to improve the process of care delivery.

Several major issues have prompted focused effort to use IT tools more effectively in healthcare. The cost of healthcare in the United States continues to rise. Despite the expenditures, healthcare providers are finding it increasingly difficult to balance budgets and grow resources to meet demand. Cost pressures are contributing to increasing staffing shortages.

In the past decade, many examples of error, waste, and inefficiency in healthcare have been identified. In 1999, the Institute of Medicine (IOM) estimated that nearly 100,000 hospitalized patients die each year from medical errors.[12] The IOM report led to increased scrutiny of the safety and efficiency of the healthcare system. In 2003, the analysis by McGlynn and others[9] documented a significant gap between the care that patients need and the care that is provided. In a sample of more than 6700 adult patients in 12 metropolitan cities, only 54.9% of patients received the recommended care.[9]

IT is a potential tool to reduce errors. A reduction in errors can result from the role of IT in managing information, its utility in standardizing care, and through its role as a vehicle to change roles and processes in an effort to reduce cost, variability, and waste. These efforts can result in improved outcomes (Fig. 23-1)

Information systems work by several mechanisms to reduce human error. The process of delivering good care is getting more difficult as the result of the sheer volume of data that clinicians must review and evaluate. This volume can range from the hundreds of data points to be analyzed from a patient's vital sign flow sheet to the thousands of new journal articles written every year that can affect management of a disease or complication. The computer can be an excellent tool to help collate, retrieve, and store this information so that it can be used effectively. Reducing the reliance on human memory can help to mitigate situations in which care is delayed or omitted.

IT can help to improve healthcare delivery by simplifying processes. It takes a lot of time to fill out multiple requisition forms to communicate with a variety of hospital departments. Using IT tools, forms can be completed and routed electronically; this can reduce time for the entire care process and improve the delivery of care. Computer systems are also highly effective in ensuring completeness of a process. Through the use of constraints or forcing functions, such as requiring that a name be filled in or dose specified in the case of a medication order, the system as a whole can be made more efficient.

Computerized systems can be used to promote the use of standard protocols or checklists to ensure that providers undertake all necessary and effective care steps. These approaches all center on the concept of decision support. Decision support

FIG. 23-1 Key drivers of healthcare information technology.

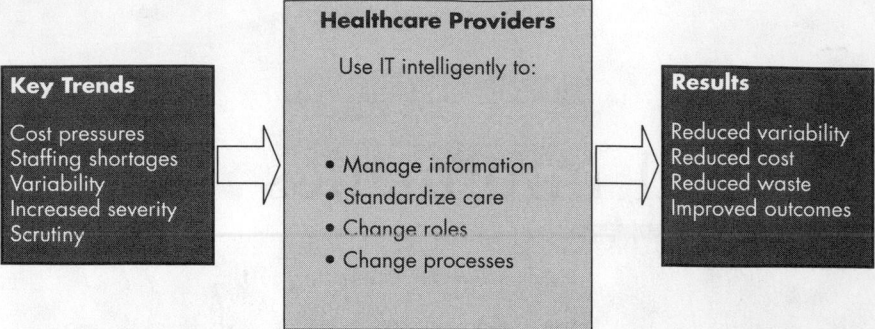

FIG. 23-1 Key drivers of healthcare information technology.

in a computerized system helps the user make the best patient care or management decisions by assembling all necessary information and by reducing the number of steps or processes to making the given decision. The effective use of these tools can decrease dependence on vigilance and reduce handoffs and redundant data entry, all of which have been shown to contribute to errors in healthcare.

IMPLEMENTION OF CLINICAL INFORMATION SYSTEMS

Despite the great promise of electronic systems and substantial financial investment in such systems, there continues to be significant variability in the success of information system implementation and adoption by clinicians. According to the Office of the National Coordinator for Health Information Technology, almost one third of electronic medical records technology implementations fail. Healthcare providers and IT experts are now beginning to understand the challenges of introducing technology into clinical workflow.

IT implementation often fails because clinical users are unprepared for the additional burden that interaction with an electronic system will place on their work patterns and clinical care delivery. In addition, the systems must be developed with adequate input from the users, and careful planning for unique hospital needs. Several high-profile implementations of computerized provider order entry (CPOE) have provided excellent case studies to teach improved approaches to IT implementation.

A large hospital in Los Angeles implemented a multimillion-dollar CPOE system with little physician input. Shortly after implementation, clinicians complained that the system was not working and patient care was being compromised. Three months after implementation, the hospital was forced to uninstall the system.

In another case, in the first 5 months following implementation of a commercially purchased CPOE system in a pediatric critical care unit at a leading children's hospital in the northeast, mortality during interfacility patient transfer more than doubled (from 2.8% to 6.6%) when compared with the mortality in the 13 months preceding CPOE implementation.[3] Several factors may have contributed to this rise. First, the system was rapidly deployed. Second, the clinical care team was not allowed to enter orders until the patient physically entered the hospital. Third, order sets were not developed to help clinicians rapidly enter common orders. Fourth,

simultaneous with the CPOE implementation, the hospital dispensing process for medications was changed. All of these factors directly affected patient care.

A second children's hospital in the northwest installed the same commercial CPOE system. When the effects of the implementation system on the northwest children's hospital was studied by Del Beccaro and others,[2] they found no difference in mortality in the preimplementation and postimplementation periods.

The Agency for Healthcare Research and Quality (AHRQ) calls for careful and thoughtful implementation of CPOE systems. Koppel's study of CPOE systems, funded by the AHRQ,[7] found two key problem areas in implementation:
- Fragmentation of data among each hospital's various information systems
- Interface problems between people and machines, particularly when the computer forced people to work in a way that differed from clinical work routines

People, Process, and Technology

Unlike simple electronic tools that automate a single task, the introduction of clinical IT involves a dynamic set of interactions that all have to be managed effectively. The categories of people, process, and technology each introduce different challenges and factors that must be addressed for successful IT implementation and adoption.

The people involved in IT implementation include individuals and groups with an interest in the project. It is clear in the previous example of the large Los Angeles hospital that the primary users of the CPOE system, the clinicians, had inadequate input during the design or implementation process. Unfortunately, clinician input is often inadequate in IT implementation projects; however, this might not result from the specific exclusion of clinicians by the project team. The clinical environment is demanding and often the clinicians who have the most clinical experience and insight are unable to break away from their clinical responsibilities to participate in the process.

It is essential to acknowledge the challenge of clinical user involvement and to develop strategies to address it. Administrative leaders must acknowledge that time devoted to large implementation projects is important, and these leaders should consider compensating participant staff for involvement in such projects. Institutions that have taken this approach have seen significant improvements in clinician commitment and engagement.

The clinicians who participate in and lead implementation projects should possess several key skills. Technical expertise is not an essential skill, and it often can be a distraction. Foremost, the clinician must have the respect of and credibility with his or her peers. The value of peer-to-peer education, advocacy, and persuasion cannot be overstated. Healthcare providers learn best from colleagues rather than from didactic sessions. The clinician must also have a good understanding of the actual clinical workflow that will be affected. It is this understanding that allows the implementation team to identify potential pitfalls and obstacles that can derail a project plan.

The involved clinician must be able to work collaboratively with colleagues from a variety of clinical and nonclinical disciplines. The clinician must help the project team understand clinical realities and also must understand the capabilities and limitations of the technology. The clinician should be able to help the group make the correct adjustments and appropriate compromises so that the technology can be easily adopted and used effectively.

The likelihood that a person will use new technology depends to some extent on individual factors. A known predictor of technology adoption is the confidence that an individual has the ability to use the tool effectively. This concept is called *self-efficacy*. Healthcare workers with low computer self-efficacy often have difficulty adapting their workflow to incorporate the use of computers.

Different units in the same hospital will have drastically different acceptance of the same technology as the result of differences in staff perceptions regarding the ease of technology use and also the result of differences in staff attitudes about changes in their practice. Gender and age play important roles in determining these perceptions and attitudes. Karsh[4] found that male users valued the usefulness of a tool, whereas female users felt that ease of use was more valuable. Older users focused more on social and process issues, whereas younger users focused more on the effects of the tool on task performance. Therefore before implementing any new technology, planners should evaluate characteristics of potential users and of the potential technology itself.

In order for technology to contribute to improvements in process, planners must be knowledgeable about all aspects of the process. Planners must evaluate and understand the rationale for each discrete step and each task in the process, and they must understand the communication needs at every level. Too often, introduction of new technology (e.g., an electronic system), even if it is designed to mimic existing workflow, will exacerbate a variety of poor processes that were previously not identified as problematic. Simply stated, if there is a bad process, then the introduction of technology can, at best, automate that bad process. The act of implementing an informatics solution can be the impetus to redesign and improve workflow or at least identify where the technology may exacerbate poor workflow.

Hospital policies and procedures are often reviewed for guidance when the evaluation of workflow reveals significant variability or a clear breach of appropriate standards. During this phase, it is important to note that the clinicians often adapt a given process to deliver care within the constraints or flaws of an existing system. The plan should address the gap between clinical practice and existing policy. IT implementation will not be successful if technology is used in an attempt to force compliance with standards that clinicians have already rejected. Before attempting to implement a technology solution, planners must revisit the rationale for the existing standards, gain consensus with the clinicians, and redefine the process with all stakeholders. Administrative leadership is a key element in advocating for changes in policies and procedures while maintaining compliance with external regulations and accreditation standards.

Technology itself can introduce problems or complications that can produce a variety of unintended consequences. The staff members at the northeast children's hospital pediatric critical care unit (mentioned previously) discovered the limitations of CPOE technology that only allowed order entry after the patient arrived in the unit. The technology was a potential contributor to delays in care associated with increased mortality after deployment of the CPOE system.

The usability of the technology will obviously affect adoption and success. In general, consumers have high expectations for a good user experience as the result of advances in the consumer world and the effects of Internet capabilities in everyday lives. Unfortunately, many healthcare technology tools are not able to offer the robust features that are prevalent in the consumer world.

Technology accessibility can have a significant effect on the success of informatics tools used in the hospital environment. Too often, projects underestimate the number and types of devices that will be needed to effectively use the tools in a given workflow. Because most IT tools are accessed via a computer, it may be challenging to have a sufficient number of devices available to meet the demand of end users. Whereas the cost of devices has dramatically decreased in recent years, the physical environment, the cost of appropriate mounts or carts, and the need for mobility are parameters that may complicate or prevent successful implementation.

In order for good tools to be useful, clinicians must be able to access a computer at the time or in the place the tool is needed to deliver good care. This is of particular relevance in the critical care setting, where bedside clinicians require immediate access to a computer in the patient's room to use technology solutions, such as bar-coded medication administration. Use of a mobile computer allows significant flexibility for the provider within the room, but satisfaction greatly diminishes if the provider is expected to move the device from room to room when caring for more than one patient. Mounted computers are useful in the hallways and common desk areas in patient care units, but they may be less accessible in a critical care room, where the provider is often surrounded by a lot of other equipment.

Evaluating any informatics tool across the categories of people, process, and technology can provide important information. The implementation and adoption of any technology is enhanced when this information is included in the analysis and project plan.

Best Practices

A set of best practices have been identified that can increase the chances of successful implementation and adoption of information technology tools.

Executive Commitment

The commitment of hospital administrators is a key determinant of successful implementation. Their leadership provides the necessary energy and resources for engagement of many disciplines in the hospital. When specific obstacles or major controversies arise, an executive sponsor who has been involved throughout the process can provide the guidance and resources necessary to continue moving forward.

Identified Project Leaders

Clinical informatics projects require coordination of many people and management of a variety of issues. It is essential to have designated leaders with the responsibility, time, and resources to navigate the project and team. Unsuccessful projects often have designated leaders who have too many other competing responsibilities.

Road Map

A high-level project plan is essential. It should indicate key milestones and deliverables from project kickoff to initial pilot through full implementation. Although this plan can be dynamic and changes should be anticipated, it should clearly show the key targets, responsible groups, and timeline.

Process Redesign

It is difficult to incorporate IT without disrupting existing workflow. Because the technology will likely change the workflow, the technology implementation plan should include time and resources to evaluate the process and to redesign some care delivery steps to take advantage of the new technology. This planned redesign allows frontline staff to see how their work will change. The plan should emphasize the priority of improved patient care, not simply the use of new tools or cost savings.

Communication Strategy

A structured communication strategy is an important element of successful implementation. The plan should identify key groups that require periodic updates. The required level of communication detail should be determined in collaboration with the executive leadership. There will always be people who believe they have received inadequate preparation and communications. An effective communication strategy ensures that key leaders and groups are knowledgeable about the goals of the project, key milestones, and their roles in the project plan.

Simulation and Pilot Testing

The active use of simulation can help find fatal flaws in any system. The closer to "real" use a simulation can be, the richer the information gained from the simulation. It is too easy to overlook glitches or potential breakdowns when testing takes place away from the clinical care setting. Ideally, frontline staff should assist in the simulation and be asked about their perceptions and concerns as to the utility of the tool. This interaction can provide insights into the tool and about the

people and environmental factors necessary for successful use of the new technology.

Training and Support

Investment in training and support is an integral component of successful implementation. The models of training have to be flexible for the type of technology being deployed and the type of users involved. The goal of formal training should be to target the initial education to the basics of use and steps to get out of trouble; this helps build user confidence and self-efficacy.

The creation of super-users has been effective at many institutions. Super-users are trained to be expert users in their clinical settings; they then serve as resources to their colleagues. Another key type of support is providing access to information when it is needed by users (i.e., when they encounter difficulties and questions); this can be referred to as *just in time* or *at the elbow support*. During initial implementation, support personnel may be present on the unit to help users navigate the system or answer questions. Support may also be available through an online site to verify how to perform specific tasks.

Feedback

A feedback collection system serves several important functions. End-users are more likely to persist in trying to use a system if they know that their frustrations and complaints are being heard. The feedback is also a source of valuable real-use data to help identify needed refinements to the system. Effective methods for obtaining feedback vary by clinical setting and user type, but a multipronged approach is usually best. Examples include an active help desk process, periodic user forums, complaint or suggestion buttons within the informatics tools themselves, and structured visits to clinical areas to ask about user perceptions and concerns. Through these and other methods, the clinical teams will remain engaged and committed to effective use of the tools.

Several signs can predict potential failure of a technology implementation project. These "red flags" were adapted from a study by Upperman and others[13] and are summarized in Box 23-1.

| Box 23-1 | **Red Flags for Potential Implementation Failure** |

- Ignoring anxiety from change
- Not considering the consequences of each process step
- Lack of extensive training in the preimplementation and postimplementation periods
- Inadequate access to computers
- Not understanding the system limitations
- Neglecting to communicate the possible negative effects of information technology as well as the benefits
- Communicating through outside technical consultants rather than in-house leadership

From Upperman JS, et al: The introduction of computerized physician order entry and change management in a tertiary pediatric hospital. *Pediatrics* 116: e634-e642, 2005

CLINICAL INFORMATION SYSTEMS

The focus on medical safety stimulated by the 1999 Institute of Medicine[12] report led to the formation of the Leapfrog Group for Patient Safety. This group consists of many large companies and organizations that pay for healthcare coverage for their employees. The group initially named three key practices that could significantly improve healthcare quality and safety. These three practices are:

1. Use of CPOE
2. Evidence-based hospital referral (choice of hospitals and referrals should be based on a hospital's experience and outcomes, particularly for complex procedures), and
3. Staffing of pediatric critical care units with physicians experienced in critical care medicine

Computerized Provider Order Entry

There are many reasons why CPOE is expected to improve healthcare quality and safety (Box 23-2). CPOE systems can aggregate data for clinical use. Unlike the paper ordering process, a clinician can interact with the system away from the bedside without relying on verbal or telephone orders, which can lead to potential errors. Because communication is electronic, CPOE systems immediately route orders and requisitions to ancillary departments.

A major focus of CPOE systems is improving the ordering of medications and their accuracy. Several studies have shown that the use of CPOE can significantly reduce medication errors. CPOE improves the process by virtually eliminating orders that are incomplete or illegible or have abbreviations. This improvement markedly increases the efficiency of the ordering process and diminishes communication errors.

Additional improvements in ordering medications result from safety checks that allow the system to alert the provider to patient drug allergies. Obviously, the CPOE system cannot provide alerts unless valid information about patient allergies is entered into the system. Each clinical unit must develop a standardized process for identifying patient allergies and correctly entering this information into the information system. The robustness of a given system rests on how well it facilitates this process.

Clinical Decision Support

Clinical decision support within the CPOE system can help to reduce medication errors. Standard decision support algorithms can alert a prescriber if an ordered dose falls outside a predefined range of acceptable dosing. In a pediatric setting these alerts may still be insufficient unless they factor in the effects of patient weight and age on an appropriate medication dose.

The next generation of CPOE systems is beginning to incorporate decision support. Decision support can be expanded to include parameters such as renal function, immune status, and eventually genomics and proteomics in dose alerts.

Order Sets

An order set is a group of related orders that can be presented to a clinician for selection. These orders can provide the standard approach to treating a particular disease process, such as community-acquired pneumonia, or they can consist of a common set of orders that are needed for the postoperative care of patients after common procedures such as an appendectomy. Order sets for high-volume clinical conditions can incorporate evidence-based medicine and reduce variations in care among clinicians. Order sets can also be created for relatively low-volume cases in which precision is of paramount importance. A standard order set for a transplant patient with graft-versus-host disease is an example of the need for precision. Each order set should follow a specific protocol established by institutional experts and can be available instantly for to the prescribing clinician. The order sets support delivery of optimal evidence-based care for each patient.

The percentage of total orders entered into a CPOE system though order sets is directly correlated with the adoption of the CPOE system. As more evidence-based treatment approaches are selected, the quality of care improves and benefits of the CPOE system become more apparent.

Many institutions have already developed treatment protocols in the paper ordering process. These protocols are the best place to begin designing CPOE order sets. Facilities with significant experience with CPOE have found that the energy and resources available during the implementation phase of CPOE wanes over time. During the maintenance phase of the CPOE system, it important to establish a process for periodic review and update of order sets with continued incorporation of the latest evidence from the healthcare literature to guide clinical care (Fig. 23-2)

The project team can often leverage existing hospital process improvement infrastructure to help establish a systematic process for developing order sets (Box 23-3). The first step in building the infrastructure is to identify the core team that will serve as the resource for the institution. Because order sets can exist for each of the clinical disciplines, it is important for the core team to work with key representatives of the patient care team so that the clinicians have confidence in the process and a sense of ownership of the order set content. Minimizing the time commitment by the clinicians will help retain their engagement. The core team should be responsible for coordinating meetings, collating the necessary documents, and filtering the literature. This process frees the clinicians to focus on important clinical content.

Alerts and Cross-Checks

Advances in CPOE technology include several features to promote excellence in patient care delivery. These features will be most effective if content is adjusted to match closely with the clinical context in which it is used. There must also be a

---

Box 23-2	**Key Advantages of a Computer Provider Order Entry System**

- Key data are aggregated for clinical use
- Clinician can interact with the medical record away from the bedside
- Immediate routing of orders and requisitions to ancillary departments
- Smart prompts and checks can enhance safety and quality of care

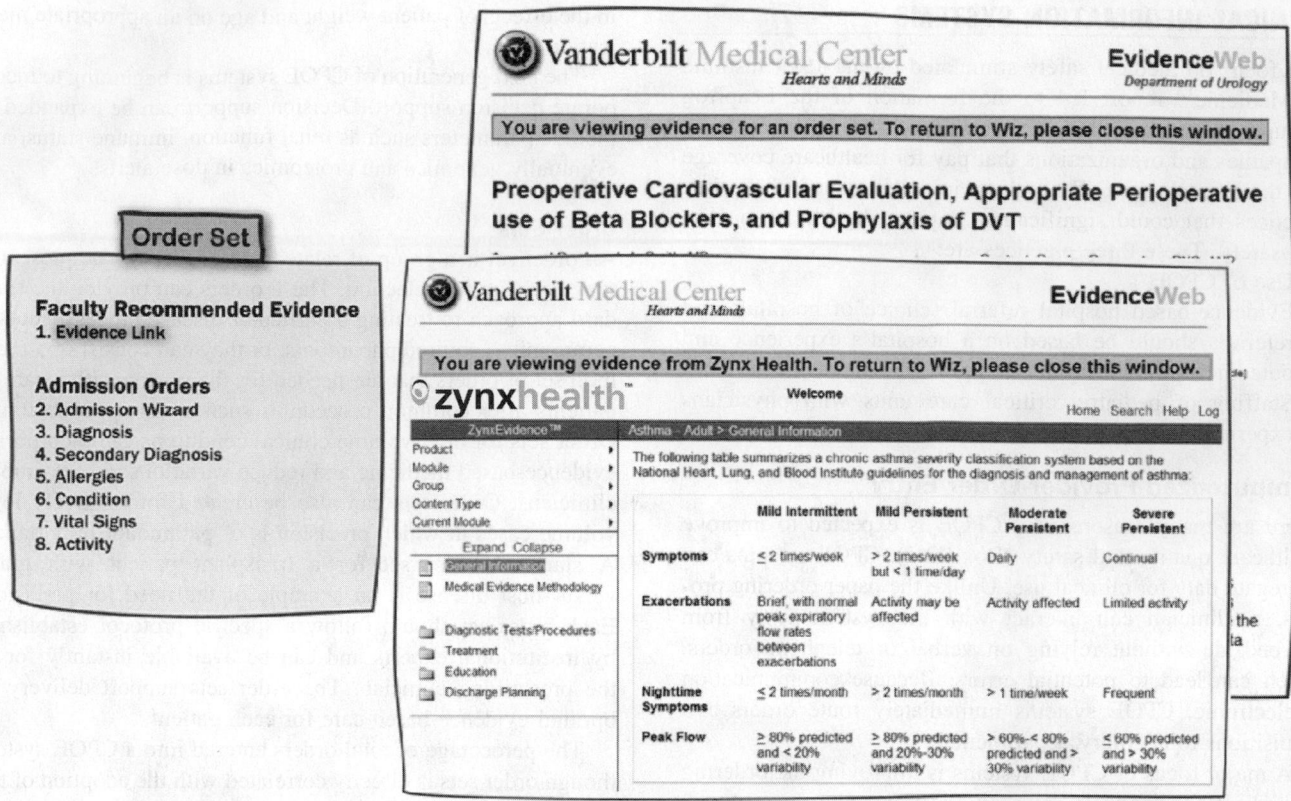

FIG. 23-2 Order sets with links. This diagram shows the relationship among traditional order sets with links to the reference material for evidence-based medicine developed by the Evidence-Based Medicine Team at the Vanderbilt University Medical Center.[11a] (Courtesy Zynx Health Incorporated, Los Angeles, CA; and Vanderbilt University Medical Center, Nashville, Tenn.)

Box 23-3 **Sample Evidence-Based Practice Process for Development of Order Sets[11a]**

Define Order Set Team
- Physician lead
- Nursing lead
- Pharmacy lead
- House staff lead
- Evidence-based practice (EBP) specialist
- Librarian consultant

Input Phase
- Clinical team and target order sets are identified.
- EBP specialist and team leads gather relevant clinical evidence.
  - Library, Zynx Health Incorporated, Cochrane database, national guidelines, medical literature
  - Core measures
- Evidence-based practice (EBP) specialist creates an evidence packet with order sets and targeted evidence.
- Initial development meeting is convened.

Development Phase
- EBP specialist and clinical team update order sets.
  - Pharmacy review
  - Relevant clinical evidence
  - Relevant core measures
- Clinical team identifies redundant or outdated order sets for cleanup.
- EBP specialist and clinical team update pathway.
- Clinical team identifies feedback data.
- Clinical team identifies relevant information for online reference portal.

Implementation Phase
- Order set creation in the CPOE system
- Pathways created for multidisciplinary use that incorporates order set data
- Evidence Web—key clinical evidence linked to order set made available in a reference portal
- Feedback obtained throughout process

CPOE, Computerized provider order entry.

---

constant balance between utility and overuse. Although prompts and reminders are viewed as helpful by clinical users, if they disrupt thought processes or are presented out of context, users will quickly develop workarounds to avoid features that are intended to be helpful or improve safety. Similar to

the consumer response to a barrage of pop-up messages during Internet use, healthcare users may develop alertfatigue and begin to cancel or close the alert feature without reviewing the content. This scenario defeats the purpose of the safety aids and should be avoided at all costs.

Some features are designed as cross-checks to ensure that every order is clinically appropriate for the patient. In the area of medication ordering, drug allergy checks and drug-drug interaction (DDI) alerts are good examples of these cross-checks. Good clinical practice requires a check to verify that a patient does not have a known allergy to a prescribed drug. Unfortunately, this check is often omitted. A variety of factors contribute to the problem; the most common is that information about the allergy is not available to the prescribing clinician at the time the medication is ordered. A CPOE system closes this gap with a drug allergy check, but it cannot eliminate the gap. The computer system is dependent on accurate entry of allergy information for every patient.

The benefit of a CPOE system is that once patient allergy information is entered, it can be helpful for every instance of medication prescription. Based on the sophistication of the CPOE algorithms, a single entered allergy can prompt an alert for any potential medication prescribed in the same general class of medications (e.g., sulfonamides or penicillin class drugs) that can trigger a reaction. It is important to note that not all allergies have the same clinical effect, and a clinician needs to have as much information as possible about the severity of the allergy to make the best clinical decision. There are times that the clinical benefit of a medication outweighs the potential for an allergic reaction.

A DDI is any situation in which one drug has the potential to increase or decrease the effect of another drug to an extent that is clinically significant. Ideally, a prescribing clinician is alerted to this possible situation during the order entry process and will be guided toward a better clinical decision. In a study by Ko and others[6] of providers and pharmacists who used the U.S. Department of Veterans Affairs CPOE system, most felt that DDI alerts increased the safety of prescribing practice. The caveat from this study was that fewer than one third of the prescribers found that the system gave the essential information necessary to make good decisions. Both the prescribers and pharmacists felt that for DDI alerts to be effective, the system should give more detailed information and should suggest appropriate alternatives.

A CPOE system can prompt providers to add corollary orders. An example is a reminder to order drug level testing if antimicrobial therapy with an aminoglycoside is ordered. The system can provide a reminder to order an activated partial thromboplastin time test if a patient is given an anticoagulant. The efficacy of these alerts depends greatly on the timing of their appearance. Alerts that open immediately and interrupt clinical thinking and workflow can be met with resistance. Providers will accept these interruptions if they indicate a gross error or potential patient harm. However alerts that serve as simple reminders are viewed as a nuisance and are often ignored.

The concept of an exit check is of great utility for alerts regarding corollary orders. Exit checks appear after the provider has completed the ordering process and is ready to exit the CPOE session. By this time, the clinician has had an opportunity to address the issues that require alerts, but the alerts appear if issues remain when the provider is ready to review the orders. Exit checks are viewed as being less intrusive to workflow, so they have had greater acceptance.

PEDIATRIC MEDICATION SAFETY

There are four steps in medication delivery: prescribing, transcribing, dispensing, and administering. Errors can occur at each step, but approximately 80% of medication errors occur at the prescribing and administering steps[1]:
- Prescribing—56% of errors
- Transcribing—6% of errors
- Dispensing—4% of errors
- Administering—34% of errors

Thus, systems focusing on reducing medication errors have focused on the prescribing and administering phases of medication delivery.

A major goal in the development of CPOE systems is improving the prescribing phase of the medication delivery process. Many studies have shown dramatic reductions in adverse drug events and medication prescribing errors with the implementation of CPOE systems.

Pediatric Medication Dosing

The use of CPOE in the pediatric population requires a special focus on dosing algorithms (Box 23-4). The process of dosing medications for the pediatric patient is distinctly different from the process used in adult patients. Pediatric medication dosing is based primarily on patient weight. In certain subpopulations, dosing differs based on the age of the patient in both chronologic and gestational terms. In neonatal patients, rapid weight changes that are significant as a percent of weight must also be considered. If weight-based dosing is used, some school-aged patients can surpass adult dosing recommendations on a milligram per kilogram basis. A CPOE system must be able to integrate these factors into appropriate decision support (Fig. 23-3).

In critical care units, the process of ordering continuous infusion medications is more complex for pediatric patients than for adults. The medications for pediatric patients are typically dosed on the basis of weight. The infusions can be prepared with standard concentrations, and the flow rate needed to deliver a specific dose varies based on the patient's weight. In the past, the concentration of the infusion varied according to the patient's weight so that the same infusion rate delivered the same dose for all patients. The latter was the basis of the classic "rule of sixes." Currently most hospitals use standard concentrations for continuous infusions.

The calculations for both standard and weight-based concentrations, such as the rule of sixes, can lead to confusion and errors. In the paper-based ordering process, prescribers often did not provide the complete information necessary for pharmacists and nurses to cross-check the calculations. A CPOE system with effective clinical decision support can

---

Box 23-4 **Key Aspects of Pediatric Medication Dosing**

- Weight-based dosing
- Age-specific algorithms
- Issues of gestational age
- Rapid weight changes
- Complex calculations for drugs that are delivered by continuous infusion

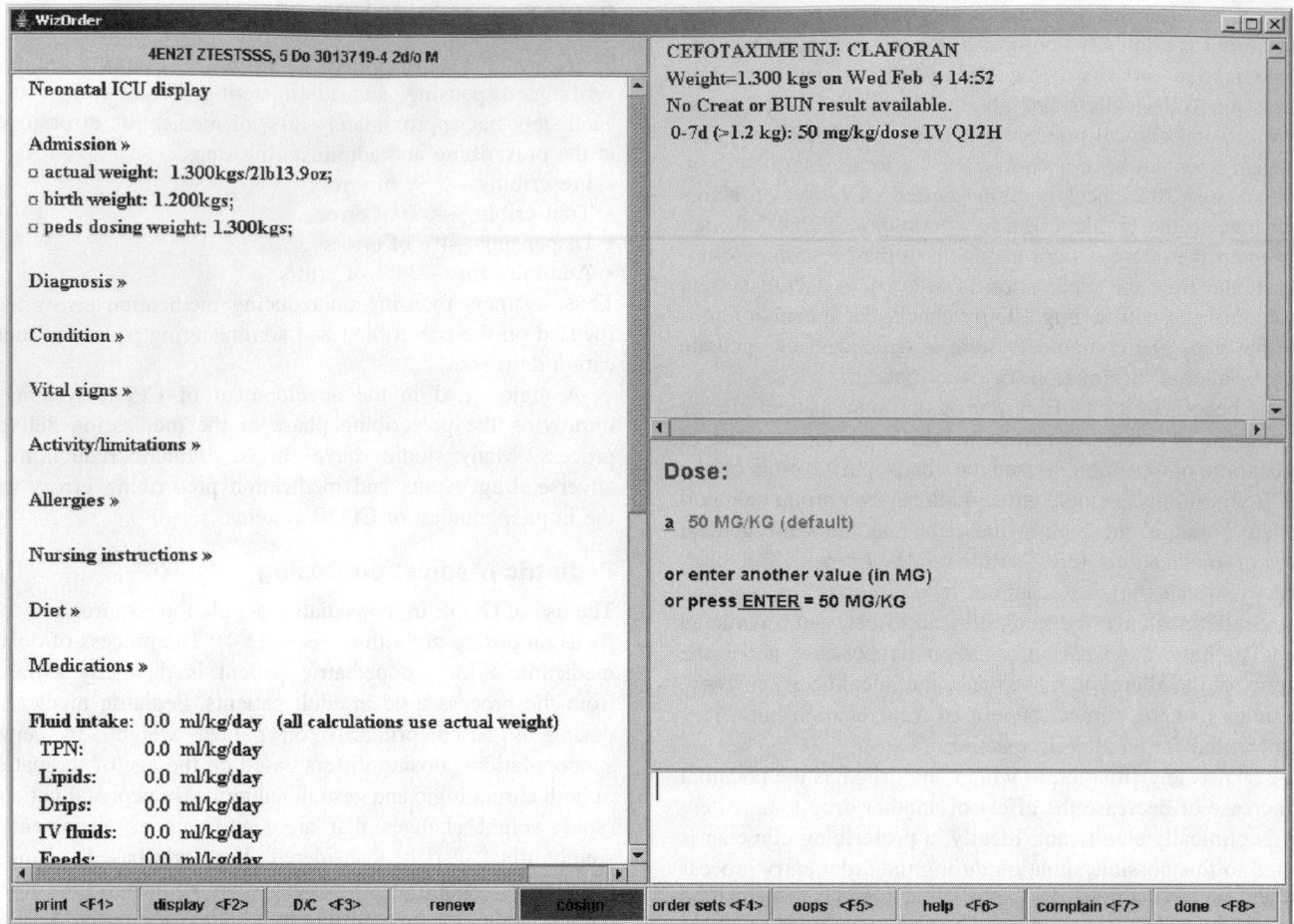

FIG. 23-3 Decision support tools. A sample view of decision support tools in a CPOE system to facilitate medication ordering for pediatric patients. (Courtesy of Vanderbilt University Medical Center, Nashville, Tenn.)

significantly improve the prescribing process for continuous infusions by performing the complex calculations, ensuring completeness of the orders, and producing a titration table against which intravenous pump settings can be compared by nurses administering the drug (Fig. 23-4). This final check by the nurse at the point of care is crucial.

Pediatric Patient Specific Decision Support

When a critical care environment transitions to an electronic ordering system, the project team should evaluate several system features and develop a standardized approach to address common pediatric dosing issues (Box 23-5).

The most basic feature of any electronic ordering system determines the types of information that must be entered before an order is accepted or completed. Many institutions require the entry of a pediatric patient's weight to increase dosing accuracy. However, in pediatric units where patients are weighed daily, especially neonatal units, this requirement could result in daily changes in medication doses that would be impractical. In addition, providers should have a consistent process regarding units used for weight (grams, pounds, kilograms) and to verify the weights entered. Providers can use a medication dosing weight, in a fashion similar to the use of dry weight for patients with renal failure. Use of a medication dosing weight allows the CPOE system to anchor the

calculations of medication doses to values that are set by the prescriber, and it also allows the clinical care team to enter patient weight values as clinically indicated.

Another important feature to address in the electronic ordering system is the process for frequent changes to therapy, such as ventilator changes and titration of continuous infusions. If the CPOE system requires a lot of time and effort to enter orders for each change, providers could resist using the system or fail to comply with order entry. It is important for unit and institutional policies to be in place to address this clinical reality.

Overall, the use of CPOE can be highly effective in reducing medication errors. The presence of advanced decision support markedly improves the utility of CPOE, especially in the care of pediatric patients.[11]

The Five Rights of Medication Administration

The core checks for appropriate medication administration are the well publicized "five rights" (Box 23-6), which are right patient, drug, dose, route, and time.

Bar-Coded Medication Administration

Bar code technology has been proposed to improve the safety of medication delivery during the medication administration phase. This technology provides an objective method to check

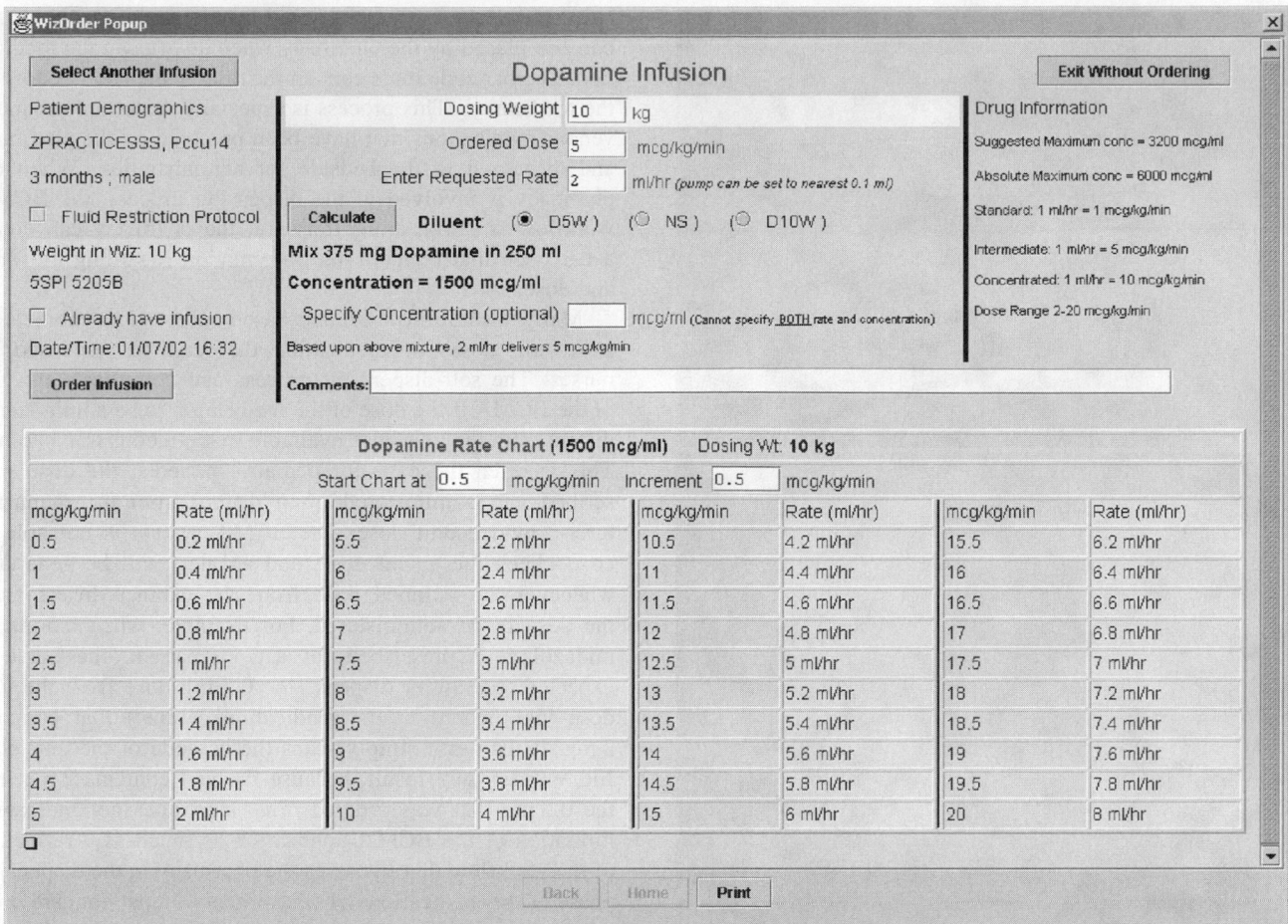

FIG. 23-4 Ordering screen for continuous infusion medications. This is an actual ordering screen for prescribing continuous infusions of drugs such as dopamine. This screen displays key features of advanced CPOE systems, such as dose and concentration calculator, dose recommendations, and titration tables to correlate dose and fluid rate. (Courtesy of Vanderbilt University Medical Center, Nashville, Tenn.)

Box 23-5	Key Features of Patient Specific Decision Support

- Provides weight- and age-specific dosing information at the time of ordering
- Menu dose options provided in mg/kg or mg depending on weight of patient
- Calculations performed by the computer
- Only intervals and doses appropriate for the specific patient are presented to the prescriber
- Doses rounded to standardized values
- Dose-check warnings provided for single doses

Box 23-6	The "Five Rights" of Medication Administration

1. Right patient
2. Right drug
3. Right dose
4. Right route
5. Right time

the patient and the accuracy of the medication during the medication administration process.

The standard process for administering medications requires mental checks of the labeling on the syringe, the medication administration record, and the patient arm band, even after the checks for propriety of drug and dose. Many medications have similar packaging and labeling that can contribute to medication errors.[5] There are tragic examples of overdose of drugs such as heparin resulting from such similarities.

The bar-coded medication administration (BCMA) system uses bar code technology to cross-check the patient's arm band bar code and the drug bar code against a system containing the medication orders for the patient to confirm that the patient should receive that drug in that dose at that time (Fig. 23-5). Alerts should be raised if the orders do not indicate a match of the drug dose, the patient, and the time. The BCMA system requires that all steps be followed and that the provider acknowledge the alerts.

BCMA technology must be incorporated into nursing workflow to be effective. There have been many anecdotes of workarounds that enable nurses to bypass the system, thereby nullifying its effectiveness as a safety check. The drug and the patient's arm band should be scanned to ensure that

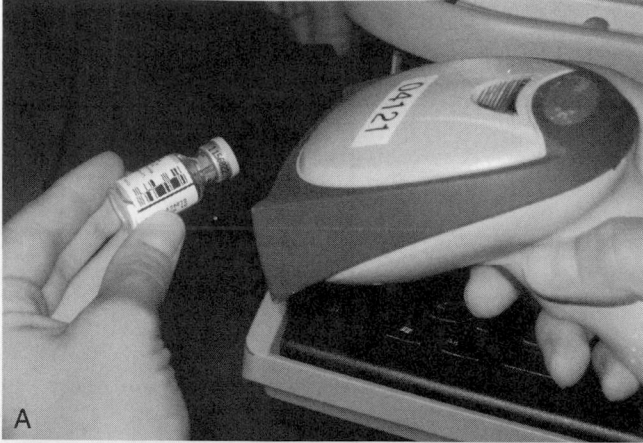

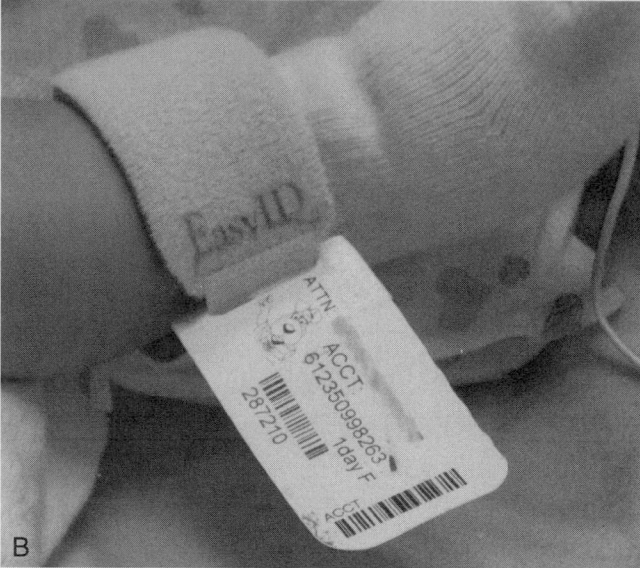

FIG. 23-5 Use of bar-code during medication administration. A, Bar-coded medication administration involves scanning the medication and B, then scanning a patient identification band.

the correct patient is receiving the correct drug in the correct dose and by the correct route at the correct time.

Implementation of BCMA technology can be successful using the principles described earlier in this chapter. BCMA systems have been used across the United States, with a variety of different vendor products. Many systems have reported near-misses when alerts from the BCMA system prevented administration of an incorrect drug or drug dose to a patient. It is difficult to determine the actual reduction in medication administration errors resulting from the BCMA technology, because few objective data exist to determine the actual medication error rate before implementation of BCMA systems.

BCMA technology is used in the pediatric setting, but several issues can complicate its implementation and effectiveness. One of the key elements in BCMA technology is the presence of a barcode on the medication to be delivered to the patient. The bar code is scanned and the drug, dose, and route of delivery are checked against the patient's medication administration record, which lists the drugs prescribed for the patient. The barcode on the medication can be the original

barcode placed on the packaging by the manufacturer or the barcode placed by the pharmacy when dispensing the medication. The bar code must contain the drug name and the dose of the medication. This process is especially important for intravenous medications that have been prepared by the pharmacy and dispensed to the bedside for administration. When the pharmacy is involved in the dispensing process, the BCMA workflow is fairly straightforward; the pharmacy can create a bar code that contains the information regarding the drug and dose.

Many institutions use unit-based medication cabinets to store unit doses of medication that can be dispensed by nurses. The self-dispensing process can complicate the use of the BCMA if the dose of the medication to be administered differs from the unit dose available in the medication cabinet. This is often the case for pediatric patients: the dose prescribed and administered often differs from the manufacturer-provided unit dose. The BCMA system is not able to cross-check the actual dose, and an alert will be generated whenever the scanned dose from the cabinet differs from the dose to be administered. For example, when 0.5 mg of midazolam is prescribed for a 5-kg patient, the nurse is expected to draw or dispense the 0.5-mg dose from the unit dose vial (stored in the medication cabinet) that contains 2 mg. If the nurse simply scans the barcode of the unit dose file, an alert will result, because the vial contains 2 mg, not the 0.5 mg that was ordered. This alert does not indicate a limitation of the BCMA application as much as a reflection of the workflow that bypasses the pharmacy in the dispensing phase of the medication delivery process. In patient care units where patient medications are obtained from medication cabinets, education of the staff is essential. The alert indicating "wrong dose" should be viewed as a safety check, reminding the nurse that the entire unit dose from the medication cabinet should not be administered to the patient. Nurses should record the drug dose actually administered to the patient.

The implementation of an electronic system will create many opportunities for improving the medication administration process. The data provided from the BCMA system can be used to focus improvement efforts and target areas of the process that require modification or enforcement of existing policies. It is essential to focus on improving the overall system rather than criticizing individual behavior. The punitive nature of medication error reporting needs to be eliminated. The goal is to create processes that prevent errors; careful study of errors can help to identify the parts of the process that should be changed or improved.

In an evaluation of BCMA use and the types of workarounds that users create, Koppel and others[8] were able to group the workarounds into three general categories:
1. Omission of process steps
2. Steps performed out of sequence
3. Unauthorized process steps
Analysis of the probable causes of these workaround categories identified five distinct issues that contributed to use of workarounds:
Technology-related causes: issues related to the BCMA application or hardware itself. For example, if the nurse must

pass the scanner over the patient or medication bar code several times before scanning is successful, or if there are frequent equipment failures, the system may be perceived as delaying or complicating medication delivery rather than enhancing it.

Task-related causes: issues related to the users workflow. For example, if the nurses are accustomed to routinely discarding drug packaging before bringing the medication to the bedside, and the bar code is located on the packaging, the nurses will have to change practice to avoid delays and rework (e.g., to retrieve the discarded package).

Organizational causes: issues related to inadequate policies, training, staffing or other areas that are governed at an organization level. For example, if the unit dose provided is consistently too large for every pediatric patient, and the nurse must always draw up a tiny fraction of that unit dose, then each time the drug is used there is an opportunity for imprecision in drug dosing or overdose.

Patient-related causes: issues related to patient level logistics. For example, if the patient's barcode is not accessible (e.g., patient is draped for a sterile procedure), providers will perform overrides or workarounds.

Environmental causes: issues related to the logistics of space, positioning, and location of key items necessary to use BCMA technology. For example, if there are insufficient bar code scanners available for the pediatric critical care unit, or if the medication cabinet and the scanners are stored in different places so that the nurse spends a great deal of time getting the medication and finding a bar code scanner, then these issues will delay medication delivery and complicate the nursing workflow.

Overall, the use of BCMA technology has great potential to improve the safety of medication administration. The effects of the safety improvements and the effects on clinical workflow and outcomes continue to be evaluated.

ELECTRONIC CLINICAL DOCUMENTATION

Many institutions are transitioning clinical documentation from the traditional paper medical record to an electronic system. Critical care units have moved to computerized charting well ahead of other in-hospital units. The large amount of monitoring data and the frequency of recording needed has provided the impetus for the move to electronic solutions.

A key benefit of electronic documentation is that the clinical team has access to charted data for review and analysis away from the bedside. This benefit is only realized if the bedside provider uses the computerized system efficiently to ensure timely data entry and appropriate communication of changes in the clinical scenario.

Traditional nursing documentation relied on narrative documentation. The transition to electronic systems will force a change in this documentation style. The shift in approach can create anxiety, confusion, and frustration. With computerized documentation solutions the nurse's clinical observations, treatment applications, and patient assessments are distributed into multiple data fields and separate documents in the electronic record; they no longer tell a story in narrative form.

The benefit of the computerized approach is that specific data elements are easier to find, and the system can manipulate the data elements for more effective data display and for analysis through the use of data queries. The electronic system should take advantage of this latter feature rather than attempt to retain the narrative form and force large amounts of free text into comment fields.

It is challenging to strike the right balance between data standardization and effective communication; this requires a thoughtful institutional approach. Implementing electronic documentation exposes the variability in nomenclature and standards among different groups of providers. If existing documentation patterns are simply translated into the electronic tools without standardization, the tools will contain many different methods of describing clinical findings, with little structure or definition. As an extreme example, one institution included 18 potential color choices to describe urine.

Excessive variability among users and providing too many choices within the data base will have a negative effect on communication. The system will be difficult for the clinician to navigate, and it will accumulate large amounts of data that will be difficult to analyze or use effectively. Communication will be more efficient and effective if data standards are created and adopted by all clinicians.

Just as in the use of CPOE for providers, electronic documentation can prompt completeness in charting by nurses (Fig. 23-6). In both the CPOE and electronic documentation, prompts must be used judiciously to minimize disruptions and support effective clinical communication, documentation, and workflow. Effective use of forcing functions requires titrating disruptions to their level of importance for clinical care. Forcing functions should be reserved to prompt entry of data that is essential either for the safety of the patient or to fulfill a regulatory requirement that all agree is a priority.

In clinical settings where charting requires frequent entry of the same data (e.g., ventilator settings in the critical care unit), many charting systems allow for the previously charted value to be automatically populated into the data field currently being charted. This feature can substantially reduce data entry time for the provider and is often touted as a key feature to improve adoption. The negative effect of this feature rests with a tendency toward inadequate review or confirmation when the clinician's time is at a premium. If the feature is used without sufficient checking, the data fields can be populated with values that do not correlate with the patient's clinical status. This same problem can arise when vital sign data are imported from clinical monitoring systems into electronic charting systems. The clinical staff should validate the data to avoid importing values that are clearly erroneous. It is important to continually educate staff about the process of documentation and the pitfalls to avoid. Audits can help to determine the need for additional staff education.

The use of electronic clinical documentation systems is expanding. The administrative and clinical leadership knowledge of these systems is improving. Balancing the user experience and the logistics of computerized documentation is becoming easier as technology advances.

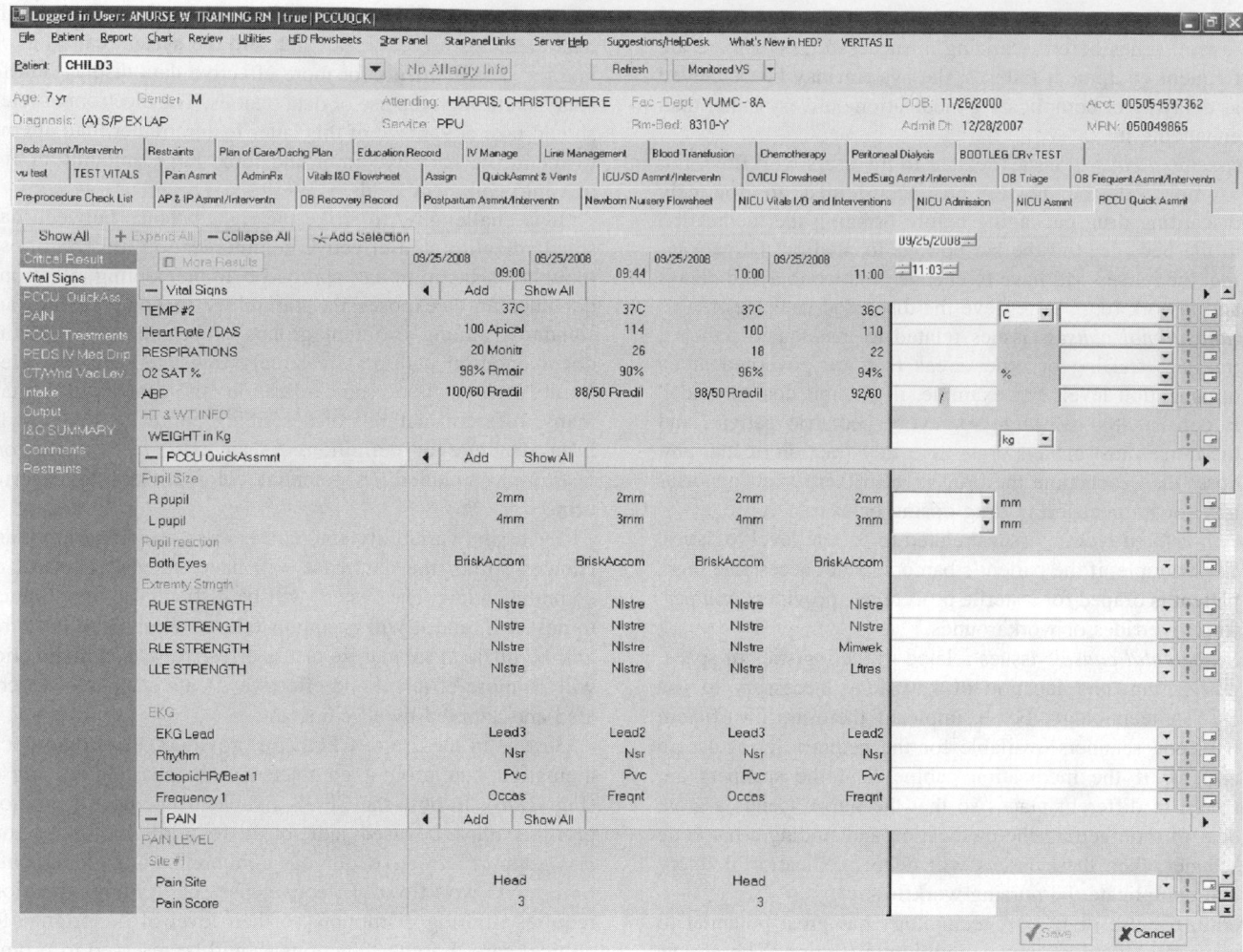

FIG. 23-6 Sample view from a nursing documentation system. Software, Horizon Expert Documentation, McKesson Provider Technologies, Atlanta, Georgia.

SUMMARY

Clinical care will continue to change with the introduction of IT. Quality of nursing care for critically ill children is dependent on the effective use of such technology and seamless integration of IT into clinical workflow. The greater the nurses' skill with the technology and the clinical care processes, the better the systems can facilitate delivery of good clinical care.

References

1. Bates DW, et al: Incidence of adverse drug events and potential adverse drug events. Implications for prevention. ADE Prevention Study Group. *J Am Med Assoc* 274:29–34, 1995.
2. Del Beccaro MA, et al: Computerized provider order entry implementation: no association with increased mortality rates in an intensive care unit. *Pediatrics* 118(1):290–295, 2006.
3. Han YY, et al: Unexpected increased mortality after implementation of a commercially sold computerized physician order entry system. *Pediatrics* 116(6):1506–1512, 2005. Erratum in: *Pediatrics* 117(2):594, 2005 Feb.
4. Karsh BT: Beyond usability: designing effective technology implementation systems to promote patient safety. *Qual Saf Health Care* 13(5):388–394, 2004.
5. Kaushal R, et al: Medication errors and adverse drug events in pediatric inpatients. *J Am Med Assoc* 285(16):2114–2120, 2001.
6. Ko Y, et al: Practitioners' views on computerized drug-drug interaction alerts in the VA system. *J Am Med Inform Assoc* 14(1):56–64, 2007.
7. Koppel R, et al: Role of computerized physician order entry systems in facilitating medication errors. *J Am Med Assoc* 293 (10):1197–1203, 2005.
8. Koppel R, et al: Workarounds to barcode medication administration systems: their occurrences, causes, and threats to patient safety. *J Am Med Inform Assoc* 15(4):408–423, 2008.
9. McGlynn EA, et al: The quality of health care delivered to adults in the United States. *N Engl J Med* 348(26):2635–2645, 2003.
10. Miller RA, et al: The anatomy of decision support during inpatient care provider order entry (CPOE): empirical observations from a decade of CPOE experience at Vanderbilt. *J Biomed Inform* 38(6):469–485, 2005.
11. Potts AL, et al: Computerized physician order entry and medication errors in a pediatric critical care unit. *Pediatrics* 113(1 Pt 1):59–63, 2004.
11a. Starmer JM, Pinson CW, Lorenzi NM: Informatics and evidence-based medicine: prescriptions for success. In Safran C, Retl S, Marin H, editors: *MedInfo 2010: partnerships for effective health solutions, 13th world congress on medical and health informatics,* Amsterdam, 2010, IOS Press.
12. The Institute of Medicine: *To err is human: building a safer health system,* Washington, DC, 1999, National Academy Press.
13. Upperman JS, et al: The introduction of computerized physician order entry and change management in a tertiary pediatric hospital. *Pediatrics* 116(5):e634–e642, 2005.

Internet Resources

American Nursing Infomatics Association: http://www.ania.org.
The Healthcare Information and Management Systems Society: http://www.himss.org.
The Leapfrog Group: http://www.leapfroggroup.org.
U.S. Department of Health and Human Services, Agency for Healthcare Research and Quality: http://www.healthit.ahrq.gov.
U.S. Department of Health and Human Services, Health Information Technology: http://www.healthit.hhs.gov.

Ethical Issues in Pediatric Critical Care

24

Ronald M. Perkin

PEARLS

- The practice of medical ethics seeks to identify and resolve competing moral claims among patients, their families, healthcare professionals, healthcare institutions, and society at large.
- Appeals to rights, such as the right of conscience, might not resolve a dispute.
- Legal considerations provide a general framework for decision making, but rarely provide a definitive answer to complex ethical questions. The law typically represents the floor, not the ceiling, of standards of morality.
- The creation of an ethical working environment in the pediatric critical care unit is a necessary precondition for addressing ethical issues raised by specific patient situations.
- The primary focus in decision making should be the interests of the child.
- Care for the critically ill child must be centered on the family.
- Informed consent is a process, not an event, and it has four key requirements: competency, disclosure, understanding, and voluntariness.
- Minors may be legally empowered to make their own decisions if they are deemed emancipated by state law or determined to be a mature minor by a judge.
- Pediatric critical care professionals should refrain from speaking about withdrawal of care. Although treatments may be withdrawn, care is never withdrawn. Care can be redirected from a focus on cure to a focus on comfort.
- The satisfaction of the patient, family, and provider may all be endangered when information is poorly delivered.
- Any medical treatment, including nutrition and hydration, can be withheld or withdrawn.

DEFINING MEDICAL ETHICS

Medical ethics is the discipline devoted to the identification, analysis, and resolution of value-based problems that arise in the care of patients.[29] The discipline is unique only because it relates to the particular dilemmas that arise in medicine, not because it embodies or appeals to some special moral principles or methodology. The practice of medical ethics seeks to identify and resolve competing moral claims among patients, their families, healthcare professionals, healthcare institutions, and society at large.

The terms *morality* and *ethics* are often used interchangeably, but most philosophers draw a distinction between the two. Morality consists of social norms of behavior that often vary among cultures. The discipline of ethics involves the development of philosophic reasons for or against a set of moral judgments. Usually the latter effort attempts to articulate and justify principles that form the foundation for rules of conduct and decision making in the face of competing moral claims.

Sources of Moral Guidance

Everyone draws on multiple sources of moral guidance, including parental and family values, cultural traditions, and religious beliefs. These sources are the roots of moral values, and they create a disposition to do the right thing. However, for many reasons these values and beliefs do not provide sufficient guidance for addressing dilemmas in clinical ethics.[50]

First, personal moral values might not address important issues in clinical ethics. Often nurses are first confronted by difficult ethical issues during education or clinical practice. Personal moral values might also offer conflicting advice on a particular situation; nurses may hold several fundamental beliefs that are in conflict. A nurse may want to alleviate the suffering of a dying infant while also respecting the sanctity of life. When nurses or other healthcare providers encounter a dilemma in clinical ethics, it is not a reflection of character or background.

The nurse's personal values and beliefs may not be sufficient to guide a dilemma in clinical ethics, because nurses have role-specific ethical obligations that go beyond their obligations as a good person. Finally, to resolve ethical dilemmas in patient care, nurses need to persuade others of their plan or recommendations, and this may require generating a consensus or compromise. Healthcare workers, patients, and family members may have different religious or cultural backgrounds than those of the patient. Clinical ethics analyze the reasons that justify a particular course of action. People can be persuaded by cogent arguments, and people with different world views can reach agreement in specific cases.

Occasionally, individuals may explain their actions as a matter of conscience: to act otherwise would make them feel guilty or ashamed or violate their sense of wholeness or integrity. Conscience involves self-reflection and judgment about whether an action is right or wrong.[9] Conscience thus arises from a fundamental commitment or intention to be moral. It unites the cognitive, conative, and emotional aspect of the moral life by a commitment to integrity or moral wholeness.[80] It is a commitment to uphold one's deepest self-identifying moral beliefs; a commitment to discern the moral features of a particular case as best one can, and to reason morally to the best of one's ability; a commitment to emotional balance in one's moral decision-making; and a commitment to make decisions according to one's moral ability and to act upon what one discerns to be the morally right course of action.[80]

In general, deeply held claims of conscience should be honored; it would strip persons of their moral agency to compel them to act in ways that violate their sense of integrity and responsibility. Claims of conscience, however, might not always resolve a dispute. Other people might cite their own conscience as a countervailing argument. Occasionally, one can believe that an act is morally wrong when it is actually permissible and vice versa.

Individuals often appeal to rights, such as a right to healthcare, to explain positions on ethical issues. To philosophers, rights are justified claims that a person can make on others or on society.[9] The language of rights is widespread, but an appeal to rights is often controversial. Other people might deny that the right exists or assert conflicting rights. Claims of rights are often used to end debates; however, the crucial issue is whether persuasive arguments support the existence of the right.[50]

Moral principles offer general values to guide us in making practical choices; several have become important focal points for discussions in medical ethics. The principle of beneficence instructs the promotion of people's well-being and nonmaleficence—to avoid harming people. The principle of distributing justice directs a fair allocation of goods, benefits, and services among those in a group, whereas the principle of social utility guides the promotion of the greatest good for the greatest number of people in a society. The principle of autonomy or self-determination prescribes that a person act to foster personal responsibility and plan his or her life to develop abilities and opportunities to flourish.

It is a mistake to suppose that moral principles simply prescribe what to do or require uniform action and conformity. First, because they are stated abstractly, they must be interpreted or specified[35]; this is done by making practical moral judgments, leaving considerable room for interpretation and disagreement from person to person or from culture to culture, even among those who agree on the importance of these principles. Second, because principles can conflict in a given situation, they sometimes have to be ranked, and people can reasonably disagree about how to do this justifiably.

Medical ethics then involve deliberation and explicit arguments to justify particular actions in specific situations. Ethics focus on the reasons why an action is considered right or wrong and asks individuals to justify their positions and beliefs by rational arguments that can persuade others.

Clinical Ethics and the Law

Through statutes, regulations, and decisions in specific cases, the law can provide guidance about what healthcare professionals can or cannot do. Therefore physicians and nurses should be familiar with the law regarding issues in clinical ethics; however, the law cannot provide definitive answers to specific ethical dilemmas. Law and ethics may conflict, and many people might regard some actions that are prohibited by law to be ethical. Similarly, some actions that are legally acceptable may not be seen as ethically permissible. In such conflicts, most healthcare professionals feel uncomfortable about simply following the letter of the law.

CLINICAL ETHICS AS AN AID TO NURSING CARE

Learning about clinical ethics can help nurses identify, understand, and resolve common ethical issues in pediatric critical care. By studying published cases, healthcare workers can gain experience in resolving specific dilemmas.[35,50] By studying cases that illustrate common ethical problems, nurses can better recognize the ethical issues they encounter. On many issues, healthcare professionals, philosophers, and the courts agree on what should be done. Clinical ethics can help to identify actions that are clearly right or wrong and those that are controversial. Subsequent sections of this chapter and information in the Chapter 24 Supplement on the Evolve Website will highlight areas of ethical agreement as well as those areas of ongoing controversy.

A systematic approach to ethical dilemmas helps to identify important considerations and fosters consistency in decisions. Clinical ethics is a practical discipline that provides a structural approach to decision making that can assist the healthcare team in identifying, analyzing, and resolving ethical issues in clinical practice.[35] Box 24-1 lists key steps to take when approaching an ethical dilemma that needs to be clarified, analyzed, and resolved.

CREATING AN ENVIRONMENT THAT SUPPORTS ETHICAL PRACTICE

On a daily basis nurses, physicians, and other members of the pediatric critical care healthcare team are faced with maintaining the delicate balance between the application of complex technological care and humane, ethical care for the critically ill pediatric patient.[74] Ethical considerations in the pediatric critical care unit often involve moments of crisis marked by disagreement over decisions, such as whether to resuscitate a patient; to withhold or withdraw "futile" treatment over a patient's or family's objections; or to allocate

---

Box 24-1 **Approach to Ethical Dilemmas**

- Identify and define the problem. Determine whether there are different ways to view the problem.
- Collect and evaluate data:
  - What is the clinical situation?
  - What is the most current and relevant data?
  - How good is the data?
- Identify the options.
- Identify potential consequences of the different options.
- Determine the policies, laws, rights, duties or values that are important. If there is conflict, which carries the most moral weight?
- Negotiate for a solution to the problem. What are the weaknesses of the solution? Is the solution consistent and universal?
- Implement the solution and evaluate the response.

limited or expensive resources, such as extracorporeal membrane oxygenation or the last pediatric critical care unit bed.

The expansion of technology combined with awareness of biologic, economic, and ethical limits to applying that technology can lead to uncertainty and conflict when it appears that providers are unable to restore a patient to the patient's previous state.[59] To address these complex issues, the pediatric critical care unit team must recognize and address the ethical issues that exist each and every day in interactions with families, patients, and fellow workers. The creation of an ethical working environment in the pediatric critical care unit is a necessary precondition for addressing ethical issues involved in cardiopulmonary resuscitation, the limitation or withdrawal of life-sustaining treatment, and conflicts in medical decision making.

An ethical work environment fosters early identification of ethical dilemmas; provides resources for ethical decision making; promotes open communication among all members of the healthcare team, including patients and families; and promotes collaborative relationships. Without a supportive, ethical environment, the healthcare system will likely cause moral distress, work dissatisfaction, and a lack of collaboration that will undermine quality patient care.

The American Association of Critical Care Nurses has recognized the inextricable links among quality of the work environment, excellent nursing practice, and patient care outcomes. The American Association of Critical Care Nurses is also committed to creating work and care environments that are safe, healing, humane, and respectful of the rights, responsibilities, needs, and contributions of all people, including patients, their families, and nurses. Six standards for establishing and sustaining healthy work environments have been identified (Box 24-2).[5]

Although the key elements are neither detailed nor exhaustive, they provide a foundation for thoughtful reflection and engaged dialogue about the realities of each work environment. Because of the interdependence of a healthy work

---

| Box 24-2 | **Key Elements for Establishing and Sustaining Healthy Work Environments** |

- Skilled Communication—Nurses must be as proficient in communication skills as they are in clinical skills.
- True Collaboration—Nurses must be relentless in pursuing and fostering true collaboration.
- Effective Decision Making—Nurses must be valued and committed partners in making policy, directing and evaluating clinical care, and leading organizational operations.
- Appropriate Staffing—Staffing must ensure the effective match between patient needs and nurse competencies.
- Meaningful Recognition—Nurses must be recognized and must recognize others for the value each brings to the work of the organization.
- Authentic Leadership—Nurse leaders must fully embrace the imperative of a healthy work environment, authentically live it and engage others in its achievement.

From American Association of Critical Care Nurses: AACN standards for establishing and sustaining healthy work environments: a journey to excellence. *Am J Crit Care* 14:187-197, 2005.

---

environment, clinical excellence, and optimal patient outcomes, adoption of these six key elements helps to optimize quality care and patient safety. These six elements are also crucial steps to ensure solid reflection on ethical dilemmas present in the pediatric critical care unit.

A frequent ethical problem in the acute care setting is a difference of opinion among the healthcare team and often involves disputes between and a nurse and a physician.[27,59,74] Such conflicts typically involve a nurse disagreeing with a physician concerning ethical issues such as the extent or invasiveness of treatment, when to stop treatment, and when not to attempt resuscitation in the event of a cardiac or respiratory arrest. In order to create an environment that supports ethical practice, a shift from a chain-of-command relationship to interdisciplinary care is required. An interdisciplinary approach seeks to blur professional boundaries and requires trust, tolerance, and a willingness to share responsibility.[74] The challenge in the pediatric critical care unit is to develop and sustain organizational and structural changes that reflect an ethical practice environment, making routine the collaborative and communicative strategies that ethical issues often require.

HOW ARE ETHICAL ISSUES IN PEDIATRICS DIFFERENT?

Children Are Different

Children are smaller than adults. This fact is obvious, but the practical and ethical implications are substantial. "The child's small size can contribute to the child's feeling intimidated by adults, even if unintentionally. Adults must physically look down at children, and children unavoidably must look up at adults. The world is largely designed for adults; so although adults sit down, children must climb up. These simple physical facts both establish and illustrate the relative imbalance of power, influence, and authority between children and adults."[10]

The relatively greater dependence and relatively lower autonomy of children present complex ethical challenges when clinical care is provided to children. Customary ethical principles of autonomy and informed consent can be different in pediatric applications. Common ethical principles such as beneficence and "do no harm" often are more multifaceted and less straightforward. Treatment objectives expressed by parents or other child caretakers can be different from the child's goals.

Healthcare professionals are ethically compelled to respect and integrate the child's expressed wishes, the parents' expressed outcomes, the child's maturational needs, and the family's cultured beliefs about family roles and child-rearing practices. Such considerations bring new ethical considerations and challenges to treatment (Box 24-3).

Children are inherently more vulnerable than most adults. Healthcare professionals have even more responsibility for ensuring ethical action than they would have with adult patients. Nurses are in a unique position to identify situations in which parental decisions or a child's actions jeopardize a child's health and well-being. Healthcare professionals are given special responsibilities in these situations because if they do not intervene, children might suffer serious, longlasting harm.

Box 24-3 **Caring for Children: Core Ethical Issues**

- Children are inherently more vulnerable than adults.
- Children's abilities are more variable and change over time.
- Children are more reliant on others and their environment.
- Ethical principles and practices in the treatment of adults must be modified in response to the child's current developmental abilities and legal status.
- Healthcare professionals must develop skills to work with families, agencies, and systems.
- Healthcare professionals must maintain an absolute commitment to the safety and well-being of the child.
- Although young children are not autonomous, their potential autonomy deserves respect.
- The primary focus in decision making should be the interests of the child.
- Healthcare professionals must constantly monitor one's own actions and motivations.
- Healthcare professionals must seek consultation and advice in difficult situations.
- Children should be given the protection of privacy.
- All persons with decisional capacity, regardless of age, have the right to make healthcare treatment decisions.

Modified from: Belitz J, Baley RA: Clinical ethics for the treatment of children and adolescents: a guide for general psychiatrists. *Psychiatr Clin N Am* 32:243–257, 2009.

Because children cannot weigh risks and benefits, compare alternatives, or appreciate the long-term consequences of decisions, they are incapable of making informed decisions. As a result, autonomy is less important in pediatrics than in adult medicine. A child's objections to beneficial medical interventions do not have the same ethical force as an adult's informed refusals. Because children are immature and vulnerable, they need an adult to make decisions for them and to protect their best interests. Parents are presumed to be the appropriate decision makers.[2]

Children must be protected from the consequences of their own unwise decisions or those of others. Indeed, it is tragic if a child dies or undergoes serious harm because a simple, effective medical treatment was not provided.

Although young children are not autonomous, their potential autonomy as future adults deserves respect. Parents influence children and shape their behavior and values, and parental values deserve great deference. However, when children reach maturity they might choose values that differ from those of their parents. Healthcare professionals may need to help ensure that parental decisions are not contrary to those of the developing young adult.

As children mature, they become capable of making informed decisions, and their involvement in care should increase. Pediatric critical care unit professionals need to provide the child with information about his or her condition and opportunities to participate in decisions about healthcare, to the extent that it is developmentally appropriate.[2]

Children also differ from one another. In a very real way, there is no such category as "children."[10] Infants differ from toddlers, who differ from preschoolers, who differ from school-aged children and adolescents. Furthermore, within any group of children there is wide variability in size, ability, psychosocial development, cognitive development, and maturity. Many children develop inconsistently in physical, cognitive, emotional, social, and moral abilities and characteristics. The individual child may progress and regress in the face of various challenges and traumas, being "childish" one day and a "young lady" or "young man" the next. Children manifest much broader developmental and individual variability than do adults. Consequently, pediatric critical care unit professionals must tailor their approaches and care to the individual state and abilities of each pediatric patient. The child's ability to engage in particular aspects of care, including its ethical aspects, or to move toward particular goals of treatment can vary with the child's immediate developmental abilities, themes, challenges, and tasks.[10]

The Family Is the Patient

Care for the critically ill child must be family-centered.[76] Family-centered care is an approach to healthcare that shapes healthcare policies, programs, facility design, and day-to-day interactions among patients, families, physicians, and other healthcare professionals. Healthcare professionals who practice family-centered care recognize the vital role that families play in ensuring the health and well-being of children and family members of all ages. These practitioners acknowledge that emotional, social, and developmental support are integral components of healthcare. They respect each child's and family's innate strengths and view the healthcare experience as an opportunity to build on these strengths, and the providers support families in their caregiving and decision-making roles. Family-centered approaches lead to better health outcomes and wiser allocation of resources as well as greater patient and family satisfaction.[4]

Family-centered care in pediatrics is based on the understanding that the family is the child's primary source of strength and support and that both the child's and the family's perspectives and information are important in clinical decision making. Family-centered practitioners are keenly aware that healthcare experiences can enhance parents' confidence in their roles and, over time, increase the competence of children and young adults to take responsibility for their own healthcare, particularly in anticipation of transition to adult service systems.

Given that the family is the child's primary source of strength and that the family's perspectives are important in clinical decision making, the pediatric critical care unit team has a moral obligation to the patient's family and a duty to increase family access to the pediatric critical care unit. Increased access to the pediatric critical care unit has also resulted in more reports of parental presence during bedside pediatric critical care unit rounds, complex procedures, and cardiopulmonary resuscitation.[16,23,63,68] All patient care units should develop written documentation for presenting the option of family presence during cardiopulmonary resuscitation (CPR) and invasive procedures. Education programs should be developed for healthcare staff to include: the benefits of the family's presence for the patient and the family, criteria for assessing the family, the role of the professional assigned as the family support person, family support methods, and contraindications for family presence.

Family meetings—when pediatric critical care unit professionals and family members join together to engage in a dialogue and devise a plan of action—are a mainstay of pediatric critical care unit clinical practice. Often the focus of these meetings is developing a consensus regarding the goals and plan of care, and they can help everyone assess the situation and participate in the development of that plan. Collaborative communication builds the foundation on which pediatric care of the highest possible quality can be created. It serves as the key factor in the solution of most ethical dilemmas.

MEDICAL DECISION MAKING

Consent or Permission from Parents or Guardians

"Parents or guardians usually have the authority to give consent or permission for their child's healthcare and participation in research. Reasons for this social policy include, first, that parents in general have the greatest knowledge about, and interest in, the well-being of their own minor children."[40] Another well-recognized reason that parents have legal authority to make these and many other decisions for their minor children is that parents or guardians must address the consequences of the choices being made. Clinicians should generally try to respect the parents' preferences because of the importance parents play in fostering the child's well-being and shaping the child's values.[40]

Parental consent, like other consents obtained in a medical setting, must be adequately informed. That is, the parent giving consent must be provided with sufficient information to understand and authorize the treatment that has been recommended. Clinicians need to reveal all information they know or should know that would be regarded as important to the parents making the decisions. Those seeking consent, for example, should provide parents with information about the diagnosis and prognosis, so that the parents understand the disease process. Reasonable alternative treatment options should also be explained, along with the nature, duration, side effects, or potential harms or benefits of the alternative options. Parents also should be told the likely consequences of no treatment. Clinicians should then test for understanding of the information, for example, by asking the parents questions about what was discussed or asking the parents to explain the procedure or treatment in general terms.

The person who gives consent must have the capacity to make decisions. The terms competent and incompetent are often reserved for legal contexts. Courts can make a determination about whether someone is competent. The presumption is that adults are legally competent and minors are not. Minors—in most parts of the United States this includes those younger than 18 years—are regarded as incompetent to make decisions about their own healthcare, especially if the decisions are momentous.[40] The reality is that many adults lack decision-making capacity, but have not been declared legally incompetent in the courts, and many legally incompetent minors have good decision-making capacity. Thus, the legal notion of competence and that of decision-making capacity should be distinguished.[40]

For the purposes of healthcare, the term *decision-making capacity* refers to an individual's ability to understand information needed to make informed consent, evaluate this information in terms of stable personal values, and use and manipulate the information in a reasonable manner.[40] For important decisions, clinicians should assess how well those giving the consent can understand the information, deliberate, and make and defend choices. It also is important that those giving consent communicate choices appropriately. These details should help clinicians decide whether parents or older minors have the capacity to make important healthcare decisions.

Consent, assent, or permission also must be given freely (i.e., voluntarily), meaning that it must not be coerced or manipulated. The fact that the parents may be distraught does not make them legally incompetent or unable to give consent. If parents are not competent or are making an inappropriate decision, clinicians may have a legal and moral duty to seek a court order so that the courts can authorize the needed intervention.

Informed consent or permission should have the following elements[40]:

1. All information or material important to the decision has been disclosed.
2. Those giving consent comprehend or understand the information that has been disclosed.
3. Those giving consent voluntarily agree to participate.
4. Those giving consent are competent to make a decision to participate.
5. Those giving consent agree to the procedure, act, intervention, or research.

In some cases informed consent can be waived, as in medical emergencies, public health emergencies, or when parents cannot be contacted.

Parents giving consent or permission should be guided by what is in the best interest of their child. Their decisions can be challenged, for example, if they endanger the child. The best interest of the child standard is one of four important standards for medical decision making; the other three are self-determination, advance directive, and presumed consent.[40] Although the best interest of the child standard is of special importance in pediatrics, each of the four standards has a role in making healthcare decisions for minors.

Assent and Self-determination

Self-determination, as a standard for healthcare decision making, applies to competent adults and to many older or emancipated minors (Table 24-1). This standard of self-determination presupposes that the person is autonomous or capable of self-determination, has informed understanding, and makes the choices voluntarily. The standard honors the basic moral principles mentioned previously; it flows from the moral principle of autonomy or self-determination and honors individual liberty; and it enables people to make choices about themselves, assess their own best interest, and develop their own capacities and life plans as they wish, as long as they do not harm others.[40]

Although the law grants full competence on the occasion of a specific birthday (e.g., 18 years of age), this practical and useful legal practice fits poorly with medical decision making. In medicine, it is more useful to view capacity as a matter of degree, and less like the "light-switch" concept found in

Table 24-1   **Glossary of Terms Related to Adolescent Medical Care**

Term	Definition
Assent	To give clear agreement, used in connection with a child's or adolescent's agreement to treatment or research participation when consent is not possible because the individual has not yet achieved adult status (see *Consent* below, which in its narrow sense can be given only by competent adults)
Bright line	Clear distinction that solves a matter in dispute in law
Capacity	Individual's ability to understand facts and consequences of a decision, communicate a choice, and appreciate the effects of that choice and alternatives; a status that is in flux and evolving in adolescents; a clinical determination that is context-sensitive
Competency	Ability to understand facts and consequences; in law, related to definitive criteria (e.g., age of majority, after which legal adulthood is attained, with the presumption of competence)
Consent	Voluntary agreement freely made without coercion or duress, and with adequate knowledge (informed); as strictly construed, can be given only by a competent adult, or in certain limited circumstances, by emancipated or mature minors; grounded in ethical principle of respect for autonomy and patient self-determination
Emancipation	Condition by which a minor is recognized as an adult for legal purposes; often triggered by certain events (e.g., marriage, military service, childbearing) or under certain conditions (e.g., adolescent living alone and financially supporting self)
Ethical	Addresses what a clinician should or should not do based on moral guiding principles; not limited to legal mandate, although often tied to certain legal rules and professional codes
Legal	Addresses what a clinician can or cannot do based on state, federal, and local laws and regulations (required; legal sanctions may follow a breach)
Mature minor	Consent authority related to context-sensitive and specific situations, or conditions in which an adolescent demonstrates a mature capacity to make decisions related to healthcare

Modified from Campbell AT: Consent, competence and confidentiality related to psychiatric conditions in adolescent medicine practice. *Adolesc Med* 17: 25-47, 2006.

the law.[40] In both law and medicine, young children are the paradigm of persons unable to make decisions for themselves. Infants are among the many incompetent and vulnerable, but minors just before the age of majority are as competent as many adults. Most young children lack the capacity, maturity, experience, or foresight to make important decisions for themselves and to determine which decisions promote their well-being and opportunities. As children gain maturity, many seek to understand important healthcare decisions being made for them, and older children may have strong opinions about their care.[12,25,82,85,87]

To acknowledge the child's emerging capacities and point of view, and to promote the child's well-being, clinicians seek the child's assent in addition to parental permission when possible.[2,40] Healthcare providers may seek the assent or agreement of children as young as 7 years. As minors become increasingly mature and competent, they should be accorded more self-determination. Children with life-threatening or chronic illnesses, for example, may want to participate in discussions and decisions about their care and find that it is a way to gain control and respect.[82] Ignoring their desires to participate can cause pain, isolation, misunderstanding, and frustration.

Assent is different from consent, because the minor's preferences need not be honored in the same way as those of adults.[40] Whether a minor's preference should be honored can depend on the probability and magnitude of the harms involved and the irreversibility of the consequences. When children cannot enhance their own well-being and opportunities, adults may have to override their decisions and not grant self-determination. The obligation to honor their wishes is not as binding as it would be for an adult.

"In many parts of the world, adults who face serious illness or death are not privy to conversations about their care, because family and clinicians believe that it is kinder to exclude them."[40] Such cultural conflicts about how to apply the principles of beneficence and nonmaleficence have the potential to cause serious problems when people travel from one country to another seeking medical care, or when patients or families from other countries receive healthcare in the United States. For example, older adolescents with serious illness may indicate a desire to discuss their prognosis and options with the medical team, while family members strongly object to telling the adolescent. Clinicians can help family members understand the importance of including the child, explaining to the family members that children understand a good deal about their diseases and even imminent death and that excluding them increases their suffering.[40] Of course, some guardians remain adamant, and clinicians may have to choose between doing what they believe is best for the patients (by informing them) and honoring parental wishes. Other clinicians find that consultations with an ethics committee can help to resolve such conflicts.

The recognition that older children can understand a great deal and be competent to participate in many decisions has been recognized recently in the literature and in social policy.[17,40] As children grow older, they are increasingly able to discuss and participate in health decisions relating to them. Some adolescents have gained authority to make healthcare decisions independently of their parents. Depending on state law, adolescents can get medical care such as contraceptives, contraceptive information and devices, abortions, and treatment for substance abuse without parental permission (i.e., legal emancipation by condition).[17]

The ideal situation is to have shared decision making and agreement among clinicians, family, and the child about what course to take. In the ordinary situation, however, parents or guardians have the authority to make decisions for the child's medical care, just as for religion and schooling, unless they endanger the child. The child's assent has been found to be increasingly important based on evidence that children with serious, chronic, or life-threatening illnesses understand a great deal and benefit from participating.[2] In addition, the importance of their assent stems from understanding that they have the competence to make important contributions to these discussions.

Age of Consent: The Mature Minor in Law

State legislation increasingly recognizes that a "light-switch" ("bright line," or purely age-related) rule regarding who is an adult may not be appropriate (see Table 24-1).[17,82] Greater flexibility is emerging in legal interpretations that allow adolescents, although they are not legal adults, to make certain healthcare decisions. One path leading to adolescent consent authority follows case (common) law, in which courts have given specific meaning and scope to adolescents being sufficiently mature (i.e., the mature minor) to provide consent to treatment.[17] This determination is subjective and is based on a case-sensitive analysis, dependent not only on the adolescent involved but also on the adolescent's condition and the risks of treatment versus no treatment.

Perhaps the clearest guideline for the mature minor doctrine came in a Tennessee Supreme Court case that established the "Rule of Sevens": (1) a minor under the age of 7 years lacks capacity; (2) a minor between 7 and 14 years of age is presumed not to have capacity, but that assumption can be rebutted (the burden is on the minor to show capacity); and (3) a minor 14 years of age or older is presumed to have capacity (the burden is on the one arguing against capacity).[18] This rule was acknowledged to be case-sensitive and not a strict standard. As reiterated by a prominent legal authority, a minor's consent should be effective if he or she is "capable of appreciating the nature, extent and probable consequences of the conduct consented to (e.g., medical treatment)," even if parental consent is "not obtained or is expressly refused."[17]

States have codified a range of situations in which sufficiently mature minors can make their own healthcare decisions, providing exceptions to the rule of parental permission for certain healthcare conditions or based on the status of the minor.[17] These statutes respond to clinician and patient concerns that a desire to seek care of a more sensitive nature (e.g., mental health or family planning services) might be impeded by a requirement for parental permission.[30]

The distinction between a mature minor and an emancipated minor has become blurred over time. Generally, mature minor consent authority relates to context-sensitive and specific situations, or conditions in which an adolescent demonstrates capacity to make decisions related to healthcare (Box 24-4), whereas emancipation represents a progression into adulthood linked with certain events that are viewed as conferring adult status. However, clinicians with specific questions are urged to consult local legal authorities for guidance.

Box 24-4	Minors as Healthcare Decision Makers: Characteristics Of Mature Minor For Healthcare

- Has experienced the illness for some time
- Understands the illness and the benefits and the burdens of treatment
- Has the ability to reason and has previously been involved in decision making about the illness
- Has a comprehension of death recognizing its personal significance and finality

Adapted from Leikin S: A proposal concerning decisions to forgo life-sustaining treatments for young people. *J Pediatr* 115:17-22, 1989.

Advance Directives and Substituted Judgment

Advance directives are used in framing healthcare decisions when the person has become incapacitated. These directives are statements made by the person who has decision-making capacity, stating how decisions should be made when they are unable to make decisions. Adults and some older children may have such directives in order to extend their control over events. Competent adults can use living wills or powers of attorney for healthcare to make known their views about how decisions should be guided and who should make decisions for them. In rare cases, minors can decide that they wish to make their views known.[40] Although such decisions are not as controlling as those of legally competent adults, they can be morally binding. "Sometimes parents and children disagree about the sort of treatment that is appropriate at the end of life, with each making what the other regards as an inappropriate request. Whenever possible, clinicians should give the requests of the older minor serious consideration and seek a consensus among the family."[40]

Substituted judgment is another rarely used standard for minors in making medical decisions, because the standard applies to those who were once able to express their views, when no advance directives were created. The standard instructs others to use their understanding of the person's views to select the option that they think the individual would have selected. Minors who are extremely sick may have expressed preferences that they hope will guide people, and such requests should receive deference if possible.

EXCEPTIONS TO PARENTS AS DECISION MAKERS

As a rule, the law protects the natural rights of parents to raise children free from unwarranted state interference, presuming that parents will act in the best interests of their children. Accordingly, parents are allowed considerable latitude for medical decisions on behalf of their children, even if the choices may not concur with the physician's recommendation. These rights are conditional on parental fulfillment of the duty to provide necessary care for minor children. Even more important than parental rights are parental responsibilities. If parents fail to provide their children with at least a minimum standard of medical care, the state can assert its interest in protecting the welfare of children by involving child protection statutes to override parental wishes.

Courts regularly uphold such interventions when parental refusals may be life threatening, even when the refusals are genuinely motivated by strong family convictions. However, when the consequences for the child are grave but not life threatening, states have differed in their willingness to intervene, reflecting the continuing struggle to balance the rights of individual children and those of family privacy. Many state child protection statutes include exemptions for parents who seek nontraditional forms of treatment based on religious convictions, although the American Academy of Pediatrics has urged states to repeal such provisions. It must be emphasized that the central principal guiding decisions should reflect the best interests of the child and not mere parental preference.

Informed Refusal of Care

Families who decline medical care for a child present the pediatric critical care unit team with an ethical dilemma: respect for the autonomy and privacy rights of the family and the importance of familial support for any therapeutic endeavor are in conflict with the duty to provide the best available care for the pediatric patient.[69] The validity of parental consent for children has been taken for granted, although the presumption that parents invariably choose in their child's best interests may at times be inaccurate. Rights are virtually never absolute and parents are not at liberty to destroy, maim, or neglect their children. The parents' authority can be contested if the parents place their children at serious risk, such as by refusing to permit the critical care team to provide life-saving interventions to a child. The pediatric critical care unit team's response to the parents' refusal of treatment will depend on the clinical circumstances, the benefits and the burdens of treatment, and the child's wishes in some cases.[24]

Parents may refuse interventions that have limited effectiveness, impose significant side effects, require chronic treatment, or are controversial. In such situations the parents' informed refusals should be decisive.[51] Refusal of such interventions might be ethically permissible even if the patient's life expectancy might be shortened.

Parents sometimes refuse treatments for life-threatening conditions, although these treatments are highly effective in restoring the child to previous health, are short term, and have few side effects.[7] It has been suggested that parents might refuse a medical recommendation for at least three categories of reasons: neglect, disagreement based on religions or other values, or inability to comply.[46] Jehovah's Witnesses commonly refuse blood transfusions for their children even when the child has suffered life-threatening hemorrhage or anemia. Similarly, Christian Scientist parents often refuse antibiotics for bacterial meningitis. Physicians who are unable to persuade parents to accept such interventions should seek a court order to administer the treatment.[52,70] A court order is important because it signifies that society believes that the parent's refusal is unacceptable.[51] As one court declared, although "parents may be free to become martyrs themselves," they are not free to "make martyrs of their children."[67]

The American Academy of Pediatrics recognizes the "important role of religion in the personal, spiritual, and social lives of many individuals and cautions physicians and other healthcare professionals to avoid unnecessary polarization when conflict over religious practices arise. Nevertheless, professionals who believe that the parental religious convictions interfere with appropriate medical care that is likely to prevent substantial harm, suffering or death should request court authorization to override parental authority or, under circumstances involving imminent threat to a child's life, intervene over parental objections."[3]

Frequently, the most difficult dilemmas arise when parents refuse interventions that are highly effective in serious illness but also highly burdensome, such as bone marrow transplantation in acute lymphocytic leukemia or combination chemotherapy in advanced cancers such as testicular carcinoma. In these situations, the child's preferences might be important. If an older child or adolescent makes an informed decision to undergo such treatment, the pediatric critical care unit team should support that decision.

If parents continue to refuse such therapy after repeated attempts at persuasion, some physicians seek court orders to compel treatment. In doing so, physicians need to account for the effects on long-term parental cooperation with the child's care. At the least, physicians should listen to the parents' objections and show respect for the parents' opinions and the ongoing responsibility of the parents for the child.

Child's Refusal of Care

In some cases children might refuse effective treatments. The physician's response should be determined by the seriousness of the clinical situation, the effectiveness and side effects of treatment, the reasons for the child's refusal, the parents' preferences regarding treatment, and the burdens of insisting on treatment. It is difficult to force adolescents to take ongoing therapies, such as insulin shots for diabetes or inhalers for asthma. The most constructive approach is to try to understand the patient's reasons for refusal, address them, and provide psychosocial support. In several cases adolescents have run away from home rather than accept cancer chemotherapy, which has significant side effects.[82] Because it is physically difficult and morally troubling to force such treatment on adolescents, these refusals have been accepted, particularly when the parents have supported the child's refusal. Sound ethical practice requires pediatric critical care unit professionals to respect the dignity of each adolescent patient by hearing and understanding the patient's discussion of values and expressed concerns about medical treatment.[82]

Baby Doe Rules

The Federal Child Abuse Amendments of 1984 and subsequent regulations, commonly called *Baby Doe Regulations,* apply to decisions to withhold medical treatment from disabled infants younger than 1 year[60]; they limit the circumstances in which interventions may be withheld.

Under these regulations, treatment other than "appropriate nutrition, hydration, or medication"[60] need not be provided if (1) the infant is chronically and irreversibly comatose; (2) the provision of such treatment would merely prolong dying, not be effective in ameliorating or correcting all of the infant's life-threatening conditions, or otherwise be futile in terms of the survival of the infant; or (3) the provision of such treatment would be virtually futile in terms of the survival of the infant, and the treatment itself under such circumstances would be inhumane. The regulations note that decisions to withhold medically indicated treatment might not be based on subjective opinions about the child's future quality of life. In addition, hospitals are encouraged to establish ethics committees, specifically infant care review committees, to advise physicians in difficult cases.

The Baby Doe Regulations have been sharply criticized.[42,43] Many terms, such as *appropriate* and *futile*, are subject to conflicting interpretations. Most importantly, parents are not included in decision making despite their customary role as surrogates. The pediatric critical care unit team should appreciate that these regulations do not require them to provide treatment that, in their judgment, is inappropriate or futile.[42]

Inappropriate Care Requests

At times, parents may request the pediatric critical care unit team to provide care that is useless or inappropriate. The pediatric critical care unit team has a duty to refuse requests that are illegal or that can cause harm, based on the moral principles of nonmaleficence. In addition, the team has a social duty to conserve resources and not provide costly, futile, or excessively burdensome interventions. The question of when treatments are futile may be disputed among families or among healthcare professionals.

Parents may request inappropriate treatment for a number of reasons (Box 24-5). Many requests for inappropriate interventions are the result of miscommunications.[40] Some of these miscommunications are embedded in social, ethnic, or religious differences. In some cases, families have unrealistic expectations, believe "everything must be done," or are "waiting for a miracle." Guilt and denial also may play a role in these irrational and unreasonable requests.[40] Clinicians should show great sensitivity and patience in helping families come to terms with a diagnosis or prognosis.

In some cases, families have a general mistrust of the healthcare system; this mistrust may appear to be vindicated

Box 24-5	**Potential Reasons That Parents Request Inappropriate Care**

- Denial of death
- Belief in miracles
- Avoidance of helpless feelings
- Religious beliefs
- Unique goals
- Guilt
- Influence of a relative or friend
- Parental disagreement
- Inadequate information
- Not enough time to digest information
- Inconsistent or contradictory information
- Distrust of healthcare providers
- Lack of confidence in medical diagnosis or prognosis
- Belief that more can be done
- Secondary gain

by an unexpected and bleak prognosis.[40] The family's request for inappropriate treatment may be an expression of this mistrust. It is sometimes helpful to include someone whom the family can trust, such as a minister or family member with a healthcare background, who can help the family understand. In rare cases, the disagreement is truly a value disagreement in which family members may, for example, see maintaining someone in a persistent vegetative state as a positive value, whereas the clinicians do not. In these and other cases, healthcare professionals should maintain professional integrity and personal morality, but may find other clinicians willing to accept the families' decisions. Substantial literature[15,29,69,40] exists on how to respond to such situations, when to override parental requests, and the dangers of using decisions about what treatments are futile as mechanisms for rationing healthcare.

In general, it is important for the pediatric critical care unit professional to remember that most demands for inappropriate interventions are likely to be the result of poor communication and inadequate understanding. The pediatric critical care unit team must spend the time necessary to approach the specific ethical dilemma (see Box 24-1). Discussion with an ethics committee or an ethics consultant may help clarify the facts and points at issue and return the child to the central role, a role sometimes lost during heated disagreements.

ETHICS OF COMMUNICATION

The ethical dimensions of communication are expressed in the relationships that healthcare providers develop with their patients, society, and ultimately themselves.[31] Society expects that patients will be treated with honesty and with respect for their autonomy. For pediatric patients who cannot speak for themselves, parents will be sought to address the best interests of the child. Depending on the relevant cognitive development of the child, however, his or her understanding and voice will be sought, whether it is to allow for information and education, to acquire individual assent, or to obtain real informed consent. All of these measures reflect the principle of respect, generally characterized in the adult setting as respect for autonomy.

The satisfaction of the patient, family, and provider may all be endangered when information is delivered poorly. The ethical dimensions of patient-provider communication represent the principles of beneficence, nonmaleficence, autonomy, justice, and utility. Their practical application is represented in the four domains of veracity (truth-telling), privacy, confidentiality, and fidelity.[31]

Truth-Telling

Codes of medical ethics have traditionally ignored the obligations and virtues of veracity. The Hippocratic oath does not address veracity, nor does the Declaration of Geneva of the World Medical Association. As recently as 1980, the Code of Medical Ethics of the American Medical Association made no mention of veracity or truth-telling as either an obligation or a virtue, giving physicians unrestricted discretion about what to disclose to their patients; this changed in the 1997 edition of the code.[6]

In medicine, there is a long and distinguished tradition of providing less than the whole (unvarnished) truth.[36,47,48] In *The Silent World of Doctor and Patient,* Katz shows that, from the time of Hippocrates until the late twentieth century, doctors routinely withheld the truth from patients and vigorously defended the morality of their decisions to do so.[36] The arguments for withholding the truth varied. Some of the arguments were centered on the patient, arguing that the truth might be too difficult to bear. "Reassure the patient and declare his safety, even though you may not be certain of it," wrote Isaac Israeli, a ninth-century physician, "for by this you will strengthen his Nature."[36] Other arguments focused on the physician and his moral obligation to foster hope. Thomas Percival, writing in the late eighteenth century, counseled doctors, "The physician should be the minister of hope and comfort to the sick."[36] Some of the arguments were economic, contending that doctors who admitted uncertainty would frighten and discourage patients and would soon go out of business. None of the arguments were apologetic.[47]

Following this ancient moral tradition, doctors learned to withhold potentially stressful information, to conceal bleak diagnoses, and not to discuss the risk of treatments or procedures. In doing so, doctors were following the moral maxim of either saying nice things or saying nothing at all.

In light of this history, recent moral sentiment that the physician should tell the patient the truth—the whole truth, no matter how horrible it might be or how ill-prepared the patient might be—represents one of those mysterious changes in morality that occur from time to time, whereby something that was once thought morally intolerable is suddenly thought of as morally obligatory.[47] When noting such a moral watershed, it is important to ask why the change occurred. Generally, it is not that morality itself changes. Instead, historical circumstances change so that people must react differently to new situations and reevaluate conventional moral wisdom.[47]

There are many reasons for the changes in attitude toward truth telling among physicians.[31] Such reasons may include the availability of more treatment options, improved rates of survival, fear of malpractice suits, involvement of multiple team members in hospitals, altered societal attitudes about medicine in general, greater attention to patients' rights, and increased recognition by physicians that communication is an effective means of enhancing patient understanding and compliance with healthcare.[31]

The obligation of veracity is based on the respect owed to others and is therefore rooted deeply in the principle of respect for patient autonomy.[2,31,48] This obligation is the primary justification and basis for rules of disclosure in informed consent. The obligation of veracity exists even when consent is not an issue, and it is the guiding precept of the duty of respect toward others. Veracity is closely related to the obligations of fidelity and promise keeping.

When any two parties communicate, there is an implicit promise that both will speak truthfully and that they will not deceive each other.[31] A patient becomes part of a contract, or a covenant, by entering into the therapeutic relationship. Although children may not legally be allowed to enter into formal contracts independent from their parents or guardians, the implied promise remains important. Such a contract includes the patient's right to have his or her wishes respected regarding diagnosis, prognosis, and treatment procedures. Cultural beliefs may affect the patient's wishes, as might limitations on a family's desire for full disclosure and informed consent.

Discerning the patient's and family's wishes can require experience, skill, listening, and time. In this truth-telling process, the health professional also expects to gain the right to truthful disclosures from the patient. Relationships between healthcare professionals and the patients and their parents ultimately depend on communication and trust. With respect to children, such dependence can be frustrating; although children are generally more honest and forthright than adults, they may act to protect their parents.[31]

There are certain culture-specific situations in which adult patients prefer not to receive complete information about their diagnosis and prognosis. Whether these feelings hold true for the children from these cultures has not been formally studied. Respect for autonomy suggests that cultural factors must be represented when considering disclosure to patients. Pellegrino warns against the use of assaultive truthfulness, suggesting that to "thrust the truth on a patient who expects to be buffered against news of impending death is a gratuitous and harmful misinterpretation of the moral foundations for respect for autonomy."[62]

Parents of children and adolescents occasionally request that the physician not disclose a diagnosis or prognosis to the young patient. Such a request creates an ethical dilemma for the practitioner; the conflict between a duty to respect the parents' wishes and a duty to tell the truth to the child.[78]

The authority of parents to direct the flow of information to the child and to organize and provide appropriate systems of emotional support is well recognized in pediatric care. Parents are regarded as moral agents for their children; pediatricians perceive that the integrity of the patient's family is necessary to sustain and nurture the child. Still, parental authority cannot be absolute. A "best interest" standard that extends beyond parents' wishes is recognized in nontreatment decisions for severely ill neonates and children, in the treatment of children whose parents have religious objection to usual care, and in the confidential care of adolescents.[78]

If there is a moral justification for lying to the patient or willfully hiding the truth, it must have a strength that overrides the principle of veracity derived from basic human respect. People deserve to be told the truth, and circumstances must be morally persuasive when considering deviating from this basic moral duty.[31] One must ask whether concealing the diagnosis, not using the name of the disease, and not speaking to the child about prognosis will do more harm than good.

A related subject to truth-telling is the disclosure of medical error. This discussion is included in the Chapter 24 Supplement on the Evolve Website.

Confidentiality

The importance of confidentiality in medical practice has been acknowledged since ancient times.[41] Respecting patients' confidentiality usually promotes the moral principle of beneficence or the patients' best interest. If patients are assured of confidentiality, they are more likely to be candid. Moreover, because privacy is what each of us wants for ourselves, it is only just to extend it to others. In addition, it is fair to adopt this policy of respecting confidentiality because, in a sense, patients own the information about themselves, and confidentiality honors their privacy and rights to control this information. If some information about the patient is released, such as a genotype for a late-onset genetic disease, it has the potential to cause harm through discrimination, labeling, or loss of self-esteem.

The social utility of respecting patients' confidentiality is also acknowledged in policies allowing physicians to avoid testifying about patients' revelations to them in healthcare settings. Confidentiality can be as important for minors as it is for adults. Minors, for example, may seek medical care as a safe haven to express how they have been intentionally injured or exploited.

Concerns about confidentiality create a major barrier to effective healthcare for many adolescents.[13] Adolescents are more likely to seek healthcare and to disclose personal information when they believe that the information will be kept confidential.

The clinician's duty to maintain confidentiality, however, is not absolute. The presumption in favor of confidentiality can be overruled if there is a greater duty at stake or if there is a recognized exception.[41] For example, an exception to the duty to maintain confidentiality is to protect a third party, as in intentional injury to children. If clinicians suspect that someone is abusing a child, they have a legal and moral duty to override confidentiality because a greater duty—the duty to protect the child—is present. In addition, there may be a duty to override confidentiality if there is a need to protect a patient from himself or herself; there may be such a duty if the minor is suicidal. There also may be a duty to protect the community that is greater than the duty to maintain someone's confidentiality, such as a duty to report communicable diseases or gunshot wounds, regardless of the patient's wishes.[41]

Breaking Bad News

Although breaking bad news is difficult and stressful for everyone, being uninformed is even more stressful for patients and families.[14,31] One of the most common complaints of patients and families is the lack of accuracy, clarity, and consistency in the information provided.[31] Family members indicate a willingness and desire to receive bad news as long as it is empathetically communicated.[31]

The diagnosis and prognosis associated with chronic conditions often provide confirmation of what was already suspected, so confirmation of the diagnosis frequently provides relief and reduction of anxiety. Reactions to bad news in the setting of an acute event are much more dramatic. In either case, accurate information allows a shifting of the goals of medical intervention and allows the patient, family and friends the support and opportunity to adjust to the new information. Effective and compassionate communication may even allow a child to be discharged from the critical care unit to die at home, or to die in a more private area of the hospital.

Sometimes, in response to their own pain, medical caregivers communicate the news of a bad prognosis in a brief encounter and may use technical terms to soften the blow, avoid the conversation altogether, or wait until the child is unconscious. Research on breaking bad news does not support the use of these techniques. Further discussion of this important topic is covered in Chapter 3.

WITHHOLDING AND WITHDRAWING THERAPY

Advances in pediatric critical care medicine have led to ethical issues of profound concern to all pediatric intensivists and nurses. One of the most striking developments in the past several years is that most children admitted to a pediatric critical care unit die after a decision is made to withhold or withdraw life-sustaining treatments.[21,26,81,83] It is important that all healthcare professionals in the pediatric critical care unit be competent in end-of-life decision making and palliative care.

The decision to forgo life-sustaining treatment is made for up to 60% of terminally ill children[83]; 80% of the deaths that occur in the neonatal critical care unit are preceded by decisions to limit, withhold, or withdraw life support.[39] Faced with decisions that challenge the very essence of the parenting role, parents of children in the pediatric critical care unit for whom withdrawal of life support has been recommended need to hear assurances that the healthcare team has not made the recommendation lightly.

The decision making at the end-of-life in the pediatric critical care unit is a dynamic process.[26] Certainly, there must be acknowledgment of the value of the child and the child's life, and acknowledgement of the sorrow of lifelong pain that such decisions evoke for parents.[28] Parents also need to be assured that their child will not suffer and that all efforts will be made to control symptoms and allow the family to be with the child as much as desired and feasible. Pediatric critical care unit professionals must refrain from speaking about "withdrawal of care." Although treatments may be withdrawn, care is never withdrawn. Care may be redirected from a focus on cure to a focus on comfort.

Despite extensive literature covering the ethical and legal aspects of withdrawal of therapy, little attention has been given to determining the optimal methods to withdraw it.[72] Despite the lack of data on optimal management of some aspects of withdrawing life-sustaining treatments, a consensus exists regarding the ethical and clinical principles that should guide this care (Box 24-6).

Box 24-6	**Principles of Withdrawing Life-Sustaining Treatments**

- The goal of withdrawing life-sustaining treatments is to remove treatments that are no longer desired, no longer beneficial, or do not provide comfort to the patient.
- Withholding life-sustaining treatments is morally and legally equivalent to withdrawing them.
- Actions whose sole goal are to hasten death are morally and legally problematic.
- Any treatment can be withheld or withdrawn.
- Withdrawal of life-sustaining treatment is a medical procedure.

Modified from Rubenfield GD: Withdrawing life-sustaining treatment in the intensive care unit. *Respir Care* 45:1399-1407, 2000.

Understanding that the goal of withdrawing life-sustaining treatments is to remove unwanted treatments rather than to hasten death is essential in clarifying the distinction between active euthanasia (providing drugs or toxins that hasten death) and death that accompanies the withdrawal of life support in the pediatric critical care unit. There is no doubt that withdrawing unwanted life-sustaining treatments, compared with continuing them, will hasten death; however, ethicists draw a line between withdrawing life-sustaining treatments when the expected but unintended effect is to hasten death and providing a treatment with the sole intent of hastening death.

The withdrawal of life-sustaining treatments is a clinical procedure, and it merits the same meticulous preparation and expectation of quality that pediatric critical care unit professionals provide when they perform procedures to initiate life support. Recommendations for the steps pediatric critical care unit professionals could take when withdrawing life-sustaining therapy are provided in the Chapter 24 Supplement on the Evolve Website.

By providing a familiar framework to guide clinical practice and by proposing a protocol for the procedure, we hope to improve the quality of care to patients at the end of life. The Chapter 24 Supplement on the Evolve Website also includes information about withdrawing life-sustaining treatment in children with inflicted trauma and special considerations in the care of the dying adolescent.

The Do-Not-Attempt-Resuscitation (DNAR) Order

The do-not-attempt-resuscitation (DNAR) order is often the focal point for controversy surrounding limitations in life-sustaining treatments. DNAR orders are unique. They are the only physician's order that is focused exclusively upon what will not be done, rather than what will be done.

The concept of doing less than everything possible to preserve the life of the patient is not new. The Hippocratic corpus advises physicians "to refuse to treat those who are overmastered by their diseases, realizing that in such cases medicine is powerless."[15] Even the earliest researchers in the field of resuscitation recognized that CPR should be used only in circumstances of reversible cardiac arrest. Unfortunately, no clear criteria exist for determining when cardiac arrest is irreversible.

In the absence of any clear guidelines for withholding CPR, by the early 1970s CPR was widely regarded as a mandatory procedure for any patient experiencing a cardiorespiratory arrest. Physicians practicing in hospitals therefore faced a dilemma; clearly it was wrong to perform CPR on patients who were imminently dying of a terminal disease, yet there was little precedent in medicine for allowing patients to die when procedures were available that might prolong life, even if only for a brief period of time.

Over the past 30 years, DNAR orders have become increasingly accepted, such that the Joint Commission requires healthcare institutions to have DNAR policies. More recently, however, it has become evident that a simple DNAR order fails to address the complexity of decision making for terminally ill patients.

In most hospitals, DNAR orders are written by the attending physician in the doctor's orders sheets. These orders are often vague and can leave substantial opportunity for miscommunication and error. Does "attempted resuscitation" refer to treatment of an acute cardiac arrest (intubation and ventilation, chest compressions, cardioversion, and medications), or does it also include "do not intubate" conditions such as respiratory failure from a pneumonia? Should patients with DNAR orders receive hand ventilation and suctioning for airway secretions, be treated with antibiotics, or given tube feedings? Should they be excluded from admission to the critical care unit, or denied palliative surgery? The answers to these questions are almost never clear in the interpretation of a simple DNAR order.

In response to these concerns, many institutions have adopted procedure-specific DNAR orders. This approach is intended to reduce much of the ambiguity surrounding DNAR orders. The greatest advantage of the procedure-directed DNAR order is its clarity. This type of order must be supplemented with a detailed note in the chart explaining the justifications for the order and documenting the discussions between the clinicians and the patient or surrogate. By focusing on procedures, the form addresses in concrete terms exactly what will or will not be done in the event of a cardiorespiratory arrest. For example, Mittelberger and others[56] found that the number of ambiguous DNAR orders was decreased from 88% to 7% after implementation of a procedure-specific DNAR order form. Two other studies have also documented improved communication among physicians and nurses after adopting procedure-specific DNAR order forms.[32,61]

DNAR replaced the older term *do not resuscitate* (DNR).[57] DNAR presupposes that there is no guarantee that resuscitation attempts are going to be successful. This shift in terminology arose partly in response to the realization that the general public had a falsely optimistic perception of the success of resuscitation. The term DNAR is not, however, specific enough to stand alone; it also requires specific orders.[57]

Another controversy concerns whether it is necessary for physicians to obtain the consent for DNAR orders from the patient or the patient's family.[11,79] Many hospitals address this issue in internal hospital policies.[54] Some hospitals, however, have adopted policies that permit physicians to write DNAR orders without the permission, or sometimes without the knowledge, of the patient or family. The presumption behind this approach is the view that CPR is a medical therapy and that physicians are uniquely qualified to determine whether and when a medical therapy is indicated. These policies are often referred to as *CPR-not-indicated policies*.[84]

However, this development in DNAR orders should be viewed with caution. Physicians have a long history of seeing complex situations from a uniquely medical perspective, ignoring important factors related to the patient's values and preferences. Rarely is the question of whether to perform CPR purely a medical issue. Often the patient's or family's denial of impending death can be overcome by proper counseling, whereas simply using the physician's authority to overrule the family's wishes can be profoundly destructive to the patient-physician relationship.

There has been a recent call to modify the standard terminology further and replace the term DNAR with the term *allow natural death* (AND).[38,57] Rather than emphasizing that something is being withheld, AND focuses on the benefits of allowing a natural process to take place. Although it initially seems to be a mere semantic issue, medical centers that have changed the terminology report easier conversations with patients and families about response to the end of life.[57] It must be acknowledged that in the highly technologic environment, such as the pediatric critical care unit, the concept of "natural" death is rendered virtually meaningless.[20]

Not surprisingly, patients with DNAR orders often believe they have been abandoned by their caregivers. Indeed, it is often the case that physicians do in fact spend less time caring for patients who have DNAR orders. This is not appropriate, as patients with DNAR orders often need more attention in terms of aggressive palliative care than patients who are not imminently dying (see Chapter 3).

In addition, DNAR orders tend to be concerned with only a small fraction of the issues that arise with dying patients. Often the question of whether resuscitation should be attempted is actually peripheral to the more important questions surrounding the use of less dramatic interventions.

In discussing resuscitation, the pediatric critical care unit professional must remember that DNAR does not connote *do not respect*. By empathetic and compassionate communication, resuscitation decisions can be made that are right for the patient and the patient's quality of life.

Withdrawal of Medically Provided Nutrition and Hydration

During the last two decades there has been a gradual consensus emerging in both law and ethics that medical nutrition and hydration can be withheld or withdrawn by the same standards that apply to other life-sustaining treatments. Specifically, it can be withheld or withdrawn after an analysis of the balance between the benefits and burdens of providing the therapy.[22,34,49,53,58,66,77]

Whereas this consensus has achieved wide acceptance among healthcare professionals caring for adult patients, professionals who care for children have been more reluctant to accept this approach.[34,44,49] Decisions about the technologic administration or withdrawal of nutrition and hydration from a terminally ill child are among the most ethically troublesome that pediatric healthcare professionals face. Part of the reason for this difficulty may be the view that nutrition and feeding is such a basic and fundamental aspect of the care provided to children.

Providing food is deeply symbolic of nurturing, caring, and commitment in the human experience.[44] The dilemma centers on whether food and fluids, provided by gastric and enteral tubes or parenteral administration, preserves life or prolongs death. Expert opinions range across the spectrum: from the belief that withholding or withdrawing food and fluids is active euthanasia to a perspective that administered nutrition and hydration will increase the dying persons' discomfort and only delay the inevitable. Despite the fact that artificial nutrition and hydration is viewed by a majority of the U.S. Supreme Court[44] as medical therapy that may be withheld, it is administered to a significant number of terminally ill patients.

During the course of an illness, a patient often loses the ability to receive, desire, or require nutrition or hydration by natural means. When a patient can no longer receive food and fluids normally, artificial nutrition or hydration are medical treatments that can benefit the patient by helping the patient to maintain proper nutrition and fluid and electrolyte balance. Because inadequate nutrition and hydration can result in death, artificial nutrition and hydration can also benefit the patient by supporting life. On the other hand, artificial nutrition or hydration can sometimes cause harm to the patient. Although healthy people feel hunger when they are deprived of food and thirst when they are deprived of fluids, patients who are dying may no longer feel hunger and thirst. During the body's natural dying process, the body starts to shut down and the patient may lose the desire for food or fluids. Because artificial hydration and nutrition may cause harm to the patient, feeding a dying patient can sometimes do more harm than good.

Clinical experience, validated by research, has demonstrated that imminently dying persons experience loss of appetite and a natural process of dehydration. Organ systems function less efficiently until they fail, and the desire to eat and drink is lost.[44] Clinical observations of hospice patients' final stages indicate that most terminally ill patients do not experience hunger and often exhibit isotonic dehydration. Benefits from end-stage dehydration include the release of endogenous opioids and the analgesic affect of ketosis.[44] There is decreased urine output, diminishing incontinence; lessened edema, decreasing the risk of pressure ulcers; and reduced pulmonary and gastric secretions, relieving congestion, coughing, and vomiting.[44] With total parenteral nutrition, the adverse effects of fluid overload, local bleeding and infection, and sepsis may be significant and shorten life while diminishing its quality.

Oral feedings by mouth, to the extent possible, are a part of comfort care for the imminently dying patient, but in most cases the aggressive use of parenteral nutrition or feeding tubes is not. The benefits are outweighed by undue burdens and complications when measured against quality of life.

Some healthcare providers may be concerned that withholding or withdrawing artificial nutrition or hydration is the same as starving a patient, but this is usually not the case in a patient who is dying. When a dying patient, or his or her surrogate decision maker, decides to forgo artificial nutrition or hydration, the patient's disease is the cause of death. From a medical perspective, withholding or withdrawing artificial nutrition or hydration from a dying patient is no different from the decision to forgo any other medical treatment, such as mechanical ventilation, which may prolong death.

Artificial nutrition and hydration are medical treatments that have no necessary connection to caring. Patients who are not receiving artificial nutrition or hydration may still be provided with adequate care. The medical and nursing staff can still provide a great deal of palliative care for the dying patient that does not involve the administration of artificial nutrition and hydration.

The American Academy of Pediatrics has recently concluded that the withdrawal of medically administered fluids and nutrition for pediatric patients is ethically acceptable in limited circumstances.[22] As always, when particularly difficult or controversial decisions are being considered, consultation with experts in ethics is strongly recommended.

THERE IS A COST OF CARING

The pediatric critical care unit is a stressful environment because of high patient acuity, morbidity and mortality, daily confrontations with ethical dilemmas, and a tension-charged atmosphere.[1] The cumulative effect on the pediatric critical care unit professional can include significant caregiver suffering.[55,65,71,73] Several concepts—burnout, compassion fatigue, moral distress and posttraumatic stress disorder (PTSD)—are related to the concept of caregiver suffering.

Burnout is "a state of physical, emotional, and mental exhaustion caused by long-term involvement in emotionally demanding situations."[64] Burnout syndrome has been identified in a high percentage of pediatric critical care unit nurses and nursing assistants.[65] Burnout syndrome emerges gradually and is the result of emotional exhaustion and job stress. In contrast, compassion fatigue is characterized by a sense of helplessness, confusion, and isolation from supporters, which can have a more rapid onset and resolution than burnout.[73]

After exposure to a traumatic event, individuals with PTSD experience symptoms of persistent recollections, avid reminders of the events, and have symptoms of increased arousal.[86] Critically ill patients, adult and pediatric, who survive their hospitalization can have symptoms of PTSD.[19,33,37,75] In addition, a high percentage of family members of pediatric critical care unit patients report PTSD symptoms.[8,45,55] Critical care nurses have also been reported to have PTSD symptoms.[55]

Moral distress occurs when an individual is unable to translate his or her moral choice into action.[73] As previously mentioned, acting in a manner contrary to personal or professional values undermines the individual's sense of integrity. When healthcare professionals cannot live up to their personal values by acting in an ethical manner, their suffering is compounded by moral distress.[73] Caregiver suffering takes a toll on the individual healthcare professional and on the workplace, causing decreased productivity, more sick days, and higher nursing turnover.[55]

Recommendations for protecting pediatric critical care unit professionals from the cumulative and complicated effects of caregiver suffering include three tiers of strategies: personal, professional, and organizational.[71] In caring for the caregivers, the challenge for healthcare organizations lies in developing respect and care for their employees in the same way that they require their employees to care for patients. Further information regarding signs, symptoms, and treatment of caregiver suffering can be found in the Chapter 24 Supplement on the Evolve Website.

References

1. Acker KH: Do critical care nurses face burnout, PTSD, or is it something else? Getting help for the helpers. *AACN Clin Issues Crit Care Nurs* 4:558–565, 1993.
2. American Academy of Pediatrics, Committee on Bioethics: Informed consent, parental permission, and assent in pediatric practice. *Pediatrics* 95:314–317, 1995.
3. American Academy of Pediatrics, Committee on Bioethics: Religious objections to medical care. *Pediatrics* 99:279–281, 1997.
4. American Academy of Pediatrics, Committee on Hospital Care: Family-centered care and the pediatrician's role. *Pediatrics* 112 (3):691–696, 2003.
5. American Association of Critical Care Nurses: AACN standards for establishing and sustaining healthy work environments: a journey to excellence. *Am J Crit Care* 14(3):187–197, 2005.
6. American Medical Association, Council on Ethical and Judicial Affairs: *Code of Medical Ethics: current opinions with annotations,* Chicago, 1997, American Medical Association.
7. Asser SM, Swan R: Child fatalities from religion motivated medical treatment. *Pediatrics* 101:625–629, 1998.
8. Azoulay E, et al: Risk of post-traumatic stress symptoms in family members of intensive care unit patients. *Am J Respir Crit Care Med* 171:987–994, 2005.
9. Beauchamp TL, Childress JF: *Principles of biomedical ethics,* ed 4, New York, 1994, Oxford University Press.
10. Belitz J, Baley RA: Clinical ethics for the treatment of children and adolescents: a guide for general psychiatrists. *Psychiatr Clin N Am* 32:243–257, 2009.
11. Blackhall LJ: Must we always use CPR? *N Engl J Med* 317:1281–1285, 1987.
12. Bluebond-Langer M: *The private world of dying children,* Princeton, NJ, 1978, Princeton University Press.
13. Brindis C, et al: Adolescents' access to health services and clinical preventive health care: crossing the great divide. *Pediatric Annals* 31:575–581, 2002.
14. Buckman R: *How to break bad news: a guide for health care professionals,* Baltimore, 1992, Johns Hopkins University Press.
15. Burns JP, Truog RD: Ethical controversies in pediatric critical care. *New Horizons* 5:72–84, 1997.
16. Cameron MA, Schleien CL, Morris ML: Parental presence on pediatric intensive care rounds. *J Pediatr* 155:522–528, 2009.
17. Campbell AT: Consent, competence and confidentiality related to psychiatric conditions in adolescent medicine practice. *Adolesc Med* 17:25–47, 2006.
18. Cardwell v. Bechtol, 724 S.W.2d 739 (Tenn. 1987).
19. Colville G: The psychological impact on children of admission to intensive care. *Pediatr Clin N Am* 55:605–616, 2008.
20. Copnell B: Death in the pediatric ICU: caring for children and families at the end of life. *Crit Care Nurs Clin N Am* 17:349–360, 2005.
21. Deviator D, Latour JM, Tissieres P: Forgoing life-sustaining or death-prolonging therapy in the pediatric ICU. *Pediatr Clin N Am* 55:791–804, 2008.
22. Dickema DS, Botken JR: Clinical report: forgoing medically provided nutrition and hydration in children. *Pediatrics* 124 (2):813–822, 2009.
23. Dingeman RS, et al: Parent presence during complex invasive procedures and cardiopulmonary resuscitation: a systematic review of the literature. *Pediatrics* 120:842–854, 2007.
24. Fleishman AR, et al: Caring for gravely children. *Pediatrics* 101:625–629, 1998.
25. Freyer DR: Care of the dying adolescent: special considerations. *Pediatrics* 113(2):381–388, 2004.
26. Garros D, Rosychuk RJ, Cox PN: Circumstances surrounding end-of-life in a pediatric intensive care unity. *Pediatrics* 112:e371–e379, 2003.
27. Granulspacher GP, Howell JD, Young MJ: Perception of ethical problems by nurses and doctors. *Arch Intern Med* 146:577–578, 1986.
28. Greig-Midlane H: The parents' perspective on withdrawing treatment. *BMJ* 323:390–395, 2001.
29. Hardart GE, DeVictor DJ, Traog RD: Ethics. In Nichols DG, editor: *Rogers textbook of pediatric intensive care,* Philadelphia, 2008, Lippincott Williams & Wilkins, pp 180–194.
30. Hartman RG: Coming of age: devising legislation for adolescent medical decision-making. *Am J Law Med* 28:409–453, 2002.
31. Hays RM, et al: Communication at the end of life. In Carter BS, Levetown M, editors: *Palliative care for infants, children, and adolescents,* Baltimore, 2004, The Johns Hopkins University Press, pp 112–140.
32. Heffner JE, Barbieri C, Casey K: Procedure-specific do-not-resuscitate orders—effect on communication of treatment limitations. *Arch Intern Med* 156:793–797, 1994.

33. Hobbie WL, et al: Symptoms of post-traumatic stress in young adult survivors of childhood cancer. *J Clin Oncol* 18:4060–4066, 2000.

34. Johnson J, Mitchell C: Responding to parental requests to forego pediatric nutrition and hydration. *J Clin Ethics* 11:128–135, 2000.

35. Jonsen AR, Siegler M, Winslade WJ: *Clinical ethics: a practical approach to ethical decisions in clinical medicine,* New York, 1992, McGraw-Hill, Inc.

36. Katz J: *The silent world of doctor and patient,* New York, 1984, Free Press.

37. Kenardy JA, Spence SH, McLeod AC: Screening for post-traumatic stress disorder in children after accidental injury. *Pediatrics* 118 (3):1002–1009, 2006.

38. Knox C, Vereb JA: Allow natural death: a more humane approach to discussing end-of-life directives. *J Emerg Nurs* 31(6):560–561, 2005.

39. Kopelman AE: Understanding, avoiding and resolving end-of-life conflicts in the NICU. *Mount Sinai J Med* 73(3):580–586, 2006.

40. Kopelman LM: Ethical and legal issues. In Perkin RM, Newton DA, Swift J, Anas N, editors: *Pediatric hospital medicine: textbook of inpatient management,* Philadelphia, 2008, Lippincott Williams & Wilkins, pp 39–47.

41. Kopelman L: Confidentiality. In Perkin RM, Newton D, Swift J, Anas N, editors: *Pediatric hospital medicine: textbook of inpatient management,* Philadelphia, 2008, Lippincott Williams & Wilkins, pp 43–44.39.

42. Kopelman LM: Are the 21 year old Baby Doe Rules misunderstood or mistaken? *Pediatrics* 115:797–802, 2005.

43. Kopelman LM, Irons TG, Kopelman AE: Neonatologists judge the "Baby Doe" regulations. *N Engl J Med* 318:677–683, 1988.

44. Kyba FC: Legal and ethical issues in end-of-life care. *Crit Care Nurs Clin N Am* 14:141–155, 2002.

45. Landolt MA, et al: Post-traumatic stress disorder in paediatric patients and their patients: an exploratory study. *J Paediatr Child Health* 34:539–543, 1998.

46. Lantos JD: Treatment refusal, noncompliance, and the pediatrician's responsibilities. *Ped Ann* 18:255–260, 1989.

47. Lantos JD: Should we always tell children the truth? *Perspect Biol Med* 40(1):78–92, 1996.

48. Leiken S: An ethical issue in pediatric cancer care: nondisclosure of a fatal prognosis. *Pediatr Ann* 10(10):401–407, 1981.

49. Levi BH: Withdrawing nutrition and hydration from children: legal, ethical, and professional issues. *Clin Pediatr* 42:139–145, 2003.

50. Lo B: *Resolving ethical dilemmas: a guide for clinicians,* Philadelphia, 2005, Lippincott Williams & Wilkins, pp 4–9.

51. Lo B: *Resolving ethical dilemmas: a guide for clinicians,* Philadelphia, 2005, Lippincott Williams & Wilkins, pp 235–242.

52. Macklin R: Consent, coercion and conflict of rights. *Perspect Biol Med* 20:365–366, 1977.

53. McCann RM, Hall WJ, Groth-Juncker A: Comfort care for terminally ill patients: the appropriate use of nutrition and hydration. *JAMA* 272:1263–1266, 1994.

54. McClung JA, Kamer RS: Legislating ethics: implications of New York's do-not-resuscitate law. *N Engl J Med* 323:270–272, 1990.

55. Meader ML, et al: Increased prevalence of post-traumatic stress disorder symptoms in critical care nurses. *Am J Respir Crit Care Med* 175:693–697, 2007.

56. Mittelberger JA, et al: Impact of procedure-specific do-not-resuscitate order form on documentation of do not resuscitate orders. *Arch Intern Med* 153:228–232, 1993.

57. Morrison W, Berkowitz I: Do not attempt resuscitation orders in pediatrics. *Pediatr Clin N Am* 54:757–771, 2007.

58. Nelson RM: Ethics in the intensive care unit: creating an ethical environment. *Crit Care Clin* 13(3):691–701, 1997.

59. Nelson LJ, et al: Forgoing medically provided nutrition and hydration in pediatric patients. *J Law Med Ethics* 23:33–46, 1994.

60. Nondiscrimination on the basis of handicap; procedures and guidelines relating to healthcare for handicapped infants—HHS. Final rules. *Fed Regist* 50:14879–14892, 1985.

61. O'Toole EE, et al: Evaluation of a treatment limitation policy with a specific treatment-limiting order page. *Arch Intern Med* 154:425–432, 1994.

62. Pelligrino E: Is truth telling to the patient a cultural artifact? *JAMA* 268:1734–1735, 1992.

63. Phipps LM, et al: Assessment of parental presence during bedside pediatric intensive care unit rounds: effect on duration, teaching and privacy. *Pediatr Crit Care Med* 8:220–224, 2007.

64. Pines AM, Aronson E: *Career burnout: causes and cures,* New York, 1988, Free Press.

65. Poncet MC, et al: Burnout syndrome in critical care nursing staff. *Am J Respir Crit Care Med* 175:698–704, 2007.

66. Porta N, Frader J: Withholding hydration and nutrition in newborns. *Theor Med Bioeth* 28:443–451, 2007.

67. Prince v. Massachusetts, 321 U.S.; 158 (1944).

68. Pruitt LM, et al: Parental presence during pediatric invasive procedures. *J. Pediatr Health Care* 22:120–127, 2008.

69. Ridgway D: Court-mediated disputes between physicians and families over the medical care of children. *Arch Pediatr Adoles Med* 158(9):891–896, 2004.

70. Rosen P: Religious freedom and forced transfusion of Jehovah's Witness children. *J Emerg Med* 14:241–243, 1996.

71. Rourke MT: Compassion fatigue in pediatric palliative care providers. *Pediatr Clin N Am* 54:631–644, 2007.

72. Rubenfield GD: Withdrawing life-sustaining treatment in the intensive care unit. *Respir Care* 45(11):1399–1407, 2000.

73. Rushton CH: The other side of caring: caregiver suffering. In Carter BS, Levetown M, editors: *Palliative care for infants, children and adolescents,* Baltimore, 2004, The Johns Hopkins University Press, pp 220–243.

74. Rushton CH, Brooks-Brunn J: Environments that support ethical practice. *New Horiz* 5(1):20–29, 1997.

75. Schelding G, et al: Health-related quality of life and post-traumatic stress disorder in survivors of the acute respiratory distress syndrome. *Crit Care Med* 26:651–659, 1998.

76. Schexnayder SM, Bryant PHI, Fiser DH: The family is the patient. In Fuhrman BP, Zimmerman JS, editors: *Pediatric critical care,* St Louis, 1998, Mosby, pp 38–42.

77. Schwarte AM: Withdrawal of nutritional support on the terminally ill. *Crit Care Nurs Clin N Am* 14:193–196, 2002.

78. Sigman GS, Kraut J, LaPluma J: Disclosure of a diagnosis to children and adolescents when parents object: a clinical ethics analysis. *AJDC* 147:764–768, 1993.

79. Snider GL: The do-not-resuscitate order: ethical and legal imperative or medical decision. *Am Rev Respir Dis* 143:665–674, 1991.

80. Sulmasy DP: What is conscience and why is respect for it important? *Theor Med Bioeth* 29:135–149, 2008.

81. Tan GH, et al: End-of-life decisions and palliative care in a children's hospital. *J Palliat Med* 9(2):332–342, 2006.

82. Traugott I, Alpers A: In their own hands: adolescents refusal of medical treatment. *Arch Pediatr Adolesc Med* 151(9):922–927, 1997.

83. Vose LA, Nelson RM: Ethical issues surrounding limitation and withdrawal of support in the pediatric intensive care unit. *J Intensive Care Med* 14:220–230, 1999.

84. Waisel DB, Truog RD: The cardiopulmonary resuscitation-not-indicated order: futility revisited. *Ann Intern Med* 122:304–308, 1995.

85. Weir RF, Peters C: Affirming the decisions adolescents make about life and death. *Hasting Cent Rep* 27(6):29–40, 1997.

86. Yehunda R: Post-traumatic stress disorder. *N Engl J Med* 346:108–114, 2002.

87. Zawistowski CA, Frader JE: Ethical problems in pediatric critical care: consent. *Crit Care Med* 31(suppl 5), S407–S410, 2003.

Appendices

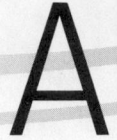

Continuous Infusion Dose Charts ("Drip Charts")

The following charts enable determination of the mcg/kg per minute dose provided by flow rates of 1 to 15 mL/h continuous infusion of drugs mixed to concentrations of 10, 200, 400, 500, 1000, and 1600 mcg/mL. The tables reflect the dose, rounded to the tenth of a decimal place.

The bedside nurse is responsible for drugs administered, so he or she must verify the dose given, even if the drugs are mixed by the pharmacy and administered through computerized infusion systems. The formula used to determine dose administered is:

$$\text{INFUSION RATE} \atop \text{mL/hour} = \frac{\text{WEIGHT(kg)} \times \text{DOSE} \times 60\,\text{min/hour}}{\text{CONCENTRATION}},$$

$$\text{Infusion Rate(mL/hour)} = \frac{\text{wt(kg)} \times \text{dose(mcg/kg per min)} \times 60\,\text{min/hour}}{\text{Concentration(mcg/mL)}}.$$

Drugs administered by continuous infusion are typically titrated to patient response. The goal of therapy is to maximize therapeutic effects while minimizing side and toxic effects. Although every effort has been made to verify the accuracy of these tables, the bedside nurse should verify the dose using the preceding formula and check against the physician or provider order, relevant institutional protocols, and the drug dose recommended.

Table A1 Dose in mcg/kg per Minute with Drug Concentration of 10 mcg/mL (1 mg/100 mL)*

		Weight (kg)											
		2	3	4	5	6	7	8	9	10	11	12	13
Flow Rate (mL/h)	1	0.08	0.055	0.042	0.033	0.028	0.024	0.021	0.019	0.017	0.015	0.014	0.013
	2	0.16	0.11	0.08	0.07	0.056	0.05	0.042	0.04	0.03	0.03	0.03	0.026
	3	0.25	0.17	0.125	0.1	0.08	0.07	0.06	0.06	0.05	0.045	0.04	0.04
	4	0.33	0.22	0.17	0.13	0.11	0.1	0.08	0.07	0.07	0.06	0.056	0.05
	5	0.42	0.28	0.21	0.17	0.14	0.12	0.11	0.09	0.08	0.08	0.07	0.065
	6	0.50	0.33	0.25	0.2	0.17	0.14	0.13	0.11	0.1	0.09	0.08	0.08
	7	0.58	0.39	0.29	0.23	0.19	0.17	0.15	0.13	0.12	0.11	0.10	0.09
	8	0.67	0.44	0.33	0.27	0.22	0.19	0.17	0.15	0.13	0.12	0.11	0.10
	9	0.75	0.5	0.38	0.3	0.25	0.21	0.19	0.17	0.15	0.14	0.125	0.12
	10	0.83	0.55	0.42	0.33	0.28	0.24	0.21	0.19	0.17	0.15	0.14	0.13
	11	0.91	0.6	0.46	0.36	0.31	0.26	0.23	0.2	0.18	0.17	0.15	0.14
	12	1	0.67	0.5	0.4	0.33	0.29	0.25	0.22	0.2	0.18	0.17	0.15
	13	1.08	0.72	0.54	0.43	0.36	0.31	0.27	0.24	0.22	0.2	0.18	0.17
	14	1.16	0.78	0.58	0.47	0.39	0.33	0.29	0.26	0.23	0.21	0.19	0.18
	15	1.25	0.83	0.63	0.5	0.42	0.36	0.315	0.28	0.25	0.23	0.21	0.19

*Values expressed represent mcg/kg per minute. Most numbers have been rounded up or down to the second or third decimal place. If numbers are within five hundredths of a decimal place of a whole number, they have been rounded up to the whole number.

Table A1   **Dose in mcg/kg per Minute with Drug Concentration of 10 mcg/mL (1 mg/100 mL)***

						Weight (kg)							
14	**15**	**16**	**17**	**18**	**19**	**20**	**21**	**22**	**23**	**24**	**25**		
0.012	0.011	0.01	0.009	0.009	0.009	0.008	0.008	0.008	0.007	0.007	0.007	1	
0.024	0.02	0.02	0.018	0.018	0.017	0.017	0.016	0.015	0.014	0.014	0.013	2	
0.036	0.03	0.03	0.029	0.028	0.026	0.025	0.024	0.023	0.022	0.02	0.02	3	
0.05	0.04	0.04	0.039	0.037	0.035	0.033	0.032	0.03	0.03	0.028	0.27	4	
0.06	0.056	0.05	0.049	0.046	0.044	0.042	0.040	0.038	0.036	0.035	0.033	5	
0.07	0.067	0.06	0.058	0.056	0.053	0.05	0.048	0.045	0.04	0.042	0.04	6	
0.08	0.078	0.07	0.069	0.065	0.06	0.058	0.056	0.053	0.051	0.049	0.047	7	
0.095	0.09	0.08	0.078	0.074	0.07	0.067	0.064	0.06	0.058	0.056	0.053	8	
0.11	0.1	0.09	0.088	0.083	0.08	0.075	0.07	0.068	0.065	0.062	0.06	9	
0.12	0.11	0.1	0.098	0.093	0.09	0.08	0.08	0.076	0.072	0.07	0.067	10	Flow Rate (mL/h)
0.13	0.12	0.11	0.108	0.10	0.097	0.09	0.09	0.08	0.08	0.076	0.073	11	
0.14	0.13	0.12	0.118	0.11	0.106	0.10	0.095	0.09	0.087	0.083	0.08	12	
0.16	0.14	0.13	0.127	0.12	0.114	0.11	0.10	0.1	0.094	0.09	0.087	13	
0.17	0.16	0.14	0.137	0.13	0.12	0.117	0.11	0.11	0.10	0.097	0.09	14	
0.18	0.17	0.15	0.147	0.14	0.132	0.125	0.12	0.114	0.11	0.104	0.1	15	

*Values expressed represent mcg/kg per minute. Most numbers have been rounded up or down to the second or third decimal place. If numbers are within five hundredths of a decimal place of a whole number, they have been rounded up to the whole number.

Table A2   **Dose in mcg/kg per Minute with Drug Concentration of 200 mcg/mL (20 mg/100 mL)***

Flow Rate (mL/h)	Weight (kg)											
	2	**3**	**4**	**5**	**6**	**7**	**8**	**9**	**10**	**11**	**12**	**13**
1	1.7	1.1	0.8	0.7	0.6	0.5	0.4	0.4	0.3	0.3	0.3	0.3
2	3.3	2.2	1.7	1.3	1.1	1	0.8	0.7	0.7	0.6	0.6	0.5
3	5	3.3	2.5	2	1.7	1.4	1.3	1.1	1	0.9	0.8	0.8
4	6.7	4.4	3.3	2.7	2.2	1.9	1.7	1.5	1.3	1.2	1.1	1
5	8.4	5.6	4.2	3.3	2.8	2.4	2.1	1.9	1.7	1.5	1.4	1.3
6	10	6.7	5	4	3.3	2.9	2.5	2.2	2	1.8	1.7	1.5
7	11.7	7.8	5.8	4.7	3.9	3.3	2.9	2.6	2.3	2.1	2	1.8
8	13.4	8.9	6.7	5.3	4.4	3.8	3.3	3	2.7	2.4	2.2	2.1
9	15	10	7.5	6	5	4.3	3.8	3.3	3	2.7	2.5	2.3
10	16.7	11.1	8.3	6.7	5.5	4.8	4.2	3.7	3.3	3	2.8	2.6
11	18.3	12.2	9.2	7.3	6	5.2	4.6	4.1	3.7	3.3	3.1	2.8
12	20	13.3	10	8	6.7	5.7	5	4.4	4	3.6	3.3	3.1
13	21.7	14.4	10.8	8.7	7.2	6.2	5.4	4.8	4.3	3.9	3.6	3.3
14	23.4	15.5	11.7	9.3	7.8	6.7	5.8	5.2	4.7	4.2	3.9	3.6
15	25	16.7	12.5	10	8.3	7.1	6.3	5.6	5	4.5	4.2	3.8

*Values expressed represent mcg/kg per minute. Numbers have been rounded up or down to the first decimal place. If numbers are within five hundredths of a decimal place of a whole number, they have been rounded up to the whole number.

Table A3   **Dose in mcg/kg per Minute with Drug Concentration of 400 mcg/mL (40 mg/100 mL)***

Flow Rate (mL/h)	Weight (kg)											
	2	**3**	**4**	**5**	**6**	**7**	**8**	**9**	**10**	**11**	**12**	**13**
1	3.3	2.2	1.7	1.3	1.1	1	0.8	0.7	0.7	0.6	0.6	0.5
2	6.7	4.4	3.3	2.7	2.2	1.9	1.7	1.5	1.3	1.2	1.1	1
3	10	6.7	5	4	3.3	2.9	2.5	2.2	2	1.8	1.7	1.5
4	13.3	8.9	6.7	5.3	4.4	3.8	3.3	3	2.7	2.4	2.2	2
5	16.7	11.1	8.3	6.7	5.5	4.8	4.2	3.7	3.3	3	2.8	2.6
6	20	13.3	10	8	6.7	5.7	5	4.4	4	3.6	3.3	3.1
7	23.3	15.6	11.7	9.3	7.8	6.7	5.8	5.2	4.7	4.2	3.9	3.6
8	26.7	17.8	13.3	10.7	8.9	7.6	6.7	5.9	5.3	4.8	4.4	4.1
9	30	20	15	12	10	8.6	7.5	6.7	6	5.5	5	4.6
10	33.3	22.2	16.7	13.3	11.1	9.5	8.3	7.4	6.7	6.1	5.6	5.1
11	36.7	24.4	18.3	14.7	12.2	10.5	9.2	8.1	7.3	6.7	6.1	5.6
12	40	26.7	20	16	13.3	11.4	10	8.9	8	7.3	6.7	6.2
13	43.3	28.9	21.6	17.3	14.4	12.4	10.8	9.6	8.7	7.9	7.2	6.7
14	46.7	31.1	23.3	18.7	15.6	13.3	11.7	10.4	9.3	8.5	7.8	7.2
15	50	33.3	25	20	16.7	14.3	12.5	11.1	10	9.1	8.3	7.7

*Values expressed represent mcg/kg per minute. Numbers have been rounded up or down to the first decimal place. If numbers are within five hundredths of a decimal place of a whole number, they have been rounded up to the whole number.

Table A2 **Dose in mcg/kg per Minute with Drug Concentration of 200 mcg/mL (20 mg/100 mL)***

					Weight (kg)							
14	**15**	**16**	**17**	**18**	**19**	**20**	**21**	**22**	**23**	**24**	**25**	
0.2	0.2	0.2	0.2	0.2	0.2	0.2	0.2	0.2	0.1	0.1	0.1	1
0.5	0.4	0.4	0.4	0.4	0.4	0.3	0.3	0.3	0.3	0.3	0.3	2
0.7	0.7	0.6	0.6	0.6	0.5	0.5	0.5	0.5	0.4	0.4	0.4	3
1	0.9	0.8	0.8	0.7	0.7	0.7	0.6	0.6	0.6	0.6	0.5	4
1.2	1.1	1	1	0.9	0.9	0.8	0.8	0.8	0.7	0.7	0.7	5
1.4	1.3	1.3	1.2	1.1	1.1	1	1	0.9	0.9	0.8	0.8	6
1.7	1.5	1.5	1.4	1.3	1.2	1.2	1.1	1.1	1	1	0.9	7
1.9	1.8	1.7	1.6	1.5	1.4	1.3	1.3	1.2	1.2	1.1	1.1	8
2.1	2	1.9	1.8	1.7	1.6	1.5	1.4	1.4	1.3	1.3	1.2	9
2.4	2.2	2.1	2	1.9	1.8	1.7	1.6	1.5	1.5	1.4	1.3	10
2.6	2.4	2.3	2.2	2	1.9	1.8	1.7	1.7	1.6	1.5	1.5	11
2.9	2.7	2.5	2.4	2.2	2.1	2	1.9	1.8	1.7	1.7	1.6	12
3.1	2.9	2.7	2.6	2.4	2.3	2.2	2.1	2	1.9	1.8	1.7	13
3.3	3.1	2.9	2.7	2.6	2.5	2.3	2.2	2.1	2	1.9	1.9	14
3.6	3.3	3.1	2.9	2.8	2.6	2.5	2.4	2.3	2.2	2.1	2	15

Flow Rate (mL/h)

*Values expressed represent mcg/kg per minute. Numbers have been rounded up or down to the first decimal place. If numbers are within five hundredths of a decimal place of a whole number, they have been rounded up to the whole number.

Table A3 **Dose in mcg/kg per Minute with Drug Concentration of 400 mcg/mL (40 mg/100 mL)***

					Weight (kg)							
14	**15**	**16**	**17**	**18**	**19**	**20**	**21**	**22**	**23**	**24**	**25**	
0.5	0.4	0.4	0.4	0.4	0.4	0.3	0.3	0.3	0.3	0.3	0.3	1
1	0.9	0.8	0.8	0.7	0.7	0.7	0.6	0.6	0.6	0.6	0.5	2
1.4	1.3	1.3	1.2	1.1	1.1	1	1	0.9	0.9	0.8	0.8	3
1.9	1.8	1.7	1.6	1.5	1.4	1.3	1.3	1.2	1.2	1.1	1.1	4
2.4	2.2	2.1	2	1.9	1.8	1.7	1.6	1.5	1.5	1.4	1.3	5
2.9	2.7	2.5	2.4	2.2	2.1	2	1.9	1.8	1.7	1.7	1.6	6
3.3	3.1	2.9	2.7	2.6	2.5	2.3	2.2	2.1	2	1.9	1.9	7
3.8	3.6	3.3	3.1	3	2.8	2.7	2.5	2.4	2.3	2.2	2.1	8
4.3	4	3.8	3.5	3.3	3.2	3	2.9	2.7	2.6	2.5	2.4	9
4.8	4.4	4.2	3.9	3.7	3.5	3.3	3.2	3	2.9	2.8	2.7	10
5.2	4.9	4.6	4.3	4.1	3.9	3.7	3.5	3.3	3.2	3.1	2.9	11
5.7	5.3	5	4.7	4.4	4.2	4	3.8	3.6	3.5	3.3	3.2	12
6.2	5.8	5.4	5.1	4.8	4.6	4.3	4.1	3.9	3.8	3.6	3.5	13
6.7	6.2	5.8	5.5	5.2	4.9	4.7	4.4	4.2	4.1	3.9	3.7	14
7.1	6.7	6.3	5.9	5.6	5.3	5	4.8	4.5	4.4	4.2	4	15

Flow Rate (mL/h)

*Values expressed represent mcg/kg per minute. Numbers have been rounded up or down to the first decimal place. If numbers are within five hundredths of a decimal place of a whole number, they have been rounded up to the whole number.

Table A4   **Dose in mcg/kg per Minute with Drug Concentration of 500 mcg/mL (50 mg/100 mL)***

						Weight (kg)							
		2	**3**	**4**	**5**	**6**	**7**	**8**	**9**	**10**	**11**	**12**	**13**
	1	4.2	2.8	2.1	1.7	1.4	1.2	1	0.9	0.8	0.8	0.7	0.6
	2	8.3	5.6	4.2	3.3	2.8	2.4	2.1	1.9	1.7	1.5	1.4	1.3
	3	12.5	8.3	6.2	5	4.2	3.6	3.1	2.8	2.5	2.3	2.1	1.9
	4	16.7	11.1	8.3	6.7	5.6	4.8	4.2	3.7	3.3	3	2.8	2.6
	5	20.8	13.9	10.4	8.3	6.9	6	5.2	4.6	4.2	3.8	3.5	3.2
	6	25	16.7	12.5	10	8.3	7.1	6.3	5.6	5	4.5	4.2	3.8
Flow Rate (mL/h)	7	29.2	19.4	14.6	11.7	9.7	8.3	7.3	6.5	5.8	5.3	4.9	4.5
	8	33	22.2	16.7	13.3	11.1	9.5	8.3	7.4	6.7	6.1	5.6	5.1
	9	37.5	25.0	18.7	15	12.5	10.7	9.4	8.3	7.5	6.8	6.2	5.8
	10	41.7	27.8	20.8	16.7	13.9	11.9	10.4	9.3	8.3	7.6	6.9	6.4
	11	45.8	30.6	22.9	18.3	15.3	13.1	11.5	10.2	9.2	8.3	7.6	7.1
	12	50	33.3	25	20	16.7	14.3	12.5	11	10	9.1	8.3	7.7
	13	54.2	36.1	27.1	21.7	18.1	15.5	13.5	12	10.8	9.8	9	8.3
	14	58.3	38.9	29.2	23.3	19.4	16.7	14.6	13	11.7	10.6	9.7	9
	15	62.5	41.7	31.2	25	20.8	17.9	15.6	13.9	12.5	11.4	10.4	9.6

*Values expressed represent mcg/kg per minute. Numbers have typically been rounded up or down to the first decimal place. If numbers are within five hundredths of a decimal place of a whole number, they have been rounded up to the whole number.

Table A5   **Dose in mcg/kg per Minute with Drug Concentration of 1000 mcg/mL (100 mg/100 mL)***

						Weight (kg)							
		2	**3**	**4**	**5**	**6**	**7**	**8**	**9**	**10**	**11**	**12**	**13**
	1	8.3	5.6	4.2	3.3	2.8	2.4	2.1	1.9	1.7	1.5	1.4	1.3
	2	16.7	11.1	8.3	6.7	5.6	4.8	4.2	3.7	3.3	3.0	2.8	2.6
	3	25	16.7	12.5	10	8.3	7.1	6.2	5.6	5.0	4.5	4.2	3.8
	4	33.3	22.2	16.7	13.3	11.1	9.5	8.3	7.4	6.7	6.1	5.6	5.1
	5	41.7	27.8	20.9	16.7	13.9	11.9	10.4	9.3	8.3	7.6	6.9	6.4
	6	50	33.3	25	20	16.7	14.3	12.5	11.1	10	9.1	8.3	7.7
Flow Rate (mL/h)	7	58.3	38.9	29.2	23.3	19.4	16.7	14.6	13	11.7	10.6	9.7	9
	8	66.7	44.4	33.3	26.7	22.2	19	16.7	14.8	13.3	12.1	11.1	10.3
	9	75	50	37.5	30	25	21.4	18.7	16.7	15	13.6	12.5	11.5
	10	83.3	55.6	41.7	33.3	27.8	23.8	20.8	18.5	16.7	15.2	13.9	12.8
	11	91.7	61	45.9	36.7	30.6	26.2	22.9	20.4	18.3	16.7	15.3	14.1
	12	100	66.7	50	40	33.3	28.6	25	22.2	20.0	18.2	16.7	15.4
	13	108.3	72.2	54.2	43.3	36.1	31	27.1	24.1	21.7	19.7	18.1	16.7
	14	116.7	77.8	58.3	46.7	38.9	33.3	29.2	25.9	23.3	21.2	19.4	17.9
	15	125	83.3	62.5	50	41.7	35.7	31.2	27.8	25.0	22.7	20.8	19.2

*Values expressed represent mcg/kg per minute. Numbers have been rounded up or down to the first decimal place. If numbers are within hundredths of a decimal place of a whole number, they have been rounded up to the whole number.

Table A4 Dose in mcg/kg per Minute with Drug Concentration of 500 mcg/mL (50 mg/100 mL)*

					Weight (kg)							
14	**15**	**16**	**17**	**18**	**19**	**20**	**21**	**22**	**23**	**24**	**25**	Flow Rate (mL/h)
0.6	0.6	0.5	0.5	0.5	0.4	0.4	0.4	0.4	0.4	0.3	0.3	1
1.2	1.1	1	1	0.9	0.9	0.8	0.8	0.8	0.7	0.7	0.7	2
1.8	1.7	1.6	1.5	1.4	1.3	1.3	1.2	1.1	1.1	1	1	3
2.4	2.2	2.1	2	1.9	1.8	1.7	1.6	1.5	1.4	1.4	1.3	4
3.0	2.8	2.6	2.5	2.3	2.2	2.1	2	1.9	1.8	1.7	1.7	5
3.6	3.3	3.1	2.9	2.8	2.6	2.5	2.4	2.3	2.2	2.1	2.0	6
4.2	3.9	3.6	3.4	3.2	3.1	2.9	2.8	2.7	2.5	2.4	2.3	7
4.8	4.4	4.2	3.9	3.7	3.5	3.3	3.2	3	2.9	2.8	2.7	8
5.4	5	4.7	4.4	4.2	3.9	3.8	3.6	3.4	3.3	3.1	3	9
6	5.6	5.2	4.9	4.6	4.4	4.2	4	3.8	3.6	3.5	3.3	10
6.5	6.1	5.7	5.4	5.1	4.8	4.6	4.4	4.2	4	3.8	3.7	11
7.1	6.7	6.2	5.9	5.6	5.3	5	4.8	4.5	4.3	4.2	4.0	12
7.7	7.2	6.8	6.4	6	5.7	5.4	5.2	4.9	4.7	4.5	4.3	13
8.3	7.8	7.3	6.9	6.5	6.1	5.8	5.6	5.3	5.1	4.9	4.7	14
8.9	8.3	7.8	7.3	7	6.6	6.3	6	5.7	5.4	5.2	5	15

*Values expressed represent mcg/kg per minute. Numbers have typically been rounded up or down to the first decimal place. If numbers are within five hundredths of a decimal place of a whole number, they have been rounded up to the whole number.

Table A5 Dose in mcg/kg per Minute with Drug Concentration of 1000 mcg/mL (100 mg/100 mL)*

					Weight (kg)							
14	**15**	**16**	**17**	**18**	**19**	**20**	**21**	**22**	**23**	**24**	**25**	Flow Rate (mL/h)
1.2	1.1	1	1	0.9	0.9	0.8	0.8	0.8	0.7	0.7	0.7	1
2.4	2.2	2.1	2	1.9	1.8	1.7	1.6	1.5	1.4	1.4	1.3	2
3.6	3.3	3.1	2.9	2.8	2.6	2.5	2.4	2.3	2.2	2.1	2	3
4.8	4.4	4.2	3.9	3.7	3.5	3.3	3.2	3	2.9	2.8	2.7	4
6	5.6	5.2	4.9	4.6	4.4	4.2	4	3.8	3.6	3.5	3.3	5
7.1	6.7	6.3	5.9	5.6	5.3	5	4.8	4.5	4.3	4.2	4	6
8.3	7.8	7.3	6.9	6.5	6.1	5.8	5.6	5.3	5.1	4.9	4.7	7
9.5	8.9	8.3	7.8	7.4	7	6.7	6.3	6.1	5.8	5.6	5.3	8
10.7	10	9.4	8.8	8.3	7.9	7.5	7.1	6.8	6.5	6.2	6	9
11.9	11.1	10.4	9.8	9.3	8.8	8.3	7.9	7.6	7.2	6.9	6.7	10
13.1	12.2	11.5	10.8	10.2	9.6	9.2	8.7	8.3	8	7.6	7.3	11
14.3	13.3	12.5	11.8	11.1	10.5	10	9.5	9.1	8.7	8.3	8	12
15.5	14.4	13.5	12.7	12	11.4	10.8	10.3	9.8	9.4	9	8.7	13
16.7	15.6	14.6	13.7	13	12.3	11.7	11.1	10.6	10.1	9.7	9.3	14
17.9	16.7	15.6	14.7	13.9	13.2	12.5	11.9	11.4	10.9	10.4	10	15

*Values expressed represent mcg/kg per minute. Numbers have been rounded up or down to the first decimal place. If numbers are within hundredths of a decimal place of a whole number, they have been rounded up to the whole number.

Table A6   **Dose in mcg/kg per Minute with Drug Concentration of 1600 mcg/mL (160 mg/100 mL)***

Flow Rate (mL/h)	Weight (kg)											
	2	**3**	**4**	**5**	**6**	**7**	**8**	**9**	**10**	**11**	**12**	**13**
1	13.3	8.9	6.7	5.3	4.4	3.8	3.3	3	2.7	2.4	2.2	2.1
2	26.7	17.8	13.3	10.7	8.9	7.6	6.7	5.9	5.3	4.8	4.4	4.1
3	40.1	26.7	20	16	13.3	11.4	10	8.9	8	7.2	6.7	6.2
4	53.3	35.6	26.7	21.3	17.8	15.2	13.3	11.9	10.7	9.7	8.9	8.2
5	66.7	44.4	33.3	26.7	22.2	19	16.7	14.8	13.3	12.1	11.1	10.3
6	80	53.3	40	32	26.7	22.9	20	17.8	16	14.5	13.3	12.3
7	93.3	62.2	46.7	37.3	31.1	26.7	23.3	20.7	18.7	17	15.6	14.4
8	106.7	71.1	53.3	42.7	35.6	30.5	26.7	23.7	21.3	19.4	17.8	16.4
9	120	80	60	48	40	34.3	30	26.7	24	21.8	20	18.5
10	133.3	88.9	66.7	53.3	44.4	38.1	33.3	29.6	26.7	24.2	22.2	20.5
11	146.7	97.8	73.3	58.7	48.9	41.9	36.7	32.6	29.3	26.7	24.4	22.6
12	160	106.7	80	64	53.3	45.7	40	35.6	32	29.1	26.7	24.6
13	173.3	115.6	86.7	69.3	57.8	49.5	43.3	38.5	34.7	31.5	28.9	26.7
14	186.7	124.4	93.3	74.7	62.2	53.3	46.7	41.5	37.3	33.9	31.1	28.7
15	200	133.3	100	80	66.7	57.1	50	44.4	40	36.3	33.3	30.8

*Values expressed represent mcg/kg per minute. Numbers have been rounded up or down to the first decimal place. If numbers are within hundredths of a decimal place of a whole number, they have been rounded up to the whole number.

Table A6   **Dose in mcg/kg per Minute with Drug Concentration of 1600 mcg/mL (160 mg/100 mL)***

					Weight (kg)								
14	**15**	**16**	**17**	**18**	**19**	**20**	**21**	**22**	**23**	**24**	**25**		
1.9	1.8	1.7	1.6	1.5	1.4	1.3	1.3	1.2	1.2	1.1	1.1	1	
3.8	3.6	3.3	3.1	3	2.8	2.7	2.5	2.4	2.3	2.2	2.1	2	
5.7	5.3	5	4.7	4.4	4.2	4	3.8	3.6	3.5	3.3	3.2	3	
7.6	7.1	6.7	6.3	5.9	5.6	5.3	5.1	4.8	4.6	4.4	4.3	4	
9.5	8.9	8.3	7.8	7.4	7	6.7	6.3	6.1	5.8	5.6	5.3	5	
11.4	10.7	10	9.4	8.9	8.4	8	7.6	7.3	7	6.7	6.4	6	
13.3	12.4	11.7	11	10.4	9.8	9.3	8.9	8.5	8.1	7.8	7.5	7	
15.2	14.2	13.3	12.5	11.9	11.2	10.7	10.2	9.7	9.3	8.9	8.5	8	
17.1	16	15	14.1	13.3	12.6	12	11.4	10.9	10.4	10	9.6	9	
19	17.8	16.7	15.7	14.8	14	13.3	12.7	12.1	11.6	11.1	10.7	10	
21	19.6	18.3	17.3	16.3	15.4	14.7	14	13.3	12.8	12.2	11.7	11	
22.9	21.3	20	18.8	17.8	16.8	16	15.2	14.5	13.9	13.3	12.8	12	
24.8	23.1	21.7	20.4	19.3	18.2	17.3	16.5	15.8	15.1	14.4	13.9	13	
26.7	24.9	23.3	22	20.7	19.6	18.7	17.8	17	16.2	15.6	14.9	14	
28.6	26.7	25.1	23.5	22.2	21	20	19	18.2	17.4	16.7	16	15	Flow Rate (mL/h)

*Values expressed represent mcg/kg per minute. Numbers have been rounded up or down to the first decimal place. If numbers are within hundredths of a decimal place of a whole number, they have been rounded up to the whole number.

Conversion Factors to Système International (SI) Units

Table B1 Conversion Factors to SI Units for Some Biochemical Components of Blood*

Component	Range in Units as Typically Reported	Conversion Factor	Normal range in SI units, Molecular Units, International Units, or Decimal Fractions
Acetoacetic acid (S)	0.2-1.0 mg/dL	98	19.6-98.0 µmol/L
Acetaminophen	*Therapeutic:* 10-30 mcg/mL		*Therapeutic:* 86-200 µmol/L
	Toxic: >200 mcg/mL		*Toxic:* >1300 µmol/L
Acetone (S)	0.3-2.0 mg/dL	172	51.6-344.0 µmol/L
Albumin (S)	3.2-4.5 g/dL	10	32-45 g/L
Ammonia (P)	20-120 mcg/dL	0.588	11.7-70.5 µmol/L
Amylase (S)	60-160 Somogyi units/dL	1.85	111-296 U/L
Base, total (S)	145-160 mEq/L	1	145-160 mmol/L
Bicarbonate (P)	21-28 mEq/L	1	21-28 mmol/L
Bile acids (S)	0.3-3.0 mg/dL	10	3-30 mg/L
		2.547	0.8-7.6 µmol/L
Bilirubin, total	*Cord, premature or full-term:* <2 mg/dL *0-1 day:* <8.7 (full-term) or <8 (preterm) mg/dL *1-2 days:* <11.5 (full-term) or <12 (preterm) mg/dL *2-5 days:* <12 (full-term) or <16 (preterm) mg/dL *Beyond 5 days:* <10 (full-term) or <20 (preterm) mg/dL		*Cord, premature or full-term:* <34 µmol/L *0-1 day:* <149 (full-term) or <137 (preterm) µmol/L *1-2 days:* <197 (full-term) or <205 (preterm) µmol/L *2-5 days:* <205 (full-term) or <274 (preterm) µmol/L *Beyond 5 days:* <171 (full-term) or <340 (preterm) µmol/L
Bilirubin, direct (conjugated) (S)	Up to 0.3 mg/dL	17.1	Up to 5.1 µmol/L
Blood gases (B)			
PCO₂ arterial	35-40 mm Hg	0.133	4.66-5.32 kPa
PO₂	95-100 mm Hg	0.133	12.64-13.30 kPa
C-reactive protein (CRP)	0-0.5 mg/dL		0-0.5 mg/dL
Calcium (ionized)	*Cord:* 5-6 mg/dL *Newborn 3-24 h:* 4.2-5.1 mg/dL *24-48 h:* 4.0-4.7 mg/dL *Beyond 48 h:* 4.8-5.3 mg/dL or 2.24-2.64 mEq/L	0.25	*Cord:* 1.25-1.5 mmol/L *Newborn 3-24 h:* 1.07-1.27 mmol/L *24-48 h:* 1.00-1.17 mmol/L *Beyond 48 h:* 1.12-1.33 mmol/L
Calcium, total	*Cord:* 9-11.5 mg/dL *Newborn 3-24 h:* 9.0-10.6 mg/dL *24-48 h:* 7.0-12.0 mg/dL *4-7 day:* 9.0-10.9 mg/dL *Child:* 8.8-10.8 mg/dL	0.25	*Cord:* 2.25-2.88 mmol/L *Newborn 3-24 h:* 2.3-2.65 mmol/L *24-48 h:* 1.75-3.0 mmol/L *4-7 days:* 2.25-2.73 mmol/L *Child:* 2.2-2.70 mmol/L
Chloride, serum	95-103 mEq/L	1	95-103 mmol/L

Continued

Table B1   **Conversion Factors to SI Units for Some Biochemical Components of Blood*—cont'd**

Component	Range in Units as Typically Reported	Conversion Factor	Normal range in SI units, Molecular Units, International Units, or Decimal Fractions
Chloride, sweat	*Normal:* <40 mEq/L		*Normal:* <40 mmol/L
	Marginal (asthma, Addison's disease, malnutrition): 40-60 mEq/L		*Marginal (asthma, Addison's disease, malnutrition):* 40-60 mmol/L
	Cystic fibrosis: >60 mEq/L		*Cystic fibrosis:* >60 mmol/L
Creatine (S)	0.1-0.4 mg/dL	76.3	7.6-30.5 µmol/L
Creatinine (S)	0.6-1.2 mg/dL	88.4	53-106 µmol/L
Creatinine clearance (P)	107-139 mL/min	0.0167	1.78-2.32 mL/s
Fatty acids (total) (S)	8-20 mg/dL	0.01	0.08-2.00 mg/L
Fibrinogen (P)	200-400 mg/dL	0.01	2.00-4.00 g/L
Gamma globulin (S)	0.5-1.6 g/dL	10	5-16 g/L
Globulins (total) (S)	2.3-3.5 g/dL	10	23-35 g/L
Glucose (fasting) (S)	70-110 mg/dL	0.055	3.85-6.05 mmol/L
Insulin	4.24 µIU/mL	0.0417	0.17-1.00 mcg/L
(radioimmunoassay) (P)	0.20-0.84 mcg/L	172.2	35-145 pmol/L
Iodine, BEI (S)	3.5-6.5 mcg/dL	0.079	0.28-0.51 µmol/L
Iodine, PBI (S)	4.0-8.0 mcg/dL	0.079	0.32-0.63 µmol/L
Iron, total (S)	60-150 mcg/dL	0.179	11-27 µmol/L
Iron-binding capacity (S)	300-360 mcg/dL	0.179	54-64 µmol/L
17-Ketosteroids (P)	25-125 mcg/dL	0.01	0.25-1.25 mg/L
Lactic dehydrogenase (S)	80-120 units at 30 °C	0.48	38-62 U/L at 30 °C
	Lactase → pyruvate: 100-190 U/L at 37 °C	1	100-190 U/L at 37 °C
Lactate (arterial)	5-14 mg/dL		0.5-1.6 mmol/L
Lipase (S)	0-1.5 U/mL (Cherry-Crandall)	278	0-417 U/L
Lipids (total) (S)	400-800 mg/dL	0.01	4.00-8.00 g/L
Cholesterol	150-250 mg/dL	0.026	3.9-6.5 mmol/L
Triglycerides	75-165 mg/dL	0.0114	0.85-1.89 mmol/L
Phospholipids	150-380 mg/dL	0.01	1.50-3.80 g/L
Free fatty acids	9.0-15.0 mM/L	1	9.0-15.0 mmol/L
Nonprotein nitrogen (S)	20-35 mg/dL	0.714	14.3-25.0 mmol/L
Phosphatase (P)			
Acid (unit/dL)	Cherry-Crandall	2.77	0-5.5 U/L
	King-Armstrong	1.77	0-5.5 U/L
	Bodansky	5.37	0-5.5 U/L
Alkaline (units/dL)	King-Armstrong	1.77	30-120 U/L
	Bodansky	5.37	30-120 U/L
	Bessey-Lowry-Brock	16.67	30-120 U/L
Phosphorus inorganic (S)	3.0-4.5 mg/dL	0.323	0.97-1.45 mmol/L
Potassium (P)	3.0-5.0 mEq/L	1	3.0-5.0 mmol/L
Proteins, total (S)	6.0-7.8 g/dL	10	60-78 g/L
Albumin	3.2-4.5 g/dL	10	32-45 g/L
Globulin	2.3-3.5 g/dL	10	23-35 g/L
Sodium (P)	135-145 mEq/L	1	135-145 mmol/L
Testosterone			
Male (S)	300-1200 ng/dL	0.035	10.5-42.0 nmol/L
Female	30-95 ng/dL	0.035	1.0-3.3 nmol/L
Thyroid tests (S)			
Thyroxine (T_4)	4-11 mcg/dL	12.87	51-142 nmol/L
T_4 expressed as iodine	3.2-7.2 mcg/dL	79.0	253-569 nmol/L
T_3 resin uptake	25-38% relative uptake	0.01	0.25-0.38% relative uptake
TSH (S)	10 µU/mL	1	$<10^{-3}$ IU/L
Urea nitrogen (S)	8-23 mg/dL	0.357	2.9-8.2 mmol/L
Uric acid (S)	2.6 mg/dL	59.5	0.120-0.360 mmol/L
Vitamin B_{12} (S)	160-950 pg/mL	0.74	118-703 pmol/L

Modified from Hockenberry MJ and Wilson D (Eds): *Wong's Nursing Care of Infants and Children*, ed 9, Philadelphia, Elsevier, 2011.
*This is a selected (not a complete) list of biochemical components. The ranges listed may differ from those accepted in some laboratories and are shown to illustrate the conversion factor and the method of expression in SI molecular units.

| Table B2 | Equivalent Values of kPa and mm Hg Units* |

kPa	0.1	0.2	0.3	0.4	0.5	0.6	0.7	0.8	0.9
mm Hg	0.75	1.5	2.25	3	3.75	4.5	5.25	6	6.75
kPa			mm Hg			kPa			mm Hg
1			7.5			21			158
2			15.0			22			165
3			22.5			23			172
4			30.0			24			180
5			37.5			25			188
6			45.0			26			195
7			52.5			27			202
8			60.0			28			210
9			67.5			29			218
10			75.0			30			225
11			82.5			31			232
12			90.0			32			240
13			97.5			33			248
14			105			34			255
15			112			35			262
16			120			36			270
17			128			37			278
18			135			38			285
19			142			39			292
20			150			40			300

*From World Health Organization: *The SI for the health professions,* Geneva, 1977, The Organization, p. 40.

| Table B3 | Some Hematology Values |

Component	Normal Range in Units as Customarily Reported	Conversion Factor	Normal Range in SI Units, Molecular Units, International Units, or Decimal Fractions
Red cell volume (male)	25-35 mL/kg body weight	0.001	0.025-0.035 L/kg body weight
Hematocrit	40-50%	0.01	0.40-0.50
Hemoglobin	13.5-18.0 g/dL	10	135-180 g/L
Hemoglobin	13.5-18.0 g/dL	0.155	2.09-2.79 mmol/L
RBC count	$4.5\text{-}6 \times 10^6$ μL	1	$4.6\text{-}6 \times 10^{12}$/L
WBC count	$4.5\text{-}10 \times 10^3$ μL	1	$4.5\text{-}10 \times 10^9$/L
Mean corpuscular volume	80-96 μm^3	1	80-96 fL

Pediatric Weight Conversions

Table C1 Conversion of Pounds to Kilograms for Pediatric Weights

Pounds*	0	1	2	3	4	5	6	7	8	9
0	0.00	0.45	0.90	1.36	1.81	2.26	2.72	3.17	3.62	4.08
10	4.53	4.98	5.44	5.89	6.35	6.80	7.35	7.71	8.16	8.61
20	9.07	9.52	9.97	10.43	10.88	11.34	11.79	12.24	12.70	13.15
30	13.60	14.06	14.51	14.96	15.42	15.87	16.32	16.78	17.23	17.69
40	18.14	18.59	19.05	19.50	19.95	20.41	20.86	21.31	21.77	22.22
50	22.68	23.13	23.58	24.04	24.49	24.94	25.40	25.85	26.30	26.76
60	27.21	27.66	28.22	28.57	29.03	29.48	29.93	30.39	30.84	31.29
70	31.75	32.20	32.65	33.11	33.56	34.02	34.47	34.92	35.38	35.83
80	36.28	36.74	37.19	37.64	38.10	38.55	39.00	39.46	39.93	40.37
90	40.82	41.27	41.73	42.18	42.63	43.09	43.54	43.99	44.45	44.90
100	45.36	45.81	46.26	46.72	47.17	47.62	48.08	48.53	48.98	49.44
110	49.89	50.34	50.80	51.25	51.71	52.16	52.61	53.07	53.52	53.97
120	54.43	54.88	55.33	55.79	56.24	56.70	57.15	57.60	58.06	58.51
130	58.96	59.42	59.87	60.32	60.78	61.23	61.68	62.14	62.59	63.05
140	63.50	63.95	64.41	64.86	65.31	65.77	66.22	66.67	67.13	67.58
150	68.04	68.49	68.94	69.40	69.85	70.30	70.76	71.21	71.66	72.12
160	72.57	73.02	73.48	73.93	74.39	74.84	75.29	75.75	76.20	76.65
170	77.11	77.56	78.01	78.47	78.92	79.38	79.83	80.28	80.74	81.19
180	81.64	82.10	82.55	83.00	83.46	83.91	84.36	84.82	85.27	85.73
190	86.18	86.68	87.09	87.54	87.99	88.45	88.90	89.35	89.81	90.26
200	90.72	91.17	91.62	92.08	92.53	92.98	93.44	93.89	94.34	94.80

*Note: The clinician should find the correct ten pound increment in the first column, then move across the row to find the correct single pound column (e.g., to convert 44 pounds, find the 40 row in the first column, then move across that row to the 4 column, to find 19.95 kg).

Table C2 Conversion of Pounds and Ounces to Grams for Pediatric Weights

Pounds	Kilograms	Pounds	Kilograms	Ounces	Kilograms	Ounces	Kilograms
1	0.454	9	4.082	1	0.028	9	0.255
2	0.907	10	4.536	2	0.057	10	0.283
3	1.361	11	4.990	3	0.085	11	0.312
4	1.814	12	5.443	4	0.113	12	0.340
5	2.268	13	5.897	5	0.142	13	0.369
6	2.722			6	0.170	14	0.397
7	3.175			7	0.198	15	0.425
8	3.629			8	0.227		

Conversion of Fahrenheit Temperatures to Celsius

°F	°C	°F	°C	°F	°C	°F	°C	°F	°C
95.0	35.0	97.3	36.3	99.9	37.7	102.2	39.0	104.5	40.3
95.2	35.1	97.5	36.4	100.0	37.8	102.4	39.1	104.8	40.4
95.4	35.2	97.9	36.6	100.2	37.9	102.6	39.2	105.0	40.6
95.6	35.3	98.0	36.7	100.4	38.0	102.7	39.3	105.2	40.7
95.8	35.4	98.2	36.8	100.6	38.1	102.9	39.4	105.4	40.8
96.0	35.6	98.4	36.9	100.8	38.2	103.3	39.6	105.6	40.9
96.3	35.7	98.6	37.0	100.9	38.3	103.4	39.7	105.8	41.0
96.4	35.8	98.8	37.1	101.2	38.4	103.6	39.8	106.0	41.1
96.6	35.9	99.0	37.2	101.5	38.6	103.8	39.9	106.2	41.2
96.8	36.0	99.1	37.3	101.7	38.7	104.0	40.0	106.4	41.3
97.0	36.1	99.3	37.4	101.8	38.8	104.2	40.1	106.5	41.4
97.2	36.2	99.7	37.6	102.0	38.9	104.4	40.2	106.9	41.6

$°C = (°F - 32) \times 5/9$. Temperature equivalents have been rounded up or down to the nearest first decimal place (tenth of a degree).

For Hypothermic Patients (Temperatures below 95° F/35° C)

°F	°C	°F	°C	°F	°C	°F	°C	°F	°C
82.4	28.0	84.9	29.4	87.4	30.8	90.0	32.2	92.5	33.6
82.6	28.1	85.1	29.5	87.6	30.9	90.1	32.3	92.7	33.7
82.8	28.2	85.3	29.6	87.8	31.0	90.3	32.4	92.8	33.8
82.9	28.3	85.5	29.7	88.0	31.1	90.5	32.5	93.0	33.9
83.1	28.4	85.6	29.8	88.2	31.2	90.7	32.6	93.2	34.0
83.3	28.5	85.8	29.9	88.3	31.3	90.9	32.7	93.4	34.1
83.5	28.6	86.0	30.0	88.5	31.4	91.0	32.8	93.6	34.2
83.7	28.7	86.2	30.1	88.7	31.5	91.2	32.9	93.7	34.3
83.8	28.8	86.4	30.2	88.9	31.6	91.4	33.0	93.9	34.4
84.0	28.9	86.5	30.3	89.0	31.7	91.6	33.1	94.1	34.5
84.2	29.0	86.7	30.4	89.2	31.8	91.8	33.2	94.3	34.6
84.4	29.1	86.9	30.5	89.4	31.9	91.9	33.3	94.5	34.7
84.6	29.2	87.0	30.6	89.6	32.0	92.1	33.4	94.6	34.8
84.7	29.3	87.3	30.7	89.8	32.1	92.3	33.5	94.8	34.9

$°C = (°F - 32) \times 5/9$. Temperature equivalents have been rounded up or down to the nearest first decimal place (tenth of a degree).

Index

Note: Page numbers followed by *b* indicate boxes, *f* indicate figures and *t* indicate tables.

Pediatric Emergency Department Supplies*

Color on Broselow pediatric tape	Gray 3-5 kg Infant	Pink 6-7 kg Infant	Red 8-9 kg Infant	Purple 10-11 kg Toddler	Yellow 12-14 kg Small Child	White 15-19 kg Child	Blue 19-23 kg Child	Orange 24-29 kg Large Child	Green 30-36 kg + Young Adult
Resuscitation Bag	Infant/Child	Infant/Child	Infant/Child	Child	Child	Child	Child	Child/Adult	Adult
O₂ mask	Infant	Infant/Pediatric	Pediatric	Pediatric	Pediatric	Pediatric	Pediatric	Adult	Adult
Oral airway (mm)	Small child (50 mm)	Small child (50 mm)	Small child (50 mm)	Child (60 mm)	Child (60 mm)	Child (60 mm)	Child/small adult (70 mm)	Child/small adult (80 mm)	Small adult (80 mm)
Laryngoscope blade	0 straight	1 straight	1 straight	1 straight	2 straight	2 straight	2 straight or curved	2 straight or curved	3 straight or curved
ET tubes (mm Internal Diameter [I.D.])	2.5-3.0 uncuffed	3.0 cuffed 3.5 uncuffed	3.0 mm cuffed 3.5 mm uncuffed	3.5 mm cuffed 4.0 mm uncuffed	4.0 mm cuffed 4.5 mm uncuffed	4.5 mm cuffed 5.0 mm uncuffed	5.0 cuffed 5.5 mm uncuffed	6.0 mm cuffed	6.5 mm cuffed
ET tube length (cm at lip)	9-10.5	10.5-11	10.5-11 cm	11-12 cm	13.5 cm	15 cm	16.5 cm	17-18 cm	18.5-19.5 cm
Stylet	6 Fr		6 Fr.	6 Fr.	6 Fr.	6 Fr.	14 Fr.	14 Fr.	14 Fr.
Suction catheter	6-8 Fr	6-8 Fr	8 Fr.	10 Fr.	10 Fr.	10 Fr.	10 Fr.	10 Fr.	10-12 Fr.
BP cuff	Neonatal/ Infant	Infant/Child	Infant/Child	Child	Child	Child	Child	Adult	Adult
IV: Catheter	22-24 G	22-24 G	22-24 G	20-24 G	18-22 G	18-22 G	18-20 G	18-20 G	16-20 G
NG tube	5-8 Fr	5-8 Fr	5-8 Fr.	8-10 Fr.	10 Fr.	10-12 Fr.	12-14 Fr.	14-18 Fr.	18 Fr.
Urinary catheter	5 Fr	5-8 Fr	8 Fr.	8-10 Fr.	10 Fr.	10-12 Fr.	10-12 Fr.	12 Fr.	12 Fr.
Chest tube	10-12 Fr	10-12 Fr	10-12 Fr.	16-20 Fr.	20-24 Fr.	20-24 Fr.	24-32 Fr.	28-32 Fr.	32-38 Fr.

*Adapted from the Broselow Pediatric Resuscitation Tape. Reproduced with permission of Jim Broselow, Broselow Medical Technologies, Hickory, North Carolina. All rights reserved.

Estimated Normal Maintenance Caloric Requirements for Infants and Children

Age	Kcal/kg per 24 hours
0-6 months	90-110
6-12 months	80-100
12-36 months	75-90
4-10 years	65-75
>10 years, male	40-55
>10 years, female	38-50

Nutrient	Percent of total daily calories	
Carbohydrates	40-70	Combined 85-88
Fat	20-50	
Protein	7-15	

Estimated Circulating Blood Volume in Children

Age	Blood Volume (mL/kg)
Neonate	80-85
Infant	75-80
Child	70-75
Adolescent, adult	65-70

Formulas for Estimating Daily Maintenance Fluid and Electrolyte Requirements for Children

	Daily Requirements	Hourly Requirements
Fluid Requirements Estimated from Weight*		
Newborn (up to 72 h after birth)	60-100 mL/kg (newborns are born with excess body water)	–
Up to 10 kg	100 mL/kg (can increase up to 150 mL/kg to provide caloric requirements if renal and cardiac function are adequate)	4 mL/kg
11-20 kg	1000 mL for the first 10 kg + 50 mL/kg for each kg over 10 kg	40 mL for first 10 kg + 2 mL/kg for each kg over 10 kg
21-30 kg	1500 mL for the first 20 kg + 25 mL/kg for each kg over 20 kg	60 mL for first 20 kg + 1 mL/kg for each kg over 20 kg
Fluid Requirements Estimated from Body Surface Area (BSA)		
Maintenance	1500 mL/m^2 BSA	–
Insensible losses	300-400 ML/m^2 BSA	–
Electrolytes		
Sodium (Na)	2-4 mEq/kg	–
Potassium (K)	1-2 mEq/kg	–
Chloride (Cl)	2-3 mEq/kg	–
Calcium (Ca)	0.5-3 mEq/kg	–
Phosphorous (Phos)	0.5-2 mmol/kg	–
Magnesium (Mg)	0.4-0.9 mEq/kg	–

*The "maintenance" fluids calculated by these formulas must only be used as a starting point to determine the fluid requirements of an individual patient. If intravascular volume is adequate, children with cardiac, pulmonary, or renal failure or increased intracranial pressure should generally receive less than these calculated "maintenance" fluids. The formula utilizing body weight generally results in a generous "maintenance" fluid total.

Normal Heart Rates in Children*

Age	Awake Heart Rate (beats/min)	Sleeping Heart Rate (beats/min)
Neonate	100-205	90-160
Infant	100-180	90-160
Toddler	98-140	80-120
Preschooler	80-120	65-100
School-age child	75-118	58-90
Adolescent	60-100	50-90

*Always consider the patient's normal range and clinical condition. Heart rate will normally increase with fever or stress.

Normal Respiratory Rates in Children*

Age	Rate (breaths/min)
Infant	30-53
Toddler	22-37
Preschool	20-28
School-age	18-25
Adolescent	12-20

*Consider the patient's normal range. The child's respiratory rate is expected to increase in the presence of fever or stress.
Data from Felming S, et al: Normal ranges of heart rate and respiratory rate in children from birth to 18 years of age: a systemic review of observational studies. *Lancet* 377:1011-1018, 2011.

Normal Blood Pressures in Children

Age	Systolic Pressure (mm Hg)*	Diastolic Pressure (mm Hg)*	Mean Arterial Pressure (mm Hg)[†]	Systolic Hypotension (mm Hg)[‡]
Birth (12 h, <1000 g)	39-59	16-36	28-42[§]	<40-50
Birth (12 h, 3 kg)	60-76	31-45	48-57	<50
Neonate (96 h)	67-84	35-53	45-60	<60
Infant (1-12 mo)	72-104	37-56	50-62	<70
Toddler (1-2 yr)	86-106	42-63	49-62	<70 + (2 × Age in years)
Preschool (3-5 yr)	89-112	46-72	58-69	<70 + (2 × Age in years)
School age (6-7 yr)	97-115	57-76	66-72	<70 + (2 × Age in years)
Preadolescent (10-12 yr)	102-120	61-80	71-79	<90
Adolescent (12-15 yr)	110-131	64-83	73-84	<90

Data from Gemelli M and others: Longitudinal study of blood pressure during the 1st year of life. *Eur J Pediatr* 149:318-320, 1990; Versmold H, et al. Aortic blood pressure during the first 12 hours of life in infants with birth weight 610-4220 gms. *Pediatrics* 67:107, 1981; Haque IU, Zaritsky AL. Analysis of the evidence for the lower limit of systolic and mean arterial pressure in children. *Pediatr Crit Care* 8:138-144, 2007; and National Heart, Lung and Blood Institute: *Fourth report on the diagnosis, evaluation, and treatment of high blood pressure in children and adolescents*, National Heart, Lung and Blood Institute, Bethesda, MD, May, 2004 (available on line: http://www.nhlbi.nih.gov/guidelines/hypertension/child.tbl.htm).
*Systolic and diastolic blood pressure ranges assume 50th percentile for height for children 1 year and older, and are consistent with the Pediatric Advanced Life Support Course (Chameides, L et al: Pediatric advanced life support provider manual. Dallas, 2011, American Heart Association).
[†]Mean arterial pressures (Diastolic pressure + [Difference between systolic and diastolic pressures ÷ 3]) for 1 year and older, assuming 50th percentile for height.
[‡]Threshold for hypotension in children 1-10 years old from Pediatric Advanced Life Support Course (Chameides, L et al: Pediatric advanced life support provider manual. Dallas, 2011, American Heart Association).
[§]Approximately equal to postconception age in weeks (may add 5 mm Hg).